Transtubular Potassium Gradient

$$TTKG = U_k \times P_{osm}/U_{osm} \times P_k$$

Should be ≥7 if hyperkalemic and normal K excretion.

Fractional Excretion of Magnesium

$$FeMg = U_{mg} \times P_{cr}/P_{mg} \times U_{cr} \times 100$$

Normal 3% to 5%.

Tubular Phosphate Reabsorption

$$\%TRP = \left(1 - \frac{U_{Ph} \times P_{Cr}}{P_{Ph} \times U_{Cr}}\right) \times 100$$

Usually >80% (higher in infants).

Hemodialysis Single Pool Kt/V_{urea}

$$spKt/V = -\text{Log n } (R - 0.008t) + (4 - 3.5R)UF/BW$$

R is the ratio of predialysis urea to post dialysis urea, *t* is the time of dialysis in hours, and *BW* is body weight in kg.

Normalized Protein Catabolic Rate

$$nPCR = 5.43 \times G/V + 0.17$$

G(mg/min) = (day 2 predialysis BUN × predialysis *V*) – (day 1 postdialysis BUN × postdialysis *V*)/*T*.

G is the urea generation rate.

V is total body water estimated from 0.58 × body weight, and *T* is time in minutes from the end of the dialysis treatment to the beginning of the next dialysis treatment.

GFR ($ml/min/1.73m^2$) = K × Ht cms/P_{creat}

K = constant	Cr mg/dl	Cr μmol/L
LBW ≤1 year	0.33	29.2
Full-term infants ≤1 year	0.45	39.8
Children 2–12	0.55	48.6
Females 13–31	0.55	48.6
Males 13–21	0.70	61.9

Bladder Volume = [Age(yrs) +2] × 30

KDOQI RECOMMENDATIONS

Ca
Maintain in normal range

PO_4
CKD stage 5, >12 years: 1.13-1.78 mmol/L (3.5-5.5 mg/dl)
1-12 years: 1.33-2.0 mmol/L (4.0-6.0 mg/dl)

PTH
CKD stage 4: 70-110 pg/ml
CKD stage 5: 200-300 pg/ml

Ca × PO_4
>12 yrs: maintain <4.4 $mmol^2/L^2$ (55 mg^2/dl^2)
≤12 yrs: <5.4 $mmol^2/L^2$ (65 mg^2/dl^2)

Hb
11.0-13.0 g/dl

Hemodialysis
$spKt/V_{urea}$ > 1.4 × 3/week

Peritoneal Dialysis
$spKt/V_{urea}$ ≥ 2.0 weekly

Comprehensive Pediatric Nephrology

Comprehensive Pediatric Nephrology

Edited by
Denis F. Geary MB, MRCP(UK), FRCPC
Professor of Paediatrics
University of Toronto
Chief, Division of Nephrology
The Hospital for Sick Children
Toronto, Ontario
Canada

Franz Schaefer MD
Professor of Pediatrics
Chief, Division of Pediatric Nephrology
Center for Pediatric and Adolescent Medicine
University of Heidelberg
Heidelberg
Germany

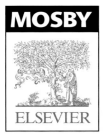

MOSBY
ELSEVIER

MOSBY
ELSEVIER

1600 John F. Kennedy Blvd.
Ste 1800
Philadelphia, PA 19103-2899

COMPREHENSIVE PEDIATRIC NEPHROLOGY ISBN: 978-0-323-04883-5

Notice

Knowledge and best practice in this field are constantly changing. As new research and experience broaden our knowledge, changes in practice, treatment and drug therapy may become necessary or appropriate. Readers are advised to check the most current information provided (i) on procedures featured or (ii) by the manufacturer of each product to be administered, to verify the recommended dose or formula, the method and duration of administration, and contraindications. It is the responsibility of the practitioner, relying on their own experience and knowledge of the patient, to make diagnoses, to determine dosages and the best treatment for each individual patient, and to take all appropriate safety precautions. To the fullest extent of the law, neither the Publisher nor the Editors assumes any liability for any injury and/or damage to persons or property arising out of or related to any use of the material contained in this book.

Library of Congress Cataloging-in-Publication Data

Comprehensive pediatric nephrology / [edited by] Denis F. Geary, Franz Schaefer.—1st ed.
p. ; cm.
ISBN 978-0-323-04883-5
1. Pediatric nephrology. I. Geary, Denis F. II. Schaefer, Franz.
[DNLM: 1. Kidney Diseases. 2. Child. 3. Urologic Diseases. WS 320 C737 2008]
RJ476.K5C66 2008
618.92'61—dc22

2007041984

Acquisitions Editor: Adrianne Brigido
Developmental Editor: Arlene Chappelle
Project Manager: Mary B. Stermel
Design Direction: Ellen Zanolle
Marketing Manager: Todd Liebel

Cover image courtesy of Norman Rosenblum.

R

Printed in China.

Last digit is the print number: 9 8 7 6 5 4 3 2 1

Sig, Nicki, Allie, Keith, Susanne, Julia, and Marie: For too many years we have spent too many hours at work, instead of being home like normal fathers. We hope this book explains in some small way what we have been trying to do.

Contributors

Juan J. Alcon MD
Pediatrc Nephrology Unit
Hospital General
University of Valencia
Valencia, Spain
41: Epidemiology and Consequences of Childhood Hypertension

Stephen I. Alexander MD, BS
Department of Nephrology
The Children's Hospital at Westmead
Westmead, Australia
15: Steroid-Sensitive Nephrotic Syndrome

Joao Guilherme Amaral MD
Assistant Professor
Image Guided Therapy Centre—Diagnostic Imaging
The Hospital for Sick Children
Toronto, Ontario
Canada
69: Pediatric Interventional Radiology

Alessandro Amore MD
Nephrology, Dialysis and Transplantation
Regina Margherita University Children's Hospital
Turin, Italy
18: IgA Nephropathy

Sharon Phillips Andreoli MD
Byron P. and Frances D. Hollett Professor of Pediatrics
Director, Division of Nephrology
James Whitcomb Riley Hospital for Children
Indianapolis, Indiana
25: Hemolytic Uremic Syndrome

Walter S. Andrews MD
Professor of Surgery
University of Missouri–Kansas City School of Medicine
Director of Pediatric Transplant
Department of Surgery
The Children's Mercy Hospitals and Clinics
Kansas City, Missouri
54: Peritoneal Dialysis Access

Christoph Aufricht MD
Universitäts-Klinik für Kinder und Jugendheilkunde
Vienna, Austria
37: Obstructive Genitourinary Disorders

Fred E. Avni MD, PhD
Professor of Radiology
Head, Department of Medical Imaging
Hôpital Erasme
Université Libre de Bruxelles
Brussels, Belgium
4: Antenatal Assessment of Kidney Morphology and Function

Arvind Bagga MD, FIAP, FAMS
Professor of Pediatrics
Division of Nephrology
All India Institute of Medical Sciences
Ansari Nagar
New Delhi, India
21: Rapidly Progressive Glomerulonephritis

Aysin Bakkaloglu MD
Department of Pediatric Nephrology
Hacettepe University
Sihhiye
Ankara, Turkey
24: Wegener's Granulomatosis, Microscopic Polyangiitis, and Childhood Polyarteritis Nodosa

Donald L. Batisky MD
Children's Hospital
Ohio State University
Columbus, Ohio
44: Treatment of Childhood Hypertension

Mary Bauman RN
Clinical Nurse Coordinator
Haemostasis/Thrombosis Program
The Hospital for Sick Children
Toronto, Ontario
Canada
26: Disordered Hemostasis and Renal Disorders

Jan Ulrich Becker MD
Institute of Pathology
University Clinic Essen
Essen, Germany
16: Steroid-Resistant Nephrotic Syndrome

Carsten Bergmann MD
Department of Human Genetics
Aachen University
Aachen, Germany
5: Genetics: Basic Concepts and Testing
9: Polycystic Kidney Disease: ADPKD and ARPKD

Alberto Bettinelli MD
Department of Pediatrics
San Leopoldo Mandic Hospital
Merate, Lecco
Italy
27: Differential Diagnosis and Management of Fluid, Electrolyte, and Acid–Base Disorders

Mario G. Bianchetti MD
Department of Pediatrics
Ospedale San Giovanni
Bellinzona, Switzerland
27: Differential Diagnosis and Management of Fluid, Electrolyte, and Acid–Base Disorders

Douglas L. Blowey MD
Associate Professor of Pediatrics and Pharmacology
Children's Mercy Hospitals and Clinics
Kansas City, Missouri
64: Drug Use and Dosage in Renal Failure

Detlef Böckenhauer MD, PhD
Consultant Paediatric Nephrologist
Great Ormond Street Hospital
London, United Kingdom
28: Fanconi Syndrome
32: Diabetes Insipidus

Patrick D. Brophy MD
C. S. Mott Children's Hospital
Ann Arbor, Michigan
39: Acute Renal Failure: Prevention, Causes, and Investigation

Deepa H. Chand MD, MHSA
Section Head
Pediatric Nephrology
Cleveland Clinic Foundation
Cleveland, Ohio
56: Hemodialysis Vascular Access: Complications and Outcomes

Pierre Cochat MD
Département de Pédiatrie and Inserm
Hospices Civils de Lyon and Université de Lyon
Hôpital Edouard Herriot
Lyon, France
58: Demographics of Pediatric Renal Transplantation

Bairbre Connolly MD, MB, FRCP(C)
Medical Director
Image Guided Therapy
The Hospital for Sick Children
Toronto, Ontario
Canada
69: Pediatric Interventional Radiology

Rosanna Coppo MD
Nephrology, Dialysis and Transplantation
Regina Margherita University Children's Hospital
Turin, Italy
18: IgA Nephropathy

Jonathan C. Craig MD, PhD
Centre for Kidney Research
The Children's Hospital at Westmead
Westmead, Australia
35: Diagnosis and Management of Urinary Tract Infections

Dagmar Csaicsich MD
Universitäts-Klinik für Kinder und Jugendheilkunde
Vienna, Austria
37: Obstructive Genitourinary Disorders

Laura Cuzzolin BSD
Department of Public Health
Section of Pharmacology
University of Verona
Verona, Italy
65: Causes and Manifestation of Nephrotoxicity

Vikas R. Dharnidharka MD
Division of Pediatric Nephrology
University of Florida College of Medicine
Gainesville, Florida
62: Prevention and Treatment of Infectious Complications in Pediatric Renal Allograft Recipients

Anne M. Durkan MD
Division of Nephrology
The Hospital for Sick Children
Toronto, Ontario
Canada
60: Acute Allograft Dysfunction

Allison A. Eddy MD
Division Head, Pediatric Nephrology
The Children's Hospital and Regional Medical Center
Seattle, Washington
34: Interstitial Nephritis

Thomas Eggermann PhD
Department of Human Genetics
Aachen University
Aachen, Germany
5: Genetics: Basic Concepts and Testing

Vassilios Fanos MD
Neonatal Intensive Care Unit
University of Cagliari
Cagliari, Italy
65: Causes and Manifestation of Nephrotoxicity

Guido Filler MD, PhD, FRCPC
Children's Hospital of Eastern Ontario
Ottawa, Ontario
Canada
68: Extracorporeal Therapies for Poisoning

Geoffrey M. Fleming MD, FAAP
Fellow, Pediatric Critical Care Medicine
Department of Pediatrics and Communicable Diseases
University of Michigan
Ann Arbor, Michigan
39: Acute Renal Failure: Prevention, Causes, and Investigation

Susan L. Furth MD, PhD
Associate Professor, Pediatrics and Epidemiology
Johns Hopkins University School of Medicine
Welch Center for Prevention, Epidemiology and Clinical Research
Baltimore, Maryland
52: Psychosocial and Ethical Issues in Children with Chronic Kidney Disease

Rasheed Gbadegesin MD
Fellow
Department of Pediatrics
University of Michigan Hospital
Ann Arbor, Michigan
12: Nephrotic Syndrome

Denis F. Geary MB, MRCP(UK), FRCPC
Professor of Paediatrics
University of Toronto
Chief, Division of Nephrology
The Hospital for Sick Children
Toronto, Ontario
Canada
53: Dialysis Modality Choice and Initiation in Children
57: Pediatric Hemodialysis Prescription, Efficacy, and Outcome

Arlene C. Gerson PhD
Division of Pediatric Nephrology
Johns Hopkins University School of Medicine
Baltimore, Maryland
52: Psychosocial and Ethical Issues in Children with Chronic Kidney Disease

Debbie S. Gipson MD, MSPH
Assistant Professor
Departments of Medicine and Pediatrics
University of North Carolina—Chapel Hill
UNC Kidney Center
Chapel Hill, North Carolina
47: Neurodevelopmental Issues in Chronic Renal Disease

Stuart L. Goldstein MD
Associate Professor of Pediatrics
Baylor College of Medicine
Medical Director, Renal Dialysis Unit and Pheresis Service
Texas Children's Hospital
Houston, Texas
40: Management of Acute Renal Failure

Manjula Gowrishankar MD, FRCPC
Associate Professor
Department of Pediatrics
Divisional Director, Pediatric Nephrology
University of Alberta
Stollery Children's Hospital
University of Alberta Hospitals
Edmonton, Alberta
Canada
31: Renal Tubular Acidosis

Nicole Graf MBBS, FRCPA
Staff Histopathologist
Department of Histopathology
The Children's Hospital at Westmead
Sydney, New South Wales
Australia
15: Steroid-Sensitive Nephrotic Syndrome

Larry A. Greenbaum MD, PhD
Division Director, Pediatric Nephrology
Emory University and Children's Healthcare of Atlanta
Atlanta, Georgia
49: Anemia in Chronic Renal Disease

Jaap W. Groothoff MD, PhD
Department of Paediatric Nephrology
Emma Children's Hospital AMC
Academic Medical Centre
Amsterdam, The Netherlands
63: Malignancy after Pediatric Renal Transplantation

Sanjeev Gulati MBBS, MD
Department of Nephrology
Sanjay Gandhi Post Graduate Institute of Medical Sciences
Lucknow, India
19: Membranous Nephropathy

Charlotte Hadtstein MD
Department of Pediatric Nephrology
Hospital for Pediatric and Adolescent Medicine
Heidelberg, Germany
42: Investigation of Hypertension in Childhood

Dieter Haffner MD
Professor and Chairman
Department of Pediatrics
University Children's Hospital
Rostock, Germany
46: Growth and Puberty in Chronic Kidney Disease

Michelle Hall MD
Associate Professor of Pediatrics
Head, Department of Pediatric Nephrology
Hôpital Universitaire des Enfants—Reine Fabiola
Université Libre de Bruxelles
Brussels, Belgium
4: Antenatal Assessment of Kidney Morphology and Function

Christine Harrison PhD
Director, Bioethics Program
The Hospital for Sick Children
Toronto, Ontario
Canada
52: Psychosocial and Ethical Issues in Children with Chronic Kidney Disease

Diane Hébert MD, FRCPC
Division of Nephrology
Department of Paediatrics
The Hospital for Sick Children
Toronto, Ontario
Canada
58: Demographics of Pediatric Renal Transplantation

Elisabeth M. Hodson MBBS, FRACP
Head, Department of Nephrology
The Children's Hospital at Westmead
Sydney, New South Wales
Australia
15: Steroid-Sensitive Nephrotic Syndrome

Stephen Hooper PhD
Department of Psychology
University of North Carolina
Chapel Hill, North Carolina
47: Neurodevelopmental Issues in Chronic Renal Disease

Bernd Hoppe MD
Professor of Pediatrics
Division of Pediatric Nephrology
University Children's Hospital
Cologne, Germany
33: Urolithiasis and Nephrocalcinosis in Childhood

Daljit K. Hothi MBBS, MRCPCH
Division of Nephrology
The Hospital for Sick Children
Toronto, Ontario
Canada
57: Pediatric Hemodialysis Prescription, Efficacy, and Outcome

Peter F. Hoyer MD
Professor of Pediatrics
Director and Chair
Children's Hospital
University Clinic Essen
Essen, Germany
16: Steroid-Resistant Nephrotic Syndrome

Julie R. Ingelfinger MD
Deputy Editor
The New England Journal of Medicine
Boston, Massachusetts
43: Etiology of Childhood Hypertension

Khalid Ismaili MD
Associate Chief
Perinatal and Pediatric Nephrology
Hôpital Universitaire des Enfants—Reine Fabiola
Brussels, Belgium
4: Antenatal Assessment of Kidney Morphology and Function

Clifford E. Kashtan MD
Professor of Pediatrics
University of Minnesota
Minneapolis, Minnesota
14: Alport Syndrome and Thin Basement Membrane Disease

Yukihiko Kawasaki MD
Department of Pediatrics
Fukushima Medical University School of Medicine
Fukushima City, Japan
23: Henoch-Schönlein Nephritis

Antoine E. Khoury MD
Division of Urology
Department of Surgery
University of Toronto
The Hospital for Sick Children
Toronto, Ontario
Canada
37: Obstructive Genitourinary Disorders

Martin Konrad MD
Universitäts-Kinderklinik
Bern, Switzerland
30: Disorders of Magnesium Metabolism

Alok Kumar MD
Department of Nephrology
Sanjay Ganchi Post Graduate Institute of Medical Sciences
Lucknow, India
19: Membranous Nephropathy

Valerie Langlois MD, FRCPC
Division of Nephrology
The Hospital for Sick Children
Toronto, Ontario
Canada
2: Laboratory Evaluation at Different Ages

Perry Yew-Weng Lau MBBS(S), MRCPCH(UK)
Department of Pediatrics
National University Hospital
Singapore
10: Hematuria and Proteinuria

Ernst Leumann MD
Professor Emeritus
Department of Nephrology
University Children's Hospital
Zurich, Switzerland
33: Urolithiasis and Nephrocalcinosis in Childhood

Xiaomei Li MD
Renal Division
Department of Medicine
First Hospital and Institute of Nephrology
Peking University
Beijing, People's Republic of China
67: Nephrotoxicity of Herbal Remedies

Christoph Licht MD
Division of Nephrology
The Hospital for Sick Children
Toronto, Ontario
Canada
17: Membranoproliferative Glomerulonephritis

Ruth Lim MD
Division of Radiology
The Hospital for Sick Children
Toronto, Ontario
Canada
1: Imaging the Pediatric Urinary Tract

Armando J. Lorenzo MD, FRCSC
Division of Urology
Department of Surgery
University of Toronto
The Hospital for Sick Children
Toronto, Ontario
Canada
37: Obstructive Genitourinary Disorders

Kera E. Luckritz DO
Pediatric Nephrology Fellow
Department of Pediatrics
Children's Hospital and Regional Medical Center
Seattle, Washington
34: Interstitial Nephritis

Empar Lurbe MD
Pediatric Nephrology Unit
Hospital General
University of Valencia
Valencia, Spain
41: Epidemiology and Consequences of Childhood Hypertension

John D. Mahan MD
Children's Hospital
Ohio State University
Columbus, Ohio
44: Treatment of Childhood Hypertension

Robert Mak MD, PhD
Division of Pediatric Nephrology
Oregon Health and Science University
Portland, Oregon
48: Nutritional Challenges in Pediatric Chronic Kidney Disease

Stephen D. Marks MBChB, MSc, MRCP, DCH, FRCPCH
Consultant Paediatric Nephrologist
Renal Unit
Great Ormond Street Hospital for Children
London, United Kingdom
22: Lupus Nephritis

M. Patricia Massicotte MD, MSc, FRCPC
Children's Hospital
University of Alberta, Edmonton
Edmonton, Alberta
Canada
26: Disordered Hemostasis and Renal Disorders

Ranjiv Mathews MD
Associate Professor
Division of Pediatric Urology
The Johns Hopkins School of Medicine
Brady Urological Institute
Baltimore, Maryland
36: Vesicoureteral Reflux

Tej K. Mattoo MD, DCH, FRCP(UK)
Professor of Pediatrics
Wayne State University School of Medicine
Chief, Pediatric Nephrology and Hypertension
Children's Hospital of Michigan
Detroit, Michigan
36: Vesicoureteral Reflux

Heather Maxwell MBc, MBChB, FRCP
Department of Paediatric Nephrology
Royal Hospital for Sick Children
Glasgow, United Kingdom
61: Chronic Renal Transplant Dysfunction

Otto Mehls MD
Department of Pediatric Nephrology
Hospital for Pediatric and Adolescent Medicine
Heidelberg, Germany
50: Disorders of Bone Mineral Metabolism in Chronic Kidney Disease

Anette Melk MD, PhD
Department of Pediatric Nephrology
Hospital for Pediatric and Adolescent Medicine
Heidelberg, Germany
3: Tools for Renal Tissue Analysis
59: Immunosuppression in Pediatric Kidney Transplantation

Michael Mengel MD
Alberta Transplant Applied Genomic Centre
Edmonton, Alberta
Canada
17: Membranoproliferative Glomerulonephritis

Shina Menon MD
Research Fellow in Pediatric Nephrology
All India Institute of Medical Sciences
Ansari Nagar
New Delhi, India
21: Rapidly Progressive Glomerulonephritis

Dawn S. Milliner MD
Division of Nephrology
Mayo Clinic
Rochester, Minnesota
33: Urolithiasis and Nephrocalcinosis in Childhood

Mark Mitsnefes MD
Division of Nephrology and Hypertension
Children's Hospital Medical Center
Cincinnati, Ohio
51: Cardiovascular Disease in Pediatric Chronic Kidney Disease

Alicia M. Neu MD
Associate Professor
Department of Pediatrics
Medical Director, Pediatric Dialysis and Kidney Transplantation
The Johns Hopkins University School of Medicine
Baltimore, Maryland
62: Prevention and Treatment of Infectious Complications in Pediatric Renal Allograft Recipients

Patrick Niaudet MD
Service de Néphrologie Pédiatrique
Hôpital Necker-Enfants Malades
Paris, France
11: Nephritic Syndrome

Richard Nissel MD
Department of Pediatrics
University Hospital
Rostock, Germany
46: Growth and Puberty in Chronic Kidney Disease

Beate Ermisch-Omran MD
Department of Pediatrics and Adolescent Medicine
Albert-Ludwigs-University Freiburg
Freiburg, Germany
8: Nephronophthisis and Medullary Cystic Kidney Disease

Heymut Omran MD
Professor
Department of Pediatrics and Adolescent Medicine
Albert-Ludwigs-University Freiburg
Freiburg, Germany
8: Nephronopthisis and Medullary Cystic Kidney Disease

Seza Ozen MD
Department of Pediatric Nephrology
Hacettepe University
Sihhiye
Ankara, Turkey
24: Wegener's Granulomatosis, Microscopic Polyangiitis, and Childhood Polyarteritis Nodosa

Francesco Perfumo MD
Nephrology, Dialysis, and Transplantation Unit
G. Gaslini Institute
Genoa, Italy
55: Pediatric Peritoneal Dialysis Prescription

Veronique Phan MD
Department of Pediatrics
Sainte-Justine Hospital
Montreal, Quebec
Canada
39: Acute Renal Failure: Prevention, Causes, and Investigation

Maury Pinsk MD, FRCPC
Assistant Professor
Department of Pediatrics
Division of Pediatric Nephrology
University of Alberta
Stollery Children's Hospital
Edmonton, Alberta
Canada
31: Renal Tubular Acidosis

Tino D. Piscione MD, PhD, FRCP(C)
Division of Nephrology
The Hospital for Sick Children
Toronto, Ontario
Canada
6: Structural and Functional Development of the Kidney

Uwe Querfeld MD
Department of Pediatric Nephrology
Charité—Universitätsmedizin Berlin
Berlin, Germany
51: Cardiovascular Disease in Pediatric Chronic Kidney Disease

Ian John Ramage MBChB, MPCP(UK)
Consultant Paediatric Nephrologist
Renal Unit
Royal Hospital for Sick Children
Glasgow, Scotland
56: Hemodialysis Vascular Access: Complications and Outcomes

Josep Redon MD
Hypertension Clinic, Internal Medicine
Hospital Clinico
University of Valencia
Valencia, Spain
41: Epidemiology and Consequences of Childhood Hypertension

Lisa A. Robinson MD, FRCPC
Division of Nephrology
The Hospital for Sick Children
Toronto, Ontario
Canada
60: Acute Allograft Dysfunction

Renee F. Robinson PharmD, MPH
Children's Hospital
Ohio State University
Columbus, Ohio
44: Treatment of Childhood Hypertension

Norman D. Rosenblum MD, FRCP(C)
Division of Nephrology
The Hospital for Sick Children
Toronto, Ontario
Canada
7: Disorders of Kidney Formation

Remi Salomon MD, PhD
Hopital Necker
Paris, France
7: Disorders of Kidney Formation

Gagandeep K. Sandhu MD
CARE Program
Department of Pediatrics
Stollery Children's Hospital
University of Alberta
Edmonton, Alberta
Canada
66: Complementary and Alternative Treatments for Renal Diseases

Franz Schaefer MD
Professor of Pediatrics
Chief, Division of Pediatric Nephrology
Center for Pediatric and Adolescent Medicine
University of Heidelberg
Heidelberg
Germany
45: Progression of Chronic Kidney Disease and Renoprotective Therapy in Children

Claus P. Schmitt MD
Department of Pediatric Nephrology
Hospital for Pediatric and Adolescent Medicine
Heidelberg, Germany
50: Disorders of Bone Mineral Metabolism in Chronic Kidney Disease

Cornelis H. Schröder MD, PhD, FASN
Professor of Pediatric Nephrology
UMC Utrecht
Utrecht, The Netherlands
53: Dialysis Modality Choice and Initiation in Children

Donna Secker MSc, RD
Dietitian
Department of Clinical Dietetics and Division of Nephrology
The Hospital for Sick Children
Toronto, Ontario
Canada
48: Nutritional Challenges in Pediatric Chronic Kidney Disease

Afroze Ramzan Sherali MBBS
Professor of Paediatrics
Head, Department of Paediatric Nephrology
National Institute of Child Health
Karachi, Pakistan
67: Nephrotoxicity of Herbal Remedies

Jennifer Dart Yin Sihoe BMBS(Nottm), FRCSEd(Paed), FHKAM(Surg)
Specialist in Paediatric Surgery
Division of Paediatric Surgery and Paediatric Urology
Department of Surgery
Prince of Wales Hospital
Shatin, New Territories
Hong Kong
38: Voiding Disorders

William E. Smoyer MD
Robert C. Kelsch Professor
Pediatric Nephrology Division
University of Michigan Health System
C. S. Mott Children's Hospital
Ann Arbor, Michigan
12: Nephrotic Syndrome

Hitoshi Suzuki MD
Department of Pediatrics
Fukushima Medical University School of Medicine
Fukushima City, Fukushima
Japan
23: Henoch-Schönlein Nephritis

Velibor Tasic MD, PhD
Professor
Department of Pediatric Nephrology
University Children's Hospital
Skopje, Macedonia
20: Postinfectious Glomerulonephritis

Burkhard Tönshoff MD, PhD
Professor of Pediatrics and Pediatric Nephrology
Vice Chairman, Department of Pediatrics I
University Children's Hospital
Heidelberg, Germany
59: Immunosuppression in Pediatric Kidney Transplantation

Jeffrey Traubici MD
Department of Diagnostic Imaging
The Hospital for Sick Children
Toronto, Ontario
Canada
1: Imaging the Pediatric Urinary Tract

Kjell Tullus MD, PhD, FRCPCH
Honorary Senior Lecturer
Nephro-urology
Institute of Child Health
Consultant Paediatric Nephrologist
Great Ormond Street Hospital for Children
London, United Kingdom
22: Lupus Nephritis

William G. van't Hoff BSc, MD, FRCPCH
Consultant Paediatric Nephrologist
Great Ormond Street Hospital
London, United Kingdom
28: Fanconi Syndrome

Priya S. Verghese MBBS
Pediatric Nephrology Fellow
Department of Pediatrics
Children's Hospital and Regional Medical Center
Seattle, Washington
34: Interstitial Nephritis

Enrico Eugenio Verrina MD
Department of Pediatric Nephrology and Dialysis
G. Gaslini Institute
Genoa, Italy
55: Pediatric Peritoneal Dialysis Prescription

Udo Vester MD
Department of Pediatric Nephrology, Gastroenterology, Endocrinology, and Transplant Medicine
Universitätsklinikum Essen
Universität Duisburg-Essen
Essen, Germany
16: Steroid-Resistant Nephrotic Syndrome

Sunita Vohra MD, FRCPC, MSc
University of Alberta
Stollery Children's Hospital
Edmonton, Alberta
Canada
66: Complementary and Alternative Treatments for Renal Diseases

Siegfried Waldegger MD
Professor
Department of Pediatrics
Philipps University of Marburg
Marburg, Germany
29: Bartter, Gitelman, and Related Syndromes

Bradley A. Warady MD
Professor of Pediatrics
University of Missouri–Kansas City School of Medicine
Chief, Section of Pediatric Nephrology
Director, Dialysis and Transplantation
The Children's Mercy Hospitals and Clinics
Kansas City, Missouri
54: Peritoneal Dialysis Access

Aoife Waters MRCPI
Division of Nephrology
The Hospital for Sick Children
Toronto, Ontario
Canada
6: Structural and Functional Development of the Kidney

Nicholas J. A. Webb DM, FRCP, FRCPCH
Department of Paediatric Nephrology
Royal Manchester Children's Hospital
Manchester, United Kingdom
61: Chronic Renal Transplant Dysfunction

Stefanie Weber MD
Department of Pediatric Nephrology
Children's University-Hospital Heidelberg
Heidelberg, Germany
13: Hereditary Nephrotic Syndrome

Gabrielle Williams BSc, PhD
Centre for Kidney Research
The Children's Hospital at Westmead
Westmead, Australia
35: Diagnosis and Management of Urinary Tract Infections

Sik-Nin Wong MBBS, FRCPCH, FRCP(Edin & Glasg), FHKCPaed, FHKAM(Paed)
Honorary Clinical Associate Professor
Department of Pediatrics
University of Hong Kong
Consultant
Department of Paediatrics and Adolescent Medicine
Tuen Mun Hospital
Tuen Mun, New Territories
Hong Kong
38: Voiding Disorders

Elke Wühl MD
Department of Pediatric Nephrology
Hospital for Pediatric and Adolescent Medicine
Heidelberg, Germany
42: Investigation of Hypertension in Childhood
45: Progression of Chronic Kidney Disease and Renoprotective Therapy in Children

Li Yang MD
Renal Division
Department of Medicine
First Hospital and Institute of Nephrology
Peking University
Beijing, People's Republic of China
67: Nephrotoxicity of Herbal Remedies

Hui-Kim Yap MBBS, MD
Department of Pediatrics
National University Hospital
Singapore
10: Hematuria and Proteinuria

Chung-Kwong Yeung MBBS, MD, FRCSE, FRCSG, FRACS, FACS, FHKAM(Surg), DCH(Lond & Irel)
Professor
Chair, Division of Paediatric Surgery and Paediatric Urology
Director, Minimally Invasive Surgical Skills Centre
Department of Surgery
Chinese University of Hong Kong
Prince of Wales Hospital
Shatin, New Territories
Hong Kong
38: Voiding Disorders

Verna Yiu MD, FRCPC
Associate Professor
Divisional Director, Pediatric Nephrology
Department of Pediatrics
University of Alberta
Edmonton, Alberta
Canada
26: Disordered Hemostasis and Renal Disorders

Klaus Zerres MD
Department of Human Genetics
Aachen University
Aachen, Germany
9: Polycystic Kidney Disease: ADPKD and ARPKD

Lothar Bernd Zimmerhackl MD
Professor and Chairman
Department of Pediatrics I
Medical University Innsbruck
Innsbruck, Austria
25: Hemolytic Uremic Syndrome

Preface

Initially, when approached by Elsevier to consider editing a textbook of Pediatric Nephrology, the intention was to emphasize the clinical content and target our readership accordingly. When further elaborating on appropriate contents of a contemporary clinical textbook, we soon realized that excellence of clinical care is not accomplished only by a review of clinical skills and diagnostic techniques, but demands an understanding of the underlying pathogenesis of disease as well as of recent scientific advances that have affected or will soon affect clinical disease management. Indeed, it may be more relevant than ever to insert some fundamentals of basic research into the physiopathology of pediatric kidney disorders for a thorough, up-to-date understanding of the clinical context. Hence, we felt there was a real need for a book on "Comprehensive Pediatric Nephrology."

The principal objective of this textbook is to provide this comprehensive information in a concise manner so that it is easily understood and useful to all pediatric nephrologists, irrespective of whether their primary interest is scientific or clinical. In addition, we hope this book will also be of value to general pediatricians and pediatric urologists, and that it will serve as an educational tool for trainees in our specialty.

Contributors to this book were deliberately selected to provide international perspectives. Authorship of several chapters was specifically chosen to represent different geographical regions, recognizing that treatments for the same disease may vary significantly between different continents. The choice of coauthors from different geographic locations, sometimes with different native languages, inevitably increased the complexity of the editorial process, but we hope that readers will appreciate the confluence of varied expertise that resulted. We are certainly grateful to our colleagues who collaborated so successfully in this manner.

Similarly, authorship for several chapters represented varied clinical specialties, specifically to include the opinions of each. Thus, the chapters on vesicoureteral reflux and obstructive and voiding disorders were coauthored by nephrologists and urologists, because we recognize that each specialty has specific, and sometimes different, expertise to approach these problems. The input from our urological colleagues was essential to meet our commitment to provide a comprehensive review of those topics. The contribution of colleagues with expertise in nutritional care, child psychology, human genetics, and bioethics were similarly valuable and reflect the necessity of a dedicated team approach to optimize the care of children with complex renal disorders.

The growing use of traditional and complementary medicines in pediatric nephrology is recognized by the inclusion of two chapters dedicated to improving our understanding of this subject. Although use of these medications or alternative remedies may be frowned upon by many pediatric nephrologists, it is important that we acknowledge the reality of their widespread use. Without condoning their use, it is important to know what our patients are consuming and to consider their potential effects when the clinical conditions change. A basic knowledge of the putative benefits and recognized side-effects of these products is essential.

Our work has been greatly facilitated by Susan Pioli and Arlene Chappelle at Elsevier, and Edit Stroganoff in Heidelberg, who kept us organized. We are truly grateful for their help.

Finally, we must also pay tribute to the colleagues with whom we interact daily, with whom we wrestle over complex clinical decisions, in whose laboratories the therapeutics of tomorrow are undergoing investigation, who provide superb day-to-day care for all of our patients, and who have alleviated our editorial burden by taking some of our clinical workload on their shoulders.

Denis F. Geary

Franz Schaefer

Contents

SECTION I: TOOLS OF INVESTIGATION IN PEDIATRIC NEPHROLOGY

CHAPTER 1 Imaging the Pediatric Urinary Tract

Jeffrey Traubici and Ruth Lim

Imaging plays an important role in the diagnosis and follow-up of many diseases of the pediatric urinary tract.[1-3] In the pediatric age group both congenital and acquired diseases of the urinary tract are assessed using a number of different modalities, and in many cases it is the imaging study that offers a diagnosis or at least narrows the differential diagnosis. Radiography, excretory urography, fluoroscopy, sonography, computed tomography (CT), magnetic resonance imaging (MRI), and nuclear medicine have all been used to assess the urinary tract, each possessing its own relative strengths and weaknesses. In many cases a combination of two or more modalities will be necessary to narrow the differential diagnosis. It is of fundamental importance not only to know the most appropriate modality for the investigation of a particular patient but also to understand the risks and benefits associated with the various available modalities. Several of those used in urinary tract imaging employ ionizing radiation. It has long been understood that exposure to radiation has deleterious effects, with recent evidence suggesting a strong association between exposure to radiation (particularly at doses reached in CT) and subsequent development of neoplastic disease.[4] Other risks to be considered relate to the administration of intravenous contrast agents and mainly involve contrast-induced nephropathy and adverse contrast reactions.[5-7] Finally, because some children will require sedation or general anesthesia in order to perform an examination, the risk associated with the anesthesia must also be considered.[8,9]

This chapter serves as an overview of these imaging modalities and presents examples of their application in the evaluation of children with nephropathy.

ULTRASOUND

Sonography has become an important part of the pediatric imaging armamentarium—perhaps the most important. Its strengths are many. To begin, it does not use ionizing radiation. In addition, ultrasound does not require administration of intravenous contrast agents, although several ultrasound contrast agents have been recently developed that can increase the accuracy of the imaging examination.[10] Furthermore, sedation is rarely required.

The most common indications for sonographic imaging of the kidneys include urinary tract infection,[11-13] follow-up of antenatally diagnosed hydronephrosis, evaluation of a palpable mass, assessment for vascular abnormalities, screening of patients at known risk for developing renal neoplasms (for instance, Beckwith-Wiedemann syndrome), and assessment for possible obstruction. Ultrasound can also assess other findings noted on antenatal imaging, such as renal agenesis, ectopia, dysplasia, or mass.

The ultrasound examination can be tailored in many ways to suit the patient and clinical situation. A patient who is upset or frightened can be scanned lying next to a parent or in the arms of a parent, which can help alleviate anxiety. Coupled with a calm and reassuring environment and various distractions (for example, toys, music, or videos), this setting often allows for the performance of a satisfactory diagnostic study. The need for sedation is extremely rare but may be considered on a case-by-case basis.

The patient can be scanned in various positions (supine, prone, or decubitus) depending on the scenario. In some situations the examination can be repeated after an intervention has been performed to determine whether it was successful or resulted in a complication. One can study the urinary tract before or after voiding, after placement of a bladder catheter, ureteral stent, or nephrostomy catheter, or after biopsy. These repeated examinations can be done without concern for the effects of radiation.

By and large the small body habitus of children allows for excellent imaging of the urinary tract. There are cases of larger teenagers and obese children in which imaging of the urinary system can be suboptimal. Scanning of the kidneys is performed mainly with curved array transducers for assessment of kidney length and status of the renal parenchyma, pelvocaliceal system, ureter, and bladder. These images can be supplemented with images obtained with a high-resolution linear transducer, which offers a superior level of spatial resolution but is limited in the depth to which it can penetrate. For that reason high-resolution sonography is particularly well suited to neonates, infants, and younger children.

The kidneys are ovoid organs that typically lie in the renal fossae, although they can be ectopic. Their lengths can be measured and compared with published nomograms[14-16] (Figure 1-1). Growth of the kidneys can be followed on serial examinations. However, it is important when assessing growth to keep in mind that the kidney can occasionally be overmeasured or undermeasured depending on the circumstances of the examination. Retardation in growth can be a sign of ongoing insult such as scarring associated with vesicoureteral reflux.[17]

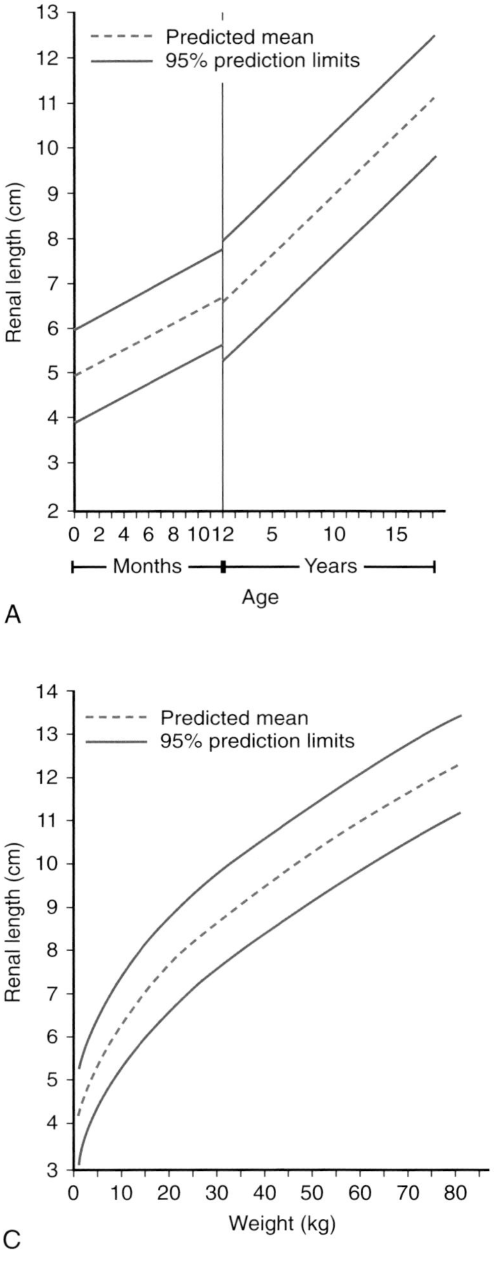

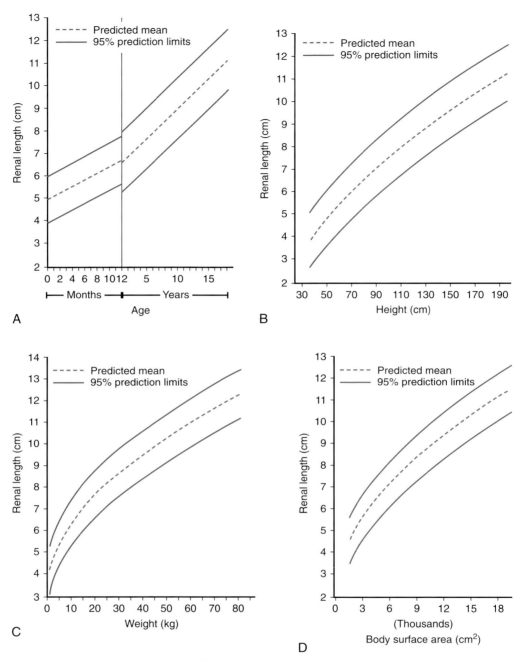

Figure 1-1 Nomograms delineate the predicted mean and 95% prediction limits of renal length as a function of age **(A),** height **(B),** weight **(C),** and total body surface area **(D).**

In healthy children there is a difference in echogenicity between normal renal cortex and the medullary pyramids, with the former more echogenic and the latter more hypoechoic (Figure 1-2). This difference, termed *corticomedullary differentiation,* is more pronounced in the neonatal period when the cortex is slightly more echogenic than in later childhood.[18] The echogenicity of the renal cortex can be compared with an internal and adjacent standard—that being the liver. One must, however, ensure that this reference (the liver) is normal. The pattern of normal renal echogenicity varies during childhood. In the neonate the renal cortex can be isoechoic or even hyperechoic compared with the liver (Figure 1-3), and the corticomedullary differentiation can be pronounced. By the time a child is several months of age, the renal cortex should be hypoechoic compared with the echogenicity of the liver.[18,19] The pyramids, particularly in neonates, can be so hypoechoic that they can be mistaken for a dilated collecting system. There are exceptions to the hypoechogenicity of the renal pyramids, the majority of which relate to disease states (that is, medullary nephrocal-

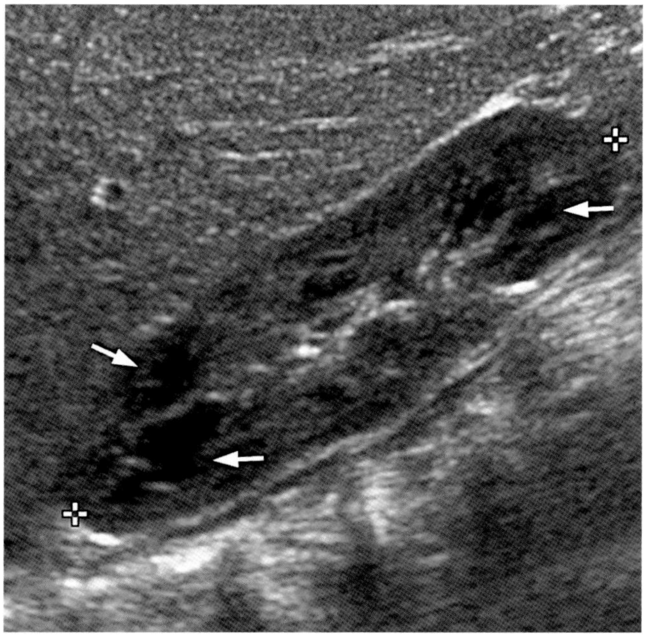

Figure 1-2 Ultrasound of the normal kidney *(length indicated by calipers)* demonstrates renal pyramids that are nearly anechoic *(arrows)* and can be mistaken for dilatation of the renal collecting system.

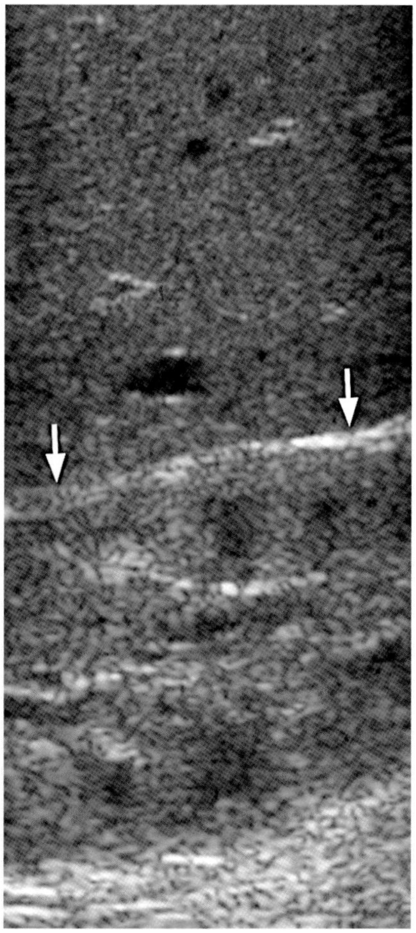

Figure 1-3 Ultrasound of the normal neonatal kidney in which the renal cortex is more echogenic than the adjacent liver. This can be a normal finding in neonates. After several months the renal cortex should be less echogenic than the liver.

cinosis) or interventions (that is, Lasix administration). The most common exception, however, seen in many neonates, may be the transient increase in echogenicity, which has been attributed to precipitation of Tamm Horsfall proteins.[20] Additionally there may be lobulation of the renal outline, especially in neonates. This should not be confused with scarring. Normal lobulation tends to be seen in the portion of the cortex between pyramids, whereas focal scarring tends to occur in portions of the cortex directly overlying the pyramid.

The renal collecting system can be assessed both qualitatively and quantitatively regarding the degree of dilatation. Measurement of pelvic dilatation can be assessed at the level of the renal hilum—or just beyond it in the case of an extrarenal pelvis. A full bladder can exaggerate the degree of dilatation. It is therefore useful to assess the pelvic diameter after voiding if the urinary bladder is overdistended. If the ureter is dilated, its diameter can be assessed along its course, although it can be visualized most reliably proximally and distally (Figure 1-4). The midportion of the ureter is often obscured by overlying bowel gas. The thickness of the wall of the ureter or bladder can also be assessed. Thickening of the urothelium anywhere along the urinary tract can be associated with, though is not pathognomonic for, infection or inflammation. Urolithiasis can be diagnosed as an echogenic focus with distal acoustic shadowing.[21] The degree of obstruction caused by a calculus can also be assessed with sonography.

Color Doppler and pulsed Doppler interrogation can be used to assess vascularity of the kidneys. The study can assess the vessels from the main renal arteries and veins through the arcuate vessels in the renal parenchyma. Indications for Doppler evaluation include suspicion of renal arterial or venous thrombosis,[22] arterial stenosis,[23] trauma,[24] infection,[25] acute tubular necrosis, and transplant rejection, although the role of rejection in evaluation remains controversial.[26]

VOIDING CYSTOURETHROGRAPHY

Voiding cystourethrography (VCUG) is the study of choice for diagnosing vesicoureteral reflux and assessing the anatomy of the bladder and urethra. Indications for this investigation include urinary tract infection,[13] antenatally or postnatally diagnosed hydronephrosis, and suspected posterior urethral valves, among others. A catheter is placed into the bladder using aseptic technique. At most institutions sedation is not administered. In our experience, the examination can be performed without sedation in the vast majority of children, given proper explanation and reassurance. Water-soluble contrast is instilled into the bladder under the pressure of gravity until pressure within the bladder induces micturition. The amount of contrast used will vary according to the patient's age and bladder capacity. At some institutions a single cycle of filling and voiding is performed. At others, two or three cycles are the routine.[27] This method, termed *cyclic VCUG*,

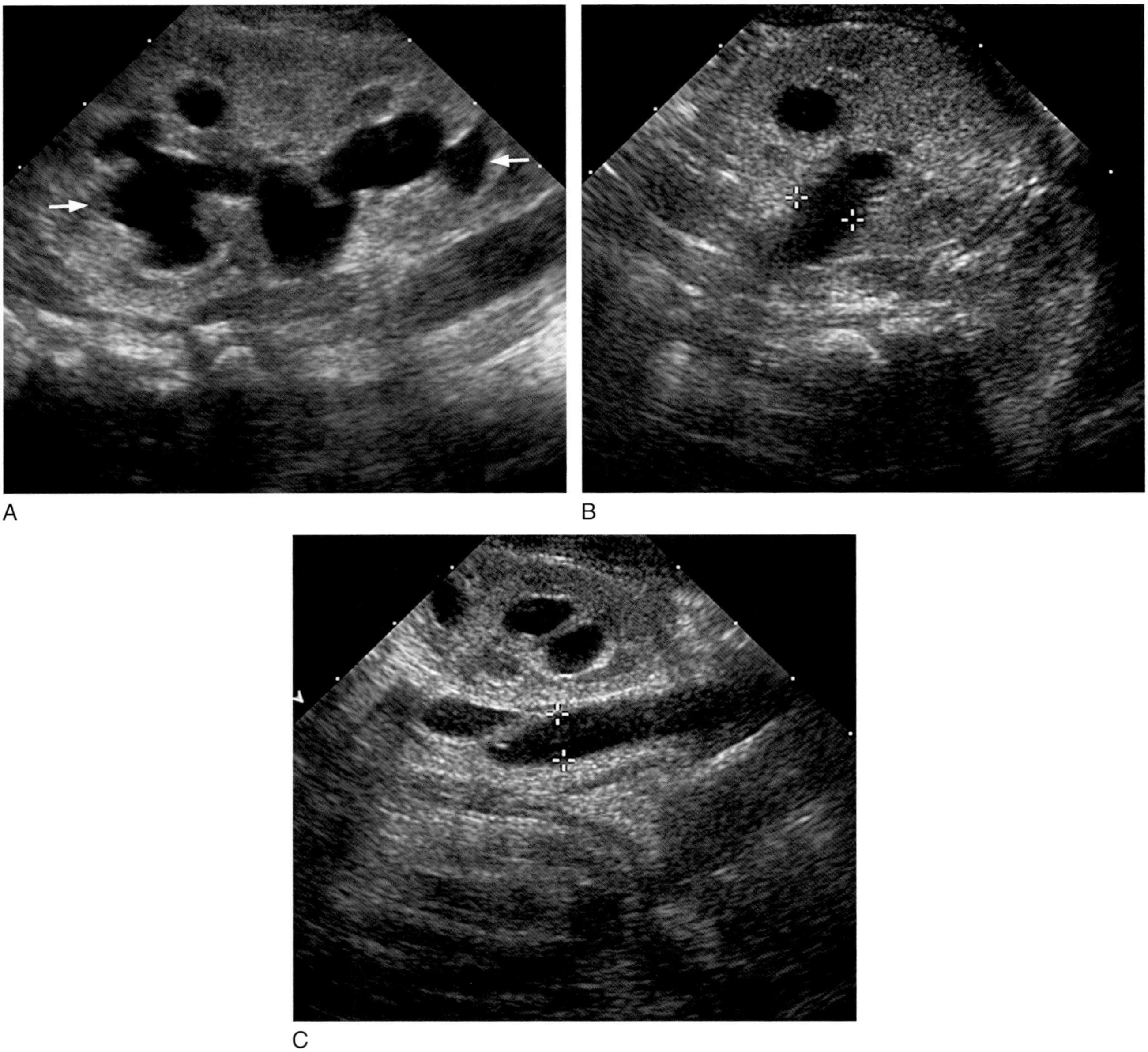

Figure 1-4 **A,** Ultrasound of the kidney in the longitudinal plane demonstrates moderate pelvocaliceal dilatation *(arrows)*. **B,** In the transverse plane the renal pelvis is measured with respect to its maximal AP diameter *(calipers)*. **C,** Scanning along the flank, one can often visualize the ureter if it is dilated *(calipers)*.

has demonstrated greater sensitivity in detecting reflux but results in a higher radiation dose than does the single-cycle method.

Exact views obtained will vary from institution to institution but all will include images of the bladder that will allow for assessment of its wall characteristics and structural abnormalities such as diverticula, ureteroceles, or urachal abnormalities. These images should also show if there is any reflux into the ureters. Images of the urethra are obtained during voiding either with the catheter in place or after its removal. Whether the urethra is imaged with a catheter in place or not depends on the institution and the individual radiologist. At our institution an image of the urethra is obtained with the catheter in place as well as after its removal, thus giving an image of the urethra in cases where the child stops voiding just as the catheter is removed. An image of the renal fossae will assess for any reflux to the level of the kidney, characterize the collecting system anatomy (duplex or not), and assign a grade to that reflux.[28]

Here, as with the other modalities, the study is tailored to the individual child. The bladder can be filled via a suprapubic catheter or a Mitrofanoff if present. If a child is unable to void naturally, the bladder can be drained via the catheter in situ. If the child is reticent to void, warm water applied to the perineum can induce voiding. Despite a variety of maneuvers, there are children who will not void on the fluoroscopy table. In these cases the micturition phase of the study is not possible and the sensitivity of the study to detect reflux is diminished. In some institutions an image is taken after the child has been permitted to void in the bathroom.

Complications related to the study can occur and are similar to those encountered in any catheterization of the bladder, with infection and trauma being the most common. We have encountered cases of urinary retention postprocedure.

NUCLEAR MEDICINE

Nuclear medicine is a modality that comprises a variety of examinations for evaluating the pediatric urinary tract. Nuclear medicine techniques differ from other imaging modalities in that they focus on function rather than detailed anatomic structure. As a result, nuclear imaging plays an important complementary role to other modalities, particularly in the structural evaluation obtained with ultrasound.

The physical principles of nuclear imaging also differ from those of other modalities. Rather than passing x-rays through the patient as is done with fluoroscopy, radiography, and CT, nuclear medicine introduces a radioactive tracer into the patient's body. A camera is then positioned adjacent to the patient and images are created by the emitted gamma rays. Depending on the specific examination being performed, the radiopharmaceutical can be injected intravenously to be extracted by the kidneys or can be instilled via catheter into the bladder. Radiation doses in nuclear medicine examinations of the urinary tract are lower than those encountered in CT and fluoroscopy.

Most pediatric patients are either cooperative about lying still on the imaging table or are infants small enough to be safely restrained. Therefore the majority of patients will not require any form of sedation when undergoing a nuclear medicine examination. However, if it is anticipated that a child will have difficulty lying still for at least 30 minutes, sedation should be considered. Occasionally general anesthesia may be necessary.

Urinary tract imaging accounts for more than half of the examinations performed in a typical pediatric nuclear medicine department. The most common indications for nuclear renal imaging examinations include urinary tract infection, antenatally or postnatally detected hydronephrosis, or suspected impairment of renal function.

OVERVIEW OF RADIOPHARMACEUTICALS

Technetium-99m (99mTc) is the radionuclide (gamma-emitting isotope) used to label the overwhelming majority of radiopharmaceuticals in urinary tract imaging. It emits a 140 keV gamma ray and has a physical half-life of 6 hours.

Technetium-99m pertechnetate is the base form of 99mTc that is obtained from a portable generator unit found in any nuclear medicine radiopharmacy. With commercially available labeling kits, 99mTc-pertechnetate can be used to label other pharmaceuticals. Additional radiopharmaceuticals routinely used in nuclear urinary tract imaging are described in the following sections.

Glomerular Filtration Agents

99mTc-diethylenetriaminepentaacetic acid (DTPA) is used to calculate glomerular filtration function. Measuring its rate of extraction from plasma via serial blood sampling provides an accurate estimate of the glomerular filtration rate (GFR). Approximately 90% of DTPA is filtered by the kidneys into the urine within 4 hours after intravenous injection.[29] Renal imaging can also be performed using 99mTc-DTPA, providing additional information on excretion and drainage, as well as the ability to plot dynamic renogram curves.

51Cr-ethylenediaminetetraacetate (EDTA) is also used in calculating GFR and is the standard GFR agent used in Europe. Because of better radioisotope binding, 51Cr-EDTA produces slightly higher values for GFR than does 99mTc-DTPA. However, this difference is small (5% or less) and is not considered clinically relevant.[30] Renal imaging is not performed with 51Cr-EDTA because it does not emit gamma rays suitable for imaging.

Tubular Secretion Agents

99mTc-mercaptoacetyltriglycine (MAG3) is injected intravenously and cleared predominantly (95%) by the renal tubules.[29] The extraction fraction of MAG3 is more than twice that of DTPA, resulting in a higher target-to-background ratio. For this reason image quality is more satisfactory with 99mTc-MAG3 than with 99mTc-DTPA, particularly in the setting of impaired renal function or urinary obstruction. 99mTc-MAG3 has become the radiopharmaceutical of choice for performing functional renal imaging (except when performing GFR measurement), which can be used to assess renal function, detect obstructive uropathy, and evaluate renal transplant allografts. Clearance of MAG3 by the kidneys is proportional to effective renal plasma flow.

Iodine-123- and iodine-131-orthoiodohippuran (OIH) have been used for nuclear renal imaging. Use of 123I-OIH and 131I-OIH in clinical imaging, however, has been replaced by 99mTc-MAG3, which produces nearly identical renogram time-activity curves. Furthermore, 99mTc-MAG3 provides markedly better image resolution than 131I-OIH and is less expensive than 123I-OIH.

Renal Cortical Agents

99mTc-dimercaptosuccinic acid (DMSA) binds to the sulfylhydryl groups of the proximal renal tubules after filtration.[29] It is usually the cortical imaging agent of choice, because only 10% is excreted into the urine during the first several hours after intravenous injection. Therefore 99mTc-DMSA produces excellent high-resolution images of the renal cortex without interference from urinary activity.

99mTc-glucoheptonate (GH) is cleared by the kidneys through both tubular secretion and glomerular filtration, with 10% to 15% remaining bound to the renal tubules 1 hour after injection. Therefore early imaging can be performed to evaluate renal perfusion, urinary excretion, and drainage. Late imaging at 1 to 2 hours will visualize the renal cortex. 99mTc-DMSA is the preferred cortical imaging agent because its cortical binding is much higher than that of 99mTc-GH.

DIRECT RADIONUCLIDE CYSTOGRAM

Direct radionuclide cystography (DRC) detects vesicoureteral reflux (VUR) with great sensitivity. It is used as a complementary modality to VCUG.[31-33] Typically, patients who present with a first-time febrile urinary tract infection or with newly discovered hydronephrosis initially undergo VCUG to diagnose reflux.[34] DRC is then used as a follow-up examination to determine if reflux has resolved or is persistent, including postoperative evaluation after ureteral reimplantation surgery. Additionally, DRC is commonly performed as a primary screening examination to detect reflux in asymptomatic patients with a small kidney or solitary kidney, or who have a family history of VUR.

VCUG vs. DRC

Since image acquisition during DRC is continuous, it is more sensitive in detecting brief, intermittent episodes of VUR that may be missed with VCUG. DRC is also more sensitive in detecting small amounts of VUR because there is no interference with the images from overlying stool and bowel gas as there is with VCUG. Additionally, and importantly, the radiation dose to the patient is approximately $^{1}/_{100}$ of the dose received during VCUG.[35]

DRC, however, provides little anatomic detail and is not effective in detecting structural abnormalities such as ureteroceles, ectopic ureteral insertions, bladder diverticula, urethral abnormalities including posterior urethral valves, or duplicated collecting systems. These structural abnormalities require VCUG and sometimes ultrasound to be adequately demonstrated.

DRC is performed in much the same manner as VCUG. The bladder is catheterized with a 5 to 8 French catheter and drained of urine, which is usually sent for microbiology culture. The bladder is then instilled with a 99mTc radiopharmaceutical, which can be any of 99mTc-pertechnetate, 99mTc-DTPA, or 99mTc-sulphur colloid. The patient lies supine on the imaging table with the camera positioned posteriorly. Continuous dynamic images are acquired while the bladder is filling and while the patient voids on the table. The bladder capacity is recorded, and radioactivity count data can subsequently be used to calculate the postvoid residual bladder volume. As they do with VCUG, some institutions may choose to perform a cyclic DRC with two or three cycles of bladder filling and thereby increase sensitivity in detecting reflux.

A DRC examination is considered positive for reflux when radiotracer can be seen in the ureter, renal pelvis, or both in one or both kidneys (Figure 1-5). VUR can occur during the bladder-filling phase or the voiding phase, and the tracer may or may not clear completely from the renal pelvis at voiding completion. The severity of reflux is usually characterized by one of the following: minimal = reflux into ureter only; moderate = reflux reaches renal pelvis; or severe = reflux reaches renal pelvis with dilatation of the pelvis and/or ureter. Minimal reflux is difficult to detect on DRC, and false-negative examinations are not uncommon when reflux reaches only the distal ureter. However, this minimal form of reflux usually resolves early in childhood, and the false-negative examinations are of dubious clinical significance.

INDIRECT RADIONUCLIDE CYSTOGRAM

An alternative test for detecting VUR is the indirect radionuclide cystogram (IRC).[36-45] This examination should be reserved for children in whom bladder catheterization is impossible[46] and who are above age 3.[35] To perform IRC, it is necessary to inject 99mTc-MAG3 intravenously. Continuous dynamic images of the kidney and bladder are obtained during bladder filling and voiding (Figure 1-6). The patient must remain motionless during imaging and can void on command after the bladder has filled. Regions of interest are drawn over the intrarenal collecting systems and the ureters, and time-activity curves are plotted. A sudden increase in activity in the renal pelvis and ureter indicates the presence of VUR (Figure 1-6).

There is ongoing debate as to whether direct or indirect radionuclide cystography is the preferable examination for detecting VUR. In theory, IRC is the better physiologic mimicker, with slow antegrade filling of the bladder. In contrast, DRC involves rapid retrograde bladder filling via a catheter, which some believe induces artificial reflux. Others assert that this higher sensitivity of DRC, as great as 95%,[47] is an advantage, and that comparison between DRC results and prior VCUG results is more valid when the same method of bladder filling is used. Proponents of DRC also point out that patients with impaired renal function may have insufficient excretion of radiotracer during IRC, which results in lower sensitivity, ranging between 32% and 81% according to the literature.[37,40,47-49] In practice there is also a high rate of IRC failure because of some children's inability to remain motionless during voiding or to void at all during image acquisition.[46] In cases of a negative IRC examination, subsequent DRC or VCUG is required to confidently exclude VUR.[35]

RENAL CORTICAL SCAN

Cortical scintigraphy with 99mTc-DMSA is a highly sensitive examination used for detecting both acute lesions (pyelonephritis) and late sequelae (parenchymal scarring) in children with urinary tract infections. It is important to understand that acute lesions of pyelonephritis can take as long as 6 months to resolve scintigraphically. Therefore permanent scarring can only be reported when the DMSA scan is performed at least 6 months after the acute infection. If less than 6 months have elapsed since the infection, any defects seen on DMSA scan should be interpreted as either resolving pyelonephritis or as a potential scar. Thus it is not routinely recommended that a renal cortical scintigraphy be performed within 6 months of an acute infection unless there is an acute need to document renal involvement, because a repeat scan will likely be needed later to exclude permanent scarring.[13,35,50-52] When requesting a DMSA scan, it is helpful for the referring physician to note the date of the most recent urinary tract infection.

Renal scarring tends to occur at the upper and lower poles of the kidney because of the round-shaped orifices of the compound papillae at these locations. The simple papillae at the midpoles have slitlike orifices that are less prone to reflux of infected urine. Renal defects are reported as unilateral or bilateral, single or multiple, small or large, and having or not having loss of volume. Permanent scarring tends to cause loss of volume, whereas acute infection does not. If present, a dilated renal pelvis can also be visualized (Figure 1-7). DMSA cortical scintigraphy is more sensitive than intravenous

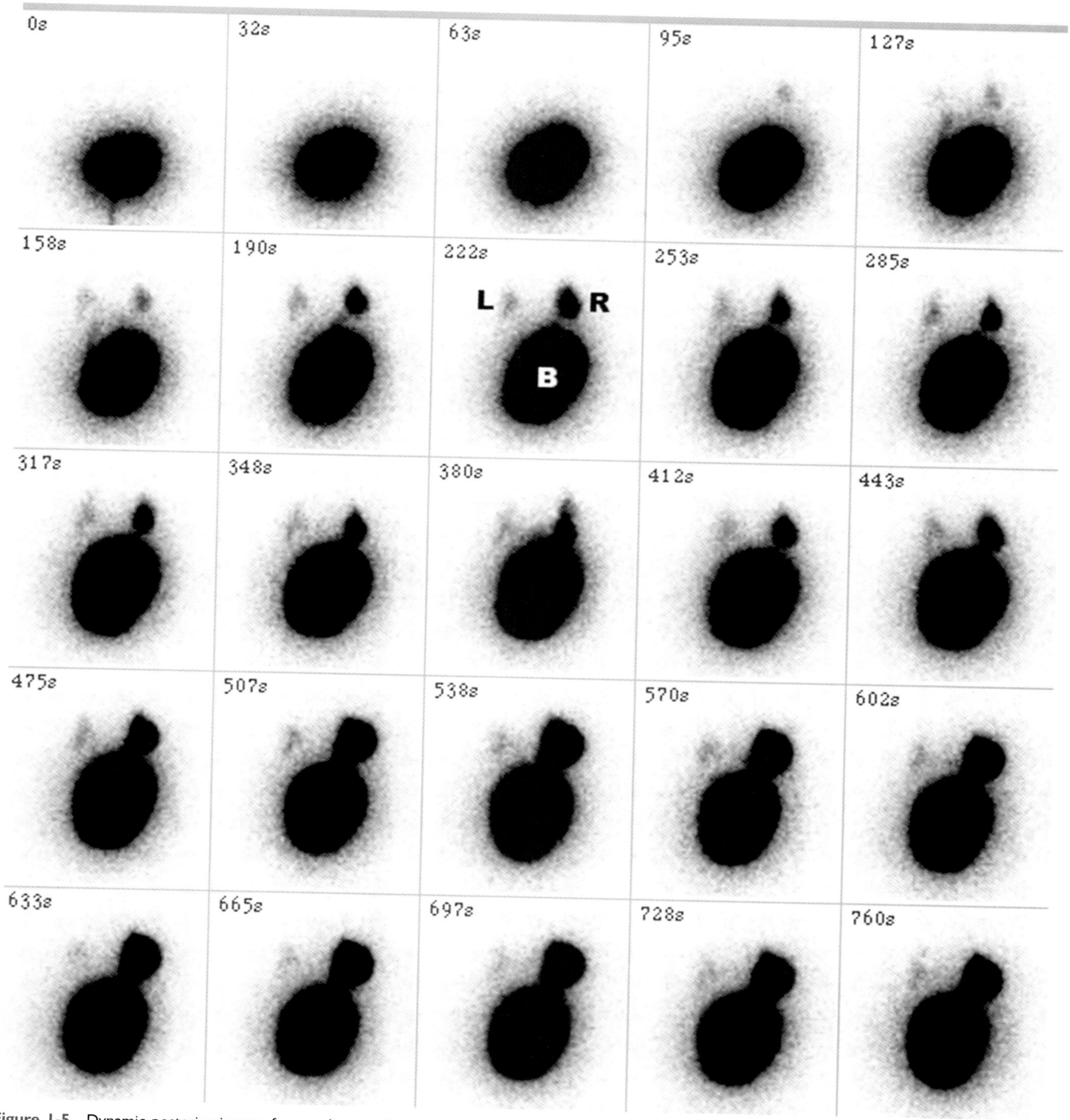

Figure 1-5 Dynamic posterior images from a direct radionuclide cystogram (DRC). This patient demonstrates bilateral vesicoureteral reflux that occurs during bladder *(B)* filling. The left-sided reflux *(L)* is moderate, and the right-sided reflux *(R)* is severe and compatible with a dilated intrarenal collecting system and ureter.

pyelography and ultrasound for detection of both acute lesions and permanent scarring.[25,51,53,54]

Other causes of cortical defects on DMSA scan include renal cysts and masses. Normal variations in appearance of the renal cortex can include indentation by the adjacent spleen, fetal lobulations, columns of Bertin, duplex kidney, and malrotated kidney. Renal cortical scans are often useful in confirming diagnoses of horseshoe kidney, ectopic kidney, or cross-fused renal ectopia when ultrasound is equivocal (Figure 1-8).

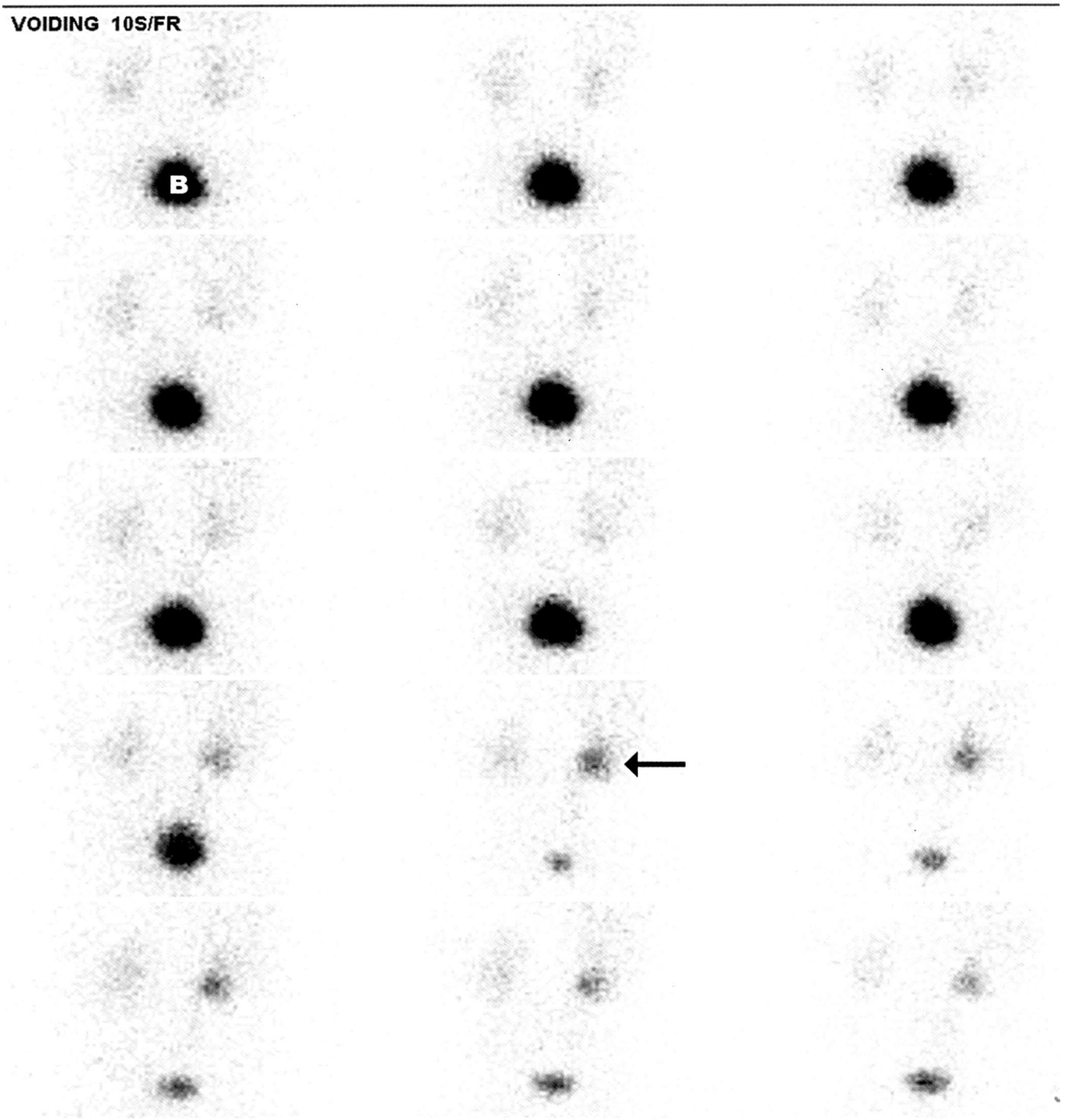

A

Figure 1-6 **A,** Dynamic posterior images from an indirect radionuclide cystogram (IRC). Initially there is normal drainage of radiotracer activity from the intrarenal collecting systems bilaterally. However, during bladder *(B)* voiding, there is a sudden and dramatic increase in the radiotracer activity in the right renal pelvis *(arrow)*, consistent with vesicoureteral reflux.

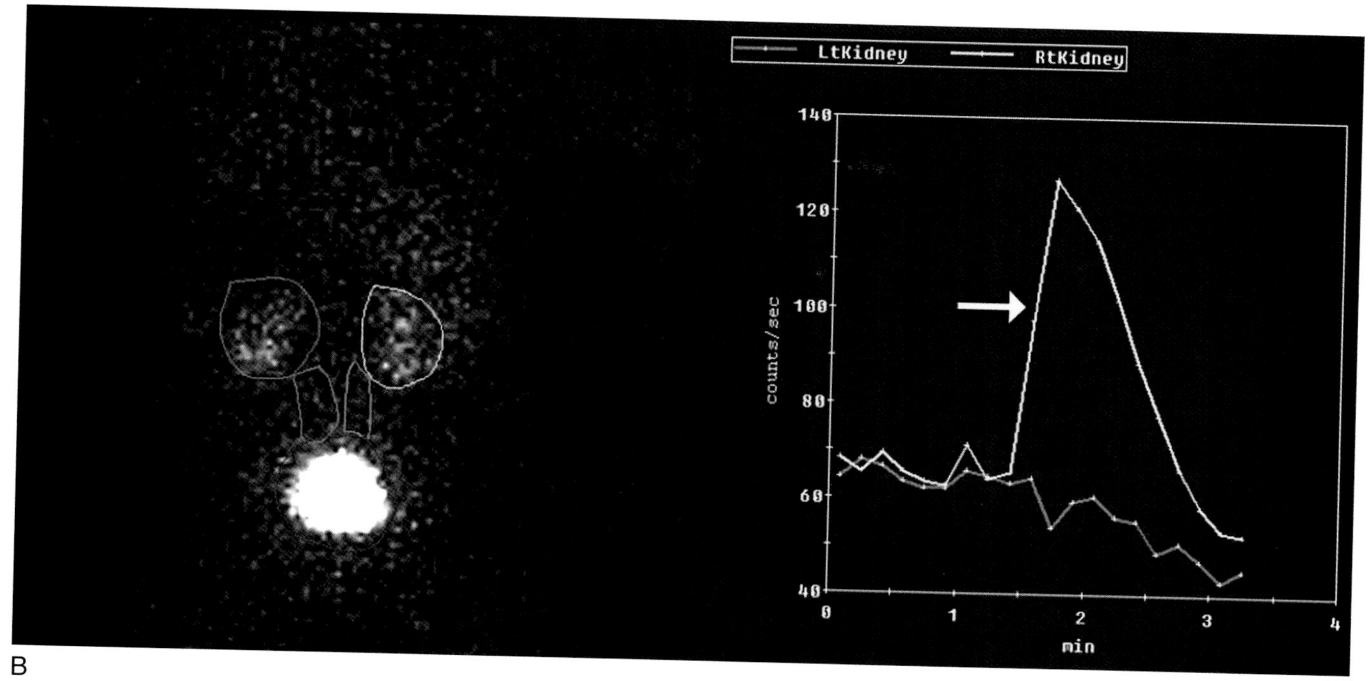

Figure 1-6, cont'd B, Dynamic renogram curve confirms this finding; a sudden increase in activity in the right renal pelvis is observed *(arrow)*. There is no evidence of reflux in the left kidney.

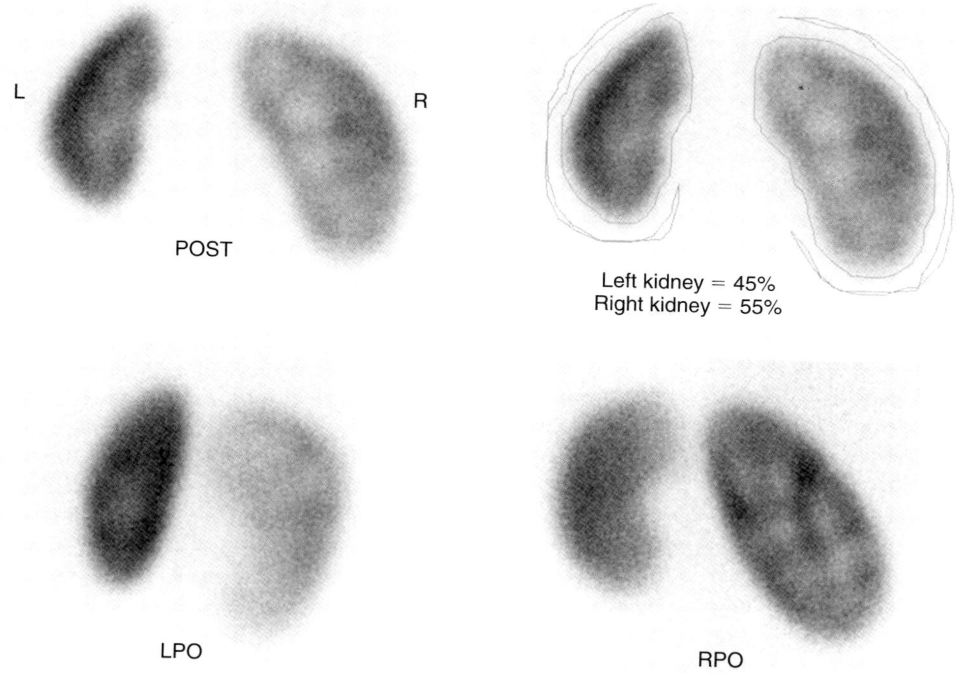

Figure 1-7 DMSA renal cortical scan in a patient with right hydronephrosis. The right kidney is asymmetrically large and demonstrates areas of central photopenia corresponding to the enlarged renal pelvis and calyces. The left kidney is normal. The differential function of the kidneys remains within normal limits (left 45%, right 55%).

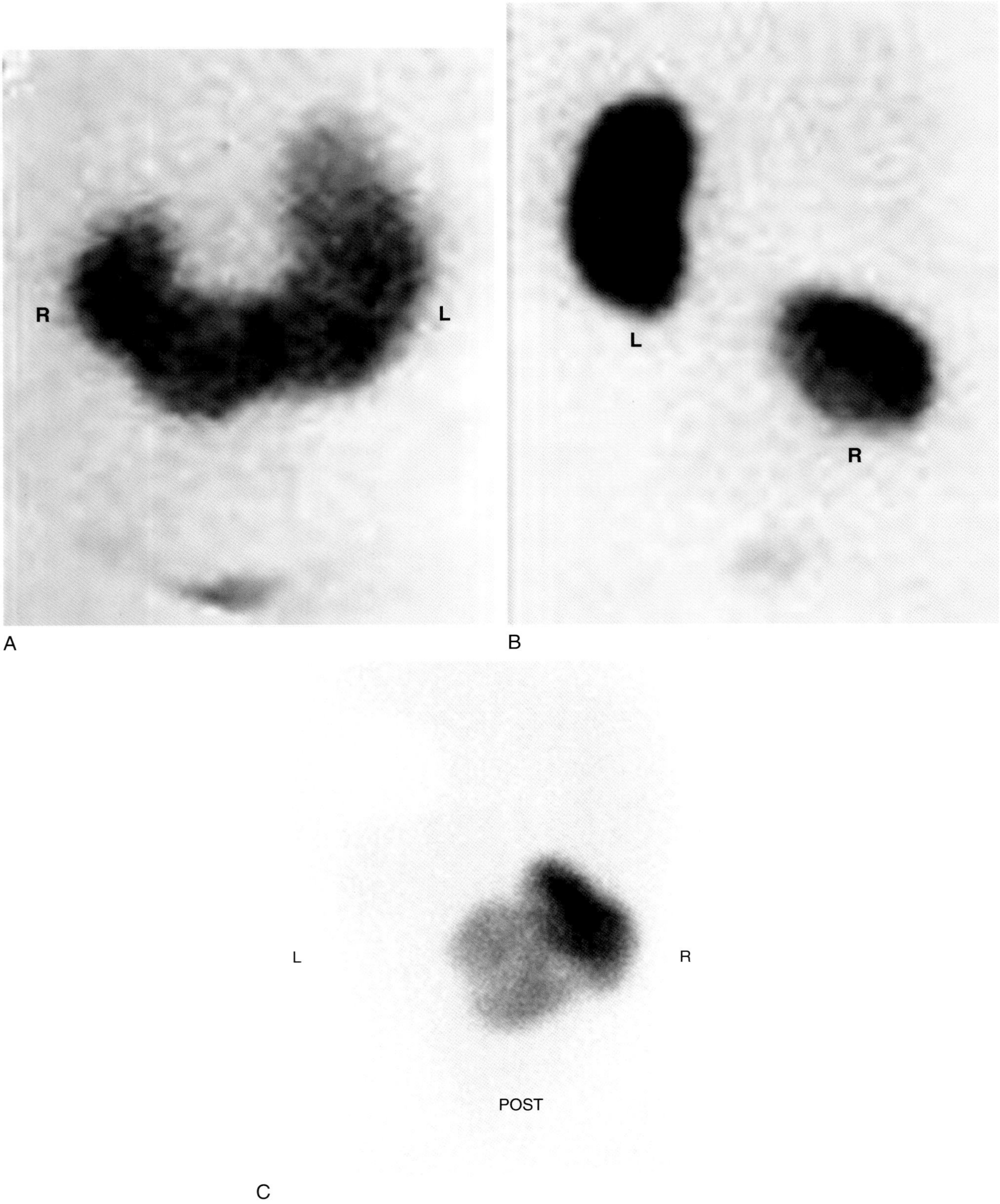

Figure 1-8 DMSA renal cortical scans in three different patients with anatomic renal variants. **A,** Anterior image of a horseshoe kidney. **B,** Posterior image of a pelvic ectopic right kidney. The left kidney is normal. **C,** Posterior image of cross-fused renal ectopia.

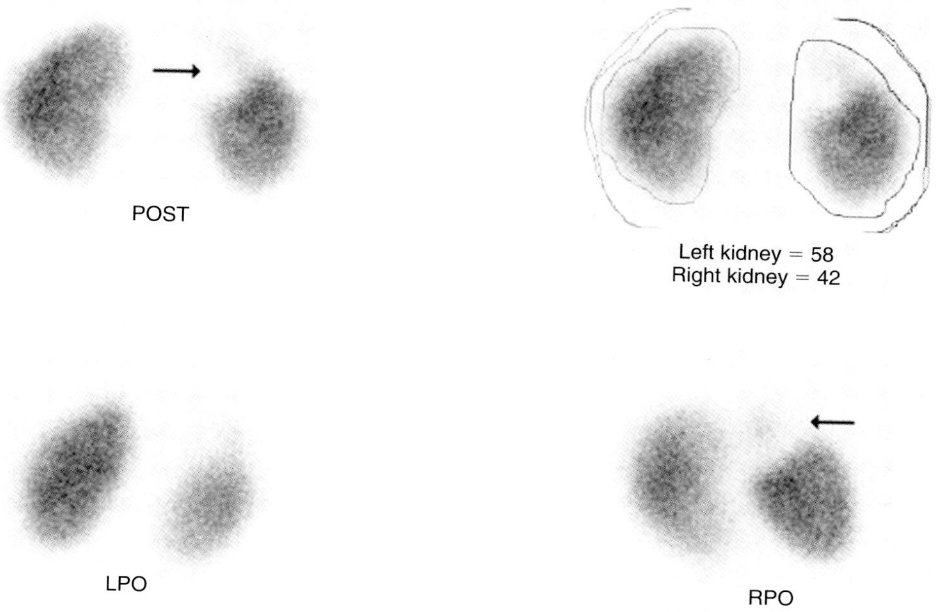

Figure 1-9 DMSA renal cortical scan in the posterior *(POST)*, left posterior oblique *(LPO)*, and right posterior oblique *(RPO)* projections. This patient has a large cortical defect *(arrows)* that represents an extensively scarred upper-pole moiety in a duplex kidney. The left kidney is normal. The differential function of the kidneys is at the outer limits of normal (left 58%, right 42%), suggesting that the remaining right lower-pole moiety has hypertrophied to somewhat compensate for the loss of upper-pole function.

Images are acquired 2 to 3 hours after injection of 99mTc-DMSA. Planar images are acquired in the posterior and right and left posterior oblique positions (Figure 1-9). In infants, additional pinhole images may be acquired that offer higher spatial resolution (Figure 1-10). In older, sufficiently cooperative children, additional single photon emission computed tomography (SPECT) images may be acquired, again improving spatial resolution[55-59] (Figure 1-11). The utility of these additional views is not yet precisely known.[60,61] Although they have been shown to improve sensitivity for detecting very small cortical defects, there is concern about the many false-positive results they have produced.[62] Furthermore, what risk these small defects pose for long-term clinical sequelae (such as hypertension and renal failure) is the subject of continued debate.[63-65]

FUNCTIONAL RENAL IMAGING AND RENOGRAPHY

Functional renal imaging uses dynamic image acquisition to evaluate renal perfusion, uptake, excretion, and drainage of radiotracer by the urinary system. Renography refers to the process of plotting the radiotracer activity in the urinary system as a function of time, resulting in renogram curves. The potential amount of information that can be acquired with functional renal imaging is large. Abnormal perfusion can suggest arterial stenosis or occlusion. Delayed uptake and excretion of radiotracer suggest parenchymal disease or dysfunction. Poor drainage of radiotracer into the bladder can suggest obstructive uropathy or overcompliance of the collecting system. Functional renal imaging can be custom-tailored for specific clinical problems. For example, a diuretic challenge can be administered to evaluate for urinary obstruction, as later described under Diuretic Renogram.

Although 99mTc-DTPA is widely used for functional renal imaging, 99mTc-MAG3 is preferred because of its higher extraction fraction and better target-to-background ratio. This advantage is particularly important in patients with impaired renal function or urinary obstruction, and also in very young patients with immature renal function.

Immediately after injection of radiotracer, imaging of renal perfusion can be performed. The patient lies supine, with the camera positioned posteriorly. Radiotracer activity should reach the kidneys about 1 second after the tracer bolus in the abdominal aorta passes the renal arteries; there should be symmetric perfusion of the kidneys.[66] Over the next 20 to 30 minutes, imaging of renal function takes place. Maximal parenchymal activity is normally seen 3 to 5 minutes after injection (T_{max}).[67] Urinary activity in the renal pelvis is typically seen 2 to 4 minutes (cortical transit time) after injection; however, there is no widespread consensus as to what constitutes a normal cortical transit time.[68] There should be prompt drainage of tracer into the urinary bladder, with less than half of the activity at T_{max} remaining in the renal pelvis 8 to 12 minutes after injection ($T_{1/2}$).[67]

Renogram curves are generated by plotting the activity within regions of interest drawn around each kidney. The renogram is a graphic representation of the uptake, excretion, and drainage phases of renal function, and the curves for each kidney should be reasonably symmetric. Patients should be

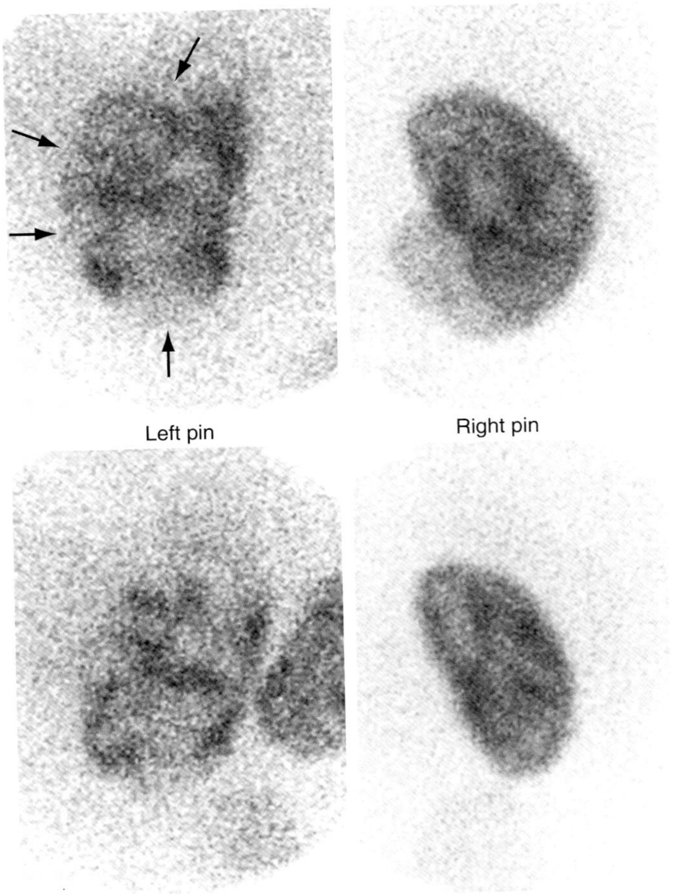

Figure 1-10 DMSA renal cortical scan images obtained with a pinhole collimator. This patient demonstrates numerous defects in the left kidney involving the upper, mid, and lower poles *(arrows)*. The right kidney is normal.

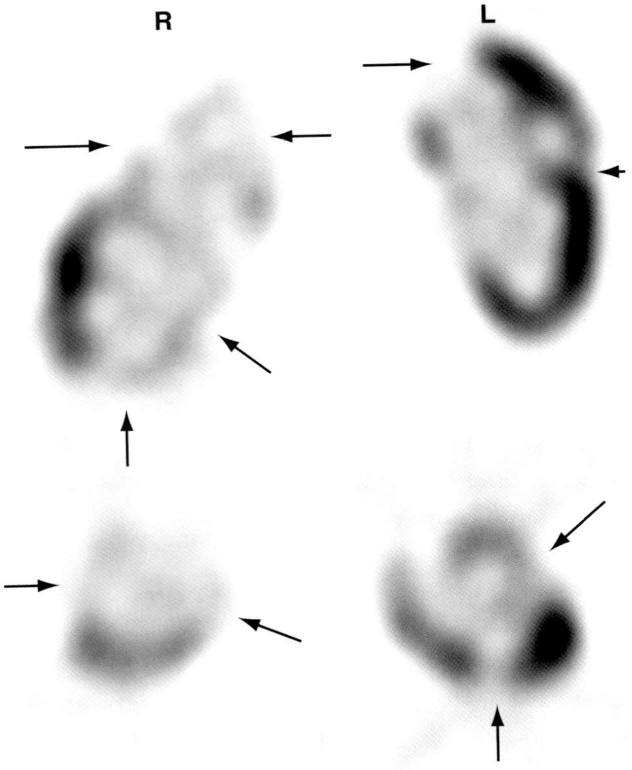

Figure 1-11 DMSA renal cortical scan images obtained with SPECT. This patient demonstrates numerous cortical defects in both kidneys *(arrows)*. The right kidney is more extensively scarred than the left kidney.

well hydrated, preferably with intravenous fluids, when functional renal imaging is performed, because dehydration will result in an abnormal renogram with globally delayed function and slow drainage.

DIURETIC RENOGRAM

In the setting of urinary collecting system dilatation not due to vesicoureteral reflux, the possibility of urinary tract obstruction must be considered. Diuretic renography, performed with furosemide, is useful in determining the presence of a high-grade obstruction at the ureteropelvic junction (UPJ) or the ureterovesical junction (UVJ). Diuretic renography is commonly used to evaluate the results of surgery in patients who have undergone pyeloplasty for ureteropelvic junction obstruction.

Diuretic renography is performed in the same manner as dynamic renal imaging (described earlier), with the additional step of administering intravenous furosemide to cause maximal urine flow through the collecting system. The dose of furosemide is usually 1 mg/kg, with a maximum dose of 40 mg.[69] The timing of the furosemide administration varies among institutions, being that several diuretic protocols have been described, validated, and debated in the literature.[35,70,71] The most commonly used protocols are F+20 (furosemide given 20 minutes after radiotracer if normal spontaneous drainage has not occurred[72]—a protocol endorsed by the American Society of Fetal Urology), F-15 (furosemide injected first, followed 15 minutes later by radiotracer—a widely used European standard),[69] and F0 (radiotracer and furosemide injected one immediately following the other).[73,74]

Bladder catheterization is not always necessary but should be performed in patients who are not toilet-trained or who have known hydroureter, vesicoureteral reflux, bladder dysfunction, or posterior urethral valves. In this particular subset of patients, back pressure from urine in the bladder may cause a false-positive result.

The patient lies supine, with the camera positioned posteriorly, and dynamic images are acquired from the time of radiotracer injection for approximately 20 minutes. In the case of the F+20 protocol, imaging is performed for an additional 20 minutes after injection of furosemide.

In the absence of obstruction, there is rapid drainage of radiotracer from the renal pelvis into the bladder to a minimal residual after 20 minutes. In quantitative terms, a drainage half-time, $T_{1/2}$, of less than 10 minutes usually means the absence of obstruction (Figure 1-12).

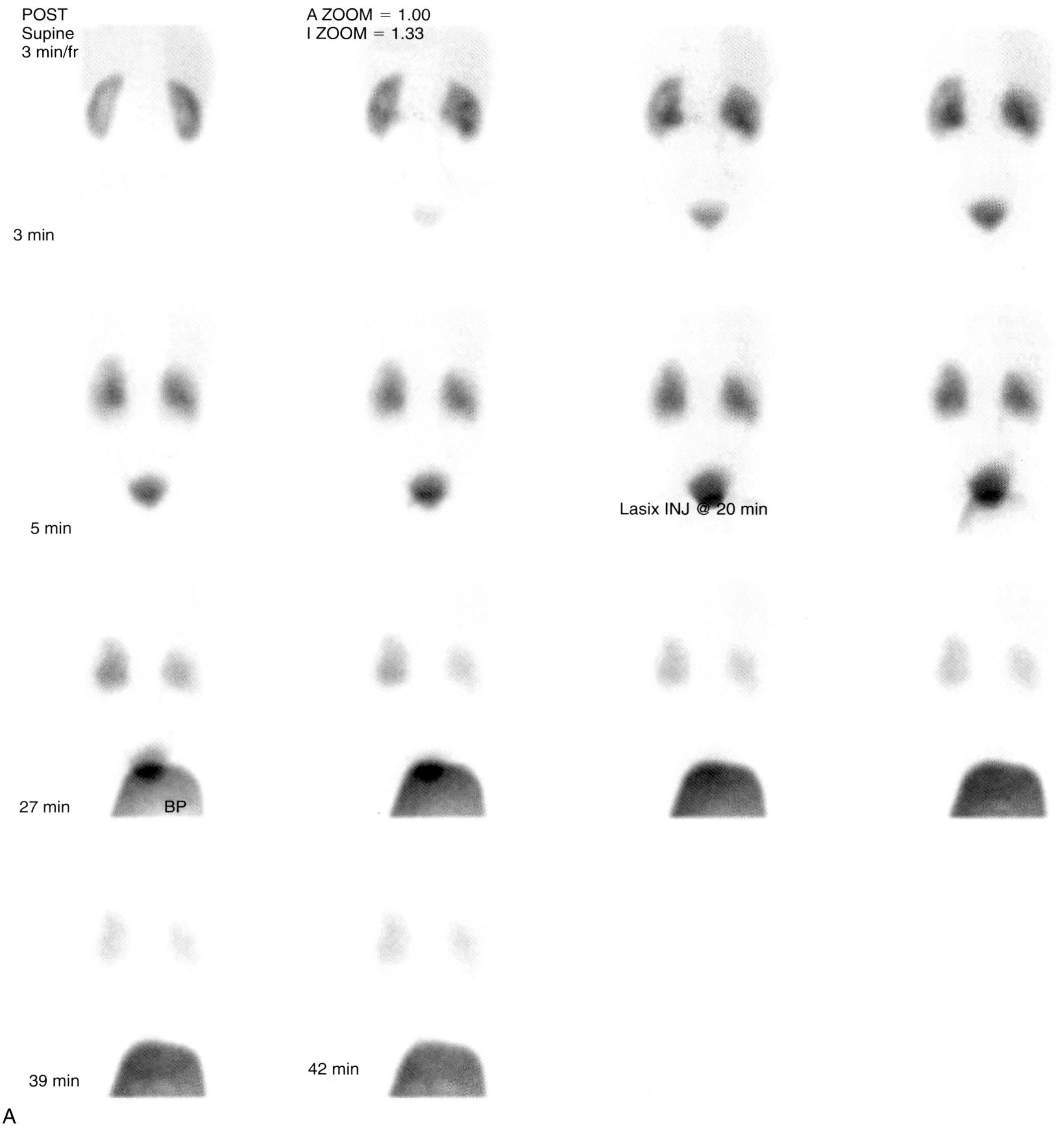

Figure 1-12 Diuretic MAG3 scan in a patient with bilateral hydronephrosis. **A,** After injection of MAG3, dynamic imaging demonstrates radiotracer accumulating in bilateral dilated intrarenal collecting systems, and there is some spontaneous drainage of tracer into the bladder. After injection of furosemide at 20 minutes (F+20 protocol), bilateral collecting systems drain rapidly as the patient voids into a bedpan *(BP)*.

Continued

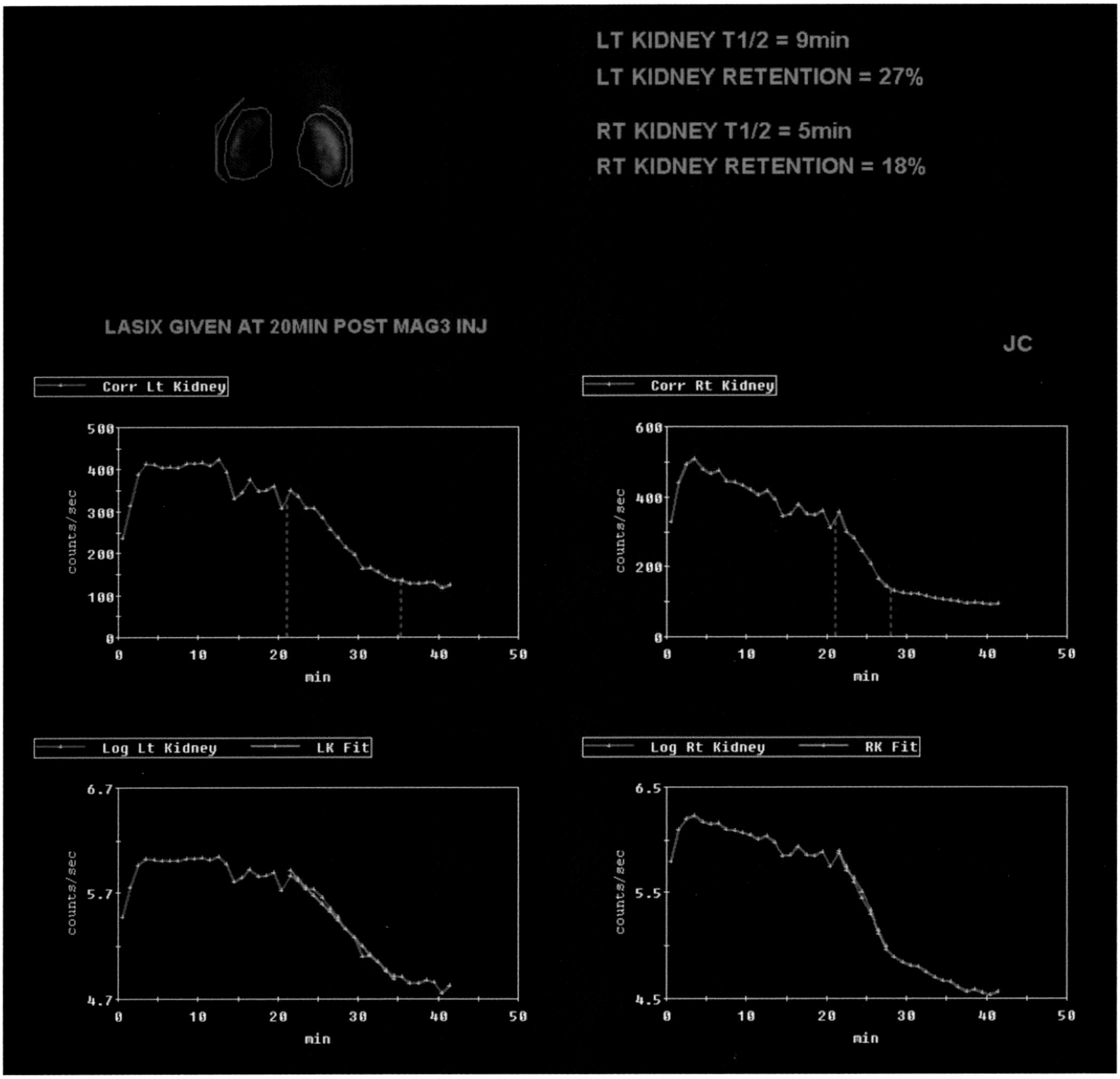

B

Figure 1-12, cont'd **B,** The renogram curve is a graphic representation of the renal activity. The calculated drainage half-time ($T_{1/2}$) of both kidneys is within normal limits, indicating the absence of a high-grade urinary obstruction.

In an obstructed system, the drainage of radiotracer from the collecting system will be slow. In this case, a $T_{1/2}$ of greater than 20 minutes indicates obstruction (Figure 1-13). $T_{1/2}$ ranging between 10 and 20 minutes is usually considered an equivocal result, and a follow-up examination is typically performed to see if the drainage normalizes or becomes frankly obstructed.

The above drainage parameters are used when analyzing a region of interest drawn around the renal pelvis, when UPJ obstruction is suspected. These values can also be applied to the ureter and to a region of interest combining the ureter and renal pelvis when UVJ obstruction is suspected.

If at the end of dynamic imaging there remains a large amount of radiotracer in the renal pelvis, ureter, or both, it is useful to have the patient void, if possible, in an upright position and follow with a final static image. Sometimes the postural/gravitational effect will cause additional drainage to occur.[35]

Pitfalls are common when interpreting diuretic renography. Poor renal function from prolonged, severe obstruction can result in poor accumulation of radiotracer in the collecting system, making the renogram difficult or impossible to interpret. A very dilated, overly compliant, but nonobstructed collecting system may have a prolonged $T_{1/2}$ because the capacious collecting system easily accommodates a large urine volume.[69,71] This reservoir effect can be observed in the setting of primary megaureter and in patients who have undergone successful pyeloplasty for UPJ obstruction.

COMPUTED TOMOGRAPHY

Although rarely the initial imaging modality in the workup of urinary tract disease, CT does contribute significantly to the imaging of children with suspected urinary tract disorders. Indications include neoplasia,[75] trauma,[76,77] severe infections,[78] and occasionally complex questions regarding anatomy[79] (although MRI often would be the preferred modality). Ultrasound may be the mainstay of imaging urolithiasis, but CT can be useful in cases that on ultrasound are equivocal or nondiagnostic.

CT allows for cross-sectional imaging of the urinary tract, and has the ability to reconstruct images in any plane for analysis. CT also provides excellent resolution of urinary tract structures. The addition of intravenous contrast to CT imaging allows for even greater accuracy in detecting disease. Newer generations of CT technology provide higher spatial and temporal resolution, and examinations can often be done without need of sedation or general anesthesia, which may be required for MRI.

On unenhanced scans the kidneys demonstrate attenuation similar to the normal liver or spleen. They are surrounded by a variable amount of retroperitoneal fat depending on the age and health status of the patient. Administration of contrast results in a reliable pattern of enhancement beginning in the renal cortex, followed by enhancement of the renal pyramids and later by opacification of the renal pelvocaliceal system, ureter, and bladder.

The contrast resolution of CT also allows for detection of hydronephrosis, renal calcifications (Figure 1-14), and diseases extending into the perirenal fat without the need for intravenous contrast. With the addition of intravenous contrast, however, one can detect individual lesions of the renal parenchyma, such as cysts, tumors, or nephroblastomatosis; focal areas of diminished enhancement, such as foci of pyelonephritis or contusion (Figure 1-15); and global abnormalities of enhancement, such as in renal artery stenosis or thrombosis.

Issues of contrast allergy and contrast-induced nephropathy relate more to the iodinated compounds administered in CT than to other contrast agents used in diagnostic imaging. It is important to consider these issues when ordering a CT examination and to discuss the indications and risks with the radiologist involved. Strategies for reducing the risk of adverse contrast reactions include considering an alternative imaging modality, performing a noncontrast-enhanced CT, or using premedication (typically corticosteroids and antihistamines). Risk factors for contrast-induced nephropathy include the following:

- Renal impairment
- Congestive heart failure
- Diabetes mellitus
- Dehydration/volume depletion
- Nephrotoxic drugs (NSAIDs, ACE inhibitors, aminoglycosides, metformin)
- Dose, frequency, and route of contrast media administration
- Comorbid events
- Hypotension, hypertension, sepsis, and cardiac disease
- Structural kidney disease or damage

In addition to alternative modalities or performing a noncontrast CT, one should consider strategies for reducing the risk of contrast-induced nephropathy, which include reducing the administered volume of contrast, using an isoosmolar contrast medium, and administering IV fluids before and after administration of contrast. Prophylactically administered *N*-acetylcysteine has been shown to reduce contrast-induced nephropathy in certain adult populations; however, it is not routinely used at our institution because its benefit has not been proven in the pediatric population.

In diagnostic imaging CT contributes significantly to the radiation dose imparted to patients, and its deleterious effects are becoming better understood. Recent evidence points to a potential and likely increased risk of cancer in patients who undergo examinations that use ionizing radiation, particularly CT.[4,80] The risk is believed to be highest in children, who have the greatest intrinsic sensitivity to these effects and who have a longer lifespan in which to manifest these effects.

MAGNETIC RESONANCE IMAGING

MRI, like ultrasound, is uniquely suited to the imaging of children in that the child is not exposed to ionizing radiation. Although energy is imparted during performance of MRI, it has not been shown to have the deleterious potential of CT. For that reason MRI is often preferred over CT for children. At the same time, the length of examination and reliance on a cooperative and still patient may mean that in some situations, particularly in children younger than 5 or 6 and in those with developmental delay or claustrophobia, sedation or general anesthesia must be administered and the child

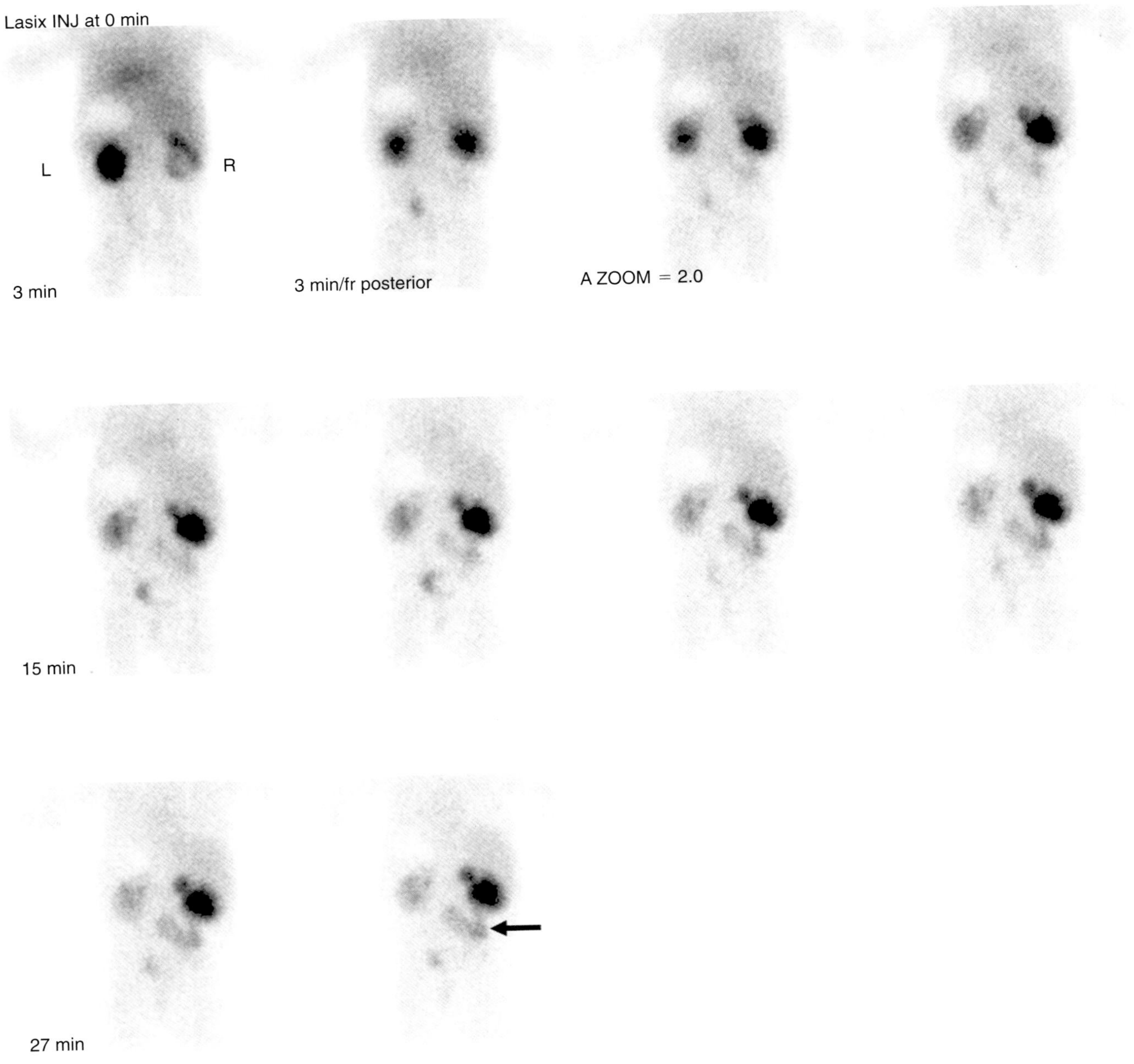

Figure 1-13 Diuretic MAG3 scan in a patient with right hydronephrosis. In this patient, MAG3 and furosemide were injected at the same time (F0 protocol). **A,** Dynamic imaging demonstrates normal drainage of radiotracer from the left intrarenal collecting system. However, the right kidney shows progressive accumulation of tracer in a dilated intrarenal collecting system and also in a dilated right ureter *(arrow)*, suggestive of urinary obstruction at the ureterovesical junction (UVJ).

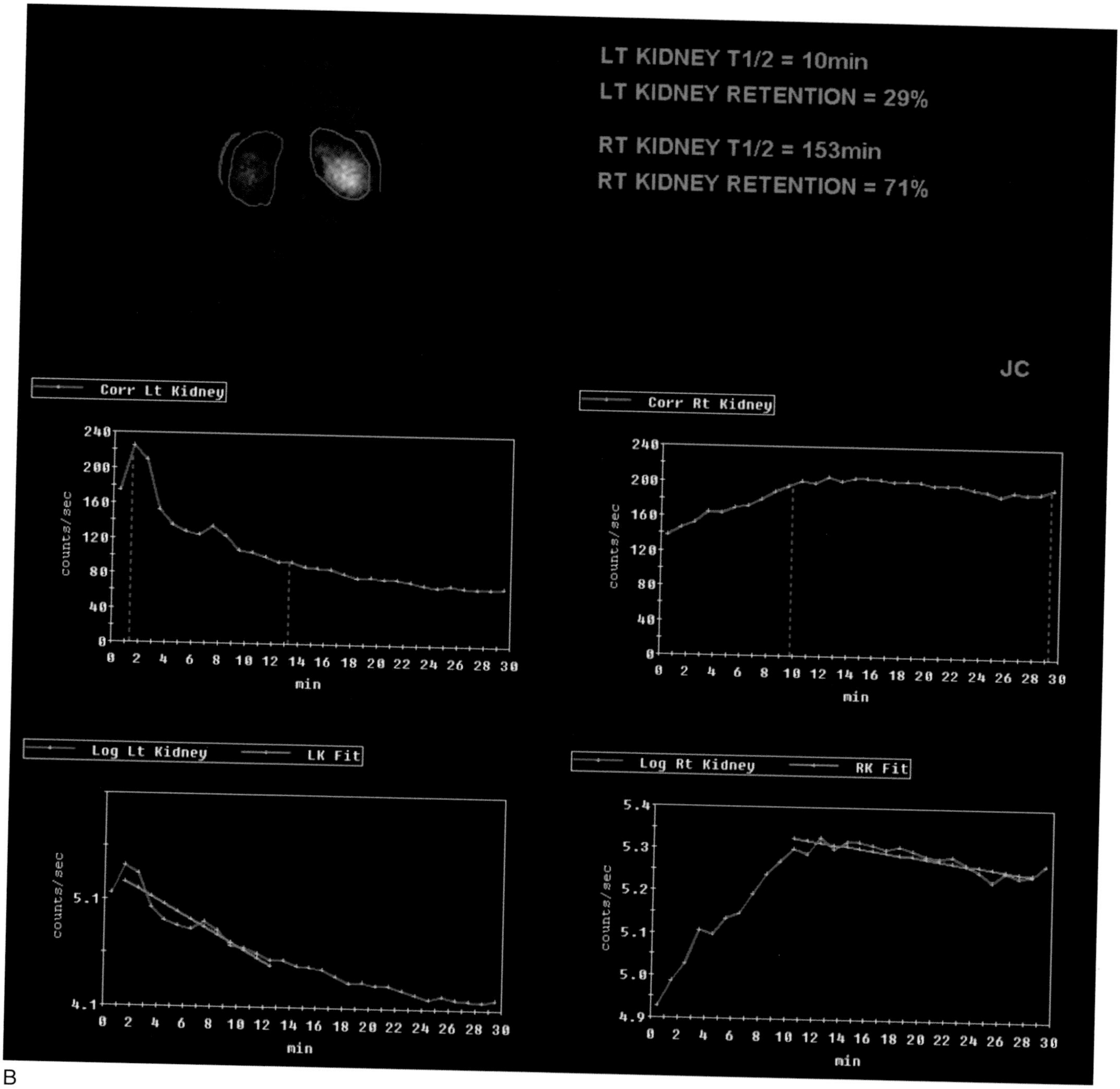

B

Figure 1-13, cont'd **B,** Renogram curve shows an abnormally prolonged $T_{1/2}$ = 153 minutes of the intrarenal collecting system, compatible with high-grade obstruction. A renogram curve plotted from a region of interest drawn around the right ureter *(not shown)* also demonstrates a prolonged $T_{1/2}$, supportive of obstruction at the UVJ.

Continued

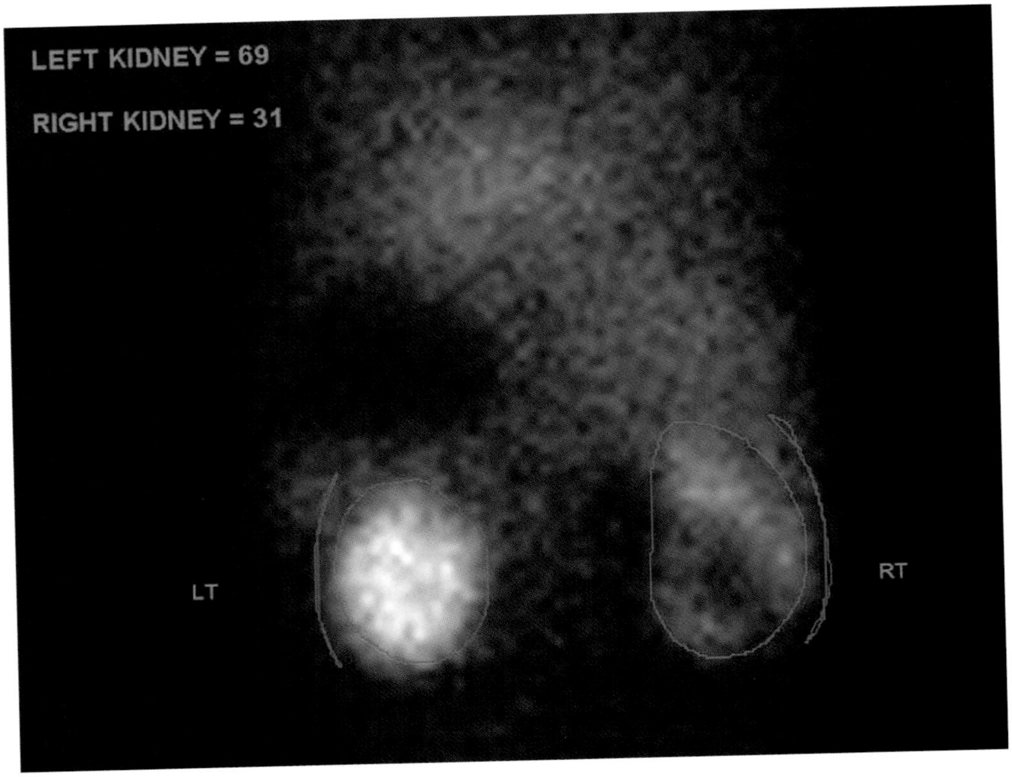

C

Figure 1-13, cont'd **C,** Differential renal function is abnormally asymmetric (left 69%, right 31%), suggesting that parenchymal damage occurred as a result of the urinary obstruction.

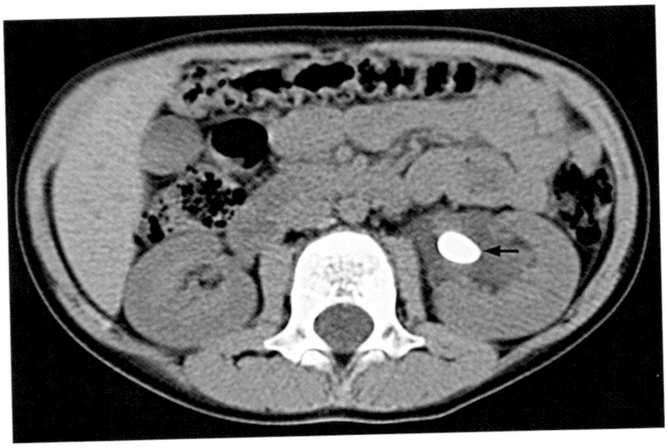

Figure 1-14 Unenhanced CT at the level of the kidneys demonstrates a calculus *(arrow)* in the left renal pelvis with some pelvic dilatation.

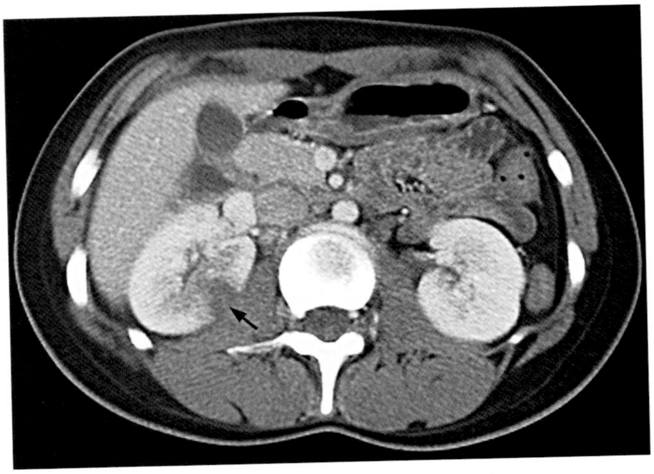

Figure 1-15 Enhanced CT at the level of the kidneys demonstrates an area in the posteromedial aspect of the right kidney with diminished enhancement *(arrow)*, consistent with the clinical suspicion of pyelonephritis.

carefully monitored.[81] In addition, access to an MR scanner remains limited in some regions of the world.

The superior tissue characterization of MRI makes it a powerful tool in assessing diseases of the urinary tract. Here, too, intravenous contrast can be administered to help in arriving at the correct diagnosis. Although generally considered safe, adverse reactions to gadolinium-based MRI contrast agents can occur, but these reactions are by and large mild. Severe reactions have been reported with MR contrast agents.[82] Recent reports have also demonstrated that gadolinium-based contrast agents have the potential to be nephrotoxic.[83] In addition, recent reports have described an association between administration of gadolinium-based contrast agents and the development of nephrogenic fibrosing

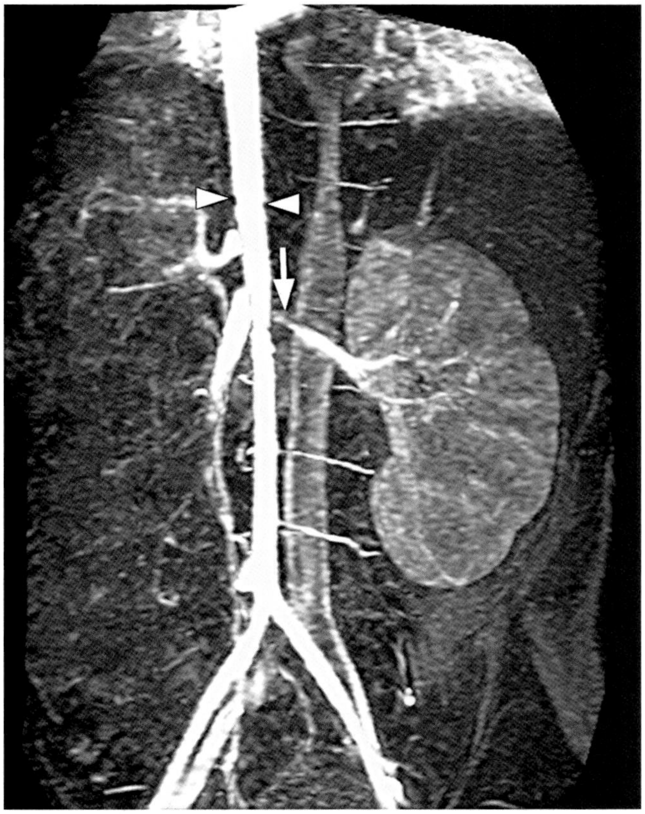

Figure 1-16 Magnetic resonance angiography (MRA) demonstrates irregularity of the aortic wall and a stenosis of the proximal aspect of the main renal artery supplying a solitary kidney. This patient was known to have neurofibromatosis.

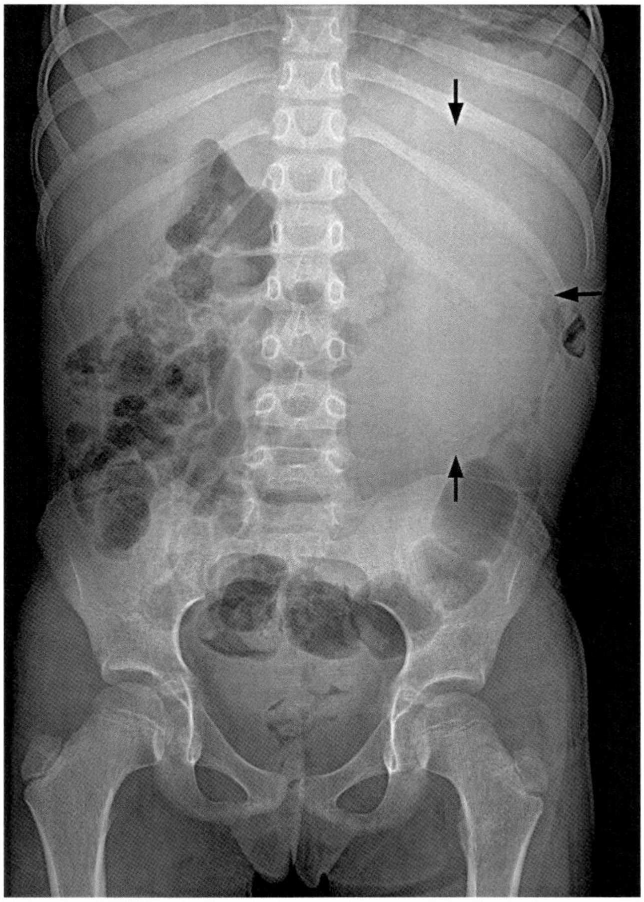

Figure 1-17 Radiograph of the abdomen demonstrates soft-tissue density in the region of the left renal fossa with displacement of bowel *(arrows)*. A renal cell carcinoma was discovered on cross-sectional imaging.

dermopathy, a condition described in patients with kidney disease who have indurated and erythematous plaques of the skin though other organ systems are also involved.[84] MRI is particularly well suited in assessing neoplasms and tumorlike conditions of the kidneys,[85,86] including nephroblastomatosis.[86] MR can assist in lesion characterization by demonstrating necrosis and hemorrhage in lesions such as Wilms' tumor or renal cell carcinoma. Areas of fat can be demonstrated in angiomyolipomas.[87,88] The demonstration of calcification, however, is not as reliable with MRI as it is with CT.

As in adults, MR can be applied in the assessment of renal arteries and renal veins in children. Bland (nontumor) thrombosis can readily be demonstrated as can tumor extension into the vessels.[89,90] Renal artery stenosis can be assessed in the investigation of hypertension[91-94] (Figure 1-16), although the role of MR in renal artery stenosis has been questioned in adult studies.[95] Also, MR angiography can be limited in children because of the small size of their arteries. MRI has been applied, too, in the assessment of infection[96-98] and trauma.[99,100]

The ability of MR to assess fluid-containing structures has been demonstrated and has allowed for MR urography (MRU) in assessing the renal collecting systems both in terms of anatomical abnormalities (congenital and acquired),[101-103] and more recently in terms of demonstrating the level and degree of obstruction.[104,105] Research into the more functional applications of MRI in the urinary tract is ongoing.

RADIOGRAPHY

Radiography is the oldest modality used in the evaluation of urinary tract disease, but its utility is limited. The normal urinary tract is not sufficiently distinct from other abdominal and pelvic structures to be properly evaluated using radiography alone. There may, however, be cases in which there is sufficient retroperitoneal fat to outline the kidneys on plain radiographs and even assess their relative sizes. A renal mass or severely hydronephrotic kidney might be detected by the presence of a soft tissue mass, calcification or fat, and displacement of adjacent structures (Figure 1-17). A full bladder can also be seen as a midline structure in the pelvis, which will occasionally displace bowel loops out of the pelvis (Figure 1-18).

Calculi in the urinary collecting system can at times be seen on radiography depending on their composition[106-108] (Figure 1-19). Nephrocalcinosis, cortical or medullary, can also be detected depending on the degree of involvement.[109] In instances of renal failure, particularly if chronic, there may

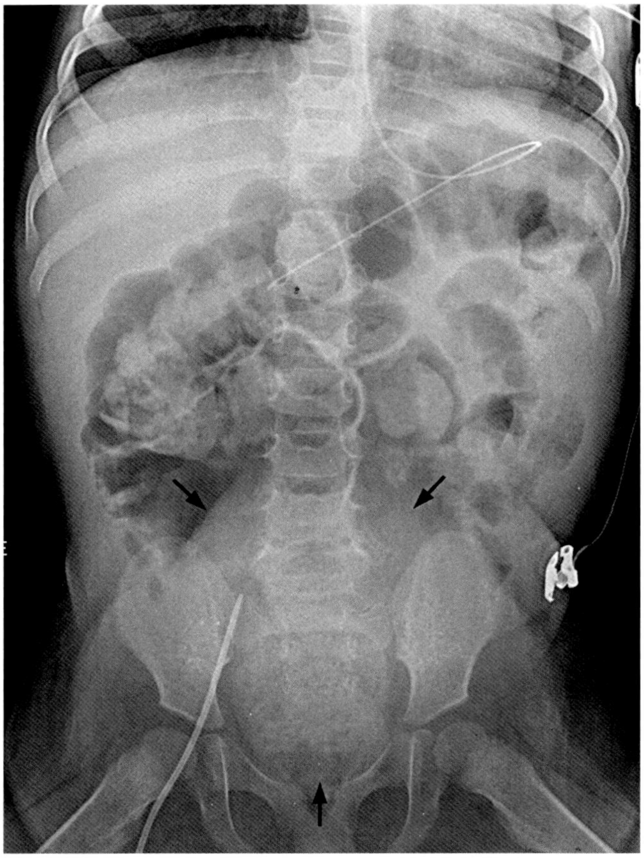

Figure 1-18 Radiograph of the abdomen demonstrates soft tissue in the pelvis displacing bowel out of the pelvis *(arrows)*. Ultrasound demonstrated that a full bladder was the cause of the imaging findings.

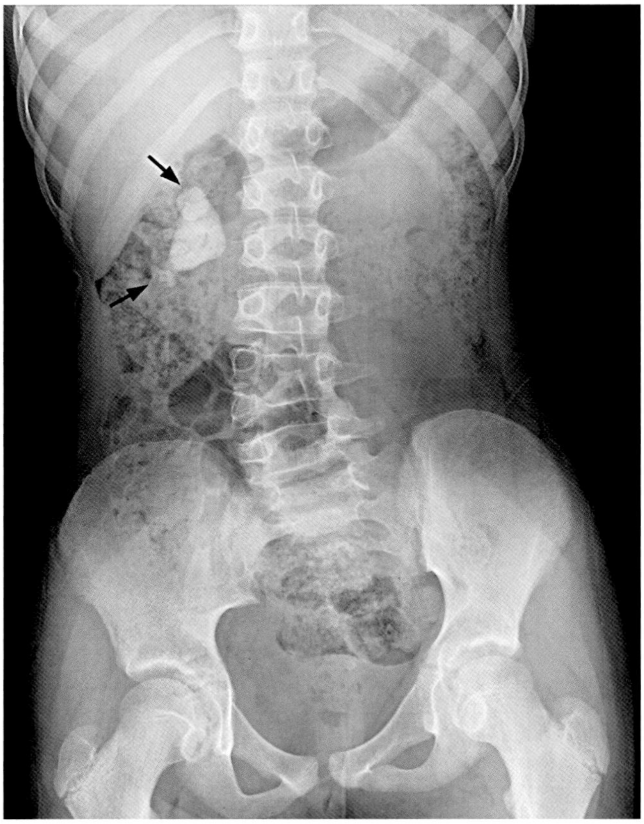

Figure 1-19 Radiograph of the abdomen demonstrates a calcific density in the region of the right renal fossa *(arrows)*. A staghorn calculus was found on ultrasound. Incidental note was made of a tripediculate vertebra in the lower lumbar spine.

be signs of renal osteodystrophy on radiography, and in fact radiography remains the mainstay of imaging osseous changes associated with renal failure.[110]

Radiographs can also be beneficial in determining the correct positioning of various drainage catheters and stents. Ureteral stents in particular can migrate, thereby mitigating their effectiveness. Most catheters and stents are sufficiently radioopaque to be visible on radiographs (Figure 1-20).

Overall, however, the role of radiography has largely been supplanted by the cross-sectional imaging modalities (ultrasound, CT, and MRI) and by nuclear medicine.

EXCRETORY UROGRAPHY

Excretory urography (intravenous pyelography) relies on the administration of intravenous contrast to enhance the urinary tract and thereby have it stand out against the remainder of the abdominal tissues.[111-114] As other modalities have been applied to the study of urinary tract disorders, use of excretory urography has fallen off sharply. Ultrasound, CT, MRI, and nuclear medicine have to a degree replaced excretory urography.[115-118] At this point, if used at all, excretory urography is performed to delineate and characterize the anatomy of the urinary tract. Congenital variants in ureteral anatomy including ectopic ureters and collecting system duplication can be delineated in this manner. For instance, urinary dribbling in girls remains in many institutions and for many urologists an indication for excretory urography in assessing for variant insertion of the ureter.[119,120] Diseases of the urothelium and papillary necrosis can also be accurately diagnosed and followed with excretory urography.[121]

Certainly if excretory urography is performed, care must be taken with respect to administration of intravenous contrast. Issues of nephrotoxicity and allergy to intravenous contrast must be considered. To minimize radiation dose, the number of radiographs obtained as part of the study should be kept to a minimum but without sacrificing the diagnostic performance of the test.

RETROGRADE URETHROGRAPHY

Though retrograde urethrography is an examination not frequently performed, there are indications for this study that have remained constant for many years. In the setting of suspected trauma to the male urethra, retrograde urethrography is still the study of choice to assess for a disrupted urethra.[122] One can also assess for other urethral abnormalities both congenital (anterior urethral valves and diverticula)

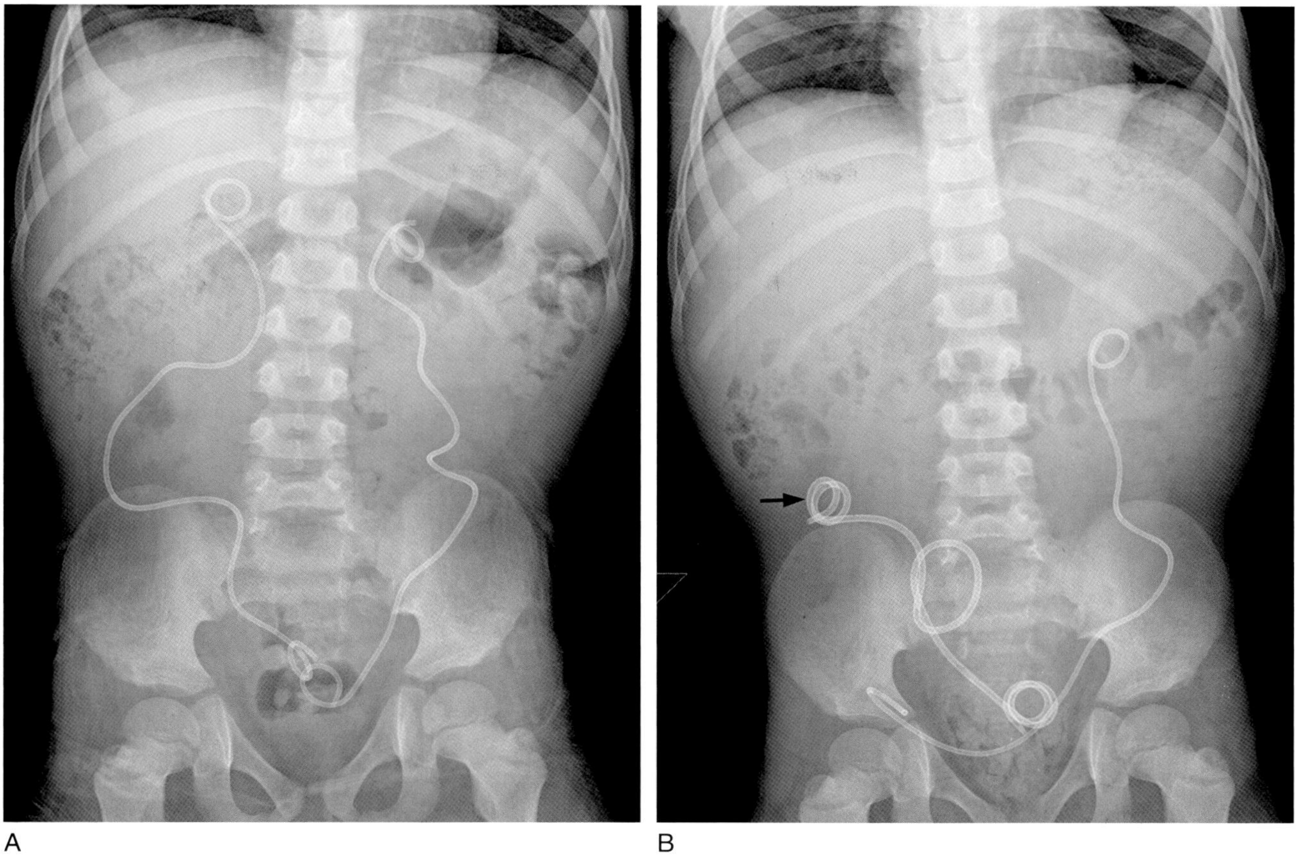

Figure 1-20 **A,** Radiograph of the abdomen demonstrates double J stents overlying the urinary tracts. Proximal and distal loops overlie the renal pelves and bladder, respectively, although the ureteral courses appear tortuous. **B,** Several days later, both stents have changes in position most evident on the right, where the proximal aspect of the stent appears to be in the right ureter *(arrow)*.

and acquired (posttraumatic, postsurgical, or infectious)[123-125] (Figure 1-21). The study involves placement of a balloon-tipped catheter into the distal urethra and careful inflation of a balloon in the fossa navicularis. Images of the urethra are taken in an oblique projection during a hand injection of water-soluble contrast. Due to the presence of the external sphincter, the posterior urethra is usually not assessed as part of this study but rather can be imaged during voiding after filling the bladder directly.

APPLICATIONS OF DIAGNOSTIC IMAGING

Diseases of the Neonate

With the increase in antenatal imaging (ultrasound and to a much lesser degree MRI) and the detection of abnormalities prenatally, there has been a commensurate increase in postnatal imaging in the workup of antenatal findings. The most common indication for assessment of the urinary tract in these situations is the follow-up of antenatally diagnosed pelvocaliceal dilatation, ectopia, agenesis, or dysplasia. The pathologies encountered in these children range from mild to severe to life threatening. The initial examination will almost always be an ultrasound to determine the presence of two kidneys, their location, and the status of the parenchyma and collecting system. An increase in parenchymal echogenicity or loss of corticomedullary differentiation can be signs of renal abnormality. Parenchymal loss, scarring, and cyst formation can be other signs of renal damage.

In many institutions the initial postnatal ultrasound is done after the first week of life so as not to miss hydronephrosis due to the relatively dehydrated state of the newborn and collapsed collecting system. If dilatation is present and involves only the pelvocaliceal system, then there may be obstruction at the ureteropelvic junction[126] (Figure 1-22). If the ureter is also dilated, the obstruction may be at the ureterovesical junction.[127] If the bladder is distended and perhaps trabeculated, the obstruction may involve the bladder outlet or urethra (Figure 1-23).[128] At the same time any degree of pelvocaliceal or ureteral dilatation can be due to vesicoureteral reflux.

The presence of a duplex collecting system can be inferred on ultrasound when the renal sinus echo complex is interrupted by a band of renal cortical tissue, though it can be difficult to distinguish this pattern from a prominent column of Bertin.[129] The presence of a duplex collecting system may be associated with obstruction (usually of the upper moiety) and/or reflux (usually of the lower moiety) according to the Meyer-Weigert rule. This rule states that the upper moiety is drained by a ureter that inserts ectopically, and the lower moiety is drained by a ureter that inserts orthotopically, with the former often obstructed by a ureterocele and the latter

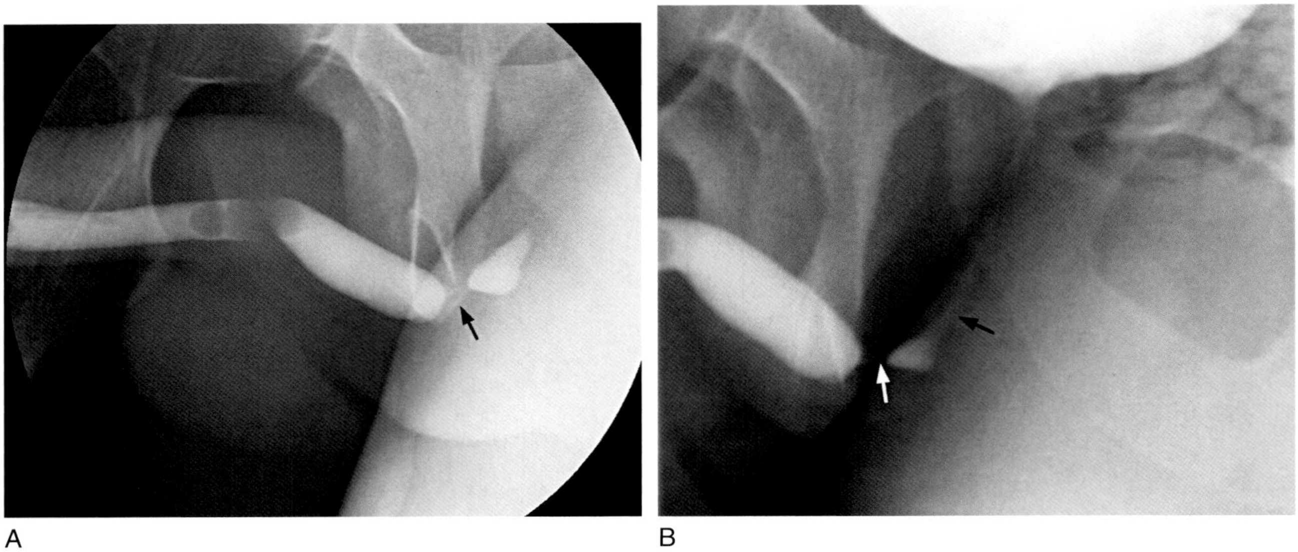

Figure 1-21 **A,** Retrograde urethrogram demonstrates a stricture of the bulbous urethra *(arrow)* posttrauma (straddle injury). **B,** In order to precisely determine the length and degree of the stricture, the bladder was filled via a suprapubic tube. With voiding and simultaneous retrograde urethrography, one can precisely delineate the stricture length and severity. Posterior urethra *(black arrow)*. Stricture *(white arrow)*.

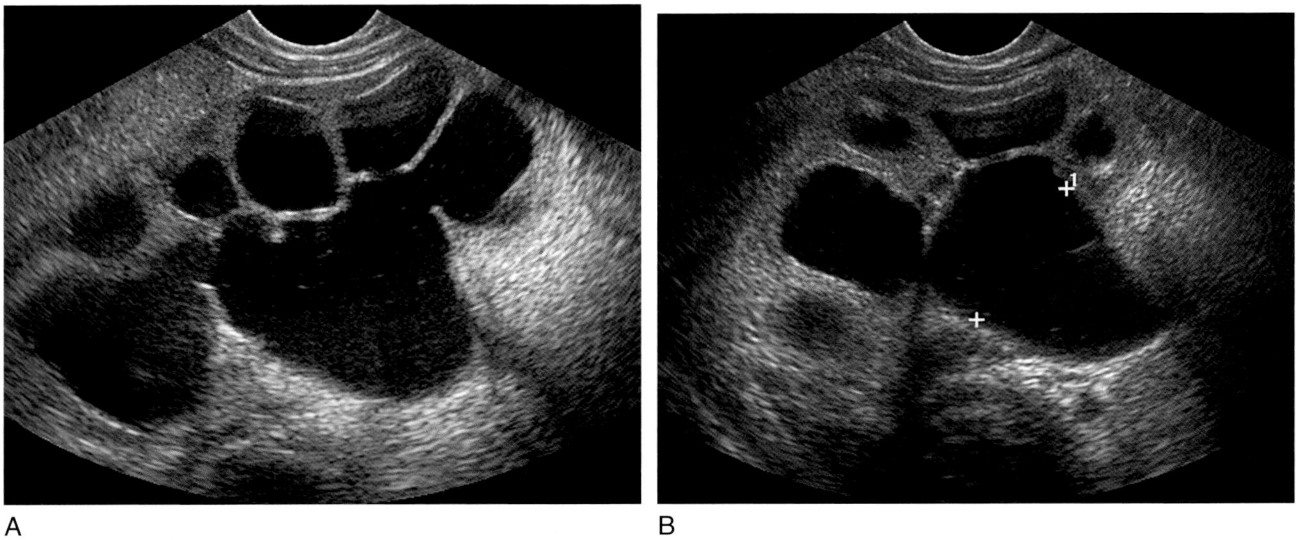

Figure 1-22 Longitudinal **(A)** and transverse **(B)** images of the kidney demonstrate a dilated collecting system with no ureteral dilatation noted in this patient, in whom diuretic renal scintigraphy confirmed severe obstruction at the ureteropelvic junction. Calipers measure the renal pelvis on the transverse image.

demonstrating reflux. These entities (obstruction and reflux) can coexist in the same patient. With respect to ureteroceles, the diagnosis can be made on almost any modality, though most commonly on ultrasound or VCUG.[130] One must bear in mind that not all ectopic ureters end in a ureterocele. Similarly, not all ureteroceles are ectopic. Ureteroceles at the normal ureterovesical junction are termed *orthotopic* or *simple ureteroceles* and like ectopic ureteroceles can be obstructive or nonobstructive.[131]

Thereafter the workup of a dilated collecting system may vary among institutions. In brief, the investigations assess for the known pathologies that affect the neonate and infant. If the dilatation is indeed determined to be present and persistent on postnatal ultrasound, a VCUG can assess for vesicoureteral reflux and its degree. The VCUG can also assess for urethral obstruction due to posterior urethral valves in a male. If the child is found not to have reflux or valves, nuclear medicine diuretic renography can assess for any degree and level of obstruction.

A number of other congenital abnormalities can be diagnosed in the antenatal or neonatal period. Failure of the ureteric bud to join the metanephric blastema is thought to be the inciting factor in the development of the multicystic dysplastic kidney (MCDK). In this case normal renal parenchyma is not present. Rather, the kidney is replaced by multiple noncommunicating cysts with dysplastic parenchymal

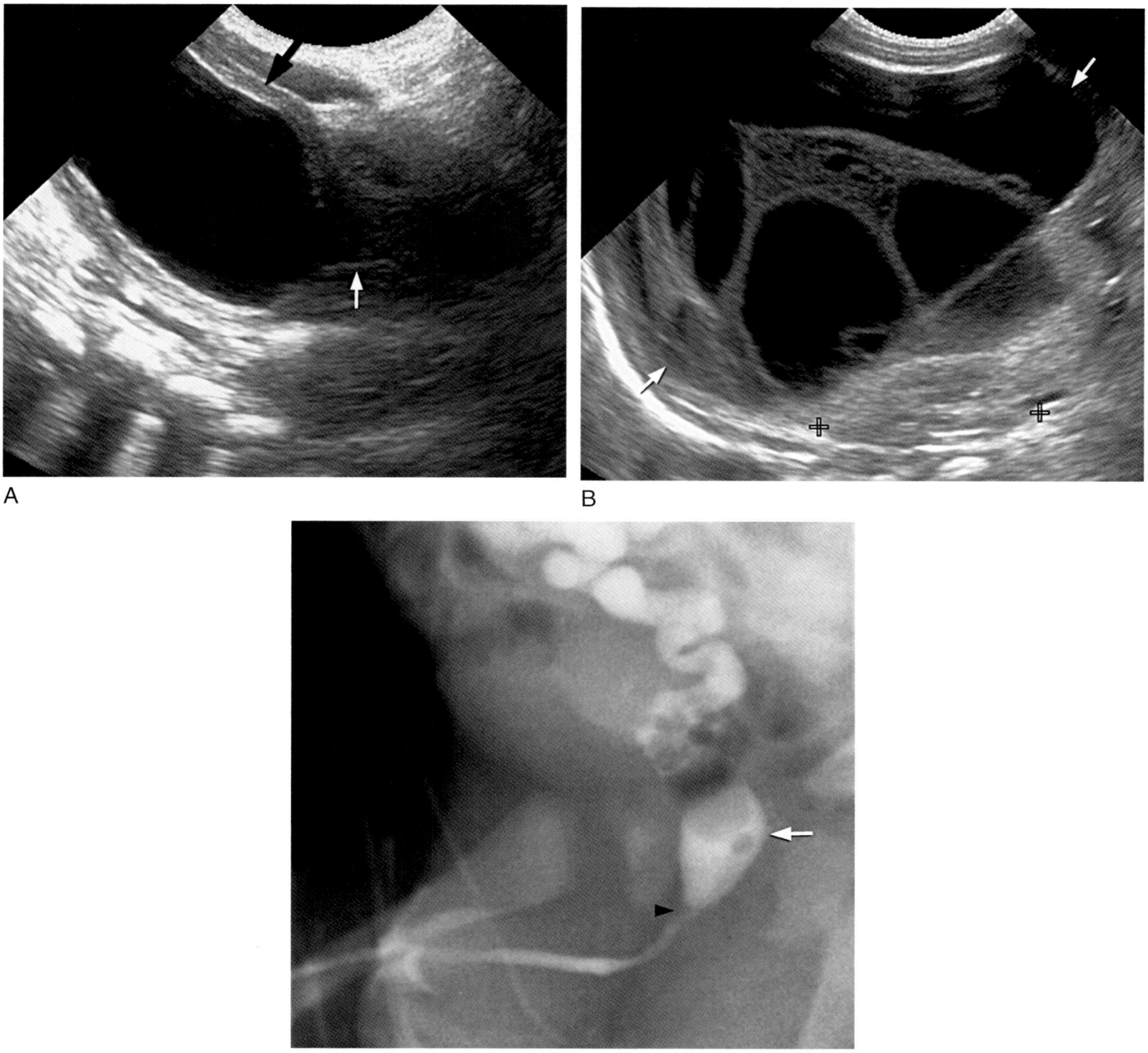

Figure 1-23 **A,** Ultrasound of the bladder in the longitudinal plane demonstrates thickening of the bladder wall *(black arrow)* and dilatation of the posterior urethra just beyond the bladder neck *(white arrow)* in this patient with posterior urethral valves. **B,** In the same patient a complex-appearing urinoma *(arrows)* is seen adjacent to an abnormally echogenic kidney *(calipers)*. **C,** Voiding cystourethrogram confirms dilatation of the posterior urethra *(white arrow)* to the level of obstruction *(black arrowhead)* just distal to the verumontanum. Vesicoureteral reflux into a tortuous ureter is also present.

tissue.[132] Demonstration of the lack of communication among the cysts differentiates this process from pelvocaliceal dilatation. Imaging can also demonstrate renal agenesis, ectopia, horseshoe, and cross-fused kidneys. Again, ultrasound is the preferred initial imaging modality, although in some cases the findings are discovered incidentally on other modalities (including DMSA).

Conditions affecting the renal vasculature in the neonate, including thrombosis of the renal arteries or veins, can be assessed with Doppler imaging of the vessels and the kidneys. Associated thrombosis of the aorta and inferior vena cava (IVC) can also be assessed. If a central catheter is present, its position can best be assessed with radiographs of the abdomen, although the catheters can certainly be resolved with ultrasound as well. If a thrombus has occurred, recanalization can be assessed sonographically after anticoagulation or thrombolysis. Occasionally residual thrombus can calcify and be visible as a linear hyperechoic structure along the vessel wall either in the major vessels or within the renal parenchyma. Follow-up renal ultrasound can also assess for any long-term sequelae of thrombosis, such as atrophy, abnormal parenchymal echogenicity, or cyst formation.

Vesicoureteral Reflux and Infection

The topic of vesicoureteral reflux and infections of the urinary tract will be discussed more fully in subsequent chapters. There are numerous contributions that can be made by imaging in these conditions. Again, ultrasound, VCUG, and nuclear medicine will be the modalities most used to assess for findings of obstruction or reflux—although findings can be seen with other modalities. Typically ultrasound will be used to look for signs suggesting obstruction or reflux, as well as assessing for signs of either acute infection or sequelae of previous infection (focal scarring or global volume loss). DMSA renal cortical scintigraphy remains the most sensitive modality for detection of pyelonephritis and scars. In the case of global volume loss, the contralateral kidney may undergo hypertrophy. VCUG will assess for the presence of reflux, whether it occurs in early filling or with voiding, and its grade. The system of the International Reflux Study in Children classifies reflux into five grades (Figure 1-24). Reflux into the ureter is classified as grade I. When contrast fills the intrarenal collecting system but without dilatation, it is classified as grade II. Grades III-V demonstrate progressive dilatation of the ureter, pelvis, and calyces.[28] VCUG also assesses the anatomy of any opacified structure, and the renal collecting system can be assessed for duplication. Parenchymal loss can be inferred by the opacification of the intrarenal system if the calyces appear convergent. The bladder can be assessed for thickening and trabeculation, and diverticulation and urachal opacification can be seen in some cases. Valves, diverticulae, and the overall morphology of the urethra, particularly in males, can also be assessed.

In cases of known VUR, follow-up evaluation can be performed with direct radionuclide cystogram to assess for resolution or persistence of reflux. In the case of a hydronephrotic kidney and a negative VCUG, a diuretic renogram can be used to evaluate for the presence of urinary tract obstruction.

There can be imaging findings for acute infection as well. With diffuse infection of the renal parenchyma, the entire kidney may be enlarged.[133] This enlargement may be reflected in an increase in renal length, although the entire volume should be assessed to detect increases in transverse diameter. Infection can also involve a portion of the kidney and can simulate a renal mass.[134] The echogenicity of the affected region can be increased or decreased.[135,136] Increased echogenicity of the renal sinus has also been described.[137] The urothelial wall of the pelvis, ureter, or bladder can be thickened. One can also look at the qualitative appearance of the fluid in the urinary tract. Echogenic debris in the collecting system can suggest, though it is not pathognomonic for, infection.

Infected areas of the kidney are often relatively hypoperfused and may demonstrate diminished enhancement after the administration of intravenous contrast on CT or MRI and diminished flow on Doppler interrogation on ultrasound (Figure 1-15). However, the area can also be hyperperfused on sonography. Acute pyelonephritis will appear as cold defects on DMSA renal cortical scan. If cortical defects persist beyond 6 months after clinical resolution of the acute infection, they are considered to be permanent scars that can predispose to renal failure and hypertension.

Fungal infection of the kidneys represents a special situation in which imaging can play an important role. In patients who are immunosuppressed or have indwelling catheters, ultrasound may demonstrate infection of the renal paren-

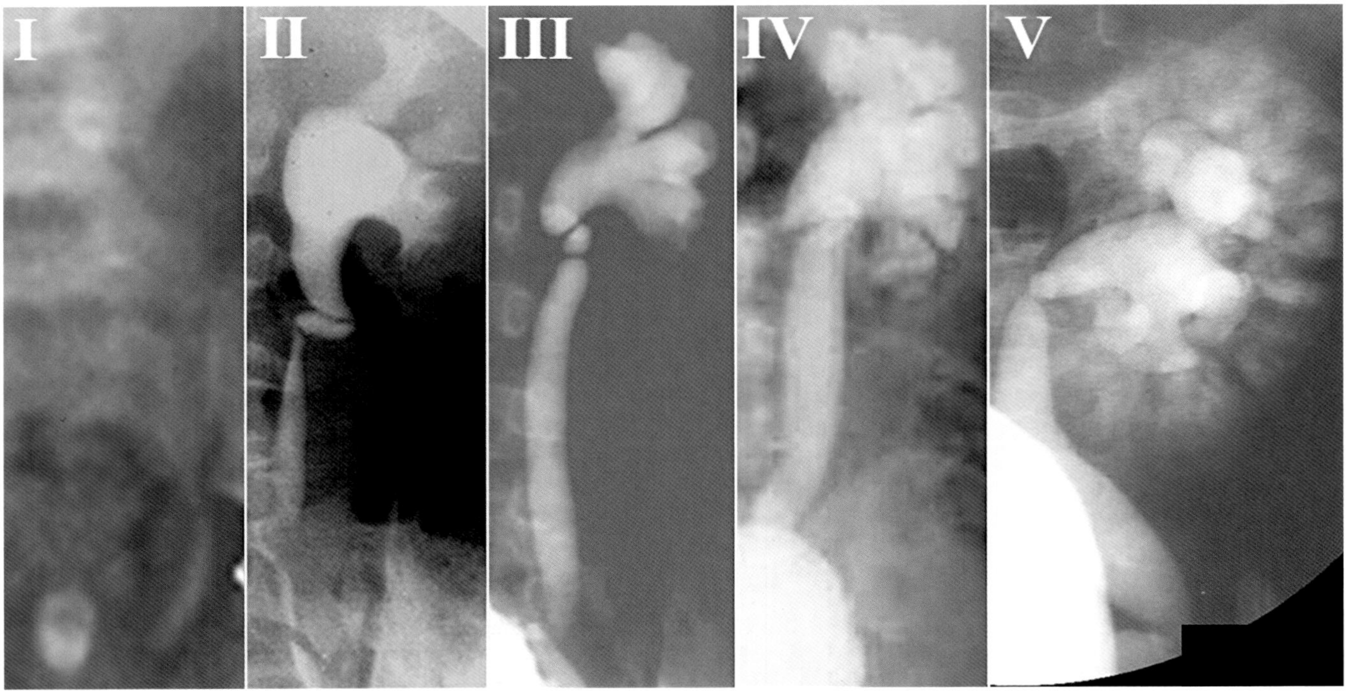

Figure 1-24 International Grading System of vesicoureteral reflux, illustrating VCUG grades I through V.

chyma and assess for the presence of fungal balls of the collecting systems.

Neoplasm

Most renal neoplasms in children present as a palpable mass detected by the parent or physician. In cases such as these the mass is often large and the first imaging modality requested is an ultrasound, though occasionally a radiograph might be obtained first. Ultrasound can suggest the renal origin of an abdominal mass by demonstrating extension of renal tissue around the mass—the so-called claw sign (Figure 1-25). It can likewise differentiate solid from cystic or necrotic areas and demonstrate if any hemorrhage or calcification is present. Ultrasound is also useful in determining whether the tumor

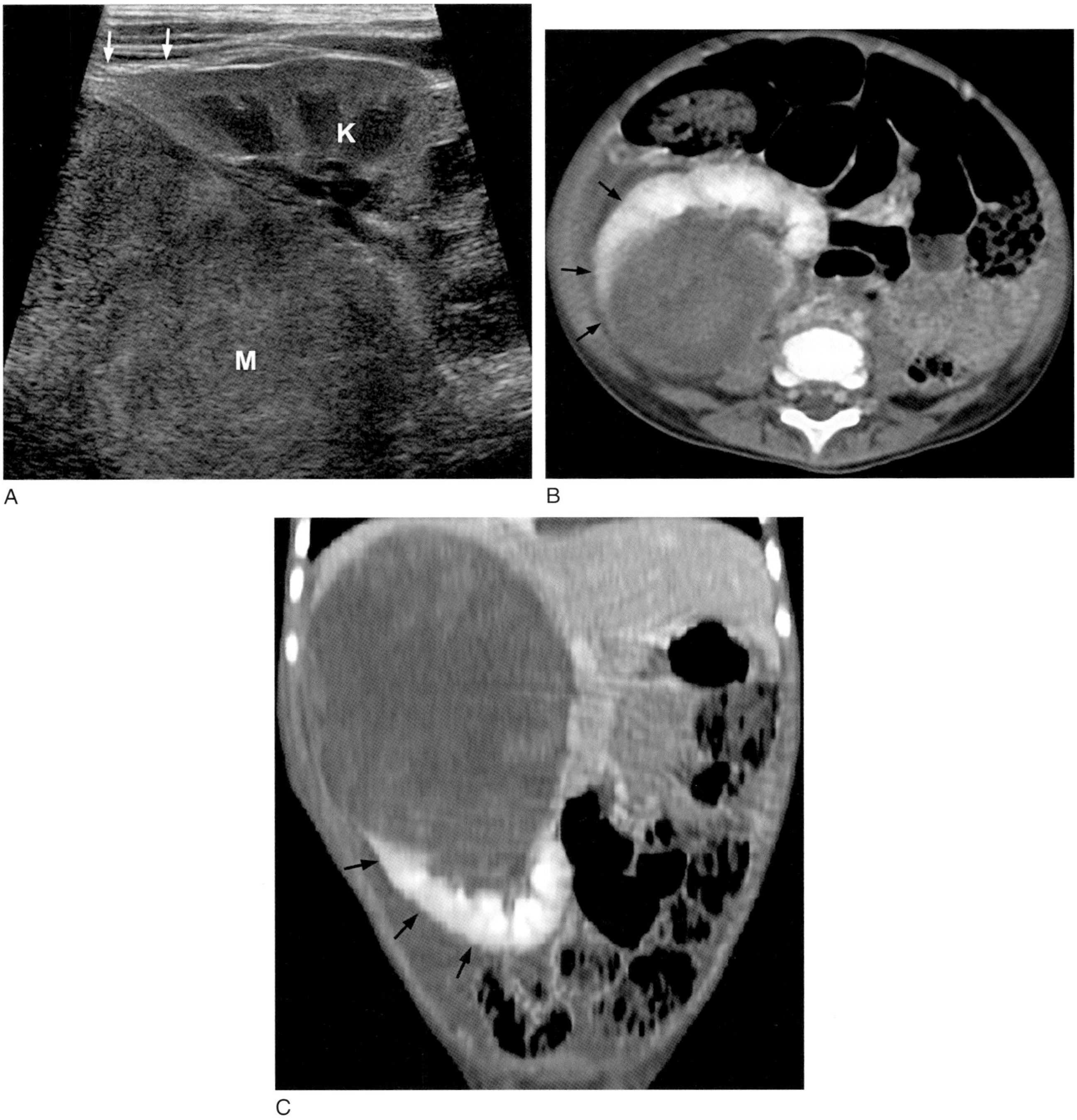

Figure 1-25 **A,** Ultrasound of the kidney demonstrates a mass arising from the kidney. A rim of renal tissue surrounds a portion of the mass—an appearance termed *claw sign*. *K*, Kidney; *M*, mass. **B, C,** CT axial images and coronal reformations demonstrate presence of a claw sign *(arrows)*, confirming the renal origin of this mass, found to be Wilms' tumor.

involves the renal vein or IVC or extends into the heart. Once it is determined that a tumor is present, CT or MRI can be used to better assess the size, extent, and involvement with adjacent structures. Although CT and MRI would be roughly equivalent in assessing the primary renal mass, CT is the modality of choice to assess the lungs for metastatic disease. If the tumor has a propensity to metastasize elsewhere, then appropriate imaging modalities, such as CT of the brain, bone scan, or MIBG scan, can be performed.

Trauma

Imaging of trauma to the urinary tract has been studied extensively and remains a topic of debate.[138] In the acute setting, the imaging evaluation of the injured child is determined by the extent and type of injury, as well as by the practice of the particular institution.[76,139] In some institutions evaluation of trauma to the abdomen begins with sonography of the abdomen to assess for free fluid and obvious visceral injuries.[140,141] At other institutions CT is the modality of choice in the initial assessment.[34,77,138] The decision as to which modality is used depends on the clinical situation. Ultrasound has a high sensitivity in detecting intraperitoneal fluid; however, in the setting of trauma, the presence of fluid is not an absolute indication for surgery. At the same time, there can be injury to the urinary tract without the presence of free fluid.[142] CT, on the other hand, can accurately assess for the presence of free fluid while assessing the solid and hollow viscera of the abdomen.

Sonography can depict a renal laceration or contusion as a focal area of abnormal echotexture. The area can be hypoechoic, isoechoic, or hyperechoic to the remainder of the kidney depending on the contents of the area and the stage of the evolution of the injury. Sonography can also depict the quality and amount of perirenal fluid (blood, urine, or both) and follow the appearance to assess whether the collection is diminishing, remaining stable, or increasing. Doppler interrogation of the kidneys can assess both for areas of the renal parenchyma that are ischemic due to vascular interruption and for arterial or venous thrombosis and pseudoaneurysm formation. Renal vascular injury can also be visualized with nuclear medicine functional renal imaging, with nonperfused regions of the kidney appearing as cold defects.

As mentioned, CT is the current modality of choice in assessing abdominal trauma in children and offers much in the evaluation of urinary tract trauma. The appearance of the kidneys and particularly their patterns of enhancement on CT can allow for the diagnosis of renal contusions and lacerations. Areas devoid of enhancement, particularly if they appear geographically, suggest infarction. Perinephric and/or periureteral fluid can also be assessed. Delayed imaging may show disruption of the collecting system if dense contrast is seen outside of the collecting system on delayed images (Figure 1-26). CT cystography has also been used to assess for injuries to the urinary bladder and urethra.

In the past, intravenous urography was used extensively in the evaluation of urinary tract trauma but is seldom used today. However, fluoroscopic studies (retrograde urethrography and cystography) are still used extensively for imaging bladder and urethral injury.

Renal Failure

The appearance of the kidneys in cases of renal failure has been touched on in other parts of this chapter. There may be findings on imaging that give a clue to the etiology of the disease if it is not yet known. In some cases the failing kidneys will appear normal despite meticulous imaging. In many cases, however, there will be some detectable abnormality that will at least suggest a renal abnormality. In acute renal failure the kidneys may appear normal or increased in size on ultrasound, and there may be an increase in parenchymal echogenicity. Diminution or loss of corticomedullary differ-

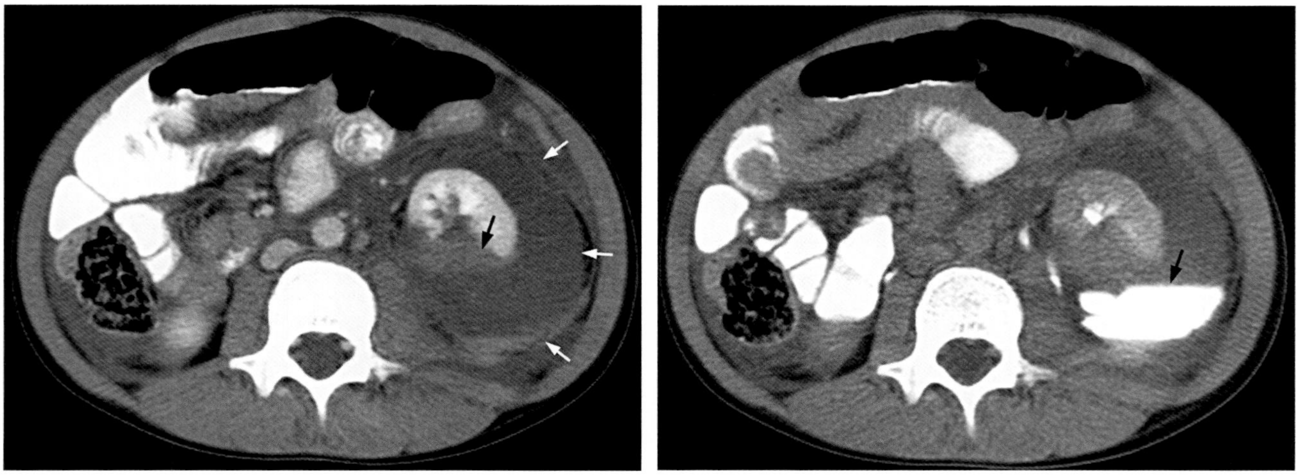

A B

Figure 1-26 **A,** Enhanced CT demonstrates a large perinephric hematoma around the left kidney *(white arrows)* and a portion of the posterior aspect of the kidney that demonstrates diminished enhancement consistent with an area of laceration/contusion *(black arrow)*. **B,** Delayed images obtained through the same area demonstrate accumulation of the intravenous contrast in the perinephric space *(arrow)*, confirming an injury to the renal collecting system.

entiation may also be present. If the changes involve mainly the cortex, then the corticomedullary differentiation may be accentuated. In chronic renal failure the kidneys tend to be small and echogenic, with diminished corticomedullary differentiation. Scarring and dysplastic cysts may be present depending on the etiology of the renal insult.

Differential Renal Function

Differential renal function refers to the percentage of total renal function contributed by each kidney. During nuclear medicine functional renal imaging, renal uptake measured between 1 and 2 minutes after radiotracer injection is used to calculate differential renal function, also known as split function or relative function. Differential renal function can also be calculated based on renal uptake measured on DMSA cortical scan images. In general, unilaterally reduced function to less than 44% to 45%[60] is considered abnormal; however, cutoff values anywhere from 40% to 45% are widely used.[35,70,143-147]

Differential function should be measured based on images acquired immediately before radiotracer enters the collecting system. Occasionally the function in one kidney may be so delayed that its parenchyma is not yet visualized by the time the contralateral kidney has begun excretion of tracer. In this situation an accurate differential function measurement is not possible.

Anatomic abnormalities are another potential source of error. Attenuation effects due to severe hydronephrosis, a large renal cyst or mass, or an ectopically positioned kidney may artifactually lower the differential function value of the affected kidney. These attenuation effects can be reduced to some degree by using geometric mean correction techniques. In the case of a duplicated collecting system, the kidney can be divided into upper- and lower-pole regions of interest so that the relative contribution of each moiety can be reported.

Glomerular Filtration Rate

Either 51Cr-EDTA or 99mTc-DTPA can be used to calculate GFR (see earlier discussion under Glomerular Filtration Agents). If 99mTc-DTPA is used, functional renal imaging and calculation of differential renal function can also be performed (Figure 1-27). Measurement of GFR is also discussed in Chapter 2.

Renal Transplant Evaluation

Imaging of the renal allograft has become an integral part of renal transplantation, particularly in the immediate postoperative period. Given its noninvasive character, sonography is a mainstay of allograft imaging and can be performed in the operating room if the surgeon requests. The location of the allograft in the iliac fossa allows for close examination using gray-scale and Doppler techniques. Sonography can assess for the overall echogenicity of the kidney and the presence of corticomedullary differentiation. It can also accurately assess the degree of hydronephrosis. In addition, sonography plays an important role in assessing for perinephric fluid collections. When large, these collections may compromise drainage of urine, or blood flow to and from the kidney.

Doppler techniques can assess for renal artery or renal vein thrombosis or thrombus in the vessels to which the renal artery and vein are anastomosed. It can also assess for other causes of compromise to flow, such as stenosis or kinking of the vessel. In addition, Doppler interrogation of the allograft can detect arteriovenous fistulae, a not uncommon complication of allograft biopsy.[148]

Although sonography can assess for signs of acute and chronic rejection, the role of Doppler interrogation of the allograft remains controversial,[26] and clinical findings and biopsy remain the mainstay of diagnosis. Later complications such as stone formation and neoplasm, including posttransplant lymphoproliferative disorder (PTLD), can also be assessed with imaging (ultrasound, CT, or MRI).

Nuclear medicine functional renal scintigraphy is another modality liberally utilized in many institutions. Patients who have undergone renal transplantation typically have renal scintigraphy performed within 24 hours after surgery to assess the baseline perfusion and function of the allograft. The camera is positioned anteriorly in these patients to better image the kidney in the iliac fossa. If renal function deteriorates or postoperative complications are suspected, follow-up imaging can be performed and used for comparison.

During the perfusion phase, radiotracer should reach the renal allograft at almost the same time it is seen in the iliac vessels. The uptake, excretion, and drainage phases should appear similar to those of a normal native kidney, with maximal parenchymal activity at 3 to 5 minutes. Tracer should be seen in the bladder 4 to 8 minutes postinjection[67] (Figure 1-28).

Possible complications of renal transplantation include acute tubular necrosis (ATN), rejection, cyclosporine toxicity, urinoma, urinary obstruction, lymphocele, hematoma, and arterial or venous thrombosis.[149-156]

Acute tubular necrosis is characterized by preserved renal perfusion but also by progressive parenchymal retention of radiotracer with decreased or absent urine production (Figure 1-29). It typically resolves within a few weeks after transplantation. ATN occurs more commonly in cadaveric transplants than in living-related donor transplants, and is related to the elapsed time between harvesting and transplantation. Cyclosporine toxicity has an appearance similar to ATN but differs in time course and occurs many weeks after transplantation. It usually resolves after withdrawal of cyclosporine therapy.

Rejection is characterized by poor perfusion and poor excretion of radiotracer. Hematoma, urinoma, and lymphocele can appear as a photopenic defect on early blood pool images. A sufficiently large urine leak may result in extrarenal accumulation of radiotracer. Vascular occlusion will appear as a large reniform photopenic region. Urinary obstruction will appear as accumulation of radiotracer in the renal pelvis with poor drainage into the bladder. Postural drainage maneuvers and diuretic challenge should be considered when urinary obstruction is suspected.[152,157]

Text continued on p. 33

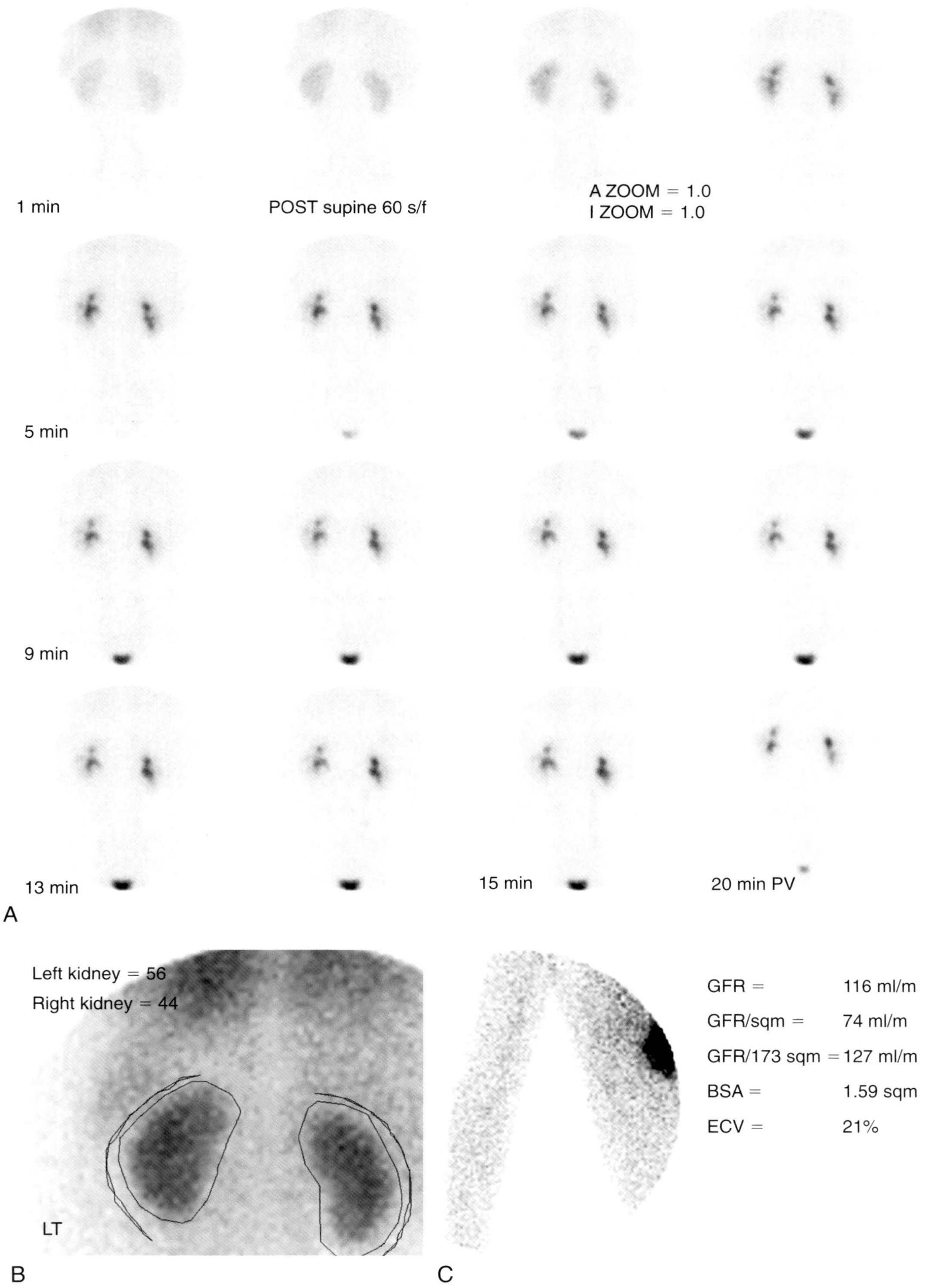

Figure 1-27 DTPA GFR calculation. When 99mTc-DTPA is used to calculate GFR, dynamic renal imaging and differential function calculation can also be performed. **A,** Dynamic renal imaging performed immediately after injection of radiotracer demonstrates normal uptake, excretion, and drainage in both kidneys. **B,** Differential renal function is symmetric and normal (left 56%, right 44%). **C,** Static image of the injection site in the antecubital fossa demonstrates that no extravasation of tracer has occurred. Calculations based on serial blood plasma sampling demonstrate normal GFR (GFR/1.73 m^2 = 127 ml/min).

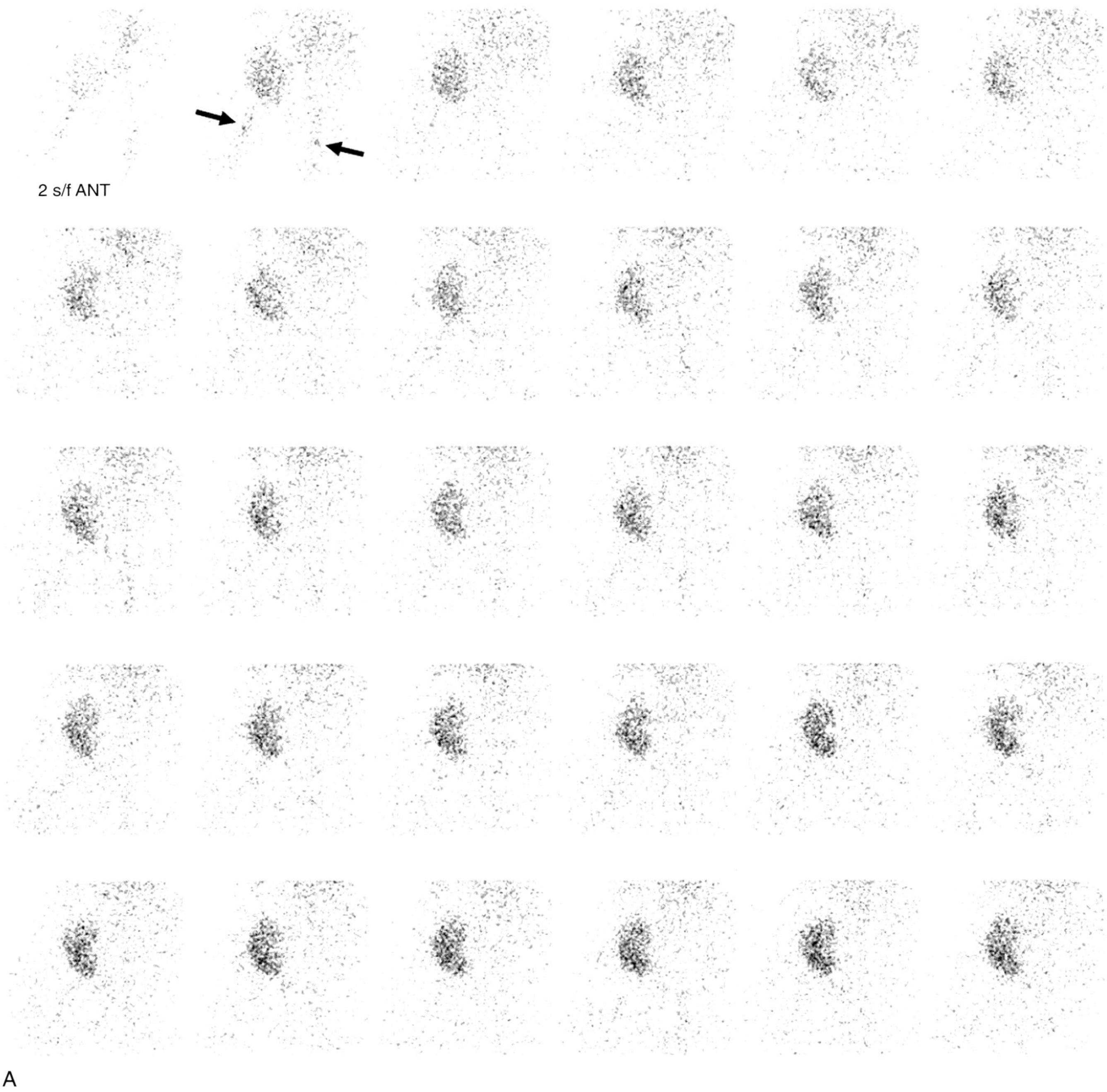

Figure 1-28 Normal MAG3 renal transplant scan. **A,** Perfusion phase imaging demonstrates radiotracer reaching the renal allograft at the same time the iliac arteries *(arrows)* are visualized.

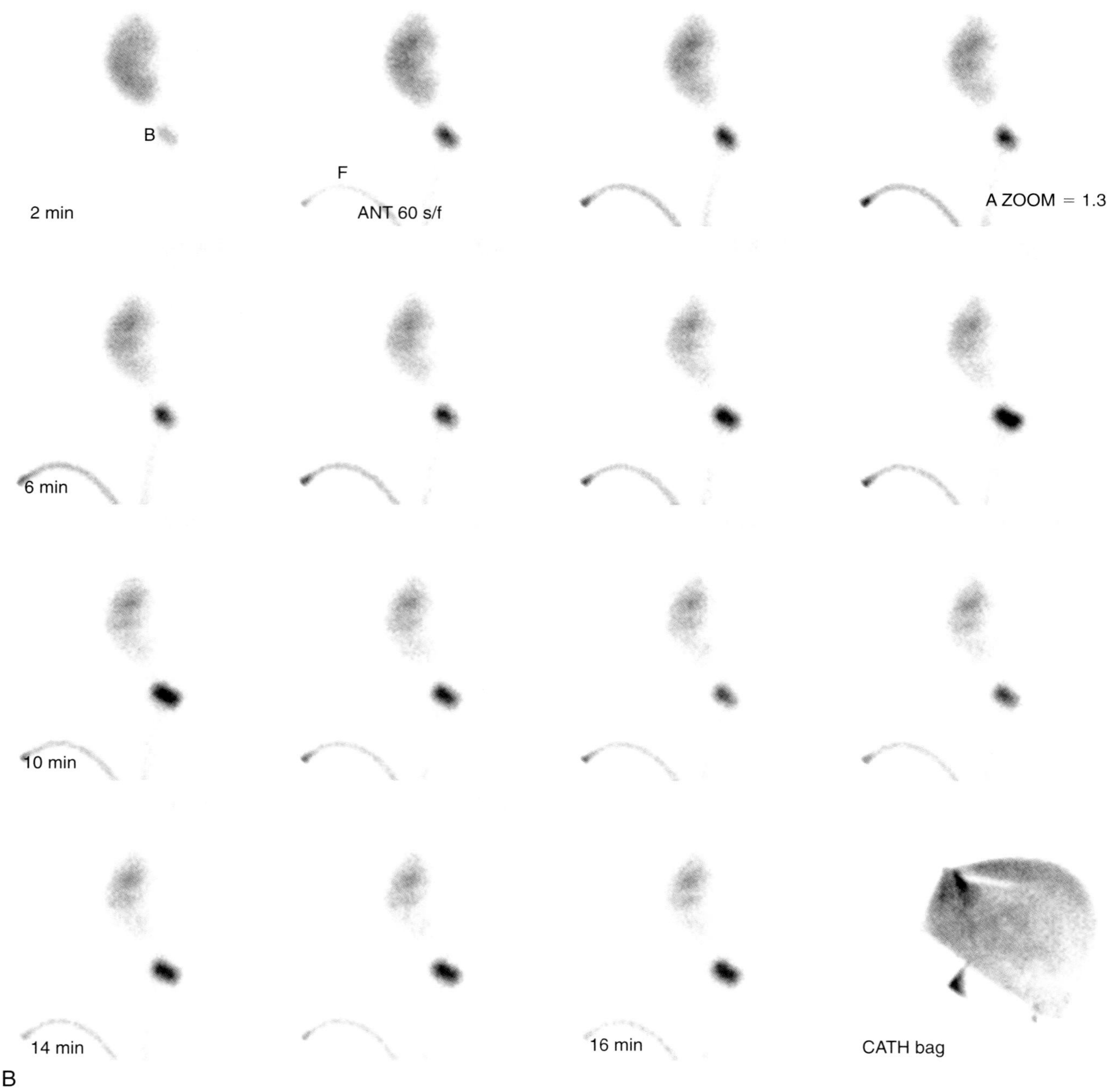

Figure 1-28, cont'd **B,** There is normal uptake, excretion, and drainage of radiotracer, with activity seen in the bladder *(B)* and Foley catheter *(F)* by 2 to 3 minutes postinjection. No parenchymal defects or urine extravasation are seen.

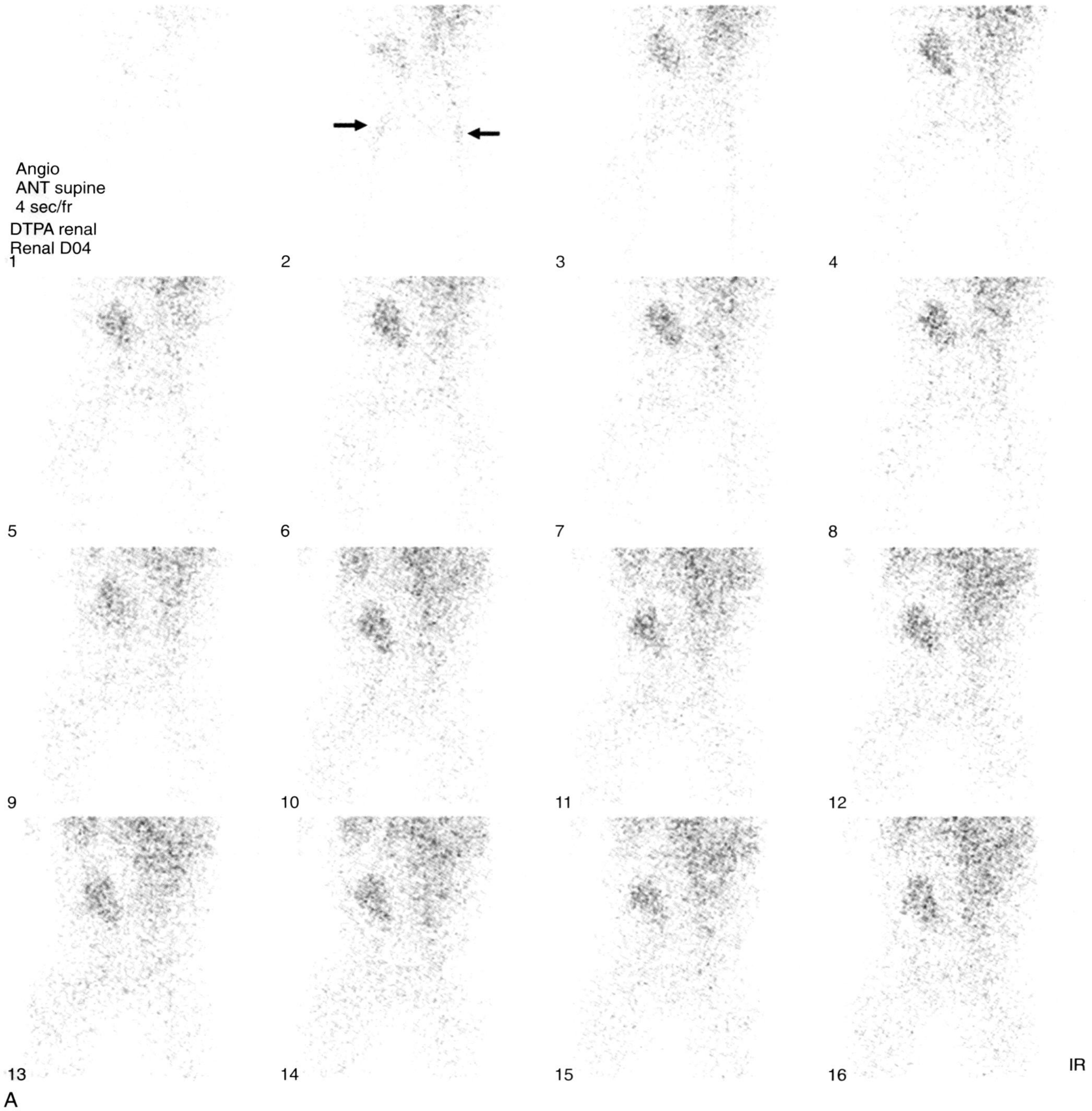

Figure 1-29 Renal transplant scan in a patient with acute tubular necrosis (ATN). **A,** Perfusion phase images show relatively preserved perfusion, with radiotracer reaching the renal allograft at the same time as the iliac arterial vessels *(arrows)*.

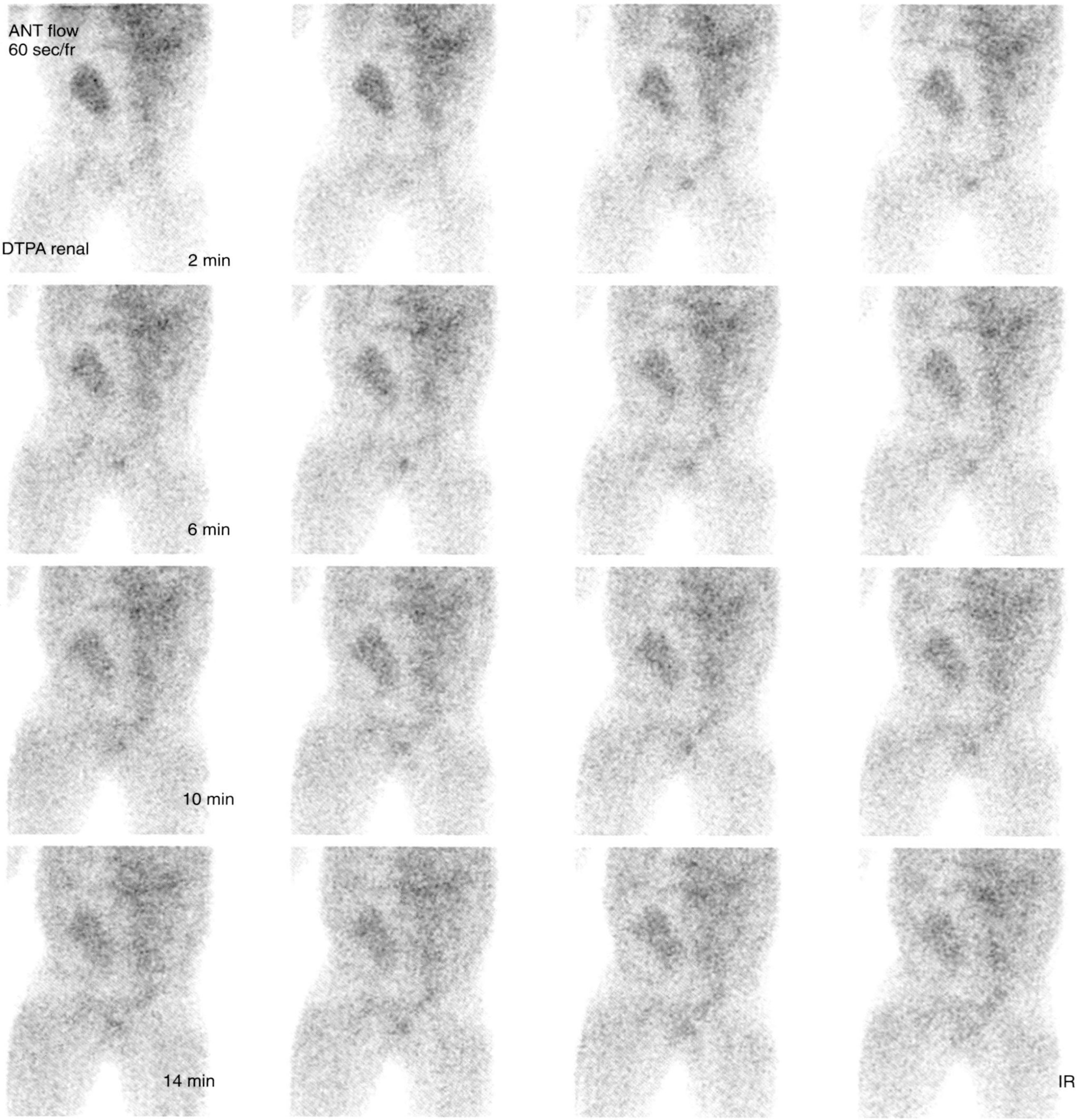

B

Figure 1-29, cont'd **B,** There is relatively preserved uptake into the renal parenchyma without focal defect. However, there is poor clearance of tracer from soft tissues, and there is no detectable excretion of tracer into the renal pelvis, ureter, or bladder consistent with ATN.

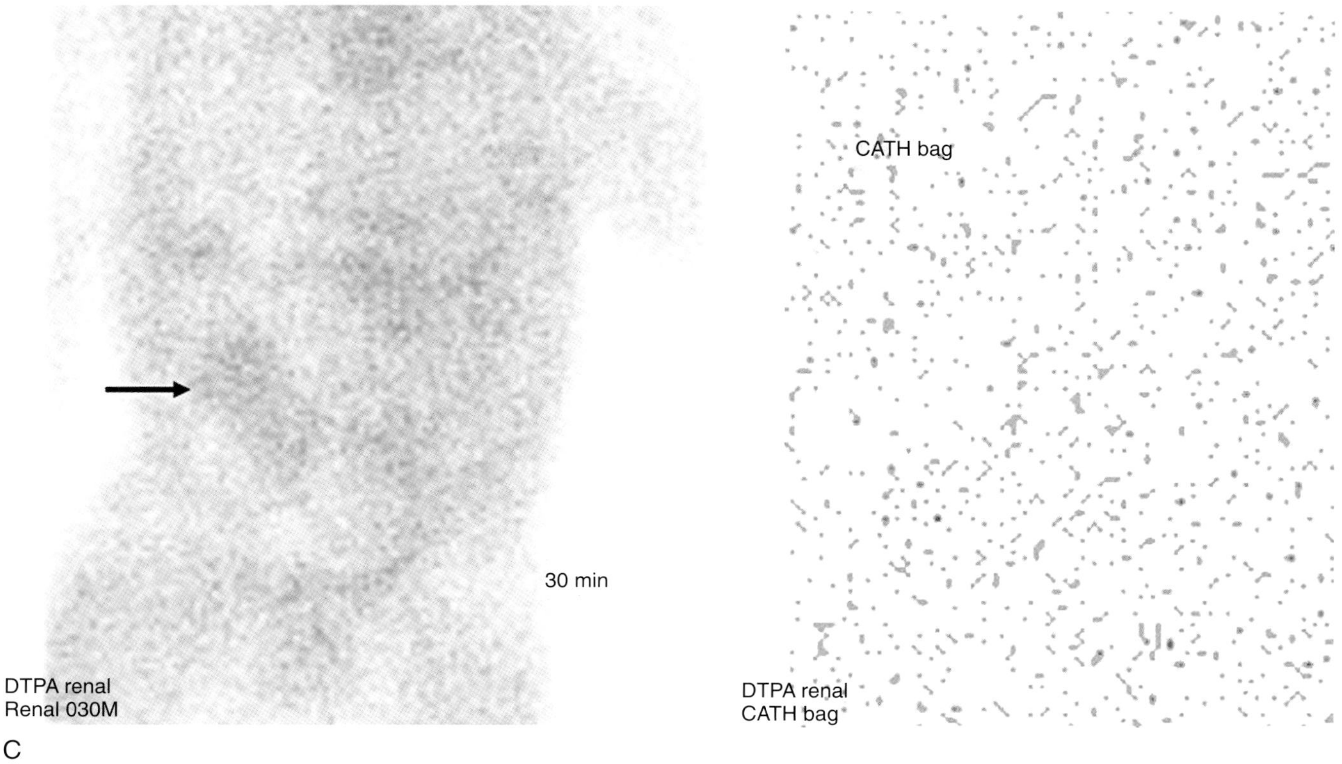

Figure 1-29, cont'd **C,** Delayed images obtained 30 minutes postinjection show prolonged retention of radiotracer in soft tissues and kidney parenchyma *(arrow)*. There continues to be no excretion of radiotracer into the urinary collecting system, and no urine activity is detected in the Foley catheter bag *(right)*.

Renal Cystic Diseases

Cysts in the kidney can be seen at any age in the pediatric group and can be associated with a wide array of disease states, as well as sporadically and unassociated with other pathologies. Differentiating a renal cyst from a caliceal diverticulum can be difficult but may be assessed using a modality such as CT or MR in which contrast is administered, because contrast will fill a diverticulum but not a cyst.

A number of systems for classification of cysts have been proposed and are discussed elsewhere in this book. Cysts of the kidneys can be broadly divided into those with hereditary causes and those with nonhereditary causes. In some cases the imaging appearance can point to an etiology and in others it cannot. Simple renal cysts can be seen in children just as in adults, though the reported incidence is as low as 0.2%.[158] Solitary cysts can also be seen as the sequela of previous insult to the kidney, such as trauma or infection. In most cases of solitary cysts, the remainder of the kidney appears normal.

On ultrasound a renal cyst will appear anechoic with an imperceptible wall. Increased through transmission can be seen deep to the cyst. On CT the cyst will have an attenuation equal to or near that of simple fluid and will again have an imperceptible wall. There should be little or no change in the attenuation of the cyst after contrast administration. If there is enhancement (either on CT or MRI) or any other complex feature to the structure, one should consider the possibility that what appears to be cystic may in fact be a neoplastic lesion that requires further evaluation.

Imaging has proven useful in the evaluation of nonhereditary renal cystic disease including multicystic dysplastic kidney,[159] solitary simple and acquired cysts,[158] and medullary sponge kidney.[160] Imaging has also proven its utility in the evaluation of hereditary cystic renal disease both in the diagnosis and in follow-up. Several authors have described the specific features of these renal cystic diseases. Autosomal dominant polycystic kidney disease (ADPKD) can appear in childhood and evolve as the child grows. The kidney may look normal at first or there may be cysts on the initial examination. As the child develops, the cysts may increase in number and size[161] (Figure 1-30). Autosomal recessive polycystic kidney disease (ARPKD) can have findings that are best seen when the kidneys are assessed with a high-resolution transducer. Macroscopic cysts, dilated tubules, crystal deposition, preservation of a normal-appearing cortical rim, and overall nephromegaly have been described in children with ARPKD.[162] In juvenile nephronophthisis, cysts are seen in the medullary pyramids.[163] The appearance of glomerulocystic disease is one of enlarged and hyperechoic kidneys with cortical cysts particularly in the periphery.[164]

In these scenarios imaging can assess not only the cysts but also associated findings. Examples include assessing for angiomyolipomas in children with tuberous sclerosis or for liver disease in children with ARPKD.

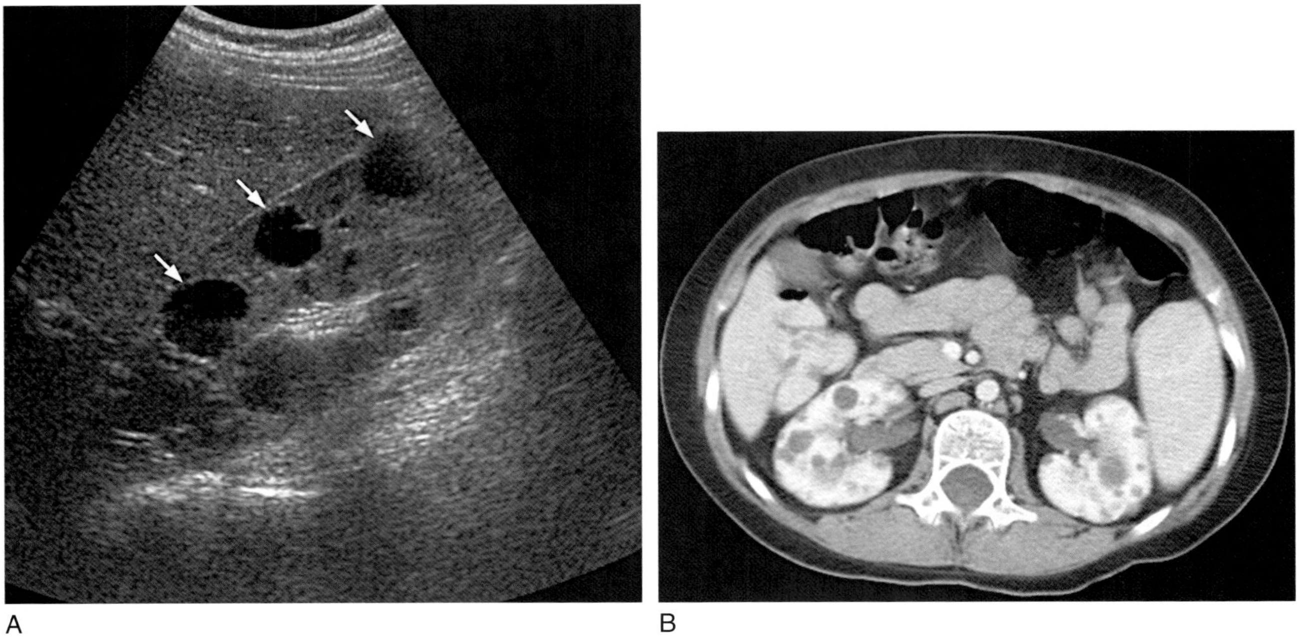

Figure 1-30 **A,** Ultrasound of the right kidney demonstrates multiple cysts *(arrows)* in a patient with autosomal dominant polycystic kidney disease. **B,** Enhanced CT in the same patient demonstrated multiple cysts of varying sizes scattered throughout both kidneys.

Nephrocalcinosis, Urolithiasis, and Miscellaneous Calcifications

A number of imaging findings in the pediatric urinary tract have been classified under the broad term *renal calcification.* Most are detected on ultrasound by virtue of the fact that ultrasound is the modality most commonly used and the most sensitive to early and subtle calcification.

Urolithiasis can be relatively easy to diagnose with imaging and with ultrasound in particular. Renal stones can range from a few millimeters in a renal calyx to several centimeters in filling the renal pelvis (staghorn calculus) (Figure 1-31). They are detected most reliably when present in the kidney or bladder but can also be seen in the ureter when they are not obscured by overlying bowel gas. They appear as echogenic foci, often with distal acoustic shadowing. When small they can be difficult to differentiate from vessels or portions of renal sinus fat, particularly if distal shadowing is not present. Renal stones can be assessed in terms of their size and any associated collecting system dilatation. As stated previously, ultrasound remains the modality of choice for imaging urolithiasis in children, with CT performed when the ultrasound examination is equivocal or nondiagnostic.

Nephrocalcinosis can also be assessed with imaging, ultrasound often being the modality of choice. Although cortical nephrocalcinosis can be seen, it is a rare finding in children.[165] Medullary nephrocalcinosis is well described in children and can be accurately diagnosed and followed—again preferably with ultrasound. The appearance is typically one of echogenic pyramids, often outlining the rim of the pyramid and a normal-appearing cortex (Figure 1-32). A pattern of peripheral increased echogenicity followed by progression toward the center of the pyramid has been described as the Anderson-Carr progression of nephrocalcinosis.[109]

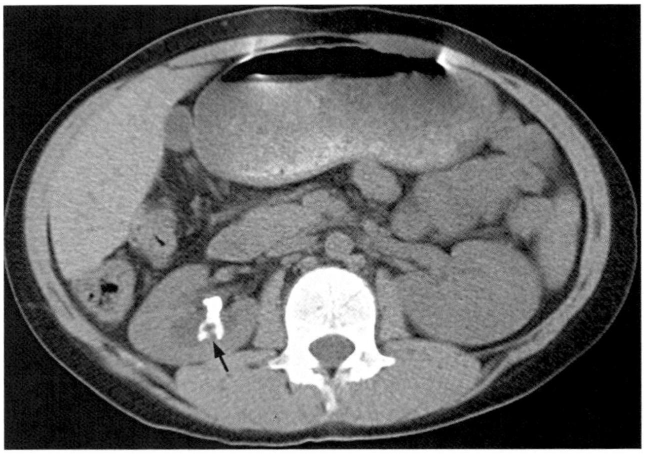

Figure 1-31 Unenhanced CT demonstrates a calculus *(arrow)* in the right renal collecting system extending into the calyces. The attenuation differences between calculi and the renal parenchyma are sufficient to allow for the diagnosis of urolithiasis without the administration of intravenous contrast.

Lastly, with the improvement in high-resolution imaging of kidneys in children, smaller echogenic foci are being detected. Although the precise etiology of these findings is still being worked out, they almost certainly represent small or early deposition of calcified or crystalline material. This deposition can be in the pelvocaliceal system, in the normal nephron, or in a pathologically dilated portion of the nephron.[162]

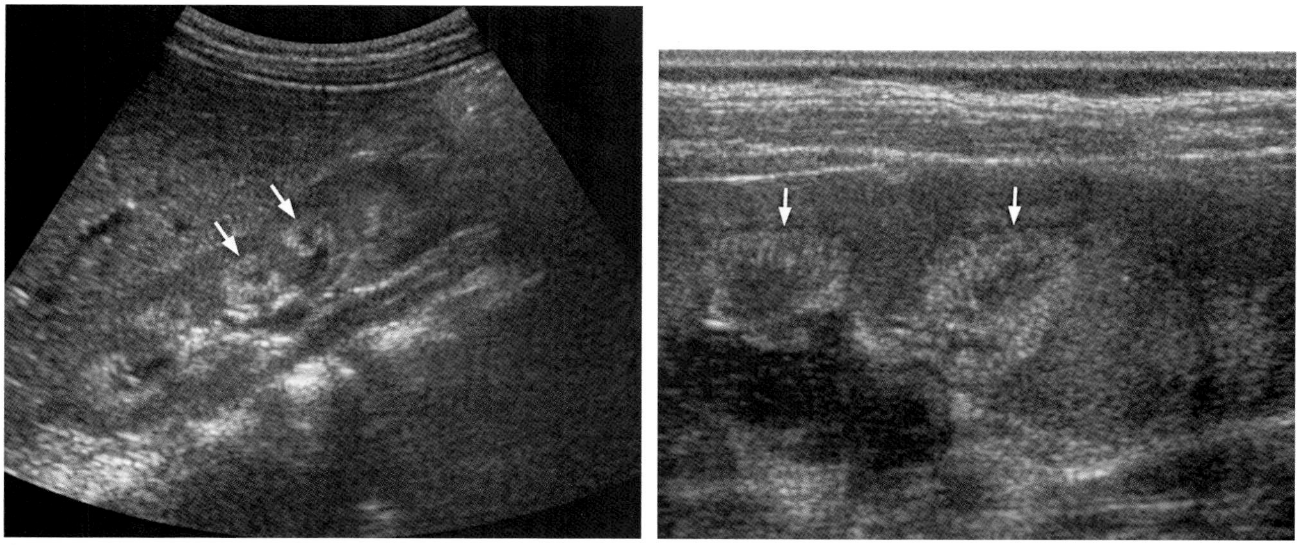

Figure 1-32 **A,** Ultrasound of the right kidney demonstrates increased echogenicity of the periphery of the renal pyramids. The renal cortex is normal. **B,** High-resolution image demonstrates this pattern of echogenicity, known as the Anderson-Carr progression of nephrocalcinosis, to better advantage.

CONCLUSION

The role of radiology in the diagnosis and treatment of diseases of the urinary tract has evolved over many decades. While modalities such as radiography and excretory urography have diminished in utility, newer modalities and their refinements, such as ultrasound, computed tomography, magnetic resonance imaging, and nuclear medicine, have reached the forefront. What remains constant is the close collaboration required among radiologists, nephrologists, and urologists in the care of children with nephropathies.

ACKNOWLEDGMENT

The authors express their gratitude to Dr. Paul Babyn and Dr. Martin Charron for their valuable assistance in the preparation and review of this chapter.

REFERENCES

1. Kirks DR, Griscom NT: *Practical pediatric imaging: diagnostic radiology of infants and children*, ed 3, Philadelphia, 1998: Lippincott-Raven.
2. Aaronson IA, Cremin BJ: *Clinical paediatric uroradiology*, Edinburgh; New York, 1984: Churchill Livingstone.
3. Kuhn JP et al: *Caffey's pediatric diagnostic imaging*, ed 10, vol 2, Philadelphia, 2004: Mosby.
4. Brenner D et al: Estimated risks of radiation-induced fatal cancer from pediatric CT, *Am J Roentgenol* 176(2):289-96, 2001.
5. Morcos SK, Thomsen HS: Adverse reactions to iodinated contrast media, *Eur Radiol* 11(7):1267-75, 2001.
6. Lameier NH: Contrast-induced nephropathy—prevention and risk reduction, *Nephrol Dial Transplant* 21(6):i11-23, 2006.
7. McClennan BL: Adverse reactions to iodinated contrast media. Recognition and response, *Invest Radiol*, 29(suppl)1:S46-50, 1994.
8. Malviya S et al: Sedation and general anaesthesia in children undergoing MRI and CT: adverse events and outcomes, *Br J Anaesth* 84(6):743-48, 2000.
9. Frush DP, Bisset GS III, Hall SC: Pediatric sedation in radiology: the practice of safe sleep, *AJR Am J Roentgenol* 167(6):1381-87, 1996.
10. Robbin ML: Ultrasound contrast agents: a promising future, *Radiol Clin North Am* 39(3):399-414, 2001.
11. Peratoner L et al: Kidney length and scarring in children with urinary tract infection: importance of ultrasound scans, *Abdom Imaging* 30(6):780-85, 2005.
12. Dacher JN et al: Imaging strategies in pediatric urinary tract infection, *Eur Radiol* 15(7):1283-88, 2005.
13. Practice parameter: the diagnosis, treatment, and evaluation of the initial urinary tract infection in febrile infants and young children. American Academy of Pediatrics. Committee on Quality Improvement. Subcommittee on Urinary Tract Infection. *Pediatrics*, 103(4 Pt 1): 843-52, 1999.
14. Chen JJ et al: The renal length nomogram: multivariable approach, *J Urol* 168(5):2149-52, 2002.
15. Blane CE et al: Sonographic standards for normal infant kidney length, *AJR Am J Roentgenol* 145(6):1289-91, 1985.
16. Rosenbaum DM, Korngold E, Teele RL: Sonographic assessment of renal length in normal children, *AJR Am J Roentgenol* 142(3):467-69, 1984.
17. Ginalski JM, Michaud A, Genton N: Renal growth retardation in children: sign suggestive of vesicoureteral reflux? *AJR Am J Roentgenol* 145(3):617-19, 1985.
18. Hricak H et al: Neonatal kidneys: sonographic anatomic correlation, *Radiology* 147(3):699-702, 1983.
19. Haller JO, Berdon WE, Friedman AP: Increased renal cortical echogenicity: a normal finding in neonates and infants, *Radiology* 142(1):173-74, 1982.
20. Starinsky R et al: Increased renal medullary echogenicity in neonates, *Pediatr Radiol* 25(suppl)1:S43-5, 1995.
21. Nimkin K et al: Urolithiasis in a children's hospital: 1985-1990, *Urol Radiol* 14(3):139-43, 1992.
22. Ricci MA, Lloyd DA: Renal venous thrombosis in infants and children, *Arch Surg* 125(9):1195-99, 1990.
23. Brun P et al: Value of Doppler ultrasound for the diagnosis of renal artery stenosis in children, *Pediatr Nephrol* 11(1):27-30, 1997.

24. Fang YC et al: A case of acute renal artery thrombosis caused by blunt trauma: computed tomographic and Doppler ultrasonic findings, *J Formos Med Assoc* 92(4):356-58, 1993.
25. Hitzel A et al: Color and power Doppler sonography versus DMSA scintigraphy in acute pyelonephritis and in prediction of renal scarring, *J Nucl Med* 43(1):27-32, 2002.
26. Sharma AK et al: Utility of serial Doppler ultrasound scans for the diagnosis of acute rejection in renal allografts, *Transpl Int* 17(3):138-44, 2004.
27. Fotter R: Pediatric uroradiology. *Medical radiology,* Berlin; New York, 2001, Springer.
28. Lebowitz RL et al: International system of radiographic grading of vesicoureteric reflux. International Reflux Study in Children, *Pediatr Radiol* 15(2):105-09, 1985.
29. Mettler FA, Guiberteau MJ: *Essentials of nuclear medicine imaging,* ed 5, Philadelphia, 2006, Saunders Elsevier.
30. Fleming JS et al: Guidelines for the measurement of glomerular filtration rate using plasma sampling, *Nucl Med Commun* 25(8):759-69, 2004.
31. Unver T et al: Comparison of direct radionuclide cystography and voiding cystourethrography in detecting vesicoureteral reflux, *Pediatr Int* 48(3):287-91, 2006.
32. Sukan A et al: Comparison of direct radionuclide cystography and voiding direct cystography in the detection of vesicoureteral reflux, *Ann Nucl Med* 17(7):549-53, 2003.
33. Fettich J et al: Guidelines for direct radionuclide cystography in children, *Eur J Nucl Med Mol Imaging* 30(5):B39-44, 2003.
34. Carpio F, Morey AF: Radiographic staging of renal injuries, *World J Urol* 17(2):66-70, 1999.
35. Piepsz A, Ham HR: Pediatric applications of renal nuclear medicine, *Semin Nucl Med* 36(1):16-35, 2006.
36. Peters AM, Morony S, Gordon I: Indirect radionuclide cystography demonstrates reflux under physiological conditions, *Clin Radiol* 41(1):44-47, 1990.
37. Gordon I, Peters AM, Morony S: Indirect radionuclide cystography: a sensitive technique for the detection of vesico-ureteral reflux, *Pediatr Nephrol* 4(6):604-06, 1990.
38. Gordon I: Indirect radionuclide cystography—the coming of age, *Nucl Med Commun,* 10(7):457-58, 1989.
39. Pollet JE, Sharp PF, Smith FW: Comparison of "direct" and "indirect" radionuclide cystography, *J Nucl Med* 26(12):1501-02, 1985.
40. Bower G et al: Comparison of "direct" and "indirect" radionuclide cystography, *J Nucl Med* 26(5):465-68, 1985.
41. Pollet JE et al: Intravenous radionuclide cystography for the detection of vesicorenal reflux, *J Urol* 125(1):75-78, 1981.
42. Conway JJ, Kruglik GD: Effectiveness of direct and indirect radionuclide cystography in detecting vesicoureteral reflux, *J Nucl Med* 17(02):81-83, 1976.
43. Conway JJ et al: Direct and indirect radionuclide cystography, *J Urol* 113(5):689-93, 1975.
44. Conway JJ, Belman AB, King LR: Direct and indirect radionuclide cystography, *Semin Nucl Med* 4(2):197-211, 1974.
45. Gordon I et al: Guidelines for indirect radionuclide cystography, *Eur J Nucl Med* 28(3):BP16-20, 2001.
46. Mandell GA et al: Procedure guideline for radionuclide cystography in children. Society of Nuclear Medicine, *J Nucl Med* 38(10):1650-54, 1997.
47. De Sadeleer C et al: How good is technetium-99m mercaptoacetyltriglycine indirect cystography? *Eur J Nucl Med* 21(3):223-27, 1994.
48. Corso A, Ostinelli A, Trombetta MA: "Indirect" radioisotope cystography after the furosemide test: its diagnostic efficacy compared to "direct" study, *Radiol Med (Torino)* 78(6):645-48, 1989.
49. Vlajkovic M et al: Radionuclide voiding patterns in children with vesicoureteral reflux, *Eur J Nucl Med Mol Imaging* 30(4):532-37, 2003.
50. Hoberman A et al: Imaging studies after a first febrile urinary tract infection in young children, *N Engl J Med* 348(3):195-202, 2003.
51. Stokland E et al: Imaging of renal scarring, *Acta Paediatr Suppl* 88(431):13-21, 1999.
52. Goldraich NP, Goldraich IH: Update on dimercaptosuccinic acid renal scanning in children with urinary tract infection, *Pediatr Nephrol* 9(2):221-26; discussion 227, 1995.
53. Mastin ST, Drane WE, Iravani A: Tc-99m DMSA SPECT imaging in patients with acute symptoms or history of UTI. Comparison with ultrasonography, *Clin Nucl Med* 20(5):407-12, 1995.
54. Majd M et al: Acute pyelonephritis: comparison of diagnosis with 99mTc-DMSA, SPECT, spiral CT, MR imaging, and power Doppler US in an experimental pig model, *Radiology* 218(1):101-08, 2001.
55. Applegate KE et al: A prospective comparison of high-resolution planar, pinhole, and triple-detector SPECT for the detection of renal cortical defects, *Clin Nucl Med* 22(10):673-78, 1997.
56. Cook GJ, Lewis MK, Clarke SE: An evaluation of 99Tcm-DMSA SPET with three-dimensional reconstruction in 68 patients with varied renal pathology, *Nucl Med Commun* 16(11):958-67, 1995.
57. Yen TC et al: A comparative study of evaluating renal scars by 99mTc-DMSA planar and SPECT renal scans, intravenous urography, and ultrasonography, *Ann Nucl Med* 8(2):147-52, 1994.
58. Takeda M et al: Value of dimercaptosuccinic acid single photon emission computed tomography and magnetic resonance imaging in detecting renal injury in pediatric patients with vesicoureteral reflux. Comparison with dimercaptosuccinic acid planar scintigraphy and intravenous pyelography, *Eur Urol* 25(4):320-25, 1994.
59. Mouratidis B, Ash JM, Gilday DL: Comparison of planar and SPECT 99Tcm-DMSA scintigraphy for the detection of renal cortical defects in children. *Nucl Med Commun* 14(2):82-86, 1993.
60. Piepsz A et al: Consensus on renal cortical scintigraphy in children with urinary tract infection. Scientific Committee of Radionuclides in Nephrourology, *Semin Nucl Med* 29(2):160-74, 1999.
61. Itoh K et al: Qualitative and quantitative evaluation of renal parenchymal damage by 99mTc-DMSA planar and SPECT scintigraphy. *Ann Nucl Med* 9(1):23-28, 1995.
62. Craig JC et al: How accurate is dimercaptosuccinic acid scintigraphy for the diagnosis of acute pyelonephritis? A meta-analysis of experimental studies, *J Nucl Med* 41(6):986-93, 2000.
63. Chiou YY et al: Renal fibrosis: prediction from acute pyelonephritis focus volume measured at 99mTc dimercaptosuccinic acid SPECT, *Radiology* 221(2):366-70, 2001.
64. Yen TC et al: Identification of new renal scarring in repeated episodes of acute pyelonephritis using Tc-99m DMSA renal SPECT, *Clin Nucl Med* 23(12):828-31, 1998.
65. Yen TC et al: Technetium-99m-DMSA renal SPECT in diagnosing and monitoring pediatric acute pyelonephritis, *J Nucl Med* 37(8):1349-53, 1996.
66. Mettler FA, Guiberteau MJ: *Essentials of nuclear medicine imaging,* ed 5, Philadelphia, 2006, Saunders Elsevier.
67. Mettler FA, Guiberteau MJ: *Essentials of nuclear medicine imaging,* ed 5, Philadelphia, 2006, Saunders Elsevier.
68. Ell PJ, Gambhir SS: *Nuclear medicine in clinical diagnosis and treatment,* ed 3, Edinburgh, Churchill Livingstone.
69. Mandell GA et al: Procedure guideline for diuretic renography in children. Society of Nuclear Medicine, *J Nucl Med* 38(10):1647-50, 1997.
70. Rossleigh MA: Renal cortical scintigraphy and diuresis renography in infants and children, *J Nucl Med* 42(1):91-95, 2001.
71. McCarthy CS et al: Pitfalls and limitations of diuretic renography, *Abdom Imaging* (1):78-81, 1994.
72. Conway JJ, Maizels M: The "well tempered" diuretic renogram: a standard method to examine the asymptomatic neonate with hydronephrosis or hydroureteronephrosis. A report from combined meetings of The Society for Fetal Urology and members of The Pediatric Nuclear Medicine Council—The Society of Nuclear Medicine, *J Nucl Med* 33(11):2047-51, 1992.
73. Donoso G et al: 99mTc-MAG3 diuretic renography in children: a comparison between F0 and F+20, *Nucl Med Commun* 24(11):1189-93, 2003.
74. Wong DC, Rossleigh MA, Farnsworth RH: F+0 diuresis renography in infants and children, *J Nucl Med* 40(11):1805-11, 1999.
75. Lowe LH et al: Pediatric renal masses: Wilms tumor and beyond, *Radiographics* 20(6):1585-603, 2000.
76. Buckley JC, McAninch JW: The diagnosis, management, and outcomes of pediatric renal injuries, *Urol Clin North Am* 33(1):33-40, 2006.
77. McAleer IM, Kaplan GW: Pediatric genitourinary trauma, *Urol Clin North Am* 22(1):177-88, 1995.

78. Dacher JN et al: Rational use of CT in acute pyelonephritis: findings and relationships with reflux, *Pediatr Radiol* 23(4):281-85, 1993.
79. Tunaci A, Yekeler E: Multidetector row CT of the kidneys, *Eur J Radiol* 52(1):56-66, 2004.
80. Slovis TL: Children, computed tomography radiation dose, and the As Low As Reasonably Achievable (ALARA) concept, *Pediatrics* 112(4):971-72, 2003.
81. Volle E, Park W, Kaufmann HJ: MRI examination and monitoring of pediatric patients under sedation, *Pediatr Radiol* 26(4):280-81, 1996.
82. Li A et al: Acute adverse reactions to magnetic resonance contrast media—gadolinium chelates, *Br J Radiol* 79(941):368-71, 2006.
83. Akgun H et al: Are gadolinium-based contrast media nephrotoxic? A renal biopsy study, *Arch Pathol Lab Med* 130(9):1354-57, 2006.
84. Sadowski EA et al: Nephrogenic systemic fibrosis: risk factors and incidence estimation, *Radiology*, 243(1):148-57, 2007.
85. Hoffer FA Magnetic resonance imaging of abdominal masses in the pediatric patient, *Semin Ultrasound CT MR* 26(4):212-23, 2005.
86. Rohrschneider WK et al: US, CT and MR imaging characteristics of nephroblastomatosis, *Pediatr Radiol* 28(6):435-43, 1998.
87. Israel GM et al: The use of opposed-phase chemical shift MRI in the diagnosis of renal angiomyolipomas, *AJR Am J Roentgenol* 184(6):1868-72, 2005.
88. Pretorius ES, Wickstrom ML, Siegelman ES: MR imaging of renal neoplasms, *Magn Reson Imaging Clin N Am* 8(4):813-36, 2000.
89. Ramchandani P et al: Impact of magnetic resonance on staging of renal carcinoma. *Urology* 27(6):564-68, 1986.
90. Hallscheidt PJ et al: Preoperative staging of renal cell carcinoma with inferior vena cava thrombus using multidetector CT and MRI: prospective study with histopathological correlation, *J Comput Assist Tomogr* 29(1):64-68, 2005.
91. Kim D et al: Abdominal aorta and renal artery stenosis: evaluation with MR angiography, *Radiology* 174(3 Pt 1):727-31, 1990.
92. Zhang H, Prince MR: Renal MR angiography, *Magn Reson Imaging Clin N Am* 12(3):487-503, vi, 2004.
93. Schoenberg SO et al: Renal MR angiography: current debates and developments in imaging of renal artery stenosis, *Semin Ultrasound CT MR* 24(4):255-67, 2003.
94. Marcos HB, Choyke PL: Magnetic resonance angiography of the kidney, *Semin Nephrol* 20(5):450-55, 2000.
95. Vasbinder GB et al: Accuracy of computed tomographic angiography and magnetic resonance angiography for diagnosing renal artery stenosis, *Ann Intern Med* 141(9):674-82; discussion 682, 2004.
96. Kovanlikaya A et al: Comparison of MRI and renal cortical scintigraphy findings in childhood acute pyelonephritis: preliminary experience, *Eur J Radiol* 49(1):76-80, 2004.
97. Weiser AC et al: The role of gadolinium enhanced magnetic resonance imaging for children with suspected acute pyelonephritis, *J Urol* 169(6):2308-11, 2003.
98. Leonidas JC, Berdon WE: MR imaging of urinary tract infections in children, *Radiology* 210(2):582-84, 1999.
99. Ku JH et al: Is there a role for magnetic resonance imaging in renal trauma? *Int J Urol* 8(6):261-67, 2001.
100. Marcos HB, Noone TC, Semelka RC: MRI evaluation of acute renal trauma, *J Magn Reson Imaging* 8(4):989-90, 1998.
101. Cohen HL et al: Congenital abnormalities of the genitourinary system, *Semin Roentgenol* 39(2):282-303, 2004.
102. Rohrschneider WK et al: Functional and morphologic evaluation of congenital urinary tract dilatation by using combined static-dynamic MR urography: findings in kidneys with a single collecting system, *Radiology* 224(3):683-94, 2002.
103. Nolte-Ernsting CC, Adam GB, Gunther RW: MR urography: examination techniques and clinical applications, *Eur Radiol* 11(3):355-72, 2001.
104. Karabacakoglu A et al: Diagnostic value of diuretic-enhanced excretory MR urography in patients with obstructive uropathy, *Eur J Radiol* 52(3):320-27, 2004.
105. Grattan-Smith JD, Jones RA: MR urography in children, *Pediatr Radiol*, 36(11):1119-32, 2006.
106. Paulson DF et al: Pediatric urolithiasis, *J Urol* 108(5):811-14, 1972.
107. Breatnach E, Smith SE: The radiology of renal stones in children, *Clin Radiol* 34(1):59-64, 1983.
108. Day DL, Scheinman JI, Mahan J: Radiological aspects of primary hyperoxaluria, *AJR Am J Roentgenol* 146(2):395-401, 1986.
109. Patriquin H, Robitaille P: Renal calcium deposition in children: sonographic demonstration of the Anderson-Carr progression, *AJR Am J Roentgenol* 146(6):1253-56, 1986.
110. Jevtic V: Imaging of renal osteodystrophy, *Eur J Radiol* 46(2):85-95, 2003.
111. Lebowitz RL: Urography in children: when should it be done? 1. Infection, *Postgrad Med* 64(4):63-72, 1978.
112. Lebowitz RL: Urography in children: when should it be done? 2. Conditions other than infection, *Postgrad Med* 64(5):61-70, 1978.
113. American Academy of Pediatrics: Committee on Radiology: Excretory urography for evaluation of enuresis, *Pediatrics* 65(1):A49-50, 1980.
114. Lebowitz RL: Excretory urography in children, *AJR Am J Roentgenol* 163(4):990, 1994.
115. Sourtzis S et al: Radiologic investigation of renal colic: unenhanced helical CT compared with excretory urography, *AJR Am J Roentgenol* 172(6):1491-94, 1999.
116. McNicholas MM et al: Excretory phase CT urography for opacification of the urinary collecting system, *AJR Am J Roentgenol* 170(5):1261-67, 1998.
117. O'Malley ME et al: Comparison of excretory phase, helical computed tomography with intravenous urography in patients with painless haematuria, *Clin Radiol* 58(4):294-300, 2003.
118. Borthne AS et al: Pediatric excretory MR urography: comparative study of enhanced and non-enhanced techniques, *Eur Radiol* 13(6):1423-27, 2003.
119. Pollack HM, Banner MP: Current status of excretory urography. A premature epitaph? *Urol Clin North Am* 12(4):585-601, 1985.
120. Carrico C, Lebowitz RL: Incontinence due to an infrasphincteric ectopic ureter: why the delay in diagnosis and what the radiologist can do about it, *Pediatr Radiol* 28(12):942-49, 1998.
121. Smith H et al: Routine excretory urography in follow-up of superficial transitional cell carcinoma of bladder, *Urology* 34(4):193-96, 1989.
122. Kawashima A et al: Imaging of urethral disease: a pictorial review, *Radiographics* 24(suppl 1):S195-216, 2004.
123. Yoder IC, Papanicolaou N: Imaging the urethra in men and women, *Urol Radiol* 14(1):24-28, 1992.
124. Pavlica P, Barozzi L, Menchi I: Imaging of male urethra, *Eur Radiol* 13(7):1583-96, 2003.
125. Sclafani SJ, Becker, JA: Radiologic diagnosis of extrarenal genitourinary trauma, *Urol Radiol* 7(4):201-10, 1985.
126. Grignon A et al: Ureteropelvic junction stenosis: antenatal ultrasonographic diagnosis, postnatal investigation, and follow-up, *Radiology* 160(3):649-51, 1986.
127. Wood BP et al: Ureterovesical obstruction and megaloureter: diagnosis by real-time US, *Radiology* 156(1):79-81, 1985.
128. Gilsanz V, Miller JH, Reid BS: Ultrasonic characteristics of posterior urethral valves, *Radiology* 145(1):143-45, 1982.
129. Mascatello VJ et al: Ultrasonic evaluation of the obstructed duplex kidney, *AJR Am J Roentgenol* 129(1):113-20, 1977.
130. Nussbaum AR et al: Ectopic ureter and ureterocele: their varied sonographic manifestations, *Radiology* 159(1):227-35, 1986.
131. Griffin J, Jennings C, MacErlean D: Ultrasonic evaluation of simple and ectopic ureteroceles, *Clin Radiol* 34(1):55-57, 1983.
132. Strife JL et al: Multicystic dysplastic kidney in children: US follow-up, *Radiology* 186(3):785-88, 1993.
133. Edell SL, Bonavita JA: The sonographic appearance of acute pyelonephritis, *Radiology* 132(3):683-85, 1979.
134. Rosenfield AT et al: Acute focal bacterial nephritis (acute lobar nephronia), *Radiology* 132(3):553-61, 1979.
135. Bjorgvinsson E, Majd M, Eggli KD: Diagnosis of acute pyelonephritis in children: comparison of sonography and 99mTc-DMSA scintigraphy, *AJR Am J Roentgenol* 157(3):539-43, 1991.
136. Farmer KD, Gellett LR, Dubbins PA: The sonographic appearance of acute focal pyelonephritis: 8 years experience, *Clin Radiol* 57(6):483-87, 2002.

137. Dacher JN et al: Renal sinus hyperechogenicity in acute pyelonephritis: description and pathological correlation, *Pediatr Radiol* 29(3):179-82, 1999.
138. Stein JP et al: Blunt renal trauma in the pediatric population: indications for radiographic evaluation, *Urology* 44(3):406-10, 1994.
139. John SD: Trends in pediatric emergency imaging, *Radiol Clin North Am* 37(5):995-1034, vi, 1999.
140. Rose JS: Ultrasound in abdominal trauma, *Emerg Med Clin North Am* 22(3):581-99, vii, 2004.
141. Soudack M et al: Experience with focused abdominal sonography for trauma (FAST) in 313 pediatric patients, *J Clin Ultrasound* 32(2):53-61, 2004.
142. Taylor GA, Sivit CJ: Posttraumatic peritoneal fluid: is it a reliable indicator of intraabdominal injury in children? *J Pediatr Surg* 30(12):1644-48, 1995.
143. Pieretti R, Gilday D, Jeffs R: Differential kidney scan in pediatric urology, *Urology* 4(6):665-8, 1974.
144. Mandell GA et al: Procedure guideline for renal cortical scintigraphy in children, Society of Nuclear Medicine, *J Nucl Med* 38(10):1644-46, 1997.
145. Clausen TD, Kanstrup IL, Iversen J: Reference values for 99mTc-MAG3 renography determined in healthy, potential renal donors, *Clin Physiol Funct Imaging* 22(5):356-60, 2002.
146. Schofer O et al: Technetium-99m mercaptoacetyltriglycine clearance: reference values for infants and children, *Eur J Nucl Med* 22(11):1278-81, 1995.
147. Tsukamoto E et al: Validity of 99mTc-DMSA renal uptake by planar posterior-view method in children, *Ann Nucl Med* 13(6):383-87, 1999.
148. Gainza FJ et al: Evaluation of complications due to percutaneous renal biopsy in allografts and native kidneys with color-coded Doppler sonography, *Clin Nephrol* 43(5):303-08, 1995.
149. Morin F, Cote I: Tc-99m MAG3 evaluation of recipients with en bloc renal grafts from pediatric cadavers, *Clin Nucl Med* 25(8):579-84, 2000.
150. Tulchinsky M, Malpani AR, Eggli DF: Diagnosis of urinoma by MAG3 scintigraphy in a renal transplant patient, *Clin Nucl Med* 20(1):80-81, 1995.
151. Carmody E et al: Sequential Tc 99m mercaptoacetyl-triglycine (MAG3) renography as an evaluator of early renal transplant function, *Clin Transplant* 7(3):245-49, 1993.
152. Cohn DA, Gruenewald S: Postural renal transplant obstruction: a case report and review of the literature, *Clin Nucl Med* 26(8):673-76, 2001.
153. Goodear M, Barratt L, Wycherley A: Intraperitoneal urine leak in a patient with a renal transplant on Tc-99m MAG3 imaging, *Clin Nucl Med* 23(11):789-90, 1998.
154. Mange KC et al: Focal acute tubular necrosis in a renal allograft, *Transplantation* 64(10):1490-92, 1997.
155. Dubovsky EV, Russell CD, Erbas B: Radionuclide evaluation of renal transplants, *Semin Nucl Med* 25(1):49-59, 1995.
156. Dubovsky EV, Russell CD: Radionuclide evaluation of renal transplants, *Semin Nucl Med* 18(3):181-98, 1988.
157. Nankivell BJ et al: Diagnosis of kidney transplant obstruction using Mag3 diuretic renography, *Clin Transplant* 15(1):11-18, 2001.
158. McHugh K et al: Simple renal cysts in children: diagnosis and follow-up with US, *Radiology* 178(2):383-85, 1991.
159. Stuck KJ, Koff SA, Silver TM: Ultrasonic features of multicystic dysplastic kidney: expanded diagnostic criteria, *Radiology* 143(1):217-21, 1982.
160. Patriquin HB, O'Regan S: Medullary sponge kidney in childhood, *AJR Am J Roentgenol* 145(2):315-19, 1985.
161. Pretorius DH et al: Diagnosis of autosomal dominant polycystic kidney disease in utero and in the young infant, *J Ultrasound Med* 6(5):249-55, 1987.
162. Traubici J, Daneman A: High-resolution renal sonography in children with autosomal recessive polycystic kidney disease, *AJR Am J Roentgenol* 184(5):1630-33, 2005.
163. Garel LA et al: Juvenile nephronophthisis: sonographic appearance in children with severe uremia, *Radiology* 151(1):93-5, 1984.
164. Fredericks BJ et al: Glomerulocystic renal disease: ultrasound appearances, *Pediatr Radiol* 19(3):184-86, 1989.
165. Wilson DA, Wenzl JE, Altshuler GP: Ultrasound demonstration of diffuse cortical nephrocalcinosis in a case of primary hyperoxaluria, *AJR Am J Roentgenol* 132(4):659-61, 1979.

CHAPTER

2 Laboratory Evaluation at Different Ages

Valerie Langlois

Laboratory evaluation is a major component in the assessment for renal disease in children. Because clinical examination rarely provides sufficient information to establish a diagnosis, nephrologists rely heavily on laboratory evaluation. Knowing the indications for each test and the normal reference ranges is important for the clinician. This chapter reviews the tests for renal disease most commonly used in clinical practice.

ASSESSMENT OF RENAL FUNCTION

Urine Analysis

The value of urine analysis in the evaluation of kidney disease should not be underestimated. Important information can be learned from this simple, quick, and inexpensive test. Many commercially available reagent strips can screen for pH, specific gravity, protein, blood, glucose, ketone, leukocytes, and nitrites in the urine. Urine specimens should be fresh and clean-voided midstream in older children.

Depending on the concentration of urine, its color varies from pale yellow to amber. Red or tea-colored urine suggests the presence of blood, hemoglobin, myoglobin, porphyrin, or nonpathologic pigments (beets, food color) or medication. Blue to green suggests the presence of biliverdin or *Pseudomonas* infection.

Urine is normally clear, but can be cloudy in the presence of leukocytes, epithelial cells, bacteria, or precipitation of amorphous phosphate or amorphous urate. Unusual urine odor can lead to the diagnosis of rare metabolic disorders such as maple syrup urine disease (maple syrup odor), phenylketonuria (musty odor), or hypermethioninemia (fishy odor).

Specific gravity (SG) reflects the concentrating and diluting ability of the kidney. In normal conditions, it reflects a person's hydration status. However, in abnormal kidneys, a very low SG may represent a concentrating defect. SG can also be used to distinguish prerenal states from intrinsic renal disease. It usually ranges from 1 : 001 to 1 : 035 and can be measured with a urinometer, a refractometer, or more commonly, reagent strips. The reagent strip test is based on pKa change of certain polyelectrolytes in relation to ionic concentration.[1]

Urinary pH usually ranges from 5.0 to 8.0 depending on the acid–base balance of the body and can be estimated using the reagent test strip. However, precise measurements should be obtained with a pH meter from a fresh urine specimen ideally collected directly in a sealed syringe from a urine catheter to avoid contact with air. Urinary pH is important in diagnosing renal tubular acidosis and monitoring in the treatment or prevention of urinary stones.

Glucose is not usually present in the urine. It is freely filtered at the level of the glomerulus and reabsorbed in the proximal tubule by way of a sodium-coupled active transport mechanism. Glucosuria can be seen when the serum glucose is above the renal threshold or due to isolated renal glucosuria or proximal tubular disorder such as Fanconi syndrome. Normal values for maximal tubular glucose reabsorption (TmG) in children vary from 254-401 mg/min/1.73 m^2 (14-22 mmol/min/1.73 m^2).[2] Glucosuria can usually be detected in the urine when plasma glucose concentration is greater than 180-200 mg/dl (10-11 mmol/L).[3]

Reagent test strips are usually impregnated with the enzyme glucose oxidase and only detect glucose. Other sugars such as galactose, lactose, fructose, and mannose can be detected by a copper reduction test such as Clinitest tablets (Ames Co.).

Ketone bodies are formed during the catabolism of fatty acids and include acetoacetic acid, beta-hydroxybutyric acid, and acetone. Reagent strips for ketones based on a color reaction with sodium nitroprusside are sensitive for acetoacetic acid but will not detect beta-hydroxybutyric acid and acetone. One of the most significant disorders in which ketones are produced is diabetic ketoacidosis. All three ketones are present in the urine with this illness, and screening for acetoacetic acid only is sufficient. Ketones can also be found in glycogen storage disease, starvation, high-fat diets, and hyperthyroidism.

The presence of leukocytes in the urine suggests urinary tract infection or acute glomerulonephritis. Strip tests detect leukocyte esterase, an enzyme found in neutrophils.

The nitrite test indicates the presence of bacteria capable of reducing dietary nitrate to nitrite, such as *Escherichia coli*, *Enterobacter*, *Citrobacter*, *Klebsiella*, and *Proteus* species. For this to occur, the urine must have incubated in the bladder for a minimum of 4 hours.[1] A negative nitrite test does not mean the absence of bacterial infection since the urine may not have remained in the bladder long enough, the urine might not contain nitrate, or the infection was caused by a bacteria that does not form nitrite.

Hematuria is defined as the presence of more than five red blood cells (RBCs) per high power field in a centrifuged urine or positive dipstick test for blood. Reagent strips detect RBCs, myoglobin, and hemoglobin. Presence of RBCs can only be confirmed by microscopic evaluation. The supernatant of a centrifuged urine containing RBCs will be clear yellow as opposed to pink if the urine contains hemoglobin or myoglobin. The morphology of the cells can help determine their origin. Presence of dysmorphic RBCs suggests glomerular hematuria.

Urine Microscopy

Microscopic evaluation of fresh urine is extremely valuable in the evaluation of renal disease. The presence of casts, cells, and crystals should be sought. Although hyaline and granular casts can be seen in normal states, cellular casts are pathologic. Red blood cell casts are pathognomonic of glomerular disease and white blood cell casts can be seen with interstitial nephritis or postinfectious glomerulonephritis.

Crystals are rarely seen in fresh urine but appear after the urine stands for a period. Uric acid, calcium oxalate, amorphous urate, cystine, tyrosine, leucine, and cholesterol are usually found in acid urine. Uric acid and calcium oxalate can be seen in normal and pathological conditions. Amorphous urates are of no clinical significance. Cystine, tyrosine, leucine, and cholesterol crystals are always relevant. Cystine crystals are related to cystinuria, whereas leucine crystals can be associated with maple syrup urine disease, methionine malabsorption syndrome (oasthouse urine disease), and serious liver disease. Tyrosine crystals also occur in serious liver disease, tyrosinosis, and oasthouse urine disease. The presence of cholesterol crystals can indicate excessive tissue breakdown or nephritic or nephrotic conditions.[1]

Triple phosphate, calcium carbonate, ammonium biurate, amorphous phosphates, and calcium-phosphate crystals are usually found in alkaline urine. Calcium carbonate and amorphous phosphate are of no clinical significance.

Urinary Protein Excretion

In a normal state, most of the filtered low molecular weight (MW) proteins (MW < 40,000) are reabsorbed in the proximal tubules. Proteins of higher molecular weight such as albumin (MW = 60,000) are filtered in smaller amounts. Tamm-Horsfall proteins are secreted by the tubular cells in the ascending thick limb of the loop of Henle and are the main proteins found in normal urine.

In disease states, increased amounts of protein can be found in the urine and may reflect damage to the glomerular barrier (glomerular proteinuria) or defective tubular reabsorption (tubular proteinuria).

In glomerular proteinuria, albumin predominates in the urine. The selectivity index is sometimes used to compare the clearance of high molecular weight protein (HMWP) such as immunoglobulin G (IgG), haptoglobin, alpha-2 microglobulin, and immunoglobulin M (IgM) with the clearance of albumin. The loss of the charge selectivity of the glomerular basement membrane allows passage of albumin but not HMWP, which results in highly selective proteinuria. If there is injury to the size-selective barrier, the proteinuria becomes less selective. Minimal change nephrotic syndrome usually has a high selectivity index.

Beta-2 microglobulin, alpha-1 microglobulin, and retinol-binding protein are used as markers of tubular proteinuria.

The Clinical Practice Guidelines for Chronic Kidney Disease in Children and Adolescents published by the National Kidney Foundation's Kidney Disease Outcomes Quality Initiative (NKF-K/DOQI)[4] recommends that untimed "spot" urine samples be used to detect and monitor proteinuria in children and adolescents. It is not usually necessary to obtain timed urine collections. Standard urine dipstick tests can be used to detect increased total urine proteins, and albumin-specific dipstick tests are acceptable in detecting microalbuminuria, which refers to albumin excretion above the normal range but below the level of detection in standard urine dipstick tests. Urine protein-to-creatinine or urine albumin-to-creatinine ratio should be measured within 3 months of a positive dipstick test to confirm proteinuria or albuminuria. Postpubertal children with diabetes of 5 or more years should have urine albumin measured by albumin-specific dipstick or albumin-to-creatinine ratio.[4] A novel dipstick, Multistix PRO, analyzes the concentration of both urinary protein and creatinine semiquantitatively in 60 seconds and correlates well with quantitative urinary protein-to-creatinine ratio.[5]

False-positive dipstick tests for proteinuria can result from prolonged immersion of the reagent strip, alkaline urine, or presence of pyuria, bacteriuria, or mucoprotein.[6]

Twenty-four-hour urine collections have long been the gold standard for quantification of urine protein excretion. However, collection in young children often requires catheterization and is not practical. A review of published studies done between 1970 and 2002 showed that the urine protein-to-creatinine ratio correlates highly with 24-hour urine collection.[7]

Twenty-four-hour urine protein excretion rates of less than 4 $mg/m^2/hr$ and more than 40 $mg/m^2/hr$ are considered in the normal and nephrotic range, respectively. A urinary microalbumin excretion rate of less than 20 μg/min is considered normal. Reference values for urinary protein and albumin excretion are found in Table 2-1.

In 2006, Mori et al.[8] showed that the urine protein-to-creatinine ratio varies according to body size and body composition reflecting muscle mass and suggested that evaluation of urine protein-to-creatinine ratio should also consider body height. Kim et al.[9] proposed urine protein-to-osmolality ratio as an alternative test to 24-hour urinary protein excretion. However, normal urinary protein-to-osmolality ratios have to be defined in normal children.

Standard urine dipstick tests are more sensitive in detecting albumin than in detecting low molecular weight proteins. Screening for low molecular weight proteins can be done with the sulfosalicylic acid test. The addition of acid to the supernatant of a centrifuged urine will cause cloudiness in the presence of any protein in the urine. A negative reagent strip test with a positive sulfosalicylic test is suggestive of low molecular weight proteinuria. Urine protein electrophoresis can confirm the diagnosis. A false-positive sulfosalicylic test can be produced by a large dose of contrast material, penicillin, cephalosporin, sulfonamide metabolites, and high uric acid concentration.[6]

TABLE 2-1 **Reference Values for Urinary Protein and Albumin Excretion**

	Timed Urine Collection for Protein (mg/m²/hr)	Spot Urine Protein/ Creatinine mg/mg (mg/mmol)	Spot Urine Albumin/ Creatinine mg/g (mg/mmol)
Normal Range			
6-24 months	<4	<0.5 (<50)	
>24 months	<4	<0.2 (<20)	<30 (<3)
Nephrotic	>40	>2.0 (>200)	

GFR, Glomerular filtration rate.
Source: Modified from Hogg RJ et al: National Kidney Foundation's Kidney Disease Outcomes Quality Initiative clinical practice guidelines for chronic kidney disease in children and adolescents: evaluation, classification, and stratification. *Pediatrics* 111(6):1416-21, 2003; and Hogg RJ et al.: Evaluation and management of proteinuria and nephrotic syndrome in children: recommendations from a pediatric nephrology panel established at the National Kidney Foundation conference on proteinuria, albuminuria, risk, assessment, detection, and elimination (PARADE). *Pediatrics* 105(6):1242-49, 2005.

TABLE 2-2 **NKF-K/DOQI Classification of the Stages of Chronic Kidney Disease**

Stage	Description	GFR (ml/min/1.73 m²)
1	Kidney damage with normal or increased GFR	>90
2	Kidney damage with mild reduction of GFR	60-89
3	Moderate reduction of GFR	30-59
4	Severe reduction of GFR	15-29
5	Kidney failure	<15

GFR, Glomerular filtration rate.
Source: Modified from Hogg RJ et al: National Kidney Foundation's Kidney Disease Outcomes Quality Initiative clinical practice guidelines for chronic kidney disease in children and adolescents: evaluation, classification, and stratification. *Pediatrics* 111(6):1416-21, 2003.

Glomerular Filtration

Glomerular filtration rate (GFR) is the most commonly used measure of kidney function. The NKF-K/DOQi guidelines for chronic kidney disease (CKD) in children and adolescents recommend establishing the presence of CKD on the basis of the presence of kidney damage and level of GFR (See Table 2-2 for NKF-K/DOQI classification of the stages of CKD.)

GFR can be quantified by measuring the clearance rate of a substance from the plasma. The substance, often referred to as the marker, can be endogenous or exogenous. It must have a stable plasma concentration and should be filtered, not reabsorbed, secreted, synthesized, or metabolized, by the kidney so that the filtered substance x = the excreted substance x.

The renal clearance of the substance x *(Cx)* can be obtained by multiplying the urinary concentration of substance x *(Ux)* times the urinary flow rate in ml/min *(V)* divided by the plasma concentration of substance x *(Px)*.

$$Cx = (Ux \times V) \div Px$$

Inulin

Urinary inulin clearance is considered the gold standard for measuring GFR because inulin has all the properties of an ideal marker. It is freely filtered by the glomerulus, is not secreted or reabsorbed in the tubules, and is not synthetized or metabolized by the kidney.

Urinary Inulin Clearance

Measurement of urinary inulin clearance requires a constant intravenous infusion to maintain a constant level of inulin over 3 to 4 hours. After an equilibration period, timed urinary specimens and plasma are collected every 30 minutes, and urinary and plasma inulin are measured to calculate urinary inulin clearance. The mean clearance of 4 or 5 measurements determines the patient's GFR. Urinary catheterization in young children is often required. To avoid this cumbersome procedure, two methods of plasma inulin clearance have been developed: the continuous infusion method and the single bolus method.

Plasma Inulin Clearance: Continuous Infusion Method

The continuous infusion method is based on the concept that once a marker has reached a steady state in the plasma and the volume of distribution is saturated, the rate of elimination of the marker will equal the rate of infusion (RI).

The clearance of the marker can then be measured[10] as follows:

$$Cx = RIx \div Px$$

Because the equilibration can take more than 12 hours in certain situations, a bolus injection can be given before the infusion to reach the steady state more rapidly.

Plasma Inulin Clearance: Single Bolus Injection Method

After a single bolus injection, 10 to 12 blood samples are collected up to 240 minutes after injection. The inulin concentration measurements are then used to construct a plasma concentration versus time curve (plasma disappearance curve). Plasma clearance of inulin can be calculated by dividing the dose by the area under the plasma concentration/time curve. This method has been shown to give accurate results in adults.[11] Van Rossum et al. developed and validated sampling strategies to minimize the number of blood samples taken, making the process more acceptable for children. They concluded that two (at 90 and 240 minutes) to four (at 10, 30, 90, and 240 minutes) samples allow accurate prediction of inulin clearance in pediatric patients.[12] The single bolus

TABLE 2-3 Normal GFR in Neonates, Children and Adolescents (adapted from references [4] and [14])

Age	Mean GFR ± SD (ml/min/1.73 m²)
29-34 weeks GA 1 week postnatal age	15.3 ± 5.6
29-34 weeks GA 2-8 week postnatal age	28.7 ± 13.8
29-34 weeks GA >8 week postnatal age	51.4
1 week term males and females	41 ± 15
2-8 weeks term males and females	66 ± 25
>8 weeks term males and females	96 ± 22
2-12 years (males and females)	133 ± 27
13-21 years (males)	140 ± 30
13-21 years (females)	126 ± 22

GA, Gestational age; *GFR*, glomerular filtration rate; *SD*, standard deviation. Source: Adapted from Hogg RJ et al: National Kidney Foundation's Kidney Disease Outcomes Quality Initiative clinical practice guidelines for chronic kidney disease in children and adolescents: evaluation, classification, and stratification. *Pediatrics* 111(6):1416-21, 2003; and Schwartz GJ, Brion LP, Spitzer A: The use of plasma creatinine concentration for estimating glomerular filtration rate in infants, children, and adolescents. *Pediatr Clin North Am* 34(3):571-90, 1987.

injection method tends to overestimate GFR (average 9.7 ml/min 1.73 m^2), but the difference between the two methods becomes smaller at lower GFR (<50 ml/min/1.73 m^2).[13]

Measurement of inulin clearance remains the gold standard for assessing GFR, However, most laboratories cannot routinely measure inulin, which makes this test impractical.

Creatinine Clearance

Creatinine clearance (Ccr) measurement has been widely used and correlates well with inulin clearance within the normal range of GFR.[14] Creatinine is an amino acid derivative produced in muscle cells. It is freely filtered, and about 10% of the creatinine found in urine is secreted by the proximal tubules. Tubular secretion varies among and within individuals.[15] As GFR declines, the percentage of secreted creatinine increases; therefore Ccr at low GFR will significantly overestimate true GFR.[16] Normal values for GFR for different age groups are found in Table 2-3.

Ccr can be calculated from a 24-hour urine collection and a blood sample as

$$Ccr = \frac{U_{vol} \times Ucr \times 1.73}{1440 \times Pcr \times BSA} \text{ ml/min/1.73m}^2$$

where U_{vol} = 24-hr urine volume, Ucr = urinary creatinine concentration, Pcr = serum creatinine concentration (plasma and urine creatinine expressed in the same units), and BSA = body surface area in m^2. The constants 1.73 and 1440 indicate the standardized adult body surface area and the number of minutes in a day.

Nuclear GFR

GFR can be accurately measured using a radioactive tracer such as chromium 51 (^{51}Cr) EDTA or technetium 99m (^{99m}Tc) diethylenetriaminepentaacetate (DTPA) in children. The most accurate method is based on the plasma disappearance curve after a single bolus injection, fitted by a double exponential curve. The clearance of the radiotracer is given by the injected dose divided by the area under the curve.[17] The initial "fast" curve represents the diffusion of the radiotracer in its distribution volume, whereas the late, slow, exponential curve represents its renal clearance. The two-compartment model requires serial blood sampling to obtain an accurate plasma disappearance curve. In general, the more blood samples acquired over time, the more accurate the calculated GFR value will be. However, to avoid obtaining too many blood samplings, two simplified methods have been proposed for routine clinical use in children[18]: the slope intercept method and the distribution volume method.

The Slope Intercept Method

The slope intercept method requires two blood samples acquired 2 and 4 hours postinjection and is based on the determination of the late exponential curve. An algorithm must be used to correct for overestimation of the clearance because this method neglects the early exponential curve. Late blood sampling (between 5 and 24 hours) may be needed for patients with renal clearance below 10-15 ml/min/1.73 m^2.

The Distribution Volume Method

The distribution volume method requires only one blood sample at 2 hours postinjection. It appears to be valid for children of any age except those with very poor renal function (GFR <30 ml/min/1.73 m^2).[17]

A major limitation of these methods is the presence of significant edema. In this situation, the disappearance of the tracer will be influenced by its diffusion into an expanded extracellular volume and artifactually elevating the calculated GFR. Infiltration of the radiotracer at the injection site can also cause artifactual elevation of GFR.

The effective dose of radiation is approximately 0.011 mSv/examination regardless of the age of the child for Cr-EDTA and twice as high with low GFR (<10 min/1.73 m^2), and 0.1 mSv/examination for Tc-DTPA.[17] The background equivalent radiation time (BERT) for an effective dose of 0.01 mSv is 1.5 days.

Additional uses of ^{99m}Tc-DTPA are discussed in Chapter 1.

Equations Predicting GFR

The need for simple and rapid determination of GFR in clinical practice led to the development of several equations to estimate GFR. Those most commonly used in pediatrics are the Schwartz formula[19] and the Counahan formula.[20]

In the classical clearance formula, the numerator Ucr × V is the excretion rate of creatinine; in steady state this must equal the rate of production. Since the rate of production is a function of muscle mass, Schwartz tested different parameters of body size to provide the best correlation with GFR measured by Ccr. The body length appeared to have the best correlation.

Schwartz formula:

$$GFR\ (\text{ml/min/1.73 m}^2) = K \times Ht \div Pcr$$

TABLE 2-4 **Mean K Value for Schwartz Formula**

	Cr mg/dl	Cr μmol/L
Low birth weight infants ≤1 year	0.33	29.2
Full term infants ≤1 year	0.45	39.8
Children 2-12 years	0.55	48.6
Females 13-21 years	0.55	48.6
Males 13-21 years	0.70	61.9

Source: Adapted from Schwartz GJ, Brion LP, Spitzer A: The use of plasma creatinine concentration for estimating glomerular filtration rate in infants, children, and adolescents. *Pediatr Clin North Am* 34(3):571-90, 1987.

TABLE 2-5 **Reference Intervals for Cystatin C (modified from reference [94])**

	Reference Intervals
Preterm infants	1.34-2.57
Full-term infants	1.36-2.23
>8 days-1 year	0.75-1.87
>1-3 years	0.68-1.90
>3-16 years	0.51-1.31

Source: Adapted from Harmoinen A et al: Reference intervals for cystatin C in pre- and full-term infants and children. *Pediatr Nephrol* 15(1-2):105-08, 2000.

where K = constant determined by regression analysis provided in Table 2-4 for different ages, Ht = height in cm, and Pcr = plasma creatinine.

Counahan formula:

$$\text{GFR (ml/min/1.73 m}^2) = 38 \times \text{Ht (cm)} \div \text{Pcr } (\mu\text{mol/L})$$

or

$$0.43 \times \text{Ht (cm)} \div \text{Pcr (mg/dl)}$$

In recent years other investigators have attempted to develop predictive equations.

Mattman et al.[21] proposed the British Columbia's Children's Hospital 2 (BCCH2) formula, which provides an estimate of GFR independent of height or weight but requires the local laboratory to derive a constant. Their modeling was developed assuming that "true GFR" was the one measured by DTPA two-point single injection method.

Leger et al.[22] used Cr EDTA as the true GFR and proposed a predictive equation using body weight (BW), height, and Pcr.

$$\text{GFR} = [56.7 \times \text{BW (kg)} + 0.142 \times \text{length}^2 \text{ (cm)}] \div \text{Pcr } (\mu\text{mol/L})$$

In Leger's series, this equation was more precise than the Schwartz formula.

The Schwartz formula remains the most widely accepted and used equation in practice.

Iohexol

Iohexol is a safe, nonionic, low osmolar contrast agent (MW 821 Da). It is eliminated exclusively by the kidneys, where it is filtered but not secreted, metabolized, or reabsorbed. It has less than 2% binding to protein. Therefore it makes an ideal marker of GFR and a good alternative to radiotracers, which are not suitable for some patients and require special handling, storage, and disposal.

Iohexol and iothalamate have similar kinetic profiles, but iohexol has a lower allergic potential.[23]

Clearance of iohexol correlates well with measured inulin clearance.[23,24] Gaspari et al.[23] showed a highly significant correlation between GFR measured by the plasma clearance of iohexol (using a two-compartment open model) and the GFR measured by urinary inulin clearance. A pilot study for children with chronic kidney disease showed that GFR can be measured accurately using a four-point iohexol plasma disappearance curve.[25]

Cystatin C

Cystatin C is a low molecular weight protein (13.36 KD) member of the cystatin superfamily of cysteine protease inhibitors. It is produced by all nucleated cells and exhibits a stable production rate. Cystatin C is freely filtered by the glomerulus and metabolized after tubular reabsorption.[26]

Cystatin C is influenced less by age, gender, and muscle mass than creatinine is.[27] Levels decline from birth to age 1, then remain stable until about 50 years of age. Normal values for cystatin C are given in Table 2-5. Cystatin C has been found by some to be influenced by age, gender, cigarette smoking, high C reactive protein,[28] steroid use,[29] and thyroid disorders.[30]

For the same cystatin C level, transplant recipients have a GFR 19% higher than patients with native kidney disease. The inflammation or immunosuppressive therapy associated with transplant may increase cystatin C production, leading to an underestimation of GFR.[26]

A meta-analysis published in 2002 concluded that cystatin C appears to be a better marker of GFR than Scr.[31] However, controversies remain.

Several cystatin C-based equations have been reported to predict GFR. There is no consensus as to which should be used.

Larsson et al.[32] and Grubb et al.[33] determined GFR by measuring the plasma clearance of iohexol and used the results to calculate an equation to convert cystatin C levels to GFR levels.

Larsson's equation:

$$\text{GFR (ml/min)} = 99.43 \times \text{cystatin C (mg/L)}^{-1.5837}$$

Grubb's equation:

$$\text{GFR (ml/min)} = 89.12 \times \text{cystatin C (mg/L)}^{-1.675}$$

For pediatric patients, Filler[34] determined GFR by ^{99}Tc-DTPA single injection technique and derived an equation to predict GFR based on cystatin C measurement.

Filler's equation:

$$\text{Log (GFR)} = 1.962 + [1.123 \times \log (1/\text{cystatin C})]$$

GFR (ml/min/1.73 m^2)
Cystatin C (mg/L)

One pediatric study[35] showed that for children with CKD stages 3-5, the intrapatient coefficient of variation of cystatin C was significantly lower than that of Scr and proposed that cystatin C is a better tool for longitudinally monitoring patients with advanced CKD.

ASSESSMENT OF TUBULAR FUNCTION

Fluid filtered by the glomerulus (plasma ultrafiltrate) enters the proximal tubule where 60% to 65% of the filtrate will be reabsorbed.[3] In disorders of the proximal tubule, excessive amounts of the solutes will be found in the urine. The fractional excretion of sodium and tubular reabsorption of phosphate can be used to assess the integrity of the proximal tubules. Detection of glucosuria and aminoaciduria can also be indicative of proximal tubular disorder in certain situations.

FRACTIONAL EXCRETION OF SODIUM

Fractional excretion of sodium (FeNa) is one of the most commonly used tests for tubular integrity. There is no "normal" for fractional excretion of sodium. It must be interpreted in the context of each patient's sodium and volume status.

In the face of extracellular volume contraction, the appropriate response will be conservation of sodium and water. Therefore the fractional excretion of sodium will be low, usually with a FeNa of less than 1% in children and less than 2.5% in neonates. The urinary sodium concentration will be less than 20 mEq/L in children and less than 30 mEq/L in neonates. If tubular damage such as in acute tubular necrosis has occurred, the fractional excretion of sodium will be inappropriately elevated. FeNa will be more than 2% in children and more than 2.5% in neonates. Urinary sodium will generally be more than 30 mEq/L.

FeNa can be calculated as follows:

$$\text{FeNa} = \frac{U_{Na} \times Pcr}{P_{Na} \times Ucr} \times 100$$

where U_{Na} = urinary concentration of sodium, Pcr = plasma creatinine, P_{Na} = plasma sodium, and Ucr = urinary creatinine.

Tubular Reabsorption of Phosphate

Usually 85% to 95% of phosphate is reabsorbed in the proximal tubule.[3] Phosphate transport is primarily regulated by the plasma phosphate concentration and parathyroid hormone, which alter the $Na^{\pm}$ phosphate carrier activity.

Tubular reabsorption of phosphate (TRP) percentage can be calculated as follows:

$$\text{TRP\%} = 1 - \left(\frac{U_{PO_4} \times Pcr}{P_{PO_4} \times Ucr} \right) \times 100$$

where U_{PO_4} = urinary concentration of phosphate, Pcr = plasma creatinine, P_{PO_4} = plasma concentration of phosphate, and Ucr = urinary concentration of creatinine.

TRP percentage varies with age. It remains high until age 15 in girls and age 14 in boys; thereafter it decreases steadily to adult levels. Reference ranges for children between ages 6 and 18 were published by Kruse.[36] In clinical practice, a value greater than 85% is usually considered normal. Low TRP percentage can be found with high parathyroid hormone (PTH) states or proximal tubular disorders.

The renal tubular maximum reabsorption rate of phosphate to glomerular filtration rate (TmP/GFR) using phosphate infusion was initially described by Bijvoet.[37] Phosphate infusion was originally used for diagnosing hypercalcemia, parathyroid disorders, and renal handling of phosphate. Although it is no longer used for evaluating hypercalcemia, it can still help in evaluating hypophosphatemia. Normograms and algorithms were derived from the initial infusion data and can be used more easily.[38]

Glucosuria

Filtered glucose is usually almost completely reabsorbed in the three segments of the proximal tubule. Glucose is transported across the apical membrane by secondary active transport depending on the sodium electrochemical gradient generated by the Na-K ATPase. Two sodium-glucose transporters are found in the proximal tubule. The SGLT2 in the early proximal tubule has a high capacity and low affinity for glucose, and the SGLT1 found in segments 2 and 3 have high affinity and low capacity.

The plasma glucose at which glucose reabsorption is maximal is called the threshold for glucose, and the transport capacity when the threshold is reached is called the maximal tubular glucose reabsorption (TmG).

In the presence of glucosuria, it is important to determine the serum glucose concentration. The normal threshold for glucose is 180-200 mg/dl (10-11 mmol/L). Isolated glucosuria with an elevated serum glucose suggests diabetes.

The presence of isolated glucosuria with a normal serum glucose concentration usually results from familial renal glucosuria. Mutations of the SGLT2 coding gene in this disorder were first described by Santer et al.[39]

Transtubular Potassium Gradient

Potassium is secreted in the late distal and cortical collecting tubules.

The transtubular potassium gradient (TTKG) is an indirect index of the activity of the potassium secretory process in the cortical distal nephron and reflects the action of aldosterone. It is an important component in the evaluation of hyperkalemia and hypokalemia.

It can be calculated using the formula proposed by West[40]:

$$\text{TTKG} = \frac{UK \div Uosm/Posm}{PK} \text{ or } \frac{UK \times Posm}{PK \times Uosm}$$

where UK = urinary potassium concentration, Uosm = urinary osmolality, Posm = plasma osmolality, and PK = plasma potassium.

The urinary sodium concentration should be greater than 25 mmol/L to ensure that insufficient sodium delivery is not limiting potassium secretion.

The luminal potassium of the terminal cortical collecting duct is estimated by dividing the urinary potassium by the urine/plasma osmolality since the luminal K concentration is influenced by water removal in the medullary segments. The serum potassium is an estimate of the peritubular potassium concentration.

TTKG appears to be a good indicator of aldosterone activity in normal children and in children with hypoaldosteronism and pseudohypoaldosteronism.[41] The expected value of TTKG is less than 2.5 during hypokalemia and greater than 7 during hyperkalemia.

Aminoaciduria

In the normal state, most amino acids are reabsorbed in the proximal tubule. Sodium-dependent cotransporters are responsible for transporting glycine and glutamine, whereas sodium-independent carriers are responsible for transporting neutral amino acids (leucine, isoleucine, and phenylalanine) and cystine and dibasic amino acids (ornithine, arginine, and lysine). A mutation in the gene *SCL3A1*, which encodes a protein responsible for transporting cystine and the dibasic amino acids, is the cause of the classical form of cystinuria (type I/I).

The cyanide-nitroprusside test is an easy way to detect urinary amino acids, which contain a free sulfhydryl group or disulfide bond such as cystine, cysteine, homocystine, and homocysteine, and should be performed in the evaluation of nephrolithiasis.[1] Generalized aminoaciduria is usually associated with Fanconi syndrome.

URINE ANION GAP

The urine anion gap is an indirect measurement of ammonium production by the distal nephron. Because ammonium is not routinely measured in most laboratories, clinicians needed an index of ammonium secretion to use in the evaluation of normal anion gap metabolic acidosis. This was initially proposed by Goldstein et al.[42] and its clinical usefulness was also shown later by Batlle et al.[43]

If ammonium is present, the sum of sodium and potassium will be less than the chloride since ammonium is an unmeasured cation. This test presupposed that the chloride is the predominant anion in the urine balancing the positive charge in urine NH_4^+.

Therefore the urine anion gap can be calculated by the equation

$$\text{Urine anion gap} = (\text{Na} + \text{K}) - \text{Cl}$$

The urine anion gap cannot be used in volume depletion with urine sodium concentration of less than 25 mmol/L or when there is increased excretion of unmeasured anions such as ketoacids or hippurate.

Urine Osmolar Gap

When the urine anion gap is positive, one cannot conclude on the presence or absence of NH_4^+ in the urine, because NH_4^+ may be excreted with an anion other than chloride. The urine ammonium concentration can be estimated by calculating the urine osmolar gap. This concept was initially developed by Halperin et al.[44] Calculating the urine osmolar gap requires measuring the urine osmolality and estimating the calculated urine osmolality.

$$\text{Calculated urine osmolality} = 2\ (\text{Na} + \text{K}) + \text{urea} + \text{glucose}$$

where Na, K, urea, and glucose are expressed in mmol/L or

$$\text{Calculated urine osmolality} = 2\ (\text{Na} + \text{K}) + (\text{glucose} \div 18) + (\text{urea} \div 2.8)$$

where Na, K are expressed in mmol/L and glucose and urea in mg/dl.

The gap between the measured and calculated urine osmolality should largely represent ammonium salts. Clinical cases are reviewed in Chapter 31.

Urine-Blood $P\text{CO}_2$

Urine-blood $P\text{CO}_2$ (U-B $P\text{CO}_2$) can be used for evaluating normal anion gap metabolic acidosis with a positive urine anion gap to differentiate between deficient ammonium production versus impaired hydrogen secretion.[45,46] The $P\text{CO}_2$ should be measured in alkaline urine. With adequate hydrogen secretion in the distal tubule, the hydrogen will couple with HCO_3 to form H_2CO_3 and then dissociate into CO_2 and H_2O.

Kim et al.[47] recently evaluated the diagnostic value of the urine-blood $P\text{CO}_2$ in patients diagnosed as having H^+-ATPase defect dRTA based on reduced urinary NH_4^+ and absolute decrease in H^+-ATPase immunostaining in intercalated cells. U-B $P\text{CO}_2$ during sodium bicarbonate loading was less than 30 mmHg in all patients with H^+-ATPase defect dRTA. Therefore a U-B $P\text{CO}_2$ of 30 mmHg or more in a patient with metabolic acidosis suggests that this is not a problem related to H^+ secretion.

General Biochemistry

Plasma Sodium

The reference range for plasma sodium varies with the patient's age and the method of measurement used. Most of the reference ranges published are derived from values of hospitalized children. However, because details of the underlying disease have not always been provided,[48,49] the ranges are of uncertain clinical value. Conventional clinical practice suggests that the normal range for plasma sodium is between 135 and 145.

Hyponatremia is the result of excess free water or sodium loss. The former is usually associated with expanded extracellular fluid, whereas the latter is often seen with volume contraction. Hyponatremia with normal plasma osmolality is usually the result of hyperlipidemia, hyperproteinemia, or hyperglycemia unless measured with an ion-specific electrode. Most laboratories now measure plasma sodium with ion-specific electrodes, and the measurement will not be affected by hyperlipidemia or hyperproteinemia. In the presence of hyperglycemia, every 3.4 mmol/L (62 mg/dl) increment in glucose will reduce plasma sodium by 1 mmol/L (mEq/L) because of water shifting from the intracellular space to the extracellular space.

Hypernatremia is usually secondary to water deficit either because of poor intake or increased water loss such as in diabetes insipidus or diabetes mellitus. Salt intoxication is a less common cause of hypernatremia.

Plasma Potassium

Potassium is an intracellular cation with 98% of body potassium located intracellularly.

Cell potassium concentration is around 140 mmol/L, whereas the normal range for plasma potassium varies between 3.2 and 6.2 mmol/L depending on age. Reference ranges vary with the method used and age of the child. In infants, the upper limit of normal can be as high as 6.2. The upper limit then progressively comes down to about 5.0 to reach the "adult" level.[49]

Hyperkalemia can be the result of intracellular to extracellular shift in the presence of acidosis, beta-blocker use, cellular breakdown, decreased excretion in renal failure, hypoaldosteronism or pseudohypoaldosteronism, and less commonly, increased potassium intake.

Hypokalemia is mostly seen in renal tubular disorders such as Fanconi syndrome, Bartter syndrome, and Gitelman syndrome and in hyperaldosteronism.

Plasma Creatinine

Pcr is often used to assess the level of renal function. During the early neonatal period, Pcr reflects the maternal creatinine. It then decreases to 0.4 mg/dl (35 μmol/L) by the middle of the second postnatal week in full-term infants.[14] After this initial decline, Pcr remains relatively stable for the first 2 years, reflecting proportional increases in GFR and muscle mass. Pcr then increases progressively to attain levels of about 0.9 ± 0.2 mg/dl (79 ± 18 μmol/L) in males and 0.7 ± 0.2 mg/dl (62 ± 18 μmol/L) in females.[14]

Total Carbon Dioxide and Bicarbonate (HCO_3^-)

Total CO_2 content of blood, plasma, or serum is composed of bicarbonate, dissolved CO_2 and carbonic acid (H_2CO_3). Since the sum of dissolved CO_2 and H_2CO_3 contributes little to the total CO_2 content (TCO_2), TCO_2 is a close approximation of bicarbonate concentration, which makes up to 96% to 99% of the total CO_2 content.[50]

HCO_3^- results obtained from blood gas analyzer are a calculated parameter. First, pH and PCO_2 are measured, and then HCO_3 is calculated using the Henderson-Hasselbalch equation

$$pH = pKa + \log[(HCO_3^-) \div (0.03 \times PCO_2)]$$

pKa is usually equal to 6.1

Discrepant values from calculated arterial bicarbonate and measured venous total CO_2 can be seen especially in acutely ill pediatric patients who are prone to large fluctuations in pK1.[51]

The reference range for total CO_2 varies between 17 and 31 mEq/L depending on age.

Total CO_2 and bicarbonate are reduced in the presence of acidosis. K/DOQI clinical practice guidelines for bone metabolism and disease in children with CKD[52] recommends that the serum level of total CO_2 be measured. Serum levels of total CO_2 should be maintained at or above 22 mmol/L in children over age 2 and at 20 mmol/L or above in neonates and infants.

Serum Calcium, Phosphorus, and Calcium-Phosphorus Product

Evaluation of serum calcium, phosphorus, and calcium-phosphorus product is reviewed in detail in the recent guidelines published by K/DOQI.[52] Representative normal values for serum phosphorus, ionized calcium, and total calcium can be found in Table 2-6.

In CKD, serum levels of phosphorus should be maintained at or above the age-appropriate lower limits and no higher than the age-appropriate upper limits. For children with CKD stage 5, the serum level of phosphorus should be maintained between 3.5 and 5.5 mg/dl (1.13-1.78 mmol/L) during adolescence and at 4 to 6 mg/dl (1.29-1.94 mmol/L) between ages 1 and 12.

Calcium in blood exists in three fractions: protein-bound calcium, free (ionized) calcium, and calcium complexes.

Total measured calcium should be corrected if serum albumin is abnormal to reflect the ionized calcium. The following formulas can be used:

$$\text{Corrected calcium (mg/dl)} = \text{total calcium (mg/dl)} + 0.8 \times [4 - \text{serum albumin (g/dl)}]$$

$$\text{Corrected calcium (mmol/L)} = [\text{total calcium (mmol/L)} - (\text{albumin (g/L)} \div 40)] + 1$$

Ionized calcium is affected by pH since hydrogen ion displaces calcium from albumin. A fall of 0.1 unit in pH will cause approximately a 0.1 mEq/L rise in the concentration of ionized calcium.

Because serum-ionized calcium is not routinely measured in most places, K/DOQI guidelines are based on corrected

TABLE 2-6 **Normal Values for Serum Phosphorus, Blood Ionized Calcium Concentrations**

Age	SERUM PHOSPHORUS mg/dl	SERUM PHOSPHORUS mmol/L*	Blood-Ionized Calcium (mmol/L)	TOTAL CALCIUM mg/dl	TOTAL CALCIUM mmol/L†
0-3 months	4.8-7.4	1.55-2.39	1.22-1.40	8.8-11.3	2.20-2.83
1-5 years	4.5-6.5	1.45-2.10	1.22-1.32	9.4-10.8	2.35-2.70
6-12 years	3.6-5.8	1.16-1.87	1.15-1.32	9.4-10.3	2.35-2.57
13-20 years	2.3-4.5	0.74-1.45	1.12-1.30	8.8-10.2	2.20-2.55

* Serum phosphorus converted from mg/dl to mmol/L using a factor of 0.3229.
† Serum calcium converted from mg/dl to mmol/L using a factor of 0.250.
Source: Adapted from K/DOQI clinical practice guidelines for bone metabolism and disease in children with chronic kidney disease. *Am J Kidney Dis* 46(4), 2005.

total calcium. Levels should be maintained within normal range for the laboratory used and preferably toward the lower end in CKD stage 5.

The serum calcium–phosphorus product should be maintained at less than 55 mg^2/dl^2 (<4.4 $mmol^2/L^2$) in adolescents over age 12 and at less than 65 mg^2/dl^2 (<5.2 $mmol^2/L^2$) in younger children.

Urinary Calcium

Measurement of calcium excretion should be part of the evaluation of patients with hematuria, nephrocalcinosis, and renal stones, and can often be useful when assessing children with frequency, dysuria, urgency, and recurrent urinary tract infections.[53] Urinary calcium excretion varies with age, being highest during infancy and reaching its nadir during puberty.

Hypercalciuria is usually defined as a urinary calcium excretion of more than 4 mg/kg/day (0.1 mmol/kg/day), based on a study by Ghazali and Barratt.[54] However, several authors have studied urinary calcium excretion and published slightly different reference ranges in their study population.[55-59]

Spot urinary calcium-to-creatinine ratios (usually collected from second-morning-fasting urine specimens) correlate well with 24-hour calcium excretion, especially for children with normal muscle mass. They can be used for clinical purposes, although they may be affected by factors such as recent dietary calcium intake.[60] Sodium, protein, phosphorus, potassium, and glucose intake can also affect calcium excretion. Published reference ranges for urinary calcium-to-creatinine ratios vary in different geographic locations (Table 2-7). More details on these values can be found in Chapter 33.

For children with reduced muscle mass, it has been reported that a urinary calcium-to-osmolality ratio greater than 0.25 (mg/L)/(mOsm/kgH_2O) predicts hypercalciuria with better sensitivity and specificity than does urine calcium-to-creatinine ratio.[61,62]

Unlike with adults, there is no apparent seasonal variation of urinary calcium-to-creatinine ratio in children.[63]

TABLE 2-7 **Normal Values for the Random UCa/Cr Ratio (mg/mg) in Children in Different Geographic Locations reproduced from [58]**

Age	*n*	95th Percentile	Country	Ref.
<7 months	103	0.86	New Hampshire, USA	9
8-18 months	40	0.60		
19 months-6 years	41	0.42		
Adults	31	0.22		
1 month-1 year	79	0.81	Switzerland	10
1-2 years	48	0.56		
2-3 years	41	0.50		
3-5 years	54	0.41		
5-7 years	40	0.30		
7-10 years	50	0.25		
10-14 years	51	0.24		
14-17 years	47	0.24		
2-6 years	32	0.63*	Sweden	11
7-10 years	79	0.42*		
11-18 years	42	0.35*		
6-17.9 years	564	0.22	Germany	12
6-13 years	220	0.26	Argentina	13
8-15 years	208	0.15	Northern India	14
7-10 years	345	0.14	Taiwan	15
11-14 years	340	0.10		
15-18 years	387	0.21		
11-15 years (girls)†	46	0.21	Maryland, USA	16
11-15 years (boys)†	51	0.18		

* 97th percentile.
† African American.
Source: So NP et al: Normal urinary calcium/creatinine ratios in African-American and Caucasian children. *Pediatr Nephrol* 16(2):133-39, 2001.

Urinary Sodium Excretion and Hypercalciuria

Measurement of urinary sodium excretion plays a valuable part in evaluating children with hypercalciuria. Polito et al. found that urinary sodium excretion and 24-hour urinary sodium/potassium (U Na/K) excretion was higher in children with hypercalciuria.[64] Urinary sodium excretion was 4 ± 2.4 mmol/kg/day in hypercalciuric children compared with 2.7 mmol/kg/day in ex-hypercalciuric children. Fasting U Na/K was 3 ± 1.6 versus 2.1 ± 1 mmol/mmol and 24-hour U Na/K 4.2 ± 3.9 versus 2.8 ± 1.5 mmol/mmol in hypercalciuric versus ex-hypercalciuric children.

Reduction of sodium and increased potassium intake can affect the degree of calciuria. Therefore measurement of urinary potassium and sodium excretion can guide therapeutic interventions.

Urinary Magnesium

Magnesium is a known stone inhibitor, because it forms complexes with oxalate and reduces supersaturation. Thirty-nine percent of children with calcium-oxalate stones in one series had hypomagnesuria defined as magnesium excretion of less than 1.2 mg/kg/24 hr.[65] As for urinary calcium, magnesium/creatinine ratios can be used. Urinary reference limits can be found in Table 2-8.

Urinary Citrate Excretion

Citrate inhibits calcium-oxalate and calcium-phosphate crystal nucleation, growth, and aggregation. In normal circumstances, citrate is freely filtered at the glomerulus with a 65%-to-90% reabsorption rate. Systemic acidosis, potassium depletion, starvation, and acetazolamide therapy are each known to decrease urinary citrate. In one study, hypocitraturia defined as citrate excretion less than 320 mg/1.73 m^2/24 hr (<1.7 mmol/1.73 m^2/24 hr) was observed in 60.6% of children with calcium-oxalate stones.[65] However, as detailed in Chapter 33, for clinical purposes urinary citrate excretion should usually exceed 150 mg/1.73 m^2/24 hr (0.8 mmol/1.73 m^2/24 hr).

Hypocitraturia is a major risk factor for nephrocalcinosis in very low birth weight infants[66] and after kidney transplantation.[67]

TABLE 2-8 **Urinary Reference Limits for Magnesium/Creatinine**

	Urinary Mg/Cr mol/mol (mg/mg)	
Age (years)	***5th percentile***	***95th percentile***
1 mo–1 yr	0.4 (0.10)	2.2 (0.48)
1-2	0.4 (0.09)	1.7 (0.37)
2-3	0.3 (0.07)	1.6 (0.34)
3-5	0.3 (0.07)	1.3 (0.29)
5-7	0.3 (0.06)	1.0 (0.21)
7-10	0.3 (0.05)	0.9 (0.18)
10-14	0.2 (0.05)	0.7 (0.15)
14-17	0.2 (0.05)	0.6 (0.13)

Source: Adapted from Matos V et al: Urinary phosphate/creatinine, calcium/creatinine, and magnesium/creatinine ratios in a healthy pediatric population. *J Pediatr* 131(2):252-57, 1997.

Urinary Oxalate

Urinary oxalate excretion is significantly increased in primary hyperoxaluria type I (PHI) and type II (PH2) and in secondary hyperoxaluria. In the primary forms, there is excessive endogenous production of oxalate caused by a deficiency of hepatic alanine:glyoxylate aminotransferase (AGT), which catalyzes the peroxisomal conversion of glyoxylate to glycine in PHI and deficiency of cytosolic glyoxylate reductase (GR), an enzyme that catalyzes the reduction of glyoxylate and hydroxypyruvate as well as the dehydrogenation of glycerate in PH2.[68] The secondary forms may result from increased intestinal absorption of oxalate secondary to malabsorptive states or impaired vitamin status.

Reference values for urinary oxalate/creatinine can be found in Chapter 33.

Patients suspected of having abnormalities in oxalate metabolism should have more extensive studies including measurement of urinary oxalate, glycolate, and l-glycerate, and in some cases liver biopsy, to assess the activity of AGT and GR enzyme. Further information concerning genetic diagnosis of primary hyperoxaluria is included in Chapter 33.

Elevated urinary oxalate and glycolate are associated with PHI; however, normal glycolate is found in 25% of subjects with PHI. Elevated urinary oxalate and l-glycerate are typically found in PH2, although l-glycerate is not always detected.[68]

Urinary Uric Acid

Increased urinary uric acid excretion can present with microscopic hematuria, abdominal and/or flank pain, dysuria, gravel, and macroscopic hematuria. About half of patients with hyperuricosuria (HU) will have microlithiasis on ultrasonography.[69] HU is usually defined by urine uric acid concentration corrected for Ccr higher than 0.53 mg/dl of GFR (0.03 mmol/L GFR).[70]

It can be calculated using the formula

$$\frac{\text{Urate excreted}}{\text{GFR}} = \frac{U_{UA} \times \text{Pcr}}{\text{Ucr}}$$

where U_{UA} = urine uric acid concentration, Pcr = plasma creatinine concentration, and Ucr = urine creatinine concentration.

The excretion varies with age, being highest in infants. Reference values for urinary urate excretion can be found in Chapter 33.

Renin-Angiotensin System

Renin is a proteolytic enzyme predominantly formed and stored in the juxtaglomerular cells of the kidney. Renal hypoperfusion and increased sympathetic activity are the major physiologic stimuli to renin secretion.[3] When released in the circulation, renin cleaves angiotensinogen to produce a decapeptide, angiotensin I. Angiotensin I is then converted to an octapeptide, angiotensin II, by the angiotensin I–converting enzyme. Angiotensin II is a potent vasoconstrictor and promotes salt and water retention. The converting enzyme is located primarily in the lung, but angiotensin II can be synthesized at a variety of sites, including the kidney, luminal membrane of vascular endothelial cells, adrenal gland, and brain. Angiotensin II promotes renal salt and water reabsorp-

TABLE 2-9 Assessment of the Renin-Angiotensin-Aldosterone System

	PRA	PAC	PAC/PRA	BP	Potassium
Primary hyperaldosteronism	Decreased	Increased	Very High (>20-50)	High	Low
GRA	Decreased	Increased	High	High	N or low
Renin-secreting tumor	Increased	Increased		High	Low
Bartter syndrome	Increased	Increased		Normal	Low
Renovascular disease	Increased	Increased	<10	High	N or low
Apparent mineralocorticoid excess, Cushing, licorice ingestion	Low	Low		High	Low

BP, Blood pressure; *GRA,* glucocorticoid remediable hypertension; *N,* normal; *PRA,* plasma renin activity; *PAC,* plasma aldosterone concentration.

TABLE 2-10 Geometric Mean and Observed Range of Plasma Renin Activity and Plasma Aldosterone Concentration in Supine Controls

Age (Years)	No. of Subjects	Mean Sodium Excretion (mmol/kg^{-1}/day)	SUPINE PLASMA RENIN ACTIVITY (NG AI L^{-1} H^{-1}) Mean	Observed Range	SUPINE PLASMA ALDOSTERONE CONCENTRATION (PMOL/L) Mean	Observed Range
<1	18	1.2	1459	472-3130	788	164-2929
1-4	18	3.8	757	110-2610	294	69-946
5-9	24	2.5	417	131-834	147	28-616
10-15	19	2.5	321	55-899	211	72-577
Adult	9	2.1	85	22-311	230	39-422

Conversion: SI to traditional units—Aldosterone: 1 pmol/L ≈ 0.036 ng/100 ml.
Source: Dillon MJ, Ryness JM: Plasma renin activity and aldosterone concentration in children. *Br Med J* 4(5992):316-19, 1975.

tion by stimulation of sodium reabsorption in the early proximal tubule and indirectly by activating aldosterone biosynthesis in the zona glomerulosa of the adrenal cortex.

Measurement of plasma renin activity may not reflect the tissue activity of the local renin-angiotensin system.

Assessment of the renin-angiotensin-aldosterone system may be required in the evaluation of hypokalemia/hyperkalemia, adrenal insufficiency, and hypertension (Table 2-9).

Renin

Renin release is dependent on renal tubular sodium concentration, renal perfusion pressure, and beta-adrenergic vascular tone. The enzymatic activity of renin can be measured and is expressed as the amount of angiotensin I generated per unit of time.

"Normal" values for plasma renin activity (PRA) highly depend on sodium intake, time of day, posture and age, and method used. PRA varies inversely with age in infants and children. Reference values derived from PRA measurement in 79 children ages 1 month to 15 years and in the supine position were published in 1975[71] and can be found in Table 2-10.

Renal vein renin sampling may be used to predict feasibility of correcting the hypertension or to identify which kidney contributes to the hypertension. When the ratio of renal vein renin from the diseased kidney (R) to renal vein renin from the normal or less-diseased contralateral kidney (RC) is above 1.5 (R/RC >1.5), there is a great probability that blood pressure will be improved after surgery.[72] However, this test should usually be interpreted in conjunction with renal angiography and not be used on its own to determine therapy because of its poor specificity.[73]

Aldosterone

Aldosterone is synthesized in the zona glomerulosa of the adrenal gland. It regulates electrolyte excretion and intravascular volume mainly through its effects on the distal tubules and cortical collecting ducts of the kidneys in which it acts to increase sodium reabsorption and potassium excretion.[74]

Aldosterone is measured by radioimmunoassay. As is the case with renin levels, it depends on sodium intake, posture, and time of the day. Serum aldosterone concentration will be highest at awakening and lowest shortly after sleep. Reference ranges for plasma aldosterone concentration can be found in Table 2-10.

Hyperaldosteronism should be sought in children with hypertension, hypokalemia, and metabolic alkalosis.[75]

Plasma Aldosterone Concentration to Plasma Renin Activity Ratio

The ratio of Plasma Aldosterone Concentration (PAC) to Plasma Renin Activity (PRA) is used as a screening tool for diagnosis of hyperaldosteronism. Both random PAC and PRA should be measured in the morning, preferably at 8 o'clock.

Patients should have stopped using aldosterone receptor antagonists, ACE inhibitors, and angiotensin receptor blockers for 3 to 6 weeks. The mean normal value is 4-10 compared with more than 30-50 in adult patients with primary hyperaldosteronism.[76]

Complement

The complement system consists of at least 30 plasma membrane proteins that provide an innate defense against microbes and an adjunct to humoral immunity.[77,78] The complement system is divided into three major pathways: classical, lectin, and alternative. The classical pathway is activated by the binding of C1q to the Fc portion of antibody. The lectin pathway is activated by the binding of lectin, which has a structure similar to C1q, to a sugar residue on the surface of a pathogen. The alternative pathway, which is an amplification loop for C3 activation, is activated by polysaccharide antigens, aggregated IgA, injured cells, or endotoxins. Plasma factors H and I are important complement regulators of the alternative pathway.

Each of these pathways of complement activation leads to the deposition of an activated C3 fragment (C3b), inducing the final steps of the complement cascade that includes opsonization, phagocytosis, induction of inflammation, and formation of the membrane attack complex (MAC) and cytolysis.[77-79]

A fourth pathway by which thrombin can directly activate C5 and thus the terminal complement cascade was recently identified.[80] However, the significance of this pathway in the pathogenesis of disease remains unclear.

Evaluation of the complement system will help in the diagnosis of glomerulonephritis. Concentration of the C3 and C4 proteins can be measured by immunological methods. CH50 is a functional assay of the classical pathway. All nine components (C1 through C9) are required to have a normal CH50, which assesses the ability of the patient's serum to lyse sheep erythrocyte optimally sensitized with rabbit antibody.

Glomerular disease associated with activation of the classical pathway will typically have a low C4 and C3, whereas disease associated with activation of the alternative pathway will have a low C3 and normal C4 (Table 2-11).

The CH50 is useful in diagnosing hypocomplementemic states (for example, congenital C2 deficiency) that would be missed if only C3 and C4 were done.

The normal range for serum C3 varies considerably from laboratory to laboratory[81]; therefore no normal values are provided in this chapter.

Serial assessment of complements can also be helpful in monitoring disease activity in immune complex mediated diseases such as lupus. Change in C3 is sensitive to change in disease activity.[81] C4 is less likely to change because one or more C4 null genes are common in systemic lupus erythematosus (SLE); therefore patients in remission can continue to have low C4.

Mutations of the complement regulatory protein factor H and factor I have been linked to atypical HUS and membranoproliferative disease and will be discussed in their individual chapters.

Antineutrophil Cytoplasmic Antibodies

Antineutrophil cytoplasmic antibodies (ANCA) are IgG autoantibodies directed against constituents of primary granules of neutrophils and monocytes lysosomes. They were first described in 1982 in patients with pauci-immune glomerulonephritis.[82] Indirect immunofluorescence (IIF) and enzyme-linked immunosorbent assay (ELISA) are the techniques most widely used to detect ANCA. With IIF, two major immunostaining patterns can be seen: the granular cytoplasmic pattern with central accentuation, known as C-ANCA, and the perinuclear pattern, which is defined as perinuclear fluorescence with nuclear extension and known as P-ANCA. Diffuse, flat cytoplasmic staining without interlobular accentuation can also be seen and is known as a C-ANCA (atypical). Atypical ANCA includes all other neutrophil-specific or monocyte-specific IIF reactivity, most commonly a combination of cytoplasmic and perinuclear fluorescence. Proteinase 3 and myeloperoxidase are two antigenic targets known to be associated with vasculitis. The cytoplasmic pattern usually suggests the presence of serum proteinase 3 ANCA (PR3-ANCA), whereas perinuclear pattern with nuclear extension will usually be associated with myeloperoxidase ANCA (MPO-ANCA).

ELISA is used to identify the presence of myeloperoxidase and proteinase 3 ANCA.[83]

Antibodies to a number of azurophilic granule proteins (lactoferrin, elastase, cathepsin G, bactericidal permeability inhibitor, catalase, lysozyme, and more) can cause a P-ANCA staining pattern. The ELISA will determine the specific antibody responsible.

ANCA measurement should be taken only for patients suspected of having vasculitis. Clinical indications for ANCA testing can be found in the International Consensus Statement on Testing and Reporting of Antineutrophil Cytoplasmic Antibodies.[83] Compliance with guidelines for ANCA testing would decrease the number of false-positives, which could lead to misdiagnosis and potentially harmful treatments.[84]

Wegener's granulomatosis, microscopic polyangiitis, Churg-Strauss syndrome, renal-limited vasculitis, and drug-induced ANCA-associated vasculitis are associated with positive ANCA. Figure 2-1 shows the value of ANCA in the diagnosis of vasculitis.[85]

TABLE 2-11 **Complement Activity for the Differential Diagnosis of Glomerulonephritis**

	C3	C4	CH50	Associated Disease
Activation of classical pathway	Low	Low	Low	SLE, MPGN type I, cryoglobulinemia, chronic infections
Activation of alternative pathway	Low	Normal		MPGN type II, postinfectious GN
Activation of lectin pathway	Normal	Normal		IgA

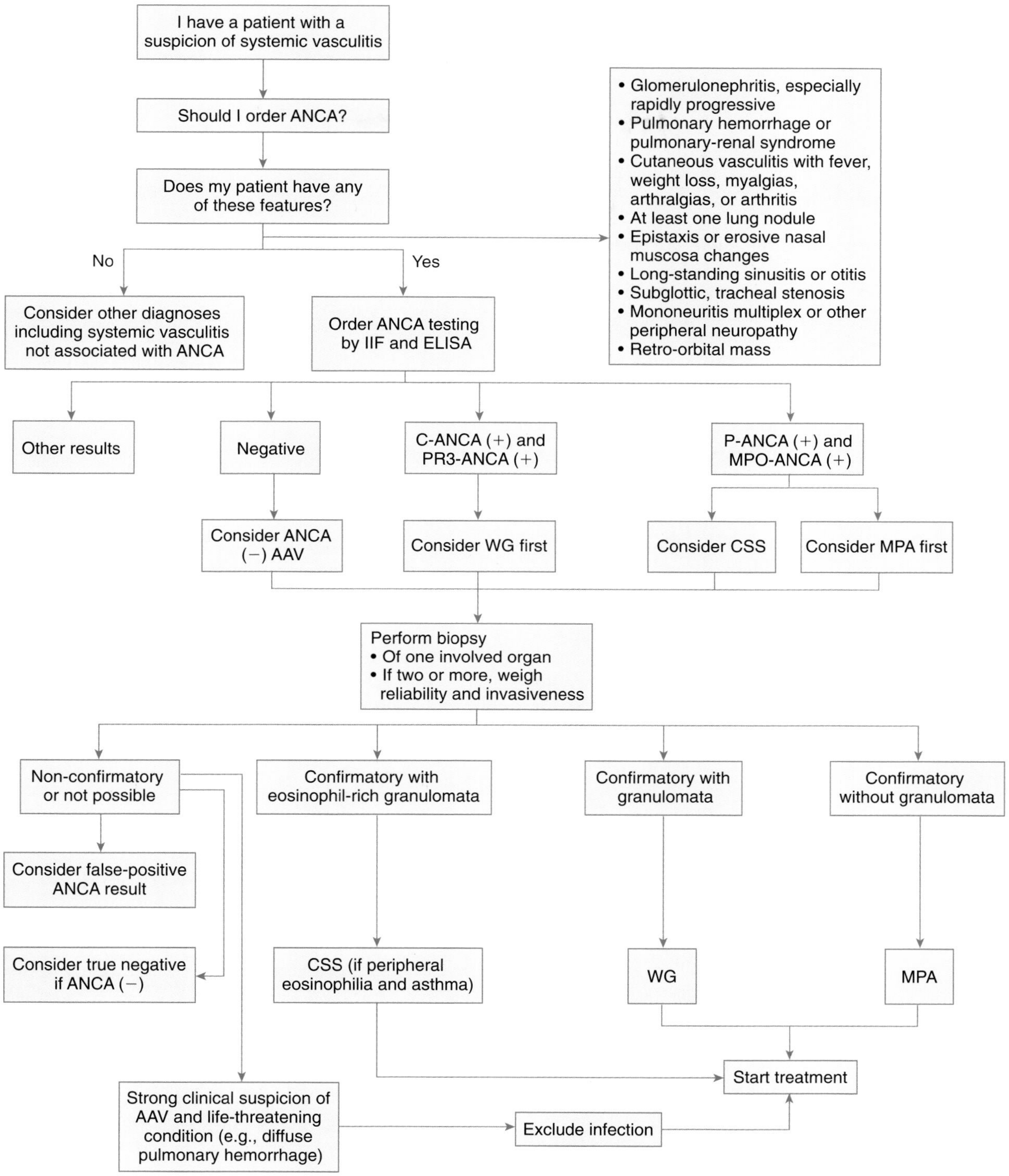

Figure 2-1 Value of ANCA in the clinical approach to ANCA-associated vasculitides. *AAV,* ANCA-associated vasculitides; *CSS,* Churg-Strauss syndrome; *ENT,* ear, nose, and throat; *IIF,* indirect immunofluorescence; *MPA,* microscopic polyangiitis; *WG,* Wegener's granulomatosis. (Reproduced from Bosch X, Guilabert A, Font J: Antineutrophil cytoplasmic antibodies, *Lancet* 368(9533):404-18, 2006.)

A recent systematic review on the value of serial ANCA determination for monitoring patients was inconclusive.[86] Although it is not generally recommended that a patient in clinical remission whose titers are elevated be treated prophylactically, such a patient should be followed closely.[85]

ANCA can also be positive in nonvasculitic diseases such as antiglomerular basement membrane disease and inflammatory bowel disease and in autoimmune disorders.

Antinuclear Antibodies and Anti–Double-Stranded DNA (Anti-dsDNA)

Antinuclear antibodies (ANAs) are autoantibodies directed against chromatin and its individual components, including double-stranded DNA and histones and some ribonucleoproteins.[87] Although ANAs are frequently found in children without a rheumatic disease,[88] they have been associated with several systemic autoimmune diseases, including SLE, scleroderma, mixed connective tissue disease, polymyositis/dermatomyositis, rheumatoid arthritis, Sjögren syndrome, drug-induced lupus, discoid lupus, and pauciarticular juvenile chronic arthritis. They are also occasionally seen in autoimmune diseases of the thyroid, liver, and lungs, in chronic infectious diseases such as mononucleosis, hepatitis C infection, subacute bacterial endocarditis, tuberculosis, and HIV, and in some lymphoproliferative disorders.

Different types of ANA are known and classified on the basis of their target antigens. Antibodies can be directed against double-stranded DNA, individual nuclear histones, nuclear proteins, and RNA-protein complex. Because some of these antibodies are more specific for a particular disease, they are helpful tests for diagnosis. They are also used for monitoring disease activity.

In most laboratories, antinuclear antibodies are measured by an indirect immunofluorescence assay using the human epithelial cell tumor line (HEp-2 cells) as the antigenic substrate. Different staining patterns can be seen that reflect the presence of antibodies to one or a combination of nuclear antigens. These patterns are neither sensitive nor specific for a single disease.

The titer of antinuclear antibodies can be helpful clinically. A negative ANA makes a diagnosis of SLE or mixed connective tissue disease very unlikely. ANAs in the sera of normal healthy childhood population using HEp-2 cells as substrate was reported as 6%[1,18] at screening dilutions of 1 : 20 in one study[89] and at 16%[15,90] in another.[91] In healthy adults, ANA titers above 1 : 40 are found in 32%, above 1 : 80 in 13%, and above 1 : 320 in 3%.[92]

The presence of very high titer (above 1 : 640) should raise suspicion of an autoimmune disease. If no diagnosis is made, the patient should be followed closely. Lower titers with no clinical sign or symptoms of disease are much less worrisome.

Anti–double-stranded DNA (anti-dsDNA) is relatively specific for SLE and fluctuates with disease activity.

Antinucleosome antibody is the earliest marker for the diagnosis of SLE. It is also a superior marker of lupus nephritis.[87] Among patients with SLE, the prevalence of antinucleosome antibodies was higher in those with renal disease (58%) compared with those without nephritis (29%).[93]

Antibodies to the Smith antigen, which is a nuclear nonhistone protein, are specific for SLE but insensitive.

REFERENCES

1. Graff SL. In Biello LA, editor: *A handbook of routine urinalysis*, Philadelphia, 1983, Lippincott Williams & Wilkins.
2. Brodehl J, Franken A, Gellissen K: Maximal tubular reabsorption of glucose in infants and children, *Acta Paediatr Scand* 61(4):413-20, 1972.
3. Rose B. In Dereck JJ and Muza N, editors: *Clinical physiology of acid-base and electrolyte disorders*, New York, 1994, McGraw-Hill.
4. Hogg RJ et al: National Kidney Foundation's Kidney Disease Outcomes Quality Initiative clinical practice guidelines for chronic kidney disease in children and adolescents: evaluation, classification, and stratification, *Pediatrics* 111(6):1416-21, 2003.
5. Kaneko K et al: Simplified quantification of urinary protein excretion using a novel dipstick in children, *Pediatr Nephrol* 20(6):834-36, 2005.
6. Ettenger RB: The evaluation of the child with proteinuria, *Pediatr Ann* 23(9):486-94, 1994.
7. The CARI guidelines. Urine protein as diagnostic test: evaluation of proteinuria in children, *Nephrology (Carlton)* 9(suppl 3):S15-19, 2004.
8. Mori Y et al: Urinary creatinine excretion and protein/creatinine ratios vary by body size and gender in children, *Pediatr Nephrol* 21(5):683-87, 2006.
9. Kim HS et al: Quantification of proteinuria in children using the urinary protein-osmolality ratio, *Pediatr Nephrol* 16(1):73-76, 2001.
10. Cole BR et al: Measurement of renal function without urine collection. A critical evaluation of the constant-infusion technic for determination of inulin and para-aminohippurate, *N Engl J Med* 287(22):1109-14, 1972.
11. Florijn KW et al: Glomerular filtration rate measurement by "single-shot" injection of inulin, *Kidney Int* 46(1):252-59, 1994.
12. van Rossum LK et al: Optimal sampling strategies to assess inulin clearance in children by the inulin single-injection method, *Clin Chem* 49(7):1170-79, 2003.
13. van Rossum LK et al: Determination of inulin clearance by single injection or infusion in children, *Pediatr Nephrol* 20(6):777-81, 2005.
14. Schwartz GJ, Brion LP, Spitzer A: The use of plasma creatinine concentration for estimating glomerular filtration rate in infants, children, and adolescents, *Pediatr Clin North Am* 34(3):571-90, 1987.
15. Levey AS: Measurement of renal function in chronic renal disease, *Kidney Int* 38(1):167-87, 1990.
16. Atiyeh BA, Dabbagh SS, B Gruskin AB: Evaluation of renal function during childhood, *Pediatr Rev* 17(5):175-80, 1996.
17. Piepsz A et al: Guidelines for glomerular filtration rate determination in children, *Eur J Nucl Med* 28(3):BP31-36, 2001.
18. Blaufox MD et al: Report of the Radionuclides in Nephrourology Committee on renal clearance, *J Nucl Med* 37(11):1883-90, 1996.
19. Schwartz GJ et al: A simple estimate of glomerular filtration rate in children derived from body length and plasma creatinine, *Pediatrics* 58(2):259-63, 1976.
20. Counahan R et al: Estimation of glomerular filtration rate from plasma creatinine concentration in children, *Arch Dis Child* 51(11):875-78, 1976.
21. Mattman A et al: Estimating pediatric glomerular filtration rates in the era of chronic kidney disease staging, *J Am Soc Nephrol* 17(2):487-96, 2006.
22. Leger F et al: Estimation of glomerular filtration rate in children, *Pediatr Nephrol* 17(11):903-07, 2002.

23. Gaspari F et al: Plasma clearance of nonradioactive iohexol as a measure of glomerular filtration rate, *J Am Soc Nephrol* 6(2):257-63, 1995.
24. Stake G et al: The clearance of iohexol as a measure of the glomerular filtration rate in children with chronic renal failure, *Scand J Clin Lab Invest* 51(8):729-34, 1991.
25. Schwartz GJ et al: Glomerular filtration rate via plasma iohexol disappearance: pilot study for chronic kidney disease in children, *Kidney Int* 69(11):2070-77, 2006.
26. Rule AD et al: Glomerular filtration rate estimated by cystatin C among different clinical presentations, *Kidney Int* 69(2):399-405, 2006.
27. Finney H, Newman DJ, Price CPP: Adult reference ranges for serum cystatin C, creatinine and predicted creatinine clearance, *Ann Clin Biochem* 37(1):49-59, 2000.
28. Knight EL et al: Factors influencing serum cystatin C levels other than renal function and the impact on renal function measurement, *Kidney Int* 65(4):1416-21, 2004.
29. Cimerman N et al: Serum cystatin C, a potent inhibitor of cysteine proteinases, is elevated in asthmatic patients, *Clin Chim Acta* 300(1-2):83-95, 2000.
30. Wiesli P et al: Serum cystatin C is sensitive to small changes in thyroid function, *Clin Chim Acta* 338(1-2):87-90, 2003.
31. Dharnidharka VR, Kwon C, Stevens G: Serum cystatin C is superior to serum creatinine as a marker of kidney function: a meta-analysis, *Am J Kidney Dis* 40(2):221-26, 2002.
32. Larsson A et al: Calculation of glomerular filtration rate expressed in mL/min from plasma cystatin C values in mg/L, *Scand J Clin Lab Invest* 64(1):25-30, 2004.
33. Grubb A et al: A cystatin C-based formula without anthropometric variables estimates glomerular filtration rate better than creatinine clearance using the Cockcroft-Gault formula, *Scand J Clin Lab Invest* 65(2):153-62, 2005.
34. Filler G, Lepage N: Should the Schwartz formula for estimation of GFR be replaced by cystatin C formula? *Pediatr Nephrol* 18(10):981-85, 2003.
35. Sambasivan AS, Lepage N, Filler G: Cystatin C intrapatient variability in children with chronic kidney disease is less than serum creatinine, *Clin Chem* 51(11):2215-16, 2005.
36. Kruse K, Kracht U, Gopfert G: Renal threshold phosphate concentration (TmPO4/GFR), *Arch Dis Child* 57(3):217-23, 1982.
37. Bijvoet OL: Relation of plasma phosphate concentration to renal tubular reabsorption of phosphate, *Clin Sci* 37(1):23-36, 1969.
38. Walton RJ, Bijvoet OL: Nomogram for derivation of renal threshold phosphate concentration, *Lancet* 2(7929):309-10, 1975.
39. Santer R et al: The molecular basis of renal glucosuria: mutations in the gene for a renal glucose transporter (SGLT2), *J Inherit Metab Dis* 23(suppl 1):178, 2000.
40. West ML et al: Development of a test to evaluate the transtubular potassium concentration gradient in the cortical collecting duct in vivo, *Miner Electrolyte Metab* 12(4):226-33, 1986.
41. Rodriguez-Soriano J, Ubetagoyena M, Vallo A: Transtubular potassium concentration gradient: a useful test to estimate renal aldosterone bio-activity in infants and children, *Pediatr Nephrol* 4(2):105-10, 1990.
42. Goldstein MB et al: The urine anion gap: a clinically useful index of ammonium excretion, *Am J Med Sci* 292(4):198-202, 1986.
43. Batlle DC et al: The use of the urinary anion gap in the diagnosis of hyperchloremic metabolic acidosis, *N Engl J Med* 318(10):594-99, 1988.
44. Halperin ML et al: The urine osmolal gap: a clue to estimate urine ammonium in "hybrid" types of metabolic acidosis, *Clin Invest Med* 11(3):198-202, 1988.
45. Halperin ML et al: Studies on the pathogenesis of type I (distal) renal tubular acidosis as revealed by the urinary PCO_2 tensions, *J Clin Invest* 53(3):669-77, 1974.
46. DuBose TD Jr, Caflisch CR: Validation of the difference in urine and blood carbon dioxide tension during bicarbonate loading as an index of distal nephron acidification in experimental models of distal renal tubular acidosis, *J Clin Invest* 75(4):1116-23, 1985.
47. Kim S et al: The urine-blood PCO gradient as a diagnostic index of H(+)-ATPase defect distal renal tubular acidosis, *Kidney Int* 66(2):761-67, 2004.
48. Ghoshal AK, Soldin SJ: Evaluation of the Dade Behring Dimension RxL: integrated chemistry system-pediatric reference ranges, *Clin Chim Acta* 331(1-2):135-46, 2003.
49. Soldin BC, Wong EC, editors: *Pediatric reference ranges*, ed 4, Washington, 2003, AACC Press.
50. Garfinkel HB, Gelfman N: Bicarbonate, not 'CO2', *Arch Intern Med* 143(11):2063-64, 1983.
51. Kost GJ, Trent JK, Saeed D: Indications for measurement of total carbon dioxide in arterial blood, *Clin Chem* 34(8):1650-52, 1988.
52. K/DOQI Clinical practice guidelines for bone metabolism and disease in children with chronic kidney disease, *Am J Kidney Dis* 46(4), 2005.
53. Biyikli NK, Alpay H, Guran T: Hypercalciuria and recurrent urinary tract infections: incidence and symptoms in children over 5 years of age, *Pediatr Nephrol* 20(10):1435-88, 2005.
54. Ghazali S, Barratt TM: Urinary excretion of calcium and magnesium in children, *Arch Dis Child* 49(2):97-101, 1974.
55. Moore E et al.: Idiopathic hypercalciuria in children: prevalence and metabolic characteristics, *Journal of Pediatrics* 92(6):906-10, 1978.
56. Sorkhi H, Haji Aahmadi M: Urinary calcium to creatinin ratio in children, *Indian J Pediatr* 72(12):1055-56, 2005.
57. De Santo NG et al: Population based data on urinary excretion of calcium, magnesium, oxalate, phosphate and uric acid in children from Cimitile (southern Italy), *Pediatr Nephrol* 6(2):149-57, 1992.
58. So NP et al: Normal urinary calcium/creatinine ratios in African-American and Caucasian children, *Pediatr Nephrol* 16(2):133-39, 2001.
59. Vachvanichsanong P, Lebel L, Moore ES: Urinary calcium excretion in healthy Thai children, *Pediatr Nephrol* 14(8-9):847-50, 2000.
60. Butani L, Kalia A: Idiopathic hypercalciuria in children—how valid are the existing diagnostic criteria? *Pediatr Nephrol* 19(6):577-82, 2004.
61. Richmond W et al: Random urine calcium/osmolality in the assessment of calciuria in children with decreased muscle mass, *Clin Nephrol* 64(4):264-70, 2005.
62. Mir S, Serdaroglu E: Quantification of hypercalciuria with the urine calcium osmolality ratio in children, *Pediatr Nephrol* 20(11):1562-65, 2005.
63. Hilgenfeld MS et al: Lack of seasonal variations in urinary calcium/creatinine ratio in school-age children, *Pediatr Nephrol* 19(10):1153-55, 2004.
64. Polito C et al: Urinary sodium and potassium excretion in idiopathic hypercalciuria of children, *Nephron* 91(1):7-12, 2002.
65. Tefekli A et al: Metabolic risk factors in pediatric and adult calcium oxalate urinary stone formers: is there any difference? *Urol Int* 70(4):273-77, 2003.
66. Sikora P et al: Hypocitraturia is one of the major risk factors for nephrocalcinosis in very low birth weight (VLBW) infants, *Kidney Int* 63(6):2194-99, 2003.
67. Stapenhorst L et al: Hypocitraturia as a risk factor for nephrocalcinosis after kidney transplantation, *Pediatr Nephrol* 20(5):652-56, 2005.
68. Rumsby G: Biochemical and genetic diagnosis of the primary hyperoxalurias: a review, *Mol Urol* 4(4):349-54, 2000.
69. La Manna A et al: Hyperuricosuria in children: clinical presentation and natural history, *Pediatrics* 107(1):86-90, 2001.
70. Stapleton FB, Nash DA: A screening test for hyperuricosuria, *J Pediatr* 102(1):88-90, 1983.
71. Dillon MJ, Ryness JM: Plasma renin activity and aldosterone concentration in children, *Br Med J* 4(5992):316-19, 1975.
72. Dillon MJ, Shah V, Barratt TM: Renal vein renin measurements in children with hypertension, *Br Med J* 2(6131):168-70, 1978.
73. Goonasekera CD et al: The usefulness of renal vein renin studies in hypertensive children: a 25-year experience, *Pediatr Nephrol* 17(11):943-49, 2002.
74. White PC: Disorders of aldosterone biosynthesis and action, *N Engl J Med* 331(4):250-58, 1994.
75. Whitworth JA: Mechanisms of glucocorticoid-induced hypertension, *Kidney Int* 31(5):1213-24, 1987.
76. Blumenfeld JD et al: Diagnosis and treatment of primary hyperaldosteronism, *Ann Intern Med* 121(11): 877-85, 1994.

77. Walport MJ: Complement. First of two parts, *N Engl J Med* 344(14):1058-66, 2001.
78. Walport MJ: Complement. Second of two parts, *N Engl J Med* 344(15):1140-44, 2001.
79. Thurman JM, Holers VM: The central role of the alternative complement pathway in human disease, *J Immunol* 176(3):1305-10, 2006.
80. Huber-Lang M et al: Generation of C5a in the absence of C3: a new complement activation pathway, *Nat Med* 12(6):682-87, 2006.
81. Hebert LA, Cosio FG, Neff JC: Diagnostic significance of hypocomplementemia, *Kidney Int* 39(5):811-21, 1991.
82. Davies DJ et al: Segmental necrotising glomerulonephritis with antineutrophil antibody: possible arbovirus aetiology? *Br Med J (Clin Res Ed)*285(6342):606, 1982.
83. Savige J et al: International Consensus Statement on Testing and Reporting of Antineutrophil Cytoplasmic Antibodies (ANCA), *Am J Clin Pathol* 111(4):507-13, 1999.
84. Mandl LA et al: Using antineutrophil cytoplasmic antibody testing to diagnose vasculitis: can test-ordering guidelines improve diagnostic accuracy? *Arch Intern Med* 162(13):1509-14, 2002.
85. Bosch X, Guilabert A, Font J: Antineutrophil cytoplasmic antibodies, *Lancet* 368(9533):404-18, 2006.
86. Birck R et al: Serial ANCA determinations for monitoring disease activity in patients with ANCA-associated vasculitis: systematic review, *Am J Kidney Dis* 47(1):15-23, 2006.
87. Saisoong S, Eiam-Ong S, Hanvivatvong O: Correlations between antinucleosome antibodies and anti-double-stranded DNA antibodies, C3, C4, and clinical activity in lupus patients, *Clin Exp Rheumatol* 24(1):51-58, 2006.
88. Malleson PN, Sailer M, Mackinnon MJ: Usefulness of antinuclear antibody testing to screen for rheumatic diseases, *Arch Dis Child* 77(4):299-304, 1997.
89. Haynes DC et al: Autoantibody profiles in juvenile arthritis, *J Rheumatol* 13(2):358-63, 1986.
90. Hogg RJ et al: Evaluation and management of proteinuria and nephrotic syndrome in children: recommendations from a pediatric nephrology panel established at the National Kidney Foundation conference on proteinuria, albuminuria, risk, assessment, detection, and elimination (PARADE), *Pediatrics* 105(6):1242-49, 2005.
91. Cabral DA et al: Persistent antinuclear antibodies in children without identifiable inflammatory rheumatic or autoimmune disease, *Pediatrics* 89(3):441-44, 1992.
92. Tan EM et al: Range of antinuclear antibodies in "healthy" individuals, *Arthritis Rheum* 40(9):1601-11, 1997.
93. Cervera R et al: Anti-chromatin antibodies in systemic lupus erythematosus: a useful marker for lupus nephropathy, *Ann Rheum Dis* 62(5):431-34, 2003.
94. Harmoinen A et al: Reference intervals for cystatin C in pre- and full-term infants and children, *Pediatr Nephrol* 15(1-2):105-08, 2000.
95. Matos V et al: Urinary phosphate/creatinine, calcium/creatinine, and magnesium/creatinine ratios in a healthy pediatric population, *J Pediatr* 131(2):252-57, 1997.

CHAPTER 3

Tools for Renal Tissue Analysis

Anette Melk

The gold standard for renal tissue analysis is the renal biopsy. It is routinely performed to allow histologic diagnoses of renal diseases and to determine the extent of damage in native and allograft kidneys. However, there has been controversy over the use and interpretation of renal biopsies. Issues among different observers include sampling errors and reproducibility. More importantly, histopathologic assessment has failed to predict progression or regression of renal diseases, thus reducing the value of renal biopsies as a guide for clinical therapeutic approaches. Because of this, researchers have always tried new methods in order to add more validity and prognostication. Needle biopsies were already being performed in the 1930s, but renal biopsies were not introduced as a clinical diagnostic tool until the 1960s, when Jones silver stain and the new techniques of electron microscopy (EM) and immunofluorescence (IF) became available. In the 1970s immunohistologic methods were applied to identify, localize, and semiquantify immune deposits, extracellular matrix proteins, and cellular infiltrates. Developments in the late 1980s and 1990s focused on methods to measure RNA and DNA. With the ongoing advances in renal imaging, this noninvasive, indirect technique may become the ultimate way of analyzing renal tissue in the future.

RENAL BIOPSY

Procedure

In children, renal biopsies were performed with open exposure of the kidney until White in England in 1962 and Metcoff in the United States in 1970 described a modified needle biopsy procedure for children, including infants. Today percutaneous renal biopsies in children are done under ultrasound guidance and have become routine.

Despite differences in details, the procedures for a renal biopsy are relatively standardized. In preparation for the biopsy the patient and parents are informed about the possible risks of the biopsy and the potential therapeutic consequences. For safety, laboratory values are obtained, including hemoglobin, platelet count, prothrombin time, partial thromboplastin time, and bleeding time if uremic. In addition, serum creatinine, electrolytes, and urine dipstick analysis may be used as baseline parameters in case of complications. Before performing the biopsy, the nephrologist should be aware of the patient's renal anatomy. Most commonly, ultrasound examination is used to exclude contraindications such as single kidneys, small kidneys, and large cysts.

Small children receive general anesthesia. In larger children the procedure can be safely performed with mild sedation to facilitate patient cooperation, but many centers use general anesthesia even in these children. Briefly, the patient is placed in a prone position with a foam roll under the upper part of the abdomen. The kidneys are localized by ultrasound from the back. The kidney with the lower pole that is easiest to reach, in most cases the right kidney, is then chosen for biopsy. The exact position of the kidney during inspiration is determined, and after marking the intended entry of the needle on the skin, the skin is cleaned with an antiseptic solution. If the patient is only sedated, the skin, subcutaneous tissue, and muscle are infiltrated with a local anesthetic. After a small incision is made, the needle, mounted on a semiautomated, spring-loaded biopsy gun is carefully introduced under ultrasound guidance until the kidney is almost reached. Manually operated needles have been widely replaced by biopsy guns because they are easier to use and have lower complication rates. The patient is then advised to take a breath and hold the air. In case of general anesthesia, the anesthesist will hold the patient in deep inspiration. The needle is quickly advanced to the capsule of the kidney and the biopsy is taken (Figure 3-1). Ideally the entire procedure is followed on the ultrasound screen to visualize the path of the biopsy needle.

After the procedure the patient usually stays in bed for 24 hours with compression of the puncture site. However, during the past several years, renal biopsies have been performed on an outpatient basis, where stable patients are discharged after about 8 hours.[1] To assure brisk diuresis the patient receives a glucose–sodium chloride solution intravenously and/or is asked to drink a lot of water. Urine is collected in single portions and examined with urine dipsticks. Hemoglobin levels and ultrasound controls are performed in most centers after 4 to 6 hours and after 24 hours. Blood pressure and heart rate controls must be done hourly.

The primary complication is macroscopic hematuria, which is seen in 0.8% to 12% of biopsies performed in pediatric patients. Other complications may include subcapsular or perirenal hematoma, infection, possible need for transfusion, and pain requiring medication. Arteriovenous fistulas have been diagnosed more often in recent years because of improved Doppler ultrasound technique. Table 3-1 provides

TABLE 3-1 **Complications of Percutaneous Biopsies in Native Kidneys**

	A (7/1969-4/1974)	B (5/1974-5/1985)	C (6/1985-3/1990)	D (4/1990-6/1992)	E (7/1992-12/1996)	All Periods
Needle	Silverman	TruCut	TruCut	Biopty	Biopty	
Localization of kidney	Radiocontrast imaging	Radiocontrast imaging	Prebiopsy ultrasound	Prebiopsy ultrasound	Ultasound guidance	
Microhematuria	21.7	32.5	26.3	47.0	40.3	30.9
Macrohematuria	2.7	16.7	15.8	8.3	4.4	9.6
Hemoglobin loss 20%	0	1.5	4.3	0	3.2	1.6
Ultrasound Examination						
No hematoma detected			67.7	53.4	44.2	53
Hematoma possible			13.8	8.6	14.2	12.7
Hematoma verified			18.5	37.9	41.6	34.3

* Rate of complications did not significantly differ during periods—A through E.
From Feneberg R, Schaefer F, Zieger B, Waldherr R, Mehls O, Schärer K: Percutaneous renal biopsy in children: a 27-year experience, *Nephron* 79(4):438-46, 1998.

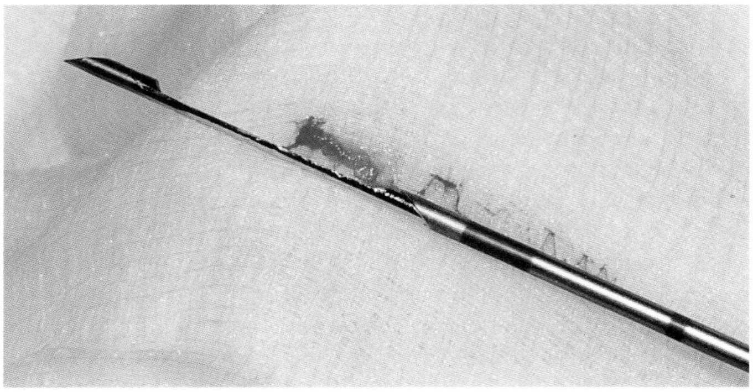

Figure 3-1 Renal biopsy specimen. (From Johnson RJ, Feehally J, editors: *Comprehensive clinical nephrology*, ed 2, Philadelphia, 2003, Elsevier)

TABLE 3-2 **Minimum Number of Glomeruli Necessary to Assume a Given Percent Involvement in the Kidney***

	Number of Abnormal Glomeruli in a Biopsy		
Biopsy size	80%†	50%†	20%†
8	8 (100)	7 (88)	3 (38)
10	10 (100)	8 (80)	4 (40)
12	12 (100)	9 (75)	5 (42)
15	14 (93)	11 (73)	6 (40)
20	19 (95)	14 (70)	7 (35)
25	23 (92)	17 (68)	9 (36)
30	28 (93)	20 (66)	10 (33)
35	32 (91)	23 (66)	11 (31)
40	36 (90)	26 (65)	12 (30)

* $p = 0.05$ (one-tailed).
† Percent involvement of the kidney sought.

on overview of the most frequent complications of different biopsy techniques over 3 decades.[2]

Processing Biopsy Specimens

Adequate processing and interpretation of the specimen is as important as accurate performance of the biopsy.[3,4] Before fixation, each core should be examined by light microscopy (LM) with tenfold magnification for the presence and number of glomeruli. This examination should lead to a decision as to whether more renal tissue is needed. One should take into account the number of glomeruli and the suspected disease process. It cannot be emphasized enough that adequacy of sample size is crucial for the validity of a biopsy specimen. To diagnose a focal disease process such as focal segmental glomerulosclerosis (FSGS), recognition of a single abnormal glomerulus is required. Making this diagnosis depends on the fraction of affected glomeruli per kidney, as well as the glomeruli present in a given biopsy specimen. The same holds true for assessment of the extent of a disease with variable pathologic involvement among glomeruli. Corwin and colleagues have published estimates on the minimum number of abnormal glomeruli that need to be present in a biopsy core containing a given number of glomeruli in order to infer with 95% confidence that a disease process involves 20%, 50%, or 80% of the kidney (Table 3-2).[5]

Appropriate fixation of the biopsy should be done as soon as possible because small cores can dry out quickly. Choice of fixatives should be discussed with the local renal pathologist. In pediatric renal diseases, LM alone can be insufficient to make a diagnosis. Therefore, specimens for IF and EM should be obtained. Because of its superior morphology, some renal pathologists prefer fixation with Bouin's alcohol picrate solution. This, however, may lead to problems if immunohistochemistry (IHC) staining needs to be performed. Fixation with paraformaldehyde or buffered formalin (4%, pH 7.2-7.4) followed by paraffin embedding is therefore common practice in most pathology departments. For IF, renal tissue should be "snap-frozen" in liquid nitrogen or placed in tissue transport media or isotonic sodium chloride solution if being transported to the laboratory immediately. Specimens for EM are usually fixed in a solution containing 0.1% to 3% glutaraldehyde. LM specimens should be sectioned at a thickness of 2 μm or less by an experienced technician. Subtle pathologic changes are more easily detected in thinner sections, thus section thickness is an important issue for glomerular pathology especially when assessing for cellularity. A variety of histochemical stains are used to evaluate renal biopsies (Figure 3-2). Typically biopsy specimens are stained with hematoxylin and eosin (H&E), periodic acid-Schiff (PAS), or periodic acid-methenamine silver (Jones silver) and Masson's trichrome. H&E is used for general morphology and reference, whereas the other three stains provide a clear distinction of extracellular matrix from cytoplasm. Depending on indication, Congo red stain (amyloid), Kossa stain (calcifications), elastic tissue stain (loss of elasticity in arteries, arterial thickening), and other stains are used. IF uses fluorescein-labeled antibodies to detect and localize immunoglobulins (IgA, IgG, IgM) and their light chains (κ, λ), components of the classical or alternative complement pathways (C1q, C3c, C4), albumin, and fibrinogen. In transplant biopsies, staining for C4d, a fragment within the complement pathway, has become a major diagnostic tool in antibody-mediated rejection.[6] The pattern of a fluorescence-positive stain should be noted, such as mesangial versus capillary staining and linear or granular staining. The granular pattern has an EM counterpart and corresponds to extracellular, electron-dense masses. EM studies do not need to be part of the routine workup of every kidney biopsy. However, EM plays an important diagnostic role in more than 50% of cases and is essential for a correct diagnosis in up to 25%. Even though it is sometimes possible to omit EM after evaluation of LM and IF, specimens for EM studies should always be procured. EM can localize deposits (mesangial, subendothelial, or subepithelial). EM is also able to detect changes in cell structure (for example, fusion of podocyte foot process and podocyte vacuolization) and alterations of the basement membrane (thickening, thinning, splicing, duplication, and other irregularities). The definite diagnosis of, for example, minimal change nephropathy, Alport's disease, or thin basement membrane disease requires EM.[7,8]

Histopathologic Assessment

Abnormalities in renal structures can occur in all four compartments of the kidneys: glomeruli, tubules, interstitium, and vasculature. Specific pathologic changes with certain diseases are discussed in later chapters; this chapter provides a general overview on the various histopathologic features that can be encountered while reading a biopsy.[3,4,9]

Glomerular changes are the primary pathologic event in many renal diseases. If glomeruli are affected, one must decide whether these changes are diffuse (almost all glomeruli are involved) or whether the disease process is focal (only some glomeruli are involved). When assessing single glomeruli, one should also determine whether the disease process involves only part of the glomerulus (segmental) or the whole glomerulus (global). *Glomerular sclerosis* refers to an increase in extracellular material such as hyaline within the mesangium that leads to compression of the capillaries. The capillary basement membrane has a wrinkled appearance, and adhesions to Bowman's capsule are found. Depending on its expansion, the sclerotic lesion can be either segmental or global. *Hypercellularity* refers to an increased number of cells, such as mesangial, endothelial, or inflammatory, in the mesangial space. Glomerular diseases involving hypercellularity are often called *proliferative*. Changes of the basement membrane that can be seen by LM involve thickening of the basement membrane and basement membrane double layering. Whereas glomerular sclerosis is caused by the accumulation of basement membrane material, hypercellularity is understood to be caused by peripheral interposition of mesangial material. Severe glomerular diseases show the formation of crescents, which are located in the urinary space of the glomerulus and consist of cells and extracellular material. The proportion of glomeruli affected by crescents is of enormous prognostic importance in acute glomerulonephritis/vasculitis. The most subtle glomerular damage is effacement of foot process and refers to the loss of normal podocyte morphology with an undivided cytoplasmic mass covering the basement membrane. Effacement of foot process cannot be seen by LM but is easily found with EM.

Tubular cells can show various signs of damage, which include loss of brush border (in proximal tubules), flattening of the tubular epithelium, detachment of tubular cells from the basement membrane, necrosis, and apoptosis. Mitosis of tubular cells is often found as a sign of repair after an episode of acute tubular necrosis. When necrosis is chronic, tubular changes occur as tubular atrophy, in which the tubules have a reduced diameter and a thickened basement membrane. Tubular atrophy is often accompanied by interstitial fibrosis. In a diseased kidney, areas with normal tubules and atrophic tubules can occur. Another type of tubular pathology is the accumulation of droplets containing various pathologic substances. This can occur in patients with heavy proteinuria or with various storage diseases.

Interstitial changes are edema, fibrosis, and infiltration by inflammatory cells. Edema indicates acute diseases, whereas fibrosis is the sequelae of chronic renal damage. In both cases tubules are no longer sitting back to back but are separated by interstitial material. The degree of interstitial fibrosis is of prognostic importance in chronic kidney diseases. In many instances, the degree of interstitial fibrosis found in a primary glomerular disease is a more powerful predictor of outcome than are glomerular changes. Infiltration of inflammatory cells can be the cause of renal diseases such as acute interstitial nephritis or acute transplant rejection, but an interstitial infiltrate can also be a solely accompanying phenomenon, as in fibrosis.

Finally, the renal vasculature can show pathologic changes. The most subtle vascular damage is fibrous intimal thickening. Overall, the vessel walls can be thickened and hyalinized, in extreme cases leading to complete obstruction of the vessels. In specific renal diseases, thrombosis of renal vessels of different sizes can occur, as well as inflammation of the vascular wall.

PROTEIN ANALYSIS

The classical way of analyzing protein in renal tissue is with IF or IHC. Both techniques use antisera or antibodies directed

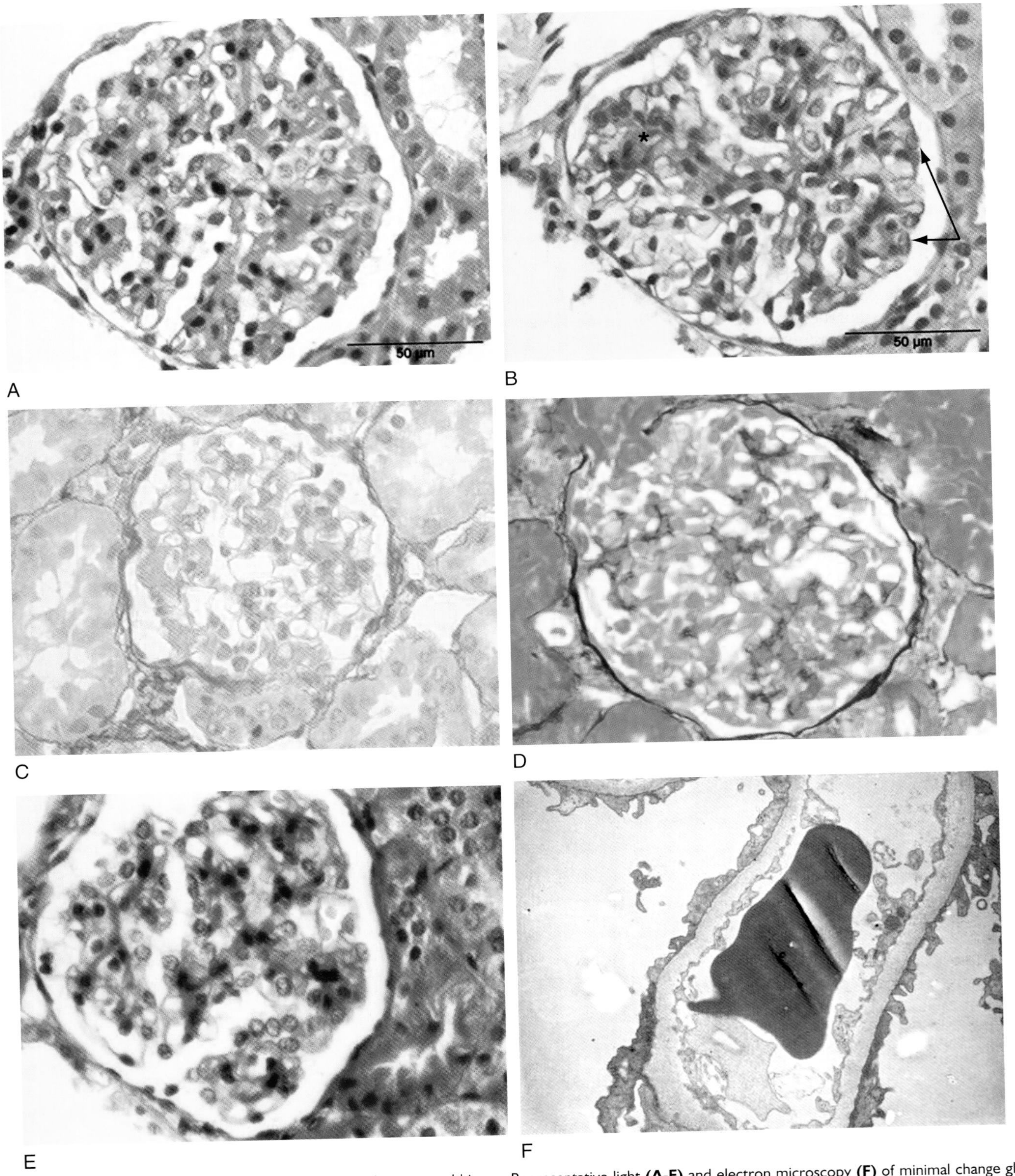

Figure 3-2 Overview of different stainings used to evaluate a renal biopsy. Representative light **(A-E)** and electron microscopy **(F)** of minimal change glomerulopathy (MCGN) with mild hypercellularity. **A,** Hematoxylin and eosin stain (H&E). The H&E stain is the workhorse of pathology; it is useful to first get an idea about glomerular changes such as proliferation and matrix deposition. In MCGN, the glomerulus shows a slightly increased number of mesangial cells, open capillaries, no evidence of intracapillary or extracapillary proliferation, and normal thickness of glomerular basement membrane (GBM). **B,** Periodic acid-Schiff (PAS) stain: PAS staining is useful in analyzing changes in glomerular cell number and GBM in more detail. In MCGN, mild segmental hypercellularity (*) and normal thickness of GBM without any irregularities is seen. Some podocytes *(arrows)* are slightly enlarged and appear detached from the GBM. **C,** Sirius red stain (fibrous tissue stain): This fibrous tissue stain is useful in analyzing the amount of fibrous tissue (fibrosis) of glomeruli and most importantly the interstitial tissue (interstitial fibrosis). In MCGN, a normal amount of fibrous tissue is found in Bowman's capsule and no increase in mesangial matrix is visible. **D,** Silver stain: This stain is most useful in detecting thickening and irregularities of the GBM. In MCGN, no thickening and spike formation is seen. **E,** Acid fuchsin-orange G stain (SFOG): This stain is used to detect protein deposition (that is, immune complex formation), which appears in bright red within the mesangial matrix or the GBM. In MCGN, no immune deposits are present. **F,** Electron microscopy of a capillary loop shows typical changes in MCGN (that is, normal thickness of GBM with no evidence of immune complex deposition) but with effacement of podocyte foot processes and loss of endothelial fenestration. (Pictures courtesy Prof. Dr. K. Amann, Erlangen.)

against the protein of interest. IF requires native tissue without fixation, whereas IHC can be performed in formalin-fixed tissues. Because fixatives can mask protein epitopes, antigen-retrieval steps become necessary, especially for nuclear antigens. Detection and visualization of primary antibody bound to paraffin sections is usually achieved with an avidin-biotin-peroxidase system. There are certain advantages and disadvantages with both methods. IF is a technically easy and quick procedure: processing, sectioning, and staining can be performed in 1 to 2 hours. Even though the cost of the prodecure is low, storage cost can be expensive. A vast range of suitable antibodies is available and background staining is generally not problematic. However, because frozen sections do not provide good morphology, an additional sample for assessment of histopathologic details is required. IHC can be done using the same tissue as used for LM. It provides much better morphologic details than IF and reveals a permanent staining. IHC is highly sensitive because of the possibility to enhance the signal by certain amplifiers, but it can be technically challenging (for example, it has a higher background staining) and expensive.

Examples of IF have been given above as they are used in the standard workup of biopsy specimens. Some pathology centers prefer to use IHC even for the standard workup because of its ability to store and archive the slides for future comparison. IHC is also used to detect viral antigens, especially in allograft biopsies, even though polymerase chain reaction (PCR) techniques are currently taking over because of their higher sensitivity. Examples of viruses that are detected include cytomegalovirus (CMV) and BK polyomavirus. The typical CMV inclusions found in smudgy tubular cells with enlarged nuclei are direct evidence of CMV tissue invasiveness but have only been found in less than 1% of transplant patients with CMV disease. A similar tubular histology with inclusions as seen with CMV is also suggestive for BK virus.[10] In addition, a pleomorphic infiltrate with lymphocytes, plasma cells, and polymorphonuclear cells (PMNs) is very suspicious for viral infection, especially BK virus nephropathy. CMV can be evaluated by using an antibody directed against CMV immediate-early antigen, whereas a monoclonal antibody directed against the BK virus large T antigen is most commonly used for detection of BK virus. In case expansile/dysplastic plasma cells are found in the interstitium of an allograft biopsy specimen, staining for Epstein-Barr virus (EBV) may be useful to make the diagnosis of posttransplant lymphoproliferative disorder (PTLD), because most but not all PTLDs are EBV positive.

New technical advances in protein analysis include various proteomic tools, but none is used for the routine workup of renal biopsies. Protein arrays are comparable to the DNA microarray technology. Protein-based chips directly measure the level of proteins in tissues using fluorescence-based imaging. The most popular arrays currently rely on antibody-antigen interactions, which can also detect antigen-protein interactions. The potential of antibody arrays is currently limited by the availability of antibodies that have both high specificity (to eliminate cross reactions with nonspecific proteins within the sample) and high affinity for the target of interest (to allow detection of small quantities within a sample). An additional challenge of protein array technology is the ability to preserve proteins in their biologically active shape and form. Another proteomic technology to analyze protein mixtures quantitatively is known as surface-enhanced laser desorption/ionization time-of-flight (SELDI-TOF). Solubilized tissue or body fluids in volumes as small as 0.1 μl are directly applied to varied chemical and biochemical surfaces that allow differential capture of proteins based on their intrinsic properties. The bound proteins are laser desorbed and ionized for mass spectrometry (MS) analysis. Masses of proteins ranging from small peptides of less than 1000 Da to proteins of greater than 300 kDa are calculated based on time-of-flight. Since mixtures of proteins will be analyzed within different samples, a unique sample fingerprint or signature will result for each sample tested. Consequently, patterns of masses rather than actual protein identifications are produced by SELDI analysis. Examples for the experimental use of SELDI-TOF in nephrology are urinary protein analysis for the identification of patients with urolithiasis and the prediction of renal allograft rejection.

RNA ANALYSIS

Methods that measure RNA in small biopsy samples have been applied to analyze diseased native kidneys as well as renal allografts. The sensitivity of RT-PCR exceeds that of Northern blotting and RNA protection assays by a hundredfold to a thousandfold and has therefore become the leading tool in recent years. RT-PCR studies have been performed investigating a large variety of genes such as chemokines, cytokines, growth factors, and extracellular matrix proteins.[11] Even though strong associations have been seen for certain genes with specific diseases, none of those genes has yet made it into routine diagnostics.

High throughput gene expression technologies emerged in the mid-1990s, and a number of different microarray platforms are available. Two-color array platforms employ clones or oligonucleotides that are spotted onto glass slides, and two differentially labeled cDNA samples are hybridized together on an array. On one-color platforms such as the Affymetrix GeneChip, a single sample is hybridized to each array. The amount of agreement or variation across the different platforms is an important issue for researchers. Several studies have compared different platforms without coming to a consensus. Some claim a significant divergence across technologies; others find the level of concordance acceptable. It seems, however, that gene chip technology is emerging as the one most utilized, because the method is highly standardized and the chips are commercially available, allowing for comparison and exchange of data between different laboratories. The major challenge of any of these platforms that analyze genome-wide RNA expression remains the extraction of biological insight from such information. Ideally, one would like to recognize specific patterns or pathways involved in certain diseases (Figure 3-3). This may become easier with new developments in analytical methods such as gene set enrichment analysis, which focuses on gene sets—groups of genes that share common biological function, chromosomal location, or regulation.

So far, microarray studies in native kidneys and in renal transplants have shown that transcript levels may serve to

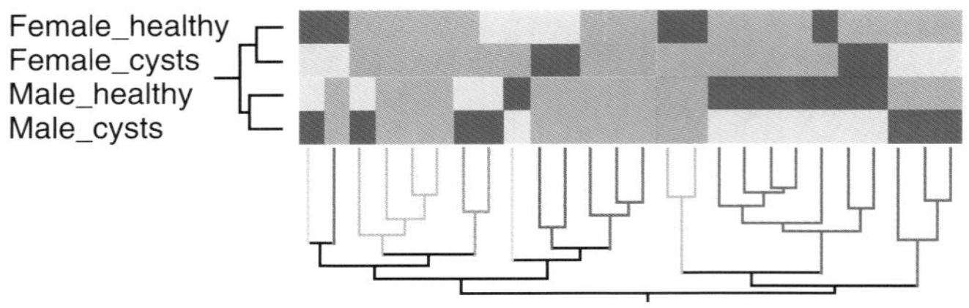

Figure 3-3 Typical dendrogram used in gene array analysis. Hierarchical cluster of genes that are differentially expressed based on gender (male/female) or disease state (normal vs. cystic kidneys) in kidneys from 36-day-old PKD*Mhm rats. The color from blue to orange reflects increasing gene expression. (Picture courtesy Dr. Li, Mannheim.)

complement histopathologic findings, thereby providing a more accurate prognosis and thus the application of individualized therapeutic regimens. One example is the identification by Sarwal and colleagues[12] of a group of pediatric transplant patients who had undergone severe acute rejection with resistance to antirejection therapy. This group segregated on the array and was found to show high expression of CD20, a B-cell marker.

The kidney has several compartments that contribute or respond differently to a disease or injury; their signals may be underestimated or even missed. Manual dissection, sieving, or laser capture microdissection (LCM) have been used to allow researchers to compare glomeruli with tubulointerstitium or to study rare cells.[13] During LCM, cells are isolated after exposure to an infrared laser that melts a thermosensitive polymer film that encapsulates the specific cells of interest. The film holding the captured cells is then transferred to a tube, where an extraction buffer is used to remove the cells for further molecular analysis. Recently LCM of fixed renal tissue has been proposed, providing a tool for analysis of archival tissue. However, the challenge is the retrieval of sufficient high-quality material for which frozen material is superior.

The combination of LCM and novel RNA amplification protocols with a thousandfold linear amplification efficiency is able to generate gene profiles that are specific for a certain nephron segment. This approach has been used to generate expression profiles of single glomeruli derived from renal biopsies showing lupus nephritis.[14] The study revealed considerable kidney-to-kidney heterogeneity, whereas glomerulus-to-glomerulus variation within a kidney was less marked.

Again, none of these novel techniques has found its way into clinical diagnostics yet.

DEOXYRIBONUCLEIC ACID ANALYSIS

Detection of viral DNA by PCR using sequence-specific primers has been described for a large panel of viruses such as CMV, BK virus, EBV, Coxsackie B viruses, parvovirus B19, hepatitis B virus, and human immunodeficiency virus. Because this approach is highly sensitive, it can be performed even with small sample sizes. Ordinarily DNA is isolated out of a somewhat thicker section cut from the formalin-fixed, paraffin-embedded specimen. For most viruses only a qualitative result is reported, that is, whether the virus is present or not. More recently, reliable methods to quantitate viral DNA in tissue specimens have become available, and first experiments have been performed using these new techniques for quantification of BK and JC polyomaviruses in the kidney. However, at present it seems that viral load may be better measured in urine than in tissue, perhaps because a urine sample represents the entire kidney.

Comparative genomic hybridization (CGH) is a molecular cytogenetics technique that enables comprehensive, genome-wide screening of DNA sequence copy number changes. It is used to characterize chromosomal abnormalities for a gain (duplication, insertion, or amplification) or net loss (deletion of material). For a CGH experiment, two genomic DNA samples are simultaneously hybridized in situ to normal human metaphase spreads and detected with different fluorochromes. This technique has been used by several groups to determine DNA copy number alterations associated with clinical outcome in Wilms' tumor specimens. Tumor DNA that contains extra copies of genetic material will bind to the corresponding chromosome on the metaphase spread. Tumor DNA that lacks a portion of normal DNA will cause more binding of normal DNA to their corresponding DNA on the metaphase spread. Another approach is a single nucleotide polymorphism (SNP) chip-based method for profiling DNA methylation. This technique is able to simultaneously detect aberrations in DNA copy number and loss of heterozygosity, making it a generally useful approach for combined genetic and epigenetic profiling in tissue samples from cancer patients. To date, Wilms' tumor specimens have only been used for validation experiments by comparing them with methylation-sensitive Southern blotting.

INDIRECT MEASUREMENTS

The kidney is an excellent organ for indirect measurements in that a urine sample not only represents material from the entire kidney but is also easily and noninvasively accessible. The value of proteinuria measurements for clinical nephrology is undoubted, but proteinuria is not specific for a certain disease. Ideally one would like to develop screens for one or a few markers that are highly sensitive and specific for a disease and could be used as diagnostic tools. Because RNA can be extracted from cells shed into the urine, some of the novel RNA-detecting technologies discussed in earlier paragraphs have been applied to urine. Urinary messenger RNA (mRNA) measurements for certain cytotoxic T-cell genes (granzyme B and perforin) and for FOXP3, a specification and functional factor for regulatory T lymphocytes, have been postulated to detect or predict the outcome of acute rejection in renal allograft recipients.[15] The mRNA expression of podocyte markers, such as nephrin and podocin, in urine was found to be significantly different among proteinuric disease categories (diabetic glomerulosclerosis, IgA nephropathy, minimal change disease, and membranous nephropathy) and correlated with the rate of decline in renal function.

Imaging methods used as indirect tools to evaluate renal tissue have been discussed elsewhere. However, novel near-infrared reflectance confocal microscopy is an outlook to future technical developments in imaging.[16] This technique provides high-resolution optical sectioning through intact tissues without the use of exogenous fluorescent stains. Structures are separated based on their natural differences in refractivity. In experimental studies in rat kidneys, it was possible to identify structures such as tubules, glomeruli, interstitium, and vasculature as well as intracellular details. It is conceivable that with further developments such a technique will be applied during surgical intervention, in transplantation, and for rapid tissue assessment.

Even though the complication rate with renal biopsies is low, taking a biopsy is still an invasive procedure. Therefore the future development of new techniques should aim for indirect and noninvasive methods to assess the status of a kidney in vivo to minimize the need for renal biopsies.

REFERENCES

1. Sweeney C, Geary DF, Hebert D, Robinson L, Langlois V: Outpatient pediatric renal transplant biopsy—is it safe? *Pediatr Transplant* 10(2):159-61, March 2006.
2. Feneberg R, Schaefer F, Zieger B, Waldherr R, Mehls O, Schärer K: Percutaneous renal biopsy in children: a 27-year experience, *Nephron* 79(4):438-46, 1998.
3. Amann K, Haas CS: What you should know about the work-up of a renal biopsy, *Nephrol Dial Transplant* 21:1157-61, 2006.
4. Fogo A: Approach to renal biopsy, *Am J Kid Dis* 42(4):826-36, 2003.
5. Corwin HL, Schwartz MM, Lewis EJ: The importance of sample size in the interpretation of the renal biopsy, *Am J Nephrol* 8:85-89, 1988.
6. Racusen LC, Colvin RB, Solez K, Mihatsch MJ, Halloran PF et al: Antibody-mediated rejection criteria—an addition to the Banff 97 classification of renal allograft rejection, *Am J Transplant* 3(6):708-14, 2003.
7. Pirson Y: Making the diagnosis of Alport's syndrome, *Kidney Int* 56:760-75, 1999.
8. Morita M, White RH, Raafat F, Barnes JM, Standring DM: Glomerular basement membrane thickness in children. A morphometric study, *Ped Nephrol* 2:190-95, 1988.
9. Racusen LC, Solez K, Colvin RB, Bonsib SM, Castro MC et al: The Banff 97 working classification of renal allograft pathology, *Kidney Int* 55:713-23, 1999.
10. Drachenberg CB, Papadimitriou JC: Polyomavirus-associated nephropathy: update in diagnosis, *Transpl Infect Dis* 8:68-75, 2006.
11. Schmid H, Cohen CD, Henger A, Schlondorff D, Kretzler M: Gene expression analysis in renal biopsies, *Nephrol Dial Transplant* 19:1347-51, 2004.
12. Sarwal M, Chua MS, Kambham N, Hsieh SC, Satterwhite T et al: Molecular heterogeneity in acute renal allograft rejection identified by DNA microarray profiling, *N Engl J Med* 349(2):125-38, 2003.
13. Emmert-Buck MR, Bonner RF, Smith PD, Chuaqui RF, Zhuang Z et al: Laser capture microdissection, *Science* 274:921-22, 1996.
14. Peterson KS, Huang JF, Zhu J, D'agati V, Liu X et al: Characterization of heterogeneity in the molecular pathogenesis of lupus nephritis from transcriptional profiles of laser-captured glomeruli, *J Clin Invest* 113:1722-33, 2004.
15. Muthukumar T, Dadhania D, Ding R, Snopkowski C, Naqvi R et al: Suthanthiran RNA for FOXP3 in the urine of renal-allograft recipients, *N Engl J Med* 353(22): 2342-51, 2005.
16. Campo-Ruiz V, Lauwrs GY, Anderson RR, Delgado-Baeza E, Gonzalez S: Novel virtual biopsy of the kidney with near infrared, reflectance confocal microscopy: a pilot study in vivo and ex vivo, *J Urol* 175:327-36, 2006.

CHAPTER

4 Antenatal Assessment of Kidney Morphology and Function

Khalid Ismaili, Fred E. Avni, and Michelle Hall

Today obstetrical two-dimensional ultrasound (US) is part of routine antenatal care in most countries of the western hemisphere. In many European countries, three sonographic examinations are performed, one in each trimester.[1] In other countries, including the United States and Canada, only a second-midtrimester examination is performed routinely, with first-trimester or third-trimester examinations performed only when there is a specific indication.[2] The more systematic use of obstetrical US has led to the discovery of many fetal abnormalities, among which uronephropathies make up one of the largest groups of congenital anomalies amenable to neonatal care, representing 0.2% to 2% of all newborns.[1] Over the next few years, the addition of three-dimensional US scanning and magnetic resonance imaging (MRI) will be another step forward and will certainly improve the ability to detect and define these structural renal abnormalities.[3] In addition, dramatic changes have occurred in the management of these children, since nowadays, uronephropathies are mostly found in asymptomatic patients and the treatment applied is mainly preventive. Also, the antenatal detection and postnatal follow-up have brought new data on the natural history of many uronephropathies.[4-6]

THE NORMAL URINARY TRACT

Bladder

Urine starts to be produced during the ninth week of fetal life. At that stage, the urine is collected in the bladder, which can be visualized as a fluid-filled structure within the fetal pelvis around the ninth or tenth week. During the second and third trimester, the fetus normally fills and partially or completely empties the bladder approximately every 25 minutes and the cycle can be monitored during the sonographic examination.[7] The bladder can easily be located by its outline of umbilical arteries, which are clearly identifiable on color Doppler.

Kidneys

Endovaginal probes can be used to visualize fetal anatomic structures earlier than with transabdominal US. Thus the fetal kidneys can be demonstrated at around 11 weeks endovaginally and around 12 to 15 weeks with transabdominal probes. During the first trimester the kidneys appear as hyperechoic oval structures at both sides of the spine (their hyperechogenicity can be compared with that of the liver or spleen).[8] This echogenicity will progressively decrease and during the third trimester the cortical echogenicity will always be less than that of the liver or spleen. Simultaneously with the decrease of echogenicity, corticomedullary differentiation will appear around 14 to 15 weeks. It should always be demonstrated in fetuses older than 18 weeks (Figure 4-1). Prominent pyramids should not be misinterpreted as calyceal dilatation.

Growth of the fetal kidneys can be evaluated throughout pregnancy. As a rule, a normal kidney grows at about 1.1 mm per week of gestation.

EVIDENCE OF NORMALLY FUNCTIONING URINARY TRACT

Besides visualization of the bladder and normal kidneys, assessment of the urinary tract should include an evaluation of the amniotic fluid volume. After 14 to 15 weeks, two thirds of the amniotic fluid is produced by fetal urination and one third by pulmonary fluid. A normal volume of amniotic fluid is mandatory for proper development of the fetal lung. This can be confirmed by measuring thoracic diameters or thoracic circumference.[9]

ULTRASOUND FINDINGS AS EVIDENCE OF ABNORMAL FETAL KIDNEY AND URINARY TRACT

Abnormal US appearance of the kidneys as a pathophysiological base of congenital renal malformation has been described extensively.[10,11] Anomalies of the urinary system detected in utero are numerous; they can include anomalies of the kidney itself, of the collecting system, of the bladder, and of the urethra. In addition, they can be isolated or in association with anomalies of other systems. Therefore the sonographic examination should be as meticulous as possible to visualize the associated features. These findings, among others, will determine the prognosis.

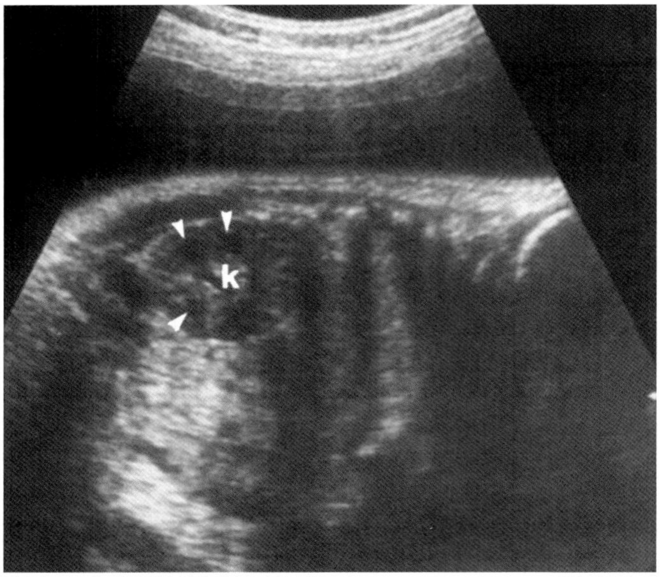

Figure 4-1 Normal fetal kidney (third trimester). Sagittal scan of the kidney (k). Corticomedullary differentiation is clearly visible (arrowheads).

Abnormal Renal Number

Bilateral renal agenesis is part of Potter's syndrome and is incompatible with extrauterine life. The diagnosis is based on the absence of renal structure and the presence of oligohydramnios after 15 weeks of gestation. Pulmonary hypoplasia is invariably associated and leads to death from respiratory failure soon after birth. In this context, enlarged globular adrenals should not be mistaken for kidneys.[12] Use of color Doppler may help localize the renal arteries and subsequently the kidneys.[13]

Unilateral renal agenesis is more common (1 in 500 pregnancies) and usually has no significant consequence on postnatal life. The pathogenesis of renal agenesis is mostly failure of formation of the metanephros. In addition, interruption in vascular supply and regression of a multicystic dysplastic kidney (MCDK) may also lead to renal agenesis in the fetal period.[14] An investigation after birth is necessary to confirm the status of the remnant kidney and to look for possible associated anomalies.[15] These anomalies can occur in both contiguous structures (such as vertebrae, genital organs, intestines, or anus) and noncontiguous structures (such as limbs, heart, trachea, ear, or central nervous system).[16]

Abnormal Renal Location

Ectopic kidney, especially in the pelvic area, is part of the differential diagnosis of the "empty renal fossa" in the fetus and may represent 42% of these cases.[15] Other possibilities, such as horseshoe or crossed fused kidneys, can also be detected in utero, and the diagnosis is usually achievable thanks to the demonstration of a typical corticomedullary differentiation.[17] An ectopic kidney is usually small and somewhat malrotated with numerous small blood vessels and associated ureteric anomalies. Ectopic kidneys may be asymptomatic, but complications from ureteral obstruction, infection, and calculi are common. Therefore at birth, the anomaly has to be confirmed by US or by MRI and voiding cystourethrography (VCUG) in complex cases.

Abnormal Renal Echogenicity

Hyperechogenicity of the fetal kidney is defined by comparison with the adjacent liver or spleen. This is difficult to assess in the first and second trimester, because the kidney is "physiologically" hyperechoic (or isoechoic at the end of the second trimester) to the liver. It is easier to characterize after 28 weeks, when the renal cortex should be hypoechoic compared with the liver and spleen.[8] Increased echogenicity of the renal parenchyma is nonspecific and occurs as a response to different changes in renal tissue.[18] Interstitial infiltration, sclerosis, and multiple microscopic cortical and medullary cysts may account for hyperechogenicity even in the absence of macrocysts. The detection of hyperechoic kidneys represents a difficult diagnostic challenge.[19] The differential diagnosis must be based on kidney size, corticomedullary differentiation, the presence of macrocysts, the degree of dilatation of the collecting system, and the amount of amniotic fluid.[20,21] The diagnosis must also take into account the familial history and the presence of associated anomalies. So far, the outcome of fetal hyperechoic kidneys can only be predicted accurately in severe cases with significant oligohydramnios.[19,21] For some patients, the characteristic US patterns will appear immediately after birth or even later. A follow-up is therefore mandatory. It should be stressed that some cases remain unsolved and have to be considered as normal variants.[18] Table 4-1 provides information on the spectrum of renal disorders associated with fetal hyperechoic kidneys.

Abnormal Renal Size

Measurements of the kidneys must be systematic whenever an anomaly of the urinary tract or amniotic fluid volume is suspected. It is therefore important to have standards for renal measurements that cover the complete gestational age range, because renal pathology often presents late in pregnancy.[22] Small kidneys most often correspond to hypodysplasia or kidneys damaged from obstructive uropathy or high-grade vesicoureteral reflux (VUR).[23,24] Enlarged kidneys may be related to urinary tract dilatation, renal cystic diseases, or tumoral involvement.

Urinary Tract Dilatation

Fetal renal pelvis dilatation is a frequent abnormality that has been observed in 4.5% of pregnancies.[25] Pyelectasis and pelviectasis are defined as dilatation of the renal pelvis, whereas pelvicaliectasis and hydronephrosis include dilatation of calyces. In practice, these terms are interchanged and used as descriptions of a dilated renal collecting system regardless of etiology.[26]

The third-trimester threshold value for the anteroposterior (AP) renal pelvis diameter of 7 mm is certainly the best prenatal criterion for both the screening of urinary tract dilatation and the selection of patients needing postnatal investigation.[22,25] Yet a 4-mm threshold for AP pelvis diameter during the second trimester of pregnancy should be considered a warning sign, because this finding may reveal a significant urologic abnormality in 12% of cases.[25]

TABLE 4-1 Conditions Associated with Hyperechoic Kidneys

	Kidney Size	Amniotic Fluid Volume	Renal Cysts	Collecting System	Associated Abnormalities	Inheritance	Alternative Prenatal Diagnosis
Obstruction	−2 to 0 SD	Normal or reduced	Cortical <1 cm	Dilated	No	Sporadic	MRI
Bilateral MCDK	Variable	Reduced	Variable sizes, mostly large	Not seen	Variable if syndromic	Sporadic	MRI
Renal vein thrombosis	0 to 2 SD	Normal	No	Not seen	Thrombus in the inferior vena cava	Sporadic	Doppler
ARPKD	2 to 4 SD	Reduced	Small medullary	Not seen	Lung hypoplasia	AR	Genetics
ADPKD	0 to 2 SD	Normal or reduced	Subcapsular and medullary	Not seen	No	AD	Genetics
Glomerulocystic dysplasia	0 to 2 SD	Variable	Small cortical	Not seen	Variable if syndromic	Variable	Genetics (*HNFβ1*)
Bardet-Biedl syndrome	2 to 4 SD	Variable	No or medullary	Not seen	Polydactyly	AR	Genetics
Beckwith-Wiedemann syndrome	2 SD	Normal or increased	No or medullary	±	Macrosome, omphalocele	AD or dysomy	Genetics
Perlman syndrome	2 SD	Normal or reduced	No	±	Macrosome	AR	—
Nephrocalcinosis	Variable	Normal	No	Not seen	No	Sporadic	—
Normal variant	0 to 2 SD	Normal or increased	No	±	No	Sporadic	—

AD, Autosomal dominant; *AR*, autosomal recessive; *ARPKD*, autosomal recessive polycystic kidney disease; *ADPKD*, autosomal dominant polycystic kidney disease; *HNF-1β*, hepatocyte nuclear factor-1β; *MCDK*, multicystic dysplastic kidney; *MRI*, magnetic resonance imaging.

TABLE 4-2 Incidence of Uronephropathies in Neonates with Antenatally Diagnosed Renal Pelvis Dilatation

Authors (ref. no.)	Year	Threshold Value of Renal Pelvis (mm)	Total	Abnormal (%)	UPJS (%)	VUR (%)	Megaureter (%)	Mild Dilatation (%)	Kidney (%)	Duplex Other (%)	(%) Undergoing Surgery
Dudley et al. (32)	1997	5	100	64	3	12	3	43	4	7	3
Stocks et al. (33)	1996	4-7	27	70	22	22		26			11
Jaswon et al. (34)	1999	5	104	45	4	22		8		4	1
Ismaili et al. (29)	2004	4-7	213	39	13	11	7	18*	5	3	3

UPJS, Uretero-pelvic junction stenosis; *VUR*, vesicoureteral reflux.
*In this study mild and transient dilatations were considered as nonsignificant findings.

There are several theories that account for the visibility of the renal pelvis during pregnancy. The distension of the urinary collecting system may simply be a dynamic and physiologic process.[27] Persutte et al. found the size of the fetal renal collecting system to be highly variable over a 2-hour period.[28] The tendency of renal pelvis dilatation to resolve spontaneously is supported by normal postnatal renal appearances reported in 36% to 80% of cases followed up after birth.[29,30] However, prenatally detected renal pelvis dilatation may be an indicator of significant urinary tract pathologies.[31] The likelihood of having a clinically significant uropathy is directly proportional to the severity of hydronephrosis.[26] A summary of the literature describing the postnatal uronephropathies found in neonates who presented with fetal renal pelvis dilatation is given in Table 4-2. The incidence and type of pathology vary considerably between studies, reflecting the differences in prenatal criteria and the variability in postnatal assessment. The two main pathologies found are pelviureteric junction stenosis and VUR. US is the first examination to perform after birth.[35] In babies with fetal renal pelvis dilatation, the presence of persistent renal pelvis dilatation or other ultrasonographic abnormalities (such as calyceal or ureteral dilatation, pelvic or ureteral wall thickening, or absence of the corticomedullary differentiation) and signs of renal dysplasia (such as small kidney, thinned or hyperechoic cortex, or cortical cysts) should determine the need for further inves-

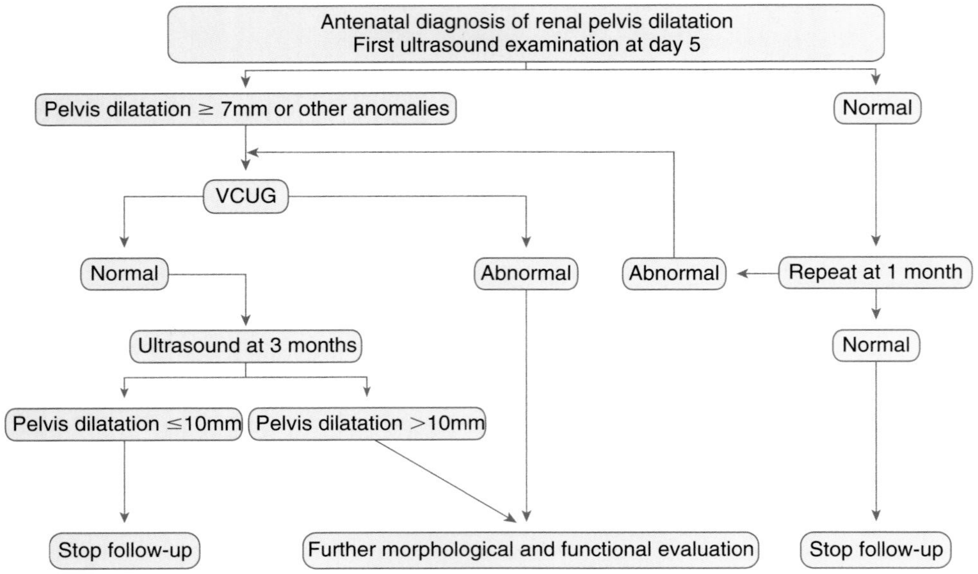

Figure 4-2 Algorithm of a rational postnatal imaging strategy in infants with mild to moderate fetal renal pelvis dilatation.

tigation.[36,37] In cases where the urinary tract appears normal on neonatal ultrasound examinations, no further evaluation is needed.[29] Based on our experience,[29,36,38] we propose an algorithm for a rational postnatal imaging strategy (Figure 4-2). Using this algorithm, we found that very few abnormal cases escaped the workup and that the risk of complications was very low.

Renal Cysts

Renal cystic diseases should be suspected not only in the case of obvious macrocysts but also in the case of hyperechoic kidneys.[24] Cysts may be present in one or both kidneys. Their origin may be genetic, and they may occur as an isolated anomaly or as part of a syndrome. Familial history is of great importance for the diagnosis.[39]

Obstructive renal dysplasia and MCDK are the most common entities in which macrocysts can be detected. Obstructive renal dysplasia is associated with urinary tract obstruction that may have resolved at the time of diagnosis, leaving the cystic sequelae behind as sole evidence that urinary flow impairment ever existed.[8] In this condition, the cysts measure less than 1 cm and are located within the hyperechoic cortex.[20] MCDK is discussed further under Renal Causes of Fetal Renal Abnormalities in this chapter. Although rare, isolated cortical cysts may be seen in utero. They may persist after birth or regress spontaneously.[40]

The most frequent genetically transmitted cystic renal diseases are the autosomal recessive and dominant polycystic kidney diseases (also discussed under Renal Causes of Fetal Renal Abnormalities). Abnormalities of the hepatocyte nuclear factor-1β (HNF-1β) encoded by the *TCF2* gene are typically associated with bilateral cortical renal microcysts and also with other renal parenchymal abnormalities, including MCDK and renal dysplasia.[41] Indeed, HNF-1β plays an important role in the early phases of kidney development.[42] It has a close relationship with other cystic diseases and may be a major factor in cystogenesis.[43] Cystic kidneys can also be part of many syndromes (Tables 4-1 and 4-3) that present associated anomalies that are sometimes typical of the underlying pathology.

Renal Tumors

Fetal renal tumors occur only rarely. Mesoblastic nephroma represents the most common congenital renal neoplasm.[52] It is a solitary hamartoma with a usually benign course. Mesoblastic nephroma appears as a large, solitary, predominantly solid, retroperitoneal mass arising and not separable from the adjacent normal kidney. It does not have a well-defined capsule and may sometimes appear as a partially cystic tumor,[8] although in the case of a tumor with multiple cysts, an MCDK should be considered first. It frequently coexists with polyhydramnios, although the reason for this association remains unclear.[52] Wilms' tumor is exceptionally rare in the fetus and may be indistinguishable from mesoblastic nephroma on imaging.[53] Another differential diagnosis to include is nephroblastomatosis, which appears either as hyperechoic nodule(s) or as a diffusely enlarged hyperechoic kidney.[54] Renal tumors have to be differentiated from adrenal tumors and from intraabdominal sequestrations.[55]

Bladder Abnormalities

Nonvisualization of the bladder in the setting of oligohydramnios indicates strong evidence of bilateral severe renal abnormality with decreased urine production. It is, however, important to carry out the examination for 60 minutes before stating its nonvisualization.

An enlarged bladder (above 3 cm in the second trimester and above 6 cm in the third trimester) suggests a bladder outlet obstruction. In the second trimester, a bladder enlargement may result from posterior urethral valve, urethral atresia, or urethral stenosis, or be part of a prune belly sequence. The degree of oligohydramnios, associated urinary tract dilatation, and renal dysplasia are variable, but the prognosis is often poor. During the third trimester an obstruc-

TABLE 4-3 **Syndromes with Cystic Renal Disease**

	Renal Cysts	Associated Abnormalities	Inheritance	Reference
Meckel-Gruber syndrome	Medullary	Encephalocele, brain/cardiac anomalies, cleft lip/palate, polydactyly	AR	(44)
Trisomy 9	Medullary	Mental retardation, intrauterine growth retardation, cardiac anomalies, joint contractures, prominent nose, sloping forehead	Chromosomal	(45)
Trisomy 13	Medullary	Mental retardation, intrauterine growth retardation, cardiac anomalies, cleft lip/palate, polydactyly	Chromosomal	(45)
Trisomy 18	Medullary	Mental retardation, intrauterine growth retardation, cardiac anomalies, small face, micrognathia, overlapping digits	Chromosomal	(45)
Bardet-Biedl syndrome	No or medullary	Polysyndactyly, obesity, mental retardation, pigmented retinopathy, hypogonadism	AR	(46)
Zellweger syndrome	Medullary	Hypotonia, seizures, failure to thrive, distinctive face, hepatosplenomegaly	AR	(47)
Ivemark syndrome	No or medullary	Polysplenia, complex heart disease, midline anomalies, situs inversus	Sporadic, AR	(48)
Beckwith-Wiedemann syndrome	Medullary	Overgrowth, macroglossia, omphalocele, hepatoblastoma, Wilms' tumor	Sporadic, AD	(49)
Jeune's syndrome	Medullary	Narrow chest, short limbs, polydactyly, periglomerular fibrosis	AR	(50)
Tuberous sclerosis	Medullary	Mental retardation, seizures, facial angiofibroma, angiomyolipoma, hypopigmented spots, cardiac rhabdomyomas, cerebral hamartomas	AD	(51)

AD, Autosomal dominant; *AR*, autosomal recessive.

tive origin has to be differentiated from other causes of bladder enlargement, such as massive VUR and megacystis-microcolon-intestial hypoperistalsis (MMH) syndrome.[56]

Nonvisualization of the bladder with an otherwise normal sonogram probably is not clinically significant. However, it may occur with bladder or cloacal exstrophy as well as other abnormalities that alter the appearance of the bladder.[57] In the case of bladder exstrophy, no bladder is seen between the two umbilical arteries; instead, a small mass is seen below the umbilical insertion of the cord. Bladder exstrophy is a difficult sonographic diagnosis since some fluid may be trapped between the open bladder and the thighs; this may be misinterpreted as a normal bladder.[58]

ASSESSMENT OF FETAL RENAL FUNCTION

In utero, excretion of nitrogenous waste products and regulation of fetal fluid and electrolyte balance as well as acid-base homeostasis are maintained by the interaction of the placenta and maternal blood.[59] Thus the placenta functions as an in vivo dialysis unit. Prenatally, several parameters have been used in the evaluation of fetal renal function. However, since fetal homeostasis depends on the integrity of the placenta, it is very difficult to assess the functional status of the fetal kidney. Furthermore, changes in the volume or composition of fetal urine may in many instances reflect the condition of the placenta rather than the condition of the fetal kidney.[60] However, exact diagnosis of renal abnormalities and accurate prediction of the renal function after birth are important tasks, because different renal diseases may require different approaches and therapies. Therefore in addition to using fetal renal sonography to determine potential fetal renal anatomical abnormalities, one must be able to assess function as accurately as possible.

Amniotic Fluid Volume

During the first trimester of gestation, the placenta (chorion and amniotic membrane) is the principal source of amniotic fluid, but after 15 weeks, fetal kidneys produce the majority of amniotic fluid. Therefore assessment of the quantity of amniotic fluid after 15 weeks constitutes the first step in evaluating the fetal urinary tract. Abnormal amounts of amniotic fluid must alert the sonographer to search diligently for renal and urinary tract anomalies.[61] Assessing amniotic fluid volume is difficult and mostly subjective. However, the four-quadrant sum of amniotic fluid pockets (amniotic fluid index) provides a reproducible method for assessing amniotic fluid volume with interobserver and intraobserver variation of 3% to 7%.[62]

Various cutoff criteria have been suggested for determination of oligohydramnios by the amniotic fluid index, including less than 1st percentile,[63] or 5th percentile for gestational age.[62] Oligohydramnios of whatever cause typically compresses and twists the fetus, thus leading to a recurrent pattern of abnormalities that has been called the oligohydramnios sequence.[16] Oligohydramnios may be caused by decreased production of fetal urine from bilateral renal agenesis or dysplasia, or by reduced egress of urine into the amniotic fluid due to urinary obstruction. Other causes may be fetal death, growth retardation, rupture of the membranes, or postterm gestation (Table 4-4).

In cases of bilateral obstructive uropathy, a recent study found the evaluation of amniotic fluid by the amniotic fluid

TABLE 4-4 **Causes of Oligohydramnios and Polyhydramnios**

	Origin	Pathologies
Oligohydramnios	Uronephropathy	Bilateral renal agenesis Bilateral renal dysplasia Autosomal recessive polycystic kidney disease Bilateral obstructive uropathy Bilateral high-grade reflux Bladder outlet obstruction
	Other	Premature rupture of membranes Placental insufficiency Fetal death Fetal growth retardation Twin-to-twin transfusion (twin donor) Maternal drug intake: prostaglandin synthase inhibitors, angiotensin-converting enzyme inhibitors, cocaine Postmaturity syndrome
Polyhydramnios	Uronephropathy	Renal tumors, especially mesoblastic nephroma Bartter syndrome Congenital nephrotic syndrome Alloimmune glomerulonephritis
	Other	Maternal diabetes Maternal drug intake: lithium, Multiple gestations Twin-to-twin transfusion (twin recipient) Fetal infections: rubella, cytomegalovirus, toxoplasmosis Fetal gastrointestinal obstructions: esophageal atresia, duodenal atresia, gastroschisis Fetal compressive pulmonary disorders: diaphragmatic hernia, pleural effusions, cystic adenomatoid malformations, narrow thoracic cage Neuromuscular conditions: anencephaly, myotonic dystrophy Cardiac anomalies Hematologic anomalies (fetal anemia) Hydrops fetalis Fetal chromosome abnormalities: trisomy 21, trisomy 18, trisomy 13 Syndromic conditions: Beckwith-Wiedemann syndrome, achondroplasia No evident cause

index to be the most reproducible and inexpensive method for predicting renal function after birth.[64] The study also showed that an amniotic fluid index less than the 5th percentile was generally associated with an adverse perinatal outcome. Yet an amniotic fluid index between the 5th and 25th percentiles should be taken as a warning sign since it may be a subtle indication of renal impairment, especially early in gestation when ultrasonographic signs of renal dysplasia may not be present and when fetal urinalysis is not available.[64]

Finally, one of the most devastating consequences of oligohydramnios, especially before 24 weeks' gestation, is pulmonary hypoplasia.[9] Traditional explanations suggest that oligohydramnios causes pulmonary hypoplasia either by compression of the fetal thorax[65] or by encouraging lung liquid loss via the trachea.[66] However, since several morphogenetic pathways governing renal development are shared with lung organogenesis, some reports suggest that abnormal lung dysplasia may precede the advent of oligohydramnios in fetuses with intrinsic defects of renal parenchymal development.[67]

Polyhydramnios, also referred to as hydramnios, is defined as a high level of amniotic fluid. Because the normal values for amniotic fluid volumes increase during pregnancy, this definition will depend on the gestational age of the fetus. During the last 2 months of pregnancy, polyhydramnios usually refers to amniotic fluid volumes greater than 1700 to 1900 ml. Severe cases are associated with much greater fluid volume excesses. The two major causes of polyhydramnios are reduced fetal swallowing or absorption of amniotic fluid, and increased fetal urination (Table 4-4). Increased fetal urination is typically observed in maternal diabetes mellitus, but it may be associated with fetal renal diseases such as mesoblastic nephroma,[52] Bartter syndrome,[68] congenital nephrotic syndrome,[69] and alloimmune glomerulonephritis.[70]

Fetal Urine Biochemical Markers

Fetal urine biochemistry was introduced about 20 years ago as an additional test to improve prediction of perinatal death and renal failure at birth.[71] Thereafter, investigators started to establish reference ranges with gestation for different biochemical parameters of fetal urine.[72] Fetal urine biochemistry is currently used especially in dilated uropathies because of technical difficulties in sampling fetal urines from a nondilated urinary tract, as seen in the majority of nephropathies. Sodium is the most widely used fetal urinary marker, although other compounds such as calcium, chloride, and β_2-microglobulin may also be of interest; prognostic values of these markers are outlined in Table 4-5. Most studies related to the analysis of fetal urine agree on some points[77]: (1)

TABLE 4-5 **Fetal Urine Biochemical Markers by Groups of Outcome**

	Normal Limits (73)	Good Prognosis (74, 75)	Postnatal Moderate Renal Failure after 1 Year (76, 77)	Poor Prognosis (Neonatal Death or Termination of Pregnancy) (75, 76)
Na+	75-100 mmol/L	<100 mmol/L	59 mmol/L (54-65)	121 mmol/L (100-140)
Ca++	2 mmol/L		2 mmol/L (1.5-2.5)	2 mmol/L (1.5-2.5)
Cl-		<90 mmol/L	57 mmol/L (52-62)	98 mmol/L (85-111)
β_2 microglobulin	<4 mg/L	<6 mg/L	6.77 mg/L (4.16-9.37)	19.5 mg/L (11-28)
Cystatin C		<1 mg/L	0.47 mg/L (0.05-4.75)	4.1 mg/L (0.45-13.1)
Osmolarity	<200 mOsm/L	<210 mOsm/L		

TABLE 4-6 **Fetal Serum Biochemical Markers by Groups of Outcome**

	Normal Values (78)	Normal Values (79)	Bilateral Hypoplasia and Dysplasia (80)	Bilateral Uropathies (79)
	Controls	Controls	Good prognosis	Neonatal death or termination of pregnancy
β_2 microglobulin	4.28 mg/L (2.95-6.61)	3.2 mg/L (1.5-4.7)	3.2 mg/L (1.5-3.7)	7 mg/L (5.1-10.6)
Cystatin C	1.67 mg/L (1.12-2.06)		1.43 mg/L (1.09-1.86)	

fetuses with renal damage (dysplasia) show increased urinary concentrations of solutes, (2) urinary sodium and calcium yield the best accuracy among measurable electrolytes, (3) β_2-microglobulin and cystatin C allow better accuracy than the measurement of any single electrolyte, and (4) the accuracy of the proposed parameters are, however, far from perfect.

Fetal Blood Sampling

Fetal blood sampling probably poses greater risks than urine sampling, but it allows measurement of a better index of fetal glomerular filtration rate (GFR).[77] In the fetus, creatinine cannot be used as a marker of GFR because it crosses the placenta and is cleared by the mother. This is not the case with β_2-microglobulin and cystatin C, which have been used to predict renal function in uropathies, in bilateral hypoplasia, and in hyperechogenic kidneys (Table 4-6). This technique is promising, especially in cases where fetal urine is difficult to sample. However, it is unlikely that β_2-microglobulin and cystatin C will overcome the limitations associated with fetal urinalysis.[77] The only take-home message of clinical interest would be that fetal serum β_2-microglobulin is helpful only when extreme values are found (less than 3.5 mg/L, good outcome; more than 5 mg/L, poor outcome).[80]

Ultrasound-Guided Renal Biopsies

Although ultrasound-guided renal biopsy would theoretically allow precise definition of the extent of renal damage in obstructed and primarily dysplastic kidneys,[81] this approach is limited by its invasiveness and high rate of failure in obtaining an adequate sample.[77] Furthermore, a focal needle aspiration is not representative of the whole kidney parenchyma since renal dysplasia is patchily distributed.

SPECIFIC RENAL AND URINARY TRACT PATHOLOGIES

Causes of fetal abnormal kidney and urinary tract may be considered as prerenal, renal, and postrenal.

Prerenal Causes of Fetal Renal Abnormalities

Intrauterine Growth Restriction

Intrauterine growth restriction caused by placental insufficiency is often associated with oligohydramnios because of the reduced urine production rate in these fetuses. This phenomenon is probably due to chronic hypoxemia, which leads to the brain-sparing redistribution of oxygenated blood away from nonvital peripheral organs such as the kidneys.[59] As a consequence, fetal renal medullary hyperechogenicity may develop between the twenty-fourth and thirty-seventh weeks of gestation due to tubular blockage caused by Tamm-Horsfall protein precipitation and may be a sign of hypoxic renal insufficiency.[82] Intrauterine growth retardation complicated by renal medullary hyperechogenicity suggests a more serious state, because these fetuses have a higher risk of pathological postnatal clinical outcome: 8% of neonatal mortality, 36% of fetal distress leading to cesarean section, 64% of transfer to intensive care unit, and 24% of perinatal infection.[82]

Renal Vein Thrombosis

Renal vein thrombosis is the most common vascular condition in the newborn kidney and represents 0.5 in 1000 admissions to neonatal intensive care units.[83] Factors predisposing a neonate to renal vein thrombosis include dehydration, sepsis, birth asphyxia, maternal diabetes, polycythemia, and the presence of indwelling umbilical venous catheter.[84] In addi-

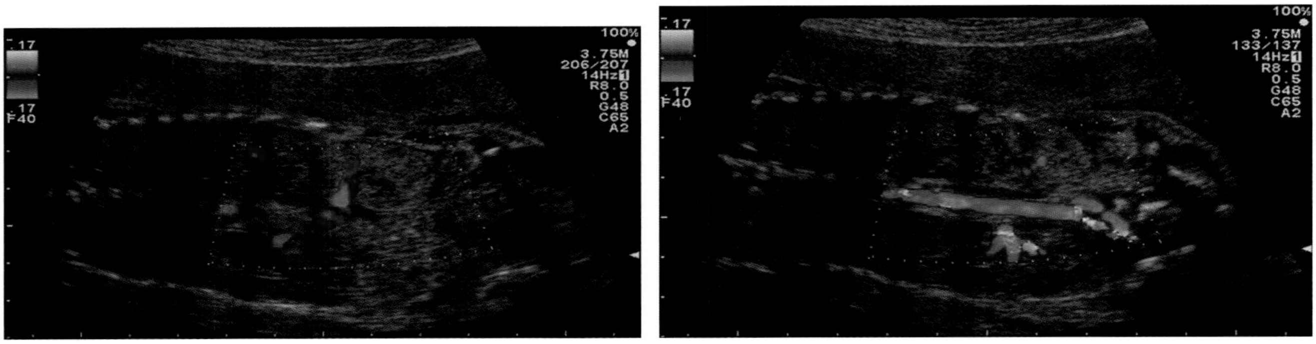

A B

Figure 4-3 Renal vein thrombosis (third trimester). Sagittal color Doppler US scan of the right kidney **(A).** Intrarenal and renal venous flows are almost absent in comparison with the normal left kidney **(B).**

tion, prothrombotic abnormalities may be present in more than 40% of these babies and include protein C or S deficiency, factor V Leiden, lupus anticoagulant, and antithrombin III deficiency.[85] Renal vein thrombosis may also occur in utero; the origin of the thrombosis, however, is not always obvious. Sonographically, the fetal kidney appears somewhat enlarged; the cortex may appear hyperechoic and without corticomedullary differentiation. Pathognomonic vascular streaks may be visible in the interlobar areas. Thrombus in the inferior vena cava is a usual association.[8] Color Doppler US may be used in addition to gray-scale examination in the assessment of renal vein thrombosis (Figures 4-3, *A*, and 4-3, *B*). In the early stages of renal vein thrombosis, intrarenal and renal venous flow and pulsatility may be absent and renal arterial diastolic flow may be decreased, with a raised resistive index. Collateral vessels develop rapidly, and in most cases there are no consequences on further renal development.[86] After birth, the hyperechoic streaks and the thrombus are calcified. This feature helps differentiate antenatal from postnatal onset of the renal vein thrombosis.[86]

The Twin-to-Twin Transfusion Syndrome

The twin-to-twin transfusion syndrome complicates 10% to 15% of monochorionic twin pregnancies.[87] The etiology of this condition is not completely understood but is thought to result from an unbalanced fetal blood supply through the placental vascular shunts, with the larger twin being the recipient and the smaller twin the donor.[88] The twin-to-twin transfusion syndrome is defined as presentation with the oligopolihydramnios sequence (that is, the deepest vertical pool being 2 cm or less in the donor's sac and 8 cm or more in the recipient's sac).[87] Additional phenotypic features in the donor include a small or nonvisible bladder and abnormal umbilical artery Doppler with absent or reverse end-diastolic frequencies. In addition to the neonatal complications of growth restriction, up to 30% of donors have renal failure or renal tubular dysgenesis or both due to the chronic renal hypoperfusion state in utero.[87] In the recipient, confirmatory features include large bladder, cardiac hypertrophy, and eventually hydrops. Risk of renal failure in the recipient twin is considerably smaller than in the donor twin. This can be seen as one fetus dying and vascular resistance dropping significantly to cause reversed blood transfusion from the recipient twin to the dead fetus, resulting in hypovolemia and anemia in the live fetus.[89]

Maternal Drug Intake

Some drugs taken by the mother can impair fetal renal function or produce congenital renal anomalies.

Angiotensin-Converting Enzyme Inhibitors Angiotensin-converting enzyme inhibitors (ACEIs) can severely affect renal development and function when used in the second and third trimesters of pregnancy and can lead to tubular dysgenesis, oligohydramnios, growth restriction, neonatal anuria, or stillbirth.[90] Until recently, information derived from a limited number of studies in animals and analysis of case reports showed no adverse fetal effects linked to the use of these drugs in the first trimester.[91] However, a study reported by Cooper et al. has shown that almost 9% of children whose mothers were prescribed ACEIs during the first trimester (but not later in pregnancy) had major congenital anomalies (cardiovascular, central nervous system, and renal malformations), a rate 2.7 times that among unexposed infants.[92] The renal anomalies are thought to be caused first by a direct action of ACEIs on the fetal renin-angiotensin system that reduces the concentration of angiotensin II, and then by secondary fetoplacental ischemia resulting from maternal hypotension and a drop of fetal-placental blood flow.[59]

Angiotensin II Receptor Antagonists (ARBs) Many reports have described fetal abnormalities that are strikingly similar to those produced by maternal treatment with ACEIs, in association with maternal use of ARBs.[93,94] As for ACEIs, maternal treatment with ARBs should be avoided.[94] Maternal treatment with ACEIs combined with sartans (ARBs) should be avoided.[94]

Nonsteroidal Antiinflammatory Drugs Cyclooxygenase type 1 (COX-1) inhibitors such as indomethacin, the most common nonsteroidal antiinflammatory drug (NSAID) used as a tocolytic, definitely reduce urine output and may lead to oligohydramnios and renal dysfunction.[59] It was hoped that cyclooxygenase type 2 (COX-2) inhibitors would target COX-2 activity and potentially spare COX-1–specific fetal side effects. However, human fetal kidneys have been shown to have an increased expression of COX-2 compared with adult kidneys, suggesting that COX-2 is constitutively expressed in the human fetal kidney.[59] Experience with sulindac and nimesulide has therefore been linked with both constriction of the ductus arteriosus and oligohydramnios.[95]

Cocaine Maternal cocaine use adversely influences fetal renal function by hypoperfusion and thus influences the fetal renin-angiotensin system. It is also associated with oligohydramnios and other fetal vascular complications, leading to a higher renal artery resistance index and a significant decrease in urine output.[96] However, and contradicting a widely held belief,[97] a recent prospective, large-scale, blinded, and systematic evaluation for congenital anomalies in prenatally cocaine-exposed children did not identify any increase in the number or consistent pattern of genitourinary tract malformations.[98]

Immunosuppressive Medications During Pregnancy When the field of transplantation was first developing, physicians worried about the potential effects of immunosuppressive medications on the child-to-be and considered pregnancy ill-advised for patients taking these medications.[99] Despite early concerns, approximately 14,000 births among women with transplanted organs have been reported worldwide.[100] Although some immunosuppressive drugs such as azathioprine, cyclosporine, and mycophenolate mofetil (MMF) have been found to be teratogenic in animals, registry records and case reports to date have found no unifying patterns of malformations in children of recipients of solid organs.[101] However, maternal use of MMF has been discouraged by the European transplantation community because questions continue as to whether MMF is associated with higher risks of fetal malformations.[102] Therefore European best practice guidelines recommend that women receiving MMF transition to another agent and wait 6 weeks before they attempt to conceive.[103]

Renal Causes of Fetal Renal Abnormalities

Multicystic Dysplastic Kidney

Multicystic dysplastic kidney (MCDK) is a prominent example of an accident of renal development. These kidneys contain bizarrely shaped tubules surrounded by a stroma that includes undifferentiated and metaplastic (for example, smooth muscle and cartilage) cells. Data collected by Liebeschuetz[104] put the prevalence of MCDK at 1 in 2400 live births, which is far higher than older reports.[105] MCDK is usually unilateral and presents typical US pattern: multiple noncommunicating cysts of varying size and nonmedial location of the largest cyst, absence of normal renal sinus echoes, and absence of normal renal parenchyma.[106] MCDK may also develop in the upper part of a duplex system or be located in an ectopic position. The prognosis for unilateral isolated MCDK is good, but meticulous examination of the contralateral kidney is essential because there is a high incidence of associated pathologies, many of which may not be detected until birth.[4,107] The distinction between MCDK and cystic renal dysplasia associated with urinary tract obstruction may be difficult, especially in the absence of hydronephrosis. This distinction, although helpful in terms of diagnosis, may be somewhat artificial in terms of prognosis, since in either case the affected kidney has minimal or no functional capacity.

Autosomal Recessive Polycystic Kidney Disease (ARPKD)

ARPKD has an incidence of 1 in 20,000 live births and may cause fetal and neonatal death in severe cases. Mutations in the *PKHD1* gene are usually demonstrated in this disease.[108] Yet since some patients survive the neonatal period with few or slight symptoms, additional genes are probably involved.[109] The disease is characterized by marked elongation of the collecting tubules that expand into multiple small cysts. The cystic dilatation of the tubules is variable and predominates in the medulla. The outer cortex is spared since it contains no tubules. The classical in utero pattern of ARPKD includes markedly enlarged (+4 SD) hyperechoic kidneys without corticomedullary differentiation. This appearance can be observed in the second trimester. The patterns may evolve and the size of the kidneys may continuously increase during the third trimester. Oligohydramnios and lung hypoplasia may be present, and therefore the prognosis is extremely poor.

Another presentation of ARPKD is reversed corticomedullary differentiation with large kidneys (+2 to +4 SD) (Figure 4-4). This finding is probably related to increased interfaces within the medullae and to the presence of material within the dilated tubules.[109] It is an important observation since there are few other causes of reversed corticomedullary differentiation. The liver involvement typical of the condition is usually impossible to demonstrate in utero. The differential diagnosis includes the glomerulocystic type of autosomal dominant polycystic kidney disease, Bardet-Biedl syndrome in which polydactyly is present,[46] and other rare entities such as bilateral renal tumors, medullary sponge kidney, bilateral nephroblastomatosis, Finnish-type nephrosis, medullary cystic disease, or congenital metabolic diseases (that is, glycogen storage disease or tyrosinosis). Oligohydramnios and absence of urine within the bladder would favor ARPKD over all of these rare entities.

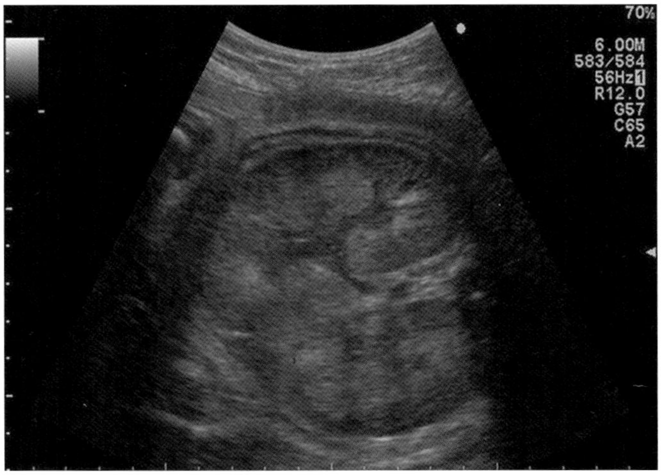

Figure 4-4 Autosomal recessive polycystic kidney disease. Sagittal scan through the kidneys that appear large (+3 SD), with reversed corticomedullary differentiation due to hyperechoic medulla, third trimester.

Autosomal Dominant Polycystic Kidney Disease

Autosomal dominant polycystic kidney disease (ADPKD) is a common hereditary kidney disease, with 1 in 1000 people carrying the gene. The pathological abnormality consists of cystic dilatation of all parts of the nephron, which causes the kidneys to enlarge as the cortex and medulla become replaced by cysts, thus leading to end-stage renal failure. There are two major types of ADPKD: type I is caused by mutations in the *PKD1* gene on chromosome 16p13.3 and accounts for 85% to 90% of cases,[110] and type II is caused by mutations in the *PKD2* gene on chromosome 4q21-22 and accounts for 10% to 15% of cases.[111] One or more other genes (type III) are likely involved since some obvious cases have none of these mutations. Although the age of clinical onset of this disorder is typically in the third to fifth decade of life, early manifestations during childhood or during the prenatal period have been reported.[112,113] There may be two different presentations in utero. In most cases the kidneys are not grossly enlarged, but the corticomedullary differentiation is increased because of cortical hyperechogenicity. In this type of ADPKD, cysts are unusual in utero; they will develop after birth. Markedly enlarged kidneys resembling ARPKD are another pattern that can be encountered in utero and suggests the glomerulocystic type of ADPKD. In this presentation of the disease, some subcortical cysts may appear in utero and renal failure may appear at birth.[109]

Renal Hypoplasia and Dysplasia

Renal dysplasia refers to abnormal differentiation or organization of cells in the renal parenchyma and is characterized histologically by the presence of primitive ducts and nests of metaplastic cartilage.[23,24] Hypoplasia is a reduction of the number of nephrons in small kidneys (below –2 SD).[23] Hypoplasia may coexist with dysplasia and the diagnosis is inferred from the hyperechoic appearance on US caused by the lack of normal renal parenchyma and structurally abnormal small kidneys (Figure 4-5).[23,24] As in most cases the diagnosis is made by ultrasound examination. The spectrum of renal dysplasia includes inherited or congenital causes of renal hypoplasia, renal adysplasia, cystic dysplasia, oligomeganephronic hypoplasia, reflux nephropathy, and obstructive renal dysplasia.[23] Cases with oligohydramnios have the poorest outcome.[114] After birth, the prognosis depends on the remaining renal function at 6 months of age. Infants with a GFR below 15 ml/min/1.73 m^2 are at higher risk for early renal replacement therapy.[23]

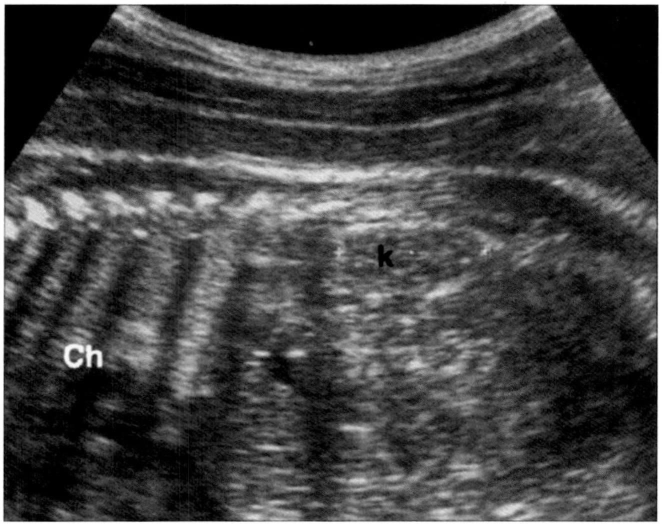

Figure 4-5 Renal hypoplasia (third trimester). Sagittal scan through the right kidney *(k)*, 20 mm between crosses (–3 SD). *Ch*, Chest.

Congenital Nephrotic Syndrome

Congenital nephrotic syndrome is defined as proteinuria leading to clinical symptoms during the 3 months after birth. Infantile nephrotic syndrome manifests later, in the first year of life. These classifications, however, are arbitrary because the majority of early-onset nephrotic syndrome diseases range from fetal life to several years of age.

Congenital nephrotic syndrome of the Finnish type (CNF) is characterized by autosomal recessive inheritance and is caused by mutations in the nephrin gene *(NPHS1)*.[115] The incidence is 1 in 8200 births in Finland, but it occurs worldwide. Most infants are born prematurely, with low birth weight for gestational age. The placenta is enlarged, weighing more than 25% of the birth weight. Edema is present at birth or appears within a few days due to severe nephrotic syndrome. In utero, the possible development of hydrops fetalis and increased nuchal translucency reflects massive proteinuria paralleled by a relatively high urine output.[116,117] Because the main part of amniotic fluid α-fetoprotein is derived from fetal urine, high values reflect intrauterine proteinuria.[118] If the α-fetoprotein concentration is 250,000 to 500,000 μg/L, and especially if there is another child with CNF in the family, it is highly suggestive of CNF.

Podocin gene *(NPHS2)* mutations have also been reported in patients with congenital nephrotic syndrome.[119] However, the severity of the disease is variable and may occur at birth, in childhood, or later in adulthood. Patients with podocin mutants that are retained in the endoplasmic reticulum, such as the R138Q mutant, are associated with the earliest onset of the disease.[119]

Pierson syndrome is a rare, lethal, autosomal recessive entity that includes congenital nephrotic syndrome attributable to diffuse mesangial sclerosis, in association with distinct eye abnormalities clinically characterized by bilateral microcoria.[120] The defective gene *(LAMB2)* has been localized to chromosome 3p21 and leads to a lack of laminin-2, an important component of the glomerular and other basement membranes.[121] In utero, fetuses may present, as in CNF, with hydrops fetalis and increased nuchal translucency. However, these findings are inconstant because severe renal failure may be already present in these fetuses, leading to early regression of urine output, oligohydramnios, and sometimes consecutive pulmonary hypoplasia.[120] Fetal kidneys appear impressively more hyperechoic than those reported in fetuses with CNF.[122]

Other cases of prenatally diagnosed congenital nephrotic syndrome have been reported, including isolated, sporadic, or familial diffuse mesangial sclerosis,[117,123] secondary nephrotic syndrome due to CMV or other intrauterine infections,[124] and massive proteinuria in offsprings of mothers with homozygous deficiency for the metallomembrane endopeptidase.[70]

Postrenal Causes of Fetal Renal Abnormalities

Dilatations of the renal pelvis, calyces, and ureters are the principal signs of impaired urinary flow on antenatal ultrasound scanning.

Ureteropelvic Junction Stenosis

Pelviureteric junction stenosis occurs in 13% of children with antenatally diagnosed renal pelvis dilatation[29] and is characterized by obstruction at the level of the junction between the renal pelvis and the ureter (Figure 4-6). The anatomical basis for obstruction includes intrinsic stenosis or valves, peripelvic fibrosis, or crossing vessels.[125] Sonographic diagnosis depends on the demonstration of a dilated renal pelvis in the absence of any dilatation of ureter or bladder (Figure 4-6). It should be particularly suspected when moderate (10 to 15 mm) or severe (greater than 15 mm) dilatation is seen in these circumstances.[26] Prognosis may be poor in bilateral cases associated with oligohydramnios and hyperechoic parenchyma. Postnatal management of these children remains controversial among the nephrourologic community.[126] Expectancy and close follow-up[127] have progressively gained wide acceptance, although the surgical attitude, either systematic within the first months of life or on the basis of variable morphological or functional parameters, is still the current attitude for many clinicians.[128] However, the final outcome, being when these children have reached old age, is remote.

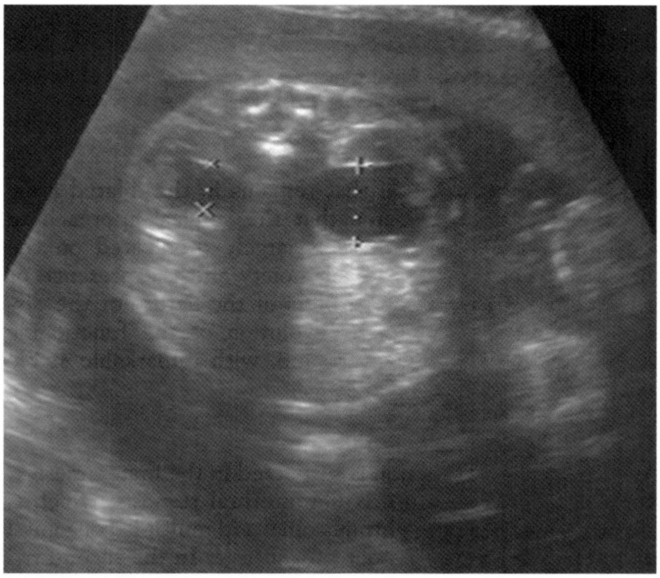

Figure 4-6 Bilateral asymmetrical pelvicalyceal dilatation (case of uretopelvic junction stenosis), third trimester. Transverse scan through fetal abdomen: marked left (20 mm) and moderate right (10 mm) dilatation.

Vesicoureteric Reflux (VUR)

VUR is defined as the retrograde flow of urine from the bladder upward within the ureter, sometimes extending into the renal pelvis, calyces, and collecting ducts. Fetal renal pelvis dilatation can signal the presence of VUR in 11%[29] to 30%[129] of cases, with the lower figure being more realistic. Making a precise diagnosis of VUR in utero is difficult, except in the rare cases that may have intermittent renal collecting system dilatation during real-time scanning (Figure 4-7).[130] The arguments surrounding the importance of diagnosing all cases of neonatal VUR center on the perceived magnitude of the risks of infection and functional decline. However, current evidence suggests that only patients with grades IV to V disease are at high risk of serious adverse outcome and delayed resolution.[131] Although some children with prenatal VUR may already have renal lesions, namely congenital dysplasia due to high-grade disease, VUR related to fetal renal pelvis dilatation was found in a large prospective study to be low grade in 74% of cases with a high rate of 2-year spontaneous resolution (91%).[6] Therefore it is unclear whether low-grade reflux detected antenatally is clinically significant. It is also unclear whether asymptomatic antenatally detected VUR and symptomatic postnatal VUR are the same pathologies.[26]

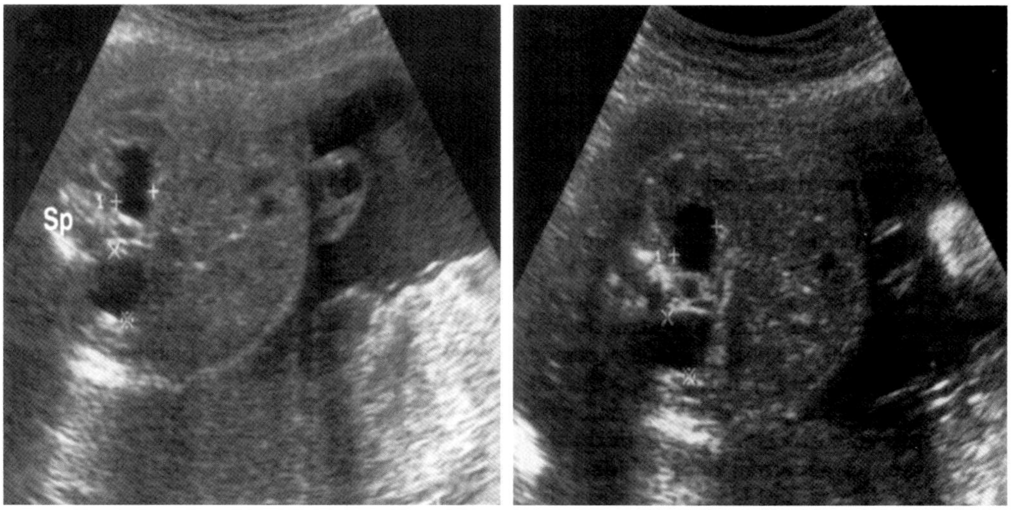

Figure 4-7 Fetal vesicoureteral reflux—transverse scans of the fetal abdomen. Intermittent renal collecting system dilatation during the same antenatal ultrasound examination due to vesicoureteral reflux. *Sp*, Spine.

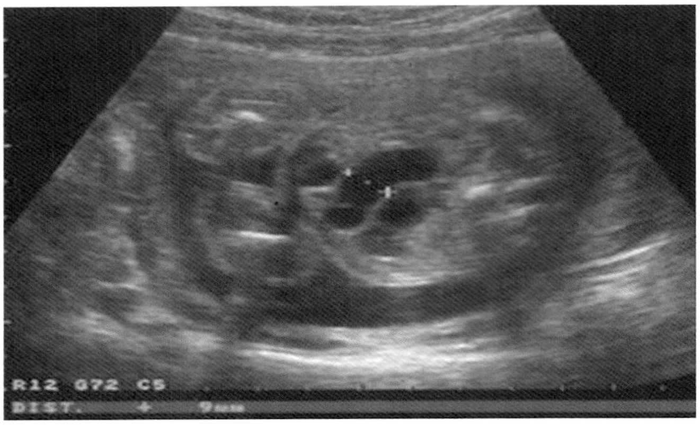

Figure 4-8 Megaureter. In utero dilatation of the right ureter (third trimester). Transverse scan of the fetal abdomen showing a serpentine fluid-filled structure. The ureter measures 9 mm (between the crosses).

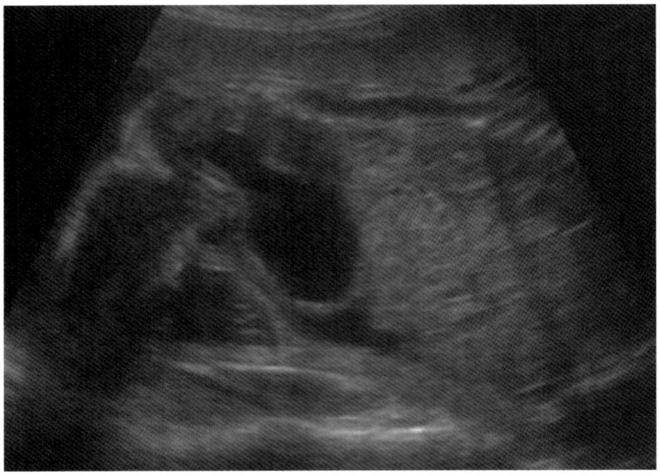

Figure 4-9 Megabladder (third trimester). Huge enlargement of the fetal bladder due to posterior urethral valves. The keyhole sign is present.

Ureterovesical Junction Obstruction (Megaureter)

The ureter may be dilated because of obstruction at the level of the junction between it and the bladder or as a result of nonobstructive causes, including high-grade reflux. Other secondary causes of megaureter should be suspected, such as neurogenic bladder or posterior urethral valves, because specific treatment strategies should be directed toward the underlying condition. Under normal conditions the ureter is not visualized in utero. Megaureter should be suspected in the presence of a serpentine fluid-filled structure with or without dilatation of the renal pelvis and calices (Figure 4-8). Prognosis of primary megaureter is generally good since most cases resolve spontaneously between ages 12 and 36 months.[132] However, in children with high-grade hydronephrosis or a retrovesical ureteral diameter of greater than 1 cm, the condition may resolve slowly and may require surgery.[132]

Duplex Kidneys

Duplication of the renal collecting system is characterized by the presence of a kidney having two pelvic structures with two ureters that may be completely or partially formed.[133] Many cases have no renal impairment and should be considered as normal variants.[29] However, a proportion of duplex kidneys may be associated with significant pathology, usually due to the presence of VUR or obstruction. Fetal urinary tract dilatations are related to complicated renal duplication in 4.7% of cases.[29] VUR usually involves only the lower pole ureter in 90% of cases. Compared to single-system reflux, duplex-system VUR tends to be of a higher grade with a high incidence of lower pole dysplasia.[5,134] Obstructive ureteroceles are associated with the upper pole ureter in 80% of cases, although obstruction of the upper pole may also occur secondary to isolated vesicoureteric junction obstruction.[133] In utero, duplex kidneys are highly suspected in the presence of two separate noncommunicating renal pelves, dilated ureters, cystic structures within one pole, and echogenic cyst in the bladder, representing ureterocele.[135] After birth, the classical radiological workup of abnormal duplex kidneys is based on US and VCUG.[136] The aim of US is to confirm the diagnosis, whereas VCUG is performed to detect VUR and to evaluate the ureterocele. Isotope studies are mandatory to determine renal function that remains in the dilated renal moiety. Most people agree that the surgical approach to complicated duplex systems is largely predicated on the function of the affected renal moiety and the presence or absence of function.[136] Regardless of the nature of the diseased moiety, however, the evolution of the functioning moiety seems favorable over time, with remarkable stable split renal function around 40%.[5]

Bladder Outlet Obstruction

When bladder obstruction is suspected in the first trimester, the most common cause is fibrourethral stenosis, which is mainly associated with chromosomal and multiple congenital anomalies and carries a poor prognosis.[137] In the second trimester the most common cause of lower urinary tract obstruction in male fetuses is posterior urethral valves, which are tissue leaflets fanning distally from the prostatic urethra to the external urinary sphincter. The failure of the bladder to empty during an extended examination and the presence of abnormal kidneys and oligohydramnios must raise suspicion of posterior urethral valves. On occasion the valve may be seen as an echogenic line and the dilated posterior urethra may take the aspect of a keyhole (Figure 4-9). The bladder wall is usually thick at this stage, and in extreme cases in utero rupture has also been observed with extravasation of urine, resulting in urinary ascites. This phenomenon is usually thought to be a protective pop-off mechanism. However, in many cases there is only a partial obstruction, and amniotic fluid volume can be maintained throughout pregnancy. In some cases spontaneous rupture of valves appears to occur in utero with the reappearance of cyclical emptying of the bladder. The most reliable prognostic indicators of poor renal functional status are presentation before 24 weeks, oligohydramnios, increased cortical echogenicity, and the absence of corticomedullary differentiation.

The prognosis in severe cases is often relatively easy to predict, and perinatal death will occur following pulmonary hypoplasia and renal failure.[138] In partial obstruction, however, the outcome is less predictable, and late morbidity most commonly takes the form of end-stage renal failure, which affects 15% to 30% of individuals during childhood.[139] Once the prognosis has been determined as accurately as possible, management of these cases should be performed in a fetal medicine and pediatric surgery reference center. In each new case the great variability of presentation makes participation of different specialists necessary in the difficult decision-making process. Various options should be discussed, including in utero follow-up with planned postnatal management, termination of pregnancy, and occasionally, in utero therapy.

It may appear reasonable to imagine that an antenatal intervention to relieve the obstruction after diagnosis may restore amniotic fluid levels, thereby allowing normal pulmonary maturation. Whether early intervention may prevent progressive renal deterioration or improve long-term renal outcomes, however, remains to be determined. A variety of in utero therapeutic approaches to bladder outflow obstruction have been tried. The open surgical technique of fetal vesicostomy has now been abandoned due to significant fetal loss, premature uterine contractions, and maternal morbidity.[140] Vesicoamniotic shunting is performed with US guidance using a pigtail shunt, which when inserted leaves one end in the fetal bladder and the other in the amniotic space. The morbidity of this technique is high, with a perinatal mortality of 53% and shunt complications of 45%.[73] Furthermore, end-stage renal failure was present in 40% of those children who survived.[73] Direct endoscopic ablation of the valves is a more recent technique and requires the introduction of an endoscope into the fetal bladder, leading to ablation of the valves either by laser, saline irrigation, or mechanical disruption using guide wire.[141,142] Direct visualization of the valves, however, is difficult, and it may be hard to avoid damage to surrounding tissues. Unfortunately, experience with these techniques does not support any advantage in terms of postnatal bladder dynamics or renal function improvement.

REFERENCES

1. Wiesel A, Queisser-Luft A, Clementi M, Bianca S, Stoll C; EUROSCAN Study Group: Prenatal detection of congenital renal malformation by fetal ultrasonographic examination: An analysis of 709,030 births in 12 European countries, *Eur J Med Genet* 48:131-44, 2005.
2. Toiviainen-Salo S, Garel L, Grignon A, Dubois J, Rypens F, Boisvert J, Perreault G, Decarie JC, Filiatrault D, Lapierre C, Miron MC, Bechard N: Fetal hydronephrosis: is there hope for consensus? *Pediatr Radiol* 34:519-29, 2004.
3. Cassart M, Massez A, Metens T, Rypens F, Lambot MA, Hall M, Avni FE: Complementary role of MRI after sonography in assessing bilateral urinary tract anomalies in the fetus, *AJR Am J Roentgenol* 182:689-95, 2004.
4. Avni EF, Thoua Y, Lalmand B, Didier F, Droulle P, Schulman CC: Multicystic dysplastic kidney: natural history from in utero diagnosis and postnatal follow-up, *J Urol* 138:1420-24.
5. Ismaili K, Hall M, Ham H, Piepsz A: Evolution of individual renal function in children with unilateral complex renal duplication, *J Pediatr* 147:208-12, 2005.
6. Ismaili K, Hall M, Piepsz A, Wissing KM, Collier F, Schulman C, Avni FE: Primary vesicoureteral reflux detected among neonates with a history of fetal renal pelvis dilatation: A prospective clinical and imaging study, *J Pediatr* 148:222-27, 2006.
7. Rabinowitz R, Peters MT, Vya S, Campbell S, Nicolaides KH: Measurement of fetal urine production in normal pregnancy by real-time ultrasonography, *Am J Obstet Gynecol* 161:1264-66, 1989.
8. Avni EF, Garel L, Hall M, Rypens F: Perinatal approach in anomalies of the urinary tract, adrenals and genital system. In Avni FE, editor: *Perinatal Imaging. From Ultrasound to MR Imaging,* Berlin Heidelberg New York, 2002, Springer.
9. Thomas IF, Smith DW: Oligohydramnios: cause of the nonrenal features of Potter's syndrome including pulmonary hypoplasia, *J Pediatr* 84:811-15, 1974.
10. Cuckow PM, Nyirady P, Winyard PJ: Normal and abnormal development of the urogenital tract, *Prenat Diagn* 21:908-16, 2001.
11. Zhou Q, Cardoza JD, Barth R: Prenatal sonography of congenital renal malformations, *AJR Am J Roentgenol* 173:1371-76, 1999.
12. Bronshtein M, Amit A, Achiron R, Noy I, Blumenfeld Z: The early prenatal sonographic diagnosis of renal agenesis: Techniques and possible pitfalls, *Prenat Diagn* 14:291-97, 1994.
13. Sepulveda W, Staggianis KD, Flack NJ, Fisk NM: Accuracy of prenatal diagnosis of renal agenesis with color flow imaging in severe second-trimester oligohydramnios, *Am J Obstet Gynecol* 173:1788-92, 1995.
14. Mesrobian HG, Rushton HG, Bulas D: Unilateral renal agenesis may result from in utero regression of multicystic renal dysplasia, *J Urol* 150:793-94, 1993.
15. Chow JS, Benson CB, Lebowitz RL: The clinical significance of an empty renal fossa on prenatal sonography, *J Ultrasound Med* 24:1049-54, 2005.
16. Limwongse C, Clarren SK, Cassidy SB: Syndromes and malformations of the urinary tract. In Barratt TM, Avner ED, Harmon WE, editors: *Pediatric Nephrology,* ed 2, Philadelphia, 1999, Lippincott Williams and Wilkins.
17. Jeanty P, Romero R, Kepple D, Stoney D, Coggins T, Fleischer AC: Prenatal diagnoses in unilateral empty renal fossa, *J Ultrasound Med* 9:651-54, 1990.
18. Estroff JA, Mandell J, Benacerraf BR: Increased renal echogenicity in the fetus, *Radiology* 181:135-39, 1991.
19. Tsatsaris V, Gagnadoux MF, Aubry MC, Gubler MC, Dumez Y, Dommergues M: Prenatal diagnosis of bilateral isolated fetal hyperechogenic kidneys. Is it possible to predict long term outcome? *BJOG* 109:1388-93, 2002.
20. Kaefer M, Peters CA, Retik AB, Benacerraf BB: Increased renal echogenicity: A sonographic sign for differentiating between obstructive and nonobstructive etiologies of in utero bladder distension, *J Urol* 158:1026-29, 1997.
21. Mashiach R, Davidovits M, Eisenstein B, Kidron D, Kovo M, Shalev J, Merlob P, Verdimon D, Efrat Z, Meizner I: Fetal hyperechogenic kidney with normal amniotic fluid volume: A diagnostic dilemma, *Prenat Diagn* 25:553-58, 2005.
22. Chitty LS, Altman DG: Charts of fetal size: Kidney and renal pelvis measurements, *Prenat Diagn* 23:891-97, 2003.
23. Ismaili K, Schurmans T, Wissing M, Hall M, Van Aelst C, Janssen F: Early prognostic factors of infants with chronic renal failure caused by renal dysplasia, *Pediatr Nephrol* 16:260-64, 2001.
24. Winyard P, Chitty L: Dysplastic and polycystic kidneys: diagnosis, associations and management, *Prenat Diagn* 21:924-35, 2001.
25. Ismaili K, Hall M, Donner C, Thomas D, Vermeylen D, Avni EF: Results of systematic screening for minor degrees of fetal renal pelvis dilatation in an unselected population, *Am J Obstet Gynecol* 188:242-46, 2003.
26. Ismaili K, Hall M, Piepsz A, Alexander M, Schulman C, Avni EF: Insights into the pathogenesis and natural history of fetuses with renal pelvis dilatation, *Eur Urol* 48:207-14, 2005.
27. Sherer DM: Is fetal hydronephrosis overdiagnosed? *Ultrasound Obstet Gynecol* 16:601-06, 2000.
28. Persutte WH, Hussey M, Chyu J, Hobbins JC: Striking findings concerning the variability in the measurement of the fetal renal collecting system, *Ultrasound Obstet Gynecol* 15:186-90, 2000.

29. Ismaili K, Avni EF, Wissing KM, Hall M: Long-term clinical outcome of infants with mild and moderate fetal pyelectasis: validation of neonatal ultrasound as a screening tool to detect significant nephrouropathies, *J Pediatr* 144:759-65, 2004.
30. Sairam S, Al-Habib A, Sasson S, Thilaganathan B: Natural history of fetal hydronephrosis diagnosed on mid-trimester ultrasound, *Ultrasound Obstet Gynecol* 17:191-96, 2001.
31. Chudleigh T: Mild pyelectasis, *Prenat Diagn* 21:936-41, 2001.
32. Dudley JA, Haworth JM, McGraw ME, Frank JD, Tizzard EJ: Clinical relevance and implications of antenatal hydronephrosis, *Arch Dis Child* 76:F31-34, 1997.
33. Stocks A, Richards D, Frentzen B, Richard G: Correlation of prenatal renal pelvic anteroposterior diameter with outcome in infancy, *J Urol* 155:1050-52, 1996.
34. Jaswon MS, Dibble L, Puri S, Davis J, Young J, Dave R, Morgan H: Prospective study of outcome in antenatally diagnosed renal pelvis dilatation, *Arch Dis Child* 80:F135-8, 1999.
35. De Bruyn R, Gordon I: Postnatal investigation of fetal renal disease, *Prenat Diagn* 21:984-91, 2001.
36. Ismaili K, Avni EF, Hall M. Results of systematic voiding cystourethrography in infants with antenatally diagnosed renal pelvis dilation, *J Pediatr* 141:21-24, 2002.
37. Moorthy I, Joshi N, Cook JV, Warren M: Antenatal hydronephrosis: negative predictive value of normal postnatal ultrasound, a 5-year study, *Clin Radiol* 58:964-70, 2003.
38. Avni EF, Ayadi K, Rypens F, Hall M, Schulman CC: Can careful ultrasound examination of the urinary tract exclude vesicoureteric reflux in the neonate? *Br J Radiol* 70:977-82, 1997.
39. Friedman W, Vogel M, Dimer JS, Luttkus A, Buscher U, Dudenhausen JW: Prenatal differential diagnosis of cystic renal disease and urinary tract obstruction: anatomic pathologic, ultrasonographic and genetic findings, *Eur J Obstet Gynecol Reprod Biol* 89:127-33, 2000.
40. Blazer S, Zimmer EZ, Blumenfeld Z, Zelikovic I, Bronshtein M: Natural history of fetal simple cysts detected early in pregnancy, *J Urol* 162:812-14, 1999.
41. Ulinski T, Lescure S, Beaufils S, Guigonis V, Decramer S, Morin D, Clauin S, Deschênes G, Bouissou F, Bensman A, Bellanné-Chantelot C: Renal phenotypes related to hepatocyte nuclear factor-1β (TCF2) mutations in a pediatric cohort, *J Am Soc Nephrol* 17:497-503, 2006.
42. Coffinier C, Thepot D, Babinet C, Yaniv M, Barra J: Essential role for the homeoprotein vHNF1/HNF1beta in visceral endoderm differentiation, *Development* 126:4785-94, 1999.
43. Hiesberger T, Shao X, Gourley E, Reinmann A, Pontoglio M, Igarashi P: Role of the hepatocyte nuclear factor-1β (HNF-1β) C-terminal domain in PKHD1 (ARPKD) gene transcription and cystogenesis, *J Biol Chem* 280:10578-86, 2005.
44. Blankenberg TA, Ruebner BH, Ellis WG, Bernstein J, Dimmick JE: Pathology of renal and hepatic anomalies in Meckel syndrome, *Am J Med Genet* 3(suppl):395-410, 1987.
45. Jones KL: *Smith's Recognizable Patterns of Human Malformation*, ed 2, Philadelphia: 1997, WB Saunders.
46. Cassart M, Eurin D, Didier F, Guibaud L, Avni EF: Antenatal renal sonographic anomalies and postnatal follow-up of renal involvement in Bardet-Biedl syndrome, *Ultrasound Obstet Gynecol* 24:51-54, 2004.
47. Moser AB, Rasmussen M, Naidu S, Watkins PA, McGuinness M, Hajra AK, Chen G, Raymond G, Liu A, Gordon D: Phenotype of patients with peroxisomal disorders subdivided into sixteen complementation groups, *J Pediatr* 127:13-22, 1995.
48. Larson RS, Rudolff MA, Liapis H, Manes JL, Davila R, Kissane J: The Ivemark syndrome: prenatal diagnosis of an uncommon cystic renal lesion with heterogeneous associations, *Pediatr Nephrol* 9:594-98, 1995.
49. Elliott M, Bayly R, Cole T, Temple IK, Maher ER: Clinical features and natural history of Beckwith-Wiedemann syndrome: presentation of 74 new cases, *Clin Genet* 46:168-74, 1994.
50. Brueton LA, Dillon MJ, Winter RM: Ellis van Creveld syndrome, Jeune syndrome and renal-hepatic-pancreatic dysplasia: separate entities or disease spectrum? *J Med Genet* 27:252-55, 1990.
51. Bernstein J, Robbins TO: Renal involvement in tuberous sclerosis, *Ann N Y Acad Sci* 615:36-49, 1991.
52. Leclair MD, El-Ghoneimi A, Audry G, Ravasse P, Moscovici J, Heloury Y; French Pediatric Urology Study Group: The outcome of prenatally diagnosed renal tumors, *J Urol* 173:186-89, 2005.
53. Bove KE: Wilms' tumor and related abnormalities in the fetus and newborn, *Semin Perinatol* 23:310-18, 1999.
54. Ambrosino MM, Hernanz-Schulman M, Horii SC, Raghavendra BN, Genieser NB: Prenatal diagnosis of nephroblastomatosis in two siblings, *J Ultrasound Med* 9:49-51, 1990.
55. Daneman A, Baunin C, Lobo E, Pracros JP, Avni F, Toi A, Metreweli C, Ho SS, Moore L: Disappearing suprarenal masses in fetuses and infants, *Pediatr Radiol* 27: 675-81, 1997.
56. Muller F, Dreux S, Vaast P, Dumez Y, Nisand I, Ville Y, Boulot P, Guibourdenche J; the Study Group of the French Fetal Medicine Society: Prenatal diagnosis of Megacystis-Microcolon-Intestinal hypoperistalsis syndrome: contribution of amniotic fluid digestive enzyme assay and fetal urinalysis, *Prenat Diagn* 25:203-09, 2005.
57. Wood BP: Cloacal malformations and extrophy syndromes, *Radiology* 177:326-27, 1990.
58. Gearhart JP, Ben-Chaim J, Jeffs RD, Sanders RC: Criteria for the prenatal diagnosis of classic bladder extrophy, *Obstet Gynecol* 85:961-64, 1995.
59. Vanderheyden T, Kumar S, Fisk NM: Fetal renal impairment, *Semin Neonatol* 8:279-89, 2003.
60. Spitzer A: The current approach to the assessment of fetal renal function: fact or fiction? *Pediatr Nephrol* 10:230-35, 1996.
61. Hobbins JC, Romero R, Grannum P, Berkovitz RL, Cullen M, Mahony M: Antenatal diagnosis of renal anomalies with ultrasound. I. Obstructive uropathy, *Am J Obstet Gynecol* 148:868-77, 1984.
62. Moore TR, Cayle JE: The amniotic fluid index in normal human pregnancy, *Am J Obstet Gynecol* 162:1168-73, 1990.
63. Phelan JP, Smith CV, Broussard A, Small M: Amniotic fluid volume assessment by four-quadrant technique at 32-42 weeks' gestation, *J Reprod Med* 32:540-42, 1987.
64. Zaccara A, Giorlandino C, Mobili L, Brizzi C, Bilancioni E, Capolupo I, Capitanucci ML, De Genaro M: Amniotic fluid index and fetal bladder outlet obstruction. Do we really need more? *J Urol* 174:1657-60, 2005.
65. Peters CA, Reid LM, Docimo S, Luetic T, Carr M, Retik AB, Mandell J: The role of the kidney in lung growth and maturation in the setting of obstructive uropathy and oligohydramnios, *J Urol* 146:597-600, 1991.
66. Laudy JA, Wladimiroff JW: The fetal lung. 1: Developmental aspects, *Ultrasound Obstet Gynecol* 16:284-90, 2000.
67. Smith NP, Losty PD, Connell MG, Meyer U, Jesudason EC: Abnormal lung development precedes oligohydramnios in transgenic murine model of renal dysgenesis, *J Urol* 175:783-86, 2006.
68. Proesmans W, Devlieger H, Van Assche A, Eggermont E, Vandenberghe K, Lemmens F, Sieprath P, Lijnen P: Bartter's syndrome in two siblings. Antenatal and neonatal observations, *Int J Pediatr Nephrol* 6:63-70, 1985.
69. Männikkö M, Kestilä M, Lenkkeri U, Alakurtti H, Holmberg C, Leisti J, Salonen R, Aula P, Mustonen A, Peltonen L, Tryggvason K: Improved prenatal diagnosis of the congenital nephrotic syndrome of the Finnish type based on DNA analysis, *Kidney Int* 51:868-72, 1997.
70. Nortier J, Debiec H, Tournay Y, Mougenot B, Noel JC, Deschodt-Lackman MM, Janssen F, Ronco P: Neonatal disease in neutral endopeptidase alloimmunization: lessons for immunological monitoring, *Pediatr Nephrol* 21:1399-405, 2005.
71. Glick PL, Harrisson MR, Golbus MS, Adzick NS, Filly RA, Callen PW, Mahony PS: Management of the fetus with congenital hydronephrosis. II: prognosis criteria and selection for treatment, *J Pediatr Surg* 20:376-87, 1985.
72. Burghard R, Pallacks R, Gordjani N, Leititis JU, Hackeloer BJ, Brandis M: Microproteins in amniotic fluid as an index of changes in fetal renal function during development, *Pediatr Nephrol* 1:574-80, 1997.
73. Coplen DE: Prenatal intervention for hydronephrosis, *J Urol* 157:2270-77, 1997.
74. Crombleholme TM, Harrisson MR, Golbus MS, Longaker MT, Langer JC, Callen PW, Anderson RL, Goldstein RB, Filly RA: Fetal intervention in obstructive uropathy: prognostic indicators and efficacy of intervention, *Am J Obstet Gynecol* 162:1239-44, 1990.

75. Muller F, Bernard MA, Benkirane A, Ngo S, Lortat-Jacob S, Oury JF, Dommergues M: Fetal urine Cystatin C as a predictor of postnatal renal function in bilateral uropathies, *Clin Chem* 45:2292-93, 1995.
76. Muller F, Dommergues M, Mandelbrot L, Aubry MC, Nihoul-Féketé C, Dumez Y: Fetal urinary biochemistry predicts postnatal renal function in children with bilateral obstructive uropathies, *Obstet Gynecol* 82:813-20, 1993.
77. Nicolini U, Spelzini F: Invasive assessment of fetal renal abnormalities: urinalysis, fetal blood sampling and biopsy, *Prenat Diagn* 21:964-69, 2001.
78. Bökenkamp A, Dieterich C, Dressler F, Mühlhaus K, Gembruch U, Bald R, Kirschstein M: Fetal serum concentrations of cystatin C and β2-microglobulin as predictors of postnatal kidney function, *Am J Obstet Gynecol* 185:468-75, 2001.
79. Dommergues M, Muller F, Ngo S, Hohlfeld P, Oury JF, Bidat L, Mahieu-Caputo D, Sagot P, Body G, Favre R, Dumez Y: Fetal serum β2-microglobulin predicts postnatal renal function in bilateral uropathies, *Kidney Int* 58:312-16, 2000.
80. Muller F, Dreux S, Audibert F, Chabaud JJ, Rousseau T, D'Hervé D, Dumez Y, Ngo S, Gubler MC, Dommergues M: Fetal serum β2-microglobulin and cystatin C in the prediction of post-natal renal function in bilateral hypoplasia and hyperechogenic enlarged kidneys, *Prenat Diagn* 24:327-32, 2004.
81. Bunduki V, Saldanha LB, Sadek L, Miguelez J, Myiyadahira S, Zugaib M: Fetal renal biopsies in obstructive uropathy: feasibility and clinical correlations—preliminary results, *Prenat Diagn* 18:101-09, 1998.
82. Suranyi A, Retz C, Rigo J, Schaaps JP, Foidart JM: Fetal renal hyperechogenicity in intrauterine growth retardation: importance and outcome, *Pediatr Nephrol* 16:575-80, 2001.
83. Schmidt B, Andrew M: Neonatal thrombosis: report of a prospective Canadian and International Registry, *Pediatrics* 96:939-43, 1995.
84. Hibbert J, Howlett DC, Greenwood KL, MacDonald LM, Saunders AJ: The ultrasound appearances of neonatal renal vein thrombosis, *BJR* 70:1191-94, 1997.
85. Marks SD, Massicotte P, Steele BT, Matsell DG, Filler G, Shah PS, Perlman M, Rosenblum ND, Shah VS: Neonatal renal venous thrombosis: Clinical outcomes and prevalence of prothrombotic disorders, *J Pediatr* 146:811-16, 2005.
86. Lalmand B, Avni EF, Nasr A, Katelbant P, Struyven J: Perinatal renal vein thrombosis: US demonstration, *J Ultrasound Med* 9:437-42, 1990.
87. Wee LY, Fisk NM: The twin-twin transfusion syndrome, *Semin Neonatol* 7:187-202, 2002.
88. Talbert DG, Bajoria R, Sepulveda W, Bower S, Fisk NM: Hydrostatic and osmotic pressure gradients produce manifestations of fetofetal transfusion syndrome in a computerized model of monochorial twin pregnancy, *Am J Obstet Gynecol* 174:598-608, 1996.
89. Chiang MC, Lien R, Chao AS, Chou YH, Chen YJ: Clinical consequences of twin-to-twin transfusion, *Eur J Pediatr* 162:68-71, 2003.
90. Sedman AB, Kershaw DB, Bunchman TE: Recognition and management of angiotensin converting enzyme inhibitor fetopathy, *Pediatr Nephrol* 9:382-85, 1995.
91. Friedman JM: ACE inhibitors and congenital anomalies, *N Engl J Med* 354:2498-2500, 2006.
92. Cooper WO, Hernandez-Diaz S, Arbogast PG, Dudley JA, Dyer S, Gideon PS, Hall K, Ray WA: Major congenital malformations after first-trimester exposure to ACE inhibitors, *N Engl J Med* 354:2443-51, 2006.
93. Lambot MA, Vermeylen D, Noel JC: Angiotensin-II-receptor inhibition in pregnancy, *Lancet* 357:1619-20, 2001.
94. Alwan S, Polifka JE, Friedman JM: Angiotensin II receptor antagonist treatment during pregnancy, *Birth Defects Research* 73:123-30, 2005.
95. Loudon JA, Groom KM, Bennett PR: Prostaglandin inhibitors in preterm labour, *Best Pract Clin Obstet Gynecol* 17:731-44, 2003.
96. Mitra SC, Ganesh V, Apuzzio JJ: Effect of maternal cocaine abuse on renal arterial flow and urine output in the fetus, *Am J Obstet Gynecol* 171:1556-59, 1994.
97. Greenfield SP, Rutigliano E, Steinhardt G, Elder JS: Genitourinary tract malformations and maternal cocaine abuse, *Urology* 37:455-59, 1991.
98. Behnke M, Eyler FD, Garvan CW, Wobie K: The search for congenital malformations in newborns with fetal cocaine exposure, *Pediatrics* 107:E74, 2001.
99. Editorial: Pregnancy and renal disease, *Lancet* 2:801-02, 1975.
100. McKay DB, Josephson MA: Pregnancy in recipients of solid organs—Effects on mother and child, *N Engl J Med* 354:1281-93, 2006.
101. Ross LF: Ethical considerations related to pregnancy in transplant recipients, *N Engl J Med* 354:1313-16, 2006.
102. Le Ray C, Coulomb A, Elefant E, Frydman R, Audibert F: Mycophenolate mofetil in pregnancy after renal transplantation: a case of major fetal malformations, *Obstet Gynecol* 103:1091-94, 2004.
103. EBPG Expert Group in Renal Transplantation: European best practice guidelines for renal transplantation. Section IV.10. Long-term management of the transplant recipient—pregnancy in renal transplant recipients, *Nephrol Dial Transplant* 17(suppl 4):50-55, 2002.
104. Liebeschuetz S, Thomas R: Unilateral multicystic dysplastic kidney, *Arch Dis Child* 77:369, 1997 (letter).
105. Cochat P, Murat FJ, Guibaud L, Bouvier R, Dupin H, Cordier MP, Wacksman J: Dysplasie rénale multikystique. In Guignard JP, Simeoni U, Gouyon JB, editors: *Diagnostic anténatal et prise en charge postnatale des néphro-uropathies malformatives.* Paris, 2000, Elsevier.
106. Stuck KJ, Koff SA, Silver TM: Ultrasonic features of multicystic dysplastic kidney: expanded diagnostic criteria, *Radiology* 143:217-21, 1982.
107. Ismaili K, Avni EF, Alexander M, Schulman C, Collier F, Hall M: Routine voiding cystourethrography is of no value in neonates with unilateral multicystic dysplastic kidney, *J Pediatr* 146:759-63, 2005.
108. Ward CJ, Hogan MC, Rossetti S, Walker D, Sneddon T, Wang X, Kubly V, Cunningham JM, Bacallao R, Ishibashi M, Milliner DS, Torres VE, Harris PC: The gene mutated in autosomal recessive polycystic kidney disease encodes a large, receptor-like protein, *Nat Genet* 30:259-69, 2002.
109. Avni FE, Garel L, Cassart M, Massez A, Eurin D, Didier F, Hall M, Teele RL: Perinatal assessment of hereditary cystic renal diseases: the contribution of sonography, *Pediatr Radiol* 36:405-14, 2006.
110. Wilson PD: Polycystic kidney disease, *N Engl J Med* 350:151-64, 2004.
111. Mochizuki T, Wu G, Hayashi T, Xenophontos SL, Veldhuisen B, Saris JJ, Reynolds DM, Cai Y, Gabow PA, Pierides A, Kimberling WJ, Breuning MH, Deltas CC, Peters DJ, Somlo S: PKD2, a gene for polycystic kidney disease that encodes an integral membrane protein, *Science* 272:1339-42, 1996.
112. Brun M, Maugey-Laulom B, Eurin D, Didier F, Avni EF: Prenatal sonographic patterns in autosomal dominant polycystic kidney disease: a multicenter study, *Ultrasound Obstet Gynecol* 24:55-61, 2004.
113. McDermot KD, Saggar-Malik AK, Economides DL, Jeffrey S: Prenatal diagnosis of autosomal dominant polycystic kidney disease (PKD1) presenting in utero and prognosis for very early onset disease, *J Med Genet* 35:13-16, 1998.
114. Avni EF, Thoua Y, Van Gansbeke D, Matos C, Didier F, Droulez P, Schulman CC: The development of hypodysplastic kidney, *Radiology* 164:123-25, 1985.
115. Kestilä M, Lenkkeri U, Lamerdin J, McCready P, Putaala H, Ruotsalainen V, Morita T, Nissinen M, Herva R, Kashtan CE, Peltonen L, Holmberg C, Olsen A, Tryggvason K: Positionally cloned gene for a novel glomerular protein—nephrin—is mutated in congenital nephrotic syndrome, *Mol Cell* 1:575-82, 1998.
116. Huttunen NP: Congenital nephrotic syndrome of Finnish type, Study of 75 cases, *Arch Dis Child* 51:344-48, 1996.
117. Souka AP, Skentou H, Geerts L, Bower S, Nicolaides KH: Congenital nephrotic syndrome presenting with increased nuchal translucency in the first trimester, *Prenat Diagn* 22:93-95, 2002.
118. Rapola J: Why is congenital nephrotic syndrome associated with a rise in the concentration of alpha-fetoprotein in the amniotic fluid? *Pediatr Nephrol* 4:206, 1990.

119. Weber S, Gribouval O, Esquivel EL, Morinière V, Tête MJ, Legendre C, Niaudet P, Antignac C: NPHS2 mutation analysis shows genetic heterogeneity of steroid-resistant nephrotic syndrome and low post-transplant recurrence, *Kidney Int* 66:571-79, 2004.
120. Mark K, Reis A, Zenker M: Prenatal findings in four consecutive pregnancies with fetal Pierson syndrome, a newly defined congenital nephrosis syndrome, *Prenat Diagn* 26:262-66, 2006.
121. Zenker M, Aigner T, Wendler O, Tralau T, Müntefering H, Fenski R, Pitz S, Schumacher V, Royer-Pokora B, Wühl E, Cochat P, Bouvier R, Kraus C, Mark K, Madlon H, Dötch J, Rascher W, Maruniak-Chudek I, Lennert T, Neumann LM, Reis A: Human laminin beta 2 deficiency causes congenital nephrosis with mesangial sclerosis and distinct eye abnormalities, *Hum Mol Genet* 13:2625-32, 2004.
122. Northrup M, Mendez-Castillo A, Brown JC, Frazier S, Luger AM: Congenital nephrotic syndrome, Finnish type: sonographic appearance and pathologic correlation, *J Ultrasound Med* 22:1097-99, 2003.
123. Habib R, Loirat C, Gubler MC, Niaudet P, Bensman A, Levy M, Broyer M: The nephropathy associated with male pseudohermaphroditism and Wilms' tumor (Drash syndrome): a distinctive glomerular lesion—report of 10 cases, *Clin Nephrol* 24:269-78, 1985.
124. Besbas N, Bayrakci US, Kale G, Cengiz AB, Akcoren Z, Akinci D, Kilic I, Bakkaloglu A: Cytomegalovirus-related congenital nephrotic syndrome with diffuse mesangial sclerosis, *Pediatr Nephrol* 21:740-42, 2006.
125. Mouriquand P, Whitten M, Pracros JP: Pathophysiology, diagnosis and management of prenatal upper tract dilatation, *Prenat Diagn* 21:942-51, 2001.
126. Ismaili K, Avni FE, Wissing KM, Piepsz A, Aubert D, Cochat P, Hall M: Current management of infants with fetal renal pelvis dilatation: a survey by French-speaking pediatric nephrologists and urologists, *Pediatr Nephrol* 19:966-71, 2004.
127. Ulman I, Jayanthi VR, Koff SA: The long-term follow-up of newborns with severe unilateral hydronephrosis initially treated nonoperatively, *J Urol* 164:1101-05, 2000.
128. Subramaniam R, Kouriefs C, Dickson AP: Antenatally detected pelvi-ureteric junction obstruction: concerns about conservative treatment, *BJU Int* 84:335-38, 1999.
129. Marra G, Barbieri G, Moioli C, Assael BM, Grumieri G, Caccamo ML: Mild fetal hydronephrosis indicating vesicoureteric reflux, *Arch Dis Child* 70:F147-50, 1994.
130. Weinberg B, Yeung N: Sonographic sign of intermittent dilatation of the renal collecting system in ten patients with vesicoureteral reflux, *J Clin Ultrasound* 26:65-68, 1998.
131. Garin EH, Campos A, Homsy Y: Primary vesicoureteral reflux: review of current concepts, *Pediatr Nephrol* 12:249-56, 1998.
132. McLellan DL, Retik AB, Bauer SB, Diamond DA, Atala A, Mandell J, Lebowitz RL, Borer JG, Peters CA: Rate and predictors of spontaneous resolution of prenatally diagnosed nonrefluxing megaureter, *J Urol* 168:2177-80, 2002.
133. Whitten SM, Wilcox DT: Duplex systems, *Prenat Diagn* 21:952-57, 2001.
134. Peppas DS, Skoog SJ, Canning DA, Belman AB: Nonsurgical management of primary vesicoureteric reflux in complete ureteral duplication. Is it justified? *J Urol* 146:1594-95, 1991.
135. Avni FE, Dacher JN, Stallenberg B, Collier F, Hall M, Schulman CC: Renal duplications: the impact of perinatal US on diagnosis and management, *Eur Urol* 1991; 20: 43-48, 1991.
136. Decter RM: Renal duplication and fusion anomalies, *Pediatr Clin North Am* 44:1323-41, 1997.
137. Favre R, Kohler M, Gasser B, Muller F, Nisand I: Early fetal megacystis between 11 and 15 weeks of gestation, *Ultrasound Obstet Gynecol* 14:402-06, 1991.
138. Housley HT, Harrisson MR: Fetal urinary tract abnormalities. Natural history, pathophysiology, and treatment, *Urol Clin North Am* 25:63-73, 1998.
139. Dinneen MD, Duffy PG: Posterior urethral valves, *Br J Urol* 78:275-81, 1996.
140. Holmes N, Harrison MR, Baskin LS: Fetal surgery for posterior urethral valves: long term postnatal outcomes, *Pediatrics* 108: 36-42, 2001.
141. Quintero RA, Hume R, Smith C, Johnson MP, Cotton DB, Romero R, Evans M: Percutaneous fetal cystoscopy and endoscopic fulguration of posterior urethral valves, *Am J Obstet Gynecol* 172:206-09, 1995.
142. Agarwal SK, Fisk NM: In utero therapy for lower urinary tract obstruction, *Prenat Diagn* 21: 970-76, 2001.

CHAPTER 5

Genetics: Basic Concepts and Testing

Carsten Bergmann and Thomas Eggermann

The purpose of this chapter is to give readers a rough overview of genetics and of testing genetic disturbances. Details of specific renal disease–related mutations and appropriate testing for individual renal disorders can be found in the chapters discussing those conditions. We cannot, of course, cover the organization and structure of DNA and its translation into protein in detail. Instead we will review patterns of inheritance and how alteration and variation in DNA may lead to disease, and how these alterations can be detected in the laboratory. Given its goal, this chapter is not extensively referenced, nor should it be viewed by the more highly motivated or demanding reader as a replacement for one of the excellent textbooks on molecular and medical genetics recommended at the end of this chapter.[1-4]

Genetics has become increasingly important in everyday life and in routine diagnostic testing. Thus it is crucial to increase interdisciplinary efforts for the benefit of each individual patient. In general, genetic testing should be preceded by counseling the affected person or family. Genetic counseling can be regarded as an educational process that seeks to help affected and at-risk individuals understand the nature of the genetic disorder, its transmission, and the options open to them in management and family planning. Only well-informed patients can make decisions concerning what is best for them in their current situation.

STRUCTURE OF THE HUMAN GENOME AND GENE STRUCTURE

Genetics (from the Greek *genno, γεννώ,* give birth) is the science of genes, heredity, and the variation of organisms. Each gene contains the information necessary for synthesizing the amino-acid sequences in proteins; that is, a certain gene carries the instructions for a specific function. Although we all have the same genes, there are different versions of them, called alleles, that determine the expression of the final phenotype or physical appearance. For example, whereas most people have genes that give them eye pigment, there are multiple alleles for specific eye colors. Each person has a particular combination of alleles for eye color, hair color, etc., that makes that person genetically unique.

The number of different genes each human possesses has long been discussed and remains a matter of debate. However, it is evident that the final number is much lower than initially thought; currently people act on the assumption of there being about 20,000 to 30,000 genes or even a bit less.

There are two general types of genes in the human genome: noncoding RNA genes and protein-coding genes. Noncoding RNA genes represent 2% to 5% of the total and encode functional RNA molecules. Many of these RNAs are involved in the control of gene expression, particularly protein synthesis. They have no overall conserved structure.

Protein-coding genes represent the majority of the total and are expressed in two stages: transcription and translation (Figure 5-1).

In the transcription process the gene is copied to produce an RNA molecule (a primary transcript) with essentially the same sequence as the gene. Most human genes are divided into exons and introns, and only the exons carry information required for protein synthesis. Most primary transcripts are therefore processed by a complex mechanism called splicing to remove intron sequences and generate a mature transcript or messenger RNA (mRNA) that only contains exons.

In the translation stage, also known as protein synthesis (Figure 5-1), three nucleotides are required to specify one amino acid (codon). The chain of amino acids must fold up to generate the final tertiary structure of the protein.

Several genes are expressed in all cells all of the time. These so-called housekeeping genes are essential for very basic cellular functions. Other genes are expressed in particular cell types or at particular stages of development (in a temporospatially tightly regulated manner); one gene can therefore encode a large number of different transcripts. This differential gene expression is achieved by regulating transcription and translation. All genes are surrounded by DNA sequences that control their expression. For instance, proteins called transcription factors bind to these sequences and can switch the genes on or off. Gene expression is therefore controlled by the availability and activity of a multitude of different transcription factors. Of course, transcription factors are proteins themselves and regulated by other transcription factors, finally constituting a complex regulatory hierarchy. For example, a direct transcriptional hierarchy has recently been demonstrated for hepatocyte nuclear factor 1-beta *(HNF1β/TCF2)* and various cystic kidney disease genes (*UMOD, PKHD1,* and *PKD2*).[5] Mutations in these genes cause a wide range of cystic kidney diseases, which are described in detail in other chapters of this book.[6] The some-

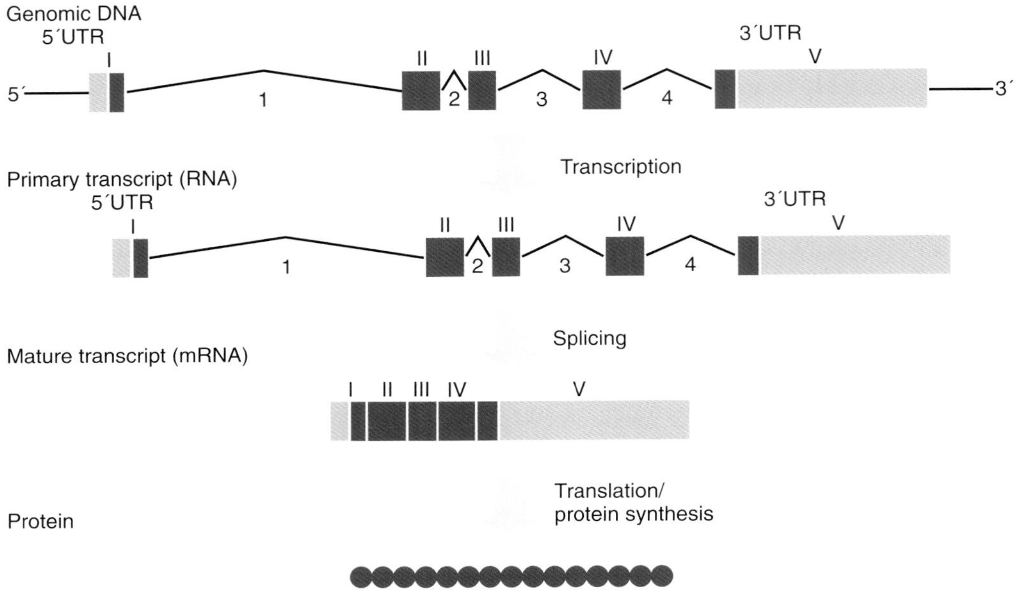

Figure 5-1 Simplified overview of gene structure and expression. A protein-coding gene is defined by the extent of the primary transcript. The promoter and any other regulatory elements are usually outside the gene. The gene itself is divided into different types of sequences. The coding region *(red)* is the information used to define the sequence of amino acids in the protein. The untranslated regions *(white)* are found in the mRNA but are not used to define the protein sequence; they are often regulatory in nature. Finally, introns *(black lines in between)* are found in the primary transcript but spliced out of the mRNA. They may interrupt the coding and untranslated regions. A precursor RNA (primary transcript) is constructed from the gene sequence and then processed with removal of the introns by splicing. Spliced RNAs contain only exonic sequences from which the protein is synthesized.

times overlapping phenotypes of different disease entities are just beginning to be understood by interdependencies on protein level within this complex network.

Genes show incredible diversity in size and organization and have no typical structure. There are, however, several conserved features. The boundaries of a protein-encoding gene are defined as the points at which transcription begins and ends. The core of the gene is the coding region, which contains the nucleotide sequence that is eventually translated into the sequence of amino acids in the protein. The coding region begins and ends with specific codons. On either side of the coding region are DNA sequences that are transcribed but are not translated. These untranslated regions (UTRs), or noncoding regions, often contain regulatory elements that control protein synthesis.

VARIATIONS AND MUTATIONS IN THE HUMAN GENOME

Human inherited diseases are based on alterations (mutations) in the DNA and are transferred from generation to generation (germline mutations). Mutations are the raw fuel that drives evolution. They can be the direct cause of a pathologic phenotype but can also result in just an increased susceptibility to disease. Mutations often arise as copying errors in DNA replication. These variations include large-scale chromosome aberrations with loss or gain of chromosomal segments or whole chromosomes, and small-scale mutations. It is important to stress that not every base change necessarily indicates a disease-causing mutation, and it is therefore crucial to carefully evaluate the pathogenicity of each identified variation.

Chromosomal disturbances are frequently associated with syndromic features such as short stature, microcephaly, organ malformations (often including urogenital malformations), and intellectual deficits. Typical pediatric nephrology patients often, though not necessarily, display a kidney-specific phenotype for which small-scale mutations are most relevant. Thus in the following sections we will refer solely to mutations affecting single base pairs or small-scale deletions and duplications. An overview of different types of single-base substitutions in polypeptide-encoding DNA is given in Figure 5-2.

This classification, however, is somewhat simplified. In genetic testing it may be difficult to prove the pathogenicity of specific mutations, especially if they are silent (or neutral, e.g., the substitution of functionally similar amino acids). In this case they are difficult to differentiate from nonpathogenic polymorphic genetic variants.

MENDELIAN INHERITANCE

Given the diploid character of the human genome, most alleles exist in duplicate. An organism is called homozygous if both alleles of a gene are identical, and it is heterozygous if the alleles are different. In diploid organisms a dominant allele on one chromosome will mask the expression of a recessive gene on the other. In contrast, a recessive phenotype appears only when the organism carries the recessive allele on both parental chromosomes. Rare exceptions might

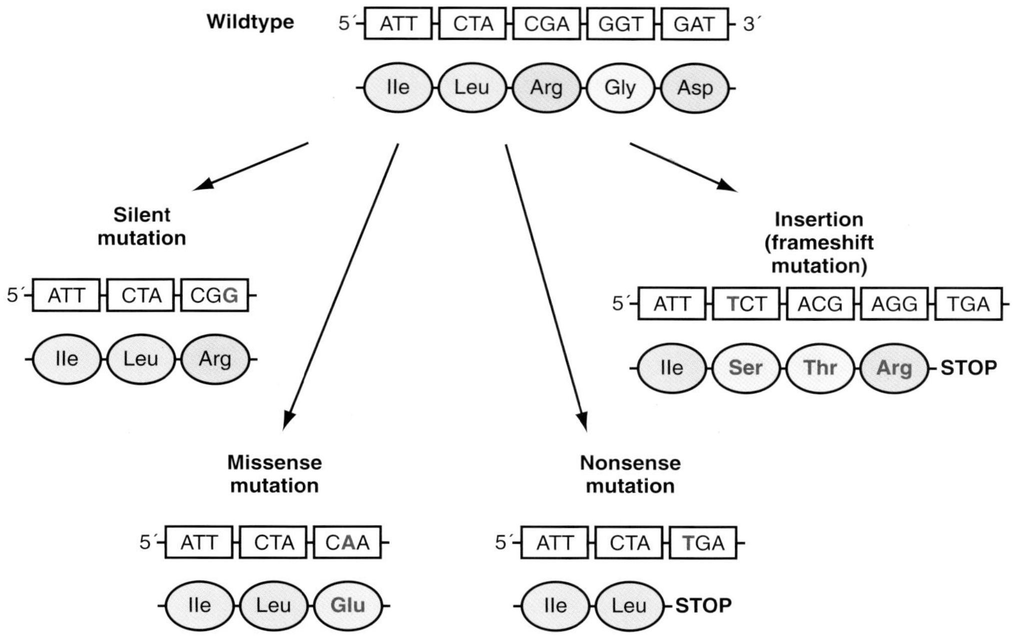

Figure 5-2 Illustration of the most frequent types of single nucleotide mutations and their functional consequences.

be cases in which heterozygous carriers of a recessive allele display a diminished phenotypic manifestation; strictly speaking, according to Gregor Mendel's principles these cases should not be termed *recessive.*

Autosomal Dominant Inheritance

Autosomal dominant inheritance means that the gene carrying a mutation is located on one of the autosomes (chromosome pairs 1 through 22). This means that males and females are equally likely to inherit the mutation. When a parent has a dominant disease due to a germline gene mutation, there is a 50% chance that any child the parent has will also inherit the mutation and the same clinical disorder. The gender of the children does not matter and the chance is 50/50 for each pregnancy.

Simplistically, *dominant* means that having a germline mutation in just one of the two copies of a particular gene is all that is needed for a person to have a trait, such as an increased risk of developing cancer. However, important characteristics of dominant gene mutations can include variable expressivity and reduced penetrance, sometimes making it difficult and confusing for patients and doctors dealing with these issues. *Variable expressivity* means that some people carrying a dominant mutation have milder or more severe symptoms than others with this mutation. In addition, which body systems the mutation affects can vary greatly as can the age at which the disease starts, even in the same family, that is, among family members who all bear the identical germline mutation. The issue of variable expression of a dominant disease merges with the term *reduced penetrance,* which means that a person carries the dominant germline mutation but does not develop any signs of disease until natural death.

The concept of reduced penetrance is particularly important in the case of autosomal dominant cancer susceptibility genes. If a person has inherited a cancer susceptibility gene, it does not mean that cancer will automatically develop. It simply means that the individual has inherited a mutation in a gene that gives that person a greater chance of developing cancer than the general population (i.e., someone without the mutation). For instance, 5% to 10% of all breast and ovarian cancers are assumed to be familial with autosomal dominant inheritance.[7] About 50% of these cases are caused by mutations in the *BRCA1* and *BRCA2* genes. However, it is important to know that the penetrance figures for *BRCA1* are currently assumed to be maximally 60% for breast cancer and 40% for ovarian cancer, whereas in *BRCA2* the penetrance is about 40% for breast cancer and 10% for ovarian cancer. Of course, these risk figures are higher than respective common lifetime risks in the general population; however, they are also far from 100% (complete penetrance) and make genetic counseling particularly complex with respect to surveillance programs and therapeutic/surgical interventions.

In contrast, complete and full penetrance is documented, for example, in autosomal dominant polycystic kidney disease (ADPKD), which is often regarded as a neoplasm in disguise.[8,9] "Full penetrance" means that each person who carries the dominant germline mutation will develop some features of the disease during his or her life. However, there is striking phenotypic variability (i.e., variable expressivity) not only interfamilially but even within the same family, indicating that modifying genes, environmental factors, and/or other mechanisms considerably influence the clinical course in ADPKD. This topic is described in detail in Chapter 9.

Autosomal Recessive Inheritance

Autosomal recessive inheritance means that the disease-related gene is located on one of the autosomes, with males and females equally affected. *Recessive* means that both copies of the gene must have a mutation in order for a person to have the trait. One copy of the mutation is inherited from the mother and the other from the father. A person who has only one recessive gene mutation is said to be a "carrier" for the trait or disease but usually does not have any health problems from carrying it. Most people do not know they carry a recessive gene mutation for a disease until they have a child with the disease. Once parents have had a child with a recessive disease, there is a one in four (25%) chance with each subsequent pregnancy for another child to be born with the same disorder. This means that there is a three out of four (75%) chance for another child not to have the disease.

In contrast to dominant inheritance in which the disease has usually already appeared in the parents' and grandparents' generation, the birth of a child with a recessive condition is often a complete surprise to a family, since in most cases there is no previous family history of the condition. Many autosomal recessive conditions occur this way. It is estimated that all people carry several recessive alleles in the heterozygous state that when present on both chromosomes cause genetic diseases. Thus the chance of having a child with a recessive disorder happens only when both parents carry the same or an allelic recessive mutation. Clearly, consanguineous parents with a common ancestor and common recessive alleles have a higher risk for producing children with autosomal recessive disorders than do nonconsanguineous couples. For first-degree cousins, the autosomal recessive disease risk in offspring is assumed to be doubled.

X-linked Inheritance

The third basic pattern of inheritance of genes is called X-linked inheritance, which means that the gene alteration causing the trait or the disorder is not located on one of the 22 autosomes but on the X chromosome. Females have two X chromosomes, whereas males have one X and one Y. Mutations in X-chromosome genes can be recessive or dominant. Their expression in females and males is usually not the same because almost all genes on the Y chromosome do not pair up with the genes on the X. In general, X-linked recessive mutations are expressed in females only if a female has two copies of the mutation (one on each X chromosome). However, for males, if their only copy of the X chromosome contains a mutation, they will have the trait or disorder. In simple terms, this is because in males the failure of this X chromosomal gene cannot be counteracted by an intact copy.

X-linked dominant disease expression in females is further complicated by their X-inactivation pattern, that is, the ratio by which the mutation-bearing X chromosome is active and the "healthy" X chromosome is inactive, or vice versa. Notably the X-inactivation pattern can vary among different organs of the female. Accordingly the disease spectrum caused by X-linked dominant mutations in females is wide and ranges from asymptomatic carriers to severely affected individuals in whom the disorder is equally expressed, as in afflicted males. A union between a healthy father and a carrier mother (conductor) has four possible outcomes, each with a 25% chance of occurring: an affected son, a healthy son, a carrier daughter (with all considerations just given), or a healthy daughter. This pattern can be explained as the father contributing only normal X chromosomes to his daughters and the Y chromosome obligatorily to his sons, and the carrier mother passing or not passing on the abnormal X. In cases where the father is affected with an X-linked disorder the situation is clear: all his daughters will inherit the X-disease chromosome from him and will be obligate carriers, whereas all his sons will be healthy (at least not affected by the X-linked disease in question). There can be no male-to-male transmission of disease in X-linked inheritance.

NONMENDELIAN INHERITANCE

Multifactorial Disorders and Digenic, Oligogenic, and Polygenic Inheritance

The majority of congenital malformations and common adult diseases presumably result from genetic interaction with complex environmental factors, the exact mechanisms of which are still poorly understood. Multifactorial or so-called part-genetic traits may be discontinuous (with distinct phenotypes, such as diabetes mellitus) or continuous (with a lack of distinct phenotypes, such as height). However, each trait is determined by the interaction of a number of genes at different loci, each with a small but additive effect, together with environmental factors. Information about the degree of genetic and environmental factors often comes from studies of twins. Consistently higher concordance rates in monozygotic twins than in dizygotic twins suggest involvement of genetic factors. However, concordance rates below unity imply environmental components to etiology. Typical examples of these multifactorial disorders are essential hypertension and diabetes mellitus other than the neonatal and early-onset forms, such as MODY (Maturity Onset Diabetes of the Young), that usually follow mendelian or epigenetic inheritance patterns.[10]

Of general interest is the genetic determination of continuous characters such as hair and skin color under the assumption of additive polygeny, which means that each of several genes adds a "dose" of pigment when present in the dominant form but not when recessive. When plotted on a graph, the possible genotypes for this trait would yield a bell-shaped, normal curve (Gaussian distribution), with most of the animals being intermediate and a "tail" out toward the extremes on both sides. Traits such as pigment modifiers, height, some kinds of coat texture in animals, and intelligence are easy to visualize as additive traits. Quantitative trait loci (QTLs) is a term often used for quantitative or continuous characters (height, weight, etc.).

For discontinuous multifactorial traits, the risk within affected families is raised above the general population risk, but the risk within an affected family is low in comparison with mendelian traits and rapidly falls toward the general population risk in more distant relatives. Thus in practice, the patient with a discontinuous multifactorial trait is often the only affected individual in that family.

Mitochondrial (Matrilineal) Inheritance

So far in this chapter we have focused on nuclear-encoded DNA. However, mitochondria contain their own small genome and also have their own machinery for protein synthesis. Mitochondria are important for energy production, and different tissues vary in the extent to which they rely on this process. The central nervous system, eye, heart, skeletal muscle, kidney, and endocrine glands are particularly reliant and hence are the main organs and tissues involved in mitochondrial diseases. Each cell has hundreds or thousands of mitochondria in the cytoplasm and each mitochondrion possesses about 10 copies of the circular mitochondrial chromosome. The mitochondrial genome is small but highly mutable compared with nuclear DNA (approximately tenfold higher), probably because its DNA replication is more error prone and the number of replications is much higher. It consists of a single circular double helix of 16,500 bases that encodes a small number of proteins and RNA molecules required for oxidative phosphorylation. It should be noted that the majority of proteins and RNA molecules required for mitochondrial function are actually encoded in chromosomal DNA and have to be imported from the cell nucleus. In principle, mitochondrial diseases result from mutations in genes that specify mitochondrial products or mitochondrial DNA expression. In contrast to most nuclear genes, mitochondrial genes do not have introns, and genetic information is extremely densely packed, with more than 90% of the sequence representing coding DNA.

Diseases of the mitochondrial genome (see the MITOMAP database for details at www.mitomap.org) are almost always maternally transmitted, given that sperm rarely contribute mitochondria during fertilization (paternally derived mitochondrial variants have almost never been detected in children). Thus a mitochondrially inherited condition can affect both sexes; however, it is passed on only by affected mothers (called *matrilineal inheritance*).

As mitochondria are randomly dispersed into daughter cells during cell division, the proportion of DNA molecules carrying a variant mutation may differ largely between mother and offspring and even in the same individual among different cells and tissues. It may be 100% or 0% (homoplasmy) or any intermediate ratio (heteroplasmy). Conclusively, variable phenotypic expressivity is a hallmark of mitochondrial disorders and makes the severity of the disease in offspring difficult to predict.

Genomic Imprinting and Epigenetic Inheritance

Mutations in the coding sequence of genes have a well-established role in the determination of phenotypic diversity and pathological conditions. However, in recent years allele expression has been recognized to be largely dependent on modification of the DNA or chromatin structure due to DNA methylation, that is, the covalent modification of cytosine, and posttranslational modification of histones such as methylation, acetylation, phosphorylation, and ubiquitinilation.[11] All these mechanisms of gene regulation are termed *epigenetic modifications* and can be disturbed by genomic imprinting disturbances, germline epimutations, and epigenetic polymorphisms secondary to or mediated by aberrant DNA methylation, histone modification, or both.

Genomic imprinting describes a parent-of-origin-dependent mechanism through which a subset of genes is expressed from only one allele (Figure 5-3). For some imprinted genes, one parental allele is totally silenced, whereas in others the imprinting signal is tissue specific, which leads to biallelic expression in some tissues and monoallelic expression in others. Disturbances of imprinting signals of specific genes might have profound consequences. Meanwhile, several human imprinting disorders such as Prader-Willi syndrome or Angelman syndrome have been identified.[12-14] In these patients an imbalanced expression of imprinted genes due to deletions or altered DNA methylation marks can be observed.

Genomic imprinting is typically reversible through successive generations: the inherited imprints are erased in primordial germ cells, and, within each generation, new imprints are reset during gametogenesis and maintained throughout development. However, single cases of inheritance of epigenetic marks unchanged through the germline—a so-called transgenerational inheritance—have been observed and provide a

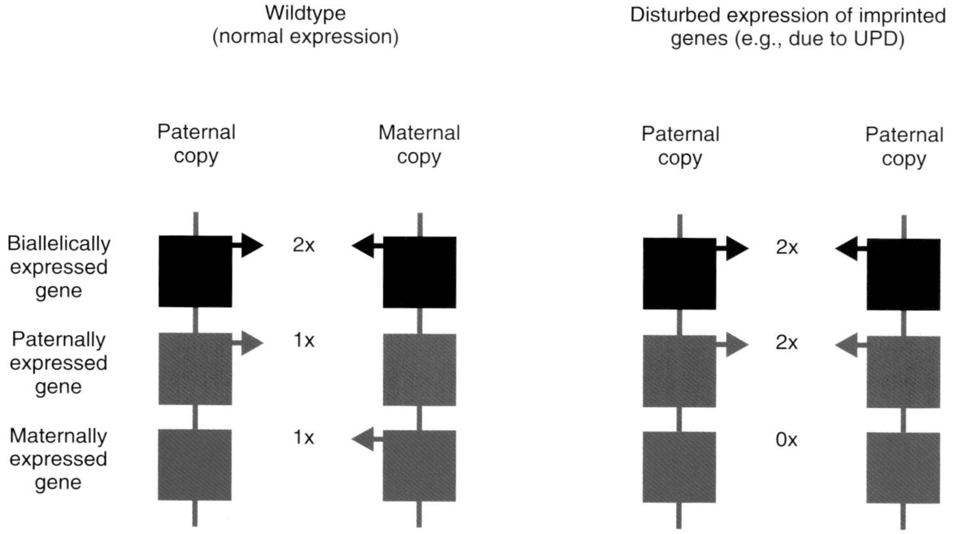

Figure 5-3 Conceivable consequences of epigenetic disturbances on the expression of maternally or paternally imprinted genes. *UPD*, Uniparental disomy—inheritance of both copies of a chromosome from one parent instead of one pair from each parent.

new mechanism for phenocopying of genetic disease.[15,16] The mosaicism and nonmendelian inheritance of epigenetic marks produce patterns of disease risk that resemble those of polygenic or complex traits.

PRINCIPLES OF GENETIC TESTING

Genetic testing aims to identify genetic alterations in patients suffering from an inherited disease. Because several types of mutations unambiguously cause clinical features, whereas others do not or their pathogeneity is not obvious, specialized knowledge of human genetics is crucial for the appropriate interpretation and communication of results.

Basic Techniques in Molecular Genetics

The majority of genetic testing procedures are widely used in medical genetics; however, genetic testing differs from other laboratory analyses in important ways.

The key technologies in molecular genetic analysis are those that aim to identify DNA sequence variations. The first step in genetic testing is extraction of a patient's nucleic acid (DNA or, in rare instances, RNA). The subsequent specific testing procedures nearly always include the polymerase chain reaction (PCR) as the most important basic technique in identifying a sequence variation. PCR allows the in vitro amplification of a single DNA molecule and the enrichment of the DNA fragment of interest. Because of the sensitivity of PCR, a wide range of tissue samples can be analyzed; these include blood samples, buccal scrapes, amniocytes and chorionic villi, hair, or semen from living individuals, but PCR also allows the analysis of archived pathological specimens and Guthrie cards to type dead individuals.

After amplification, PCR products are almost always separated by gel electrophoresis. This electrophoresis can simply be used to separate nucleic fragments by size to demonstrate deletions or insertions, but amplified fragments can also be electrophoresed under specific conditions to differentiate between wild-type genomic sequences and fragments carrying mutations. Such methods include prescreening techniques such as single-strand conformation polymorphism analysis (SSCA), denaturing gradient gel electrophoresis (DGGE), denaturing high performance liquid chromatography (DHLPC), or heteroduplex analysis, which result in abnormal electrophoretic patterns, indicating that a small-scale mutation is present although not defining the nature of this alteration. More information can be obtained by direct sequencing, that is, the analysis of a DNA sequence base by base. Of course, DNA sequencing represents the gold standard of DNA analysis, but it is often time consuming and expensive, particularly with large genes. Therefore a prescreening of DNA samples by the aforementioned nonspecific techniques may be indicated to identify those exons/fragments that indeed harbor genetic alterations. DNA sequencing can then be used to identify the alteration. In addition to DNA sequencing as the gold standard for detecting small-scale mutations, numerous other techniques such as restriction fragment length polymorphisms (RFLPs) or amplification-refractory mutation specific PCR approaches (ARMS) have been developed to identify known mutations. These tests are highly specific but only allow for analysis of specific variants.

Specific assays such as DNA sequencing, RFLPs, or ARMS are of course helpful in cases of genetic diseases with a restricted and well-known spectrum of mutations. However, these targeted approaches fail to give reasonable results in diseases with a high number of "private" mutations such as in autosomal recessive polycystic kidney disease (ARPKD), in which many families carry their own point mutations. Routine diagnostic procedures often consist of a mixture of techniques, including specific tests to cover frequent mutations and screening assays to detect unknown variants.

Another problem with these techniques is that they cover only small-scale fragments: the majority of routine PCR-based tests allow the analysis of genomic sequences with a maximum length of about 500 to 1000 bp. Thus it is noteworthy that gross alterations such as multiexon deletions or duplications are most likely not detectable by standard PCR screening methods, which do not allow quantification. Therefore additional assays to quantify the DNA copy number of the gene of interest have become more and more important in molecular genetics. The significance of DNA copy number variations has been recently and impressively illustrated for genetic testing of the renal cysts and diabetes syndrome (RCAD, or MODY5). RCAD/MODY5 is caused by mutations in the transcription factor *HNF1β/TCF2*. However, as recently shown, a significant proportion of patients do not carry a point mutation but rather a large deletion not detectable by DNA sequencing.[17-20] Meanwhile several reliable strategies for determination of DNA copy numbers have been developed, including Real-Time PCR, quantitative multiplex PCR of short fluorescent fragments (QMPSF), and multiplex ligation probe amplification (MLPA).[21]

Linkage Analysis and Its Limitations

Identification of a pathogenic mutation in a patient with an inherited disease is not always possible. The reasons for this can be multiple: (a) the genomic localization of a gene responsible for an inherited disease is known but not the gene itself, (b) the gene is large and the mutation detection rate is low, and (c) the time to identify a pathogenic mutation is limited, possibly because of an ongoing pregnancy of the index patient's mother.

However, genetic testing in families asking about the risk for further children and relatives can sometimes be offered without knowing the causative mutation in the family. In some situations an indirect genotyping approach, called a *linkage analysis*, can be performed (Figures 5-4, 5-5). Linkage is based on the combined transmission of physically closely linked genomic segments. Prerequisites for linkage analysis are that the genomic localization of the gene is known, that polymorphic markers are available, that the clinical diagnosis is correct, and that DNA samples of numerous family members including the index patient can be obtained. As a consequence, the inheritance of a polymorphic marker indirectly indicates the transmission of a pathogenic mutation in a pedigree. However, linkage analysis always results in probable risk estimations but never allows an absolutely secure conclusion. One reason for this limitation is that recombination events might disturb linkage of a polymorphic marker and the disease locus, possibly leading to an incorrect result.

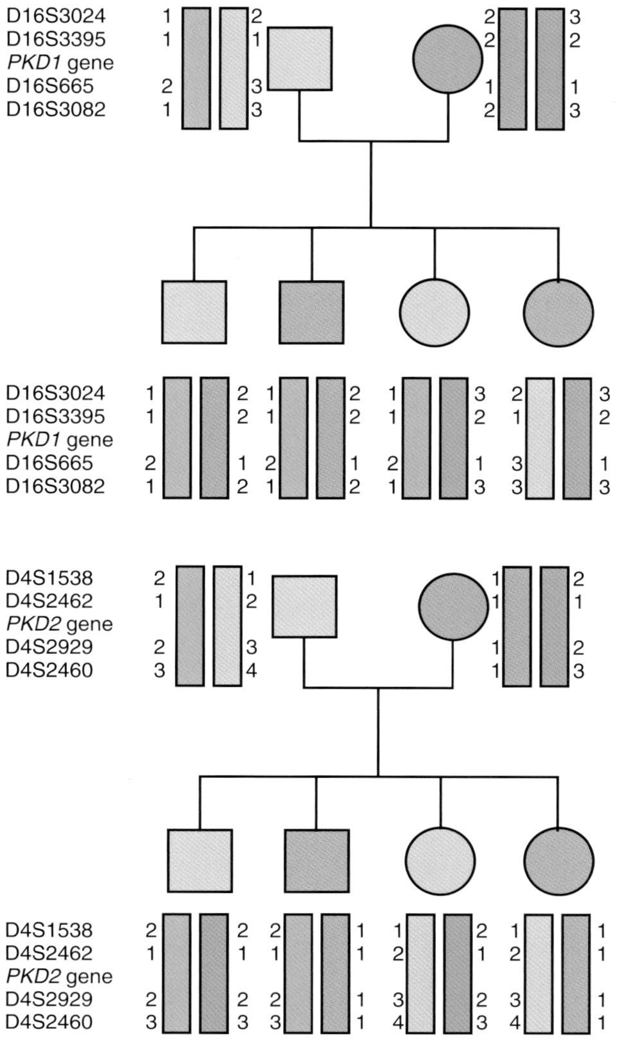

Figure 5-4 Linkage analysis for *PKD1* and *PKD2* in a family with ADPKD. The affected mother *(red circle)* transmitted the disease to two of her four children (one son and one daughter with red symbol, respectively). The disease haplotype of the mother is reddened. Linkage is compatible with *PKD2* (lower pedigree), it can be excluded for *PKD1* (upper pedigree) in this family for two reasons. First, the two affected children inherited different maternal haplotypes, and second, the eldest healthy son inherited the same maternal haplotype as his affected brother.

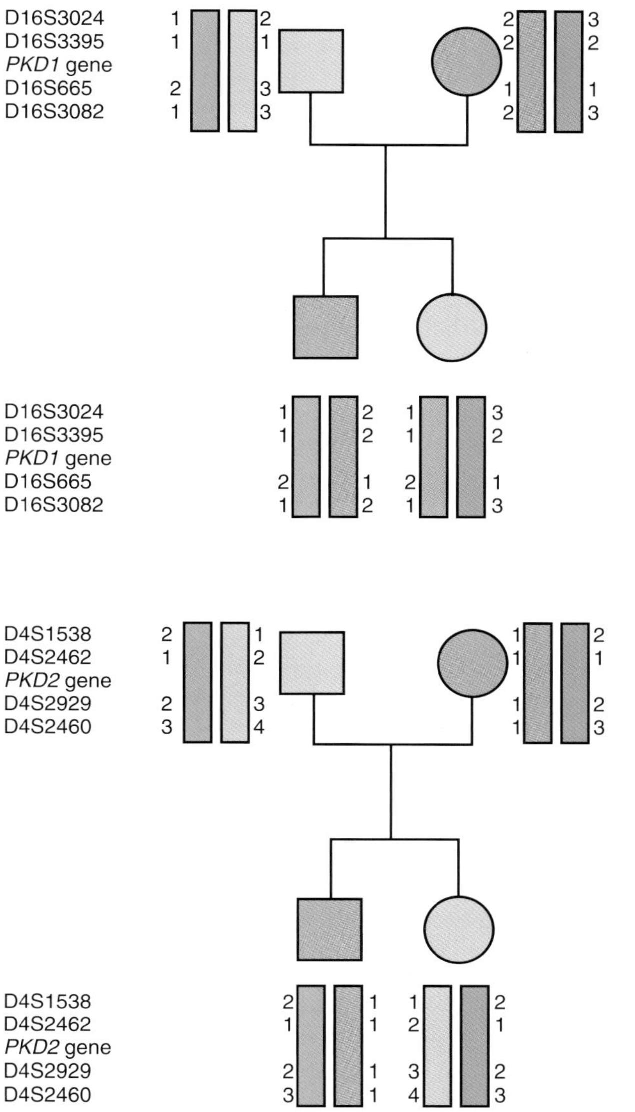

Figure 5-5 Linkage analysis for *PKD1* and *PKD2* in a family with ADPKD. In contrast to the pedigree shown in Figure 5-4, linkage analysis in this small family is not very meaningful. Principally, this family is compatible with linkage to both *PKD* loci. If further family members with known disease status are available for analysis, they should be included in the linkage analysis to increase its information.

Another limitation is caused by heterogeneity of a disease. Three types of heterogeneity can be distinguished:

1. Locus heterogeneity, in which the same clinical phenotype can result from mutations at any one of several different loci (e.g., nephronophthisis or Bardet-Biedl syndrome)[6,22]
2. Allelic heterogeneity (multiple allelism), in which many different mutations within a given gene can be seen in different patients with a certain genetic condition (e.g., the genes known for ARPKD and ADPKD)[9,23,24]
3. Clinical heterogeneity, in which mutations in the same gene produce two or more different diseases (e.g., pleiotropic effects of *NPHP6/CEP290* mutations resulting in nephronophthisis, Senior-Loken syndrome, Joubert syndrome, Meckel-Gruber syndrome, or Leber congenital amaurosis)[25-31]

It is worth noting that many disorders show all three types of heterogeneity.

Linkage analysis can be further hampered by "simple" technical problems: the family may be too small to provide reasonable data (Figure 5-5); in cases of consanguinity the molecular markers might be noninformative; and last but not least, not all family members necessary for linkage are available.

Association Studies

Although the phenotypes of most mendelian disorders are mainly caused by alterations in one single gene, it is now generally accepted that modifying genes, other genetic mechanisms (e.g., epigenetic alterations), and environmental factors considerably influence the clinical course. As outlined earlier, in some cases there is a smooth transition toward multifactorial inheritance patterns. These patterns can be observed for most complex diseases (e.g., asthma or vesicoureteral reflux) in which the interactions between genetic changes and environmental exposures are clearly evident. Genetic variation in one or more genes can increase the individual susceptibility for a disease, but genetic variability often implies unpredictable or poorly predictable vulnerability. Among the 3.2 billion base pairs in the human genome, less than 1% uniquely identifies each human being. Single nucleotide polymorphisms (SNPs) are predicted to occur at least about every 300 bp. Although only a portion of these SNPs will result in amino acid changes, SNPs provide the genetic diversity that, at least in part, underlies the variable susceptibility for environmental stimuli and the variable risk of disease development and progression. Association studies aim to detect such susceptibility factors.[32] Association is not a specifically genetic phenomenon; rather, it is simply a statistical statement about the co-occurrence of alleles or phenotypes. Allele A is associated with disease D if people who have D also have A significantly more often than would be predicted from the individual frequencies of D and A in the population.

In monogenic diseases, the characterization of a causative gene may be difficult, but it is usually obvious when one has succeeded and detected mutations in this gene in patients afflicted with the disease under investigation. For complex diseases it is generally less clear and sometimes difficult to distinguish true susceptibility factors from irrelevant or less relevant DNA polymorphisms.[33] However, identification of susceptibility factors for a disease will greatly advance our understanding of its pathogenesis and hopefully improve its middle- and long-term treatment. In turn, identification of mendelian disease genes will also offer new insights into the pathogenesis and treatment options for complex disorders.

Technical progress will definitely make population screening easier, but one always has to ask whether such screening is worthwhile, cost-effective, and ethically acceptable. An ability to define genetic susceptibility might greatly assist in identifying relevant lifestyle factors, for example. It is essential when identifying somebody at risk that this information be of some real value for the individual.

GENETIC TESTING IN CLINICAL PRACTICE

Genetic testing is usually applied in the following situations: (a) to confirm a clinical diagnosis and, if possible, to support a directed therapy; (b) to test the carriership for an autosomal recessive or X-chromosomal pathogenic allele (heterozygosity testing); (c) prenatal testing; and (d) predictive testing.

Genetic confirmation of a clinical diagnosis is a common indication. However, as previously mentioned, only a well-directed analysis of single genes based on the clinical diagnosis is meaningful. Currently, screening of all known human genes is not possible due to lack of applicable techniques and the huge amount of information that prevents reasonable interpretation.

Because many clinical symptoms are not specific for a distinct monogenic entity, mutations in different genes contributing to the etiology of a disease also have to be considered. Thus a detailed clinical description is a prerequisite for a well-directed genetic testing algorithm. Missing or nonspecific information such as "renal dysplasia" is not helpful and often leads to ambiguous results. Nevertheless it must be mentioned that a genetic test can confirm a clinical diagnosis only by a positive test result. In case of a negative finding, the diagnosis cannot be definitely excluded by the available genetic data. This inability to exclude a specific genetic disease is based on the fact that the mutation detection rate for a gene almost never reaches 100%.

There are several reasons for the inability to detect mutations in a considerable proportion of chromosomes in a certain gene. Missing mutations may reside in regions that are not routinely screened, such as alternatively spliced exons, regulatory elements, or introns distant from the splice donor and acceptor sites, but that may lead to aberrant splicing. Moreover, some of the changes currently categorized as nonpathogenic may ultimately turn out to be disease associated. Alternatively, other mutational mechanisms, for example, gross deletions/duplications or genomic rearrangements, usually cannot be excluded by PCR-based mechanisms. Furthermore, the sensitivity of the applied screening method has to be considered when evaluating genetic testing.

The most reliable testing for carriership can be offered to relatives of patients with a previously proven pathogenic mutation(s). In this situation the respective mutation(s) can be confirmed or excluded in the person seeking genetic counseling. However, the situation is more complex when an unambiguously pathogenic mutation cannot be detected in the family's index patient. As explained earlier, linkage analysis might often be an appropriate tool to further narrow the risk estimation; however, the limitations of linkage analysis have to be considered carefully. In cases where an index patient was not tested by molecular techniques because genetic tests were not available at the time of the patient's death and DNA from the patient was not archived, testing the parents might be helpful to indirectly confirm or corroborate the clinical diagnosis and to detect the causative mutation(s). Finally, these results might be useful in determining risk for other relatives.

Just as in carrier testing, identification of the causative mutation(s) is often a prerequisite for a reliable prenatal diagnosis. If the index patient's mutation(s) is known, fetal DNA extracted from chorionic villus sampling (CVS) or amniocytes can be tested for the respective mutation(s). Whether CVS or amniocentesis (AC) is offered to a family depends on the type of genetic disease and its recurrence risk. Moreover, the applied procedure may also depend on the fetal position at the time of biopsy. All these issues should be discussed in detail with the parents in advance and usually require an interdisciplinary approach, including gynecologists and clinical geneticists given that this discussion should also reflect possible results and consequences for a current pregnancy. Regarding this point, it is important to mention that not only the best-case but also the worst-case scenario should be discussed in advance with the parents and should be embedded in genetic counseling. Limitations of prenatal testing include a possible contamination of fetal DNA with maternal tissue, leading to a false-negative result. To circumvent this problem and to confirm the results of direct genetic testing, a prenatal genetic test should always be accompanied by an indirect linkage analysis for molecular markers closely flanking the gene of interest or located within the respective gene. Prenatal genetic testing is complex and demands an interdisciplinary diagnostic approach; thus an intensive precedent discussion and coverage of all clinical and molecular aspects are required.

Predictive genetic testing is used to predict future risk of disease in an asymptomatic person. In contrast to conventional medical diagnostic tests that define something about the patient's current condition, a predictive genetic test informs only about a future condition that may or may not develop in the tested individual. Predictive genetic testing often raises issues of privacy, independence, insurability, and discrimination, and the test results may have severe emotional consequences. Therefore the possible consequences should be discussed with the patient and/or relatives before testing, and genetic counseling also provided to ultimately allow for informed decision making.

With rare exceptions (such as cases in which a test result has direct therapeutic implications for the patient), predictive testing should not be performed in children and adolescents under 18. The identified risk may be very high (e.g., a positive test for some autosomal dominantly inherited disorders) yet often contains a component of uncertainty, not only about whether a specific condition will develop, but also about when it may appear and how severe it will be. These uncertainties contrast with the presentation of predictive genetic testing in popular media, which often fosters an illusion that genetic risk is highly predictable and definitive in all aspects that may be relevant to the patient.

Predictive genetic testing also frequently has direct implications for family members. Thus concern for relatives may be a motivating factor for a patient wanting to undergo such testing. On the other hand, some patients may resist participating in testing because they prefer not to have information about their genetic risk.

The value of a predictive test depends on the nature of the disease for which testing is being carried out, how effective treatment is, and the cost and efficacy of screening and surveillance measures. Given that the clinical utility of predictive genetic testing for different diseases varies considerably, it is of utmost importance to be aware of the usefulness and complexity of a specific predictive genetic test in advance of testing. Undoubtedly predictive genetic testing is recommended when early identification of individuals at risk of a specific condition will lead to reduced morbidity and mortality through targeted screening, surveillance, and prevention. In addition, the utility of a given predictive genetic test may also change over time as knowledge grows, new strategies for prevention are developed, and costs change. Overall, the complexity of these factors mandates discussions about testing and interdisciplinary approaches that are closely tailored to the testing context and the individual's needs and preferences.

GLOSSARY OF TERMS

Alleles	Alternative forms of a gene at the same locus
Alternative splicing	Formation of diverse mRNAs through differential splicing of an mRNA precursor
Anticipation	Occurrence of a genetic disorder at earlier age of onset and/or at increased severity in successive generations
Autosome	Any chromosome (1-22) other than the sex chromosomes X and Y
cDNA	DNA sequence that contains only exonic sequences and was made from an mRNA molecule
Centimorgan	Length of DNA that on average has 1 crossover per 100 gametes
Cis	Location of two genes/changes on the same chromosome
Codon	Three consecutive bases/nucleotides in DNA/RNA that specify an amino acid
Compound	Individual with two different mutant alleles at a locus
Concordant	Both members of a twin pair show the trait
Consanguineous	Mating between individuals who share at least one common ancestor
Conservation	Sequence similarity for genes present in two distinct organisms or for gene families; can be detected by measuring the sequence similarity at the nucleotide (DNA or RNA) or amino acid (protein) level
Crossover	Exchange of genetic material between homologous chromosomes during meiosis
Digenic inheritance	Two genes interacting to produce a disease phenotype
Diploid	Chromosome number of somatic cells
Discordant	Only one member of a twin pair shows the trait
Disomy, uniparental	Inheritance of both copies of a chromosome from one parent instead of one from each parent
Domain	Segment of a protein associated with a specialized structure or function
Dominant	Trait expressed in the heterozygote
Downstream	Sequence that is distal or 3′ from the reference point
Empiric risk	Recurrence risk based on experience rather than calculation
Epigenetics	Term describing nonmutational phenomena (e.g., methylation and acetylation) that modify the expression of a gene

Euchromatin	Majority of nuclear DNA that remains relatively unfolded during most of the cell cycle and is therefore accessible to transcriptional machinery
Exon	Segment of a gene (usually protein coding) that remains after splicing of the primary RNA transcript
Expressivity	Variation in the severity of a genetic trait
Genotype	Genetic constitution of the organism; usually refers to a particular pair of alleles the individual carries at a given locus of the genome
Germline	Cell lineage resulting in eggs or sperm
Germline mutation	Any detectable, heritable variation in the lineage of germ cells transmitted to offspring while those in somatic cells are not
Gonadal (germline) mosaicism	Occurrence of more than one genetic constitution in the precursor cells of eggs or sperm
Haplotype	Group of nearby, closely linked alleles inherited together as a unit
Heterochromatin	Chromosomal regions that remain tightly folded during the entire cell cycle
Heterozygote	Person with one normal and one mutant allele at a given locus on a pair of homologous chromosomes
Homozygote	Person with identical alleles at a given locus on a pair of homologous chromosomes
Imprinting	Parent-specific expression or repression of genes or chromosomes in offspring
Intron	Segment of a gene transcribed into the primary RNA transcript but excised during exon splicing, thus does not code for a protein
Isodisomy, uniparental	Inheritance of two copies of one homologue of a chromosome from one parent, with loss of the corresponding homologue from the other parent
Karyotype	Classified chromosome complement of an individual or a cell
Lyon hypothesis (X inactivation)	Principle of inactivation of one of the two X chromosomes in normal female cells (first proposed by Dr. Mary Lyon)
Mendelian	Following patterns of inheritance originally proposed by Gregor Mendel
Monogenic disorder	Caused by mutations in a single gene
Mosaicism	Occurrence of more than one genetic constitution arising in an individual after fertilization
Multifactorial disorder	Caused by the interaction of multiple genetic and environmental factors
Mutation	Change from the normal to an altered form of a particular gene that has harmful; pathogenic effects
Oligogenic inheritance	Character that is determined by a small number of genes acting together
Penetrance	Frequency with which a genotype manifests itself in a given phenotype
Phenotype	Visible expression of the action of a particular gene; the clinical picture resulting from a genetic disorder
Pleiotropy	Multiple effects of a single gene
Polymerase chain reaction (PCR)	Amplification of DNA using a specific technique that allows analysis of minute original amounts of DNA
Polymorphism	Usually used for any sequence variant present at a frequency greater than 1% in a population
Recessive	A trait expressed only when both alleles at a given genetic locus are altered
Recombination	Separation of alleles that are close together on the same chromosome by crossing over of homologous chromosomes at meiosis
SNP (single nucleotide polymorphism)	Usually used for any sequence variant present at a frequency greater than 1% in a population
Somatic	Involving the body cells rather than the germline
Syndrome, genetic	Nonrandom combination of features
Teratogen	Any agent causing congenital malformations
Trans	Location of two genes/changes on opposite chromosomes of a pair
Transcription	Production of mRNA from the DNA template
Translation	The process by which protein is synthesized from an mRNA sequence
Trinucleotide repeat	Repeated sequence of three bases (e.g., CAG) expanded and unstable in a group of genetic disorders (see also Anticipation)

REFERENCES

1. Harper PS: *Practical genetic counselling*, ed 6, 2004, Oxford, Oxford University Press.
2. Lewin B: *Genes VII*, Oxford, Oxford University Press, 2000.
3. Lewis R: *Human genetics—concepts and applications*, ed 6, 2005, WCB McGraw-Hill.
4. Strachan T, Reid AP: *Human molecular genetics*, ed 3, New York, 2004, Garland Science Publishing.
5. Gresh L, Fischer E, Reimann A et al: A transcriptional network in polycystic kidney disease, *EMBO J* 23:1657-68, 2004.
6. Hildebrandt F, Otto E: Cilia and centrosomes: a unifying pathogenic concept for cystic kidney disease? *Nat Rev Genet* 6:928-40, 2005.
7. Sivell S, Iredale R, Gray J, Coles B: Cancer genetic risk assessment for individuals at risk of familial breast cancer, *Cochrane Database Syst Rev* 2:CD003721, 2007.
8. Torres VE, Harris PC, Pirson Y: Autosomal dominant polycystic kidney disease, *Lancet* 369:1287-301, 2007.
9. Rossetti S, Harris PC: Genotype-phenotype correlations in autosomal dominant and autosomal recessive polycystic kidney disease, *J Am Soc Nephrol* 18:1374-80, 2007.
10. Hattersley AT: Molecular genetics goes to the diabetes clinic, *Clin Med* 5:476-81, 2005.
11. Lewis A, Reik W: How imprinting centres work, *Cytogenet Genome Res* 113:81-89, 2006.
12. Maher E, Reik W: Beckwith-Wiedemann syndrome: imprinting in clusters revisited, *J Clin Invest*105:247-52, 2000.
13. Abu-Amero S, Monk D, Apostolidou S et al: Imprinted genes and their role in human fetal growth, *Cytogenet Genome Res* 113:262-70, 2006.
14. Horsthemke B, Buiting K: Imprinting defects on human chromosome 15, *Cytogenet Genome Res* 113:292-99, 2006.
15. Gosden RG, Feinberg AP: Genetics and epigenetics: nature's pen-and-pencil set, *N Engl J Med* 356:731-33, 2007.
16. Hitchins MP, Wong JJ, Suthers G et al: Inheritance of a cancer-associated MLH1 germ-line epimutation, *N Engl J Med* 356:697-705, 2007.
17. Bellanne-Chantelot C, Clauin S, Chauveau D et al: Large genomic rearrangements in the hepatocyte nuclear factor-1beta (TCF2) gene are the most frequent cause of maturity-onset diabetes of the young type 5, *Diabetes* 54:3126-32, 2005.
18. Edghill EL, Bingham C, Ellard S, Hattersley AT: Mutations in hepatocyte nuclear factor-1beta and their related phenotypes, *J Med Genet* 43:84-90, 2006.
19. Ulinski T, Lescure S, Beaufils S et al: Renal phenotypes related to hepatocyte nuclear factor-1beta (TCF2) mutations in a pediatric cohort, *J Am Soc Nephrol* 17:497-503, 2006.
20. Decramer S, Parant O, Beaufils S et al: Anomalies of the TCF2 gene are the main cause of fetal bilateral hyperechogenic kidneys, *J Am Soc Nephrol* 18:923-33, 2007.
21. Schouten P, McElgunn CJ, Waaijer R et al: Relative quantification of 40 nucleic acid sequences by multiplex ligation-dependent probe amplification, *Nucleic Acids Res* 30:e57, 2002.
22. Tobin JL, Beales PL: Bardet-Biedl syndrome: beyond the cilium, *Pediatr Nephrol*, 2007.
23. Bergmann C, Senderek J, Küpper F et al: PKHD1 mutations in autosomal recessive polycystic kidney disease (ARPKD), *Hum Mutat* 23:453-63, 2004.
24. Bergmann C, Senderek J, Windelen E et al: Clinical consequences of PKHD1 mutations in 164 patients with autosomal-recessive polycystic kidney disease (ARPKD), *Kidney Int* 67:829-48, 2005.
25. Sayer JA, Otto EA, O'Toole JF et al: The centrosomal protein nephrocystin-6 is mutated in Joubert syndrome and activates transcription factor ATF4, *Nat Genet* 38:674-81, 2006.
26. Valente EM, Silhavy JL, Brancati F et al: Mutations in CEP290, which encodes a centrosomal protein, cause pleiotropic forms of Joubert syndrome, *Nat Genet* 38:623-25, 2006.
27. Den Hollander AI, Koenekoop RK, Yzer S et al: Mutations in the CEP290 (NPHP6) gene are a frequent cause of Leber congenital amaurosis, *Am J Hum Genet* 79:556-61, 2006.
28. Perrault I, Delphin N, Hanein S et al: Spectrum of NPHP6/CEP290 mutations in Leber congenital amaurosis and delineation of the associated phenotype, *Hum Mutat* 28:416, 2007.
29. Baala L, Audollent S, Martinovic J et al: Pleiotropic effects of *CEP290 (NPHP6)* mutations extend to Merkel syndrome, *Am J Hum Genet* 81:170-79, 2007.
30. Brancati F, Barrano G, Silhavy JL et al: *CEP290* mutations are frequently identified in the oculo-renal form of Joubert syndrome-related disorders, *Am J Hum Genet* 81:104-13, 2007.
31. Frank V, den Hollander AI, Ortiz Brüchle N et al: Mutations of the *CEP290* gene encoding a centrosomal protein cause Meckel-Gruber syndrome, *Hum Mutat* 29:45-52, 2007.
32. Altshuler D, Daly M, Kruglyak L: Guilt by association, *Nature Genet* 38:729-39, 2000.
33. Pritchard JK: Are rare variants responsible for susceptibility to complex diseases? *Am J Hum Genet* 69:124-37, 2001.

CHAPTER 6

Structural and Functional Development of the Kidney

Tino D. Piscione and Aoife M. Waters

The kidney presents in the highest degree the phenomenon of sensibility; the power of reacting to various stimuli in a direction which is appropriate for the survival of the organism; a power of adaptation which almost gives one the idea that its component parts must be endowed with intelligence.

E. H. Starling, 1909

As recognized by Starling, the mammalian kidney, through evolution, has developed adaptive regulatory mechanisms such as conservation of water, excretion of waste, maintenance of electrolytes, and acid-base homeostasis. As a result, such regulatory function requires the coordinate development of specific cell types within a precise pattern so that body fluid composition can be closely monitored and regulated. The developmental program that controls this precise patterning is a highly dynamic process involving interplay between genetic and cellular factors. Defects in developmental programming of the kidney result in a spectrum of structural and functional disorders that are discussed in other chapters in this book. To provide a framework for understanding the developmental origins of these disorders, the structural and functional development of the kidney is outlined here.

PART 1: ANATOMIC DEVELOPMENT OF THE KIDNEY

Tino D. Piscione

OVERVIEW OF HUMAN KIDNEY DEVELOPMENT

Human kidney development begins at the fifth week of gestation.[1] The first functioning nephrons are formed by week 9. By 32 to 34 weeks, nephrogenesis is completed after which no new nephron units are formed.[2,3] In humans that suffer fetal or perinatal renal injury, the developing kidney is not capable of compensating for irreversible nephron loss by either accelerating the rate of nephron formation ex utero in infants born prematurely or by de novo generation of nephrons once nephrogenesis is completed.[2,4] Consequently the number of functioning nephrons formed at 32 to 34 weeks' gestation may have important implications for long-term renal outcome.

There is increasing evidence that the number of nephrons formed at birth is a determinant of renal function later in life. This concept is supported by the association of renal failure in humans with oligomeganephronia[5,6] and by the demonstration of reduced glomerular number in humans with primary hypertension and chronic kidney disease.[7,8] Quantitative analyses in humans and rodents using stereologic methods of glomerular counting in renal autopsy specimens have revealed a direct relationship between birth weight and glomerular number.[9,10] The latter data are consistent with the Barker hypothesis, which proposes that adult disease has fetal origins and is based on epidemiologic studies showing a correlation between birth weight and the incidence of cardiovascular disease.[11,12] Consequently mechanisms that control structural and functional kidney development are likely to be crucial for programming long-term, as well as short-term, renal survival.

MORPHOLOGIC STAGES OF HUMAN KIDNEY DEVELOPMENT

Our understanding of the morphologic stages of human kidney development is largely based on histologic descriptions of microdissected human fetal kidney autopsy specimens performed by Edith Potter and Vitoon Osathanondh.[1,13,14] Their seminal work was complemented by analyses of mouse kidney development performed by Lauri Saxen.[15] These studies revealed conserved mechanisms of nephrogenesis between humans and mice, and formed the basis for utilizing the murine embryonic kidney as an ideal system to study mammalian kidney development. Advances in human genomics and mammalian developmental genetics have further accelerated the tempo of new discovery in the field of developmental nephrology. Consequently this research has resulted in a clearer understanding of the original morphologic descriptions of kidney development and the identification of key regulators of nephrogenesis (reviewed in[16,17]). The morphologic stages of mammalian kidney development are summarized in the following section. Cellular events that underlie these morphologic changes are discussed in Part 2 under Sodium Transport in the Developing Kidney. Current knowledge of genetic and molecular regulation is then reviewed in Potassium Transport in the Developing Kidney, also in Part 2.

OVERVIEW OF MAMMALIAN KIDNEY MORPHOGENESIS

The mammalian kidney derives from two parts of the metanephros, its embryonic precursor. The first part is the ureteric bud, which originates as an epithelial outgrowth of the wolffian duct. The ureteric bud gives rise to the collecting duct (CD) system, including cortical and medullary CDs, renal calyces, renal pelvis, ureter, and trigone of the bladder.[2,15] Development of the CD system involves an embryonic process termed *branching morphogenesis,* defined as the formation of branched tubules.[18] As a developmental process, branching morphogenesis is essential in the formation of several tissues, including kidney, lung, mammary tissue, exocrine pancreas, and salivary glands (reviewed in[18]). In kidney development, renal branching morphogenesis may be considered a sequence of related events, which include (1) outgrowth of the ureteric bud, (2) iterative branching of the ureteric bud and derivation of its daughter CDs, (3) patterning of the cortical and medullary CD system, and (4) formation of the pelvicalyceal system.

The second part of the metanephros that forms the mammalian kidney is the metanephric mesenchyme. Metanephric mesenchyme originates as undifferentiated cells located in the posterior intermediate mesoderm adjacent to the metanephric duct. Differentiation of metanephric mesenchyme gives rise to all epithelial cell types that make up the mature nephron, including the visceral and parietal epithelium of the glomerulus, the proximal convoluted tubule, the ascending and descending limbs of the loops of Henle, and the distal convoluted tubule.[2,15] Metanephric mesenchymal differentiation involves a process termed *mesenchymal-epithelial transformation (MET).* MET results in conversion of loosely associated, nonpolarized mesenchymal cells into tightly associated, polarized epithelial cells that form primitive tubules. Further differentiation of epithelial cell types within these primitive tubules occurs in a spatially organized proximal-distal pattern, resulting in formation of the glomerular and tubular segments of the mature nephron.

Ureteric Bud Induction

Genetic and molecular control of ureteric bud outgrowth are discussed in greater detail in the section "Ureteric Bud Induction" later in the chapter. Here we focus on morphogenetic events of ureteric bud induction, such as the number and position of ureteric buds that form at the onset of kidney development.

Ureteric bud formation may be considered the initial step in mammalian kidney development (Figure 6-1, *A*). The ureteric bud forms as an outgrowth of the wolffian duct in response to external cues provided by surrounding metanephric mesenchyme. The wolffian duct, also known as the mesonephric or nephric duct, is a paired embryonic epithelial tubule extending in an anterior-posterior orientation on either side of the midline. It is divided into three segments—the pronephros, mesonephros, and metanephros. At its anterior end the pronephros forms the renal anlage in fish[19] and frogs[20] but degenerates in mammals. The midportion of the wolffian duct, the mesonephros, gives rise to male reproductive organs, including the rete testis, efferent ducts, epididymis, vas deferens, seminal vesicle, and prostate.[21] In females the mesonephric portion of the wolffian duct degenerates. The caudal portion, the metanephros, gives origin to the ureteric bud on its lateral aspect. The posterior segment of the duct communicates with the cloaca to form the trigone of the bladder.[21]

Ureteric bud formation is initiated at week 5 of human fetal gestation and at embryonic day 10.5 (E10.5) in mice. Signals from the metanephric mesenchyme induce the ureteric bud to form, elongate, and invade the mesenchyme. Failure to induce ureteric bud outgrowth results in renal agenesis, which occurs unilaterally or bilaterally if the ureteric bud fails to form on one or both wolffian ducts, respectively.[16] Additional signals are required to restrict the number of ureteric buds induced to form from the wolffian duct, as revealed by the demonstration of severe renal and urogenital malformations in humans and mice when ectopic outgrowth of multiple ureteric buds from a single wolffian duct is observed.[22] Moreover, the relative position of ureteric bud outgrowth from the wolffian duct appears to be crucial to formation of a single ureter and competent vesicoureteral junction. A relationship between ectopic positioning of ureteric bud outgrowth and vesicoureteral reflux is largely supported by evidence from Mackie and Stephens, who described defects in vesicoureteral junction formation in patients with ureteral duplications.[23] On the basis of their observations, they postulated that when outgrowth of the ureteric bud occurs at an ectopic site, the final site of the ureteral orifice in the bladder will be ectopic.[23] These data are supported by phenotypic analyses of mice with mutations in *Bmp4,*[24] *Robo2,*[25] and components of the renin-angiotensin cascade,[26,27] which show ureteral duplications or vesicoureteral reflux and demonstrate ectopic placement of ureteric bud formation on the wolffian duct.

Renal Branching Morphogenesis

Renal branching morphogenesis commences between the fifth and sixth week of gestation[2] in humans, and at E11.5 in mice[15] when the ureteric bud invades the metanephric mesenchyme and forms a T-shaped, branched structure (Figure 6-1, *B*). This T-shaped structure subsequently undergoes further iterative branching events (Figure 6-1, C) to generate approximately 15 generations of branches. In human kidney development, the first 9 generations of branching are completed by approximately 15 weeks' gestation.[2] During this time new nephrons are induced through reciprocal inductive interactions between the newly formed tips of the ureteric bud and surrounding metanephric mesenchyme. By week 20 to 22 of gestation, ureteric bud branching is completed, and the remainder of CD development occurs by extension of peripheral (or cortical) segments and remodeling of central (or medullary) segments.[2] During these final stages new nephrons form predominantly through the induction of

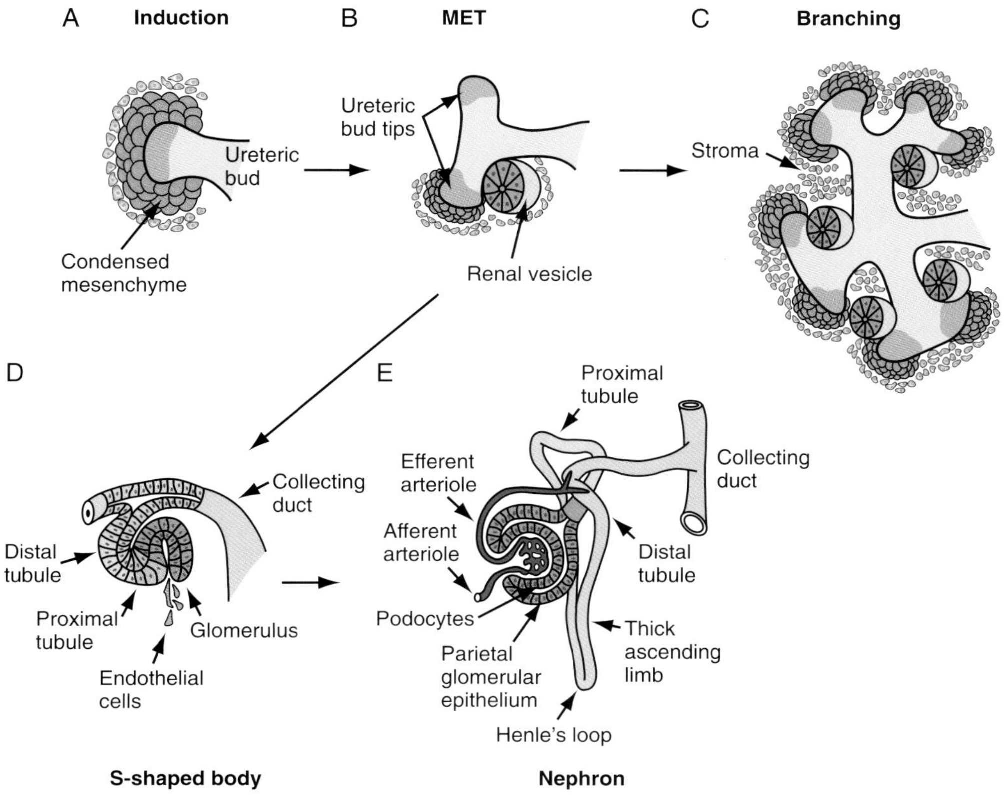

Figure 6-1 Stages of nephrogenesis. **A,** Induction of the metanephric mesenchyme by the ureteric bud promotes aggregation of condensed mesenchyme around the tip of the ureteric bud. **B,** Polarized renal vesicles subsequently develop as the mesenchyme undergoes epithelial transition. Fusion of renal vesicles occurs with the collecting ducts. **C,** Stromal cells secrete factors that influence cell fate choices in neighboring nephrogenic structures and collecting ducts. **D,** A cleft forms in the renal vesicle, giving rise to the comma-shaped body. The development of the S-shaped body involves formation of a proximal cleft that is subsequently invaded by angioblasts and starts the process of glomerulogenesis **(E).** (Image redrawn from Dressler GR: The cellular basis of kidney development, *Annu Rev Cell Dev Biol* 22:509-29, 2006.)

approximately four to seven nephrons around the tips of terminal CD branches that have completed their branching program while retaining the capacity to induce new nephron formation.[2,15]

Throughout renal branching morphogenesis, the branching ureteric bud recapitulates a patterned, morphogenetic sequence. This sequence includes (1) expansion of the advancing ureteric bud branch at its leading tip (called the *ampulla*), (2) division of the ampulla causing the formation of new ureteric bud branches, and (3) elongation of the newly formed branch segment. Analysis of renal branching morphogenesis in organ culture systems employing kidneys of transgenic mice expressing the fluorescent reporter (known as enhanced green fluorescent protein, or EGFP) in the ureteric bud lineage have been informative regarding the sequence and pattern of branching events that occur following the formation of the initial T structure.[28,29] Accordingly, all terminal branching begins with formation of a swollen ampulla at the tip, expanding to two to three times the diameter of the parental trunk before it is clear how many daughter segments will be generated. The majority of bifurcations are symmetric wherein the ampulla flattens and extends in two opposite directions, resulting in terminal bifurcation. However, trifid branching (i.e., three daughter branches arising from one ampulla) and lateral branching (i.e., de novo branch formation arising from a ureteric bud truncal segment) resulting in asymmetric branching have also been described.[28] When asymmetric branching occurs, the ampulla first grows in one direction, forming an L rather than a T shape. In the case of a trifurcation, the ampulla forms three distinct humps, each of which forms a new segment. Regression of trifid branches is frequently observed,[28,30] suggesting that dynamic remodeling occurs during renal branching morphogenesis. Morphometric analyses of individual branch growth parameters reveal a conserved hierarchic pattern of diminishing final length achieved for successive ureteric bud branch generations such that sixth generation branches are shorter than fifth generation branches, etc.[28] However, in kidney organ culture, asymmetric branching has been described in which branches forming in the posterior region of kidney explants elongate at a slower growth rate compared with branches formed in anterior regions.[31] Presumably, mechanisms that promote asymmetric renal branching morphogenesis may be crucial to achieving the final nonspheric shape attained by the fully formed kidney.

Corticomedullary Patterning and Formation of the Pelvicalyceal System

Between weeks 22 and 34 of human fetal gestation,[2] or E15.5-birth in mice,[15] morphologic changes result in the establishment of peripheral (i.e., cortical) and central (i.e., medullary) domains in the developing kidney. The renal cortex, which represents 70% of total kidney volume at birth,[30] becomes organized as a relatively compact, circumferential rim of tissue surrounding the periphery of the kidney. The renal medulla, which represents 30% of total kidney volume at birth,[30] has a modified cone shape with a broad base contiguous with cortical tissue. The apex of the cone is formed by convergence of CDs in the inner medulla and is termed *papilla*.

Distinct morphologic differences emerge between CDs located in the medulla and those located in the renal cortex during this stage of kidney development. Medullary CDs are organized into elongated, relatively unbranched linear arrays that converge centrally in a region devoid of glomeruli. In contrast, CDs located in the renal cortex continue to induce metanephric mesenchyme. The specification of cortical and medullary domains is essential for the eventual function of the mature CD system. The most central segments of the CD system formed from the first five generations of ureteric bud branching undergo remodeling by increased growth and dilation of these tubules to form the pelvis and calyces (reviewed in[32]).

The developing renal cortex and medulla exhibit distinct axes of growth. The renal cortex grows along a circumferential axis, resulting in a tenfold increase in volume while preserving compact organization of cortical tissue around the developing kidney.[30] In this manner, differentiating glomeruli and tubules maintain their relative position in the renal cortex with respect to the external surface of the kidney, or renal capsule. The preservation of this spatial relationship between developing nephrons and the renal capsule appears to be crucial, as revealed by defective nephron development in mice that fail to form a renal capsule.[33] In contrast to the circumferential pattern of growth exhibited by the developing renal cortex, the developing renal medulla expands 4.5-fold in thickness along a longitudinal axis perpendicular to the axis of cortical growth.[30] This pattern of renal medulla growth is largely due to elongation of outer medullary CDs.[30] The development of a medullary zone coincides with the appearance of stromal cells between the seventh and eighth generations of ureteric bud branches.[30] It is suggested that stromal cells provide stimulatory cues to promote the growth of medullary CDs.[30] Additional support for this hypothesis is provided by analyses of mutant mice lacking functional expression of stromal transcription factors Pod1 and Foxd1,[34-36] which demonstrate defects in medullary CD patterning.

Mesenchymal-Epithelial Transformation

MET is initiated when the ureteric bud invades the metanephric mesenchyme (Figure 6-1). Upon contact with the ureteric bud, the mesenchyme condenses to form a discrete zone four-to-five-cells thick around the ampulla of the advancing ureteric bud, termed *cap condensate*.[37,38] Near the junction of the ampulla and its corresponding ureteric bud truncal segment, a localized cluster of cells separates from the cap condensate and forms an oval mass, called a *pretubular aggregate*. Formation of the pretubular aggregate may be considered a primordial event in nephron development (or nephronogenesis) since cells within this cluster acquire an epithelial cellular phenotype, including a columnar shape and a basement membrane.[37] Simultaneously with epithelialization, an internal cavity forms within the pretubular aggregate, at which point the structure is called a *renal vesicle*. The renal vesicle subsequently forms a connection with its neighboring ureteric bud ampulla, permitting the ureteric bud lumen to communicate with the internal cavity of the renal vesicle.

Archetypal organ culture experiments have demonstrated that isolated metanephric mesenchyme undergoes apoptosis unless induced by coculture with ureteric bud rudiments or a heterologous inducer (e.g., spinal cord).[15,39] These data suggest that the default program for metanephric mesenchyme development is death unless induction occurs.[37] Furthermore, removal of the inducer following induction did not prevent further differentiation of the mesenchyme,[37] which suggests that the developmental program for MET, once initiated, is not dependent on cues continuously supplied by the ureteric bud. The observation that induced metanephric mesenchymal cells may contain all the information necessary to form new nephrons without need for further support from the ureteric bud has led to speculation that induced metanephric mesenchymal cells may represent a nephrogenic stem cell population.

Stromal cells are comprised of interstitial cells that secrete extracellular matrix and growth factors, and are thought to provide a supportive framework around the developing nephrons and collecting system. Prevailing theories regarding the developmental origin of stromal cells include their development as a separate lineage within the metanephric mesenchyme[40,41] or their migration into the developing kidney as neural crest precursors.[42,43] During nephronogenesis and renal branching morphogenesis, stromal cells are found surrounding developing nephrons and ureteric bud branches. As the renal cortex and medulla become morphologically distinct regions, stromal cells become defined geographically and molecularly into two separate populations: cortical stroma, which form interstitium between induced nephrons and express *Foxd1*, *Raldh2*, *Rarα*, and *Rarβ2;* and medullary stroma, which form interstitium between medullary CDs and express *Fgf7*, *Pod1*, and *Bmp4*. Key roles for stromal cells in kidney development are suggested by the demonstration of defects in renal branching morphogenesis and nephronogenesis in mutant mice lacking stromal-expressed genes.[24,33,35,44-46] By birth, many medullary stromal cells have undergone apoptosis and the space they once occupied is filled by developing loops of Henle.[47] Once nephrogenesis is complete, stromal cells differentiate into a diverse population that includes fibroblasts, lymphocyte-like cells, and pericytes.[47,48]

Proximal and Distal Tubule Morphogenesis

All epithelial cell types of the nephron, including glomerular and tubular cells, originate from multipotential precursors residing in renal vesicles.[41,49] Nephron segmentation into glomerular and tubular domains is initiated by the sequential formation of two clefts in the renal vesicle[2] (Figure 6-1, *D*). Creation of a lower cleft, termed *vascular cleft*, heralds formation of the comma-shaped body. The comma-shaped body is a transient structure that rapidly undergoes morphogenetic conversion into an S-shaped structure (termed *S-shaped body*) upon generation of an upper cleft. The S-shaped body is characterized by three segments or limbs. The middle and upper limbs give rise to the tubular segments of the mature nephron. Whereas the middle limb of the S-shaped body gives rise to the proximal convoluted tubule,[2] the descending and ascending limbs of the loops of Henle and the distal convoluted tubule originate from the upper limb of the S-shaped body[2,15] (Figure 6-1, *E*). As the vascular cleft broadens and deepens, the lower limb of the S-shaped body forms a cup-shaped unit. Epithelial cells lining the inner wall of this cup will make up the visceral glomerular epithelium, or podocytes. Cells lining the outer wall of the cup will form parietal glomerular epithelium, or Bowman's capsule. Morphogenetic stages of glomerular development, including the formation of the glomerular endocapillary tuft, are discussed in the section Glomerulogenesis, later in the chapter.

All parts of the developing nephron become larger as they mature. However, the most striking changes consist of increased tortuosity of the proximal convoluted tubule and elongation of the loop of Henle.[2] Cellular maturation of the proximal tubule involves transition from columnar to cuboidal epithelium, elaboration of apical and basal microvilli, and gradual increase in tubular diameter and length.[50] The human kidney at birth shows marked heterogeneity in proximal tubule length as one progresses from the outer cortex to the inner cortex.[51] Uniformity in proximal tubule length is achieved by 1 month of life and continues to lengthen at a uniform rate. Prospective cells of the loop of Henle are thought to be first positioned at the junctional region of the middle and upper limbs of the S-shaped body near the vascular pole of the glomerulus, where it will form the macula densa.[52] The descending and ascending limbs of the presumptive loop of Henle are first recognizable as a U-shaped structure in the periphery of the developing renal cortex, termed the *nephrogenic zone*.[52,53] Maturation of the primitive loop involves elongation of both ascending and descending limbs through the corticomedullary boundary. Continued maturation involves differentiation of descending and ascending limb epithelia, resulting in a gradual decrease in cell height.[54] Development of the presumptive distal tubule involves elongation of the connecting piece that joins with the ureteric bud/CD.

Longitudinal growth of the medulla contributes to lengthening of the loops of Henle such that all but a small percentage of them extend below the corticomedullary junction in full-term newborn infants.[2] As the kidney grows postnatally, the loops of Henle further elongate and reach the inner two thirds of the renal medulla in the mature kidney. There the loops of Henle contribute to the kidney's urine-concentrating mechanism through differential transport of urine solutes along its ascending limb, resulting in generation of an interstitial medullary tonicity gradient. Maintenance of this gradient is functionally coupled to urine concentration by rendering a favorable gradient for water reabsorption from CDs. Functional development of the kidney's urine-concentrating mechanism is dependent on elongation of the loops of Henle during nephrogenesis, because longer loops are more capable of generating steeper medullary tonicity gradients, which favor urine-concentrating capacity. In the extremely premature fetus, the loops of Henle are short due to the relative distance between the renal capsule and the renal papilla. Consequently the urine-concentrating capacity of the premature kidney is limited by generation of a shallow medullary tonicity gradient.

Glomerulogenesis

During embryonic development, formation of the lower limb of the S-shaped body heralds the onset of glomerulogenesis[2,55] (Figure 6-2, *A*). The vascular cleft provides an entry point to which progenitor endothelial and mesangial cells are recruited.[56] Cells residing along the inner surface of the lower S-shaped body limb represent nascent podocytes (Figure 6-2, *B*). At this stage immature podocytes are proliferative and exhibit a columnar shape, apical cell attachments, and a single-layer basement membrane.[55]

Development of the glomerular capillary tuft is a dynamic process involving recruitment and proliferation of endothelial and mesangial cell precursors, formation of a capillary plexus, and concomitant assembly of podocytes and mesangial cells distributed around the newly formed capillary loops.[55] The origin of endothelial and mesangial cell precursors is the subject of ongoing controversy. Experimental evidence involving autologous transplantation of embryonic kidney rudiments into adult renal cortex suggests that glomerular endothelial precursors, or angioblasts, and mesangial precursors originate from a unique subpopulation of induced metanephric mesenchyme that do not differentiate along epithelial or stromal lineages.[56-58] However, an alternate theory is provided using evidence that glomerular capillaries originate from ingrowth of primitive sprouts from external vessels through experiments involving engraftment of rodent fetal kidneys onto avian chorioallantoic membrane.[59] These latter experiments reveal that developing glomeruli are populated by cells that derive from both donor and recipient tissues, supporting the potential role of angiogenesis in glomerular capillary tuft development.

Although clear cause-and-effect relationships are not known, recruitment of angioblasts and mesangial precursors into the vascular cleft results in deformation of the lower S-shaped body limb into a cuplike structure[2] (Figure 6-2). Formation of a primitive vascular plexus occurs at this so-called capillary loop stage. Podocytes of capillary loop stage glomeruli lose mitotic capacity[60] and begin to demonstrate complex cellular architecture, including the formation of actin-based cytoplasmic extensions, or foot processes, and the formation of specialized intercellular junctions, termed *slit diaphragms*.[61,62] Subsequent development of the glomerular capillary tuft involves extensive branching of capillaries and formation of endothelial fenestrae.[2] Mesangial cells, in turn, populate the core of the tuft and provide structural support to capillary loops through the deposition of extracellular matrix.[63,64] The full complement of glomeruli in the fetal human kidney is attained by 32 to 34 weeks, when nephrogenesis ceases.[2] At birth, superficial glomeruli, which are chronologically the last to be formed, are significantly smaller than juxtamedullary glomeruli, which are the earliest formed glomeruli.[51] Subsequent glomerular development involves hypertrophy, and glomeruli reach adult size by $3^1/_2$ years of age.[51]

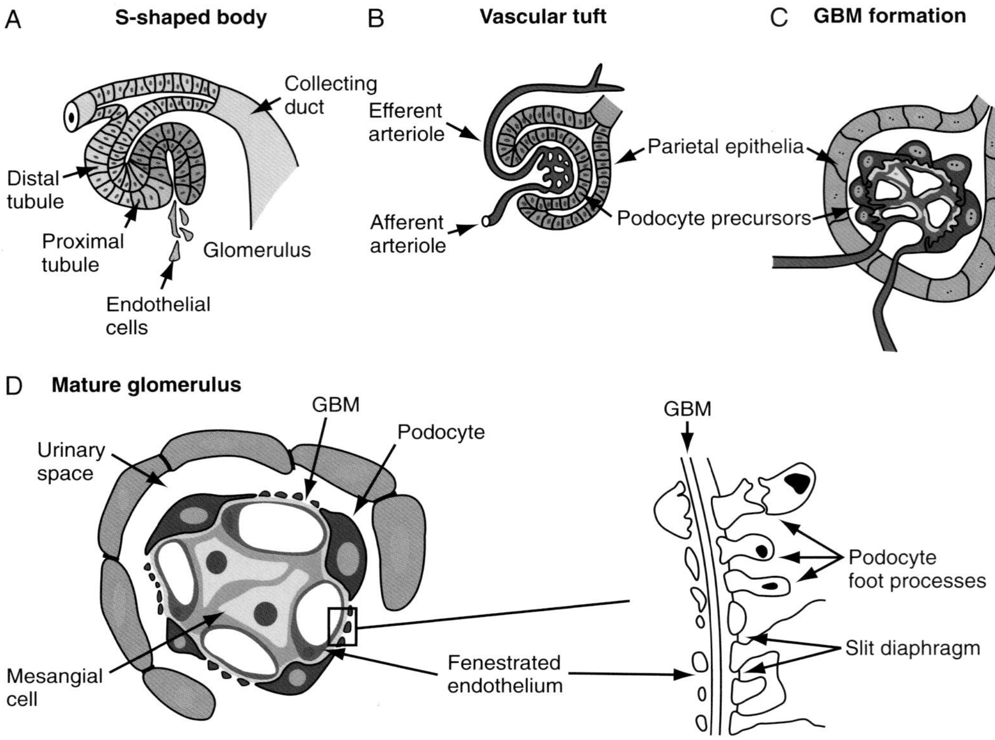

Figure 6-2 Glomerular development. **A,** Endothelial cells are recruited into the cup-shaped glomerular precursor region of the S-shaped body, forming a primitive vascular tuft. (From Pichel JG et al: Defects in enteric innervation and kidney development in mice lacking GDNF, *Nature* 382:73-76, 1996.) **B,** Podocyte precursors contact invading endothelial cells and begin to differentiate. In turn, endothelial cells form a primitive capillary plexus (capillary loop stage). (From Schuchardt A et al: Defects in the kidney and enteric nervous system of mice lacking the tyrosine kinase receptor Ret, *Nature* 367:380-383, 1994.) **C,** An interposed glomerular basement membrane forms between podocytes and endothelial cells. Parietal epithelial cells encapsulate the developing glomerulus. **D,** Elaboration of podocyte primary and secondary cellular processes accompanies podocyte differentiation and formation of the glomerular filtration barrier. *Inset,* A high magnification electron micrograph showing the fenestrated endothelium, podocyte foot processes, and slit diaphragms located between the interdigitating foot processes. (Image redrawn from Dressler GR: The cellular basis of kidney development, *Annu Rev Cell Dev Biol* 22:509-29, 2006.)

CELLULAR EVENTS IN KIDNEY MORPHOGENESIS

Overview

Epithelial morphogenesis involves temporal and spatial coordination of multiple cellular activities such as cell proliferation, apoptosis, changes in cell shape, and cell migration.[65] Despite their importance to epithelial development, little is known how these cellular events are coupled during renal branching morphogenesis and nephron development. In the following section, spatial and temporal patterns of cell proliferation and apoptosis during renal CD development and nephron morphogenesis are reviewed. Evidence that regulation of these cellular events is essential for normal morphogenesis is highlighted.

Roles of Cell Proliferation in Kidney Development

During renal branching morphogenesis, cell proliferation is highly conspicuous at the tips of the ureteric bud/CD branches where inductive and branching events occur.[66] In contrast, cell proliferation is detected at lower levels in the medulla and renal papilla.[66]

The relationship between cell proliferation and branch induction is the subject of ongoing research. Localized cell proliferation appears to contribute to evagination of the ureteric bud from the wolffian duct and formation of ampullae. During ureteric bud induction, proliferation rates are highest on the side of the wolffian duct where the ureteric bud forms.[67] As the ureteric bud generates new branches, proliferation rates are higher in branch tips than in trunks.[67-69]

During nephronogenesis, epithelial progenitors that comprise the proximal and distal tubular segments of the developing nephron demonstrate cell proliferation throughout much of their development.[70] In contrast, podocyte maturation coincides with a loss of mitotic activity and cell cycle blockade.[60] The limited capacity of mature podocytes to undergo cell proliferation has important implications concerning the glomerular response to injury, because damaged podocytes cannot compensate for loss of function by way of regeneration. Moreover, escape from cell-cycle blockade in mature podocytes has been associated with severe changes in glomerular cytoarchitecture and a rapidly progressive decline in renal function, as demonstrated by the deleterious course of idiopathic collapsing and human immunodeficiency virus (HIV) nephropathies.[71]

Roles for Apoptosis in Kidney Development

Soluble factors are essential for preventing a default program for apoptosis within the metanephric mesenchyme. For example, isolated metanephric mesenchyme undergoes cell death in the absence of inductive cues;[39] however, mesenchymal cells are rescued from apoptosis in the presence of growth factors (e.g., EGF, FGF2, BMP7)[72-74] and when exposed to a native (e.g., isolated ureteric bud) or heterologous (e.g., isolated spinal cord tissue) inducer.[73,75] Inhibition of mesenchymal apoptosis by pharmacologic or genetic manipulation causes defects in ureteric bud branching and nephrogenesis,[26,76] suggesting that alterations of metanephric mesenchymal apoptosis disrupt important functional interactions between mesenchymal and epithelial cells. Possible roles for apoptosis in metanephric mesenchyme include regulation of metanephric size through elimination of cells yet to respond to inductive signals, establishment of tissue boundaries between cell populations induced to enter developmental programs of epithelial or stromal determination, or elimination of cells that secrete inhibitory factors that block differentiation of developing nephrons and CDs.[66,77]

In the developing collecting system, apoptosis is infrequently detected in the tips and trunks of the branching ureteric bud.[66] At later stages of embryonic and postnatal kidney development, apoptosis is prominent in the medullary regions of the rat CD system that give rise to the calyces and renal pelvis and renal papilla.[66] The prominence of apoptosis in the region of the rat-developing kidney that eventually forms the renal pelvis suggests a potential role for apoptosis in remodeling the first three to five generations of the branched ureteric bud/developing CD system. The extent to which apoptosis contributes to this morphogenetic process, however, is unknown. Other suggested roles for medullary apoptosis include elimination of medullary interstitial cells as a mechanism for making room for new blood vessel ingrowth.[78]

In contrast to metanephric mesenchyme that undergoes apoptosis in the absence of an inducer, isolated ureteric bud cells do not demonstrate apoptosis when cultured ex vivo in growth factor-free basal medium.[79] The mechanism underlying cellular preservation in this context is unclear and may reflect an intrinsic survival tendency imparted to ureteric bud–derived cells by cellular factors such as the establishment of basement membrane, cell polarity, and junctional complex formation. Thus in contrast to metanephric mesenchyme, the occurrence of apoptosis in the ureteric bud lineage is more likely to result as a developmentally regulated cellular event than by default from lack of survival factors.

Evidence that cell survival is spatially regulated during renal branching morphogenesis is provided by several studies in which dysregulated apoptosis and cell proliferation are associated with defective CD development. For example, increased branched ureteric bud cell proliferation and subsequent medullary CD cell apoptosis were observed in *Gpc3 null* mice that exhibit profound cystic degeneration of the medullary CD system,[80,81] suggesting that altered spatiotemporal patterns of CD cell proliferation and apoptosis may be a crucial mechanism underlying the CD dysplasia observed in these mutant mice. Also, increased apoptosis was associated with CD cyst formation in mice mutated for genes associated with cell survival, including *bcl2*[82] and *AP-2*.[83] Moreover, apoptosis was a prominent feature of dilated CDs in experimental models of fetal and neonatal urinary tract obstruction.[84,85] These data suggest a causal relationship between CD apoptosis and two frequent features of renal dysplasia—cystogenesis and urinary tract dilation. It is unclear from these studies, however, whether excessive CD apoptosis is a primary event in collecting system dilation or cyst formation in dysplastic or obstructed kidneys.[86]

GENETIC AND MOLECULAR CONTROL OF KIDNEY MORPHOGENESIS

Overview

Development of the mammalian kidney is controlled by reciprocal inductive interactions between the metanephric mesenchyme and the ureteric bud. Signals that promote and direct ureteric bud branching morphogenesis originate from all derivative cell types of the metanephric mesenchyme, including induced and uninduced mesenchyme,[39,75,87] stromal cells,[33,35,44,45,88] and angioblasts,[89,90] as well as the ureteric bud itself.[69] Similarly, metanephric mesenchyme responds to inductive cues supplied by the ureteric bud to initiate mesenchyamalepithelial transformation.[17,72,91,92] Subsequent patterning and differentiation of nephrogenic cell types are highly dependent on factors supplied by developing epithelial[93,94] and stromal cells.[33,36,95]

The molecular and genetic control of kidney morphogenesis is the subject of several recent comprehensive reviews.[17,92,96-98] Mutational analyses in mice have yielded much insight into the role of several genes and molecular pathways that function as key variables in nephrogenesis subprograms, such as ureteric bud induction and outgrowth, ureteric bud branching, spatial patterning of the collecting system, nephronogenesis including segmental differentiation, and lower urinary tract development. The phenotypes resulting from murine gene mutations (e.g., failed ureteric bud outgrowth and ectopic ureteric bud outgrowth) serve as paradigms for renal malformations (namely, renal agenesis and duplex kidney) that predict roles for corresponding human gene mutations in the pathogenesis of these conditions (Table 6-1). The following sections focus on major phenotypes generated by mutations in several genes that exhibit their roles at discrete stages in nephrogenesis.

Ureteric Bud Induction

Defects in ureteric bud induction are likely to underlie human malformation phenotypes that result in complete absence of nephrogenesis (e.g., unilateral or bilateral renal aplasia), or in ectopic formation of the kidney (e.g., duplex kidney).

Transcriptional Control of Ureteric Bud Outgrowth

Phenotypic analyses of mice with targeted gene deletions or tissue-specific mutational inactivation of conditional alleles have been informative regarding the roles of several transcription factor genes for induction of ureteric bud outgrowth, including *Eya1*,[99] *Six1*,[100] *Pax2*,[101,102] *Wt1*,[103] *Sall1*,[104] and *Lim1*.[105,106] *Pax2*,[107] *Lim1*,[108] and the tyrosine kinase receptor *Ret*[109] are expressed in the murine wolffian duct before the onset of ureteric bud induction. *Sall1*,[104] *Six1*,[100] *Eya1*[99,110] and the secreted peptide growth factor *Gdnf*[111] are expressed in intermediate mesoderm in the presumptive metanephric mesenchyme. *Wt1* expression is induced in the metanephric

TABLE 6-1 Mouse Mutations Exhibiting Defects in Kidney Morphogenesis and Predominant Accompanying Renal Phenotypes

Mutant Gene	Morphogenetic Defect	Predominant Mutant Renal Malformation Phenotype
	Failed ureteric bud outgrowth	
Metanephric mesenchyme derived		Renal aplasia
Eya1		
Gdnf		
Odd1		
Sall1		
Six1		
Wt1		
Ureteric bud derived		
Emx2		
Gfrα1		
Hoxa11/Hoxd11/Hoxc11		
Hs2st		
Itgα8		
Lim1		
Pax2		
Ret		
	Ectopic ureteric bud outgrowth	
Bmp4		Duplex collecting system
Foxc1		
Robo2		
Slit2		
Spry1		
	Decreased ureteric bud branching	
Fgfr2		Renal hypoplasia, renal dysplasia
Foxd1		
Pod1		
Raldh2		
Rarα/Rarβ2		
Spry2		
Wnt11		
	Defective renal medulla formation	
Fgf7		Medullary dysplasia
Fgf10		
Gpc3		
$p57^{KIP2}$		
Agt		Hydronephrosis
Agtr1		
Agtr2		
Bmp4		
Bmp5		
	Defective tubulogenesis	
Bmp7		Renal hypoplasia, renal dysplasia
Brn1		
Fgf8		
Pod1		
Lim1		
Notch1		
Notch2		
Psen1/ Psen2		
Rbpsuh		
Wnt4		
Wnt9b		
	Defective glomerulogenesis	
Jag1		Glomerular malformation
Notch2		
Pdgfβ		
Pdgfrβ		
Pod1		
Vegf		Loss of glomerular filtration selectivity
Col4α3/Col4α4/Col4α5		
Lamb		
Lmx1β		
Mafβ		
Wt1		

mesenchyme at the onset of ureteric bud induction.[103] *Pax2*[112] and *Lim1*[105] are also expressed in induced metanephric mesenchyme and nephrogenic derivatives. Homozygous deletion in any of the aforementioned genes in mice causes ureteric bud outgrowth failure, and results in bilateral renal agenesis or severe renal dysgenesis with variable penetrance depending on the gene involved. Shared features of these mutant phenotypes include arrest of ureteric bud induction, arrest of mesenchymal-epithelial induction, and attenuation or loss of GDNF-RET signaling[113] (discussed following). The morphogenetic mechanism responsible for ureteric bud outgrowth failure in each mutant is different, however. For example, *Pax2* mutants fail to form the posterior wolffian duct from which the ureteric bud derives.[102] In contrast, *Lim1*[105,114] and *Sall1*[104] mutants initiate, but do not complete, ureteric bud induction. *Wt1* mutants also exhibit failed ureteric bud induction and show apoptosis of the metanephric mesenchyme.[103] The morphogenetic role of *Wt1* is further revealed by tissue recombination experiments that examine the inductive capacities of *Wt1* mutant and wild-type isolated ureteric bud and metanephric mesenchyme. These studies show that isolated metanephric mesenchyme explants from *Wt1* knockout mice are neither competent in responding to inductive signals from wild-type ureteric buds nor able to induce growth and branching of isolated wild-type ureteric bud explants.[103,115] On the other hand, *Sall1*-deficient mesenchyme, which expresses *Wt1*, responds to a heterologous inducer (e.g., *Sall1* $(^{-/-})$ spinal cord) in ex vivo tissue recombination experiments,[104] suggesting that *Sall1* functions downstream of *Wt1* in a genetic regulatory cascade. Taken together, these data suggest that *Wt1* is required in metanephric mesenchyme to initiate the developmental program for MET, which, in turn, mediates the provision of cues for ureteric bud induction. In contrast, *Sall1* likely regulates the inductive potential of these mesenchymal cells.

The Role of GDNF-RET Signaling

Genes encoding the peptide growth factor glial-derived neurotrophic factor *(Gdnf)*,[116] its tyrosine kinase receptor *Ret*,[117] and its coreceptor *Gfrα1*[118] are recognized as crucial regulators of ureteric bud outgrowth. Targeted mutagenesis of *Gdnf* in mice causes bilateral renal aplasia due to ureteric bud outgrowth failure[119,120] (Figure 6-3, *A*). Similarly, homozygous deletion of *Ret* or *Gfrα1* cause the same defect[117,121,122] (Figure 6-3, *B*), indicating a crucial role for GDNF-RET-GFRα1 signaling in early murine renal branching morphogenesis. In 20% to 40% of $Gdnf^{-/-}$ or $Ret^{-/-}$ mutant offspring, the aplastic renal phenotype is not fully penetrant and initial ureteric bud outgrowth is evident,[117,119] indicating that ureteric bud outgrowth is not under the exclusive control of GDNF-RET signaling. Other molecular pathways likely to play important roles in ureteric bud induction include signaling through integrins as revealed by the demonstration in mice that approximately 50% of embryos deficient in the $\alpha 8$ integrin gene show termination of ureteric bud outgrowth at the point of contact with the metanephric mesenchyme.[123] Likewise, 100% of mice with a homozygous null mutation in the gene heparan sulfate 2-sulfotransferase *(Hs2st)*,[124] which is involved in proteoglycan synthesis, show a similar phenotype, supporting the role of heparan sulfate proteoglycans in ureteric bud induction.

In vitro and in vivo data support the role of GDNF-RET signaling in ureteric bud cell proliferation. In vitro, GDNF stimulates cell proliferation in cultured primary ureteric bud cells,[125] as well as in CDs of whole kidney explants.[67,126] GDNF does not, however, stimulate cell proliferation in isolated ureteric bud explants, although it does promote ureteric bud cell survival by inhibiting apoptosis.[116] Thus even though GDNF may exert direct inhibitory effects on apoptosis, it may require the presence of other factors for its proliferative effects in the ureteric bud lineage.

Regulation of GDNF-RET Expression and Function

Stemming from the importance of the GDNF-RET signaling axis in early kidney development, considerable attention has been given to identifying genes that regulate the expression and function of *Gdnf* and *Ret*, and to defining a genetic regulatory cascade during renal development. Before kidney development, *Gdnf* is expressed along the anteroposterior length of the intermediate mesoderm parallel to the wolffian duct.[116] Likewise, *Ret* is expressed throughout the wolffian duct at this stage.[109] At the time of ureteric bud induction, *Gdnf* expression is restricted to the posterior intermediate mesoderm in proximity to the site of ureteric bud outgrowth, which marks the metanephric mesenchyme. In vitro studies involving the application of GDNF-soaked agarose beads demonstrate that the entire length of the wolffian duct is competent to respond to ectopic GDNF and initiate the morphogenetic program for ureteric bud branching.[116,126] These data suggest that for a single ureteric bud to form, the spatial activity of GDNF-RET signaling must be tightly regulated. The demonstration of renal malformations including duplex kidney and hydronephrosis in transgenic mice that ectopically express *Gdnf* or *Ret* throughout the length of the wolffian duct further underscores the importance of posterior restriction of GDNF-RET signaling activity to establishing normal renal number and form.[127,128]

Positive regulation of *Gdnf* expression. Functional and genetic evidence support the role of three transcription factor genes expressed in intermediate mesoderm—*Eya1*, *Six1*, and *Pax2*—in a molecular cascade that promotes *Gdnf* expression during kidney development (Figure 6-4). *Eya1* and *Six1* are placed at the top of this cascade based on the loss of *Gdnf* expression in mice mutant for either *Eya1* or *Six1*.[129] *Eya1* is expressed in an overlapping domain with *Gdnf* in the presumptive metanephric mesenchyme at the time of ureteric bud outgrowth.[99] *Eya1* knockout mice exhibit renal agenesis resulting from failed ureteric bud outgrowth.[99] Since *Gdnf* is not expressed in the metanephric mesenchyme of $Eya1^{-/-}$ mutant kidneys, the renal defect in *Eya1* null mutants is thought to be due to lack of GDNF-RET signaling. *Six1* null mice, which also show failed ureteric bud induction and subsequent apoptosis of the mesenchyme,[100] demonstrate normal levels of *Eya1* expression, placing *Eya1* upstream of *Six1*. *Pax2* expressed in the intermediate mesoderm lies upstream of *Gdnf* by directly activating its transcription.[112] *Eya1* null mice show normal *Pax2* expression,[99] yet *Pax2* expression is lost in *Six1* mutant mice.[100] These data suggest that *Six1* may not be essential for inducing *Pax2* expression

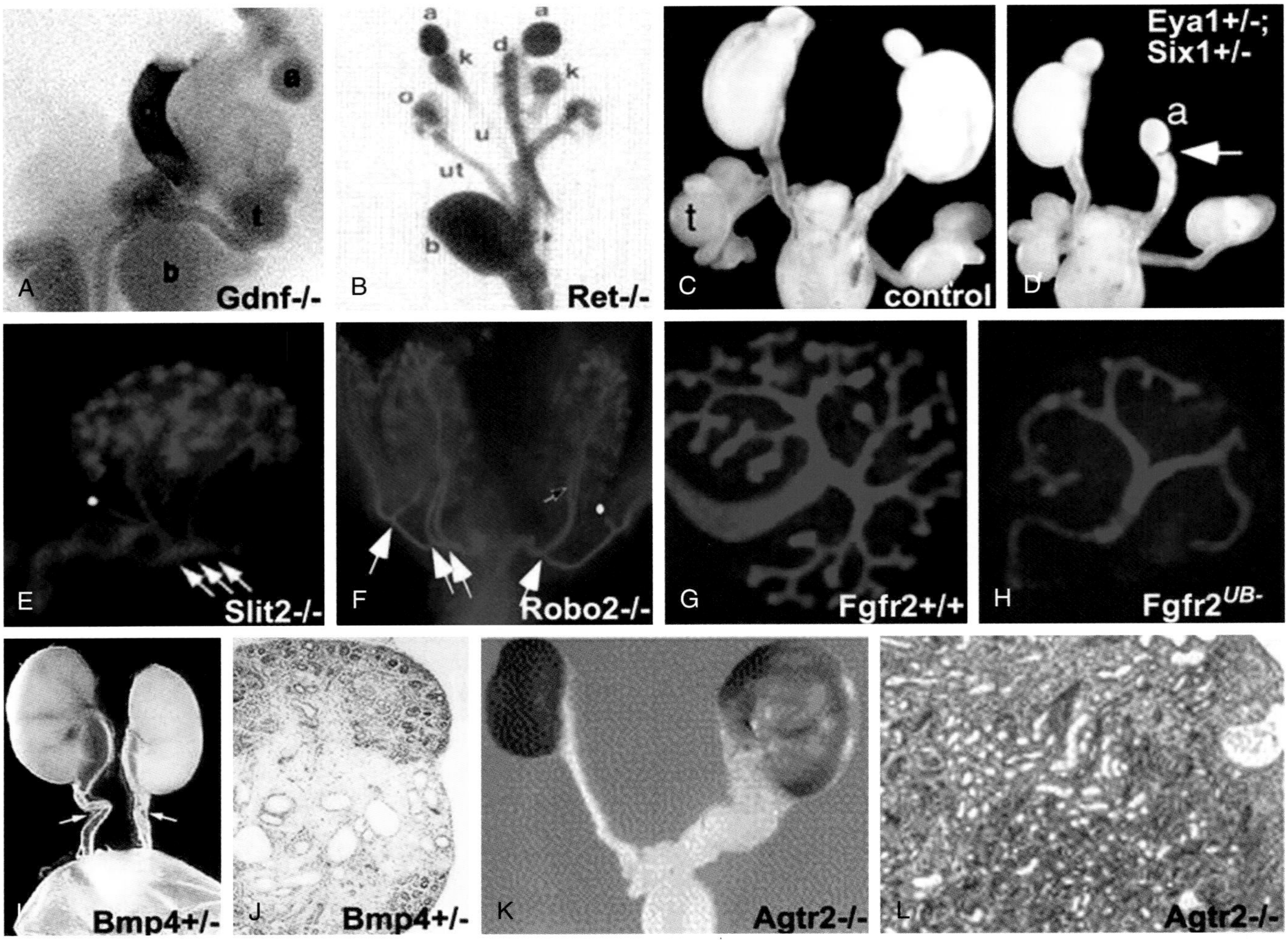

Figure 6-3 Representative kidney phenotypes of mice having targeted or conditional gene mutations with effects on renal branching morphogenesis. **A,** Bilateral renal agenesis in *Gdnf* null mutants. [119] **B,** Severe bilateral renal hypoplasia in *Ret* null mutants.[117] **C, D,** Unilateral renal agenesis *(white arrow)* in *Eya1/Six1* double heterozygous mutant mice (**C,** wild-type control).[100] **E, F,** Multiple ectopic ureters *(white arrows)* are shown in *Slit2* and *Robo2* knockout mice as revealed by transgenic expression of EGFP in ureteric bud–derived cells.[25] **G, H,** Decreased ureteric bud branching is shown in mice following conditional *Fgfr2* inactivation in ureteric bud derivatives.[225] **I, J,** *Bmp4* heterozygous mice show a spectrum of renal malformations including severe bilateral hydronephrosis (**I,** *white arrows)* and cystic dysplasia **(J).**[24] **K, L,** *Agtr2* null mutant mice show severe hydronephrosis (**K,** right kidney) and medullary dysplasia **(L).**[26] Images shown were obtained from original papers as noted with permission. *a,* Adrenal gland; *b,* bladder; *d,* dorsal aorta; *k,* kidney; *o,* ovary; *t,* testis; *u,* ureter; *ut,* uterine horn.

in the intermediate mesoderm but may be required to maintain its expression in developing mesenchyme during the initial stages of nephrogenesis.

In addition to *Eya1*, *Six1*, and *Pax2*, other activators of *Gdnf* expression have been identified, including the paralogous genes *Hoxa11*, *Hoxc11*, and *Hoxd11*. Compound inactivation of at least two of these genes causes renal aplasia and loss of *Gdnf* and *Six2* expression.[130] Since *Eya1* and *Pax2* expression are normal in hox compound mutant mice, it has been suggested that hox genes maintain *Gdnf* expression by cooperating with *Eya1* to induce *Six1 and Six2* expression.[129] An additional regulatory mechanism for the maintenance of *Gdnf* expression in uninduced mesenchyme involves *Emx2*, a transcription factor expressed in the wolffian duct.[131] *Emx2* null mice exhibit bilateral renal agenesis due to failure of the ureteric bud to form its first branch following induction.[131] Morphogenetic arrest in these mutants is associated with downregulation of ureteric bud markers *Ret*, *Pax2*, and *Lim1*, as well as *Gdnf* in the metanephric mesenchyme. Tissue recombination experiments between isolated wild-type and mutant *Emx2* kidney rudiments reveal that the mutant ureteric bud is incompetent to induce metanephric mesenchyme.[131] These data suggest *Emx2* may be important in the nascent ureteric bud for providing cues to maintain *Gdnf* expression in the mesenchyme and sustain ureteric bud branching morphogenesis (Figure 6-4).

Negative regulation of *Gdnf* expression. Negative regulation is a conserved mechanism that counterbalances stimulatory processes and controls branch number, position, and shape in developing organ systems that feature branching morphogenesis as a fundamental process, including lung and kidney.[18] In the developing kidney, at least three genes—*Foxc1*, *Slit2*, and *Robo2*—are involved in restricting *Gdnf* expression to the posterior intermediate mesoderm, which

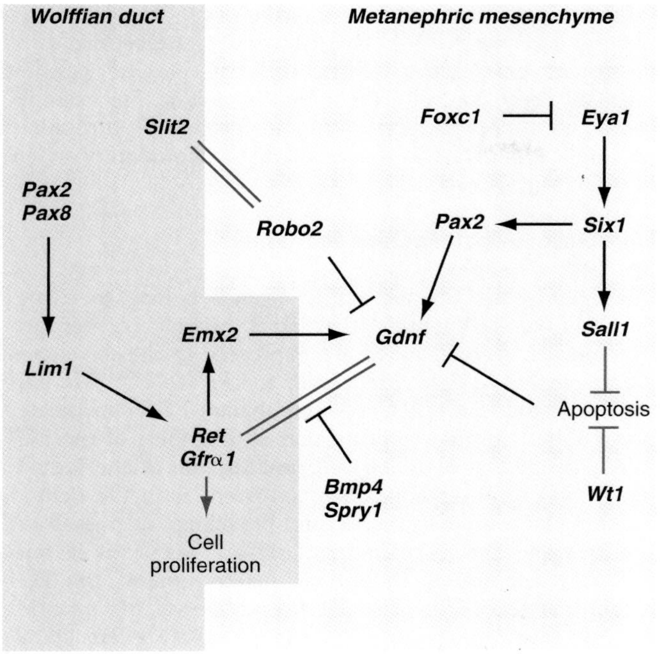

Figure 6-4 Schematic diagram showing genetic regulation of Gdnf-Ret signaling axis during ureteric bud induction. *Black arrows*, Positive regulation; *black T*, negative regulation; *blue double lines*, ligand-receptor interaction; *green arrow*, stimulatory cellular effect; *red T*, inhibitory cellular effect.

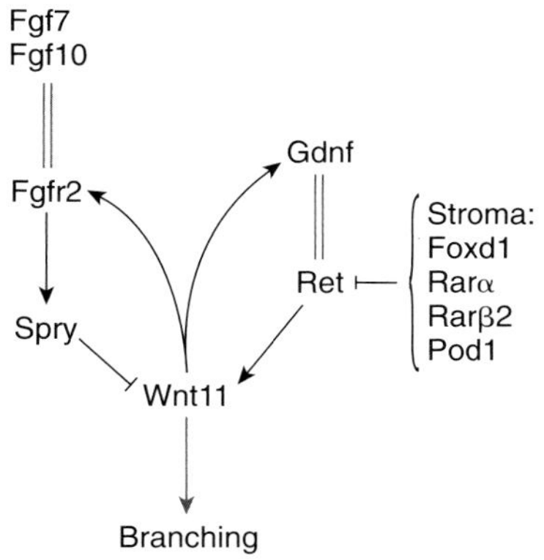

Figure 6-5 Schematic diagram showing genetic regulation of Gdnf-Ret signaling axis during early renal branching morphogenesis. *Black arrows*, Positive regulation; *black T*, negative regulation; *blue double lines*, ligand-receptor interaction; *green arrow*, stimulatory cellular effect.

may function in a negative regulatory mechanism of renal branching morphogenesis (Figure 6-4). Demonstration of ectopic ureteric bud formation, multiple ureters and hydroureter, and anterior expansion of *Gdnf* expression in *Foxc1*, *Slit2*, or *Robo2* homozygous null mutant mice supports this conclusion.[25,132] *Foxc1* encodes a transcription factor expressed in an overlapping domain with *Gdnf* in the intermediate mesoderm.[132] The mechanism of defective renal branching morphogenesis in *Foxc1*$^{-/-}$ mutant mice is thought to result from an anterior expansion of *Eya1* and *Gdnf* expression in the intermediate mesoderm, leading to ectopic GDNF stimulation of wolffian duct budding.[132] The secreted protein SLIT2 and its receptor ROBO2 are encoded by genes best known for their roles in axon guidance, functioning as chemorepellents that cause axons or migrating cells to move away from the source of SLIT2.[133,134] In the developing kidney, *Slit2* is primarily expressed in the wolffian duct, whereas *Robo2* is detected in a complementary pattern in the nephrogenic mesenchyme.[135] In *Slit2* and *Robo2* mutant mice (Figure 6-3, *E, F*), *Gdnf* expression is also expanded anteriorly in the posterior intermediate mesoderm; however, this expansion occurs independent of alterations in the expression of *Foxc1*, *Eya1*, and *Pax2*.[25] Consequently, SLIT2 and ROBO2 are likely to function in a parallel mechanism that restricts GDNF-RET activity during ureteric bud outgrowth.

Negative regulation of *Ret* expression. When the ureteric bud begins to invade the metanephric mesenchyme, *Ret* expression becomes spatially restricted to the tips of ureteric bud branches.[109] The demonstration of defective branching morphogenesis in transgenic mice that ectopically express *Ret* throughout the CD system[127] underscores the importance of regulating *Ret* expression spatially during kidney development. *Ret* expression is partly under the control of four transcription factors expressed by cells of the stromal lineage—*Rarα, Rarβ2, Foxd1*, and *Pod1* (Figure 6-5). RARα and RARβ2, members of the retinoic acid receptor (RAR) and retinoid X receptor (RXR) families of transcription factors, are both expressed in stromal cells surrounding induced mesenchyme and *Ret*-expressing ureteric bud branch tips.[44] *Rarα*$^{-/-}$;*Rarβ2*$^{-/-}$ double mutant mice have small kidneys characterized by a decreased number of ureteric bud branches and loss of normal cortical stromal patterning between induced nephrons.[44] In the CDs of *Rarα*$^{-/-}$;*Rarβ2*$^{-/-}$ double mutant mice, *Ret* expression is downregulated whereas *Gdnf* expression in the metanephric mesenchyme is maintained. The renal defect in these mice can be rescued by overexpressing a *Ret* transgene in the ureteric bud lineage,[88] suggesting a role for stromal cell-derived, retinoid-mediated signals in maintaining *Ret* expression during renal branching morphogenesis.

The forkhead/winged helix transcription factor *Foxd1* and the basic helix loop helix transcription factor *Pod1* have roles in regulating the spatially restricted pattern of *Ret* expression during CD development. *Foxd1* is most strongly expressed in the developing kidney in the cortical, or subcapsular, stroma.[33,35] In contrast, *Pod1* is most abundant in medullary stromal cells.[46,136] Homozygous deletion of either *Foxd1* or *Pod1* results in decreased renal branching morphogenesis and misexpression of *Ret* throughout the developing collecting system.[35,46] These data suggest that stromal cues expressed under the control of *Foxd1* and *Pod1* are involved in inhibiting *Ret* expression in the truncal segments of the developing ureteric bud. It is not clear from the analyses of these mutants whether secreted stromal factors directly block *Ret* expression in CDs. Because *Foxd1* and *Pod1* mutants show additional defects in nephron morphogenesis[35,46] (see "Early Nephron Segmentation" later in this chapter), these stromal genes may indirectly control *Ret* expression through the production of nephron-derived factors that act secondarily on CD cells to inhibit *Ret* expression.

Feedback loops involved in regulation of GDNF-RET signaling. The gene *Spry1* (*Sprouty1*) is implicated in a negative feedback loop involving GDNF-RET signaling and its downstream effector, *Wnt11* (Figure 6-5). *Spry1* is expressed along the length of the wolffian duct, with highest levels of expression in the posterior duct.[137] Loss of *Spry1* function in mice results in renal malformations including multiple ureters, multiplex kidneys, and hydroureter.[137,138] *Spry1*$^{-/-}$ mutants exhibit ectopic ureteric bud induction and show increased expression of *Gdnf* in the metanephric mesenchyme, expanded expression of GDNF-RET target genes such as *Wnt11*, and increased sensitivity to GDNF in metanephric culture. WNT11, a secreted protein, is expressed in ureteric bud tips.[126,139] Loss of *Wnt11* in mice results in reduced levels of GDNF in the metanephric mesenchyme and reduced ureteric bud branching morphogenesis, suggesting that it functions to maintain *Gdnf* expression in the metanephric mesenchyme.[140] The role of *Spry1* as a negative regulator of renal branching morphogenesis is further supported by the demonstration of decreased ureteric bud branching in transgenic mice that ectopically express human *SPRY2*, a related homolog, throughout the wolffian duct.[141]

A second example of negative feedback in renal branching morphogenesis involves secreted growth factors belonging to the bone morphogenetic protein (BMP) family. Several BMPs, including *Bmp2, 4, 5, 6,* and *7* and their receptors, are expressed in the developing kidney in distinct but partially overlapping domains.[142-145] Kidney organ culture studies have revealed inhibitory roles for BMP2, 4, and 7 in ureteric bud branching morphogenesis.[31,146-148] However, convincing evidence that BMPs modulate ureteric bud outgrowth in vivo is provided only for *Bmp4*.[24] Mice heterozygous for *Bmp4* exhibit ectopic or duplicated ureteric buds and show renal phenotypes that mimic the human syndrome, congenital anomalies of the kidney and urinary tract (CAKUT), a pleiotropic condition that features a spectrum of renal malformations including hypodysplastic kidneys, hydroureteronephrosis, and ureteral duplications[149,150] (Figure 6-3, *I-J*). *Bmp4* is expressed in stromal cells immediately adjacent to the wolffian duct and the early ureteric bud.[24,142] The abnormal sites of ureteric bud outgrowth in *Bmp4*$^{+/-}$ mice led to the proposal that BMP4 may suppress ureteric induction by antagonizing the local effect of GDNF-RET signaling at the preferential site of induction on the wolffian duct.[24] Support for this hypothesis is provided by the demonstration that BMP4 can block the ability of GDNF to induce ureteric bud outgrowth from wolffian duct in vitro.[112,151] Exogenous BMP4 also inhibits further ureteric bud branching in vitro in an asymmetric manner,[31,146] suggesting that BMP4 may have additional roles in three-dimensional growth of the ureteric bud/collecting system.

Early Renal Branching Morphogenesis

GDNF and Parallel Signaling Mechanisms

In addition to its role as a potent stimulus for ureteric bud induction, GDNF is shown in vivo and in vitro to be a strong stimulus for subsequent ureteric bud branching.[126,128] The ability of GDNF to induce ureteric bud branching in vivo is revealed by the demonstration of multiple branched ureteric buds in transgenic mice that express *Gdnf* ectopically in the wolffian duct lineage.[128] Although these data demonstrate in vivo that the wolffian duct is competent to respond to GDNF along its entire length, in vitro studies show that recombinant GDNF is not sufficient to induce robust branching in isolated ureteric bud culture.[116,152] These latter data suggest that other factors cooperate with GDNF-RET in parallel signaling mechanisms to control ureteric bud branching. For example, WNT11[139,140] and the heparin-binding protein pleiotrophin[153] are implicated as factors that facilitate the stimulatory actions of GDNF in this process.

Fibroblast Growth Factors and Other Secreted Peptides

Fibroblast growth factor (FGF) ligands belong to a large family of secreted peptides that signal through receptor tyrosine kinases. Several FGFs are expressed in the developing kidney, including *Fgf2, Fgf7, Fgf8,* and *Fgf10*.[45,154,155] In vitro studies testing the effects of recombinant FGFs on isolated ureteric bud cultures indicate that all members of the FGF family support growth and cell proliferation of the ureteric bud.[154] These observations are consistent with the demonstration of decreased ureteric bud branching, decreased cell proliferation, and increased ureteric bud apoptosis in mice following conditional mutational inactivation of the FGF receptor gene *Fgfr2* in the ureteric bud lineage[156] (Figure 6-3, *G, H*). Interestingly, FGF family members exert unique spatial effects on ureteric bud cell proliferation in vitro. For example, FGF10 preferentially stimulates cell proliferation at the ureteric bud tips, whereas FGF7 induces cell proliferation in a nonselective manner throughout the developing CD system.[154] These data suggest that multiple FGF family members may function in complex morphogenetic programs that control three-dimensional growth of the developing CD system. FGF7 is also shown to induce the expression of the Sprouty gene *Spry2*, in developing CDs in vitro.[141] Consequently, *Fgf7* may also participate with *Spry2* in a feedback loop that controls ureteric bud branching by regulating *Gdnf* and *Wnt11* expression (Figure 6-5).

Several other secreted peptides including hepatocyte growth factor (HGF), transforming growth factor alpha (TGFα), epidermal growth factor (EGF), and FGF1 stimulate branching morphogenesis in vitro.[154,157-159] However, in vivo evidence does not support essential roles for these factors in early kidney development since kidney development is normal when genes encoding these proteins are mutated in mice.[160-162] Consequently, other mechanisms may compensate for their loss of function during kidney development.

GDNF, FGF7, and TGF-β have been shown to promote the expression of tissue inhibitors of metalloproteinases (TIMPs) from cultured ureteric bud cells.[163,164] TIMPS regulate the local activity of extracellular matrix metalloproteases (MMPs) that are implicated in altering the composition of metanephric extracellular matrix to facilitate branch initiation. This concept is supported by the demonstration that TIMPs block ureteric bud branching in vitro.[163,165] Consequently, growth factors may play an important role in regulating the local activity of matrix-degrading proteases by controlling TIMP expression.

Medullary Patterning and Formation of the Pelvicalyceal System

Regional specification of cortical and medullary domains of the renal CD system (also known as corticomedullary patterning) is a relatively late event in kidney development. At least four soluble growth factor genes (*Fgf7, Fgf10, Bmp4,* and *Bmp5*), one proteoglycan gene (*Gpc3*), one cell cycle regulatory gene (*p57(KIP2)*), and molecular components of the renin-angiotensin axis (*Agt, Agtr1, Agtr2*) are implicated in medullary CD morphogenesis as revealed by the demonstration of predominant defects in renal medulla development in mutant mice.

The kidneys of *Fgf7* null mice are phenotypically characterized by marked underdevelopment of the papilla, the innermost portion of the medulla.[45] Similarly, *Fgf10* null kidneys exhibit modest medullary dysplasia at E19.5, characterized by reduced numbers of loops of Henle and medullary CDs, increased medullary stromal cells, and enlargement of the renal calyx.[166] Cellular responses to FGFs are modulated through interactions with sulfated glycosaminoglycan (S-GAG) side chains of cell surface proteoglycans.[167] Syndecans and glypicans are heparan sulfate proteoglycans expressed in developing CDs,[81,168] and their expression is required for normal CD growth and branching.[124,169] Moreover, treatment of embryonic kidney explants with pharmacologic inhibitors of sulfated proteoglycan synthesis leads to loss of *Wnt11* expression at the ureteric bud branch tips,[139] suggesting that sulfated proteoglycans interact with multiple mechanisms that control ureteric bud branching.

Functional and genetic evidence in humans and mice demonstrate that glypican-3 (GPC3), a glycosylphosphotidylinositol (GPI)–linked cell surface heparan sulfate proteoglycan, is required for normal patterning of the medulla.[80,81] Medullary dysplasia in the *Gpc3*-deficient mouse arises from overgrowth of the ureteric bud and CDs due to increased cell proliferation in the ureteric bud lineage early during development,[80] with subsequent destruction of these elements due to apoptosis.[81] The defect is thought to be caused by an altered cellular response of GPC3-deficient CD cells to growth factors along an evolutionarily conserved mechanism.[170,171] Evidence in support of this hypothesis is provided by the augmented stimulatory effect of exogenous FGF7 on CD growth and branching in cultured kidney explants and CD cell lines derived from GPC3-deficient mice.[81]

Defective renal medulla formation in *Gpc3* null mutant mice illustrates the importance of tightly regulated cell proliferation and apoptosis in this process. Additional support for this concept is provided by the phenotypic analysis of mice carrying a null mutation for *p57(KIP2)*, a cell cycle regulatory gene. *p57(KIP2)* knockout mice show medullary dysplasia characterized by a decreased number of inner medullary CDs, in addition to abdominal, skeletal, and adrenal defects.[172] Genetic studies in humans and mice suggest a potential functional interaction between *p57(KIP2)* and the insulin-like growth factor-2 (*IGF2*) gene in the regulation of cell proliferation during the formation of the renal medulla. For example, phenotypic features of mice with *p57(KIP2)* null mutations are exhibited by approximately 15% of individuals with Beckwith-Wiedemann syndrome, a heterogeneous disorder characterized by somatic overgrowth and renal dysplasia.[173] Genetic linkage studies in humans with this disorder have mapped the disease to chromosome 11p15.5, which harbors loci for *p57(KIP2)* and for *IGF2* and *H19*, a gene with effects on maternal imprinting of other regional loci. Murine *H19* mutations result in enhanced *Igf2* expression but do not cause renal dysplasia.[174] However, $H19;^{-/-}$ $p57(KIP2)^{-/-}$ double knockout mice exhibit elevated serum levels of IGF2 and more severe renal dysplasia than that observed in *p57(KIP2)* single knockout mice.[175] These findings support an additional mechanism for the cause of renal medullary dysplasia resulting from dysregulated stimulation of cell proliferation through the inactivation of p57(KIP2) and overexpression of IGF2.

The phenotypic spectrum exhibited by *Bmp4* heterozygous mutant mice includes hydronephrosis and hydroureter,[24] signifying that *Bmp4* may play additional roles in renal branching morphogenesis that involve formation of the ureter and renal pelvis. Support for this concept is provided by the finding in kidney explants that recombinant BMP4 induces smooth muscle actin, an early marker for smooth muscle differentiation, in periureteric mesenchymal cells.[146] Moreover, mice mutant for *Bmp5* show similar defects in renal pelvis and ureter development,[176] suggesting that these BMPs may function via overlapping mechanisms. Consistent with a role for BMP signaling in the development of these anatomic structures is the demonstrated mRNA expression profiles for *Bmp4* and *Bmp5* in mesenchymal cells lining the ureter and the developing renal pelvis,[24,142,144] and BMP receptors *Alk3* and *Alk6* in neighboring CDs.[24]

Mutations in genes encoding components of the renin-angiotensin axis, best known for their role in controlling renal hemodynamics, also cause abnormalities in the development of the renal calyces and pelvis. Mice homozygous for a null mutation in the angiotensinogen (*Agt*) gene encoding the corresponding angiotensin precursor demonstrate progressive widening of the calyx and atrophy of the papillae and underlying medulla.[177] Identical defects occur in homozygous mutants for the angiotensin receptor-1 (*Agtr1*) gene.[178] The underlying defect in these mutants appears to be decreased cell proliferation of the smooth muscle cell layer lining the renal pelvis, resulting in decreased thickness of this layer in the proximal ureter. Mutational inactivation of *Agtr2* results in a range of anomalies including vesicoureteral reflux, duplex kidney, renal ectopia, ureteropelvic or ureterovesical junction stenoses, renal dysplasia or hypoplasia, multicystic dysplastic kidney, or renal agenesis[26] (Figure 6-3, *K, L*). Null mice demonstrate a decreased rate of apoptosis of the cells around the ureter, suggesting that *Agtr2* also plays a role in morphogenetic remodeling of the ureter.

Mesenchymal-Epithelial Transformation

Induction of Metanephric Mesenchyme

Regional specification of metanephric mesenchyme at the posterior intermediate mesoderm requires function of the transcription factor Odd-skipped 1 (*Odd1*).[179] Induction of mesenchyme by the ureteric bud causes mesenchymal condensation at the ureteric bud tip. Morphologically, condensed mesenchyme is termed a *cap condensate*, and its formation is genetically marked by upregulated expression of transcription factors *Wt1*,[103] *Sall1*,[104] *Pax2*,[107] and *Pod1*,[46] and by expression of transmembrane molecules cadherin-11[180] and α8 integrin.[123]

Seminal experiments involving isolated kidney rudiments cultured ex vivo established the role of ureteric bud–derived secreted factors in providing inductive cues for condensed mesenchyme to undergo epithelial differentiation.[39] The isolation of ureteric bud cell lines has facilitated the identification of several secreted factors that function individually or in combination to cause mesenchymal-epithelial conversion and tubulogenesis in vitro, including FGF2,[181] leukemia inhibitory factor (LIF),[91,182,183] transforming growth factor-β2 (TGFβ2),[183,184] and growth/differentiation factor-11 (GDF-11).[183,185]

Tubulogenesis

Formation of pretubular aggregates heralds the beginning of tubulogenesis during kidney development. Wnt genes play a key role in epithelial conversion, as suggested by the observation that cells expressing Wnt proteins are potent inducers of tubulogenesis in isolated metanephric mesenchyme.[186,187] A genetic requirement for *Wnt4* in MET and early tubulogenesis is revealed by the demonstration of nephrogenesis arrest at the cap condensate stage in mice mutant for *Wnt4* (Figure 6-6, *A*, *B*). *Wnt9b*, expressed in cap condensates, is also necessary for tubulogenesis and acts upstream of *Wnt4* in this developmental program.[188] The effects of Wnt signals are modulated by mesenchymal-derived secreted Wnt binding proteins, secreted frizzled-related proteins (sFRPs). sFRPs antagonize the actions of *Wnt4* and *Wnt9b* by binding secreted Wnt proteins in vitro and preventing them from activating membrane-bound Wnt receptors.[189]

BMPs and FGFs are believed to play a crucial role in regulating the size of the epithelial precursor population within the developing metanephric mesenchyme. In vitro studies show that *Bmp7* inhibits mesenchymal apoptosis and, in conjunction with FGF2, maintains the competence of mesenchyme to respond to inductive signals. However, the combined effects of BMP7 and FGF2 in kidney organ culture block tubulogenesis.[73] This in vitro observation has led to the speculation that *Bmp7* functions in a mechanism with FGF2 that balances mesenchymal differentiation and renewal.[96] Consistent with this hypothesis is the demonstration in *Bmp7*-deficient mice of developmental arrest and rudimentary kidneys without inhibiting the differentiation of already induced cells, which is likely due to failure to expand and renew the epithelial precursor population[190,191] (Figure 6-6, C, *D*).

Early Nephron Segmentation

Proximal-distal patterning of nephron epithelial cell fate, as reflected by the formation of tubular and glomerular cell fate domains, is a crucial step in nephron segmentation. Glomerular versus tubular cell fate decision making appears to be regulated by external cues provided by neighboring stromal cells. This is revealed in experiments involving isolated rat renal vesicles cultured in the presence of stromal-derived conditioned medium.[95] Although the molecular identity of these stromal-derived factors is still unknown, analysis of chimeric mice reveal that normal glomerular epithelial differentiation requires the function of *Pod1* in neighboring stromal cells.[36] Thus *Pod1* may be involved in the transcriptional regulation of stromal factors that promote podocyte cell fate determination during early nephron segmentation.

Two transcription factors expressed at the renal vesicle stage, *Lim1* and *Brn1*, appear to be involved in initiating proximal-distal nephron epithelial cell fate patterning during nephrogenesis. Whereas *Lim1* is uniformly expressed in renal vesicles,[105] *Brn1* expression is initiated in renal vesicles in a more spatially restricted pattern.[53] Conditional knockout of *Lim1* in metanephric mesenchyme causes developmental arrest at the renal vesicle stage, and results in loss of *Brn1* expression in these structures[105] (Figure 6-6, *E*). In contrast, targeted deletion of *Brn1* resulting in loss of metanephric mesenchyme *Brn1* expression does not prevent the early stages of nephron morphogenesis but blocks formation of the loop of Henle at an early developmental stage and suppresses terminal differentiation of distal nephron epithelia.[53] Taken together, these data suggest that *Brn1* functions downstream of *Lim1* in a genetic hierarchy that establishes proximal and distal cell fates. An additional role for *Lim1* in specifying podocyte cell fate is revealed by the analysis of *Lim1* chimeric mutant mice.[105]

In vivo and in vitro data support a model whereby the mechanism for patterning glomerular and tubular cell fates along the proximal-distal axis of the S-shaped body is dependent on negative feedback between *Wt1* and *Pax2*.[192-194] During early kidney development, the mRNA expression patterns of *Pax2* and *Wt1* in nephrogenic epithelial structures become restricted in S-shaped bodies such that the expression domain of *Pax2* is complementary to the corresponding domain for *Wt1*. *Wt1* expression is restricted to glomerular epithelial precursors, which give rise to podocytes later in glomerular development.[195] In contrast, *Pax2* expression is restricted to that portion that gives rise to tubular epithelial precursors of the proximal and distal nephron segments, and is later repressed in differentiated tubular epithelium.[93,196] The precise roles for *Wt1* or *Pax2* in nephron epithelial differentiation is not evident from the analyses of renal phenotypes in mice with targeted *Wt1* or *Pax2* mutations since these mutants fail to form kidneys.[102,103] However, evidence from transgenic mice that overexpress PAX2 in all nephrogenic cell types illustrates the importance of spatially restricting *Pax2* expression during early nephronogenesis since these mice exhibit dysplastic kidneys and show defective differentiation of both tubular and glomerular epithelia.[197] The secreted factor, *Fgf8*, also appears to be important for survival of tubular precursors as revealed by the degeneration of S-shaped bodies in mice where *Fgf8* has been conditionally inactivated in metanephric mesenchyme.[93]

Genetic evidence in mice suggests that the process for selecting which nephrogenic progenitors will comprise the proximal portion of the developing nephron (i.e., the podocytes and proximal convoluted tubule) is dependent on Notch signaling.[198-200] Conditional knockout of *Notch2* and *Rbpsuh*, but not *Notch1*, in metanephric mesenchyme before nephron segmentation results in complete lack of both proximal tubule and glomerular epithelia[199] (Figure 6-6, *F*, *G*). Similar effects were observed in mutant mice when presenilin-mediated Notch activation was abrogated by mutagenesis of *Psen1* and *Psen2*,[200] and in cultured metanephroi when Notch signaling was blocked following treatment with the γ-secretase inhibitor DAPT.[198]

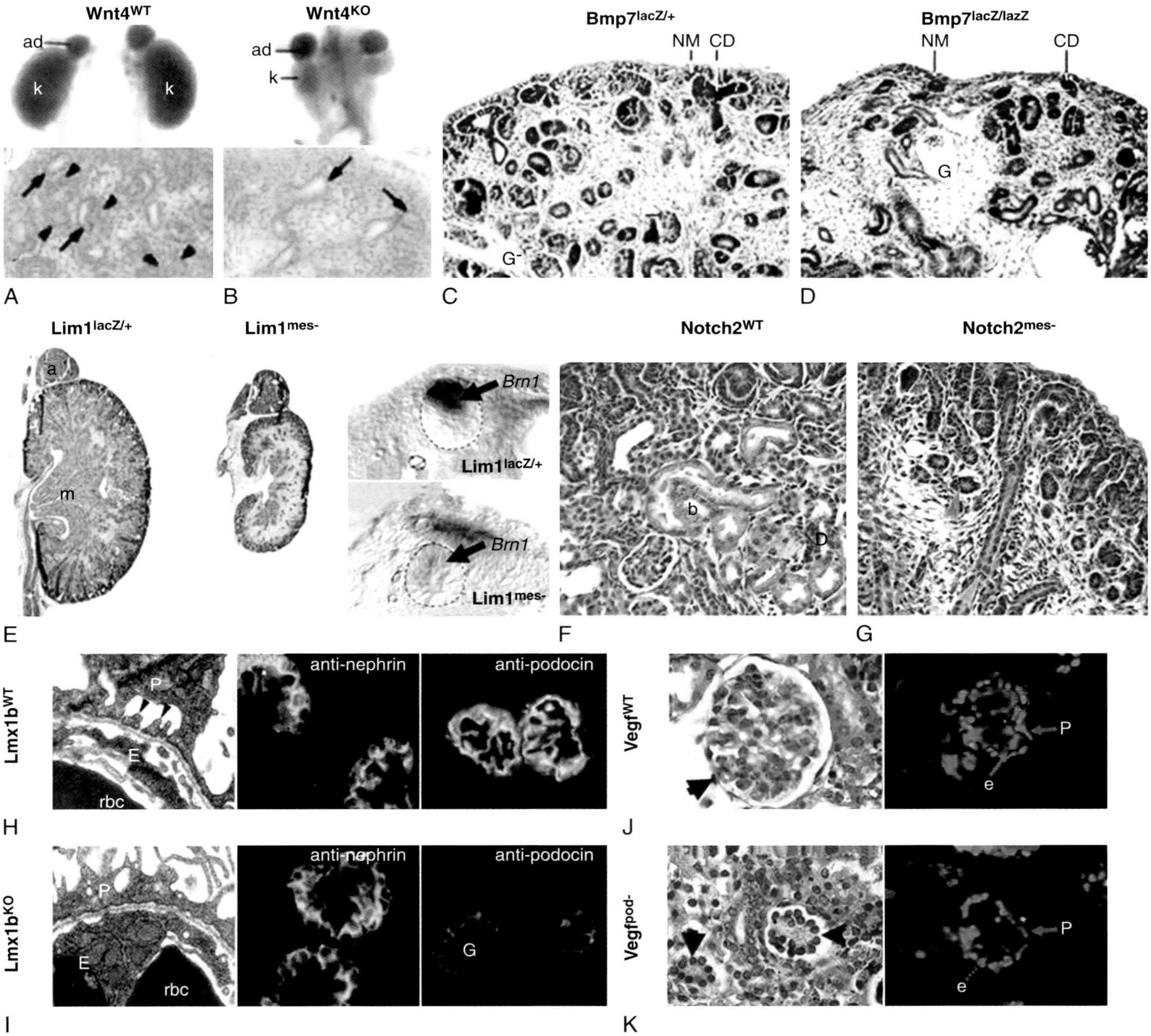

Figure 6-6 Representative kidney phenotypes of mice having targeted or conditional gene mutations with effects on tubulogenesis and glomerulogenesis. Images shown were obtained from original papers as noted with permission. **A, B,** *Wnt4* null mutant mice show bilateral renal hypoplasia (**B,** *upper panel*) and defective MET on light microscopy (**B,** *lower panel*).[226] *Black arrows,* Collecting ducts; *black arrowheads,* mesenchyme-derived nephrogenic tissue elements. **C, D,** *Bmp7* knockout mice **(D)** show decreased formation of new nephrons and abnormal glomerulogenesis *(black G)*.[227] Blue staining **(C,D)** denotes expression of lacZ under the control of the *Bmp7* promoter. **E,** Conditional inactivation of *Lim1* in metanephric mesenchyme result in small, dysplastic kidneys (**E,** *middle panel*). Loss of *Brn1* mRNA expression in renal vesicles (**E,** *lower-right panel*) suggests an early patterning defect in *Lim1*-deficient mesenchyme. Blue staining in **E** *(left panel and upper-right panel)* denotes lacZ expression under the control of the Lim1 promoter. **F, G,** Conditional knockout of *Notch2* in metanephric mesenchyme **(G)** blocks formation of proximal tubules and glomeruli.[199] *Green arrow,* Proximal tubule; *green arrowhead,* distal tubule; *blue arrowhead,* collecting duct. **H, I,** *Lmx1b* null mutant mice **(I)** show defective glomerulogenesis as revealed by podocyte foot process fusion on electron microscopy.[203] Nephrin protein is detected in podocytes of *Lmx1b*-deficient mice (**H** and **I,** *middle panels*). Podocin levels are markedly reduced in *Lmx1b* mutant mice (**H** and **I,** *right panels*). *Black arrowheads,* Foot processes. **J, K,** Conditional knockout of *Vegf* in podocytes causes severe glomerular defects **(K).**[216] Double staining for podocytes (**J** and **K,** *right panels; green cells, P*) and endothelial cells (**J** and **K,** *right panels; red cells,* e) reveals defective endothelial survival in *Vegf* conditional mutants (**K,** *right panel*).

Glomerulogenesis

Podocyte terminal differentiation. Podocytes are a population distinct from other cells in developing nephrons during the transition from S-shaped body to glomerulus.[55] Functional and genetic evidence support the role of Notch signaling in determining podocyte cell fate early in nephron development.[198,200] Additional roles for the Notch receptor gene *Notch2* and its ligand *Jagged1* at later stages of glomerular capillary tuft assembly are revealed by the analysis of compound mutant mice that show avascular glomeruli or aneurysmal defects in glomerular capillary tuft formation.[201]

Following podocyte cell fate determination, transcription factors *Wt1*, *Pod1*, *Lmx1b*, and *Mafb* have important roles in podocyte terminal differentiation through the analysis of mutant phenotypes. Loss of function mutations in *Pod1*, *Lmx1b*, and *Maf2b* cause podocyte defects in mice that become evident at the capillary loop stage (in the case of *Pod1*) or later (in the case of *Lmx1b* and *Maf2b*)[46,202,203] (Figure 6-6, *H*, *I*). In humans, *LMX1b* mutations are identified in patients with nail-patella syndrome, which is associated with focal segmental glomerulosclerosis.[204] The role of Wt1 in podocyte differentiation is not revealed by mouse knockout studies, because $Wt1^{-/-}$ mutant mice fail to develop kidneys. However, a role for *Wt1* in podocyte differentiation is suggested by the identification of *WT1* mutations in humans with Denys-Drash syndrome and Frasier syndrome,[205-207] which are inherited disorders associated with mesangial sclerosis, a form of glomerular disease characterized by defects in podocyte differentiation.[208] Demonstration of an identical glomerular phenotype in mice with targeted *Wt1* mutations genetically similar to the *WT1* mutation in humans with the aforementioned syndromes[209-212] serves as additional support that *Wt1* has important roles in podocyte differentiation.

Glomerular capillary tuft development. Several signaling systems are involved in the recruitment of endothelial and mesangial precursors and in the formation and assembly of the glomerular capillary tuft. Vascular endothelial growth factor (VEGF) is secreted by podocyte precursors of early S-shaped bodies.[213] VEGF promotes recruitment of angioblasts into the vascular cleft.[214] This process is under tight regulatory control as suggested by the demonstration of severe glomerular defects in mice when the gene dosage of *Vegf* is genetically manipulated[215,216] (Figure 6-6, *J*, *K*). The local effects of VEGF are likely modulated by angiopoietin-1 and -2, which are expressed by podocytes and mesangial cells, respectively.[217] Recruitment of mesangial cells is under the guidance of platelet-derived growth factor (PDGF)-BB, expressed by endothelial cells, that binds to its receptor, PDGF receptor-β (PDGFRβ).[218] The function of this axis is required for proliferation and assembly of glomerular capillaries and mesangium as revealed by the absence of glomerular capillary tufts in mice deficient in either *Pdgfβ* or *Pdgfrβ*.[219,220]

During the S-shaped stage, podocyte progenitors express a primitive glomerular basement membrane predominantly composed of laminin-1, and α-1 and α-2 subchains of type IV collagen.[221] During glomerular development, composition of the glomerular basement membrane undergoes transition as laminin-1 is replaced by laminin-11, and α-1 and α-2 type IV collagen chains are replaced by α-3, α-4, and α-5 subchains.[221] As demonstrated in several mouse models, failure of these changes results in severe structural and functional defects.[222-224]

PART I REFERENCES

1. Osathanondh V, Potter EL: Development of human kidney as shown by microdissection, *Arch Path* 82:391-402, 1966.
2. Potter EL: *Normal and abnormal development of the kidney*, Chicago, 1972, Year Book Medical Publishers Inc.
3. Hinchliffe SA, Sargent PH, Howard CV et al: Human intrauterine renal growth expressed in absolute number of glomeruli assessed by the disector method and Cavalieri principle, *Lab Invest* 64(6):777-84, 1991.
4. Rodriguez MM, Gomez AH, Abitbol CL et al: Histomorphometric analysis of postnatal glomerulogenesis in extremely preterm infants, *Pediatr Dev Pathol* 7(1):17-25, 2004.
5. Brenner BM, Chertow GM: Congenital oligonephropathy and the etiology of adult hypertension and progressive renal injury, *Am J Kidney Dis* 23(2):171-75, 1994.
6. Brenner BM, Mackenzie HS: Nephron mass as a risk factor for progression of renal disease, *Kidney Int Suppl* 63:S124-27, 1997.
7. Keller G, Zimmer G, Mall G et al: Nephron number in patients with primary hypertension, *N Engl J Med* 348(2):101-08, 2003.
8. Hoy WE, Hughson MD, Singh GR et al: Reduced nephron number and glomerulomegaly in Australian Aborigines: a group at high risk for renal disease and hypertension, *Kidney Int* 70(1):104-10, 2006.
9. Hughson M, Farris AB 3rd, Douglas-Denton R et al: Glomerular number and size in autopsy kidneys: the relationship to birth weight, *Kidney Int* 63(6):2113-22, 2003.
10. Manalich R, Reyes L, Herrera M et al: Relationship between weight at birth and the number and size of renal glomeruli in humans: a histomorphometric study, *Kidney Int* 58(2):770-73, 2000.
11. Barker DJ, Osmond C, Golding J et al: Growth in utero, blood pressure in childhood and adult life, and mortality from cardiovascular disease, *BMJ* 298(6673):564-67, 1998.
12. Barker DJ, Eriksson JG, Forsen T et al: Fetal origins of adult disease: strength of effects and biological basis, *Int J Epidemiol* 31(6):1235-39, 2002.
13. Osathanondh V, Potter EL: Development of human kidney as shown by microdissection. II. Renal pelvis, calyces, and papillae, *Arch Pathol* 76:277-89, 1963.
14. Osathanondh V, Potter EL: Development of human kidney as shown by microdissection. III. Formation and interrelationship of collecting tubules and nephrons, *Arch Pathol* 76:66-78, 1963.
15. Saxen L: *Organogenesis of the kidney*, Cambridge, 1987, Cambridge University Press.
16. Piscione TD, Rosenblum ND: The malformed kidney: disruption of glomerular and tubular development, *Clin Genet* 56(5):343-58, 1999.
17. Piscione TD, Rosenblum ND: The molecular control of renal branching morphogenesis: current knowledge and emerging insights, *Differentiation* 70(6):227-46, 2002.
18. Hu MC, Rosenblum ND: Genetic regulation of branching morphogenesis: lessons learned from loss-of-function phenotypes, *Pediatr Res* 54(4):433-38, 2003.
19. Drummond IA, Majumdar A, Hentschel H et al: Early development of the zebrafish pronephros and analysis of mutations affecting pronephric function, *Development* 125:4655-67, 1998.
20. Vize PD, Seufert DW, Carroll TJ et al: Model systems for the study of kidney development: use of the pronephros in the analysis of organ induction and patterning, *Dev Biol* 188:189-204, 1997.

21. Staack A, Donjacour AA, Brody J et al: Mouse urogenital development: a practical approach, *Differentiation* 71(7):402-13, 2003.
22. Woolf AS, Winyard PJ: Molecular mechanisms of human embryogenesis: developmental pathogenesis of renal tract malformations, *Pediatr Dev Pathol* 5(2):108-29, 2002.
23. Mackie GG, Stephens FD: Duplex kidneys: a correlation of renal dysplasia with position of the ureteral orifice, *J Urol* 114:274-80, 1975.
24. Miyazaki Y, Oshima K, Fogo A et al: Bone morphogenetic protein 4 regulates the budding site and elongation of the mouse ureter, *J Clin Invest* 105:863-73, 2000.
25. Grieshammer U, Le M, Plump AS et al: SLIT2-mediated ROBO2 signaling restricts kidney induction to a single site, *Dev Cell* 6(5):709-17, 2004.
26. Nishimura H, Yerkes E, Hohenfellner K et al: Role of the angiotensin type 2 receptor gene in congenital anomalies of the kidney and urinary tract, CAKUT, of mice and men, *Molecular Cell* 3:1-10, 1999.
27. Tsuchida S, Matsusaka T, Chen X et al: Murine double nullizygotes of the angiotensin type 1A and 1B receptor genes duplicate severe abnormal phenotypes of angiotensinogen nullizygotes, *J Clin Invest* 101:755-60, 1998.
28. Watanabe T, Costantini F: Real-time analysis of ureteric bud branching morphogenesis in vitro, *Dev Biol* 271(1):98-108, 2004.
29. Lin Y, Zhang S, Tuukkanen J et al: Patterning parameters associated with the branching of the ureteric bud regulated by epithelial-mesenchymal interactions, *Int J Dev Biol* 47(1):3-13, 2003.
30. Cebrian C, Borodo K, Charles N et al: Morphometric index of the developing murine kidney, *Dev Dyn* 231(3):601-08, 2004.
31. Cain JE, Nion T, Jeulin D et al: Exogenous BMP-4 amplifies asymmetric ureteric branching in the developing mouse kidney in vitro, *Kidney Int* 67(2):420-31, 2005.
32. Al-Awqati Q, Goldberg MR: Architectural patterns in branching morphogenesis in the kidney, *Kidney Int* 54:1832-42, 1998.
33. Levinson RS, Batourina E, Choi C et al: Foxd1-dependent signals control cellularity in the renal capsule, a structure required for normal renal development, *Development* 132(3):529-39, 2005.
34. Bard J: A new role for the stromal cells in kidney development, *BioEssays* 18(9):705-07, 1996.
35. Hatini V, Huh SO, Herzlinger D et al: Essential role of stromal mesenchyme in kidney morphogenesis revealed by targeted disruption of Winged Helix transcription factor BF-2, *Genes Dev* 10:1467-78, 1996.
36. Cui S, Schwartz L, Quaggin SE: Pod1 is required in stromal cells for glomerulogenesis, *Dev Dyn* 226(3):512-22, 2003.
37. Bard JB: Growth and death in the developing mammalian kidney: signals, receptors and conversations, *Bioessays* 24(1):72-82, 2002.
38. Klein G, Langegger M, Goridis C et al: Neural cell adhesion molecules during embryonic induction and development of the kidney, *Development* 102(4):749-61, 1998.
39. Grobstein C: Morphogenetic interaction between embryonic mouse tissues separated by a membrane filter, *Nature* 172:869-71, 1953.
40. Al-Awqati Q, Oliver JA: Stem cells in the kidney, *Kidney Int* 61(2):387-95, 2002.
41. Oxburgh L, Chu GC, Michael SK et al: TGFbeta superfamily signals are required for morphogenesis of the kidney mesenchyme progenitor population, *Development* 131(18):4593-605, 2004.
42. Sainio K, Nonclercq D, Saarma M et al: Neuronal characteristics in embryonic renal stroma, *Int J Dev Biol* 38(1):77-84, 1994.
43. Sariola H, Holm K, Henke-Fahle S: Early innervation of the metanephric kidney, *Development* 104(4):589-99, 1998.
44. Mendelsohn C, Batourina E, Fung S et al: Stromal cells mediate retinoid-dependent functions essential for renal development, *Development* 126:1139-48, 1999.
45. Qiao J, Uzzo R, Obara-Ishihara T et al: FGF-7 modulates ureteric bud growth and nephron number in the developing kidney, *Development* 126:547-54, 1999.
46. Quaggin SE, Schwartz L, Cui S et al: The basic-helix-loop-helix protein pod1 is critically important for kidney and lung organogenesis, *Development* 126:5771-83, 1999.
47. Cullen-McEwen LA, Caruana G, Bertram JF: The where, what and why of the developing renal stroma, *Nephron Exp Nephrol* 99(1): e1-8, 2005.
48. Lemley KV, Kriz W: Anatomy of the renal interstitium, *Kidney Int* 39(3):370-81, 1991.
49. Herzlinger D, Koseki C, Mikawa T et al: Metanephric mesenchyme contains multipotent stem cells whose fate is restricted after induction, *Development* 114(3):565-72, 1992.
50. Evan AP, Gattone VH 2nd, Schwartz GJ: Development of solute transport in rabbit proximal tubule. II. Morphologic segmentation, *Am J Physiol* 245(3):F391-407, 1983.
51. Fetterman GH, Shuplock NA, Philipp FJ et al: The growth and maturation of human glomeruli and proximal convolutions from term to adulthood: Studies by microdissection, *Pediatrics* 35:601-19, 1965.
52. Neiss WF: Histogenesis of the loop of Henle in the rat kidney, *Anat Embryol (Berl)* 164(3):315-30, 1982.
53. Nakai S, Sugitani Y, Sato H et al: Crucial roles of Brn1 in distal tubule formation and function in mouse kidney, *Development* 130(19):4751-59, 2003.
54. Neiss WF, Klehn KL: The postnatal development of the rat kidney, with special reference to the chemodifferentiation of the proximal tubule, *Histochemistry* 73(2):251-68, 1981.
55. Kreidberg JA: Podocyte differentiation and glomerulogenesis, *J Am Soc Nephrol* 14(3):806-14, 2003.
56. Robert B, St John PL, Hyink DP et al: Evidence that embryonic kidney cells expressing flk-1 are intrinsic, vasculogenic angioblasts, *Am J Physiol* 271(3 Pt 2):F744-53, 1996.
57. Hyink DP, Tucker DC, St John PL et al: Endogenous origin of glomerular endothelial and mesangial cells in grafts of embryonic kidneys, *Am J Physiol* 270(5 Pt 2):F886-99, 1996.
58. Ricono JM, Xu YC, Arar M et al: Morphological insights into the origin of glomerular endothelial and mesangial cells and their precursors, *J Histochem Cytochem* 51(2):141-50, 2003.
59. Sariola H, Ekblom P, Lehtonen E et al: Differentiation and vascularization of the metanephric kidney grafted on the chorioallantoic membrane, *Dev Biol* 96(2):427-35, 1993.
60. Nagata M, Nakayama K, Terada Y et al: Cell cycle regulation and differentiation in the human podocyte lineage, *Am J Pathol* 153(5):1511-20, 1998.
61. Garrod DR, Fleming S: Early expression of desmosomal components during kidney tubule morphogenesis in human and murine embryos, *Development* 108(2):313-21, 1990.
62. Pavenstadt H, Kriz W, Kretzler M: Cell biology of the glomerular podocyte, *Physiol Rev* 83(1):253-307, 2003.
63. Ekblom P: Formation of basement membranes in embryonic kidney: an immunohistological study, *J Cell Biol* 91:1-10, 1981.
64. Sariola H, Timpl R, von der Mark K et al: Dual origin of glomerular basement membrane, *Dev Biol* 101:86-96, 1984.
65. Karihaloo A, Nickel C, Cantley LG: Signals which build a tubule, *Nephron Exp Nephrol* 100(1):e40-45, 2005.
66. Coles HSR, Burne JF, Raff MC: Large-scale normal cell death in the developing rat kidney and its reduction by epidermal growth factor, *Development* 117:777-84, 1993.
67. Michael L, Davies JA: Pattern and regulation of cell proliferation during murine ureteric bud development, *J Anat* 204(4):241-55, 2004.
68. Fisher CE, Michael L, Barnett MW et al: Erk MAP kinase regulates branching morphogenesis in the developing mouse kidney, *Development* 128(21):4329-38, 2001.
69. Meyer TN, Schwesinger C, Bush KT et al: Spatiotemporal regulation of morphogenetic molecules during in vitro branching of the isolated ureteric bud: toward a model of branching through budding in the developing kidney, *Dev Biol* 275(1):44-67, 2004.
70. Robillard J, Porter C, Jose P: Structure and function of the developing kidney. In Holliday M, Barratt T, Avner E, editors: *Pediatric nephrology*, Philadelphia, 1994, Williams & Williams.
71. Barisoni L, Kriz W, Mundel P et al: The dysregulated podocyte phenotype: a novel concept in the pathogenesis of collapsing idiopathic focal segmental glomerulosclerosis and HIV-associated nephropathy, *J Am Soc Nephrol* 10(1):51-61, 1999.
72. Barasch J, Qiao J, McWilliams G et al: Ureteric bud cells secrete multiple factors, including bFGF, which rescue renal progenitors from apoptosis, *Am J Physiol* 273:F757-67, 1997.
73. Dudley AT, Godin RE, Robertson EJ: Interaction between FGF and BMP signaling pathways regulates development of metanephric mesenchyme, *Genes Dev* 13:1601-13, 1999.

74. Koseki C, Herzlinger D, Al-Awqati Q: Apoptosis in metanephric development, *J Cell Biol* 119(5):1327-33, 1992.
75. Grobstein C: Inductive interaction in the development of the mouse metanephros, *J Ex Zool* 130:319-40, 1955.
76. Araki T, Saruta T, Okano H et al: Caspase activity is required for nephrogenesis in the developing mouse metanephros, *Exp Cell Res* 248(2):423-29, 1999.
77. Winyard PJD, Nauta J, Lirenman DS et al: Deregulation of cell survival in cystic and dysplastic renal development, *Kidney Int* 49:135-46, 1996.
78. Loughna S, Landels E, Woolf AS: Growth factor control of developing kidney endothelial cells, *Exp Nephrol* 4(2):112-18, 1996.
79. Perantoni AO, Williams CL, Lewellyn AL: Growth and branching morphogenesis of rat collecting duct anlagen in the absence of metanephrogenic mesenchyme, *Differentiation* 48:107-13, 1991.
80. Cano-Gauci DF, Song H, Yang H et al: Glypican-3-deficient mice exhibit developmental overgrowth and some of the renal abnormalities typical of Simpson-Golabi-Behmel syndrome, *J Cell Biol* 146:255-64, 1999.
81. Grisaru S, Cano-Gauci D, Tee J et al: Glypican-3 modulates BMP- and FGF-mediated effects during renal branching morphogenesis, *Dev Biol* 231:31-46, 2001.
82. Sorenson CM, Rogers SA, Korsmeyer SJ et al: Fulminant metanephric apoptosis and abnormal kidney development in bcl-2-deficient mice, *Am J Physiol* 268:F73-F81, 1995.
83. Moser M, Pscherer A, Roth C et al: Enhanced apoptotic cell death of renal epithelial cells in mice lacking transcription factor AP-2ß, *Genes Dev* 11:1938-48, 1997.
84. Chevalier RL: Growth factors and apoptosis in neonatal ureteral obstruction, *J Am Soc Nephrol* 7:1098-105, 1996.
85. Tarantal AF, Han VK, Cochrum KC et al: Fetal rhesus monkey model of obstructive renal dysplasia, *Kidney Int* 59:446-56, 2001.
86. Frisch SM, Francis H: Disruption of epithelial cell-matrix interactions induces apoptosis. *J Cell Biol* 124:619-26, 1994.
87. Erickson RA: Inductive interactions in the development of the mouse metanephros, *J Exp Zool* 169(1):33-42, 1968.
88. Batourina E, Gim S, Bello N et al: Vitamin A controls epithelial/mesenchymal interactions through Ret expression, *Nat Genet* 27:74-78, 2001.
89. Gao X, Chen X, Taglienti M et al: Angioblast-mesenchyme induction of early kidney development is mediated by Wt1 and Vegfa, *Development* 132(24):5437-49, 2005.
90. Tufro-McReddie A, Norwood VF, Aylor KW et al: Oxygen regulates vascular endothelial growth factor-mediated vasculogenesis and tubulogenesis, *Dev Biol* 183(2):139-49, 1997.
91. Barasch J, Yang J, Ware CB et al: Mesenchymal to epithelial conversion in rat metanephros is induced by LIF, *Cell* 99(4):377-86, 1999.
92. Shah MM, Sampogna RV, Sakurai H et al: Branching morphogenesis and kidney disease, *Development* 131(7):1449-62, 2004.
93. Grieshammer U, Cebrian C, Ilagan R et al: FGF8 is required for cell survival at distinct stages of nephrogenesis and for regulation of gene expression in nascent nephrons, *Development* 132(17):3847-57, 2005.
94. Perantoni AO, Timofeeva O, Naillat F et al: Inactivation of FGF8 in early mesoderm reveals an essential role in kidney development, *Development* 132(17):3859-71, 2005.
95. Yang J, Blum A, Novak T et al: An epithelial precursor is regulated by the ureteric bud and by the renal stroma, *Dev Biol* 246(2):296-310, 2002.
96. Dressler GR: The cellular basis of kidney development, *Annu Rev Cell Dev Biol* 22:509-29, 2006.
97. Costantini F: Renal branching morphogenesis: concepts, questions, and recent advances, *Differentiation* 74(7):402-21, 2006.
98. Yu J, McMahon AP, Valerius MT: Recent genetic studies of mouse kidney development, *Curr Opin Genet Dev* 14(5):550-57, 2004.
99. Xu P-X, Adams J, Peters H et al: Eya1-deficient mice lack ears and kidneys and show abnormal apoptosis of organ primordial, *Nat Genet* 23:113-17, 1999.
100. Xu PX, Zheng W, Huang L et al: Six1 is required for the early organogenesis of mammalian kidney. *Development* 130(14):3085-94, 2003.
101. Rothenpieler UW, Dressler GR: Pax-2 is required for mesenchyme-to-epithelium conversion during kidney development, *Development* 119:711-20, 1993.
102. Torres M, Gomez-Pardo E, Dressler GR et al: Pax-2 controls multiple steps of urogenital development, *Development* 121:4057-65, 1995.
103. Kreidberg JA, Sariola H, Loring JM et al: WT-1 is required for early kidney development. *Cell* 74:679-91, 1993.
104. Nishinakamura R, Matsumoto Y, Nakao K et al: Murine homolog of SALL1 is essential for ureteric bud invasion in kidney development, *Development* 128:3105-15, 2001.
105. Kobayashi A, Kwan KM, Carroll TJ et al: Distinct and sequential tissue-specific activities of the LIM-class homeobox gene Lim1 for tubular morphogenesis during kidney development, *Development* 132(12):2809-23, 2005.
106. Tsang TE, Shawlot W, Kinder SJ et al: Lim1 activity is required for intermediate mesoderm differentiation in the mouse embryo, *Dev Biol* 223(1):77-90, 2000.
107. Dressler GR, Deutsch U, Chowdhury K et al: Pax-2, a new murine paired-box-containing gene and its expression in the developing excretory system, *Development* 109:787-95, 1990.
108. Fujii T, Pichel JG, Taira M et al: Expression patterns of the murine LIM class homeobox gene lim1 in the developing brain and excretory system, *Dev Dyn* 1:73-83, 1994.
109. Pachnis V, Mankoo B, Costantini F: Expression of the c-ret protooncogene during mouse embryogenesis, *Development* 119:1005-17, 1993.
110. Kalatzis V, Sahly I, El-Amraoui A et al: Eya1 expression in the developing ear and kidney: towards the understanding of the pathogenesis of Branchio-Oto-Renal (BOR) syndrome, *Dev Dyn* 213:486-99, 1998.
111. Hellmich HL, Kos L, Cho ES et al: Embryonic expression of glial cell-line derived neurotrophic factor (GDNF) suggests multiple developmental roles in neural differentiation and epithelial-mesenchymal interactions, *Mech Dev* 54:95-105, 1996.
112. Brophy PD, Ostrom L, Lang KM et al: Regulation of ureteric bud outgrowth by Pax2-dependent activation of the glial derived neurotrophic factor gene, *Development* 128:4747-56, 2001.
113. Costantini F, Shakya R: GDNF/Ret signaling and the development of the kidney, *Bioessays* 28(2):117-27, 2006.
114. Shawlot W, Behringer RR: Requirement for Lim1 in head-organizer function, *Nature* 374:425-30, 1995.
115. Donovan MJ, Natoli TA, Sainio K et al: Initial differentiation of the metanephric mesenchyme is independent of WT1 and the ureteric bud, *Dev Genet* 24:252-62, 1999.
116. Sainio K, Suvanto P, Davies J et al: Glial-cell-line-derived neurotrophic factor is required for bud initiation from ureteric epithelium, *Development* 124:4077-87, 1997.
117. Schuchardt A, D'Agati V, Larsson-Blomberg L et al: Defects in the kidney and enteric nervous system of mice lacking the tyrosine kinase receptor, *Ret Nature* 367:380-83, 1994.
118. Enomoto H, Araki T, Jackman A et al: GFRα1-deficient mice have deficits in the enteric nervous system and kidneys, *Neuron* 21:317-24, 1998.
119. Pichel JG, Shen L, Sheng HZ et al: Defects in enteric innervation and kidney development in mice lacking GDNF, *Nature* 382:73-76, 1996.
120. Sanchez MP, Silos-Santiago I, Frisen J et al: Renal agenesis and the absence of enteric neurons in mice lacking GDNF, *Nature* 382:70-73, 1996.
121. Schuchardt A, D'Agati V, Pachnis V et al: Renal agenesis and hypodysplasia in ret-k-mutant mice result from defects in ureteric bud development, *Development* 122:1919-29, 1996.
122. Cacalano G, Farinas I, Wang LC et al: GFRalpha1 is an essential receptor component for GDNF in the developing nervous system and kidney, *Neuron* 21:53-62, 1998.
123. Müller U, Wang D, Denda S et al: Integrin α8β1 is critically important for epithelial-mesenchymal interactions during kidney morphogenesis, *Cell* 88:603-13, 1997.
124. Bullock SL, Fletcher JM, Beddington RSP et al: Renal agenesis in mice homozygous for a gene trap mutation in the gene encoding heparan sulfate 2-sulfotransferase, *Genes Dev* 12:1894-906, 1998.

125. Towers PR, Woolf AS, Hardman P: Glial cell line-derived neurotrophic factor stimulates ureteric bud outgrowth and enhances survival of ureteric bud cells in vitro, *Exp Nephrol* 6:337-51, 1998.
126. Pepicelli CV, Kispert A, Rowitch D et al: GDNF induces branching and increased cell proliferation in the ureter of the mouse, *Dev Biol* 192:193-98, 1997.
127. Srinivas S, Wu Z, Chen C-M et al: Dominant effects of RET receptor misexpression and ligand-independent RET signaling on ureteric bud development, *Development* 126:1375-86, 1999.
128. Shakya R, Jho EH, Kotka P et al: The role of GDNF in patterning the excretory system, *Dev Biol* 283(1):70-84, 2005.
129. Brodbeck S, Englert C: Genetic determination of nephrogenesis: the Pax/Eya/Six gene network, *Pediatr Nephrol* 19(3):249-55, 2004.
130. Wellik DM, Hawkes PJ, Capecchi MR: Hox11 paralogous genes are essential for metanephric kidney induction, *Genes Dev* 16(11):1423-32, 2002.
131. Miyamoto N, Yoshida M, Kuratani S et al: Defects of urogenital development in mice lacking Emx2, *Development* 124:1653-64, 1997.
132. Kume T, Deng K, Hogan BL: Murine forkhead/winged helix genes Foxc1 (Mf1) and Foxc2 (Mfh1) are required for the early organogenesis of the kidney and urinary tract, *Development* 127:1387-95, 2000.
133. Tessier-Lavigne M, Goodman CS; The molecular biology of axon guidance, *Science* 274:1123-33, 1996.
134. Brose K, Bland KS, Wang KH et al: Slit proteins bind Robo receptors and have an evolutionarily conserved role in repulsive axon guidance, *Cell* 96:795-806, 1999.
135. Piper M, Georgas K, Yamada T et al: Expression of the vertebrate Slit gene family and their putative receptors, the Robo genes, in the developing murine kidney, *Mech Dev* 94:213-17, 2000.
136. Quaggin SE, Vanden Heuvel GB, Igarashi P. Pod-1, a mesoderm-specific basic-helix-loop-helix protein expressed in mesenchymal and glomerular epithelial cells in the developing kidney, *Mech Dev* 71:37-48, 1998.
137. Basson MA, Akbulut S, Watson-Johnson J et al: Sprouty1 is a critical regulator of GDNF/RET-mediated kidney induction, *Dev Cell* 8(2):229-39, 2005.
138. Basson MA, Watson-Johnson J, Shakya R et al: Branching morphogenesis of the ureteric epithelium during kidney development is coordinated by the opposing functions of GDNF and Sprouty1, *Dev Biol* 299(2):466-77, 2006.
139. Kispert A, Vainio S, Shen L et al: Proteoglycans are required for maintenance of Wnt-11 expression in the ureter tips, *Development* 122:3627-37, 1996.
140. Majumdar A, Vainio S, Kispert A et al: Wnt11 and Ret/Gdnf pathways cooperate in regulating ureteric branching during metanephric kidney development, *Development* 130(14):3175-85, 2003.
141. Chi L, Zhang S, Lin Y et al: Sprouty proteins regulate ureteric branching by coordinating reciprocal epithelial Wnt11, mesenchymal Gdnf and stromal Fgf7 signalling during kidney development, *Development* 131(14):3345-56, 2004.
142. Dudley AT, Robertson EJ: Overlapping expression domains of bone morphogenetic protein family members potentially account for limited tissue defects in BMP7 deficient embryos, *Dev Dyn* 208:349-62, 1997.
143. Godin RE, Robertson EJ, Dudley AT: Role of BMP family members during kidney development, *Int J Dev Biol* 43:405-11, 1999.
144. Dewulf N, Verschueren K, Lonnoy O et al: Distinct spatial and temporal expression patterns of two type 1 receptors for bone morphogenetic proteins during mouse embryogenesis, *Endocrinology* 136:2652-63, 1995.
145. Verschueren K, Dewulf N, Goumans MJ et al: Expression of type I and type IB receptors for activin in midgestation mouse embryos suggests distinct functions in organogenesis, *Mech Dev* 52:109-23, 1995.
146. Raatikainen-Ahokas A, Hytonen M, Tenhunen A et al: Bmp-4 affects the differentiation of metanephric mesenchyme and reveals an early anterior-posterior axis of the embryonic kidney, *Dev Dyn* 217:146-58, 2000.
147. Piscione TD, Yager TD, Gupta IR et al: BMP-2 and OP-1 exert direct and opposite effects on renal branching morphogenesis. *Am J Physiol* 273:F961-75, 1997.
148. Piscione TD, Phan T, Rosenblum ND: BMP7 controls collecting tubule cell proliferation and apoptosis via Smad1-dependent and -independent pathways, *Am J Physiol* 280:F19-33, 2001.
149. Pope JC IV, Brock JW III, Adams MC et al: How they begin and how they end: classic and new theories for the development and deterioration of congenital anomalies of the kidney and urinary tract, CAKUT. *J Am Soc Nephrol* 10:2018-28, 1999.
150. Ichikawa I, Kuwayama F, Pope JC et al: Paradigm shift from classic anatomic theories to contemporary cell biological views of CAKUT, *Kidney Int* 61(3):889-98, 2002.
151. Bush KT, Sakurai H, Steer DL et al: TGF-beta superfamily members modulate growth, branching, shaping, and patterning of the ureteric bud, *Dev Biol* 266(2):285-98, 2004.
152. Qiao J, Sakurai H, Nigam SK: Branching morphogenesis independent of mesenchymal-epithelial contact in the developing kidney, *Proc Natl Acad Sci USA* 96:7330-35, 1999.
153. Sakurai H, Bush KT, Nigam SK: Identification of pleiotrophin as a mesenchymal factor involved in ureteric bud branching morphogenesis, *Development* 128:3283-93, 2001.
154. Qiao J, Bush KT, Steer DL et al: Multiple fibroblast growth factors support growth of the ureteric bud but have different effects on branching morphogenesis, *Mech Dev* 109(2):123-35, 2001.
155. Cancilla B, Davies A, Cauchi JA et al: Fibroblast growth factor receptors and their ligands in the adult rat kidney, *Kidney Int* 60(1):147-55, 2001.
156. Poladia DP, Kish K, Kutay B et al: Role of fibroblast growth factor receptors 1 and 2 in the metanephric mesenchyme, *Dev Biol* 291(2):325-39, 2006.
157. Barros EJG, Santos OFP, Matsumoto K et al: Differential tubulogenic and branching morphogenetic activities of growth factors: implications for epithelial tissue development, *Proc Natl Acad Sci USA* 92:4412-4416, 1995.
158. Cantley LG, Barros EJG, Gandhi M et al: Regulation of mitogenesis, motogenesis, and tubulogenesis by hepatocyte growth factor in renal collecting duct cells, *Am J Physiol* 267:F271-80, 1994.
159. Montesano R, Soriano JV, Pepper MS et al: Induction of epithelial branching tubulogenesis in vitro, *J Cell Physiol* 173:152-61, 1997.
160. Bladt F, Riethmacher D, Isenmann S et al: Essential role for the c-met receptor in the migration of myogenic precursor cells into the limb bud, *Nature* 376:768-71, 1995.
161. Threadgill DW, Dlugosz AA, Hansen LA et al: Targeted disruption of mouse EGF receptor: effect of genetic background on mutant phenotype, *Science* 269:230-34, 1995.
162. Uehara Y, Minowa O, Mori C et al: Placental defect and embryonic lethality in mice lacking hepatocyte growth factor/scatter factor, *Nature* 373(6516):702-05, 1995.
163. Barasch J, Yang J, Qiao JY et al: Tissue inhibitor of metalloproteinase-2 stimulates mesenchymal growth and regulates epithelial branching during morphogenesis of the rat metanephros, *J Clin Invest* 103:1299-307, 1999.
164. Sakurai H, Nigam SK: In vitro branching tubulogenesis: implications for developmental and cystic disorders, nephron number, renal repair, and nephron engineering, *Kidney Int* 54:14-26, 1998.
165. Pohl M, Sakurai H, Bush KT et al: Matrix metalloproteinases and their inhibitors regulate in vitro ureteric bud branching morphogenesis, *Am J Physiol* 279:F891-900, 2000.
166. Ohuchi H, Hori Y, Yamasaki M et al: FGF10 acts as a major ligand for FGF receptor 2 IIIb in mouse multi-organ development, *Biochem Biophys Res Commun* 277:643-49, 2000.
167. Bonneh-Barkay D, Shlissel M, Berman B et al: Identification of glypican as a dual modulator of the biological activity of fibroblast growth factors, *J Biol Chem* 272:12415-21, 1997.
168. Bernfield M, Hinkes MT, Gallo RL: Developmental expression of the syndecans: possible function and regulation, *Development Suppl*:205-12,1993.
169. Davies J, Lyon M, Gallagher J et al: Sulphated proteoglycan is required for collecting duct growth and branching but not nephron formation during kidney development, *Development* 121:1507-17, 1995.

170. Jackson SM, Nakato H, Sugiura M et al: Dally, a *Drosophila* glypican, controls cellular responses to the TGF-ß-related morphogen, Dpp, *Development* 124:4113-20, 1997.
171. Tsuda M, Kamimura K, Nakato H et al: The cell-surface proteoglycan dally regulates wingless signalling in *Drosophila, Nature* 400:276-80, 1999.
172. Zhang P, Liégeois NJ, Wong C et al: Altered cell differentiation and proliferation in mice lacking p57KIP2 indicates a role in Beckwith-Wiedemann syndrome, *Nature* 387:151-58, 1997.
173. Hatada I, Ohashi H, Fukushima Y et al: An imprinted gene p57KIP2 is mutated in Beckwith-Wiedemann syndrome, *Nat Genet* 14:171-73, 1996.
174. Leighton PA, Ingram RS, Eggenschwiler J et al: Disruption of imprinting caused by deletion of the H19 gene region in mice, *Nature* 375:34-39, 1995.
175. Caspary T, Cleary MA, Perlman EJ et al: Oppositely imprinted genes p57(Kip2) and Igf2 interact in a mouse model for Beckwith-Wiedemann syndrome, *Genes Dev* 13(23):3115-24, 1999.
176. Green MC: Mechanism of the pleiotropic effects of the short-ear mutant gene in the mouse, *J Exp Zool* 176:129-50, 1968.
177. Niimura F, Labostky PA, Kakuchi J et al: Gene targeting in mice reveals a requirement for angiotensin in the development and maintenance of kidney morphology and growth factor regulation, *J Clin Invest* 96:2947-54, 1995.
178. Miyazaki Y, Tsuchida S, Nishimura H et al: Angiotensin induces the urinary peristaltic machinery during the perinatal period, *J Clin Invest* 102:1489-97, 1998.
179. James RG, Kamei CN, Wang Q et al: Odd-skipped related 1 is required for development of the metanephric kidney and regulates formation and differentiation of kidney precursor cells, *Development* 133(15):2995-3004, 2006.
180. Cho EA, Patterson LT, Brookhiser WT et al: Differential expression and function of cadherin-6 during renal epithelium development, *Development* 125(5):803-12, 1998.
181. Karavanov AA, Karavanova I, Perantoni A et al: Expression pattern of the rat Lim-1 homeobox gene suggests a dual role during kidney development, *Int J Dev Biol* 42:61-66, 1998.
182. Stewart CL, Kaspar P, Brunet LJ et al: Blastocyst implantation depends on maternal expression of leukaemia inhibitory factor, *Nature* 359(6390):76-79, 1992.
183. Plisov SY, Yoshino K, Dove LF et al: TGF beta 2, LIF and FGF2 cooperate to induce nephrogenesis, *Development* 128(7):1045-57, 2001.
184. Sanford LP, Ormsby I, Gittenberger-de Groot AC et al: TGFβ2 knockout mice have multiple developmental defects that are non-overlapping with other TGFβ knockout phenotypes, *Development* 124:2659-70, 1997.
185. McPherron AC, Lawler AM, Lee SJ: Regulation of anterior/posterior patterning of the axial skeleton by growth/differentiation factor 11, *Nat Genet* 22(3):260-64, 1999.
186. Herzlinger D, Qiao J, Cohen D et al: Induction of kidney epithelial morphogenesis by cells expressing wnt-1, *Dev Biol* 166:815-18, 1994.
187. Kispert A, Vainio S, McMahon AP: Wnt-4 is a mesenchymal signal for epithelial transformation of metanephric mesenchyme in the developing kidney, *Development* 125:4225-34, 1998.
188. Carroll TJ, Park JS, Hayashi S et al: Wnt9b plays a central role in the regulation of mesenchymal to epithelial transitions underlying organogenesis of the mammalian urogenital system, *Dev Cell* 9(2):283-92, 2005.
189. Yoshino K, Rubin JS, Higinbotham KG et al: Secreted Frizzled-related proteins can regulate metanephric development, *Mech Dev* 102(1-2):45-55, 2001.
190. Dudley AT, Lyons KM, Robertson EJ: A requirement for bone morphogenetic protein-7 during development of the mammalian kidney and eye, *Genes Dev* 9:2795-807, 1995.
191. Luo G, Hofmann C, Bronckers AL et al: BMP-7 is an inducer of nephrogenesis, and is also required for eye development and skeletal patterning, *Genes Dev* 9:2808-20, 1995.
192. Majumdar A, Lun K, Brand M et al: Zebrafish no isthmus reveals a role for pax2.1 in tubule differentiation and patterning events in the pronephric primordial, *Development* 127(10):2089-98, 2000.
193. Wallingford JB, Carroll TJ, Vize PD: Precocious expression of the Wilms' tumor gene xWT1 inhibits embryonic kidney development in Xenopus laevis, *Dev Biol* 202(1):103-12, 1998.
194. Ryan G, Steele-Perkins V, Morris JF et al: Repression of Pax-2 by WT1 during normal kidney development, *Development* 121(3):867-75, 1995.
195. Pelletier J, Schalling M, Buckler AJ et al: Expression of the Wilms' tumor gene WT1 in the murine urogenital system, *Genes Dev* 5:1345-56, 1991.
196. Dressler GR, Douglass EC: Pax-2 is a DNA-binding protein expressed in embryonic kidney and Wilms tumor, *Proc Natl Acad Sci USA* 89:1179-83, 1992.
197. Dressler GR, Wilkinson JE, Rothenpieler UW et al: Deregulation of Pax-2 expression in transgenic mice generates severe kidney abnormalities, *Nature* 362:65-67, 1993.
198. Cheng HT, Miner JH, Lin M et al: Gamma-secretase activity is dispensable for mesenchyme-to-epithelium transition but required for podocyte and proximal tubule formation in developing mouse kidney, *Development* 130(20):5031-42, 2003.
199. Cheng HT, Kim M, Valerius MT et al: Notch2, but not Notch1, is required for proximal fate acquisition in the mammalian nephron, *Development* 134(4):801-11, 2007.
200. Wang P, Pereira FA, Beasley D et al: Presenilins are required for the formation of comma- and S-shaped bodies during nephrogenesis, *Development* 130(20):5019-29, 2003.
201. McCright B, Gao X, Shen L et al: Defects in development of the kidney, heart and eye vasculature in mice homozygous for a hypomorphic Notch2 mutation, *Development* 128:491-502, 2001.
202. Sadl V, Jin F, Yu J et al: The mouse Kreisler (Krml1/MafB) segmentation gene is required for differentiation of glomerular visceral epithelial cells, *Dev Biol* 249(1):16-29, 2002.
203. Miner JH, Morello R, Andrews KL et al: Transcriptional induction of slit diaphragm genes by Lmx1b is required in podocyte differentiation, *J Clin Invest* 109(8):1065-72, 2002.
204. Dreyer SD, Zhou G, Baldini A et al: Mutations in LMX1B cause abnormal skeletal patterning and renal dysplasia in nail patella syndrome, *Nature Genet* 19:47-50, 1998.
205. Barbaux S, Niaudet P, Gubler M-C et al: Donor splice-site mutations in WT1 are responsible for Frasier syndrome, *Nature Genet* 17:467-70, 1997.
206. Klamt B, Koziell A, Poulat F et al: Frasier syndrome is caused by defective alternative splicing of WT1 leading to an altered ratio of WT1+/-KTS splice isoforms, *Hum Mol Genet* 7:709-14, 1998.
207. Coppes MJ, Liefers GJ, Higuchi M et al: Inherited WT1 mutation in Denys-Drash syndrome, *Cancer Res* 52(21):6125-28, 1992.
208. Yang Y, Jeanpierre C, Dressler GR et al: WT1 and PAX-2 podocyte expression in Denys-Drash syndrome and isolated diffuse mesangial sclerosis, *Am J Pathol* 154(1):181-92, 1999.
209. Gao F, Maiti S, Sun G et al: The Wt1+/R394W mouse displays glomerulosclerosis and early-onset renal failure characteristic of human Denys-Drash syndrome, *Mol Cell Biol* 24(22):9899-910, 2004.
210. Patek CE, Little MH, Fleming S et al: A zinc finger truncation of murine WT1 results in the characteristic urogenital abnormalities of Denys-Drash syndrome, *Proc Natl Acad Sci USA* 96(6):2931-36, 1999.
211. Hammes A, Guo JK, Lutsch G et al: Two splice variants of the Wilms' tumor 1 gene have distinct functions during sex determination and nephron formation, *Cell* 106(3):319-29, 2001.
212. Guo JK, Menke AL, Gubler MC et al: WT1 is a key regulator of podocyte function: reduced expression levels cause crescentic glomerulonephritis and mesangial sclerosis, *Hum Mol Genet* 11(6):651-59, 2002.
213. Kitamoto Y, Tokunaga H, Tomita K: Vascular endothelial growth factor is an essential molecule for mouse kidney development: glomerulogenesis and nephrogenesis. *J Clin Invest* 99(10):2351-57, 1997.
214. Tufro A, Norwood VF, Carey RM et al: Vascular endothelial growth factor induces nephrogenesis and vasculogenesis, *J Am Soc Nephrol* 10(10):2125-34, 1999.
215. Eremina V, Cui S, Gerber H et al: Vascular endothelial growth factor a signaling in the podocyte-endothelial compartment is

required for mesangial cell migration and survival, *J Am Soc Nephrol* 17(3):724-35, 2006.
216. Eremina V, Sood M, Haigh J et al: Glomerular-specific alterations of VEGF-A expression lead to distinct congenital and acquired renal diseases, *J Clin Invest* 111(5):707-16, 2003.
217. Woolf AS, Yuan HT: Angiopoietin growth factors and Tie receptor tyrosine kinases in renal vascular development, *Pediatr Nephrol* 16(2):177-84, 2001.
218. Lindahl P, Hellström M, Kalén M et al: Paracrine PDGF-B/PDGF-Rß signaling controls mesangial cell development in kidney glomeruli, *Development* 125:3313-22, 1998.
219. Leveen P, Pekny M, Gebre-Medhin S et al: Mice deficient for PDGF B show renal, cardiovascular, and hematological abnormalities, *Genes Dev* 8:1875-87, 1994.
220. Soriano P: Abnormal kidney development and hematological disorders in PDGF ß-receptor mutant mice, *Genes Dev* 8:1888-96, 1994.
221. Miner JH, Sanes JR: Collagen IV alpha 3, alpha 4, and alpha 5 chains in rodent basal laminae: sequence, distribution, association with laminins, and developmental switches, *J Cell Biol* 127(3):879-91, 1994.
222. Miner JH, Li C: Defective glomerulogenesis in the absence of laminin alpha5 demonstrates a developmental role for the kidney glomerular basement membrane, *Dev Biol* 217(2):278-89, 2000.
223. Miner JH, Sanes JR: Molecular and functional defects in kidneys of mice lacking collagen alpha 3(IV): implications for Alport syndrome, *J Cell Biol* 135(5):1403-13, 1996.
224. Noakes PG, Miner JH, Gautam M et al: The renal glomerulus of mice lacking s-laminin/laminin ß2: nephrosis despite molecular compensation by laminin ß1, *Nature Genet* 10:400-06, 1995.
225. Zhao H, Kegg H, Grady S et al: Role of fibroblast growth factor receptors 1 and 2 in the ureteric bud, *Dev Biol* 276(2):403-15, 2004.
226. Stark K, Vainio S, Vassileva G et al: Epithelial transformation of metanephric mesenchyme in the developing kidney regulated by Wnt-4, *Nature* 372:679-83, 1994.
227. Oxburgh L, Dudley AT, Godin RE et al: BMP4 substitutes for loss of BMP7 during kidney development, *Dev Biol* 286(2):637-46, 2005.

PART 2: FUNCTIONAL DEVELOPMENT OF THE NEPHRON

Aoife M. Waters

GENERAL OVERVIEW OF ANTENATAL, PERINATAL, AND POSTNATAL FLUID AND ELECTROLYTE HOMEOSTASIS

Fluid and electrolyte homeostasis in the fetus is controlled by the placenta. As a result, the placenta receives a significant proportion of the fetal cardiac output (33%), whereas the fetal kidneys receive only 2.5% even in late gestation.[1] Urine production begins at approximately 10 weeks of gestation and coincides with the acquisition of the first capillary loops by the inner medullary metanephric nephrons. Thereafter, hourly fetal urine production increases from 5 ml at 20 weeks to approximately 50 ml at 40 weeks.[2] By 20 weeks' gestation, fetal urine production contributes to over 90% of amniotic fluid volume.[3] Severe oligohydramnios due to abnormal fetal renal function in the second trimester can result in pulmonary hypoplasia and in severe cases, Potter's syndrome.[4]

At birth, the newborn consists largely of water, with total body water making up 75% of body weight at full term. Total body water is even higher in preterm infants, making up to 80% to 85% of body weight.[5] Adaptation to the extrauterine environment involves an increase in glomerular filtration with an immediate postnatal natriuresis. High circulating levels of atrial natriuretic peptide (ANP) are responsible for the postnatal physiological natriuresis.[6] Fetal creatinine clearance is low but increases with gestational age (Figure 6-7). In addition, a progressive increase in renal tubular resorptive capacity occurs with concomitant glomerular maturation during fetal development.[7,8] Further maturation of tubular function occurs postnatally.[7] Changes include an increase in resorptive surface area, an increase in transporter number, and maturation of function, along with further modification of paracrine regulatory mechanisms.[7] In the following section we discuss the developmental changes that occur in the perinatal nephron, which are necessary for extrauterine adaptation.

GLOMERULAR FUNCTION IN THE FETAL, PERINATAL, AND POSTNATAL PERIOD

Glomerular filtration is the transudation of plasma across the glomerular filtration barrier (GFB) and is the first step in the formation of urine (Figure 6-8). Filtration depends on both Starling's forces and an adequate renal blood flow.[9] The total glomerular filtration rate (GFR) is the sum of the GFR of each single functioning nephron, SNGFR [where $SNGFR = (k \times S) \times (\Delta P - \Delta\pi)$]. ΔP is the hydrostatic pressure difference between the glomerular capillary pressure (P_{GC}) and the hydrostatic pressure in Bowman's space (P_{BS}). $\Delta\pi$ is the oncotic pressure difference between the glomerular capillary pressure (π_{GC}) and the oncotic pressure in Bowman's space (π_{BS}). K_f is the product of the hydraulic permeability of glomerular capillary walls (k) and the surface area available for filtration, (S), ($K_f = k \times S$). Here we will discuss the functional development of glomerular filtration in the perinatal period.

Fetal GFR

During nephrogenesis, an increase in renal mass parallels an increase in fetal GFR.[10] Indeed, fetal GFR correlates well with both gestational age and body weight (Figure 6-7).[10] Preterm infants of 30 weeks' gestational age have a creatinine clearance of less than 10 ml/min/1.73 m^2 within the first 24 to 40 hours of birth,[11] whereas creatinine clearance in term infants is higher and ranges between 10 and 40 ml/min/1.73 m^2.[12] All four determinants of SNGFR contribute in varying degrees to the maturational increase in GFR.[13] Mean arterial pressure increases during fetal development with a concomitant increase in P_{GC}.[14] An increase in renal plasma flow leads to a further increase in SNGFR.[15] In addition, plasma oncotic pressure also rises with advancing gestational age.[16] However, the increase in P_{GC} is greater than that observed for π_{GC}, favoring ultrafiltration.

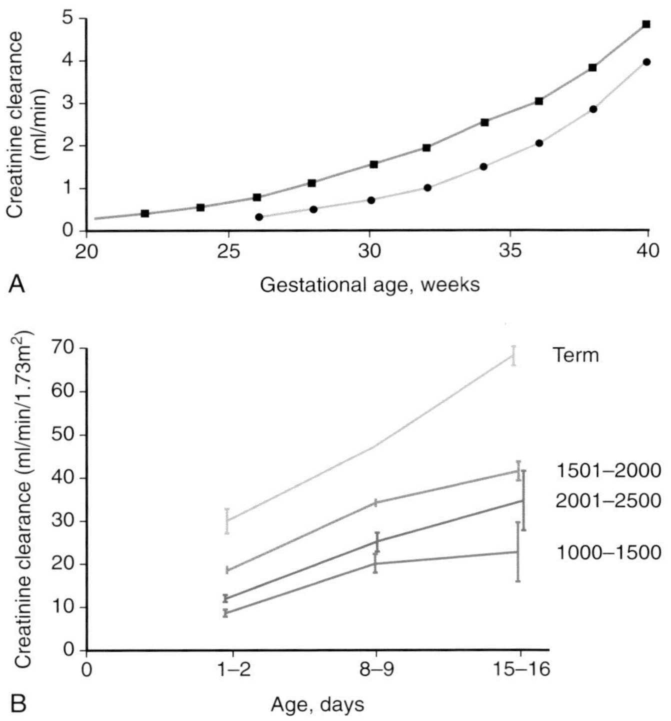

Figure 6-7 Creatinine clearance (C_{Cr}) for human fetuses from 20 weeks (■) and corresponding preterm neonates (●). Creatinine clearance correlates well with gestational age **(A)** and body weight **(B)**. (From Haycock GB: Development of glomerular filtration and tubular sodium reabsorption in the human fetus and newborn, *Br J Urol* 81(suppl 2):33-38, 1998.)

Fetal renal blood flow can be measured by Doppler ultrasound techniques and increases from 20 ml/min at 25 weeks' gestation to more than 60 ml/min at 40 weeks.[11] Fetal renal blood flow is low due to high renal vascular resistance (RVR).[17] RVR depends on arteriolar tone and on the number of resistance vessels. As nephrogenesis proceeds, an increase in the number of glomerular vessels is observed, and in preterm infants born before 36 weeks' gestation, the postnatal fall in RVR can in part be attributable to new nephron formation.[17] Concomitantly, a redistribution of renal blood flow occurs from the inner medullary nephrons to the more superficial cortical nephrons. Total GFR increases as a result of an increase in SNGFR arising from newly formed superficial cortical glomeruli.[13,18]

Assessment of fetal glomerular function is possible by measuring fetal serum cystatin C or β_2-microglobulin. Fetal serum cystatin C is independent of gestational age and has been shown to have a high specificity (92%) for the prediction of postnatal kidney dysfunction. Reference intervals were calculated in a study of 129 cordocenteses involving 54 fetuses without renal disease.[19] Mean serum cystatin C levels were 1.6 mg/L, with 2.0 mg/L being the upper limit of normal; in the same study, fetal serum β_2-microglobulin decreased significantly with gestational age and the upper limit could be calculated from 7.19(mg/L) − [0.052(mg/L) × gestational age (weeks)]. In the same study, serum β_2-microglobulin was demonstrated to have a higher sensitivity (87%) than cystatin C in predicting postnatal renal dysfunction. Both tests may therefore be used to assess fetal glomerular function in antenatally diagnosed renal malformations.

Neonatal GFR

A rapid rise in creatinine clearance occurs in term infants over the first 4 days of life (Figure 6-7, *B*). Preterm infants also experience a rise in creatinine clearance, which occurs more slowly than in term neonates.[20] Overall, a doubling of GFR is seen over the first 2 weeks of life in term infants and reaches adult values by 2 years of age.[21,22] Postnatally the mean arterial pressure increases, and consequently an increase in glomerular hydraulic pressure occurs, resulting in an increase in GFR. A dramatic postnatal fall in RVR with redistribution of intrarenal blood flow from the juxtamedullary nephrons to the superficial cortical nephrons also contributes to increased GFR in the postnatal period. The fraction of cardiac output supplying the neonatal kidneys increases to 15% to 18% over the first 6 weeks of life.[23] An increase in the area available for glomerular filtration also contributes to the increase in GFR seen postnatally.[13] Glomerular size, GBM surface area, and capillary permeability to macromolecules all contribute to postnatal increase in GFR.[24] Changes in both afferent and efferent arteriolar tone also contribute to the maturation of glomerular filtration. A decrease in renal vasoconstrictors and activation of renal vasodilators occurs over the first 2 weeks of life and are discussed in the following section.

Vasoregulatory Mechanisms of the Neonatal Kidney

Renal Vasoconstrictors in the Developing Nephron

Renin-angiotensin system (RAS). Regulation of renal blood flow and glomerular filtration is controlled by the renin-angiotensin system (RAS). Angiotensin II is a potent vasoconstrictor of the efferent arteriole, which results in an increase in P_{GC} and therefore GFR. Both plasma renin activity and angiotensin II levels are high in the neonate. Renal angiotensin converting enzyme (ACE) levels are higher than adult levels in the first 2 weeks of life, and expression is localized to the proximal tubules and capillaries in the developing human kidney.[25,26] Expression of angiotensinogen and ACE increases during late gestation and peaks after birth.[26,27] Also, the number of angiotensin type 1 (AT1) receptors are twice that of adult levels at 2 weeks of age.[28] AT2 receptors, on the other hand, are more abundant in the fetal kidney, with progressive downregulation during fetal maturation. In contrast, AT1 receptors undergo upregulation as the fetal kidney matures.[29] Animal studies have shown that angiotensin II constricts the fetal renal arteries via the AT1 receptor, and during fetal life plays an important role in controlling the resistance of the umbilical arteries and thus the total fetal peripheral vascular resistance.[30] In newborn lambs, maintenance of arterial pressure and baroreceptor control of heart rate and renal sympathetic nerve activity is controlled by circulating and endogenous angiotensin II.[31] Therefore the RAS plays a significant role in maintaining blood pressure, as well as vascular resistance in the developing fetus.

Indeed, the importance of the fetal RAS is highlighted by case reports of ACE fetopathy with the use of angiotensin converting enzyme inhibitors (ACEIs) in pregnancy. Maternal ACEIs can result in decreased placental perfusion, fetal hypo-

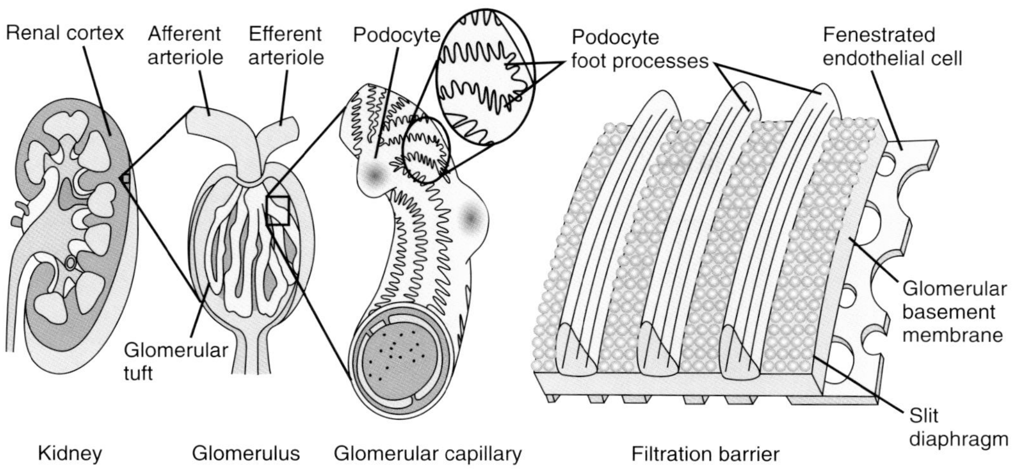

Figure 6-8 Glomerular filtration barrier. The glomerular filtration barrier is composed of multiple layers that block the passage of plasma macromolecules and maintain plasma oncotic pressure. Each capillary loop is lined by a fenestrated capillary endothelium. Outside this endothelial lining lies the porous glomerular basement membrane, which is attached to highly dynamic epithelial cells called *podocytes*. Each podocyte has interdigitating foot processes with neighboring podocytes and are connected to each other by a platform of signaling molecules called the *slit diaphragm*. The slit diaphragm is the major barrier to filtration of plasma macromolecules. (Redrawn with permission from Tryggvason K, Wartiovaara J: How does the kidney filter plasma? *Physiology 20:96-101, 2005.*)

tension, oligohydramnios, and neonatal renal failure.[32] Recently mutations in genes coding for renin, angiotensinogen, ACE, and AT1 have been described in autosomal recessive renal tubular dysgenesis and fetal hypotension.[33] Both inherited and acquired defects of the RAS, therefore, can alter fetal renal hemodynamics with deleterious effects on renal development.

Renal nerves and catecholamines. High RVR in the perinatal period can be partly attributed to increased renal sympathetic nerve activity (through α1 receptor stimulation) and rising circulating catecholamine levels.[34] Renal sympathetic nerves cause renal vasoconstriction, primarily of the afferent arteriole, which results in decreased P_{GC} and decreased GFR (Figure 6-9).[35] Renal sympathetic nerve activity increases immediately after birth in sheep, and plasma epinephrine and norepinephrine increase severalfold immediately following birth.[36,37] A fall in catecholamine levels subsequently occurs over the first few days of life.[38] Renal denervation in maturing piglets has been shown to increase RBF, demonstrating the role of renal nerves in maintaining high RVR. Renin release is also stimulated by the sympathetic nervous system. Rodent studies have shown that renin-containing cells and nerve fibers are detected at 17 days' gestation in close spatial relationship along the main branches of the renal artery.[39] Innervation of these cells follows the centrifugal pattern of renin distribution and nephrovascular development. The density and organization of nerve fibers increases with age along the arterial vascular tree.[39] The high RVR observed in the perinatal period most likely results from an interplay between increased sympathetic nerve activity and high plasma renin levels.

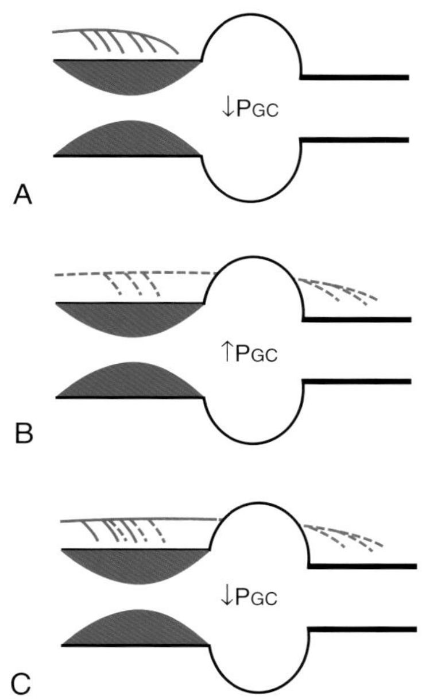

Figure 6-9 The renal nerves constrict the renal vasculature, causing decreases in renal blood flow and glomerular filtration. **A,** Afferent arteriolar vasoconstriction: decreased P_{GC}. **B,** Efferent arteriolar vasoconstriction: increased P_{GC}. **C,** Decreased P_{GC} is observed when afferent arteriolar vasoconstriction is greater than efferent arteriolar vasoconstriction. (Redrawn with permission from Denton KM, Luff SE, Shweta A, Anderson WP: Differential neural control of glomerular ultrafiltration, *Clinl Exp Pharmacol Physiol* 31:380-86, 2004.)

Endothelin. Endothelin (ET) is a potent vasoconstrictor secreted by the endothelial cells of renal vessels, mesangial cells, and distal tubular cells in response to angiotensin II, bradykinin (BK), epinephrine, and shear stress.[40] Renal vasomotor tone is exquisitely sensitive to endothelin. An increase in RVR occurs following ET-induced contraction of glomerular arterioles (afferent more than efferent) with a subsequent reduction in GFR.[40] In the early postnatal period, ET is elevated in term and preterm neonates. A reduction in ET levels then occurs after the first week of life.[41] Newborn rat kidneys have a higher number of ET receptors than do adult rat kidneys. A comparable binding affinity for ET has also been shown.[42] In addition, ET can cause vasodilation. Activation of ET_B receptors on the vascular endothelium evokes the release of vasodilators. The renal vasculature of fetal renal lambs reacts with vasodilation to low doses of ET, which may be due to the secondary release of nitric oxide (NO) that blunts the vasoconstrictor effects of ET.[43,44] Endothelin may therefore have both vasoconstrictor effects and vasodilatory effects on the neonatal kidney.

Renal Vasodilators in the Developing Nephron

Prostaglandins. Prostaglandin E_2 (PGE_2), PGD_2, and PGI_2, the major prostaglandins, increase RBF by stimulating afferent arteriolar vasodilation, free water clearance, urine flow, and natriuresis. PGs are synthesized by the fetal and neonatal kidney.[45] Alterations in the synthetic and catabolic activity of renal prostaglandins occur with advancing gestational and postnatal age. Concomitant alterations in RBF, GFR, water, and electrolyte excretion occur, suggesting an important role for PGs in renal function development.

Newborns have high circulating levels of PGs that counteract the highly activated vasoconstrictor state of the neonatal microcirculation.[46] PG synthesis inhibitors can have a deleterious renal vasoconstrictor effect in the immature kidney. Long-term maternal indomethacin treatment may decrease fetal urine output enough to alter amniotic fluid volume.[47] Severe renal impairment leading to fetal or neonatal death has been reported with the use of PG synthesis inhibitors such as indomethacin.[48] Renal dysfunction depends in part on dosage, timing of therapy, and the cardiovascular and renal status of the infant before treatment.[49] Recent rodent studies with targeted gene disruption have shown that cyclooxygenase type-2 (COX-2) is necessary for late stages of nephrogenesis and that deficiency of COX-2 activity leads to pathologic changes in cortical architecture and eventually renal failure.[50] Therefore both the RAS and PGs are important in controlling renal hemodynamics and nephrogenesis.

Nitric oxide. NO plays a major role in maintaining basal renal vascular tone in the mature kidney. Through activation of its second messenger cGMP, NO results in vasodilation, modification of renin release, and change in GFR.[51] NO also plays an important role in maintaining glomerular filtration in the developing kidney. Animal studies have shown that inhibition of NO synthesis by infusion with L-arginine analogs significantly decreases GFR in the developing kidney but not in the adult kidney.[52-54] Treatment with angiotensin receptor blockers abolishes the decrease in GFR observed in developing kidneys treated with L-arginine analogs.[54] Therefore NO plays a critical role in the developing kidney by counterregulating the vasoconstricting effects of angiotensin II and protecting the immature kidney.

Kallikrein-kinin system. BK is a vasodilator and diuretic peptide produced by the action of kallikrein (KK), an enzyme produced by the CD epithelial cells. Activation of the BK-2 receptor by BK stimulates NO and PG production, resulting in vasodilation and natriuresis. An endogenous kallikrein-kinin system is expressed in the developing kidney with higher neonatal expression than that found in adult kidneys.[55,56] Renal expression and urinary excretion of KK rise rapidly in the postnatal period, with excretion of KK correlating well with the rise in RBF.[57,58] Blockade of the BK-2 receptor results in renal vasoconstriction in newborn rabbits, demonstrating the renal vasodilatory action of BK in the neonatal kidney.[59]

Disordered Vasoregulatory Mechanisms

Vasomotor nephropathy (VMNP) is defined as renal dysfunction due to reduced renal perfusion, with the preterm infant being particularly vulnerable.[60] Main causes of neonatal acute renal failure include prerenal mechanisms such as hypotension, hypovolemia, hypoxemia, and neonatal septicemia. Hypotension can independently stimulate vasoconstrictive mediators such as angiotensin II, cause renal vasoconstriction and hypoperfusion, and further reduce neonatal GFR. Treatment of neonatal hypotension often involves inotropic support such as dopamine. Dopamine has a direct effect on renal function via renal dopaminergic receptors located in the renal arteries, glomeruli, and proximal and distal tubules.[61] At low doses (0.5-2 μg/kg/min) dopamine causes renal vasodilation and increases GFR and electrolyte excretion.[62] In neonatal intensive care units, higher doses of dopamine (6-10 μg/kg/min) are used to achieve systemic cardiovascular effects. Such doses have an opposite effect on renal function, causing renal vasoconstriction and reduction in sodium and water excretion.[62] Hypoxemia reduces renal blood flow and GFR. In a study of severely asphyxiated neonates, 61% developed acute renal failure.[63] Hypoxemia stimulates ET, ANP, and PG release. In addition, mechanical ventilation can reduce venous return and cardiac output, sometimes resulting in renal hypoperfusion and renal dysfunction.[60] Neonatal VMNP can therefore result from disturbances of glomerular hemodynamics through a complex interplay of renal vasoregulatory mechanisms.

WATER TRANSPORT IN THE DEVELOPING KIDNEY

Term neonates can dilute their urine to osmolalities as low 50 mosm/L, which is similar to adult values.[64] However, the ability to excrete a water load is limited by the neonate's low GFR. As a result, neonates have a higher total body water content than adults do, making up 75% of body weight at full term and 80% to 85% in preterm infants between 26 and 31 weeks' gestation.[5] Under normal physiologic conditions, the kidneys have to excrete this water load during the first week of life.[65] Therefore maximal concentrating abilities are not necessary at birth and in fact are low in the neonatal period. A progressive increase in concentrating capacity occurs postnatally, and in term infants reaches adult levels by the first month of life (Figure 6-10).[66] In the premature neonate, concentrating capacity is maximal at about 500 mosm/L for a more prolonged period,[67] which places the sick premature infant at greater risk for serious disturbances in water and electrolyte homeostasis.[68] Reasons for limited concentrating capacity include diminished responsiveness of the CDs to antidiuretic hormone (ADH), anatomic immaturity of the renal medulla, and decreased medullary concentration of sodium chloride (NaCl) and urea.[69,70] Each of these components is discussed in detail in the following section.

Antidiuretic Hormone in the Development of Water Transport

Normal ADH Physiology

ADH exerts its antidiuretic effect in the CD via the V_2 receptor on the basolateral membrane of the principal and inner medullary CD cells.[71,72] Binding of ADH to the V_2 receptor

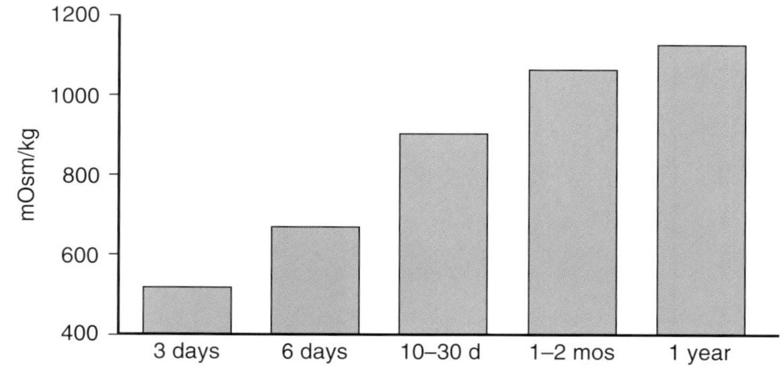

Figure 6-10 Renal concentrating capacity increases in the postnatal period in the term infant, reaching adult values by the first month of life. (From Polacek E, Vocel J, Neugebauerova L, Sebkova M, Vechetova E: The osmotic concentrating ability in healthy infants and children, *Arch Dis Child* 40:291-295, 1965.)

results in activation of adenylcyclase, increased cAMP, and activation of protein kinase A. Subsequent phosphorylation of the cytoplasmic COOH terminus at serine 256 of the aquaporin-2 (AQ2) water channel occurs and results in the insertion of AQ2 into the apical or luminal membrane of the CD cells.[73-75] Water enters the cells via AQ2 and exits the cell via the AQ3 and AQ4 water channels located on the basolateral membrane of the CD cells.[76] Water reabsorption depends on a hypertonic medullary interstitium, which drives water from the luminal fluid across the tubular epithelium.[77]

Development of Water Transport in the Collecting Duct

Low neonatal urinary concentrating capacity is not attributed to low ADH levels. During labor, ADH levels are elevated, which is consistent with the raised intracranial pressure and hypoxemia acting as stimuli for ADH release.[78] Despite adequate ability to secrete ADH, no correlation exists between ADH levels and urine osmolality in the first 3 weeks of life.[79] ADH stimulation of the neonatal cortical collecting duct (CCD) results in a lower permeability response to water than that seen in the adult.[80,81] Response to ADH improves with aging. Similarly, studies have shown that the concentrating capacity is even lower in infants who have sustained neonatal asphyxia.[82] V_2 receptor mRNA expression is observed in rodents as early as day 16 of gestation in cells of the developing medullary and CCD.[83] Rodent studies have shown that the number of V_2 receptors does not change during the first 2 weeks of life. By the fifth week of life, the number of receptors is similar to adult levels.[84] However, the low response of the immature kidney to ADH is more likely to be due to immaturity of the intracellular second messenger systems than to inadequate receptor number. ADH-binding sites precede the onset of adenylcyclase responsiveness.[85] In addition, ADH-stimulation of adenylcyclase generation is markedly lower in the neonatal period and is only about one third that of the cAMP response seen in the adult CCD.[86] However, even when cAMP generation is rescued using cAMP analogs, the hydraulic permeability of isolated, microperfused rabbit CCD remains low.[87] Intracellular phosphodiesterases degrade cAMP. Indeed, an increase in phosphodiesterase IV and inhibition of the production of cAMP by PGE2 acting through EP3 receptors (PGE2 receptor subtype localized to the CCD and inner medullary CD) has been shown to inhibit adenylcyclase generation on ADH stimulation. Therefore cAMP inhibition likely accounts for the immature kidney's reduced response to ADH.[88,89]

AQ2 levels (mRNA and protein) are lower in early postnatal life and reach maximal expression at 10 weeks of age (Figure 6-11).[90] AQ2 trafficking can be appropriately stimulated by dehydration and DDAVP in the immature kidney while the urine osmolality remains low.[90] Glucocorticoids regulate AQ2 expression and increase expression of both AQ2 protein and mRNA in the infant and not in the adult.[91] Expression of AQ3 and AQ4 does not change significantly after birth and therefore does not seem to play a role in the maturation of water transport in the CD.[92]

Tonicity of the Developing Medullary Interstitium

In addition to low CD responsiveness to ADH, two other factors are responsible for the low concentrating capacity of the neonatal nephron. Neonatal medullary interstitium has a low tonicity, which is due to a low concentration of NaCl and urea.[93] Factors such as low protein intake, low sodium transport by the thick ascending loop of Henle (TAL),[94] immaturity of the medullary architecture with shorter loops of Henle,[95,96] and alterations in urea transport[97] all contribute to the lower tonicity of the medullary interstitium. Activity of the sodium-potassium ATPase (Na^+-K^+-ATPase) in the TAL increases after birth, with the most pronounced increase in activity occurring between the second and third week of life; this correlates well with increased urine-concentrating capacity.[98] In addition, the loops of Henle elongate and penetrate the medulla, forming tubulovascular units that are completed by the fourth postnatal week in rodents.[99]

Over the first 3 weeks of life, the medulla/cortex urea ratio has been shown to increase in newborn rabbits.[93] A striking increase in the number of urea transporters occurs during the first 2 weeks of life in rodents.[97] Urea transporters prevent the loss of urea from the medulla into the circulation, thereby ensuring a high concentration of urea in the medullary interstitium. Renal concentrating capacity depends on dietary protein intake,[93] and infants fed on high-protein diets show a significant improvement in urinary concentrating capacity.[82,100]

In summary, the neonatal kidney's ability to concentrate urine depends on a number of steps involving the ADH-signal transduction pathway (Figure 6-12), the maturation of Henle's loop, and tonicity of the medullary interstitium.

Postnatal Urine Flow

Oliguria is the most helpful sign of renal impairment in the neonate, and a delay in the first void in a newborn may signal a renal disorder. Preterm neonates void earlier than term or

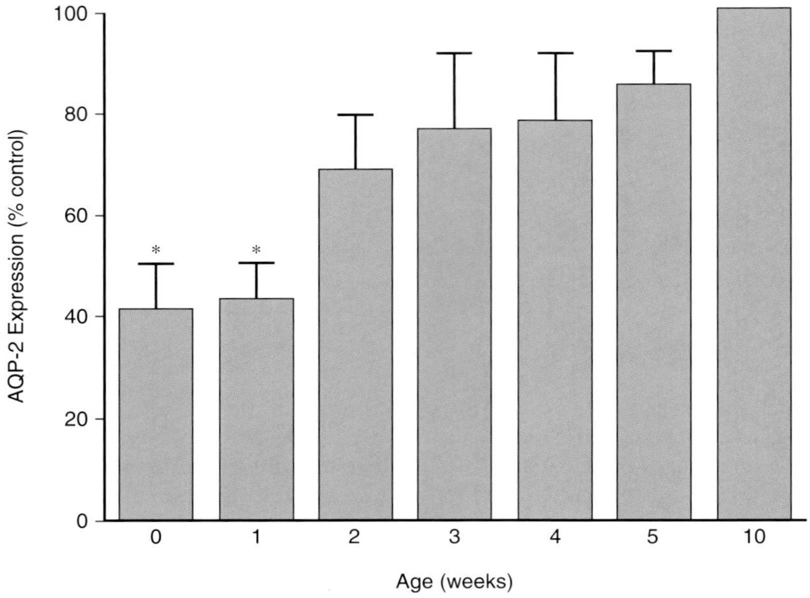

Figure 6-11 Aquaporin-2 (AQ2) expression between 0 and 10 weeks of age. An increase in protein expression occurs in the postnatal period. (From Bonilla-Felix, M: Development of water transport in the collecting duct, *Am J Physiol Renal Physiol* 287(6):F1093-101, 2004.)

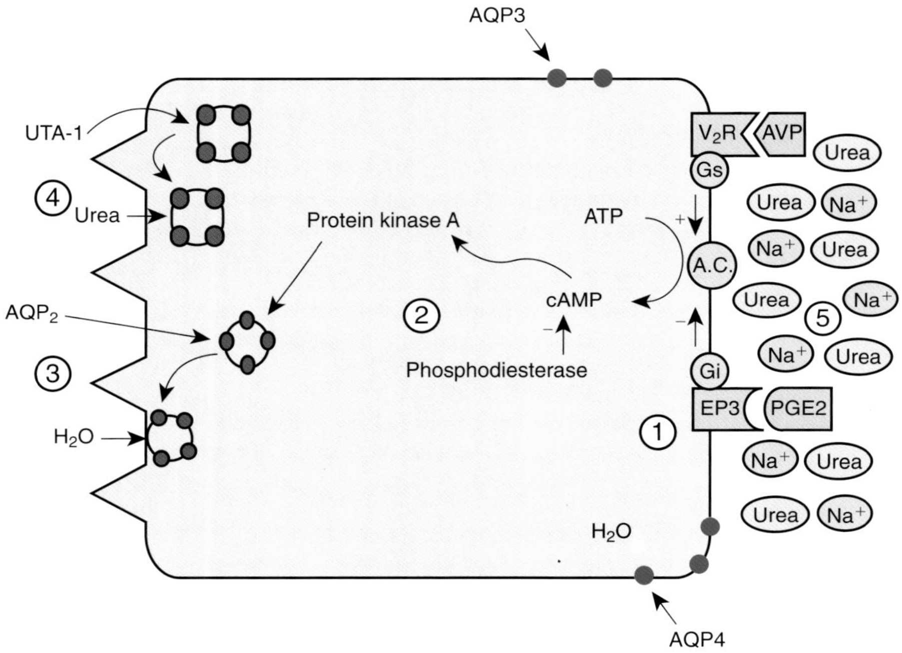

Figure 6-12 Mechanisms responsible for the immature kidney's response to ADH. *1,* Inhibition of cAMP generation by PGE_2 through EP3 receptor; *2,* rapid degradation of formed cAMP resulting from increased phosphodiesterase activity; *3,* low expression of AQP2 during early postnatal life; *4,* low expression of UTA-1 during early postnatal life; *5,* low concentration of urea and sodium in the medullary interstitium resulting from low rates of sodium transport, low dietary protein intake, and low expression of urea transporters. (Redrawn with permission from Bonilla-Felix, M: Development of water transport in the collecting duct, *Am J Physiol Renal Physiol* 287(6):F1093-110, 2004.)

postterm neonates,[101] and the majority of normal newborns void within the first 24 hours of life regardless of gestational age. Therefore any neonate who remains anuric beyond the first day of life should be evaluated for renal insufficiency. Factors that determine urine output include water balance, solute load, and renal concentrating ability.

Minimum urine volume (L) = Urine solutes to be excreted/urine osmolality (max)

As a result, a neonate receiving the usual renal solute load (7-15 mosm/kg/day) with a maximal renal concentrating capacity of 500 mosm/kg would require a minimal urine output of approximately 1 ml/kg per hour to remain in solute balance. Since acute renal failure results in progressively positive solute balance, a urine-flow rate of less than 1 ml/kg per hour has become an accepted criterion for the determination of oliguria in the neonate.

SODIUM TRANSPORT IN THE DEVELOPING KIDNEY

Adaptation to the extrauterine environment involves a physiologic natriuresis in the immediate postnatal period, with preterm infants losing up to 16% of birth weight in the first 3 days of life and term infants losing slightly less.[102] Human neonates remain in negative sodium balance for the first 4 days

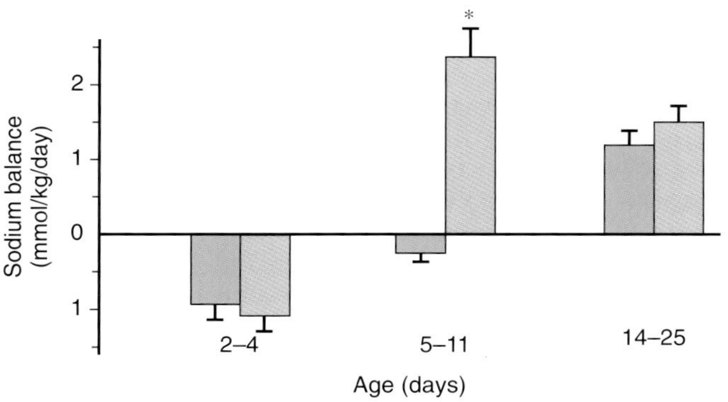

Figure 6-13 Net external sodium balance for preterm infants in the first 3 weeks of life. ▨ Control infants; ▨ sodium-supplemented infants, 4-5 mEq/kg/day; (*) $p < 0.0005$ vs. controls. In the first 2 to 4 days after birth, infants undergo natriuresis regardless of sodium intake, whereas by 1 week, supplemented infants achieve positive sodium balance sooner than controls. (From Al-Dahhan J, Haycock GB, Nichol B, Chantler C, Stimmle L: Sodium homeostasis in term and preterm neonates. III. Effect of salt supplementation, *Arch Dis Child* 59:945-50, 1984; copyright 1984 by Blackwell Science, Inc.)

of life and then shift to a positive sodium balance by the second and third weeks of life (Figure 6-13).[103] Sodium conservation occurs because sodium is essential for neonatal growth. In contrast to term neonates, preterm infants of less than 35 weeks' gestation do not tolerate sodium deprivation, and hyponatremia may develop because of tubular immaturity and sodium wasting.[104] For this reason sodium supplementation is important. Sodium requirements for a term newborn range from 1 to 1.5 mEq/kg daily, whereas requirements for a preterm neonate range from 3 to 5 mEq/kg daily. Sodium supplementation in the preterm infant enhances the cumulative weight gain following the initial postnatal diuresis.[103] The following section addresses the mechanisms involved in the postnatal natriuresis and the factors involved in the neonatal transition from negative to positive sodium balance.

Early Postnatal Natriuresis

High perinatal circulating levels of ANP have been implicated in the immediate postnatal natriuresis seen in both term and preterm infants.[6] ANP is a natriuretic hormone produced within cardiac myocytes and released by stretch of the atrial wall. At birth, pulmonary vascular resistance falls and left atrial venous return increases, stimulating the release of ANP. ANP exerts a number of physiologic effects, including natriuresis, diuresis, inhibition of renin and aldosterone release, vasorelaxation, and an increase in GFR and vascular permeability.[105]

ANP binds to physiological active receptors, resulting in an increase in intracellular cGMP.[106] As a result, inhibition of sodium transport occurs across the apical membranes of renal tubular epithelial cells, which leads to natriuresis. Plasma ANP concentration decreases with maturation.[107,108] A fall in right atrial volume occurs over the first 4 days of life, with parallel reductions in ANP concentration and urinary cGMP excretion.[109] In addition, a decrease in cGMP production per ANP-binding site has been shown to occur rapidly in the suckling period in neonatal rats.[110] Therefore sodium excretion is reduced after the first few postnatal days and the neonatal kidney subsequently aims to conserve sodium.

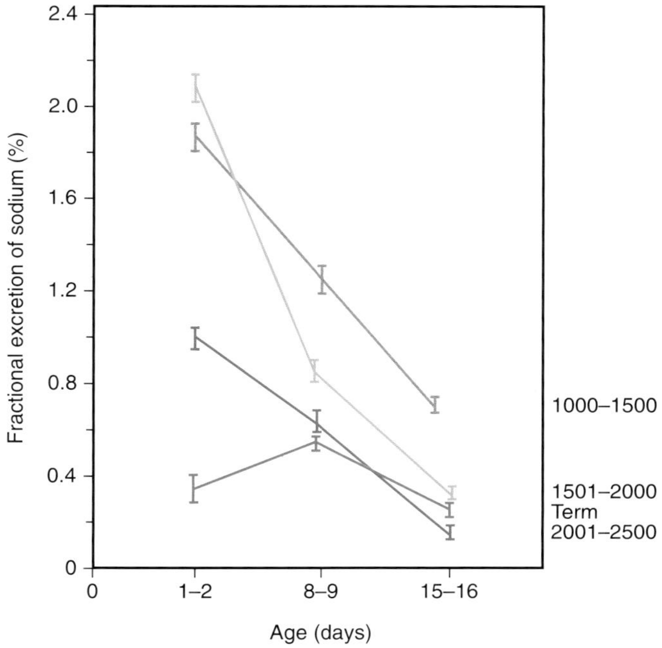

Figure 6-14 Fractional excretion of sodium during the first 2 weeks of life in preterm and term infants. Sodium is conserved despite an increase in GFR. (From Chevalier RL: The moth and the aspen tree: sodium in early postnatal development, *Kidney Int* 59(5):1617-25, 2001.)

Neonatal Transition to Positive Sodium Balance

A reduction in the fractional excretion of sodium occurs after the first week of life with fractions below 1% in the majority of infants (Figure 6-14).[111] Factors contributing to decreased fractional excretion of sodium include maturation of sodium transport mechanisms in the postnatal nephron, in addition to high circulating levels of angiotensin II, catecholamines, glucocorticoids, and a reduction in ANP. Each of these factors is discussed in the following section.

Maturation of Sodium Transport Mechanisms in the Developing Nephron

A progressive maturation of each tubular segment occurs in the postnatal kidney.[112] Each tubular segment is described separately here.

Proximal tubule. Solute transport in the neonatal proximal tubule is similar to that in the adult and follows both chloride and bicarbonate reabsorption. Several animal studies have shown an increase in the activity of the sodium/hydrogen (Na^+-H^+) exchanger during neonatal maturation.[113,114] In addition, an increase in activity of the chloride/formate exchanger has also been shown to occur.[115] Na^+-K^+-ATPase function plays a key role in proximal tubular sodium reabsorption with a progressive functional maturation occurring from birth (Figure 6-15).[116,117] Posttranslational increase in the $\alpha 1$ and $\beta 1$ subunits of the Na^+-K^+-ATPase transporter occurs immediately after birth in guinea pigs.[118]

Thick ascending limb of loop of Henle. Sodium chloride transport in the thick ascending limb of loop of Henle (TALH) occurs by paracellular and transcellular pathways via the apical sodium-potassium-2-chloride cotransporter (Na^+-$2Cl^-$-K^+) and the Na^+-H^+ type 3 exchangers. The Na^+-K^+-ATPase

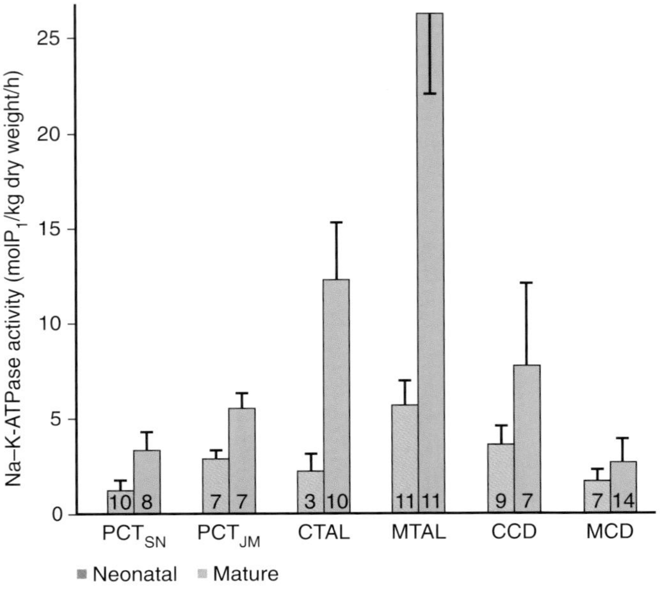

Figure 6-15 Na^+-K^+-ATPase activity in the neonatal and adult nephron. The Na^+-K^+-ATPase activity is lower in the neonate than in the adult. (Reproduced from Schmidt U, Horster M: Na-K-activated ATPase: activity maturation in rabbit nephron sygments dissected in vitro. *Am J Physiol* 233(1):F55-60, 1977.)

transporter controls sodium extrusion via the basolateral cell membrane. Transcription of Na^+-$2Cl^-$-K^+ cotransporter is observed early in development, before the onset of filtration in the descending loop of Henle. Physiologic studies, however, show that Na^+-$2Cl^-$-K^+ cotransporter is unlikely to be functional until postnatally, because low reabsorptive capacity has been shown for this segment in early postnatal life.[94] Compared with expression in adults, expression of all these transporters is lower in neonates.[119-122] Postnatally a five-to-tenfold increase in activity of the Na^+-K^+-ATPase cotransporter occurs and is greater than that seen in other tubular segments (Figure 6-15).[116,123] Na^+-K^+-ATPase consists of two subunits—a catalytic and a regulatory subunit. Both the α1 and β1 isoforms are present in the mature kidney. On the other hand, the α1 subunit is detected early in fetal life, whereas the β1 subunit is detected only after birth. Interestingly the β2 isoform is expressed in the fetal kidney, and in contrast to the adult, Na^+-K^+-ATPase is expressed on both the apical and basolateral cell membranes. After birth the β2 isoform is downregulated and the α1 and β1 isoforms are upregulated.[124] Heterodimerization of the α1 and β1 isoforms is essential for Na^+-K^+-ATPase function. Treatment with glucocorticoids increases mRNA synthesis of both subunits of the Na^+-K^+-ATPase transporter. During postnatal life a 20% increase in sodium reabsorption occurs along this segment and reflects functional maturation of the transporters themselves, as well as their regulatory mechanisms. An increase in resorptive surface area also contributes to increased sodium reabsorption.

Distal tubule. In the distal tubule the sodium chloride cotransporter (Na^+-Cl^-) is the major sodium influx cotransporter. In the mature nephron, Na^+-Cl^- is expressed along the entire distal tubule, starting beyond the Na^+-$2Cl^-$-K^+-expressing postmacular segment and ending at the transition into the collecting tubules.[125] During development, Na^+-Cl^- mRNA is detected in distal tubular segments before expression of Na^+-$2Cl^-$-K^+ mRNA and sodium-phosphate type 2 cotransporter $2Na^+$-Pi type II mRNA expression. Later in development, Na^+-Cl^- expression proceeds gradually into the postmacula segment of the TALH.[121]

Cortical collecting duct. Fine-tuning of sodium reabsorption occurs in the CCD where the amiloride-sensitive epithelial sodium channel (ENaC) plays an important role. ENaC is located on the apical membrane of distal tubular, cortical, and outer medullary CD cells.[126] ENaC consists of three subunits—α, β, and γ. Rodent studies show that the amount of total renal embryonic rat ENaC subunit mRNA is low but increases from rodent gestation days 16 to 19.[127] After birth an increase in α ENaC mRNA expression is observed, whereas β- and γ-ENaC mRNA expression decreases.[128] In the immature kidney, the greatest expression is seen in the terminal CD for all three subunits. As the kidney matures, expression in the cortical distal nephron increases and is complete by the ninth postnatal day in rodents.[129] Endogenous glucocorticoids do not appear to have any effect on prenatal maturation of ENaC in the kidney.[130] In the CCD, Na^+-K^+-ATPase is also expressed on the basolateral cell membrane.

Tracer uptake assays of individual CCDs have shown that activity of the Na^+-K^+-ATPase increases within the same time that it takes for maturation of net transepithelial sodium and potassium reabsorption.[131] Sodium resorptive capacity of the CCD increases immediately after birth and reflects an increase in expression of ENaC, as well as Na^+-K^+-ATPase.[132]

Developmental Paracrine Regulation of Renal Sodium Excretion

Renin angiotensin aldosterone system (RAAS). Studies have shown that RAAS is involved in neonatal renal tubular sodium reabsorption. Acute volume expansion in neonatal rat pups results in natriuresis and AT1 blockade attenuates the natriuretic response, demonstrating that angiotensin II mediates sodium reabsorption via the ATI receptor.[133] The proximal tubule is the likely site of sodium reabsorption, because angiotensin II augments sodium reabsorption in the proximal tubule in adult rats during volume contraction.[134] In addition, angiotensin II stimulates aldosterone, which stimulates sodium reabsorption in the TALH in mice, as well as the distal tubule and the CD. Preterm neonates without sodium supplementation demonstrate markedly increased plasma renin and aldosterone activity compared with their sodium supplemented counterparts, which indicates that the neonatal RAAS is involved in sodium homeostatic mechanisms.[135]

Catecholamines

Catecholamines stimulate NaCl and water reabsorption by the proximal tubule, ascending limb of Henle's loop, distal tubule, and CD. Circulating plasma catecholamines are high in the neonatal period and then fall over the first few days of life (see section on development of glomerular filtration). Catecholamines stimulate an increase in renin release, which promotes sodium reabsorption. In addition, dopamine acting via the D2 receptor in preterm neonates enhances sodium reabsorption in the proximal tubule.[136]

Glucocorticoids and Thyroid Hormone

Plasma cortisol levels increase markedly after birth.[137] Maturation of the Na^+-H^+ exchanger occurs under the influence of glucocorticoids as demonstrated by the attenuated postnatal increase of Na^+-H^+ exchanger activity, protein, and mRNA abundance in the brush border of proximal tubular cells of adrenalectomized newborn rodents.[138] Glucocorticoids also play a role in the maturation of transporters along the entire nephron.[139,140]

Thyroid hormone plays a role in the maturation of the paracellular pathways of sodium reabsorption.[141] Hypothyroid animals have paracellular tubular chloride permeability to that seen in the mature nephron. In addition, thyroid hormone, which increases sharply after birth, plays a role in the regulation of the Na^+-K^+-ATPase activity.[142]

Fractional Excretion of Sodium

In the oliguric term neonate (urine flow less than 1 ml/kg/hr), fractional excretion of sodium of less than 2.5% suggests a prerenal cause such as volume depletion, hypoalbuminemia, or reduced cardiac output.[143] The criterion of 2.5% is valid after the first 10 days of life in the low birth weight newborn after the period of postnatal natriuresis.[111] In addition, very low birth weight infants have greater fractional sodium excretion due to immaturity of the sodium reabsorptive capacity.[144]

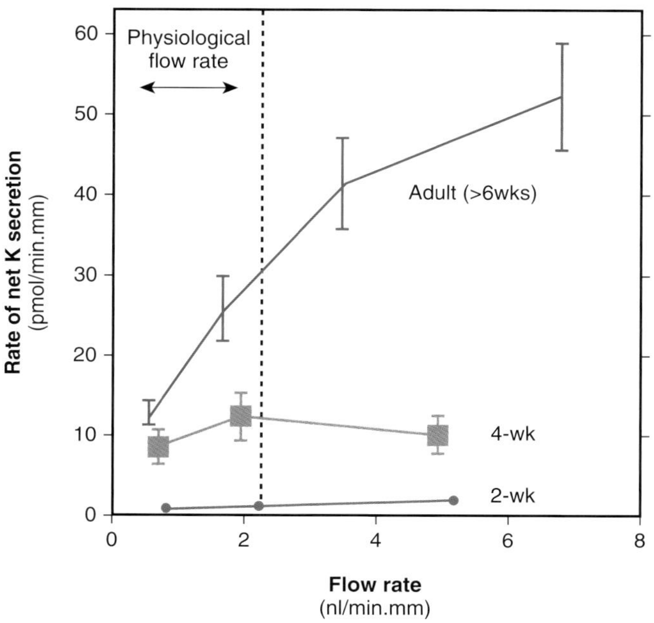

Figure 6-16 Net potassium secretion in maturing rabbits. (From Zhou H, Satlin LM: Renal potassium handling in healthy and sick newborns, *Semin Perinatol* 28(2):103-11, 2004.)

POTASSIUM TRANSPORT IN THE DEVELOPING KIDNEY

Like sodium, potassium is critical for somatic growth, and an increase in total body potassium content is associated with growth.[145] In contrast to adults, neonates greater than 30 weeks' gestational age must maintain a positive potassium balance.[145,146] Premature newborns, as a result, tend to have higher plasma potassium concentrations than children.[146] In utero the placenta transports potassium from the mother to the fetus.[147] Interestingly, potassium levels greater than 6.5 mmol/L are observed in 30% to 50% of very low birth weight infants in the first 48 hours in the absence of potassium intake and not after 72 hours.[148] A shift from the intracellular to the extracellular fluid compartment, as a result of sodium-potassium (Na^+-K^+) pump failure and/or a limited renal potassium excretory capacity, has been postulated to account for this increase.[149,150]

Renal potassium excretion is determined by the rate of potassium excretion by the principal cells of the distal tubule and CD. Net potassium secretion cannot be detected in microperfused CCD of newborn rabbits until after the third week of life (Figure 6-16),[151] and flow-stimulated transport is not detected until after the first postnatal month.[152]

Maturation of Potassium Transport Mechanisms in the Developing Nephron

Maturation of tubular transport mechanisms for each tubular segment is discussed in the following sections.

Proximal Tubule and Loop of Henle

In the mature nephron, 65% of the filtered potassium load is reabsorbed passively in the proximal tubule[153] and only 10% reaches the early distal tubule. In contrast, 35% of filtered potassium load reaches the distal tubule of the newborn rat.[154] Therefore postnatal maturation of the TALH is required for further potassium reabsorption. Indeed, both the diluting capacity and Na^+-K^+-ATPase activity increase after birth.[98,116] As discussed earlier, transcription of NKCC2 is observed early in development, before the onset of filtration in the descending loop of Henle, but is unlikely to be functional until postnatally in view of the low reabsorptive capacity shown for this segment in early postnatal life.[94] Apical ROMK (renal outer medullary potassium) channel has been detected in the TALH at an earlier developmental stage compared to the CCD. Functional analyses on ROMK in the developing TALH have not been performed.

Cortical Collecting Duct

As shown in rodent studies, in the fully differentiated CCD, two types of potassium channels are involved in potassium secretion: (1) the ROMK channel, which mediates potassium secretion under baseline conditions,[155,156] and (2) the maxi-K^+ channel, which mediates flow-stimulated potassium secretion.[157] ROMK has only been shown in principal cells of the CCD. Maxi-K^+ exists in both the principal and intercalated cells of the CCD.[157] In isolated CCDs of neonatal rabbits, apical ROMK channels are not detected in the first 7 days of life, and subsequently a threefold increase in the number of ROMK channels is seen in the principal cells of CCD between the third and fifth week of life and follows 1 week after an increase in ENaC activity is detected.[158,159] Also, expression of ROMK protein on apical cell membranes of the TALH and occasional CCD in the inner cortex and outer medulla is detected by indirect immunofluorescence studies in 1-week-old animals.[160] By 3 weeks of age, expression increases to involve the middle and outer CCDs.[160]

Maxi-K^+ channels mediate flow-stimulated K^+ secretion and do not appear to be functional in 4-week-old rabbits subjected to a sixfold increase in tubular flow rate.[152] However, a small but significant increase in net potassium secretion after 5 weeks of age is observed. An associated increase in mRNA and protein expression of the maxi-K^+ channel α subunit is seen on the apical surface of the CCD intercalated cells.[152]

In addition to potassium excretion, potassium reabsorption also occurs in the distal nephron via the apical hydrogen-potassium (H^--K^+-ATPase). Fluorescent functional assays identify significant H^+-K^+-ATPase activity on apical cell membranes of neonatal intercalated cells,[161] suggesting that neonatal CDs have a capacity to retain potassium. Indeed, a longitudinal prospective study of fractional potassium excretion in infants 23 to 31 weeks' gestational age demonstrated that despite a threefold increase of filtered potassium, the renal excretion fell by half between 26 and 30 weeks.[145] This study supports the idea that the developing kidney has the capacity for potassium reabsorption.

Regulation of Potassium Balance in the Neonate

Table 6-2 illustrates the factors that acutely regulate plasma potassium in the neonate. Despite high circulating levels of aldosterone, the immature kidney displays an insensitivity to aldosterone.[146] In adult and neonatal rats, the number of mineralocorticoid receptors, the receptor affinity, and degree of hormone-receptor nuclear binding is similar.[162] Aldosterone insensitivity may result from immature intracellular signal transduction mechanisms. Aldosterone insensitivity in the immature kidney is supported by the low transtubular potassium gradients (TTKG) reported in 27-week gestational age infants compared with 30-week infants followed over the first 5 days of postnatal life.[163] However, the low TTKG may also reflect a low secretory ability. Glucocorticoids have a significant effect on potassium balance in extremely low birth rate infants during the first week of life. Infants whose mothers received a full course of prenatal steroids had no hyperkalemia (>6.5 mmol/L) and a less-negative potassium balance at the end of the first week of life.[164] Several studies have shown that glucocorticoids upregulate the expression of the Na^+-K^+-ATPase,[165] resulting in a decreased potassium shift from the intracellular to extracellular compartments.

TABLE 6-2 Neonatal Potassium Regulation

	Effect on Cell Uptake of K^+
Physiologic	
Plasma K concentration	
↑	↑
↓	↓
Insulin	
Catecholamines	
α-agonists	↓
β-agonists	↑
Pathologic	
Acid-base balance	
Acidosis	↓
Alkylosis	↑
Hyperosmolality	↑ cell efflux
Cell breakdown	↑ cell efflux

Adapted from Zhou H, Satlin LM: Renal potassium handling in healthy and sick newborns, *Semin Perinatol* 29(2):103-11, 2004.

ACID-BASE REGULATION IN THE DEVELOPING KIDNEY

Term neonates have a lower bicarbonate concentration than adults (Figure 6-17).[166,167] In the low birth weight newborn, total bicarbonate may be as low as 15 mmol/L during the early postnatal period and is within normal limits.[166] Bicarbonate gradually increases with increasing GFR. Misdiagnosis of renal tubular acidosis may occur if one does not take into account the physiologically low plasma bicarbonate in neonates. In addition, neonates need to excrete 2-3 mEq/kg/day of acid because of their high protein intake and formation of new bone. The neonate has a reduced ability to respond to an acid load, whereas ammoniagenesis and titratable acidity mature after 4 to 6 weeks in the low birth weight newborn.[168] Renal regulation of acid–base balance undergoes complex changes during development, which is discussed in detail in a later section.

Proximal Tubule Handling of Bicarbonate in the Neonate

Bicarbonate reabsorption in the proximal tubule in the neonate is one third that of the adult[169] and is due to lower activity of similar transporters present in the adult.[170] In the mature nephron, the number of apical sodium-hydrogen ion type 3 (NHE3) antiporters is lower, with about one third the activity of its adult counterpart.[113] In the neonate, the H^+-ATPase does not appear to be active, whereas the basolateral Na^+-K^+-ATPase has about one half of the activity as in adults.[171] Similarly the carbonic anhydrase (CA) type IV isoform, which is expressed on the brush border of proximal tubular epithelial cells, has a lower activity in the developing nephron of rabbits. During maturation, however, activity does increase and parallels an increase in proximal tubular bicarbonate reabsorption.[172] Ammoniagenesis occurs in the neonatal kidney but at a much lower rate than in adults.[173,174] Glutamine and activity of the deaminating enzyme glutaminase are lower in the neonatal kidney, whereas glutaminate, an inhibitor of glutaminase, is higher. As a result, neonates cannot generate the same amount of ammonia during an acid load and take longer to recover their acid–base balance.

Thick Ascending Limb of Henle's Loop

Although transcription of Na^+-$2Cl^-$-K^+ is observed early in development, Na^+-$2Cl^-$-K^+ is unlikely to be functional until postnatally, because a low reabsorptive capacity has been shown for this segment in early postnatal life.[94] As discussed earlier, expression of the TALH transporters is lower in the neonate.[119-122] As a result, bicarbonate and ammonium reabsorption occur at a lower rate compared to the adult. A postnatal five-to-tenfold increase in activity of the Na^+-K^+-ATPase cotransporter has been shown and is greater than that seen in other tubular segments (Figure 6-15).[116-123]

Cortical Collecting Duct

Microperfusion studies of neonatal rabbit kidneys demonstrate a low capacity to secrete acid compared with their adult controls.[175] The neonatal number of intercalated cells is

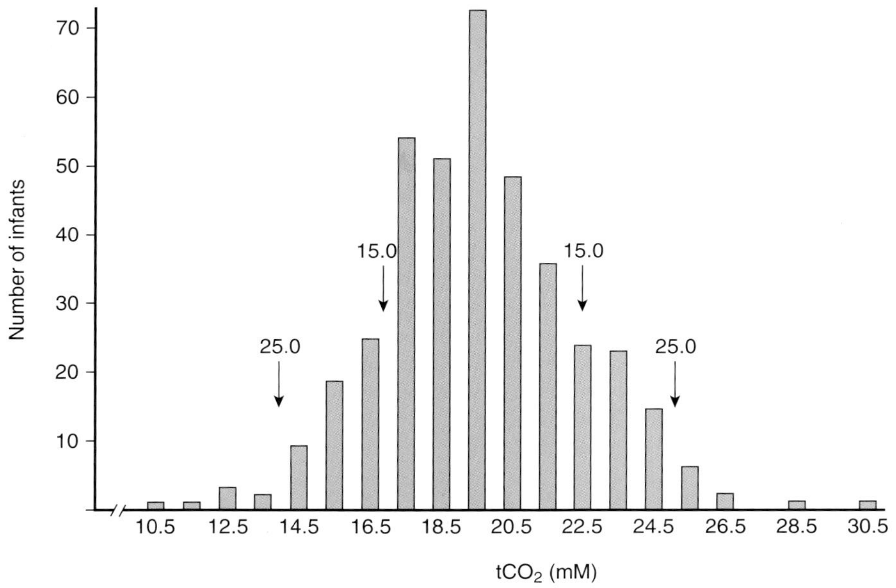

Figure 6-17 Frequency distribution of serum total bicarbonate (tCO_2) in low birth weight neonates during first month of life. Mean is approximately 20 mM, but normal range ±2 standard deviations (SD) is 14.5 to 24.5 mM. (Reprinted with permission from Schwartz GJ, Haycock GB, Edelmann CM Jr, Spitzer A: Late metabolic acidosis: a reassessment of the definition, *J Pediatr* 95(1):102-07, 1997.)

half that of the adult.[176-178] In addition, lower levels of the CA type II isoform have been shown in neonatal rat kidneys.[178-179] The CA type II isoform is important for the function of the α intercalated cell and may be indicative of the increase in acid-secreting capability of the developing CCD.

Regulation of Maturational Acid–Base Homeostatic Mechanisms

Glucocorticoids

Glucocorticoids can stimulate bicarbonate reabsorption, and a developmental increase in circulating cortisol levels precedes the observed increase in bicarbonate reabsorption.[180] Pregnant rabbits injected with glucocorticoids give birth to neonatal rabbits with proximal tubular bicarbonate reabsorption rates similar to that of adults.[180] An increase in NHE3 antiporters occurs with prenatal glucocortocoids.[181] Adrenalectomy prevents this maturational increase in NHE3 antiporter expression at both the level of protein and mRNA. Therefore the maturational increase in glucocorticoids is responsible for the postnatal increase seen in proximal tubule acidification.

RENAL CALCIUM HANDLING IN THE DEVELOPING KIDNEY

Higher calcium and phosphorus levels are required for the growing skeleton in the fetus.[182-183] The placenta actively transports calcium by a calcium pump in the basal membrane to maintain a high fetal/maternal calcium ratio.[184] Elevated fetal calcium suppresses PTH release.[185] PTH is the main regulator of calcium metabolism after birth. Circulating fetal calcium levels increase with advancing gestational age, and at term the fetus is hypercalcemic relative to the maternal levels.[186] Serum calcium levels fall over the first 24 hours in the absence of the placenta. As a result, PTH secretion is stimulated[187] but the response to falling calcium is not sufficient such that a physiologic nadir of serum calcium occurs in the first 2 days of life. Although this nadir is still within the adult range, it represents a significant decrease compared with fetal levels.[185] Term infants typically achieve normal serum calcium levels by the second week of life, with typical circulating concentrations of ionized calcium in neonates being in the range of 1 to 1.5 mmol/L (2-3 mEq/L).[188] After birth the kidney plays an important role in calcium and phosphorus homeostasis. The amount of calcium excreted increases over the first 2 weeks of life,[189] and normal calcium/creatinine values, as outlined in Chapter 2, are accordingly higher in infants. The most common cause of hypercalciuria in the neonate is iatrogenic. The risk of nephrocalcinosis is increased when calciuric drugs such as frusemide and glucocorticoids are administered. As a result, neonates with bronchopulmonary dysplasia are at increased risk for developing nephrocalcinosis. Substituting frusemide with thiazide diuretics, however, reduces this risk.

In the mature nephron, calcium reabsorption in the proximal tubule occurs by the paracellular (80%) and transcellular (20%) pathways. Calcium diffuses across an apical cell membrane into the cell and down its electrochemical gradient via Ca^{2+} channels. Calcium is extruded across the basolateral cell membrane via the $3Na^{+}Ca2^{+}$ antiporter and a $Ca2^{+}$-ATPase. Little is known about the ontogeny of such transporters in the developing nephron. In the distal nephron, active calcium reabsorption occurs through the highly Ca^{2+}-selective TRPV5 channel and binds to calbindin/D28K. The calbindin/D28K ferries Ca^{2+} to the basolateral $3Na^{+}Ca2^{+}$ exchanger (NCX1) and the plasma membrane ATPase (PMCA1b), extruding calcium into the blood compartment. Expression of TRPV6, calbindin/D9K, TRPV5, and calbindin/D28K have been shown at 18 days' gestation in fetal mouse kidneys.[190] TRPV6 reaches a maximum level at 1 week of age and then decreases to less than 10% of TRPV5 expression, suggesting a possible role for TRPV6 during developmental regulation of calcium homeostasis. Expression of TRPV5 and calbindin/D28K peak at the third postnatal week and then fall.[190] Further functional studies are required to ascertain the response and ontogeny of the calcium transport proteins in the developing kidney.

RENAL PHOSPHATE HANDLING IN THE DEVELOPING KIDNEY

Phosphate is of critical importance to body functions particularly during periods of growth. Neonates excrete only 60% of intestinally absorbed phosphate and have a higher phosphate concentration than that of adults.[191] In neonates, the transtubular reabsorption of phosphate is high: they reabsorb 99% of the filtered load of phosphate on the first day of life and 90% by the end of the first week.[192] Micropuncture studies performed on guinea pig neonatal proximal tubules demonstrate a higher phosphate reabsorption rate than in adult guinea pigs.[193] Reabsorption does not occur through the $2Na^+$-Pi IIa antiporter but rather through its developmental isoform, the $2Na^+$-Pi IIc antiporter, the expression of which is higher in weaning animals and has a reduced function in adults.[194]

Regulation of Renal Phosphate Handling in the Developing Kidney

Increased phosphate reabsorption in the early postnatal period is thought to be multifactorial. Parathyroidectomy in immature rats results in a greater increase in maximal tubular phosphate reabsorption than in mature rats, suggesting a role for PTH in neonatal phosphaturia.[195] However, a decline in resorptive capacity is also observed with age in the presence of parathyroid glands, suggesting an enhanced capacity of the immature tubule to reabsorb phosphate. In addition, responsiveness to PTH increases threefold during the first few weeks of life, suggesting a maturation of second messenger systems.[196] In the mature nephron, PTH and Klotho are phosphaturic hormones. PTH may inhibit proximal tubular uptake by internalizing $2Na^+$-Pi cotransporters from the brush border membrane to the subapical compatment.[197] Klotho causes phosphaturia by inhibition of $2NA^+$-Pi cotransporters via altering glycosylation of $2NA^+$-Pi cotransporter type IIa in the brush border.[198] Future research will provide an interesting insight into the ontogeny of Klotho and fibroblast growth factor-23 (FGF-23), a phosphaturic hormone, during maturation of renal phosphate transport systems.

Growth hormone (GH) has also been shown to upregulate $2Na^+$Pi symporter in micropuncture studies performed on 4-week-old rat proximal tubules, an effect that is independent of PTH.[199,200] Developmental differences in the expression of GH receptors have not been shown, and therefore the mechanism enhancing the GH effect is unknown. Both GH and IGF-1 mRNA have been localized to apical membranes of proximal tubular epithelial cells, suggesting a role of the GH/IGF-1 axis in Pi reabsorption.[201]

MAGNESIUM HANDLING IN THE DEVELOPING KIDNEY

In the adult kidney 80% of total serum magnesium is filtered and more than 95% is reabsorbed along the nephron.[202] Also, in the adult kidney the proximal tubule reabsorbs 15% to 20% of the filtered magnesium, whereas in the developing kidney 70% of the filtered magnesium is absorbed in the proximal tubule.[203] A maturational decrease in paracellular permeability at the level of the tight junction has been suggested as a reason for the decline in proximal magnesium reabsorption. From early childhood on, the majority of magnesium transport (70% of the filtered load) occurs in the loop of Henle, whereas the distal convoluted tubule reabsorbs 5% to 10% of the filtered magnesium. Transport in the TALH is passive and paracellular, driven by a lumen-positive transepithelial voltage and involves paracellin-1, a member of the claudin family involved in tight junction formation.[204] Active and transcellular reabsorption of magnesium occurs in the DCT and probably through the apical TRPM6 channel.[205] Ontogeny of the TRPM6 channel and its family members and paracellin-1 requires further research.

RENAL GLUCOSE HANDLING IN THE DEVELOPING KIDNEY

In the mature nephron more than 99% of filtered glucose is reabsorbed.[206] Glucosuria is more common among neonates.[207] Maximum tubular reabsorption of glucose is lower in preterm and term infants than in adults.[208] Age-related differences in glucose transport activity correlate with differences in sodium conductance. Changes in membrane permeability to sodium affect membrane potential, a factor that modifies glucose reabsorption. Therefore factors such as an increase in cell membrane surface area, in basolateral Na^+-K^+-ATPase, increased density of transporter proteins, and the development of new nephrons are implicated in the increase in glucose resorptive capacity observed as the fetus matures.[209-211]

RENAL AMINO ACID HANDLING IN THE DEVELOPING KIDNEY

Amino acids are reabsorbed in the proximal one third of the proximal tubule in an active, sodium-dependent process.[212] Specific amino acid transport systems on the luminal cell membrane reabsorb the amino acids by secondary active transport against an uphill concentration gradient, along with sodium. Aminoaciduria is frequently observed in the neonate. Factors include decreased activity of the amino acid-sodium cotransporter, increased Na^+/H^+ exchange at the luminal membrane, and decreased activity of the Na^+-K^+/ATPase at the basolateral membrane.[213] Of note, not all the amino acids are wasted to the same degree.[213] Developmental differences have been shown for the amino acid system and the glycine transporter systems.[214,215]

ASSESSMENT OF RENAL FUNCTIONAL MATURATION

Either glomerular or tubular indicators can measure renal functional maturation. Glomerular function is assessed by serum creatinine levels, urinary microalbumin, immunoglobulin G, and GFR. Tubular function can be assessed by the fractional excretion of sodium or urinary α_1-microglobulin and urinary levels of other tubular proteins normally reabsorbed by the proximal tubule, such as N-acetyl-β-D-glucosaminidase (NAG) and β_2-microglobulin.[216,217] All markers have been closely associated with gestational age. A decrease in urinary tubular proteins occurs with increasing gestational age.[218] Tables 6-3 and 6-4 illustrate reference ranges for electrolytes in both preterm and term infants.

TABLE 6-3 **Serum Electrolyte Values in Preterm Infants (Birth Weight 1500-1750 g)**[219]

	AGE 1 WEEK			AGE 3 WEEKS			AGE 5 WEEKS			AGE 7 WEEKS		
Parameter	**Mean**	**SD**	**Range**	**Mean**	**SD**	**Range**	**Mean**	**SD**	**Range**	**Mean**	**SD**	**Range**
Sodium (mmol/L)	139.6	±3.2	133-146	136.3	±2.9	129-142	136.8	±2.5	133-148	137.2	±1.8	133-142
Potassium (mmol/L)	5.6	±0.5	4.6-6.7	5.8	±0.6	4.5-7.1	5.5	±0.6	4.5-6.6	5.7	±0.7	4.6-7.1
Chloride (mmol/L)	108.2	±3.7	100-117	108.3	±3.9	102-116	107	±3.5	100-115	107	±3.3	101-115
CO_2 (mmol/L)	20.3	±2.8	13.8-27.1	18.4	±3.5	12.4-26.2	20.4	±3.4	12.5-26.1	20.6	±3.1	13.7-26.9
Phosphate (mmol/L)	2.5	±0.4	1.7-3.5	2.4	±0.2	2.0-2.8	2.3	±0.2	1.8-2.6	2.2	±0.3	1.4-2.6
Total calcium (mmol/L)	2.3	±0.3	1.5-2.9	2.4	±0.1	2.0-2.8	2.4	±0.1	2.2-2.6	2.4	±0.2	2.2-2.7
BUN* (mmol/L)	3.3	±1.9	1.1-9.1	4.8	±2.8	0.7-11.2	4.7	±2.5	0.7-9.5	4.8	±2.4	0.9-10.9

**BUN*, Blood, urea, nitrogen.
Conversions: phosphate (mg/dl) to mmol/L: multiplied by 0.3229; calcium (mg/dl) to mmol/L: multiplied by 0.25; BUN (mg/dl) to mmol/L: multiplied by 0.357.

TABLE 6-4 Serum Electrolyte Values in Term Infants

Parameter	Units	Age	Range	Comment
Sodium[220]	mmol/L	0-1 week 1-4 weeks	133-146 134-144	
Potassium[220]	mmol/L	0-1 week 1-4 weeks	3.2-5.5 (plasma) 3.4-6.0 (plasma)	Plasma potassium is 10% lower than serum potassium, because potassium is released from platelets during coagulation
Phosphate[221]	mmol/L	1-2 days 2-3 days 3-4 days 4-6 days 6-12 days	2.03-2.66 1.89-2.92 1.83-2.68 1.67-2.68 1.54-2.90	Affected by type of milk fed, being generally higher in formula-fed babies
Bicarbonate[215]	mmol/L	1 hour 24 hours 7 days	16.8-21.6 17.6-22.8 19.2-24.4	Arterial
Magnesium[222]	mmol/L	1 day 3 days 5 days 7-28 days	0.72-1.00 0.81-1.05 0.78-1.02 0.65-1.00	
Calcium total[221,223]	mmol/L	1-2 days 2-3 days 3-4 days 4-6 days 6-12 days	2.18-2.48 2.14-2.64 2.22-2.55 2.25-2.68 2.26-2.69	Interpret with albumin concentration
Calcium-ionized[222]		1 day 3 days 5 days	1.05-1.37 1.10-1.44 1.20-1.48	

SUMMARY

Adaptation to the extrauterine environment involves an increase in both glomerular and renal tubular maturation. Even for very low birth weight infants, the capacity for postnatal homeostatic adaptation is remarkable. Changes in resorptive surface area, transporter number, and functional development of second messenger systems all contribute to the maturational effect of neonatal kidney function.

PART 2 REFERENCES

1. Rudolph AM, Heymann MA, Teramo KAW, Barrett CT, Raiha NCR: Studies on the circulation of the previable human fetus, *Pediat Res* 5:452-65, 1971.
2. Rabinowitz R, Peters MT, Vyas S, Campbell S, Nicolaides KH: Measurement of fetal urine production in normal pregnancy by real-time ultrasonography, *Am J Obstet Gynecol* 161(5):1264-66, 1989.
3. Vanderheyden T, Kumar S, Fisk NM: Fetal renal impairment, *Semin Neonatol* 8(4):279-89, 2003.
4. Potter E: Bilateral renal agenesis, *J Pediatr* 29:68, 1946.
5. Friis-Hansen B: Water distribution in the foetus and newborn infant, *Acta Paediatr Scand Suppl* 305:7-11, 1983.
6. Tulassay T, Seri I, Rascher W: Atrial natriuretic peptide and extracellular volume contraction after birth, *Acta Paediatr Scand* 76(3):444-46, 1987.
7. Baum M, Quigley R, Satlin L: Maturational changes in renal tubular transport, *Curr Opin Nephrol Hypertens* 12(5):521-26, 2003.
8. Nicolini U, Spelzini F: Invasive assessment of fetal renal abnormalities: urinalysis, fetal blood sampling and biopsy, *Prenat Diagn* 21(11):964-69, 2001.
9. Pappenheimer JR: Permeability of glomerulomembranes in the kidney, *Klin Wochenschr* 33(15-16):362-65, 1955.
10. Kleinman LI, Lubbe RJ: Factors affecting the maturation of renal PAH extraction in the new-born dog, *J Physiol* 223(2):411-18, 1972.
11. Veille JC, Hanson RA, Tatum K, Kelley K: Quantitative assessment of human fetal renal blood flow, *Am J Obstet Gynecol* 169(6):1399-402, 1993.
12. Chevalier RL: Developmental renal physiology of the low birth weight pre-term newborn, *J Urol* 156(2 Pt 2):714-19, 1996.
13. Spitzer A, Edelmann CM, Jr: Maturational changes in pressure gradients for glomerular filtration, *Am J Physiol* 221(5):1431-35, 1971.
14. Ichikawa I, Maddox DA, Brenner BM: Maturational development of glomerular ultrafiltration in the rat, *Am J Physiol* 236(5):F465-71, 1979.
15. Aperia A, Herin P: Development of glomerular perfusion rate and nephron filtration rate in rats 17-60 days old, *Am J Physiol* 228(5):1319-25, 1975.
16. Allison ME, Lipham EM, Gottschalk CW: Hydrostatic pressure in the rat kidney, *Am J Physiol* 223(4):975-83, 1972.
17. Gruskin AB, Edelmann CM, Jr, Yuan S: Maturational changes in renal blood flow in piglets, *Pediatr Res* 4(1):7-13, 1970.
18. Aperia A, Broberger O, Herin P, Joelsson I: Renal hemodynamics in the perinatal period. A study in lambs, *Acta Physiol Scand* 99(3):261-69, 1997.
19. Bokenkamp A, Dieterich C, Dressler F, Muhlhaus K, Gembruch U, Bald R et al: Fetal serum concentrations of cystatin C and beta2-microglobulin as predictors of postnatal kidney function, *Am J Obstet Gynecol* 185(2):468-75, 2001.

20. Aperia A, Broberger O, Elinder G, Herin P, Zetterstrom R: Postnatal development of renal function in pre-term and full-term infants, *Acta Paediatr Scand* 70(2):183-87, 1981.
21. Bueva A, Guignard JP: Renal function in preterm neonates, *Pediatr Res* 36(5):572-77, 1994.
22. Guignard JP, Torrado A, Da Cunha O, Gautier E: Glomerular filtration rate in the first three weeks of life, *J Pediatr* 87(2):268-72, 1975.
23. Paton JB, Fisher DE, DeLannoy CW, Behrman RE: Umbilical blood flow, cardiac output, and organ blood flow in the immature baboon fetus, *Am J Obstet Gynecol* 117(4):560-66, 1973.
24. Fetterman GH, Shuplock NA, Philipp FJ, Gregg HS: The growth and maturation of human glomeruli and proximal convolutions from term to adulthood: studies by microdissection, *Pediatrics* 35:601-19, 1965.
25. Wolf G: Angiotensin II and tubular development, *Nephrol Dial Transplant* 17(suppl 9):48-51, 2002.
26. Yosipiv IV, El-Dahr SS: Developmental biology of angiotensin-converting enzyme, *Pediatr Nephrol* 12(1):72-79, 1998.
27. Niimura F, Okubo S, Fogo A, Ichikawa I: Temporal and spatial expression pattern of the angiotensinogen gene in mice and rats, *Am J Physiol* 272(1 Pt 2):R142-47, 1997.
28. Tufro-McReddie A, Harrison JK, Everett AD, Gomez RA: Ontogeny of type 1 angiotensin II receptor gene expression in the rat, *J Clin Invest* 91(2):530-37, 1993.
29. Kakuchi J, Ichiki T, Kiyama S, Hogan BL, Fogo A, Inagami T et al: Developmental expression of renal angiotensin II receptor genes in the mouse, *Kidney Int* 47(1):140-47, 1995.
30. Segar JL, Barna TJ, Acarregui MJ, Lamb FS: Responses of fetal ovine systemic and umbilical arteries to angiotensin II, *Pediatr Res* 49(6):826-33, 2001.
31. Segar JL, Minnick A, Nuyt AM, Robillard JE: Role of endogenous ANG II and AT1 receptors in regulating arterial baroreflex responses in newborn lambs, *Am J Physiol* 272(6 Pt 2):R1862-73, 1997.
32. Robillard JE, Weismann DN, Gomez RA, Ayres NA, Lawton WJ, VanOrden DE: Renal and adrenal responses to converting-enzyme inhibition in fetal and newborn life, *Am J Physiol* 244(2):R249-56, 1983.
33. Lacoste M, Cai Y, Guicharnaud L, Mounier F, Dumez Y, Bouvier R et al: Renal tubular dysgenesis, a not uncommon autosomal recessive disorder leading to oligohydramnios: role of the renin-angiotensin system, *J Am Soc Nephrol* 17(8):2253-63, 2006.
34. Nakamura KT, Matherne GP, McWeeny OJ, Smith BA, Robillard JE: Renal hemodynamics and functional changes during the transition from fetal to newborn life in sheep, *Pediatr Res* 21(3):229-34, 1987.
35. DiBona GF, Kopp UC: Neural control of renal function, *Physiol Rev* 77(1):75-197, 1997.
36. Buckley NM, Brazeau P, Gootman PM, Frasier ID: Renal circulatory effects of adrenergic stimuli in anesthetized piglets and mature swine, *Am J Physiol* 237(6):H690-95, 1979.
37. Smith FG, Smith BA, Guillery EN, Robillard JE: Role of renal sympathetic nerves in lambs during the transition from fetal to newborn life, *J Clin Invest* 88(6):1988-94, 1991.
38. Segar JL, Mazursky JE, Robillard JE: Changes in ovine renal sympathetic nerve activity and baroreflex function at birth, *Am J Physiol* 267(5 Pt 2):H1824-32, 1994.
39. Pupilli C, Gomez RA, Tuttle JB, Peach MJ, Carey RM: Spatial association of renin-containing cells and nerve fibers in developing rat kidney, *Pediatr Nephrol* 5(6):690-95, 1991.
40. Naicker S, Bhoola KD: Endothelins: vasoactive modulators of renal function in health and disease, *Pharmacol Ther* 90(1):61-88, 2001.
41. Mattyus I, Zimmerhackl LB, Schwarz A, Brandis M, Miltenyi M, Tulassay T: Renal excretion of endothelin in children, *Pediatr Nephrol* 11(4):513-21, 1997.
42. Abadie L, Blazy I, Roubert P, Plas P, Charbit M, Chabrier PE et al: Decrease in endothelin-1 renal receptors during the 1st month of life in the rat, *Pediatr Nephrol* 10(2):185-89, 1996.
43. Bogaert GA, Kogan BA, Mevorach RA, Wong J, Gluckman GR, Fineman JR et al: Exogenous endothelin-1 causes renal vasodilation in the fetal lamb, *J Urol* 156(2 Pt 2):847-53, 1996.
44. Semama DS, Thonney M, Guignard JP: Role of endogenous endothelin in renal haemodynamics of newborn rabbits, *Pediatr Nephrol* 7(6):886-90, 1993.
45. Gleason CA: Prostaglandins and the developing kidney, *Semin Perinatol* 11(1):12-21, 1987.
46. Guignard JP, Gouyon JB, John EG: Vasoactive factors in the immature kidney, *Pediatr Nephrol* 5(4):443-46, 1991.
47. Cantor B, Tyler T, Nelson RM, Stein GH: Oligohydramnios and transient neonatal anuria: a possible association with the maternal use of prostaglandin synthetase inhibitors, *J Reprod Med* 24(5):220-23, 1980.
48. Simeoni U, Messer J, Weisburd P, Haddad J, Willard D: Neonatal renal dysfunction and intrauterine exposure to prostaglandin synthesis inhibitors, *Eur J Pediatr* 148(4):371-73, 1989.
49. Marpeau L, Bouillie J, Barrat J, Milliez J: Obstetrical advantages and perinatal risks of indomethacin: a report of 818 cases, *Fetal Diagn Ther* 9(2):110-15, 1994.
50. Jensen BL, Stubbe J, Madsen K, Nielsen FT, Skott O: The renin-angiotensin system in kidney development: role of COX-2 and adrenal steroids, *Acta Physiol Scand* 181(4):549-59, 2004.
51. Bachmann S, Mundel P: Nitric oxide in the kidney: synthesis, localization, and function, *Am J Kidney Dis* 24(1):112-29, 1994.
52. Bogaert GA, Kogan BA, Mevorach RA: Effects of endothelium-derived nitric oxide on renal hemodynamics and function in the sheep fetus, *Pediatr Res* 34(6):755-61, 1993.
53. Ballevre L, Solhaug MJ, Guignard JP: Nitric oxide and the immature kidney, *Biol Neonate* 70(1):1-14, 1996.
54. Solhaug MJ, Wallace MR, Granger JP: Nitric oxide and angiotensin II regulation of renal hemodynamics in the developing piglet, *Pediatr Res* 39(3):527-33, 1996.
55. El-Dahr SS, Figueroa CD, Gonzalez CB, Muller-Esterl W: Ontogeny of bradykinin B2 receptors in the rat kidney: implications for segmental nephron maturation, *Kidney Int* 51(3):739-49, 1997.
56. El-Dahr SS: Spatial expression of the kallikrein-kinin system during nephrogenesis, *Histol Histopathol* 19(4):1301-10, 2004.
57. El-Dahr SS, Chao J: Spatial and temporal expression of kallikrein and its mRNA during nephron maturation, *Am J Physiol* 262(5 Pt 2):F705-11, 1992.
58. Robillard JE, Lawton WJ, Weismann DN, Sessions C: Developmental aspects of the renal kallikrein-like activity in fetal and newborn lambs, *Kidney Int* 22(6):594-601, 1982.
59. Toth-Heyn P, Guignard JP: Endogenous bradykinin regulates renal function in the newborn rabbit, *Biol Neonate* 73(5):330-36, 1998.
60. Toth-Heyn P, Drukker A, Guignard JP: The stressed neonatal kidney: from pathophysiology to clinical management of neonatal vasomotor nephropathy, *Pediatr Nephrol* 14(3):227-39, 2000.
61. Felder RA, Felder CC, Eisner GM, Jose PA: The dopamine receptor in adult and maturing kidney, *Am J Physiol* 257(3 Pt 2):F315-27, 1989.
62. Seri I: Cardiovascular, renal, and endocrine actions of dopamine in neonates and children, *J Pediatr* 126(3):333-44, 1995.
63. Karlowicz MG, Adelman RD: Nonoliguric and oliguric acute renal failure in asphyxiated term neonates, *Pediatr Nephrol* 9(6):718-22, 1995.
64. Rodriguez-Soriano J, Vallo A, Castillo G, Oliveros R: Renal handling of water and sodium in infancy and childhood: a study using clearance methods during hypotonic saline diuresis, *Kidney Int* 20(6):700-04, 1981.
65. Rodriguez G, Ventura P, Samper MP, Moreno L, Sarria A, Perez-Gonzalez JM: Changes in body composition during the initial hours of life in breast-fed healthy term newborns, *Biol Neonate* 77(1):12-16, 2000.
66. Polacek E, Vocel J, Neugebauerova L, Sebkova M, Vechetova E: The osmotic concentrating ability in healthy infants and children, *Arch Dis Child* 40:291-95, 1965.
67. Sujov P, Kellerman L, Zeltzer M, Hochberg Z: Plasma and urine osmolality in full-term and pre-term infants, *Acta Paediatr Scand* 73(6):722-26, 1984.
68. Day GM, Radde IC, Balfe JW, Chance GW: Electrolyte abnormalities in very low birthweight infants, *Pediatr Res* 10(5):522-26, 1976.
69. Bonilla-Felix M: Development of water transport in the collecting duct, *Am J Physiol Renal Physiol* 287(6):F1093-101, 2004.

70. Edelmann CM, Barnett HL, Troupkou V: Renal concentrating mechanisms in newborn infants. Effect of dietary protein and water content, role of urea, and responsiveness to antidiuretic hormone, *J Clin Invest* 39:1062-69, 1960.
71. Grantham JJ, Burg MB: Effect of vasopressin and cyclic AMP on permeability of isolated collecting tubules, *Am J Physiol* 211(1):255-59, 1996.
72. Sands JM, Nonoguchi H, Knepper MA: Vasopressin effects on urea and H2O transport in inner medullary collecting duct subsegments, *Am J Physiol* 253(5 Pt 2):F823-32, 1987.
73. Fushimi K, Uchida S, Hara Y, Hirata Y, Marumo F, Sasaki S: Cloning and expression of apical membrane water channel of rat kidney collecting tubule, *Nature* 361(6412):549-52, 1993.
74. Fushimi K, Sasaki S, Marumo F: Phosphorylation of serine 256 is required for cAMP-dependent regulatory exocytosis of the aquaporin-2 water channel, *J Biol Chem* 272(23):14800-04, 1997.
75. Nielsen S, Chou CL, Marples D, Christensen EI, Kishore BK, Knepper MA: Vasopressin increases water permeability of kidney collecting duct by inducing translocation of aquaporin-CD water channels to plasma membrane, *Proc Natl Acad Sci U S A* 92(4):1013-17, 1995.
76. Liu H, Wintour EM: Aquaporins in development—a review, *Reprod Biol Endocrinol* 3:18, 2005.
77. Knepper MA, Nielsen S, Chou CL, DiGiovanni SR: Mechanism of vasopressin action in the renal collecting duct, *Semin Nephrol* 14(4):302-21, 1994.
78. Hadeed AJ, Leake RD, Weitzman RE, Fisher DA: Possible mechanisms of high blood levels of vasopressin during the neonatal period, *J Pediatr* 94(5):805-08, 1979.
79. Rees L, Forsling ML, Brook CG: Vasopressin concentrations in the neonatal period, *Clin Endocrinol (Oxf)* 12(4):357-62, 1980.
80. Siga E, Horster MF: Regulation of osmotic water permeability during differentiation of inner medullary collecting duct, *Am J Physiol* 260(5 Pt 2):F710-16, 1991.
81. Horster MF, Zink H: Functional differentiation of the medullary collecting tubule: influence of vasopressin, *Kidney Int* 22(4):360-65, 1982.
82. Svenningsen NW, Aronson AS: Postnatal development of renal concentration capacity as estimated by DDAVP-test in normal and asphyxiated neonates, *Biol Neonate* 25(3-4):230-41, 1974.
83. Ostrowski NL, Young WS 3rd, Knepper MA, Lolait SJ: Expression of vasopressin V1a and V2 receptor messenger ribonucleic acid in the liver and kidney of embryonic, developing, and adult rats, *Endocrinology* 133(4):1849-59, 1993.
84. Ammar A, Roseau S, Butlen D: Postnatal ontogenesis of vasopressin receptors in the rat collecting duct, *Mol Cell Endocrinol* 86(3):193-203, 1992.
85. Rajerison RM, Butlen D, Jard S: Ontogenic development of antidiuretic hormone receptors in rat kidney: comparison of hormonal binding and adenylate cyclase activation, *Mol Cell Endocrinol* 4(4):271-85, 1976.
86. Bonilla-Felix M, John-Phillip C: Prostaglandins mediate the defect in AVP-stimulated cAMP generation in immature collecting duct, *Am J Physiol* 267(1 Pt 2):F44-48, 1994.
87. Bonilla-Felix M, Vehaskari VM, Hamm LL: Water transport in the immature rabbit collecting duct, *Pediatr Nephrol* 13(2):103-07, 1999.
88. Quigley R, Chakravarty S, Baum M: Antidiuretic hormone resistance in the neonatal cortical collecting tubule is mediated in part by elevated phosphodiesterase activity, *Am J Physiol Renal Physiol* 286(2):F317-22, 2004.
89. Negishi M, Sugimoto Y, Hayashi Y, Namba T, Honda A, Watabe A et al: Functional interaction of prostaglandin E receptor EP3 subtype with guanine nucleotide-binding proteins, showing low-affinity ligand binding, *Biochim Biophys Acta* 1175(3):343-50, 1993.
90. Bonilla-Felix M, Jiang W: Aquaporin-2 in the immature rat: expression, regulation, and trafficking, *J Am Soc Nephrol* 8(10):1502-09, 1997.
81. Yasui M, Marples D, Belusa R, Eklof AC, Celsi G, Nielsen S et al: Development of urinary concentrating capacity: role of aquaporin-2, *Am J Physiol* 271(2 Pt 2):F461-68, 1996.
92. Yamamoto T, Sasaki S, Fushimi K, Ishibashi K, Yaoita E, Kawasaki K et al: Expression of AQP family in rat kidneys during development and maturation, *Am J Physiol* 272(2 Pt 2):F198-204, 1997.
93. Forrest JN, Jr., Stanier MW: Kidney composition and renal concentration ability in young rabbits, *J Physiol* 187(1):1-4, 1966.
94. Horster M: Loop of Henle functional differentiation: in vitro perfusion of the isolated thick ascending segment, *Pflugers Arch* 378(1):15-24, 1978.
95. Cha JH, Kim YH, Jung JY, Han KH, Madsen KM, Kim J: Cell proliferation in the loop of Henle in the developing rat kidney, *J Am Soc Nephrol* 12(7):1410-21, 2001.
96. Liu W, Morimoto T, Kondo Y, Iinuma K, Uchida S, Imai M: "Avian-type" renal medullary tubule organization causes immaturity of urine-concentrating ability in neonates, *Kidney Int* 60(2):680-93, 2001.
97. Kim YH, Kim DU, Han KH, Jung JY, Sands JM, Knepper MA et al: Expression of urea transporters in the developing rat kidney, *Am J Physiol Renal Physiol* 282(3):F530-40, 2002.
98. Zink H, Horster M: Maturation of diluting capacity in loop of Henle of rat superficial nephrons, *Am J Physiol* 233(6):F519-24, 1997.
99. Speller AM, Moffat DB: Tubulo-vascular relationships in the developing kidney, *J Anat* 123(Pt 2):487-500, 1977.
100. Edelmann CM Jr, Barnett HL, Stark H: Effect of urea on concentration of urinary nonurea solute in premature infants, *J Appl Physiol* 21(3):1021-25, 1966.
101. Clark DA: Times of first void and first stool in 500 newborns, *Pediatrics* 60(4):457-59, 1977.
102. Hansen JD, Smith CA: Effects of withholding fluid in the immediate postnatal period, *Pediatrics* 12(2):99-113, 1953.
103. Al-Dahhan J, Haycock GB, Nichol B, Chantler C, Stimmler L: Sodium homeostasis in term and preterm neonates. III. Effect of salt supplementation, *Arch Dis Child* 59(10):945-50, 1984.
104. Engelke SC, Shah BL, Vasan U, Raye JR: Sodium balance in very low-birth-weight infants, *J Pediatr* 93(5):837-41, 1978.
105. Goetz KL: Physiology and pathophysiology of atrial peptides, *Am J Physiol* 254(1 Pt 1):E1-15, 1988.
106. Chevalier RL: Atrial natriuretic peptide in renal development, *Pediatr Nephrol* 7(5):652-56, 1993.
107. Weil J, Bidlingmaier F, Dohlemann C, Kuhnle U, Strom T, Lang RE: Comparison of plasma atrial natriuretic peptide levels in healthy children from birth to adolescence and in children with cardiac diseases, *Pediatr Res* 20(12):1328-31, 1986.
108. Kikuchi K, Shiomi M, Horie K, Ohie T, Nakao K, Imura H et al: Plasma atrial natriuretic polypeptide concentration in healthy children from birth to adolescence, *Acta Paediatr Scand* 77(3):380-84, 1988.
109. Bierd TM, Kattwinkel J, Chevalier RL, Rheuban KS, Smith DJ, Teague WG et al: Interrelationship of atrial natriuretic peptide, atrial volume, and renal function in premature infants, *J Pediatr* 116(5):753-59, 1990.
110. Semmekrot B, Chabardes D, Roseau S, Siaume-Perez S, Butlen D: Developmental pattern of cyclic guanosine monophosphate production stimulated by atrial natriuretic peptide in glomeruli microdissected from kidneys of young rats, *Pflugers Arch* 416(5):519-25, 1990.
111. Ross B, Cowett RM, Oh W: Renal functions of low birth weight infants during the first two months of life, *Pediatr Res* 11(11):1162-64, 1977.
112. Spitzer A: The role of the kidney in sodium homeostasis during maturation, *Kidney Int* 21(4):539-45, 1982.
113. Baum M: Neonatal rabbit juxtamedullary proximal convoluted tubule acidification, *J Clin Invest* 85(2):499-506, 1990.
114. Guillery EN, Karniski LP, Mathews MS, Robillard JE: Maturation of proximal tubule Na+/H+ antiporter activity in sheep during transition from fetus to newborn, *Am J Physiol* 267(4 Pt 2):F537-45, 1994.
115. Guillery EN, Huss DJ: Developmental regulation of chloride/formate exchange in guinea pig proximal tubules, *Am J Physiol* 269(5 Pt 2):F686-95, 1995.
116. Schmidt U, Horster M: Na-K-activated ATPase: activity maturation in rabbit nephron segments dissected in vitro, *Am J Physiol* 233(1):F55-60, 1997.
117. Fukuda Y, Bertorello A, Aperia A: Ontogeny of the regulation of Na+, K(+)-ATPase activity in the renal proximal tubule cell, *Pediatr Res* 30(2):131-34, 1991.

118. Guillery EN, Huss DJ, McDonough AA, Klein LC: Posttranscriptional upregulation of Na(+)-K(+)-ATPase activity in newborn guinea pig renal cortex, *Am J Physiol* 273(2 Pt 2):F254-63, 1997.
119. Biemesderfer D, Rutherford PA, Nagy T, Pizzonia JH, Abu-Alfa AK, Aronson PS: Monoclonal antibodies for high-resolution localization of NHE3 in adult and neonatal rat kidney, *Am J Physiol* 273(2 Pt 2):F289-99, 1997.
120. Igarashi P, Vanden Heuvel GB, Payne JA, Forbush B 3rd: Cloning, embryonic expression, and alternative splicing of a murine kidney-specific Na-K-Cl cotransporter, *Am J Physiol* 269(3 Pt 2):F405-18, 1995.
121. Schmitt R, Ellison DH, Farman N, Rossier BC, Reilly RF, Reeves WB et al: Developmental expression of sodium entry pathways in rat nephron, *Am J Physiol* 276(3 Pt 2):F367-81, 1999.
122. Bachmann S, Bostanjoglo M, Schmitt R, Ellison DH: Sodium transport-related proteins in the mammalian distal nephron—distribution, ontogeny and functional aspects, *Anat Embryol (Berl)* 200(5):447-68, 1999.
123. Rane S, Aperia A: Ontogeny of Na-K-ATPase activity in thick ascending limb and of concentrating capacity, *Am J Physiol* 249(5 Pt 2):F723-28, 1985.
124. Burrow CR, Devuyst O, Li X, Gatti L, Wilson PD: Expression of the beta2-subunit and apical localization of Na+-K+-ATPase in metanephric kidney, *Am J Physiol* 277(3 Pt 2):F391-403, 1999.
125. Obermuller N, Bernstein P, Velazquez H, Reilly R, Moser D, Ellison DH et al: Expression of the thiazide-sensitive Na-Cl cotransporter in rat and human kidney, *Am J Physiol* 269(6 Pt 2):F900-10, 1995.
126. Duc C, Farman N, Canessa CM, Bonvalet JP, Rossier BC: Cell-specific expression of epithelial sodium channel alpha, beta, and gamma subunits in aldosterone-responsive epithelia from the rat: localization by in situ hybridization and immunocytochemistry, *J Cell Biol* 127(6 Pt 2):1907-21, 1994.
127. Vehaskari VM, Hempe JM, Manning J, Aviles DH, Carmichael MC: Developmental regulation of ENaC subunit mRNA levels in rat kidney, *Am J Physiol* 274(6 Pt 1):C1661-66, 1998.
128. Horster M: Embryonic epithelial membrane transporters, *Am J Physiol Renal Physiol* 279(6):F982-96, 2000.
129. Watanabe S, Matsushita K, McCray PB Jr, Stokes JB: Developmental expression of the epithelial Na+ channel in kidney and uroepithelia, *Am J Physiol* 276(2 Pt 2):F304-14, 1999.
130. Nakamura K, Stokes JB, McCray PB Jr: Endogenous and exogenous glucocorticoid regulation of ENaC mRNA expression in developing kidney and lung, *Am J Physiol Cell Physiol* 283(3):C762-72, 2002.
131. Constantinescu AR, Lane JC, Mak J, Zavilowitz B, Satlin LM: Na(+)-K(+)-ATPase-mediated basolateral rubidium uptake in the maturing rabbit cortical collecting duct, *Am J Physiol Renal Physiol* 279(6):F1161-68, 2000.
132. Vehaskari VM. Ontogeny of cortical collecting duct sodium transport, *Am J Physiol* 267(1 Pt 2):F49-54, 1994.
133. Chevalier RL, Thornhill BA, Belmonte DC, Baertschi AJ: Endogenous angiotensin II inhibits natriuresis after acute volume expansion in the neonatal rat, *Am J Physiol* 270(2 Pt 2):R393-97, 1996.
134. Quan A, Baum M: Endogenous angiotensin II modulates rat proximal tubule transport with acute changes in extracellular volume, *Am J Physiol* 275(1 Pt 2):F74-78, 1998.
135. Sulyok E, Nemeth M, Tenyi I: Relationship between the postnatal development of the renin-angiotensin-aldosterone system and electrolyte and acid-base status of the NaCl-supplemented premature infants. In *The Kidney During Development: Morphogenesis and Function* (Spitzer A, editor). New York, Masson, 1982, p. 273.
136. Sulyok E: Dopaminergic control of neonatal salt and water metabolism, *Pediatr Nephrol* 2(1):163-65, 1988.
137. Magyar DM, Fridshal D, Elsner CW, Glatz T, Eliot J, Klein AH et al: Time-trend analysis of plasma cortisol concentrations in the fetal sheep in relation to parturition, *Endocrinology* 107(1):155-59, 1980.
138. Gupta N, Tarif SR, Seikaly M, Baum M: Role of glucocorticoids in the maturation of the rat renal Na+/H+ antiporter (NHE3), *Kidney Int* 60(1):173-81, 2001.
139. Guillery EN, Karniski LP, Mathews MS, Page WV, Orlowski J, Jose PA et al: Role of glucocorticoids in the maturation of renal cortical Na+/H+ exchanger activity during fetal life in sheep, *Am J Physiol* 268(4 Pt 2):F710-17, 1995.
140. Celsi G, Nishi A, Akusjarvi G, Aperia A: Abundance of Na(+)-K(+)-ATPase mRNA is regulated by glucocorticoid hormones in infant rat kidneys, *Am J Physiol* 260(2 Pt 2):F192-97, 1991.
141. Shah M, Quigley R, Baum M: Maturation of proximal straight tubule NaCl transport: role of thyroid hormone, *Am J Physiol Renal Physiol* 278(4):F596-602, 2000.
142. McDonough AA, Brown TA, Horowitz B, Chiu R, Schlotterbeck J, Bowen J et al: Thyroid hormone coordinately regulates Na+-K+-ATPase alpha- and beta-subunit mRNA levels in kidney, *Am J Physiol* 254(2 Pt 1):C323-29, 1988.
143. Mathew OP, Jones AS, James E, Bland H, Groshong T: Neonatal renal failure: usefulness of diagnostic indices, *Pediatrics* 65(1):57-60, 1980.
144. Siegel SR, Oh W: Renal function as a marker of human fetal maturation, *Acta Paediatr Scand* 65(4):481-85, 1976.
145. Delgado MM, Rohatgi R, Khan S, Holzman IR, Satlin LM: Sodium and potassium clearances by the maturing kidney: clinical-molecular correlates, *Pediatr Nephrol* 18(8):759-67, 2003.
146. Sulyok E, Nemeth M, Tenyi I, Csaba IF, Varga F, Gyory E et al: Relationship between maturity, electrolyte balance and the function of the renin-angiotensin-aldosterone system in newborn infants, *Biol Neonate* 35(1-2):60-65, 1979.
147. Serrano CV, Talbert LM, Welt LG: Potassium deficiency in the pregnant dog, *J Clin Invest* 43:27-31, 1964.
148. Lorenz JM, Kleinman LI, Markarian K: Potassium metabolism in extremely low birth weight infants in the first week of life, *J Pediatr* 131(1 Pt 1):81-86, 1997.
149. Stefano JL, Norman ME, Morales MC, Goplerud JM, Mishra OP, Delivoria-Papadopoulos M: Decreased erythrocyte Na+,K(+)-ATPase activity associated with cellular potassium loss in extremely low birth weight infants with nonoliguric hyperkalemia, *J Pediatr* 122(2):276-84, 1993.
150. Sato K, Kondo T, Iwao H, Honda S, Ueda K: Internal potassium shift in premature infants: cause of nonoliguric hyperkalemia, *J Pediatr* 126(1):109-13, 1995.
151. Satlin LM: Postnatal maturation of potassium transport in rabbit cortical collecting duct, *Am J Physiol* 266(1 Pt 2):F57-65, 1994.
152. Woda CB, Miyawaki N, Ramalakshmi S, Ramkumar M, Rojas R, Zavilowitz B et al: Ontogeny of flow-stimulated potassium secretion in rabbit cortical collecting duct: functional and molecular aspects, *Am J Physiol Renal Physiol* 285(4):F629-39, 2003.
153. Giebisch G. Renal potassium transport: mechanisms and regulation, *Am J Physiol* 274(5 Pt 2):F817-33, 1998.
154. Lelievre-Pegorier M, Merlet-Benichou C, Roinel N, de Rouffignac C: Developmental pattern of water and electrolyte transport in rat superficial nephrons, *Am J Physiol* 245(1):F15-21, 1983.
155. Frindt G, Palmer LG: Low-conductance K channels in apical membrane of rat cortical collecting tubule, *Am J Physiol* 256(1 Pt 2): F143-51, 1989.
156. Wang WH, Schwab A, Giebisch G: Regulation of small-conductance K+ channel in apical membrane of rat cortical collecting tubule, *Am J Physiol* 259(3 Pt 2):F494-502, 1990.
157. Pacha J, Frindt G, Sackin H, Palmer LG: Apical maxi K channels in intercalated cells of CCT, *Am J Physiol* 261(4 Pt 2):F696-705, 1991.
158. Satlin LM, Palmer LG: Apical Na+ conductance in maturing rabbit principal cell, *Am J Physiol* 270(3 Pt 2):F391-97, 1996.
159. Satlin LM, Palmer LG: Apical K+ conductance in maturing rabbit principal cell, *Am J Physiol* 272(3 Pt 2):F397-404, 1997.
160. Zolotnitskaya A, Satlin LM: Developmental expression of ROMK in rat kidney, *Am J Physiol* 276(6 Pt 2):F825-36, 1999.
161. Hunter M, Lopes AG, Boulpaep EL, Giebisch GH: Single channel recordings of calcium-activated potassium channels in the apical membrane of rabbit cortical collecting tubules, *Proc Natl Acad Sci USA* 81(13):4237-39, 1984.
162. Stephenson G, Hammet M, Hadaway G, Funder JW: Ontogeny of renal mineralocorticoid receptors and urinary electrolyte responses in the rat, *Am J Physiol* 247(4 Pt 2):F665-71, 1984.

163. Rodriguez-Soriano J, Ubetagoyena M, Vallo A: Transtubular potassium concentration gradient: a useful test to estimate renal aldosterone bio-activity in infants and children, *Pediatr Nephrol* 4(2):105-10, 1990.
164. Omar SA, DeCristofaro JD, Agarwal BI, LaGamma EF: Effect of prenatal steroids on potassium balance in extremely low birth weight neonates, *Pediatrics* 106(3):561-67, 2000.
165. Celsi G, Wang ZM, Akusjarvi G, Aperia A: Sensitive periods for glucocorticoids' regulation of Na+,K(+)-ATPase mRNA in the developing lung and kidney, *Pediatr Res* 33(1):5-9, 1993.
166. Schwartz GJ, Haycock GB, Edelmann CM Jr, Spitzer A: Late metabolic acidosis: a reassessment of the definition, *J Pediatr* 95(1):102-07, 1997.
167. Edelmann CM, Soriano JR, Boichis H, Gruskin AB, Acosta MI: Renal bicarbonate reabsorption and hydrogen ion excretion in normal infants, *J Clin Invest* 46(8):1309-17, 1967.
168. Kerpel-Fronius E, Heim T, Sulyok E: The development of the renal acidifying processes and their relation to acidosis in low-birth-weight infants, *Biol Neonate* 15(34):156-68, 1970.
169. Schwartz GJ, Evan AP: Development of solute transport in rabbit proximal tubule. I. HCO-3 and glucose absorption, *Am J Physiol* 245(3):F382-90, 1983.
170. Baum M, Quigley R: Ontogeny of proximal tubule acidification, *Kidney Int* 48(6):1697-704, 1995.
171. Schwartz GJ, Brown D, Mankus R, Alexander EA, Schwartz JH: Low pH enhances expression of carbonic anhydrase II by cultured rat inner medullary collecting duct cells, *Am J Physiol* 266(2 Pt 1): C508-14, 1994.
172. Winkler CA, Kittelberger AM, Watkins RH, Maniscalco WM, Schwartz GJ: Maturation of carbonic anhydrase IV expression in rabbit kidney, *Am J Physiol Renal Physiol* 280(5):F895-903, 2001.
173. Goldstein L: Renal ammonia and acid excretion in infant rats, *Am J Physiol* 218(5):1394-98, 1970.
174. Goldstein L: Ammonia metabolism in kidneys of suckling rats, *Am J Physiol* 220(1):213-17, 1971.
175. Mehrgut FM, Satlin LM, Schwartz GJ: Maturation of HCO3-transport in rabbit collecting duct, *Am J Physiol* 259(5 Pt 2):F801-08, 1990.
176. Kim J, Tisher CC, Madsen KM: Differentiation of intercalated cells in developing rat kidney: an immunohistochemical study, *Am J Physiol* 266(6 Pt 2):F977-90, 1994.
177. Satlin LM, Matsumoto T, Schwartz GJ: Postnatal maturation of rabbit renal collecting duct. III. Peanut lectin-binding intercalated cells, *Am J Physiol* 262(2 Pt 2):F199-208, 1992.
178. Satlin LM, Schwartz GJ: Postnatal maturation of rabbit renal collecting duct: intercalated cell function, *Am J Physiol* 253(4 Pt 2): F622-35, 1987.
179. Karashima S, Hattori S, Ushijima T, Furuse A, Nakazato H, Matsuda I: Developmental changes in carbonic anhydrase II in the rat kidney, *Pediatr Nephrol* 12(4):263-68, 1998.
180. Baum M, Quigley R. Prenatal glucocorticoids stimulate neonatal juxtamedullary proximal convoluted tubule acidification, *Am J Physiol* 261(5 Pt 2):F746-52, 1991.
181. Baum M, Moe OW, Gentry DL, Alpern RJ: Effect of glucocorticoids on renal cortical NHE-3 and NHE-1 mRNA, *Am J Physiol* 267(3 Pt 2):F437-42, 1994.
182. David L, Anast CS: Calcium metabolism in newborn infants. The interrelationship of parathyroid function and calcium, magnesium, and phosphorus metabolism in normal, "sick," and hypocalcemic newborns, *J Clin Invest* 54(2):287-96, 1974.
183. Moniz CF, Nicolaides KH, Tzannatos C, Rodeck CH: Calcium homeostasis in second trimester fetuses, *J Clin Pathol* 39(8):838-41, 1986.
184. Care AD: The placental transfer of calcium, *J Dev Physiol* 15(5):253-57, 1991.
185. Kovacs CS, Kronenberg HM: Maternal-fetal calcium and bone metabolism during pregnancy, puerperium, and lactation, *Endocr Rev* 18(6):832-72, 1997.
186. Hsu SC, Levine MA: Perinatal calcium metabolism: physiology and pathophysiology, *Semin Neonatol* 9(1):23-36, 2004.
187. Saggese G, Baroncelli GI, Bertelloni S, Cipolloni C: Intact parathyroid hormone levels during pregnancy, in healthy term neonates and in hypocalcemic preterm infants, *Acta Paediatr Scand* 80(1):36-41, 1991.
188. Wandrup J, Kroner J, Pryds O, Kastrup KW: Age-related reference values for ionized calcium in the first week of life in premature and full-term neonates, *Scand J Clin Lab Invest* 48(3):255-60, 1988.
189. Karlen J, Aperia A, Zetterstrom R: Renal excretion of calcium and phosphate in preterm and term infants, *J Pediatr* 106(5):814-19, 1985.
190. Song Y, Peng X, Porta A, Takanaga H, Peng JB, Hediger MA et al: Calcium transporter 1 and epithelial calcium channel messenger ribonucleic acid are differentially regulated by 1,25 dihydroxyvitamin D3 in the intestine and kidney of mice, *Endocrinology* 144(9):3885-94, 2003.
191. Brodehl J, Gellissen K, Weber HP: Postnatal development of tubular phosphate reabsorption, *Clin Nephrol* 17(4):163-71, 1982.
192. Hohenauer L, Rosenberg TF, Oh W: Calcium and phosphorus homeostasis on the first day of life, *Biol Neonate* 15(12):49-56, 1970.
193. Kaskel FJ, Kumar AM, Feld LG, Spitzer A: Renal reabsorption of phosphate during development: tubular events, *Pediatr Nephrol* 2(1):129-34, 1988.
194. Segawa H, Kaneko I, Takahashi A, Kuwahata M, Ito M, Ohkido I et al: Growth-related renal type II Na/Pi cotransporter, *J Biol Chem* 277(22):19665-72, 2002.
195. Haramati A, Mulroney SE, Webster SK: Developmental changes in the tubular capacity for phosphate reabsorption in the rat, *Am J Physiol* 255(2 Pt 2):F287-91, 1988.
196. Imbert-Teboul M, Chabardes D, Clique A, Montegut M, Morel F: Ontogenesis of hormone-dependent adenylate cyclase in isolated rat nephron segments, *Am J Physiol* 247(2 Pt 2):F316-25, 1984.
197. Forster IC, Henando N, Biber J, Murer H: Proximal tubular handling of phosphate: a molecular perspective, *Kidney Int* 70(9):1548-59, 2006.
198. Hu MC, Zhang J, Shi M, Rosenblatt K, Baum M et al: Klotho is a phosphaturic hormone: in vivo evidence, *J Am Soc Nephrol* 17:105A, 2005.
199. Mulroney SE, Lumpkin MD, Haramati A: Antagonist to GH-releasing factor inhibits growth and renal Pi reabsorption in immature rats, *Am J Physiol* 257(1 Pt 2):F29-34, 1989.
200. Woda CB, Halaihel N, Wilson PV, Haramati A, Levi M, Mulroney SE: Regulation of renal NaPi-2 expression and tubular phosphate reabsorption by growth hormone in the juvenile rat, *Am J Physiol Renal Physiol* 287(1):F117-23, 2004.
201. Hammerman MR, Karl IE, Hruska KA: Regulation of canine renal vesicle Pi transport by growth hormone and parathyroid hormone, *Biochim Biophys Acta* 603(2):322-35, 1980.
202. Konrad M, Schlingmann KP, Gudermann T: Insights into the molecular nature of magnesium homeostasis, *Am J Physiol Renal Physiol* 286(4):F599-605, 2004.
203. De Rouffignac C, Quamme G: Renal magnesium handling and its hormonal control, *Physiol Rev* 74(2):305-22, 1994.
204. Simon DB, Lu Y, Choate KA, Velazquez H, Al-Sabban E, Praga M et al: Paracellin-1, a renal tight junction protein required for paracellular Mg2+ resorption, *Science* 285(5424):103-06, 1999.
205. Voets T, Nilius B, Hoefs S, van der Kemp AW, Droogmans G, Bindels RJ et al: TRPM6 forms the Mg2+ influx channel involved in intestinal and renal Mg2+ absorption, *J Biol Chem* 279(1):19-25, 2004.
206. Rossi R, Danzebrink S, Linnenburger K, Hillebrand D, Gruneberg M, Sablitzky V et al: Assessment of tubular reabsorption of sodium, glucose, phosphate and amino acids based on spot urine samples, *Acta Paediatr* 83(12):1282-86, 1994.
207. Arant BS Jr: Developmental patterns of renal functional maturation compared in the human neonate, *J Pediatr* 92(5):705-12, 1978.
208. Brodehl J, Franken A, Gellissen K: Maximal tubular reabsorption of glucose in infants and children, *Acta Paediatr Scand* 61(4):413-20, 1972.
209. Beck JC, Lipkowitz MS, Abramson RG: Characterization of the fetal glucose transporter in rabbit kidney. Comparison with the adult brush border electrogenic Na+-glucose symporter, *J Clin Invest* 82(2):379-87, 1988.
210. LeLievre-Pegorier M, Geloso JP: Otogeny of sugar transport in fetal rat kidney, *Biol Neonate* 38(1-2):16-24, 1980.

211. Robillard JE, Sessions C, Kennedy RL, Smith FG Jr: Maturation of the glucose transport process by the fetal kidney, *Pediatr Res* 12(5):680-84, 1978.
212. Silbernagl S: The renal handling of amino acids and oligopeptides, *Physiol Rev* 68(3):911-1007, 1988.
213. Zelikovic I, Chesney RW: Development of renal amino acid transport systems, *Semin Nephrol* 9(1):49-55, 1989.
214. Baerlocher KE, Scriver CR, Mohyuddin F: The ontogeny of amino acid transport in rat kidney. II. Kinetics of uptake and effect of anoxia, *Biochim Biophys Acta* 249(2):364-72, 1971.
215. Baerlocher KE, Scriver CR, Mohyuddin F: The ontogeny of amino acid transport in rat kidney. I. Effect on distribution ratios and intracellular metabolism of proline and glycine. *Biochim Biophys Acta* 249(2):353-63, 1971.
216. Muller F, Dommergues M, Bussieres L, Lortat-Jacob S, Loirat C, Oury JF et al: Development of human renal function: reference intervals for 10 biochemical markers in fetal urine, *Clin Chem* 42(11):1855-60, 1996.
217. Ojala R, Ala-Houhala M, Harmoinen AP, Luukkaala T, Uotila J, Tammela O: Tubular proteinuria in pre-term and full-term infants, *Pediatr Nephrol* 21(1):68-73, 2006.
218. Awad H, el-Safty I, el-Barbary M, Imam S: Evaluation of renal glomerular and tubular functional and structural integrity in neonates, *Am J Med Sci* 324(5):261-66, 2002.
219. Thomas JL, Reichelderfer TE: Premature infants: analysis of serum during the first seven weeks, *Clin Chem* 14(3):272-80, 1968.
220. Greeley C, Snell J, Colaco et al: Pediatric reference ranges for electrolytes and creatinine, *Pediatric Laboratory Medicine* 11/3, 1993.
221. Thalme B: Calcium, chloride, cholesterol, inorganic phosphorus and total protein in blood plasma during the early neonatal period studied with ultramicrochemical methods, *Acta Paediatr* 51:649-60, 1962.
222. Nelson N, Finnstrom O, Larsson L: Plasma ionized calcium phosphate and magnesium in preterm and small for gestational age infants, *Acta Paediatr Scand* 78(3):351-57, 1989.
223. Mayne PD, Kovar IZ: Calcium and phosphorus metabolism in the premature infant, *Ann Clin Biochem* 28(Pt.2):131-42, 1991.

CHAPTER 7

Disorders of Kidney Formation

Norman D. Rosenblum and Remi Salomon

Developmental abnormalities of the renal tract account for 30% to 50% of end-stage renal disease in children.[1] Approximately one half of such cases are associated with lower urinary tract abnormalities. Together these abnormalities constitute a spectrum of phenotypes, namely congenital abnormalities of the kidney and urinary tract (CAKUT). In this chapter we review renal malformations and abnormalities of kidney location. We discuss the epidemiology of these abnormalities, their etiologies and clinical manifestations, and aspects of clinical management.

CLASSIFICATION AND DEFINITION OF RENAL MALFORMATIONS

The malformed kidney is classified by its gross and microscopic anatomical features. A generally accepted classification scheme consists of:

- Renal agenesis
- Simple renal hypoplasia
- Renal dysplasia
- Renal dysplasia/hypoplasia (hypodysplasia)

Malformations can be either unilateral or bilateral. Renal agenesis refers to congenital absence of the kidney and ureter. Simple renal hypoplasia is defined as a small kidney with a reduced number of nephrons and normal renal architecture. Renal dysplasia is defined by the presence of malformed kidney tissue elements. Characteristic microscopic abnormalities include abnormal differentiation of mesenchymal and epithelial elements, a decreased number of nephrons, loss of corticomedullary differentiation, and the presence of dysplastic elements including cartilage and bone (Figure 7-1). Dysplastic kidneys range in size from large distended kidneys with multiple large cysts to small kidneys with or without cysts. A small dysplastic kidney without macroscopic cysts is often classified clinically as a hypoplastic/dysplastic kidney since pathological examination, which provides a means to distinguish between simple hypoplasia and dysplasia, is not commonly performed during life. The multicystic dysplastic kidney (MCDK) is an extreme form of renal dysplasia.

EPIDEMIOLOGY OF RENAL MALFORMATION

The incidence of renal and urinary tract malformations is 0.3 to 1.6 per 1000 liveborn and stillborn infants.[2] Lower urinary tract abnormalities are found in about 50% of affected patients and include vesicoureteral reflux (25%), ureteropelvic junction obstruction (11%), and ureterovesical junction obstruction (11%).[3] Renal malformations are commonly detected in the antenatal period and account for 20% to 30% of all anomalies detected.[4] In the prenatal period, upper urinary tract dilatation is the most frequent abnormality detected. Renal malformations, other than mild antenatal pelviectasis, occur in association with nonrenal malformations in about 30% of cases.[2] There are more than 100 syndromes associated with renal and urinary tract malformations[5] (Table 7-1). Bilateral renal agenesis occurs in 1 in 3000 to 1 in 10,000 births. Males are affected more often than females. Unilateral renal agenesis has been reported with a prevalence of 1 in 1000 autopsies. The incidence of unilateral dysplasia is 1 in 3000 to 5000 births (1 in 3640 for the MCDK) compared with 1 in 10,000 for bilateral dysplasia.[6] The male-to-female ratio for bilateral and unilateral renal dysplasia is 1.32 : 1 and 1.92 : 1, respectively.[7] Nine percent of first-degree relatives of patients with bilateral renal agenesis or bilateral renal dysgenesis have some type of renal malformation.[8] The incidence of renal ectopia is 1 in 1000 autopsies, but the clinical recognition is estimated to be only 1 in 10,000 patients.[9] Males and females are equally affected. Renal ectopia is bilateral in 10% of cases; when unilateral, there is a slight predilection for the left side. The incidence of fusion anomalies is estimated to be about 1 in 600 infants.[10]

ABNORMAL MOLECULAR SIGNALING IN THE MALFORMED KIDNEY

Human renal development is complete by 34 weeks' gestation. Thus by definition, renal malformation is a problem of disordered renal embryogenesis. The morphological, cellular, and genetic events that underlie normal renal development are reviewed in Chapter 6. Perturbations in ureteric bud outgrowth, branching morphogenesis, and induction of nephrogenesis are thought to underlie the majority of the malformations described in humans.

Failure of ureteric bud outgrowth and invasion of the metanephric blastema are events antecedent to renal agenesis or severe renal dysgenesis. Studies in the mouse embryo, a model of human renal development, have identified genes that control ureteric bud outgrowth. Some of these genes are mutated in human renal malformations also characterized by agenesis or severe dysgenesis.[11] Here we highlight how some

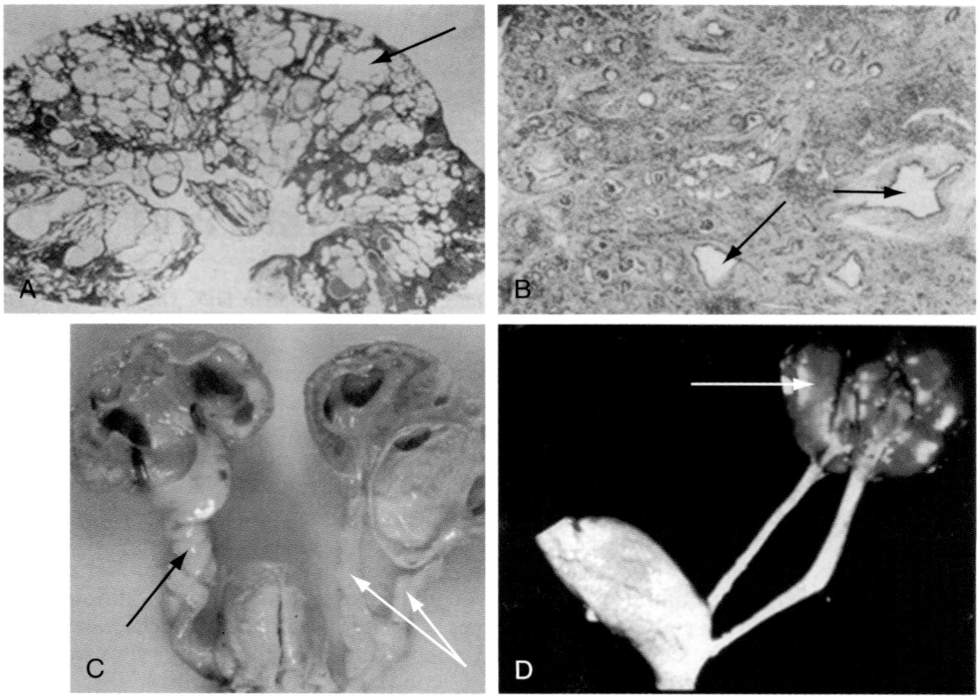

Figure 7-1 Anatomical features of human renal and lower urinary tract malformations. **A,** MCDK characterized by numerous cysts (arrow) distorting the renal architecture. **B,** Dysplastic renal tissue demonstrating lack of recognizable nephron elements, dilated tubules, large amounts of stromal tissue, and primitive ducts (arrows) characterized by epithelial tubules with fibromuscular collars. **C,** Ureteral duplication (right, white arrows) and dilated ureter (left, black arrow) associated with a ureterocele. All ureters are obstructed at the level of the bladder and are associated with hydronephrosis. **D,** Crossed fused ectopia with fused orthotopic and heterotopic kidneys (arrow).

TABLE 7-1 **Most Frequent Syndromes, Chromosomal Abnormalities, and Metabolic Disorders with Renal or Urinary Tract Malformation**

Syndromes	Chromosomal Abnormalities	Metabolic Disorders
Beckwith-Wiedemann	Trisomy 21	Peroxysomal
Cerebrooculorenal	Klinefelter	Glycosylation defect
CHARGE	DiGeorge, 22q11	Mitochondriopathy
DiGeorge	45, XO (Turner)	Glutaric aciduria type II
Ectrodactyly, ectodermal dysplasia, and cleft lip/palate	(XXY) Klinefelter	Carnitine palmitoyl transferase II deficiency
Ehlers-Danlos	Tri 9 mosaic, Tri 13, Tri 18, del 4q, del 18q, dup 3q, dup 10q	
Fanconi pancytopenia	Triploidy	
Fraser		
Fryns		
Meckel		
Marfan		
MURCS association		
Oculoauriculovertebral (Goldenhar)		
Oculo-facial-digital (OFD)		
Pallister-Hall		
Renal cysts and diabetes		
Simpson-Golabi-Behmel (SGBS)		
Tuberous sclerosis		
Townes-Brocks		
VATER		
WAGR		
Williams-Beuren		
Zellweger (cerebrohepatorenal)		

genes serve to stimulate or limit ureteric bud outgrowth and how these functions are related to the genesis of human diseases.

Sonic hedgehog (SHH) is a secreted protein that controls a variety of critical processes during embryogenesis. In mammals, SHH acts to control gene transcription via three members of the GLI family of transcription factors, GLI1, GLI2, and GLI3. Frameshift mutations in GLI3 that result in the expression of a short, truncated form of GLI3 are found in humans with Pallister-Hall syndrome (PHS) (OMIM # 126510) and renal agenesis or dysplasia.[12] A pathogenic role for truncated GLI3 was demonstrated in mice engineered such that the normal *GLI3* allele was replaced with the truncated isoform. These mice are characterized by renal agenesis or dysplasia similar to humans with PHS.[13] Subsequent analysis of renal embryogenesis in mice deficient in SHH and GLI3 provides the basis for a model that suggests that the truncated form of GLI3 represses genes that are required for the initiation of renal development. These genes include *PAX2* and *SALL1* (see text that follows).[14]

Glial cell derived neurotrophic factor (GDNF) is expressed in the metanephric blastema and interacts with its cell surface receptor, RET, expressed on the surface of ureteric bud cells. Mutational inactivation of *Gdnf* in mice causes bilateral renal agenesis due to failure of ureteric bud outgrowth. Expression of GDNF is positively controlled by genes in which mutations have been associated with human syndromes characterized by renal agenesis or renal dysplasia. *EYA1*, a transcription factor, is mutated in humans with branchio-oto-renal (BOR) syndrome and unilateral or bilateral renal agenesis or severe dysplasia.[15] *EYA1* is expressed in metanephric mesenchyme cells in the same spatial and temporal pattern as GDNF. Mice with EYA1 deficiency also demonstrate renal agenesis and failure of GDNF expression.[16] EYA1 functions in a molecular complex that consists, in part, of SIX1. Mutations in *SIX1* are also associated with BOR syndrome,[17] and mutational inactivation of *Six1* in mice results in renal agenesis or severe dysgenesis.[18] The gene encoding SALL1 is mutated in patients with Townes-Brock syndrome (TBS) and renal agenesis or dysplasia (OMIM # 107480)[19] and also in patients that lack extrarenal features of TBS.[20] Like GDNF and EYA1, SALL1 is expressed in the metanephric mesenchyme prior to and during ureteric bud invasion. Mutational inactivation of *Sall1* in mice causes renal agenesis or severe dysgenesis and a marked decrease in GDNF expression.[21] Thus both EYA1 and SALL1 function upstream of GDNF to positively regulate its expression, thereby controlling ureteric bud outgrowth.

The timing and location of ureteric bud outgrowth from the Wolffian duct is a critical determinant of normal metanephric development. A pathogenic role for abnormal ureteric bud outgrowth from the Wolffian duct was first hypothesized on the basis of the clinical-pathological observation that abnormal insertion of the ureter into the lower urinary tract is frequently associated with a duplex kidney. Moreover, the renal parenchyma associated with a ureter with ectopic insertion into the bladder is frequently dysplastic.[22] Investigation of mice with CAKUT has revealed mechanisms that control the site of ureteric bud outgrowth. FOXC1 is a transcription factor that is expressed in a spatial and temporal pattern in the metanephric mesenchyme similar to that of GDNF. Homozygous *Foxc1* null mutant mice exhibit renal abnormalities consisting of ureteric duplication, hydroureter, and ectopic ureteric buds. Remarkably, these mice demonstrate an anterior expansion of the spatial expression domain of *Gdnf*.[23] These findings demonstrate that inhibition of GDNF expression is required to determine the position and number of ureteric bud outgrowths.

Ureteric bud branching within the metanephric mesenchyme is controlled by genetic and nutritional factors. The number of ureteric bud branches elaborated is considered a major determinant of final nephron number since ureteric bud branch tips induce discrete subsets of metanephric mesenchyme cells to undergo nephrogenesis. *PAX2* is exemplary of genes that control ureteric bud branching. *PAX2* is a paired-box–type transcription factor and is mutated in patients with renal-coloboma syndrome (RCS) (OMIM # 120330). Interestingly, *PAX2* mutations are also found in patients with renal hypoplasia or dysplasia without extrarenal symptoms.[20] During renal development, PAX2 is expressed in the Wolffian duct, the ureteric bud, and in metanephric blastema cells induced by ureteric bud branch tips. Mice with a *Pax2* mutation identical in type to that found in humans with RCS exhibit decreased ureteric bud branching and renal hypoplasia. Investigation of the mechanisms controlling abnormal ureteric bud branching in a murine model of RCS ($Pax2^{1Neu}$) revealed that increased ureteric bud cell apoptosis decreases the number of ureteric bud branches and glomeruli formed. Remarkably, rescue of ureteric bud cell apoptosis normalizes the mutant phenotype.[24]

Ureteric bud branching is also controlled by vitamin A and its signaling effectors. Expression of RET, the receptor for GDNF, is controlled by members of the retinoic acid receptor family of transcription factors that function in the vitamin A signaling pathway. These members, including RAR alpha and RAR beta2, are expressed in stromal cells surrounding *Ret*-expressing ureteric bud branch tips.[25,26] Mice deficient in these receptors exhibit a decreased number of ureteric bud branches and diminished expression of *Ret*. These observations are consistent with the finding that vitamin A deficiency during pregnancy causes renal hypoplasia in the fetus.[27] Thus, genetic and nutritional factors interact to control ureteric bud branching and nephrogenesis. The number of nephrons is likely determined by a complex combination of factors including genetic variants, environmental events, and stochastic factors. This could explain the variable number of nephrons in humans, which ranges from approximately 230,000 to 1,800,000.[28] Loss-of-function mutations in some developmental genes account for a severe reduction in the number of nephrons leading to renal insufficiency. In other cases the glomerular filtration rate is normal, but a correlation has been found between the number of nephrons and the occurrence of arterial hypertension later in life (see Chapter 43).

HUMAN RENAL MALFORMATIONS WITH A DEFINED GENETIC ETIOLOGY

Renal congenital malformations are more often sporadic than familial and isolated rather than associated with other mal-

TABLE 7-2 Human Gene Mutations Exhibiting Defects in Renal Morphogenesis

Primary Disease	Gene	Kidney Phenotype	References
Alagille syndrome	*JAGGED1*	Cystic dysplasia	81
Apert syndrome	*FGFR2*	Hydronephrosis	82
Beckwith-Wiedemann syndrome	*p57^{KIP2}*	Medullary dysplasia	83
Branchio-oto-renal (BOR) syndrome	*EYA1, SIX1*	Unilateral or bilateral agenesis/dysplasia, hypoplasia, collecting system anomalies	15
Campomelic dysplasia	*SOX9*	Dysplasia, hydronephrosis	84, 85
Duane-radial ray (Okihiro) syndrome	*SALL4*	UNL agenesis, VUR, malrotation, cross fused ectopia, pelviectasis	86
Fraser syndrome	*FRAS1*	Agenesis, dysplasia	87
Hypothyroidism, sensorineural deafness, and renal anomalies (HDR) syndrome	*GATA3*	Dysplasia	88
Kallmann syndrome	*KAL1, FGFR1, PROK2, PROK2R*	Agenesis	89
Mammary-ulnar syndrome	*TBX3*	Dysplasia	90
Pallister-Hall syndrome	*GLI3*	Dysplasia	12, 14
Renal-coloboma syndrome	*PAX2*	Hypoplasia, vesicoureteral reflux	44
Renal tubular dysgenesis	RAS components	Tubular dysplasia	73
Renal cysts and diabetes syndrome	*HNF-1β*	Dysplasia, hypoplasia	91
Simpson-Golabi-Behmel syndrome	*GPC3*	Medullary dysplasia	92
Smith-Lemli-Opitz syndrome	*7-hydroxy-cholesterol reductase*	Agenesis, dysplasia	93
Townes-Brocks syndrome	*SALL1*	Hypoplasia, dysplasia, VUR	19
Zellweger syndrome	*PEX1*	VUR, cystic dysplasia	94

formations. However, familial cases and extrarenal symptoms are sometimes unrecognized. A careful evaluation of family history reveals a clustering of isolated or syndromic urinary tract and renal malformations in more than 10% of cases. Familial aggregation of renal malformations in a subset of patients suggests that genetic events might be involved. Knowledge of the most frequent syndromes, a careful clinical examination, and appropriately selected investigations are critical to the clinical approach to these disorders.

Mutations in more than 30 genes have been identified in children with renal development anomalies, generally as part of a multiorgan syndrome (Table 7-2). Some of these syndromes and their associated genes are described here. The most frequent syndromes in which renal malformations are encountered are listed in Table 7-1 and Table 7-2. For a complete list of syndromes featuring renal malformations, see McKusick's Online Mendelian Inheritance in Man at http://www.ncbi.nlm.nih.gov/omim.

Genetic Causes of Syndromic Human Renal Malformations

Branchio-oto-renal Syndrome

The association of branchial (B), otic (O), and renal (R) anomalies was first described by Fraser and Melnick.[29,30] Major diagnostic criteria consist of hearing loss (93% to 98%), branchial defects (49% to 68.5%), ear pits (82% to 83.5%), and renal anomalies (38% to 67%).[31,32] The association of these three major features defines the classical BOR syndrome (OMIM # 113650). Yet many patients have only one or two of these major features in association with other minor features such as external ear anomalies, preauricular tags, or other facial abnormalities (Table 7-3). Hearing loss can be conductive, sensorineural, or mixed.

TABLE 7-3 Major and Minor Criteria for the Diagnosis of BOR Syndrome

Major Features	Minor Features
Deafness	External ear anomalies
Branchial anomalies	Preauricular tags
Preauricular pits	Other facial anomalies
Renal malformations	Cataract, lacrymal duct stenosis

The frequency of BOR syndrome has been estimated at 1 in 40,000 births.[33] The transmission is autosomal dominant with incomplete penetrance and variable expressivity. Renal malformations include unilateral or bilateral renal agenesis and hypodysplasia, as well as malformation of the lower urinary tract including vesicoureteral reflux, pyeloureteral obstruction, and ureteral duplication. Different renal malformations can be observed in the same family; moreover, some individuals have normal kidneys (Bronchiootic [BO] syndrome, OMIM # 120502). Other infrequent abnormalities have been described in patients with BOR syndrome. These include aplasia of the lacrimal ducts, congenital cataract, and anterior segment anomalies.[29,30] Characteristic temporal bone findings include cochlear hypoplasia (four fifths of normal size with only two turns), dilation of the vestibular aqueduct, bulbous internal auditory canals, deep posterior fossae, and acutely angled promontories.[31]

In 1992, linkage analysis in a large BOR family led to the definition of a locus on chromosome 8.[34] Five years later, the corresponding gene *EYA1* was identified.[15] This gene encodes for a non–DNA-binding transcription cofactor. Another causative gene, *SIX1*, encodes for a transcription factor that interacts with EYA1.[17] These two transcription factors control the expression of PAX2 and GDNF in the metanephric mesenchyme.[35] The EYA1 protein contains a highly conserved region called the eyes absent homologous region, which is encoded within exons 9-16, the site of most mutations identified to date. More than 50 different mutations have been identified. A comprehensive list of all *EYA1* mutations can be found on the University of Iowa website (http://www.medicine.uiowa.edu/pendredandbor/). Importantly, direct sequencing techniques will miss large deletions, duplications, and chromosome rearrangements, which have been estimated to comprise 20% to 25% of *EYA1* mutations.[36] If direct sequencing is negative, it is then necessary to use other techniques that allow the detection of these rearrangements.

The wide spectrum of phenotypic features associated with *EYA1* mutations complicates the approach to making a diagnosis of BOR syndrome.[32] A reasonable approach is to limit analysis of *EYA1* to families in which at least one member fulfills the criteria for classical BOR syndrome (Table 7-3). Investigations should include a family history and an examination of relatives for preauricular pits, lacrimal duct stenosis, and branchial fistulae and/or cysts. Hearing studies and renal ultrasound should be performed in all first-degree relatives.

Molecular testing can confirm the diagnosis and provide genetic recurrence risk information to families. However, variability of the phenotype even with the same mutation does not permit accurate prediction of the disease severity. In some families the same mutation is associated with renal malformation in some individuals but not in others. This discrepancy might be explained by stochastic factors that impact the formation of the kidneys or by other unlinked genetic events that may act in synergy with the EYA1 protein during nephrogenesis. Recently such a complex inheritance was found in a BOR family in which the proband harbored not only a heterozygous *EYA1* mutation, but also mutations in the *GDNF* and *RET* genes (see the RET/GDNF signaling pathway below). *SIX1* heterozygous mutation seems less frequent than the *EYA1* mutation, having been reported in five kindreds as of 2006.[17]

Renal-Coloboma Syndrome

Renal-coloboma syndrome (RCS), also named papillorenal syndrome, is an autosomal dominant congenital anomaly characterized by the association of renal hypoplasia, vesicoureteric reflux, and optic nerve coloboma.[37] A wide range of renal malformations can be observed in RCS. Oligomeganephronic hypoplasia, renal dysplasia, and vesicoureteric reflux are the most frequent malformations, but multicystic dysplasia[38] and pelviureteric junction obstruction have also been described.[20,38,39] Similarly, the ocular phenotype is extremely variable. The most common finding is an optic disc pit associated with vascular abnormalities and cilioretinal arteries, with mild visual impairment limited to blind-spot enlargement.[40] In other cases the only ocular anomaly is optic nerve dysplasia with an abnormal vessel pattern and no functional consequence (Figure 7-2). In contrast, a large coloboma of the optic nerve or of the chorioretina and the morning glory anomaly can be responsible for a severe visual impairment.[41] Coloboma and the related anomalies are probably the consequence of an incomplete closure of the embryonic fissure of the optic cup. Other extrarenal manifestations can include sensorineural hearing loss, joint laxity, Arnold-Chiari malformation, and seizures of unknown cause.[42,43] In addition to its expression in the metanephros and in the optic fissure, *PAX2* is also expressed in the hindbrain during its development. However, neurological symptoms are not usually present in RCS.

PAX2 is expressed in the mesonephros and in the metanephros during the very early stages of renal development. In 1995, Sanyanusin et al. reported heterozygous mutations in

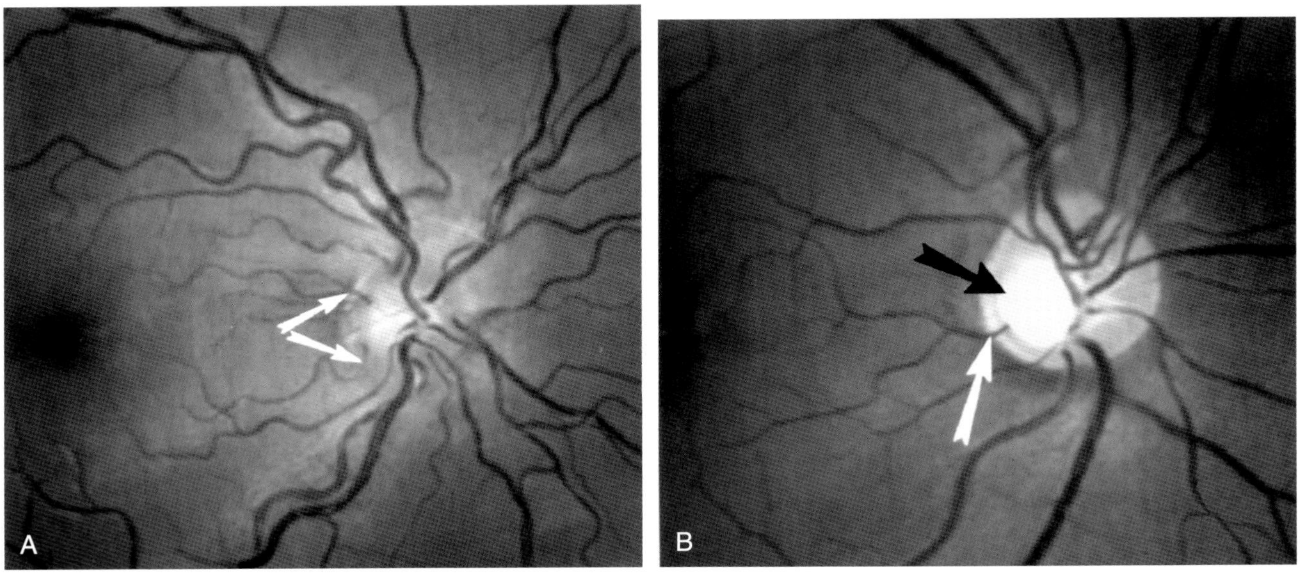

Figure 7-2 Optic disk appearance in two patients with RCS and PAX2 mutations. **A,** Characteristic features of optic disk coloboma with a deep temporal excavation (arrows). **B,** The optic disk is dysplastic, with thickening (black arrow) and emergence of abnormal vessels (white arrow).

TABLE 7-4 **Renal Cyst and Diabetes Syndrome**

Main features*	Large hyperechoic fetal kidneys Renal hypodysplasia with cortical microcysts Diabetes mellitus (MODY5)	
Occasional features	Genital malformations	Female: vaginal aplasia, rudimentary or bicornuate uterus Male: epididymal cysts, atresia of the vas deferens, asthenospermia, hypospadias
	Hyperuricemia, rarely gout (reduced fractional excretion of uric acid) Moderate elevation of liver enzymes Subclinical defect of exocrine pancreatic functions	

* Age at onset and severity of these symptoms are highly variable.

two RCS families.[44] Since then, more than 30 mutations have been reported, most of them lying in the second and third exons. Other gene(s) are probably also responsible for this syndrome since *PAX2* mutations are not found in approximately 50% of RCS patients. The *PAX2* gene is located on chromosome 10q24-25; it encodes a transcription factor that belongs to the paired-box family of homeotic genes. Most of the mutations are located in exons 2 and 3, which encode the DNA-binding domain.* Importantly, the RCS phenotype is highly variable even in patients harboring the same *PAX2* mutation, suggesting that modifier genes might be implicated. A *SIX1* mutation has been found in association with a *PAX2* mutation in two siblings with severe renal hypodysplasia that led to renal insufficiency during childhood and optic nerve coloboma. Interestingly, their father, who harbored only the *PAX2* mutation, had a mild renal malformation with late-onset renal insufficiency and no ocular defect.[20]

Optic nerve coloboma occurs frequently as an isolated anomaly or as a feature of other multiorgan syndromes such as CHARGE association, COACH syndrome, and acro-renal-ocular syndrome. Because optic nerve coloboma and related disorders can be easily misdiagnosed, the prevalence of RCS is probably underestimated. It is wise to examine the fundus in every patient with renal hypodysplasia and conversely to perform renal ultrasound and serum creatinine in every patient with optic nerve coloboma.

Renal Cysts and Diabetes Syndrome

Mutations in the *TCF2* gene encoding the transcription factor HNF-1β were initially found in patients with diabetes type MODY5.[45,46] Diabetes mellitus is present in approximately 60% of all cases reported, usually occurs before age 25, and is often associated with pancreatic atrophy.[47-49] In some patients a subclinical deficiency of pancreatic exocrine functions has been demonstrated.[47] More than 80 families with *TCF2* mutations have been reported as of 2006. Additional features have been described, including a wide spectrum of renal phenotypes (Table 7-4). The presence of cysts is the most consistent feature of the renal phenotype, leading to the name *renal cysts and diabetes (RCAD) syndrome*. The cysts are usually cortical, bilateral, and small.[50] Mutations in the *TCF2* gene have also been found in association with a variety of renal development disorders such as renal hypoplasia and dysplasia, MCDKs, renal agenesis, horseshoe kidneys, and pelviureteric junction obstruction, as well as clubbing and tiny diverticulae of the calyces.[51-53] When histology is available, the most specific finding is the presence of cortical glomerular cysts with dilatation of the Bowman spaces (glomerulocystic dysplasia).[54] Other nonspecific lesions such as cystic renal dysplasia, interstitial fibrosis, or oligomeganephronia have also been reported. Antenatal presentation with enlarged hyperechoic kidneys seems to be a common finding.[55]

Various genital tract malformations have been reported, mostly in females. These include vaginal aplasia, rudimentary uterus, bicornuate urterus, uterus didelphys, and double vagina. In males, hypospadias, epididymal cysts, and agenesis of the vas deferens have been reported.[47] These genital anomalies have been described in approximately 10% to 15% of patients with *TCF2* mutations but might be underestimated especially in the pediatric series. Reduced fractional excretion of uric acid (less than 15%) and hyperuricemia is observed in some cases and is usually asymptomatic. Moderate elevation of liver enzymes is a common finding, but severe hepatopathy has not been reported. Ovarian cancer and renal chromophobe-cell cancer were reported in one patient. A fortuitous association is possible, but further investigation in patients with *TCF2* mutations may be worthwhile since HNF-1α inactivation has been recently associated with hepatic tumors.[56]

HNF-1β is a homeotic transcription factor involved in the development of the pancreas, kidneys, liver, and intestine. More than 50 mutations have been reported, most of which are located in the first four exons that encode the DNA-binding domain. In more than one third of the cases, the gene is entirely deleted.[48,50] Such alterations are not detected by conventional amplification and screening methods. There is no correlation between the type of mutation and the phenotype. Importantly, deletions are frequently not transmitted by the parents but appear *de novo* in the proband. Analysis of *TCF2* can thus be recommended not only in patients with a family history of RCAD syndrome but also in cases with renal cysts when polycystic disease or nephronophthisis is unlikely. The presence of cortical bilateral cysts is probably the most typical finding. Reduced uric acid fractional excretion, elevation of liver enzymes, glucose intolerance, and abnormalities of the genital tract should be systemically sought and *TCF2* analyzed if one of these symptoms is

* http://pax2.hgu.mrc.ac.uk

present. As with other syndromes, phenotypic variability can be observed between families and also in family members with the same mutation, which suggests a role for environmental and genetic factors.

Kallmann Syndrome

Kallmann syndrome (KS) is defined by the presence of hypogonadotropic hypogonadism and deficiency of the sense of smell (anosmia or hyposmia).[57,58] Some affected individuals exhibit unilateral renal agenesis (about one third), cleft lip and/or palate, selective tooth agenesis, bimanual synkinesis, and hearing impairment.[59] Other renal urinary tract malformations including duplex systems, hydronephrosis, and vesicoureteric reflux have been rarely reported. Anosmia/hyposmia is related to the absence or hypoplasia of the olfactory bulbs and tracts. Hypogonadism is due to a deficiency in gonadotropin-releasing hormone (GnRH). The GnRH-synthesizing neurons migrate during development from the olfactory epithelium to the forebrain along the olfactory nerve pathway.[60,61] KS is genetically heterogeneous. Four genes with mutations in affected patients have been identified. These include *KAL1*, an X-chromosome encoded gene that gives rise to anosmin-1; *FGFR1* (fibroblast growth factor receptor 1), mutated in autosomal dominant forms of KS[62]; *PROK2* (prokineticin-2); and *PROK2R* (prokineticin-2 receptor).[63] Mutations in these four genes have been found in 14% *(KAL1)*, 7% *(FGFR1)*, 7% *(PROKR2)*, and 2% *(PROK2)* of KS patients, but renal anomalies have been reported only in patients with *KAL1* mutations.[64]

Townes-Brocks Syndrome and VATER/VACTERL Associations

Townes-Brocks syndrome (TBS) is an autosomal dominant malformation syndrome characterized by imperforate anus, preaxial polydactyly and/or triphalangeal thumbs, external ear defects, sensorineural hearing loss, and, less frequently, kidney, urogenital, and heart malformations.[65,66] Intelligence is usually normal. REAR (renal-ear-anal-radial) syndrome is another term used to describe this condition.[67] The presentation of TBS is highly variable within and between affected families.

TBS features overlap those seen in VATER association (anal, radial, and renal malformations). However, TBS is not usually characterized by tracheoesophageal fistula or vertebral anomalies. Ear anomalies and deafness are not typical of VATER. VACTERL with hydrocephalus, reported as an X-linked or autosomal recessive condition, may include radial, cardiac, and renal anomalies and imperforate anus along with other VATER features. Some of these patients have Fanconi anemia. The gene mutated in human TBS is *SALL1*, a member of the Spalt family that is required for the normal development of the limbs, nervous system, kidney, and heart.[19] VATER association is usually sporadic and there is no recognized teratogen or chromosomal abnormality.

Tubular Dysgenesis and Mutations of RAS System Elements

Renal tubular dysgenesis (RTD) is a severe perinatal disorder characterized by absence or paucity of differentiated proximal tubules, early severe oligohydramnios, and perinatal death. The latter is usually due to pulmonary hypoplasia and skull ossification defects.[68-70] This condition has also been described in clinical conditions associated with renal ischemia, including twin-to-twin transfusion syndrome, major cardiac malformations, severe liver diseases, and fetal or infantile renal artery stenosis,[71] and in fetuses exposed in utero to angiotensin-converting enzyme inhibitors (ACEIs) or angiotensin II (AngII) receptor antagonists.[72] Mutations in the genes that encode components of the renin-angiotensin system have been identified in some families.[73]

The RET/GDNF Signaling Pathway

The protooncogene *RET*, a tyrosine kinase receptor, and its ligand, GDNF, play a pivotal role during early nephrogenesis and enteric nervous system development. Activating *RET* mutations cause multiple endocrine neoplasia, whereas inactivating mutations lead to Hirschsprung disease. Recently two *RET* mutations (Y791F and S649L) were found in patients with renal hypodysplasia (RHD) living in central European countries. These mutations reportedly predispose humans to the emergence of medullary thyroid carcinoma (MTC). None of the patients or their carrier relatives had clinical evidence of MTC at the time of the study. A low penetrance of RHD was suggested by minimal or no renal phenotypes in most carrier relatives. A *GDNF* mutation and a previously described *EYA1* mutation in addition to the *RET* Y791F mutation was observed in a patient with BOR syndrome. RHD was limited to the single family member heterozygous for all three mutations.

GENETIC CAUSES OF ISOLATED (NONSYNDROMIC) RENAL MALFORMATION

In the majority of children with renal malformation, neither a syndrome nor a Mendelian pattern of inheritance is obvious. It appears that in a substantial proportion of such cases genes that control nephrogenesis are mutated. A recent study on a cohort of 100 patients with renal hypodysplasia and renal insufficiency demonstrated that 16% of them had mutations in one gene encoding for a transcription factor. The majority of mutations were identified in *TCF2* (HNF-1β) (especially in the subset with kidney cysts) and *PAX2*. *EYA1* and *SALL1* mutations were found in single cases.[20] Some of the mutations that were identified in these genes were *de novo* mutations, explaining the sporadic appearance of RHD. Careful analysis of patients with *TCF2* and *PAX2* mutations revealed the presence of extrarenal symptoms in only half, supporting previous reports that *TCF2* and *PAX2* mutations can be responsible for isolated renal tract anomalies or at least CAKUT malformations with minimal extrarenal features.[39,50] This study demonstrates that subtle extrarenal symptoms in syndromal RHD can easily be missed. Genetic testing in children with RHD should be preceded by a thorough clinical evaluation for extrarenal symptoms, including eye, ear, and metabolic anomalies. The presence of nonrenal anomalies increases the likelihood of detecting a specific genetic abnormality (Table 7-5). In addition, mutations in genes that are usually associated with syndromes can occur in patients with isolated RHD.

TABLE 7-5 Clinical Indications to Search for a Renal Anomaly

Exposure to teratogens	ACE inhibitors and angiotensin receptor blockers Alcohol Alkylating agents Cocaine Thrimethadione Vitamin A congeners
Findings on physical examination	High imperforate anus Abnormal external genitalia Supernumerary nipples Preauricular pits and ear tags, cervical cysts or fistula Hearing loss Aniridia Coloboma or optic disk dysplasia Hemihypertrophy
Other	Glucose intolerance

CLINICAL APPROACH TO RENAL MALFORMATION

The majority of renal malformations are now diagnosed antenatally, largely because of the widespread use and sensitivity of fetal ultrasound. The sensitivity of prenatal ultrasound screening for renal malformations is about 82%, and the mean time at which these malformations are detected is 23 weeks' gestation.[2] In general, urinary tract malformations detected antenatally are isolated and present as mild hydronephrosis with no therapeutic consequences. Parents should be reassured (see Chapter 37). In contrast, bilateral forms of renal agenesis, severe dysgenesis, bilateral ureteric obstruction, or obstruction of the bladder outlet or the urethra can cause severe oligohydramnios as early as 18 weeks. Because amniotic fluid is critical to lung development, oligohydramnios as early as the second trimester can result in lung hypoplasia, a potentially fatal disorder. The oligohydramnios sequence, termed Potter's syndrome, in its most severe form consists of a typical facial appearance characterized by pseudoepicanthus, recessed chin, posteriorly rotated flattened ears and flattened nose, as well as decreased fetal movement, musculoskeletal features including clubfoot and clubhand, hip dislocation, joint contractures, and pulmonary hypoplasia. The renal prognosis can be evaluated antenatally. Poor outcome can be predicted when there is severe oligohydramnios and small and hyperechogenic kidneys. Amniotic fluid analysis may be of help in some cases. Antenatal diagnosis and assessment of the renal prognosis are important for consideration of early termination in cases of fatal (or eventually severe) renal disease and for preparing parents and medical staff for the likelihood of neonatal renal insufficiency. Other organ malformations should be sought carefully, and a karyotype should be done if they are detected.

The clinical presentation of renal malformation in the postnatal period depends on the amount of functioning renal mass, the presence of bilateral urinary tract obstruction, and the occurrence of urinary tract infection. Bilateral renal agenesis or severe dysplasia is likely to show soon after birth, with decreased renal function. This may be accompanied by oliguria. Alternatively, patients may have a flank mass or an asymptomatic abnormality detected by renal imaging.

A detailed history and careful physical examination should be carried out on all infants with an antenatally detected renal malformation (Table 7-5). An early (within 24 hours of life) renal ultrasound is recommended for newborns with a history of oligohydramnios, progressive antenatal hydronephrosis, distended bladder on antenatal sonograms, or bilateral severe hydroureteronephrosis. In male infants, a distended bladder and bilateral hydroureteronephrosis may be secondary to posterior urethral valves, a condition that requires immediate renal imaging and clinical intervention. In general, unilateral anomalies do not require urgent investigation after birth. Renal ultrasound for unilateral hydronephrosis is not recommended within the first 72 hours of life because urine output gradually increases over the first 24 to 48 hours of life as renal plasma flow and glomerular filtration rate increase.[74] Thus the degree of urinary tract dilatation can be underestimated during this period of transition.

Clinical Approach to Specific Malformations

Unilateral Renal Agenesis

A diagnosis of unilateral renal agenesis depends on the certainty that a second kidney does not exist in the pelvis or some other ectopic location. Since absence of one kidney induces compensatory hypertrophy in the existing kidney, the presence of a large kidney on one side suggests the possibility of unilateral renal agenesis. Since unilateral agenesis is associated with contralateral urinary tract abnormalities including ureteropelvic junction obstruction and vesicoureteral reflux in 20% to 40% of cases,[75] imaging of the contralateral side is suggested. Management of affected patients involves determining the functional status of the contralateral kidney. If the contralateral kidney is normal, the long-term renal functional outcome is excellent. However, some studies have revealed that a substantial proportion of patients will develop proteinuria and hypertention in the long term. It is therefore reasonable to propose that individuals with a single functioning kidney should have their blood pressure measured and urine tested for protein periodically throughout life.

Renal Hypoplasia

Unless associated with other malformations, renal hypoplasia can be asymptomatic. Unilateral hypoplasia is often discovered incidentally during an abdominal sonogram or other imaging study. In contrast, patients with bilateral renal hypoplasia are at risk for decreased renal function and chronic kidney disease.

Renal Dysplasia

The dysplastic kidney is generally smaller than normal. However, cystic elements can contribute to large kidney size, the most extreme example being the MCDK (see following section). During the antenatal period, unilateral disease is likely to be discovered as an incidental finding. This may also be the case for bilateral renal dysplasia unless it is associated with oligohydramnios. After birth, bilateral renal dysplasia may limit glomerular filtration, causing renal failure that is usually progressive. Postnatal ultrasonography of the dysplastic kidney is characterized by increased echogenicity, loss of corticomedullary differentiation and cortical cysts. Renal dysplasia is strongly associated with dilatation of the upper and lower urinary tract, and vesicoureteric reflux and posterior urethral valves.[76] Accordingly, imaging of the lower urinary tract should be performed to determine whether these abnormalities are present.

Multicystic Dysplastic Kidney

The MCDK presents by ultrasonagraphy as a large cystic nonreniform mass in the renal fossa and by palpation as a flank mass. The MCDK is nonfunctional, a condition that can be demonstrated by imaging with MAG3 or DTPA radionuclide scanning. The MCDK is usually unilateral. If bilateral, it is fatal. Complications of MCDK include hypertension (0.01% to 0.1%). Wilms' tumor and renal cell carcinoma have also been described in MCDK, but the incidence of malignant complications is not significantly different from the general population.[77] In 25% of cases the contralateral urinary tract is abnormal. Contralateral abnormalities can include rotational or positional anomalies, renal hypoplasia, vesicoureteric efflux, and ureteropelvic junction obstruction.[6] Contralateral UPJ obstruction occurs in 5% to 10% of cases.

Gradual reduction in renal size and eventual resolution of the mass of the MCDK is common. At two years an involution in size by ultrasound has been noted in up to 60% of affected kidneys. Complete disappearance of the MCDK can occur in a minority of patients (3% to 4%) by the time of birth, and in 20% to 25% by two years. Increase in the size of MCDK can be seen in some cases. The contralateral kidney shows compensatory hypertrophy by ultrasound evaluation.

Management of patients with MCDK has shifted from routine nephrectomy to observation and medical therapy. Because of the risk of associated anomalies in the contralateral kidney, the possibility of VUR should be evaluated and blood pressure should be measured. Renal ultrasound is generally recommended at an interval of 3 months for the first year of life and then every 6 months up to involution of the mass, or at least up to five years. Compensatory hypertrophy of the contralateral kidney is expected and should be monitored by renal ultrasound. Medical therapy is usually effective in treating hypertension in the small number of affected patients, but nephrectomy may be curative in resistant cases.

Renal Ectopia

Normally the kidneys lie on either side of the spine in the lumbar region and are located in the retroperitoneal renal fossae. Rapid caudal growth during embryogenesis results in migration of the developing kidney from the pelvis to the retroperitoneal renal fossa. With ascension comes a 90° rotation from a horizontal to a vertical position with the renal hilum finally directed medially. Migration and rotation are complete by 8 weeks of gestation.

Simple congenital ectopy refers to a low-lying kidney that failed to ascend normally. It most commonly lies over the pelvic brim or in the pelvis and is termed a pelvic kidney. Less commonly, the kidney may lie on the contralateral side of the body, a state known as crossed ectopy without fusion. Clinical presentation can be asymptomatic or symptomatic. Asymptomatic presentation is when the ectopic kidney has been diagnosed coincidentally such as might occur during routine antenatal sonography. Symptomatic presentation occurs with urinary tract infections. Symptoms such as abdominal pain or fever may be present. On examination an abdominal mass may be palpable. Other presenting features include hematuria, incontinence, renal insufficiency, and hypertension.[9] A high incidence of urological abnormalities has been associated with renal ectopia. Vesicoureteral reflux is the most common, occurring in 20% of crossed renal ectopia and 30% of simple renal ectopia. In bilateral simple renal ectopia, there is a higher incidence of VUR, occurring in 70% of cases. Other associated urological abnormalities include contralateral renal dysplasia (4%), cryptorchidism (5%), and hypospadias (5%).[9] Reduced renal function is commonly observed by radionuclide scan in the ectopic kidney. Female genital anomalies such as agenesis of the uterus and vagina[78] or unicornuate uterus[79] have also been associated with ectopic kidneys. Other anomalies described include adrenal, cardiac, and skeletal anomalies. Clinical assessment should therefore include a careful physical examination for other anomalies. Renal ultrasonography can help with diagnosis and defining the underlying anatomy. A VCUG should be undertaken, particularly if there is hydronephrosis, given the risk of VUR and obstruction. A DMSA scan is also recommended to assess for differential renal function.

Renal Fusion

Renal fusion is defined as the fusion of two kidneys. The most common fusion anomaly is the horseshoe kidney, in which fusion occurs at one pole of each kidney, usually the lower pole. The fused kidney may lie in the midline (symmetrical horseshoe kidney), or the fused part may lie lateral to the midline (asymmetric horseshoe kidney). In a crossed fused ectopic kidney, the kidney from one side has crossed the midline to fuse with the kidney on the other side. Fusion is thought to occur before the kidneys ascend from the pelvis to their normal dorsolumbar position, usually between the fourth and ninth week of gestation. As a result, fusion anomalies seldom assume the high position of normal kidneys. The blood supply may therefore come from vessels such as the iliac arteries. Abnormal rotation is also associated with early fusion of the developing kidneys. The pelvis of each kidney lies anteriorly, and the ureter therefore traverses over the isthmus of a horseshoe kidney or the anterior surface of the fused kidney. Ureteric compression may occur due to external compression caused by a traversing aberrant artery. The majority of patients may be asymptomatic. Some, however, develop obstruction that presents with loin pain or hematuria and may be associated with urinary tract infections due to urinary stasis or vesicoureteric reflux. Renal calculi may occur in up to 20% of cases.[80] Other associated urological anomalies include ureteral duplication, ectopic ureter, and retrocaval ureter. Genital anomalies such as bicornuate and/or septate uterus, hypospadias, and undescended testis have also been described. Associated nonrenal anomalies involve the gastrointestinal tract (anorectal malformations such as imperforate anus, malrotation, and Meckel diverticulum), the central nervous system (neural tube defects), and the skeleton (rib defects, clubfoot, or congenital hip dislocation). Investigations should include static imaging (renal ultrasound), functional imaging (DMSA scan), and a VCUG.

REFERENCES

1. Seikaly MG, Ho PL, Emmett L, Fine RN, Tejani, A: Chronic renal insufficiency in children: the 2001 Annual Report of the NAPRTCS, *Pediatr Nephrol* 18:796-804, 2003.
2. Wiesel A, Queisser-Luft A, Clementi M, Bianca S, Stoll, C: Prenatal detection of congenital renal malformations by fetal ultrasonographic examination: an analysis of 709,030 births in 12 European countries, *Eur J Med Genet* 48:131-44, 2005.
3. Piscione TD, Rosenblum N: The malformed kidney: disruption of glomerular and tubular development, *Clin Genet* 56:343-58, 1999.
4. Queisser-Luft A, Stolz G, Wiesel A, Schlaefer K, Spranger J: Malformations in newborn: results based on 30,940 infants and fetuses from the Mainz congenital birth defect monitoring system (1990-1998), *Arch Gynecol Obstet* 266:163-67, 2002.
5. Limwongse C, Cassidy SB: Syndromes and malformations of the urinary tract. In Avner ED, Harmon WE, Naudet P, editors: *Pediatric Nephrology*, Philadelphia, 2004, Williams & Wilkins.
6. Winyard P, Chitty L: Dysplastic and polycystic kidneys: diagnosis, associations and management, *Prenat Diagn* 21:924-35, 2001.
7. Harris J, Robert E, Kallen B: Epidemiologic characteristics of kidney malformations, *Eur J Epidemiol* 16:985-92, 2000.
8. Roodhooft AM, Jason MD, Birnholz JC, Holmes LB: Familial nature of congenital absence and severe dysgenesis of both kidneys, *N Engl J Med* 310:1341-44, 1984.
9. Guarino N et al: The incidence of associated urological abnormalities in children with renal ectopia, *J Urol* 172:1757-59, 2004.
10. Weizer AZ et al: Determining the incidence of horseshoe kidney from radiographic data at a single institution, *J Urol* 170:1722-26, 2003.
11. Hu MC, Rosenblum ND: Genetic regulation of branching morphogenesis: lessons learned from loss-of-function phenotypes, *Pediatr Res* 54:433-38, 2003.
12. Kang S, Graham JM, Jr, Olney AH, Biesecker LG: GLI3 frameshift mutations cause autosomal dominant Pallister-Hall syndrome, *Nat Genet* 15:266-68, 1997.
13. Bose J, Grotewold L, Ruther U: Pallister-Hall syndrome phenotype in mice mutant for Gli3, *Hum Mol Genet* 11:1129-35, 2002.
14. Hu MC et al: GLI3-dependent transcriptional repression of Gli1, Gli2 and kidney patterning genes disrupts renal morphogenesis, *Development* 133:569-78, 2006.
15. Abdelhak S et al: A human homologue of the *Drosophila eyes absent* gene underlies Branchio-Oto-Renal (BOR) syndrome and identifies a novel gene family, *Nature Gen* 15:157-64, 1997.
16. Xu PX et al: Eya1-deficient mice lack ears and kidneys and show abnormal apoptosis of organ primordia, *Nature Genet* 23:113-17, 1999.
17. Ruf RG et al: SIX1 mutations cause branchio-oto-renal syndrome by disruption of EYA1-SIX1-DNA complexes, *Proc Natl Acad Sci U S A* 101:8090-95, 2004.
18. Xu PX et al: Six1 is required for the early organogenesis of mammalian kidney, *Development* 130:3085-94, 2003.
19. Kohlhase J, Wischermann A, Reichenbach H, Froster U, Engel W: Mutations in the SALL1 putative transcription factor gene cause Townes-Brocks syndrome, *Nature Genet* 18:81-83, 1998.
20. Weber S et al: Prevalence of mutations in renal developmental genes in children with renal hypodysplasia: results of the ESCAPE study, *J Am Soc Nephrol* 17:2864-70, 2006.
21. Nishinakamura R et al: Murine homolog of SALL1 is essential for ureteric bud invasion in kidney development, *Development* 128:3105-15, 2001.
22. Schwarz RD, Stephens FD, Cussen LJ: The pathogenesis of renal dyplasia III. Complete and incomplete urinary obstruction, *Invest Urol* 19:101-03,1981.
23. Kume T, Deng K, Hogan BLM: Murine forkhead/winged helix genes Foxc1 (Mf1) and Foxc2 (Mfh1) are required for the early organogenesis of the kidney and urinary tract, *Development* 127:1387-95, 2000.
24. Dziarmaga A, Eccles M, Goodyer P: Suppression of ureteric bud apoptosis rescues nephron endowment and adult renal function in Pax2 mutant mice, *J Am Soc Nephrol* 17:1568-75, 2006.
25. Mendelsohn C, Batourina E, Fung S, Gilbert T, Dodd, J: Stromal cells mediate retinoid-dependent functions essential for renal development, *Development* 126:1139-48, 1999.
26. Batourina E et al: Vitamin A controls epithelial/mesenchymal interactions through Ret expression, *Nature Genet* 27:74-78, 2001.
27. Leliévre-Pégorier M et al: Mild vitamin A deficiency leads to inborn nephron deficit in the rat, *Kidney Int* 54:1455-62, 1998.
28. Nyengaard JR, Bendtsen TF: Glomerular number and size in relation to age, kidney weight, and body surface in normal man, *Anat Rec* 232:194-201, 1992.
29. Fraser FC, Ling D, Clogg D, Nogrady B: Genetic aspects of the BOR syndrome—branchial fistulas, ear pits, hearing loss, and renal anomalies, *Am J Med Genet* 2:241-52, 1978.
30. Melnick M, Bixler D, Silk K, Yune H, Nance WE: Autosomal dominant branchiootorenal dysplasia, *Birth Defects Orig Artic Ser* 11:121-28, 1975.
31. Chen A et al: Phenotypic manifestations of branchio-oto-renal syndrome, *Am J Med Genet* 58:365-70, 1995.
32. Chang EH et al: Branchio-oto-renal syndrome: the mutation spectrum in EYA1 and its phenotypic consequences, *Hum Mutat* 23: 582-89, 2004.
33. Fraser FC, Sproule JR, Halal F: Frequency of the branchio-oto-renal (BOR) syndrome in children with profound hearing loss, *Am J Med Genet* 7: 341-49, 1980.
34. Kumar S et al: Autosomal dominant branchio-oto-renal syndrome—localization of a disease gene to chromosome 8q by linkage in a Dutch family, *Hum Mol Genet* 1:491-95, 1992.
35. Sajithlal G, Zou D, Silvius D, Xu PX: Eya1 acts as a critical regulator for specifying the metanephric mesenchyme, *Dev Biol* 284:323-36, 2005.
36. Vervoort VS et al: Genomic rearrangements of EYA1 account for a large fraction of families with BOR syndrome, *Eur J Hum Genet* 10:757-66, 2002.
37. Weaver RG et al: Optic nerve coloboma associated with renal disease, *Am J Med Genet* 29:597-605, 1988.
38. Fletcher J et al: Multicystic dysplastic kidney and variable phenotype in a family with a novel deletion mutation of PAX2, *J Am Soc Nephrol* 16:2754-61, 2005.
39. Salomon R et al: PAX2 mutations in oligomeganephronia, *Kidney Int* 59:457-62, 2001.
40. Dureau P et al: Renal coloboma syndrome, *Ophthalmology* 108:1912-16, 2001.
41. Parsa CF et al: Redefining papillorenal syndrome: an underdiagnosed cause of ocular and renal morbidity, *Ophthalmology* 108:738-49, 2001.
42. Schimmenti LA et al: Further delineation of renal-coloboma syndrome in patients with extreme variability of phenotype and identical PAX2 mutations, *Am J Hum Genet* 60:869-78, 1997.
43. Eccles MR, Schimmenti LA: Renal-coloboma syndrome: a multi-system developmental disorder caused by PAX2 mutations, *Clin Genet* 56:1-9, 1999.
44. Sanyanusin P et al: Mutation of the *PAX2* gene in a family with optic nerve colobomas, renal anomalies and vesicoureteral reflux, *Nature Genet* 9:358-63, 1995.
45. Coffinier C, Thepot D, Babinet C, Yaniv M, Barra J: Essential role for the homeoprotein vHNF1/HNF1beta in visceral endoderm differentiation, *Development* 126:4785-94, 1999.
46. Kolatsi-Joannou M et al: Hepatocyte nuclear factor-1beta: a new kindred with renal cysts and diabetes and gene expression in normal human development, *J Am Soc Nephrol* 12:2175-80, 2001.
47. Bellanne-Chantelot C et al: Clinical spectrum associated with hepatocyte nuclear factor-1beta mutations, *Ann Intern Med* 140:510-17, 2004.
48. Bellanne-Chantelot C et al: Large genomic rearrangements in the hepatocyte nuclear factor-1beta (TCF2) gene are the most frequent cause of maturity-onset diabetes of the young type 5, *Diabetes* 54:3126-32, 2005.
49. Edghill EL, Bingham C, Ellard S, Hattersley AT: Mutations in hepatocyte nuclear factor-1beta and their related phenotypes, *J Med Genet* 43:84-90, 2006.

50. Ulinski T et al: Renal phenotypes related to hepatocyte nuclear factor-1beta (TCF2) mutations in a pediatric cohort, *J Am Soc Nephrol* 17: 497-503, 2006.
51. Lindner TH et al: A novel syndrome of diabetes mellitus, renal dysfunction and genital malformation associated with a partial deletion of the pseudo-POU domain of hepatocyte nuclear factor-1beta, *Hum Mol Genet* 8:2001-08, 1999.
52. Bingham C et al: Mutations in the hepatocyte nuclear factor-1beta gene are associated with familial hypoplastic glomerulocystic kidney disease, *Am J Hum Genet* 68:219-24, 2001.
53. Bingham C et al: Solitary functioning kidney and diverse genital tract malformations associated with hepatocyte nuclear factor-1beta mutations, *Kidney Int* 61:1243-51, 2002.
54. Rizzoni G et al: Familial hypoplastic glomerulocystic kidney. A new entity? *Clin Nephrol* 18:263-68, 1982.
55. Decramer S et al: Anomalies of the TCF2 gene are the main cause of fetal bilateral hyperechogenic kidneys, *J Am Soc Nephrol,* 2007.
56. Rebouissou S et al: Germline hepatocyte nuclear factor 1alpha and 1beta mutations in renal cell carcinomas, *Hum Mol Genet* 14:603-14, 2005.
57. Kallmann FJ, Schoenfeld WA, Barrera SE: The genetic aspects of primary eunuchoidism, *Am J Ment Defic* 48:303-36, 1944.
58. De Morsier G: Median craioencephalic dysraphias and olfactogenital dysplasia, *World Neurol* 3:485-506, 1962.
59. Tsai PS, Gill JC: Mechanisms of disease: Insights into X-linked and autosomal-dominant Kallmann syndrome, *Nat Clin Pract Endocrinol Metab* 2:160-71, 2006.
60. Naftolin F, Harris GW, Bobrow M: Effect of purified luteinizing hormone releasing factor on normal and hypogonadotrophic anosmic men, *Nature* 232:496-97, 1971.
61. Schwanzel-Fukuda M, Bick D, Pfaff DWL: Luteinizing hormone-releasing hormone (LHRH)-expressing cells do not migrate normally in an inherited hypogonadal (Kallmann) syndrome, *Brain Res Mol Brain Res* 6:311-26, 1989.
62. Dode C et al: Loss-of-function mutations in FGFR1 cause autosomal dominant Kallmann syndrome, *Nat Genet* 33: 463-65, 2003.
63. Dode C et al: Kallmann syndrome: mutations in the genes encoding prokineticin-2 and prokineticin receptor-2, *PLoS Genet* 2:e175, 2006.
64. Dode C et al: Novel FGFR1 sequence variants in Kallmann syndrome, and genetic evidence that the FGFR1c isoform is required in olfactory bulb and palate morphogenesis, *Hum Mutat* 28:97-98, 2007.
65. Townes PL, Brocks ER: Hereditary syndrome of imperforate anus with hand, foot, and ear anomalies, *J Pediatr* 81:321-26, 1972.
66. O'Callaghan M, Young ID: The Townes-Brocks syndrome, *J Med Genet* 27:457-61, 1990.
67. Kurnit DM, Steele MW, Pinsky L, Dibbins A: Autosomal dominant transmission of a syndrome of anal, ear, renal, and radial congenital malformations, *J Pediatr* 93:270-73, 1978.
68. Allanson JE, Hunter AG, Mettler GS, Jimenez C: Renal tubular dysgenesis: a not uncommon autosomal recessive syndrome: a review, *Am J Med Genet* 43:811-14, 1992.
69. McFadden DE, Pantzar JT, Van Allen MI, Langlois S: Renal tubular dysgenesis with calvarial hypoplasia: report of two additional cases and review, *J Med Genet* 34:846-48, 1997.
70. Kumar D, Moss G, Primhak R, Coombs R: Congenital renal tubular dysplasia and skull ossification defects similar to teratogenic effects of angiotensin converting enzyme (ACE) inhibitors, *J Med Genet* 34:541-55, 1997.
71. Mahieu-Caputo D et al: Twin-to-twin transfusion syndrome. Role of the fetal renin-angiotensin system, *Am J Pathol* 156:629-36, 2000.
72. Barr M, Jr, Cohen MM, Jr: ACE inhibitor fetopathy and hypocalvaria: the kidney-skull connection, *Teratology* 44:485-95, 1991.
73. Gribouval O et al: Mutations in genes in the renin-angiotensin system are associated with autosomal recessive renal tubular dysgenesis, *Nat Genet* 37:964-68, 2005.
74. Bueva A, Guignard JP: Renal function in preterm neonates, *Pediatr Res* 36:572-77, 1994.
75. Krzemien G, Roszkowska-Blaim M, Kostro I et al: Urological anomolies in children with renal agenesis of multicystic dysplastic kidney, *J Appl Genet* 46:171, 2006.
76. Shibata S, Nagata M: Pathogenesis of human renal dysplasia: an alternative scenario to the major theories, *Pediatr Int* 45:605-09, 2003.
77. Kuwertz-Broeking E, Brinkmann OA, Von Lengerke HJ et al: Unilateral multicystic dysplastic kidney experience in children, *BJU Int* 93:388, 2004.
78. D'Alberton A, Reschini E, Ferrari N, Candiani P: Prevalence of urinary tract abnormalities in a large series of patients with uterovaginal atresia, *J Urol* 126:623-24, 1981.
79. Fedele L, Bianchi S, Agnoli B, Tozzi L, Vignali M: Urinary tract anomalies associated with unicornuate uterus, *J Urol* 155:847-48, 1996.
80. Raj GV, Auge BK, Assimos D, Preminger GM: Metabolic abnormalities associated with renal calculi in patients with horseshoe kidneys, *J Endourol* 18:157-61, 2004.
81. Oda T et al: Mutations in the human Jagged1 gene are responsible for Alagille syndrome, *Nature Genet* 16:235-42, 1997.
82. Wilkie AOM et al: Apert syndrome results from localised mutations of FGFR2 and is allelic with Crouzon syndrome, *Nature Genet* 9:165-72, 1996.
83. Hatada I et al: An imprinted gene p57KIP2 is mutated in Beckwith-Wiedemann syndrome, *Nat Genet* 14:171-73, 1996.
84. Wagner T et al: Autosomal sex reversal and compomelic dysplasia are caused by mutations in and around the SRY-related gene SOX9, *Cell* 79:1111-20, 1994.
85. Houston CS et al: The Campomelic syndrome: review, report of 17 cases and follow-up on the currently 17-year-old boy first reported by Maroteaux et al in 1971, *Am J Med Genet* 15:3-28, 1998.
86. Sakaki-Yumoto M et al: The murine homolog of SALL4, a causative gene in Okihiro syndrome, is essential for embryonic stem cell proliferation, and cooperates with Sall1 in anorectal, heart, brain and kidney development, *Development* 133:3005-13, 2006.
87. McGregor L et al: Fraser syndrome and mouse blebbed phenotype caused by mutations in FRAS1/Fras1 encoding a putative extracellular matrix protein, *Nat Genet* 34:203-08, 2003.
88. Van Esch H et al: GATA3 haplo-insufficiency causes human HDR syndrome, *Nature* 406:419-22, 2000.
89. Franco B et al: A gene deleted in Kallmann's syndrome shares homology with neural cell adhesion and axonal path-finding molecules, *Nature* 353:529-36, 1991.
90. Bamshad M et al: Mutations in human TBX3 alter limb, apocrine and genital development in ulnar-mammary syndrome, *Nat Genet* 16:311-15, 1997.
91. Bohn S et al: Distinct molecular and morphogenetic properties of mutations in the human HNF1beta gene that lead to defective kidney development, *J Am Soc Nephrol* 14:2033-41, 2003.
92. Pilia G et al: Mutations in GPC3, a glypican gene, cause the Simpson-Golabi-Behmel overgrowth syndrome, *Nature Genet* 12:241-47, 1996.
93. Tint GS et al: Defective cholesterol biosynthesis associated with the Smith-Lemli-Opitz Syndrome, *N Engl J Med* 330:107-13, 1994.
94. Preuss N et al: PEX1 mutations in complementation group 1 of Zellweger spectrum patients correlate with severity of disease, *Pediatr Res* 51:706-14, 2002.

CHAPTER

8 Nephronophthisis and Medullary Cystic Kidney Disease

Heymut Omran and Beate Ermisch-Omran

THE NEPHRONOPHTHISIS/MEDULLARY CYSTIC DISEASE COMPLEX

The nephronophthisis complex comprises a genetically heterogenous group of renal cystic disorders that have an autosomal recessive inheritance pattern. The term *autosomal dominant medullary cystic kidney disease* (MCKD) has been used for a disease indistinguishable by pathological means from recessive juvenile nephronophthisis.[1,2] Initially, besides the different inheritance pattern, the main discriminating feature between recessive and dominant disease conditions was thought to be a different age of onset for terminal renal failure. However, renal failure may also occur in recessive disease variants during late adulthood. Because of their morphological similarities, the term *nephronophthisis/medullary cystic disease complex* has been used to summarize this group of diseases.[3]

NEPHRONOPHTHISIS

Fanconi et al. introduced the term *familial juvenile nephronophthisis* to describe a disease characterized by autosomal recessive inheritance, a defect in urinary concentrating capacity, severe anemia, and progressive renal failure that leads to death before puberty.[4,5] Renal histology is characterized by disintegrated tubular basement membranes, tubular atrophy and cyst formation, and a sclerosing tubulointerstitial nephropathy (Figure 8-1).[6,7] Corticomedullary cysts occur late in the disease process[8] and are only a facultative finding (Figure 8-2). Thus, although nephronophthisis has been referred to as cystic kidney disorder, cysts are not a hallmark of the disease.

Nephronophthisis can be associated with extrarenal disease manifestations including ocular motor apraxia, retinitis pigmentosa, Leber congenital amaurosis, coloboma of the optic nerve, cerebellar vermis aplasia, liver fibrosis, cranioectodermal dysplasia, cone-shaped epiphyses, asphyxiating thoracic dysplasia (Jeune's syndrome), Ellis-van Creveld syndrome, and rarely *situs inversus*.[9,10] These extrarenal disease manifestations are not encountered in dominant MCKD and may help direct genetic testing. Several genes involved in the pathogenesis of nephronophthisis have been identified to date that are responsible for infantile (type 2, *NPHP2*), juvenile (type 1, *NPHP1*; type 4, *NPHP4*; type 5, *NPHP5*; type 6, *NPHP6*; Joubert syndrome; and *AHI1*), and adolescent (type 3, *NPHP3*) forms differing in the onset of end-stage renal disease.[10-19] The clinical course and renal phenotype are similar in most forms of nephronophthisis, which are referred to here as "classical nephronophthisis" variants. The only exception is infantile nephronophthisis (nephronophthisis type 2), which is characterized by a distinct clinical course and pathology and is therefore addressed separately in this chapter. Clinical and diagnostic findings of the various nephronophthisis variants are summarized in Table 8-1.

Extrarenal Disease Manifestations

Senior-Løken Syndrome

Senior-Løken syndrome refers to the association of nephronophthisis and retinal degeneration.[20,21] Two variants of retinal disorders have been described. Leber congenital amaurosis, the most severe variant, is a clinically and genetically heterogeneous retinal disorder that occurs in infancy and is accompanied by profound visual loss, nystagmus, poor pupillary reflexes, and either a normal retina or varying degrees of atrophy and pigmentary changes.[22-24] The electroretinogram is extinguished or severely reduced.[25] Leber congenital amaurosis is inherited as an autosomal recessive trait and several genetic defects have been identified in isolated cases.

A milder variant also associated with nephronophthisis is referred to as tapetoretinal degeneration. Usually patients suffer from severe tubelike restriction of visual fields and night blindness. Funduscopy reveals various degrees of atrophic and pigmentary retinal alterations.

Joubert Syndrome

Joubert syndrome is an autosomal recessive disorder clinically characterized by muscular hypotonia evolving into cerebellar ataxia, mental retardation, abnormal neonatal breathing pattern (alternating tachypnea and/or apnea), and/or unusual eye movements. The abnormal eye movements often comprise oculomotor apraxia or difficulty with smooth eye pursuits and horizontal saccades, with jerking head thrusting and nystagmus.[26] Joubert syndrome is characterized by the molar tooth sign, a distinctive radiological finding that reflects a complex malformation of the midbrain and hindbrain, consisting of increased interpeduncular distance at the

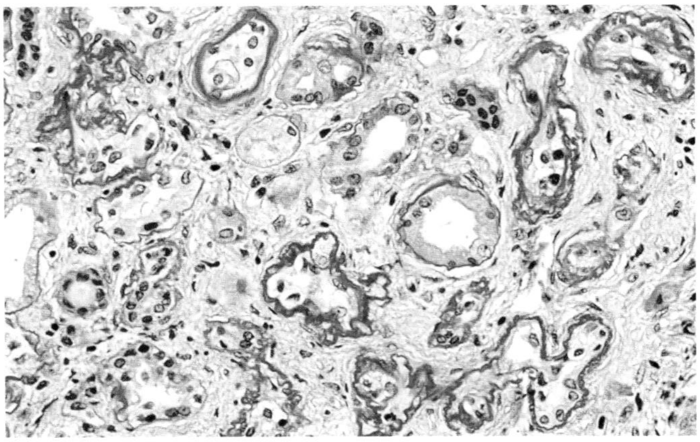

Figure 8-1 PAS-stained renal biopsy specimen depicting characteristic findings of "classical nephronophthisis" comprising tubular basement alterations with irregular thickening and thinning, tubular atrophy, and cystic dilatation of tubules.

pontomesencephalic junction, cerebellar vermis hypoplasia, and thickened, straight, and elongated superior cerebellar peduncles that resemble a molar tooth on axial magnetic resonance imaging (Figure 8-3).[27]

Cogan Syndrome

Congenital ocular motor apraxia type Cogan is characterized by impairment of horizontal voluntary eye movements, ocular attraction movements, and optokinetic nystagmus.[28] Compensation for the defective horizontal eye movements is accomplished through jerky movements of the head. The disease is not progressive, and older patients may be able to compensate by an overshooting thrust of the eyeballs rather than by head jerks. The condition can improve with age.

RHYNS Syndrome

Hedera and Gorski[29] reported two brothers with retinitis pigmentosa, growth hormone deficiency, and acromelic

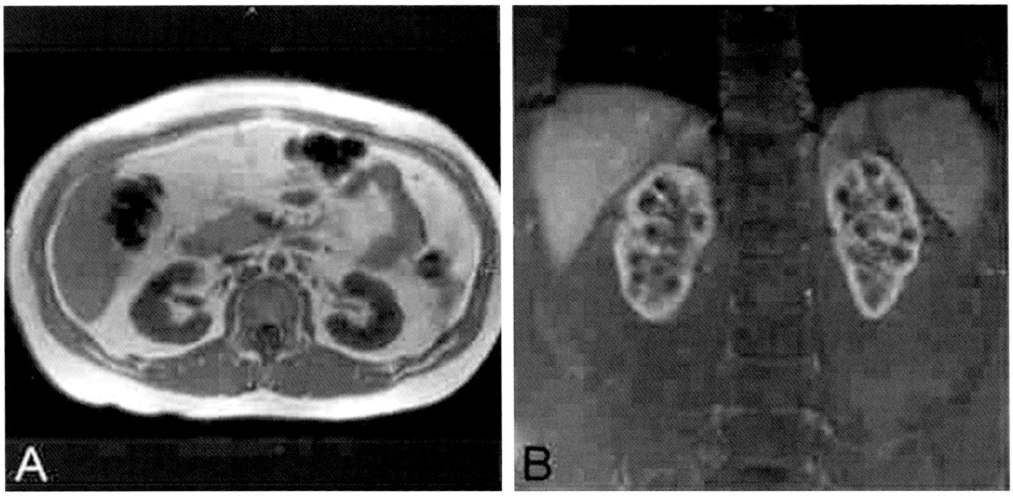

Figure 8-2 Magnetic resonance tomography findings of the kidneys in a patient with nephronophthisis type 1. Note the prominent cysts at the corticomedullary junction on axial **(A)** and coronal **(B)** images.

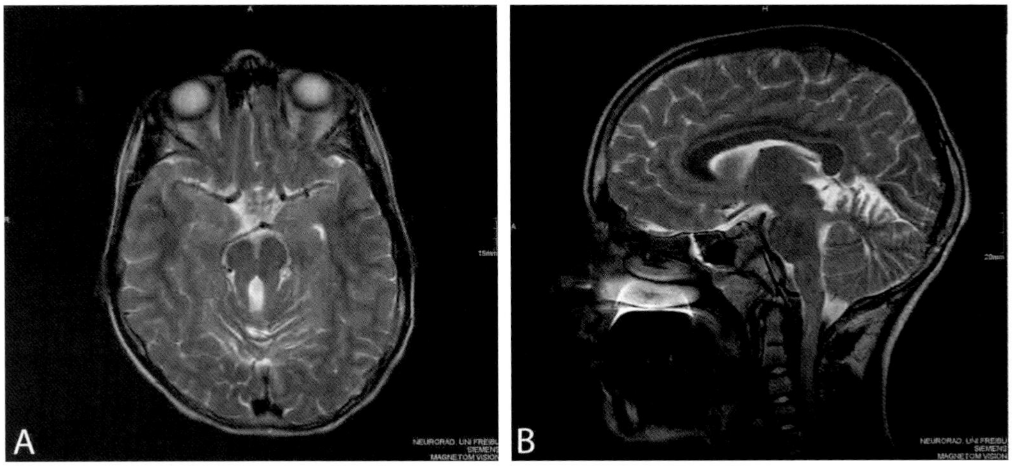

Figure 8-3 Cranial magnetic resonance tomography findings in a patient with Joubert syndrome. **A,** Axial T2-weighted image at the pontine level shows thickened superior cerebellar peduncles and umbrella-shaped fourth ventricle, giving the appearance of a molar tooth. **B,** Sagittal T2-weighted image demonstrates prominent superior cerebellar peduncles running horizontally toward the brain stem and cerebellar atrophy.

TABLE 8-1 **Clinical and Diagnostic Findings in Genetically Characterized Nephronophthisisis Variants (Autosomal Recessive Inheritance)**

					NEPHRONOPHTHISIS ASSOCIATED WITH EXTRARENAL MANIFESTATIONS							
Nephronophthisis Variants (Genes and Loci)	**Age at ESRD (Years)**	**Histology**	**Pathology**	**Isolated NPHP**	**Joubert Syndrome**	**Severe Retinal Degeneration**	**Tapeto-Retinal Degeneration**	**Cogan Syndrome**	**Liver Fibrosis**	**Situs Inversus**	**Other Symptoms**	**Isolated Joubert Syndrome**
NPHP1/JBTS4 (2q12-q13)	7-29 (median 13)	TIN,TBM, TA,TCD	≤ kidneys CMC +/–	Yes	Yes	No	Yes	Yes	No	No	No	No
NPHP3 (3q21-q22)	11-47 (median 19)	TIN,TBM, TA,TCD	≤ kidneys CMC +/–	Yes	No	No	Yes	No	Yes	No	No	No
NPHP4 (1p36)	6-35	TIN,TBM, TA,TCD	≤ kidneys CMC +/–	Yes	No	Yes	Yes	Yes	No	No	No	No
NPHP5 (3q21)	6-32 (median 15)	TIN,TBM, TA,TCD	≤ kidneys CMC +/–	No	No	Yes	No	No	No	No	No	No
NPHP6/JBTS5 (12q21)	5-17 (median 12)	TIN,TBM, TA,TCD	≤ kidneys CMC +/–	No	Yes	Yes	Yes	No	No	No	Microphthalmos, elevated liver enzymes	Yes
JBTS1 (9q34)	Not known	Not known	Not known	No	Not known	No	No	No	No	No	No	Yes
JBTS2 (11p11-q12)	15-17	TIN,TBM, TA,TCD	≤ kidneys CMC +/–	No	Yes	No	No	Yes	No	No	Bilateral ptosis, strabismus	Yes
JBTS3/AHI1 (6q23)	>16	TIN,TBM, TA,TCD	≤ kidneys CMC +/–	No	Yes	No	Yes	No	No	No	Polymicrogyria, coloboma	Yes
NPHP2/INV (9q22-q31)	1-5	TIN, cortical microcysts	Enlarged kidneys	Yes	No	Yes	No	No	No	Yes	Ventricular septal defect	No

CMC, Cysts predominantly located at the corticomedullary junction; *ESRD,* end-stage renal disease; ≤ *kidneys,* small or normal size; *TA,* tubular atrophy; *TBM,* tubular basement membrane alterations; *TCD,* tubular cystic dilatation; *TIN,* tubulointerstital nephropathy.

skeletal dysplasia. They proposed for this clinical picture the acronym RHYNS (retinitis pigmentosa, hypopituitarism, nephronophthisis, and skeletal dysplasia). They assumed an autosomal recessive mode of inheritance. However, since all four known cases were male, an X-linked mode of inheritance cannot be excluded.

Mainzer-Saldino Syndrome

The association of cone-shaped phalangeal epiphyses and nephronophthisis has been referred to as Mainzer-Saldino syndrome.[30,31] Many of those affected had additional retinitis pigmentosa and some had ataxia and hepatic fibrosis.[32,33]

Boichis Disease

The association of nephronophthisis and hepatic fibrosis has been referred to as Boichis disease. Other associated findings are retinal degeneration.[34-36]

Nephronophthisis Variants

Nephronophthisis Type I (NPHP I)

Genetics and Etiology In juvenile nephronophthisis the responsible gene *(NPHP1)*, which is localized on chromosome 2q12-q13,[37-38] has been identified by positional cloning.[11,12] Large homozygous deletions of this gene are a major cause of juvenile nephronophthisis.[39] Nephronophthisis type 1 (OMIM #256100) accounts for 27% to 62% of nephronophthisis cases and is one of the most frequent genetic causes of end-stage renal disease in children and young adults.[40,41] In the majority (94%) of NPHP1 patients, large homozygous deletions of approximately 290 kb involving the *NPHP1* locus (on chromosome 2q12-q13) can be detected, whereas only some patients carry point mutations in combination with a heterozygous deletion.[40] *NPHP1* encodes nephrocystin, a 733-amino-acid protein with an N-terminal coiled-coil domain, an adjacent Src homology 3 (SH3) domain flanked by two highly acidic E-rich domains, and a conserved nephrocystin homology domain that encompasses the C-terminal two thirds of the protein.[11,12] A number of protein interaction partners, including $p130^{CAS}$, proline-rich tyrosine kinase 2 (Pyk2), and tensin, have been identified that are supposed to function in focal adhesion complexes or at sites of cell-cell contact in polarized MDCK cells.[42,43] In addition, the proteins involved in nephronophthisis types 2, 3, and 4 have been shown to associate with nephrocystin, suggesting assembly into a large multiprotein complex.[10,14,15,44] Recent findings suggest that this protein complex is localized at the ciliary base (transition zone) and plays a functional role in motile (e.g., respiratory cilia) and immotile cilia (e.g., renal monocilia, connecting cilia of the photoreceptor).[45,46] Interestingly this expression can be used to demonstrate nephrocystin deficiency in patients with *NPHP1* deletions through an analysis of ciliated nasal respiratory cells obtained by simple, noninvasive nasal brushings (Figure 8-4).[46]

Clinical Features Life table analysis for juvenile nephronophthisis indicates that terminal renal failure is reached between as early as 7 to at least 29 years of age. In the latter patient, however, end-stage renal disease did not occur during the observation period. Thus it is still conceivable that a few individuals with homozygous *NPHP1* deletions do not experience renal failure at all. However, the median age of onset of terminal renal failure was 13.1 years (quartiles are 75%, 17.3 years; 25%, 11.3 years).[47] Recently Bollee et al. (2006) confirmed that *NPHP1* mutations can not only cause renal failure during childhood but also during adulthood.[48] They reported four adults with chronic renal failure at ages 19, 22, 22, and 25, respectively. It is important to note that renal imaging revealed no (n = 2) or only one (n = 2) cortical cyst. Therefore cysts at the corticomedullary junction are not an obligatory finding in juvenile nephronophthisis. Other clinical manifestations such as polyuria and secondary enuresis might be a hint for the diagnosis but are only facultative findings in the disease. Proteinuria and hypertension are not typically found in nephronophthisis. However, these symptoms might develop especially when renal function deteriorates. In the four patients reported by Bollee et al.,[48] proteinuria ranged from 0.2 g to 1.6 g per day. So far no recurrence of the disease has been reported following renal transplantation.

The most common extrarenal disease manifestation in patients with juvenile nephronophthisis is tapetoretinal degeneration. It is usually a milder type of retinitis pigmentosa. Some patients may not even complain of any symptoms, although specific retinal changes can be detected by a funduscopic ophthalmologic examination. Other extrarenal manifestations such as cerebellar ataxia with vermis aplasia and mental retardation (Joubert syndrome) and ocular motor apraxia type Cogan (Cogan syndrome) have been reported only in rare, individual cases.[26,49]

Nephronophthisis Type 3

Genetics and Etiology Based on clinical symptoms, renal pathology, and genetic findings in a large consanguineous 340-member Venezuelan kindred, a new distinct disease variant, adolescent nephronophthisis, was identified.[50] A total genome scan of linkage analysis was conducted, and a gene locus for adolescent nephronophthisis was localized to a region of homozygosity by descent on chromosome 3q within a critical genetic interval of 2.4 cM.[50] Fluorescence in situ hybridization experiments refined the chromosomal assignment of nephronophthisis type 3 *(NPHP3)* to chromosome 3q21-q22.[51]

Synteny between the human *NPHP3* locus on chromosome 3q and the *pcy* locus on mouse chromosome 9 has been demonstrated by human-mouse synteny analysis based on expressed genes, providing the first evidence of synteny between a human and a spontaneous murine renal cystic disease.[51] Renal pathology observed in the recessive *pcy* mouse model of late-onset polycystic kidney disease comprised tubular basement membrane changes, tubular atrophy and dilatation, and sclerosing tubulointerstitial nephropathy, as well as renal cyst development at the corticomedullary junction resembling human adolescent nephronophthisis.[51] Demonstration of synteny suggested that both diseases are caused by recessive mutations of homologous genes.

Additional linkage analyses showed that some families with Senior-Løken syndrome also inherited the disease through a mutated gene residing in the same chromosomal region.[52] Subsequently, recessive mutations in the *NPHP3* gene were identified in patients with adolescent nephro-

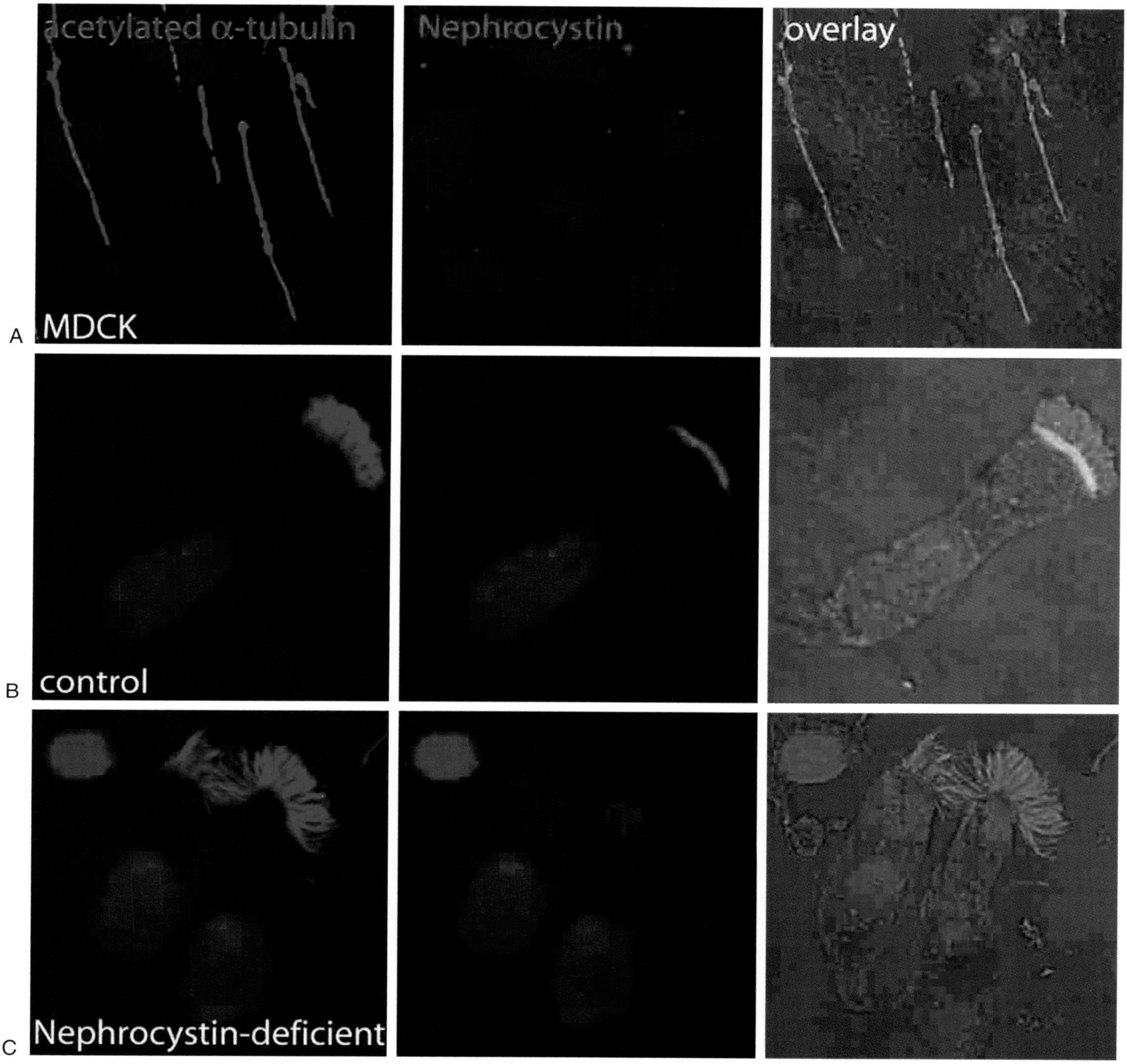

Figure 8-4 High-resolution immunofluorescence microscopy of Madin-Darby canine kidney (MDCK) cells and human respiratory cells. Nuclei are stained blue. **A,** Renal monocilia of MDCK cells are stained with α-tubulin (green). Nephrocystin (red) specifically localizes to the ciliary transition zone at the ciliary base. **B,** Motile respiratory cilia of control cells are stained with α-tubulin (green). Nephrocystin (red) also specifically localizes to the ciliary transition zone at the ciliary base. **C,** In respiratory cells of nephronophthisis patients with homozygous *NPHP1* deletions, nephrocystin is absent from the entire cell. Microscope settings of the red channel were adjusted to visualize background staining.

nophthisis.[15] *NPHP3* encodes a novel 1330-amino-acid protein, which interacts with nephrocystin. In the adult kidney, specific gene expression in distal tubules located at the corticomedullary border was observed, which corresponds to the site of cyst formation in adolescent nephronophthisis. Expression in retina and liver is in agreement with associated tapetoretinal degeneration or hepatic fibrosis in patients carrying *NPHP3* mutations. In addition, a homozygous missense mutation in *Nphp3* was found to be most likely responsible for the polycystic kidney disease *(pcy)* mouse phenotype.[15]

Clinical Features Onset of terminal renal failure occurs in adolescent nephronophthisis significantly later (median 19 years, quartile borders 16.0 and 25.0 years) than in juvenile nephronophthisis.[50] Clinical signs of adolescent nephronophthisis consist of renal symptoms such as polyuria, polydipsia, secondary enuresis, severe anemia, and progressive renal failure.[50] Renal morphology is characterized by cysts at the corticomedullary junction. Renal histology shows the characteristic triad of irregularly thickened tubular basement membranes, atrophy and dilatation of tubules, and sclerosing tubulointerstitial nephropathy.[50]

In some patients with adolescent nephronophthisis carrying *NPHP3* mutations, extrarenal disease manifestations such as tapetoretinal degeneration or hepatic fibrosis have been reported.[15]

Nephronophthisis Type 4

Genetics and Etiology Schuermann et al. (2002) localized a gene locus for nephronophthisis type 4 *(NPHP4)* to chromosome 1p36 using a homozygosity mapping strategy in a large consanguineous pedigree of German ancestry.[53] After reduction of the critical genetic interval, recessive mutations in the *NPHP4* gene were identified.[13,14] *NPHP4* is a 30-exon gene with one untranslated first exon and encodes a protein that has been referred to as nephrocystin-4 and nephroretinin.[13,14] Mutational analysis in a large cohort of 250 unrelated patients with nephronophthisis, Cogan syndrome, or Senior-Løken syndrome identified in only six families (2.4%) biallelic mutations, indicating that *NPHP4* mutations are only responsible for a small number of nephronophthisis cases. Based on similar mutational phenotypes, interaction of nephrocystin-4 with nephrocystin was suspected and confirmed, indicating that both proteins function in the same signaling pathway.[14] Consistent with these findings, nephrocystin-4/nephrocystin has been recently sublocalized to identical subcellular compartments (cilia and centrosomes).[44] In addition, expression and phenotype analysis of the nephrocystin-1 and nephrocystin-4 homologs in *Caenorhabditis elegans* revealed redundant phenotypes suggestive of a distinct role in sensory cilia.[54-56]

Clinical Features In most patients reported thus far with *NPHP4* mutations, no extrarenal disease manifestation has been documented. In a study where eight families with *NPHP4* mutations were reported, associated retinal disease was present in only two families.[13] In one family the three affected individuals suffered from the most severe variant of retinal disease (Leber congenital amaurosis). End-stage renal disease was reached at 6 to 35 years of age (median 22 years). In another study reporting eight families with *NPHP4* mutations, end-stage renal disease occurred at a mean age of 12.7 years (range 6 to 20 years). Interestingly, three affected siblings from one family had Cogan syndrome, characterized by defective or absent horizontal voluntary eye movements. Lesions located in the frontal oculogyric center as well as vermis cerebellar hypoplasia were associated with this syndrome.[14] Retinal degeneration was not reported in these families.[14] Screening of a large cohort of nephronophthisis cases identified an individual with associated Usher syndrome (retinal degeneration and sensory hearing deficit).[41] The histological picture shows the same characteristic features as those known for classical nephronophthisis variants. To date, no recurrence of the renal disease has been reported in renal transplants.[57]

Nephronophthisis Type 5

Genetics and Etiology Using a homozygosity mapping strategy in a consanguineous kindred from Turkey with three children exhibiting the typical clinical features of Senior-Løken syndrome, a novel gene locus distinct from the *NPHP3* locus on chromosome 3q21.1 was found.[16] Truncating mutations in a novel protein with "IQ calmodulin binding domains" were identified. No missense mutations were observed. The nephronophthisis type 5 *(NPHP5)* gene spans 65 kb and consists of 15 exons. Like other nephrocystin proteins, nephrocystin-5 was also localized to primary cilia. In addition, nephrocystin-5 was found to specifically localize to connecting cilia of photoreceptor cells, where it interacts with RPGR and the Ca^{2+}-binding protein calmodulin.[16]

Clinical Features *NPHP5* mutations have so far been detected only in patients with Senior-Løken syndrome with early severe retinal degeneration (Leber congenital amaurosis). Thus nephronophthisis patients without any early retinal disease should not be screened for *NPHP5* mutations. In 21 patients with *NPHP5* mutations, end-stage renal disease ranged between 6 and 32 years (median 15 years).

Nephronophthisis Type 6

Genetics and Etiology Using genetic mapping and positional candidate strategy in a newly identified mouse mutant "rd16," an in-frame deletion in a novel centrosomal protein CEP290 leading to early-onset retinal degeneration was identified.[58] In parallel, recessive mutations in the 55-exon *CEP290*, also referred to as the *NPHP6* (nephronophthisis type 6) gene, located on chromosome 12q21 were identified in five families with variable neurological, retinal, and renal manifestations.[19,59] *CEP290* expression was detected mostly in proliferating cerebellar granule neuron populations and showed centrosome and ciliary localization, linking Joubert syndrome–related and retinal disorders to other human ciliopathies. CEP290 interacts with and modulates the activity of ATF4, a transcription factor implicated in cAMP-dependent renal cyst formation.[19] In addition, abrogation of its function in zebrafish recapitulates the renal, retinal, and cerebellar phenotypes of Joubert syndrome.[19]

Clinical Features The phenotype associated with *CEP290* mutations is mainly characterized by the neurological and neuroradiological features of Joubert syndrome associated with severe retinal and renal involvement.[19,59] All examined patients suffered from Joubert syndrome and congenital blindness or other forms of early retinitis pigmentosa. Two patients had associated renal involvement due to nephronophthisis manifesting at 15 and 17 years of age.[59] Two younger patients had abnormal renal sonography with demonstration of cortical renal cysts and/or reduced cortico-medullary differentiation. Other rare clinical findings included microphthalmos and elevated liver enzymes.[59] In a larger patient series (n = 12), end-stage renal disease was reached at a median age of 12 years but occurred as early as 5 years of age.[19]

Various Types of Joubert Syndrome

Joubert Syndrome Type I

Genetics and Etiology Upon applying a homozygosity mapping strategy, a gene locus for Joubert syndrome type 1 *(JBTS1)* was localized to chromosome 9q34.[60] However, the responsible gene has not yet been identified.

Clinical Features Saar et al. (1999) reported two families with linkage to the *JBTS1* locus.[60] All four affected children from the first family had hypotonia and severe developmental delay (motor and mental retardation), and two of them had ataxia. All four had oculomotor abnormalities from early infancy and jerky eye movements with impairment of smooth pursuit and saccades. On neuroimaging, the patients had absent posterior lobe of vermis, with a small and deformed anterior lobe. Breathing patterns in the neonatal period were normal. The two affected children from the other family showed, in infancy, abnormal jerky eye movements and impairment of smooth pursuit and saccades. Both affected children were severely retarded and hypotonic. Neuroimaging revealed absent posterior lobe of vermis, with a small and deformed anterior lobe. No comments regarding renal involvement were given.

Joubert Syndrome Type 2

Genetics and Etiology In a large consanguineous family with Joubert syndrome and nephronophthisis, a gene locus referred to as *JBST2* (Joubert syndrome type 2) has been mapped to the pericentromeric region of chromosome 11 (11p11.2-q12.3).[61] Gene identification is under way.

Clinical Features All four patients reported by Valente et al.[61] had nystagmus and ocular motor apraxia, with impairment of smooth pursuit and saccades. One patient also had bilateral ptosis and strabismus. Neonatal irregular breathing was not reported. Head circumference was within normal values and no dysmorphic features were present. All patients had developmental delay and moderate-to-severe psychomotor retardation, hypotonia with well-preserved deep tendon reflexes, and truncal ataxia. Magnetic resonance imaging of the brain revealed cerebellar vermian aplasia and the molar tooth sign. Two of four affected children developed chronic renal failure at the respective ages of 15 and 17 years. Clinical history (polyuria and polydipsia) and histology were consistent with classical nephronophthisis. Renal sonography revealed increased echogenicity and normal corticomedullary differentiation. No renal cysts were noted.[61]

Joubert Syndrome Type 3

Genetics and Etiology In several families with Joubert syndrome, some with cortical polymicrogyria recessive frameshift and missense mutations in the *AHI1* gene were identified.[17,62] *AHI1* is located on chromosome 6q23 within the Joubert syndrome type 3 *(JBTS3)* locus and consists of 31 exons, encoding the Jouberin protein. Screening of 117 Joubert syndrome patients revealed mutations in only 15% of cases.[63] Jouberin is an alternatively spliced signaling molecule that contains seven Trp-Asp (WD) repeats, an SH3 domain, and numerous SH3-binding sites. The gene is expressed strongly in embryonic hindbrain and forebrain, suggesting that AHI1 is required for both cerebellar and cortical development.[17]

Clinical Features In addition to classical findings of Joubert syndome, some patients with *AHI1* mutations had retinal degeneration, polymicrogyria, and coloboma.[17,18,63] Renal involvement (nephronophthisis) occurred in only a subset of these patients but may have been severe enough to cause renal failure.[18,63] One patient reached end-stage renal disease at age 16, and two patients beyond age 20. It is important to note that most patients with *AHI1* mutations are still too young to determine whether or not they might develop renal failure.

Joubert Syndrome Type 4

Because mutations of the *NPHP1* gene are also a rare cause of Joubert syndrome, as explained previously, the *NPHP1* gene has also been referred to as *JBTS4* (Joubert syndrome type 4). Screening of 117 Joubert syndrome patients revealed mutations in *NPHP1* in just 2% of cases, indicating that *NPHP1* is only a minor contributor in the pathogenesis of this disorder.[63]

Joubert Syndrome Type 5

Because mutations of the *NPHP6 (CEP290)* gene cause obligatory Joubert syndrome, as mentioned earlier, the *NPHP6* gene has been also referred to as *JBTS5* (Joubert syndrome type 5).

Infantile Nephronophthisis (Nephronophthisis Type 2)

Genetics and Etiology

The *inv* mouse model features multiorgan defects including renal cysts, altered left-right laterality, and hepatobiliary duct malformations transmitted in an autosomal recessive manner. The respective gene was identified and is referred to as *inv* encoding inversin.[64,65] Affected mice usually die of renal and liver failure in early postnatal life. Because the clinical phenotype of *inv* mice resembles that of infantile nephronophthisis, candidate gene analysis was performed in the human orthologous gene called *INV* or *NPHP2*. In addition, the human *NPHP2* gene mapped exactly to chromosomal site (9q22-q31), where previously a gene locus for infantile nephronophthisis was localized.[66] Indeed, subsequently in a small number of patients with infantile nephronophthisis with and without *situs inversus*, mutations in the 16-exon *NPHP2* gene were identified.[10] Localization to renal monocilia and demonstration of interaction of nephrocystin and inversin strongly indicate that both proteins function in a large multiprotein complex. Recent findings indicate that inversin functions as a switch between distinct Wnt signaling pathways.[67]

Clinical Features

Infantile nephronophthisis differs from classical nephronophthisis variants in many respects. Infantile nephronophthisis (NPHP2, OMIM # 602088) is characterized by an early disease onset that might start before birth or in early infancy. Infantile nephronophthisis leads to terminal renal failure within the first five years of life.[10,66,68,69] Whereas kidney size in classical nephronophthisis variants is normal or small, in infantile nephronophthisis the kidneys are typically enlarged. Patients often suffer from hypertension and may show acute renal failure. In patients with *NPHP2* mutations, end-stage renal disease was reached between the first and fifth year of life. Interestingly, one patient had associated *situs inversus* and ventricular septal defect of the heart. Another patient with homzygous *NPHP2* mutations suffered from retinitis pigmentosa already present at the age of 2.[70]

Morphologically this type of hereditary tubulointerstitial nephropathy differs from juvenile nephronophthisis by the presence of cortical microcysts and by the absence of medullary cysts and typical tubular basement membrane changes.[69]

Etiology of Cyst Formation in Nephronophthisis

Cilia Hypothesis

Cilia dysfunction has been implicated in diverse human disorders.[71] Various cystic kidney disorders are associated with dysfunction of renal monocilia (see Chapter 9), which are localized on the epithelial surface of nephron segments where they extend into the lumen of the kidney tubules and possibly act as fluid flow or chemosensors.[72,73] Proteins involved in renal monocilia function include the ciliary proteins polycystin-1, polycystin-2, and fibrocystin (mutated in autosomal dominant and autosomal recessive polycystic kidney disease, respectively), as well as various BBS proteins mutated in Bardet-Biedl syndrome, which localize to the basal bodies of cilia.[74] Furthermore, as outlined in this paragraph, all nephrocystin proteins analyzed thus far localize either to cilia or the ciliary base, indicating that cilia function is essential in preserving renal architecture and integrity (Figure 8-4).[75]

Recent molecular findings indicate that disruption of BBS proteins perturbs planar cell polarity in vertebrates[76] and that altered regulation of Wnt signaling contributes to cystic kidney disease.[67]

MEDULLARY CYSTIC KIDNEY DISEASE

Medullary cystic kidney disease (MCKD) is a progressive tubulointerstitial nephropathy with autosomal dominant inheritance that leads to end-stage renal disease in late adulthood.[3] Two loci for the autosomal dominant disease, MCKD1 on chromosome 1q[77] and MCKD2 on chromosome 16p[78] have been reported. Clinical symptoms are similar in both MCKD variants. Small corticomedullary cysts may develop over the course of the disease but are not a prerequisite for the diagnosis. Kidney size is normal or slightly reduced. Renal histological findings include tubular basement membrane disintegration, tubular atrophy with cyst development, and interstitial round cell infiltration associated with fibrosis, all of which resemble the findings observed in classical nephronophthisis (Figure 8-1). Thus imaging and histological findings cannot confirm diagnosis, and analysis of the clinical and pedigree data is mandatory to establish correct diagnosis. Clinical and diagnostic findings are summarized in Table 8-2.

Medullary Cystic Kidney Disease Type I

Genetics and Etiology

In a large Cypriotic kindred the *MCKD1* locus was mapped to chromosome 1q21-q23.1.[77] Detailed mutational analyses in 23 kindreds showing evidence for linkage to the *MCDK1* locus has not yet identified the responsible gene.[79]

Clinical Features

Six large Cypriot families including 186 family members who permitted the localization of the MCKD1 gene have been carefully examined.[80] Males and females were equally affected. The disease led to end-stage renal disease at a mean age of 53.7 years, ranging from 36 to 80 years. Hypertension was found in 51% of those affected. Using ultrasonography, cysts were detected in 40% of tested gene carriers. Mainly corticomedullary or medullary cysts but also cortical cysts were reported. Approximately half of the gene carriers had normal-size kidneys with no cysts, whereas 11% had small kidneys with increased echogenicity but without cysts. Overall 60% had no cysts, limiting the diagnostic value of renal cysts at least in the early stages of this disease. Another study incorporating data from 128 affected individuals (23 kindreds) showed that end-stage renal disease can occur within a wider age range (5 to 76 years).[79] Renal biopsy was

TABLE 8-2 **Clinical and Diagnostic Findings in Medullary Cystic Kidney Disease Variants (Autosomal Recessive Inheritance)**

Medullary Cystic Kidney Disease Variants (Genes and Loci)	Age at ESRD (Years)	Hyper-Tension	Renal Imaging	Histology	Hyperuricemia/ Gouty Arthritis	Extrarenal Manifes-tations	Allelic Disorders
MCKD1 (1q21-q23.1)	5-76 (median 32) 36-80 (median 54)	~50%	60% no cysts 10% increased echogenicity Normal or small kidneys	TIN, TBM, TA, TCD,	~40%	Absent	Not known
MCKD2/UMOD (16p11-p13)	16-54 (median 31)	~50%	~ 50% no cysts Normal or small kidneys	TIN, TBM, TA, TCD	~40-50%	Absent	Glomerulocystic kidney disease Familial juvenile hyperuricemic nephropathy

ESRD, End-stage renal disease; *TA*, tubular atrophy; *TBM*, tubular basement membrane alterations; *TCD*, tubular cystic dilatation; *TIN*, tubulointerstitial nephropathy.

performed in affected patients from 15 families and confirmed previous histological findings of classical nephronophthisis. Interestingly, hyperuricemia and hypertension were not frequent findings and occurred in 8 (34%) and 13 (56%) families, respectively.

Medullary Cystic Kidney Disease Type 2

Genetics and Etiology

Medullary cystic kidney disease type 2 (MCKD2) and familial juvenile hyperuricemic nephropathy (FJHN) are both autosomal dominant renal diseases characterized by juvenile onset of hyperuricemia, gout, and progressive renal failure. Clinical features of both conditions vary in presence and severity. Genetic linkage studies have localized genes for both conditions to overlapping regions of chromosome 16p11-p13.[78,81] These clinical and genetic findings suggest that these conditions may be allelic. Subsequently four dominant uromodulin *(UMOD)* gene mutations that segregate with the disease phenotype in three families with FJHN and in one family with MCKD2 were identified.[82] *UMOD* encodes the Tamm-Horsfall protein (THP), which is expressed primarily at the luminal side of renal epithelial cells of the thick ascending loop of Henle and of early distal convoluted tubules. THP is the most abundant protein in the urine of humans.[83] Exon 4, which encodes EGF-like protein domains, appears to be a hot spot for *UMOD* mutations.[83] Another gene for FJHN residing on chromosome 16p11 remains to be identified.[84] Interestingly, allelism of glomerulocystic kidney disease variant can also be demonstrated by detection of *UMOD* mutations.[85] This disease is characterized by cystic dilatation of Bowman's space and the initial proximal convoluted tubule. In addition, clinical features similar to MCKD and FJHN such as hyperuricemia and impairment of urine-concentrating ability can be observed.

Clinical Features

FJHN has been discriminated from MCKD mainly by the absence of renal cysts. However, Hart et al. could show that both disorders are allelic, which explains why some but not all affected individuals within the same pedigree exhibit renal cysts.[82] In addition, as detailed previously, renal cysts are not an obligatory finding in MCKD.

In an Italian kindred with 10 affected individuals enabling gene localization of the *MCKD2* locus, 5 had hyperuricemia and 2 had gouty arthritis. End-stage renal disease was reached at a median of 31 years, ranging from 16 to 54 years.[78]

Wolf et al.[83] reported three families with *UMOD* mutations. Six of 12 affected family members also had hyperuricemia. End-stage renal disease occurred between 29 and 60 years. In all families, renal imaging by magnetic resonance imaging or ultrasound revealed suspicious results with small kidneys, reduced parenchyma, or cysts. In all cases renal histology was compatible with MCKD, depicting microcysts in 4 out of 12 cases and in the others dilated or atrophic tubules, global sclerosis, extensive tubulointerstitial atrophy with fibrosis, and signs of chronic diffuse inflammation.

Recently in a large Spanish kindred with *UMOD* mutations, an individual with recessive (bi-allelic) *UMOD* mutations was identified.[86] The homozygous individual survived to adulthood and had an earlier onset of hyperuricemia and faster progression to end-stage renal disease than did heterozygous individuals.

THERAPY

So far no specific therapy correcting the genetic or functional defect in nephronophthisis or MCKD is available. Thus the mainstay of therapy is management of chronic renal failure as outlined in Section 11. In contrast to other inherited or acquired systemic disorders such as focal segmental glomerulosclerosis or IgA nephropathy, renal allografts are not at risk for recurrence of the primary disease in nephronophthisis or MCKD patients.

The novel molecular insights into the pathogenesis of the disorders may allow testing of novel therapeutic strategies to slow renal failure. The demonstration that mutations of orthologous genes cause nephronophthisis and the cystic kidney phenotype in the *pcy*-mouse strain facilitates the testing of such novel therapeutic interventions.[15] Interventional studies in *pcy* mice have shown a slowing of disease progression with dietary modifications such as protein restriction and soy protein application, as well as with administration of methylprednisolone and vasopressin receptor 2 antagonists.[87] Future clinical studies will have to prove the efficacy of these therapeutic concepts in human disease.

Acknowledgment

We are grateful to Heike Olbrich and Manfred Fliegauf for the preparation of tables and figures and for their continuous support.

REFERENCES

1. Goldman SH, Walker SR, Merigan TCJ, Gardner KDJ, Bull JM: Hereditary occurrence of cystic disease of the renal medulla, *N Engl J Med* 274:984-92, 1966.
2. Strauss MB, Sommers SC: Medullary cystic disease and familial juvenile nephronophthisis, *N Engl J Med* 277:863-64, 1967.
3. Gardner KD: Cystic diseases of the kidney: a perspective on medullary cystic disease, *Birth Defects Orig Artic Ser* 10:29-31, 1974.
4. Fanconi G, Hanhart E, Albertini A, Uhlinger E, Dolivo G, Prader A: Die familiäre juvenile Nephronophthise, *Helv Paediatr Acta* 6:1-49, 1951.
5. Smith C, Graham J: Congenital medullary cysts of kidneys with severe refractory anemia, *Am J Dis Child* 69:369-77, 1945.
6. Waldherr R, Lennert T, Weber HP, Fodisch HJ, Scharer K: The nephronophthisis complex: A clinicopathologic study in children, *Virchows Arch [Pathol Anat]* 394:235-54, 1982.
7. Zollinger HU, Mihatsch MJ, Edefonti A, Gaboardi F, Imbasciati E, Lennert T: Nephronophthisis (medullary cystic disease of the kidney). A study using electron microscopy, immunofluorescence, and a review of the morphological findings, *Helv Paediatr Acta* 35:509-30, 1980.

8. Blowey DL, Querfeld U, Geary D, Warady BA, Alon U: Ultrasound findings in juvenile nephronophthisis, *Pediatr Nephrol* 10:22-24, 1996.
9. Hildebrandt F, Omran H: New insights: nephronophthisis-medullary cystic kidney disease, *Pediatr Nephrol* 16:168-76, 2001.
10. Otto EA, Schermer B, Obara T, O'Toole JF, Hiller KS, et al: Mutations in INVS encoding inversin cause nephronophthisis type 2, linking renal cystic disease to the function of primary cilia and left-right axis determination, *Nat Genet* 34:413-20, 2003.
11. Hildebrandt F, Otto E, Rensing C, Nothwang HG, Vollmer M, et al: A novel gene encoding an SH3 domain protein is mutated in nephronophthisis type 1, *Nat Genet* 17:149-53, 1997a.
12. Saunier S, Calado J, Heilig R, Silbermann F, Benessy F, et al: A novel gene that encodes a protein with a putative src homology 3 domain is a candidate gene for familial juvenile nephronophthisis, *Hum Mol Genet* 6:2317-23, 1997.
13. Otto E, Hoefele J, Ruf R, Mueller AM, Hiller KS, et al: A gene mutated in nephronophthisis and retinitis pigmentosa encodes a novel protein, nephroretinin, conserved in evolution, *Am J Hum Genet* 71:1161-67, 2002.
14. Mollet G, Salomon R, Gribouval O, Silbermann F, Bacq D, et al: The gene mutated in juvenile nephronophthisis type 4 encodes a novel protein that interacts with nephrocystin, *Nat Genet* 32:300-05, 2002.
15. Olbrich H, Fliegauf M, Hoefele J, Kispert A, Otto E, et al: Mutations in a novel gene, NPHP3, cause adolescent nephronophthisis, tapeto-retinal degeneration and hepatic fibrosis, *Nat Genet* 34:455-59, 2003.
16. Otto EA, Loeys B, Khanna H, Hellemans J, Sudbrak R, et al: Nephrocystin-5, a ciliary IQ domain protein, is mutated in Senior-Løken syndrome and interacts with RPGR and calmodulin, *Nat Genet* 37:282-88, 2005.
17. Dixon-Salazar T, Silhavy JL, Marsh SE, Louie CM, Scott LC, et al: Mutations in the AHI1 gene, encoding jouberin, cause Joubert syndrome with cortical polymicrogyria, *Am J Hum Genet* 75:979-87, 2004.
18. Utsch B, Sayer JA, Attanasio M, Pereira RR, Eccles M, et al: Identification of the first AHI1 gene mutations in nephronophthisis-associated Joubert syndrome, *Pediatr Nephrol* 21:32-35, 2006.
19. Sayer JA, Otto EA, O'Toole JF, Nurnberg G, Kennedy MA, et al: The centrosomal protein nephrocystin-6 is mutated in Joubert syndrome and activates transcription factor ATF4, *Nat Genet* 38:674-81, 2006.
20. Løken AC, Hanssen O, Halvorsen S, Jølster NJ: Hereditary renal dysplasia and blindness, *Acta Paediatr* 50:177-84, 1961.
21. Senior B, Friedmann AI, Braudo JL: Juvenile familial nephropathy with tapetoretinal degeneration: a new oculo-renal dystrophy, *Am J Ophthalmol* 52:625-33, 1961.
22. Leber T: Über Retinitis pigmentosa und angeborene Amaurose. Albrecht von Graefe's, *Arch Klin Exp Ophthalmol* 15:1-25, 1869.
23. Leber T: Über anormale Formen der Retinitis pigmentosa, *Arch für Ophthalmol* 17:314-41, 1871.
24. François J: Leber's congenital tapeto-retinal degeneration, *Int Ophthalmol Clin* 8:929-47, 1968.
25. Franceschetti A, Dieterle P: L'importance diagnostique de l'electrorétinogramme dans le dégénérescences tapéto-rétinennes avec rétrécissement du champ visuel et héméralopie, *Conf Neurol* 14:184-86, 1954.
26. Parisi MA, Bennett CL, Eckert ML, Dobyns WB, Gleeson JG, et al: The NPHP1 gene deletion associated with juvenile nephronophthisis is present in a subset of individuals with Joubert syndrome, *Am J Hum Genet* 75:82-91, 2004.
27. Maria BL, Quisling RG, Rosainz LC, Yachnis AT, Gitten JC, et al: Molar tooth sign in Joubert syndrome: clinical, radiologic, and pathologic significance, *J Child Neurol* 14:368-76, 1999.
28. Cogan DG: Heredity of congenital ocular motor apraxia, *Trans Am Acad Ophthal Otolaryng* 76:60-63, 1972.
29. Hedera P, Gorski JL: Retinitis pigmentosa, growth hormone deficiency, and acromelic skeletal dysplasia in two brothers: possible familial RHYNS syndrome, *Am J Med Genet* 101:142-45, 2001.
30. Mainzer F, Saldino RM, Ozonoff MB, Minagi H: Familial nephropathy associated with retinitis pigmentosa, cerebellar ataxia and skeletal abnormalities, *Am J Med* 49:556-62, 1970.
31. Giedion, A: Phalangeal cone shaped epiphysis of the hands (PhCSEH) and chronic renal disease: the conorenal syndromes, *Pediat Radiol* 8:32-38, 1979.
32. Popovic-Rolovic M, Calic-Perisic N, Bunjevacki G, Negovanovic D: Juvenile nephronophthisis associated with retinal pigmentary dystrophy, cerebellar ataxia, and skeletal abnormalities, *Arch Dis Child* 51:801-03, 1976.
33. Robins DG, French TA, Chakera TM: Juvenile nephronophthisis associated with skeletal abnormalities and hepatic fibrosis, *Arch Dis Child* 51:799-801, 1976.
34. Boichis H, Passwell J, David R, Miller H: Congenital hepatic fibrosis and nephronophthisis: a family study, *Quart J Med* 42:221-33, 1973.
35. Proesmans W, Van Damme B, Macken J: Nephronophthisis and tapetoretinal degeneration associated with liver fibrosis, *Clin Nephrol* 3:160-64, 1975.
36. Delaney V, Mullaney J, Bourke E: Juvenile nephronophthisis, congenital hepatic fibrosis and retinal hypoplasia in twins, *Quart J Med* 186:281-96, 1978.
37. Antignac C, Arduy CH, Beckmann JS, Benessy F, Gros F, et al: A gene for familial juvenile nephronophthisis (recessive medullary cystic kidney disease) maps to chromosome 2p, *Nat Genet* 3:342-45, 1993.
38. Hildebrandt F, Singh-Sawhney I, Schnieders B, Centofante L, Omran H, et al: Mapping of a gene for familial juvenile nephronophthisis: refining the map and defining flanking markers on chromosome 2. APN Study Group, *Am J Hum Genet* 53:1256-61, 1993.
39. Konrad M, Saunier S, Heidet L, Silbermann F, Benessy F, et al: Large homozygous deletions of the 2q13 region are a major cause of juvenile nephronophthisis, *Hum Mol Genet* 5:367-71, 1996.
40. Hildebrandt F, Rensing C, Betz R, Sommer U, Birnbaum S, Imm A, et al: Arbeitsgemeinschaft fur Paediatrische Nephrologie (APN) Study Group: Establishing an algorithm for molecular genetic diagnostics in 127 families with juvenile nephronophthisis, *Kidney Int* 59:434-45, 2001.
41. Hoefele J, Sudbrak R, Reinhardt R, Lehrack S, Hennig S, et al: Mutational analysis of the NPHP4 gene in 250 patients with nephronophthisis, *Hum Mutat* 25:411, 2005.
42. Donaldson JC, Dempsey PJ, Reddy S, Bouton AH, Coffey RJ, Hanks SK: Crk-associated substrate p130(Cas) interacts with nephrocystin and both proteins localize to cell-cell contacts of polarized epithelial cells, *Exp Cell Res* 256:168-78, 2000.
43. Benzing T, Gerke P, Hopker K, Hildebrandt F, Kim E, Walz G: Nephrocystin interacts with Pyk2, p130(Cas), and tensin and triggers phosphorylation of Pyk2, *Proc Natl Acad Sci U S A* 98:9784-89, 2001.
44. Mollet G, Silbermann F, Delous M, Salomon R, Antignac C, Saunier S: Characterization of the nephrocystin/nephrocystin-4 complex and subcellular localization of nephrocystin-4 to primary cilia and centrosomes, *Hum Mol Genet* 14:645-56, 2005.
45. Schermer B, Hopker K, Omran H, Ghenoiu C, Fliegauf M, et al: Phosphorylation by casein kinase 2 induces PACS-1 binding of nephrocystin and targeting to cilia, *EMBO J* 24:4415-24, 2005.
46. Fliegauf M, Horvath J, von Schnakenburg C, Müller D, Thumfart J, et al: Nephrocystin specifically localizes to the transition zone of renal and respiratory cilia and is absent in nephronophthisis patients with NPHP1 deletions, *J Am Soc Nephrol* (in press).
47. Hildebrandt F, Strahm B, Nothwang HG, Gretz N, Schnieders B, et al: Molecular genetic identification of families with juvenile nephronophthisis type 1: rate of progression to renal failure. APN Study Group. Arbeitsgemeinschaft fur Padiatrische Nephrologie, *Kidney Int* 51:261-69, 1997b.
48. Bollee G, Fakhouri F, Karras A, Noel LH, Salomon R, et al: (Nephronophthisis related to homozygous NPHP1 gene deletion as a cause of chronic renal failure in adults, *Nephrol Dial Transplant* 21:2660–63, 2006.
49. Betz R, Rensing C, Otto E, Mincheva A, Zehnder D, et al: Children with ocular motor apraxia type Cogan carry deletions in the gene (NPHP1) for juvenile nephronophthisis, *J Pediatr* 136:828-31, 2000.
50. Omran H, Fernandez C, Jung M, Häffner K, Fargier B, et al: Identification of a new gene locus for adolescent nephronophthisis, on

chromosome 3q22 in a large Venezuelan pedigree, *Am J Hum Genet* 66:118-27, 2000.
51. Omran H, Häffner K, Burth S, Fernandez C, Fargier B, et al: Human adolescent nephronophthisis: Gene locus synteny with polycystic kidney disease in pcy mice, *J Am Soc Nephrol* 12:107-13, 2001.
52. Omran H, Sasmaz G, Häffner K, Volz A, Olbrich H, et al: Identification of a gene locus for Senior-Løken syndrome in the region of the nephronophthisis type 3 gene, *J Am Soc Nephrol* 13:75-79, 2002.
53. Schuermann MJ, Otto E, Becker A, Saar K, Ruschendorf F, et al: Mapping of gene loci for nephronophthisis type 4 and Senior-Løken syndrome, to chromosome 1p36, *Am J Hum Genet* 70:1240-46, 2002.
54. Wolf MT, Lee J, Panther F, Otto EA, Guan KL, Hildebrandt F: Expression and phenotype analysis of the nephrocystin-1 and nephrocystin-4 homologs in *Caenorhabditis elegans*, *J Am Soc Nephrol* 16:676-87, 2005.
55. Jaureguia AR, Barr MM. Functional characterization of the C. elegans nephrocystins NPHP-1 and NPHP-4 and their role in cilia and male sensory behaviors, *Experimental Cell Research* 305:333-42, 2005.
56. Winkelbauer ME, Schafer JC, Haycraft CJ, Swoboda P, Yoder BK: The C. elegans homologs of nephrocystin-1 and nephrocystin-4 are cilia transition zone proteins involved in chemosensory perception, *J Cell Sci* 118:5575-87, 2005.
57. Hoefele J, Otto E, Felten H, Kuhn K, Bley TA, et al: Clinical and histological presentation of 3 siblings with mutations in the NPHP4 gene, *Am J Kidney Dis* 43:358-64, 2004.
58. Chang B, Khanna H, Hawes N, Jimeno D, He S, et al: In-frame deletion in a novel centrosomal/ciliary protein CEP290/NPHP6 perturbs its interaction with RPGR and results in early-onset retinal degeneration in the rd16 mouse, *Hum Mol Genet* 15:1847-57, 2006.
59. Valente EM, Silhavy JL, Brancati F, Barrano G, Krishnaswami SR, et al: Mutations in CEP290, which encodes a centrosomal protein, cause pleiotropic forms of Joubert syndrome, *Nat Genet* 38:623-25, 2006.
60. Saar K, Al-Gazali L, Sztriha L, Rueschendorf F, Nur-E-Kamal M, et al: Homozygosity mapping in families with Joubert syndrome identifies a locus on chromosome 9q34.3 and evidence for genetic heterogeneity, *Am J Hum Genet* 65:1666-71, 1999.
61. Valente EM, Salpietro DC, Brancati F, Bertini E, Galluccio T, et al: Description, nomenclature, and mapping of a novel cerebello-renal syndrome with the molar tooth malformation, *Am J Hum Genet* 73:663-67, 2003.
62. Ferland RJ, Eyaid W, Collura RV, Tully LD, Hill RS, et al: Abnormal cerebellar development and axonal decussation due to mutations in AHI1 in Joubert syndrome, *Nat Genet* 36:1008-13, 2004.
63. Parisi MA, Doherty D, Eckert ML, Shaw DW, Ozyurek H, et al: AHI1 mutations cause both retinal dystrophy and renal cystic disease in Joubert syndrome, *J Med Genet* 43:334-39, 2006.
64. Mochizuki T, Saijoh Y, Tsuchiya K, Shirayoshi Y, Takai S, et al: Cloning of inv, a gene that controls left/right asymmetry and kidney development, *Nature* 395:177-81, 1998.
65. Morgan D, Turnpenny L, Goodship J, Dai W, Majumder K, et al: Inversin, a novel gene in the vertebrate left–right axis pathway, is partially deleted in the inv mouse, *Nat Genet* 20:149-56, 1998.
66. Haider NB, Carmi R, Shalev H, Sheffield VC, Landau D: A Bedouin kindred with infantile nephronophthisis demonstrates linkage to chromosome 9 by homozygosity mapping, *Am J Hum Genet* 63:1404-10, 1998.
67. Simons M, Gloy J, Ganner A, Bullerkotte A, Bashkurov M, et al: Inversin, the gene product mutated in nephronophthisis type II, functions as a molecular switch between Wnt signaling pathways, *Nat Genet* 37:537-43, 2005.
68. Bodaghi E, Honarmand MT, Ahmadi M: Infantile nephronophthisis, *Int J Pediatr Nephrol* 8:207-10, 1987.
69. Gagnadoux MF, Bacri JL, Broyer M, Habib R: Infantile chronic tubulo-interstitial nephritis with cortical microcysts: variant of nephronophthisis or new disease entity? *Pediatr Nephrol* 3:50-55, 1989.
70. O'Toole JF, Otto EA, Frishberg Y, Hildebrandt F: Retinitis pigmentosa and renal failure in a patient with mutations in INVS, *Nephrol Dial Transplant* 21:1989-91, 2006.
71. Ibanez-Tallon I, Heintz N, Omran H: To beat or not to beat: roles of cilia in development and disease, *Hum Mol Genet* 12:R27-35, 2003.
72. Nauli SM, Alenghat FJ, Luo Y, Williams E, Vassilev P, et al: Polycystins 1 and 2 mediate mechanosensation in the primary cilium of kidney cells, *Nat Genet* 33:129-37, 2003.
73. Watnick T, Germino G: From cilia to cyst, *Nat Genet* 34:355-56, 2003.
74. Badano JL, Teslovich TM, Katsanis N: The centrosome in human genetic disease, *Nat Rev Genet* 6:194-205, 2005.
75. Hildebrandt F, Otto E: Cilia and centrosomes: a unifying pathogenic concept for cystic kidney disease? *Nat Rev Genet* 6:928-40, 2005.
76. Ross AJ, May-Simera H, Eichers ER, Kai M, Hill J, et al: Disruption of Bardet-Biedl syndrome ciliary proteins perturbs planar cell polarity in vertebrates, *Nat Genet* 37:1135-40, 2005.
77. Christodoulou K, Tsingis M, Stavrou C, Eleftheriou A, Papapavlou P, et al: Chromosome 1 localization of a gene for autosomal dominant medullary cystic kidney disease, *Hum Mol Genet* 7:905-11, 1998.
78. Scolari F, Puzzer D, Amoroso A, Caridi G, Ghiggeri GM, et al: Identification of a new locus for medullary cystic disease, on chromosome 16p12, *Am J Hum Genet* 64:1655-60, 1999.
79. Wolf MT, Mucha BE, Hennies HC, Attanasio M, Panther F, et al: Medullary cystic kidney disease type 1: mutational analysis in 37 genes based on haplotype sharing, *Hum Genet* 119:649-58, 2006.
80. Stavrou C, Koptides M, Tombazos C, Psara E, Patsias C, et al: Autosomal-dominant medullary cystic kidney disease type 1: clinical and molecular findings in six large Cypriot families, *Kidney Int* 62:1385-94, 2002.
81. Kamatani N, Moritani M, Yamanaka H, Takeuchi F, Hosoya T, Itakura M: Localization of a gene for familial juvenile hyperuricemic nephropathy causing underexcretion-type gout to 16p12 by genome-wide linkage analysis of a large family, *Arthritis Rheum* 43:925-29, 2000.
82. Hart TC, Gorry MC, Hart PS, Woodard AS, Shihabi Z, et al: Mutations of the UMOD gene are responsible for medullary cystic kidney disease 2 and familial juvenile hyperuricaemic nephropathy, *J Med Genet* 39:882-92, 2002.
83. Wolf MT, Mucha BE, Attanasio M, Zalewski I, Karle SM, et al: Mutations of the Uromodulin gene in MCKD type 2 patients cluster in exon 4, which encodes three EGF-like domains, *Kidney Int* 64:1580-87, 2003.
84. Stiburkova B, Majewski J, Hodanova K, Ondrova L, Jerabkova M, et al: Familial juvenile hyperuricaemic nephropathy (FJHN): linkage analysis in 15 families, physical and transcriptional characterisation of the FJHN critical region on chromosome 16p11.2 and the analysis of seven candidate genes, *Eur J Hum Genet* 11:145-54, 2003.
85. Rampoldi L, Caridi G, Santon D, Boaretto F, Bernascone I, et al: Allelism of MCKD, FJHN and GCKD caused by impairment of uromodulin export dynamics, *Hum Mol Genet* 12:3369-84, 2003.
86. Rezende-Lima W, Parreira KS, Garcia-Gonzalez M, Riveira E, Banet JF, Lens XM: Homozygosity for uromodulin disorders: FJHN and MCKD-type 2, *Kidney Int* 66:558-63, 2004.
87. Torres VE: Therapies to slow polycystic kidney disease, *Nephron Exp Nephrol* 98:e1-e7, 2004.

CHAPTER

9 Polycystic Kidney Disease: ADPKD and ARPKD

Carsten Bergmann and Klaus Zerres

Cystic kidney diseases (CKDs) are a clinically and genetically heterogeneous group of disorders that may present in utero or be clinically silent well into adulthood. Progressive fibrocystic renal changes are often accompanied by hepatobiliary changes or sometimes other extrarenal abnormalities (e.g., pancreatic cysts or retinitis pigmentosa).[1] The number of diseases with renal cysts suggests they are a somewhat nonspecific kidney response to a wide array of genetic and nongenetic aberrations. Although there are still more questions than answers, substantial progress has been made in unraveling the etiology of CKDs. As a prerequisite, CKD genes and their encoded proteins have been identified, providing investigators with essential tools for analyzing the molecular and cellular mechanisms that underlie these diseases. In spite of different genetic entities, recent findings have proven the cystogenic process to share common phenotypic abnormalities.[2] These are compatible with cellular dedifferentiation and reexpression of proteins usually found during developmental stages, increased proliferation and apoptosis rates, disorganization of the extracellular matrix, and aberrant protein-sorting and fluid-transport characteristics. It has also been shown that most CKD proteins colocalize in multimeric complexes at distinct subcellular epithelial sites, and compelling evidence suggests that cilia play a central pathogenic role.[3] Overall, these findings point to common pathogenic pathways for most CKDs regardless of the underlying disease entity. This may provide a molecular basis for the perplexing clinical observation that similar or even identical phenotypes can result from mutations in different genes. Recently several promising trials have further extended our understanding of the pathophysiology of CKD and may have the potential for rational personalized therapies in future years.[2]

CLASSIFICATION AND DIFFERENTIAL DIAGNOSIS OF CYSTIC KIDNEY DISEASES

In their seminal studies, Osathanondh and Potter systematically classified renal cystic diseases into four distinct types.[4] Potter syndrome type I is referred to as autosomal recessive polycystic kidney disease (ARPKD), type II as renal cystic dysplasia, type III as autosomal dominant polycystic kidney disease (ADPKD), and type IV occurs when a long-standing obstruction in either the kidney or ureter leads to cystic kidneys or hydronephrosis. Particularly types II, III, and IV can be part of many syndromes. While this classification still has a great impact for concise pathoanatomical description, it is hardly to be reconciled with clinical and genetic entities.

Accurate diagnosis is essential in both managing patients with CKD and counseling their families. When an effort is made to classify the wide array of CKDs, it may be reasonable to first distinguish between acquired and inherited forms. Knowledge about the family history and the clinical picture, together with the location and morphology of the cysts and any possible extrarenal manifestations, should help in making a diagnosis. Sometimes cytogenetic studies may be useful in excluding a chromosomal aberration.

Inherited CKDs mainly include ADPKD and ARPKD, glomerulocystic kidney disease (GCKD), and entities comprising the medullary cystic kidney disease–nephronophthisis complex. Notably, cystic kidneys are an important feature of numerous genetic syndromes such as the dominant disorders tuberous sclerosis, branchio-oto-renal syndrome and von Hippel-Lindau disease or the recessively inherited Meckel-Gruber, Bardet-Biedl, and Zellweger syndromes (Table 9-1). This chapter focuses on the polycystic kidney diseases ADPKD and ARPKD; a thorough discussion of other entities can be found in later sections of this book. We aim to summarize the current state of knowledge of structure and function of genes and proteins underlying polycystic kidney disease, to explore the cellular pathophysiology and clinical consequences of changes in mutant genes, and to discuss potential therapeutic approaches.

AUTOSOMAL DOMINANT POLYCYSTIC KIDNEY DISEASE

Epidemiology and Morphology

ADPKD is the most common inherited renal disease and one of the most common Mendelian human disorders, with a frequency of 1/400-1000.[5,6] This approximates to about 12.5 million affected individuals worldwide. After diabetes mellitus and hypertension, ADPKD is the single most common cause of end-stage renal disease (ESRD); about 5% to 10% of all patients requiring renal replacement therapy (kidney transplant or dialysis) are affected by ADPKD. Overall,

TABLE 9-1 **Selection of Syndromes with Cystic Kidney Disease**

Disease	OMIM Number	Mode of Inheritance	Gene/Locus	Clinical Hallmarks
ARPKD with facial and skeletal anomalies	263210	AR	Unknown	Polycystic kidneys and congenital hepatic fibrosis identical with *PKHD1*-linked ARPKD; in addition, skeletal anomalies (brachymelia, butterfly vertebrae, distinctive shape of iliac bones) and facial anomalies (microbrachycephaly, hypertelorism, epicanthic folds, anteverted nares)
Bardet-Biedl syndrome	209900	AR/digenic/triallelic	Highly heterogeneous (*BBS1-12* genes known); further loci to be expected	Obesity, hypogonadism, retinal degeneration, cognitive impairment, polydactyly, renal dysfunction
Branchio-oto-renal syndrome	113650	AD (highly variable expression)	*EYA1* gene 8q13.3; *SIX1* gene 14q23; *SIX5* gene 19q13.3	Branchial cysts/fistulae, external ear malformations, preauricular pits, hearing loss, renal anomalies
CDG (congenital disorders of glycosylation) syndrome	212065	AR	Highly heterogeneous (many genes known); further loci to be expected	Disorders of almost all organs and systems reported (e.g., isolated cystic kidney disease and congenital hepatic fibrosis), often with mental retardation (but not mandatory); should be considered in any child with unexplained clinical syndrome
Ellis-van Creveld syndrome	225500	AR	*EVC1* and *EVC2* genes 4p16	Chondroectodermal dysplasia with short limbs, short ribs, postaxial polydactyly, dysplastic nails and teeth, congenital cardiac defects
Jeune syndrome (asphyxiating thoracic dystrophy)	208500	AR	*IFT80* gene 3q26.1; Locus mapped 15q13	Severely constricted thoracic cage with respiratory insufficiency, rhizomelia, postaxial polydactyly, cystic kidneys, congenital hepatic fibrosis
Meckel-Gruber syndrome	249000	AR	*MKS1* gene 17q23.2; *MKS2* locus 11q13; *MKS3* gene 8q22.1; *MKS4/CEP290* gene 12q21.3; *MKS5/RPGRIP1L* gene 16q12.2; Further loci to be expected	Cystic kidneys, anomalies of central nervous system (typically occipital meningoencephalocele; occasionally Dandy-Walker malformation, hydrocephalus, etc.), postaxial polydactyly, fibrocystic liver changes
RCAD (renal cysts and diabetes) syndrome	137920	AD (highly variable expression, often spontaneous mutations)	*TCF2/HNF1β* gene 17q12	Highly variable renal spectrum (e.g., hypoplastic glomerulocystic kidneys), maturity-onset diabetes of the young (MODY), genital tract abnormalities, hyperuricemia, abnormal liver function
Short rib polydactyly syndromes	263530	AR	Unknown; SRPS type III patients with *EVC1* mutations reported	Group of severe, often lethal, skeletal dysplasias characterized by hypoplastic thorax, short ribs, short limbs, polydactyly, and visceral abnormalities. Phenotypic overlap (e.g., with Ellis-van Creveld syndrome demonstrated by *EVC1* mutations in SRPS type III patients) and controversy as to whether the different SRPS variants are due to variable expression or to genetic heterogeneity.
Tuberous sclerosis	191100	AD (~50% spontaneous mutations)	*TSC1* gene (Hamartin) 9q34; *TSC2* gene (Tuberin) 16p13.3	Neurocutaneous syndrome (phacomatosis), hamartomas in multiple organs, angiofibromas, mental retardation, seizures, hypomelanotic macules/"ash leaf" spots, retinal phakomas or plaquelike hamartomas, diverse renal manifestations (angiomyolipomas, renal cell carcinomas, polycystic kidney disease)
Von Hippel-Lindau disease	193300	AD	*VHL* gene 3p25.3	Hemangioblastoma (retinal, cerebellar, and spinal), renal cell carcinoma, pheochromocytoma
Zellweger (cerebro-hepato-renal) syndrome	214100	AR	Highly heterogeneous (many genes known, involved in peroxisome biogenesis); further loci to be expected	Peroxisomal biogenesis disorder with highly variable clinical spectrum: craniofacial features (large anterior fontanel with widely spaced sutures; broad, full forehead; flat occiput; etc.), neurological aberrations (profound hypotonia, depressed neonatal and deep tendon reflexes, seizures), ocular abnormalities (congenital clouding/cataracts, glaucoma, etc.), calcific stippling of patellae and other bones, enlarged fibrotic liver, cystic kidneys

AD, Autosomal dominant; *AR*, autosomal recessive; *ARPKD*, autosomal recessive polycystic kidney disease.

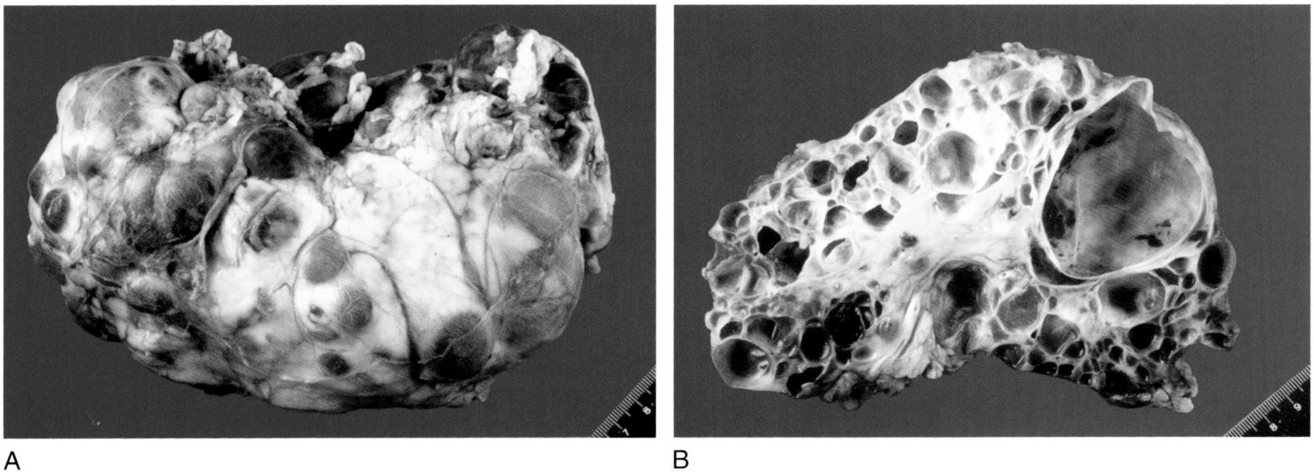

Figure 9-1 **A,** Macroscopic appearance of advanced-stage ADPKD showing an enlarged kidney with multiple cysts almost completely replacing the renal parenchyma. **B,** On cut section, multiple cysts in the cortex and medulla can be seen that vary considerably in appearance and size, from a few millimeters to several centimeters in diameter.

the disease is a major health care issue of socioeconomic interest.

Histopathologically, renal cysts are fluid-filled epithelia-lined dilated saccular lesions that generally arise from tubular segments. ADPKD is characterized by the formation and progressive enlargement of renal cysts in all segments of the nephron. In contrast to ARPKD, in which the cysts usually remain connected with the tubular lumen, in ADPKD the enlarging cystic dilations may become disconnected from the tubular space. Renal cysts in ADPKD vary considerably in size and appearance, from a few millimeters to diameters of many centimeters (Figure 9-1).

Clinical Course and Treatment

ADPKD is a systemic disorder with profound extrarenal cystic and noncystic complications, which are summarized in Table 9-2. Among the most important extrarenal manifestations commonly seen in adults are cysts in other epithelial organs (especially in the liver and pancreas) and cardiovascular abnormalities. In pediatric patients, however, extrarenal ADPKD features are only rarely observed.

Renal Involvement Despite significant extrarenal disease burden in many ADPKD patients, the kidneys are usually the center of interest. Although there are currently no disease-specific treatment options, it is crucial, as with other forms of chronic kidney disease, to prevent and effectively manage complications such as arterial hypertension and urinary tract infections to slow progression to ESRD. Renal insufficiency and ESRD in ADPKD are treated with standard medical management of chronic renal failure and renal replacement therapy as outlined in other chapters of this book.

About 95% of all carriers show ultrasonographic evidence of ADPKD at the age of 20, and almost every patient at age 30. Less clear is the proportion of carriers that can already be identified by ultrasound in childhood. However, these cases usually do not show an onset of clinical symptoms until adulthood and have to be differentiated from those with an early-manifesting clinical course. In a study by the Denver Polycystic Kidney Disease Research Group, approximately 60% of children younger than 5 and 75% to 80% of children 5 to 18 with a *PKD1* mutation had renal cysts detectable by ultrasound.[7] Bear and colleagues proposed a rate of false-negative ultrasonographic diagnosis of about 35% below the age of 10 years.[8] In general, the finding of even one renal cyst should alert the clinician to the possibility of ADPKD, because simple cysts are extremely rare in childhood.[9] Ravine et al. found no prevalence in individuals age 15 to 29.[10] Thus in children with a 50% risk of ADPKD, the finding of one cyst is considered diagnostic.

TABLE 9-2 **Frequency of Extrarenal Manifestations in ADPKD**

Manifestation	Frequency
Gastrointestinal	
Hepatic cysts	~50% (increases with age)
Pancreatic cysts	~7%
Colonic diverticula	80% of patients with ESRD
Congenital hepatic fibrosis	Rare
Cholangiocarcinoma	Rare
Cardiovascular	
Valve abnormalities	~25%
Intracranial aneurysms	~8%
Thoracic/abdominal aneurysms	Unknown
Miscellaneous	
Arachnoid cysts	~5%
Ovarian/testicular cysts	Unknown

Source: Modified according to Gabow PA: Autosomal dominant polycystic disease. *N Engl J Med* 329(5):332-42, 1993.

A recent study by the CRISP (Consortium for Radiologic Imaging Studies of Polycystic Kidney Disease) consortium on a total of 241 ADPKD patients showed that renal and cyst volumes increase at a relatively uniform rate (per affected individual), with an average increase in kidney volume of 5.3% a year.[11] Greater renal enlargement was associated with a more rapid decrease in renal function. Chronic renal failure presents in about 50% of patients by the age of 60. On average, PKD2 is regarded to be significantly milder than PKD1, with a 15-to-20-years-later median age of onset of ESRD (53 vs. 69 years) and a lower prevalence of arterial hypertension and urinary tract infections.[12] These authors did not identify any sex influence for PKD1; however, females affected by PKD2 were found to have a significantly longer median survival (71.0 vs. 67.3 years) than males. Another study corroborated these findings by a later mean age of onset of ESRD (76.0 vs. 68.1 years) in PKD2 females.[13]

Early-Onset ADPKD Clinical symptoms do not usually arise until the middle decades. However, there is striking phenotypic variability not just interfamilially but even within the same family, indicating that modifying genes, environmental factors, and/or other mechanisms later discussed influence the clinical course in ADPKD considerably.[14,15] In line with this, a small proportion of ADPKD patients show an early-manifesting clinical course. Early manifestation in ADPKD is usually defined as clinical symptoms (e.g., arterial hypertension, proteinuria, or impaired renal function) occurring before the age of 15. Among these are cases with significant perinatal/neonatal morbidity and mortality sometimes indistinguishable from those with severe ARPKD. Conflicting data exist on the concise incidence of early-manifesting ADPKD cases that may result in reduced fitness and thus may equal the portion of autosomal dominant spontaneous *PKD* mutations. While most authors propose a figure of 1% to 2%,[16,17] Sweeney and Avner suggest a prevalence of up to 5%.[18] Given the prevalence rates for ADPKD (1/400-1000) and ARPKD (1/20,000), one can surmise that among children with PKDs in departments of pediatric nephrology, the total number of patients with early-onset ADPKD is about the same as those with ARPKD.

Independent of the exact prevalence figure for early-onset ADPKD, affected families with early-manifesting offspring have a high recurrence risk of almost 50% for the birth of a child with a similar clinical course.[19] Of special importance for genetic counseling of those pedigrees is that the aforementioned risk does not apply solely to parents of the severely affected index case, but also to offspring of affected siblings of the respective parent carrying the same germline mutation.[20-22]

Although these findings clearly corroborate a common familial modifying background for such early and severe disease expression, conclusive data regarding underlying mechanisms are still lacking and a matter of ongoing research. The most seriously discussed mechanisms are anticipation, imprinting, and the segregation of modifying genes. Anticipation denotes the progressively earlier appearance and increased severity of a disorder in successive generations. Whereas this mechanism has been well established for many neurological diseases (e.g., fragile X syndrome, spastic paraplegia, and myotonic dystrophy), only weak arguments exist for ADPKD. Fick et al. suggested an unstable mutation as a plausible explanation responsible for 53% of the informative 86 families of their study that demonstrated anticipation defined as a 10-year-earlier onset of ESRD in offspring compared with their affected parent.[23] However, the types of mutations identified so far provide no hint for unstable DNA in ADPKD. Furthermore, several groups failed to find any evidence of anticipation.[24-26] In the study by Geberth et al.,[25] the median difference in age at renal death in 74 parent-offspring pairs was 0 years, ranging from below 26.3 to above 27.2 years. There was no deviation from normal (Gaussian) distribution according to the Shapiro-Wilk test. Moreover, the proposal of anticipation was rebutted by MacDermot et al., who described a family in which the clinical presentation of ADPKD was impossible to reconcile with anticipation.[26] The gene carrier in generation I showed more severe clinical symptoms than his offspring in generation II, whereas in generation III the affected father of two affected fetuses presenting in utero was asymptomatic.

Similarly inconsistent are data available for imprinting mechanisms. Imprinting denotes the differential expression of genetic material depending on whether the genetic material has been inherited from the mother or father. Bear et al. were first to postulate an influence of genetic imprinting on disease progression in ten Newfoundland pedigrees linked to *PKD1*.[8] Age of onset of ESRD was significantly earlier in persons inheriting the disease from their mothers than from their fathers (50.5 vs. 64.8 years, $p = 0.004$). A statistically significant predominance of affected mothers transmitting the mutant gene was corroborated by two larger series of families with early-onset ADPKD.[19,23] In our survey of 64 families that included 79 children with early-onset ADPKD, a statistically significant maternal predominance was observed (M : F = 41 : 23).[19] In the study by Fick et al.,[23] the mutation was transmitted maternally in 65% of the 52 parent-offspring pairs with ESRD anticipation. Even though these findings are in line with a genetic imprinting effect in terms of an earlier onset and accelerated progression of ADPKD in cases of a maternally inherited gene, they cannot fully explain early-onset ADPKD in every case because paternal transmission has been frequently observed (ref. 26 and own unpublished data).

Segregation of a modifying allele being inherited from the unaffected parent is an intriguing hypothesis. The recurrence risk of about 25% for similarly early-onset ADPKD in sibships[19] fits this hypothesis and is further supported by the low incidence of in utero presentation of ADPKD in second-degree relatives in these families. Single case reports in the literature of second degree relatives also affected by early-onset ADPKD may thus be explained by chance segregation of a modifying gene in these families.[20-22] However, two additional pedigrees with very unusual transmission of early-onset ADPKD may raise some suspicion as to the accuracy of this hypothesis.[16,27] In one of these families an affected mother had four offspring with in utero onset PKD by two different, unrelated husbands.[16] In the other pedigree, early-onset of ADPKD was reported in mother and daughter.[27] Thus in these families, it would have had to be presumed that every affected parent carried a rare modifying allele to fit this theory. Therefore at present, any mechanism just discussed cannot sufficiently explain early-onset ADPKD and requires further examination.

Clinical Spectrum of Children with ADPKD The clinical spectrum of children with ADPKD varies widely and can range from fetuses with prenatal ultrasonographic evidence of massively enlarged kidneys and oligohydramnios/anhydramnios who may die perinatally from respiratory insufficiency to fully asymptomatic children with renal cysts noted more or less accidentally on ultrasound. In general the single most useful investigation in the evaluation of a child with early onset of cystic renal disease of unknown underlying disease entity might be ultrasound of the parents.[28] If ADPKD is clinically suspected and the parents are younger than 30, the grandparents should be considered for renal ultrasound.[29] Notably, a negative family history does not exclude the possibility of ADPKD in that the affected parent may well have a clinically silent disease. Given the autosomal dominant mode of inheritance the recurrence risk for a further affected child is 50%. In cases of normal parental renal ultrasound at age 30 and trusted paternity, a spontaneous mutation has to be discussed, but the recurrence risk is negligible except for the rare case of germline mosaicism in one parent. As a matter of course, in those cases differential diagnoses such as ARPKD should be considered as well.

Two large, longitudinal studies on ADPKD children conducted at the University of Colorado demonstrated that severe renal enlargement at a young age and/or hypertension were risk factors for accelerated renal growth.[30,31] To use renal enlargement as a marker for disease progression is clinically relevant, because many symptoms such as pain, hematuria, proteinuria, stones, and hypertension are associated with large kidneys. Furthermore, these authors confirmed that a large cyst number in early childhood is a predictor for faster structural progression. Conclusively, larger kidneys are associated with increased morbidity and more rapid progression to ESRD.

Intriguingly, in children with ADPKD, renal involvement is commonly asymmetric (including asymmetric kidney enlargement) and even unilateral in a minority at early stages of the disease.[32] As with ARPKD, the kidneys can present as large and hyperechoic bilateral masses with decreased corticomedullary differentiation. Whereas the ultrasonographic kidney pattern in ADPKD and ARPKD often becomes quite similar and hard to distinguish with ongoing disease,[33-35] the radiographic features in early disease course are often easier to distinguish. Unlike ARPKD, in which the cysts are usually fusiform and tiny, often impressing as pepper-salt pattern on ultrasound, ADPKD kidneys are frequently characterized by macrocysts even in small children.[36]

Although a significant proportion of adult ADPKD patients experience at least one episode of gross hematuria that is known to be a risk factor for the progression of renal disease,[37-39] hematuria is not as common in children and occurs in only about 10% of affected children at a mean age of 9.[30]

Arterial Hypertension Arterial hypertension in the first months of life may occur more often in patients with ARPKD; however, it is also common in pediatric ADPKD patients with normal renal function.[17,26,40] Hypertension should be identified as early as possible and aggressively treated, particularly in children under 12 who have more than 10 renal cysts.[41] This is consistent with data emerging from clinical studies of adult ADPKD.[42] The precise pathogenesis of hypertension in PKD remains to be elucidated; at least in part it appears to be mediated by activation of the intrarenal renin-angiotensin-aldosterone system (RAAS), reduced renal blood flow, and increased sodium retention.[43,44] However, there is controversial data concerning whether RAAS is activated in the first place, or at least inappropriately activated with respect to the prevailing blood pressure and sodium state.[45] Several studies have postulated that the aforementioned link between structural severity and hypertension is due to the upregulation of the RAAS.[46-48] Renin was found to be overexpressed in tubulocystic ADPKD epithelia.[49] Larger kidneys with a greater number of cysts may predispose for arterial hypertension through excess renal angiotensin II production. This hypothesis is corroborated by the finding of high renin concentrations in cyst fluid and the ability of cystic epithelia to synthesize renin.[49] In turn, angiotensin II acts as a growth factor for renal tubular cells and boosts the mitogenic actions of epidermal growth factor (EGF), which may further sustain faster renal growth in hypertensive children with enlarged kidneys.[50-53] However, a recent study by Doulton et al. found that activation of the classic circulating RAAS was no greater in hypertensive ADPKD patients than in individuals with essential hypertension.[54] This finding softens the argument that RAAS blockade is obligatory in ADPKD, although the issues of potentially activated intrarenal RAAS systems and the potential effects of RAAS blockade on cardiovascular events remain unresolved. An impressive lowering of blood pressure and an amplified antihypertensive effect of ACE inhibition by sodium restriction was noted in both renal patients and controls. Although this study questions the superiority of RAAS blockade over other antihypertensive drug classes in ADPKD, RAAS blockade may have important specific effects on the kidney tissue level.

Intracerebral Aneurysms Among cardiovascular comorbidities, intracerebral aneurysms (ICAs) play a significant role. However, the usefulness of screening for ICAs in patients known to be affected with ADPKD is a matter of ongoing debate.[55,56] A prevalence of about 8% of asymptomatic ICAs has been estimated in several large prospective series.[57-59] This figure is four to five times above the rate found in the general population.[60] Pirson et al. concluded in their comprehensive review that the prevalence of asymptomatic ICAs is about 6% in ADPKD patients in the absence of a positive family history of ICA or SAH (subarachnoid hemorrhage) and approximately 16% in those patients with a family history.[55]

Magnetic resonance (MR) angiography is the first-choice screening test; it does not require intravascular administration of contrast material and carries essentially no risk.[55] However, before any intervention, intraarterial angiography is necessary and carries a 5% risk of complications, including a 0.5% risk of permanent neurologic deficit in the general population.[61-66] When considering the elective treatment outcome for unruptured ICAs, one has to distinguish between surgical clipping and endovascular coil embolization. In a meta-analysis of 61 studies including 2460 patients that was published between 1966 and 1996 on clipping unruptured ICAs, mortality was 2.6% and morbidity was 10.9%. In more recent years, postoperative mortality and morbidity were significantly lower for nongiant aneurysms and aneurysms with an anterior location.[67] A meta-analysis of 90 cases electively treated by coil embolization reported no deaths related to the procedure and a 6.7% rate of permanent complications.[68] A more recent comparison of two groups of patients considered candidates for either procedure revealed mortality rates of 1% and 2% and a significant worsening in neurologic function in 25% and 8% of the patients treated by surgical clipping or endovascular coiling, respectively.[69] However, the lower mortality and morbidity rates of embolization should be weighed against the uncertainty of its long-term efficacy given that total obliteration of the ICA can usually be obtained in only about 40% of cases.[55]

The decision to screen and/or intervene in the ADPKD population is a challenging issue that must take a couple of aspects into account in every case. Fortunately, aneurysm rupture is not common among children and adolescents with ADPKD. Mariani et al. pointed out that there is little chance of detecting an ICA before age 30 and thus do not recommend screening before the third decade.[70] Chapman and Guay-Woodford tend toward consideration of screening at the age of 20.[71] General recommendations do not exist for adults with ADPKD either; however, the approach suggested by Pirson et al. may represent a balanced and reasonable view.[55] In their opinion, patients without family history of ICA should not be screened unless they firmly request it. In contrast, the risks of harboring an asymptomatic ICA and the pros and cons of screening should be explained in detail to individuals with a positive family history. In case of negative screening, the need for further periodic screening every 3 to 5 years remains, given that tiny ICAs may have been missed; however, for the moment the patient can be reassured. The same applies to individuals with an ICA less than 5 mm in diameter, although reevaluation at yearly intervals, smoking cessation, and strict control of hypertension and hyperlipidemia are recommended. While every ICA greater than 10 mm in diameter should be appropriately treated, the treatment of ICAs 5 to 10 mm in diameter is being increasingly discussed among specialists, particularly in young patients with an ICA treatable by coil embolization, considering that more than 50% of ruptured ICAs in ADPKD are larger than 10 mm in diameter.[65]

Liver Cysts Simple, mostly solitary hepatic cysts are common, with a prevalence of 2.5% to 10% among the general population.[72,73] These cysts must not be confused with hepatic cysts observed in about 50% of all patients with ADPKD. They usually gain in size and number as they do in the kidney. Their prevalence increases from about 20% in the third decade to approximately 75% in the seventh decade of life.[74] Women, especially those who have used hormones, been pregnant, or both, are usually more often and more severely affected.[74] There are some ADPKD families in whom hepatic cysts can be predominant with multiple cysts throughout the liver but who have very few renal cysts. Nevertheless, these cases have to be distinguished from autosomal dominant polycystic liver disease (PCLD), which is different from ADPKD at the phenotypic and genotypic level and is characterized by lack of renal cysts and progressive development of multiple (usually more than 20) liver cysts. Two separate genes, *PRKCSH* and *SEC63*, have been identified as causing familial PCLD.[75,76]

Regardless of the underlying entity, the pathogenesis, manifestations, and management of hepatic cysts are similar. Liver cysts usually arise from progressive dilatation of abnormal ducts in biliary hamartomas.[77,78] Hamartomas are the result of a ductal plate malformation (DPM) of small intrahepatic bile ducts. These bile ducts have lost continuity with the remaining biliary tree, explaining the noncommunicating nature of the cysts.[79] The smooth transition between various disease entities is illustrated by the fact that DPM is usually associated with congenital hepatic fibrosis (CHF) and hyperplastic biliary ducts. All these histologic findings are mandatory in ARPKD[80] and have also been described in ADPKD patients.[81-83]

Liver cysts rarely result in clinical problems and complications are much less common than with renal cysts. Usually hepatic, pancreatic, or ovarian cysts are not observed before puberty; however, there are single case reports of affected children in the first year of life.[84,85] If those children develop cyst infection, typical symptoms are right upper-quadrant pain, fever with leukocytosis, and a rise in liver enzymes.[86] In these cases surgical drainage is often recommended, because antibiotics alone may be ineffective.[87] To differentiate a complicated from an uncomplicated hepatic cyst, magnetic resonance imaging is the most sensitive technique and first-choice screening test. The massively enlarged liver secondary to hepatic cysts results in disabling discomfort in some patients. These individuals may benefit from percutaneous cyst decompression with alcohol sclerosis when one or a few large cysts are present.[85] Occasionally, more aggressive surgical intervention with fenestration, partial hepatectomy, or both may be required. A full review of the surgical management of adult PCLD is given by Tan and colleagues.[88] Further complications might result from hemorrhage into a cyst, which may cause severe acute abdominal pain, fever, and/or elevated liver enzymes, and possibly mimic acute cholecystitis or hepatic abscess.[89] Exceptionally rare is a ruptured cyst that gives rise to hemoperitoneum.

Genetics

Marquardt is thought to be the first to postulate genetic heterogeneity of PKDs, stating: "In surviving individuals, cystic kidneys are inherited dominantly. In non-viable individuals, cystic kidneys are recessive."[90] It took more than 35 years from that point of view before Blyth and Ockenden demonstrated in a systemic analysis that the age at presentation alone is not a reliable criterion for defining genetic heterogeneity.[91] Parental renal ultrasound, however, is still the most important classification criterion in most cases for distinguishing between ARPKD and ADPKD.

As the name implies, ADPKD is transmitted in an autosomal dominant, fully penetrant fashion, that is, virtually all individuals who inherit a mutated *PKD* germline allele will develop sonographically detectable renal cysts by age 30. The majority of ADPKD patients (about 85%) carries a germline mutation in the *PKD1* gene on chromosome 16p13.3,[92,93] whereas about 15% harbor a mutation in the *PKD2* gene on chromosome 4q21.[94] A further, yet-to-be-identified ADPKD locus has been proposed in a few reports concerning possibly unlinked families. One such pedigree was identified as having bilineal inheritance of both *PKD1* and *PKD2* germline mutations.[95]

PKD1 *and* PKD2 *Genes and Their Encoded Polycystin-1 and Polycystin-2 Proteins*

PKD1 is a large gene with a longest open reading frame (ORF) transcript of 46 exons predicted to encode a 4302 amino acid multidomain integral membrane glycoprotein (polycystin-1). *PKD2* has 15 exons encoding a 5.3 kb transcript that is translated into a 968 aa protein (polycystin-2). In keeping with the systemic nature of ADPKD, the two polycystins are widely expressed in tissues other than kidney. The systemic character is further emphasized by mouse models with homozygous *Pkd1* or *Pkd2* mutations.[96-99] Some of these mice are embryonic lethal and display severe cardiovascular anomalies along with renal and pancreatic cysts. The expression of polycystin-1 and polycystin-2 is developmentally regulated, with highest levels during late fetal and early neonatal life. Renal expression is highest in distal tubule and collecting-duct epithelial cells. Notably, the majority of cysts in ADPKD originates from collecting ducts, which is of importance for therapeutic approaches discussed later.

According to Knudson's two-hit model of tumorigenesis, second-hit mutation and resulting loss of heterozygosity (LOH) have been proposed as the mechanism that underlie cyst formation in ADPKD. Considerable intrafamilial phenotypic variation, focal cyst formation with evidence of epithelial cell clonality within individual cysts, as well as the detection of somatic mutations (occasionally transheterozygous in *PKD1* and *PKD2*, respectively) in cells lining renal and hepatic cysts are all in keeping with this theory.[100-104] However, it is apparent that this mechanism with a germline mutation to one allele and a somatic mutation to the other cannot fully explain cystogenesis. Patients and mice have been described that carry a germline *PKD1* and *PKD2* mutation (double heterozygotes) and thus are to be regarded as "homozygously" affected in every cell of the organism.[95,105] Contrary to the two-hit theory, not every renal tubular cell or nephron in these individuals gives rise to a cyst, and the clinical course is not substantially more severe than in cases with either mutation alone. Therefore the second-hit mutation to the other *PKD* gene may act as a modifying factor that boosts the risk of cyst development and/or drives cyst progression rather than initiates cyst events. A similar mechanism might be responsible for the severe clinical course with early-onset ADPKD along with tuberous sclerosis in most patients harboring a large genomic deletion in 16p13.3 that encompasses the *PKD1* and *TSC2* genes.[106] A possible synergistic functional link between polycystin-1 and the *TSC2* protein tuberin is indicated by the role tuberin plays in trafficking polycystin-1 to the lateral cell membrane.[107,108] Regarding the mechanisms underlying cystogenesis in ADPKD, it is worth noting that increased as well as decreased polycystin-1 expression may result in cyst formation. Lantinga-van Leeuwen and colleagues recently demonstrated that haploinsufficiency of *Pkd1* itself suffices to elicit a cystic phenotype.[109] Thus, taking all data into consideration, the two-hit model of cyst formation initially proposed for ADPKD is an attractive but no longer tenable theory in explaining the complex process of cystogenesis.

As shown in Figure 9-2, the predicted structure of polycystin-1 and polycystin-2 indicates that they are glycosylated integral membrane proteins. There is growing evidence that the polycystins are among the key players in the pathogenesis of cystic kidney disease. Polycystin-2 is predicted to have six transmembrane passes with cytoplasmic N- and C-termini. It is believed to function as a divalent cation channel, particularly involved in cellular Ca^{2+}, signaling belonging to the transient receptor potential (TRP) protein superfamily.[110] Polycystin-2 has been shown to interact with HAX-1 and α-actinin among other proteins,[111-113] and thus may be crucial for cytoskeletal organization, cell adhesion, proliferation, and migration. Notably, the ARPKD protein polyductin/fibrocystin has recently been demonstrated as another binding partner of polycystin-2, as well as of the calcium-modulating cyclophilin ligand CAML, a protein also known to be involved in Ca^{2+} signaling.[114,115]

Polycystin-1 is a huge integral membrane glycoprotein with an extensive aminoterminal extracellular region, 11 transmembrane passes, and a short 200 aa cytoplasmic carboxy-terminus. The intracellular C-terminus is predicted to contain several different potential phosphorylation sites and is supposed to mediate protein interactions by, for example, a heterotrimeric G-protein activation site and a coiled-coil domain that has been demonstrated to interact with the C-terminus of polycystin-2.[116-118] Notably, further renal cystoproteins, such as the nephrocystins, the Bardet-Biedl proteins BBS2 and BBS7, and the OFD1 (orofaciodigital syndrome type 1) protein, are predicted to contain putative coiled-coil domains too, even though this motif may be less specific and often found in proteins involved in protein-protein interactions.[1] Many of the structural motifs present in the large extracellular portion of polycystin-1, such as 16 copies of the immunoglobulinlike PKD domain, 2 cysteine-flanked leucine-rich repeats, the WSC homology domain (a cell-wall integrity and stress response component), and a C-type lectin domain, are putatively involved in protein-protein or protein-carbohydrate interactions. Thus polycystin-1 is believed to form multiprotein complexes at the cell membrane with functions in cell-cell and/or cell-matrix interactions via a possible role as receptor for currently unidentified ligands. Moreover, polycystin-1 is involved in mechanosensation and intracellular signal transduction.

PKD1/PKD2 *Mutation Spectrum and Routine Diagnostic Testing*

It must be emphasized that mutation screening in ADPKD is cumbersome and not a routine diagnostic test. Usually ADPKD is diagnosed clinically and ultrasonographically. As mentioned previously, about 95% of all carriers show ultrasonographic evidence of ADPKD by the age of 20 and almost every patient by age 30. Thus mutation analysis can usually be restricted to a few families. The main arguments

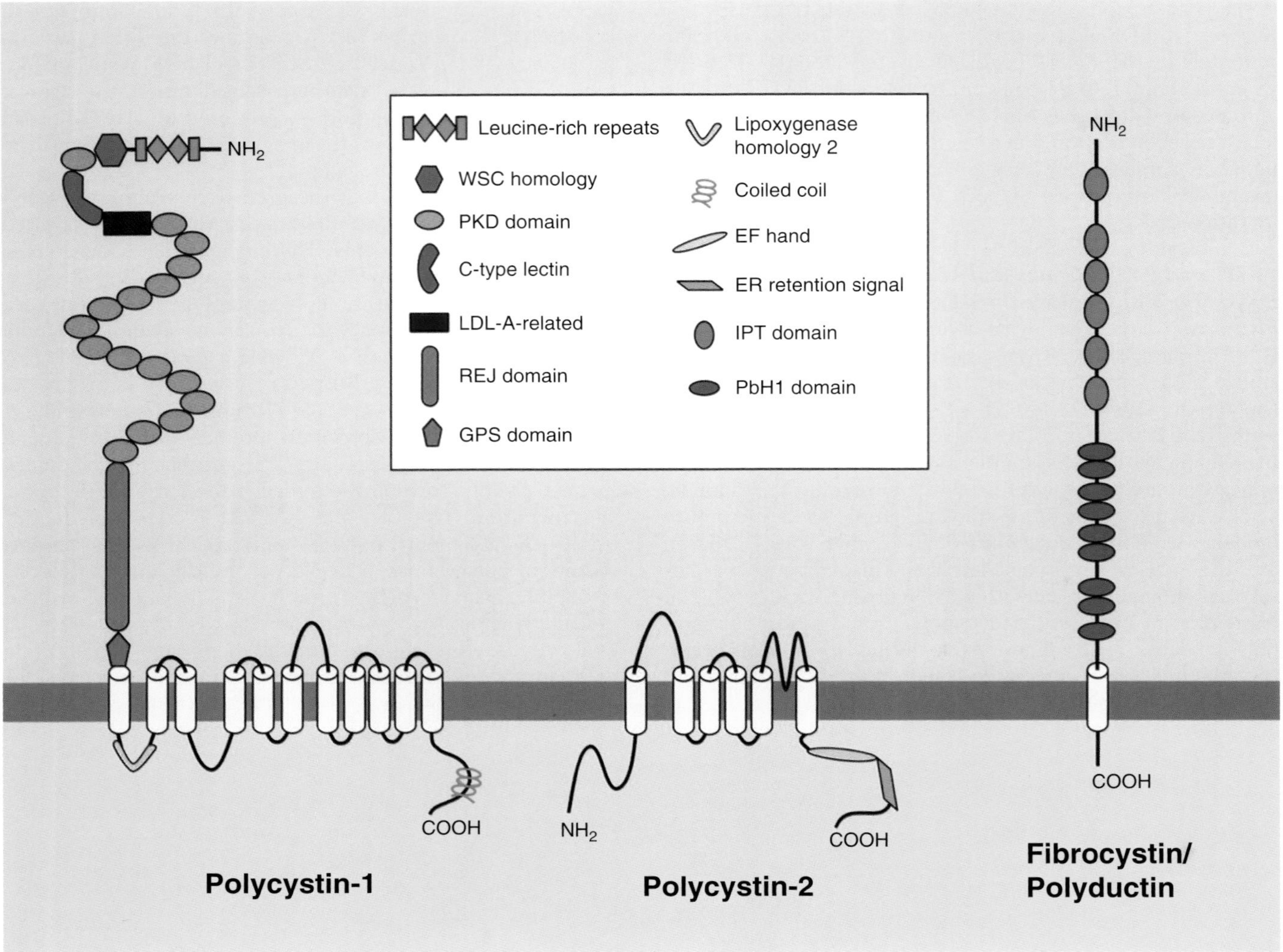

Figure 9-2 Structures of polycystin-1, polycystin-2, and fibrocystin/polyductin. Dark blue line indicates the membrane bilayer. Pink background indicates cytosol. Blue background indicates extracellular space or ER lumen. Protein motifs are identified in the figure legend. Light gray cylinders represent putative transmembrane segments. Only the membrane-bound form of fibrocystin/polyductin is shown. Structures are not drawn to scale. (From Igarashi P, Somlo S: Genetics and pathogenesis of polycystic kidney disease. *J Am Soc Nephrol* 13:2384-98, 2002.)

in favor of mutation analysis may be (1) donor screening of a relative willing to donate a healthy kidney with ambiguous ultrasonographic findings in the donor's kidneys and/or younger than age 30, (2) a request for prenatal diagnosis (PND) in families with early-onset ADPKD, or (3) to assess the recurrence risk for offspring of affected individuals without a family history of ADPKD. Mutation analysis of the *PKD1* gene is complicated by genomic duplication of the first 33 exons at 6 other sites on chromosome 16p. Many of these pseudogenes are expressed as mRNA transcripts but probably do not encode proteins. Both *PKD1* and *PKD2* mutations are scattered throughout the genes' coding regions, exhibiting marked allelic heterogeneity with most mutations being unique to single families (private mutations).[119,120] The majority of mutations presumably truncate the resulting protein and thus is assumed to be pathogenic; however, a considerable proportion of changes are novel amino acid substitutions that are difficult to evaluate with respect to their significance.

Genotype-Phenotype Correlations

Overall, the analysis of ESRD in affected persons within one family carrying the same mutation shows a wide range of variability that clearly illustrates the limitations of possible genotype-phenotype correlations.[121] Although no definite genotype-phenotype correlations have been identified for *PKD2*,[13,122] certain interdependencies have been set up in *PKD1* as to mutations 5′ to the median are associated with a slightly earlier age at onset of ESRD (53 vs. 56 years).[123] Moreover, the median position of the *PKD1* mutation was found to be further 5′ located in families with a vascular phenotype of intracranial aneurysms and subarachnoid hemorrhage.[124] However, for genetic counseling and the prediction of the outcome of an individual patient, these genotype-phenotype correlations are only of limited value. As outlined in detail previously, a positive family history for intracranial aneurysm or SAH is considered a strong risk factor for intracranial aneurysms and warrants further diagnostic testing (e.g., MR angiography).[55]

AUTOSOMAL RECESSIVE POLYCYSTIC KIDNEY DISEASE

Epidemiology and Morphology

ARPKD is much rarer than its dominant counterpart with a proposed incidence among Caucasians of about 1 in 20,000 live births corresponding to a carrier frequency of approximately 1 in 70 in nonisolated populations. The exact incidence is unknown since published studies vary in the cohorts of patients examined (e.g., autopsied patients vs. moderately affected patients followed by pediatricians), and some severely affected babies may die perinatally without a definitive diagnosis. Isolated populations may have higher prevalences, such as an incidence of 1 in 8000 in Finland reported by Kääriänen.[16] As mentioned before, among children with PKDs in departments of pediatric nephrology, the total number of patients with ARPKD equals the quantity of individuals affected with early-onset ADPKD. Among cases from departments of pediatric pathology, ARPKD with severe intrauterine manifestation outranks early-onset ADPKD.

Histologic changes can vary depending on the age of presentation and the extent of cystic involvement. However, usually ARPKD can be reliably diagnosed pathoanatomically.[125,126] Principally, the kidneys are symmetrically enlarged (up to 10 times normal size) in affected neonates and retain their reniform contour (Figure 9-3, Table 9-3). Macroscopically, the cut surface demonstrates the cortical extension of fusiform or cylindrical spaces arranged radially throughout the renal parenchyma from medulla to cortex (Figure 9-4). Invariable histological manifestations are fusiform dilations of renal collecting ducts and distal tubuli lined by columnar or cuboidal epithelium that usually remain in contact with the urinary system (unlike ADPKD), whereas glomerular cysts (as in ADPKD) or dysplastic elements (e.g., cartilage, as in Meckel-Gruber syndrome) are usually not evident in ARPKD kidneys (Figure 9-5). During early fetal development, a transient phase of proximal tubular cyst formation has been identified that is largely absent by birth, however.[127] As mentioned previously, with advancing clinical course and development of larger renal cysts accompanied by interstitial fibrosis, ARPKD kidney structure may increasingly resemble the pattern observed in ADPKD.[34] Liver changes are obligatory for ARPKD and characterized by dysgenesis of the hepatic portal triad attributable to defective remodeling of the ductal plate with hyperplastic biliary ducts and CHF (Figure 9-6).[77] These hepatobiliary changes subsumed as DPM are present from early (first trimester) embryonic development on and lead to progressive portal fibrosis. At later stages, fibrous septa may link different portal tracts by intersecting the hepatic parenchyma, often leading to portal hypertension; however, the remaining liver parenchyma usually develops normally. Thus liver enzymes, except for cholestasis parameters that are sometimes elevated, are characteristically not increased. As extensively discussed for ADPKD, liver cysts usually arise from DPM and biliary ectasia, and there obviously exist smooth transitions to extensive dilations of both intrahepatic and extrahepatic bile ducts and forms such as Caroli disease/syndrome.[77]

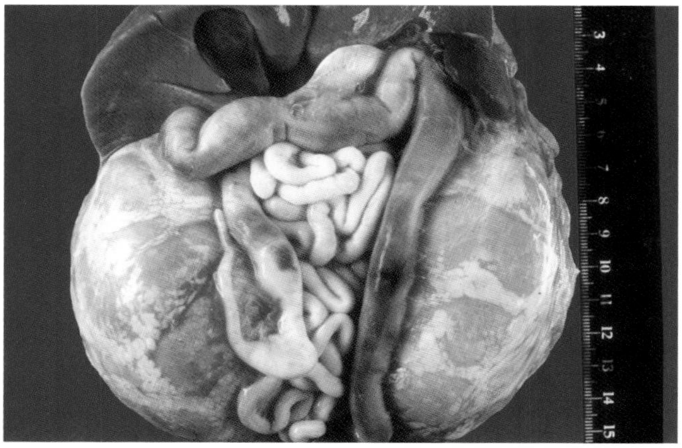

Figure 9-3 Abdominal situs of an ARPKD patient with symmetrically enlarged kidneys that maintain their reniform configuration.

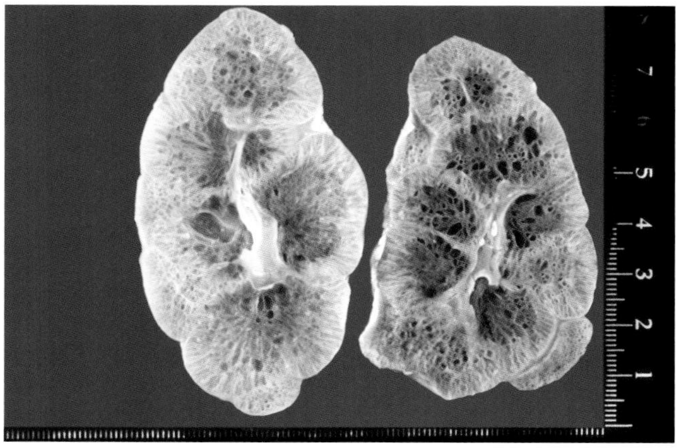

Figure 9-4 Cross-section of ARPKD kidneys reveals the cortical extension of fusiform or cylindrical spaces arranged radially throughout the renal parenchyma from medulla to cortex.

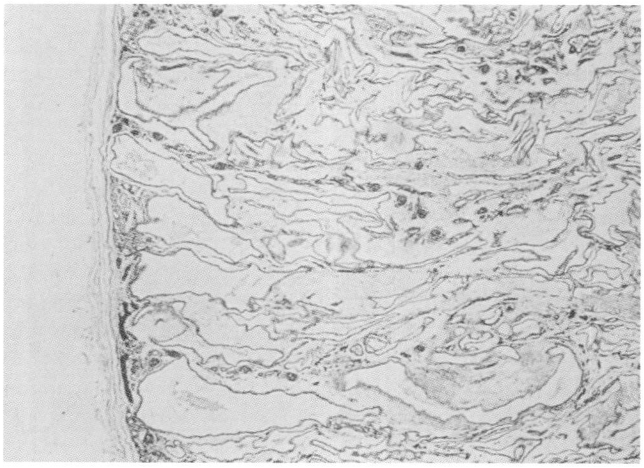

Figure 9-5 Microscopically, fusiform dilations of renal collecting ducts and distal tubuli lined by columnar or cuboidal epithelium can be observed in ARPKD. These dilated collecting ducts run perpendicular to the renal capsule.

TABLE 9-3 Characteristics of Autosomal Recessive and Dominant Polycystic Kidney Diseases

	ARPKD	ADPKD
Synonyms	Infantile polycystic kidney disease Potter type I	Adult polycystic kidney disease Potter type III
Incidence	~1:20,000	1:400-1,000 (~2% early manifesting)
Pathology of Kidneys		
Macroscopy	Massively, symmetrically enlarged kidneys (reniform)	Generally enlarged (also reniform), but usually to a lesser extent
Location of cysts	Dilated collecting ducts and distal tubuli	Cysts in all parts of the nephron (including glomerulus)
Ultrasound and diameter of cysts	At onset, typical pepper-salt pattern in ultrasound; increased echogenicity of renal parenchyma throughout cortex and medulla due to tiny, sometimes invisible, cysts (usually < 2 mm); with advancing age, up to several cm similar to ADPKD pattern	Cysts of different size in cortex and medulla (usually several larger cysts in adults); at onset often small, however, sometimes already several cm early in childhood
Pathology of liver	Mandatory: ductal plate malformation/congenital hepatic fibrosis with hyperplastic biliary ducts and portal fibrosis (may impress as Caroli disease)	"Liver cysts" common in adults, but rare in children. Occasionally, ductal plate malformation/ congenital hepatic fibrosis
Associated anomalies	Rarely pancreatic cysts and/or fibrosis; single case reports with intracranial aneurysms	Pancreatic cysts and/or cysts in other epithelial organs; intracranial aneurysms in ~8%, familially clustered
Main clinical manifestations	Peri-/neonatal period: respiratory distress (in 30%-50%). With prolonged survival renal insufficiency, portal hypertension, and other comorbidities (highly variable)	General onset 3rd-5th decade, with arterial hypertension, proteinuria, hematuria, and/or renal insufficiency, ~2% early manifestation in childhood (rarely with perinatal respiratory distress)
Risk for siblings	25%	50% (except in rare cases of spontaneous mutation with virtually no risk)
Risk for own children	<1% (unless unaffected parent is related to his/her affected partner, or ARPKD is known in the unaffected partner's family)	50% (also for patients with a spontaneous mutation)
Manifestation in affected family members	Often similar clinical course in siblings (in ~20% gross intrafamilial variability)	Variable, however, often similar within the same family; in case of early manifestation, ~50% recurrence risk
Parental kidneys	No alterations	Usually one affected parent with cysts in both kidneys (unless parents are too young/<30 years), except for in rare cases of spontaneous mutation
Prognosis	In perinatal cases with respiratory distress, usually poor; for those surviving the neonatal period, much better, with renal death in ~15% in childhood, often with severe complications due to portal hypertension and esophageal varices; if possible, transplantation (often combined kidney-liver TX)	In early-manifesting cases, often better than in ARPKD; in "adult" cases, chronic renal failure in ~50% by age of 60 years; and median age of ESRD onset (53 vs. 69 years in PKD1 vs. PKD2)

ADPKD, Autosomal dominant polycystic kidney disease; *ARPKD*, autosomal recessive polycystic kidney disease; *TX*, transplantation.

Clinical Course and Treatment

While ADPKD is usually a disease of adults, with no more than 2% to 5% of patients displaying an early manifesting clinical course, ARPKD is typically an infantile disease. However, the clinical spectrum is much more variable than generally presumed.[128] Nevertheless, despite dramatic advances in neonatal and intensive care over the past decades, the short-term and long-term morbidity and mortality of ARPKD remain substantial. Ages at diagnosis and initial clinical features are listed in Table 9-4, which summarizes results of various clinical studies on ARPKD. Notably, these studies differ widely in their selection criteria of patients and their mode of data analysis. Patients in our studies[129,130] and those in Guay-Woodford's and Desmond's survey[131] were mostly recruited from departments of pediatric nephrology. As a consequence, individuals with an early lethal form of ARPKD were underrepresented. Gagnadoux et al.[132] and Capisonda et al.[133] reported clinical outcomes of patients from specialized single centers. Most of the individuals in the study by Roy et al.[134] had previously been reported by Kaplan et al., who exclusively included patients with pathoanatomically proven CHF.[135] Kääriäinen et al. analyzed data obtained mainly from Finnish death registers.[136] Inclusion criteria in the study by Cole et al. were diagnosis within the first year of life and survival of the neonatal period.[137]

Overall, the majority of ARPKD cases are identified late in pregnancy or at birth. Severely affected fetuses display a "Potter" oligohydramnios phenotype with pulmonary hypoplasia, a characteristic facies, and contracted limbs with clubfeet. As many as 30% to 50% of affected neonates die from

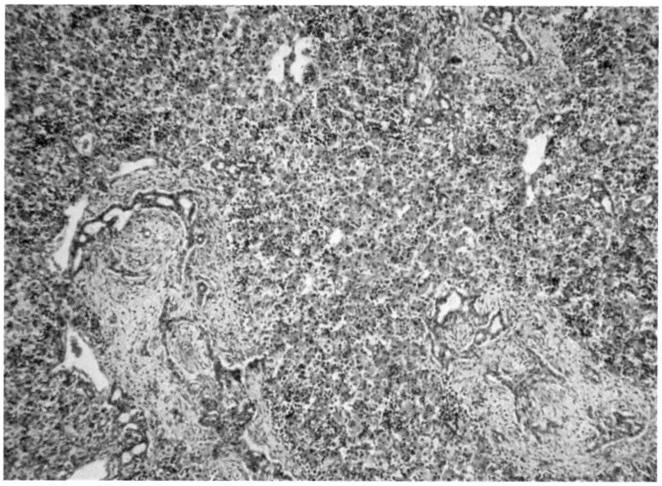

Figure 9-6 Obligatory hepatobiliary changes in ARPKD subsumed as ductal plate malformation (DPM) and characterized by dysgenesis of the hepatic portal triad with hyperplastic biliary ducts and congenital hepatic fibrosis (CHF).

respiratory insufficiency shortly after birth. The respiratory distress in these severely affected children is mainly caused by the massively enlarged kidneys and a critical degree of pulmonary hypoplasia, which is an accompaniment of in utero renal dysfunction leading to oligohydramnios/anhydramnios. Renal failure is rarely a cause of neonatal demise. Hyponatremia related to a urine dilution defect is often present in the newborn period, but usually resolves over time.[129,131,135] Advances in mechanical ventilation and other supportive measures, as well as further improvements in renal replacement therapies, have increased the survival rates of ARPKD patients, with some of them reaching adulthood. Somewhat surprisingly, several patients carrying two convincing *PKHD1* mutations were recently reported who were clinically asymptomatic until advanced adulthood and may have a normal life expectancy (ref. 128 and own unpublished data). Although these cases suggest some sort of alertness, overall they may be exceptions to the rule, because usually a wide range of associated comorbidities evolve in ARPKD, including systemic hypertension, ESRD, and clinical manifestations of CHF.[130,131,134] Thus ARPKD is an important cause of renal-related and liver-related morbidity and mortality in children with a still severely diminished life expectancy. In our recent study of almost 200 ARPKD patients with known *PKHD1* mutation status, survival rates of those who survived the first month of life were 94% at 5 years and 92% at 10 years of age,[130] while Dell and Avner reported a 10-year survival rate of 82% for patients who survived the first year of life.[138]

Chronic renal failure was first detected at a mean age of 4 years in patients of our recent survey, which included mainly patients from departments of pediatric nephrology.[130] Infants with ARPKD may have a transient improvement in their glomerular filtration rate (GFR) resulting from renal maturation in the first 6 months of life.[139] However, a progressive but highly variable decrease in renal function subsequently occurs. The management of children with declining renal function should follow the standard guidelines established for chronic renal insufficiency in other pediatric patients.[139] In our study,[130] ESRD occurred in 29% of patients at 10 years and 58% at 20 years, which is much lower than figures reported by previous studies that proposed rates of approximately 50% of ARPKD patients who progressed to ESRD within the first decade of life.[134,137] Renal transplantation is the treatment of choice for individuals with ESRD. In case of massively enlarged kidneys, native nephrectomies may be warranted to allow allograft placement.

Arterial hypertension usually develops in the first few months of life and affects up to 80% of children with ARPKD (Table 9-4). Hypertension can be difficult to control in these children and may require multidrug treatment; however, it should be treated early and aggressively, with blood pressure carefully monitored to prevent sequelae of hypertension (e.g., cardiac hypertrophy or congestive heart failure) and deterioration of renal function. Therapies with angiotensin converting enzyme (ACE) inhibitors are the treatment of choice. Other drugs that are generally effective include calcium channel blockers, AT II receptor inhibitors, beta-blockers (particularly in those patients with signs of CHF and portal hypertension), and diuretics (especially loop agents).[131,140] As previously discussed for ADPKD, the pathophysiology of hypertension in ARPKD is not clearly understood. Although peripheral vein renin values are not usually elevated in hypertensive ARPKD patients, the pathogenesis of hypertension appears to be mediated, at least in part, by dysregulation of renal sodium transport and activation of the RAAS that lead to increased intravascular volume.[135]

By ultrasound, children with ARPKD typically are found to have characteristically large, bilateral echogenic kidneys with poor corticomedullary differentiation; macrocysts are uncommon in small infants although they may be observed with advanced clinical course when ultrasonographic patterns of ARPKD and ADPKD oftentimes adjust and become hard to differentiate.[33-35] Data for kidney length measured by ultrasound related to age among the patients of our recent study revealed that 92% had a kidney length above or on the 97th centile for age, respectively +2 standard deviation (SD) scores.[130] In no case was the kidney size decreased, ranging from 0 to +17 SDs. No correlations were observed between kidney length and renal function or between kidney length and duration of the disease.

In keeping with generally prolonged survival in ARPKD, for many patients hepatobiliary complications come to dominate the clinical picture. Although hepatocellular function is usually preserved, these individuals develop sequelae of portal hypertension and may show hematemesis or melena resulting from bleeding esophageal varices and/or hypersplenism with consequent pancytopenia. Primary management of variceal bleeding may include endoscopic approaches such as sclerotherapy or variceal banding. In some patients portosystemic shunting or liver–kidney transplantation (sequential or combined) should be considered a viable therapeutic option. A serious, potentially lethal complication in ARPKD is ascending suppurative cholangitis that may cause fulminant hepatic failure. It always requires diligent evaluation with aggressive antimicrobial treatment. Notably, ARPKD patients

TABLE 9-4 **Summary of Findings Obtained in Clinical Studies of ARPKD Patients**

	Bergmann et al. (2005)	Guay-Woodford and Desmond (2003)	Capisonda et al. (2003)	Roy et al. (1997)	Zerres et al. (1996)	Gagnadoux et al. (1989)	Kaplan et al. (1989)	Kääriäinen et al. (1988)	Cole et al. (1987)
Patients (n)	186 (164)	166	31	52	115	33	55	73 (18 neonatal survivors)	17
Age at diagnosis	23% prenatal 31% < 1 mo 16% 1-12 mo 30% > 1 yr	46% prenatal 27% < 1 mo 11% 1-12 mo 16% > 1 yr	32% prenatal 23% < 1 mo 19% 1-12 mo 26% > 1 yr	85% < 1 yr 15% > 1 yr	10% prenatal 41% < 1 mo 23% 1-12 mo 26% > 1 yr	33% < 1 mo 55% 1-18 mo 12% 6-11 yr	42% < 1 mo 42% 1-12 mo 16% < 1 yr	72% < 1 mo 6% < 1 yr 22% > 1 yr	100% 1-12 mo (inclusion criteria)
Renal function	86% GFR < 3rd percentile for age Median age CRF 4.0 yr 29% ESRD (by 10 yr)	42% GFR < 3rd percentile for age 13% ESRD	51% GFR < 80 ml/min/1.73 m^2 16% ESRD	33% ESRD (by 15 yr)	72% GFR < 3rd percentile for age 10% ESRD	42% GFR < 80 ml/min/1.73 m^2 21% ESRD	58% SC > 100 μmol/ml	82% GFR < 90 ml/min/1.73 m^2	35% GFR < 40 ml/min/1.7 m^2 29% ESRD
Kidney length	92% > 2 SD	NA	NA	NA	68% > 2 SD	100% > 2 SD	NA	NA	NA
Hypertension (% on drug treatment)	76% (80% M/72% F) medication started at median age of 3 yr (53% during first 6 mo)	65%	55%	60% (by 15 yr)	70%	76%	65%	61%	100% (drug treatment or BP > 95th percentile)
Growth retardation	16% < 2 SD (23% M/10% F)	24% < 2 SD	NA	NA	25% < 2 SD	18% < 4 SD	NA	6% < 2.5 SD	NA
Anemia	14% (9% M/19% F)	NA	NA	NA	NA	NA	NA	NA	NA
Evidence of portal hypertension	44% (41% M/47% F)† 38% splenomegaly 15% esophageal varices 2% ascites	15%	37%	23% (8/35)	46%	39%	47%	50% (hepatomegaly)	35%
Survival rate	1 yr: 85% 5 yr: 84% 10 yr: 82%	1 yr: 79% 5 yr: 75%	1 yr: 87% 9 yr: 80%	NA	1 yr: 89% 3 yr: 88%	1 yr: 91%	1 yr: 79% 10 yr: 51% 15 yr: 46%	1 yr: 19%	1 yr: 88%
Death rate in the first year of life	15%	8%	13%	26%	9%	9%	24%	22%	12%

BP, Blood pressure; *ESRD*, end-stage renal disease; *NA*, not available; *SD*, standard deviation.

*Based on sonographic evidence of hepatomegaly, splenomegaly, and directional reversal of portal vein flow, or clinical, radiological, or endoscopic evidence of esophageal varices or ascites.

†Manifestation of clinical signs of congenital hepatic fibrosis was positively correlated with age. In 87%, increased echogenicity of the liver has been reported (89% M/84% F). Cystic changes of the liver probably representing Caroli's disease with dilated larger intrahepatic bile ducts have been noted in 27 individuals, equaling 16% of the total cohort (17% M/15% F). Within this survey only two boys exhibited impaired hepatocellular function (1%), underscoring that liver function is usually retained in ARPKD. In six patients (4 M/2 F) liver transplantation (LTX) was performed (mean age 13.8 yr). In four cases it was done in parallel with NTX (combined LNTX).

may not display the typical clinical findings of cholangitis; thus every patient with unexplained recurrent sepsis, particularly with gram-negative organisms, should be critically evaluated for this diagnosis.[141]

Another aspect depicted in recent clinical studies on ARPKD was the renal-hepatobiliary morbidity pattern.[130,131] Although most patients usually show uniform disease progression, individual ARPKD patients present with an organ-specific phenotype, that is, either an (almost) exclusive renal phenotype or a predominant or mere liver phenotype. In accordance, it could be demonstrated that *PKHD1* mutations can cause isolated CHF or Caroli disease (ref. 130, 142 and own unpublished data). Noteworthy is that two transgenic mouse models for *Pkhd1* display an isolated liver phenotype without any renal involvement.[143,144]

Genetics

Given the autosomal recessive mode of inheritance, the recurrence risk for subsequent pregnancies of parents of an affected child is 25%. Overall, males and females seem to be affected equally. As indicated by formal genetics, unaffected siblings harbor a two-thirds risk of being a carrier of ARPKD. However, most healthy siblings, other close relatives, and patients themselves seeking genetic counseling for their own family planning can be reassured. The risk for their own children having ARPKD will be comparably low when neither the partner is related to the index family nor a case of ARPKD is known in the partner's pedigree (for offspring of patients, 1 in 140; for offspring of patients' healthy siblings, 1 in 420; for offspring of patients' healthy uncles or aunts, 1 in 560, when using a heterozygosity rate of 1 in 70, respectively).

On the basis of age at presentation and relative degrees of renal and hepatic involvement, Blyth and Ockenden stratified ARPKD patients into four phenotypic entities (perinatal, neonatal, infantile, and juvenile).[90] In keeping with their theory, they hypothesized four distinct genes to be responsible for ARPKD. Doubts on the correctness of this hypothesis arose when affected sibships with significant discordance in disease onset and manifestation were discovered.[145-147] These observations prompted us to propose that the entire spectrum of ARPKD is caused by multiple allelism in a single gene.[148] We could confirm this hypothesis by mapping the gene underlying ARPKD to the short arm of chromosome 6 and demonstrating that all phenotypic variants are compatible with linkage to this single locus.[149,150]

PKHD1 *Gene and Polyductin/Fibrocystin Protein*

In 2002, two groups independently identified the sequence of the *PKHD1* gene providing the basis for direct genotyping.[151,152] *PKHD1* is among the largest disease genes characterized to date in the human genome, extending over a genomic segment of at least 470 kb and including a minimum of 86 exons. Both *PKHD1* and its murine ortholog undergo a complex and extensive pattern of alternative splicing, generating transcripts highly variable in size. In accordance with the disease phenotype, the gene is highly expressed in the fetal and adult kidney and at lower levels in the liver.[152,153] Weak expression is present in other tissues also, among them the pancreas and arterial wall. The longest *PKHD1* transcript contains 67 exons with an ORF composed of 66 exons (ATG start codon in exon 2) that encodes a protein of 4074 amino acids (aa).

The predicted full-length protein (polyductin/fibrocystin) represents a novel putative integral membrane protein with a signal peptide at the amino terminus of its extensive, highly glycosylated extracellular domain, a single transmembrane (TM)-spanning segment, and a short cytoplasmic C-terminal tail (192 aa) containing potential protein kinase A phosphorylation sites (Figure 9-2). The putative ~3860 aa extracellular portion contains several IPT (immunoglobulinlike, plexin, transcription factor) and IPT-like domains that can be found in cell surface receptors and in the Rel family of transcription factors. Between the IPT domains and the TM segment, multiple PbH1 (parallel beta-helix 1) repeats are present, a motif that can be observed in polysaccharidases and may bind to carbohydrate moieties such as glycoproteins on the cell surface and/or in the basement membrane. Based on the structural features of the deduced protein and on the human ARPKD phenotype, polyductin/fibrocystin might be involved in cellular adhesion, repulsion, and proliferation. In addition, the domain and structural analyses suggest that the *PKHD1* potential products may be involved in intercellular signaling and function as receptor, ligand, and/or membrane-associated enzyme.[152]

In common with most other cystoproteins, polyductin has been shown to be localized to primary cilia with concentration in the basal body area.[154-159] The lack of a clear polyductin homologue in C. *elegans* and in other phyla suggests that this protein has been a relatively late evolutionary addition to the ancestral polycystin pathway. However, this hypothesis awaits experimental clarification. It is well known that kidney development constitutes a classic model of mesenchymal epithelial transformation. By immunoprobing human metanephroi and kidney epithelial lines, it was demonstrated that during acquisition of epithelial polarity, polyductin localizes to the apical zone of nephron precursor cells and then to basal bodies at the origin of primary cilia in fully differentiated epithelia. These striking patterns of subcellular localization and the known interactions with polycystin-2 and CAML place polyductin at key sites where it may play roles not only in microtubule organization as a characteristic centrosomal function, but also in mechanosensation of urine flow as an ascribed primary ciliary function.

Recent data suggest the existence of different, partly secreted polyductin isoproteins and Notch-like posttranslational processing.[154-161] However, it is unknown how many alternative *PKHD1* transcripts are actually translated into protein and have biological function(s). In case various mRNAs are translated, the *PKHD1* gene may encode numerous distinct polypeptides differing in size and amino acid sequence. This attractive hypothesis is supported by different lines of evidence. First, multiple bands could have been detected in western blot analysis of diverse groups.[154-158] Moreover, Masyuk and colleagues showed the translation of different, partly secreted polyductin isoproteins in cholangiocytes.[159] Kaimori et al. detected the expected full-length polyductin product (>400 kDa) and a C-terminally tagged 80-90 kDa product in the plasma membrane when using a cell surface biotinylation assay.[160] Intriguingly, Hiesberger and coworkers could demonstrate that regulated intramembrane proteolysis (RIP) is induced by primary cilia-dependent Ca^{2+} signaling and generates a C-terminal polyductin fragment that can signal directly to the nucleus.[161] Finally, it will be important to establish which isoforms are essential for renal and hepatobiliary integrity to better understand the role of polyductin in the etiology of ARPKD. The distribution of mutations over the entire *PKHD1* gene suggests that the longest ORF transcript is necessary for proper polyductin function in the kidney and liver. Thus it might be proposed that a critical amount of the full-length protein is required for normal function. Alternatively, however, it could be hypothesized that mutations disrupt a critical functional stoichiometric or temporal balance between the different protein products that is normally maintained by elaborate, tightly regulated splicing patterns. In light of the complex splicing pattern and multiple transcripts, the identification of *PKHD1* mutations is one means to decipher those exons whose presence in a transcript is essential for the function of polyductin.

PKHD1 *Mutation Spectrum and Routine Diagnostic Testing*

The large size of *PKHD1*, its presumably complex pattern of splicing, and lack of knowledge of the encoded protein's function(s) pose significant challenges to DNA-based diagnostic testing. Further requirements for investigation are set by the extensive allelic heterogeneity, with a high level of missense mutations and private mutations in "nonisolate" populations.[130,142,162-167] Thus it was crucial to set up a locus-specific database for *PKHD1* (http://www.humgen.rwth-aachen.de). By now, about 350 different *PKHD1* mutations (mostly point mutations and small deletions/duplications/insertions) on approximately 900 mutated alleles are listed in this database along with all known presumably nonpathogenic sequence variants.

Remarkably, mutation detection rates of about 80% for the entire clinical spectrum of ARPKD patients ranging from individuals with perinatal demise to moderately affected adults have been shown.[130,165-167] The power of *PKHD1* mutation analysis is further strengthened by the observation that in more than 95% of families screened, at least one mutation could be identified. However, the molecular defect still remains to be determined in a considerable proportion of chromosomes. The major cause of missing mutations may be limited sensitivity of the screening method even though denaturing high-performance liquid chromatography (DHPLC) that has been mainly applied has been shown to be efficient and effective in analyzing large genes. Moreover, some silent exonic changes and a subset of adjacent intronic sequence variations may also have an effect on PKHD1 splicing, for example, by affecting splice enhancer or silencer sites (ESE/ISE or ESS/ISS).[168] However, functional and mRNA studies are usually needed to prove any possible pathogenic effect of such changes.[169] We recently showed that missing mutations alternatively reside in regulatory elements and that genomic rearrangements occur in the *PKHD1* gene (ref. 170 and own unpublished data). In patients without a detectable *PKHD1* mutation, misdiagnosis of ARPKD has to be considered even though evidence for genetic heterogeneity has been found in only a small subset of families (own unpublished data).

The most common mutation, c.107C>T (p.Thr36Met) in exon 3, has been described in each *PKHD1* mutation study reported to date and accounts for approximately 15% to 20% of mutated alleles.[164] There are conflicting data as to whether it is an ancestral change or occurs because of a frequent mutational event. Ultimately it cannot be excluded that some of the mutated c.107C>T alleles represent a founder effect in the central European population where it is particularly frequent.[171] However, there is compelling evidence that c.107C>T constitutes a mutational "hotspot," most likely a result of methylation-induced deamination of the mutagenic CpG dinucleotide.[172] In a recent study, c.107C>T was identified on various haplotypes in a multitude of obviously unrelated families of different ethnic origins.[130] Convincingly, patients of a nonconsanguineous Finnish family homozygous for c.107C>T were shown to harbor differing haplotypes. Further evidence of recurrence and against a common ancestral origin of mutated c.107C>T alleles was demonstrated by diverse haplotypes among two German-Austrian pedigrees that carried the same set of missense mutations (c.107C>T + c.7264T>G).[130]

Except for c.107C>T (p.Thr36Met), there are no mutational hotspots, but marked allelic heterogeneity at *PKHD1*, with the majority of mutations unique to a single family in "nonisolate" populations. Given the size of the *PKHD1* gene and the absence of mutational hotspots, *PKHD1* molecular testing can be a time-consuming, labor-intensive process. However, diagnostic testing has recently been simplified by the characterization of an algorithm for *PKHD1* that allows for detection of most mutations by analysis of only a subset of fragments and facilitates robust *PKHD1* mutation analysis in a routine diagnostic setting.[173] Overall, this algorithm is an efficient and economical approach for mutation analysis of the large and complex *PKHD1* gene.

Genotype-Phenotype Correlations

Setting up genotype-phenotype correlations for *PKHD1* is hampered by multiple allelism and the high rate of different compound heterozygotes. Genotype-phenotype correlations can be drawn for the type of mutation rather than for the site of individual mutations.[162] All patients carrying two truncating mutations display a severe phenotype with perinatal or neonatal demise, whereas patients surviving the neonatal period bear at least one missense mutation. Although the converse does not apply and some missense changes are obviously as devastating as truncating mutations, missense changes are more frequently observed among patients with a moderate clinical course, and chain-terminating mutations are more commonly associated with a severe phenotype. No significant clinical differences could be observed between patients with two missense mutations and those harboring a truncating mutation in trans; thus the milder mutation obviously defines the phenotype.[130]

Loss of function probably explains the uniformly early demise of patients carrying two truncating alleles. This "frameshift rule," based on the assumption that a truncated ORF will always constitute a null mutation, has also been postulated to be responsible for the generally uniform phenotype in Duchenne muscular dystrophy (DMD) caused by dystrophin mutations that cause premature translation termination.[174] This uniformity is probably attributable to ablation of the message by nonsense-mediated decay (NMD). Regarding polyductin, a critical amount of the full-length protein seems necessary for normal function that obviously cannot be compensated with alternative isoforms that might be generated by reinitiation of translation at a downstream ATG codon as a possible mechanism for the evasion of NMD.

In contrast, missense mutations and small, inframe deletions may have more variable effects on the protein's function, as exemplified by the diversity observed in patients with Becker muscular dystrophy carrying dystrophin mutations that leave the ORF in register. Phenotypic diversity also reflects the variable extent to which different *PKHD1* missense mutations might compromise the function and/or abundance of the mutant protein. Although some may result in hypomorphic alleles with reduced function allowing for a clinically milder course, others might represent loss-of-function variants. As depicted by discordant siblings (see following), phenotypes cannot be simply explained on the basis of the genotype but likely depend on the background of other genes,[175,176] epigenetic factors (e.g., alternative splicing),[177,178] and environmental influences as well. Such modifiers will probably have their greatest impact on the phenotype in the setting of hypomorphic missense changes and may explain, at least in part, the highly variable clinical course resulting from missense mutations; they are less likely to be relevant in null alleles.

Phenotypes may further be influenced by the location and character of amino acid substitutions. It might thus be reasonable to categorize *PKHD1* missense mutations into severe and moderate/mild changes as done for various other disorders.[179,180] Such correlations, however, are hampered for *PKHD1* by significant multiple allelism and the high rate of different compound heterozygotes. Nevertheless, the bulk of mutational data identified since cloning of *PKHD1* allowed us to start categorizing missense mutations carefully.[130] In line with the "frameshift rule" previously outlined, termination-type mutations represent loss-of-function alleles with a uniform effect on phenotype. Thus one would expect the position and character of the missense change to determine the clinical course in compound heterozygotes with one truncating and one missense mutation. *PKHD1* missense mutations have only been classified in case of recurrence in at least two unrelated families either homozygously or in compound with a truncating mutation on the other parental allele. Nevertheless, as a matter of course, conclusions should be dealt with tentatively, given that this concept represents a simplified view and the dataset is limited.

Phenotypic Variability Among Affected Siblings

It is well known that affected sibships are valuable in setting up genotype-phenotype correlations. While the majority of sibships displays comparable clinical courses, about 20% of ARPKD multiplex pedigrees exhibit gross intrafamilial phenotypic variability with perinatal/neonatal demise in one and survival into childhood or even adulthood in another affected sib (ref. 147 and own unpublished data of more than 100 ARPKD multiplex pedigrees). An even higher proportion of 20 out of 48 sibships (42%) was present in our recent survey among families with at least one neonatal survivor per family, but this figure was biased by the study design.[130] After the study was adjusted for differing family sizes, the risk for perinatal demise of a further affected child was 37% (22 perinatally deceased children from a total of 59 patients excluding the moderately affected index cases). For genetic counseling, this rate is alarming given that our study cohort was representative for the spectrum of patients followed by departments of pediatric nephrology. Of course, phenotype categorization into severe and moderate is a simplified and artificial view considering the much better prognosis for patients who survive the most critical neonatal period. For instance, survival of an individual might depend on available intensive care facilities or birth order if the parents are aware of ARPKD risk. Overall, some alertness is warranted in predicting the clinical outcome of a further affected child. However, what is clearly depicted by discordant siblings is that phenotypes cannot be explained simply on the basis of the *PKHD1* genotype. Characterizing those putative modifying factors will be one of the major challenges for future studies.

Prenatal Diagnosis

Given the recurrence risk of 25%, the often devastating course of early manifestations of ARPKD and a usually comparable clinical course among affected siblings, many parents of ARPKD children seek early and reliable PND to guide future family planning. Typically ARPKD patients are identified by ultrasound only late in pregnancy or at birth. However, even with state-of-the-art technology, fetal sonography, performed at the time when termination of pregnancy (TOP) is usually performed, frequently fails to detect enlargement and increased echogenicity of kidneys or oligohydramnios secondary to poor fetal urine output.[181-183] Therefore an early and reliable PND for ARPKD in at-risk families is only feasible by molecular genetic analysis. This became feasible for families with confirmed diagnosis of ARPKD in the index patient in 1994, when *PKHD1* was mapped to chromosome 6p.[149] In fact, almost all patients with typical ARPKD are currently known to be linked to this locus. However, a haplotype-based linkage analysis represents an indirect approach with its inherent limitations. As a matter of course, access to the DNA from a previous affected sibling is necessary. Moreover, the reliability of this test is predicated on a correct diagnosis of ARPKD in the family's proposed index patient. Thus linkage analysis cannot be offered in families where (1) no DNA of an affected child or fetus is available, (2) in cases without proven pathoanatomical diagnosis (at least liver biopsy), (3) in individuals with diagnostic doubts, and (4) in patients with heterozygous haplotypes despite parental consanguinity. In these cases mutation analysis of the *PKHD1* gene should be performed as the basis for PND and genetic counseling.[165,184]

PATHOMECHANISMS UNDERLYING CYST FORMATION

Primary Cilia

To unravel the still widely unknown molecular pathomechanisms of CKDs, it is crucial to further characterize the involved proteins and signaling pathways. To understand genetic interaction, it needs to be modeled at the cellular

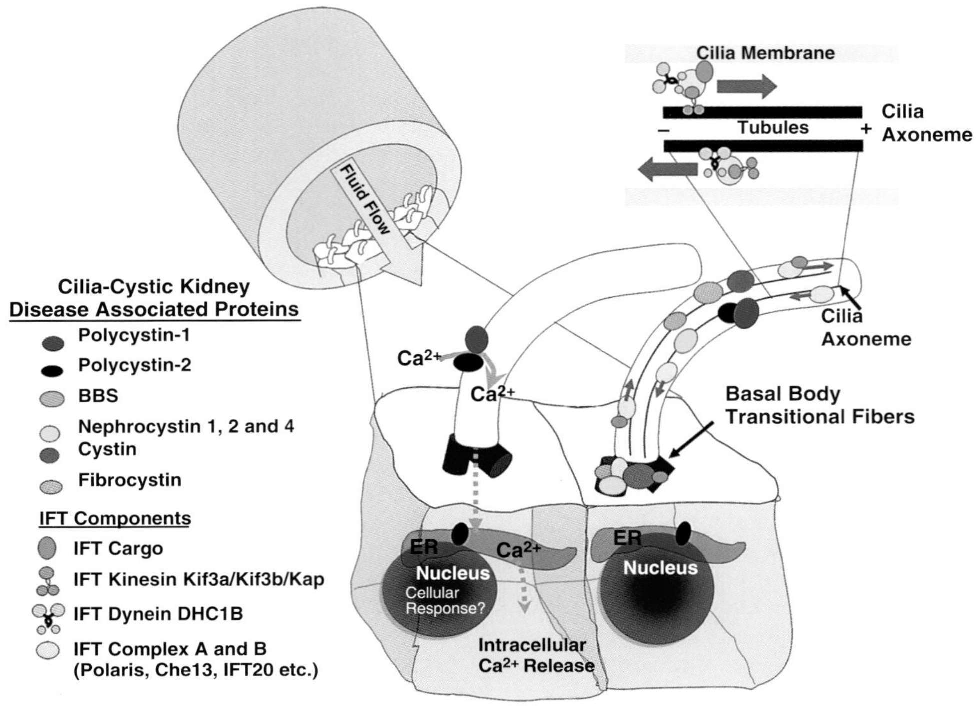

Figure 9-7 Primary cilia function in tubules as sensors for fluid flow. *Top left:* example of a single ductal tubule (kidney, liver, pancreas) where cilia extend from the surface of epithelial cells into the extracellular lumen. *Bottom right:* enlarged view showing that ductal epithelial cell cilia consist of cystic kidney disease-associated proteins. The polycystins are thought to form a complex required for the flow-mediated calcium entry in response to deflection of the axoneme. This subsequently results in release of internal calcium stores from the endoplasmic reticulum (ER), possibly mediated by polycystin-2. Furthermore, it has recently been shown that the COOH-terminal region of polycystin-1 is cleaved where it translocates to the nucleus in response to duct obstruction. Whether this cleavage of polycystin-1 occurs in the cilia or in another location in the cell has yet to be determined. In addition to the polycystins, many other proteins involved in renal cystic disorders in mice or humans have been located to the cilium or basal body. These include proteins responsible for nephronophthisis, Bardet-Biedl syndrome (BBS), and autosomal recessive polycystic kidney disease (ARPKD) in humans and several genes shown to be critical in cyst development in murine models. All types of cilia are formed and maintained using a process known as intraflagellar transport (IFT) *(inset, top right)*. (From Davenport JR, Yoder BK: An incredible decade for the primary cilium: a look at a once-forgotten organelle. *Am J Physiol Renal Physiol* 289:F1159-69, 2005.)

level. As mentioned previously, it is noteworthy that most, if not all, cystoproteins, among them polycystin-1, polycystin-2, and polyductin, appear colocalized to primary cilia and their associated cellular organisms as basal bodies and centrosomes (Figure 9-7).[1,3] This puts the primary cilium at the center of a putative common network of cystoproteins in which these proteins may interact with each other and converge into the same signaling cascades. The importance of primary renal cilia as critical organelles for architectural homeostasis of the kidney might be partly explained by their function in sensing environmental cues such as tubular luminal flow. This, in turn, triggers transient Ca^{2+} currents that may regulate intracellular signaling pathways that control physiologic cell function. Among these mechanosensoric and chemosensoric functions is the control of proliferative and apoptotic mechanisms.[185] In line with this, many studies have shown the cellular phenotype of renal cysts to be compatible with dedifferentiation, characterized by increased proliferation and apoptosis, altered protein sorting, changed secretory features, and disorganization of the extracellular matrix.[2] The protein complex of polycystin-1 and polycystin-2 has been demonstrated to mediate mechanosensation in vivo in the primary cilium of kidney epithelial cells. Accordingly, activation of Ca^{2+} channels initiates a strong increase of intracellular Ca^{2+} that is further propagated by the release of Ca^{2+} from intracellular stores.[186-188] The central role of primary cilia in CKD pathogenesis is further stressed by animal models for PKD. The *Pck* rat (with disrupted *Pkhd1*) and orpk-mouse (with a mutation in the *Tg737* gene encoding polaris) both display shortened, stunted cilia lacking protein expression. Even more convincingly, a conditional knockout mouse for the ciliary motor protein Kif3A in renal collecting ducts developed PKD.[189]

Signaling Pathways

In terms of maintaining a differentiated kidney epithelium with controlled fluid secretion and cell proliferation, a highly coordinated crosstalk between Ca^{2+} and cAMP as second messengers is critical.[190,191] Growth factors act through tyrosine kinase receptors and Ras proteins on the MAPK/ERK-signaling pathway and finally lead to cell proliferation.[192] The importance of the MAPK-signaling cascade in the pathogenesis of PKD is further emphasized by increased renal levels of phosporylated Raf-1 and ERK in orthologous animal models for PKD and the development of PKD in H-Ras transgenic mice.[193,194] In keeping, activation of JNK and AP-1 could be demonstrated for ADPKD.[195,196] Moreover, in a recent study ARL6, as a member of the Ras family of small GTP-binding proteins, was identified to be responsible for one form of the Bardet-Biedl syndrome.[197] Besides the aforementioned signaling cascades, there is compelling evidence for further pathways underlying PKD. Whereas a potential role of the Wnt-signaling pathway has been proposed for years in ADPKD,[198] a predominant importance has been shown in the pathogenesis of other CDKs only recently.[199-201]

An influence of the polycystins on JAK-STAT signaling may have been first demonstrated by Bhunia and coworkers.[202] In accordance, polycystin-1 binds and activates the JAK2-kinase dependent on polycystin-2 as a cofactor. Subsequently STAT1 becomes activated, homodimerizes, translocates to the nucleus, and favors the transcription of the cyclin-dependent kinase inhibitor p21 (cip1/waf1). This in turn causes a cell cycle arrest in the G0/G1-phase with terminal differentiation of the cell. It has been shown that polycystin-1 undergoes RIP (Regulated Intramembranous Proteolysis), which results in nuclear translocation of its cytoplasmic tail.[203] It was recently demonstrated that the polycystin-1 tail interacts with the transcription factor STAT6 and the coactivator P100, and stimulates STAT6-dependent gene expression.[204] Intriguingly, STAT6 usually localizes to primary cilia of renal epithelial cells; however, termination of apical fluid flow results in its nuclear translocation. Cyst-lining cells in ADPKD exhibit elevated levels of nuclear STAT6, P100, and the polycystin-1 cytoplasmic tail. Exogenous expression of the human polycystin-1 tail resulted in renal cyst formation in zebrafish embryos. Conclusively, the study by Low et al. identified a novel mechanotransductory ciliary pathway that involves polycystin-1, modifies gene expression, and is inappropriately activated in ADPKD.[204]

TREATMENT PROSPECTS

For patients affected by CKDs, there is currently no curative treatment option to slow, ameliorate, or even regress the clinical course. However, recent animal studies have identified potential approaches to influence the disease process by targeting downstream cellular changes (Table 9-5).[2,205] Increased expression of vasopressin V_2 receptor, *c-myc*, and epidermal growth factor receptor (EGFR) in cystic kidneys has led to the most promising therapeutic approaches delineated as follows.

Vasopressin V_2 Receptor Antagonists

Vasopressin V_2 receptor (V_2R) antagonists may be closest to approval as therapeutic agents against disease progression in PKD. The concept is based on the common characteristic of all forms of CKD to be unable to concentrate urine properly. Most probably as an attempt to compensate this inability, V_2R mRNA expression is upregulated in CKD kidneys.[206,207] Vasopressin, the major adenylcyclase agonist in the principal cells of renal collecting ducts, induces cAMP generation. Given the central role that Ca^{2+} and cAMP play in the pathogenesis of PKD, therapeutic approaches should aim at increasing intracellular Ca^{2+} concentration, reducing renal cAMP, or both. Studies directed at the inhibition of renal cAMP accumulation by V_2R antagonist administration have been performed in several orthologous animal models of human PKD.[206-210] Significant amelioration of disease progression was demonstrated in every tested model. Administration of the V_2R antagonist OPC31260 in the *pcy* mouse even caused regression of already established renal cystic pathology, with

TABLE 9-5 **Therapeutic Interventions in Animal Models of CKD**

	Cy/+ Rat (Han:SPRD)	*Pck* Rat	*orpk* Mouse	*bpk* Mouse	*cpk* Mouse	*pcy* Mouse	*Pkd2 ws25/–* Mouse	*Pkd1–/–* Mouse
Vasopressin V_2R antagonists		+			+	+	+	
PPAR γ agonist Pioglitazone								+
EGFR tyrosine kinase inhibitors	+	0/–	+	+				
EGF				+	+			
TACE				+				
Taxol/paclitaxel	0/–		0/–		+	0/–		
c-myc antisense oligonucleotides					+			
Caspase inhibitor IDN-8050	+							
Rapamycin	+				+			
Methylprednisolone	+					+		
ACE inhibitors	+	0/–						
MMP inhibitor	+							
Low-protein diet	+					+		
Lipid-lowering drugs	+					+		
Amiloride	+	0/–						
MEK inhibitor PD184352 (CI-1040)						+		

+, Positive effect on the disease; 0/–, no or negative effect on the disease.

decreased proliferation, apoptosis, and interstitial fibrosis. The V_2R antagonist OPC41061 (Tolvaptan), which has proven effective in rodent models orthologous to human ADPKD, ARPKD, and nephronophthisis, has successfully completed Phase II clinical trials and is undergoing extended clinical testing in Phase III trials.[208-210] V_2R antagonist administration to humans has not resulted in adverse effects except for the expected mild-to-moderate thirst that was well tolerated by all the subjects.[211] An ambivalent feature of V_2R antagonization is the almost exclusive expression of the V_2R in renal collecting duct principal cells and endothelial cells. Whereas this warrants specificity and safety of the drug, it also implicates that extrarenal manifestations of PKD will not be targeted.

C-myc Antisense Oligonucleotides

The systemic character of most forms of CKD and the renoselectivity of V_2R antagonists require other therapeutic approaches to treat extrarenal disease manifestations. In view of the dedifferentiated cellular phenotype of renal cysts, many investigators consider PKD a neoplastic disorder that should be treated like any other cancer.[212] Accordingly, chemotherapeutic agents such as *c-myc* antisense oligonucleotides and EGFR tyrosine kinase inhibitors have been employed in animal models of PKD. The first cancer chemotherapeutic drug tested in a PKD mouse model was taxol, a microtubule stabilizing agent that was found to promote survival in *cpk* mutants.[213] Since *cpk* mice bear a mutation in the ciliary protein cystin, taxol's protective effect may actually reside in the restoration of cilia function. However, later studies on taxol in other rodent models of CKD were disillusioning and failed to show efficacy.[214,215]

Several lines of evidence support a causative role of the oncogene *c-myc* in renal cyst formation: *c-myc* transgenic mice develop PKD, whereas this phenotype disappears in revertant *c-myc* transgenic mice.[216,217] *C-myc* is overexpressed in rodent PKD models[218-220] as well as in human ADPKD.[221] Inhibition of *c-myc* overexpression by specific antisense oligonucleotides in *cpk mice* resulted in a striking amelioration of both renal and hepatobiliary pathology.[222,223] The efficacy of *c-myc* antisense oligonucleotides in PKD animal models has stipulated clinical trials, which are ongoing in humans with ADPKD.

EGFR Tyrosine Kinase Inhibitors

There are conflicting data on the exact role of EGF and EGFR in PKD and the usefulness of this pathway as a therapeutic target. The rationale for using these agents is the increased expression of EGFR in cystic renal and hepatobiliary epithelia[224-227] and decreased EGF expression in these tissues.[224,228-230] The wide array of EGF family members activating the EGFR (e.g., TGFα) may explain this apparent discrepancy in expression data. Although EGF and EGFR tyrosine kinase inhibitors have been shown to be effective in several animal models of PKD,[231-236] a setback occurred with the recent failure to demonstrate a protective effect in the *Pck* rat.[237]

Rapamycin and Other Therapeutic Approaches

Two recent studies on the immunosuppressant and potent antiproliferative agent rapamycin yielded promising results in animal models of PKD.[238,239] Rapamycin decreased proliferation of cystic and noncystic tubules, markedly inhibited renal enlargement and cystogenesis, and prevented the loss of kidney function. Furthermore, another study by the same group demonstrated that use of the caspase inhibitor IDN-8050 reduced tubular apoptosis and proliferation and slowed the disease progression in the Han:SPRD rat model of PKD.[240] Conclusively, there is increasing evidence that both epithelial cell apoptosis and proliferation are dysregulated in PKD and represent major mechanisms for cyst growth.

The approach to use immunosuppressants may appear logical given the chronic interstitial inflammatory infiltrate found in essentially all forms of CKD. In accordance, an earlier study on methylprednisolone retarded the progression of PKD in rodents.[241] However, caution may be indicated in light of the extensive data on glucocorticoid-induced PKD in neonatal mammals.[242]

Recently the long-acting somatostatin analogue octreotide was administered for 6 months in a small cohort of ADPKD patients with mild-to-moderate renal insufficiency.[243] Octreotide was well tolerated in the majority of patients and found to inhibit renal enlargement. This therapeutic concept is based on the inhibition of cAMP-generated chloride secretion by the tubular epithelium lining the cysts. Noteworthy is that octreotide is also effective in women with polycystic ovary syndrome.[244] The long-term renoprotective efficacy of this agent will need to be verified in large-scale trials.

CONCLUSIONS AND FUTURE DIRECTIONS

Although there are currently no established effective therapies for any of the diseases discussed, our understanding of CKD is increasing rapidly, and the results of seminal interventional studies in animal models are promising. Even though curative therapies for patients with CKD have yet to surface, effective slowing of disease progression appears within reach as a remarkable therapeutic first step.

In the search for new therapeutic targets for CKD, continuing to unravel the molecular mechanisms underlying the largely variable phenotype of these conditions will be of utmost importance. Novel molecular technologies in conjunction with classical genetics hold promise in providing further insight into the logic of signaling networks and identifying new powerful and specific therapeutic targets.

Acknowledgments

This work performed in our laboratory was supported by grants from the Deutsche Forschungsgemeinschaft (DFG) (KZ and CB), the German-Israeli Foundation (GIF) (CB), and the START program of the medical faculty of Aachen University (CB). CB is a recipient of a scholarship of the German Kidney Foundation (Deutsche Nierenstiftung).

REFERENCES

1. Hildebrandt F, Otto E: Cilia and centrosomes: a unifying pathogenic concept for cystic kidney disease? *Nat Rev Genet* 6(12):928-40, 2005.
2. Harris PC, Torres VE: Understanding pathogenic mechanisms in polycystic kidney disease provides clues for therapy, *Curr Opin Nephrol Hypertens* 15(4):456-63, 2006.
3. Simons M, Walz G: Polycystic kidney disease: Cell division without a c(l)ue? *Kidney Int* 70:854-64, 2006.
4. Osathanondh V, Potter EL: Pathogenesis of polycystic kidneys, *Archives of Pathology, Chicago*, 77:459-509, 1964.
5. Wilson PD: Polycystic kidney disease, *N Engl J Med* 350:151-64, 2004.
6. Igarashi P, Somlo S: Genetics and pathogenesis of polycystic kidney disease, *J Am Soc Nephrol* 13:2384-98, 2002.
7. Gabow PA, Kimberling WJ, Strain JD et al: Utility of ultrasonography in the diagnosis of autosomal dominant polycystic kidney disease in children, *J Am Soc Nephrol* 8(1):105-10, 1997.
8. Bear JC, Parfrey PS, Morgan JM et al: Autosomal dominant polycystic kidney disease: new information for genetic counselling, *Am J Med Genet* 43(3):548-53, 1992.
9. McHugh K, Stringer DA, Hebert D, Babiak CA: Simple renal cysts in children: diagnosis and follow-up with US, *Radiology* 178(2):383-85, 1991.
10. Ravine D, Gibson RN, Donlan J, Sheffield LJ: An ultrasound renal cyst prevalence survey: specificity data for inherited renal cystic diseases, *Am J Kidney Dis* 22(6):803-07, 1993.
11. Grantham JJ, Torres VE, Chapman AB et al: Volume progression in polycystic kidney disease, *N Engl J Med* 354(20):2122-30, 2006.
12. Hateboer N, v Dijk MA, Bogdanova N et al: Comparison of phenotypes of polycystic kidney disease types 1 and 2. European PKD1-PKD2 Study Group, *Lancet* 353:103-07, 1999.
13. Magistroni R, He N, Wang K et al: Genotype-renal function correlation in type 2 autosomal dominant polycystic kidney disease, *J Am Soc Nephrol* 14:1164-74, 2003.
14. Paterson AD, Magistroni R, He N et al: Progressive loss of renal function is an age-dependent heritable trait in type 1 autosomal dominant polycystic kidney disease, *J Am Soc Nephrol* 16:755-62, 2005.
15. Persu A, Duyme M, Pirson Y et al: Comparison between siblings and twins supports a role for modifier genes in ADPKD, *Kidney Int* 66:2132-36, 2004.
16. Kaariainen H: Polycystic kidney disease in children: a genetic and epidemiological study of 82 Finnish patients, *J Med Genet* 24(8):474-81, 1987.
17. Sedman A, Bell P, Manco-Johnson M et al: Autosomal dominant polycystic kidney disease in childhood: a longitudinal study, *Kidney Int* 31(4):1000-05, 1987.
18. Sweeney WE Jr, Avner ED: Molecular and cellular pathophysiology of autosomal recessive polycystic kidney disease (ARPKD), *Cell Tissue Res* 326:671-85, 2006.
19. Zerres K, Rudnik-Schoneborn S, Deget F: Childhood onset autosomal dominant polycystic kidney disease in sibs: clinical picture and recurrence risk. German Working Group on Paediatric Nephrology (Arbeitsgemeinschaft fur Padiatrische Nephrologie), *J Med Genet* 30(7):583-88, 1993.
20. Ross DG, Travers H: Infantile presentation of adult-type polycystic kidney disease in a large kindred, *J Pediatr* 87(5):760-63, 1975.
21. Zerres K, Hansmann M, Knopfle G, Stephan M: Prenatal diagnosis of genetically determined early manifestation of autosomal dominant polycystic kidney disease? *Hum Genet* 71(4):368-69, 1985.
22. Gal A, Wirth B, Kaariainen H et al: Childhood manifestation of autosomal dominant polycystic kidney disease: no evidence for genetic heterogeneity, *Clin Genet* 35(1):13-19, 1989.
23. Fick GM, Johnson AM, Gabow PA: Is there evidence for anticipation in autosomal-dominant polycystic kidney disease? *Kidney Int* 45(4):1153-62, 1994.
24. Torra R, Darnell A, Botey A et al: Interfamilial and intrafamilial variability of clinical expression in autosomal dominant polycystic kidney disease. Vimercate, Italy, abstract meeting on ADPKD, 1994.
25. Geberth S, Ritz E, Zeier M, Stier E: Anticipation of age at renal death in autosomal dominant polycystic kidney disease (ADPKD)? *Nephrol Dial Transplant* 10(9):1603-06, 1995.
26. MacDermot KD, Saggar-Malik AK, Economides DL, Jeffery S: Prenatal diagnosis of autosomal dominant polycystic kidney disease (PKD1) presenting in utero and prognosis for very early onset disease, *J Med Genet* 35(1):13-16, 1998.
27. Fick GM, Johnson AM, Strain JD et al: Characteristics of very early onset autosomal dominant polycystic kidney disease, *J Am Soc Nephrol* 3(12):1863-70, 1993.
28. Ogborn MR: Polycystic kidney disease—a truly pediatric problem, *Pediatr Nephrol* 8(6):762-67, 1994.
29. Bear JC, McManamon P, Morgan J, et al: Age at clinical onset and at ultrasonographic detection of adult polycystic kidney disease: data for genetic counselling, *Am J Med Genet* 18(1):45-53, 1984.
30. Fick-Brosnahan GM, Tran ZV, Johnson AM et al: Progression of autosomal-dominant polycystic kidney disease in children, *Kidney Int* 59(5):1654-62, 2001.
31. Shamshirsaz A, Bekheirnia RM, Kamgar M et al: Autosomal-dominant polycystic kidney disease in infancy and childhood: progression and outcome, *Kidney Int* 68(5):2218-24, 2005.
32. Fick-Brosnahan G, Johnson AM, Strain JD, Gabow PA: Renal asymmetry in children with autosomal dominant polycystic kidney disease, *Am J Kidney Dis* 34(4):639-45, 1999.
33. Nicolau C, Torra R, Badenas C et al: Sonographic pattern of recessive polycystic kidney disease in young adults. Differences from the dominant form, *Nephrol Dial Transplant* 15:1373-78, 2000.
34. Avni FE, Guissard G, Hall M et al: Hereditary polycystic kidney diseases in children: changing sonographic patterns through childhood, *Pediatr Radiol* 32:169-74, 2002.
35. Nahm AM, Henriquez DE, Ritz E: Renal cystic disease (ADPKD and ARPKD), *Nephrol Dial Transplant* 17:311-14, 2002.
36. Zerres K: Genetics of cystic kidney diseases. Criteria for classification and genetic counselling, *Pediatr Nephrol* 1(3):397-404, 1987.
37. Gabow PA, Duley I, Johnson AM: Clinical profiles of gross hematuria in autosomal dominant polycystic kidney disease, *Am J Kidney Dis* 20(2):140-43, 1992.
38. Gabow PA, Johnson AM, Kaehny WD et al: Factors affecting the progression of renal disease in autosomal-dominant polycystic kidney disease, *Kidney Int* 41(5):1311-19, 1992.
39. Johnson AM, Gabow PA: Identification of patients with autosomal dominant polycystic kidney disease at highest risk for end-stage renal disease, *J Am Soc Nephrol* 8(10):1560-67, 1997.
40. Gagnadoux MF, Habib R, Levy M, et al: Cystic renal diseases in children, *Adv Nephrol Necker Hosp* 18:33-57, 1989.
41. Avner ED: Childhood ADPKD: answers and more questions, *Kidney Int* 59(5):1979-80, 2001.
42. Davis ID, MacRae Dell K, Sweeney WE, Avner ED: Can progression of autosomal dominant or autosomal recessive polycystic kidney disease be prevented? *Semin Nephrol* 21(5):430-40, 2001.
43. Chapman AB, Schrier RW: Pathogenesis of hypertension in autosomal dominant polycystic kidney disease, *Semin Nephrol* 11(6):653-60, 1991.
44. Harrap SB, Davies DL, Macnicol AM, et al: Renal, cardiovascular and hormonal characteristics of young adults with autosomal dominant polycystic kidney disease, *Kidney Int* 40(3):501-08, 1991.
45. Ritz E: Hypertension in autosomal dominant polycystic kidney disease: is renin acquitted as a culprit? *J Hypertens* 24(6):1023-25, 2006.
46. Chapman AB, Johnson A, Gabow PA, Schrier RW: The renin-angiotensin-aldosterone system and autosomal dominant polycystic kidney disease, *N Engl J Med* 323(16):1091-96, 1990.
47. Watson ML, Macnicol AM, Allan PL, Wright AF: Effects of angiotensin converting enzyme inhibition in adult polycystic kidney disease, *Kidney Int* 41(1):206-10, 1992.
48. Wang D, Strandgaard S: The pathogenesis of hypertension in autosomal dominant polycystic kidney disease, *J Hypertens* 15(9):925-33, 1997.

49. Torres VE, Donovan KA, Scicli G, et al: Synthesis of renin by tubulocystic epithelium in autosomal-dominant polycystic kidney disease, *Kidney Int* 42(2):364-73, 1992.
50. Ichikawi I, Harris RC: Angiotensin actions in the kidney: renewed insight into the old hormone, *Kidney Int* 40(4):583-96, 1991.
51. Rosenberg ME, Hostetter TH: Effect of angiotensin II and norepinephrine on early growth response genes in the rat kidney, *Kidney Int* 43(3):601-09, 1993.
52. Wolf G, Neilson EG: Angiotensin II as a hypertrophogenic cytokine for proximal tubular cells, *Kidney Int Suppl* 39:S100-07, 1993.
53. Chatterjee PK, Weerackody RP, Mistry SK et al: Selective antagonism of the AT1 receptor inhibits angiotensin II stimulated DNA and protein synthesis in primary cultures of human proximal tubular cells, *Kidney Int* 52(3):699-705, 1997.
54. Doulton TW, Saggar-Malik AK, He FJ, et al: The effect of sodium and angiotensin-converting enzyme inhibition on the classic circulating renin-angiotensin system in autosomal-dominant polycystic kidney disease patients, *J Hypertens* 24(5):939-45, 2006.
55. Pirson Y, Chauveau D, Torres V: Management of cerebral aneurysms in autosomal dominant polycystic kidney disease, *J Am Soc Nephrol* 13:269-76, 2002.
56. Gibbs GF, Huston J 3rd, Qian Q et al: Follow-up of intracranial aneurysms in autosomal-dominant polycystic kidney disease, *Kidney Int* 65:1621-27, 2004.
57. Chapman AB, Rubinstein D, Hughes R et al: Intracranial aneurysms in autosomal dominant polycystic kidney disease, *N Engl J Med* 327(13):916-20, 1992.
58. Huston J 3rd, Torres VE, Sulivan PP et al: Value of magnetic resonance angiography for the detection of intracranial aneurysms in autosomal dominant polycystic kidney disease, *J Am Soc Nephrol* 3(12):1871-77, 1993.
59. Ruggieri PM, Poulos N, Masaryk TJ, et al: Occult intracranial aneurysms in polycystic kidney disease: screening with MR angiography, *Radiology* 191(1):33-39, 1994.
60. Rinkel GJ, Djibuti M, Algra A, van Gijn J: Prevalence and risk of rupture of intracranial aneurysms: a systematic review, *Stroke* 29(1):251-56, 1998.
61. Bederson JB, Awad IA, Wiebers DO, et al: Recommendations for the management of patients with unruptured intracranial aneurysms: A statement for healthcare professionals from the Stroke Council of the American Heart Association, *Circulation* 102(18):2300-08, 2000.
62. Schievink WI, Torres VE, Piepgras DG, Wiebers DO: Saccular intracranial aneurysms in autosomal dominant polycystic kidney disease, *J Am Soc Nephrol* 3(1):88-95, 1992.
63. Chauveau D, Pirson Y, Verellen-Dumoulin C et al: Intracranial aneurysms in autosomal dominant polycystic kidney disease, *Kidney Int* 45(4):1140-46, 1994.
64. International Study of Unruptured Intracranial Aneurysms Investigators: Unruptured intracranial aneurysms—risk of rupture and risks of surgical intervention, *N Engl J Med* 339(24):1725-33, 1998.
65. Chauveau D, Pirson Y, Le Moine A et al: Extrarenal manifestations in autosomal dominant polycystic kidney disease, *Adv Nephrol Necker Hosp* 26:265-89, 1997.
66. Belz MM, Hughes RL, Kaehny WD et al: Familial clustering of ruptured intracranial aneurysms in autosomal dominant polycystic kidney disease, *Am J Kidney Dis* 38(4):770-06, Oct 2001.
67. Raaymakers TW, Rinkel GJ, Limburg M, Algra A: Mortality and morbidity of surgery for unruptured intracranial aneurysms: a meta-analysis, *Stroke* 29(8):1531-38, 1998.
68. Brilstra EH, Rinkel GJ, van der Graaf Y et al: Treatment of intracranial aneurysms by embolization with coils: a systematic review, *Stroke* 30(2):470-76, 1999.
69. Johnston SC, Wilson CB, Halbach VV et al: Endovascular and surgical treatment of unruptured cerebral aneurysms: comparison of risks, *Ann Neurol* 48(1):11-19, 2000.
70. Mariani L, Bianchetti MG, Schroth G, Seiler RW: Cerebral aneurysms in patients with autosomal dominant polycystic kidney disease—to screen, to clip, to coil? *Nephrol Dial Transplant* 14(10):2319-22, 1999.
71. Chapman AB, Guay-Woodford LM: *The family and ADPKD*. The Polycystic Kidney Research (PKR) Foundation 38-39, 1997.
72. Mathieu D, Vilgrain V, Mahfouz AE et al: Benign liver tumors, *Magn Reson Imaging Clin N Am* 5:255-88, 1997.
73. Cheung J, Scudamore CH, Yoshida EM: Management of polycystic liver disease, *Can J Gastroenterol* 18:666-70, 2004.
74. Torres VE: Polycystic kidney disease: guidelines for family physicians, *Am Fam Physician* 53(3):847-48, 850, 1996.
75. Drenth JP, te Morsche RH, Smink R et al: Germline mutations in PRKCSH are associated with autosomal dominant polycystic liver disease, *Nat Genet* 33(3):345-47, 2003.
76. Davila S, Furu L, Gharavi AG, et al: Mutations in SEC63 cause autosomal dominant polycystic liver disease, *Nat Genet* 36(6):575-77, 2004.
77. Desmet VJ: Ludwig symposium on biliary disorders—part I. Pathogenesis of ductal plate abnormalities, *Mayo Clin Proc* 73:80-89, 1998.
78. Qian Q, Li A, King BF et al: Clinical profile of autosomal dominant polycystic liver disease, *Hepatology* 37:164-71, 2003.
79. Lazaridis KN, Strazzabosco M, Larusso NF: The cholangiopathies: disorders of biliary epithelia, *Gastroenterology* 127:1565-77, 2004.
80. Cobben JM, Breuning MH, Schoots C et al: Congenital hepatic fibrosis in autosomal-dominant polycystic kidney disease, *Kidney Int* 38(5):880-85, 1990.
81. Lipschitz B, Berdon WE, Defelice AR, Levy J: Association of congenital hepatic fibrosis with autosomal dominant polycystic kidney disease. Report of a family with review of literature, *Pediatr Radiol* 23(2):131-33, 1993.
82. Tamura H, Kato H, Hirose S, et al: An adult case of polycystic kidney disease associated with congenital hepatic fibrosis, *Nippon Jinzo Gakkai Shi* 36(8):962-67, 1994.
83. Milutinovic J, Schabel SI, Ainsworth SK: Autosomal dominant polycystic kidney disease with liver and pancreatic involvement in early childhood, *Am J Kidney Dis* 13(4):340-44, 1989.
84. Everson GT: Hepatic cysts in autosomal dominant polycystic kidney disease, *Mayo Clin Proc* 65(7):1020-25, 1990.
85. Telenti A, Torres VE, Gross JB Jr, et al: Hepatic cyst infection in autosomal dominant polycystic kidney disease, *Mayo Clin Proc* 65(7):933-42, 1990.
86. McDonald MI, Corey GR, Gallis HA, Durack DT: Single and multiple pyogenic liver abscesses. Natural history, diagnosis and treatment, with emphasis on percutaneous drainage, *Medicine (Baltimore)* 63(5):291-302, 1984.
87. Torres VE, Rastogi S, King BF, et al: Hepatic venous outflow obstruction in autosomal dominant polycystic kidney disease, *J Am Soc Nephrol* 5(5):1186-92, 1994.
88. Tan YM, Ooi LL, Mack PO: Current status in the surgical management of adult polycystic liver disease, *Ann Acad Med Singapore* 31(2):217-22, 2002.
89. Torres VE: Treatment of polycystic liver disease: one size does not fit all, *Am J Kidney Dis* 49:725-28, 2007.
90. Marquardt W: Cystennieren, Cystenleber, und Cystenpancreas bei zwei Geschwistern, Thesis University of Tübingen, 1935.
91. Blyth H, Ockenden BG: Polycystic disease of kidney and liver presenting in childhood, *J Med Genet* 8(3):257-84, 1971.
92. The International Polycystic Kidney Disease Consortium: Polycystic kidney disease: the complete structure of the PKD1 gene and its protein, *Cell* 81:289-98, 1995.
93. Hughes J, Ward CJ, Peral B et al: The polycystic kidney disease 1 (PKD1) gene encodes a novel protein with multiple cell recognition domains, *Nat Genet* 10:151-60, 1995.
94. Mochizuki T, Wu G, Hayashi T et al: PKD2, a gene for polycystic kidney disease that encodes an integral membrane protein, *Science* 272:1339-42, 1996.
95. Pei Y, Paterson AD, Wang KR et al: Bilineal disease and trans-heterozygotes in autosomal dominant polycystic kidney disease, *Am J Hum Genet* 68:355-63, 2001.
96. Lu W, Peissel B, Babakhanlou H et al: Perinatal lethality with kidney and pancreas defects in mice with a targeted Pkd1 mutation, *Nat Genet* 17:179-81, 1997.
97. Boulter C, Mulroy S, Webb S et al: Cardiovascular, skeletal, and renal defects in mice with a targeted disruption of the Pkd1 gene, *Proc Natl Acad Sci USA* 98:12174-79, 2001.

98. Lu W, Shen X, Pavlova A et al: Comparison of Pkd1-targeted mutants reveals that loss of polycystin-1 causes cystogenesis and bone defects, *Hum Mol Genet* 10:2385-96, 2001.
99. Kim K, Drummond I, Ibraghimov-Beskrovnaya O, Klinger K et al: Polycystin 1 is required for the structural integrity of blood vessels, *Proc Natl Acad Sci USA* 97:1731-36, 2000.
100. Qian F, Watnick TJ, Onuchic LF, Germino GG: The molecular basis of focal cyst formation in human autosomal dominant polycystic kidney disease type I, *Cell* 87(6):979-87, 1996.
101. Brasier JL, Henske EP: Loss of the polycystic kidney disease (PKD1) region of chromosome 16p13 in renal cyst cells supports a loss-of-function model for cyst pathogenesis, *J Clin Invest* 99(2):194-99, 1997.
102. Watnick TJ, Torres VE, Gandolph MA, et al: Somatic mutation in individual liver cysts supports a two-hit model of cystogenesis in autosomal dominant polycystic kidney disease, *Mol Cell* 2(2):247-51, 1998.
103. Watnick T, He N, Wang K et al: Mutations of PKD1 in ADPKD2 cysts suggest a pathogenic effect of trans-heterozygous mutations, *Nat Genet* 25(2):143-44, 2000.
104. Koptides M, Mean R, Demetriou K et al: Genetic evidence for a trans-heterozygous model for cystogenesis in autosomal dominant polycystic kidney disease, *Hum Mol Genet* 9(3):447-52, 2000.
105. Wu G, Tian X, Nishimura S et al: Trans-heterozygous Pkd1 and Pkd2 mutations modify expression of polycystic kidney disease, *Hum Mol Genet* 11(16):1845-54, 2002.
106. Brook-Carter PT, Peral B, Ward CJ et al. Deletion of the TSC2 and PKD1 genes associated with severe infantile polycystic kidney disease—a contiguous gene syndrome, *Nat Genet* 8(4):328-32, 1994.
107. Ong AC, Harris PC, Biddolph S, et al: Characterisation and expression of the PKD-1 protein, polycystin, in renal and extrarenal tissues, *Kidney Int* 55(5):2091-116, 1999.
108. Kleymenova E, Ibraghimov-Beskrovnaya O, Kugoh H et al: Tuberin-dependent membrane localization of polycystin-1: a functional link between polycystic kidney disease and the TSC2 tumor suppressor gene, *Mol Cell* 7(4):823-32, 2001.
109. Lantinga-van Leeuwen IS, Dauwerse JG, Balde HJ et al: Lowering of Pkd1 expression is sufficient to cause polycystic kidney disease, *Hum Mol Genet* 13:3069-77, 2004.
110. Köttgen M, Benzing T, Simmen T et al: Trafficking of TRPP2 by PACS proteins represents a novel mechanism of ion channel regulation, *EMBO J* 24:705-16, 2005.
111. Gallagher AR, Cedzich A, Gretz N et al: The polycystic kidney disease protein PKD2 interacts with Hax-1, a protein associated with the actin cytoskeleton, *Proc Natl Acad Sci USA* 97:4017-22, 2000.
112. Li Y, Montalbetti N, Shen PY et al: Alpha-actinin associates with polycystin-2 and regulates its channel activity, *Hum Mol Genet* 14:1587-603, 2005.
113. Li Y, Wright JM, Qian F et al: Polycystin 2 interacts with type-I IP3 receptor to modulate intracellular Ca2+ signaling, *J Biol Chem* 280:41258-306, 2006.
114. Wang S, Zhang J, Nauli S et al: Fibrocystin is associated with Polycystin-2 and regulates intracellular calcium, *J Am Soc Nephrol* 15, ASN Renal Week abstracts issue, 2004.
115. Nagano J, Kitamura K, Hujer KM et al: Fibrocystin interacts with CAML, a protein involved in Ca(2+) signaling, *Biochem Biophys Res Commun* 338:880-89, 2005.
116. Qian F, Boletta A, Bhunia AK et al: Cleavage of polycystin-1 requires the receptor for egg jelly domain and is disrupted by human autosomal-dominant polycystic kidney disease 1-associated mutations, *Proc Natl Acad Sci USA* 99:16981-86, 2002.
117. Qian F, Germino FJ, Cai Y et al: PKD1 interacts with PKD2 through a probable coiled-coil domain, *Nat Genet* 16:179-83, 1997.
118. Hanaoka K, Qian F, Boletta A et al: Co-assembly of polycystin-1 and -2 produces unique cation-permeable currents, *Nature* 408: 990-94, 2000.
119. Rossetti S, Strmecki L, Gamble V et al: Mutation analysis of the entire PKD1 gene: genetic and diagnostic implications, *Am J Hum Genet* 68:46-63, 2001.
120. Rossetti S, Chauveau D, Walker D et al: A complete mutation screen of the ADPKD genes by DHPLC, *Kidney Int* 61:1588-99, 2000.
121. Ritz E, Zeier M, Waldherr R: Progression to renal insufficiency. In Watson ML, Torres VE, editors: *Polycystic Kidney Disease,* Oxford, UK, 1996, Oxford University Press.
122. Hateboer N, Veldhuisen B, Peters D et al: Location of mutations within the PKD2 gene influences clinical outcome, *Kidney Int* 57:1444-51, 2000.
123. Rossetti S, Burton S, Strmecki L et al: The position of the polycystic kidney disease 1 (PKD1) gene mutation correlates with the severity of renal disease, *J Am Soc Nephrol* 13:1230-37, 2002.
124. Rossetti S, Chauveau D, Kubly V et al: Association of mutation position in polycystic kidney disease 1 (PKD1) gene and development of a vascular phenotype, *Lancet* 361:2196-201, 2003.
125. Guay-Woodford LM: Autosomal recessive polycystic kidney disease: clinical and genetic profiles. In Watson ML, Torres VE, editors: *Polycystic Kidney Disease,* Oxford, UK, 1996, Oxford University Press.
126. Zerres K, Rudnik-Schöneborn S, Senderek J et al: Autosomal recessive polycystic kidney disease (ARPKD), *J Nephrol* 16:453-58, 2003.
127. Nakanishi K, Sweeney WE Jr, Zerres K et al: Proximal tubular cysts in fetal human autosomal recessive polycystic kidney disease, *J Am Soc Nephrol* 11(4):760-63, 2000.
128. Adeva M, El-Youssef M, Rossetti S et al: Clinical and molecular characterization defines a broadened spectrum of autosomal recessive polycystic kidney disease (ARPKD), *Medicine (Baltimore)* 85(1):1-21, 2006.
129. Zerres K, Rudnik-Schöneborn S, Deget F et al: Autosomal recessive polycystic kidney disease in 115 children: clinical presentation, course and influence of gender, *Acta Paediatr* 85:437-45, 1996.
130. Bergmann C, Senderek J, Windelen E et al: Clinical consequences of PKHD1 mutations in 164 patients with autosomal recessive polycystic kidney disease (ARPKD), *Kidney Int* 67:829-48, 2005.
131. Guay-Woodford LM, Desmond RA: Autosomal recessive polycystic kidney disease: the clinical experience in North America, *Pediatrics* 111:1072-80, 2003.
132. Gagnadoux MF, Habib R, Levy M et al: Cystic renal diseases in children, *Adv Nephrol Necker Hosp* 8:33-57, 1989.
133. Capisonda R, Phan V, Traubuci J et al: Autosomal recessive polycystic kidney disease: outcomes from a single-center experience, *Pediatr Nephrol* 18:119-126, 2003.
134. Roy S, Dillon MJ, Trompeter RS, Barratt TM: Autosomal recessive polycystic kidney disease: long-term outcome of neonatal survivors, *Pediatr Nephrol* 11:302-306, 1997.
135. Kaplan BS, Fay J, Shah V et al: Autosomal recessive polycystic kidney disease, *Pediatr Nephrol* 3:43-49, 1989.
136. Kääriäinen H, Koskimies O, Norio R: Dominant and recessive polycystic kidney disease in children: evaluation of clinical features and laboratory data, *Pediatr Nephrol* 2:296-302, 1998.
137. Cole BR, Conley SB, Stapleton FB: Polycystic kidney disease in the first year of life, *J Pediatr* 111:693-99, 1987.
138. Dell K, Avner E: Autosomal recessive polycystic kidney disease gene reviews; genetic disease online reviews at gene tests-gene clinics. University of Washington, Seattle, 2003.
139. Warady BA, Alexander SR, Watkins S, et al: Optimal care of the pediatric end-stage renal disease patient on dialysis, *Am J Kidney Dis* 33(3):567-83, 1999.
140. Jafar TH, Stark PC, Schmid CH et al: ACE Inhibition in Progressive Renal Disease (AIPRD) Study Group. The effect of angiotensin-converting-enzyme inhibitors on progression of advanced polycystic kidney disease, *Kidney Int* 67(1):265-71, 2005.
141. Kashtan CE, Primack WA, Kainer G et al: Recurrent bacteremia with enteric pathogens in recessive polycystic kidney disease, *Pediatr Nephrol* 13(8):678-82, 1999.
142. Rossetti S, Torra R, Coto E et al: A complete mutation screen of PKHD1 in autosomal-recessive polycystic kidney disease (ARPKD) pedigrees, *Kidney Int* 64:391-403, 2003.
143. Moser M, Matthiesen S, Kirfel J et al: A mouse model for cystic biliary dysgenesis in autosomal recessive polycystic kidney disease (ARPKD), *Hepatology* 41:1113-21, 2005.

144. Tao B, Garcia-Gonzales M, Onuchic LF, Eicher EM, Germino GG, Guay-Woodford LM: Evidence that Pkhd1 has a complex transcriptional profile in a new spontaneous mouse model of ARPKD, *J Am Soc Nephrol* 16, ASN Renal Week abstracts issue, 2005.
145. Chilton SJ, Cremin BJ: The spectrum of polycystic disease in children, *Pediatr Radiol* 11(1):9-15, 1981.
146. Kaplan BS, Kaplan P, de Chadarevian JP et al: Variable expression of autosomal recessive polycystic kidney disease and congenital hepatic fibrosis within a family, *Am J Med Genet* 29(3):639-47, 1988.
147. Deget F, Rudnik-Schoneborn S, Zerres K: Course of autosomal recessive polycystic kidney disease (ARPKD) in siblings: a clinical comparison of 20 sibships, *Clin Genet* 47(5):248-53, 1995.
148. Zerres K, Volpel MC, Weiss H: Cystic kidneys. Genetics, pathologic anatomy, clinical picture, and prenatal diagnosis, *Hum Genet* 68(2):104-35, 1984.
149. Zerres K, Mucher G, Bachner L et al: Mapping of the gene for autosomal recessive polycystic kidney disease (ARPKD) to chromosome 6p21-cen, *Nat Genet* 7(3):429-32, 1994.
150. Guay-Woodford LM, Muecher G, Hopkins SD et al: The severe perinatal form of autosomal recessive polycystic kidney disease maps to chromosome 6p21.1-p12: implications for genetic counseling, *Am J Hum Genet* 56(5):1101-07, 1995.
151. Ward CJ, Hogan MC, Rossetti S et al: The gene mutated in autosomal recessive polycystic kidney disease encodes a large, receptor-like protein, *Nat Genet* 30:259-69, 2002.
152. Onuchic LF, Furu L, Nagasawa Y et al: PKHD1, the Polycystic Kidney and Hepatic Disease 1 gene, encodes a novel large protein containing multiple immunoglobulin-like plexin-transcription-factor domains and parallel beta-helix 1 repeats, *Am J Hum Genet* 70: 1305-17, 2002.
153. Nagasawa Y, Matthiesen S, Onuchic LF et al: Identification and characterization of Pkhd1, the mouse orthologue of the human ARPKD gene, *J Am Soc Nephrol* 13(9):2246-58, 2002.
154. Ward CJ, Yuan D, Masyuk TV et al: Cellular and subcellular localization of the ARPKD protein; fibrocystin is expressed on primary cilia, *Hum Mol Genet* 12:2703-10, 2003.
155. Masyuk TV, Huang BQ, Ward CJ et al: Defects in cholangiocyte fibrocystin expression and ciliary structure in the PCK rat, *Gastroenterology* 125:1303-10, 2003.
156. Zhang MZ, Mai W, Li C et al: PKHD1 protein encoded by the gene for autosomal recessive polycystic kidney disease associates with basal bodies and primary cilia in renal epithelial cells, *Proc Natl Acad Sci USA* 101:2311-16, 2004.
157. Wang S, Luo Y, Wilson PD et al: The autosomal recessive polycystic kidney disease protein is localized to primary cilia, with concentration in the basal body area, *J Am Soc Nephrol* 15:592-602, 2004.
158. Menezes LF, Cai Y, Nagasawa Y et al: Polyductin, the PKHD1 gene product, comprises isoforms expressed in plasma membrane, primary cilium, and cytoplasm, *Kidney Int* 66:1345-55, 2004.
159. Masyuk TV, Muff MA, Huang BQ et al: Functional implications of topographical distribution of fibrocystin in cholangiocytes, *J Am Soc Nephrol* 16, ASN Renal Week abstracts issue, 2005.
160. Kaimori JY, Nagasawa Y, Garcia-Gonzales MA et al: The PKHD1 product, polyductin/fibrocystin, undergoes notch-like posttranslational processing, *J Am Soc Nephrol* 16, ASN Renal Week abstracts issue, 2005.
161. Hiesberger T, Gourley E, Ward CJ et al: Primary cilia-dependent Ca2+ signalling induces the proteolytic cleavage and nuclear translocation of fibrocystin, *J Am Soc Nephrol* 16, ASN Renal Week abstracts issue, 2005.
162. Bergmann C, Senderek J, Sedlacek B et al: Spectrum of mutations in the gene for autosomal recessive polycystic kidney disease (ARPKD/PKHD1), *J Am Soc Nephrol* 14:76-89, 2003.
163. Furu L, Onuchic LF, Gharavi A et al: Milder presentation of recessive polycystic kidney disease requires presence of amino acid substitution mutations, *J Am Soc Nephrol* 14:2004-14, 2003.
164. Bergmann C, Senderek J, Küpper F et al: PKHD1 mutations in autosomal recessive polycystic kidney disease (ARPKD), *Hum Mutat* 23:453-63, 2004.
165. Bergmann C, Senderek J, Schneider F et al: PKHD1 mutations in families requesting prenatal diagnosis for autosomal recessive polycystic kidney disease (ARPKD), *Hum Mutat* 23:487-95, 2004.
166. Sharp AM, Messiaen LM, Page G et al: Comprehensive genomic analysis for PKHD1 mutations in ARPKD cohorts, *J Med Genet* 42:336-49, 2005.
167. Losekoot M, Haarloo C, Ruivenkamp C et al: Analysis of missense variants in the PKHD1-gene in patients with autosomal recessive polycystic kidney disease (ARPKD), *Hum Genet* 25:1-22, 2005.
168. Baralle D, Baralle M: Splicing in action: assessing disease causing sequence changes, *J Med Genet* 42:737-48, 2005.
169. Bergmann C, Frank V, Küpper F et al: Functional analysis of PKHD1 splicing in autosomal recessive polycystic kidney disease (ARPKD), *J Hum Genet* 51:788-93, 2006.
170. Bergmann C, Küpper F, Schmitt CP et al: Multi-exon deletions of the PKHD1 gene cause autosomal recessive polycystic kidney disease (ARPKD), *J Med Genet* 42:e63, 2005.
171. Consugar MB, Anderson SA, Rossetti S, et al: Haplotype analysis improves molecular diagnostics of autosomal recessive polycystic kidney disease, *Am J Kidney Dis* 45(1):77-87, 2005.
172. Cooper DN, Krawczak M. *Human Gene Mutation*, Oxford, UK, 1993. BIOS Scientific Publishers Limited.
173. Bergmann C, Küpper F, Dornia C et al: Algorithm for efficient PKHD1 mutation screening in autosomal recessive polycystic kidney disease (ARPKD), *Hum Mutat* 25:225-31, 2005.
174. Muntoni F, Torelli S, Ferlini A: Dystrophin and mutations: one gene, several proteins, multiple phenotypes, *Lancet Neurol* 2(12): 731-40, 2003.
175. Guay-Woodford LM, Wright CJ, Walz G, Churchill GA: Quantitative trait loci modulate renal cystic disease severity in the mouse bpk model, *J Am Soc Nephrol* 11:1253-60, 2006.
176. Sommardahl C, Cottrell M, Wilkinson JE et al: Phenotypic variations of orpk mutation and chromosomal localization of modifiers influencing kidney phenotype, *Physiol Genomics* 21:127-34, 2001.
177. Modrek B, Lee C: A genomic view of alternative splicing, *Nat Genet* 30:13-19, 2002.
178. Nissim-Rafinia M, Kerem B. Splicing regulation as a potential genetic modifier, *Trends Genet* 18:123-27, 2002.
179. White PC, Speiser PW: Congenital adrenal hyperplasia due to 21-hydroxylase deficiency, *Endocr Rev* 21:245-91, 2000.
180. Salvatore F, Scudiero O, Castaldo G: Genotype-phenotype correlation in cystic fibrosis: the role of modifier genes, *Am J Med Genet* 111:88-95, 2002.
181. Zerres K, Hansmann M, Mallmann R, Gembruch U: Autosomal recessive polycystic kidney disease. Problems of prenatal diagnosis, *Prenat Diagn* 8:215-29, March 1988.
182. Reuss A, Wladimiroff JW, Stewart PA, Niermeijer MF: Prenatal diagnosis by ultrasound in pregnancies at risk for autosomal recessive polycystic kidney disease, *Ultrasound Med Biol* 16:355-59, 1990.
183. Zerres K, Mücher G, Becker J et al: Prenatal diagnosis of autosomal recessive polycystic kidney disease (ARPKD): molecular genetics, clinical experience, and fetal morphology, *Am J Med Genet* 76:137-144, 1988.
184. Zerres K, Senderek J, Rudnik-Schöneborn S: New options for prenatal diagnosis in autosomal recessive polycystic kidney disease (ARPKD) by mutation analysis of the PKHD1 gene, *Clin Genet* 66:53-57, 2004.
185. Zhang Q, Taulman PD, Yoder BK: Cystic kidney diseases: all roads lead to the cilium. Physiology (Bethesda) 19:225-30, 2004.
186. Praetorius HA, Spring KR: Bending the MDCK cell primary cilium increases intracellular calcium, *J Membr Biol* 184:71-79, 2001.
187. Pazour GJ, Rosenbaum JL: Intraflagellar transport and cilia-dependent diseases, *Trends Cell Biol* 12:551-55, 2002.
188. Nauli SM, Alenghat FJ, Luo Y, Williams E, Vassilev P, Li X, Elia AE, Lu W, Brown EM, Quinn SJ, Ingber DE, Zhou J: Polycystins 1 and 2 mediate mechanosensation in the primary cilium of kidney cells, *Nat Genet* 33:129-37, 2003.
189. Lin F, Hiesberger T, Cordes K et al: Kidney-specific inactivation of the KIF3A subunit of kinesin-II inhibits renal ciliogenesis and produces polycystic kidney disease, *Proc Natl Acad Sci USA* 100:5286-91, 2003.

190. Belibi FA, Reif G, Wallace DP et al: AMP promotes growth and secretion in human polycystic kidney epithelial cells, *Kidney Int* 66:964-73, 2004.
191. Yamaguchi T, Wallace DP, Magenheimer BS et al: Calcium restriction allows cAMP activation of the B-Raf/ERK pathway, switching cells to a cAMP-dependent growth-stimulated phenotype, *J Biol Chem* 279:40419-30, 2004.
192. Peyssonnaux C, Eychene A: The Raf/MEK/ERK pathway: new concepts of activation, *Biol Cell* 93:53-62, 2001.
193. Gilbert E, Morel A, Tulliez M et al: In vivo effects of activated H-ras oncogene expressed in the liver and in urogenital tissues, *Int J Cancer* 73:749-56, 1997.
194. Schaffner DL, Barrios R, Massey C et al: Targeting of the rasT24 oncogene to the proximal convoluted tubules in transgenic mice results in hyperplasia and polycystic kidneys, *Am J Pathol* 142:1051-60, 1993.
195. Parnell SC, Magenheimer BS, Maser RL et al: Polycystin-1 activation of c-Jun N-terminal kinase and AP-1 is mediated by heterotrimeric G proteins, *J Biol Chem* 227:19566-72, 2002.
196. Le Hang N, van der Wal A, van der Bent P et al: Increased activity of activator protein-1 transcription factor components ATF2, c-Jun, and c-Fos in human and mouse autosomal dominant polycystic kidney disease, *J Am Soc Nephrol* 16 (9):2724-31, Sep 2005.
197. Fan Y, Esmail MA, Ansley SJ et al: Mutations in a member of the Ras superfamily of small GTP-binding proteins causes Bardet-Biedl syndrome, *Nat Genet* 36:989-93, 2004.
198. Kim E, Arnould T, Sellin LK et al: The polycystic kidney disease 1 gene product modulates Wnt signalling, *J Biol Chem* 274:4947-53, 1999.
199. Germino GG: Linking cilia to Wnts, *Nat Genet* 2005;37:455-57, 2005.
200. Simons M, Gloy J, Ganner A et al: Inversin, the gene product mutated in nephronophthisis type II, functions as a molecular switch between Wnt signaling pathways, *Nat Genet* 37:537-43, 2005.
201. Ross A, May-Simera H, Eichers ER et al: Disruption of Bardet-Biedl syndrome ciliary proteins perturbs planar cell polarity in vertebrates, *Nat Genet* 37:1135-40, 2005.
202. Bhunia AK, Piontek K, Boletta A et al: PKD1 induces p21(waf1) and regulation of the cell cycle via direct activation of the JAK-STAT signaling pathway in a process requiring PKD2, *Cell* 109:157-68, 2002.
203. Chauvet V, Tian X, Husson H et al: Mechanical stimuli induce cleavage and nuclear translocation of the polycystin-1 C terminus, *J Clin Invest* 114:1433-43, 2004.
204. Low SH, Vasanth S, Larson CH et al: Polycystin-1, STAT6, and P100 function in a pathway that transduces ciliary mechanosensation and is activated in polycystic kidney disease, *Dev Cell* 10:57-69, 2006.
205. Gattone VH 2nd: Emerging therapies for polycystic kidney disease, *Curr Opin Pharmacol* 5:535-42, 2005.
206. Gattone VH 2nd, Wang X, Harris PC, Torres VE: Inhibition of renal cystic disease development and progression by a vasopressin V2 receptor antagonist, *Nat Med* 9:1323-26, 2003.
207. Torres VE, Wang X, Qian Q et al: Effective treatment of an orthologous model of autosomal dominant polycystic kidney disease, *Nat Med* 10:363-64, 2005.
208. Wang X, Gattone VH 2nd, Harris PC, Torres VE: Effectiveness of vasopressin V2 receptor antagonists OPC-31260 and OPC-41061 on polycystic kidney disease development in the PCK rat, *J Am Soc Nephrol* 16:846-51, 2005.
209. Gattone VH 2nd, Kinne Q, Torres VE: Efficacy of OPC-41061 in the treatment of murine nephronophthisis, *J Am Soc Nephrol* 2005 (in press).
210. Wang X, Gattone VH 2nd, Somlo S et al: Effectiveness of vasopressin V2 receptor antagonist OPC-41061 on polycystic kidney disease development in Pkd2 WS25/– mice, *J Am Soc Nephrol* 2005 (in press).
211. Ohnishi A, Orita Y, Takagi N et al: Aquaretic effect of a potent, orally active, nonpeptide V2 antagonist in men, *J Pharmacol Exp Ther* 272:546-51, 1995.
212. Grantham JJ: Lillian Jean Kaplan International Prize for advancement in the understanding of polycystic kidney disease. Understanding polycystic kidney disease: a systems biology approach, *Kidney Int* 64:1157-62, 2003.
213. Woo DD, Miao SY, Pelayo JC et al: Taxol inhibits progression of congenital polycystic kidney disease, *Nature* 368:750-53, 1994.
214. Sommardahl CS, Woychik RP, Sweeney WE et al: Efficacy of taxol in the orpk mouse model of polycystic kidney disease, *Pediatr Nephrol* 11:728-33, 1997.
215. Martinez JR, Cowley BD, Gattone VH 2nd et al: The effect of paclitaxel on the progression of polycystic kidney disease in rodents, *Am J Kidney Dis* 29:435-44, 1997.
216. Trudel M, D'Agati V, Costantini F: C-myc as an inducer of polycystic kidney disease in transgenic mice, *Kidney Int* 39:665-71, 1991.
217. Trudel M, Chretien N, D'Agati V: Disappearance of polycystic kidney disease in revertant c-myc transgenic mice, *Mamm Genome* 5:149-52, 1994.
218. Cowley BD Jr, Smardo FL Jr, Grantham JJ, Calvet JP: Elevated c-myc protooncogene expression in autosomal recessive polycystic kidney disease, *Proc Natl Acad Sci USA* 84:8394-98, 1987.
219. Gattone VH 2nd, Kuenstler KA, Lindemann GW et al: Renal expression of a transforming growth factor-alpha transgene accelerates the progression of inherited, slowly progressive polycystic kidney disease in the mouse, *J Lab Clin Med* 127:214-22, 1996.
220. Harding MA, Gattone VH 2nd, Grantham JJ, Calvet JP: Localization of overexpressed c-myc mRNA in polycystic kidneys of the cpk mouse, *Kidney Int* 41:317-25, 1992.
221. Husson H, Manavalan P, Akmaev VR et al: New insights into ADPKD molecular pathways using combination of SAGE and microarray technologies, *Genomics* 84:497-510, 2004.
222. Ricker JL, Mata JE, Iversen PL, Gattone VH: c-myc antisense oligonucleotide treatment ameliorates murine ARPKD, *Kidney Int* 61:125-31, 2002.
223. Gattone VH 2nd, Ricker JR: Interventions in polycystic kidney disease using antisense oligonucleotide, *FASEB J* 16:A1097, 2002.
224. Gattone VH, Ricker JL, Trambaugh CM, Klein RM: Multiorgan mRNA misexpression in murine autosomal recessive polycystic kidney disease, *Kidney Int* 62:1560-69, 2002.
225. Orellana SA, Sweeney WE, Neff CD, Avner ED: Epidermal growth factor receptor expression is abnormal in murine polycystic kidney, *Kidney Int* 47:490-99, 1995.
226. Sweeney WE Jr, Avner ED: Functional activity of epidermal growth factor receptors in autosomal recessive polycystic kidney disease, *Am J Physiol* 275:F387-94, 1998.
227. Nauta J, Sweeney WE, Rutledge JC, Avner ED: Biliary epithelial cells from mice with congenital polycystic kidney disease are hyperresponsive to epidermal growth factor, *Pediatr Res* 37:755-63, 1995.
228. Gattone VH 2nd, Andrews GK, Niu FW et al: Defective epidermal growth factor gene expression in mice with polycystic kidney disease, *Dev Biol* 138:225-30, 1990.
229. Cowley BD Jr, Rupp JC: Abnormal expression of epidermal growth factor and sulfated glycoprotein SGP-2 messenger RNA in a rat model of autosomal dominant polycystic kidney disease, *J Am Soc Nephrol* 6:1679-81, 1995.
230. Weinstein T, Hwang D, Lev-Ran A et al: Excretion of epidermal growth factor in human adult polycystic kidney disease, *Isr J Med Sci* 33:641-42, 1997.
231. Dell KM, Nemo R, Sweeney WE Jr et al: A novel inhibitor of tumor necrosis factor-alpha converting enzyme ameliorates polycystic kidney disease, *Kidney Int* 60:1240-48, 2001.
232. Sweeney WE, Chen Y, Nakanishi K et al: Treatment of polycystic kidney disease with a novel tyrosine kinase inhibitor, *Kidney Int* 57:33-40, 2000.
233. Torres VE, Sweeney WE Jr, Wang X et al: EGF receptor tyrosine kinase inhibition attenuates the development of PKD in Han : SPRD rats, *Kidney Int* 64:1573-79, 2003.
234. von Vigier RO, Sweeney WE Jr, Murcia NS et al: Receptor tyrosine kinase inhibition attenuates hepatobiliary abnormalities in a murine model of autosomal recessive polycystic kidney disease, *J Am Soc Nephrol* 15:57A, 2004.
235. Gattone VH 2nd, Lowden DA, Cowley BD Jr: Epidermal growth factor ameliorates autosomal recessive polycystic kidney disease in mice, *Dev Biol* 169:504-10, 1995.

236. Nakanishi K, Gattone VH 2nd, Sweeney WE, Avner ED: Renal dysfunction but not cystic change is ameliorated by neonatal epidermal growth factor in bpk mice, *Pediatr Nephrol* 16:45-50, 2001.
237. Torres VE, Sweeney WE Jr, Wang X et al: Epidermal growth factor receptor tyrosine kinase inhibition is not protective in PCK rats, *Kidney Int* 66:1766-73, 2004.
238. Tao Y, Kim J, Schrier RW, Edelstein CL: Rapamycin markedly slows disease progression in a rat model of polycystic kidney disease, *J Am Soc Nephrol* 16:46-51, 2005.
239. McKee B, Perrone R, Gattone VH 2nd: Rapamycin ameliorates murine polycystic kidney disease, *Fed Proc* 19:A194, 2005.
240. Tao Y, Kim J, Faubel S et al: Caspase inhibition reduces tubular apoptosis and proliferation and slows disease progression in polycystic kidney disease, *Proc Natl Acad Sci U S A* 102:6954-59, 2005.
241. Gattone VH 2nd, Cowley BD Jr, Barash BD et al: Methylprednisolone retards the progression of inherited polycystic kidney disease in rodents, *Am J Kidney Dis* 25:302-13, 1995.
242. Ogborn MR, Crocker JF: Na-K ATPase activity in murine glucocorticoid induced polycystic kidney disease in vivo, *Clin Invest Med* 16:22-28, 1993.
243. Ruggenenti P, Remuzzi A, Ondei P et al: Safety and efficacy of long-acting somatostatin treatment in autosomal-dominant polycystic kidney disease, *Kidney Int* 68:206-16, 2005.
244. Gambineri A, Patton L, De Iasio R et al: Efficacy of octreotide-LAR in dieting women with abdominal obesity and polycystic ovary syndrome, *J Clin Endocrinol Metab* 90:3854-62, 2005.

CHAPTER 10

Hematuria and Proteinuria

Hui-Kim Yap and Perry Yew-Weng Lau

In children, the presence of blood or protein in urine may be just a normal, transient finding that usually accompanies a nonspecific viral infection. However, it can sometimes be an indicator of a kidney or urinary tract disorder. Macroscopic hematuria or an incidental finding of hematuria or proteinuria on urine dipstick examination is often alarming for parents, causing them to bring their child to medical attention. The presence of hematuria without proteinuria is generally not indicative of serious pathology except in the case of calculi, malignancies, and in some regions of the world, schistosomiasis. On the other hand, the presence of proteinuria is a more important diagnostic and prognostic marker of significant glomerular disease, as well as chronic kidney disease.

HEMATURIA

In a normal person, very few red blood cells are excreted into the urine; rather, they are believed to pass into the urine via the glomerulus. The pliability of the red blood cells allows them to squeeze through the capillary basement membrane. The normal red blood cell excretion rate can be greater after exercise. Glomerular inflammation results in damage to the capillary endothelium and glomerular basement membrane, resulting in increased passage of red blood cells into the urinary space. Macroscopic hematuria is visible to the naked eye, whereas microscopic hematuria is usually detected by a urine dipstick test during routine examinations or by microscopic examination of the urine sediment.

A very small quantity of blood can discolor the urine. If fresh blood is present in the urine, the urine will be pink or red. If left standing even in the bladder, the urine will develop a hazy smoke or brown color. The brown color comes from the metheme derivative of the oxidized heme pigment. Some pigments and crystals, when present at a significant concentration, will cause color changes in the urine that can be misinterpreted as hematuria. Discoloration of urine can be due to intravascular hemolysis, rhabdomyolysis, metabolic disorders, or a number of foods and drugs (Table 10-1).

Definition

The definition of hematuria is based on urine microscopic examination findings of red blood cells of more than 5/μL in a fresh uncentrifuged midstream urine specimen[1] or more than 3 red blood cells/high-power field in the centrifuged sediment from 10 ml of freshly voided midstream urine. However, there is controversy as to the number of red blood cells required for diagnosis of microscopic hematuria. Some investigators have used a definition of greater than 2 red blood cells/high-power field in 12 ml of a midstream urine specimen spun at 1500 RPM for 5 minutes.[2] Others have used a definition of 10 red blood cells/high-power field in a midstream urine collection.[3] A study using more stringent criteria has greater positive predictive value regarding the presence of disease but loses some negative predictive value. Regardless of the criterion used, important cofactors to consider when a child has hematuria include the presence of proteinuria, urinary casts, hypertension, a family history of renal disease, and other clinical or laboratory findings that suggest renal or urinary tract disease.

Urine Dipstick

The urine dipstick utilizes the peroxidase-like activity of hemoglobin present in the urine. The hemoglobin peroxidase activity converts the chromogen tetramethylbenzidine incorporated in the dipstick into an oxidized form, resulting in a green-blue color. It is important to follow the manufacturer's instructions for dipstick use closely. The dipstick should be dipped briefly in the urine and excess fluid tapped off. Strict attention should then be paid to the interval indicated on the container before comparing the resulting color with the color chart. Delayed readings may produce false-positive results. The test depends on free hemoglobin that comes from hemolysis of the red blood cells in the urine. It is assumed that when there is significant hematuria, some of the red blood cells will always lyse and sufficient free hemoglobin will be released to cause a positive test. The test is very sensitive and can detect as little as 150 μg/L of free hemoglobin.

False-positive results can occur in hemoglobinuria following intravascular hemolysis or in myoglobinuria after rhabdomyolysis. False-positive results can also be due to the presence of oxidizing agents in the urine, such as hypochlorite and microbial peroxidases associated with urinary tract infection. Conversely, false-negative results can be due to the presence of large amounts of reducing agents such as ascorbic acid or urine with high specific gravity, in which case the dipstick test is less sensitive.

TABLE 10-1 Causes of Discoloration of Urine

Dark yellow or orange urine	Normal concentrated urine Drugs such as rifampicin
Dark brown or black urine	Bile pigments Methemoglobinemia Alanine, cascara, resorcinol Alkaptonuria, homogentesic acid, melanin, thymol, tyrosinosis
Red or pink urine	Red blood cells (hematuria) Free hemoglobin (hemoglobinuria) Myoglobin (myoglobinuria) Porphyrins Urates in high concentration (may produce pinkish tinge) Foods (e.g., beetroot, blackberries, red dyes) Drugs (e.g., benzene, chloroquine, desferoxamine, phenazopyridine, phenolphthalein)

Because of the sensitive nature of the urine dipstick test, it is unwise to investigate on the basis of a trace reading. Similarly, a child with a dipstick reading of 1+ on one occasion and negative readings on subsequent dipstick testing is unlikely to benefit from further investigations. Only if the urine dipstick reading for blood is persistently 1 or more is further evaluation warranted. In clinical practice it is important to confirm hematuria with urine microscopic examination. An absence of red blood cells in the urine with a positive dipstick reaction may suggest hemoglobinuria or myoglobinuria.

Urine Microscopy

Microscopic examination of the urine sediment is important in diagnosing and evaluating hematuria. When abundant, red blood cells are easy to identify by their characteristic biconcave disc appearance under microscopy. When scanty, they become distorted in the urine and difficult to differentiate from other unidentified small objects. Urine centrifugation is one way to solve this problem. After centrifugation and removal of supernatant, the deposit is resuspended in the remaining urine and examined under the microscope. Urine microscopic examination can have false-negative results when the urine is of low specific gravity or has an alkaline pH. These conditions result in red blood cells hemolyzing rapidly in standing urine, producing a positive urine dipstick test due to the free hemoglobin but without the characteristic red blood cells seen under microscopy.

Morphology of the red blood cells can help identify the origin of bleeding.[4,5] Red blood cells from the lower urinary tract maintain their morphology, whereas those from the glomeruli show great variation in shape, size, and hemoglobin content because of shearing stress on their surface when passing from the capillary lumens through gaps in the glomerular basement membrane into the urinary space.[6] Phase-contrast microscopy on freshly voided urine allows this differentiation. Red blood cells that are more than 90% to 95% isomorphic (i.e., of normal size and shape) are most commonly from the lower urinary tract. If more than 30% of dysmorphic red blood cells (blebs, budding, and segmental loss of membrane with reduction in red cell volume) are present, the hematuria is more likely to be of glomerular origin.[7]

The presence of casts or crystals in the urine can also be helpful in locating the origin of bleeding. Red blood cell casts are always pathologic and usually suggest glomerulonephritis. They should be examined on fresh urine or acidic urine stored at 4°C, because red blood cell casts disintegrate readily in alkaline urine, taking on a granular appearance. Hence the finding of granular casts in association with hematuria may indicate that the blood originated in the kidneys. When white blood cells are also present in the urine, infection and interstitial or glomerular inflammatory disorders should be considered. Interstitial nephritis is even more likely if Wright stain of the urine shows the presence of eosinophils. On urinalysis, infections and poststreptococcal nephritis often show neutrophils. Hyaline casts are associated with proteinuria, and a few such casts may be found in concentrated early-morning samples from healthy people. If a child has other findings that suggest nephrolithiasis, the shape of the crystals may help identify the chemical nature of the calculi. Calcium oxalate crystals may point to hypercalciuria.

Etiology

Hematuria may originate from the glomeruli, renal tubules and interstitium, or urinary tract (including collecting systems, ureters, bladder, and urethra). A practical approach is to determine whether the hematuria is of glomerular or nonglomerular origin. The various causes of hematuria in children are listed in Table 10-2. In children, the source of bleeding is more often from the glomeruli than from the urinary tract. The four different clinical presentations of hematuria are as follows:

1. Child with red or dark-colored urine
2. Child with lower urinary tract symptoms
3. Child with clinical features of acute glomerulonephritis
4. Asymptomatic child with incidental finding of microscopic hematuria on urine dipstick

These presentations will be considered separately because the approach is different in each scenario even though the causes may overlap.

Child with Red or Dark-Colored Urine

The first step in the evaluation is to exclude red discoloration of urine due to certain foods or drugs, hemoglobinuria, and myoglobinuria (Table 10-1). A urine microscopic examination is essential to confirm that the discoloration is due to red blood cells. Macroscopic hematuria of glomerular origin is usually described as brown, tea-colored, or cola-colored, whereas that of lower urinary tract origin (bladder and urethra) is usually pink or red.

Causes of gross hematuria in children include the following:

1. Acute glomerulonephritis if edema and hypertension are also present
2. Urinary tract infection, hemorrhagic cystitis, urethritis, perineal irritation, urolithiasis, or hypercalciuria (conditions usually accompanied by voiding symptoms such as dysuria, frequency, and urgency)

TABLE 10-2 Causes of Hematuria in Children

Glomerular		**Nonglomerular**
Familial benign hematuria (thin basement membrane disease)	Glomerulonephritis (GN)	Urinary tract infection
Nonfamilial benign hematuria	Primary GN	Hypercalciuria
	Postinfectious acute GN	Renal calculi
	Membranoproliferative GN	Trauma
	Membranous nephropathy	Exercise
	Rapidly progressive GN	Chemical cystitis such as cyclophosphamide
	IgA nephropathy	Coagulopathy
	Secondary GN	Vascular malformations
	Systemic lupus erythematosus	Nutcracker syndrome
	Henoch-Schönlein purpura	Malignancy
	Polyarteritis nodosa	Renal: nephroblastoma
	Wegener granulomatosis	Bladder: rhabdomyosarcoma
	Hemolytic uremic syndrome	Menarche
	Hereditary nephritis (Alport syndrome)	Factitious
	Renal vein thrombosis	
	Interstitial nephritis	
	Cystic renal disease	

3. Exercise-induced hematuria
4. Trauma
5. Coagulopathy
6. Malignancy
7. Recurrent gross hematuria suggestive of IgA nephropathy, familial benign hematuria, nutcracker syndrome, or Alport syndrome

Exercise-induced hematuria is a transient hematuria that appears immediately after severe exercise such as long-distance running and usually disappears within 48 hours. This is due to an excess in red cell excretion and is benign.

Trauma sufficient to cause hematuria is usually associated with an obvious history such as traumatic urethral catheterization or abdominal injury. Cases of radiologic evaluation of hematuria after abdominal trauma with a finding of previously unsuspected obstructed urinary tract such as pelviureteric junction stenosis have been reported.

Children with bleeding disorders such as hemophilia or thrombocytopenia commonly have microscopic hematuria and may also develop gross hematuria. Sickle cell hemoglobinopathy can result in hematuria by causing infarction of the renal collecting systems.[8]

Urinary tract tumors are rare. Children with nephroblastoma can have microscopic but rarely macroscopic hematuria. More commonly, nephroblastomas are discovered following evaluation of abdominal distension or abdominal masses. Rhabdomyosarcoma of the bladder is extremely rare and usually presents with voiding symptoms in addition to macroscopic hematuria.

The nutcracker phenomenon refers to compression of the left renal vein between the aorta and superior mesenteric artery before the left renal vein joins the inferior vena cava. This leads to left renal vein hypertension that may result in rupture of the thin-walled vein into the renal calyceal fornix, with the clinical presentation of intermittent gross or microscopic hematuria. This phenomenon with its associated symptoms of unilateral hematuria and left flank pain is known as the nutcracker syndrome. It occasionally presents as a varicocele in boys or abnormal menstruation in pubertal girls as a result of the development of venous varicosities of the gonadal vein.[9] This syndrome also occurs in relatively young and previously healthy patients with an asthenic habitus. Using Doppler ultrasonography to examine the left renal vein, Okada et al. suggested that the nutcracker syndrome might be one of the important causes of gross or microscopic hematuria with a relatively high prevalence.[10] Magnetic resonance angiography is required to demonstrate the dilated left renal vein after passing between the aorta and superior mesenteric artery. Controversy exists regarding the treatment of nutcracker syndrome. Spontaneous resolution of hematuria in children with nutcracker syndrome has been reported following an increase in body mass index.[10,11]

Children with IgA nephropathy, familial benign hematuria, or Alport syndrome can have macroscopic hematuria at the time of, or 1 or 2 days following, an upper respiratory tract infection—a phenomenon known as synpharyngitic hematuria. The urine may be normal between bouts of hematuria, but a considerable proportion of these children have persistent microscopic hematuria between attacks of gross hematuria. A family history is important to help distinguish between Alport syndrome and familial benign hematuria.

In the diagnostic workup for a child showing painless gross hematuria, the absence of significant proteinuria or red blood cell casts is an indication for a renal and bladder ultrasound to exclude malignancy or cystic renal disease. If investigations reveal the presence of a tumor, structural urogenital abnormality, or urinary calculus, a urologic referral is required. Cystoscopy may also be required in cases of children with recurrent nonglomerular macroscopic hematuria of unknown cause.

Child with Associated Lower Urinary Tract Symptoms

Hematuria with accompanying dysuria, frequency, urgency, or flank or abdominal pain may suggest a diagnosis of urinary tract infection, hypercalciuria, or nephrolithiasis.

One third of urinary tract infections have associated hematuria, although this is usually microscopic in nature. Urinary tract infections are mainly caused by bacteria, but viruses, fungi, and parasites are potential etiologic agents. Acute hemorrhagic cystitis is characterized by gross hematuria and symptoms of bladder inflammation and is associated with adenovirus type 11 and type 21. Macroscopic hematuria usually resolves by 5 days, and microscopic hematuria may persist for 2 or 3 days longer.[12]

Schistosomiasis (bilharziasis) is an important cause of hematuria that should be considered in natives of tropical Africa and Middle Eastern countries and also in immigrants from these areas.[13] It is contracted by swimming in lakes and ponds infested with snails that are infected by the flatworm *Schistosoma haematobium*. Eggs of the flatworm that become trapped in the bladder and lower urinary tract cause an intense granulomatous inflammatory reaction that results in hematuria. In developing countries tuberculosis of the urinary tract is another cause of hematuria, both microscopic and macroscopic, especially in children with prolonged ill health.[14]

Nephrolithiasis is rare in children, with a reported incidence rate between 0.13 and 0.94 cases per 1000 hospital admissions of children.[15] It can present with hematuria alone or hematuria with colic. Pain can be caused by a renal stone or clots of blood passing down the ureter. An association between hematuria and hypercalciuria has been reported in children with asymptomatic macroscopic or microscopic hematuria without signs of renal stones.[16] Children with hypercalciuria may have accompanying irritative urinary symptoms such as dysuria, frequency, and urgency, as well as increased urinary excretion of calcium despite normal serum calcium levels. The urine calcium over creatinine ratio in a single urine specimen is a useful index of calcium excretion for screening and monitoring purposes. In a large study, the 97th-percentile level of urinary calcium over creatinine ratio in children eating an unrestricted diet was 0.69 mmol/mmol.[17]

Child with Clinical Features of Acute Glomerulonephritis

Acute nephritic syndrome is characterized by a sudden onset of macroscopic hematuria accompanied by hypertension, oliguria, edema, and varying degrees of renal insufficiency due to acute glomerular injury. The majority of cases of acute nephritic syndrome have a postinfectious etiology, most commonly following infection with group A β-hemolytic streptococcal infection of throat or skin. It is important to identify acute nephritic syndrome in a child with hematuria because immediate and appropriate management can prevent morbidity and mortality caused by uncontrolled hypertension, fluid overload, and renal insufficiency (see Chapter 11).

Asymptomatic Child with Incidental Finding of Microscopic Hematuria on Urine Dipstick

Increased use of the urine dipstick test to screen for urinary tract infection in a febrile child or in children during routine school health examinations in many countries has resulted in the detection of asymptomatic microscopic hematuria. However, because microscopic hematuria and mild proteinuria may appear transiently during fever, illness, or extreme exertion, it is not practical or cost-effective to extensively investigate every child to find the cause of microscopic hematuria. One possible approach is to repeat the urine dipstix test and microscopic urinalysis twice within 2 weeks following the initial result. If the hematuria resolves, no further tests are required. If microscopic hematuria persists on at least two of the three consecutive samples, then further evaluation is required.[18]

The common diagnoses in children with persistent microscopic hematuria without proteinuria are benign familial hematuria, idiopathic hypercalciuria, IgA nephropathy, and Alport syndrome. Benign familial hematuria, also known as thin basement membrane nephropathy (TBMN), is the most common cause of persistent microscopic hematuria in children. It may be inherited in an autosomal dominant or autosomal recessive manner. The red blood cells in the urine may be dysmorphic and there may be red blood cell casts. Occasionally, frank hematuria occurs with an upper respiratory tract infection. Proteinuria, progressive renal insufficiency, hearing deficits, or eye abnormalities almost never occur in patients with TBMN or in their family members. The main histologic finding is thinning of glomerular basement membrane. A renal biopsy is usually not indicated if TBMN is suspected unless there are atypical features that suggest IgA nephropathy or Alport syndrome.

Mass urine screening programs in school children have reported a prevalence of isolated microscopic hematuria in 0.21% to 0.94%.[19-21] Of those children subsequently referred for evaluation of persistent microscopic hematuria, a glomerular pathology was the most likely cause among 22.2% to 52.3% based on either phase-contrast microscopy or renal biopsy findings.[19,21-23]

Clinical Approach

In approaching a child with hematuria, we should ensure that serious conditions are not missed, avoid unnecessary and expensive laboratory tests, reassure the family, and provide guidelines for further studies if there is a change in the child's course. Obtaining a careful history and physical examination is the crucial first step in the evaluation.

History

Knowing both the timing of urinary changes in terms of days or hours and the associated symptoms is beneficial. Patients should be asked about recent trauma, exercise, passage of urinary stones, recent respiratory or skin infections, and intake of medications (including over-the-counter medications and calcium or vitamin D supplementation) or herbal compounds. Associated symptoms to look for should include fever, dysuria, urinary frequency and urgency, back pain, skin rashes, joint symptoms, and face and leg swelling. Predisposing illnesses such as sickle cell disease or trait should be noted. Family history should be searched for documented hematuria, hypertension, renal stones, renal failure, deafness, and coagulopathy. For girls in the peripubertal period, a history of menarche is useful. With sexually active teenagers, the social history should take into account all recent sexual activity and any known exposure to sexually transmitted diseases since cystitis and urethritis can present with hematuria.

Physical Examination

The presence or absence of hypertension and edema suggesting acute nephritic syndrome determines how urgent and extensive the diagnostic evaluation should be. Associated rashes or arthritis may indicate hematuria due to systemic lupus erythematosus or Henoch-Schönlein nephritis. The presence of fever or loin pain may point to pyelonephritis. A palpable and ballotable renal mass will require radiologic investigations to exclude hydronephrosis, polycystic kidney, or renal tumor.

Investigations

Investigations for causes of hematuria can be extensive. Tailoring an evaluation according to the type of clinical presentation reduces unnecessary laboratory and radiologic investigations (Figure 10-1). The first step is to confirm hematuria with urine microscopic examination. If the child has associated fever or irritative urinary symptoms, a urine culture should be studied to rule out urinary tract infection. For children with an incidental finding of microscopic hematuria during illness or after exertion, further evaluation is required only if there is persistent microscopic hematuria on at least two of three consecutive samples.

The next step in the evaluation is to determine the site of bleeding. Two investigations that are necessary once hematuria is confirmed are urine tests for protein and urine phase-contrast microscopy to examine the red blood cell morphology. Hematuria (gross or microscopic) associated with significant dysmorphic red blood cells, in particular acanthocytes (ring forms with vesicle-shaped protrusions),[24] and proteinuria indicate glomerular bleeding. It is important to remember that some proteinuria may also be present in nonglomerular causes of macroscopic hematuria. However, the proteinuria usually does not exceed 2+ (1 g/L) on dipstick examination if the only source of protein is from extraglomerular bleed. Therefore a child with proteinuria 2+ or

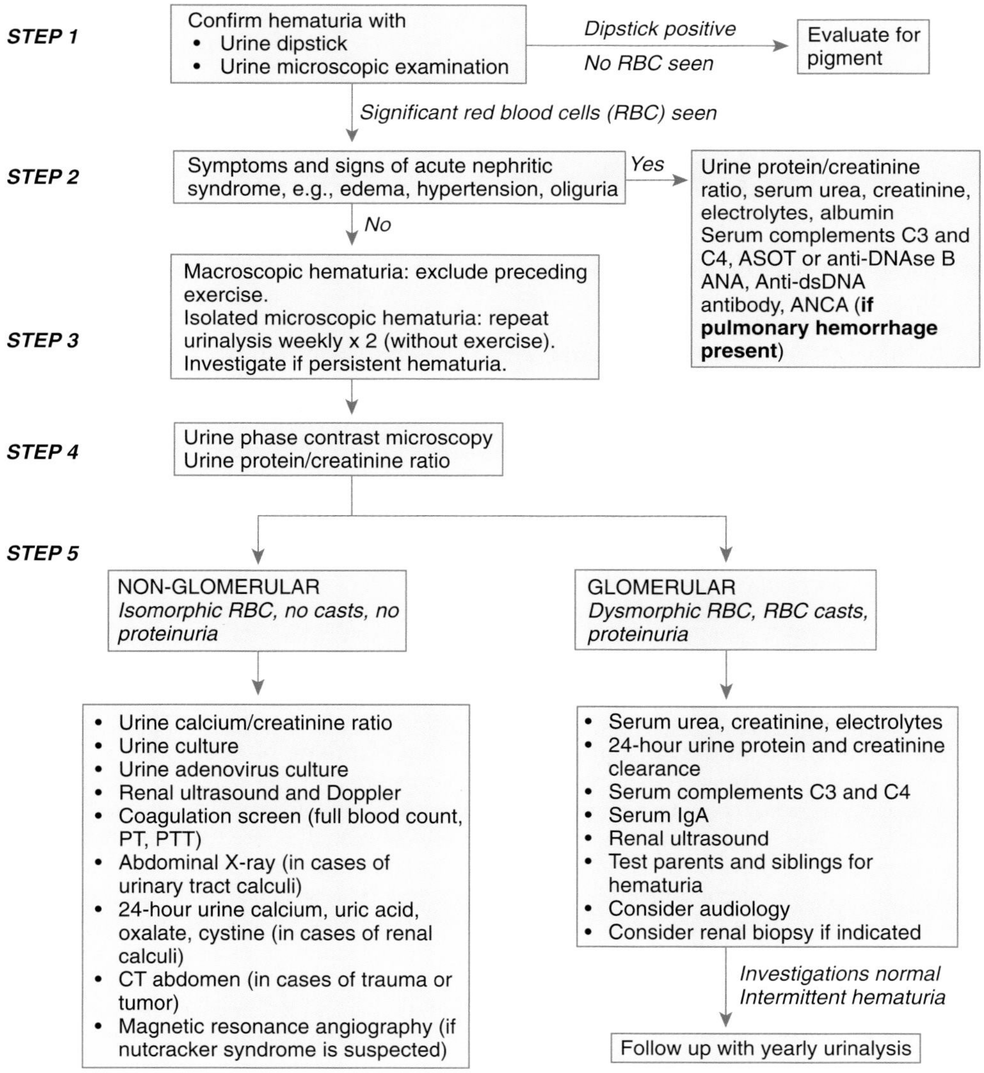

Figure 10-1 Algorithm for investigating hematuria.

more should be investigated for glomerulonephritis. Similarly, red blood cell casts, if present, are highly specific for glomerulonephritis.

Renal function needs to be determined in children with glomerular pathology. If there is significant proteinuria, the serum albumin should be measured. In addition, laboratory investigations for the cause should be performed. These include serum complements C3 and C4, antistreptolysin O titers (ASOTs) or antiDNAse B, antinuclear antibodies (ANAs), anti-double-stranded DNA (dsDNA) antibody, antineutrophil cytoplasmic antibodies (ANCAs), IgA levels, hepatitis B surface antigen, and viral titers if appropriate. Serum IgA levels are increased in 30% to 50% of adult patients but in only 8% to16% of children with IgA nephropathy.[25] In countries where IgA nephropathy is a significant cause of glomerulonephritis, 10% to 35% of children undergoing renal biopsy for isolated hematuria were found to have IgA nephropathy.[25,26] Clinical presentations should be considered when deciding the type of investigations required. For example, a preceding sore throat, pyoderma, or impetigo and the presence of edema, hypertension, and proteinuria suggest poststreptococcal glomerulonephritis. Serum ASOT and complement C3 levels would suffice in this case. If these tests are not informative, then further investigations are warranted to rule out other causes. An audiologic examination may help detect high-frequency sensorineural hearing deficit in Alport syndrome. Renal ultrasound is useful in determining the size of the kidneys as a guide to chronicity and also in diagnosing polycystic kidneys that are associated with glomerular hematuria.

Hematuria associated with mainly isomorphic red blood cells, absence of red blood cell casts and absence of proteinuria indicate a nonglomerular cause. Urine calcium over creatinine ratio should be taken to rule out hypercalciuria. A renal ultrasound and abdominal X-ray are indicated if urinary tract calculi are suspected. When a urinary tract calculus is identified, a complete assessment of the urinary constituents associated with stone risk is needed. In rare cases renal ultrasound may detect hydronephrosis or nephroblastoma as a cause of the hematuria. When there is a family history of bleeding diathesis, a coagulation screen may be necessary. A CT scan of the abdomen and pelvis may be required if there is a history of abdominal trauma followed by gross hematuria. If nutcracker syndrome is suspected in a child with recurrent gross hematuria, Doppler sonography can be used as a diagnostic tool, followed by magnetic resonance angiography for confirmation.

Cystoscopy in children seldom reveals the cause of hematuria but should be done when preliminary investigations have failed to find a cause and when bladder or urethral pathology is a consideration because of accompanying voiding symptoms. Initial hematuria suggests a urethral origin, whereas terminal hematuria is indicative of a bladder cause. Vascular malformations in the bladder have been detected via cystoscopy. In the rare instance where a bladder mass is noted on ultrasound, cystoscopy is also indicated. Cystoscopy to lateralize the source of bleeding is best performed during active bleeding.

An asymptomatic child with an incidental finding of persistent microscopic hematuria often poses the greatest dilemma regarding the extent of investigations and follow-up. The most common diagnoses in children with persistent microscopic hematuria without proteinuria and hypertension are benign persistent or benign familial hematuria, idiopathic hypercalciuria, IgA nephropathy, and Alport syndrome. In communities where postinfectious GN is common, subclinical disease is also a typical cause of persistent microscopic hematuria. It is worthwhile to screen family members for microscopic hematuria. If they are found to have incidental asymptomatic microscopic hematuria without proteinuria, benign familial hematuria is likely the cause and more extensive evaluation is not necessary. The yield of renal ultrasonography for evaluation of the asymptomatic child with microscopic hematuria remains unproven.[27] It is important to follow up these patients yearly to ensure that they have not developed proteinuria, because benign familial hematuria can be an early manifestation of Alport syndrome.

Indications for Renal Biopsy

Although renal biopsy is usually not indicated in isolated glomerular hematuria, it should be considered in cases of hematuria where the following are found:

- Association with significant proteinuria except in post-streptococcal glomerulonephritis
- Association with persistent low serum complement C3
- Association with unexplained azotemia
- A systemic disease with proteinuria, such as systemic lupus erythematosus, Henoch-Schönlein purpura, and ANCA-positive vasculitis
- A family history of significant renal disease suggestive of Alport syndrome
- Recurrent gross hematuria of unknown etiology
- Persistent glomerular hematuria and the parents are anxious about the diagnosis and prognosis

PROTEINURIA

It is well established that proteinuria is associated with progressive renal disease.[28] In recent years proteinuria has been increasingly recognized as a mediator of progressive renal insufficiency in both adults and children,[29-31] as well as a risk factor for cardiovascular disease.[32-34] On the other hand, proteinuria can also be a transient finding in children that occurs during times of stress, including exercise, fever, and dehydration, and does not denote renal disease.

Renal Handling of Proteins

Plasma proteins can cross the normal glomerular barrier relative to their molecular size and charge. Larger plasma proteins such as globulins are virtually excluded from the normal glomerular filtrate, whereas smaller proteins like albumin are filtered in low concentrations. Molecular charge plays an important role in determining glomerular permeability to macromolecules. This is due to the presence of negatively charged sialoproteins that line the surfaces of the glomerular endothelial and epithelial cells, as well as glycosaminoglycans present in the glomerular basement membrane. Hence negatively charged molecules are less able to cross the glomerulus than are neutral molecules of identical size. On the other hand, positively charged molecules have enhanced clearances.

After crossing the glomerular barrier, almost all of the filtered proteins are reabsorbed by the proximal tubule. Under normal conditions approximately 60% of protein in normal urine is derived from plasma protein. Albumin predominates and constitutes about 40% of the filtered urinary protein. The rest of the urinary proteins are globulins, peptides, enzymes, hormones, and partially degraded plasma proteins. The proteins are degraded in the tubular cells by lysosomal enzymes to low molecular weight fragments and amino acids. Excretion of these low molecular weight proteins results from a balance between the amount filtered and the amount reabsorbed.

Forty percent of normal urinary protein is of tissue rather than plasma origin, and consists of a heterogenous group of numerous proteins, many of which are glycoproteins. Some of these are derived from cells lining the urinary tract and have the potential of being important diagnostic indicators. The major protein in this group is Tamm-Horsfall protein or uromodulin, a major constituent of urinary casts.[35] It is excreted in amounts of 30 to 60 mg per day in adults and is secreted into the urine mainly at the thick ascending limb of the loop of Henle.

Excess urinary protein loss can result from increased permeability of the glomeruli to the passage of serum proteins (glomerular proteinuria), decreased reabsorption of proteins by the renal tubules (tubular proteinuria), or increased secretion of tissue protein into the urine (secretory proteinuria). Additionally, increased excretion of low molecular weight proteins may be due to marked overproduction of the protein, resulting in the filtered load exceeding the normal proximal reabsorptive capacity (overflow proteinuria).

Measurement of Proteinuria in Children

The normal rate of protein excretion in the urine is less than 4 mg/m^2 per hour or less than 150 mg/1.73 m^2 per day throughout childhood in both boys and girls.[36] Abnormal proteinuria is defined as 4 to 40 mg/m^2 per hour, and more than 40 mg/m^2 per hour is defined as nephrotic range proteinuria (Table 10-3).

Urine Dipstick

The urine dipstick is an excellent screening test for the presence of proteinuria.[36] The dipstick is impregnated with the dye tetrabromophenol blue, buffered to pH 3.5. At a constant pH, the binding of protein to this dye results in the development of a blue color proportionate to the amount of protein present. If urine is protein-free, the dipstick is yellow. The color changes from yellow to yellow-green to green to green-blue with increasing concentrations of protein. The dipstick can be read as negative; trace; or 1+, 2+, 3+, and 4+, which corresponds to insignificant; less than 0.2 g/L, 0.3 g/L, 1 g/L, 3 g/L; and greater than 20 g/L concentrations, respectively.

The dipstick test, however, has a few limitations. For instance, observer error can occur during interpretation of the color of the dipstick. False-positive and false-negative results for protein can also occur. If the dipstick is kept in the urine too long, the buffer may leach out, producing a false-positive test. Additionally, false-positive tests can occur in the presence of gross hematuria, pyuria, and bacteriuria or if the urine is contaminated with antiseptics such as chlorhexidine or benzalkonium, which are often used in skin cleansing before clean catch of the urine. False-positive results may appear in urine specimens after administration of radiographic contrast such as an intravenous urogram, penicillin or cephalosporin therapy, tolbutamide, or sulfonamides.

Results of the dipstick test can be affected by the concentration and pH of urine. If the urine is very dilute, the urinary protein concentration may be reduced to a level below the sensitivity of the dipstick (0.1 to 0.15 g/L) even in patients excreting up to 1 gram of protein per day. Hence we should interpret with caution any negative dipstick result for protein in urine with a specific gravity less than 1.002. On the other hand, if the urine is highly concentrated with urine specific gravity greater than 1.025, a healthy child can register trace of protein on the dipstick, giving a false-positive result. Regarding pH of urine, very alkaline urine (pH greater than 8.0) can cause a false-positive result, whereas very acid urine (pH less than 4.5) can cause a false-negative result.

False-negative results occur in nonalbumin proteinuria. Because albumin binds better to dye than do other proteins,

TABLE 10-3 **Quantification of Proteinuria in Children**

Method	Abnormal Proteinuria	Precautions
Urine dipstick	1+ or more in a concentrated urine specimen (specific gravity ≥1.020)	False-positive if urine pH > 8.0 or specific gravity > 1.025 or tested within 24 hr of radiocontrast study
Sulfosalicylic acid test	1+ or more	False-positive with iodinated radiocontrast agents
Urine protein/creatinine ratio (U_p/U_{Cr} ratio) in spot urine	>0.02 g/mmol or >0.2 mg/mg in children >2 yr >0.06 g/mmol or >0.6 mg/mg in children 6 mo to 2 yr Nephrotic range: >0.2 g/mmol or >2 mg/mg	Protein excretion varies with child's age
Timed urine protein excretion rate	>4 mg/m^2/hr or >150 mg/1.73 m^2/24 hr Nephrotic range: >40 mg/m^2/hr or >3 g/1.73 m^2/24 hr	In an accurately collected 24-hr urine specimen, urine creatinine should be in the range of 0.13-0.20 mmol/kg or 16-24 mg/kg ideal body weight for females, and 0.18-0.23 mmol/kg or 21-27 mg/kg ideal body weight for males

the urine dipstick detects it primarily, leaving low molecular weight proteins undetected. Dipstick results correlate better with the level of albuminuria than with total proteinuria. Hence the dipstick is highly specific for albuminuria but relatively insensitive, and is unable to detect microalbuminuria associated with early glomerular injury seen in diabetic nephropathy or cardiovascular disease. A negative dipstick test for protein does not exclude the presence of low concentrations of globulins, mucoproteins, or Bence-Jones protein in urine.

Sulfosalicylic Acid Test

An alternative method for measuring urine protein by dipstick in the office in patients with questionable proteinuria is the sulfosalicylic acid precipitation of protein in urine. This technique provides a more quantitative estimate of all the proteins present, including both albumin and the low molecular weight proteins. This test is performed by mixing one part urine supernatant with three parts 3% sulfosalicylic acid, with the resultant turbidity graded as shown in Table 10-4.[37] As with the urine dipstick, iodinated radiocontrast agents can cause a false-positive result, hence the urine should not be tested for at least 24 hours after a contrast study.

Quantification of Proteinuria

Results obtained with urine dipstick testing and with quantitative 24-hour protein excretion methods correlate fairly well in most situations. As mentioned previously, the dipstick is sensitive to albumin, whereas quantitative methods detect all kinds of proteins including globulin and low molecular weight protein. For example, in multiple myeloma, large amounts of protein are excreted and yet the urine dipstick for protein is negative. Hence quantitative urinary protein measurement is necessary in such a case.

A more important reason for quantitative measurement of protein loss in urine is to determine whether the patient requires a more extensive evaluation. When sent for quantitative measurement, urine with a dipstick reading of protein 1+ was often found to contain protein within the normal acceptable range.

Quantification of proteinuria has traditionally demanded timed urine collection. Urinary protein excretion in adults is usually measured in a 24-hour urine collection, which is more accurate than spot urine protein analysis. However, 24-hour urine collection poses logistic problems, especially in young children who have yet to achieve continence at night. Timing and volume errors plus the need to correct the protein excretion rate for body surface area make this method inaccurate and cumbersome.

The other method for quantification of proteinuria is to obtain a single voided urine sample. The concentrations of both protein and creatinine are measured in the urine sample and protein levels are expressed per unit of creatinine (U_p/U_{Cr} ratio). The advantages of this method are that timed urine samples and corrections for body size are not required. The assumption is that creatinine excretion is directly related to body mass and is relatively constant throughout the day.

Many studies have found that the amount of protein excreted in a 24-hour urine correlates extremely well with the protein to creatinine ratio measured in random urine samples.[38,39] What remains debatable is whether early-morning urine samples or random samples obtained during normal activities in the day are better in reflecting renal disease. The U_p/U_{Cr} ratio is higher in samples obtained in a person in an upright position than in a recumbent position, a phenomenon known as orthostatic proteinuria.[40] Studies that included subjects with normal renal function and those with renal failure have shown that U_p/U_{Cr} ratios from daytime samples correlate better with 24-hour urine protein excretion values than do values from early-morning samples.[40] On the other hand, early-morning samples had the better correlation when data was evaluated from normal subjects and from those with renal disease that was associated with normal glomerular filtration rates.[41] In subjects with renal disease and orthostatic proteinuria, daytime U_p/U_{Cr} ratios can be misleading. Hence in the evaluation of children with possible renal disease, the first morning urine specimen is recommended for U_p/U_{Cr} ratio quantification in order to eliminate the effect of posture.

Another recommended approach is the use of U_p/U_{Cr} ratio to monitor the progress of proteinuria, with the 24-hour urine collection for protein excretion used for the initial diagnostic investigation except in children who have yet to achieve continence. Sometimes a 12-hour urine collection is done, and the protein excretion rate is then extrapolated to a 24-hour value by using the appropriate correction factor. This is useful in children who have achieved continence in the day but are still enuretic at night.

A recently developed and commercially available novel dipstick, Multistix PRO (Bayer), is able to analyze concentrations of both urinary protein and creatinine semiquantitatively in only 60 seconds. The semiquantitative U_p/U_{Cr} by

TABLE 10-4 **Sulfosalicylic Acid Test**

Grade	Appearance	Protein Concentration (g/L)
0	No turbidity	0
Trace	Slight turbidity	0.01-0.1
1+	Turbidity through which print can be read	0.15-0.3
2+	White cloud without precipitate through which heavy black lines on a white background can be seen	0.4-1
3+	White cloud with precipitate through which heavy black lines cannot be seen	1.5-3.5
4+	Flocculent precipitate	>5

Multistix PRO correlates well with both quantitative U_p/U_{Cr} and daily urinary protein excretion.[42] The Multistix PRO could help in avoiding errors and difficulties associated with timed urine collection and be useful in monitoring urinary protein excretion in children with renal diseases at the outpatient clinic.

Clinical Scenarios

Child with Intermittent Proteinuria

In intermittent proteinuria, protein is detectable in only some of the urine samples from the proteinuric child, which may be related to posture or occur at random. Orthostatic (postural) proteinuria is defined as elevated protein excretion when the subject is upright but normal protein excretion during recumbency. This occurs commonly in adolescents, with a frequency of 2% to 5%. Total urine protein excretion rarely exceeds 1 g/1.73 m^2 per day.

The postulated causes of orthostatic proteinuria are alterations in renal or glomerular hemodynamics, circulating immune complexes, and partial renal vein entrapment.[43] Long-term studies in which patients have been followed for up to 50 years have documented the benign nature of orthostatic proteinuria, although rare cases of glomerulosclerosis have been identified later in life in patients who had an initial diagnosis of orthostatic proteinuria.[44,45]

No treatment is required for children with orthostatic proteinuria. It is important to remember that patients with glomerular disease may have an orthostatic component to their proteinuria. Protein excretion in these patients is greater when they are active or upright than when they are resting. Hence orthostatic proteinuria should not be diagnosed unless the urine collected when the subject is at rest has no detectable protein.

Often, intermittent proteinuria is not related to posture. Instead, it might be found after exercise or in association with stress, dehydration, or fever, or it might occur on a random basis for which there is no obvious cause. A large proportion of healthy children may have occasional urine samples that contain protein in detectable concentrations. Although such proteinuria can be indicative of serious disease of the urinary tract, the majority of observations have shown that intermittent occurrence of protein in the urine as an isolated finding does not indicate the presence of urinary tract disease.

Child with Persistent Proteinuria

Persistent proteinuria is defined as proteinuria of 1+ or more by dipstick measurement on multiple occasions. This is abnormal and should be further investigated. Subjects who have persistent proteinuria, especially in association with additional evidence of renal disease such as microscopic hematuria, are the ones most likely to have significant pathology in the urinary tract. In a Japanese school screening study that included almost 5 million children, the prevalence of persistent isolated proteinuria was 0.07% in the 6-to-11-year age group and rose to 0.37% in 12-to-14-year-olds.[19]

The majority of persistent proteinuria cases are of glomerular origin, though nonglomerular mechanisms can also cause marked proteinuria (Table 10-5). Glomerular proteinuria may be due to the following factors:

- Increase in glomerular permeability to plasma proteins in residual nephrons in cases where there is reduction in nephron mass. This mechanism probably explains the increased proteinuria seen in patients with progressive renal disease reaching end-stage and the increased proteinuria observed in renal transplant donors.[46]

TABLE 10-5 Causes of Proteinuria in Children

	PERSISTENT PROTEINURIA	
Intermittent Proteinuria	**Glomerular**	**Tubular**
Nonpostural	Primary glomerulopathies	Hereditary
Fever	Minimal change disease	Proximal renal tubular acidosis
Exercise	Focal segmental glomerulosclerosis	Cystinosis
Emotional stress	Mesangiocapillary glomerulonephritis	Galactosemia
No known cause	Membranous nephropathy	Tyrosinemia type I
Postural (Orthostatic)	Rapidly progressive glomerulonephritis	Hereditary fructose Intolerance
	Congenital nephrotic syndrome	Wilson disease
	Secondary glomerulonephritis	Lowe syndrome
	Postinfectious glomerulonephritis	Acquired
	Lupus nephritis	Pyelonephritis
	IgA nephropathy	Interstitial nephritis
	Henoch-Schönlein nephritis	Acute tubular necrosis
	Alport syndrome	Analgesic abuse
	Hepatitis B nephropathy	Drugs such as penicillamine
	Hepatitis C nephropathy	Heavy metal poisoning (e.g., lead, cadmium, gold, mercury)
	Human immunodeficiency virus (HIV) nephropathy	Vitamin D intoxication
	Amyloidosis	
	Hemolytic uremic syndrome	
	Diabetes mellitus	
	Hypertension	
	Hyperfiltration following nephron loss	
	Reflux nephropathy	

- Loss of negative charge in the glomerular filtration barrier.[47,48] This mainly results in albuminuria. There is little increase in glomerular permeability to globulins, hence the proteinuria is highly selective. A typical example is minimal change disease.
- Direct injury to the glomerular filtration barrier. The glomerular capillary wall consists of three structural components that form the permselectivity barrier, the endothelial cells, glomerular basement membrane, and podocytes. It is now realized that the podocyte is crucial for maintenance of the glomerular filter, and disruption of the epithelial slit diaphragm finally leads to proteinuria.[49] These changes have been demonstrated in patients with nephrotic syndrome irrespective of the primary disease. Such injury increases the effective pore size in the glomeruli, resulting in an increase in the permeability of the mechanical barriers to the filtration of proteins. Hence there is an increase in filtration of albumin and also the larger proteins such as globulins. Clearance of globulins is relatively high and the proteinuria is described as nonselective.
- Changes in glomerular capillary pressure due to disease and resulting in increased filtration fraction.[29,30,50] Examples are increased filtration fraction in hyperreninemia and hyperfiltration of nephrons in the early stages of diabetic nephropathy. The resulting increased filtered load of protein overwhelms the tubular reabsorptive mechanisms, hence the excess protein appears in the urine.

Glomerular proteinuria can be classified as selective or nonselective. In selective proteinuria, there is a predominance of low molecular weight proteins such as albumin or transferrin as compared with higher molecular weight proteins characterized by IgG. The selectivity index is expressed as the clearance ratio of IgG over albumin or transferrin. An index less than 0.1 is indicative of highly selective proteinuria[51,52] and is seen in steroid-sensitive nephrotic syndrome and Finnish-type congenital nephrotic syndrome. More recent studies have shown a significant relationship between selectivity of proteinuria and tubulointerstitial damage in renal disease.[53] When proteinuria is highly selective, tubulointerstitial damage is less often seen on histology.

Nonglomerular mechanisms include tubular proteinuria, overflow proteinuria, and secretory proteinuria. Tubular proteinuria results when there is damage to the proximal convoluted tubule, which normally reabsorbs most of the filtered protein. The amount of protein in the urine due to tubular damage is usually not large and does not exceed more than 1 g/1.73 m^2 per day. Glomerular and tubular proteinuria can be distinguished by protein electrophoresis of the urine. The primary protein in glomerular proteinuria is albumin, whereas in tubular proteinuria the low molecular weight proteins migrate primarily in the α and β regions. β_2-microglobulin, α_1-microglobulin, and retinol-binding protein are the markers commonly used as the index for tubular proteinuria.[54]

Overflow proteinuria results when the plasma concentration of filterable proteins exceeds the renal threshold for that protein. This can occur even in normal renal function. Examples include monoclonal gammopathy of undetermined significance or multiple myeloma in adults (immunoglobulin light chains or Bence-Jones protein), hemoglobinuria, myoglobinuria, β_2-microglobulinemia, myelomonocytic leukemia, and sometimes following transfusions. After multiple transfusions of either albumin or whole blood, plasma albumin concentration may increase sufficiently to cause albuminuria.

In secretory proteinuria, increased excretion of tissue proteins into the urine can result in proteinuria. A typical example is excretion of Tamm-Horsfall protein in the neonatal period, accounting for the higher levels of protein excretion typically seen at this age. In urinary tract infections, mild proteinuria may be detected upon irritation of the urinary tract and increased secretion of tissue proteins into the urine. Secretory proteinuria also occurs in analgesic nephropathy and inflammation of the accessory sex glands.

Child with Nephrotic Syndrome

Nephrotic syndrome is defined as heavy proteinuria severe enough to cause hypoalbuminemia, edema, and hypercholesterolemia. Nephrotic range proteinuria is defined as greater than 40 mg/m^2 per hour or greater than 3 g/1.73 m^2 per day for timed urine collection, or random urine protein to creatinine ratio of greater than 0.2 g/mmol or 2 mg/mg. The evaluation and management of a child showing nephrotic syndrome are different from that of a child with proteinuria of nonnephrotic range. Nephrotic syndrome is discussed elsewhere in this book.

Clinical Approach to Proteinuria

Findings of proteinuria in single urine specimens in children and adolescents are relatively common. In large-school screening programs, the prevalence of isolated proteinuria on a single urine screen ranged from 1.2% to 15% of children.[21,55,56] Findings of persistent proteinuria on repeated urine testing are much less common. When proteinuria is detected, it is important to determine whether it is transient, orthostatic, or persistent in type. It is also important to exclude acute nephritic or nephrotic syndrome, because these conditions demand urgent investigations and treatment.

History

One should inquire about symptoms of renal failure or glomerulonephritis (edema, hematuria, polyuria, or nocturia), and connective tissue disorders (including rashes and joint pain). A history of recurrent urinary tract infections may suggest reflux nephropathy. Intake of drugs that may be associated with proteinuria, such as nonsteroidal antiinflammatory medications, should also be discussed. Finally, a family history of polycystic kidney disease, renal failure, or deafness should be obtained.

Physical Examination

Examination may reveal evidence of renal failure, such as growth failure, anemia, and renal osteodystrophy. Blood pressure must be measured because hypertension is an important prognostic indicator in chronic kidney disease. Presence of raised jugular venous pressure, hepatomegaly, and edema suggest that the child may be fluid-overloaded because of acute nephritic syndrome or renal impairment, requiring urgent diuresis. Signs of nephrotic syndrome to look for include generalized edema, ascites, pleural effusion, and scrotal edema (in males). Associated signs of systemic illnesses, such as palpable purpuric rash on the lower limbs suggesting Henoch-Schönlein purpura and joint swelling suggesting connective tissue disorders, should be sought. Palpable flank masses may suggest hydronephrosis or polycystic kidney disease.

Investigations

Isolated proteinuria is benign in the vast majority of children and can be transient and postural; hence it is inappropriate to extensively investigate all children found to have proteinuria. A step-by-step approach is recommended to evaluate isolated proteinuria in an asymptomatic child. However, if the child has signs and symptoms that suggest renal disease, a detailed investigation should be started early. Similarly, if the initial urine dipstick test shows the presence of hematuria in addition to proteinuria, a detailed evaluation for renal disease should be performed. Microscopic hematuria is the most common indicator of a glomerular lesion in a proteinuric patient. The existence of hematuria with proteinuria carries a more serious connotation than does proteinuria alone. Investigations including renal biopsy of school children with persistent hematuria and proteinuria have found that 25% to 60% had evidence of a glomerulopathy,[22,57] especially in those with heavy proteinuria greater than 1 g/L.[22]

In an asymptomatic child, the first step is to determine whether the proteinuria is persistent (Figure 10-2). Most children found to have proteinuria on urine dipstick screening do not have renal disease and the proteinuria will resolve on repeat testing.[19] If proteinuria of 1+ or more persists on two subsequent dipstick tests at weekly intervals, further investigations are required. If proteinuria is absent on subsequent testing, the initial proteinuria may be transient and related to fever, severe exercise, or emotional stress, with no further investigations required. The parents and patient should be reassured, and as a precaution, a urine dipstick test for protein can be repeated in 3 to 6 months. If proteinuria on dipstick recurs or is persistent, the next step is to quantify the amount of proteinuria.

The two methods used to quantify proteinuria are spot urine protein to creatinine ratio and 24-hour urinary total protein collection. A spot urine specimen is more convenient to obtain than a 24-hour urine collection. For spot urine protein to creatinine ratio, an early-morning urine specimen is recommended to exclude orthostatic proteinuria. In orthostatic proteinuria, morning samples are negative for protein and evening samples may contain varying concentrations of protein. The 24-hour urinary total protein is normal or mildly elevated. If orthostatic proteinuria is suspected, one way to prove this is to provide the family with urine dipsticks and instruct them to test their child's urine. The child's urine is tested two times a day for 1 week, with the first sample voided in the morning as soon as the child wakes up and the last voided in the evening before the child goes to sleep. It is important for the child to remain supine in bed throughout the night so that the morning sample consists of urine formed in the recumbent position. The evening sample will consist of urine formed in the upright position. If the urine dipstick is persistently negative in the morning and positive in the evening, orthostatic proteinuria is likely. No further investigations are required, and the urine should be rechecked for proteinuria in 1 year as a precaution.

If spot urine protein to creatinine ratio is more than 0.02 g/mmol or 0.2 mg/mg, it is advisable to confirm the presence of significant proteinuria with a 24-hour urinary total protein collection. After excluding transient and orthostatic proteinuria and if the 24-hour urinary total protein is greater than 0.3 g/1.73 m^2 per day, it is useful to evaluate for renal disease. Urinary protein excretion less than 0.3 g/1.73 m^2 per day is associated with regression of proteinuric chronic nephropathies,[58] suggesting that investigations are only necessary above this level. The suggested workup includes the following:

Urine Examination Microscopic examination of the fresh urine sample for blood, casts, and crystals is required. A clean catch urine sample for culture may be necessary to rule out occult urinary tract infection, especially if there is a history of recurrent fevers in infancy.

If a tubular disorder or interstitial nephritis is suggested from the history or urinary findings of eosinophils, measurement of urinary excretion of β_2-microglobulin, α_1-microglobulin, and retinol-binding protein, each a marker of tubular proteinuria, can be helpful. Tubular proteinuria is suspected if the urinary excretion of β_2-microglobulin, α_1-microglobulin, and retinol-binding protein exceeds 0.04, 2.2, and 0.024 mg/mmol creatinine or 4×10^{-4}, 0.022, and 2.4×10^{-4} mg/mg creatinine, respectively.[54]

Blood Examination Renal function with serum urea, creatinine, and electrolytes should be assessed. Creatinine clearance gives a more accurate picture of renal function than serum creatinine alone. A reduction in renal function is one of the most important indications for renal biopsy. Serum total protein and albumin should be checked because most proteinuric patients do not have decreased levels of proteins or albumin in their blood unless they have nephrotic syndrome or have had heavy proteinuria for a significant period. Hypoproteinemia may also be an indication for renal biopsy. In addition, serum cholesterol is measured as an indicator of the presence or absence of hyperlipidemia and nephrotic syndrome.

Serum levels of the third and fourth components of complement (C3 and C4) should be checked routinely because they may provide evidence of glomerulonephritis. Decreased C3 and C4 levels are seen in systemic lupus erythematosus, whereas decreased C3 with normal C4 levels are seen in mesangiocapillary (membranoproliferative) glomerulonephritis and postinfectious glomerulonephritis. ANA, anti-dsDNA antibodies, IgA levels, ASOT or antiDNAse B titers, ANCA, hepatitis B, hepatitis C, and HIV serology should be considered if the clinical setting and preliminary investigations are suggestive, because these may give a clue to the underlying etiology of the proteinuria.

Renal Imaging Renal ultrasonography is performed routinely in the evaluation of proteinuria to identify anatomic abnormalities of the kidneys or urinary tract, because they

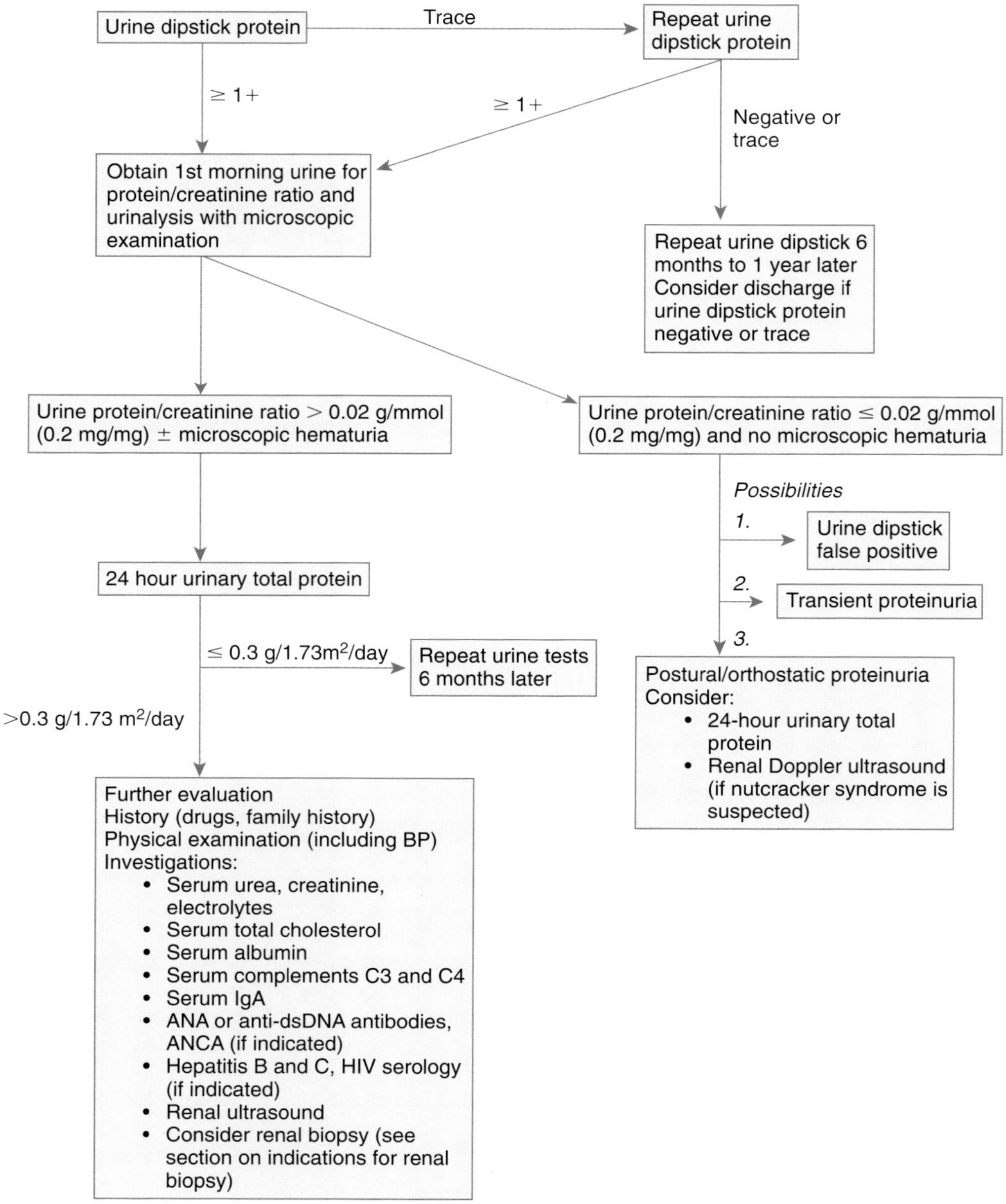

Figure 10-2 Algorithm for investigating proteinuria.

can result in a reduction of nephron mass. A significant difference in the size of kidneys may suggest underlying reflux nephropathy. If reflux nephropathy is suspected, a DMSA scan is useful to demonstrate the existence of renal scars. Renal Doppler sonography is helpful if the patient has coexisting hypertension, because proteinuria can occur in hypertensive nephropathy due to renal artery stenosis. In patients with orthostatic proteinuria, Doppler sonography of the left renal vein may be a useful screening tool for excluding the nutcracker syndrome.[59]

Audiometry Audiometry is indicated when there is a family history of nephritis, renal failure, or deafness. Deafness may be detected during later childhood in Alport syndrome and is generally associated with progressive renal disease.

If these urine and blood tests, as well as the initial renal ultrasound, are normal, and if the proteinuria is less than 1 g/1.73 m^2 per day, it is unlikely that the child has a serious renal disease. The family should therefore be reassured that the proteinuria may disappear or may persist without evidence of progressive renal failure ever developing. As the level of proteinuria is associated with outcome in chronic nephropathies,[29,58,60] it is also important to emphasize to the family that follow-up urine tests are necessary. The child should be reviewed within 3 to 6 months. If the repeat proteinuria is not significant (i.e., <1 g/1.73 m^2/day), the child's urine is then monitored twice during the subsequent year and yearly thereafter. If there is persistent significant proteinuria on follow-up, a renal biopsy may be indicated.

Indications for Renal Biopsy

Renal biopsy is indicated in the following situations:

- Persistent significant proteinuria of more than 1 g/1.73 m^2 per day. The heavier the proteinuria, the more likely a tissue diagnosis will be obtained from the renal biopsy. The exception here is the child who demonstrates typical steroid sensitive nephrotic syndrome suggestive of minimal change disease where renal biopsy is not indicated at presentation.
- Proteinuria associated with urinary sediment abnormalities. Renal biopsy is more likely to be diagnostic when proteinuria is associated with urinary sediment abnormalities than when either proteinuria or hematuria are isolated abnormalities.
- Decreased glomerular filtration rate (GFR). A GFR of less than 80 ml/1.73 m^2/min is an indication for renal biopsy. The exception is a child recovering from an acute glomerulonephritis (e.g., postinfectious glomerulonephritis). In this case the GFR should be remeasured in a month, and if the GFR remains low, a renal biopsy is required.
- Persistent low C3 levels of more than 3 months. Low C3 level during the acute phase of postinfectious glomerulonephritis is not an indication for biopsy. If the C3 level remains low after 3 months, a renal biopsy is indicated.
- Evidence of a collagen vascular disease or vasculitis (such as systemic lupus erythematosus, Henoch-Schönlein purpura, or ANCA-positive vasculitis) either clinically or serologically.

Treatment Options for Significant Proteinuria in the Nonnephrotic Range

It is recognized that glomerular proteinuria may well play a role in the progression of kidney disease.[61] Proteinuria has also been identified as a risk factor for cardiovascular disease in adults and children.[32-34] Moreover, as the severity of proteinuria increases, it is associated with metabolic disturbances such as hypercholesterolemia, hypertriglyceridemia, and hypercoagulability, all of which contribute to cardiovascular disease. The question is whether proteinuria results in decreased levels of plasma proteins. The liver has considerable reserve capacity for increased production of new proteins and can often compensate for urinary losses. Only when proteinuria is heavy and chronic, exceeding the patient's ability to make new protein, might hypoproteinemia ensue such as in nephrotic syndrome.

The following are postulated mechanisms whereby proteinuria may induce renal injury:[36]

- Filtration of lipoproteins and absorption by proximal tubules may activate inflammatory pathways, causing cell injury
- Filtration of cytokines or chemokines may provoke cell proliferation, inflammatory cell infiltration, and activation of infiltrating cells
- Filtration or generation of novel antigens may function as antigen-presenting cells and initiate a cellular immune response
- Iron that is filtered into tubular fluid and bound to transferrin may be directly toxic or have indirect effects due to iron-catalyzed synthesis of reactive oxygen metabolites
- Activation of the alternative complement pathway by proximal tubules may be harmful
- Release of lysosomal enzymes into the cytoplasm of protein-reabsorbing tubules may cause damage
- Release of vasoconstricting molecules may cause ischemic tubular injury
- Interstitial fibrosis may result from the release of fibrosis-promoting factors from renal cells activated or injured by proteinuria
- The proteinaceous casts can obstruct renal tubules

Persistent significant proteinuria should be regarded seriously. Besides finding the exact cause and targeting specific therapy if possible, other treatment options include dietary protein recommendations and use of antiproteinuric medications.

Dietary Protein Recommendations

Dietary protein restrictions have been proposed in adults with chronic kidney disease to stabilize renal function.[58,62] In a small series of children with chronic renal insufficiency, some benefit from dietary protein restriction has been described.[63] However, another controlled study did not demonstrate a significant impact from protein restriction on the rate of progression in children.[31] High dietary protein intake may indeed worsen proteinuria in some patients with nephrotic syndrome. Moreover, it does not result in a higher serum albumin. Hence it is best to avoid excess dietary protein in children with proteinuric renal diseases and to provide them with the recommended daily allowance of protein for their age.[64]

Drugs with Antiproteinuric Effects

Certain classes of antihypertensive agents such as angiotensin converting enzyme inhibitors (ACEIs) and angiotensin II receptor blockers (ARBs) can reduce systemic blood pressure and provide other beneficial effects that include decreasing urinary protein excretion and the risk of renal fibrosis. In addition, renal function is better preserved in children with chronic kidney disease when lower systolic blood pressures are achieved.[65] However, the long-term benefits of ACEIs and ARBs in children and adolescents with proteinuria remain to be established. There are reports of infants born to mothers taking ACEIs during the second and third trimesters of pregnancy who developed oligohydramnios, pulmonary hypoplasia, and postnatal hypertension. Postmortem examination of these neonates showed severe glomerular and tubular malformations in the kidneys. Hence ACEIs are contraindicated during pregnancy.[66] In young infants, the safety of ACEIs and ARBs is still unknown.

Conclusion

Although investigations have been recommended in the workup for a child who shows hematuria or proteinuria, many of the cases result in normal, transient findings. Hence a stepwise evaluation is recommended to avoid unnecessary and expensive investigations and yet not miss serious conditions. Early detection and treatment of serious conditions would hopefully delay or prevent the onset of renal insufficiency. However, whereas screening programs may be able to identify hematuria and proteinuria at an early stage, the major disadvantages are cost, as well as the anxiety that may be created in parents and children where the findings are spurious or transient.

REFERENCES

1. Vehaskari VM, Rapola J, Koskimies O, Savilahti E, Vilska J, Hallman N: Microscopic hematuria in schoolchildren: epidemiology and clinicopathologic evaluation, *J Pediatr* 95:676-84, 1979.
2. Shaw ST, Jr, Poon SY, Wong ET: Routine urinalysis: is the dipstick enough? *JAMA* 253:1596-1600, 1985.
3. Dodge WF: Cost effectiveness of renal disease screening, *Am J Dis Child* 131:1274-80, 1977.
4. Fairley KF, Birch DF: Microscopic urinalysis in glomerulonephritis, *Kidney Int Suppl* 42:S9-S12, 1993.
5. Pollock C, Pei-Ling L, Győry AZ, Grigg R, Gallery ED et al: Dysmorphism of urinary red blood cells—value in diagnosis, *Kidney Int* 36:1045-49, 1989.
6. Schramek P, Moritsch A, Haschkowitz H, Binder BR, Maier M: In vitro generation of dysmorphic erythocytes, *Kidney Int* 36:72-77, 1989.
7. Shichiri M, Hosoda K, Nishio Y, Ogura M, Suenaga M et al: Red-cell-volume distribution curves in diagnosis of glomerular and non-glomerular hematuria, *Lancet* 1:908-11, 1988.
8. Pham PT, Pham PC, Wilkinson AH, Lew SQ: Renal abnormalities in sickle cell anemia, *Kidney Int* 57:1-8, 2000.
9. Hohenfellner M, Steinbach F, Schultz-Lampel D, Lampel A, Steinbach F et al: The nutcracker syndrome: new aspects of pathophysiology, diagnosis and treatment, *J Urol* 146:685-88, 1991.
10. Okada M, Tsuzuki K, Ito S: Diagnosis of the nutcracker phenomenon using two-dimensional ultrasonography, *Clin Nephrol* 49:35-40, 1998.
11. Tanaka H, Waga S: Spontaneous remission of persistent severe hematuria in an adolescent with nutcracker syndrome: seven years' observation, *Clin Exp Nephrol* 8:68-70, 2004.
12. Mufson MA, Belshe RB, Horrigan TJ, Zollar LM: Causes of acute hemorrhagic cystitis in children, *Am J Dis Child* 126:605-09, 1973.
13. Summer AP, Stauffer W, Maroushek SR, Nevins TE: Hematuria in children due to schistosomiasis in a nonendemic setting, *Clin Pediatr (Philadelphia)* 45:177-81, 2006.
14. Altintepe L, Tonbul HZ, Ozbey I, Guney I, Odabas AR, et al: Urinary tuberculosis: ten years' experience, *Ren Fail* 27:657-61, 2005.
15. Polinsky MS, Kaiser BA, Baluarte HJ, Gruskin AB: Renal stones and hypercalciuria, *Adv Pediatr* 40:353-84, 1993.
16. Stapleton FB, Roy S III, Noe HN, Jerkins G: Hypercalciuria in children with hematuria, *N Engl J Med* 310:1345-48, 1984.
17. Shaw NJ, Wheeldon J, Brocklehurst JT: Indices of intact serum parathyroid hormone and renal excretion of calcium, phosphate and magnesium, *Arch Dis Child* 65:1208-12, 1990.
18. Diven SC, Travis LB: A practical primary care approach to hematuria in children, *Pediatr Nephrol* 14:65-72, 2000.
19. Murakami M, Yamamoto H, Ueda Y, Murakami K, Yamauchi K: Urinary screening of elementary and junior high-school children over a 13-year period in Tokyo, *Pediatr Nephrol* 5:50-53, 1991.
20. Zainal D, Baba A, Mustaffa BE: Screening proteinuria and haematuria in Malaysian children, *Southeast Asian J Trop Med Public Health* 26:785-88, 1995.
21. Yap HK, Quek CM, Shen Q, Joshi V, Chia KS: Role of urinary screening programmes in children in the prevention of chronic kidney disease, *Ann Acad Med Singapore* 34:3-7, 2005.
22. Lin CY, Hsieh CC, Chen WP, Yang LY, Wang HH: The underlying diseases and follow-up in Taiwanese children screened by urinalysis, *Pediatr Nephrol* 16:232-37, 2001.
23. Cho BS, Kim SD, Choi YM, Kang HH: School urinalysis screening in Korea: prevalence of chronic renal disease, *Pediatr Nephrol* 16:1126-28, 2001.
24. Köhler H, Wandel E, Brunck B: Acanthocyturia—a characteristic marker for glomerular bleeding, *Kidney Int* 40:115-20, 1991.
25. Yoshikawa N, Iijima K, Ito H: IgA nephropathy in children, *Nephron* 83:1-12, 1999.
26. Coppo R, Gianoglio B, Porcellini G, Maringhini S: Frequency of renal diseases and clinical indication for renal biopsy in children (Report of the Italian National Registry of renal biopsies in children), *Nephrol Dial Transplant* 13:293-97, 1998.
27. Feld LG, Meyers KE, Kaplan BS, Bruder Stapleton F: Limited evaluation of microscopic hematuria in pediatrics, *Pediatrics* 102:E42, 1998.
28. Cameron JS: Proteinuria and progression in human glomerular diseases, *Am J Nephrol* 10:81-87, 1990.
29. Ruggenenti P, Perna A, Mosconi L, Pisoni R, Remuzzi G: Urinary protein excretion rate is the best independent predictor of ESRF in non-diabetic proteinuric chronic nephropathies, *Kidney Int* 53:1209-16, 1998.
30. Remuzzi G, Ruggenenti P, Benigni A: Understanding the nature of renal disease progression, *Kidney Int* 51:2-15, 1997.
31. Wingen AM, Fabian-Bach C, Schaefer F, Mehls O. Randomised, multicentre study of a low-protein diet on the progression of renal failure in children, *Lancet* 349:1117-23, 1997.
32. Grimm RH, Svendsen KH, Kasiske B, Keane WF, Wahi MM: Proteinuria is a risk factor for mortality over 10 years of follow-up: MRFIT Research Group, Multiple Risk Factor Intervention Trial, *Kidney Int Suppl* 63:S10-S14, 1997.
33. Kannel WB, Stampfer MJ, Castelli WP, Verter J: The prognostic significance of proteinuria: the Framingham Study, *Am Heart J* 108:1347-52, 1984.
34. Portman RJ, Hawkins E, Verani R: Premature atherosclerosis in pediatric renal patients: report of the Southwest Pediatric Nephrology Study Group, *Pediatr Res* 29:349A, 1991.
35. Kumar S, Muchmore A: Tamm-Horsfall protein-uromodulin (1950-1990), *Kidney Int* 37:1395-401, 1990.
36. Hogg RJ, Portman RJ, Milliner D, Lemley KV, Eddy A, Ingelfinger J: Evaluation and management of proteinuria and nephrotic syndrome in children: recommendations from a pediatric nephrology panel established at the National Kidney Foundation Conference on Proteinuria, Albuminuria, Risk, Assessment, Detection, and Elimination (PARADE), *Pediatrics* 105:1242-49, 2000.
37. Rose BD: *Pathophysiology of renal disease,* ed 2, New York, 1987, McGraw-Hill.
38. Elises JS, Griffiths PD, Hocking MD, Taylor CM, White RH: Simplified quantification of urinary protein excretion in children, *Clin Nephrol* 30:225-29, 1998.
39. Ginsberg JM, Chang BS, Matarese RA, Garella S: Use of single voided urine samples to estimate quantitative proteinuria, *N Engl J Med* 309:1543-46, 1983.
40. Houser MT, Jahn MF, Kobayashi A, Walburn J: Assessment of urinary protein excretion in the adolescent: effect of body position and exercise, *J Pediatr* 109:556-61, 1986.
41. Yoshimoto M, Tsukahara H, Saito M, Hayashi S, Haruki S et al: Evaluation of variability of proteinuria indices, *Pediatr Nephrol* 4:136-39, 1990.
42. Kaneko K, Someya T, Nishizaki N, Shimojima T, Ohtaki R, Kaneko KI: Simplified quantification of urinary protein excretion using a novel dipstick in children, *Pediatr Nephrol* 20:834-36, 2005.
43. Vehaskari VM: Mechanism of orthostatic proteinuria, *Pediatr Nephrol* 4:328-30, 1990.
44. Berns JS, McDonald B, Gaudio KM, Siegel NJ: Progression of orthostatic proteinuria to focal and segmental glomerulosclerosis, *Clin Pediatr* 25:165-66, 1986.

45. Springberg PD, Garrett LE Jr, Thompson AL Jr, Collins NF, Lordon RE, Robinson RR: Fixed and reproducible orthostatic proteinuria: results of a 20-year follow-up study, *Ann Intern Med* 97:516-19, 1982.
46. Rizvi SA, Naqvi SA, Jawad F, Ahmed E, Asghar A: Living kidney donor follow-up in a dedicated clinic, *Transplantation* 79:1247-51, 2005.
47. Chang RL, Deen WM, Robertson CR, Brenner BM: Permselectivity of the glomerular capillary wall: III. Restricted transport of polyanions, *Kidney Int* 8:212-18, 1975.
48. Takahashi S, Watanabe S, Wada N, Murakami H, Funaki S et al: Charge selective function in childhood glomerular diseases, *Pediatr Res* 59:336-40, 2006.
49. Kriz W, Kretzler M, Provoost AP, Shirato I: Stability and leakiness: opposing challenges to the glomerulus, *Kidney Int* 49:1570-74, 1996.
50. Ruggenenti P, Remuzzi G: The role of protein traffic in the progression of renal diseases, *Annu Rev Med* 51:315-27, 2000.
51. Joachim GR, Cameron JS, Schwartz M, Becker EL: Selectivity of protein excretion in patients with the nephrotic sydnrome, *J Clin Invest* 43:2332-46, 1964.
52. Cameron JS, White RHR: Selectivity of proteinuria in children with the nephrotic syndrome, *Lancet* 1:463-68, 1965.
53. Bazzi C, Petrini C, Rizza V, Arrigo G, D'Amico GA: Modern approach to selectivity of proteinuria and tubulointerstitial damage in nephrotic syndrome, *Kidney Int* 58:1732-41, 2000.
54. Bergon E, Granados R, Fernandez-Segoviano P, Miravalles E, Bergon M: Classification of renal proteinuria: a simple algorithm, *Clin Chem Lab Med* 40:1143-50, 2002.
55. Dodge WF, West EF, Smith EH, Bunce H III: Proteinuria and hematuria in school-age children: epidemiology and early natural history, *J Pediatr* 88:327-47, 1976.
56. Vehaskari VM, Rapola J: Isolated proteinuria: analysis of a school-age population, *J Pediatr* 101:661-68, 1982.
57. Hisano S, Ueda K: Asymptomatic hematuria and proteinuria: renal pathology and clinical outcome in 54 children, *Pediatr Nephrol* 3:229-34, 1989.
58. Ruggenenti P, Schieppati A, Remuzzi G: Progression, remission, regression of chronic renal diseases, *Lancet* 357:1601-08, 2001.
59. Park SJ, Lim JW, Cho BS, Yoon TY, Oh JH: Nutcracker syndrome in children with orthostatic proteinuria: diagnosis on the basis of Doppler sonography, *J Ultrasound Med* 21:39-45, 2002.
60. Perna A, Remuzzi G: Abnormal permeability to proteins and glomerular lesions: a meta-analysis of experimental and human studies, *Am J Kidney Dis* 27:34-41, 1996.
61. Williams JD, Coles GA: Proteinuria—a direct cause of renal morbidity, *Kidney Int* 45:443-50, 1994.
62. Kasiske BL, Lakatua JD, Ma JZ, Louis TA: A meta-analysis of the effects of dietary protein restriction on the rate of decline in renal function, *Am J Kidney Dis* 31:954-61, 1998.
63. Jureidini KF, Hogg RJ, van Renen MJ, Southwood TR, Henning PH: Evaluation of long-term aggressive dietary management of chronic renal failure in children, *Pediatr Nephrol* 4:1-10, 1990.
64. Uauy RD, Hogg RJ, Brewer ED, Reisch JS, Cunningham C, Holliday MA: Dietary protein and growth in infants with chronic renal insufficiency: a report from the Southwest Pediatric Nephrology Study Group and the University of California, San Francisco, *Pediatr Nephrol* 8:45-50, 1994.
65. Ellis D, Vats A, Moritz ML, Reitz S, Grosso MJ, Janosky JE: Long-term antiproteinuric and renoprotective efficacy and safety of losartan in children with proteinuria, *J Pediatr* 143:89-97, 2003.
66. Tabacova S: Mode of action: angiotensin-converting enzyme inhibition—developmental effects associated with exposure to ACE inhibitors, *Crit Rev Toxicol* 35:747-55, 2005.

CHAPTER

11 Nephritic Syndrome

Patrick Niaudet

Nephritic syndrome is a clinical syndrome defined by the association of hematuria, proteinuria, and often arterial hypertension and renal failure. Nephritic syndrome is due to glomerular injury with glomerular inflammation. Clinical presentations of nephritic syndrome include acute nephritic syndrome, syndrome of rapidly progressive glomerulonephritis, syndrome of recurrent macroscopic hematuria, and syndrome of chronic glomerulonephritis. Each presentation can be associated with several types of glomerulonephritis. Clinical presentation, family history, presence of extrarenal symptoms, results of immunologic tests, and renal histology most often identify the underlying disease. Patients with rapidly progressive glomerulonephritis need urgent histologic diagnosis and treatment to prevent irreversible renal damage.

CLASSIFICATION OF GLOMERULONEPHRITIS

Glomerulonephritis can be classified on histopathologic grounds. By light microscopy, there is no histologic lesion specific of a particular disease. The same morphologic appearance may have different clinical presentations. Whether the glomerulonephritis is primary or secondary to a systemic disease, there is always a good correlation between the histologic lesions and the prognosis. With the exception of acute poststreptococcal glomerulonephritis, this is one reason why renal biopsy is so important in a patient with glomerulonephritis.

According to the absence or presence of proliferative lesions, several disorders may be described. Membranous glomerulonephritis is the most frequent form of glomerulonephritis without cellular proliferation. It is characterized by a diffuse thickening of the glomerular basement membrane (GBM) due to the presence of deposits on the epithelial side of the GBM. These deposits are separated by spike projections of the basement membrane. There are three main types of proliferative glomerulonephritis. Endocapillary proliferative glomerulonephritis (or mesangial proliferative glomerulonephritis) is characterized by endocapillary cell proliferation without alteration of the GBM. The proliferation mainly involves mesangial cells with an increase of mesangial matrix. In addition to mesangial cell proliferation, in some cases endothelial cells may proliferate and circulating polymorphonuclear cells, as well as monocytes and macrophages, may be present. This is characteristic of acute poststreptococcal glomerulonephritis. The second type is membranoproliferative glomerulonephritis (MPGN). In addition to endocapillary cell proliferation, there is a diffuse thickening of the GBM due to the interposition of mesangial matrix between the basement membrane and the endothelial cells. By electron microscopy these two types can be described as type I with subendothelial deposits and type II with dense deposits inside the basement membrane. The third type of proliferative glomerulonephritis is endocapillary and extracapillary glomerulonephritis, where endocapillary cell proliferation is accompanied by extracapillary cell proliferation or crescents.

Immunofluorescence examination is most important for the study of glomerulonephritis. Several types of deposits may be present according to their appearance, their location, and their composition (Table 11-1). There are two types of glomerulonephritis that can only be diagnosed by immunofluorescence examination. The first is anti-GBM glomerulonephritis with linear deposits of IgG along the glomerular basement membrane. By light microscopy, the lesions most often consist of necrotizing and crescentic glomerulonephritis. The second type is IgA nephropathy with the presence of granular deposits in the mesangium that contain mainly IgA but also frequently IgG and C3. The same appearance is observed in Henoch-Schönlein purpura nephritis. By light microscopy, there are several features that define the severity of endocapillary and extracapillary cell proliferation.

In other types of glomerulonephritis, immunofluorescence examination is also helpful to define disease. The presence of humps that contain C3 on the external side of the GBM is characteristic of postinfectious glomerulonephritis. Membranous glomerulonephritis is characterized by the presence of granular deposits on the external side of the GBM that contain mainly IgG. In membranoproliferative glomerulonephritis type I, C3 deposits are found along the GBM and in the mesangial areas, often in association with IgG deposits. Voluminous deposits that only contain C3 are present in the mesangium of patients with MPGN type II. Table 11-2 shows the main types of glomerulonephritis.

ACUTE NEPHRITIC SYNDROME

The onset of acute nephritic syndrome may be sudden, with fever, headache, and abdominal pain, or more progressive, with peripheral edema, weight gain, and asthenia. Peripheral

TABLE 11-1 Immunofluorescence Microscopy in Glomerulonephritis

Deposits	Deposits	Location	Main protein	Disease
Linear	Continuous	GBM	IgG	Anti-GBM disease
Granular	Disseminated	Extramembranous	C3	Postinfectious GN
Granular	Contiguous	Extramembranous	IgG	Membranous GN
Granular	Irregular	Endomembranous	C3	MPGN type I
Granular	Nodular	Mesangial	C3	MPGN type II
Granular	Arborized pattern	Mesangial	IgA	IgA nephropathy
Granular	Irregular	Mesangial and peripheral	IgG, IgA, IgM, C3	SLE

TABLE 11-2 Classification of Glomerulonephritis

Primary glomerulonephritis	Membranous glomerulonephritis Membranoproliferative glomerulonephritis type I Membranoproliferative glomerulonephritis type II (dense deposit disease) IgA nephropathy Anti-GBM disease Idiopathic crescentic glomerulonephritis
Secondary glomerulonephritis	Poststreptococcal glomerulonephritis Other infections Henoch-Schönlein purpura Systemic lupus erythematosus Microscopic polyangiitis Wegener granulomatosus Churg-Strauss syndrome Cryoglobulinemia Rheumatic fever

edema is often moderate but may be more pronounced with anasarca. Edema and systemic hypertension are secondary to extracellular volume expansion, including vascular volume expansion. Pulmonary or cerebral oedema may complicate acute nephritic syndrome. Hypertension is often severe and may be responsible for hypertensive encephalopathy with headaches, seizures, coma, and blindness. Congestive heart failure may develop due to fluid retention and hypertension, in which case echocardiography should be performed. Oliguria is accompanied by brown urine. Proteinuria is often prominent, more than 2 g per day, and nonselective. Hematuria is constant, either microscopic or macroscopic, and higher than 200.000 per minute. There are red blood cell casts and dysmorphic red blood cells, typical of their glomerular origin. Renal blood flow and glomerular filtration rate fall, resulting in a moderate or severe increase in serum creatinine that usually normalizes within a few days.

Sometimes the clinical presentation is atypical. For instance, when patients present with oligoanuria, the differential diagnosis from acute tubular necrosis is not obvious. The diagnosis may be suspected because the patient is hypertensive and has peripheral edema, and because hematuria preceded renal failure. Renal histology shows the glomerular lesions. Other patients may have isolated macroscopic hematuria, isolated proteinuria, or isolated hypertension.

TABLE 11-3 Investigations in a Child with Acute Nephritic Syndrome or Rapidly Progressive Glomerulonephritis

Complement levels (CH50, C3, C4)
Antistreptolysin O, anti-DNAse B, antistreptokinase, anti-NADase, antihyaluronidase antibodies
IgA
Antinuclear antibodies, anti-DNA antibodies
ANCA
Anti-GBM antibodies
Serology for EBV and hepatitis B and C
Renal biopsy with light microscopy and immunofluorescence

The pathologic correlate of acute nephritic syndrome is proliferative glomerulonephritis. Proliferation is initially due to the presence of neutrophils and monocytes and later to an increase in resident glomerular cells, namely endothelial cells and mesangial cells. This inflammation may involve most glomeruli (diffuse proliferative glomerulonephritis) or may be less extensive (focal proliferative glomerulonephritis).[1]

Clinical, biologic, and histologic evaluations are necessary to identify the precise glomerular disease, and early diagnosis is important because many of the disorders respond to therapy. The clinical history and physical examination may provide evidence of a systemic disease. A recent skin or throat infection suggest poststreptococcal glomerulonephritis, whereas a facial rash and arthritis favor systemic lupus erythematosus. Laboratory investigations are also needed and can be extensive (Table 11-3). Serum complement measurement, including total hemolytic complement and C3, provides useful information for classification and follow-up of acute nephritic syndrome.

Renal biopsy is often required, and immunofluorescence microscopy examination is particularly helpful in that it may show granular deposits of immunoglobulins that define immune-complex glomerulonephritis. Linear deposition of immunoglobulins along the glomerular basement membrane is characteristic of anti-GBM disease. The absence of significant deposits of immunoglobulins defines a pauci-immune glomerulonephritis (Figure 11-1).

Most often, at least in children, acute nephritic syndrome is secondary to acute postinfectious glomerulonephritis. Acute nephritic syndrome may also be secondary to a primary

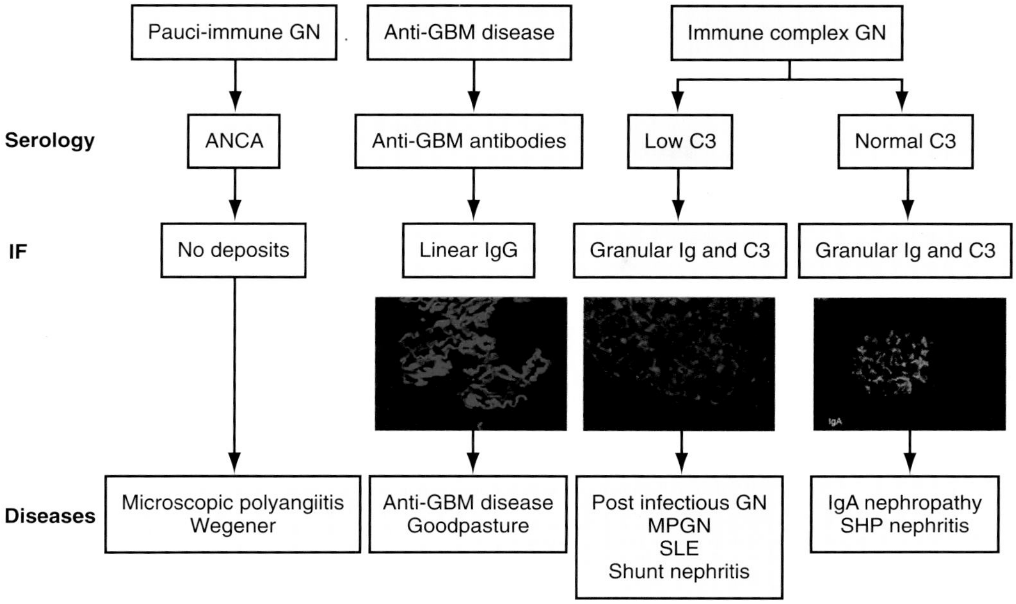

Figure 11-1 Evaluation and diagnosis of acute nephritic syndrome.

TABLE 11-4 Causes of Nephritic Syndrome in Children

Primary renal diseases	IgA nephropathy Membranoproliferative glomerulonephritis type I or type II Anti-GBM disease Idiopathic crescentic glomerulonephritis
Secondary renal diseases	Postinfectious glomerulonephritis (poststreptococcal, endocarditis, shunt nephritis) Henoch-Schönlein purpura nephritis Systemic lupus erythematosus Wegener's granulomatosis Microscopic polyangiitis

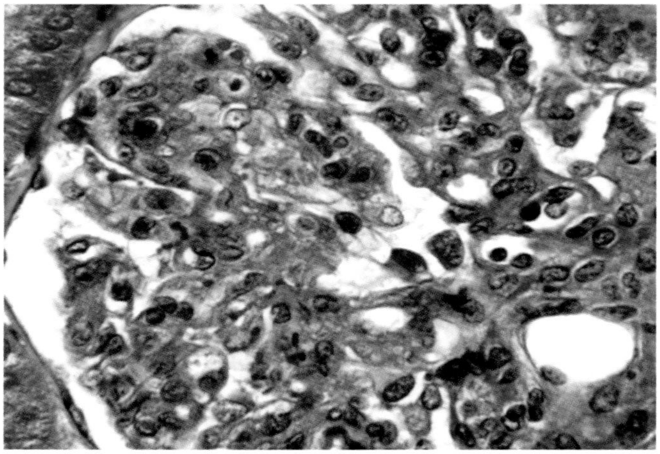

Figure 11-2 Poststreptococcal glomerulonephritis. Endocapillary proliferation and numerous red (fibrinous) extramembranous deposits (humps).

glomerulonephritis such as IgA nephropathy, anti-GBM disease, MPGN, or pauci-immune glomerulonephritis. Sometimes extrarenal symptoms indicate a secondary glomerulonephritis, such as Henoch-Schönlein purpura nephritis or lupus nephritis (Table 11-4).

The main cause of acute nephritic syndrome is acute postinfectious glomerulonephritis, which usually follows a streptococcal infection.[2] It occurs most often after an upper respiratory tract or a skin infection with a nephritogenic strain of group A2 β-hemolytic streptococcus. In a child with acute nephritic syndrome, several features suggest a diagnosis of acute poststreptococcal glomerulonephritis: a throat or skin infection in previous weeks, an increase in the antistreptolysin O and anti-DNAse antibody titers, and a marked but transient reduction of C3 and C4. The diagnosis is usually made on clinical and serologic grounds. When a renal biopsy is performed, it shows a diffuse endocapillary proliferative glomerulonephritis with numerous polynuclear cells and the presence of humps on the external side of the GBM (Figure 11-2). In most cases the prognosis is good, with complete recovery. Early complications include hypertensive encephalopathy, cardiac failure, and pulmonary edema where there is fluid overload. Except in rare cases with extensive crescent formation, serum creatinine is moderately elevated and normalizes within a few days, whereas proteinuria disappears within a few days or weeks and hematuria may last longer. Complement returns to normal within 6 to 8 weeks. In children, a renal biopsy is indicated if the infectious context is not obvious, the child presents with extrarenal symptoms, renal failure persists for more than 10 days, C3 remains low for more than 2 months, and proteinuria does not disappear after 3 to 6 months. Other infectious agents (bacterial, viral,

TABLE 11-5 Acute Glomerulonephritis and Infections

Bacterial infections	Skin or throat (*Streptococcus* group A) Endocarditis (*Staphylococcus aureus, Streptococcus viridans*) Visceral abscess (*S. aureus, Escherichia coli, Pseudomonas, Proteus mirabilis*) Shunt nephritis (*S. aureus, Staphylococcus albus, S. viridans*) Pneumonia (*Diplococcus pneumoniae, Mycoplasma*) Typhoid fever (*Salmonella typhi*)
Viral infections	Epstein-Barr virus Parvovirus B19 Varicella CMV Coxsackie Rubella Mumps Hepatitis B
Parasitic infections	*Schistosoma mansoni* *Plasmodium falciparum* *Toxoplasma gondii* *Filaria*

fungal, or parasitic) may also trigger the development of acute glomerulonephritis (Table 11-5).

Acute nephritic syndrome may be secondary to MPGN.[3] Indeed, the clinical presentation of MPGN may mimic acute postinfectious glomerulonephritis and may show following an infection. However, with MPGN, proteinuria persists, as well as a low C3. The C3 and C4 levels are decreased in MPGN type I due to the activation of both complement pathways. In MPGN type II or dense deposit disease, C3 is low but C4 is not decreased because only the alternative pathway of complement activation is involved. An IgG autoantibody (C3 nephritic factor) that binds to the C3 convertase and promotes permanent activation of the alternative pathway is present in most cases.

Few patients with IgA nephropathy present with acute nephritic syndrome. Acute nephritic syndrome may also be observed in children with anti-GBM disease and in children with vasculitis associated with ANCA, although a clinical presentation of rapidly progressive glomerulonephritis is more frequent (see later).

Acute nephritic syndrome may occur in patients with systemic disease such as Henoch-Schönlein purpura or systemic lupus erythematosus. The clinical manifestations of Henoch-Schönlein purpura include a classic tetrad of rash, arthralgias, abdominal pain, and renal disease that can occur in any order and at any time over several days to several weeks. Renal disease is usually noted within a few days to 4 weeks after the onset of systemic symptoms.[4] Urinalysis in affected patients reveals mild proteinuria with an active sediment characterized by microscopic (or macroscopic) hematuria with red cell and other cellular casts. Most patients have relatively mild disease characterized by asymptomatic hematuria and proteinuria with a normal or only slightly elevated plasma creatinine concentration. However, more marked findings may occur, including nephrotic syndrome, hypertension, and acute renal failure. On renal biopsy, the disease is characterized by the diffuse presence of granular deposits that always contain predominant IgA localized within the mesangium. By light microscopy, four patterns may be described: mesangiopathic glomerulonephritis, focal and segmental glomerulonephritis, diffuse proliferative endocapillary glomerulonephritis, and endocapillary and extracapillary glomerulonephritis.

Clinical symptoms and signs of renal involvement, which usually appear during the first years, are noted in 40% to 80% of patients with systemic lupus erythematosus.[5] Proteinuria is the most frequent abnormality. It may be moderate, but more often it is abundant when accompanied by nephrotic syndrome. Microscopic hematuria is mostly associated with proteinuria. The urinary sediment contains granular casts, often with red cells. Patients with severe nephritis are often hypertensive and have reduced renal function with an increased plasma creatinine. This occurs in up to 50% of children with lupus nephritis. Anti-double-stranded DNA antibodies are more specific to systemic lupus erythematosus (SLE) than are antinuclear antibodies. Hypocomplementemia is observed in 75% of cases at presentation. Decreased levels of CH50, C1q, and C4 are related to the activation of the classical pathway of the complement system. Renal biopsy in patients with acute nephritic syndrome commonly shows class III or class IV nephropathy (focal proliferative glomerulonephritis or diffuse proliferative glomerulonephritis) with immune deposits where IgG, mainly IgG1 and IgG3, is dominant. IgA and IgM are also present, as well as early complement components C1q and C4, along with C3. Such positivity for the three Ig classes and C1q, C4, and C3 is called *full house* and is only found in lupus nephritis. Fibrin deposits are also found, particularly in class IV biopsies.

SYNDROME OF RAPIDLY PROGRESSIVE GLOMERULONEPHRITIS

The syndrome of rapidly progressive glomerulonephritis is characterized by a subacute nephritic syndrome with deterioration of renal function.[6] Patients often have macroscopic hematuria with red blood cell casts and heavy proteinuria with nephrotic syndrome and edema. Hypertension may be less pronounced than in patients with acute nephritic syndrome. Renal failure persists, and patients may develop oligoanuria within a few days. The same biologic tests as for acute nephritic syndrome should be performed, including detection of anti-GBM antibodies, ANCA, anti-DNA antibodies, and measurement of complement fractions. Renal biopsy should be performed quickly.

The pathologic correlate of rapidly progressive glomerulonephritis is crescentic glomerulonephritis, where extracapillary proliferation involves the majority of glomeruli. The crescents are composed of monocytes and parietal epithelial cells that proliferate in the Bowman's space (Figure 11-3). Crescents may be segmental or circumferential and are initially cellular but may rapidly progress to fibrosis. The prognosis is related to the proportion of crescents, their extent (segmental or circumferential), and their content (cellular, fibrocellular, or fibrous). An immediate diagnosis and prompt treatment are necessary to prevent development of irreversible renal failure.

Rapidly progressive glomerulonephritis can occur as a primary renal disease without any sign of systemic disease. The classification is based on the results of immunofluorescence microscopy that shows the presence or absence of immune deposits. Linear deposition of IgG along the glomerular basement membrane is characteristic of anti-GBM disease. Granular deposits are observed in different primary glomerular diseases where crescents are superimposed, such as MPGN, IgA nephropathy, and membranous nephropathy. Some cases do not show immune deposits and are referred to as pauci-immune glomerulonephritis. These cases are frequently associated with antineutrophil cytoplasmic antibodies.[7]

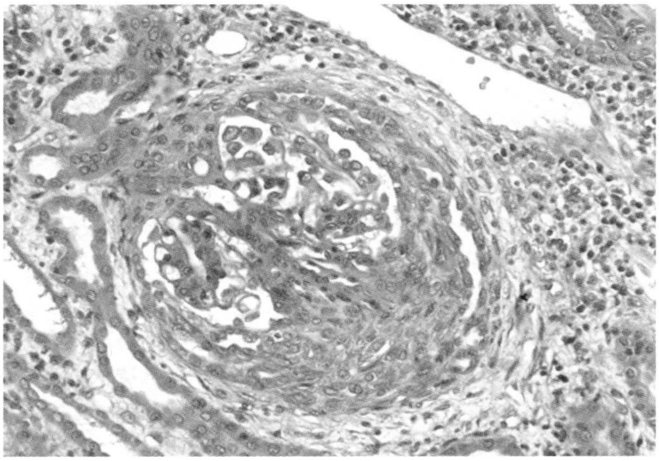

Figure 11-3 Crescentic glomerulonephritis. Circumferential fibrocellular crescent.

Anti-GBM disease is an autoimmune disease caused by circulating autoantibodies directed against the $\alpha3$ chain of type IV collagen.[8,9] This is a rare disorder that may be associated with pulmonary hemorrhage (Goodpasture syndrome) or limited to the kidney. Antibodies are bound to the GBM, accompanied by complement activation, leukocyte infiltration, ruptures of the GBM, and necrotizing proliferative glomerulonephritis with crescents. Patients have hematuria, proteinuria, and rapid deterioration of renal function. Circulating anti-GBM antibodies can be detected with indirect immunofluorescence by incubating the patient's serum with a frozen section of a normal human kidney. The antibody titer may be measured by radioimmunoassay or by enzyme-linked immunosorbent assay (ELISA). Renal biopsy shows crescentic necrotizing glomerulonephritis and linear deposition of IgG along the GBM, often with C3 deposition.

The presence of circulating antineutrophil cytoplasmic antibodies (ANCAs) is an important diagnostic clue when the renal biopsy shows pauci-immune glomerulonephritis.[10] These antibodies are detected by indirect immunofluorescence and by ELISA (Figure 11-4). A diffuse cytoplasmic staining by immunofluorescence (C-ANCA) correlates with the presence of antiproteinase-3 antibodies, whereas a perinuclear staining (P-ANCA) is observed with antimyeloperoxidase antibodies. ANCAs are observed in Wegener's granulomatosis, microscopic polyangiitis, and idiopathic necrotizing glomerulonephritis. C-ANCAs are associated with Wegener's granulomatosus with a specificity of 95%. Patients with microscopic polyangiitis may have either C-ANCAs or P-ANCAs, whereas the majority of those with necrotizing glomerulonephritis have P-ANCAs.[11] ANCAs may also be found in the serum of patients with SLE, Henoch-Schönlein purpura, or anti-GBM disease.

Rapidly progressive glomerulonephritis can also result from immune complex glomerulonephritis, which includes SLE, Henoch-Schönlein purpura nephritis, poststreptococcal glomerulonephritis, or endocarditis.

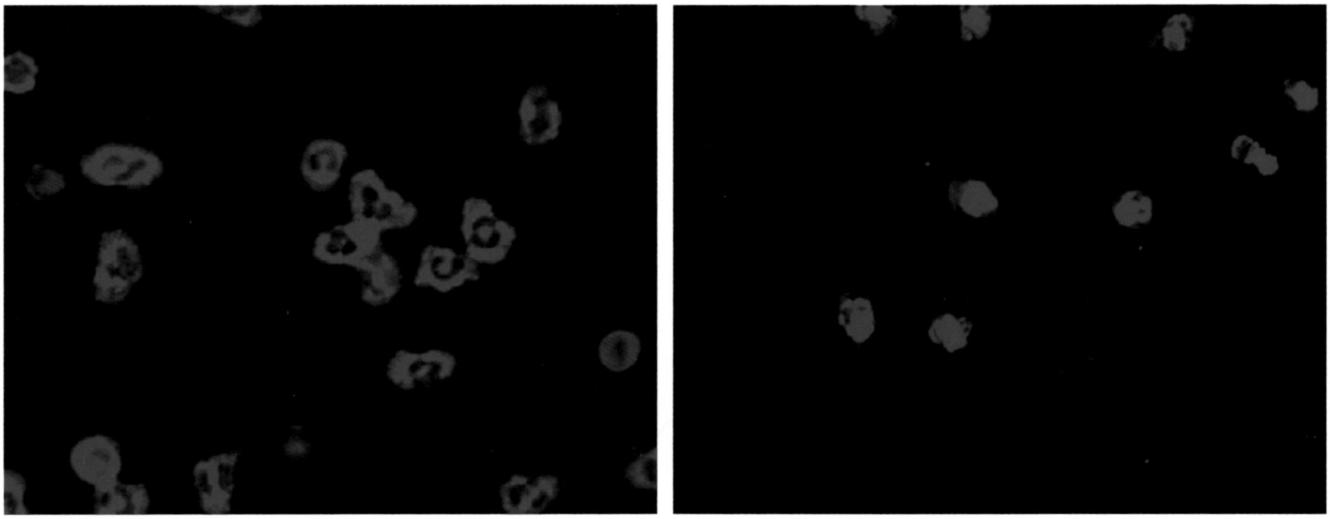

C-ANCA

P-ANCA

Figure 11-4 Pattern of immunofluorescence of C-ANCA and P-ANCA.

SYNDROME OF RECURRENT MACROSCOPIC HEMATURIA

This syndrome is characterized by transient episodes of macroscopic hematuria of 1 to 3 or more days. It often occurs 1 or 2 days following an upper respiratory tract infection. It can be accompanied by proteinuria, which may or may not persist after macroscopic hematuria has resolved. Blood pressure is usually normal.

This syndrome is often observed in children with IgA nephropathy. However, renal biopsy is necessary to confirm this diagnosis. Recurrent episodes of macroscopic hematuria may also be observed in children with Alport syndrome.

SYNDROME OF CHRONIC GLOMERULONEPHRITIS

Most human glomerulonephritis progresses at variable rates relative to chronic renal failure. Although clinical symptoms may have developed earlier and brought the child to medical attention, some children are diagnosed at a late stage of the disease with hypertension, proteinuria with or without hematuria, and progressive renal insufficiency. Renal biopsy at this stage may show nonspecific lesions of end-stage kidney disease, and it may not be possible to identify the glomerular disease that initiated the glomerular lesions. Immunofluorescence is often more helpful.

DIFFERENTIAL DIAGNOSIS

Acute nephritic syndrome secondary to acute glomerular inflammation can mimic other diseases. Children with hemolytic uremic syndrome often have macroscopic hematuria, proteinuria, hypertension, and acute renal failure but also show hemolytic anemia with schizocytes and thrombocytopenia. In addition, hemolytic uremic syndrome often follows an episode of diarrhea secondary to a verotoxin-producing strain of *Escherichia coli*. Some patients with Alport syndrome have macroscopic hematuria and proteinuria, mimicking acute nephritic syndrome. A family history, an association with hearing defects, and a renal biopsy will confirm the diagnosis.

PATHOGENESIS

Nephritic syndrome is secondary to glomerular inflammation. Several immunologic events may initiate glomerular injury.[12] The role of antibodies has been clearly demonstrated. The interaction of antibodies with antigens in situ in the glomerulus, which may or may not lead to the formation of immune complexes, is the main mechanism of glomular injury, whereas the glomerular deposition of circulating immune complexes is probably much less frequent. A cellular immune response mediated by T lymphocytes has been shown to induce glomerular injury in experimental models with an infiltration of glomeruli by circulating inflammatory cells. However, in most types of glomerulonephritis, both humoral and cellular events are involved.

Once these events have started, secondary mechanisms of glomerular injury begin with a cascade of inflammatory mediators. These mediators are responsible for an increased permeability to proteins and a decreased glomerular filtration rate. They are also responsible for structural alterations of the glomeruli with hypercellularity, thrombosis, necrosis, and crescent formation.[13,14]

Humoral Immunity

Humoral immunity is involved in many forms of glomerulonephritis, with deposition of antibodies within the kidney being the initiating event. Indeed, immunoglobulin deposition is observed in the glomeruli in many forms of glomerulonephritis. These immunoglobulins are presumed to be part of immune complexes. Circulating immune complexes may localize in the glomeruli by simple deposition. Normally, following complement activation, circulating immune complexes are cleared when they bind to the C3b receptor on erythrocytes that are then removed by the liver and spleen. In some instances circulating immune complexes may bind to the Fc receptors of mesangial cells and deposit in the glomeruli. This mechanism is probably less frequent than in situ formation of immune complexes where antibodies bind to structural components of the glomerulus or to antigens that have been trapped or planted within the glomerulus.[15] For example, autoantibodies may develop against components of the GBM and result in anti-GBM disease. These autoantibodies have been shown to be directed against an epitope located in the noncollagenous domain of the $\alpha 3$ chain of type IV collagen (the Goodpasture antigen).[9] The same antigen is also present in the alveolar basement membrane, which explains why some patients also develop pulmonary hemorrhage. Binding of the antibodies to the GBM triggers the inflammatory response, resulting in glomerulonephritis.

Autoantibodies may be directed against glomerular cell surface antigens. In the animal model of Heyman nephritis that resembles human membranous nephropathy, antibodies are directed against megalin, a member of the low-density lipoprotein receptor gene family, expressed on epithelial cells such as podocytes and the brush border of proximal tubular cells.[16,17] The rat Thy 1 model is another example of glomerulonephritis induced by antibodies directed against mesangial cell antigens.[18] Glomerular damage may also result from the interaction of antibodies directed against endothelial cell surface antigens. Exogenous antigens trapped or planted in the glomerulus may bind antibodies, resulting in the in situ formation of immune complexes. There is increasing evidence that in most types of human glomerulonephritis, immune complexes are formed in situ and do not result from the deposition of immune complexes preformed in the circulation.[12] Such mechanism may well explain glomerulonephritis related to drugs, infectious agents, or endogenous antigens such as nucleic acids or tumor antigens. These in situ formed immune complexes tend to disappear unless they enlarge and stabilize. This occurs when the immune response, which consists of a polyclonal B-cell activation, induces the formation of different antibodies such as rheumatoid factors IgM anti-IgG or anti-idiotypic antibodies that bind to the complexes. These immune complexes activate the complement cascade and trigger glomerular inflammation.

In IgA nephropathy, recent studies have shown that IgA deposition in the glomerular mesangium may be the result of an abnormal structure.[19-21] The glomerular deposits are composed of monomeric IgA1, and it has been shown that the amount of O-galactose residues in the hinge region is significantly decreased in patients with the disease. This structural anomaly may be responsible for delayed clearance of IgA1 and an increased binding of IgA1 to the mesangial cells.

Cell-Mediated Immunity

The generation of nephritogenic antibodies that initiate glomerulonephritis requires the presence of T lymphocytes. T lymphocytes may also cause glomerulonephritis in the absence of antibodies, although this mechanism is much less common, occurring in the experimental model of glomerulonephritis when CD4+ T lymphocytes from an animal immunized with GBM are transferred to a normal animal.[22]

Secondary Mediators of Glomerulonephritis

Once the primary immunologic event has taken place, a number of mediators are activated that produce the inflammatory response and lead to glomerulonephritis.[23,24]

Complement

Activation of the complement system contributes to the inflammatory response as has been demonstrated in several forms of experimental glomerulonephritis.[25,26] Also, deposition of complement components is a frequent feature of human glomerulonephritis. Complement activation generates C3b and C5a, which are small chemoattractant peptides that stimulate the release of vasoactive amines and chemotactic factors from basophils and mast cells. C5b fragments also attract neutrophils, eosinophils, and basophils to the site of injury.[18] The terminal complement components formed by C5b-C9 constitute the membrane attack complex (MAC) that can directly injure resident glomerular cells without the participation of inflammatory cells.[27] MAC can also activate the production of interleukin (IL)-8 and macrophage chemotactic protein-1 (MCP-1) by endothelial cells[28] and the production of IL-1, reactive oxygen species (ROS), and prostaglandins by mesangial cells. It also mediates endothelial cell apoptosis.[29] In contrast, the complement system allows the elimination of circulating immune complexes, preventing their deposition in the glomeruli. Complement components maintain the circulating immune complexes as soluble so they can be cleared by phagocytic cells.

Coagulation System

Activation of the coagulation cascade in the glomeruli is triggered by tissue factor and leads to the formation of thrombi. Fibrin deposition is frequently observed in necrotizing glomerulonephritis and crescentic glomerulonephritis. Intraglomerular thrombi also have proinflammatory actions. In several experimental models of glomerulonephritis, fibrinolytic agents such as ancrod or streptokinase have a beneficial effect. The role of fibrin deposition is also demonstrated in the experimental model of fibrinogen-deficient mice that are resistant to the induction of anti-GBM disease.[30]

Recruitment of Leukocytes

Infiltration of glomeruli by leukocytes is a constant feature of glomerulonephritis. Monocytes and macrophages play a major role in the inflammatory lesions. Renal injury due to these cells occurs via the release of proinflammatory cytokines such as TNFα, the recruitment of leukocytes via the release of chemokines such as MCP-1, macrophage inflammatory protein-1α and Rantes, cell proliferation via the release of macrophage colony-stimulating factor, cell death via the release of ROS,[31] and proteases that may also damage the GBM.[32,33] Circulating monocytes and macrophages are recruited in the kidney through chemokines produced locally during the inflammatory reaction.[34] Experimentally, blockade of chemokines such as macrophage chemotactic protein-1 or its receptor CCR2, or RANTES,[35-37] prevent leukocyte accumulation in the kidney. Then, macrophages migrate into the renal tissue following the interaction between cell surface adhesion molecules and their ligands on the endothelial cells.[38] This migration is regulated by chemoattractant molecules, especially chemokines.[39] Two families of chemokines have been more extensively investigated, α-chemokines and β-chemokines. α-chemokines have a common CXC structure and recruit polymorphonuclear cells. CC or β-chemokines recruit monocytes through their receptors, CCR. Proliferation of monocytes and macrophages that increases the inflammatory reaction occurs following the local production of growth factors such as the monocyte colony stimulating factor (MCSF).[40] Macrophages are important effector cells in glomerular lesions following humoral or cell-mediated immune injury.[41] They also release tissue factor that induces fibrin deposition, crescent formation, and growth factors such as transforming growth factor beta (TGFβ) and IL-1 that promote fibrosis.[42]

The main chemotactic factors for the accumulation of neutrophils in glomerulonephritis are C5a and other chemokines such as IL-8. The migration of neutrophils follows the interaction of adhesion molecules on these neutrophils with endothelial cells (selectins, integrins, ICAM-1, and VCAM). The adhesion molecules are induced following the production of cytokines and mediators of inflammation. Neutrophils may then release ROS, particularly H_2O_2, and proteolytic enzymes that contribute to glomerular damage.

Endothelial and Mesangial Cells

Glomerular endothelial cell injury occurs following antibody deposition. This injury induces cell proliferation, expression of adhesion molecules, and release of vasoctive molecules, and finally causes necrosis, apoptosis, and thrombosis.[43,44]

Mesangial cell proliferation occurs in a variety of human glomerulonephritides, including IgA nephropathy and lupus nephritis. Activation and proliferation of mesangial cells is triggered by a variety of mediators such as cytokines, growth factors, immune complexes, antibodies, and C5b. Activated mesangial cells produce proinflammatory mediators including chemokines, cytokines, ROS, prostaglandins, growth factors, and extracellular matrix components.

Role of Small Peptides

Many growth factors and cytokines are produced by both glomerular and inflammatory cells.[39,45] They bind to specific cell surface receptors and may either promote or prevent renal injury. Growth factors such as platelet-derived growth factor (PDGF), TGFβ, and vascular endothelial growth factor (VEGF) have important roles in glomerular injury, including glomerular cell proliferation, extracellular matrix deposition, and sclerosis. PDGF has a mitogenic effect on mesangial cells and is a chemoattractant that also promotes tissue repair.[46] TGFβ has an antiproliferative effect on glomerular cells and a proapoptotic action.

Interleukins are known to play an important role in the inflammatory response. IL-1, IL-8, and IL-18 have a proinflammatory action in glomerulonephritis.[47] IL-1 induces mesangial cell proliferation and promotes the synthesis of several substances. IL-8 is produced by mesangial cells and is a chemoattractant for granulocytes. Other interleukins such as IL-4, IL-10, and IL-11 have an anti-inflammatory and protective effect.

TREATMENT

Most children with acute nephritic syndrome need to be hospitalized. There is no reason to prescribe rest unless the child prefers to stay in bed. Dietary recommendations include restricting water and sodium intake. The amount of water is calculated according to weight gain and diuresis. In case of renal failure, potassium intake should also be restricted.

In case of oliguria with weight gain, loop diuretics should be prescribed. They often induce effective diuresis and consequently reduce blood volume. Furosemide at a dose of 2 mg/kgBW may be given orally or intravenously and repeated twice a day if needed.

Hypertension should be treated with antihypertensive drugs. Nifedipine may be given orally at a dose of 0.5 mg/kgBW every 6 hours. If blood pressure is not well controlled with nifedipine, the use of nicardipine as a continuous intravenous infusion at a dose of 0.5 to 2 μg/kgBW per minute is recommended.

In pulmonary edema, oxygen and loop diuretics are indicated, and when these measures are not sufficient, dialysis with ultrafiltration should be initiated. Dialysis should also be started early in children who have severe oliguria with increased serum creatinine and hyperkalemia. Peritoneal dialysis is usually preferred, starting with small volumes if there is respiratory distress.

Immunosuppressive therapies are indicated in select cases, but it should be remembered that they can have serious side effects. Furthermore, although such therapies are widely prescribed, proof of their efficacy is often missing. For example, children with heavy proteinuria, renal insufficiency, and histologic lesions of glomerular and tubulointerstitial fibrosis will not benefit and may develop life-threatening complications from these aggressive treatments. Many of these disorders are treated with a combination of steroids and cytotoxic agents. Corticosteroids are effective in several types of glomerulonephritis. They inhibit the activity of NFκB and thereby the synthesis of several cytokines such as IL-1 that promote glomerular inflammation. Plasma exchange is useful in removing anti-GBM antibodies. Cyclophosphamide, either oral or IV, decreases glomerular inflammation. More specific treatments for glomerular diseases are discussed in subsequent chapters.

Treatments to delay the progression of chronic glomerulonephritis in children should be given. These include strictly controlling blood pressure and blocking the renin-angiotensin system in children with persistent proteinuria. Recent data in adults suggest that the combination of converting enzyme inhibitors and angiotensin receptor antagonists is superior to either agent alone in the prevention of progressive disease.[48] In addition to their antihypertensive and antiproteinuric effects, these therapies may have an antifibrotic effect.[49]

REFERENCES

1. Couser WG: Glomerulonephritis, *Lancet* 353:1509-15, 1999.
2. Rodriguez-Iturbe B: Postinfectious glomerulonephritis, *Am J Kidney Dis* 35:46-48, 2000.
3. West CD: Childhood membranoproliferative glomerulonephritis: An approach to management, *Kidney Int* 29:1077-93, 1986.
4. Rai A, Nast C, Adler S: Henoch-Schonlein purpura nephritis, *J Am Soc Nephrol* 10:2637-44, 1999.
5. Niaudet P, Salomon R: Systemic lupus erythematosus. In ED Avner, WE Harmon, P Niaudet, editors: *Pediatric nephrology*, ed 5, Philadelphia, 2004, Lippincott Williams and Wilkins.
6. Jennette JC: Rapidly progressive crescentic glomerulonephritis, *Kidney Int* 63:1164-77, 2003.
7. Eisenberger U, Fakhouri F, Vanhille P, Beaufils H, Mahr A et al: ANCA-negative pauci-immune renal vasculitis: histology and outcome, *Nephrol Dial Transplant* 20:1392-99, 2005.
8. Borza DB, Netzer KO, Leinonen A, Todd P, Cervera J et al: The goodpasture autoantigen. Identification of multiple cryptic epitopes on the NC1 domain of the alpha3(IV) collagen chain, *J Biol Chem* 275:6030-37, 2000.
9. Hellmark T, Burkhardt H, Wieslander J: Goodpasture disease. Characterization of a single conformational epitope as the target of pathogenic autoantibodies, *J Biol Chem* 274:25862-68, 1999.
10. Seo P, Stone JH: The antineutrophil cytoplasmic antibody-associated vasculitides, *Am J Med* 117:39-50, 2004.
11. Hauer HA, Bajema IM, van Houwelingen HC, Ferrario F, Noel LH: Renal histology in ANCA-associated vasculitis: differences between diagnostic and serologic subgroups, *Kidney Int* 61:80-89, 2002.
12. Couser WG: Mediation of immune glomerular injury, *Clin Invest* 71:808-11, 1993.
13. Chadban SJ, Atkins RC: Glomerulonephritis, *Lancet* 365:1797-806, 2005.
14. Couser WG: Pathogenesis of glomerulonephritis, *Kidney Int Suppl* 42:S19-26, 1993.
15. Nangaku M, Couser WG: Mechanisms of immune-deposit formation and the mediation of immune renal injury, *Clin Exp Nephrol* 9:183-91, 2005.
16. Farquhar MG, Saito A, Kerjaschki D, Orlando RA: The Heymann nephritis antigenic complex: megalin (gp330) and RAP, *J Am Soc Nephrol* 6:35-47, 1995.
17. Cattran DC: Idiopathic membranous glomerulonephritis, *Kidney Int* 59:1983-94, 2001.
18. Eddy AA: Immune mechanisms of glomerular injury. In ED Avner, WE Harmon, P Niaudet, editors: *Pediatric nephrology*, ed 5, Philadelphia, 2004, Lippincott Williams and Wilkins.
19. Amore A, Cirina P, Conti G, Brusa P, Peruzzi L, Coppo R: Glycosylation of circulating IgA in patients with IgA nephropathy modulates proliferation and apoptosis of mesangial cells, *J Am Soc Nephrol* 12:1862-71, 2001.
20. Lai KN: Pathogenic IgA in IgA nephropathy: still the blind men and the elephant? *Kidney Int* 69:1102-03, 2006.
21. Xu LX, Zhao MH: Aberrantly glycosylated serum IgA1 are closely associated with pathologic phenotypes of IgA nephropathy, *Kidney Int* 68:167-72, 2005.
22. Wu J, Hicks J, Borillo J, Glass WF 2nd, Lou YH: $CD4^+$ T cells specific to a glomerular basement membrane antigen mediate glomerulonephritis, *J Clin Invest* 109:517-24, 2002.
23. Couser WG, Johnson RJ: Mechanisms of progressive renal disease in glomerulonephritis, *Am J Kidney Dis* 23:193-98, 1994.

24. Couser WG: Pathogenesis of glomerular damage in glomerulonephritis, *Nephrol Dial Transplant* 13 Suppl 1:10-15, 1998.
25. Nangaku M, Johnson RJ, Couser WG: Glomerulonephritis and complement regulatory proteins, *Exp Nephrol* 5:345-54, 1997.
26. Nangaku M: Complement regulatory proteins in glomerular diseases, *Kidney Int* 54:1419-28, 1998.
27. Brandt J, Pippin J, Schulze M, Hansch GM, Alpers CE et al: Role of the complement membrane attack complex (C5b-9) in mediating experimental mesangioproliferative glomerulonephritis, *Kidney Int* 49:335-43, 1996.
28. Kilgore KS, Schmid E, Shanley TP, Flory CM, Maheswari V et al: Sublytic concentrations of the membrane attack complex of complement induce endothelial interleukin-8 and monocyte chemoattractant protein-1 through nuclear factor-kappa B activation, *Am J Pathol* 150:2019-31, 1997.
29. Hughes J, Nangaku M, Alpers CE, Shankland SJ, Couser WG, Johnson RJ: C5b-9 membrane attack complex mediates endothelial cell apoptosis in experimental glomerulonephritis, *Am J Physiol Renal Physiol* 278:F747-57, 2000.
30. Drew AF, Tucker HL, Liu H, Witte DP, Degen JL, Tipping PG: Crescentic glomerulonephritis is diminished in fibrinogen-deficient mice, *Am J Physiol Renal Physiol* 281:F1157-63, 2001.
31. Boyce NW, Tipping PG, Holdsworth SR: Glomerular macrophages produce reactive oxygen species in experimental glomerulonephritis, *Kidney Int* 35:778-82, 1989.
32. Kaneko Y, Sakatsume M, Xie Y, Kuroda T, Igashima M et al: Macrophage metalloelastase as a major factor for glomerular injury in anti-glomerular basement membrane nephritis, *J Immunol* 170:3377-85, 2003.
33. Johnson RJ, Lovett D, Lehrer RI, Couser WG, Klebanoff SJ: Role of oxidants and proteases in glomerular injury, *Kidney Int* 45:352-59, 1994.
34. Perez de Lema G, Maier H, Nieto E, Vielhauer V, Luckow B et al: Chemokine expression precedes inflammatory cell infiltration and chemokine receptor and cytokine expression during the initiation of murine lupus nephritis, *J Am Soc Nephrol* 12:1369-82, 2001.
35. Chen S, Bacon KB, Li L, Garcia GE, Xia Y et al: In vivo inhibition of CC and CX3C chemokine-induced leukocyte infiltration and attenuation of glomerulonephritis in Wistar-Kyoto (WKY) rats by vMIP-II, *J Exp Med* 188:193-98, 1998.
36. Tang WW, Qi M, Warren JS: Monocyte chemoattractant protein 1 mediates glomerular macrophage infiltration in anti-GBM Ab GN, *Kidney Int* 50:665-71, 1996.
37. Zernecke A, Weber KS, Erwig LP, Kluth DC, Schroppel B et al: Combinatorial model of chemokine involvement in glomerular monocyte recruitment: role of CXC chemokine receptor 2 in infiltration during nephrotoxic nephritis, *J Immunol* 166:5755-62, 2001.
38. Adler S, Brady HR: Cell adhesion molecules and the glomerulopathies, *Am J Med* 107:371-86, 1999.
39. Luster AD: Chemokines—chemotactic cytokines that mediate inflammation, *N Engl J Med* 338:436-45, 1998.
40. Yang N, Isbel NM, Nikolic-Paterson DJ, Li Y, Ye R et al: Local macrophage proliferation in human glomerulonephritis, *Kidney Int* 54:143-51, 1998.
41. Boyle JJ: Human macrophages kill human mesangial cells by Fas-L-induced apoptosis when triggered by antibody via CD16, *Clin Exp Immunol* 137:529-37, 2004.
42. Floege J, Johnson RJ, Gordon K, Iida H, Pritzl P et al: Increased synthesis of extracellular matrix in mesangial proliferative nephritis, *Kidney Int* 40:477-88, 1991.
43. Kang DH, Kanellis J, Hugo C, Truong L, Anderson S et al: Role of the microvascular endothelium in progressive renal disease, *J Am Soc Nephrol* 13:806-16, 2002.
44. Segal MS, Baylis C, Johnson RJ: Endothelial health and diversity in the kidney, *J Am Soc Nephrol* 17:323-24, 2006.
45. Cybulsky AV: Growth factor pathways in proliferative glomerulonephritis, *Curr Opin Nephrol Hypertens* 9:217-23, 2000.
46. Johnson RJ, Floege J, Couser WG, Alpers CE: Role of platelet-derived growth factor in glomerular disease, *J Am Soc Nephrol* 4:119-28, 1993.
47. Atkins RC, Nikolic-Paterson DJ, Song Q, Lan HY: Modulators of crescentic glomerulonephritis, *J Am Soc Nephrol* 7:2271-78, 1996.
48. Nakao N, Yoshimura A, Morita H, Takada M, Kayano T, Ideura T: Combination treatment of angiotensin-II receptor blocker and angiotensin-converting-enzyme inhibitor in non-diabetic renal disease (COOPERATE): a randomised controlled trial, *Lancet* 361:117-24, 2003.
49. Remuzzi A, Gagliardini E, Sangalli F, Bonomelli M, Piccinelli M et al: ACE inhibition reduces glomerulosclerosis and regenerates glomerular tissue in a model of progressive renal disease, *Kidney Int* 69:1124-30, 2006.

CHAPTER

12 Nephrotic Syndrome

Rasheed Gbadegesin and William E. Smoyer

Nephrotic syndrome is a common type of kidney disease seen in children. Historically, Roelans is credited with the first clinical description of nephrotic syndrome in the late fifteenth century, whereas Zuinger later provided a detailed description of the clinical course of the disease and its importance as a cause of chronic renal failure in the presteroid era.[1] Nephrotic syndrome is characterized by massive proteinuria, hypoalbuminemia, and edema, although additional clinical features such as hyperlipidemia are also usually present. In the first few years of life, children with this condition often show periorbital swelling with or without generalized edema. The disease is due to development of structural and functional defects in the glomerular filtration barrier, resulting in its inability to restrict urinary loss of protein. Physiologically, the liver tries to compensate for the excessive loss with increased protein and lipoprotein synthesis. Nephrotic syndrome develops when the loss of protein in urine exceeds the rate of albumin synthesis in the liver, resulting in hypoalbuminemia and edema. Nephrotic syndrome may be caused by a variety of glomerular and systemic diseases, but by far the most common type in childhood is idiopathic nephrotic syndrome. Before the introduction of antibiotics, corticosteroids, and other immunosuppressive therapies, nephrotic syndrome was associated with mortality as high as 67%, usually following infections. The first significant improvement in mortality was seen in 1939 after the introduction of sulfonamides and then penicillin. The introduction of adrenocorticotropic hormone and cortisone in the 1950s contributed to an even greater decrease in mortality (to 9%), which was noted to occur in association with dramatic resolution of proteinuria.[2]

DEFINITIONS

The observations that nephrotic syndrome was responsive to corticosteroids and that its clinical course could be characterized by remission and relapse led to several further observations that remain highly relevant to both the treatment and prognosis of nephrotic syndrome today. It is estimated that about 80% of children with idiopathic nephrotic syndrome will respond to corticosteroid treatment with complete resolution of proteinuria and edema. Among this steroid-responsive group, the clinical course is variable, with up to 60% having frequent relapses or becoming dependent on steroid therapy to maintain them in remission. Based on these findings, it became important to establish some clinically relevant definitions for the diagnosis of nephrotic syndrome and to clarify various patient responses to treatment.

Nephrotic Syndrome: Diagnosis of nephrotic syndrome requires the presence of edema, massive proteinuria (>40 mg/m^2/hr or a urine protein/creatinine ratio >2.0 mg/mg), and hypoalbuminemia (<2.5 g/dl).[3,4]

Remission: Remission is characterized by a marked reduction in proteinuria (to <4 mg/m^2/hr or urine albumin dipstick of 0 to trace for 3 consecutive days) in association with resolution of edema and normalization of serum albumin to at least 3.5 g/dl.[3,4]

Relapse: Relapse is defined as recurrence of massive proteinuria (>40 mg/m^2/hr, urine protein/creatinine ratio >2.0 mg/mg, or urine albumin dipstick ≥2+ on 3 consecutive days), most often in association with recurrence of edema.[3,4]

Steroid-Sensitive Nephrotic Syndrome: Patients who enter remission in response to corticosteroid treatment alone are referred to as having steroid-sensitive nephrotic syndrome (SSNS).

Steroid-Resistant Nephrotic Syndrome: Patients who fail to enter remission after 8 weeks of corticosteroid treatment are referred to as having steroid-resistant nephrotic syndrome or (SRNS).[3,4] It should be noted, however, that significant discrepancies exist in the literature about the definition of SRNS. Whereas some authors define this state as a failure to enter remission after 4 weeks of treatment with prednisone at a dosage of 60 mg/m^2/day, others define it as failure to enter remission after 4 weeks of prednisone at a dosage of 60 mg/m^2/d followed by 4 weeks of prednisone taken on alternate days at a dosage of 40 mg/m^2/dose, or as 4 weeks of prednisone at a dosage of 60 mg/m^2/d followed by three intravenous pulses of methylprednisolone at a dosage of 1000 mg/1.73 m^2/dose.[5,6] Although these discrepancies make direct comparison of reports of the efficacy of newer treatments for nephrotic syndrome more difficult, the most important implication for patients who have been given the label SRNS is that they are at significantly higher risk for development of complications of the disease (discussed later in this chapter), as well as progression of the disease to chronic kidney disease (CKD) or end stage renal disease (ESRD).

Steroid-Dependent Nephrotic Syndrome: Some patients respond to initial corticosteroid treatment by entering complete remission but develop a relapse either while still receiving steroids or within 2 weeks of discontinuation of treatment following a steroid taper. Such patients typically require continued low-dose treatment with steroids to prevent development of relapse, and are therefore referred to as having steroid-dependent nephrotic syndrome (SDNS).[7]

Frequent Relapsing Nephrotic Syndrome: Patients in this group enter complete remission in response to steroids. They remain in remission for several weeks following discontinuation of treatment but develop frequent relapses. If relapses occur 4 or more times in any 12-month period, these patients are referred to as having frequent relapsing nephrotic syndrome (FRNS)[7]

Both SDNS and FRNS patients are at increased risk of developing complications of nephrotic syndrome and complications from frequent use of steroids and other immunosuppressive agents. Although it is not well documented, children with FRNS and SDNS can also develop CKD or ESRD. The likelihood of these risks is generally considered to fall between those for SSNS patients and the significantly increased risks for SRNS patients.

EPIDEMIOLOGY

The annual incidence of nephrotic syndrome in most countries in the Western Hemisphere is estimated to range from 2 to 7 new cases per 100,000 children,[4,8-11] and the prevalence is about 16 cases per 100,000 children.[4] There is a male preponderance among young children, at a ratio of 2:1 to females, although this gender disparity disappears by adolescence, making the incidence in adolescents and adults equal among males and females.[9,12-15]

The incidence of nephrotic syndrome has been fairly stable over the last 30 years, but there are suggestions that the histopathologic patterns may be changing. For example, reports from different parts of the world indicate an increasing occurrence of focal segmental glomerulosclerosis (FSGS) not only after adjusting for variations in renal biopsy practices but also based on the generous assumption that all patients who did not have a renal biopsy had minimal change nephrotic syndrome (MCNS).[9,12-15]

The incidence and the histologic pattern of nephrotic syndrome are also affected by geographic location and ethnic origin. In a report from the United Kingdom, idiopathic nephrotic syndrome was found to be 6 times more common in children of Asian descent living in the United Kingdom than among their European counterparts.[16] In contrast, hospital-based data from Sub-Saharan Africa suggest that idiopathic nephrotic syndrome is relatively less common among African children, where the disease is more often due to glomerular lesions induced by infectious agents.[17-19] In the United States, nephrotic syndrome appears to occur relatively proportionately among children of various ethnic backgrounds. A recent review of children diagnosed with nephrotic syndrome in Houston, Texas, revealed that the distribution of patients closely resembled the ethnic composition of the surrounding community.[12] These data in conjunction with data from African countries seem to suggest that the interaction of genetic and environmental factors is important in the pathogenesis of nephrotic syndrome. However, race appears to have an important impact on the histologic lesion associated with nephrotic syndrome. In this same study the authors found that although only 11% of Hispanic and 18% of Caucasian patients with nephrotic syndrome had FSGS, 47% of African American children had this less favorable diagnosis.[12]

Age also correlates with both the frequency of presentation and the biopsy findings associated with nephrotic syndrome. The most common age for presentation is 2 years, and 70% to 80% of cases occur in children younger than 6.[4,8] To some extent age also predicts the histologic lesion associated with nephrotic syndrome. Children diagnosed before age 6 represented 79.6% of those with MCNS compared with 50% of those with FSGS and only 2.6% of those with membranoproliferative glomerulonephritis (MPGN).[20] When these data were analyzed on the basis of renal histology, the median ages at presentation were found to be 3 years for MCNS, 6 years for FSGS, and 10 years for MPGN.[20] Thus excluding the first year of life, these data combined suggest that the likelihood of having MCNS decreases with increasing age, whereas the likelihood of having the less favorable diagnosis of FSGS or MPGN increases.[20,21]

The histologic lesion associated with nephrotic syndrome has important ramifications for the likelihood of response to steroid treatment. Although almost 80% of children diagnosed with nephrotic syndrome in a multicenter International Study of Kidney Diseases in Children (ISKDC) study entered remission following an initial 8-week course using prednisone, when these children were analyzed based on histology, steroid responsiveness was found in 93% of those with MCNS compared with only 30% of those with FSGS and 7% of those with MPGN.[5,20] In addition to histology, response to steroids also varies with geographic location and ethnicity. Whereas 80% of children in western countries will be steroid responsive, studies from South Africa, Nigeria, and more recently Ghana show that only 9% to 50% of children with nephrotic syndrome are steroid responsive.[19,22,23]

Failure to respond to steroid treatment has important ramifications for the risk of developing progressive renal failure later in life. In a multicenter evaluation of 75 children with FSGS, it was found that within 5 years after diagnosis, 21% had developed ESRD, 23% had developed CKD, and 37% had developed persistent proteinuria, whereas only 11% remained in remission.[24] Thus once a child is given the diagnosis of FSGS, the risk for development of CKD or ESRD within 5 years is almost 50%.

ETIOLOGY

Nephrotic syndrome in childhood is largely primary or idiopathic, although a small proportion of cases are secondary to infectious agents and other glomerular and systemic diseases. The etiology of nephrotic syndrome is also age dependent. Most cases appearing in the first 3 months of life are referred to as congenital nephrotic syndrome (CNS) and are due to genetic diseases. Although there has been no systematic study of the etiology of nephrotic syndrome presenting in the rest of the first year of life (3 to 12 months), there are data suggesting that up to 40% of cases during this time may also be due to genetic causes.[25] Beyond the first year of life and in the first decade, most cases are due to primary or idiopathic nephrotic syndrome, whereas the proportion of secondary nephrotic syndrome cases increases beyond the first 10 years of life.

Congenital Nephrotic Syndrome

Nephrotic syndrome appearing in the first 3 months of life is referred to as congenital nephrotic syndrome (CNS). Most cases in this age group are due to genetic causes (see Chapter 13), the majority being mutations in the gene encoding nephrin, a podocyte slit diaphragm protein. These mutations were first described in the Finnish, hence the name congenital nephrotic syndrome of the Finnish type (CNF).[26] The incidence of CNF is highest in Finland but occurs in other populations as well. Congenital nephrotic syndrome is not synonymous with CNF, because mutations in other genes encoding podocyte slit diaphragm proteins, such as podocin, can also cause early-onset nephrotic syndrome. In one series mutations in the podocin gene *(NPHS2)* were shown to be responsible for up to 40% of all cases of nephrotic syndrome occurring in the first 3 months of life.[25] Nephrotic syndrome in the first 3 months of life may also be part of multisystemic syndromes such as Pierson syndrome, nail-patella syndrome, Denys-Drash syndrome, and others (see Chapter 13), or a result of congenital infections such as syphilis and cytomegalovirus (Table 12-1).

Nephrotic Syndrome Beyond Infancy

Beyond the first year of life, most cases of nephrotic syndrome are idiopathic. The most common histologic variant is MCNS, which is responsible for more than 80% of all cases.[14] Other, less common histopathologic types in this age group include FSGS, MPGN, and mesangial proliferative glomerulonephritis (Table 12-2). Genetic disease is also responsible for some cases in this age group. In one series it was shown that mutations in *NPHS2*, inherited in an autosomal recessive manner, were responsible for 10% to 25% of all cases of familial and sporadic SRNS.[27,28] The phenotype typically associated with *NPHS2* mutations includes onset of nephrotic syndrome in early childhood, resistance to steroid treatment, predominant FSGS histopathologic findings on renal biopsy, progression to ESRD within 5 years of diagnosis, and significantly reduced risk of disease recurrence following renal transplantation.[27,28] Other genetic factors include autosomal dominant transmitted causes such as mutations in the Wilms' tumor suppressor gene *(WT1)*, *α-actinin 4*, *CD2AP*, and *TRPC6*.[29-33] Apart from those in *WT1*, most of these mutations tend to result in adult-onset disease.

Nephrotic syndrome may also be secondary to a number of systemic diseases in children. Pediatric illnesses such as systemic lupus erythematosus, especially membranous (WHO Class V) SLE; Henoch-Schönlein purpura; diabetes mellitus; and sarcoidosis may all present with nephrotic syndrome.

Infectious agents may also cause nephrotic syndrome and can be viral, bacterial, or parasitic. Although it is not yet fully understood how these agents cause nephrotic syndrome, in most cases it is probably due to an aberrant immune response to them, resulting in the formation and deposition of immune complexes in the glomerulus. The importance of these agents as a cause of nephrotic syndrome tends to parallel their prevalence in particular regions of the world. For example, hepatitis B and C are important causes of nephrotic syndrome in Hong Kong and countries in Africa.[34,35] Malaria, especially quartan malaria, is also an important cause in areas where malaria is endemic.[18] Human immunodeficiency virus (HIV), too, can cause nephrotic syndrome in both adults and children. Although the renal lesion associated with HIV can be variable, the most common histologic finding associated with HIV is FSGS, especially the collapsing variant. Although the effect of treatment of the underlying infection on the nephropathy is not well documented, but there are reports that hepatitis B–associated nephrotic syndrome may be amenable to treatment of the hepatitis.[22] A list of infectious agents associated with nephrotic syndrome is shown in Table 12-2. Other, less common causes of nephrotic syndrome include drugs such as gold, penicillamine, angiotensin converting enzyme inhibitors (ACEIs), nonsteroidal antiinflammatory drugs (NSAIDs), sickle cell disease, lymphoma, leukemia, bee stings, and various types of food allergies. In addition, nephrotic syndrome is being seen more often in children with obesity. The histologic lesion most commonly found in this setting is FSGS.

TABLE 12-1 Etiologies of Congenital Nephrotic Syndrome (0-3 Months of Age)

Genetic	Congenital nephrotic syndrome of the Finnish type (CNF) due to mutation in nephrin *(NPHS1)* gene Autosomal recessive FSGS due to mutation in podocin *(NPHS2)* gene Autosomal dominant diffuse mesangial Sclerosis (DMS) due to mutation in *WT1* gene Congenital nephrotic syndrome due to mutation in laminin β_2 gene
Syndromes	Denys-Drash syndrome due to *WT1* mutation with DMS Pierson syndrome Galloway Mowat syndrome Nail-patella syndrome due to mutation in LIM-homeodomain protein *(LMX1B)* Schimke immunoosseous dysplasia with FSGS due to mutation in *SMARCAL1* Cockayne syndrome Jeune's syndrome
Idiopathic	Minimal change nephrotic syndrome FSGS Nonsyndromic DMS
Infections	Congenital syphilis Congenital cytomegalovirus (CMV) infection Congenital toxoplasmosis

PATHOGENESIS

The central abnormality in all cases of nephrotic syndrome is the development of massive proteinuria. Although the molecular basis for this is still speculative, there is evidence in the literature that nephrotic syndrome may be a consequence of a primary glomerular defect, circulating factors, or an immunological abnormality.

Primary Glomerular Defect

One of the most important functions of the kidney is the filtration of blood by glomeruli, which allows excretion of fluid and waste products while retaining the majority of blood

TABLE 12-2 Etiologies of Nephrotic Syndrome (Beyond 3 Months of Age)

Idiopathic	Minimal change nephrotic syndrome (MCNS) Focal segmental glomerulosclerosis (FSGS) Mesangial proliferative glomerulonephritis Membranoproliferative glomerulonephritis (MPGN) Membranous nephropathy (MN) IgM nephropathy C1q nephropathy
Genetic	Autosomal recessive FSGS due to mutation in gene encoding podocin *(NPHS2)* Autosomal dominant diffuse mesangial sclerosis (DMS) due to mutation in gene encoding *WT1* Autosomal dominant FSGS due to mutation in gene encoding *α-actinin 4* Autosomal dominant FSGS due to mutation in gene encoding CD2-associated protein *(CD2AP)* Autosomal dominant FSGS due to mutation in gene encoding transient receptor potential cation channel 6 *(TRPC6)*
Infections	Hepatitis B and C HIV Malaria Schistosomiasis Filariasis
Systemic diseases	Henoch-Schönlein purpura Systemic lupus erythematosus Diabetes mellitus Sarcoidosis
Metabolic diseases	Fabry's disease Glutaric acidemia Glycogen storage disease Mitochondrial cytopathies
Hematologic and oncologic diseases	Leukemia Lymphoma (Hodgkin's most likely can lead to minimal change) Sickle cell disease
Drugs	Nonsteroidal antiinflammatory drugs (NSAIDs) Gold Penicillamine Angiotensin converting enzyme inhibitors (ACEIs) Pamidronate Interferon Mercury Heroin Lithium
Others	Bee stings (MCNS) Food allergies Obesity (usually with FSGS) Oligomeganephronia Pregnancy

proteins and all blood cells within the vasculature. This process of filtration is made possible by the glomerular filtration barrier, which is made up of specialized fenestrated endothelial cells, the glomerular basement membrane (GBM), and glomerular epithelial cells (podocytes) whose distal foot processes are attached to the GBM (Figure 12-1).[36] Neighboring podocyte foot processes are connected to each other by networks of specialized cell-cell junctions known as slit diaphragms. In addition, the GBM has an abundant supply of negatively charged heparin sulfate proteoglycan, resulting in negatively charged molecules being relatively more restricted from passage than positively charged molecules of the same size.[37] In health, molecules greater than 42 Å in diameter, or more than 200 kDa, are unable to cross the filtration barrier.[38] This restriction depends largely on the structural integrity of the podocyte foot processes and slit diaphragms, as well as the GBM charge. In nephrotic syndrome there is loss of negative charge of the GBM.[39-41] Other morphologic changes in podocytes that occur during development of nephrotic syndrome include swelling, retraction, and effacement (spreading) of the podocyte distal foot processes, vacuole formation, occurrence of occluding junctions, displacement of slit diaphragms, and detachment of podocytes from the GBM.[8-10,20]

The importance of podocyte and slit diaphragm structure to the pathogenesis of nephrotic syndrome is further reinforced by recent observations in humans and experimental animals that mutations in genes encoding some of the slit diaphragm proteins or their transcription factors can cause SRNS and/or FSGS.[26,29-33,42] These findings have been the subject of many recent reviews in the literature.[43-45] Mutations in the gene encoding the slit diaphragm protein nephrin

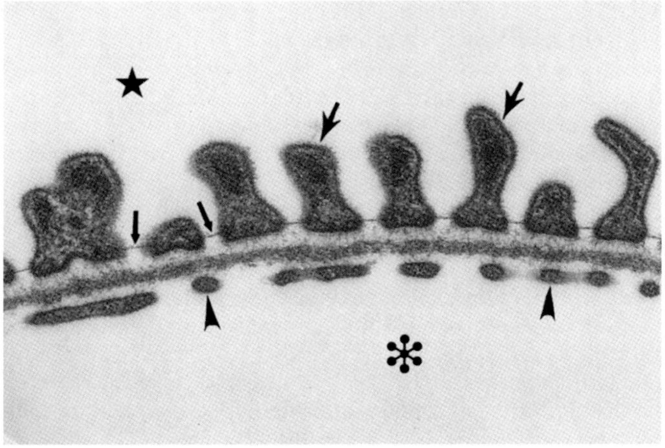

Figure 12-1 Electron micrograph of the components of the glomerular filtration barrier. During normal glomerular filtration, plasma water is filtered from the glomerular capillary lumen *(asterisk)* through the fenestrated endothelial cell layer *(arrowheads)*, then across the glomerular basement membrane (GBM) and through the slit diaphragms *(small arrows)* that bridge the filtration slits between adjacent podocyte foot processes *(large arrows)*, and finally into the urinary space *(star)* where it enters the lumen of the proximal tubule. These podocyte foot processes are normally tall and evenly spaced along the GBM, but during nephrotic syndrome they become spread out along the GBM, with apical displacement of the slit diaphragms. The layer of negatively charged glycocalyx can be seen in this image as a blurry coating on the apical surfaces of the podocyte foot processes. (Adapted with permission from Smoyer WE, Mundel P: Regulation of podocyte structure during the development of nephrotic syndrome, *J Mol Med* 76 (3-4):172-83, 1998.)

(NPHS1) causes CNF in infants.[26] In addition, mutations in *NPHS2* are estimated to be responsible for up to 25% of cases of familial and sporadic SRNS in children.[27,28] Mutations in the transcription factor suppressor gene *WT1* result in Denys-Drash syndrome and Frasier syndrome in children, although they may also cause isolated FSGS and diffuse mesangial sclerosis (DMS).[33,46,47] Mutations in other genes encoding podocyte and GBM proteins include (1) the actin-bundling protein α-actinin 4, which causes adult-onset FSGS; (2) laminin β_2, which results in Pierson syndrome; (3) CD2-associated protein (CD2AP), which results in adult-onset FSGS; (4) the LIM-homeodomain protein (encoded by *LMX1B*), which results in nail-patella syndrome; and (5) the chromatin regulator encoded by *SMARCAL1*, which results in FSGS associated with Schimke immunoosseous dysplasia.[29,48-50] This subject is discussed in greater detail in Chapter 13.

Circulating Factors

There are experimental data to support the existence of soluble mediators that may alter capillary wall permeability in nephrotic syndrome.[40,51-53] Evidence for this includes (1) development of nephrotic syndrome in newborn babies born to mothers with nephrotic syndrome who apparently transferred a soluble factor to their fetuses in utero,[52] (2) marked reduction of proteinuria following treatment with protein A immunoadsorption in various types of primary nephrotic syndromes,[54] (3) recurrence of FSGS in transplanted kidneys in patients with primary FSGS, with remission of recurrent disease induced by treatment with protein A immunoadsorption due to presumed removal of circulating factors,[55] and (4) induction of enhanced glomerular permeability in experimental animals injected with serum from patients with FSGS recurrence in transplanted kidneys.[56] Furthermore, inhibitors of glomerular permeability have also been isolated from the serum of children with FSGS and identified as components of apolipoproteins, suggesting that an imbalance between serum permeability factors and permeability inhibitors may have a pathogenic role in FSGS.[57]

Immunological Abnormality

The theory that nephrotic syndrome may be due to dysregulation of the immune system has existed for more than 30 years. There are numerous reports of abnormalities of both the humoral and cellular immune responses during relapse of nephrotic syndrome. However, the idea that nephrotic syndrome may be due to dysregualtion of T lymphocyte function was first proposed by Shalhoub and his colleagues.[51] Evidence for this includes (1) responsiveness of most forms of primary nephrotic syndrome to corticosteroids, alkylating agents, calcineurin inhibitors, and mycophenolate mofetil, all of which are known inhibitors of T lymphocyte function, (2) induction of remission of nephrotic syndrome following infections with measles and malaria, diseases known to depress cell-mediated immunity, and (3) identification of MCNS as a paraneoplastic manifestation of Hodgkin's disease and other lymphoreticular malignancies. Other reports have also suggested an important role of the cell-mediated immune system in nephrotic syndrome, including depressed cell-mediated immunity during relapses of MCNS alterations in T cell subsets during relapses,[58,59] and increased cell surface expression of IL-2 receptors on T cells, reflective of T cell activation.[59] In addition, numerous cytokines, released in part by T lymphocytes, have been reported to be variably altered during nephrotic syndrome.[60,61] It should be noted, however, that despite numerous reports, none of these cytokines has proven to be both present in the majority of cases of MCNS and able to induce significant proteinuria in experimental animals.

PATHOPHYSIOLOGY

Accumulation of fluid in the interstitial compartment, which typically manifests as facial or generalized edema, is the cardinal symptom in children with nephrotic syndrome. By definition, edematous nephrotic patients always have a total body excess of both sodium and water. The edema in nephrotic syndrome is generally presumed to result from massive proteinuria, which leads to hypoalbuminemia and retention of sodium and water to compensate for intravascular volume depletion.

The pathogenesis of edema in nephrotic syndrome can be most easily understood by analysis of the classic Starling equation, which explains the regulation of fluid movement across capillary walls[62]:

$$\begin{aligned}\text{Net filtration} &= \text{LpS } (\Delta \text{ hydraulic pressure} - \Delta \text{ oncotic pressure}) \\ &= \text{LpS } [(P_{cap} - P_{if}) - s(\pi_{cap} - \pi_{if})]\end{aligned}$$

where:

Lp = the capillary permeability

S = the surface area of the capillary wall

P_{cap} = the capillary hydrostatic pressure
P_{if} = the interstitial fluid hydrostatic fluid pressure
s = the reflection coefficient for proteins (0 = complete permeability and 1 = complete impermeability)
π_{cap} = the capillary oncotic pressure
π_{if} = the interstitial fluid oncotic pressure

In healthy patients, edema formation is prevented by a balance between forces favoring edema (capillary hydrostatic pressure [P_{cap}]) and those opposing it (capillary oncotic pressure [π_{cap}]). In the normal state, the slight tendency toward fluid accumulation in the interstitial space is counterbalanced by the lymphatics, which return this fluid to the circulation. Hypoalbuminemia develops in nephrotic patients when the rate of urinary loss of albumin exceeds the ability of the liver to synthesize it. The resultant hypoalbuminemia leads to low capillary oncotic pressure (π_{cap}), which leads to relatively unopposed capillary hydrostatic pressure (P_{cap}) and subsequent edema formation. The edema formation then results in relative intravascular volume depletion, which triggers neurohumoral compensatory mechanisms to try to replete the intravascular volume. The key mediators of these mechanisms include the sympathetic nervous system (SNS), the renin angiotensin aldosterone system (RAAS), and arginine vasopressin (AVP), with the net result being sodium and water retention by the kidney. In the setting of nephrotic syndrome, mechanoreceptors in the carotid sinus, aortic arch, left ventricle, and afferent arterioles in the glomeruli detect decreased pressure distension. This produces (1) increased SNS outflow from the central nervous system, (2) activation of the RAAS, and (3) nonosmotic release of AVP from the hypothalamus. These three changes result in peripheral vasoconstriction (increased SNS and angiotensin II), sodium retention (increased SNS, angiotensin II, and aldosterone), and water retention.

Although it is widely accepted that patients with nephrotic syndrome have an excess of total body sodium and water as a result of these compensatory mechanisms, the status of their intravascular volume is somewhat controversial. There are two hypotheses that explain the intravascular state in nephrotics: the so-called underfill hypothesis and overfill hypothesis. The underfill hypothesis (Figure 12-2) proposes the existence of a reduced effective circulating blood volume in nephrotic syndrome. It is supported by findings of low urine sodium in the setting of edema, most likely due to activation of the RAAS with resultant elevation of aldosterone levels and reduction in urinary sodium excretion. Furthermore, suppression of atrial natriuretic peptide (ANP) also contributes to low urinary sodium.[63] Additional evidence for the underfill hypothesis includes improvement in sodium excretion with albumin infusion or head-out water immersion, and decreased cardiac output and increased vascular

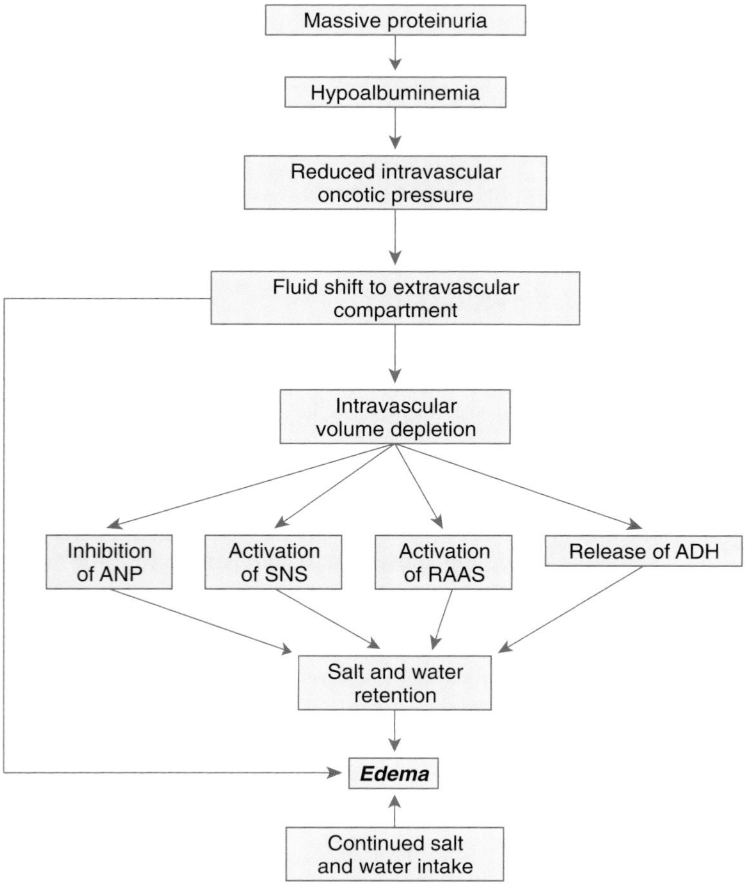

Figure 12-2 Underfill hypothesis of edema formation in nephrotic syndrome. Proposed sequence of pathophysiologic events leading to the formation of edema in nephrotic syndrome according to the underfill hypothesis. Some authors have suggested that the underfill hypothesis is seen more in human clinical disease, whereas the overfill hypothesis is seen more in animal models of nephrosis. *ADH*, Antidiuretic hormone; *ANP*, atrial natriuretic peptide; *RAAS*, renin angiotensin aldosterone system; *SNS*, sympathetic nervous system. (From Schrier RW, Fassett RG: A critique of the overfill hypothesis of sodium and water retention in the nephrotic syndrome, *Kidney Int* 53 (5):1111-17, 1998.)

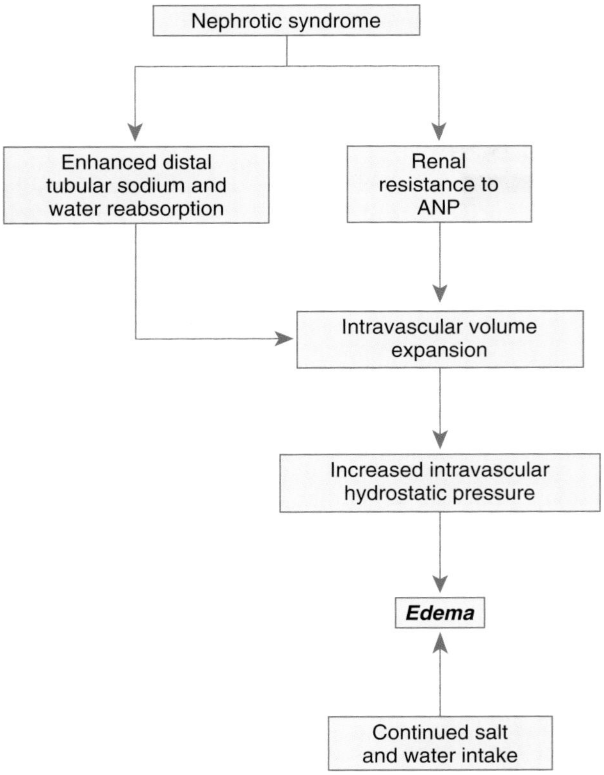

Figure 12-3 Overfill hypothesis of edema formation in nephrotic syndrome. Shown is the proposed sequence of pathophysiologic events leading to the formation of edema in nephrotic syndrome according to the overfill hypothesis. Some authors have suggested that the overfill hypothesis is seen more in animal models of nephrosis than in the human clinical setting. ANP, Atrial natriuretic peptide. (From Schrier RW, Fassett RG: A critique of the overfill hypothesis of sodium and water retention in the nephrotic syndrome, *Kidney Int* 53 (5):1111-17, 1998.)

resistance in animal models of nephrotic syndrome.[64] Findings that do not support the underfill hypothesis as the sole explanation for edema formation in nephrotic syndrome include reports of normal or increased intravascular volume in some patients and variable plasma renin levels in others.[65,66]

In contrast, the overfill hypothesis (Figure 12-3) proposes the existence of an expanded intravascular volume in nephrotic syndrome. Proponents of this hypothesis postulate that nephrotic patients have a primary defect in sodium excretion from the distal convoluted tubules, resulting in an expanded circulatory volume that then leads to suppression of the RAAS. This distal tubular sodium reabsorption has been suggested as secondary to resistance to the effects of ANP.[67] Evidence includes a finding of increased sodium reabsorption from proteinuric kidneys in a rat unilateral proteinuria kidney model,[68] as well as the finding that urinary sodium excretion is not affected by albumin infusion or head-out water immersion in some nephrotic patients.[69] Some authors have argued that the overfill hypothesis is seen more in animal models of nephrosis than in humans in the clinical setting.[70] It should be noted, however, that overfilled and underfilled states are not mutually exclusive, and that the volume status may depend on the stage of disease when a child is being evaluated. It is possible that the underfilled state may be predominant in the acute setting in which massive proteinuria causes rapid development of hypoalbuminemia and an abrupt drop in plasma oncotic pressure, whereas the overfilled state may be predominant in the chronic phase during which patients may have continuing sodium retention due to persistent low-grade hypoalbuminemia.

Because management of edema in children with nephrotic syndrome may be different for those believed to be intravascularly volume-expanded as opposed to volume-contracted, establishing whether a child is overfilled versus underfilled can be clinically important. One group has advocated measuring the fractional excretion of sodium (FE_{Na}) and the relative urinary potassium excretion $[U_K/(U_K + U_{Na})]$ to clarify the distinction.[69] Nephrotic patients with a low FE_{Na} (<1%) and high urinary potassium excretion (>60%) would be expected to have a low intravascular volume. In addition, these urinary findings have been shown to correlate with elevated plasma renin, aldosterone, norepinephrine, and vasopressin levels.[69]

CLINICAL FEATURES AND DIAGNOSIS

History and Physical Examination

The clinical diagnosis of idiopathic nephrotic syndrome is often very simple. In a child with periorbital or generalized edema, the primary care physician can quickly make this diagnosis by documenting significant proteinuria with more than 2+ albumin on urine dipstick or a spot urine protein/creatinine ratio greater than 2 mg/mg and serum albumin of less than 2.5 g/dl. In addition, a careful history should exclude possible complications and identify children with atypical presentations that might reflect other serious systemic illnesses. It should include an evaluation of any abdominal distension, which is usually due to ascites and sometimes edema of the anterior abdominal wall. Although severe distension may be accompanied by abdominal discomfort, persistent abdominal pain may be due to primary bacterial peritonitis (a potentially life-threatening complication), gut edema, or relative gut ischemia due to hypoperfusion secondary to intravascular volume depletion. Other causes of an acute abdomen should also be considered. A history of coughing or breathing difficulties or both may indicate pleural effusion. Pulmonary edema, though rarely found in idiopathic nephrotic children, should lead to consideration of secondary causes of nephrotic syndrome that might cause significant intravascular fluid retention. Although a history of gross hematuria is unusual in nephrotic syndrome, microscopic hematuria may be seen in up to 23% of patients with MCNS and in a higher percentage of patients with other histologic variants.[20] Severe intravascular volume depletion may cause acute renal failure, and some children may present with oliguria or anuria. In such cases prompt intravascular volume repletion is important to correct prerenal acute renal failure and to prevent development of acute tubular necrosis. A history of possible systemic symptoms including fevers, weight loss, night sweats, polyuria, polydipsia, hair loss, oral ulcers, rashes, abdominal pain, and joint pain or swelling should also be elicited, because they may be manifestations of systemic diseases such as systemic lupus erythematosus, Henoch-Schönlein purpura, or diabetes mellitus, which can all cause nephrotic syndrome. A medication history should also be taken in that medications such as NSAIDs, gold, and penicillamine can also cause nephrotic syndrome. The history should exclude other causes of generalized edema, such as chronic liver failure, heart failure, and malnutrition in areas of the world where clinical malnutrition is prevalent.

Regarding physical examination, blood pressure should be carefully determined in nephrotic children; it can be either low (due to intravascular volume depletion) or elevated (due to neurohumoral responses to hypovolemia, intrinsic renal causes, or occasionally renal vein thrombosis). Hypertension has been reported in up to 21% of children 6 years and under with biopsy-confirmed MCNS, and may be present in up to 50% of children with other histologic types.[20] A careful examination of the abdomen should also be performed to exclude abdominal tenderness or guarding that may be signs of bacterial peritonitis. In addition, extremities should be examined to exclude warmth, tenderness, or pain that may suggest venous thrombosis. Finally, obtaining a detailed family history is also important, because some causes of nephrotic syndrome are familial, as previously discussed.

Laboratory Evaluation

Diagnosis of nephrotic syndrome is confirmed by the triad of generalized edema, proteinuria, albuminuria (>2+ on dipstick or urine protein/creatinine ratio >2 mg/mg), and hypoalbuminemia (serum albumin <2.5 g/dl), although hypercholesterolemia is also commonly present. In addition to documenting proteinuria, urinalysis with microscopy should be carried out to look for hematuria and possible red blood cell casts. In patients with a typical presentation, serum studies should include an evaluation of complete blood count, electrolytes, blood urea nitrogen (BUN), creatinine, and albumin levels. For patients at an older age at presentation or with atypical presentation, additional serum studies to exclude secondary causes of nephrotic syndrome should include C3 and C4 complement levels; antinuclear antibody (ANA) and possibly anti-double-stranded DNA; HIV antibody; hepatitis A, B, and C serologies; and consideration of other viral serologies such as HIV antibodies.

Because immunosuppressive therapy is the mainstay of treatment for most cases of childhood nephrotic syndrome, many pediatric nephrologists recommend placing a PPD (purified protein derivative) test to screen for occult tuberculosis before instituting immunosuppression. This is particularly important in areas of the world where tuberculosis is endemic and for recent immigrants from such regions. In addition, many nephrologists obtain a varicella IgG titer before treatment to classify patients as varicella-naive or varicella-immune, which can be of great aid when suspecting or confirming varicella exposure in children who are immunocompromised during treatment. A varicella-naive patient receiving immunosuppressive treatment for nephrotic syndrome who is exposed to varicella should be treated with varicella zoster immunoglobulin (VZIG) within 96 hours of exposure if possible.[71] This passive immunization can sometimes be lifesaving due to the potential severity of a primary varicella infection in an immunocompromised host.

Renal ultrasound does not usually have a role in the evaluation of childhood nephrotic syndrome. However, in the setting of a nephrotic child who develops gross hematuria, thrombocytopenia, or unexplained persistent hypertension, a renal ultrasound should be considered to exclude possible development of renal vein thrombosis.

Renal Biopsy

More than 80% of children with idiopathic nephrotic syndrome will respond to steroid therapy by entering complete remission. Based on this statistic, an initial trial of 4 to 8 weeks of high-dose daily steroid therapy is usually prescribed in children under 10 before considering renal biopsy. In general, renal biopsy is indicated only in the setting of atypical features such as (1) age at onset (less than 1 year or more than 10), (2) SDNS or SRNS, (3) gross or persistent microscopic hematuria or presence of red cell casts, (4) abnormal serologies, or (5) significant persistent renal failure. Due to the known nephrotoxicity (interstitial fibrosis) of calcineurin inhibitors such as cyclosporine and tacrolimus, renal biopsy is also indicated before initiation of these second-line or third-line immunosuppressive agents, as well as approximately every 2 years as long as use of these medications continues.

TREATMENT OF NEPHROTIC SYNDROME

Specific Therapy

The initial treatment for new-onset nephrotic syndrome generally includes 60 mg/m^2/day (maximum 80 mg/d) of prednisone for 4 to 8 weeks, followed by 40 mg/m^2 every other day for 4 to 8 weeks, and then a gradual taper until it is discontinued.[4,14] In a recent Cochrane review, a direct correlation was reported between longer duration of steroid therapy and longer duration of remission, and an indirect correlation with frequency of relapses.[72] In patients with FRNS and SDNS, alternative agents with potential steroid-sparing effects are often used, including cyclophosphamide, levamisole, cyclosporine, tacrolimus, and mycophenolate mofetil. In patients with SRNS, however, the most commonly used agents include cyclosporine, tacrolimus, high-dose intravenous methylprednisolone, and mycophenolate mofetil (MMF), although the efficacy of almost all these agents is lower in these patients compared with FRNS or SDNS patients. A more detailed discussion of the variety of specific therapies for nephrotic syndrome in children is presented in Chapters 15 and 16.

General Management

Edema

Patients with nephrotic syndrome have increased total body fluid and sodium during active disease. General measures to control edema include salt restriction, moderate fluid restriction, and judicious use of diuretics. Dietary recommendations include maintenance of protein intake at approximately 130% to 140% of the RDA for age, as well as avoidance of saturated fats that can worsen hyperlipidemia.

Because the intravascular volume status in children with nephrotic syndrome is typically low, diuretics should generally be used only when significant intravascular depletion has been either excluded or corrected. Typically correction of intravascular depletion can be achieved by initiating intravenous 25% albumin at 1-2 g/kg/d either as a continuous infusion or divided q 6-8 hours. Albumin treatment should continue for 4 to 6 hours before initial administration of diuretics to minimize the risk of worsening any intravascular volume depletion that may be present. In general, slowly increasing the serum albumin level to approximately 2.8 g/dl adequately restores the intravascular oncotic pressure and volume, but there appears to be little additional clinical benefit to increasing the albumin level to normal values.

The most commonly used diuretic in this setting is the loop diuretic furosemide. It acts by inhibiting the sodium-potassium-2 chloride transporter in the thick ascending limb of the loop of Henle. During nephrotic syndrome, however, several factors may impair its efficacy. Because furosemide is highly protein bound, hypoalbuminemia may result in reduced delivery of albumin-bound furosemide to the proximal tubular cells for secretion into the tubular lumen. Hypoalbuminemia also causes an increased volume of distribution of furosemide due to diffusion of the free drug into the expanded interstitial compartment.[73] Another potential cause for the tubular resistance to furosemide seen during nephrotic syndrome results from massive proteinuria, leading to binding of urinary albumin to furosemide in the tubular lumen and a reduction of free drug available to act in the thick ascending limb of the loop of Henle.[73]

Measures to overcome resistance to furosemide include increased doses, coadministration with albumin, and coadministration with distal tubular diuretics. Doses ranging from 200% to 300% of normal can often achieve the desired clinical effects, although high doses in the presence of significant renal impairment may increase the risk for ototoxicity, which has been shown to be related to the peak levels.[74] Clinically effective dosing strategies for intravenous furosemide in nephrotic children with normal renal function typically range from 0.5-1 mg/kg q 6-12 hours, although reports in children with cardiac disease have shown that continuous infusion of furosemide results in a more efficient diuresis compared with intermittent administration.[75,76] Alternatively, coadministration of furosemide with albumin, which has been reported to improve furosemide efficacy by expanding the intravascular volume, resulting in improved renal perfusion and drug delivery to the kidney, is also widely used.[76,77] Another approach to improve the clinical efficacy of furosemide is coadministration with thiazides or the thiazide-type diuretic metolazone, which acts primarily in the distal tubule but has some effects on the proximal tubule.[78] When diuretics are used, physicians should watch closely for common and serious side effects of 3 agents, which include increased risk of thrombosis, electrolyte disturbances such as hypokalemia and metabolic alkalosis, hypercalciuria and nephrocalcinosis, and ototoxicity.[76]

Nonpharmacologic management of edema has also proven to be useful. Elevation of the extremities, or scrotum in cases of severe scrotal edema, to the level of the heart or higher increases the tissue hydrostatic pressure and helps redistribute edema fluid back into the intravascular space. Another safe and effective treatment, although not widely used, is head-out water immersion.[79] This treatment has been reported to have a potent diuretic and natriuretic effect, resulting in significant increases in central blood volume and urine output and reductions in plasma arginine vasopressin, renin, aldosterone, and norepinephrine levels.[79]

Hyperlipidemia

Hyperlipidemia is commonly found in children with nephrotic syndrome. The characteristic lipid profile includes elevations in total plasma cholesterol, very-low-density lipoprotein (VLDL), and low-density lipoprotein (LDL) cholesterol, triglyceride, and lipoprotein A, as well as variable alterations (more typically decreased) in high-density lipoprotein (HDL) cholesterol.[80,81] Although hyperlipidemia in children with SSNS is often transient and usually returns to normal after remission, children with SRNS refractory to therapy often have sustained hyperlipidemia. Such chronic hyperlipidemia has been associated with increased risk for cardiovascular complications and progressive glomerular damage in adults.[82-86] Thus pharmacologic treatment of hyperlipidemia in children with refractory nephrotic syndrome may reduce both the risk for cardiovascular complications later in life and the risk of disease progression.

The potential usefulness of hydroxymethylglutaryl CoA (HMG CoA) reductase inhibitors (statins) in children with SRNS has been reported in a few uncontrolled trials. One study reported a 41% reduction in cholesterol and a 44% reduction in triglyceride levels within 6 months of treatment.[87] A second study found a significant reduction within 2 to 4 months in total cholesterol (40%), LDL cholesterol (44%), and triglyceride (33%) levels, but no significant changes in HDL cholesterol levels.[88] Treatment was found to be safe, with no associated adverse clinical or laboratory events. Although the long-term safety of statins in children has not yet been established, they appear to be generally well tolerated in adults with nephrotic syndrome, with only minor side effects such as asymptomatic increases in liver enzymes, creatine kinase, and rarely diarrhea.[89]

Antiproteinuric Agents

Angiotensin converting enzyme inhibitors (ACEIs) are increasingly being used in the management of persistent proteinuria and control of hypertension in children with SRNS or SDNS. The antiproteinuric effects of ACEIs are due to their ability to reduce glomerular capillary plasma flow rate, decrease transcapillary hydraulic pressure, and alter the permselectivity of the glomerular filtration barrier.[90-92] Numerous uncontrolled studies in adult and pediatric patients with SRNS have reported significant reductions in proteinuria in response to ACEI treatment.[90-94] In addition, a recent randomized crossover trial revealed that, compared with pretreatment values, low-dose enalapril reduced the median urine albumin/creatinine ratio by 33%, whereas high-dose enalapril reduced the ratio by 52%, confirming a dose-related reduction in proteinuria in response to enalapril.[95] In some studies angiotensin receptor blockers (ARBs) have been shown to have the same effect.[96,97] Additionally, a recent metaanalysis in adults with both diabetic and nondiabetic proteinuric renal disease reported the combination of ACEIs and ARBs to be associated with a significant decrease in proteinuria without clinically meaningful changes in serum potassium or GFR.[97]

COMPLICATIONS

Infection

Intercurrent infections represent one of the most serious complications of nephrotic syndrome. Risk factors for infection include low serum IgG levels due to urinary loss of IgG, abnormal T lymphocyte function, and decreased levels of factors B (C3 proactivator) and D, each a component of the alternative complement pathway, which result in a decreased ability to opsonize encapsulated bacteria such as *Streptococcus pneumoniae*.[98,99] In addition, use of steroids and other immunosuppressive medications during relapses further increases the risk of infection.

The most common and serious type of infection is primary bacterial peritonitis, which is estimated to have an incidence of 5% in children with nephrotic syndrome.[100] Other types of infections include cellulitis, sepsis, meningitis, and pneumonia. Most infections are due to *S. pneumoniae* (peritonitis) or *Staphylococcus* (cellulitis), although infections due to gram-negative organisms such as *Escherichia coli* and *Haemophilus influenzae* may also occur.

Children with nephrotic syndrome and peritonitis typically present with fever, abdominal tenderness, and leukocytosis in the setting of overt edema and ascites. Diagnosis of peritonitis may be difficult, because some of the systemic symptoms and signs of infection can be masked by concurrent use of corticosteroids. If the diagnosis is suspected, an abdominal paracentesis is recommended and fluid should be sent for both microscopy and culture. The diagnosis can be confirmed based on the clinical features of peritonitis and a peritoneal fluid WBC count of more than 250/mm^3.[101,102] *S. pneumoniae* and *E. coli* are the most common pathogens in peritonitis, but others have been reported. Broad spectrum antibiotics should be used initially, with coverage narrowed based on culture results.

Strategies for preventing peritonitis include immunization against potential pathogens along with prophylactic antibiotics. Immunization against *Pneumococcus* is recommended, and has been shown to be more effective in children with SSNS than in those with SRNS, and in those not receiving steroids than in those receiving steroids at the time of immunization.[103] Vaccination against *Pneumococcus* has also been shown to be efficacious even in nephrotic children receiving steroids.[104] Despite this, one recent study reported after a 36-month follow-up that patients with SSNS immunized with a polyvalent pneumoccoccal vaccine had a reduction in antipneumoccoccal antibodies.[105] The 2000 American Academy of Pediatrics statement on the use of heptavalent conjugated pneumococcal vaccine recommends universal vaccination of all children up to 23 months old, with children, including those with nephrotic syndrome, ages 24 to 59 months to receive the vaccine only if they are believed to be at moderate or high risk.[106,107]

Viral infections, especially varicella, may also be life threatening in children with nephrotic syndrome. Verification of immunity to varicella, or immunization once patients are on alternate-day steroids, should be performed. If a nonimmune immunosuppressed child is exposed to varicella, passive immunization with VZIG should be performed within 96 hours of exposure to minimize the risk of serious systemic Varicella infection.

The use of prophylactic antibiotics to prevent infections in children with nephrotic syndrome is controversial. They have been recommended in a recent review, particularly for high-risk patients such as those under 2 years, those with SRNS and FRNS, and those with a previous pneumococcal infection.[108] However, some authors have questioned the potential development of resistant organisms with this approach.[109]

Thromboembolism

The risk of thromboembolic phenomenon in children with nephrotic syndrome is estimated at 1.8% to 5%,[110] with higher risk reported in children with SRNS than in those with SSNS.[111] Factors contributing to an increased risk of thrombosis during nephrotic syndrome include abnormalities of the coagulation cascade, such as increased clotting factor synthesis in the liver (factors I, II, V, VII, VIII, X, and XIII), and loss of coagulation inhibitors such as antithrombin III in the urine. Other prothrombotic risks in these children include increased platelet aggregability (and sometimes thrombocytosis), hyperviscosity resulting from increased fibrinogen levels, hyperlipidemia, prolonged immobilization, and use of diuretics. In one series, diuretics were found to be the major iatrogenic risk factor for thrombosis.[111]

The majority of episodes of thrombosis are venous in origin. The most common sites for thrombosis are the deep leg veins, ileofemoral veins, and the inferior vena cava. In addition, use of central venous catheters can further increase the risk of thrombosis. Renal vein thrombosis (RVT) can also occur and may manifest as gross hematuria with or without acute renal failure. Development of these features should prompt either renal Doppler ultrasonography or magnetic resonance angiography to rule out RVT. Pulmonary embolism is another important complication that may be fatal if not recognized early. Although rare, cerebral venous thrombosis, most commonly in the sagittal sinus, has also been reported.[112] In addition to prompting imaging studies, development of thrombosis should prompt an evaluation for possible inherited hypercoagulable states. Typical acute management of thrombosis in nephrotic children includes initial heparin infusion or low molecular weight heparin, followed by transition to warfarin for 6 months. These children should also receive prophylactic anticoagulation therapy during future relapses.[113]

Cardiovascular Disease

Development of cardiovascular disease is increasingly recognized as an important complication of nephrotic syndrome in patients with prolonged clinical courses. Risk factors include the presence of hypertension, hyperlipidemia, long-term treatment with steroids and other immunosuppressive drugs (such as cyclosporine) that can alter serum lipid levels, oxidant stress, and hypercoagulability.[14] Based on these findings, aggressive treatment of chronic hyperlipidemia and hypertension in children with SRNS or prolonged clinical courses is recommended.

Respiratory Distress

Respiratory distress may occur as a complication of nephrotic syndrome or its treatment. In the presence of severe hypoalbuminemia, pleural effusions may develop and can become clinically significant. In addition, aggressive infusion of albumin with inadequate use of diuretics may induce acute pulmonary edema due to the rapid shift of fluid from the interstitium to the intravascular compartment. Possible development of a pulmonary embolism should also be considered in any nephrotic child who develops acute tachypnea or hypoxia.

Bone Disease

Corticosteroid therapy can cause decreased bone formation and increased bone resorption, placing children with nephrotic syndrome at increased risk for developing reduced bone mineral density. Surprisingly, data to support this theoretical risk are controversial. In a recent study of nephrotic children on long-term, high-dose steroids that used dual-energy x-ray absorptiometry to assess total body and spine mineral content, Leonard et al. found no difference in whole body mineral content between patients and controls, although the bone mineral content of the spine was significantly lower in patients than in controls.[114] Another study reported that 22% of nephrotic children had reduced bone mass, although it did not take into consideration the children's height z scores and the children were not compared with normal controls.[115] A further risk factor for reduced bone mineral density is loss of vitamin D binding protein (a carrier protein for 25-hydroxyl cholecalciferol) in the urine.[116] In addition, Weng et al. reported low plasma 25-hydroxyl cholecalciferol levels in a group of children with FRNS who were in remission at the time of the study.[117] Based on these studies, the role of vitamin D supplementation in SSNS children remains somewhat unclear; however, supplementation may be beneficial for SRNS children at high risk for CKD.

Acute Renal Failure

Acute renal failure (ARF) is a relatively uncommon complication of nephrotic syndrome in children. Potential causes include (1) reduced renal perfusion, (2) acute tubular necrosis, (3) renal vein thrombosis, (4) renal interstitial edema, and (5) altered glomerular permeability. In a report of oliguric ARF that developed among children with MCNS on renal biopsy, altered glomerular permeability was found to have played a greater role than did reduced renal perfusion as a cause for ARF.[118]

Other Complications

Other complications reported in children with nephrotic syndrome include anemia, subclinical hypothyroidism, intussusception, and treatment-related side effects such as growth failure, hypertension, cataracts, and hyperlipidemia (Table 12-3).

PROGNOSIS

The single most important prognostic factor for maintenance of long-term normal renal function in nephrotic syndrome is the patient's initial response to corticosteroids. Although children who enter complete remission during an 8-week initial course of oral corticosteroids have an excellent prognosis, the prognosis for those who fail to enter remission is more guarded. Overall, close to 80% of newly diagnosed children treated with corticosteroids will achieve complete remission.[5]

TABLE 12-3 **Complications of Nephrotic Syndrome**

Infectious	Peritonitis Cellulitis Disseminated Varicella infection
Cardiovascular	Hypertension Hyperlipidemia Coronary artery disease
Respiratory	Pleural effusion Pulmonary embolism
Hematologic	Venous (more common) or arterial (less common) thrombosis Anemia
Gastrointestinal	Intussusception
Renal	Acute renal failure Renal vein thrombosis
Endocrinologic	Reduced bone mineral density Hypothyroidism, clinical and subclinical (more common in CNS)
Neurologic	Cerebral venous thrombosis
Treatment-related	
General	Infection, hypertension
Steroids	Growth impairment, reduced bone density, posterior capsular cataracts, avascular necrosis of femoral head
Alkylating agents	Hemorrhagic cystitis, dose-related oligospermia and premature ovarian failure, increased risk of malignancy
Calcineurin inhibitors	Gingival hyperplasia, hirsutism, hyperkalemia, encephalopathy
Mycophenolate mofetil (MMF)	Nausea, vomiting, diarrhea, constipation, dose-related leukopenia, headache

Steroid responsiveness varies by renal histologic type, with 93% of children with MCNS being steroid responsive compared with 56% with mesangial proliferative glomerulonephritis (IgM nephropathy in some centers), 30% with FSGS, 7% with MPGN, and 0% with membra-nous nephropathy.[5] In addition, the frequency of steroid responsiveness generally decreases with increasing age at presentation.

Among children with SSNS, relapse is common. It is estimated that 70% of children with nephrotic syndrome will experience one or more relapses. However, the frequency of relapses decreases over time. A large study of children with MCNS reported a gradual increase in the number of nonrelapsing patients over time, such that 8 years after disease onset 80% of children were relapse-free.[119] In addition, 75% of those children with no relapses in the first 6 months after treatment either had rare relapses or continued in remission for their entire clinical course. Risk factors for frequent relapses or a steroid-dependent course have not been carefully studied, but the literature suggests that an age of less than 5 years at onset and a prolonged time to initial remission are possible risk factors.[120,121] More recently Tsai et al. reported a higher incidence of the DD (homozygous deletion) genotype for the angiotensin converting enzyme (ACE) gene in SDNS and SRNS children compared with SSNS children, suggesting a potential role for ACE in regulating clinical response to steroids.[122]

Initial steroid resistance clearly identifies a subset of patients at high risk for progressive kidney disease. It is estimated that 40% to 50% of children with SRNS will progress to CKD or ESRD within 5 years of diagnosis, despite aggressive immunosuppression. Among children with nephrotic syndrome due to FSGS who progress to ESRD, renal transplantation can also pose serious challenges. Nephrotic syndrome recurs in the allograft in up to 30% of children with FSGS and leads to graft loss in about 50% of such patients.[123] Among children with FSGS due to *NPHS2* mutations, the risk for recurrence has been controversial.[27,28,124]

The introduction of antibiotics and steroids in treating nephrotic syndrome has led to a significant reduction in mortality, from 60% to 70% to less than 5%. In an ISKDC series of 521 children with nephrotic syndrome, 10 deaths were reported, resulting in a mortality rate of 1.9%.[125] Of note, 9 of these 10 children had either early relapses or SRNS and 6 (60%) died from infections, confirming infection as an important cause of mortality in nephrotic syndrome.

Nephrotic syndrome is one of the most common forms of renal disease seen in children. Although the introduction of antibiotics and refinement of immunosuppressive medications have greatly decreased mortality and improved the quality of life for children with this disease, neither the mechanism(s) of action nor the target cell for these therapies is known. In spite of this, the prognosis for long-term maintenance of normal renal function is excellent unless complete remission cannot be achieved. Hopefully our growing understanding of the pathobiology of nephrotic syndrome will lead to development of more effective therapies in the future.

REFERENCES

1. Arneil GC: The nephrotic syndrome, *Pediatr Clin North Am* 18 (2):547-59, 1971.
2. Arneil GC, Lam CN: Long-term assessment of steroid therapy in childhood nephrosis, *Lancet* 2 (7468):819-21, 1966.
3. ISKDC: The primary nephrotic syndrome in children. Identification of patients with minimal change nephrotic syndrome from initial response to prednisone, *J Pediatr* 98 (4):561-64, 1981.
4. Niaudet P: Steroid-resistant idiopathic nephrotic syndrome in children. In Avner ED, Harmon WE, Niaudet P, editors: *Pediatric nephrology*, Philadelphia, 2004, Lippincott Williams & Wilkins.
5. ISKDC: Primary nephrotic syndrome in children: clinical significances of histopathologic variants of minimal change, *Kidney Int* 20 (6):765-71, 1981.
6. Niaudet P, Gagnadoux MF, Broyer M: Treatment of childhood steroid-resistant idiopathic nephrotic syndrome, *Advances in Nephrology from the Necker Hospital* 28:43-61, 1998.
7. Schulman SL et al: Predicting the response to cytotoxic therapy for childhood nephrotic syndrome: superiority of response to corticosteroid therapy over histopathologic patterns, *J Pediatr* 113 (6):996-1001, 1988.
8. Nash MA et al: The nephrotic syndrome. In Edelmann CMJ, editor: *Pediatric kidney disease*, Boston, 1992, Little, Brown, and Company.
9. Srivastava T, Simon SD, Alon US: High incidence of focal segmental glomerulosclerosis in nephrotic syndrome of childhood, *Pediatr Nephrol* 13 (1):13-18, 1999.
10. Hogg RJ et al: Evaluation and management of proteinuria and nephrotic syndrome in children: Recommendations from a pediatric nephrology panel established at the National Kidney Foundation Conference on Proteinuria, Albuminuria, Risk, Assessment, Detection, and Elimination (PARADE), *Pediatrics* 105 (6):1242-49, 2000.
11. McEnery PT, Strife CF: Nephrotic syndrome in childhood. Management and treatment in patients with minimal change disease, mesangial proliferation, or focal glomerulosclerosis, *Pediatr Clin North Am* 29 (4):875-94, 1982.
12. Bonilla-Felix M et al: Changing patterns in the histopathology of idiopathic nephrotic syndrome in children, *Kidney Int* 55 (5):1885-90, 1999.
13. Kari JA: Changing trends of histopathology in childhood nephrotic syndrome in western Saudi Arabia, *Saudi Med J* 23 (3):317-21, 2002.
14. Eddy AA, Symons JM: Nephrotic syndrome in childhood, *Lancet* 362 (9384):629-39, 2003.
15. Filler G et al: Is there really an increase in non-minimal change nephrotic syndrome in children? *Am J Kidney Dis* 42 (6):1107-13, 2003.
16. Sharples PM, Poulton J, White RH: Steroid responsive nephrotic syndrome is more common in Asians, *Arch Dis Child* 60 (11):1014-17, 1985.
17. Coovadia HM, Adhikari M, Morel-Maroger L: Clinico-pathological features of the nephrotic syndrome in South African children, *Quarterly Journal of Medicine* 48 (189):77-91, 1979.
18. Hendrickse RG et al: Quartan malarial nephrotic syndrome. Collaborative clinicopathological study in Nigerian children, *Lancet* 1 (1761):1143-49, 1972.
19. Abdurrahman MB et al: Clinicopathological features of childhood nephrotic syndrome in northern Nigeria, *Quarterly Journal of Medicine* 75 (278):563-76, 1990.
20. ISKDC: Nephrotic syndrome in children: Prediction of histopathology from clinical and laboratory characteristics at time of diagnosis, *Kidney Int* 13:159-65, 1978.
21. Sorof JM et al: Age and ethnicity affect the risk and outcome of focal segmental glomerulosclerosis, *Pediatr Nephrol* 12 (9):764-68, 1998.
22. Bhimma R, Coovadia HM, Adhikari M: Nephrotic syndrome in South African children: changing perspectives over 20 years, *Pediatr Nephrol* (4):429-34, 1997.
23. Doe JY et al: Nephrotic syndrome in African children: lack of evidence for 'tropical nephrotic syndrome'? *Nephrol Dial Transplant* 21 (3):672-76, 2006.

24. The Southwest Pediatric Nephrology Study Group: Focal segmental glomerulosclerosis in children with idiopathic nephrotic syndrome: A report of the Southwest Pediatric Nephrology Study Group, *Kidney Int* 27:442-49, 1995.
25. Hinkes B et al: Genetic causes of nephrotic syndrome in the first year of life. American Pediatric Nephrology Meeting, 2006. Marburg.
26. Lenkkeri U et al: Structure of the gene for congenital nephrotic syndrome of the Finnish type (NPHS1) and characterization of mutations, *Am J Hum Genet* 64 (1):51-61, 1999.
27. Ruf RG et al: Patients with mutations in NPHS2 (podocin) do not respond to standard steroid treatment of nephrotic syndrome, *JASN* 15 (3):722-32, 2004.
28. Weber S et al: NPHS2 mutation analysis shows genetic heterogeneity of steroid-resistant nephrotic syndrome and low post-transplant recurrence, *Kidney Int* 66 (2):571-79, 2004.
29. Shih NY et al: Congenital nephrotic syndrome in mice lacking CD2-associated protein, *Science* 286 (5438):312-15, 1999.
30. Kaplan JM et al: Mutations in ACTN4, encoding alpha-actinin-4, cause familial focal segmental glomerulosclerosis, *Nat Genet* 24 (3):251-56, 2000.
31. Ruf RG et al: Prevalence of WT1 mutations in a large cohort of patients with steroid-resistant and steroid-sensitive nephrotic syndrome, *Kidney Int* 66 (2):564-70, 2004.
32. Winn MP et al: A mutation in the TRPC6 cation channel causes familial focal segmental glomerulosclerosis, *Science* 308 (5729): 1801-04, 2005.
33. Mucha B et al: Members of the APN Study Group. Mutations in the Wilms' tumor 1 gene cause isolated steroid resistant nephrotic syndrome and occur in exons 8 and 9, *Pediatr Res* 59 (2):325-31, 2006.
34. Wong SN, Yu EC, Chan KW: Hepatitis B virus associated membranous glomerulonephritis in children—experience in Hong Kong, *Clin Nephrol* 40 (3):142-47, 1993.
35. Bhimma R et al: Treatment of hepatitis B virus-associated nephropathy in black children, *Pediatr Nephrol* 17 (6):393-99, 2002.
36. Smoyer WE, Mundel P: Regulation of podocyte structure during the development of nephrotic syndrome, *J Mol Med* 76 (3-4):172-83, 1998.
37. White RH, Glasgow EF, Mills RJ: Clinicopathological study of nephrotic syndrome in childhood, *Lancet* 1 (7661):1353-59, 1970.
38. Brenner BM, Hostetter TH, Humes HD: Glomerular permselectivity: barrier function based on discrimination of molecular size and charge, *Am J Physiol* 234 (6):F455-60, 1978.
39. Kitano Y, Yoshikawa N, Nakamura H: Glomerular anionic sites in minimal change nephrotic syndrome and focal segmental glomerulosclerosis, *Clin Nephrol* 40 (4):199-204, 1993.
40. Carrie BJ, Salyer WR, Myers BD: Minimal change nephropathy: an electrochemical disorder of the glomerular membrane, *Am J Med* 70 (2):262-68, 1981.
41. Van den Born J et al: A monoclonal antibody against GBM heparin sulfate induces an acute selective proteinuria in rats, *Kidney Int* 41 (1):115-23, 1992.
42. Boute N et al: NPHS2, encoding the glomerular protein podocin, is mutated in autosomal recessive steroid-resistant nephrotic syndrome, *Nat Genet* 24:349-54, 2000.
43. Barisoni L, Mundel P: Podocyte biology and the emerging understanding of podocyte diseases, *Am J Nephrol* 23 (5):353-60, 2003.
44. Benzing T: Signaling at the slit diaphragm, *J Am Soc Neph* 15 (6):1382-91, 2004.
45. Tryggvason K, Patrakka J, Wartiovaara J: Hereditary proteinuria syndromes and mechanisms of proteinuria, *N Engl J Med* 354 (13):1387-401, 2006.
46. Pelletier J et al: Germline mutations in the Wilms' tumor suppressor gene are associated with abnormal urogenital development in Denys-Drash syndrome, *Cell* 67 (2):437-47, 1991.
47. Barbaux S et al: Donor splice-site mutations in WT1 are responsible for Frasier syndrome, *Nat Genet* 17 (4):467-70, 1997.
48. Morello R, Lee B: Insight into podocyte differentiation from the study of human genetic disease: nail-patella syndrome and transcriptional regulation in podocytes, *Pediatr Res* 51 (5):551-58, 2002.
49. Boerkoel CF et al: Mutant chromatin remodeling protein SMARCAL1 causes Schimke immuno-osseous dysplasia, *Nat Genet* 30 (2):215-20. Epub 2002 Jan 22.
50. Zenker M et al: Human laminin beta2 deficiency causes congenital nephrosis with mesangial sclerosis and distinct eye abnormalities, *Human Mol Genet* 13 (21):2625-32, 2004.
51. Shalhoub RJ: Pathogenesis of lipoid nephrosis: a disorder of T-cell function, Lancet 2 (7880):556-60, 1974.
52. Kemper MJ, Wolf G, Muller-Wiefel DE: Transmission of glomerular permeability factor from a mother to her child, *N Engl J Med* 344 (5):386-87, 2001.
53. Meyrier A: Mechanisms of disease: focal segmental glomerulosclerosis, *Nat Clin Prac Nephrol* 1 (1):44-54, 2005.
54. Sasdelli M et al: Cell mediated immunity in idiopathic glomerulonephritis, *Clin Ex Immunol* 46 (1):27-34, 1984.
55. Dantal J et al: Effect of plasma protein adsorption on protein excretion in kidney-transplant recipients with recurrent nephrotic syndrome, *N Engl J Med* 330 (1):7-14, 1994.
56. Savin VJ et al: Circulating factor associated with increased glomerular permeability to albumin in recurrent focal segmental glomerulosclerosis, *N Engl J Med* 334 (14):878-83, 1996.
57. Candiano G et al: Inhibition of renal permeability towards albumin: a new function of apolipoproteins with possible pathogenetic relevance in focal glomerulosclerosis, *Electrophoresis* 22 (9):1819-25, 2001.
58. Topaloglu R et al: T-cell subsets, interleukin-2 receptor expression and production of interleukin-2 in minimal change nephrotic syndrome, *Pediatr Nephrol* 8 (6):649-52, 1994.
59. Yan K et al: The increase of memory T cell subsets in children with idiopathic nephrotic syndrome, *Nephron* 79 (3):274-80, 1998.
60. Garin EH: Circulating mediators of proteinuria in idiopathic minimal lesion nephrotic syndrome, *Pediatr Nephrol* 14 (8-9):872-78, 2000.
61. Van den Berg JG, Weening JJ: Role of the immune system in the pathogenesis of idiopathic nephrotic syndrome, *Clin Sci (Lond)* 107 (2):125-36, 2004.
62. Starling EH: The fluids of the body. Chicago, Kemer Herter Lectures, 1908.
63. Usberti M et al: Considerations on the sodium retention in nephrotic syndrome. *Am J Nephrol* 15 (1):38-47, 1995.
64. Hinojosa-Laborde C, Jones SY, DiBona GF: Hemodynamics and baroreflex function in rats with nephrotic syndrome, *Am J Physiol* 267 (4 Pt 2):R953-64, 1994.
65. Geers AB et al: Plasma and blood volumes in patients with the nephrotic syndrome, *Nephron* 38 (3):170-73, 1984.
66. Dorhout Mees EJ, Geers AB, Koomans HA: Blood volume and sodium retention in the nephrotic syndrome: a controversial pathophysiological concept, *Nephron* 36 (4):201-11, 1984.
67. Vande Walle JG, Donckerwolcke RA, Koomans HA: Pathophysiology of edema formation in children with nephrotic syndrome not due to minimal change disease, *J Am Soc Nephrol* 10 (2):323-31, 1999.
68. Ichikawa I et al: Role for intrarenal mechanisms in the impaired salt excretion of experimental nephrotic syndrome, *J Clin Invest* 71 (1):91-103, 1983.
69. Vande Walle JG, Donckerwolcke RA, Koomans HA: Pathogenesis of edema formation in nephrotic syndrome, *Pediatr Nephrol* 16 (3):283-93, 2001.
70. Schrier RW, Fassett RG: A critique of the overfill hypothesis of sodium and water retention in the nephrotic syndrome, *Kidney Int* 53 (5):1111-17, 1998.
71. Pickering LK: Varicella-zoster infections. In Pickering LK, editor: *Red Book: Report of the Committee on Infectious Diseases*, American Academy of Pediatrics, Elk Grove Village, IL, 2003.
72. Hodson EM et al: Corticosteroid therapy for nephrotic syndrome in children, *Cochrane Database Syst Rev* 25 (1):CD001533, 2005.
73. Brater DC: Diuretic therapy, *N Engl J Med* 339 (6):387-95, 1998.
74. Rybak LP: Furosemide ototoxicity: clinical and experimental aspects, *Laryngoscope* 95 (9 Pt 2) (suppl 38):1-14, 1985.
75. Singh NC et al: Comparison of continuous versus intermittent furosemide administration in postoperative pediatric cardiac patients, *Crit Care Med* 20 (1):17-21, 1992.

76. Eades SK, Christensen ML: The clinical pharmacology of loop diuretics in the pediatric patient, *Pediatr Nephrol* 12 (7):603-16, 1998.
77. Haws RM, Baum M: Efficacy of albumin and diuretic therapy in children with nephrotic syndrome, *Pediatrics* 91 (6):1142-46, 1993.
78. Puschett JB: Pharmacological classification and renal actions of diuretics, *Cardiology* 84(suppl 2):4-13, 1994.
79. Rascher W et al: Diuretic and hormonal responses to head-out water immersion in nephrotic syndrome, *J Pediatr* 109 (4):609-14, 1986.
80. Querfeld U et al: Lipoprotein(a) serum levels and apolipoprotein(a) phenotypes in children with chronic renal disease, *Pediatr Res* 34 (6):772-76, 1993.
81. Querfeld U: Should hyperlipidemia in children with the nephrotic syndrome be treated? *Pediatr Nephrol* 13 (1):77-84, 1999.
82. Veverka A, Jolly JL: Recent advances in the secondary prevention of coronary heart disease, *Expert Rev of Cardiovasc Ther* 2 (6):877-89, 2004.
83. Moorhead JF, Wheeler DC, Varghese Z: Glomerular structures and lipids in progressive renal disease, *Am J Med* 87 (5N):12N-20N, 1989.
84. Keane WF: Lipids and the kidney, *Kidney Int* 46 (3):910-20, 1994.
85. Samuelsson O et al: Lipoprotein abnormalities are associated with increased rate of progression of human chronic renal insufficiency, *Nephrol Dial Transplant* 12 (9):1908-15, 1997.
86. Taal MW: Slowing the progression of adult chronic kidney disease: therapeutic advances, *Drugs* 64 (20):2273-89, 2004.
87. Coleman JE, Watson AR: Hyperlipidaemia, diet and simvastatin therapy in steroid-resistant nephrotic syndrome of childhood, *Pediatr Nephrol* 10 (2):171-74, 1996.
88. Sanjad SA, al-Abbad A, al-Shorafa S: Management of hyperlipidemia in children with refractory nephrotic syndrome: the effect of statin therapy, *J Pediatr* 130:470-74, 1997.
89. Olbricht CJ et al: Simvastatin in nephrotic syndrome. Simvastatin in Nephrotic Syndrome Study Group, *Kidney Int Suppl* 71:S113-16, 1999.
90. Trachtman H, Gauthier B: Effect of angiotensin-converting enzyme inhibitor therapy on proteinuria in children with renal disease, *J Pediatr* 112 (2):295-98, 1998.
91. Milliner DS, Morgenstern BZ: Angiotensin converting enzyme inhibitors for reduction of proteinuria in children with steroid-resistant nephrotic syndrome, *Pediatr Nephrol* 5 (5):587-90, 1991.
92. Delucchi A et al: Enalapril and prednisone in children with nephrotic-range proteinuria, *Pediatr Nephrol* 14:1088-91, 2000.
93. Prasher PK, Varma PP, Baliga KV: Efficacy of enalapril in the treatment of steroid resistant idiopathic nephrotic syndrome, *Journal Assoc Physicians India* 47:180-82, 1999.
94. Lama G et al: Enalapril: antiproteinuric effect in children with nephrotic syndrome, *Clin Nephrol* 53 (6):432-36, 2001.
95. Bagga A et al: Enalapril dosage in steroid-resistant nephrotic syndrome, *Pediatr Nephrol* 19 (1):45-50, 2004.
96. Kanda H et al: Antiproteinuric effect of ARB in lupus nephritis patients with persistent proteinuria despite immunosuppressive therapy, *Lupus* 14 (4):288-92, 2005.
97. MacKinnon M et al: Combination therapy with an angiotensin receptor blocker and an ACE inhibitor in proteinuric renal disease: a systematic review of the efficacy and safety data, *Am J Kidney Dis* 48 (1):8-20, 2006.
98. Kaysen GA: Nonrenal complications of the nephrotic syndrome, *Annu Rev Med* 45:201-10, 1994.
99. Harris RC, Ismail N: Extrarenal complications of the nephrotic syndrome, *Am J Kidney Dis* 23 (4):477-97, 1994.
100. Krensky AM, Ingelfinger JR, Grupe WE: Peritonitis in childhood nephrotic syndrome: 1970-1980, *American Journal of Diseases of Children* 136 (8):732-36, 1982.
101. Hingorani SR, Weiss NS, Watkins SL: Predictors of peritonitis in children with nephrotic syndrome, *Pediatr Nephrol* 17 (8):678-82, 2002.
102. Castellote J et al: Rapid diagnosis of spontaneous bacterial peritonitis by use of reagent strips, *Hepatology* 37 (4):893-96, 2003.
103. Spika JS et al: Serum antibody response to pneumococcal vaccine in children with nephrotic syndrome, *Pediatrics* 69 (2):219-23, 1982.
104. Wilkes JC et al: Response to pneumococcal vaccination in children with nephrotic syndrome, *Am J Kidney Dis* 2 (1):43-46, 1982.
105. Guven AG et al: Rapid decline of anti-pneumococcal antibody levels in nephrotic children, *Pediatr Nephrol* 19 (1):61-65, 2004.
106. Overturf GD: American Academy of Pediatrics. Committee on Infectious Diseases. Technical report: prevention of pneumococcal infections, including the use of pneumococcal conjugate and polysaccharide vaccines and antibiotic prophylaxis, *Pediatrics* 106 (2 Pt 1):367-76, 2006.
107. Hsu K et al: Population-based surveillance for childhood invasive pneumococcal disease in the era of conjugate vaccine, *Pediatr Infect Dis J* 24 (1):17-23, 2005.
108. McIntyre P, Craig JC: Prevention of serious bacterial infection in children with nephrotic syndrome, *J Paediatr Child Health* 34 (4):314-17, 1998.
109. Milner LS et al: Penicillin resistant pneumococcal peritonitis in nephrotic syndrome, *Arch Dis Child* 62 (9):964-65, 1987.
110. Citak A et al: Hemostatic problems and thromboembolic complications in nephrotic children, *Pediatr Nephrol* 14 (2):138-42, 2000.
111. Lilova MI, Velkovski IG, Topalov IB: Thromboembolic complications in children with nephrotic syndrome in Bulgaria (1974-1996), *Pediatr Nephrol* 15 (1-2):74-78, 2000.
112. Gangakhedkar A et al: Cerebral thrombosis in childhood nephrosis, *J Paediatr Child Health* 41 (4):221-24, 2005.
113. Andrew M et al: Guidelines for antithrombotic therapy in pediatric patients, *J Pediatr* 132 (4):575-88, 1998.
114. Leonard MB et al: Long-term, high-dose glucocorticoids and bone mineral content in childhood glucocorticoid-sensitive nephrotic syndrome, *N Engl J Med* 351 (9):868-75, 2004.
115. Gulati S et al: Longitudinal follow-up of bone mineral density in children with nephrotic syndrome and the role of calcium and vitamin D supplements, *Nephrol Dial Transplant* 20 (8):1598-603, 2005.
116. Auwerx J et al: Decreased free 1,25-dihydroxycholecalciferol index in patients with the nephrotic syndrome, *Nephron* 42 (3):231-35, 1986.
117. Weng FL et al: Vitamin D insufficiency in steroid-sensitive nephrotic syndrome in remission, *Pediatr Nephrol* 20 (1):56-63, 2005.
118. Vande Walle J et al: ARF in children with minimal change nephrotic syndrome may be related to functional changes of the glomerular basal membrane, *Am J Kidney Dis* 43 (3):399-404, 2004.
119. Tarshish P et al: Prognostic significance of the early course of minimal change nephrotic syndrome: report of the International Study of Kidney Disease in Children, *J Am Soc Nephrol* 8 (5):769-76, 1997.
120. Takeda A et al: Risk factors for relapse in childhood nephrotic syndrome, *Pediatr Nephrol* 10 (6):740-41, 1996.
121. Yap HK et al: Risk factors for steroid dependency in children with idiopathic nephrotic syndrome, *Pediatr Nephrol* 16 (12):1049-52, 2001.
122. Tsai IJ et al: Angiotensin-converting enzyme gene polymorphism in children with idiopathic nephrotic syndrome, *Am J Nephrol* 26 (2):157-62, 2006.
123. Salomon R, Gagnadoux MF, Niaudet P: Intravenous cyclosporine therapy in recurrent nephrotic syndrome after renal transplantation in children, *Transplantation* 75 (6):810-14, 2003.
124. Bertelli R et al: Recurrence of focal segmental glomerulosclerosis after renal transplantation in patients with mutations of podocin, *Am J Kidney Dis* 41 (6):1314-21, 2003.
125. ISKDC: Minimal change nephrotic syndrome in children: deaths during the first 5 to 15 years' observation, *Pediatrics* 73 (4):497-501, 1984.

CHAPTER 13

Hereditary Nephrotic Syndrome

Stefanie Weber

During the past decade, defects in various genes have been associated with the development of steroid-resistant nephrotic syndrome (SRNS) in children and adults. These genes encode for proteins that participate in the development and structural architecture of glomerular visceral epithelial cells (podocytes). This novel insight moved the podocyte with its interdigitating foot processes and slit diaphragms (SD) into the center of interest regarding the pathophysiology of proteinuria.

Whereas light microscopy shows variable aspects ranging from minimal change nephropathy to diffuse mesangial sclerosis or focal and segmental glomerulosclerosis (FSGS) (Figure 13-1), all hereditary proteinuria syndromes share a common phenotype when evaluated by electron microscopy, which uniformly demonstrates the typical flattening of the foot processes and loss of the SD. With respect to the clinical course, two entities can be distinguished: disorders of early glomerular development manifesting prenatally, directly after birth, or in early infancy, and disorders with late-onset nephrotic syndrome, typically manifesting as FSGS in adulthood. In the following sections, important genes involved in both types of manifestations are discussed.

HEREDITARY DISORDERS OF EARLY GLOMERULAR DEVELOPMENT

Podocytes develop from the nephrogenic blastema in a chain of events in conjunction with development of the renal glomeruli. First, local condensation of the mesenchyme leads to the formation of the nephron anlage, that is, the comma-shaped and the S-shaped bodies, and eventually the formation of the mature glomerulus. Podocytes are the first cells that can clearly be distinguished in this process, forming a disklike layer of epithelial cells. The subsequent differentiation to mature podocytes with interdigitating primary and secondary foot processes is associated with a general loss of ability for further proliferation. At this stage, early cell-cell contacts (adherens junctions) have developed into a specialized structure, the SD, spanning the intercellular space. The final glomerular filtration barrier is constituted by the fenestrated endothelium, the glomerular basement membrane (GBM), and interdigitating podocytes.

A number of genes are involved in these processes (Table 13-1; Figure 13-2), and *WT1* is one of the major mediators of podocyte differentation. *NPHS1* and *NPHS2* code for nephrin and podocin, respectively, two proteins that have important roles for the organization of the SD. *LAMB2* encodes laminin β2, one component of the heterotrimeric laminins that link the podocyte to the GBM. *LMX1B* encodes the transcription factor Lmx1b that in the kidney is exclusively expressed in podocytes. It is one of the crucial genes regulating gene expression during early steps of podocyte development. The most recently identified gene involved in early-onset nephrotic syndrome *NPHS3/PLCE1*, encodes for phospholipase C epsilon-1, involved in podocyte signaling processes.

WT1 Gene Mutations

Wilms' tumor is one of the most common solid tumors of childhood, occurring in 1 of 10,000 children and accounting for 8% of childhood cancers. The Wilms' tumor suppressor gene *(WT1)* was first identified in 1990.[1] *WT1* locates on chromosome 11p13 and encodes a zinc finger transcription factor that regulates the expression of many genes during kidney and urogenital development. Mutations in *WT1* were first identified in pediatric patients affected by Wilms' tumor, aniridia, genitourinary malformations, and mental retardation (WAGR syndrome).[2] These were truncating mutations, associated with complete loss of function of WT1. *WT1* mutations were also identified in patients with isolated Wilms' tumor.[3] In tumor material of isolated cases, both germline and somatic mutations have been detected. Familial Wilms' tumor forms seem to follow a dominant pattern of inheritance, with dominant germline mutations. However, in a number of these cases the classical two-hit inactivation model, with loss of heterozygosity due to a second somatic event, has been described as the underlying cause of tumor development.[4]

Subsequently, *WT1* mutations were also associated with Denys-Drash syndrome (DDS),[5] Frasier syndrome (FS),[6] and diffuse mesangial sclerosis (DMS) with isolated nephrotic syndrome (NS) (Jeanpierre et al., 1998).[7] The full picture of autosomal dominant Denys-Drash syndrome is characterized by early-onset NS, male pseudohermaphroditism, gonadal dysgenesis, and development of Wilms' tumor (in more than 90% of patients). Wilms' tumor may precede or develop after the manifestation of NS. Age at onset of NS is generally within the first months of life.[8] In rare cases enlarged and hyperechogenic kidneys are already demonstrated by prenatal ultrasound.[9] Renal histology typically presents with DMS[10] and electron microsocopy reveals foot process effacement.

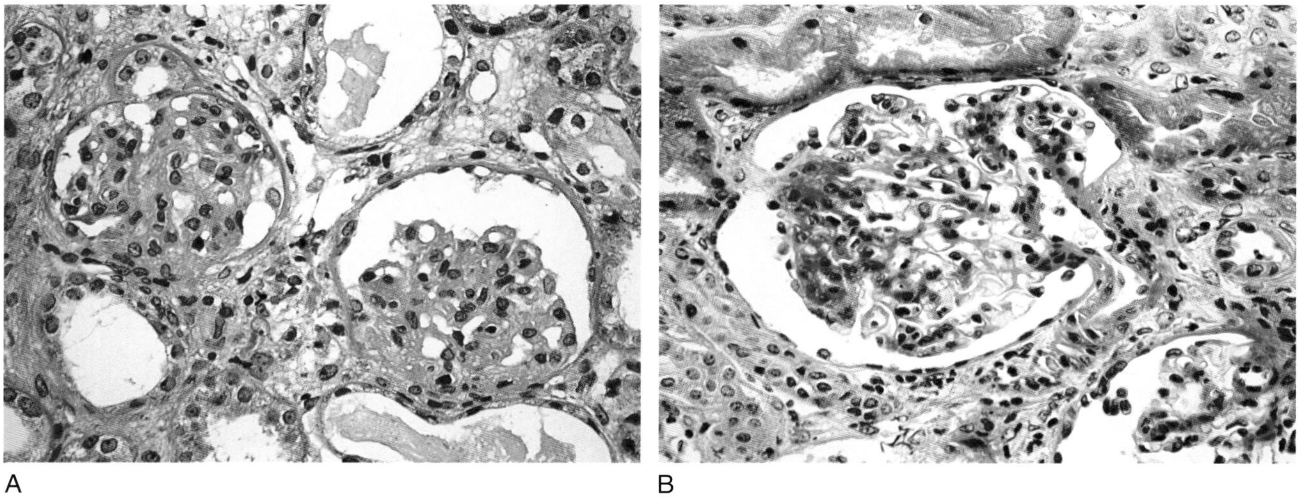

Figure 13-1 Kidney histology of a patient with diffuse mesangial sclerosis **(A)** and focal segmental glomerulosclerosis **(B)**, respectively. (Courtesy Rüdiger Waldherr, Praxis für Pathologie, Heidelberg, Germany.)

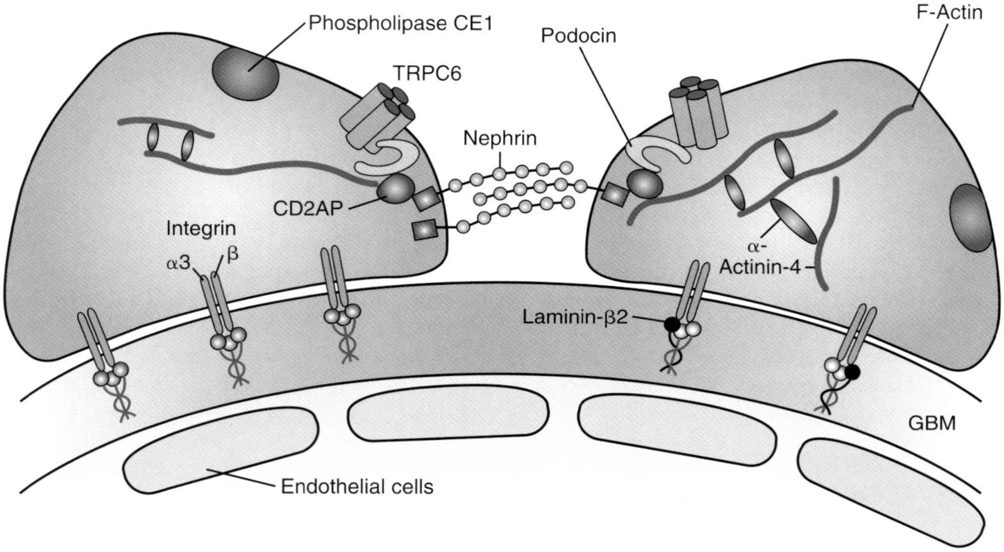

Figure 13-2 Schema of a podocyte foot process cross section depicting important components involved in hereditary nephrotic syndrome.

The NS is resistant to steroid treatment and renal function deteriorates rapidly to end-stage renal disease (ESRD) during infancy. Bilateral nephrectomy is generally advised in ESRD to prevent development of Wilms' tumor.[11] Recurrence of NS after kidney transplantation has not been observed so far.[12]

Dominant *WT1* mutations are identified in the vast majority of DDS patients. These mutations predominantly affect exons 8 and 9 of the *WT1* gene and most of them are de novo mutations not observed in the parents. Most *WT1* mutations associated with DDS are missense mutations affecting conserved amino acids of the zinc finger domains, with R394W being the most frequent mutation observed. These alterations of the zinc finger structure reduce the DNA-binding capacity of the WT1 protein.[13] A heterozygous knock-in mouse model has been created for the R394W missense mutation, presenting with DMS and male genital anomalies[14] supporting the dominant nature of the disease.

Of note is that some patients affected by *WT1* mutations in exons 8 and 9 do not display with the full picture of DDS but rather with isolated DMS. *WT1* analysis should therefore be performed in all children with isolated DMS and early-onset NS because of the high risk of Wilms' tumor development in case of a positive mutation analysis result. Close monitoring by renal ultrasound (e.g., every 6 months) is important in all children with *WT1* mutation and early-onset NS. In addition, karyotype analysis is recommended in all girls with isolated DMS to detect a possible male pseudohermaphroditism. Some patients with isolated DMS display with recessive mutations in *WT1*, with both the maternal and paternal allele being affected.[7]

TABLE 13-1 Overview on Important Disorders Causing Hereditary Nephrotic Syndromes

	Inheritance	Locus	Gene	Protein	OMIM Accession No.
Early-onset nephrotic syndrome					
Isolated DMS	AR	11p13	*WT1*	WT1	256370
Denys-Drash syndrome (typically DMS)	AD	11p13	*WT1*	WT1	194080
Frasier syndrome (typically FSGS)	AD	11p13	*WT1*	WT1	136680
Congenital nephrotic syndrome/Finnish type	AR	19q13	*NPHS1*	Nephrin	602716
Recessive familial SRNS	AR	1q25	*NPHS2*	Podocin	600995
Recessive nephrotic syndrome	AR	10q23-q24	*NPHS3/PLCE1*	PLCE1	608414
Pierson syndrome	AR	3p21	*LAMB2*	Laminin β2	609049
Nail-patella syndrome	AD	9q34.1	*LMX1B*	Lmx1b	161200
Recessive SRNS with sensorineural deafness	AR	14q24.2	*?*	?	(to follow)
Late-onset nephrotic syndrome/FSGS					
FSGS1	AD	19q13	*ACTN4*	α-Actinin 4	603278
FSGS2	AD	11q21-22	*TRPC6*	TRPC6	603965
FSGS3 (CD2AP-associated disease susceptibility)	AD	6	*CD2AP*	CD2AP	607832

AD, Autosomal dominant; *AR*, autosomal recessive; *?*, unknown.

Frasier syndrome is characterized by a progressive glomerulopathy and male pseudohermaphroditism also[15]; however, differences from DDS include later onset of proteinuria in childhood and slower deterioration of renal function. ESRD develops only in the second or third decade of life. As in DDS, proteinuria and NS are steroid resistant. Renal histology in FS patients typically shows FSGS[16]; in a minority of patients only minimal change lesions are observed. In female patients the genitourinary tract is normally developed, whereas a complete sex reversal with gonadal dysgenesis is observed in 46,XY patients. Primary amenorrhea in conjunction with NS is a typical feature of these 46,XY patients and should prompt molecular analysis of *WT1*. Although the risk of developing Wilms' tumor is low in patients with FS, gonadoblastomata developing from gonadal dysgenesis are frequently observed. After diagnosis of FS, gonadectomy is highly recommended in 46,XY patients.

In 1997 it was first demonstrated that mutations in the *WT1* gene also underly the pathogenesis of FS.[6] Notably, the class of mutations in FS differs from DDS: whereas mutations affecting the coding sequence of exons 8 and 9 cause DDS, mutations associated with FS represent donor splice-site mutations located in intron 9. Similar to DDS, these mutations occur in a heterozygous state and frequently are de novo mutations not observed in the parents. The donor splice site of intron 9 plays an important role for the generation of the KTS isoform of the WT1 protein. This isoform contains three additional amino acids (lysine-threonine-serine; KTS). It has been demonstrated that the (+) KTS/(−) KTS protein dose ratio is of high relevance for WT1 action during genitourinary and kidney development. In FS patients this ratio is markedly reduced due to the splice-site mutations.[6]

Although the pathogenicity of *WT1* mutations is beyond any doubt, there is remarkable phenotypical heterogeneity: splice-site mutations typical for FS may in some cases be found in patients with DDS[5] or isolated DMS,[17] and patients with typical DDS mutations may display with isolated FSGS[18] or Wilms' tumor without NS.[19]

NPHS1 Gene Mutations Associated with Autosomal Recessive Congenital Nephrotic Syndrome of the Finnish Type

Congenital nephrotic syndrome (CNS) of the Finnish type (CNF) is characterized by autosomal recessive inheritance and development of proteinuria in utero.[20] The responsible gene was mapped in 1994 to chromosome 19q13[21] and mutations in *NPHS1* have been subsequently identified in affected children.[22] *NPHS1* encodes for nephrin, a zipperlike protein of the glomerular SD. Typically, severe NS manifests before 3 months of age, and renal biopsy specimens show immature glomeruli, mesangial cell hypercellularity, glomerular foot process effacement, and pseudocystic dilations of the proximal tubules. NS is steroid resistant in these patients, and treatment options include albumin infusions, pharmacological interventions with ACE inhibitors and indomethacin, and ultimately unilateral or bilateral nephrectomy.[23-26]

Nephrin is exclusively expressed in podocytes at the level of the SD after full differentiation has occurred.[27] Nephrin belongs to the immunoglobulin superfamily, having a single putative transmembrane domain, a short intracellular N-terminus, and long extracellular C-terminus.[22] The extracellular C-terminus is predicted to bridge the intercellular space between the interdigitating foot processes, making nephrin a key component of the SD. Nephrin strands contribute to the porous structure of the SD, forming pores of approximately 40 nm.[28] These pores are currently believed to be partly responsible for the size selectivity of the SD and the glomerular filtration barrier.

Apart from its role as a structural protein, nephrin also appears to participate in intracellular signaling pathways maintaining the functional integrity of the podocyte.[29-31] The SD constitutes a highly dynamic protein complex that recruits signal transduction components and initiates signaling to regulate complex biologic programs in the podocyte. A number of proteins within this signaling platform were identified to interact with nephrin, among them podocin, CD2AP, and TRPC6, all of which are also associated with the development of NS when altered by gene mutations (see later). It is suggested that the plasma membrane of the filtration slit has a special lipid composition comparable to lipid rafts.[32] Lipid rafts are specialized microdomains of the plasma membrane and have a unique lipid content and a concentrated assembly of signal transduction molecules.[33] It was shown that nephrin is a lipid raft–associated protein at the SD and that podocin serves to recruit nephrin into these microdomains. Disease-causing podocin mutations fail to target nephrin into rafts, thus altering nephrin-induced signal transduction.[31] In summary, these studies confirm the extraordinary role of SD proteins in maintaining the glomerular filtration barrier.

Mutations in *NPHS1* were first identified in the Finnish population, leading to the classification of "Finnish type" CNS. Two truncating mutations were found with high frequency in affected Finnish children, suggesting an underlying founder effect in the Finnish population; they are called L41fsX90 (Fin major, truncating the majority of the protein) and R1109X (Fin minor, truncating only a short C-terminal part). In subsequent studies, *NPHS1* mutations were also identified in non-Finnish patients throughout the world, and to date more than 50 different mutations have been described. The Fin major and Fin minor mutations are only rarely observed in non-Finnish patients. Several mutational hot spots were identified affecting the immunoglobulin domains of the nephrin protein.[34] The immunoglobulin domains 2, 4, and 7 appear particularly important for gene function. In addition to the high prevalence in Finland, *NPHS1* mutations are also common among Mennonites in Pennsylvania; 8% of this population are carriers of a heterozygous mutant allele.[35]

Recent studies suggest that CNF may be a genetically heterogenous disorder: in a number of affected patients, *NPHS1* mutations were absent but in some individuals mutations were identified in *NPHS2* (see later). These patients showed the typical histologic features of CNF. However, these results are preliminary and additional studies will have to be performed that include a larger number of patients to confirm a role of *NPHS2* in CNF.

Interestingly, in rare cases a triallelic digenic modus of inheritance was observed in patients with CNS/SRNS: mutations in both *NPHS1* and *NPHS2* were identified with a total of three affected alleles (two *NPHS1* mutations and one *NPHS2* mutation or vice versa).[34] It is speculated that the additional single mutation of the second gene plays a role as a genetic modifier, possibly aggravating the clinical phenotype. These data provide evidence of a functional interrelationship between nephrin and podocin and underscore the critical role that these genes play in regulating glomerular protein filtration.

NPHS2 Gene Mutations Associated with Autosomal Recessive SRNS

The *NPHS2* gene was mapped by linkage analysis in eight families with autosomal recessive SRNS to chromosome 1q25-q31[36] and recessive mutations in *NPHS2* were identified subsequently.[37] NS in these families was characterized by steroid resistance, age at onset between 3 and 5 years, and no recurrence of proteinuria after renal transplantation. *NPHS2* mutations have never been reported in patients with SSNS. Renal histology typically shows FSGS; however, some patients present with only minimal change lesions. In some cases progression from minimal change lesions to FSGS has been demonstrated in repeat biopsies.

NPHS2 encodes for podocin, a 42 kD integral membrane protein expressed in both fetal and mature glomeruli.[37] By electron microscopy and immunogold labeling it was demonstrated that the site of expression is the SD of the podocytes. Because both protein termini are located in the cytosol and podocin is predicted to have only one membrane domain, a hairpinlike structure of the protein was proposed. Interacting with both nephrin and CD2AP, podocin appears to link nephrin to the podocyte cytoskeleton. In patients affected by recessive mutations in *NPHS2*, SD formation is impaired and the typical foot process effacement is visible. These observations suggest that podocin has an important function in maintaining the glomerular filtration barrier. The knockout of *Nphs2* in mice is associated with a phenotype highly reminiscent of the human disease, with podocyte foot process effacement, nephrotic range proteinuria, and chronic renal insufficiency.[38] Podocin, like nephrin, is localized in lipid rafts[32] and is important for recruiting nephrin to these microdomains of the plasma membrane.[31] Some mutations in *NPHS2* impair the ability of podocin to target nephrin to the rafts, especially the most frequent mutation, R138Q, identified in European patients.[31]

Up to now, more than 30 pathogenic mutations have been described in *NPHS2;* most mutations affect the stomatin domain located in the C-terminal part of the protein.[39,40] Mutations in *NPHS2* were first identified in infants with SRNS and rapid progression to ESRD.[37] Subsequently, however, it became evident that defects in podocin can be responsible for SRNS first manifesting at any age from birth to adulthood.[41-43] A partial genotype-phenotype correlation is apparent: whereas the R138Q mutation is typically associated with early-onset NS, other missense mutations (e.g., V180M, R238S) are predominantly found in patients with a later onset of SRNS.[40]

A frequent single nucleotide polymorphism (PM) in the *NPHS2* gene (R229Q) is prevalent in the heterozygous state in approximately 3% of the normal population (range 0.5% to 7%, depending on the genetic background).[44] A common flanking haplotype is associated with the R229Q PM in individuals of widespread ethnic origin, suggesting that the sequence variation arose in a common ancestor long ago.[45] R229Q is present in compound heterozygosity with a single pathogenic *NPHS2* mutation in some patients with FSGS/SRNS. NS manifests late in these individuals, suggesting a reduced pathogenicity when compared with true/nonpolymorphic *NPHS2* mutations. R229Q is therefore considered a nonneutral PM enhancing the susceptibility to FSGS in association with a second mutant *NPHS2* allele.[45] Moreover, in a large study of more than 1500 individuals of the general population, the R229Q PM was significantly associated with the prevalence of microalbuminuria, a risk factor for developing chronic renal insufficiency and cardiovascular events.[46] In vitro studies have demonstrated that R229Q podocin shows decreased binding to its interacting protein partner, nephrin.[45] These interesting findings underline the functional importance of podocin for the glomerular filtration barrier, with even subtle changes of the amino acid sequence impairing its proper function.

The role of R229Q in the homozygous state is discussed controversially, however. Some authors identified R229Q in the homozygous state in SRNS patients with no other pathogenic mutations in *NPHS2*. In several studies involving very large control groups, no healthy control individual displayed with R229Q in the homozygous state. Only one homozygous control individual was identified out of 1577 samples in the study of Pereira et al.[46] These observations strongly suggest that R229Q homzygosity is disease causing.[40] However, given an average allele frequency of 3%, the frequency of homozygous carriers should amount to 0.1% in the general population, whereas SRNS is much less frequent in demographic terms. Hence R229Q homozygosity alone cannot be sufficient to cause disease, and other genetic or nongenetic factors most likely play a modifying role in disease manifestation in homozygous carriers.

LAMB2 Gene Mutations Associated with Pierson Syndrome

Pierson syndrome is characterized by CNS caused by DMS and peculiar eye abnormalities, including a typical nonreactive narrowing of the pupils (microcoria) (Figure 13-3), but also additional lens and corneal abnormalities.[47] Recently, recessive mutations in *LAMB2* on chromosome 3p21 were identified as the underlying genetic defect.[48] *LAMB2* encodes for the protein laminin β2, one component of the trimeric laminins in the kidney that crosslink the basolateral membrane of the podocyte to the GBM. Most disease-associated alleles identified in Pierson patients were truncating mutations leading to loss of laminin β2 expression in the kidney.[48] Ocular laminin β2 expression in unaffected controls was strongest in the intraocular muscles, corresponding well to the characteristic hypoplasia of ciliary and pupillary muscles observed in affected patients. Subsequent genotype-phenotype studies revealed that some mutations in *LAMB2*, especially hypomorphic missense mutations, can be associated with a phenotypic spectrum that is much broader than previously anticipated, including isolated CNS or CNS with minor ocular changes different from those observed in Pierson syndrome.[49] Fetal ultrasound in four consecutive fetuses of a family with Pierson syndrome and positive *LAMB2* mutation analysis consistently revealed marked hyperechogenicity of the kidneys and variable degrees of pyelectasis by 15 weeks of gestation.[50] Placentas were significantly enlarged. Hydrops fetalis due to severe hypalbuminemia demonstrated by chordocentesis occurred in one fetus, and anencephaly was detected in another. Development of oligohydramnios indicated a prenatal decline of renal excretory function. From these studies it can be concluded that mutational analysis in *LAMB2* should also be considered in isolated CNS if no mutations are found in *NPHS1*, *NPHS2*, or *WT1*, and in cases with prenatal onset of nephrotic disease with typical sonomorphologic findings of the kidneys and the development of oligohydramnios.

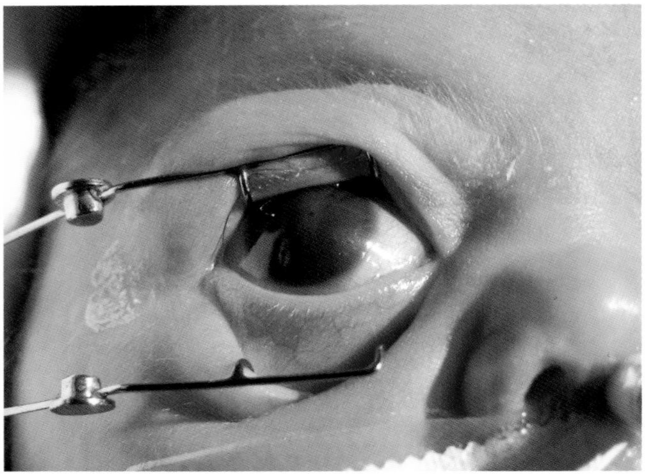

Figure 13-3 Typical aspect of a patient with Pierson syndrome and microcoria. (Courtesy Kveta Blahova, Pediatric Clinic, Charles University, Prague, Czech Republic.)

LMX1B Gene Mutations Associated with Autosomal Dominant Nail-Patella Syndrome

Nail-patella syndrome (NPS) or onychoösteodysplasia is caused by dominant mutations in the *LMX1B* gene, located on chromosome 9q34.1 and encoding the LIM-homeodomain protein Lmx1b. Lmx1b plays a central role in dorsal/ventral patterning of the vertebrate limb, and targeted disruption of Lmx1b results in skeletal defects including hypoplastic nails, absent patellae, and a unique form of renal dysplasia.[51] Prominent features of affected children are dysplasia of nails and absent or hypodysplastic patellae. In many patients, iliac horns, dysplasia of the elbows, glaucoma, and/or hearing impairment are also detected. *LMX1B* is highly expressed in podocytes, and patients can also display an involvement of the kidney comprising proteinuria, nephrotic syndrome, or renal insufficiency. Overall, nephropathy is reported in approximately 40% of affected patients (microalbuminuria or overt proteinuria)[52] but ESRD in less than 10%.[53] Interestingly, renal involvement appears significantly more frequent in females and in patients with a positive family history of NPS nephropathy.[52] In NPS patients with renal involvement, electron microscopy shows collagen fibrillike deposition in the GBM with typical lucent areas.[54] These characteristic ultrastructural changes can be present even in patients without apparent nephropathy.[55] Large genotype-phenotype studies have demonstrated that individuals with an *LMX1B* mutation located in the homeodomain show a significantly higher frequency of renal protein loss and higher values of proteinuria than subjects with mutations in the LIM domains.[52] However, no clear genotype-phenotype association is apparent for extrarenal manifestations.

Insight into Lmx1b function has been further obtained by the generation of *Lmx1b* knock-out animals.[56] In *Lmx1b*(–/–) mice the expression of GBM collagens is reduced and podocytes have a reduced number of foot processes, are dysplastic, and lack typical SD structures. Interestingly, mRNA and protein levels for CD2AP and podocin are greatly reduced in these kidneys and several *LMX1B* binding sites were identified in the putative regulatory regions of both *CD2AP* and *NPHS2* (encoding podocin).[56] These observations support a cooperative role for Lmx1b, CD2AP, and podocin in foot process and SD formation (see Figure 13-2).

PLCE1 Gene Mutations Associated with Autosomal Recessive Nephrotic Syndrome

A new gene locus for nephrotic syndrome *(NPHS3)* was recently mapped to chromosome 10q23-q24. Positional candidate genes were selected based on increased gene expression levels in a rat glomerulus differential expression database, and six different homozygous truncating mutations in six different kindreds were identified in the *PLCE1* gene.[57] Interestingly, two of the individuals with truncating *PLCE1* mutations entered remission following steroid or cyclosporin A treatment. The observation of a possible responsiveness to immunosuppression in *PLCE1* mutation carriers awaits confirmation in a larger number of affected patients.

PLCE1 codes for the enzyme phospholipase C epsilon-1, which is involved in intracellular signal transduction. *PLCE1* is widely expressed in many tissues, including the podocytes. The knock-down of *pcle1* in zebrafish is associated with the development of podocyte foot process effacement and edematous outer appearance of the fish,[57] confirming a specific role of phospholipase C epsilon-1 in the maintenance of the glomerular filtration barrier. Still, the pathogenesis of isolated podocyte damage and development of proteinuria in patients lacking phospholipase C epsilon-1 remains to be elucidated.

Recessive SRNS with Sensorineural Deafness

In 2003 Ruf et al. mapped a novel gene locus for recessive SRNS on chromosome 14q24.2 in a large consanguineous Palestinian kindred with SRNS and deafness.[58] The causative genetic defect is still unidentified.

HEREDITARY DISORDERS WITH LATE-ONSET NEPHROTIC SYNDROME

Hereditary late-onset FSGS is a heterogeneous condition generally transmitted in an autosomal dominant fashion. Three disease loci (FSGS1, FSGS2, and FSGS3) have been mapped in affected families, and as a result the responsible genetic defects have been identified.

ACTN4 Gene Mutations

In 1998 a locus for autosomal dominant late-onset FSGS (FSGS1) was mapped to chromosome 19q13 (FSGS1),[59] and mutations in *ACTN4* were identified as the underlying pathogenic cause.[60] *ACTN4* encodes for α-actinin-4, an actin-bundling protein of the cytoskeleton highly expressed in podocytes. Both a knock-down and an overexpression transgenic mouse model have been established for *Actn4*, demonstrating proteinuria and podocyte alterations. It was therefore discussed that α-actinin-4 plays an important role for the cytoskeletal function of the podocyte. Young knock-out mice present with focal areas of foot process effacement, and older animals present with diffuse effacement and globally disrupted podocyte morphology.[61] Moreover, *Actn4* was shown to be upregulated in the kidneys of different animal models of proteinuria. Human *ACTN4* mutations were identified in three different families with FSGS.[60] The clinical course in affected family members was characterized by progressively increasing proteinuria starting in adolescence and developing into FSGS and chronic renal insufficiency later in adult life. ESRD was observed in a number of affected individuals. All *ACTN4* mutations identified so far represent nonconservative amino acid substitutions affecting the actin-binding domain of α-actinin-4. In vitro studies demonstrated that mutant α-actinin-4 binds filamentous actin more strongly than wild-type protein. Based on this observation it was proposed that dominant mutations in *ACTN4* interfere with the maintenance of podocyte architecture: a proper organization of the cytoskeleton seems to be important for normal functioning of podocyte foot processes. Interestingly, however, not all mutation carriers of the families reported by Kaplan et al. displayed with a renal phenotype. The observed incomplete penetrance suggests that additional factors (genetic or nongenetic) are involved in the pathogenesis, which in conjunction with a mutation in *ACTN4* lead to the manifestation of FSGS. *ACTN4* mutations may confer disease susceptibility, as also discussed for mutations in *CD2AP* and *TRPC6*. However, mutations in *ACTN4* represent a rare cause of hereditary FSGS, accounting for approximately 4% of familial FSGS.[62]

TRPC6 Gene Mutations

In 1999 a second gene locus for autosomal dominant FSGS (FSGS2) was mapped to chromosome 11q21-q22 using a 399-member Caucasian kindred of British heritage dating back seven generations.[63] Fourteen deceased family members had suffered from ESRD, 14 living family members were on dialysis or had undergone renal transplantation, and 3 individuals were proteinuric. Six years later, the responsible gene, *TRPC6*, was identified.[64,65] *TRPC6* encodes the transient receptor potential cation channel TRPC6 that is thought to mediate capacitative calcium entry into cells. Expression analysis revealed that TRPC6 is highly expressed in the kidney and also in podocytes at the site of the SD. A dominant missense mutation was identified in the original family studied by Winn et al., and five additional families with mutations in TRPC6 were characterized by Reiser et al. Two of the missense mutations in the latter study were shown to increase the current amplitudes of TRPC6, consistent with a gain-of-function effect of the mutations. Interestingly, however, both studies describe carrier individuals with a normal renal phenotype, pointing to an incomplete penetrance of the mutations. *TRPC6* mutations have been identified in very few children; early disease onset seems to be exceptional. So far it is unknown how the dysfunction of a cation channel is related to the development of podocyte damage and loss of the glomerular filtration barrier. One hypothesis is related to the observation that MEC-2, a *C. elegans* homologue of podocin, participates in the mechanosensation of the worm. MEC-2 is physically and functionally linked to ion channels, transducing the signals of mechanosensation. Because TRPC6 interacts with podocin and nephrin at the SD, it was proposed that podocin takes part in mechanosensation processes at the glomerular filtration barrier, transducing signals to TRPC6 that in turn modulates intracellular calcium concentrations in the podocyte. Nephrin, on the other hand, is thought to stimulate different pathways of the intracellular signaling machinery. Therefore, a complex protein network involving nephrin, podocin, CD2AP, and the cation channel TRPC6 is established to maintain the SD structure of the foot process. Mutations in TRPC6 likely affect this functional network by altering the intracellular calcium concentration of the podocyte.

CD2AP Gene Mutations

In 1999, FSGS3 was shown to map to chromosome 6 and reported to be caused by haploinsufficiency for *CD2AP*.[66] *CD2AP* encodes for the CD2-associated protein CD2AP, an actin-binding protein that was originally identified as a cytoplasmic ligand of the CD2 receptor on T and natural killer cells. *CD2AP* knock-out mice presented not only with impaired immune functions but also with severe NS and FSGS, accompanied by mesangial hypercellularity and extracellular matrix deposition.[67] Electron microscopy showed the typical loss of podocyte foot process integrity with process effacement and loss of the SD structure. Screening in FSGS patients led to identification of a dominant *CD2AP* mutation (a 2-bp substitution altering the exon 7 splice acceptor site) in two adult patients with late-onset FSGS.[66] An enhanced disease susceptibility for FSGS conferred by the change in CD2AP expression was postulated as the underlying pathogenic mechanism. CD2AP interacts with nephrin and both proteins localize to lipid rafts in the plasma membrane,[32] suggesting that CD2AP is required to connect nephrin (and thus the SD) to the cytoskeleton of the podocyte. An impairment of CD2AP function might be associated with enhanced cytoskeletal fragility, predisposing to podocyte damage. Since the initial description of *CD2AP* mutations in two patients, no additional human mutations have been reported. Hence the overall role of CD2AP for human disease remains to be elucidated.

SYNDROMAL DISORDERS ASSOCIATED WITH NEPHROTIC SYNDROME

A large number of syndromes have been described on clinical grounds with patients displaying proteinuria (steroid resistant) in addition to various extrarenal manifestations. Renal histology usually reveals FSGS lesions, but DMS may also be observed. Classification of the syndromal entity is usually based on characteristic accompanying extrarenal manifestations. A genetic basis has been identified in only a minority of these syndromes. Here we discuss two important syndromes that invariably present with SRNS: Schimke syndrome and Galloway-Mowat syndrome.

Schimke Syndrome

Schimke immunoosseous dysplasia maps to chromosome 2q34-36 and is caused by recessive mutations in the *SMARCAL1* gene.[68] *SMARCAL1* encodes the SWI/SNF-related, matrix-associated, actin-dependent regulator of chromatin subfamily a-like protein 1, a protein involved in the remodeling of chromatin to change nucleosome compaction for gene regulation, replication, recombination, and DNA repair. The clinical phenotype of Schimke immunoosseous dysplasia is characterized by growth retardation caused by spondyloepiphyseal dysplasia, a slowly progressive immune defect, cerebral infarcts, skin pigmentation, and SRNS beginning in childhood. FSGS lesions are frequently observed in kidney biopsy specimens and the majority of patients progress to ESRD. However, disease severity and age at onset follow a continuum from early onset and severe symptoms, with death early in life, to later onset and mild symptoms, with survival into adulthood. Genotype-phenotype studies suggest that recessive loss-of-function mutations (frameshift, stop, and splice-site mutations) are generally associated with a more severe course of the disease, whereas some missense mutations allow retention of partial *SMARCAL1* function and thus cause milder disease.[68]

Galloway-Mowat Syndrome

Galloway-Mowat syndrome (GMS) is characterized by microcephaly and other brain anomalies, severe mental retardation, and early-onset NS (CNS).[69] Both FSGS and DMS were observed in kidney biopsies of affected individuals.[69,70] An important number of patients also show hiatus hernia. Both males and females are affected and an occurrence in siblings of the same family has been reported. These observations point to a possible autosomal recessive mode of inheritance, but no gene locus has thus far been identified. However, as different genetic research groups work hard to map the causative gene locus, new insights into the pathology of GMS can be anticipated.

CLINICAL ASPECTS

Clinical aspects of NS are discussed in detail in earlier chapters. Here we want to focus on issues specific for genetic forms of SRNS.

Therapeutic Implications

In general, therapy for SRNS is demanding. Numerous immunosuppressive agents have shown some efficacy in a fraction of the SRNS population; these include cyclophosphamide, azathioprine, cyclosporin, and mycophenolate mofetil, mostly in combination with glucocorticoids. However, genetically determined forms of SRNS have proven insensitive to immunosuppressive interventions, which is pathophysiologically explained by the presence of intrinsic defects in podocyte architecture and function. Hence it is suggested that children with hereditary SRNS, especially with *NPHS2* mutations, be spared from any form of immunosuppressive treatment. Conversely, *NPHS2* mutations have never been reported in patients with SSNS, so screening for this mutation seems not to be indicated even in patients with reduced steroid sensitivity (such as frequent relapsers or those who are steroid dependent).

Antiproteinuric pharmacological treatment with ACE inhibitors or AT1 receptor blockers is probably effective in slowing down the progression of renal insufficiency, although efficacy has not been formally proven in carriers of individual mutations.

Living-Related Donor Transplantation

Living-related kidney transplantation is generally considered the therapy of choice in pediatric patients with ESRD. However, in patients affected by SRNS caused by germline mutations in podocyte genes, several aspects need to be considered. First, it is yet unknown how kidneys of a heterozygous donor behave and develop in a recipient with recessive SRNS. Parents of affected children with recessive SRNS each carry one mutant allele that is also present in the transplanted kidney. It could be speculated that these kidneys are more easily prone to develop proteinuria if other proproteinuric factors (e.g., arterial hypertension, salt-rich diet) are superposed. So far animal models of SRNS do not support this hypothesis and comprehensive human data addressing this question are lacking. Consequences for the donor should also be considered. It is still unknown whether the prognosis of the remaining single kidney in the heterozygous parental donor is impaired by the gene mutation. Again, the remaining heterozygous kidney may be more susceptible to proteinuric disease than are single kidneys of individuals without mutations. Up to now our experience with living-related donor transplantation in hereditary SRNS is limited and does not support a restriction in affected children. Still, careful surveillance of both donor and recipient seems advisable.

In families of patients affected by autosomal dominant late-onset SRNS, only one of the parents is a carrier of the pathogenic sequence variation. Genetic testing of family members will help delineate mutation carriers in the family. If the mutation occurred as a de novo mutation in the patient, both parents are equally suitable for living-donor transplantation from a genetic point of view.

Recurrence of Nephrotic Syndrome after Renal Transplantation

Many investigators have studied the pathogenesis of increased glomerular permeability and recurrence of proteinuria after transplantation in FSGS. In general, recurrence of proteinuria after renal transplantation is observed in approximately 30% of FSGS patients.[71] This risk appears higher in children than in adult patients.[72] Affected patients display with proteinuria, which is often in the nephrotic range. Frequently, proteinuria recurs within a few days after renal transplantation. In children, the mean time to recurrent proteinuria is 14 days posttransplant.[73] Recurrence of proteinuria/FSGS following renal transplantation negatively impacts graft survival in both children and adult patients. Risk factors are an age less than 15 years, rapid progression of renal insufficiency, and diffuse mesangial proliferation in the initial biopsy of the native kidney.[74] In nonhereditary FSGS/SRNS, recurrence of proteinuria has been discussed to follow a T-cell dysfunction and production of proteinuric circulating factor(s), such as using an in vitro bioassay of glomerular permeability to albumin. Savin et al. proposed the existence of a circulating proteinuric factor that predisposes to the development of posttransplant proteinuria recurrence.[75]

In *NPHS2*-associated SRNS/FSGS, recurrence of posttransplant proteinuria is a rare phenomenon, observed in less than 10% of transplant patients.[39,40] Interestingly, the in vitro test of glomerular permeability has also shown high values in a few patients with proven recessive *NPHS2* mutations and posttransplant recurrence,[76] and an important role of circulating serum factors has been discussed to explain this phenomenon in hereditary SRNS. However, these factors were not identified in all patients with *NPHS2* mutations and with recurrence of proteinuria after transplantation.[77] Therefore, possible proteinuric factors are not the only cause of posttransplant recurrence in patients with *NPHS2* mutations.[78] The biochemical nature of proteinuric factors has yet to be determined. Identification of a homozygous truncating *NPHS2* mutation in one patient with posttransplant NS prompted the search for antipodocin antibodies, but all results were negative, excluding a de novo glomerulonephritis as the underlying cause.[40] Antipodocin antibodies were also not identifiable in patients with *NPHS2* missense mutations and posttransplant NS.

In CNF, the risk of a recurrence of proteinuria after transplantation seems to be important: it was demonstrated that especially patients affected by the Fin major mutation have a risk of approximately 25% of posttransplant NS. Subsequent studies revealed that the pathogenesis of this recurrence is related to the development of antinephrin antibodies directed against the wild-type nephrin protein residing in the transplanted kidney,[79] analogous to the anti-GBM antibodies against type IV collagen causing posttransplant de novo glomerulonephritis in patients with Alport syndrome. Treatment options of posttransplant NS in these patients are scarce; a subset of patients seems to respond to cyclophosphamide.[79]

Genetic Counseling

Positive results of mutational analysis in pediatric patients with SRNS should be followed by adequate genetic counseling. This demands close collaboration between pediatric nephrologists and human geneticists. Parents of children affected by recessive disease will have a 25% chance of giving birth to another affected child. In parents of children with dominant disease, this risk amounts to 50% (with the exception of patients with de novo mutations; the risk of recurrence in these families is very low). Parents of affected children need to be informed that treatment options are limited in hereditary SRNS and that renal function may deteriorate rapidly. Close monitoring of renal function and early treatment of complications of chronic renal insufficiency are advised. In autosomal dominant FSGS, genetic counseling might be difficult because of incomplete penetrance and variable expressivity. It seems that individual mutation carriers can be affected to differing degrees, with an obvious mild phenotype in some family members and ESRD in others. Genetic counseling is not only important for parents but also for the affected child. Children with recessive disease will transmit a heterozygous mutation to their own future children, but as long as the other parent is not a mutation carrier, all offspring will be healthy. Patients affected by dominant FSGS will transmit the pathogenic mutation in 50% of cases, but offspring carrying the mutation might also be affected by FSGS.

In some cases established genotype-phenotype correlations might be helpful to estimate the risk of a more severe clinical course. In *NPHS2*-associated SRNS, for example, some mutations have been associated with early onset and aggravated clinical course, whereas other mutations were shown to be less pathogenic.[40] For other disease entities, the analysis of clinical symptoms of other affected family members can help predict the severity of the disease: in NPS, the risk of having a child with NPS nephropathy is about 1 : 4 and the risk of having a child in whom renal failure will develop is about 1 : 10 if NPS nephropathy occurs in other family members.[53] Genetic counseling is especially important in families affected by NS with serious prognosis. In children affected by CNS with female outer appearance, mutation analysis in *WT1* is mandatory in order to rule out risk of Wilms' tumor development.

ACKNOWLEDGMENT

I would like to thank Martin Zenker (Institute of Human Genetics, University of Erlangen-Nuremberg) for his reflections on Pierson syndrome.

REFERENCES

1. Rose EA, Glaser T, Jones C et al: Complete physical map of the WAGR region of 11p13 localizes a candidate Wilms' tumor gene, *Cell* 60:405-508, 1990.
2. Gessler M, Poustka A, Cavenee W et al. Homozygous deletion in Wilms tumours of a zinc-finger gene identified by chromosome jumping, *Nature* 343:774-78, 1990.
3. Haber DA, Buckler AJ, Glaser T et al: An internal deletion within an 11p13 zinc finger gene contributes to the development of Wilms' tumor, *Cell* 61:1257-69, 1990.
4. Schumacher V, Schneider S, Figge A et al: Correlation of germ-line mutations and two-hit inactivation of the WT1 gene with Wilms tumors of stromal-predominant histology, *Proc Nat Acad Sci* 94: 3972-77, 1997.
5. Pelletier J, Bruening W, Kashtan CE et al: Germline mutations in the Wilms' tumor suppressor gene are associated with abnormal urogenital development in Denys-Drash syndrome, *Cell* 67(2):437-47, 1991.
6. Barbaux S, Niaudet P, Gubler MC et al: Donor splice-site mutations in WT1 are responsible for Frasier syndrome, *Nat Genet* 17(4):467-70, 1997.
7. Jeanpierre C, Denamur E, Henry I et al: Identification of constitutional WT1 mutations, in patients with isolated diffuse mesangial sclerosis, and analysis of genotype/phenotype correlations by use of a computerized mutation database, *Am J Hum Genet* 62(4):824-33, 1998.
8. Habib R, Gubler MC, Antignac C et al: Diffuse mesangial sclerosis: a congenital glomerulopathy with nephrotic syndrome, *Adv Nephrol Necker Hosp* 22:43-57, 1993.
9. Maalouf EF, Ferguson J, van Heyningen V et al: In utero nephropathy, Denys-Drash syndrome and Potter phenotype, *Pediatr Nephrol* 12(6):449-51, 1998.
10. Habib R, Loirat C, Gubler MC et al: The nephropathy associated with male pseudohermaphroditism and Wilms' tumor (Drash syndrome): a distinctive glomerular lesion–report of 10 cases, *Clin Nephrol* 24(6):269-78, 1985.
11. Hu M, Zhang GY, Arbuckle S et al: Prophylactic bilateral nephrectomies in two paediatric patients with missense mutations in the WT1 gene, *Nephrol Dial Transplant* 19(1):223-26, 2004.
12. Niaudet P, Gubler MC: WT1 and glomerular diseases, *Pediatr Nephrol* 21(11):1653-60, 2006.
13. Little M, Wells C. A clinical overview of WT1 gene mutations, *Hum Mutat* 9(3):209-25, 1997.
14. Gao F, Maiti S, Sun G et al: The Wt1+/R394W mouse displays glomerulosclerosis and early-onset renal failure characteristic of human Denys-Drash syndrome, *Mol Cell Biol* 24(22):9899-910, 2004.
15. Frasier SD, Bashore RA, Mosier HD: Gonadoblastoma associated with pure gonadal dysgenesis in monozygous twins, *J Pediatr* 64:740-45, 1964.
16. Gubler MC, Yang Y, Jeanpierre C et al: WT1, renal development, and glomerulopathies, *Adv Nephrol Necker Hosp* 29:299-315, 1999.
17. Denamur E, Bocquet N, Baudouin V et al: WT1 splice-site mutations are rarely associated with primary steroid-resistant focal and segmental glomerulosclerosis, *Kidney Int* 57(5):1868-72, 2000.
18. Koziell AB, Grundy R, Barratt TM et al: Evidence for the genetic heterogeneity of nephropathic phenotypes associated with Denys-Drash and Frasier syndromes, *Am J Hum Genet* 64(6):1778-81, 1999.
19. Kaplinsky C, Ghahremani M, Frishberg Y et al: Familial Wilms' tumor associated with a WT1 zinc finger mutation, *Genomics* 38(3):451-53, 1996.
20. Rapola J. Congenital nephrotic sindrome, *Pediatr Nephrol* 1(3):441-46, 1987.
21. Kestila M, Mannikko M, Holmberg C et al: Congenital nephrotic syndrome of the Finnish type maps to the long arm of chromosome 19, *Am J Hum Genet* 54: 757-64, 1994.
22. Kestila M, Lenkkeri U, Mannikko M et al: Positionally cloned gene for a novel glomerular protein—nephrin—is mutated in congenital nephrotic syndrome, *Mol Cell* 1(4):575-82, 1998.
23. Coulthard MG. Management of Finnish congenital nephrotic syndrome by unilateral nephrectomy, *Pediatr Nephrol* 3(4):451-53, 1989.
24. Holmberg C, Antikainen M, Ronnholm K et al: Management of congenital nephrotic syndrome of the Finnish type, *Pediatr Nephrol* 9(1):87-93, 1995.
25. Pomeranz A, Wolach B, Bernheim J et al: Successful treatment of Finnish congenital nephrotic syndrome with captopril and indomethacin, *J Pediatr* 126(1):140-42, 1995.
26. Kovacevic L, Reid CJ, Rigden SP: Management of congenital nephrotic syndrome, *Pediatr Nephrol* 18(5):426-30, 2003.
27. Ruotsalainen V, Ljungberg P, Wartiovaara J et al: Nephrin is specifically located at the slit diaphragm of glomerular podocytes, *Proc Natl Acad Sci U S A* 96(14):7962-67, 1999.
28. Wartiovaara J, Ofverstedt LG, Khoshnoodi J et al: Nephrin strands contribute to a porous slit diaphragm scaffold as revealed by electron tomography, *J Clin Invest* 114(10):1475-83, 2004.
29. Huber TB, Kottgen M, Schilling B et al: Interaction with podocin facilitates nephrin signaling, *J Biol Chem* 276:41543-46, 2001.
30. Huber TB, Hartleben B, Kim J et al: Nephrin and CD2AP associate with phosphoinositide 3-OH kinase and stimulate AKT-dependent signaling, *Mol Cell Biol* 23: 4917-28, 2003.
31. Huber TB, Simons M, Hartleben B et al: Molecular basis of the functional podocin-nephrin complex: Mutations in the NPHS2 gene disrupt nephrin targeting to lipid raft microdomains, *Hum Mol Genet* 12: 3397-405, 2003.
32. Schwarz K, Simons M, Reiser J et al: Podocin, a raft-associated component of the glomerular slit diaphragm, interacts with CD2AP and nephrin, *J Clin Invest* 108:1621-29, 2001.
33. Simons K, Toomre D: Lipid rafts and signal transduction, *Nat Rev Mol Cell Biol* 1:31-39, 2000.
34. Koziell A, Grech V, Hussain S et al: Genotype/phenotype correlations of NPHS1 and NPHS2 mutations in nephrotic syndrome advocate a functional inter-relationship in glomerular filtration, *Hum Mol Genet* 11(4):379-88, 2002.
35. Bolk S, Puffenberger EG, Hudson J et al: Elevated frequency and allelic heterogeneity of congenital nephrotic syndrome, Finnish type, in the old order Mennonites, *Am J Hum Genet* 65(6):1785-90, 1999.
36. Fuchshuber A, Jean G, Gribouval O et al: Mapping a gene (SRN1) to chromosome 1q25-q31 in idiopathic nephrotic syndrome confirms a distinct entity of autosomal recessive nephrosis, *Hum Molec Genet* 4:2155-58, 1995.

37. Boute N, Gribouval O, Roselli S et al: NPHS2, encoding the glomerular protein podocin, is mutated in autosomal recessive steroid-resistant nephrotic syndrome, *Nat Genet* 24(4):349-54, 2000.
38. Roselli S, Heidet L, Sich M et al: Early glomerular filtration defect and severe renal disease in podocin-deficient mice, *Mol Cell Biol* 24:550-60, 2004.
39. Ruf RG, Lichtenberger A, Karle SM et al: Patients with mutations in NPHS2 (podocin) do not respond to standard steroid treatment of nephrotic syndrome, *J Am Soc Nephrol* 15(3):722-32, 2004.
40. Weber S, Gribouval O, Esquivel EL et al: NPHS2 mutation analysis shows genetic heterogeneity of steroid-resistant nephrotic syndrome and low post-transplant recurrence, *Kidney Int* 66(2):571-79, 2004.
41. Caridi G, Bertelli R, Di Duca M et al: Broadening the spectrum of diseases related to podocin mutations, *J Am Soc Nephrol* 14(5):1278-86, 2003.
42. Caridi G, Bertelli R, Scolari F et al: Podocin mutations in sporadic focal-segmental glomerulosclerosis occurring in adulthood. *Kidney Int* 64(1):365, 2003.
43. Schultheiss M, Ruf RG, Mucha BE et al: No evidence for genotype/phenotype correlation in NPHS1 and NPHS2 mutations, *Pediatr Nephrol* 19(12):1340-48, 2004.
44. Franceschini N, North KE, Kopp JB et al: NPHS2 gene, nephrotic syndrome and focal segmental glomerulosclerosis: a HuGE review, *Genet Med* 8(2):63-75, 2006.
45. Tsukaguchi H, Sudhakar A, Le TC et al: NPHS2 mutations in late-onset focal segmental glomerulosclerosis: R229Q is a common disease-associated allele, *J Clin Invest* 110(11):1659-66, 2002.
46. Pereira AC, Pereira AB, Mota GF et al: NPHS2 R229Q functional variant is associated with microalbuminuria in the general population, *Kidney Int* 65(3):1026-30, 2004.
47. Pierson M, Cordier J, Hervouuet F et al: An unusual congenital and familial congenital malformative combination involving the eye and the kidney, *J Genet Hum* 12:184-213, 1963.
48. Zenker M, Aigner T, Wendler O et al: Human laminin beta2 deficiency causes congenital nephrosis with mesangial sclerosis and distinct eye abnormalities, *Hum Mol Genet* 13(21):2625-32, 2004.
49. Hasselbacher K, Wiggins RC, Matejas V et al: Recessive missense mutations in LAMB2 expand the clinical spectrum of LAMB2-associated disorders, *Kidney Int* 70(6):1008-12, 2006.
50. Mark K, Reis A, Zenker M: Prenatal findings in four consecutive pregnancies with fetal Pierson syndrome, a newly defined congenital nephrosis syndrome, *Prenat Diagn* 26(3):262-66, 2006.
51. Chen H, Lun Y, Ovchinnikov D et al: Limb and kidney defects in Lmx1b mutant mice suggest an involvement of LMX1B in human nail patella syndrome, *Nat Genet* 19(1):51-55, 1998.
52. Bongers EM, Huysmans FT, Levtchenko E et al: Genotype-phenotype studies in nail-patella syndrome show that LMX1B mutation location is involved in the risk of developing nephropathy, *Eur J Hum Genet* 13(8):935-46, 2005.
53. Looij BJ Jr, te Slaa RL, Hogewind BL et al: Genetic counselling in hereditary osteo-onychodysplasia (HOOD, nail-patella syndrome) with nephropathy, *J Med Genet* 25(10):682-86, 1988.
54. Browning MC, Weidner N, Lorentz WB Jr: Renal histopathology of the nail-patella syndrome in a two-year-old boy, *Clin Nephrol* 29(4):210-13, 1988.
55. Taguchi T, Takebayashi S, Nishimura M et al: Nephropathy of nail-patella syndrome, *Ultrastruct Pathol* 12(2):175-83, 1988.
56. Miner JH, Morello R, Andrews KL et al: Transcriptional induction of slit diaphragm genes by Lmx1b is required in podocyte differentiation, *J Clin Invest* 109(8):1065-72, 2002.
57. Hinkes B, Wiggins RC, Gbadegesin R et al: Positional cloning uncovers mutations in PLCE1 responsible for a nephrotic syndrome variant that may be reversible, *Nat Genet* 38(12):1397-405, 2006.
58. Ruf RG, Wolf MT, Hennies HC et al: A gene locus for steroid-resistant nephrotic syndrome with deafness maps to chromosome 14q24.2, *J Am Soc Nephrol* 14(6):1519-22, 2003.
59. Mathis BJ, Kim SH, Calabrese K et al: A locus for inherited focal segmental glomerulosclerosis maps to chromosome 19q13, *Kidney Int* 53(2):282-86, 1998.
60. Kaplan JM, Kim SH, North KN et al: Mutations in ACTN4, encoding alpha-actinin-4, cause familial focal segmental glomerulosclerosis, *Nat Genet* 24(3):251-56, 2000.
61. Kos CH, Le TC, Sinha S et al: Mice deficient in alpha-actinin-4 have severe glomerular disease, *J Clin Invest* 111(11):1683-90, 2003.
62. Weins A, Kenlan P, Herbert S et al:. Mutational and Biological Analysis of alpha-actinin-4 in focal segmental glomerulosclerosis, *J Am Soc Nephrol* 16(12):3694-701, 2005.
63. Winn MP, Conlon PJ, Lynn KL et al: Linkage of a gene causing familial focal segmental glomerulosclerosis to chromosome 11 and further evidence of genetic heterogeneity, *Genomics* 58(2):113-20, 1999.
64. Winn MP, Conlon PJ, Lynn KL et al: A mutation in the TRPC6 cation channel causes familial focal segmental glomerulosclerosis, *Science* 308(5729):1801-04, 2005.
65. Reiser J, Polu KR, Moller CC et al: TRPC6 is a glomerular slit diaphragm-associated channel required for normal renal function, *Nat Genet* 37(7):739-44, 2005.
66. Kim JM, Wu H, Green G et al: CD2-associated protein haploinsufficiency is linked to glomerular disease susceptibility, *Science* 300:1298-300, 2003.
67. Shih, NY, Li J, Karpitskii V et al: Congenital nephrotic syndrome in mice lacking CD2-associated protein, *Science* 286:312-15, 1999.
68. Boerkoel CF, Takashima H, John J et al: Mutant chromatin remodeling protein SMARCAL1 causes Schimke immuno-osseous dysplasia. *Nat Genet* 30(2):215-20, 2002.
69. Galloway WH, Mowat AP: Congenital microcephaly with hiatus hernia and nephrotic syndrome in two sibs, J Med Genet. 1968; 5(4):319-21, 1968.
70. Garty BZ, Eisenstein B, Sandbank J et al: Microcephaly and congenital nephrotic syndrome owing to diffuse mesangial sclerosis: an autosomal recessive syndrome, *J Med Genet* 31(2):121-25, 1994.
71. Artero M, Biava C, Amend W et al: Recurrent focal glomerulosclerosis: natural history and response to therapy, *Am J Med* 92(4):375-83, 1992.
72. Senggutuvan P, Cameron JS, Hartley RB et al: Recurrence of focal segmental glomerulosclerosis in transplanted kidneys: analysis of incidence and risk factors in 59 allografts, *Pediatr Nephrol* 4(1):21-28, 1990.
73. Tejani A, Stablein DH: Recurrence of focal segmental glomerulosclerosis posttransplantation: a special report of the North American Pediatric Renal Transplant Cooperative Study, *J Am Soc Nephrol* 2(12 Suppl):S258-63, 1992.
74. Habib R, Hebert D, Gagnadoux MF et al: Transplantation in idiopathic nephrosis, *Transplant Proc* 14(3):489-95, 1982.
75. Savin VJ, Sharma R, Sharma M et al: Circulating factor associated with increased glomerular permeability to albumin in recurrent focal segmental glomerulosclerosis, *N Engl J Med* 334(14):878-83, 1996.
76. Carraro M, Caridi G, Bruschi M et al: Serum glomerular permeability activity in patients with podocin mutations (NPHS2) and steroid-resistant nephrotic syndrome, *J Am Soc Nephrol* 13(7):1946-52, 2002.
77. Höcker B, Knüppel T, Waldherr R et al: Recurrence of proteinuria 10 years post-transplant in NPHS2-associated focal segmental glomerulosclerosis after conversion from cyclosporin A to sirolimus, *Pediatr Nephrol* 21(10):1476-79, 2006.
78. Bertelli R, Ginevri F, Caridi G et al: Recurrence of focal segmental glomerulosclerosis after renal transplantation in patients with mutations of podocin, *Am J Kidney Dis* 41(6):1314-21, 2003.
79. Patrakka J, Ruotsalainen V, Reponen P et al: Recurrence of nephrotic syndrome in kidney grafts of patients with congenital nephrotic syndrome of the Finnish type: role of nephrin, *Transplantation* 73(3):394-403, 2002.

CHAPTER

14 Alport Syndrome and Thin Basement Membrane Nephropathy

Clifford E. Kashtan

The diseases associated with familial glomerular hematuria can currently be divided into three categories based on the site of the causative mutation (Table 14-1). The type IV collagen disorders include Alport syndrome (AS) and thin basement membrane nephropathy (TBMN), diseases that arise from mutations in three of the six type IV collagen genes—*COL4A3*, *COL4A4*, or *COL4A5*. Mutation in *COL4A3*, *COL4A4*, or *COL4A5*, or genetic linkage to one of these loci, has been established in all investigated cases of AS. About 40% of cases of TBMN exhibit mutation in *COL4A3* or COL4A4 or linkage to one of these genes.[1] The *MYH9* disorders, Epstein syndrome and Fechtner syndrome, are characterized clinically by autosomal dominant hereditary nephritis associated with deafness and macrothrombocytopenia, and result from mutations in *MYH9*, the gene that encodes nonmuscle myosin heavy chain IIA. The third category, "unknown," includes the approximately 60% of families with TBMN in which genetic linkage to type IV collagen loci has been excluded but no other locus has been identified to date. Together, AS and TBMN account for about 30% to 50% of children with isolated glomerular hematuria seen in pediatric nephrology clinics.[2-5]

Although a mechanistic explanation for the hematuria exhibited by patients with these disorders has not been firmly established, the fact that urine of otherwise normal individuals contains red blood cells suggests that familial hematuria may represent an exaggeration of a physiologic process of intermittent rupture and repair of glomerular capillary walls. Persistent hematuria could occur because of an increased frequency of ruptures, a less efficient repair process, or both. The tensile strength of the glomerular capillary wall of a subject with AS or TBMN has never been compared experimentally with that of a normal individual. However, if anterior lenticonus is accepted as an in vivo demonstration of the consequences of a weakened basement membrane (the anterior lens capsule), then the notion that the glomerular capillary walls of AS and TBMN patients are mechanically weak and that this weakness is secondary to deficiency of certain type IV collagen proteins becomes plausible.

ALPORT SYNDROME

The first description of a family with inherited hematuria appeared in 1902 in a report by Guthrie.[6] Subsequent monographs about this family by Hurst in 1923[7] and Alport in 1927[8] established that affected individuals in this family, particularly males, developed deafness and uremia. The advent of electron microscopy led to the discovery of unique glomerular basement membrane (GBM) abnormalities in patients with AS,[9-11] setting the stage for the histochemical[12-14] and genetic[15,16] studies that resulted in the identification of type IV collagen genes as the sites of disease-causing mutations.

Etiology and Pathogenesis

Type IV Collagen Proteins, Tissue Distribution, and Genes

The type IV collagen family of proteins consists of six α chains that, while genetically distinct, share several basic structural features: a major collagenous domain of approximately 1400 residues containing the repetitive triplet sequence glycine (Gly)-X-Y, in which X and Y represent a variety of other amino acids; a C-terminal noncollagenous (NC1) domain of approximately 230 residues; and a noncollagenous *N*-terminal sequence of 15 to 20 residues. The collagenous domains each contain approximately 20 interruptions of the collagenous triplet sequence, whereas each NC1 domain contains 12 completely conserved cysteine residues. Type IV collagen molecules are heterotrimers consisting of three α chains arising from self-association of NC1 domains and folding of the collagenous domains into triple helical structures. The specificity of chain association is determined by amino acid sequences within the NC1 domains and results in three trimeric species in vivo: $\alpha1_2\alpha2$, $\alpha3\alpha4\alpha5$, and $\alpha5_2\alpha6$.[17] Unlike interstitial collagens, which lose their NC1 domains and form fibrillar networks, type IV collagen trimers form open, nonfibrillar networks through NC1-NC1 and amino-terminal interactions.

$\alpha1_2\alpha2$ Trimers are found in all basement membranes. Distribution of $\alpha3\alpha4\alpha5$ and $\alpha5_2\alpha6$ trimers is more restricted. In normal human kidneys, $\alpha3\alpha4\alpha5$ trimers are found in GBM, Bowman's capsules, and basement membranes of distal tubules, whereas $\alpha5_2\alpha6$ trimers are detectable in Bowman's capsules and basement membranes of distal tubules and collecting ducts, but not in GBM.[18,19] $\alpha5_2\alpha6$ Trimers are present in normal epidermal basement membranes (EBMs), but $\alpha3\alpha4\alpha5$ trimers are not. $\alpha3\alpha4\alpha5$ Trimers also occur in several basement membranes of the eye and of the cochlea.[20-22]

TABLE 14-1 Familial Glomerular Hematurias

	Genetic Locus	Protein Product	Renal Symptoms	ESRD	GBM Ultrastructure	Extrarenal Manifestations
Type IV Collagen Disorders						
Alport syndrome						
X-linked	*COL4A5*	α5(IV)	Hematuria, proteinuria, hypertension	All males, some females	Thinning (early), lamellation (late)	Deafness, lenticonus, perimacular flecks
Autosomal recessive	*COL4A3* *COL4A4* (biallelic)	α3(IV) α4(IV)	Hematuria, proteinuria, hypertension	All males and females	Thinning (early), lamellation (late)	Deafness, lenticonus, perimacular flecks
Autosomal dominant	*COL4A3* *COL4A4* (heterozygous)	α3(IV) α4(IV)	Hematuria, proteinuria, hypertension	Males and females (late)	Thinning (early), lamellation (late)	Deafness
Thin basement membrane nephropathy	*COL4A3* *COL4A4* (heterozygous)	α3(IV) α4(IV)	Hematuria	Rare	Thinning	Rare
MYH9 Disorders						
Epstein syndrome	*MYH9* (heterozygous)	NMMHC-IIAA[3]	Hematuria, proteinuria	Yes	Lamellation	Deafness, large platelets
Fechtner syndrome	*MYH9* (heterozygous)	NMMHC-IIAA[3]	Hematuria, proteinuria	Yes	Lamellation	Deafness, large platelets, May-Hegglin anomaly
Unknown*						
	Unknown	Unknown	Hematuria	Rare	Thinning	Rare

ESRD, End-stage renal disease; *GBM*, glomerular basement membrane; *NMMHC-IIA*, nonmuscle myosin heavy chain IIA.
* This category includes familial cases of thin basement membrane nephropathy in which mutation in *COL4A3* or *COL4A4* has been excluded, with no other locus identified.

The six type IV collagen genes are distributed in adjacent pairs on three chromosomes. The *COL4A1* and *COL4A2* genes encode the α1(IV) and α2(IV) chains, respectively, and are located on chromosome 1. *COL4A3* and *COL4A4*, which encode the α3(IV) and α4(IV) chains, reside on chromosome 2. The α5(IV) and α6(IV) chains are encoded by the *COL4A5* and *COL4A6* genes on the X chromosome. The paired genes are arranged in a 5′-5′ fashion, separated by sequences of varying length containing regulatory elements.

Genetics

AS occurs in three genetic forms: X-linked (XLAS), autosomal recessive (ARAS), and autosomal dominant (ADAS). XLAS accounts for approximately 80% of patients with the disease and results from mutations in the *COL4A5* gene. Affected males are hemizygotes who carry a single mutant *COL4A5* allele, whereas affected females are heterozygotes carrying normal and mutant alleles. About 15% of people with AS have ARAS due to mutations in both alleles of *COL4A3* or *COL4A4*. These patients may be homozygotes, with identical mutations in both alleles of the affected gene, particularly if they have consanguineous parents, or they may be compound heterozygotes, with different mutations in the two alleles. The remaining AS patients—about 5%—have ADAS due to heterozygous mutations in *COL4A3* or *COL4A4*. Most individuals with heterozygous mutations in these genes have isolated, nonprogressive microscopic hematuria associated with thin GBMs or are asymptomatic. It is not clear why some people with heterozygous mutations in *COL4A3* or *COL4A4* develop a progressive nephropathy, that is, ADAS.

Several hundred mutations, most of which are unique, have been identified in the *COL4A5* gene in patients and families with XLAS.[23] A variety of mutation types have been described: large rearrangements (~20%), small deletions and insertions (~20%), missense mutations altering a glycine residue in the collagenous domain of α5(IV) (30%), other missense mutations (~8%), nonsense mutations (~5%), and splice-site mutations (~15%).[24] The type of *COL4A5* mutation, or *COL4A5* genotype, has a significant impact on the course of XLAS in affected males.[24,25] Those with a large deletion, nonsense mutation, or a small mutation changing the mRNA reading frame have a 90% risk of developing ESRD before age 30. In contrast, 70% of patients with a splice-site and 50% of patients with a missense mutation progress to ESRD before age 30.[24] The position of a glycine substitution may impact the disease course.[25] In contrast to males with XLAS, a statistical relationship between *COL4A5* genotype and renal phenotype cannot be demonstrated in females with XLAS, perhaps because of the overwhelming influence of random X-chromosome inactivation.[26]

Clinical Manifestations

The course of AS is heavily gender dependent. Males with XLAS or ARAS inevitably develop end stage renal disease (ESRD), although in males with XLAS the rate of progression is influenced by the nature of the *COL4A5* mutation. Most females with XLAS have nonprogressive or slowly progressive renal disease, but a significant minority demonstrates progression to ESRD. The course of AS is similar in males and females with ARAS. In general, patients with ADAS progress less rapidly than do patients with XLAS or ARAS.[27]

Renal Symptoms

Persistent microscopic hematuria (MH) occurs in all males with AS regardless of genetic type and is probably present from early infancy. Approximately 95% of heterozygous females with XLAS have persistent or intermittent MH,[26] and 100% of females with ARAS have persistent MH. Episodic gross hematuria is not unusual in affected boys and girls with AS.[28]

In males with XLAS and in males and females with ARAS, proteinuria typically becomes detectable in late childhood or early adolescence and is progressive. In one large cohort of females with XLAS, 75% were found to have proteinuria, although the timing of onset was not investigated.[26]

Blood pressure in childhood is typically normal, but, like proteinuria, hypertension is common in adolescent males with XLAS or ARAS and in females with ARAS. Most females with XLAS have normal blood pressure, but hypertension may develop, particularly in those with proteinuria.

All males with XLAS eventually require renal replacement therapy, with 50% reaching ESRD by age 25, 80% by age 40, and 100% by age 60.[24] Although there is much less data available on males and females with ARAS, the epidemiology of ESRD is probably similar to XLAS males. In patients with ADAS, the age at which 50% of patients have progressed to ESRD is approximately 50 years, or twice as long as XLAS males.[27]

The risk of ESRD is much lower in XLAS females than in XLAS males, but it is by no means trivial. About 12% of XLAS females reach ESRD by age 45, 30% by age 60, and 40% by age 80.[26] Risk factors for ESRD in XLAS females include proteinuria and sensorineural deafness.[26,29]

The Alport nephropathy progresses predictably through a series of clinical phases. Phase I typically lasts from birth until late childhood or early adolescence and is characterized by isolated hematuria, with normal protein excretion and renal function. In Phase II, proteinuria is superimposed on hematuria but renal function remains normal. Patients in Phase III exhibit declining renal function in addition to hematuria and proteinuria, and those in Phase IV have ESRD. These phases have histological correlates, as described later under Renal Histopathology. The rate of passage through these phases is primarily a function of the causative mutation, at least in males with XLAS. Patients with *COL4A5* mutations that prevent production of any functional protein (deletions, nonsense mutations) proceed through these phases more rapidly than those whose mutations allow synthesis of a functional, albeit abnormal, protein (some missense mutations). Random X inactivation is probably of critical importance in determining the rate of passage in females with XLAS, although this has yet to be proven. Females with XLAS can be viewed as passing through the same phases as males, but the rate of progression is typically so slow that the journey to ESRD is not completed during the individual's lifetime.

Hearing

Hearing is normal at birth in males with XLAS and in males and females with ARAS, but bilateral impairment of perception of high-frequency sounds often becomes detectable in late childhood. Sensorineural hearing loss (SNHL) is present in 50% of XLAS males by approximately age 15, 75% by age 25, and 90% by age 40.[24] In males with missense mutations in *COL4A5*, the risk of SNHL before age 30 is 60%, whereas the risk of SNHL before age 30 in those with other types of mutations is 90%.[24]

SNHL occurs less often in females with XLAS. About 10% of XLAS females have SNHL by age 40 and about 20% by age 60.[26] The hearing deficit is progressive and extends into the range of conversational speech with advancing age. Because the deficit usually does not exceed 60-70 dB and speech discrimination is preserved, affected individuals benefit from hearing aids.

SNHL has been localized to the cochlea.[30] In control cochleae, the α3(IV), α4(IV), and α5(IV) chains are expressed in the spiral limbus, the spiral ligament, and in the basement membrane situated between the organ of Corti and the basilar membrane.[31-33] However, these chains are not expressed in the cochleae of ARAS mice,[32] XLAS dogs,[33] or men with XLAS.[22] Examination of well-preserved cochleae from men with XLAS revealed a unique zone of separation between the organ of Corti and the underlying basilar membrane, as well as cellular infiltration of the tunnel of Corti and the spaces of Nuel.[34] These changes may be associated with abnormal tuning of basilar membrane motion and hair-cell stimulation, resulting in defective hearing.

Ocular Anomalies

Abnormalities of the lens and retina are common in individuals with AS, typically becoming apparent in the second to third decade of life in XLAS males and in both males and females with ARAS. Anterior lenticonus, which is considered virtually pathognomonic for AS,[35] was present in about 15% of a large cohort of XLAS males.[24] Dot-fleck retinopathy, a characteristic alteration of retinal pigmentation concentrated in the perimacular region,[36] was also found in about 15% of this cohort.[24] Recurrent corneal erosions[37,38] and posterior polymorphous dystrophy, manifested by clear vesicles on the posterior surface of the cornea,[39] have also been described in AS patients.

The α3(IV), α4(IV), and α5(IV) chains are normal components of the anterior lens capsule and other ocular basement membranes, and mutations that interfere with the formation or deposition of α3α4α5 trimers prevent expression of these chains in the eye.[20,31] The anterior lens capsules of AS patients with anterior lenticonus are markedly attenuated, especially over the central region of the lens, and exhibit focal areas of dehiscence.[40,41] This is perhaps the clearest example of the mechanical consequences of AS mutations. It does not take much of a leap to attribute the hematuria of AS to the structural weakness of the α3α4α5-deficient glomerular capillary wall.

Leiomyomatosis

Several dozen families in which AS is transmitted in association with leiomyomas of the esophagus and tracheobronchial tree have been described.[42] Affected individuals carry X-chromosomal deletions that involve the *COL4A5* gene and terminate within the second intron of the adjacent *COL4A6* gene.[43-45] Those affected tend to become symptomatic in late childhood and may exhibit dysphagia, postprandial vomiting, epigastric or retrosternal pain, recurrent bronchitis, dyspnea, cough, or stridor. Females with the Alport syndrome–leiomyomatosis complex typically have genital leiomyomas, with clitoral hypertrophy and variable involvement of the labia majora and uterus.

Renal Histopathology

Children with AS typically show little in the way of renal parenchymal changes by light microscopy before age 5. In older patients, mesangial hypercellularity and matrix expansion may be observed. As the disease progresses, focal segmental glomerulosclerosis, tubular atrophy, and interstitial fibrosis become the predominant light microscopic abnormalities. Although some patients exhibit an increase in immature glomeruli or interstitial foam cells, these changes are not specific for AS.

Electron microscopy of renal biopsy specimens is often diagnostic, although the expression of the pathognomonic lesion is age dependent and, for those with X-linked Alport syndrome, gender dependent. The classic ultrastructural lesion is diffuse thickening of the glomerular capillary wall, accompanied by "basket weave" transformation of the lamina densa, intramembranous vesicles, scalloping of the epithelial surface of the GBM, and disappearance of podocyte foot processes (Figure 14-1). These changes are more prevalent in affected males, typically becoming prominent in late childhood and adolescence. In early childhood the predominant ultrastructural lesion in males is diffuse attenuation of the GBM. Affected females can display a spectrum of lesions, including predominantly normal-appearing GBM; focal GBM attenuation; diffuse GBM attenuation; mixed attenuation

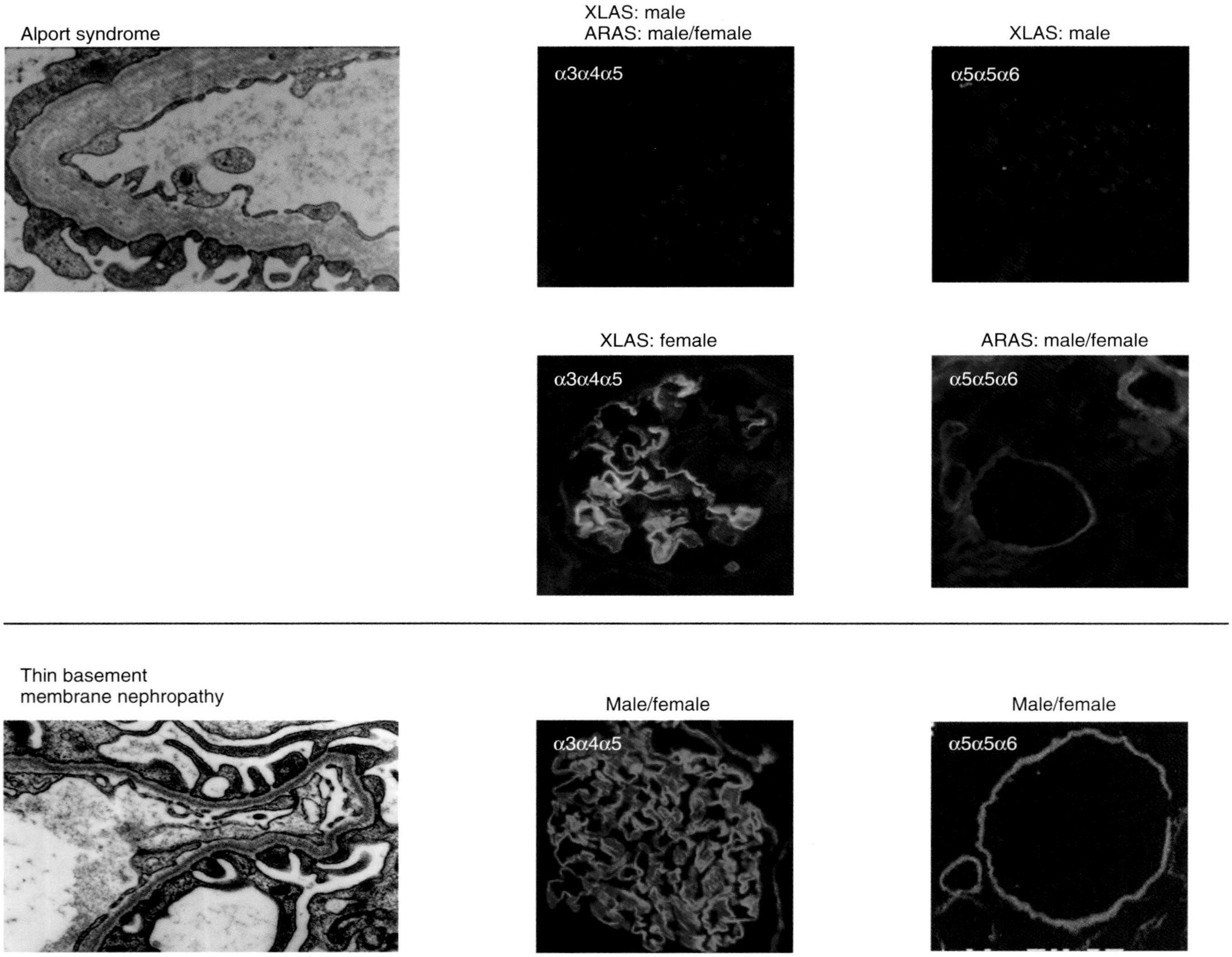

Figure 14-1 Typical findings on electron microscopy and type IV collagen immunostaining in Alport syndrome and thin basement membrane nephropathy. *ARAS*, autosomal recessive Alport syndrome; *XLAS*, X-linked Alport syndrome.

and thickening/basket weaving; and diffuse basket weaving. The extent of the GBM lesion progresses inexorably in males, although the rate of progression may be influenced by *COL4A5* genotype. Females may have static or progressive GBM lesions. X-chromosome inactivation pattern, age, and *COL4A5* genotype could all contribute to the dynamics of GBM change in affected females.

The classic GBM lesion is not found in all kindreds with AS. Adult patients who demonstrate only GBM thinning, yet have *COL4A5* mutations, have been described. Although these represent a minority of AS patients and families, they highlight the somewhat vague histological distinction between AS and TBMN. This issue is discussed further under Thin Basement Membrane Nephropathy.

Routine immunofluorescence microscopy is normal, or shows nonspecific deposition of immunoproteins, in patients with AS. In contrast, specific immunostaining for type IV collagen α chains is often diagnostic and can distinguish the X-linked and autosomal recessive forms of the disease (Figure 14-1). The utility of this approach derives from the fact that most disease-causing mutations in AS alter the expression of the α3α4α5 and $\alpha5_2\alpha6$ type IV collagen trimers in renal basement membranes. Most *COL4A5* mutations prevent expression of both trimer forms in the kidney, so that in about 80% of XLAS males, immunostaining of renal biopsy specimens for α3(IV), α4(IV), and α5(IV) chains is completely negative. About 60% to 70% of XLAS females exhibit mosaic expression of these chains, whereas in the remainder, immunostaining for these chains is indistinguishable from normal. The biallelic mutations in *COL4A3* and *COL4A4* that cause ARAS often prevent expression of α3α4α5 trimers but have no effect on expression of $\alpha5_2\alpha6$ trimers. In renal biopsy specimens from these patients, immunostaining for α3(IV) and α4(IV) chains is negative. However, although immunostaining of GBM for the α5(IV) chain is negative, because of the absence of α3α4α5 trimers, Bowman's capsules, distal tubular basement membranes, and collecting duct basement membranes are positive for α5(IV), because of the unimpaired expression of $\alpha5_2\alpha6$ trimers. Heterozygous carriers of a single *COL4A3* or *COL4A4* mutation have exhibited normal renal basement membrane immunostaining for α3(IV), α4(IV), and α5(IV) chains upon study.

The $\alpha5_2\alpha6$ trimer is a normal component of EBMs. Consequently, about 80% of males with XLAS can be diagnosed by skin biopsy on the basis of absence of α5(IV) expression in EBMs. In 60% to 70% of XLAS females there is a mosaic pattern of immunostaining for α5(IV). EBM expression of α5(IV) is normal in patients with ARAS and in subjects with heterozygous mutations in *COL4A3* or *COL4A4*.

Diagnosis and Differential Diagnosis

AS is just one potential cause of familial and sporadic glomerular hematuria. Accurate diagnosis rests on careful clinical evaluation, a precise family history, selective application of invasive diagnostic techniques, and, in appropriate patients, molecular diagnosis.

When a child with isolated hematuria has a positive family history for hematuria, an autosomal dominant pattern of inheritance, combined with a negative family history for ESRD, strongly suggests a diagnosis of benign TBMN. Less common conditions associated with familial glomerular hematuria include the autosomal dominant MYH9 disorders (Epstein syndrome and Fechtner syndrome), in which macrothrombocytopenia is a constant feature; familial IgA nephropathy; and X-linked membranoproliferative glomerulonephritis.

When family history for hematuria is negative, the differential diagnosis of isolated glomerular hematuria, or hematuria associated with proteinuria, includes IgA nephropathy, membranoproliferative glomerulonephritis, membranous nephropathy, lupus nephritis, postinfectious glomerulonephritis, and Henoch Schönlein nephritis, among others, in addition to AS and TBMN. Some of these conditions will be strongly suspected on the basis of clinical findings (e.g., rash and joint complaints), and others will be suggested by laboratory findings (e.g., hypocomplementemia).

Audiometry may be helpful in children above ages 6 to 8, especially in boys, in that high-frequency SNHL would point toward a diagnosis of AS. The presence of anterior lenticonus or the dot-fleck retinopathy may be diagnostic. However, these lesions are more prevalent in patients with advanced disease and are less likely to be present in young patients in whom diagnostic ambiguity tends to be the greatest.

Tissue studies are appropriate when clinical and pedigree information does not allow a diagnosis of benign familial hematuria and when AS cannot be ruled out by symptoms and laboratory findings. In some centers skin biopsy has become the initial invasive diagnostic procedure in patients suspected of AS, because the majority of subjects with XLAS will display abnormal expression of the α5(IV) chain in EBMs, as previously described. Normal EBM α5(IV) expression in a patient with hematuria has several possible explanations: (1) the patient has XLAS but his or her *COL4A5* mutation allows EBM expression of α5(IV); (2) the patient has ARAS or ADAS, in which α5(IV) expression is expected to be preserved; or (3) the patient has a disease other than AS. Renal biopsy would then provide the opportunity to diagnose other diseases, to examine type IV collagen α chain expression in renal basement membranes, and to evaluate GBM at the ultrastructural level.

Mutation analysis using direct sequencing is capable of identifying *COL4A5* mutations in up to 80% of males with XLAS.[46] High mutation detection rates in *COL4A3* and *COL4A4* in patients with ARAS are also possible, particularly if there is parental consanguinity. The availability of mutation analysis to clinicians varies considerably by locality. For example, mutation analysis is available in several countries in Western Europe, but there are no laboratories in the United States that currently offer such testing. An up-to-date listing of laboratories accepting specimens for type IV collagen gene analysis is available on the GeneReviews website (www.genereviews.org).

Treatment

Since there have been no controlled therapeutic trials in human AS, treatment recommendations are derived from animal studies and anecdotal clinical experience. Several therapeutic approaches have demonstrated efficacy in murine ARAS, including angiotensin interference,[47-49] inhibition of TGFβ-1,[50] chemokine receptor 1 blockade,[51] administration of bone morphogenic protein-7,[52] suppression of matrix metalloproteinases,[53] and bone marrow transplantation.[54] Angiotensin converting enzyme (ACE) inhibition also prolonged survival in a canine XLAS model.[55] Uncontrolled studies in human AS subjects have shown that ACE inhibition can reduce proteinuria, at least transiently.[56,57]

An uncontrolled study of a small group of boys and men with XLAS suggested that cyclosporine reduced proteinuria and stabilized renal function, and cyclosporine therapy prolonged survival of male dogs with XLAS.[58,59] However, results of another study suggested that cyclosporine may accelerate the development of interstitial fibrosis in AS patients.[60]

At this time, angiotensin blockade directed at suppressing proteinuria appears to be the safest option for slowing progression to ESRD in patients with AS. This approach utilizes agents that have been widely used in both children and adults with renal disease and hypertension and for which there is extensive clinical experience. Treatment of hypertension and other manifestations of advancing disease is, of course, an important component of therapy for AS.

Renal Transplantation

In general, outcomes following renal transplantation in patients with AS are excellent.[61] Clinicians involved in transplantation must address two important aspects of the disease. First, the donor selection process must avoid nephrectomy in relatives at risk for ESRD. Second, posttransplant management should provide surveillance for posttransplant anti-GBM nephritis, a complication unique to AS.

Informed donor evaluation requires familiarity with the genetics of AS and the signs and symptoms of the disease. In families with XLAS, 100% of affected males and approximately 95% of affected females exhibit hematuria. Consequently, males who do not have hematuria are not affected, and a female without hematuria has only about a 5% risk of being affected. Given an estimated 30% risk of ESRD in women with AS,[26] these women should generally be discouraged from kidney donation, even if hematuria is their only symptom.

Overt anti-GBM nephritis occurs in 3% to 5% of transplanted AS males.[62] Onset is typically within the first posttransplant year, and the disease usually results in irreversible graft failure within weeks to months of diagnosis. The risk of recurrence in subsequent allografts is high. In males with XLAS, the primary target of anti-GBM antibodies is the α5(IV) chain.[63,64] Both males and females with ARAS can develop posttransplant anti-GBM nephritis, and in these cases the primary antibody target is the α3(IV) chain.[63,65] The α3(IV) chain is also the target of Goodpasture autoantibodies, but the epitope identified by these antibodies differs from the α3(IV) epitope recognized by ARAS anti-GBM alloantibodies.[66]

THIN BASEMENT MEMBRANE NEPHROPATHY

The term *benign familial hematuria (BFH)* was historically used to describe kindreds displaying autosomal dominant transmission of isolated, nonprogressive glomerular hematuria.[67-69] Renal biopsy findings in these families are typically limited to GBM attenuation by electron microscopy. In 1996, Lemmink and colleagues were the first to report a heterozygous *COL4A4* mutation in a family with BFH.[70] *Thin basement membrane nephropathy* has gradually become the preferred term for hematuria associated with GBM attenuation, because it encompasses BFH, sporadic cases of isolated hematuria associated with thin GBM, and familial or sporadic cases of thin GBM in which hematuria is accompanied by proteinuria, hypertension, and/or renal insufficiency.

In discussing TBMN, it is important to recall that GBM thinning is a pathological description rather than a distinct, homogeneous entity (Table 14-2). GBM attenuation can result from hemizygous or heterozygous mutations in *COL4A5* (X-linked Alport syndrome, or XLAS), biallelic mutations in *COL4A3* or *COL4A4* (autosomal recessive Alport syndrome, or ARAS), heterozygous mutations in *COL4A3* or *COL4A4* (the carrier state for ARAS), or mutations at other unknown genetic loci.

It is the underlying cause of GBM attenuation that determines prognosis, perhaps in combination with remote modifier loci, rather than the GBM thinning itself. Hemizygous

TABLE 14-2 **Classification of Hematuric Conditions Associated with Thin Glomerular Basement Membranes**

	Inheritance	Clinical Features	Family History
Benign familial hematuria (BFH)	Autosomal dominant	Isolated hematuria	Positive for hematuria; negative for ESRD
Thin basement membrane nephropathy (TBMN)	Autosomal dominant or sporadic*	Isolated hematuria; some have proteinuria, HTN, CRI	May be negative for hematuria; may be positive for HTN, CRI
Alport syndrome†	XL (80%), AR (15%), AD (5%)	Isolated hematuria in young patients; proteinuria, HTN, CRI develop with age; SNHL, ocular lesions	Positive for hematuria in ~85% of XL patients and ~50% of AR patients; may be positive for SNHL, ESRD

AD, Autosomal dominant; *AR*, autosomal recessive; *CRI*, chronic renal insufficiency; *ESRD*, end-stage renal disease; *HTN*, hypertension; *SNHL*, sensorineural hearing loss; *XL*, X-linked.

* About 40% of patients/families with BFH or TBMN have mutations in *COL4A3* or *COL4A4* or exhibit linkage to these loci. The genetic loci are currently unknown in approximately 60%.

† Glomerular basement membrane thinning is often the predominant ultrastructural abnormality in children with Alport syndrome.

mutations in *COL4A5* and biallelic mutations in *COL4A3* or *COL4A4* lead to progressive GBM thickening and renal failure, whereas heterozygous mutations in *COL4A3* or *COL4A4* are usually associated with persistent GBM attenuation and a less severe outcome. Women with heterozygous mutations in *COL4A5* are arrayed across the middle of the prognostic spectrum. The range of outcomes likely reflects differences between cellular responses to complete absence of α3α4α5 trimers (ARAS and hemizygous XLAS), mixed α3α4α5-positive and α3α4α5-negative GBM (heterozygous XLAS), and homogeneous reduction in α3α4α5 content (heterozygous *COL4A3* or *COL4A4* mutations).

Etiology and Pathogenesis

The essential features of the type IV collagen protein family are discussed in the preceding section on Alport syndrome. By immunofluorescence, renal basement membranes of individuals with TBMN show no abnormalities in the expression of the type IV collagen α3-α6 chains, in contrast to patients with AS[14,71] (Figure 14-1). Since these studies have not used quantitative methodologies, it is possible that heterozygous mutations in *COL4A3* or *COL4A4* result in reduction of α3α4α5(IV) trimers in GBM.

It is assumed that the attenuated GBM of TBMN and early AS is mechanically fragile and that, as a result, the glomerular capillary wall has an increased potential for rupture at physiologic levels of intracapillary pressure. This mechanism remains theoretical in that it has never been tested in vivo or in the laboratory.

However, there is indirect evidence in support of this hypothesis. Persistent microscopic hematuria is more common in women, who have relatively thin GBM.[72] Macroscopic hematuria, intermittent or persistent, is fairly common in children with AS but tends to disappear with age, perhaps because the GBM thickens and becomes less susceptible to rupture.[28]

Does the hematuria of these conditions result from persistent ruptures at rare sites, or do ruptures occur and undergo repair[73] at multiple sites contemporaneously? If there is a process of rupture and repair, it seems unlikely that it could be responsible for the progressive GBM thickening that occurs in AS patients but not in patients with TBMN.

The results of genetic studies in TBMN families were recently summarized.[1] Identification of mutations in *COL4A3* or *COL4A4*, or demonstration of genetic linkage to these loci, has been achieved in about 40% of TBMN families. About 20 mutations in *COL4A3* and *COL4A4*, predominantly single nucleotide substitutions, have been described in TBMN families.

Clinical Manifestations

Children with TBMN typically exhibit persistent microscopic hematuria, although intermittent microhematuria may be observed. Episodic gross hematuria may occur in association with acute infection. Blood pressure, renal function, and urine protein excretion are typically normal.[3,5] Extrarenal abnormalities such as hearing loss or ocular defects are unusual and probably unrelated.

Proteinuria appear to be more common in adults with TBMN, occurring in up to 30% of patients.[74-80] About 5% to 7% of adult TBMN patients exhibit elevation in serum creatinine.[74,78,80]

Histopathology

Patients with TBMN typically exhibit diffuse thinning of the lamina densa and, perhaps as a result, of the GBM as a whole. The thickness of normal GBM is age and gender dependent. Both the lamina densa and the GBM increase rapidly in thickness between birth and 2 years of age, followed by gradual thickening throughout childhood and adolescence.[81] GBM thickness in adult men exceeds that in adult women.[82]

Because a variety of techniques have been used to measure GBM width, there is no standard definition of "thin" GBM (Figure 14-1). The cutoff value in adults ranges from 250 nm to 330 nm depending on technique.[79,83] For children, the cutoff is in the range of 200-250 nm (250 nm is within 2SD of the mean at age 11).[3,4,84]

Podocyte foot process width is normal in TBMN. Light microscopy typically shows no abnormalities, especially in children. Adult TBMN patients with renal dysfunction or hypertension may exhibit premature glomerular obsolescence.[78] Routine immunofluorescence studies are typically unremarkable.

Diagnosis and Differential Diagnosis

IgA nephropathy, TBMN, and AS are the most common causes of glomerular hematuria in the pediatric population. Careful clinical evaluation and thorough pedigree analysis can help segregate children with glomerular hematuria into those who require renal biopsy or other tissue studies and those who can be followed prospectively without the need for tissue studies. Because adults with familial hematuria may not be aware that they are affected,[76] obtaining urinalyses on parents of children with hematuria may be helpful.

In a child with isolated microscopic hematuria, a strong family history of dominantly transmitted hematuria, and a negative family history for renal failure, a clinical diagnosis of TBMN can be made and renal biopsy withheld. These children should be monitored every 1 to 2 years for development of proteinuria or hypertension and to update the family history.

In a child with GBM attenuation and a negative or limited family history, the challenge for the clinician is to distinguish TBMN and AS. Results of audiometry and ophthalmologic examination may be helpful if abnormal, but the younger the child, the less useful these tests are, given the usual natural history of hearing loss and ocular changes in AS (see preceding section). Immunostaining for type IV collagen α3, α4, and α5 chains can be particularly helpful in these situations, as discussed in an earlier section under Alport Syndrome. Unfortunately, molecular analysis of type IV collagen genes is not readily available in all areas. Current information on molecular testing for type IV collagen disorders can be obtained from the GeneReviews website (www. genereviews. org).

Treatment

Treatment is not necessary for most TBMN patients, especially children, because the course of the disorder is typically benign. Adult patients with proteinuria are theoretically candidates for angiotensin blockade, although there are no specific studies in this area.

REFERENCES

1. Rana K, Wang YY, Buzza M, Tonna S, Zhang KW et al: The genetics of thin basement membrane nephropathy, *Semin Nephrol* 25:163-70, 2005.
2. Trachtman H, Weiss R, Bennett B, Griefer I: Isolated hematuria in children: indications for a renal biopsy, *Kidney Int* 25:94-99, 1984.
3. Schroder CH, Bontemps CM, Assmann KJM, Schuurmans-Stekhoven JH, Foidart JM: Renal biopsy and family studies in 65 children with isolated hematuria, *Acta Paediatr Scand* 79:630-36, 1990.
4. Lang S, Stevenson B, Risdon RA: Thin basement membrane nephropathy as a cause of recurrent haematuria in childhood, *Histopathology* 16:331-37, 1990.
5. Piqueras AI, White RH, Raafat F, Moghal N, Milford DV: Renal biopsy diagnosis in children presenting with hematuria, *Pediatr Nephrol* 12:386-91, 1998.
6. Guthrie LG: "Idiopathic" or congenital, hereditary and familial hematuria, *Lancet* 1:1243-46, 1902.
7. Hurst AF: Hereditary familial congenital haemorrhagic nephritis occurring in sixteen individuals in three generations, *Guy's Hosp Rec* 3:368-70, 1923.
8. Alport AC: Hereditary familial congenital haemorrhagic nephritis, *Br Med J* 1:504-06, 1927.
9. Hinglais N, Grunfeld J-P, Bois LE: Characteristic ultrastructural lesion of the glomerular basement membrane in progressive hereditary nephritis (Alport's syndrome), *Lab Invest* 27:473-87, 1972.
10. Spear GS, Slusser RJ: Alport's syndrome: emphasizing electron microscopic studies of the glomerulus, *Am J Pathol* 69:213-22, 1972.
11. Churg J, Sherman RL: Pathologic characteristics of hereditary nephritis, *Arch Pathol* 95:374-79, 1973.
12. Olson DL, Anand SK, Landing BH, Heuser E, Grushkin CM, Lieberman E: Diagnosis of hereditary nephritis by failure of glomeruli to bind anti-glomerular basement membrane antibodies, *J Pediatr* 96:697-99, 1980.
13. McCoy RC, Johnson HK, Stone WJ, Wilson CB: Absence of nephritogenic GBM antigen(s) in some patients with hereditary nephritis, *Kidney Int* 21:642-52, 1982.
14. Kashtan C, Fish AJ, Kleppel M, Yoshioka K, Michael AF: Nephritogenic antigen determinants in epidermal and renal basement membranes of kindreds with Alport-type familial nephritis, *J Clin Invest* 78:1035-44, 1986.
15. Atkin CL, Hasstedt SJ, Menlove L, Cannon L, Kirschner N et al: Mapping of Alport syndrome to the long arm of the X chromosome, *Am J Hum Genet* 42:249-55, 1988.
16. Barker DF, Hostikka SL, Zhou J, Chow LT, Oliphant AR: Identification of mutations in the COL4A5 collagen gene in Alport syndrome, *Science* 248:1224-27, 1990.
17. Hudson BG: The molecular basis of Goodpasture and Alport syndromes: beacons for the discovery of the collagen IV family, *J Am Soc Nephrol* 15:2514-27, 2004.
18. Yoshioka K, Hino S, Takemura T, Maki S, Wieslander J et al: Type IV Collagen α 5 chain: normal distribution and abnormalities in X-linked Alport syndrome revealed by monoclonal antibody, *Am J Pathol* 144:986-96, 1994.
19. Peissel B, Geng L, Kalluri R, Kashtan C, Rennke HG et al: Comparative distribution of the α1(IV), α5(IV) and α6(IV) collagen chains in normal human adult and fetal tissues and in kidneys from X-linked Alport syndrome patients, *J Clin Invest* 96:1948-57, 1995.
20. Cheong HI, Kashtan CE, Kim Y, Kleppel MM, Michael AF: Immunohistologic studies of type IV collagen in anterior lens capsules of patients with Alport syndrome, *Lab Invest* 70:553-57, 1994.
21. Cosgrove D, Kornak JM, Samuelson G: Expression of basement membrane type IV collagen chains during postnatal development in the murine cochlea, *Hearing Res* 100:21-32, 1996.
22. Zehnder AF, Adams JC, Santi PA, Kristiansen AG, Wacharasindhu C et al: Distribution of type IV collagen in the cochlea in Alport syndrome, *Arch Otolaryngol Head Neck Surg* 131:1007-13, 2005.
23. Lemmink HH, Schröder CH, Monnens LAH, Smeets HJM: The clinical spectrum of type IV collagen mutations, *Hum Mutat* 9:477-99, 1997.
24. Jais JP, Knebelmann B, Giatras I, De Marchi M, Rizzoni G et al: X-linked Alport syndrome: natural history in 195 families and genotype-phenotype correlations in males, *J Am Soc Nephrol* 11:649-57, 2000.
25. Gross O, Netzer KO, Lambrecht R, Seibold S, Weber M: Meta-analysis of genotype-phenotype correlation in X-linked Alport syndrome: impact on clinical counseling, *Nephrol Dial Transpl* 17:1218-27, 2002.
26. Jais JP, Knebelmann B, Giatras I, De Marchi M, Rizzoni G et al: X-linked Alport syndrome: natural history and genotype-phenotype correlations in girls and women belonging to 195 families: a "European Community Alport Syndrome Concerted Action" study, *J Am Soc Nephrol* 14:2603-10, 2003.
27. Pochet JM, Bobrie G, Landais P, Goldfarb B, Grunfeld J-P: Renal prognosis in Alport's and related syndromes: influence of the mode of inheritance, *Nephrol Dial Transpl* 4:1016-21, 1989.
28. Gubler M, Levy M, Broyer M, Naizot C, Gonzales G et al: Alport's syndrome: a report of 58 cases and a review of the literature, *Am J Med* 70:493-505, 1981.
29. Grunfeld J-P, Noel LH, Hafez S, Droz D: Renal prognosis in women with hereditary nephritis, *Clin Nephrol* 23:267-71, 1985.
30. Wester DC, Atkin CL, Gregory MC: Alport syndrome: clinical update, *J Am Acad Audiol* 6:73-79, 1995.
31. Kleppel MM, Santi PA, Cameron JD, Wieslander J, Michael AF: Human tissue distribution of novel basement membrane collagen, *Am J Pathol* 134:813-25, 1998.
32. Cosgrove D, Samuelson G, Meehan DT, Miller C, McGee J et al: Ultrastructural, physiological, and molecular defects in the inner ear of a gene-knockout mouse model of autosomal Alport syndrome, *Hearing Res* 121:84-98, 1998.
33. Harvey SJ, Mount R, Sado Y, Naito I, Ninomiya Y et al: The inner ear of dogs with X-linked nephritis provides clues to the pathogenesis of hearing loss in X-linked Alport syndrome, *Am J Pathol* 159:1097-104, 2001.
34. Merchant SN, Burgess BJ, Adams JC, Kashtan CE, Gregory MC et al: Temporal bone histopathology in alport syndrome, *Laryngoscope* 114:1609-18, 2004.
35. Nielsen CE: Lenticonus anterior and Alport's syndrome, *Arch Ophthalmol* 56:518-30, 1978.
36. Perrin D, Jungers P, Grunfeld JP, Delons S, Noel LH, Zenatti C: Perimacular changes in Alport's syndrome, *Clin Nephrol* 13:163-67, 1980.
37. Rhys C, Snyers B, Pirson Y: Recurrent corneal erosion associated with Alport's syndrome, *Kidney Int* 52:208-11, 1997.
38. Burke JP, Clearkin LG, Talbot JF: Recurrent corneal epithelial erosions in Alport's syndrome, *Acta Ophthalmol* 69:555-57, 1991.
39. Teekhasaenee C, Nimmanit S, Wutthiphan S, Vareesangthip K, Laohapand T et al: Posterior polymorphous dystrophy and Alport syndrome, *Ophthalmology* 98:1207-15, 1991.
40. Streeten BW, Robinson MR, Wallace R, Jones DB: Lens capsule abnormalities in Alport's syndrome, *Arch Ophthalmol* 105:1693-97, 1987.
41. Kato T, Watanabe Y, Nakayasu K, Kanai A, Yajima Y: The ultrastructure of the lens capsule abnormalities in Alport's syndrome, *Jpn J Ophthalmol* 42:401-05, 1998.
42. Antignac C, Heidet L: Mutations in Alport syndrome associated with diffuse esophageal leiomyomatosis, *Contrib Nephrol* 117:172-82, 1996.
43. Antignac C, Knebelmann B, Druout L, Gros F, Deschenes G et al: Deletions in the COL4A5 collagen gene in X-linked Alport syndrome: characterization of the pathological transcripts in non-renal cells and correlation with disease expression, *J Clin Invest* 93:1195-207, 1994.
44. Zhou J, Mochizuki T, Smeets H, Antignac C, Laurila P et al: Deletion of the paired α5(IV) and α6(IV) collagen genes in inherited smooth muscle tumors, *Science* 261:1167-69, 1993.

45. Segal Y, Peissel B, Renieri A, de Marchi M, Ballabio A et al: LINE-1 elements at the sites of molecular rearrangements in Alport syndrome-diffuse leiomyomatosis, *Am J Hum Genet* 64:62-29, 1999.
46. Martin P, Heiskari N, Zhou J, Leinonen A, Tumelius T et al: High mutation detection rate in the COL4A5 collagen gene in suspected Alport syndrome using PCR and direct DNA sequencing, *J Am Soc Nephrol* 9:2291-301, 1998.
47. Gross O, Schulze-Lohoff E, Koepke ML, Beirowski B, Addicks K et al: Antifibrotic, nephroprotective potential of ACE inhibitor vs AT1 antagonist in a murine model of renal fibrosis, *Nephrol Dial Transplant* 19:1716-23, 2004.
48. Gross O, Beirowski B, Koepke ML, Kuck J, Reiner M et al: Preemptive ramipril therapy delays renal failure and reduces renal fibrosis in COL4A3-knockout mice with Alport syndrome, *Kidney Int* 63:438-46, 2003.
49. Gross O, Koepke ML, Beirowski B, Schulze-Lohoff E, Segerer S, Weber M: Nephroprotection by antifibrotic and anti-inflammatory effects of the vasopeptidase inhibitor AVE7688, *Kidney Int* 68:456-63, 2005.
50. Sayers R, Kalluri R, Rodgers KD, Shield CF, Meehan DT, Cosgrove D: Role for transforming growth factor-beta 1 in Alport renal disease progression, *Kidney Int* 56:1662-73, 1999.
51. Ninichuk V, Gross O, Reichel C, Kandoga A, Pawar RD et al: Delayed chemokine receptor 1 blockade prolongs survival in collagen 4A3-deficient miche with Alport disease, *J Am Soc Nephrol* 16:977-85, 2005.
52. Zeisberg M, Bottiglio C, Kumar N, Maeshima Y, Strutz F et al: Bone morphogenic protein-7 inhibits progression of chronic renal fibrosis associated with two genetic mouse models, *Am J Physiol Renal Physiol* 285:F1060-67, 2003.
53. Zeisberg M, Khurana M, Rao VH, Cosgrove D, Rougier JP et al: Stage-specific action of matrix metalloproteinases influences progressive hereditary kidney disease, *PLoS Med* 3:e100, 2006.
54. Sugimoto H, Mundel TM, Sund M, Xie L, Cosgrove D, Kalluri R: Bone-marrow-derived stem cells repair basement membrane collagen defects and reverse genetic kidney disease, *Proc Natl Acad Sci U S A* 103:7321-26, 2006.
55. Grodecki KM, Gains MJ, Baumal R, Osmond DH, Cotter BV, Valli VE, Jacobs RM: Treatment of X-linked hereditary nephritis in Samoyed dogs with angiotensin converting enzyme inhibitor, *J Comp Pathol* 117:209-25, 1997.
56. Cohen EP, Lemann J: In hereditary nephritis angiotensin-converting enzyme inhibition decreases proteinuria and may slow the rate of progression, *Am J Kid Dis* 27:199-203,1996.
57. Proesmans W, Van Dyck M: Enalapril in children with Alport syndrome, *Pediatr Nephrol* 19:271-75, 2004.
58. Callis L, Vila A, Carrera M, Nieto J: Long-term effects of cyclosporine A in Alport's syndrome, *Kidney Int* 55:1051-56, 1999.
59. Chen D, Jefferson B, Harvey SJ, Zheng K, Gartley CJ et al: Cyclosporine A slows the progressive renal disease of Alport syndrome (X-linked hereditary nephritis): results from a canine model, *J Am Soc Nephrol* 14:690-98, 2003.
60. Charbit M, Dechaux M, Gagnadoux M, Grunfeld J, Niaudet P: Cyclosporine A therapy in Alport syndrome, *J Am Soc Nephrol* 14:111A, 2003.
61. Kashtan CE, McEnery PT, Tejani A, Stablein DM: Renal allograft survival according to primary diagnosis: a report of the North American Pediatric Renal Transplant Cooperative Study, *Pediatr Nephrol* 9:679-84, 1995.
62. Kashtan CE: Renal transplantation in patients with Alport syndrome, *Pediatr Transpl* 10:651-57, 2006.
63. Brainwood D, Kashtan C, Gubler MC, Turner AN: Targets of alloantibodies in Alport anti-glomerular basement membrane disease after renal transplantation, *Kidney Int* 53:762-66, 1998.
64. Dehan P, Van Den Heuvel LPWJ, Smeets HJM, Tryggvason K, Foidart J-M: Identification of post-transplant anti-$\alpha5$(IV) collagen alloantibodies in X-linked Alport syndrome, *Nephrol Dial Transpl* 11:1983-88, 1996.
65. Kalluri R, van den Heuvel LP, Smeets HJM, Schroder CH, Lemmink HH et al: A COL4A3 gene mutation and post-transplant anti-$\alpha3$(IV) collagen alloantibodies in Alport syndrome, *Kidney Int* 47:1199-204, 1995.
66. Wang XP, Fogo AB, Colon S, Giannico G, Abul-Ezz SR et al: Distinct epitopes for anti-glomerular basement membrane Alport alloantibodies and Goodpasture autoantibodies within the noncollagenous domain of alpha3(IV) collagen: a Janus-faced antigen, *J Am Soc Nephrol* 16:3563-71, 2005.
67. Marks MI, Drummond KN: Benign familial hematuria, *Pediatrics* 44:590-93, 1969.
68. McConville JM, West CD, McAdams AJ: Familial and nonfamilial benign hematuria, *J Pediatr* 69:207-14, 1996.
69. Pardo V, Berian MG, Levi DF, Strauss J: Benign primary hematuria: clinicopathologic study of 65 patients, *Am J Med* 67:817-22, 1979.
70. Lemmink HH, Nillesen WN, Mochizuki T, Schröder CH, Brunner HG et al: Benign familial hematuria due to mutation of the type IV collagen $\alpha4$ gene, *J Clin Invest* 98:1114-18,1996.
71. Pettersson E, Tornroth T, Wieslander J: Abnormally thin glomerular basement membrane and the Goodpasture epitope, *Clin Nephrol* 33:105-09, 1990.
72. Dische FE, Anderson VER, Keane SJ, Taube D, Bewick M, Parsons V: Incidence of thin membrane nephropathy: morphometric investigation of a population sample, *J Clin Pathol* 43:457-60, 1990.
73. Liapis H, Foster K, Miner JH: Red cell traverse through thin glomerular basement membrane, *Kidney Int* 61:762-63, 2002.
74. Auwardt R, Savige J, Wilson D: A comparison of the clinical and laboratory features of thin basement membrane disease (TBMD) and IgA glomerulonephritis (IgA GN), *Clin Nephrol* 52:1-4, 1999.
75. Badenas C, Praga M, Tazon B, Heidet L, Arrondel C et al: Mutations in the COL4A4 and COL4A3 genes cause familial benign hematuria, *J Am Soc Nephrol* 13:1248-54, 2002.
76. Blumenthal SS, Fritsche C, Lemann J: Establishing the diagnosis of benign familial hematuria: the importance of examining the urine sediment of family members, *JAMA* 259:2263-66, 1998.
77. Goel S, Davenport A, Goode NP, Shires M, Hall CL et al: Clinical features and outcome of patients with thin and ultrathin glomerular membranes, *QJM* 88:785-93, 1995.
78. Nieuwhof CM, de Heer F, de Leeuw P, van Breda Vriesman PJ: Thin GBM nephropathy: premature glomerular obsolescence is associated with hypertension and late onset renal failure, *Kidney Int* 51:1596-601, 1997.
79. Tiebosch ATMG, Frederik PM, van Breda Vriesman PJC, Mooy JMV, van Rie H et al: Thin-basement-membrane nephropathy in adults with persistent hematuria, *N Engl J Med* 320:14-18, 1989.
80. Van Paassen P, van Breda Vriesman PJ, van Rie H, Tervaert JW: Signs and symptoms of thin basement membrane nephropathy: a prospective regional study on primary glomerular disease—The Limburg Renal Registry, *Kidney Int* 66:909-13, 2004.
81. Vogler C, McAdams AJ, Homan SM: Glomerular basement membrane and lamina densa in infants and children: an ultrastructural evaluation, *Pediatr Pathol* 7:527-34, 1997.
82. Steffes MW, Barbosa J, Basgen JM, Sutherland DER, Najarian JS, Mauer SM: Quantitative glomerular morphology of the normal human kidney, *Kidney Int* 49:82-86, 1983.
83. Dische FE: Measurement of glomerular basement membrane thickness and its application to the diagnosis of thin-membrane nephropathy, *Arch Pathol Lab Med* 116:43-49, 1992.
84. Milanesi C, Rizzoni G, Braggion F, Galdiolo D: Electron microscopy for measurement of glomerular basement membrane width in children with benign familial hematuria, *Appl Pathol* 2:199-204, 1984.

CHAPTER 15

Steroid-Sensitive Nephrotic Syndrome

Elisabeth M. Hodson, Stephen I. Alexander, and Nicole Graf

Nephrotic syndrome is characterized by massive proteinuria, hypoalbuminemia, and generalized edema. Nephrotic syndrome in children is divided into idiopathic, congenital (occurring in the first year of life), or secondary to diseases such as Henoch Schönlein nephritis or systemic lupus erythematosus. Between 1967 and 1974, the International Study of Kidney Disease in Childhood (ISKDC) enrolled 521 children age 12 weeks to 16 years with idiopathic nephrotic syndrome in order to evaluate the histopathologic, clinical, and laboratory characteristics of nephrotic syndrome in children. The renal biopsy studies demonstrated that about 80% of children had either minimal change disease (MCD 76.4%), focal and segmental glomerulosclerosis (FSGS 6.9%), or mesangioproliferative glomerulonephritis (MesPGN 2.3%).[1] Subsequently the ISKDC demonstrated that the response to corticosteroids was highly predictive of renal histology, with 93% of children with MCD achieving complete remission following an 8-week course of prednisone.[2] However, between 25% and 50% of children with MesPGN or FSGS on biopsy also responded to prednisone.[2] Now renal biopsy is generally limited to children with unusual clinical features at presentation or to children who fail to respond to corticosteroids. Because most children do not undergo renal biopsy at diagnosis, children with idiopathic nephrotic syndrome are now classified according to their initial response to corticosteroids into steroid-sensitive nephrotic syndrome (SSNS) or steroid-resistant nephrotic syndrome (SRNS). Although many children with SSNS have one or more relapses, the majority continue to respond to corticosteroids throughout their subsequent course,[3-5] and the long-term prognosis for complete resolution with normal renal function is good. This chapter is devoted to SSNS. Commonly used definitions for SSNS and SRNS are shown in Table 15-1.

EPIDEMIOLOGY

In Europe, the United States, and Australia, the overall incidence of idiopathic nephrotic syndrome is 1 to 3 per 100,000 children below age 16,[6-9] with a cumulative prevalence of 16 per 100,000 children.[7] The incidence is higher in Asian,[6,10,11] African American,[8] and Arab[12] children. In Asian children residing in northern England, the overall rates are 7.4 (95% confidence intervals [CI] 5.3-9.5) for South Asian children compared with 1.6 (95% CI 1.3-1.8) per 100,000 children per year for non–South Asian children[6] with 88% responsive to corticosteroids. In Libya an incidence of 11.6 per 100,000 children was reported,[12] with 98% responsive to corticosteroids. In African American children, rates of 2.8 to 3.6 per 100,000 per year have been reported compared with 1.8 to 2.3 in Caucasian children.[7,8]

SSNS is more common in boys than in girls, with a male/female ratio of around 2 : 1 and a peak incidence between 1 and 4 years.[1,6,7] There is a decreasing trend with increasing age in the incidence of idiopathic nephrotic syndrome overall and of the proportion with SSNS (Table 15-2). SSNS is less common in African[13] and African American children.[8] In South Africa only 7.2% of 236 African children had SSNS compared with 62% of 286 Indian children.[13] In the past 2 decades the proportion of children with idiopathic nephrotic syndrome who respond to corticosteroids appears to be falling when compared with 1978 ISKDC data.[1] Among 159 Canadian children age 6 months to 19 years, the proportion with SSNS fell from 81% between 1985 and 1993 to 65% between 1993 and 2002; this was accompanied by an increase in biopsy-documented FSGS from 11% to 25%.[14] Similar increases in FSGS have been reported from South Africa[13] and the United States.[8]

ETIOLOGY AND PATHOGENESIS

A T-Cell Disease

In 1974 a series of clinical observations led Dr. Shaloub to propose that SRNS was due to an abnormality in T-cell function.[15] Nephrotic syndrome had been observed in patients with Hodgkins lymphoma and cases of thymoma.[16,17] The disease was noted to remit in children who had measles, which led some to propose using measles as a therapeutic strategy.[18-20] A major effect of the measles virus is that it inhibits cell-mediated immunity, thereby shutting down T-cell function. Furthermore, the response of nephrotic syndrome to T-cell suppressive agents such as steroids or calcineurin inhibitors also supported their role in nephrotic syndrome.[15] These features all suggest that lymphocytes are key cells in SSNS.

A Circulating Factor

MCD appears to exist in a spectrum with FSGS. A proportion of children with MCD on clinical and histologic grounds develop FSGS.[21] In both there appears to be a circulating factor, with FSGS children being less responsive to therapeu-

TABLE 15-1 **Definitions Used in Idiopathic Nephrotic Syndrome**[124,199,209,210]

Classification	Definition
Nephrotic syndrome	Edema, proteinuria >40 mg/m^2/hr or protein/creatinine ratio >0.2 g/mmol (>2 g/g) or 50 mg/kg/day or 3-4+ on urine dipstick, hypoalbuminemia <25 g/L (<2.5 mg/100 ml)
Remission	Urinary protein excretion ≤4 mg/m^2/hr or 0-trace of protein on urine dipstick or protein/creatinine ratio <0.02 g/mmol (<0.2 g/g) for 3 consecutive days
Initial responder	Attainment of complete remission within initial 8 weeks of corticosteroid therapy
Initial nonresponder/steroid resistance	Failure to achieve remission during initial 8 weeks of corticosteroid therapy
Relapse	Urinary protein >40 mg/m^2/hr or protein/creatinine ratio >0.2 g/mmol (>2 g/g) or 2+ protein or more on urine dipstick for 3 consecutive days
Infrequent relapse	One relapse within 6 months of initial response or one to three relapses in any 12-month period
Frequent relapse	Two or more relapses within 6 months of initial response or four or more relapses in any 12-month period
Steroid dependence	Two consecutive relapses during corticosteroid therapy or within 14 days of ceasing therapy
Late nonresponder	Proteinuria for >8 weeks following one or more remissions

TABLE 15-2 **Nephrotic Syndrome in Yorkshire, UK, 1987-1998**

	STEROID-SENSITIVE NEPHROTIC SYNDROME		STEROID-RESISTANT NEPHROTIC SYNDROME		ALL PRIMARY NEPHROTIC SYNDROME	
Age Group (Years)	Incidence*	95% CI†	Incidence	95% CI	Incidence	95% CI
0-<1	0.5	0.0-1.1	0.2	0.0-0.5	0.5	0.0-1.1
1-4	4.1	3.3-5.0	0.5	0.2-0.8	4.6	3.7-5.5
5-9	1.7	1.2-2.3	0.2	0.0-0.4	1.9	1.4-2.5
10-15	0.9	0.6-1.2	0.2	0.1-0.4	1.1	0.7-1.5
Total	2.0	1.7-2.3	0.3	0.2-0.4	2.3	2.0-2.6

*Incidence per 100,000 patient years in children aged 0-15 years.
†Confidence intervals.
Reproduced from McKinney PA, Feltbower RG, Brocklebank JT, Fitzpatrick MM: Time trends and ethnic patterns of childhood nephrotic syndrome in Yorkshire, UK, *Pediatr Nephrol* 16(12):1040-44, 2001.

tic agents for various reasons. Within this group is a subset of children in which the disease resides in structural changes in the glomeruli with genetic mutations in key glomerular slit process proteins, including nephrin, podocin, Actinin 4, and WT-1. These are described elsewhere but in brief are associated with no response to steroids and progression to end-stage renal failure, and do not show evidence of a circulating factor as demonstrated by rapid recurrence of disease in a transplanted kidney. The timing of response with the return to normal function taking days to weeks is also supportive of slow podocyte recovery from an injurious cytokine. The higher rates of recurrence in children with FSGS receiving living-related kidneys suggests that there may be a degree of HLA restriction of response, which is also supported by HLA-linkage studies showing that increased incidence of disease is tied to certain alleles such as HLA B8, B13, DWQ2, DQB10301, and DR7.[22-25]

Over the years various growth factors and cytokines have been proposed as pathogenic in SSNS. The initial identification of the vascular permeability factor (VPF), now called vascular endothelial growth factor (VEGF), was thought to have identified the key protein leading to nephrotic syndrome.[26-28] However, identification of this protein in normal urine delayed further investigation of its role. More recently it has been noted to be increased in urine during relapses of nephrotic syndrome though circulating levels are unchanged, suggesting that VEGF levels reflect the concomitant proteinuria.[29,30] Recent tissue-restricted knockouts of VEGF in mice restricted to podocytes have demonstrated a key role for local VEGF in maintaining glomerular endothelial integrity and again have reinforced its importance, though perhaps more locally, in maintaining permeability.[31,32] Soluble immune response suppressor (SIRS) was also identified as a cytokine in patients with SRNS, but again the inability to consistently characterize this protein despite many mechanistic observations led to its exclusion as the likely factor.[27,28,33]

Other circulating factors have been proposed, and the development of a functional assay of glomerular permeability by Dr. Savin in the late 1990s identified a proteinuric factor that was small, highly glycosylated, and hydrophobic.[34] This appeared likely to allow fractionation of nephrotic sera, which would allow identification of the factor. Other observations that protein A columns could remove the nephrotic factor posttransplant also seemed to point to identifying features.[35]

In addition, recent induction of proteinuria in rats with transfer of serum may allow models that can identify this factor.[36]

The central role of T cells in disease has led to a number of strategies to help identify the underlying defect. The thought that the disease was caused by a low-frequency pathogenic clone has given way to a view that there is a generalized alteration in the lymphocytes that is triggered in these individuals and can then be switched off by treatment. This has been studied in several ways, including assessment of T-cell–derived cytokine responses either directly in plasma or by measurement of supernatants from activated mononuclear cells or measurement of RNA, assessment of T-cell subsets by immunophenotyping, or finally by functional assays of cell-mediated immunity.

Phenotypes of Cytokine-Secreting T Cells: Th1, Th2, Treg, and Th17

On activation, naive T cells become polarized into different subsets defined by their cytokine production and driven by the cytokine milieu in which they are activated. The initial division of T cells occurs as CD4 (originally "helper") T cells that respond to exogenous antigen presented by antigen-presenting cells in the context of MHC Class II, and CD8 (originally "effector") T cells that respond to internal antigens presented by all cells. CD4 T cells are further divided into Th1 and Th2 cells based on the cytokines they produce.[37] This was initially observed in mice, but human Th1 cells also produce cytokines such as IFN-gamma and TNF, which are used in cell-mediated immune responses. Th2 cells produce IL-4, IL-5, and IL-13, which are key to humoral immunity and are used by B cells to class switch and also act as growth factors for eosinophils.[38,39] It is now apparent that CD8 T cells can produce cytokines and be polarized to Tc1 and Tc2, expressing similar cytokines to those in CD4 Th cell subsets.[40] The observation that allergy is more common in children with nephrotic syndrome suggests that this might be a Th2 disease.[41] A subset of T cells thought to suppress activity in other T cells was originally described as suppressor T cells, and these have recently been reclassified as regulatory T cells (Tregs). They are thymically derived and express regulatory cytokines such as TGF-β and IL-10, and regulatory molecules such as CTLA-4. A key marker of these cells is expression of the transcription factor foxp3.[42-44] Interestingly there is now another T-cell subset that is an alternative to regulatory T cells, which is called the Th17 cell because it expresses the cytokine IL-17. Th17 cells are induced by IL-23 but can be generated by IL-6 and TGF-β, thus acting as an alternate pathway of development to regulatory T cells.[44,45]

In general, studies of cytokines in nephrotic syndrome have been disappointing. No clear upregulation of Th2-type cytokines has been demonstrated. Studies of serum from patients in remission show IL-1 unchanged; IL-2 normal or undetected in four of five studies; sIL-2R increased in four of six studies; IFN-gamma normal or not detected in three studies and increased in two; IL-4 normal or decreased; IL-8 normal, increased, and decreased in four studies; IL-10, IL-12, and IL-13 either normal or not detected; and TNF-α normal in three of four studies.[46] Studies of culture supernatants of stimulated mononuclear cells from children with active SSNS are also highly variable, although four studies suggest elevated IL-4, two studies elevated IL-12, and five studies elevated TNF-α. RNA measurements for specific cytokines in blood have been equally unrewarding as have those using intracellular cytokine staining.[46] Urinary reports are confounded by concurrent proteinuria, but there has been a recent report of IL-17 increased in urine of SSNS patients.[26,47] Other non–T-cell inflammatory proteins associated with SSNS include neopterin, which is produced by activated macrophages and is increased in SSNS.[48]

Molecular Studies

Other molecular strategies have been used. These include comparisons of the RNA expressed in CD2-positive cells during relapse and remission. These comparisons showed limited Th1-like and Th2-like profiles but also expression of early thymic-type genes, suggesting that the lymphocytes involved might be recent emigrants from the thymus. Other comparative arrays have shown an upregulation of TRAIL RNA but no increase in secreted TRAIL, a T-cell death effector molecule.[49,50] Other studies in FSGS renal tissue show upregulation of CD8 T-cell effector molecules.[51] Although a role for the signaling molecule NFκB has been suggested, studies find differences in expression of its components only in SRNS.[52-54] Gene linkage other than HLA linkage has shown that in familial SSNS a locus exists at 2p12-p13.2 with an logarithm of the odds (LOD) score greater than 3.0.[55] Although a number of candidate genes exist in this region, none have yet been identified in these families as causing disease.

Role of the Thymus

The expression data just mentioned, the association of nephrotic syndrome with T-cell lymphomas and thymomas, the timing of thymic involution occurring around puberty at the same time as the resolution of relapses for the majority of children with uncomplicated SSNS, and the exquisite sensitivity of thymocytes to steroids all suggest a role for early T cells or other thymically derived cells in SSNS. However, clear evidence for this is not yet available.

Role of Infection

Although there has been no exact infectious agent identified as inducing nephrotic syndrome, there is an identifiable viral prodrome in about 50% of relapse cases. Whether this merely reflects cytokine release with the initiation of nephrotic syndrome or is an initiation of the disease by a viral trigger is not clear.

Summary

Although evidence supports a role for T cells activated to secrete a permeability factor, identifying the specific T-cell changes or characterization of the factor remains a major challenge in SSNS.

HISTOPATHOLOGY

SSNS comprises a spectrum of disease that includes MCD, MesPGN (also known as diffuse mesangial hypercellularity), IgM nephropathy, and FSGS. Although these diseases are readily distinguished on biopsy, the clinical significance of the distinction remains controversial, with significant overlap in behavior and variation in morphologic diagnosis over time in a small proportion of cases. This confusion is reflected in the literature. Some studies suggest a difference in behavior between those with and those without mesangial hypercellularity in the absence of immune deposits.[56] Other studies suggest an increased risk of steroid resistance and/or development of focal sclerosing lesions with MesPGN/IgM nephropathy,[57,58] with some studies documenting transition of MCD, MesPGN, and IgM nephropathy to FSGS in frequently relapsing patients over time.[21,59] Additional studies suggest that response to therapy in cases with immune deposition is "unpredictable"[60] or variable.[61] Finally, a number of studies have failed to find any significant difference in outcomes among these categories.[62,63] Regardless of histopathology, children with disease resistant to steroids generally have a poorer outcome than those with responsive disease.[64] The ultimate prognosis for children with primary nephrotic syndrome and frequently relapsing disease associated with mesangial hypercellularity, positive immunofluorescence, or both remains difficult to predict.

Minimal Change Disease

The defining histologic feature of MCD is normal-appearing glomeruli on light microscopic examination (Figure 15-1). This assumes that the specimen has an adequate sample of glomeruli, including deep glomeruli from the juxtamedullary region of the renal cortex. Glomeruli of normal young children are generally smaller than adults', so they appear relatively hypercellular. There is no significant expansion of mesangial matrix and no increase in mesangial cellularity (either by increased numbers of mesangial cells or infiltration by inflammatory cells). The cytoplasm of the podocytes may appear to be mildly swollen or vacuolated. Glomerular capillary loops remain patent and in many cases may appear mildly dilated. The glomerular capillary walls are thin, with no evidence of basement membrane thickening. No basement membrane reduplication or epithelial spike formation is evident on examination of silver-stained sections. The presence of an occasional glomerular "tip" lesion, defined as adhesion of the tuft to the Bowman's capsule at the site of the opening of the proximal convoluted tubule, may be seen in MCD, provided the glomerulus is otherwise normal in size and cellularity.[65,66] The interstitium is normal without significant inflammation, fibrosis, or tubular atrophy. Proximal tubule epithelial cells may contain hyaline droplets consistent with protein loss.

The immunofluoresence in MCD is negative. Small amounts of IgM or C3 are considered by some to be compatible with MCD; however, any significant immune reactant, even in the setting of histologically normal glomeruli, effectively excludes this diagnosis.[60,63,64] Clinical significance of these immune-positive cases with normal histology is still controversial, and many now consider that these cases represent a spectrum of disease rather than distinct entities. Electron microscopic examination of untreated MCD shows uniform abnormality of the podocytes, with marked effacement of the foot processes over at least 50% of the glomerular capillary surface, resulting in a smooth homogenous layer of epithelial cell cytoplasm that lacks the normal interdigitation. The cytoplasm of the cells may be enlarged, with clear vacuoles and prominence of organelles. This is accompanied by microvillus transformation along the urinary surface of the podocytes (Figure 15-2). The glomerular basement membrane otherwise appears normal, as do the mesangial cells and matrix. Immune deposits are absent. These changes are commonly modified with steroid treatment, and the degree of foot process effacement may be incomplete if the biopsy is taken from a partially treated patient.

Mesangial Proliferative Glomerulopathy

Light microscopic examination of MesPGN shows generalized, diffuse mesangial cell hyperplasia, involving more than

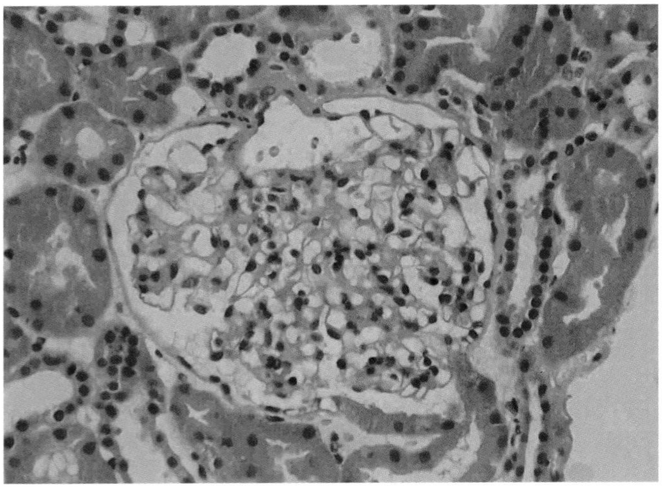

Figure 15-1 The glomerulus appears normal to light microscopic examination, with normal mesangial matrix and cellularity. Capillary loops are dilated with normal thin capillary walls. (H&E stain, ×400)

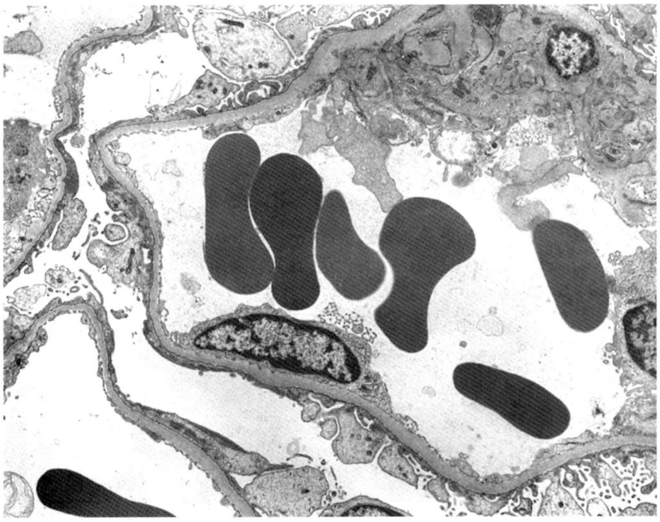

Figure 15-2 Low-power electron photomicrograph includes a capillary loop with extensive effacement of foot processes accompanied by swelling and microvillarization of podocytes. Glomerular basement membranes appear normal and no dense deposits are seen. (Courtesy Paul Kirwan, Electron Microscopy Unit, Department of Anatomical Pathology, CRGH, Concord, Sydney, Australia)

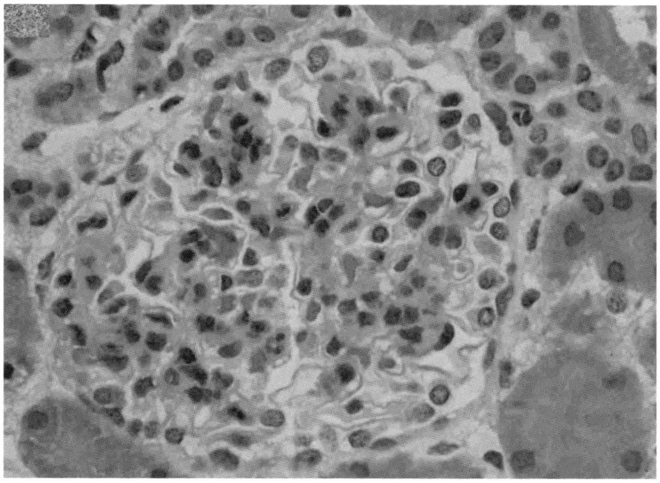

Figure 15-3 The glomerulus shows increased numbers of mesangial cells with mildly increased matrix. The capillary loops appear normal. (H&E stain, ×400)

80% of the glomeruli. Increased numbers of mesangial cell nuclei are clearly present within the mesangial matrix, which is either normal or only mildly increased (Figure 15-3). There is generally no obvious lobulation of the glomerulus, and segmental sclerosis is absent. As in MCD, glomerular basement membranes remain thin and capillary loops clearly patent. By definition, spikes are not seen in silver-stained sections. There is no significant interstitial change (either tubular atrophy or fibrosis) to suggest glomerular loss. Glomerular immaturity, characterized by hypercellularity and a layer of cuboidal epithelium along the surface of the glomerular tuft, may be seen in some cases, particularly in younger children. Recent studies have suggested that these cases may have a less favorable clinical course.[67]

Many cases of MesPGN show positive granular mesangial IgM ± C3 and very occasionally small amounts of C1q or IgG, although a proportion of cases have negative immunofluorescence. Some have considered these immune-positive cases as MesPGN, whereas others separate the positive cases into further distinct categories, most commonly IgM nephropathy. As noted earlier, these three "entities" probably represent a spectrum rather than separate diseases. On electron microscopy there is mesangial cell hyperplasia with effacement of epithelial cell foot processes and microvillus transformation of epithelial cells. Dense deposits are not typically found and the glomerular capillary basement membrane is normal.

IgM Nephropathy

IgM nephropathy shows light microscopic features that may mimic those of either MCD or MesPGN. The sampled glomeruli may appear completely normal on routine stains or may show diffuse mesangial hypercellularity. Some cases will show a combination of features, with some but not all glomeruli appearing hypercellular. As with MCD and MesPGN, segmental sclerosing lesions are not seen in an adequately sampled specimen, glomerular capillary loops remain thin walled and patent, and there is no basement membrane thickening or evidence of spike formation. Interstitial changes are absent. Granular deposits of IgM are confined to the mesangium and are generally seen in all glomeruli regardless of their histologic appearance. Lesser amounts of C3 are common, and some cases may also show small amounts of C1q or IgG. In these cases the IgM should remain as the dominant reactant. On electron microscopy there may be a mild increase in mesangial matrix. Immune deposits are often absent though some cases will show occasional small dense deposits located in paramesangial regions. Effacement of epithelial cell foot processes is usually seen to a varying degree, usually with microvillus transformation.

Focal Segmental Glomerulosclerosis

Although FSGS more commonly results in steroid-resistant disease, a proportion of cases will respond, at least initially, to steroid therapy,[68,69] and thus brief mention of the pathologic features is made here. In FSGS, segmental (involving only a portion of the tuft) and focal (involving some but not all glomeruli) sclerosis of glomeruli is present. The light microscopic changes are not specific for primary idiopathic FSGS, and other causes of segmental sclerosing lesions need to be excluded.[70] The sclerosed segments show collapse of the glomerular capillary with increase in matrix material but with variable patterns of glomerular involvement.[71] The uninvolved portion of the glomerular tuft should appear essentially normal. Idiopathic FSGS typically shows early preferential involvement of the deep juxtamedullary glomeruli so that adequate sampling of this region is needed to reduce the risk of missing a focal lesion. (This risk is estimated at 35% if only 10 glomeruli are examined, falling to a 12% risk if 20 glomeruli are examined.[68]) Even a single segmental sclerosing lesion away from the glomerular tip is sufficient to exclude a diagnosis of MCD. Clues to the presence of possible FSGS without diagnostic sclerosing lesions include abnormal glomerular enlargement, which appears to be an early indicator of the sclerotic process, and focal interstitial fibrosis and tubular atrophy (above that expected for age), which suggest glomerular loss.[68] Typically FSGS shows negative immunofluorescence though nonspecific uptake of IgM may be seen, commonly within sclerosed segments. Deposits similar to that of IgM nephropathy may also be present. On electron microscopy nonsclerosed glomeruli show epithelial cell foot process fusion, which may not be complete or as widespread as in typical untreated MCD. However, finding foot process fusion is often not helpful in making this distinction, as steroid therapy may partially restore foot processes in MCD.

CLINICOPATHOLOGIC CORRELATIONS AT PRESENTATION OF NEPHROTIC SYNDROME

Children with MCD cannot be separated on clinical features from those with FSGS or MesPGN, although they are generally younger and less likely to have hematuria, hypertension, and renal dysfunction at presentation.[1] The ISKDC found that 80% of MCD children were age 6 and under compared with 50% of FSGS children. Systolic and diastolic blood pressures were elevated at presentation in 21% and 14% of

MCD children and in 49% and 33% of FSGS children. Hematuria occurred in 23% of MCD children and in 48% of FSGS children.

CLINICAL AND LABORATORY FEATURES AT ONSET OF NEPHROTIC SYNDROME

In 30% to 50% of cases the onset of SSNS is preceded by an upper respiratory tract infection.[72,73] Clinical manifestations of allergy may be present in about 30% of SSNS children[73] compared with less than 20% of children without SSNS, but an acute allergic reaction rarely seems to be a precipitant of a relapse. The most common initial symptom in SSNS is periorbital edema, although the significance of this finding may not be realized until the child develops generalized edema and ascites.[74] Frequently periorbital edema is misdiagnosed as an allergy or as conjunctivitis. Symptoms may be present for as long as a year before diagnosis, although 78% of cases are diagnosed within a month of the first symptom. The degree of edema is variable, with some children having only mild periorbital and ankle edema whereas others have pleural effusions and gross ascites with scrotal and penile edema in boys and labial edema in girls. The rapid formation of edema with reduction in plasma volume may be associated with abdominal pain and malaise. Some children have serious infections at presentation, including peritonitis.[75] Elevated systolic and diastolic blood pressures are initially present in 5% to 20% of children with MCD, but generally hypertension does not persist.[1,72] Urinalysis shows 3-4+ protein on urinalysis. Microscopic hematuria is present at diagnosis in 20% to 30% of children but rarely persists, and macroscopic hematuria occurs in less than 1% of children with SSNS.[1,72] Serum albumin levels usually fall below 20 g/L and may be less than 10 g/L with a concomitant reduction in total protein levels. Renal function is generally normal, although serum creatinine may be elevated at presentation in association with intravascular volume depletion and, rarely, acute renal failure. Children have elevated cholesterol and triglycerides at presentation and these continue to be abnormal while the child remains nephrotic. However, measurements of lipids at presentation do not provide useful additional information that could contribute to diagnosis or management of these children. Serum electrolytes are usually within the normal range. Total serum calcium levels are low because of hypoalbuminemia, but ionized calcium levels are usually normal. Hemoglobin and hematocrit levels may be elevated at presentation in patients with reduced plasma volumes.

OUTCOME OF CHILDREN WITH SSNS

Relapse

Despite a relapsing course, the long-term prognosis for most children with SSNS is for resolution of their disease and maintenance of normal renal function. Follow-up studies of children with SSNS and MCD[3,5] indicate that 80% to 90% of children relapse one or more times. Among children who relapse, 35% to 50% relapse frequently or become steroid dependent.[3,5] Data from the ISKDC study indicated that the clinical course during follow-up could be predicted from the course during the first 6 months after treatment.[5] Of 148 children who remained in remission during the first 6 months after initial steroid therapy, 76% either never relapsed or relapsed rarely. Among 73 children who experienced one relapse in the 6 months after initial therapy, 70% ceased to relapse after a median period of 2.7 years. Among 102 children with two or more relapses in the first 6 months after initial therapy, 63% ceased to relapse after an average of 3 years, whereas 34% had become infrequent relapsers within 2 years. The proportion of children without relapse reached 80% by 8 years of follow-up.[3,5] Other studies have reported an inverse relationship between the length of a remission and risk for subsequent relapse.[76,77] Other predictors for frequent relapses and steroid dependence are upper respiratory tract infections, microscopic hematuria, and a longer time to remission after beginning treatment with prednisone.[78,79]

Five series involving 463 patients provide information on the likelihood of relapses persisting into adult life.[4,76,80-82] The duration of follow-up varied from 10 to 44 years. The proportion of patients still having relapses of nephrotic syndrome as adults varied between 7% and 42%. Lahdenkari and colleagues[80] reported a 30-year follow-up of children with SSNS first reported by Koskimies and co-workers in 1982.[3] Of 104 patients, 10% experienced episodes of SSNS as adults. The period between childhood and adult episodes was 2 to 17 years, with an average of 4.6 years (range 1 to 11 years) between adulthood episodes. Two studies with follow-up periods of 20 years reported higher relapse rates of 33% and 42% in adult patients.[4,81] The higher relapse rates probably reflect patient selection with higher proportions of frequently relapsing or steroid-dependent patients as evidenced by the need for corticosteroid-sparing therapy. In both studies adult patients with relapses had had significantly higher numbers of relapses per year in childhood, with childhood rates being 0.95 to 1.3 per year in adults with relapses compared with 0.3 to 0.42 per year among adults without relapses. Some studies[4,82] but not others[81] suggest that younger age at onset predicts a higher likelihood of continuing to relapse in adult life.

Renal Function

The majority of children with SSNS and biopsy proven or presumed MCD have a good prognosis for renal function. Only one child (0.3%) of the ISKDC series of 334 children with SSNS and MCD developed renal failure.[5] Similarly, in the five series of 463 patients,[4,76,80-82] only one patient (0.2%)[4] progressed to end-stage renal failure, indicating that the risk of end-stage renal failure among children with SSNS and MCD is very low even in children with frequently relapsing or steroid-dependent SSNS. In contrast, the prognosis for renal function in children with SSNS and IgM nephropathy or FSGS on biopsy is more guarded, with great variation in the reported numbers progressing to renal failure. Some studies[83-85] have reported that no child with SSNS and FSGS developed chronic renal failure during follow-up periods averaging about 10 years. Among Brazilian children, 12% of 42 children with SSNS and FSGS developed chronic renal failure during an average 10-year follow-up.[86] In a series of 49 children (57% African American) with SSNS and FSGS or IgM nephropathy, selected because the patients had had multiple biopsies, 37% became resistant to corticosteroids and progressed to chronic renal failure.[87]

Other Complications

Of 164 children with nephrotic syndrome seen between 1929 and 1957 and therefore treated before corticosteroids and antibiotics were regularly used, 56% recovered completely, 4% had persistent proteinuria, and 40% died, 20% of them from infections.[74] In the 1960s, 1970s, and 1980s, death rates of around 7% were reported[72,82,88] among children with SSNS. A recent study[81] reported only one death (0.7%) associated with disease among 138 children with SSNS presenting between 1970 and 2003. Reported long-term complications in 43 adults with continuing relapses included short stature (16%), obesity (5%), thromboembolism (7%), and hypertension (7%).[4] Osteoporosis was found in 7 of 11 patients studied. The risk of cardiovascular disease in adults with SSNS in childhood did not appear to differ from rates in the normal population,[89] but only 62 patients were followed up.

INDICATIONS FOR RENAL BIOPSY

Following the studies of the ISKDC, routine renal biopsy at presentation and before corticosteroid administration has been abandoned. Biopsy is reserved for nephrotic children less than 1 year of age, for those who have unusual clinical and laboratory features (macroscopic hematuria, hypertension, persistent renal insufficiency, and low C3 component of complement), for those with initial or secondary steroid resistance, and for those with frequent relapses before administration of second-line therapy. SSNS rarely presents in the first year of life and may prove difficult to differentiate at presentation from other forms of nephrotic syndrome occurring in this age group. Most pediatric nephrologists would consider biopsy necessary before using corticosteroids in children less than 1 year of age. Originally biopsies at presentation were recommended for children above 8 to 10 years[90] on the basis of the ISKDC studies. Now most pediatric nephrologists do not have a rigid upper age limit for treating children with idiopathic nephrotic syndrome without prior renal biopsy, and will give corticosteroids to children and adolescents if renal function and complements are normal, persistent hypertension is absent, and microscopic hematuria is transitory. This management is supported by retrospective studies of clinicopathologic correlations in Indian children and adolescents[91,92] in which children without two or more abnormal clinical features generally demonstrated steroid sensitivity regardless of histology. However, these data may not apply to African American adolescent populations where the incidence of MCD at 20% to 30%[93] is much lower than the 40% to 50% seen in Indian or northern European adolescents.[6,91]

Opinions differ as to whether children with SSNS should have renal biopsies before beginning corticosteroid-sparing therapies. In some centers, particularly in North America, renal biopsies are commonly carried out before using alternative therapy, whereas this practice has been largely abandoned in Europe and India. Thus a survey of North American pediatric nephrologists found that 33% and 49% of respondents would perform biopsies on children with frequently relapsing or steroid-dependent SSNS before starting alternative therapy to obtain prognostic information or because respondents believed that results would influence therapy.[94] Studies from North America have demonstrated that renal histologies (FSGS, MesPGN, and IgM nephropathy) with less favorable prognoses are common in children with frequently relapsing or steroid-dependent SSNS[95,96]; that steroid-dependent patients with MesPGN, IgM nephropathy, or FSGS are more likely to have one or more relapses after cyclophosphamide therapy compared with children with MCD[59,83]; and that African American children with FSGS are more likely to progress to chronic kidney failure.[97] In contrast, studies from Europe and India[84,92,98] have demonstrated no relationship between renal histology and the prebiopsy or postcyclophosphamide course even though MesPGN and FSGS are more common in selected series of children with frequently relapsing or steroid-dependent SSNS compared with ISKDC data.

Before a biopsy is performed on a child with frequently relapsing or steroid-dependent SSNS, it should be determined whether the benefits of this procedure outweigh the potential risk of significant hemorrhage (1%).[99] In particular, the clinician needs to know whether the renal pathology will influence the specific therapy administered and/or whether it will provide information on the likelihood of the child developing end-stage renal failure. Studies state that even if the renal biopsy shows FSGS, the most important predictor for end-stage renal failure in idiopathic nephrotic syndrome is not the renal pathology but the achievement and maintenance of remission following any therapy.[100] Thus renal biopsy before commencing corticosteroid-sparing therapy is not indicated in children who continue to achieve complete remission with corticosteroids.

MANAGEMENT OF SSNS

Treatment of the First Episode of Nephrotic Syndrome with Corticosteroids

Corticosteroids have been used to treat idiopathic nephrotic syndrome since the early 1950s. In 1956 Dr. Gavin Arneil described the successful use of 60 mg of prednisone daily in four children with idiopathic nephrotic syndrome.[101] Because of the clear net benefits of corticosteroids, no placebo-controlled trials have ever been performed on children with nephrotic syndrome. The ISKDC agreed on a standard corticosteroid regimen for the first episode of SSNS,[102] and this regimen has provided the control group against which to test other regimens of prednisone therapy. At presentation children received prednisone 60 mg/m^2/day (maximum dose 80 mg) in divided doses for 4 weeks followed by 40 mg/m^2/day (maximum 60 mg per day) in divided doses on 3 consecutive days out of 7 for 4 weeks. Subsequently a randomized controlled trial (RCT) carried out by the Arbeitsgemeinschaft für Pädiatrische Nephrologie (APN)[103-105] demonstrated that prednisone given on alternate days was more effective in maintaining remission than prednisone given on 3 consecutive days out of 7, so alternate-day prednisone dosing is generally now used. Because no significant differences in the time to remission or risk of subsequent relapse between single and divided doses of prednisone have been demonstrated,[104-106] a single daily dose is now the preferred option during daily therapy to achieve greater compliance. No RCTs have examined lower daily doses of prednisone in the initial episode of nephrotic syndrome, although in a small case series, doses of 30 mg/m^2/day led to remission durations similar to the 60 mg/m^2/day dose used by the ISKDC.[107]

Though demonstrated to be more effective than shorter durations of treatment (one trial; 60 patients; RR 1.46; 95% CI 1.01-2.12),[104,105,108] the ISDKC regimen is associated with a high relapse rate, so the efficacy of longer durations of steroids has been tested in RCTs with the aim of extending remission. In a metaanalysis of six trials that compared prednisone treatment for 2 months with periods of 3 months or more,[104,105] prednisone administration for 3 to 7 months (4 to 8 weeks at 60 mg/m^2/day and then on alternate days) reduced the risk of relapse by 30% at 12 to 24 months (six trials[109-114]; 422 patients; RR 0.70; 95% CI 0.58-0.84) (Figure 15-4, *A*), with a significant reduction also in the number of children who relapsed frequently and in the mean number of relapses per year. There were no significant differences in risks of adverse effects (Table 15-3) or in the cumulative prednisone dose (three trials[109,113,114]; 245 children; weighted mean difference 0.71; 95% CI –0.67-2.09). Further trials[105] have now demonstrated that steroid therapy for 6 months significantly reduces the risk for relapse compared with 3 months (four trials[113,115-117]; 382 children; RR 0.57; 95% CI 0.45-0.71) (Figure 15-4, *B*). No additional benefit was demonstrated in one trial of treatment for 12 months compared with 5 months.[118] These data provide evidence that prolonged corticosteroid therapy (6 months) should be given to reduce the risk for relapse following the first episode of SSNS.

There is an inverse linear relationship between the risk for relapse and duration of induction therapy, suggesting an increase in benefit with treatment up to 7 months (RR = 1.26-0.112 duration; $r^2 = 0.56$; $p = 0.03$).[105,119] With each increase of 1 month of therapy over 2 months, the relative risk for relapse falls by 11%. If the relapse rate in a population

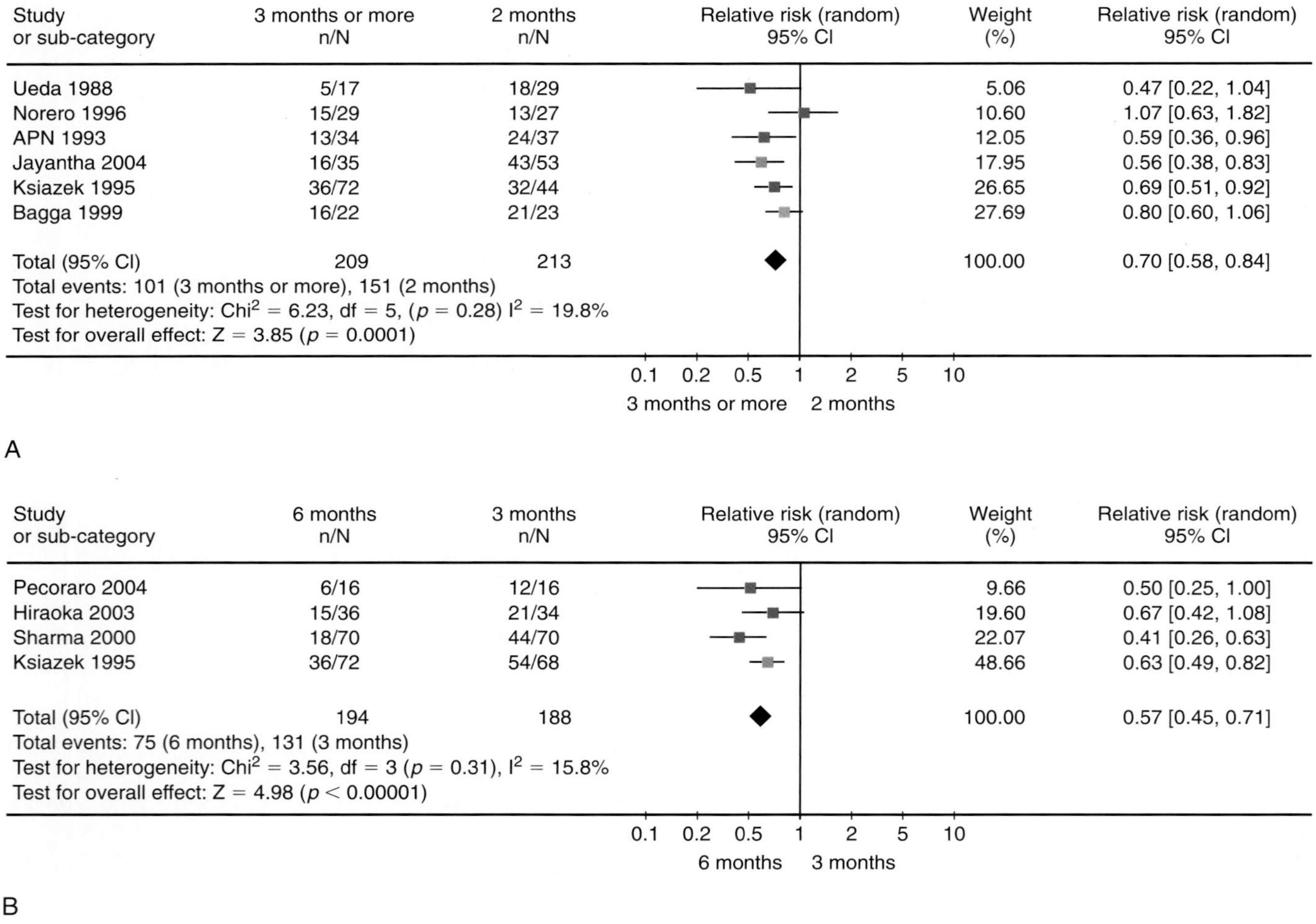
Study or sub-category
3 months or more n/N
2 months n/N
Relative risk (random) 95% CI
Weight (%)
Relative risk (random) 95% CI
Ueda 1988 5/17 18/29 5.06 0.47 [0.22, 1.04]
Norero 1996 15/29 13/27 10.60 1.07 [0.63, 1.82]
APN 1993 13/34 24/37 12.05 0.59 [0.36, 0.96]
Jayantha 2004 16/35 43/53 17.95 0.56 [0.38, 0.83]
Ksiazek 1995 36/72 32/44 26.65 0.69 [0.51, 0.92]
Bagga 1999 16/22 21/23 27.69 0.80 [0.60, 1.06]
Total (95% CI) 209 213 100.00 0.70 [0.58, 0.84]
Total events: 101 (3 months or more), 151 (2 months)
Test for heterogeneity: Chi² = 6.23, df = 5, (p = 0.28) I² = 19.8%
Test for overall effect: Z = 3.85 (p = 0.0001)
0.1 0.2 0.5 1 2 5 10
3 months or more 2 months
A
Study or sub-category
6 months n/N
3 months n/N
Relative risk (random) 95% CI
Weight (%)
Relative risk (random) 95% CI
Pecoraro 2004 6/16 12/16 9.66 0.50 [0.25, 1.00]
Hiraoka 2003 15/36 21/34 19.60 0.67 [0.42, 1.08]
Sharma 2000 18/70 44/70 22.07 0.41 [0.26, 0.63]
Ksiazek 1995 36/72 54/68 48.66 0.63 [0.49, 0.82]
Total (95% CI) 194 188 100.00 0.57 [0.45, 0.71]
Total events: 75 (6 months), 131 (3 months)
Test for heterogeneity: Chi² = 3.56, df = 3 (p = 0.31), I² = 15.8%
Test for overall effect: Z = 4.98 (p < 0.00001)
0.1 0.2 0.5 1 2 5 10
6 months 3 months
B

Figure 15-4 Metaanalyses of the relative risk (95% confidence intervals) for relapse of nephrotic syndrome by 12 to 24 months in **A,** six trials comparing prolonged prednisone therapy (3 to 7 months) with 2 months of therapy and in **B,** four trials comparing 6 months with 3 months of prednisone therapy in children with the first episode of SSNS. Results are shown ordered by trial weights. The test statistic *Z* indicates that increased duration of prednisone is significantly more effective in reducing the number of children who relapse compared with 2 or 3 months of prednisone.[105] (Reproduced from Hodson EM, Knight JF, Willis NS, Craig JC: Update of *Cochrane Database Syst Rev:* CD001533, 2004; PMID:15106158 [Review], *Cochrane Database of Syst Rev:* CD001533, 2005. Published by John Wiley & Sons, Ltd.)

TABLE 15-3 **Adverse Effects of Corticosteroids**

Adverse Effect	No. of Trials	No. of Patients	% in High-Dose Group	% in Standard Group	Risk Difference (95% Confidence Intervals)
Hypertension	7	526	11%	6.2%	0.05 (–0.03-0.06)
Ophthalmologic disorders	6	460	4.9%	5.1%	0.00 (–0.04-0.12)
Growth retardation	4	354	5.1%	11.2%	–0.02 (–0.08-0.04)
Psychologic disorders	4	293	4.6%	2.1%	0.01 (–0.03-0.06)
Cushing's syndrome	4	292	37.3%	30.6%	0.15 (–0.06-0.36)
Osteoporosis	3	233	0.81%	4.5%	–0.02 (–0.09-0.05)
Severe infections	2	172	32.7%	40.8%	–0.08 (–0.23-0.06)

Adverse effects of corticosteroids by 12 to 24 months following treatment of the first episode of steroid-sensitive nephrotic syndrome for 3 to 7 months (total prednisone induction dose 2922-5235 mg/m^2) compared with 2 months (total induction dose 2240 mg/m^2)

of children treated for 2 months is 70%, the calculated number of children relapsing by 12 to 24 months would fall by 8% for every increase by 1 month in the duration of therapy so that treatment for 6 months would reduce the risk of relapse by 32% (4% × 8%) to 38%. In populations with lower relapse rates following 2 months of therapy, the benefit of longer courses of prednisone treatment will be less.

Increased duration of corticosteroid therapy results in increased total dose of corticosteroid therapy, making the effects of duration and dose difficult to separate. Compared with the standard induction dose of prednisone of 2240 mg/m^2, administered doses of 2922 to 5235 mg/m^2 significantly reduce the risk for relapse at 12 to 24 months (seven trials[109-114,120]; 481 children; RR 0.69; 95% CI 0.59-0.81).[105] In two recent trials,[115,120] different total doses of prednisone were administered for the same duration (3 or 6 months). A metaanalysis of these studies showed that the risk of relapse was reduced by 40% with higher doses of steroids (two trials; RR 0.59; 95% CI 0.42-0.84),[105] suggesting that both increased dose and prolonged duration of corticosteroids are important in reducing the risk of relapse.

Despite the available data from RCTs, a survey of pediatric nephrologists in North America demonstrated considerable variation among respondents in their approach to the first episode of idiopathic nephrotic syndrome, although about 70% used durations of therapy exceeding the ISKDC's 8-week regimen.[121] Pediatric nephrologists have been reluctant to increase the duration of prednisone therapy, possibly because data on benefits and harms come from relatively small trials of variable quality.[105] Nevertheless these trials have provided consistent results demonstrating that increased duration and/or doses of corticosteroids reduce the risk for relapse without an increase in adverse effects. Results of a well-designed, adequately powered, and placebo-controlled RCT recently begun in the United Kingdom comparing 2 months with 4 months of prednisone therapy with an emphasis on the documentation of adverse effects are awaited.[122]

Treatment of Relapsing SSNS with Corticosteroids

The ISKDC defines relapse as recurrence of proteinuria for 3 consecutive days without reference to the presence or absence of edema (Table 15-1). Opinions differ on whether prednisone therapy should be recommenced immediately when proteinuria has persisted for 3 days to avoid the associated complications of an edematous relapse[123] or whether treatment should be deferred for several days[124] to determine whether proteinuria will resolve spontaneously. Proteinuria may remit spontaneously in 15% to 30% of relapses without commencing prednisone or increasing the dose.[125,126] Spontaneous remissions may occur after 10 to 14 days of proteinuria.[125] Narchi has argued that defining and treating relapse only on the basis of recurrence of proteinuria for 3 days could lead to children being erroneously labeled as frequent relapsers and given long-term corticosteroid therapy or corticosteroid-sparing agents unnecessarily.[126] There is no evidence that delaying treatment increases the time to subsequent remission; therefore it is reasonable to wait some days after recurrence of proteinuria before administering corticosteroids, provided the child remains well and without significant edema.

There are few data from RCTs on corticosteroid regimens for children with relapsing SSNS. Single trials have demonstrated that the risk of subsequent relapse within 2 years is reduced by 40% if children are treated for 7 months compared with 2 months of therapy,[105,127] and that children with steroid-dependent SSNS average three fewer relapses during follow-up if they receive daily rather than alternate-day therapy during intercurrent upper respiratory tract infections.[105,128] Boluses of intravenous methylprednisolone followed by oral prednisone have been proposed for relapsing SSNS. In a single RCT, no significant reduction in the risk of relapse at 1 year could be demonstrated with high-dose intravenous methylprednisolone followed by oral prednisone for 6 months compared with oral prednisone alone. However, the total dose of oral prednisone administered was higher in the control group than in the group receiving intravenous prednisone.[104,105,129]

The ISKDC proposed that relapses should be treated with daily prednisone (60 mg/m^2/day) until the child has been in remission for 3 days, followed by prednisone on 3 consecutive days out of 7 for 4 weeks. In the absence of data from RCTs, pediatric nephrologists have generally continued to treat relapses with daily prednisone (60 mg/m^2/day) until the child achieves remission, and then continued alternate-day therapy for varying durations. In two published regimens,[90,130] children with frequently relapsing SSNS are treated with daily prednisone until remission, followed by alternate-day prednisone at decreasing doses until an alternate-day dose of 10 to 30 mg/m^2 (0.3 to 1 mg/kg), which maintains remission, is reached. This dose is then continued for 12 to 24 months. This regimen is associated with a reduction in relapse rate with maintenance of growth rate. Others have reported that remission can be maintained with satisfactory growth using daily prednisone at 7.5 mg/m^2/day (0.25 mg/kg/day) for 18 months.[131]

Adverse Effects of Corticosteroids

The most frequent and important adverse effects reported in the experimental and control groups of RCTs[105] are cushingoid features and obesity (42% of 501 children in six trials); hypertension (10% of 735 children in nine trials); growth retardation (8% of 345 children in four trials); ophthalmologic disorders including posterior subcapsular cataracts[132,133] and raised intraocular pressure (6% of 655 children in eight trials); behavioral changes including aggression, inattention,[134] hyperactivity, and sleep disturbances (4% of 362 children in five trials); and osteoporosis (2% of 233 children in two trials). Taken from short-term trials, these numbers are likely to underestimate the true burden of adverse effects of corticosteroids in children with SSNS.

The current practice of using alternate-day rather than daily prednisone to maintain remission stems from early reports that growth rate was less affected by alternate-day prednisone. An RCT has demonstrated that children given alternate-day prednisone after renal transplantation grow at a better rate than those given daily prednisone.[135] Some studies of children with SSNS have reported normal growth rates,[136-138] whereas others have described reduced growth rates with delayed onset of puberty.[139,140] A recent detailed study of 56 children with frequently relapsing or steroid-dependent SSNS has clearly demonstrated the adverse effect that corticosteroids have on growth.[141] During prepubertal growth, the cohort lost 0.49 ± 0.6 of height standard deviation score (SDS), whereas 23 patients who had reached final height had lost 0.92 ± 0.8 height SDS from onset of their disease and 0.68 ± 0.7 height SDS from their target height SDS. Final height SDS was significantly lower in children who required prednisone during puberty. Partial catchup growth occurred in children permanently withdrawn from prednisone. Logistic regression revealed that prednisone treatment was the only variable associated with negative delta height SDS. Growth rates should be regularly assessed, particularly in children with frequently relapsing or steroid-dependent SSNS who are nearing their pubertal growth spurt, and corticosteroid-sparing agents considered if growth rates deteriorate.

Derangements of bone mineral metabolism may occur in patients with nephrotic syndrome and normal renal function. Vitamin D binding protein and 25-hydroxyvitamin D levels are reduced in nephrotic children,[142] whereas levels of calcium, 1.25-dihydroxyvitamin D, and parathyroid hormone levels are generally normal.[142-144] Levels of 25-hydroxyvitamin D increase in remission but remain low compared with those in healthy children.[144] Abnormalities of bone mineral metabolism are aggravated by treatment with corticosteroids. Corticosteroids reduce bone formation by inhibiting osteoblast activity and inhibiting bone matrix formation. In addition, they increase bone resorption directly and by reducing calcium absorption via inhibition of vitamin D activity with a secondary increased release of parathyroid hormone.[145,146] Low bone area and trabecular thickness with focal areas of osteoid accumulation consistent with osteopenia and abnormal mineralization have been found in children with steroid-dependent SSNS[146]; bone formation rate correlated inversely with the daily prednisone dose. Serum osteocalcin and alkaline phosphatase levels fall during corticosteroid therapy consistent with reduced bone formation.[144]

Corticosteroid therapy is associated with osteopenia (decrease in quantity of bone tissue) and osteoporosis (osteopenia with bone fragility). Trabecular bone is affected more severely than cortical bone. Vertebral crush fractures, identified on radiographs of the lateral spine, are the most common fractures seen in children treated with corticosteroids.[147] In adults, bone mass accounts for 75% to 85% of the variance in bone strength, thus measurements of bone mass can provide an indication of bone strength.[148] Dual energy x-ray absorptiometry (DXA) is widely used to assess bone mass in children with SSNS, although there is currently no evidence that densitometric data can predict the likelihood of fracture in children with osteopenia.[147] DXA measures the mass of bone mineral per projection area (grams/cm^2), which is a size-dependent measure.[147] Thus results must be corrected for height in short children to prevent underestimation of bone mineral density (BMD) in comparison with age-matched controls. Early studies of BMD in nephrotic children on corticosteroids provided conflicting results.[149,150] Two large studies of BMD in children with SSNS using different DXA scanners have recently been published. A North American cross-sectional study[151] of 60 children with SSNS who had received an average of 23 g of prednisone demonstrated that whole body bone mineral content (BMC) was increased and lumbar spine BMC was normal in children with SSNS compared with age-matched local controls when adjusted for bone area, height, age, sex, pubertal stage, and race. Nephrotic children had significantly lower Z-scores for height and higher Z-scores for weight and body mass index (BMI) compared with controls. The investigators concluded that corticosteroid-induced increases in BMI were associated with increased whole body BMC and maintenance of BMC of the spine. The increases in BMI would place added strain on the bones of these ambulant children, leading to increased mineral content and counteracting any deleterious effect of corticosteroids on bone health.[147] In contrast, in 100 nonobese Indian children with SSNS who had received 5.6 to 18 g of prednisone, 61% had low BMD levels compared with normal values from North American controls.[143] No children developed fractures. Although comparison with a non-Indian reference range will overestimate the number of children with low BMD, a nonobese population of children with SSNS is likely to be at greater risk of low BMD. These data indicate that differences in growth and body composition in different study populations and the use of appropriate control groups need to be considered when interpreting studies of bone mass in children with SSNS. Newer modalities such as peripheral quantitative computed tomography (pQCT) may prove more predictive of bone health in SSNS, because pQCT can assess cortical and trabecular bone.[145] Until data are available that show that BMD measurements lead to effective treatment and improved outcomes for bone health, routine measurements of BMD cannot be recommended in children with frequently relapsing or steroid-dependent SSNS.

Corticosteroid-associated fractures are rare in children with SSNS unlike children with chronic inflammatory disorders such as juvenile rheumatoid arthritis. In chronic inflammatory disorders, it is difficult to differentiate between the effects of corticosteroids and the effects of increased inflammatory cytokines, malnutrition, and reduced mobility on bone mass. It is possible that SSNS children who do not have these additional disease effects are at less risk of osteoporosis.[147] Recent publications have demonstrated improved BMD in SSNS children who were given vitamin D and calcium supplements, and have argued that such treatments be used routinely during prednisone therapy.[152,153] However, no data were provided to demonstrate that the response was not due to correction of preexisting vitamin D and calcium deficiency. Although further data are required to determine if calcium and vitamin D supplements have any role in preventing osteopenia in children with SSNS, it is important to ensure optimum bone health in all children with SSNS by giving adequate intakes of calcium and vitamin D based on age, adequate exercise, and maintain normal pubertal progression.[147] Bisphosphonates are widely used in adults to treat corticosteroid-induced osteoporosis, but experience with these medications in pediatric corticosteroid-associated osteoporosis is limited.[147]

Corticosteroid Sparing Agents in Frequently Relapsing and Steroid-Dependent SSNS

Alkylating agents, cyclosporin, and levamisole have been demonstrated in RCTs to be effective in reducing relapse rates in frequently relapsing and steroid-dependent SSNS. Their use is indicated in children who have significant adverse effects from prednisone therapy. Other agents including mycophenolate mofetil, tacrolimus, and vincristine are also used, but no RCTs comparing these agents with prednisone or other corticosteroid agents have been published to date. There are no data demonstrating differences in efficacy between alkylating agents, levamisole, and cyclosporin, so their use depends on availability and patient and physician preferences. However, pediatric nephrologists commonly use alkylating agents or levamisole initially and reserve cyclosporin for children who continue to relapse frequently despite these agents.

Alkylating Agents

The use of cyclophosphamide and chlorambucil in childhood nephrotic syndrome was first described in 1963[154] and 1966, respectively.[155] In RCTs, alkylating agents (oral cyclophosphamide 2 to 3 mg/kg daily or chlorambucil 0.2 mg/kg daily administered for 8 weeks) reduced the risk of relapse by 70% in frequently relapsing SSNS at 6 to 12 months after treatment (five trials[156-160]; 134 children; RR 0.32; 95% CI 0.16-0.63)[161,162] (Figure 15-5). No significant difference in efficacy between cyclophosphamide and chlorambucil could be demonstrated in a comparison trial.[161-163] In an RCT there was no significant difference in efficacy between 8 and 12 weeks of cyclophosphamide treatment,[161-164] although a study comparing treated patients with historical controls has suggested a benefit of treating for 12 weeks.[165] Many children will relapse after a course of an alkylating agent. In a systematic review of 26 studies of cyclophosphamide and chlorambucil usage in SSNS, overall relapse-free survival after 5 years was below 40%.[166] For frequently relapsing SSNS, relapse-free survivals were 72% and 36% after 2 and 5 years, respectively. For steroid-dependent children, relapse-free survivals were 40% and 24% after 2 and 5 years, respectively. Similar results were found in a single-center study of 109 children in which the

Study or sub-category	Alkylating agent n/N	Prednisone/placebo n/N	Relative risk (random) 95% CI	Weight (%)	Relative risk (random) 95% CI
Grupe 1976–CHL	0/10	11/11		5.75	0.05 [0.00, 0.71]
Chiu 1973–CPA	1/12	5/11		9.99	0.18 [0.03, 1.33]
Alatas 1978–CHL	1/5	6/6		12.31	0.20 [0.03, 1.15]
Barratt 1970–CPA	3/11	13/15		28.05	0.31 [0.12, 0.84]
ISKDC 1974–CHL	9/27	16/26		43.90	0.54 [0.29, 1.00]
Total (95% CI)	65	69		100.00	0.32 [0.16, 0.63]

Total events: 14 (Alkylating agent), 51 (Prednisone/placebo)
Test for heterogeneity: $Chi^2 = 5.69$, df = 4 ($p = 0.22$), $I^2 = 29.7\%$
Test for overall effect: Z = 3.28 ($p = 0.001$)

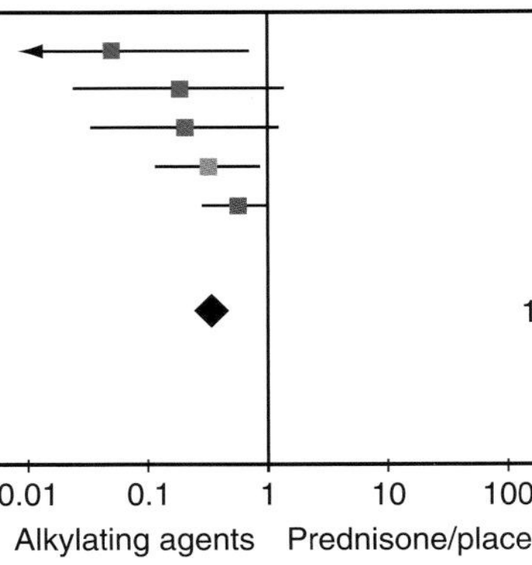

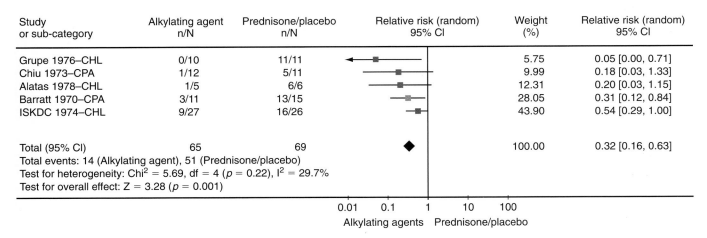

Figure 15-5 Metaanalysis of the relative risk (95% confidence intervals) for relapse of nephrotic syndrome by 6 to12 months in five trials comparing alkylating agents (cyclophosphamide [CPA] or chlorambucil [CHL]) with prednisone alone or placebo in children with relapsing steroid-sensitive nephrotic syndrome. Results are shown ordered by trial weights. The test statistic *Z* indicates that alkylating agents were significantly more effective in reducing the number of children who relapse compared with prednisone or placebo.[161] (Reproduced from Durkan A, Hodson EM, Willis NS, Craig JC: Update of *Cochrane Database Syst Rev:* CD002290, 2001; PMID:11687155O [Review], *Cochrane Database of Syst Rev:* CD002290, 2005. Published by John Wiley & Sons, Ltd.)

cumulative rate of sustained remission was 24% after 10 years, with 54% of frequently relapsing children and 17% of steroid-dependent children achieving sustained remission ($p < 0.05$).[167] Intravenous cyclophosphamide (500 mg/m^2/dose for 6 monthly doses) was more effective than oral cyclophosphamide (2 mg/kg/day for 12 weeks) in reducing the risk for relapse at 6 months (RR 0.56; 95% CI 0.33-0.92) but not at 2 years.[161,168] After pulse intravenous cyclophosphamide, sustained remissions of 6 months or more were reported in 51% of children followed for an average of 2 years with a 40% lower cumulative dose of cyclophosphamide.[169] There are little data on the efficacy of second courses of alkylating agents, although disease-free survivals may be better than the first course.[166]

Adverse effects of alkylating agents are frequent and may be severe. Latta and co-workers identified adverse effects from 38 reports involving 866 children who received 906 courses of cyclophosphamide and 638 children who received 671 courses of chlorambucil for frequently relapsing SSNS[166] (Table 15-4). They concluded that chlorambucil in the recommended dosage was potentially more toxic than cyclophosphamide because of a higher risk of infections, malignancies, and seizures. However, this conclusion was not based on comparative data from RCTs, so differences between cyclophosphamide and chlorambucil studies in patient populations cannot be excluded. Alkylating agents may reduce male fertility and cause abnormal gonadal function in men. In SSNS there is a dose-dependent relationship between the number of patients with sperm counts below 10^6 per ml and the cumulative dose of cyclophosphamide.[166] The threshold cumulative dose for safe use of cyclophosphamide remains uncertain because of individual reports of oligospermia in boys receiving less than 200 mg/kg. These data suggest that single courses of cyclophosphamide at a dosage of 2 mg/kg daily should not exceed 12 weeks (cumulative dose 168 mg/kg) and that second courses should be avoided. Data on gonadal toxicity with chlorambucil in SSNS are scarce. In male patients treated for lymphoma, total doses of 10 to 17 mg/kg led to azoospermia[170]; similar total doses are used in SSNS. Gonadal toxicity is less severe in women, with most reports observing little or no toxicity with alkylating agents in SSNS.[166]

Cyclosporin

Cyclosporin has been used to treat children with frequently relapsing or steroid-dependent SSNS since 1985.[59] Single trials[161,162,171,172] have demonstrated no significant difference in efficacy during treatment between cyclosporin and cyclophosphamide (55 children; RR 1.07; 95% CI 0.48-2.35) or cyclosporin and chlorambucil (40 children; RR 0.82; 95% CI 0.44-1.53). The majority of children treated with cyclosporin relapse when therapy is ceased. Adverse effects are significant, with 4% of children developing hypertension, 9% reduced renal function, 28% gum hypertrophy, and 34% hirsutism.[161,162] In long-term studies, remissions of 1 and 2 years are achieved in 60% and 40% of children, respectively.[173] However, many require low-dose, long-term prednisone to maintain remission despite adequate whole blood levels of cyclosporin.

Cyclosporin toxicity is well documented in children receiving this therapy outside the transplant setting,[174,175] though few studies have correlated clinical toxicity with morphologic features.[176,177] The toxic effects are essentially the same in transplant and nontransplant settings. Cyclosporin toxicity may be characterized by reduction in glomerular filtration rate with no discernible histologic abnormality, or by acute and chronic tubular changes, vascular changes, or both in the kidney. Acute changes of toxic tubulopathy are classically described as isometric vacuolation of proximal tubular epithelial cells. However, this is often a focal phenomenon and may be seen in only a small number of tubules in a biopsy sample. The vacuoles are of similar size (hence "isometric") and occur on the basis of dilation of the smooth endoplasmic reticulum of the cells. Nonspecific changes of acute tubular necrosis may be seen in some cases, with intraluminal desquamation of epithelial cells, dilatation of the tubules, and regenerative nuclear changes. Acute vascular changes may result in microvascular thrombosis and in endothelial and myocyte necrosis. Chronic vascular changes include nodular hyaline arteriopathy, which arises on the basis

TABLE 15-4 **Adverse Effects of Alkylating Agents in Children with Steroid-Sensitive Nephrotic Syndrome**

		CYCLOPHOSPHAMIDE		CHLORAMBUCIL	
Adverse Effect		**Total Assessed**	**No. (%) with Outcome**	**Total Assessed**	**No. (%) with Outcome**
Deaths	Patients	866	7 (0.8%)	625	7 (1.1%)
Malignancies	Patients	866	2 (0.2%)	534	3 (0.6%)
Seizures	Patients	866	0 (0%)	266	9 (3.4%)
Infections	Courses	609	9 (1.5%)	552	35 (6.3%)
Hemorrhagic cystitis	Courses	762	22 (2.2%)	552	0 (0%)
Leucopenia	Courses	619	210 (32.4%)	456	151 (33%)
Thrombocytopenia	Courses	214	5 (2.1%)	408	24 (5.9%)
Hair loss	Courses	736	131 (17.8%)	237	5 (2.1%)

Reproduced from Latta K, von Schnakenburg C, Ehrich JH: A meta-analysis of cytotoxic treatment for frequently relapsing nephrotic syndrome in children, *Pediatr Nephrol* 16(3):271-82, 2001.

of individual myocyte necrosis of arteriolar smooth muscle, and "striped" interstitial fibrosis and tubular atrophy that reflect focal ischemic damage. Ultimately, chronic cyclosporin nephrotoxicity can result in glomerular changes of chronic ischemia, focal and segmental glomerulosclerosis, or both.

Cyclosporin-induced tubulointerstitial lesions on renal biopsy are reported in 30% to 40% of children who have received cyclosporin for 12 months or more,[178-180] with 80% having interstitial fibrosis when treated for 4 or more years. Cyclosporin-associated arteriopathy is uncommon. Risk factors for fibrosis are total duration of cyclosporin therapy and having heavy proteinuria for more than 30 days during therapy.[178] Arteriopathy but not interstitial fibrosis improves after cyclosporin has been ceased for 12 months or more.[181] Because of these histologic changes, it is recommended that children with SSNS receive cyclosporin for periods of less than 2 years or undergo annual renal biopsies if cyclosporin is continued,[178] particularly because interstitial changes may occur in the absence of renal impairment.[174]

Cyclosporin is usually started at 5 mg/kg/day in two divided doses, with subsequent dosing altered to achieve predose blood levels of 50 to 100 ng/ml (measured by fluorescence polarization immunoassay). The cyclosporin dose, required to maintain trough levels, may be decreased by one-third by administering ketoconazole as a cyclosporin-sparing agent, providing a reduction in drug costs.[182] Glomerular filtration rate was significantly better in the group receiving ketoconazole; rates of hypertension, gum hypertrophy, and hirsutism were unchanged. Ketoconazole was well tolerated with no evidence of liver dysfunction. Recent studies in children with SSNS have demonstrated better correlations between area under the curve concentrations of cyclosporin and 2-hour postdose levels than with trough levels.[183] Using a 2-hour postdose level of 300 to 400 ng/ml to guide dosage, lower doses of cyclosporin could be used without a change in the relapse rate.[184]

Levamisole

Levamisole is an antihelminthic agent with immunomodulatory properties.[185] Its use in childhood nephrotic syndrome was first described by Tanphaichitr and co-workers in 1980,[186] and many later studies have described its benefits as well.[185] Because its manufacturer ceased production, however, levamisole is currently not available.[185] It is usually administered at 2.5 mg/kg on alternate days. Levamisole reduced the risk of relapse by 40% in comparison with prednisone alone in three trials (137 patients[187-189]; RR 0.60; 95% CI 0.45-0.79) but was ineffective in a fourth trial in which a lower total dose was given.[161,190] Efficacy of levamisole in frequently relapsing and steroid-dependent SSNS appears similar to that of cyclophosphamide as demonstrated in an RCT[191] that compared it with pulse intravenous cyclophosphamide, and in a retrospective analysis of 51 children that compared it with oral cyclophosphamide.[192] Adverse effects of levamisole are uncommon but include leucopenia, gastrointestinal effects, and occasionally vasculitis.[193,194]

Mycophenolate Mofetil

Mycophenolate mofetil (MMF) is an inhibitor of the de novo purine pathway with inhibitory effects on T lymphocyte and B lymphocyte proliferation.[195] It is increasingly being used as a corticosteroid-sparing agent in children with frequently relapsing or steroid-dependent SSNS who have already received alkylating agents and cyclosporin. Currently there are no published data from RCTs on its efficacy. Three prospective studies involving 76 children who were treated for 6 to 12 months reported a reduction in relapse rate of 50% to 75% during treatment.[195-197] Prednisone dosage could be reduced in many patients and ceased in about half the cases.[195,197] Most children relapsed when MMF was ceased. Studies have used 450 to 600 mg/m^2/day in two divided doses. Trough levels of mycophenolic acid, measured by enzymatic immunoassay, below 2.5 mcg/ml were associated with a greater risk of relapse.[197] Renal function improved on transfer from cyclosporin to MMF.[198] The main adverse effects of MMF are abdominal pain, diarrhea, anemia, leucopenia, and thrombocytopenia, although to date MMF has been well tolerated in children with SSNS, with only mild abdominal pain reported.[195,197] In children who relapse on MMF alone, a combination of cyclosporin and MMF may maintain remission with the potential for lower cyclosporin doses.[197]

Other Agents

In RCTs, no significant reduction in the risk of relapse has been demonstrated with azathioprine.[161,162,199,200] Nevertheless based on data from case series showing reduction in relapse rates, long-term use of azathioprine has been proposed for children with SSNS.[201] Mizoribine blocks purine biosynthesis pathways and is widely used in Japan for children with SSNS.[202] In case series using dosages of 3 to 5 mg/kg/day, relapse rates fell by up to 50%. However, in an RCT involving 197 children who received 4 mg/kg/day of mizoribine or placebo, there was no significant difference in relapse rates, and 16% of treated patients developed hyperuricemia.[203] In RCTs, no significant reduction in relapse rate occurred with intravenous immunoglobulin[204] or sodium cromoglycate.[205]

Tacrolimus,[206] vincristine,[207] and the ACE inhibitor captopril[208] have been reported to reduce the risk of relapse in case series. In a retrospective comparison between 20 children treated with cyclosporin or tacrolimus, no difference in the relapse rate, prednisone dose, or renal toxicity was found.[206] In 7 of 12 children with steroid-dependent SSNS, vincristine reduced the risk of relapse in the year after treatment compared with the previous year.[207] Captopril administered to 36 children with steroid-dependent SSNS in remission reduced the relapse rate and mean prednisone dose required.[208]

CONCLUSION

Although the long-term outlook for most children with SSNS is resolution of nephrotic syndrome and continuing normal renal function, approximately half will suffer multiple relapses requiring corticosteroids and one or more corticosteroid-sparing agents during the course of their disease and will also be at risk of multiple disease and treatment-related complications. In summary:

- SSNS is more common in Asian but less common in African and African American children compared with Caucasian children

- The proportion of children with idiopathic nephrotic syndrome who respond to corticosteroids appears to be decreasing
- The etiology and pathogenesis of SSNS remains largely unknown
- The outcome of SSNS is for resolution of disease and normal renal function in the majority of patients
- The first episode of SSNS should be treated with corticosteroid therapy for 6 months to reduce the risk of relapse
- Further data are required on the most effective way of treating relapsing SSNS with corticosteroids
- Prognosis for long-term renal function depends on remission of proteinuria rather than histology so that renal biopsies are not indicated before using corticosteroid-sparing therapy in children with SSNS
- There are no data demonstrating differences in efficacy between alkylating agents, cyclosporin, and levamisole, so their use depends on availability and physician and patient preference
- Data from randomized controlled trials indicate that there is no significant difference in the risk of relapse with azathioprine or mizoribine compared with prednisone alone
- Randomized controlled trials are required to determine the efficacy of mycophenolate mofetil and tacrolimus in children with relapsing SSNS

Further information on the underlying cause of SSNS is needed to guide therapy. New randomized controlled trials are required both to compare new therapies with existing therapies and to determine the optimal regimens for using corticosteroid therapy in the initial and subsequent episodes of SSNS.

REFERENCES

1. Nephrotic syndrome in children: prediction of histopathology from clinical and laboratory characteristics at time of diagnosis. A report of the International Study of Kidney Disease in Children, *Kidney Int* 13(2):159-65, 1978.
2. The primary nephrotic syndrome in children. Identification of patients with minimal change nephrotic syndrome from initial response to prednisone. A report of the International Study of Kidney Disease in Children, *J Pediatr* 98(4):561-64, 1981.
3. Koskimies O, Vilska J, Rapola J, Hallman N: Long-term outcome of primary nephrotic syndrome, *Arch Dis Child* 57(7):544-48, 1982.
4. Fakhouri F, Bocquet N, Taupin P, Presne C, Gagnadoux MF et al: Steroid-sensitive nephrotic syndrome: from childhood to adulthood, *Am J Kidney Dis* 41(3):550-57, 2003.
5. Tarshish P, Tobin JN, Bernstein J, Edelmann CM Jr: Prognostic significance of the early course of minimal change nephrotic syndrome: report of the International Study of Kidney Disease in Children, *J Am Soc Nephrol* 8(5):769-76, 1997.
6. McKinney PA, Feltbower RG, Brocklebank JT, Fitzpatrick MM: Time trends and ethnic patterns of childhood nephrotic syndrome in Yorkshire, UK, *Pediatr Nephrol* 16(12):1040-44, 2001.
7. Schlesinger ER, Sultz HA, Mosher WE, Feldman JG: The nephrotic syndrome. Its incidence and implications for the community, *Am J Dis Child* 116(6):623-32, 1968.
8. Srivastava T, Simon SD, Alon US: High incidence of focal segmental glomerulosclerosis in nephrotic syndrome of childhood, *Pediatr Nephrol* 13(1):13-18, 1999.
9. Fletcher JT, Hodson EM, Willis NS, Puckeridge S, Craig JC: Population-based study of nephrotic syndrome: Incidence, demographics, clinical presentation and risk factors, *Pediatr Nephrol* 19:C96, 2004.
10. Sharples PM, Poulton J, White RH: Steroid responsive nephrotic syndrome is more common in Asians, *Arch Dis Child* 60(11):1014-17, 1985.
11. Feehally J, Kendell NP, Swift PG, Walls J: High incidence of minimal change nephrotic syndrome in Asians, *Arch Dis Child* 60(11):1018-20, 1985.
12. Elzouki AY, Amin F, Jaiswal OP: Primary nephrotic syndrome in Arab children, *Arch Dis Child* 59(3):253-55, 1984.
13. Bhimma R, Coovadia HM, Adhikari M: Nephrotic syndrome in South African children: changing perspectives over 20 years, *Pediatr Nephrol* 11(4):429-34, 1997.
14. Filler G, Young E, Geier P, Carpenter B, Drukker A, Feber J: Is there really an increase in non-minimal change nephrotic syndrome in children? [Review], *Am J Kidney Dis* 42(6):1107-13, 2003.
15. Shalhoub RJ: Pathogenesis of lipoid nephrosis: a disorder of T-cell function, *Lancet* 2:556-60, 1974.
16. Routledge RC, Hann IM, Jones PH: Hodgkin's disease complicated by the nephrotic syndrome, *Cancer* 38:1735-40, 1976.
17. Yum MN, Edwards JL, Kleit S: Glomerular lesions in Hodgkin disease, *Arch Pathol* 99:645-49, 1975.
18. Keng KL, Kuipers F: Inoculation with measles virus in therapy of nephrotic syndrome, *Ned Tijdschr Geneeskd* 95:1806-14, 1951.
19. Lander HB: Effects of measles on nephrotic syndrome, *Am J Dis Child* 78:813-85, 1949.
20. Rosenblum AH, Lander HB, Fisher RM: Measles in the nephrotic syndrome, *J Pediatr* 35:574-84, 1949.
21. Tejani A: Morphological transition in minimal change nephrotic syndrome, *Nephron* 39(3):157-59, 1985.
22. Cambon-Thomsen A, Bouissou F, Abbal M, Duprat MP, Barthe P et al: HLA and Bf in idiopathic nephrotic syndrome in children: differences between corticosensitive and corticoresistant forms, *Pathol Biol (Paris)* 34:725-30, 1986.
23. Kobayashi T, Ogawa A, Takahashi K, Uchiyama M: HLA-DQB1 allele associates with idiopathic nephrotic syndrome in Japanese children, *Acta Paediatr Jpn* 37:293-96, 1995.
24. Lagueruela CC, Buettner TL, Cole BR, Kissane JM, Robson AM: HLA extended haplotypes in steroid-sensitive nephrotic syndrome of childhood, *Kidney Int* 38:145-50, 1990.
25. Noss G, Bachmann HJ, Olbing H: Association of minimal change nephrotic syndrome (MCNS) with HLA-B8 and B13, *Clin Nephrol* 15:172-74, 1981.
26. Brenchley PE: Vascular permeability factors in steroid-sensitive nephrotic syndrome and focal segmental glomerulosclerosis, *Nephrol Dial Transplant* 18(suppl 6):vi21-vi25, 2003.
27. Eddy AA, Schnaper HW: The nephrotic syndrome: from the simple to the complex, *Semin Nephrol* 18:304-16,1998.
28. Schnaper HW, Aune TM: Identification of the lymphokine soluble immune response suppressor in urine of nephrotic children, *J Clin Invest* 76:341-49, 1985.
29. Matsumoto K, Kanmatsuse K: Elevated vascular endothelial growth factor levels in the urine of patients with minimal-change nephrotic syndrome, *Clin Nephrol* 55:269-74, 2001.
30. Webb NJ, Watson CJ, Roberts IS, Bottomley MJ, Jones CA et al: Circulating vascular endothelial growth factor is not increased during relapses of steroid-sensitive nephrotic syndrome, *Kidney Int* 55:1063-71, 1999.
31. Eremina V, Cui S, Gerber H, Ferrara N, Haigh J et al: Vascular endothelial growth factor a signaling in the podocyte-endothelial compartment is required for mesangial cell migration and survival, *J Am Soc Nephrol* 17:724-35, 2006.
32. Eremina V, Sood M, Haigh J, Nagy A, Lajoie G et al: Glomerular-specific alterations of VEGF-A expression lead to distinct congenital and acquired renal diseases, *J Clin Invest* 111:707-16, 2003.

33. Schnaper HW, Aune TM: Steroid-sensitive mechanism of soluble immune response suppressor production in steroid-responsive nephrotic syndrome, *J Clin Invest* 79:257-64, 1987.
34. Savin VJ, Sharma R, Sharma M, McCarthy ET, Swan SK et al: Circulating factor associated with increased glomerular permeability to albumin in recurrent focal segmental glomerulosclerosis, *N Engl J Med* 334:878-83, 1996.
35. Dantal J, Bigot E, Bogers W, Testa A, Kriaa F et al: Effect of plasma protein adsorption on protein excretion in kidney-transplant recipients with recurrent nephrotic syndrome, *N Engl J Med* 330:7-14, 1994.
36. Garin EH, Laflam PF, Muffly K: Proteinuria and fusion of podocyte foot processes in rats after infusion of cytokine from patients with idiopathic minimal lesion nephrotic syndrome, *Nephron Exp Nephrol* 102:e105-e112, 2006.
37. Abbas AK, Murphy KM, Sher A: Functional diversity of helper T lymphocytes, *Nature* 383:787-93, 1996.
38. Mosmann TR, Cherwinski H, Bond MW, Giedlin MA, Coffman RL: Two types of murine helper T cell clone. I. Definition according to profiles of lymphokine activities and secreted proteins, *J Immunol* 136:2348-57, 1996.
39. Street NE, Mosmann TR: Functional diversity of T lymphocytes due to secretion of different cytokine patterns, *FASEB J* 5:171-77, 1991.
40. Sad S, Marcotte R, Mosmann TR: Cytokine-induced differentiation of precursor mouse CD8+ T cells into cytotoxic CD8+ T cells secreting Th1 or Th2 cytokines, *Immunity* 2:271-79, 1995.
41. Cambon-Thomsen A, Bouissou F, Abbal M, Duprat MP, Barthe P et al: HLA and Bf in idiopathic nephrotic syndrome in children: differences between corticosensitive and corticoresistant forms, *Pathol Biol (Paris)* 34:725-30, 1986.
42. Fehervari Z, Sakaguchi S: Development and function of CD25+CD4+ regulatory T cells, *Curr Opin Immunol* 16:203-38, 2004.
43. Hori S, Nomura T, Sakaguchi S: Control of regulatory T cell development by the transcription factor Foxp3, *Science* 299:1057-61, 2003.
44. Iwakura Y, Ishigame H: The IL-23/IL-17 axis in inflammation, *J Clin Invest* 116:1218-22, 2006.
45. Weaver CT, Harrington LE, Mangan PR, Gavrieli M, Murphy KM: Th17: an effector CD4 T cell lineage with regulatory T cell ties, *Immunity* 24:677-88, 2006.
46. Araya CE, Wasserfall CH, Brusko TM, Mu W, Segal MS et al: A case of unfulfilled expectations. Cytokines in idiopathic minimal lesion nephrotic syndrome, *Pediatr Nephrol* 21:603-10, 2006.
47. Matsumoto K, Kanmatsuse K: Increased urinary excretion of interleukin-17 in nephrotic patients, *Nephron* 91:243-49, 2002.
48. Bakr A, Rageh I, El Azouny M, Deyab S, Lotfy H: Serum neopterin levels in children with primary nephrotic syndrome, *Acta Paediatr* 95:854-56, 2006.
49. Mansour H, Cheval L, Elalouf JM, Aude JC, Alyanakian MA et al: T-cell transcriptome analysis points up a thymic disorder in idiopathic nephrotic syndrome, *Kidney Int* 67:2168-77, 2005.
50. Okuyama S, Komatsuda A, Wakui H, Aiba N, Fujishima N et al: Up-regulation of TRAIL mRNA expression in peripheral blood mononuclear cells from patients with minimal-change nephrotic syndrome, *Nephrol Dial Transplant* 20:539-44, 2005.
51. Strehlau J, Schachter AD, Pavlakis M, Singh A, Tejani A, Strom TB: Activated intrarenal transcription of CTL-effectors and TGF-beta1 in children with focal segmental glomerulosclerosis, *Kidney Int* 61:90-95, 2002.
52. Schachter AD: The pediatric nephrotic syndrome spectrum: clinical homogeneity and molecular heterogeneity, *Pediatr Transplant* 8:344-48, 2004.
53. Aviles DH, Matti V, V, Manning J, Ochoa AC, Zea AH: Decreased expression of T-cell NF-kappaB p65 subunit in steroid-resistant nephrotic syndrome, *Kidney Int* 66:60-67, 2004.
54. Valanciute A, le Gouvello S, Solhonne B, Pawlak A, Grimbert P et al: NF-kappa B p65 antagonizes IL-4 induction by c-maf in minimal change nephrotic syndrome, *J Immunol* 172:688-98, 2004.
55. Ruf RG, Fuchshuber A, Karle SM, Lemainque A, Huck K et al: Identification of the first gene locus (SSNS1) for steroid-sensitive nephrotic syndrome on chromosome 2p, *J Am Soc Nephrol* 14:1897-900, 2003.
56. Murphy WM, Jukkola AF, Roy S III: Nephrotic syndrome with mesangial-cell proliferation in children—a distinct entity? *Am J Clin Pathol* 72(1):42-47, 1979.
57. Waldherr R, Gubler MC, Levy M, Broyer M, Habib R: The significance of pure diffuse mesangial proliferation in idiopathic nephrotic syndrome, *Clin Nephrol* 10(5):171-79, 1978.
58. Zeis PM, Kavazarakis E, Nakopoulou L, Moustaki M, Messaritaki A et al: Glomerulopathy with mesangial IgM deposits: long-term follow up of 64 children, *Pediatr Int* 43(3):287-92, 2001.
59. Tejani A, Phadke K, Nicastri A, Adamson O, Chen CK et al: Efficacy of cyclophosphamide in steroid-sensitive childhood nephrotic syndrome with different morphological lesions, *Nephron* 41(2):170-73, 1985.
60. Kopolovic J, Shvil Y, Pomeranz A, Ron N, Rubinger D, Oren R: IgM nephropathy: morphological study related to clinical findings, *Am J Nephrol* 7(4):275-80, 1987.
61. Hsu HC, Chen WY, Lin GJ, Chen L, Kao SL et al: Clinical and immunopathologic study of mesangial IgM nephropathy: report of 41 cases, *Histopathology* 8(3):435-46, 1984.
62. Habib R, Girardin E, Gagnadoux MF, Hinglais N, Levy M, Broyer M: Immunopathological findings in idiopathic nephrosis: clinical significance of glomerular "immune deposits." *Pediatr Nephrol* 2(4):402-08, 1988.
63. Al Eisa A, Carter JE, Lirenman DS, Magil AB: Childhood IgM nephropathy: comparison with minimal change disease, *Nephron* 72(1):37-43, 1996.
64. Myllymaki J, Saha H, Mustonen J, Helin H, Pasternack A: IgM nephropathy: clinical picture and long-term prognosis, *Am J Kidney Dis* 41(2):343-50, 2003.
65. Haas M, Yousefzadeh N: Glomerular tip lesion in minimal change nephropathy: a study of autopsies before 1950, *Am J Kidney Dis* 39(6):1168-75, 2002.
66. Howie AJ: Pathology of minimal change nephropathy and segmental sclerosing glomerular disorders [Review], *Nephrol Dial Transplant* 18(suppl 6):vi33-38, 2003.
67. Ostalska-Nowicka D, Zachwieja J, Maciejewski J, Wozniak A, Salwa-Urawska W: The prognostic value of glomerular immaturity in the nephrotic syndrome in children, *Pediatr Nephrol* 19:633-37, 2004.
68. Ichikawa I, Fogo A: Focal segmental glomerulosclerosis [Review], *Pediatr Nephrol* 10(3):374-91, 1996.
69. Schnaper HW: Idiopathic focal segmental glomerulosclerosis [Review], *Semin Nephrol* 23(2):183-93, 2003.
70. McAdams AJ, Valentini RP, Welch TR: The nonspecificity of focal segmental glomerulosclerosis. The defining characteristics of primary focal glomerulosclerosis, mesangial proliferation, and minimal change, *Medicine* 76(1):42-52, 1997.
71. D'Agati V: Pathologic classification of focal segmental glomerulosclerosis [Review], *Semin Nephrol* 23(2):117-34, 2003.
72. Habib R, Kleinknecht C: The primary nephrotic syndrome of childhood. Classification and clinicopathologic study of 406 cases [Review], *Pathology Annual* 6:417-74, 1971.
73. Meadow SR, Sarsfield JK: Steroid-responsive and nephrotic syndrome and allergy: clinical studies, *Arch Dis Child* 56(7):509-16, 1981.
74. Arneil GC: 164 children with nephrosis, *Lancet* 2:1103-10, 1961.
75. Alwadhi RK, Mathew JL, Rath B: Clinical profile of children with nephrotic syndrome not on glucorticoid therapy, but presenting with infection, *J Paediatr Child Health* 40(1-2):28-32, 2004.
76. Lewis MA, Baildom EM, Davis N, Houston IB, Postlethwaite RJ: Nephrotic syndrome: from toddlers to twenties, *Lancet* 1(8632):255-59, 1989.
77. Takeda A, Takimoto H, Mizusawa Y, Simoda M: Prediction of subsequent relapse in children with steroid-sensitive nephrotic syndrome, *Pediatr Nephrol* 16(11):888-93, 2001.
78. Yap HK, Han EJ, Heng CK, Gong WK: Risk factors for steroid dependency in children with idiopathic nephrotic syndrome, *Pediatr Nephrol* 16(12):1049-52, 2001.

79. Constantinescu AR, Shah HB, Foote EF, Weiss LS: Predicting first-year relapses in children with nephrotic syndrome, *Pediatrics* 105(3 Pt 1):492-95, 2000.
80. Lahdenkari AT, Suvanto M, Kajantie E, Koskimies O, Kestilä M, Jalanko H: Clinical features and outcome of childhood minimal change nephrotic syndrome: is genetics involved? *Pediatr Nephrol* 20:1073-80, 2005.
81. Rüth EM, Kemper MJ, Leumann EP, Laube GF, Neuhaus TJ: Children with steroid-sensitive nephrotic syndrome come of age: long-term outcome, *J Pediatr* 147(2):202-07, 2005.
82. Trompeter RS, Lloyd BW, Hicks J, White RH, Cameron JS: Long-term outcome for children with minimal-change nephrotic syndrome, *Lancet* 1(8425):368-70, 1985.
83. Berns JS, Gaudio KM, Krassner LS, Anderson FP, Durante D et al: Steroid-responsive nephrotic syndrome of childhood: a long-term study of clinical course, histopathology, efficacy of cyclophosphamide therapy, and effects on growth, *Am J Kidney Dis* 9(2):108-14, 1987.
84. Webb NJ, Lewis MA, Iqbal J, Smart PJ, Lendon M, Postlethwaite RJ: Childhood steroid-sensitive nephrotic syndrome: does the histology matter? *Am J Kidney Dis* 27(4):484-88, 1996.
85. Cattran DC, Rao P: Long-term outcome in children and adults with classic focal segmental glomerulosclerosis, *Am J Kidney Dis* 32(1):72-79, 1998.
86. Abrantes MM, Cardosa LSB, Lima EM, Silva JMP, Diniz JS et al: Clinical course of 110 children and adolescents with primary focal segmental glomerulosclerosis, *Pediatr Nephrol* 21:482-89, 2006.
87. Ahmad H, Tejani A: Predictive value of repeat renal biopsies in children with nephrotic syndrome, *Nephron* 84(4):342-46, 2000.
88. Minimal change nephrotic syndrome in children: deaths during the first 5 to 15 years' observation. Report of the International Study of Kidney Disease in Children, *Pediatrics* 73(4):497-501, 1984.
89. Lechner BL, Bockenhauer D, Iragorri S, Kennedy TL, Siegel NJ: The risk of cardiovascular disease in adults who have had childhood nephrotic syndrome, *Pediatr Nephrol* 19:744-48, 2004.
90. Broyer M, Meyrier A, Niaudet P, Habib R: Minimal changes and focal and segmental glomerular sclerosis. In Cameron JS, Davison AM, Grunfeld JP, Kerr D, Ritz E, editors: *Oxford textbook of clinical nephrology*, Oxford, 1992, Oxford University Press.
91. Gulati S, Sural S, Sharma RK, Gupta A, Gupta RK: Spectrum of adolescent-onset nephrotic syndrome in Indian children, *Pediatr Nephrol* 16(12):1045-48, 2001.
92. Gulati S, Sharma AP, Sharma RK, Gupta A, Gupta RK: Do current recommendations for kidney biopsy in nephrotic syndrome need modifications? *Pediatr Nephrol* 17(6):404-08, 2002.
93. Baqi N, Singh A, Balachandra S, Ahmad H, Nicastri A et al: The paucity of minimal change disease in adolescents with primary nephrotic syndrome, *Pediatr Nephrol* 12(2):105-07, 1998.
94. Primack WA, Schulman SL, Kaplan BS: An analysis of the approach to management of childhood nephrotic syndrome by pediatric nephrologists, *Am J Kidney Dis* 23(4):524-27, 1994.
95. Siegel NJ, Gaudio KM, Krassner LS, McDonald BM, Anderson FP, Kashgarian M: Steroid-dependent nephrotic syndrome in children: histopathology and relapses after cyclophosphamide treatment, *Kidney Int* 19:454-59, 1981.
96. Trachtman H, Carroll F, Phadke K, Khawar M, Nicastri A et al: Paucity of minimal-change lesion in children with early frequently relapsing steroid-responsive nephrotic syndrome, *Am J Nephrol* 7(1):13-17, 1987.
97. Sorof JM, Hawkins EP, Brewer ED, Boydstun II, Kale AS, Powell DR: Age and ethnicity affect the risk and outcome of focal segmental glomerulosclerosis, *Pediatr Nephrol* 12(9):764-68, 1998.
98. Stadermann MB, Lilien MR, van de Kar NC, Monnens LA, Schroder CH: Is biopsy required prior to cyclophosphamide in steroid-sensitive nephrotic syndrome? *Clin Nephrol* 60(5):315-17, 2003.
99. White RH, Poole C: Day care renal biopsy, *Pediatr Nephrol* 10(4):408-11, 1996.
100. Gipson DS, Chin H, Presler TP, Jennette C, Massengill S et al: Differential risk of remission and ESRD in childhood FSGS, *Pediatr Nephrol* 21:344-49, 2006.
101. Arneil GC: Treatment of nephrosis with prednisolone, *Lancet* 1:409-11, 1956.
102. Arneil GC: The nephrotic syndrome [Review], *Pediatr Clin North Am* 18(2):547-59, 1971.
103. Alternate-day versus intermittent prednisone in frequently relapsing nephrotic syndrome. A report of Arbetsgemeinschaft für Pädiatrische Nephrologie, *Lancet* 1(8113):401-03, 1979.
104. Hodson EM, Knight JF, Willis NS, Craig JC: Corticosteroid therapy in nephrotic syndrome: a meta-analysis of randomised controlled trials, *Arch Dis Child* 83(1):45-51, 2000.
105. Hodson EM, Knight JF, Willis NS, Craig JC: Corticosteroid therapy for nephrotic syndrome in children. Update of *Cochrane Database Syst Rev*: CD001533, 2004; PMID:15106158 [Review], *Cochrane Database of Syst Rev*: CD001533, 2005.
106. Ekka BK, Bagga A, Srivastava RN: Single- versus divided-dose prednisolone therapy for relapses of nephrotic syndrome, *Pediatr Nephrol* 11(5):597-99, 1997.
107. Choonara IA, Heney D, Meadow SR: Low dose prednisolone in nephrotic syndrome, *Arch Dis Child* 64(4):610-11, 1989.
108. Short versus standard prednisone therapy for initial treatment of idiopathic nephrotic syndrome in children; Arbeitsgemeinschaft für Pädiatrische Nephrologie, *Lancet* 1 (8582):380-83, 1988.
109. Bagga A, Hari P, Srivastava RN: Prolonged versus standard prednisolone therapy for initial episode of nephrotic syndrome, *Pediatr Nephrol* 13(9):824-27, 1999.
110. Ueda N, Chihara M, Kawaguchi S, Niinomi Y, Nonoda T et al: Intermittent versus long-term tapering prednisolone for initial therapy in children with idiopathic nephrotic syndrome. *J Pediatr* 112(1):122-26, 1988.
111. Norero C, Delucchi A, Lagos E, Rosati P: Initial therapy of primary nephrotic syndrome in children: evaluation in a period of 18 months of two prednisone treatment schedules. Chilean Co-operative Group of Study of Nephrotic Syndrome in Children, *Rev Med Chil* 124(5):567-72, 1996.
112. Ehrich JH, Brodehl J: Long versus standard prednisone therapy for initial treatment of idiopathic nephrotic syndrome in children; Arbeitsgemeinschaft für Pädiatrische Nephrologie, *Eur J Pediatr* 152(4):357-61, 1993.
113. Ksiázek J, Wyszyńska T: Short versus long initial prednisone treatment in steroid-sensitive nephrotic syndrome in children, *Acta Paediatr* 84(8):889-93, 1995.
114. Jayantha UK: Comparison of ISKDC regime with a 7 month regime in the first attack of nephrotic syndrome, *Pediatr Nephrol* 19:C81, 2004.
115. Pecoraro C, Caropreso MR, Malgieri G, Ferretti AVS, Raddi G et al: Therapy of first episode of steroid responsive nephrotic syndrome: a randomised controlled trial, *Pediatr Nephrol* 19:C72, 2004.
116. Hiraoka M, Tsukahara H, Matsubara K, Tsurusawa M, Takeda N et al: A randomized study of two long-course prednisolone regimens for nephrotic syndrome in children, *Am J Kidney Dis* 41(6):1155-62, 2003.
117. Sharma RK, Ahmed M, Gupta A, Gulati S, Sharma AP: Comparison of abrupt withdrawal versus slow tapering regimens of prednisolone therapy in the management of first episode of steroid responsive childhood idiopathic nephrotic syndrome, *J Am Soc Nephrol* 11:97A, 2000.
118. Kleinknecht C, Broyer M, Parchoux B, Loriat C, Nivet H, Palcoux JB: Comparison of short and long treatment at onset of steroid sensitive nephrosis, *Int J Pediatr Nephrol* 3:45, 1982.
119. Hodson EM, Craig JC, Willis NS: Evidence-based management of steroid-sensitive nephrotic syndrome [Review], *Pediatr Nephrol* 20:1523-30, 2005.
120. Hiraoka M, Tsukahara H, Haruki S, Hayashi S, Takeda N et al: Older boys benefit from higher initial prednisolone therapy for nephrotic syndrome; The West Japan Cooperative Study of Kidney Disease in Children, *Kidney Int* 58(3):1247-52, 2000.
121. Lande MB, Leonard MB: Variability among pediatric nephrologists in the initial therapy of nephrotic syndrome, *Pediatr Nephrol* 14 (8-9):766-9, 2000.
122. Webb, NJ: 2006 (personal communication).
123. Brodehl J: The treatment of minimal change nephrotic syndrome: lessons learned from multicentre co-operative studies [Review], *Eur J Pediatr* 150(6):380-87, 1991.

124. Consensus statement on management and audit potential for steroid responsive nephrotic syndrome. Report of a Workshop by the British Association for Paediatric Nephrology and Research Unit, Royal College of Physicians [Review], *Arch Dis Child* 70(2):151-57, 1994.
125. Wingen AM, Müller-Wiefel DE, Scharer K: Spontaneous remissions in frequently relapsing and steroid dependent idiopathic nephrotic syndrome, *Clin Nephrol* 23(1):35-40, 1985.
126. Narchi H: Nephrotic syndrome relapse: need for a better evidence based definition, *Arch Dis Child* 89(4):395, 2004.
127. Jayantha UK: Prolonged versus standard steroid therapy for children with a relapsing course of nephrotic syndrome, *Pediatr Nephrol* 19:C99, 2004.
128. Mattoo TK, Mahmoud MA: Increased maintenance corticosteroids during upper respiratory infection decrease the risk of relapse in nephrotic syndrome, *Nephron* 85(4):343-45, 2000.
129. Imbasciati E, Gusmano R, Edefonti A, Zucchelli P, Pozzi C et al: Controlled trial of methylprednisolone pulses and low dose oral prednisone for the minimal change nephrotic syndrome, *British Medical Journal Clinical Research Ed.* 291(6505):1305-08, 1985.
130. Elzouki AY, Jaiswal OP: Long-term, small dose prednisone therapy in frequently relapsing nephrotic syndrome of childhood. Effect on remission, statural growth, obesity, and infection rate, *Clin Pediatr* 27(8):387-92, 1988.
131. Srivastava RN, Vasudev AS, Bagga A, Sunderam KR: Long-term, low-dose prednisolone therapy in frequently relapsing nephrotic syndrome, *Pediatr Nephrol* 6(3):247-50, 1992.
132. Ng JS, Wong W, Law RW, Hui J, Wong EN, Lam DS: Ocular complications of paediatric patients with nephrotic syndrome, *Clin Experiment Ophthalmol* 29(4):239-43, 2001.
133. Brocklebank JT, Harcourt RB, Meadow SR: Corticosteroid-induced cataracts in idiopathic nephrotic syndrome, *Arch Dis Child* 57(1):30-34, 1982.
134. Hall AS, Thorley G, Houtman PN: The effects of corticosteroids on behavior in children with nephrotic syndrome, *Pediatr Nephrol* 18(12):1220-23, 2003.
135. Broyer M, Guest G, Gagnadoux MF: Growth rate in children receiving alternate-day corticosteroid treatment after kidney transplantation, *J Pediatr* 120(5):721-25, 1992.
136. Saha MT, Laippala P, Lenko HL: Normal growth of prepubertal nephrotic children during long-term treatment with repeated courses of prednisone, *Acta Paediatr* 87(5):545-48, 1998.
137. Polito C, Oporto MR, Totino SF, La Manna A, Di Toro R: Normal growth of nephrotic children during long-term alternate-day prednisone therapy, *Acta Paediatr Scand* 75(2):245-50, 1986.
138. Foote KD, Brocklebank JT, Meadow SR: Height attainment in children with steroid-responsive nephrotic syndrome, *Lancet* 2(8461):917-19, 1985.
139. Rees L, Greene SA, Adlard P, Jones J, Haycock GB et al: Growth and endocrine function in steroid sensitive nephrotic syndrome, *Arch Dis Child* 63(5):484-90, 1988.
140. Donatti TL, Koch VH, Fujimura MD, Okay Y: Growth in steroid-responsive nephrotic syndrome: a study of 85 pediatric patients, *Pediatr Nephrol* 18(8):789-95, 2003.
141. Emma F, Sesto A, Rizzoni G: Long-term linear growth of children with severe steroid-responsive nephrotic syndrome, *Pediatr Nephrol* 18(8):783-88, 2003.
142. Grymonprez A, Proesmans W, Van Dyck M, Jans I, Goos G, Bouillon R. Vitamin D metabolites in childhood nephrotic syndrome, *Pediatr Nephrol* 9(3):278-81, 1995.
143. Gulati S, Godbole M, Singh U, Gulati K, Srivastava A: Are children with idiopathic nephrotic syndrome at risk for metabolic bone disease? *Am J Kidney Dis* 41(6):1163-69, 2003.
144. Biyikli NK, Emre S, Sirin A, Bilge I: Biochemical bone markers in nephrotic children, *Pediatr Nephrol* 19:869-73, 2004.
145. Bachrach LK: Bare-bones fact—children are not small adults, *N Eng J Med* 351(9):924-96, 2004.
146. Freundlich M, Jofe M, Goodman WG, Salusky IB: Bone histology in steroid-treated children with non-azotemic nephrotic syndrome, *Pediatr Nephrol* 19:400-07, 2004.
147. Munns CF, Cowell CT: Prevention and treatment of osteoporosis in chronically ill children [Review], *J Musculoskel Neuronal Interact* 5(3):262-72, 2005.
148. Schonau E: The peak bone mass concept: is it still relevant? [Review], *Pediatr Nephrol* 19:825-31, 2004.
149. Lettgen B, Jeken C, Reiners C: Influence of steroid medication on bone mineral density in children with nephrotic syndrome, *Pediatr Nephrol* 8(6):667-70, 1994.
150. Polito C, La Manna A, Todisco N, Cimmaruta E, Sessa G, Pirozzi M: Bone mineral content in nephrotic children on long-term, alternate-day prednisone therapy, *Clin Pediatr* 34(5):234-36, 1995.
151. Leonard MB, Feldman HI, Shults J, Zemel BS, Foster BJ, Stallings VA: Long-term, high-dose glucocorticoids and bone mineral content in childhood glucocorticoid-sensitive nephrotic syndrome, *N Eng J Med* 351(9):868-75, 2004.
152. Gulati S, Sharma RK, Gulati K, Singh U, Srivastava A: Longitudinal follow-up of bone mineral density in children with nephrotic syndrome and the role of calcium and vitamin D supplements, *Nephrol Dial Transplant* 20:1598-603, 2005.
153. Bak M, Serdaroglu E, Guclu R: Prophylactic calcium and vitamin D treatments in steroid-treated children with nephrotic syndrome, *Pediatr Nephrol* 21(3):350-54. 2006.
154. Coldbeck JH: Experience with alkylating agents in the treatment of children with nephrotic syndrome, *Med J Aust* 2:987-89, 1963.
155. Grupe WE, Heymann W: Cytotoxic drugs in steroid-resistant renal disease. Alkylating and antimetabolic agents in the treatment of nephrotic syndrome, lupus nephritis, chronic glomerulonephritis, and purpura nephritis in children, *American Journal of Diseases of Children* 112(5):448-58, 1966.
156. Grupe WE, Makker SP, Ingelfinger JR: Chlorambucil treatment of frequently relapsing nephrotic syndrome, *N Eng J Med* 295(14):746-49, 1976.
157. Chiu J, McLaine PN, Drummond KN: A controlled prospective study of cyclophosphamide in relapsing, corticosteroid-responsive, minimal-lesion nephrotic syndrome in childhood, *J Pediatr* 82(4):607-13, 1973.
158. Alatas H, Wirya IG, Tambunan T, Himawan S: Controlled trial of chlorambucil in frequently relapsing nephrotic syndrome in children (a preliminary report), *J Med Asso Thai* 61(suppl)1:222-28, 1978.
159. Barratt TM, Soothill JF: Controlled trial of cyclophosphamide in steroid-sensitive relapsing nephrotic syndrome of childhood, *Lancet* 2(7671):479-82, 1970.
160. Prospective, controlled trial of cyclophosphamide therapy in children with nephrotic syndrome. Report of the International Study of Kidney Disease in Children, *Lancet* 2(7878):423-47, 1974.
161. Durkan A, Hodson EM, Willis NS, Craig JC: Non-corticosteroid treatment for nephrotic syndrome in children. Update of *Cochrane Database Syst Rev*: CD002290, 2001; PMID: 116871550 [Review], *Cochrane Database of Syst Rev*: CD002290, 2005.
162. Durkan AM, Hodson EM, Willis NS, Craig JC: Immunosuppressive agents in childhood nephrotic syndrome: a meta-analysis of randomized controlled trials, *Kidney Int* 59(5):1919-27, 2001.
163. Arbeitsgemeinschaft für Pädiatrische Nephrologie: Effect of cytotoxic drugs in frequently relapsing nephrotic syndrome with and without steroid dependence, *N Eng J Med* 306(8):451-44, 1982.
164. Ueda N, Kuno K, Ito S: Eight and 12 week courses of cyclophosphamide in nephrotic syndrome, *Arch Dis Child* 65(10):1147-50, 1990.
165. Arbeitsgemeinschaft für Pädiatrische Nephrologie: Cyclophosphamide treatment of steroid dependent nephrotic syndrome: comparison of eight week with 12 week course, *Arch Dis Child* 62(11):1102-06, 1987.
166. Latta K, von Schnakenburg C, Ehrich JH: A meta-analysis of cytotoxic treatment for frequently relapsing nephrotic syndrome in children, *Pediatr Nephrol* 16(3):271-82, 2001.
167. Vester U, Kranz B, Zimmermann S, Hoyer PF: Cyclophosphamide in steroid-sensitive nephrotic syndrome: outcome and outlook, *Pediatr Nephrol* 18(7):661-44, 2003.
168. Prasad N, Gulati S, Sharma RK, Singh U, Ahmed M: Pulse cyclophosphamide therapy in steroid-dependent nephrotic syndrome, *Pediatr Nephrol* 19:494-98, 2004.
169. Gulati S, Pokhariyal S, Sharma RK, Elhence R, Kher V et al: Pulse cyclophosphamide therapy in frequently relapsing nephrotic syndrome, *Nephrol Dial Transplant* 16(10):2013-17, 2001.

170. Miller DG: Alkylating agents and human spermatogenesis, *JAMA* 217(12):1662-65, 1971.
171. Ponticelli C, Edefonti A, Ghio L, Rizzoni G, Rinaldi S et al: Cyclosporin versus cyclophosphamide for patients with steroid-dependent and frequently relapsing idiopathic nephrotic syndrome: a multicentre randomized controlled trial, *Nephrol Dial Transplant* 8(12):1326-32, 1993.
172. Niaudet P: Comparison of cyclosporin and chlorambucil in the treatment of steroid-dependent idiopathic nephrotic syndrome: a multicentre randomized controlled trial. The French Society of Paediatric Nephrology, *Pediatr Nephrol* 6(1):1-3, 1992.
173. Hulton SA, Neuhaus TJ, Dillon MJ, Barratt TM: Long-term cyclosporin A treatment of minimal-change nephrotic syndrome of childhood, *Pediatr Nephrol* 8(4):401-03, 1994.
174. Niaudet P, Broyer M, Habib R: Treatment of idiopathic nephrotic syndrome with cyclosporin A in children, *Clin Nephrol* 35 (suppl)1: S31-6, 1991.
175. Tirelli AS, Paterlini G, Ghio L, Edefonti A, Assael BM et al: Renal effects of cyclosporin A in children treated for idiopathic nephrotic syndrome, *Acta Paediatr* 82(5):463-68, 1993.
176. D'Agati VD: Morphologic features of cyclosporin nephrotoxicity [Review], *Contrib Nephrol* 114:84-110, 1995.
177. Mihatsch MJ, Thiel G, Ryffel B: Morphologic diagnosis of cyclosporine nephrotoxicity [Review], *Semin Diagn Pathol* 5(1):104-21, 1988.
178. Iijima K, Hamahira K, Tanaka R, Kobayashi A, Nozu K et al: Risk factors for cyclosporine-induced tubulointerstitial lesions in children with minimal change nephrotic syndrome, *Kidney Int* 61(5):1801-05, 2002.
179. Inoue Y, Iijima K, Nakamura H, Yoshikawa N: Two-year cyclosporin treatment in children with steroid-dependent nephrotic syndrome, *Pediatr Nephrol* 13(1):33-38, 1999.
180. Niaudet P, Habib R, Tete MJ, Hinglais N, Broyer M: Cyclosporin in the treatment of idiopathic nephrotic syndrome in children, *Pediatr Nephrol* 1(4):566-73, 1987.
181. Hamahira K, Iijima K, Tanaka R, Nakamura H, Yoshikawa N: Recovery from cyclosporine-associated arteriolopathy in childhood nephrotic syndrome, *Pediatr Nephrol* 16(9):723-27, 2001.
182. El Husseini A, El Basuony F, Mahmoud I, Donia A, Hassan N et al: Co-administration of cyclosporine and ketoconazole in idiopathic childhood nephrosis, *Pediatr Nephrol* 19:976-81, 2004.
183. Filler G: How should microemulsified Cyclosporine A (Neoral) therapy in patients with nephrotic syndrome be monitored? *Nephrol Dial Transplant* 20:1032-34, 2005.
184. Fujinaga S, Kaneko K, Takada M, Ohtomo Y, Akashi S, Yamashiro Y: Preprandial C2 monitoring of cyclosporine treatment in children with nephrotic syndrome, *Pediatr Nephrol* 20:1359-60, 2005.
185. Davin JC, Merkus MP: Levamisole in steroid-sensitive nephrotic syndrome of childhood: the lost paradise? [Review], *Pediatr Nephrol* 20:10-14, 2005.
186. Tanphaichitr P, Tanphaichitr D, Sureeratanan J, Chatasingh S: Treatment of nephrotic syndrome with levamisole, *J Pediatr* 96(3 Pt 1):490-93, 1980.
187. Dayal U, Dayal AK, Shastry JC, Raghupathy P: Use of levamisole in maintaining remission in steroid-sensitive nephrotic syndrome in children [erratum in *Nephron* 67(4):507, 1994], *Nephron* 66(4): 408-12, 1994.
188. Levamisole for corticosteroid-dependent nephrotic syndrome in childhood; British Association for Paediatric Nephrology, *Lancet* 337(8757):1555-57, 1991.
189. Rashid HU, Ahmed S, Fatima N, Khanam, A: Levamisole in the treatment of steroid dependent or frequently relapsing nephrotic syndrome in children, *Bangladesh Renal Journal* 15(1):6-8, 1996.
190. Weiss R: Randomized double-blind placebo controlled, multicenter trial of levamisole for children with frequently relapsing/steroid dependent nephrotic syndrome, *J Am Soc Nephrol* 4:289, 1993.
191. Donia AF, Ammar HM, El Agroudy A, Moustafa F, Sobh MA: Long-term results of two unconventional agents in steroid-dependent nephrotic children, *Pediatr Nephrol* 20:1420-25, 2005.
192. Alsaran K, Grisaru S, Stephens D, Arbus G: Levamisole vs. cyclophosphamide for frequently-relapsing steroid-dependent nephrotic syndrome, *Clin Nephrol* 56(4):289-94, 2001.
193. Palcoux JB, Niaudet P, Goumy P: Side effects of levamisole in children with nephrosis, *Pediatr Nephrol* 8(2):263-64, 1994.
194. Barbano G, Ginevri F, Ghiggeri GM, Gusmano R: Disseminated autoimmune disease during levamisole treatment of nephrotic syndrome, *Pediatr Nephrol* 13(7):602-03, 1999.
195. Bagga A, Hari P, Moudgil A, Jordan SC: Mycophenolate mofetil and prednisolone therapy in children with steroid-dependent nephrotic syndrome, *Am J Kidney Dis* 42(6):1114-20, 2003.
196. Hogg RJ, Fitzgibbons L, Bruick J, Bunke M, Ault B et al: Clinical trial of mycophenolate mofetil (MMF) for frequent relapsing nephrotic syndrome in children, *Pediatr Nephrol* 19:C18, 2004.
197. Mendizabal S, Zamora I, Berbel O, Sanahuja MJ, Fuentes J, Simon J: Mycophenolate mofetil in steroid/cyclosporine-dependent/resistant nephrotic syndrome, *Pediatr Nephrol* 20:914-19, 2005.
198. Ulinski T, Dubourg L, Said MH, Parchoux B, Ranchin B, Cochat P: Switch from cyclosporine A to mycophenolate mofetil in nephrotic children, *Pediatr Nephrol* 20:482-85, 2005.
199. Abramowicz M, Barnett HL, Edelmann CM Jr, Greifer I, Kobayashi O et al: Controlled trial of azathioprine in children with nephrotic syndrome. A report for the International Study of Kidney Disease in Children, *Lancet* 1(7654):959-61, 1970.
200. Barratt TM, Cameron JS, Chantler C, Counahan R, Ogg CS, Soothill JF: Controlled trial of azathioprine in treatment of steroid-responsive nephrotic syndrome of childhood, *Arch Dis Child* 52(6):462-63, 1977.
201. Hiraoka M, Tsukahara H, Hori C, Ohshima Y, Momoi T et al: Efficacy of long-term azathioprine for relapsing nephrotic syndrome, *Pediatr Nephrol* 14(8-9):776-78, 2000.
202. Honda M: Nephrotic syndrome and mizoribine in children [Review], *Pediatr Int* 44(2):210-16, 2002.
203. Yoshioka K, Ohashi Y, Sakai T, Ito H, Yoshikawa N et al: A multicenter trial of mizoribine compared with placebo in children with frequently relapsing nephrotic syndrome, *Kidney Int* 58(1):317-24, 2000.
204. Rowe PC, McLean RH, Ruley EJ, Salcedo JR, Baumgardner RA et al: Intravenous immunoglobulin in minimal change nephrotic syndrome: a crossover trial, *Pediatr Nephrol* 4(1):32-35, 1990.
205. Trompeter RS, Thomson PD, Barratt TM, Soothill JF: Controlled trial of disodium cromoglycate in prevention of relapse of steroid-responsive nephrotic syndrome of childhood, *Arch Dis Child* 53(5):430-32, 1978.
206. Sinha MD, MacLeod R, Rigby E, Clark AG: Treatment of severe steroid dependent nephrotic syndrome (SDNS) in paediatrics with tacrolimus therapy, *Pediatr Nephrol* 19:C72, 2004.
207. Kausman JY, Yin L, Jones CL, Johnstone L, Powell HR: Vincristine treatment in steroid-dependent nephrotic syndrome, *Pediatr Nephrol* 20:1416-19, 2005.
208. Jayantha UK: Captopril therapy in children with steroid dependent nephrotic syndrome and their long term follow up, *Pediatr Nephrol* 19:C98, 2004.
209. Hogg RJ, Portman RJ, Milliner D, Lemley KV, Eddy A, Ingelfinger J: Evaluation and management of proteinuria and nephrotic syndrome in children: recommendations from a pediatric nephrology panel established at the National Kidney Foundation conference on proteinuria, albuminuria, risk, assessment, detection, and elimination (PARADE), *Pediatrics* 105(6):1242-49, 2000.
210. Indian Pediatric Nephrology Group IAoP: Consensus statement on management of steroid sensitive nephrotic syndrome [Review], *Indian Pediatr* 38(9):975-86, 2001.

CHAPTER

16 Steroid-Resistant Nephrotic Syndrome

Peter F. Hoyer, Udo Vester, and Jan Ulrich Becker

DEFINITION

Among pediatric nephrologists there are two definitions of steroid-resistant nephrotic syndrome (SRNS). The definition introduced by the International Study of Kidney Disease in Children (ISKDC) and used by the Arbeitsgemeinschaft für Pädiatrische Nephrologie (APN) is widely accepted as follows[1]: *No urinary remission within 4 weeks of prednisone therapy 60 mg/m²/day*. The other definition, employed by the Society of French Speaking Pediatric Nephrologists,[2] states: *No urinary remission following 4 weeks of prednisone 60 mg/m²/day followed by three intravenous pulses of methylpredisolone*. The rationale for both definitions is the experience that almost all patients with minimal change who respond will do so within 4 weeks (Figure 16-1) and only a small percentage will respond later (often called *late responders*). It is of great importance for interpretation of clinical data and studies to know the patient's age and the definition used.

INTRODUCTION

Treatment of SRNS remains a difficult challenge in pediatric nephrology. Because of poor prognosis in the past, the majority of children have received intensive treatment regimens and many of them have been overtreated. At the moment there is no diagnostic marker for children displaying with nephrotic syndrome that can be used as a predictor of steroid responsiveness or resistance. The most important prognostic marker for children with nephrotic syndrome is their response to steroid treatment. Initial steroid treatment can be avoided only in patients with a family history of SRNS or in those who have a known gene mutation. There is an urgent need to distinguish as soon as possible those patients who may benefit from prolonged immunosuppressive treatment from those who will not benefit from such treatment and who will just suffer from its major side effects. There is emerging evidence that the majority of genetic forms of SRNS should receive symptomatic treatment only.

INCIDENCE

The incidence of SRNs varies throughout the world. As shown in Table 16-1, the incidence of minimal change versus other histologies in patients biopsied because of nephrotic syndrome varies among children and adults and among children from the Northern Hemisphere and those from Africa. There are also different patterns in South America and Asia. It should be kept in mind that these comparisons are relative, because the initial therapy with steroids cannot be compared between children and adults. Furthermore there are no data about how different pharmacogenetic backgrounds and therapeutic doses of prednisone with different pharmacokinetic and pharmacodynamic profiles influence response to treatment. In addition, race appears to have an important impact on the histology associated with nephrotic syndrome. Although the incidence of nephrotic syndrome has remained stable over the last 30 years, evidence from the literature suggests that the total number of patients with focal segmental glomerulosclerosis (FSGS) is increasing, especially in South Africa and India.[3-5] A weak predictor for the probability of FSGS as opposed to minimal change nephrotic syndrome (MCNS) is age. In children with MCNS, about 80% are diagnosed before the age of 6 compared with 50% of those with FSGS lesions in histology.

HISTOLOGY

Because nephrotic syndrome is just a clinical description, the incidence of the different histomorphologic entities (Figures 16-2 and 16-3) behind the SRNS is expected to vary according to patients' age and regional and race factors. The most dominant lesion is FSGS, although a minority of steroid-resistant patients have MCNS. There has long been a debate that MCNS may transition to FSGS in selected cases, but this hypothesis has never been proven. A major reason for misdiagnosing FSGS as MCNS is due to the sampling error in renal biopsies. Kidneys with FSGS show preferentially early involvement of only a few glomeruli in the juxamedullary area, which can easily be missed on biopsies. The risk of misdiagnosing FSGS is estimated at 35% if only 10 glomeruli are harvested, and falls to about 12% if 20 glomeruli can be examined.

FSGS is defined as loss of glomerular capillary lumina due to an increase in mesangial matrix. An important feature in FSGS is diffuse effacement of podocyte foot processes, which is subtle in primary FSGS. Secondary forms of FSGS usually show effacement of about 50% or less of foot processes. For the disease to qualify as primary FSGS, other causes for podocyte damage with segmental glomerular scarring, such as immune complex glomerulunephritis, have to be excluded by immunohistology and electron microscopy.

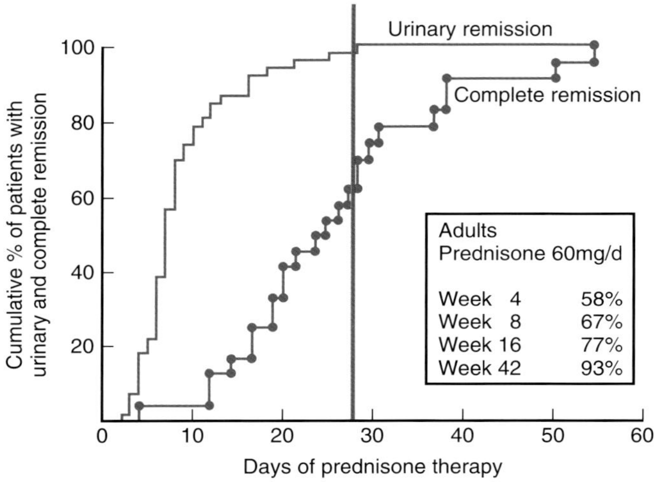

Figure 16-1 Steroid response with prednisone treatment: cumulative percentage of patients with urinary remission and serum remission. Curves demonstrate that about 50% of patients will respond within 7 to 10 days, more than 90 within 3 weeks, and almost all patients within 4 weeks. Complete remission will be achieved 2 to 3 weeks after urinary remission. In the box is percentage of adult patients in remission receiving a total dose of 60 mg/day. (From Short versus standard prednisone therapy for initial treatment of idiopathic nephrotic syndrome in children. Arbeitsgemeinschaft fur Padiatrische Nephrologie, *Lancet* 1(8582):380-83, 1998.)

TABLE 16-1 Underlying Histologies Studied in Patients with Nephrotic Syndrome in Children and Adults from Europe, the United States, and Africa

Histology	Children*	Adults*	Zimbabwe†	Durban‡
MCNS	76	20	9.2	14
FSGS	8	15	15.1	28
MemGN	7	40	15.1	41 (35 hepatitis B)
MPGN	4	7	33.6	9
Miscellaneous	5	18	17.0	5

Note: There is evidence that FSGS is more common in African children than in children from the Northern Hemisphere.
* Lewis MA, Baildom EM, Davies N, Houston IB, Postlethwaite RJ: Steroid-sensitive minimal change nephrotic syndrome. Long-term follow-up, *Contrib Nephrol* 67:226-28, 1988.
† Combined study of children and adults.[51]
‡ Study with pediatric patients.[5]

A nomenclature for idiopathic FSGS has been proposed by a group of nephropathologists.[6] It lists five precisely defined FSGS variants: collapsing, cellular, tip, perihilar, and FSGS not otherwise specified (NOS). This classification was derived from patients over 21 years of age. The glomerular disease collaborative network found FSGS not otherwise specified in 42% of the population, the perihilar variant in 26%, the tip lesion in 17%, the collapsing lesion in 11%, and the cellular variant in 3% of patients. The collapsing form was seen in over 90% of African Americans, whereas the tip lesion was most common in Caucasian patients. The degree of proteinuria was highest in the collapsing variant followed by patients with a tip lesion, and was less in patients with perihilar FSGS and those with FSGS NOS. The usefulness of such a classification is controversial, because some of the patients with tip lesions show progression to other forms. Nonetheless, use of this classification is encouraged and may help segregate specific entities from the "big basket" of FSGS.

There are no similar studies in pediatric patients. Although renal pathologists usually try to classify pediatric patients according to the aforementioned classification, its impact has not been evaluated. One recent study looked for clinical and histologic markers predicting outcome.[7] Sixty-six patients, 38 male and 28 female, were followed for at least 10 years. Multivariate analysis identified the presence of mesangial expansion ($p = 0.011$) and tip lesions ($p = 0.005$) as the independent predictors of favorable response to cytotoxic therapy, whereas the presence of renal impairment ($p = 0.008$) and extensive focal segmental sclerosis ($p = 0.025$) were independent predictors of unfavorable response.

Membranous glomerulonephritis (MGN) (Figure 16-4) is another important histomorphologic entity in patients with SRNS. In children it is much less common than FSGS compared with the adult population, in which this diagnosis is much more frequent. The list of etiologies leading to membranous nephropathy in adults is quite long, whereas in the pediatric population it is mainly secondary to hepatitis B or is idiopathic.

PATHOGENESIS

As described in earlier chapters, the key element in the pathogenesis of proteinuria in nephrotic syndrome is the podocyte. Since the discovery of a mutation in the nephrin gene in patients with congenital nephrotic syndrome of the Finnish type, the biology of the podocyte has become a center of interest. With the description of new gene mutations and altered gene products responsible for the structure function and signaling of podocytes, understanding of diseases with proteinuria has increased; however, with more knowledge, the number of questions has also increased. In general, one can distinguish two mechanisms leading to proteinuria: congenital and acquired.

During embryonic development, the outer part of the GBM is made by podocytes. Major podocytes need a full complement of proteins for building up complex structures as well as for signaling (Figure 16-5). A major function of podocytes is to perform as a buttress against the pressure of the glomerular capillaries. Any stress and functional impairment, as well as podocyte loss, may compromise the filtration barrier and lead to proteinuria.

It is logical that congenital defects may be somewhat resistant to any kind of pharmacologic treatment. In acquired diseases the major goal should be eliminating the cause of podocyte injury, as well as allowing the podocytes to recover and restoring their function after injury. Since podocytes have not been shown to replicate, any loss must be compensated by those remaining. Continuing podocyte loss may be critical below a certain threshold, which is estimated as a loss of

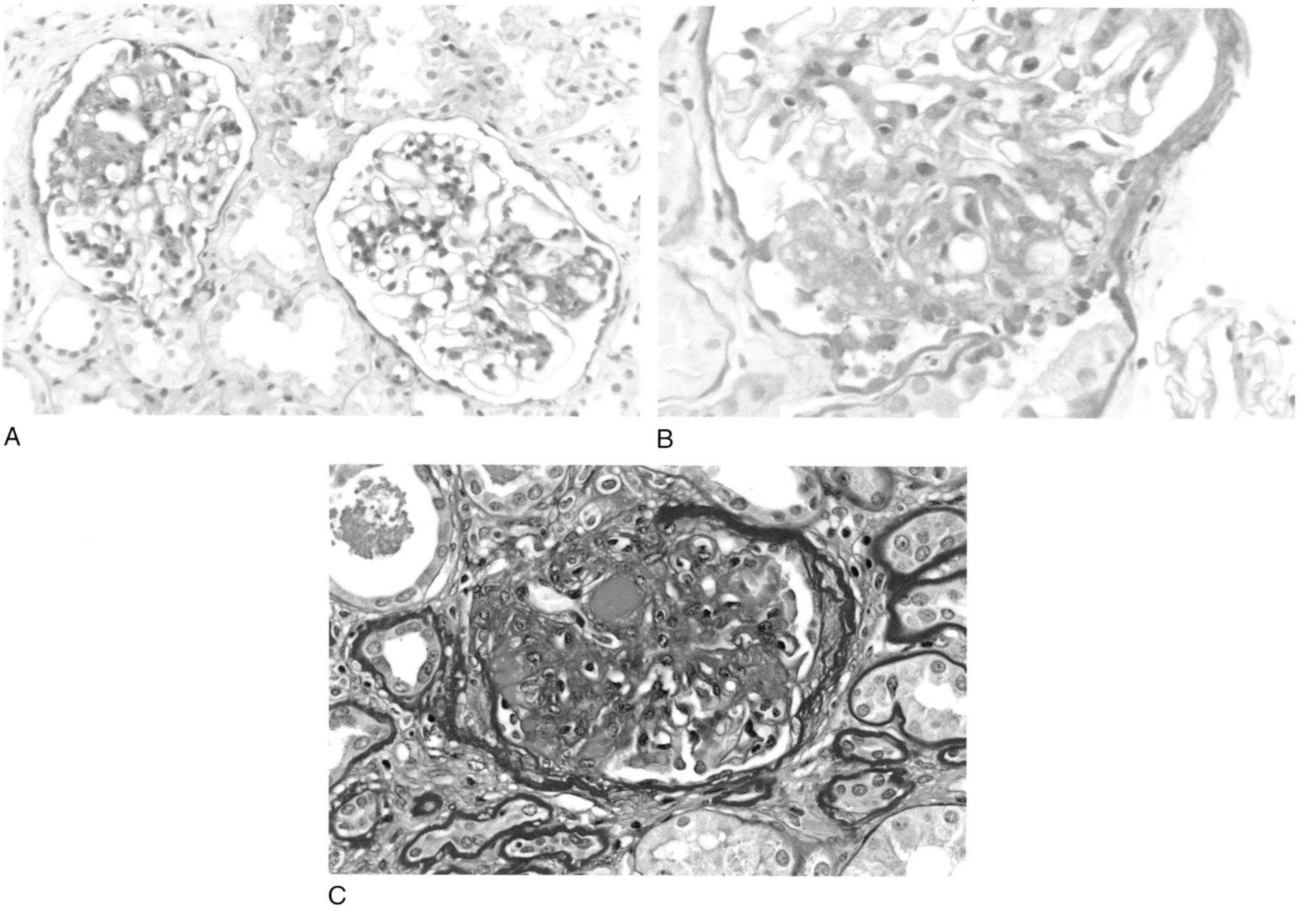

Figure 16-2 Histologies of renal biopsies of patients with steroid-resistant nephrotic syndrome. **A,** Histomorphology of FSGS NOS in a 9-year-old patient. Two glomeruli with segmental sclerosis. The right glomerulus with a recently sclerosed segment with foamy matrix at 3 o'clock, and the left glomerulus with a more mature, dense segmental sclerosis at 9 o'clock to 1 o'clock . PAS, original magnification ×200. **B,** Histomorphology of tip-lesion variant FSGS in a 19-year-old patient. The sclerosed glomerular segment at the 6 o'clock position is situated directly at the glomerulotubular junction. PAS, original magnification ×400. **C,** Histomorphology of diffuse mesangial sclerosis in Denys-Drash syndrome in a 12-year-old male patient. Mesangial proliferation with a slightly nodular appearance. PAS, original magnification ×400.

more than 20%[8,9] (Figure 16-6). As shown by Kriz[10,11] and others, a decreasing podocyte number leads to denuded GBM areas that will come into contact with the parietal epithelial cells lining Bowman's capsule by force of the intracapillary pressure. Once sclerotic lesions are established, a point of no return for these lesions is reached. Misdirected filtration (Figure 16-7) via the glomerular basement areas attached to Bowman's capsule and into the periglomerular and peritubular interstitium leads to inflammation and scarring of the renal cortex. Therefore any treatment should try to regenerate podocyte function before sclerotic lesions appear. It is amazing that the classical hypothesis of the immortal podocyte has never been questioned. The fact that a cell with such a highly developed structure should live for almost 70 years is doubtful. If there is podocyte turnover, it might be so low that it has escaped the attention of investigators. To what extent stem cells might contribute to podocyte turnover has to be studied. However, such a possibility may be attractive for future therapeutic approaches.

The inflammatory changes leading to tubulointerstitial scarring should be regarded as an important part of this disease leading to end-stage renal failure. The understanding of such processes, especially the epithelial mesenchymal transition (EMT), is of great interest. A detailed understanding may provide a rationale for specific interventions in the future. Until then, nonspecific immunosuppressive effects that dampen this process are used.

GENETICS

An overview of the variety of conditions associated with FSGS is given in Table 16-2, and recent advances in genetics and mutations associated with SRNS are covered in Chapter 13.

Recently Hinkes[12] described a new mutation leading to SRNS, called *NPHS3*. The gene product is phospholipase C epsilon (PLCE1). This mutation causes early-onset nephrotic syndrome leading to end-stage kidney disease in young children. Kidney histology of affected individuals show diffuse mesangiosclerosis (DMS). The gene product is expressed in the developing kidney in mature glomerular podocytes, which has been shown to lead to an arrest of normal glomerular

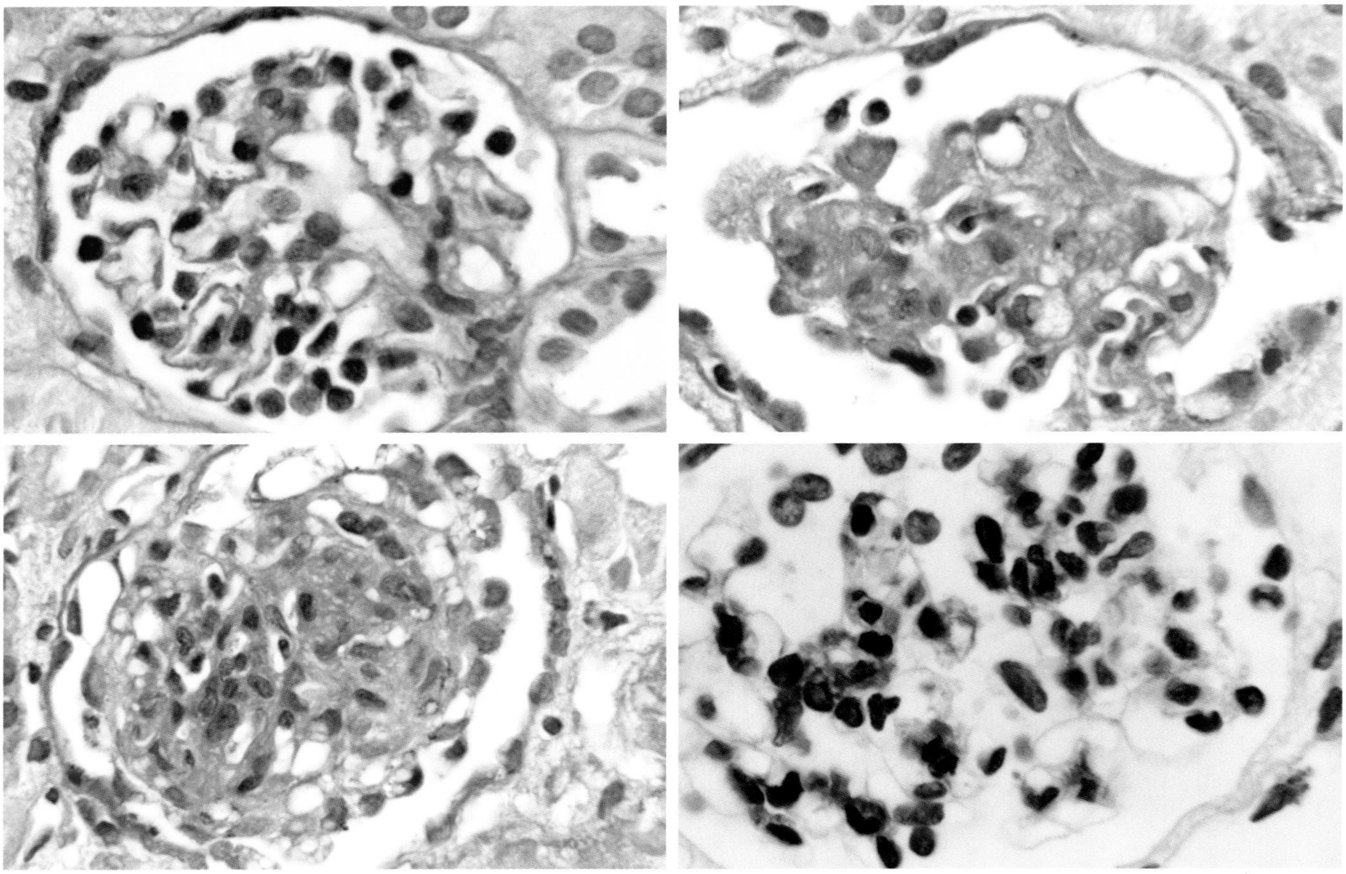

Figure 16-3 Histomorphology of mesangioproliferative IgA glomerulonephritis. This 2-year-old boy showed steroid-resistant nephrotic syndrome. Slight mesangial expansion with open capillary loops (top left) and mesangial proliferation with sclerosis in a focal and segmental fashion (bottom left and top right) are morphologically similar to primary FSGS. However, IgA-dominant mesangial immune deposits (brown, bottom right) are diagnostic of IgA glomerulonephritis. PAS and immunoperoxidase, original magnification ×600.

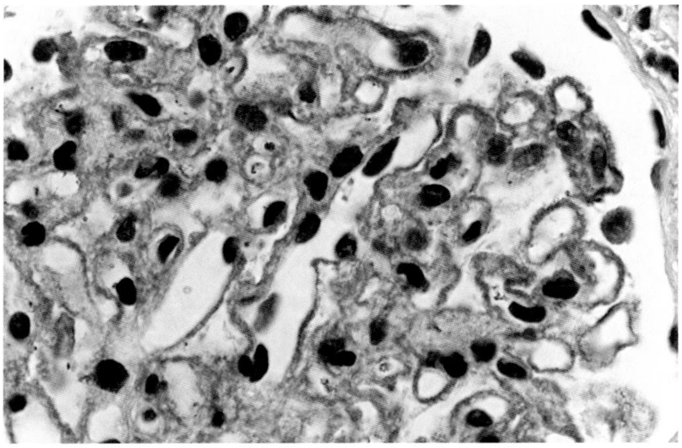

Figure 16-4 Histomorphology of membranous glomerulonephritis in a 16-year-old patient. Massive granular deposits of IgG (brown) along the glomerular basement membrane. Immunoperoxidase, original magnification ×600.

development. Interestingly, a few patients with this mutation might respond to immunosuppressive therapy.

SRNS may be part of syndromatic diseases as listed in Table 16-2 (see examples, Figures 16-8 and 16-9). Careful clinical examination is essential to rule out minor abnormalities suggestive of syndromatic forms of nephrotic syndrome to avoid unnecessary steroid treatment. In many cases, however, steroid therapy will start first and genetic investigations will be initiated only if steroid resistance has been confirmed by the classical definition. In the clinical day-to-day practice there is sometimes a tremendous delay between the request for genetic testing and when the result will be available. Because there are no markers predicting a gene defect, many patients may undergo further immunosuppressive therapy until a clear diagnosis is established. During this time, any therapy with irreversible or severe side effects should be avoided. Up to now it has been shown that immunosuppressive therapy is of no value in patients with *NPHS1*, *NPHS2*, *WT1*, and *TRPC6* mutations. Ruf et al.[13] have reported that out of 165 families with SRNS, 43 (26%) showed homozygote or compound heterozygote mutations in the *NPHS2* gene (podocin). In contrast, no mutations were found in 120 families with steroid-sensitive

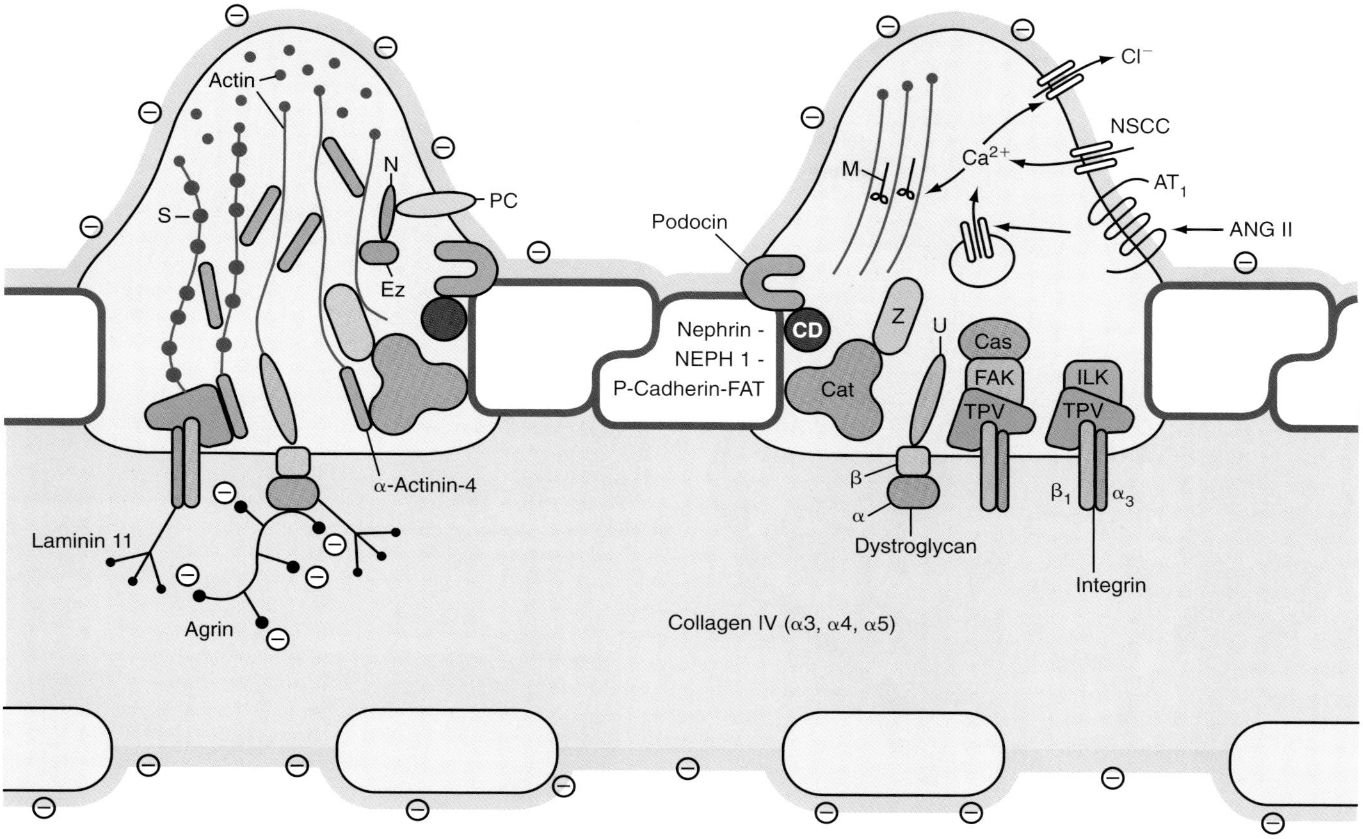

Figure 16-5 Schematic drawing of the molecular equipment of the podocyte foot processes. *Cas,* p130Cas; *Cat,* catenins; *CD,* CD2-associated protein, *Ez,* ezrin; *FAK,* focal adhesion kinase; *ILK,* integrin-linked kinase; *M,* myosin; *N,* NHERF2; *NSCC,* nonselective cation channel; *PC,* podocalyxin; *S,* synaptopodin; *TPV,* talin, paxillin, vinculin; *U,* utrophin; *Z,* ZO-1. (Redrawn from Pavenstadt[48]; [Pavenstadt modified from Endlich[49]].)

Figure 16-6 Podocyte injury and podocytopenia (modified from Mundel[9]). After injury, podocytes can undergo apoptosis or detachment or fail to proliferate. These events lead to a decrease in podocyte number (podocytopenia), which contributes to the development of progressive glomerulosclerosis. The mechanisms underlying podocytopenia are being elucidated. Apoptosis results from increased transforming growth factor-β—(TGF-β), angiotensin II, reactive oxygen species (ROS), and a decrease in the cyclin-dependent kinase (CDK) inhibitors p21 and p27. The α3β1 integrin is most likely to be critical in podocyte detachment from the underlying glomerular basement membrane (GBM). In contrast to other glomerular cells, podocytes do not typically proliferate in response to injury and cannot replace those lost by apoptosis and detachment. The inability to proliferate is secondary to increased levels of the CDK-inhibitors p21, p27, and/or p57. (Micrograph from Pavenstadt H, Kriz W, Kretzler M: Cell biology of the glomerular podocyte, *Physiol Rev* 83:253-307, 2003.)

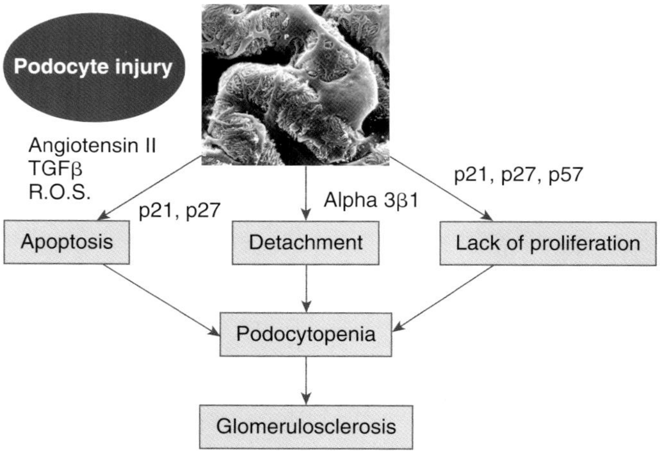

nephrotic syndrome. None of the patients with homozygous or compound heterozygous mutations in the *NPHS2* gene who were treated with cyclosporine or cyclophosphamide demonstrated complete remission of the nephrotic syndrome.

The geographic variation of *NPHS2* mutations is of importance. Maruyama et al.[14] reported that mutations in the *NPHS2* gene are uncommon in Japanese pediatric patients with SRNS.

Nongenetic FSGS

There is evidence from many clinical observations that a circulating factor targets the kidney, leading to proteinuria and glomerular sclerotic lesions. Most striking are

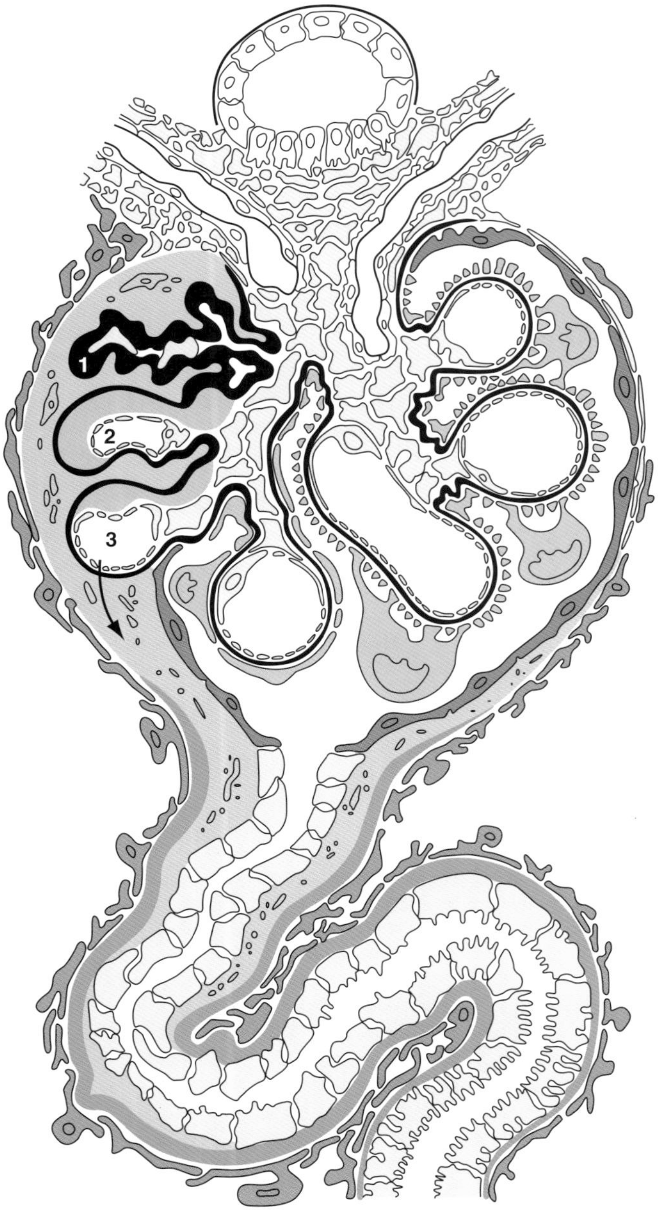

Figure 16-7 The Kriz hypothesis of misdirected filtration.[10] Schematic showing the essential feature of misdirected filtration and filtrate spreading at an intermediate stage of nephron degeneration. The GBM is shown in black; podocytes are densely stippled; parietal epithelial cells are less densely stippled; and interstitial endothelial cells are loosely stippled; and mesangial cells are hatched. The tuft adhesion contains several collapsed capillary loops. It also contains a perfused loop, which is partially hyalinized. The filtrate of this loop is delivered into a paraglomerular space that is separated from the interstitium by a layer of fibroblasts. This newly created space extends onto the outer aspect of the tubule by expanding and/or separating the tubular basement membrane from its epithelium.

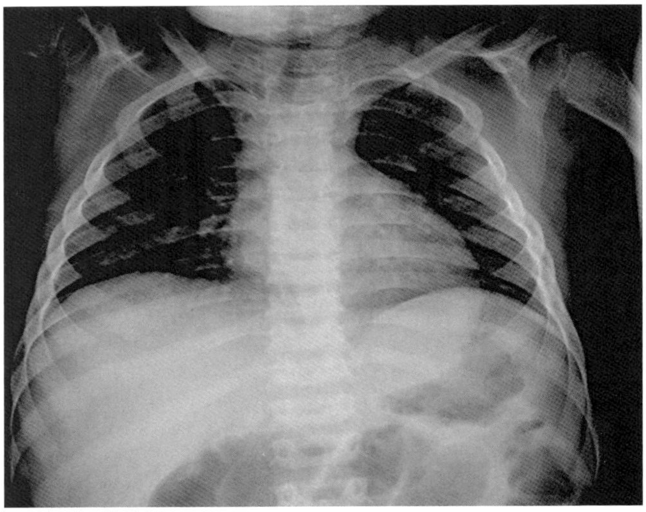

Figure 16-8 Schimke syndrome. Chest x-ray demonstrating spondyloepiphyseal dysplasia of the vertebral bodies.

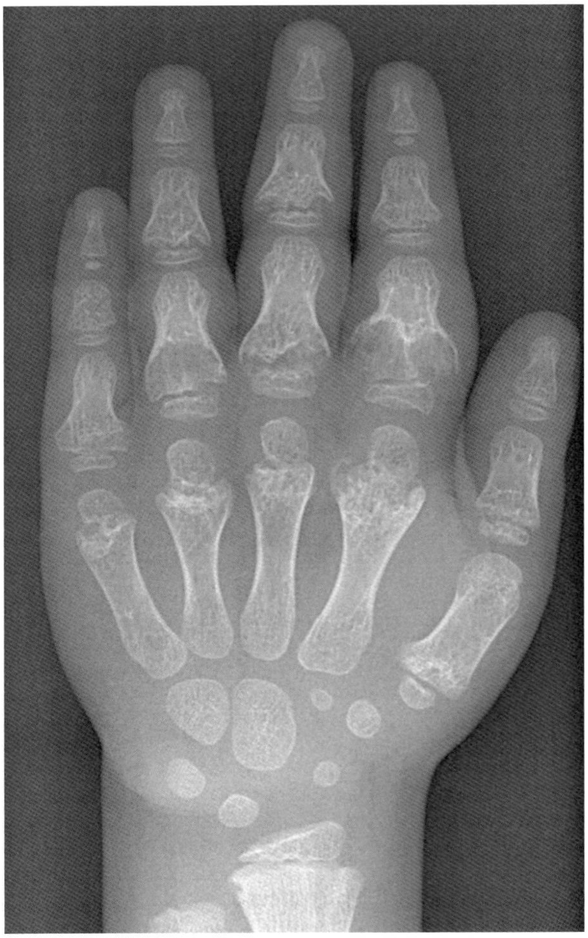

Figure 16-9 X-ray of the left hand showing enchondromatosis in a child with SRNS.

TABLE 16-2 Focal Segmental Glomerulosclerosis as Listed in OMIN PubMed

1: #603278 FOCAL SEGMENTAL GLOMERULOSCLEROSIS 1; FSGS1 Gene map locus 19q13	13: #232220 GLYCOGEN STORAGE DISEASE Ib Gene map locus 11q23
2: #603965 FOCAL SEGMENTAL GLOMERULOSCLEROSIS 2; FSGS2 Gene map locus 11q21-q22	14: *608414 PHOSPHOLIPASE C, EPSILON-1; PLCE1 Gene map locus 10q23
3: #607832 FOCAL SEGMENTAL GLOMERULOSCLEROSIS 3; FSGS3 Gene map locus Chr.6	15: #600995 NEPHROTIC SYNDROME, STEROID-RESISTANT, AUTOSOMAL RECESSIVE; SRN1 Gene map locus 1q25-q31
4: %609469 NEPHROPATHY, PROGRESSIVE, WITH DEAFNESS Gene map locus 11q24	16: *590100 TRANSFER RNA, MITOCHONDRIAL, TYROSINE; MTTY
5: *603652 TRANSIENT RECEPTOR POTENTIAL CATION CHANNEL, SUBFAMILY C, MEMBER 6; TRPC6 Gene map locus 11q21-q22	17: #607426 COENZYME Q10 DEFICIENCY Gene map locus 9p13.3, 6q21, 4q21-q22
6: *604638 ACTININ, ALPHA-4; ACTN4 Gene map locus 19q13	18: *167409 PAIRED BOX GENE 2; PAX2 Gene map locus 10q24.3-q25.1
7: +232200 GLYCOGEN STORAGE DISEASE I GLUCOSE-6-PHOSPHATASE, CATALYTIC, INCLUDED; G6PC, INCLUDED Gene map locus 17q21	19: *602716 NEPHRIN; NPHS1 Gene map locus 19q13.1
8: #242900 IMMUNOOSSEOUS DYSPLASIA, SCHIMKE TYPE Gene map locus 2q34-q36	20: %191830 UROGENITAL ADYSPLASIA, HEREDITARY
9: *604241 CD2-ASSOCIATED PROTEIN; CD2AP Gene map locus Chr.6	21: #173900 POLYCYSTIC KIDNEYS POLYCYSTIC KIDNEY DISEASE, ADULT, INCLUDED; APKD, INCLUDED Gene map locus 16p13.3-p13.12
10: *607102 WILMS TUMOR 1 GENE; WT1 Gene map locus 11p13	22: *604766 PODOCIN; NPHS2 Gene map locus 1q25-q31
11: #610725 NEPHROTIC SYNDROME, TYPE 3; NPHS3 Gene map locus 10q23	23: #609049 PIERSON SYNDROME NEPHROTIC SYNDROME, CONGENITAL, WITH OR WITHOUT OCULAR ABNORMALITIES, INCLUDED Gene map locus 3p21
12: #232240 GLYCOGEN STORAGE DISEASE Ic GLYCOGEN STORAGE DISEASE Id, INCLUDED; GSD1D, INCLUDED Gene map locus 11q23	24: %104200 ALPORT SYNDROME, AUTOSOMAL DOMINANT

observations about the recurrence of proteinuria within hours after renal transplantation in some patients who had end-stage renal failure with FSGS.

The nature of the factor has yet to be defined. Some call it the Savin factor, because major work has been carried out by Virginia Savin[15] and her group to isolate it.[16] This factor is believed to be removable by plasma separation, and anecdotal data on successful treatment after recurrence of FSGS posttransplant support this possibility. Some clinical observations point toward suppressive effects with the use of immunosuppressive drugs, especially calcineurin inhibitors. Such concepts are attractive treatment strategies; however, no reliable tests for identifying such a factor have been elaborated.

THERAPY

A review of the current literature about treatment of children with SRNS reveals that many children with familial or syndromic FSGS or with the known mutations still receive too much immunosuppressive therapy either initially or after an escalation with current available immunosuppressive drugs.

A metaanalysis of randomized controlled prospective trials in SRNS with FSGS without genetic testing demonstrates that cyclosporin may lead to a complete remission in almost one third of children. In contrast, neither oral nor intravenous cyclophosphamide demonstrates any effect on remission.

A major problem in reviewing the literature was that most studies were nonrandomized and retrospective, with low numbers of patients. In approximately two thirds of the studies, the number of patients was less than 10. Other studies have included both children and adults with MCNS and mesangial proliferation. The fact that different age groups may have different underlying diseases has been ignored. A further problem is that the steroid therapy used, as well as the definitions, did not meet the international accepted standards. Most studies focused on short-term effects, and long-term studies are lacking. In children, attention should be focused on side effects of therapy and comorbidity, such as impaired growth and body configuration.

Specific Agents

Glucocorticosteroids

In the early 1990s, Mendoza et al.[17-19] treated patients with SRNS due to FSGS with a protocol involving infusions of high doses of methylprednisolone, often in combination with oral alkylating agents. Twenty-three children have been treated in this manner, with a follow-up of 46 +/– 5 months. Twelve of them went into complete remission, six had minimal to moderate proteinuria, and four remained nephrotic. Each had a normal glomerular filtration rate. One child developed chronic renal failure and subsequently died while on dialysis. These results appear significantly better than in previous series of children with FSGS. More cases have been added to this first series, and the so-called Mendoza protocol has been used in many centers. However, a prospective randomized controlled trial has never been published. Concerns about methylprednisolone side effects left many clinicians reluctant to employ this protocol but stimulated a search for new drugs allowing steroid sparing.

The mode of action of corticosteroids was speculative and unclear until recently. Experimental data from Fujii et al.[20] may offer new insights into possible mechanisms for efficacy. Fujii demonstrated defective nephrin transport following endoplasmic reticulum-stress; that is, endoplasmic reticulum stress in podocytes may cause alteration of nephrin N-glycosylation, which may be an underlying factor in the pathogenesis of the proteinuria in nephrotic syndrome. Dexamethasone may restore this imbalance by stimulating expression of mitochondrial genes, resulting in production of ATP, which is an essential factor for proper folding machinery aided by the ER chaperones. It is unclear if there will be a place for dexamethasone in future therapeutic proposals.

Calcineurin Inhibitors

Calcineurin inhibitors have been used more in an empirical manner than on the basis of clear rationale. Cyclosporin is a calcineurin inhibitor that suppresses immune response by downregulating the transcription of various cytokine genes. The most significant of these cytokines is interleukin-2, which serves as the major activation factor for T cells in numerous immunologic processes. Cyclosporin inhibits cytokine production from T helper cells (Th1 and Th2) and also has an inhibitory effect on antigen-presenting cells (Langerhans and dendritic cells), which are the main agents of T-cell stimulation. A further effect of interleukin-2 inhibition is a reduction in B-cell activation and subsequent antibody production. Interleukin-2 levels are known to become elevated during proteinuria and to normalize during remission in adults with idiopathic nephrotic syndrome and in children with MCNS or FSGS.[21] However, this pattern of interleukin-2 activity is felt to be part of a more widespread disorder of cellular immunity that results in nephrotic syndrome rather than being causal of proteinuria.

It has been reported that cyclosporin has some antiproteinuric action on glomerular perm-selectivity to proteins that is unrelated to its immunosuppressive properties. Among these are an influence on perm-selectivity and charge selectivity, and impairment of glomerular filtration rate. These data come from various human studies[22-25] and animal models[26-28] with no immunologically mediated disease. Some studies revealed that lesions from the primary glomerular disease had either not regressed or had continued to progress.[23,24,29]

An uncontrolled trial in the early 1990s showed that about half of the patients had a stable course during cyclosporin treatment, whereas the others were resistant to the treatment (Figure 16-10). Knowledge of the various genetic and nongenetic causes of SRNS might easily explain this difference in response.

The first controlled data about efficacy of cyclosporin in SRNS came from Lieberman and Tejani[30]: they performed a randomized double-blind placebo-controlled trial of cyclosporin in 25 children with steroid-resistant idiopathic FSGS. Cyclosporin significantly reduced proteinuria and increased serum albumin levels. Interestingly, hypercholesterolemia seemed to antagonize the effect of cyclosporin, leading to the proposal to increase the dose according to cholesterol levels. This has been cited in the literature quite often, but apparently has not been translated into clinical use as discerned from review of the literature. Major concerns were the nephrotoxic side effects of cyclosporin, as well as a fear that progression of the disease might be indistinguishable from toxicity.

The French Society of Pediatric Nephrology published its experience with 65 children with steroid-resistant idiopathic nephrosis.[2] Patients were treated with cyclosporin at 150 to 200 mg/m^2 in combination with prednisone at 30 mg/m^2 daily for 1 month and on alternate days for 5 months. Renal biopsy

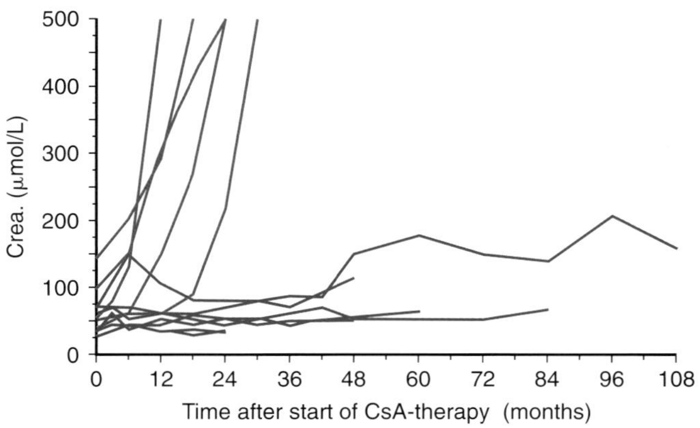

Figure 16-10 Clinical course under CsA in an unselected group of children with SRNS with FSGS lesion (our own observations before the genetic diagnoses became available). Interestingly, half of the patients improve under CsA therapy, whereas the others remain therapy resistant. This is clearly evidence for the variety of underlying diseases and an argument against uniform treatment based only on the definition "steroid resistance."

showed minimal change disease in 45 children and FSGS in 20. Twenty-seven patients achieved complete remission.

A study in adult patients[31] provided Level I evidence for efficacy of cyclosporin. In this study a 26-week regimen of cyclosporin therapy was compared with placebo in 49 patients with steroid-resistant FSGS; both groups also received low-dose prednisone. Further evidence was provided by Ponticelli et al.[32] Cyclosporin was compared to symptomatic treatment in 44 patients (adults and children) with SRNS. Eight (57%) cyclosporin-treated patients attained remission (complete or partial). Three (16%) control patients had partial remissions, but details regarding their diagnoses were incomplete. The majority of remitters had relapsed by the end of month 12 when cyclosporin was stopped.

The Arbeitsgemeinschaft für Pädiatrische Nephrologie (APN) conducted a prospective randomized trial that included children with SRNS at initial manifestation. Six months of treatment with cyclosporin (trough level 80 to 120 ng/L) versus 6 months of treatment with cyclophosphamide (6 × 500 mg/m^2) were compared. Although the goal was to involve 60 patients, the study was stopped after the inclusion of 32. A complete remission was achieved in 2 out of 15 receiving cyclosporin and in 2 out of 17 receiving cyclophosphamide; a partial remission was obtained in 7 out of 15 versus 2 out of 17. It was concluded that initial response with cyclosporin was better than with cyclophosphamide pulses (60% vs. 17%). Complete remission after week 24 was similar in both groups. In those who did not respond to cyclophosphamide, a successful remission was achieved in 45% with cyclosporin. Safety in both arms was comparable.

Recently Franz and colleagues[33] presented data that cyclosporin protects podocyte stress fibers through stabilization of synaptopodin protein expression. If this is supported by future experimental data, a nonimmunologic approach for the treatment might be envisaged.

A pilot trial of tacrolimus in the management of SRNS was published by McCauley et al. in 1993.[34] All patients except one experienced at least a 50% reduction in protein excretion at some time during tacrolimus therapy. No controlled study has been carried out, and only uncontrolled experiences have been published. Loeffler[35] reported a series of 16 patients resistant to other immunosuppressive drugs. In this mixed group he concluded that tacrolimus is an effective, well-tolerated medication for treatment-resistant forms of nephrotic syndrome in children, resulting in a complete remission rate of 81% and a partial remission rate of 13%. More data and a prospective trial are needed to confirm these promising results and to demonstrate the safety of this approach.

As of now, of the newer immunosuppressive agents only cyclosporin has been approved for use in nephrotic syndrome by licensing authorities in some countries.

An algorithm for the use of cyclosporin in SRNS (Figure 16-11) has been proposed.[35a] (Result of an expert meeting, London, 2005.)

Antiproliferative Agents

Azathioprine and vincristine have been used by some individuals but have not been widely recommended because of the lack of positive results. Cyclophosphamide has failed to prove any benefit, although many investigators have included this drug in their armamentarium. In most of the reports, drug combinations were employed that did not allow separation of single drug effects. The prospective trial of the APN mentioned earlier was stopped because of the inferiority of cyclophosphamide to cyclosporin.

Mycophenolate mofetil (MMF) has attracted investigators' interest because of its nonnephrotoxic profile. Some uncontrolled trials point toward possible benefits, but (a) the lack of control data, (b) the anecdotal character, (c) the possible selection bias in reporting, and (d) the fact that this drug has been in routine use for more than 10 years in the transplant setting but no robust data are available demonstrating any effect for prevention of posttransplant recurrence of original disease all argue against premature recommendations. One should await the results of the trial being undertaken in the United States under the auspices of the National Institutes of Health, wherein treatment with cyclosporin over 26

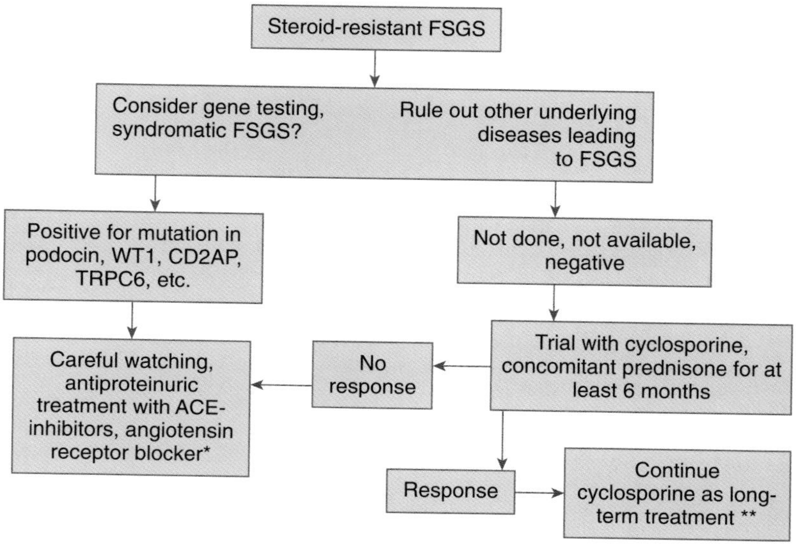

Figure 16-11 Proposed algorithm for treatment based on current knowledge (according to recommendations for the use of cyclosporin in patients with nephrotic syndrome developed by an expert meeting in London, 2005).
* The recommendation of ACE inhibitors and AT1 receptor blockers is based mainly on evidence from adult patients. Pediatric data are uncontrolled observations and the use has not been approved by licensing authorities.
** Treatment should be continued for years, but it remains unclear for exactly how long.

weeks will be compared with MMF/pulse steroids and continued for 52 weeks if response of proteinuria occurs. Both treatment arms include low-dose prednisone and ACE inhibitor therapy. Patients will be recruited at more than 130 sites in North America.

Antiproteinuric Treatment

There is strong evidence from studies in adult patients that ACE inhibitors effectively lower proteinuria in various diseases involving proteinuria.[36-41] These results have been accepted by many pediatric nephrologists as a robust argument for introducing ACE inhibitors for their patients with proteinuria. The dilemma is that in pediatric patients this has led to off-label use without proper phase II and III trials.

A large series of pediatric patients have been treated with ramipril in the Escape Trial[42]—a prospective assessment of the renoprotective efficacy of ACE inhibition and intensified blood pressure control. In this assessment, 397 children (ages 3 to 18 years) with chronic renal failure (GFR 11 to 80 ml/min/1.73 m^2) and elevated or high-normal BP received ramipril (6 mg/m^2) following a 6-month run-in period, including a 2-month washout of any previous ACE inhibitors.

Blood pressure was reduced with equal efficacy daytime and nighttime. Urinary protein excretion was reduced by 50% on average, with similar relative efficacy in patients with hypo/dysplastic nephropathies and glomerulopathies. The magnitude of proteinuria reduction depended on baseline proteinuria ($r = 0.32$, $p < 0.0001$), and was correlated with the antihypertensive efficacy of the drug ($r = 0.22$, $p < 0.001$). Small, uncontrolled trials in pediatric patients with persistant nephritic syndrome also found some reduction of proteinuria.[43-47]

The positive interpretation of a renoprotective effect of ACE inhibitors with and without AT1 receptor antagonist has made it unlikely that children are left without such treatment.

CONCLUSION

Steroid-resistant nephrotic syndrome is not a single entity. The most dominant lesion is focal segmental glomerulosclerosis (FSGS). Better understanding of the underlying diseases and mechanisms will guide future treatment. Early genetic diagnosis might help to avoid ineffective but harmful immunosuppressive therapy.

REFERENCES

1. Brodehl J, Krohn HP, Ehrich JH: The treatment of minimal change nephrotic syndrome (lipoid nephrosis): Cooperative studies of the Arbeitsgemeinschaft fur Padiatrische Nephrologie (APN), *Klin Padiatr* 194:162-65, 1982.
2. Niaudet P: Treatment of childhood steroid-resistant idiopathic nephrosis with a combination of cyclosporine and prednisone. French society of pediatric nephrology, *J Pediatr* 125:981-86, 1994.
3. Srivastava T, Simon SD, Alon US: High incidence of focal segmental glomerulosclerosis in nephrotic syndrome of childhood, *Pediatr Nephrol* 13:13-18, 1999.
4. Coovadia HM, Adhikari M, Morel-Maroger L: Clinico-pathological features of the nephrotic syndrome in South African children, *Q J Med* 48:77-91, 1979.
5. Bhimma R, Coovadia HM, Adhikari M: Nephrotic syndrome in South African children: Changing perspectives over 20 years, *Pediatr Nephrol* 11:429-34, 1997.
6. D'Agati V: Pathologic classification of focal segmental glomerulosclerosis, *Semin Nephrol* 23:117-34, 2003.
7. Abeyagunawardena AS, Sebire NJ, Risdon RA, Dillon MJ, Rees L et al: Predictors of long-term outcome of children with idiopathic focal segmental glomerulosclerosis, *Pediatr Nephrol* 22(2):215-21, 2006.
8. Wharram BL, Goyal M, Wiggins JE, Sanden SK, Hussain S et al: Podocyte depletion causes glomerulosclerosis: Diphtheria toxin-induced podocyte depletion in rats expressing human diphtheria toxin receptor transgene, *J Am Soc Nephrol* 16:2941-52, 2005.
9. Mundel P, Shankland SJ: Podocyte biology and response to injury, *J Am Soc Nephrol* 13:3005-15, 2002.
10. Kriz W: The pathogenesis of 'classic' focal segmental glomerulosclerosis—lessons from rat models, *Nephrol Dial Transplant* 18 Suppl 6:vi39-44, 2003.
11. Kriz W, Hartmann I, Hosser H, Hahnel B, Kranzlin B et al: Tracer studies in the rat demonstrate misdirected filtration and peritubular filtrate spreading in nephrons with segmental glomerulosclerosis, *J Am Soc Nephrol* 12:496-506, 2001.
12. Hinkes B, Wiggins RC, Gbadegesin R, Vlangos CN, Seelow D et al: Positional cloning uncovers mutations in PLCE1 responsible for a nephrotic syndrome variant that may be reversible, *Nat Genet* 38:1397-1405, 2006.
13. Ruf RG, Lichtenberger A, Karle SM, Haas JP, Anacleto FE et al: Patients with mutations in *NPHS2* (podocin) do not respond to standard steroid treatment of nephrotic syndrome, *J Am Soc Nephrol* 15:722-732, 2004.
14. Maruyama K, Iijima K, Ikeda M, Kitamura A, Tsukaguchi H et al: *NPHS2* mutations in sporadic steroid-resistant nephrotic syndrome in Japanese children, *Pediatr Nephrol* 18:412-16, 2003.
15. Savin VJ, Sharma R, Sharma M, McCarthy ET, Swan SK et al: Circulating factor associated with increased glomerular permeability to albumin in recurrent focal segmental glomerulosclerosis, *N Engl J Med* 334:878-83, 1996.
16. Sharma M, Sharma R, McCarthy ET, Savin VJ: The focal segmental glomerulosclerosis permeability factor: Biochemical characteristics and biological effects, *Exp Biol Med (Maywood)* 229:85-98, 2004.
17. Mendoza SA, Reznik VM, Griswold WR, Krensky AM, Yorgin PD, Tune BM: Treatment of steroid-resistant focal segmental glomerulosclerosis with pulse methylprednisolone and alkylating agents, *Pediatr Nephrol* 4:303-07, 1990.
18. Mendoza SA, Tune BM: Treatment of childhood nephrotic syndrome, *J Am Soc Nephrol* 3:889-94, 1992.
19. Mendoza SA, Tune BM: Management of the difficult nephrotic patient, *Pediatr Clin North Am* 42:1459-68, 1995.
20. Fujii Y, Khoshnoodi J, Takenaka H, Hosoyamada M, Nakajo A et al: The effect of dexamethasone on defective nephrin transport caused by er stress: A potential mechanism for the therapeutic action of glucocorticoids in the acquired glomerular diseases, *Kidney Int* 69:1350-59, 2006.
21. Tejani A, Ingulli E: Current concepts of pathogenesis of nephrotic syndrome, *Contrib Nephrol* 114:1-5, 1995.
22. Zietse R, Wenting GJ, Kramer P, Schalekamp MA, Weimar W: Effects of cyclosporin a on glomerular barrier function in the nephrotic syndrome, *Clin Sci (Lond)* 82:641-50, 1992.
23. Meyrier A, Noel LH, Auriche P, Callard P: Long-term renal tolerance of cyclosporin a treatment in adult idiopathic nephrotic syndrome. Collaborative group of the societe de nephrology, *Kidney Int* 45:1446-56, 1994.
24. Ambalavanan S, Fauvel JP, Sibley RK, Myers BD: Mechanism of the antiproteinuric effect of cyclosporine in membranous nephropathy, *J Am Soc Nephrol* 7:290-98, 1996.
25. Heering P, Schneider A, Grabensee B, Plum J: [Effect of cyclosporin a on renal function in patients with glomerulonephritis], *Dtsch Med Wochenschr* 126:1093-98, 2001.

26. Kokui K, Yoshikawa N, Nakamura H, Itoh H: Cyclosporin reduces proteinuria in rats with aminonucleoside nephrosis, *J Pathol* 166:297-301, 1992.
27. Schrijver G, Assmann KJ, Wetzels JF, Berden JH: Cyclosporin a reduces albuminuria in experimental anti-gbm nephritis independently from changes in GFR, *Nephrol Dial Transplant* 10:1149-54, 1995.
28. Desassis JF, Raats CJ, Bakker MA, van den Born J, Berden JH: Antiproteinuric effect of ciclosporin a in adriamycin nephropathy in rats, *Nephron* 75:336-41, 1997.
29. Chen H, Tang Z, Zeng C, Hu W, Wang Q et al: Pathological demography of native patients in a nephrology center in China, *Chin Med J (Engl)* 116:1377-81, 2003.
30. Lieberman KV, Tejani A: A randomized double-blind placebo-controlled trial of cyclosporine in steroid-resistant idiopathic focal segmental glomerulosclerosis in children, *J Am Soc Nephrol* 7:56-63, 1996.
31. Cattran DC, Appel GB, Hebert LA, Hunsicker LG, Pohl MA et al: A randomized trial of cyclosporine in patients with steroid-resistant focal segmental glomerulosclerosis. North America nephrotic syndrome study group, *Kidney Int* 56:2220-26, 1999.
32. Ponticelli C, Rizzoni G, Edefonti A, Altieri P, Rivolta E et al: A randomized trial of cyclosporine in steroid-resistant idiopathic nephrotic syndrome, *Kidney Int* 43:1377-84, 1993.
33. Franz S, Faul C, Mundel P: Cyclosporin protects stress fibers through stabilization of synaptopdin protein expression, *JASN* 16:109A, 2005.
34. McCauley J, Shapiro R, Ellis D, Igdal H, Tzakis A, Starzl TE: Pilot trial of fk 506 in the management of steroid-resistant nephrotic syndrome, *Nephrol Dial Transplant* 8:1286-90, 1993.
35. Loeffler K, Gowrishankar M, Yiu V: Tacrolimus therapy in pediatric patients with treatment-resistant nephrotic syndrome, *Pediatr Nephrol* 19:281-87, 2004.
35a. Cattran DC, Alexopoulos E, Heering P, Hoyer PF, Johnston A, et al: Cyclosporin in idiopathic glomerular disease associated with the nephrotic syndrome: workshop recommendations, *Kidney Int* 2007 (epub ahead of print Sep. 27).
36. MacKinnon M, Shurraw S, Akbari A, Knoll GA, Jaffey J, Clark HD: Combination therapy with an angiotensin receptor blocker and an ace inhibitor in proteinuric renal disease: A systematic review of the efficacy and safety data, *Am J Kidney Dis* 48:8-20, 2006.
37. Remuzzi G, Macia M, Ruggenenti P: Prevention and treatment of diabetic renal disease in type 2 diabetes: The BENEDICT study, *J Am Soc Nephrol* 17:S90-97, 2006.
38. Kelly DJ, Zhang Y, Cox AJ, Gilbert RE: Combination therapy with tranilast and angiotensin-converting enzyme inhibition provides additional renoprotection in the remnant kidney model, *Kidney Int* 69:1954-60, 2006.
39. Remuzzi A, Gagliardini E, Sangalli F, Bonomelli M, Piccinelli M et al: Ace inhibition reduces glomerulosclerosis and regenerates glomerular tissue in a model of progressive renal disease, *Kidney Int* 69:1124-30, 2006.
40. Song JH, Cha SH, Lee HJ, Lee SW, Park GH, Kim MJ: Effect of low-dose dual blockade of renin-angiotensin system on urinary TGF-beta in type 2 diabetic patients with advanced kidney disease, *Nephrol Dial Transplant* 21:683-89, 2006.
41. Pozzi C, Del Vecchio L, Casartelli D, Pozzoni P, Andrulli S et al: Ace inhibitors and angiotensin II receptor blockers in iga nephropathy with mild proteinuria: The ACEARB study, *J Nephrol* 19:508-14, 2006.
42. Wuhl E, Mehls O, Schaefer F: Antihypertensive and antiproteinuric efficacy of ramipril in children with chronic renal failure, *Kidney Int* 66:768-76, 2004.
43. Chiarelli F, Casani A, Verrotti A, Morgese G, Pinelli L: Diabetic nephropathy in children and adolescents: A critical review with particular reference to angiotensin-converting enzyme inhibitors, *Acta Paediatr Suppl* 425:42-45, 1998.
44. Camacho Diaz JA, Gimenez Llort A, Garcia Garcia L, Jimenez Gonzalez R: [long-term effect of angiotensin-converting inhibitors in children with proteinuria], *An Esp Pediatr* 55:219-24, 2001.
45. Srivastava RN: Isolated asymptomatic proteinuria, *Indian J Pediatr* 69:1055-58, 2002.
46. Peco-Antic A, Virijevic V, Paripovic D, Babic D: [Renoprotective effect of ramipril in children with chronic renal failure—the experience of one centre], *Srp Arh Celok Lek* 132 Suppl 1:34-38, 2004.
47. Artero M, Biava C, Amend W, Tomlanovich S, Vincenti F: Recurrent focal glomerulosclerosis: Natural history and response to therapy, *Am J Med* 92:375-83, 1992.
48. Pavenstadt H, Kriz W, Kretzler M: Cell biology of the glomerular podocyte, *Physiol Rev* 83:253-307, 2003.
49. Endlich K, Kriz W, Witzgall R: Update in podocyte biology, *Curr Opin Nephrol Hypertens* 10:331-40, 2001.

CHAPTER

17 Membranoproliferative Glomerulonephritis

Christoph Licht and Michael Mengel

Membranoproliferative glomerulonephritis (MPGN)—also referred to as mesangiocapillary glomerulonephritis—was originally described by West et al.[1] MPGN comprises a collection of morphologically related but pathogenetically distinct disorders that are characterized by glomerular hypercellularity, increased mesangial matrix, and thickening of the peripheral capillary walls. The disease is characterized by functional impairment of the glomerular basement membrane (GBM), causing progressive loss of renal function that eventually results in end-stage renal disease (ESRD). Clinical features at first manifestation are hematuria (88%), proteinuria (nephrotic range) (67%), impaired renal function (31%), and hypertension (25%) as found in a survival study by Habib et al. some 30 years ago.[2]

Traditionally MPGN is divided into three subtypes, MPGN type I, MPGN type II, and MPGN type III, based on findings made by light and electron microscopy. Whereas MPGN type I shows interposition of mesangial cells and matrix between basement membrane and endothelial cells resulting in the formation of a double-contour or tramtrack structure of subendothelial electron-dense deposits, MPGN type III shows similar electron-dense deposits both subendothelially and subepithelially. By contrast, MPGN type II or dense deposit disease (DDD) is characterized by complement-containing dense deposits within the lamina densa of the GBM.

Recent progress in the interpretation of the morphologic findings and understanding of the pathogenesis of MPGN suggests that reclassification of MPGN according to underlying pathophysiologic principles may be appropriate. Conditions associated with a membranoproliferative pattern of injury range from immune-complex-mediated diseases (idiopathic forms of MPGN—in the literature referred to as MPGN type I and MPGN type III, autoimmune diseases, chronic infections, etc.) to thrombotic microangiopathies (HUS/TTP, antiphospholipid antibody syndrome, etc.) to paraprotein deposition diseases (cryoglobulinemia type I, Waldenström macroglobulinemia, etc.).[3]

In contrast, MPGN type II/DDD seems to result from an impairment of the regulation of the alternative complement pathway, specifically from unrestricted activity of the alternative pathway C3 convertase C3bBb, and should be considered an independent disease entity.

Information about the prevalence of MPGN is scarce and differs with age and region: whereas in adults MPGN is considered one of the major causes of nephrotic syndrome, with 0.2% to 20% of all cases being primary glomerulopathies (Europe and North America),[4] the frequency in children is reported as only 6.2%.[5] In Asia, South America, and Africa, MPGN accounts for 30% to 40% of all cases of nephrotic syndrome.[4] In general, the overall incidence of MPGN continues to decrease in developed countries and remains high in developing countries.[6]

MPGN mainly affects older children and adolescents (median age about 10 years at onset of disease). Half of the patients exhibit nephrotic syndrome, and the others exhibit mild proteinuria, 20% with macrohematuria. About one third develop hypertension at onset of disease. Children with MPGN have an unfavorable prognosis and may develop ESRD in late childhood or early adolescence.[2,7,8]

CLASSIFICATION OF MEMBRANOPROLIFERATIVE GLOMERULONEPHRITIS

Pathology of Membranoproliferative Glomerulonephritis

MPGN is a morphologic pattern that is primarily defined at the light microscopic level.[9] Thus pathologists usually use the term *membranoproliferative glomerulonephritis* to refer to a general pattern of glomerular injury seen in a variety of disease processes that frequently share a common pathogenetic mechanism rather than to a more restricted meaning that addresses a particular disease entity causing characteristic clinical symptoms. Accordingly, both a pathomorphologic classification of MPGN (type I, type II, and type III) and a pathogenetic classification (idiopathic/primary versus secondary) coexist.

The membranoproliferative pattern of injury is characterized by mesangial proliferation and thickening of the peripheral GBM. Typically the thickening is due to mesangial cell interposition with double contours of the GBM.[9-11] Mesangial expansion with cell proliferation and extension into peripheral basement membranes causes a cloverleaf-like accentuation of the glomerular tuft (Figure 17-1). In the vast majority of cases these characteristic glomerular changes are the consequence of immune deposition in the glomerular capillary wall, and based on the morphologic pattern just described, the terms *mesangiocapillary glomerulonephritis* and *lobular glomerulonephritis* have been used synonymously.[12,13]

Therefore the membranoproliferative pattern of glomerular injury is nonspecific. It can occur in primary (idiopathic) and secondary forms.[3] The primary forms are subdivided into three major morphologic types (type I, type II, and type III) based on their light microscopic, immunofluorescence/immunohistochemical, and ultrastructural features (Table 17-1).[9,11] Currently type I is characterized by subendothelial deposits and can be regarded as the classical form of MPGN, whereas the presence of dense intramembranous deposits discriminates MPGN type II (i.e., DDD).[14] By light microscopy, both variants can look almost identical on the basis of their lobular appearance of the glomerular tuft, rendering the term *lobular glomerulonephritis* obsolete. The terminology became even more complicated with the description of further variants or types of MPGN. A type with many features of MPGN type I but with the additional presence of numerous electron-dense deposits on the subepithelial side of the GBMs was designated as type III MPGN by Bruckholder et al.[15-17] The situation is further complicated by the additional use of the term *MPGN type III* for another MPGN variant independently described by Anders in 1977 and Strife in 1984.[18,19]

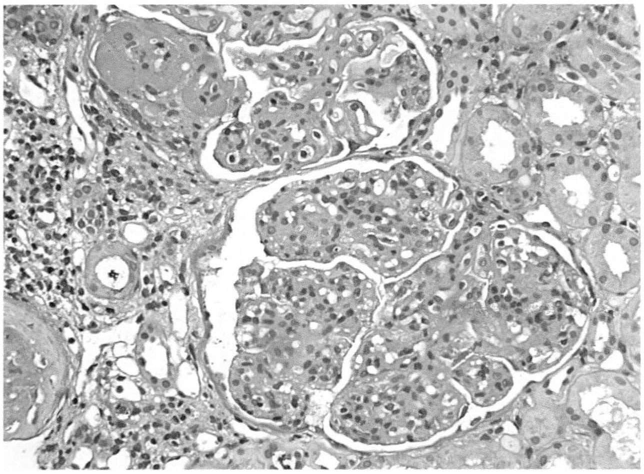

Figure 17-1 MPGN pattern of glomerular injury: The glomerular tuft shows an accentuated lobularity (cloverleaf-like) and increased cellularity of the expanded mesangium. The peripheral basement membranes are thickened. PAS stain, magnification ×200.

Secondary forms of MPGN can be related to a variety of underlying conditions or systemic diseases comprising autoimmune, infectious, neoplastic, and thrombotic disorders (Table 17-2).[3,9,10,12,13] Secondary MPGNs are more common than the primary forms. Differentiation of primary from secondary MPGN requires integral consideration of clinical and pathologic (light microscopy and immunofluorescence/immunohistochemistry, electron microscopy) findings. Most cases of secondary MPGN are seen in adults, but in children primary MPGN predominates.

Primary MPGN

Primary (idiopathic) MPGN is defined as a glomerulonephritis with a membranoproliferative pattern by light microscopy without any detectable underlying cause or systemic disease. Primary forms of MPGN are most common in older children, adolescents, and young adults. It is rarely seen in children younger than 2 years or adults older than 50 (range 6 to 35 years).[2,20] Both male and female children are equally affected.

The most common morphologic variant of primary MPGN is type I, whereas type II is extremely rare (less than 5% of all primary MPGN). Because of the various definitions and sub-subtypes of type III MPGN, its incidence varies in the literature, but most authors suggest that this heterogeneous type of MPGN is far less common than type I but slightly more common than type II.

MPGN Type I Primary MPGN type I usually has a chronic, slowly progressive course, with alternation of remission and exacerbation that is mirrored by its clinical presentation with an initially nephritic and later nephrotic syndrome. It has been diagnosed in children under 2 years, but most pediatric patients show signs of the disease after 8 years of age.[10]

TABLE 17-1 Primary MPGN—Pathological Features in Different Subtypes

Type	Light Microscopy	Immunofluorescence/ Immunohistochemistry	Electron Microscopy
I	Diffuse mesangial cell proliferation, double contours of GBM, mesangial cell interposition, cloverleaf-like accentuation of the glomerular tuft	Only C3 or C3 + IgG IgM, IgA, C1q +/–	Deposits subendothelial and mesangial
II	Variable mesangial cell proliferation, pronounced GBM thickening, rare mesangial cell interposition, and double contours	Only C3 linear in GBM Mesangial deposits	Deposits intramembranous (lamina densa)
III	Diffuse mesangial cell proliferation, double contours of GBM, mesangial cell interposition, GBM thickening	Only C3 or C3 + IgG In a granular membranous-like pattern in some cases IgM, IgA, C1q +/–	Deposits mesangial (+/–); Subendothelial; Intramembranous (+/–); Subepithelial (+/–)

GBM, Glomerular basement membrane.

TABLE 17-2 Secondary MPGN: Synopsis

Conditions Underlying Secondary MPGN	Type of MPGN*
Infectious Diseases: Bacterial/Viral/Protozoal	
Hepatitis B, C, EBV, HIV	I, III
Endocarditis/visceral abscesses	I
Infected ventriculoatrial shunts/empyema	I
Malaria, schistosomiasis, mycoplasma	I
Tuberculosis, leprosy	I, II
Epstein-Barr virus infection	I
Brucellosis	MPGN-like pattern
Systemic Immune Diseases	
Cryoglobulinemia	I, III
Systemic lupus erythematosus	I, III, II
Sjögren's syndrome	III, I
Rheumatoid arthritis	I
Heriditary deficiencies of complement components	I, II
X-linked agammaglobulinemia	MPGN-like pattern
Neoplasms/Dysproteinemias	
Plasma cell dyscrasia	MPGN-like pattern
Fibrillary and immunotactoid glomerulonephritis	MPGN-like pattern
Light chain deposition disease	MPGN-like pattern
Heavy chain deposition disease	MPGN-like pattern
Light and heavy chain deposition disease	MPGN-like pattern
Leukemias and lymphomas (with cryoglobulinemia)	I, III
Waldenström macroglobulinemia	I, III
Carcinomas, Wilms' tumor, malignant melanoma	II
Chronic Liver Disease	
Chronic active hepatitis (B, C)	I, III
Cirrhosis	I, III
Alpha-1-antitrypsin deficiency	I
Miscellaneous	
All conditions leading to thrombotic microangiopathy	MPGN-like pattern
Sickle cell disease	I
Partial lipodystrophy (mainly dense deposit disease)	II, I, III
Transplant glomerulopathy	MPGN-like pattern
Niemann-Pick disease (Type C)	II

* Listed according to frequency.

By light microscopy and low-power magnification, glomeruli show the typical accentuated lobularity of their tufts. By the time of biopsy, mesangial extension and capillary wall thickening are usually diffuse and global but can also be focal and segmental in mild cases or at early stages of glomerulonephritis. The mesangium is expanded by an apparent increase in matrix and number of mesangial cells. In severe cases with pronounced mesangial expansion, the mesangium can assume a nodular appearance similar to diabetic glomerulopathy and nodular light chain glomerulopathy on light microscopy. With disease progression, the number of mesangial cells decreases and matrix increases, finally leading to glomerulosclerosis.

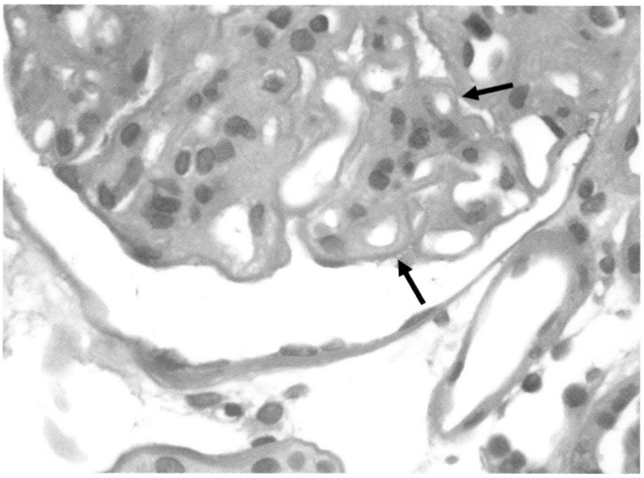

Figure 17-2 Double contours of thickened capillary walls in a case of type I MPGN. PAS stain, magnification ×630.

The glomerular capillary walls are thickened and characteristically show segmental duplication. Double contours (tramtracks) (Figure 17-2) of basement membranes are the consequence of mesangial cell interposition. During the course of inflammation, mesangial cells migrate into the peripheral capillary walls and place themselves between the glomerular endothelium and the GBM (i.e., into the subendothelial space). In this localization, mesangial cells start to synthesize new basement membrane material, forming a new layer of basement membrane at the endothelial side of the original basement membrane. Resulting double contours of peripheral capillary walls can best be seen in a silver stain but can also be appreciated in a conventional PAS stain. Mesangial interposition and double contouring can be either segmental or circumferential involving a capillary loop. In some cases inflammatory cells such as monocytes and neutrophils can increase glomerular hypercellularity. Crescents have been described for individual cases of MPGN type I. Vascular and tubulointerstitial changes are nonspecific. Depending on duration and severity of MPGN and accompanying diseases (e.g., hypertension), various degrees of tubular atrophy, interstitial fibrosis, arteriosclerosis, and nonspecific interstitial inflammation can be observed.

Immune deposits are usually seen by immunofluorescence (frozen or paraffin sections) or immunohistochemistry (paraffin sections) in the mesangium and in the peripheral capillary walls. Characteristic is a granular to pseudolinear staining pattern in peripheral capillary walls accentuating glomerular lobularity (Figure 17-3). Immune deposits are predominantly composed of immunoglobulin IgG and complement C3 but can vary in their intensity between the mesangium and the subendothelial space of capillary walls from case to case.

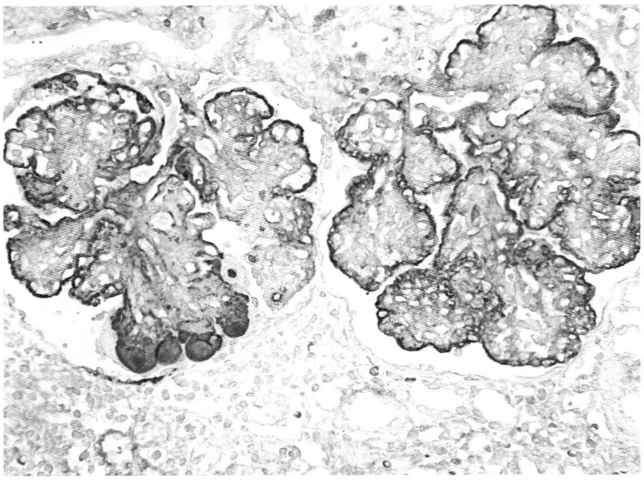

Figure 17-3 Immunohistochemistry (paraffin sections) for complement component C3 in a case of MPGN type I.

However, the staining intensity of C3 is usually greater than that of IgG, and in some cases only C3 can be found. IgA, IgM, and C1q are mostly less intense.

By electron microscopy the deposits are electron dense and found in the expanded mesangium, as well as in the widened subendothelial space of the basement membranes. Mesangial hypercellularity and mesangial cell interposition in adjacent basement membranes are typical ultrastructural features of MPGN. The interposition of mesangial cells into the subendothelial space of the basement membranes narrows the capillary lumen. Double contours of capillary walls can segmentally be appreciated and correspond to the original outer layer of the basement membrane (lamina densa and lamina rara externa) and to the newly synthesized inner neomembrane. Electron-dense deposits and mesangial cells can usually be found between these two membrane layers (Figure 17-4). Subepithelial deposits are not a typical feature in MPGN type I but rather suggest type III MPGN. On the epithelial side of the basement membrane there is usually extensive effacement of the podocyte foot processes.

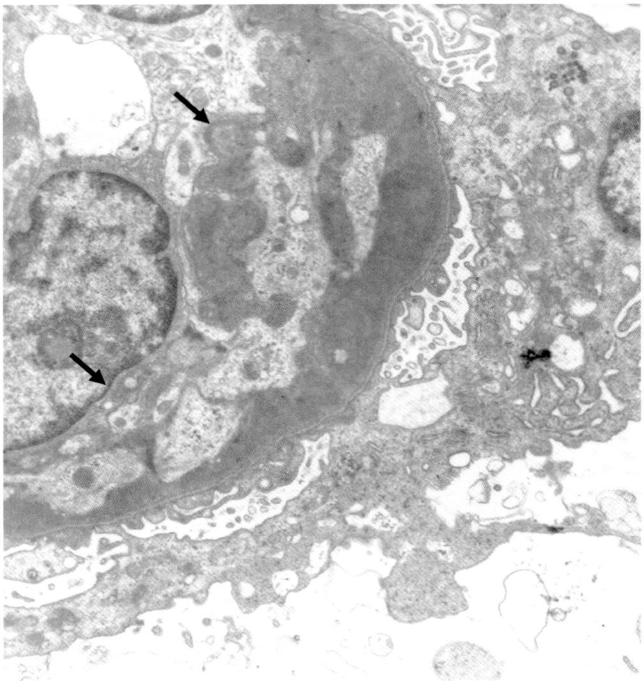

Figure 17-4 MPGN type I with large irregular electron dense deposits in the widened subendothelial space. Delicate inner layer of newly synthesized basement membrane material *(arrows)* causes double contours of the glomerular capillary wall. Electron microscopy, magnification ×8000.

MPGN Type II/Dense Deposit Disease MPGN type II/DDD is primarily a disease variant that occurs in children and young adults, with the vast majority of patients presenting at under 20 years of age. Children under the age of 5 with MPGN type II/DDD have been described as well.[10,21,22] In MPGN type II/DDD the mesangial cell proliferation is relatively mild and, in general, highly variable compared with MPGN type I cases. However, infiltration of accompanying inflammatory cells (neutrophils, histiocytes, mononuclear cells) can mask mesangial cell proliferation and lead to mesangial glomerular hypercellularity. In MPGN type II/DDD by light microscopy, peripheral capillary walls usually appear significantly thickened but only rarely show less-developed double contours (which are more frequent and more pronounced in MPGN type I). Besides GBMs, Bowman's capsule and tubular basement membranes can be thickened as well. Thickened membranes stain well with PAS and thioflavin T but frequently are found in an irregular fashion involving only segments of glomeruli, tubuli, and Bowman's capsule. In some cases crescents have been described.

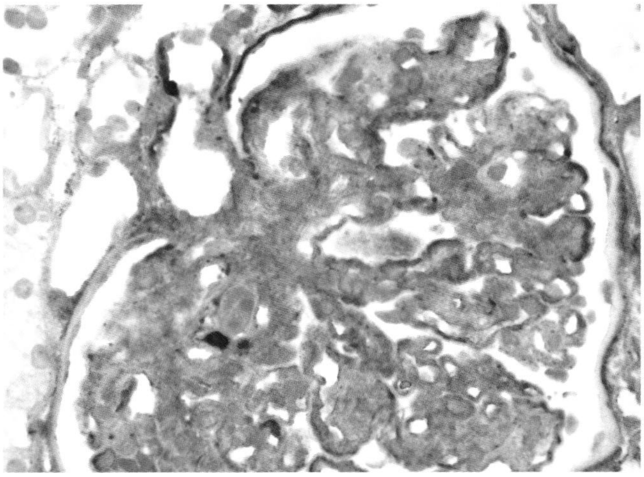

Figure 17-5 MPGN type II/DDD with segmental bandlike intramembranous C3 stain (immunohistochemistry in paraffin sections) in thickened GBM. Focal mesangial C3 stain can be appreciated.

Intramembranous deposits are usually highlighted by immunofluorescence (frozen or paraffin sections) or immunohistochemistry (paraffin section) in a distinctive pattern. Usually an intensive linear staining for C3 (Figure 17-5) in peripheral GBMs can be seen in MPGN type II/DDD. Depending on size and distribution of mesangial deposits, a corresponding C3 deposition can be observed by immuno-

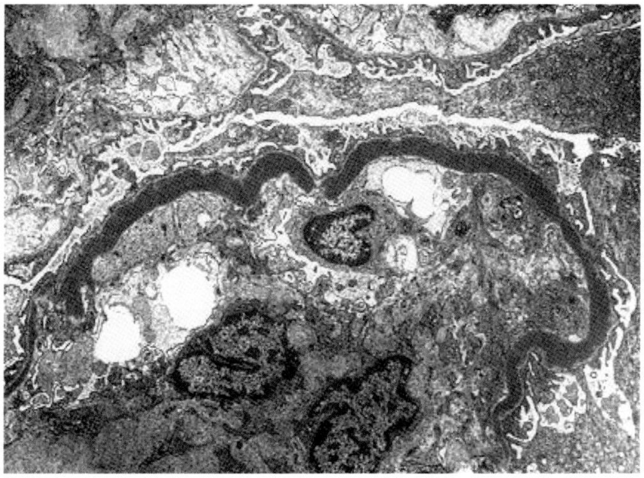

Figure 17-6 MPGN type II/DDD with bandlike electron-dense deposits in the lamina densa of a thickened GBM. Electron microscopy, magnification ×6500. (EM by Ruediger Waldherr, Heidelberg, Germany.)

fluorescence/immunohistochemistry. Immunoglobulins and C1q are usually negative or only faintly detectable.

Electron microscopy is indispensable for the definitive diagnosis of MPGN type II/DDD. The ultrastructural hallmark is a bandlike, highly electron-dense transformation of the lamina densa of the GBM by uniform amorphous deposits (Figure 17-6). These intramembranous dense deposits are usually seen segmentally and thus cause a sausage-string appearance of the basement membrane by alternating thin and thickened basement membrane segments. In the majority of cases nodular dense deposits are found in the mesangium but diffuse deposits can also be present. Similar dense deposits can be found in Bowman's capsule and tubular basement membranes. However, the exact composition of the dense deposit material is unknown.

MPGN Type III Two main morphologic variants of MPGN type III are described, one by Burkholder[17] and another by Anders and Strife.[19,23-25] However, it is still a matter of debate whether type III MPGN may simply be a variant of type I MPGN or represents an established and distinctive clinicopathologic entity.[10-12,26]

Bruckholder described a subtype simultaneously showing features of MPGN type I and membranous glomerulonephritis. Correspondingly, by light microscopy, thickened capillary walls with segmental double contours and mesangial cell interposition can be seen. By silver stain, subepithelial spikes as seen in membranous glomerulonephritis can be demonstrated with the thickened basement membranes. There can be varying degrees of mesangial cell proliferation and additional inflammation of the glomerular tuft as in type I MPGN.

The other variant of MPGN type III described independently by Anders and Strife in the late 1970s shows irregular, thickened, strongly PAS-positive basement membranes by light microscopy. By silver stain the thickened basement membranes appear to be irregular, disrupted, segmentally duplicated, or "moth eaten."

Both subtypes of MPGN type III show similar findings by immunofluorescence (frozen or paraffin sections) or immunohistochemistry (paraffin section). Usually the staining for C3 is most intense, but approximately 50% of the cases show IgG in an equal distribution but with slightly less intensity. Considerably less-intense stain is observed for IgM, IgA, and C1q. Half of the cases are positive for C3 only. Deposition of complement and immunoglobulins is found in a coarsely granular fashion, with great variability from case to case in the mesangium and in thickened peripheral capillary basements. Focal tubular basement membrane staining for C3 can be observed.

Subtyping of MPGN type III is based on electron microscopic findings. The Bruckholder variant shows electron-dense deposits at the subendothelial and subepithelial side of the GBM, as well as discrete deposits in the mesangium. Subepithelial deposits are frequently flanked by newly formed basement membrane spikes, comparable to stage II membranous glomerulonephritis. In cases with an irregular distribution of the deposits, the basement membrane can show an irregular lamellation with intermixing basement material and deposits. If basement membranes have an irregular appearance, distinction from the Strife and Anders variant can be difficult. Usually with this subtype of type III MPGN, complex deposits are found in the subendothelial space extending into the basement membrane (i.e., intramembranous deposits) but can also further enter into the subepithelial region. The deposits are distributed in an irregular fashion but are less electron dense and more ill defined than in the other variants of MPGN. In some cases the deposits have such weak electron density that they are hard to distinguish from the surrounding basement membrane.

Secondary MPGN

A great number of systemic diseases and pathognomonic conditions (Table 17-2) can have renal involvement with an MPGN-like pattern (mesangial hypercellularity with nodular expansion of the mesangium, mesangial cell interposition, or double contours of GBMs) of glomerular injury. Thus this group is quite heterogeneous but can be subdivided into subgroups as shown in Table 17-2. However, some secondary forms (such as cryoglobulinemic MPGN or MPGN due to hepatitis B and hepatitis C) apparently correspond pathogenetically, clinically, and pathohistologically to the accepted forms of MPGN previously described and are caused by immune complex-mediated mechanisms. However, some of these cases show atypical MPGN-like morphologic features, with only segmental double contours or focal mesangial cell interposition and moderate mesangial expansion on one side but predominant subendothelial C3 deposition on a background of serum hypocomplementemia on the other side. In contrast, others just resemble the morphologic MPGN pattern (thrombotic microangiopathy, transplant glomerulopathy) but have no immune-complex-related pathogenesis.

The following sections provide more details about the three major and most common variants of secondary MPGN: MPGN related to cryoglobulinemia, hepatitis B, and hepatitis C. The other forms of secondary MPGN (listed in Table 17-2) are frequently part of a spectrum of glomerular involve-

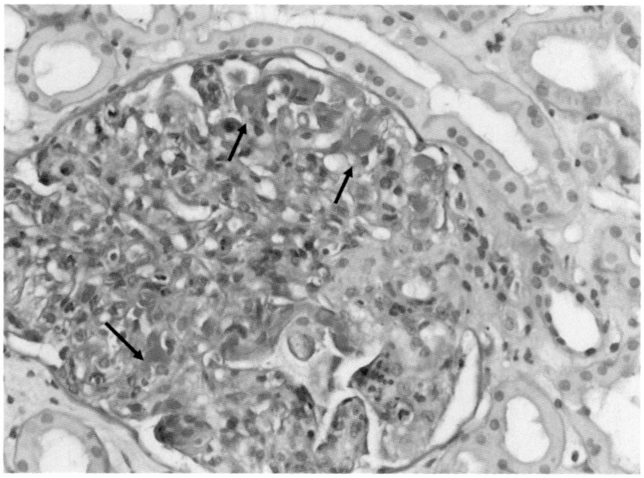

Figure 17-7 Cryoglobulinemic glomerulonephritis with diffuse proliferative, MPGN-like pattern. Numerous hyaline thrombi *(arrows)* in capillary lumina, and infiltrating inflammatory cells (predominantly neutrophils) are present. PAS stain, magnification ×400.

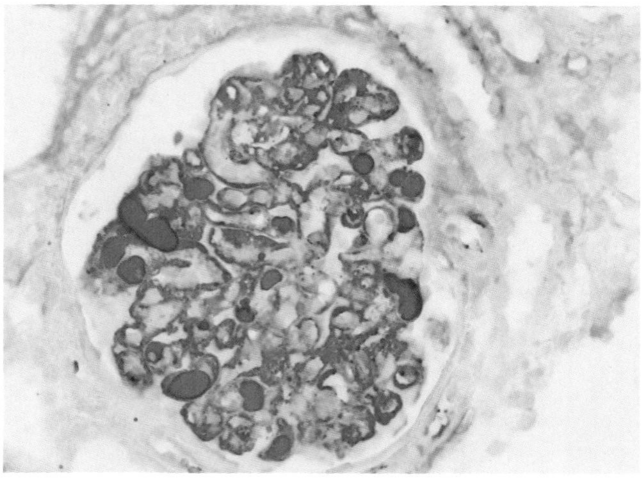

Figure 17-8 Same case as in Figure 17-7, with granular deposition of cryoglobulins in the mesangium, peripheral capillary walls, and with numerous IgM-positive capillary thrombi. Immunohistochemistry in paraffin section for IgM, magnification ×400.

ment in a large number of systemic diseases, some of which are rare and beyond the scope of this chapter. Rare variants of secondary MPGN have been reviewed in detail by Rennke.[3]

Secondary MPGN in Cryoglobulinemia Most cases of glomerulonephritis in patients with cryoglobulinemia (cryoglobulinemic MPGN) are of type I MPGN, followed by type III MPGN. Cases of predominantly endocapillary and extracapillary proliferative glomerulonephritis with segmental features of MPGN can also often be seen (Figure 17-7). Cyroglobulins can be present in various conditions and represent immunoglobulins that have the physical property of reversibly precipitating in the cold. Three types are discriminated: type 1 cryoglobulins consist of a single monoclonal immunoglobulin (IgG kappa or IgM kappa) and can be observed in association to dysproteinemias (multiple myeloma, B-cell lymphomas, Waldenström macroglobulinemia); type 2 cryoglobulins are mixed cryoglobulins with monoclonal immunoglobulin (IgM kappa) complexed to a polyclonal immunoglobulin (IgG), most frequently associated with chronic hepatitis B and hepatitis C, dysproteinemias, autoimmune diseases, or chronic infection; type 3 cryoglobulins are also mixed cryoglobulins containing two polyclonal components (IgG-IgM or IgG-IgG) and are common in autoimmune and infectious diseases. Type 2 cryoglobulins are the most frequent cause for development of glomerulonephritis, followed by type 3 and type 1.

In renal biopsy, cryoglobulin deposition is found subendothelially and intramembranously but frequently can form characteristic intracapillary hyaline thrombi (Figures 17-7 and 17-8). Membranoproliferative lobularity is often accompanied by infiltration of the glomerular tuft by numerous inflammatory cells (Figure 17-7). Infiltrating histiocytes can phagocytose the intraluminal deposits of cryoglobulins. In less than 30% of cases, small vessel vasculitis is seen in the renal biopsy, with intraluminal and intimal cryoglobulin deposits analogous to the glomerular capillaries.

By immunofluorescence (frozen or paraffin sections) or immunohistochemistry (paraffin sections), the cryoglobulinemic deposits reflect the composition of the cryoglobulins in the patient's serum. Thus in most cases of type 1 cryoglobulinemia, monoclonal IgG will be found, whereas in the setting of Waldenström macroglobulinemia, monoclonal IgM predominates. Correspondingly, in type 2 cryoglobulinemia the deposits usually stain for IgG, IgM, C3, C1q, and kappa light chains.

By electron microscopy, predominantly subendothelial cryoglobulin deposits are seen (corresponding to MPGN type I). In approximately half of the cases the deposits are segmentally organized. In type 1 cryoglobulinemia the deposits might show a fibrillar organization. In type 2 cryoglobulinemia, more frequently tubuloannular substructures (Figure 17-9) of the deposits can be found. The areas of organization usually involve some but not all of the deposits; those remaining commonly show a granular pattern.

Whereas cryoglobulinemia is a well-known condition in adults, it is extremely rare in children, and so far there are no reports in the literature of children with cryoglobulin-mediated MPGN.

Secondary MPGN in Hepatitis C Immune complex glomerulonephritis in patients with hepatitis C may or may not be associated with cryoglobulinemia in 30%.[27,28] If cryoglobulinemia is present, the glomerulonephritis is termed *cryoglobulinemic glomerulonephritis.* If not, the appropriate term is *hepatitis C–associated glomerulonephritis.* In cases with cryoglobulins, the pathogenesis of glomerulonephritis is based on the cryoglobulins themselves. For patients with hepatitis C without cryoglobulins, the presumed pathogenesis involves glomerular deposition of immune complexes in the setting of chronic hepatitis antigenemia. Because glomerulonephritis is a late renal manifestation of hepatitis C infection (up to 10 or more years after infection), it is rarely seen in children.

Renal biopsy in most cases of hepatitis C–associated glomerulonephritis shows MPGN type I, followed by MPGN

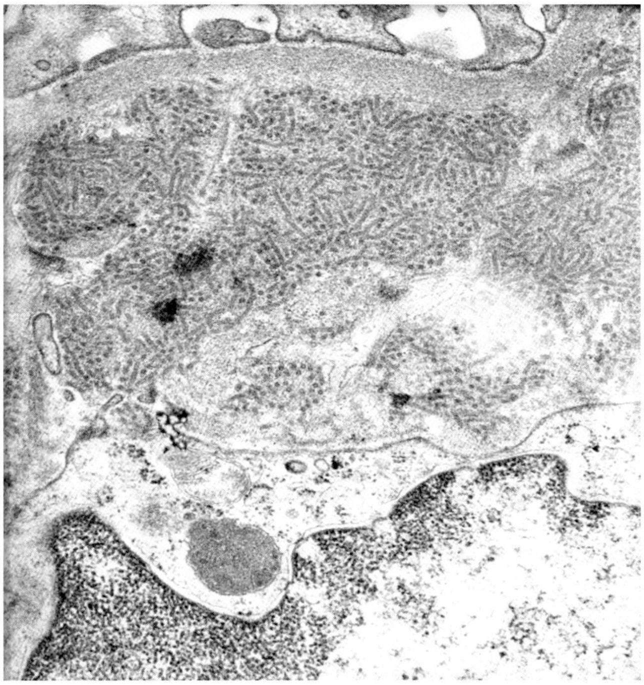

Figure 17-9 Organized deposits in type 2 cryoglobulinemia. Electron microscopy, magnification ×12,500.

type III and membranous glomerulonephritis, as well as diffuse proliferative variants of immune complex glomerulonephritis. In transplant patients, especially those with chronic hepatitis C infection, the MPGN pattern of glomerular injury may be indistinguishable from chronic transplant glomerulopathy.

Immunofluorescence (frozen or paraffin sections) or immunohistochemistry (paraffin sections) usually shows capillary wall and mesangial deposition of large amounts of predominantly IgG, IgM, and C3. However, staining intensity can vary from case to case and there are cases lacking IgG.

Depending on the histologic pattern of glomerulonephritis, deposits are seen by electron microscopy in the mesangium, as well as in a subendothelial and/or subepithelial localization, but rarely intramembranously. As a sign of chronic viral infection, tubuloreticular inclusions can be found in the endoplasmic reticulum of glomerular endothelial cells.

Secondary MPGN in Hepatitis B Hepatitis B–associated glomerulonephritis is more common in children than in adults. Similarly to hepatitis C patients, those with chronic hepatitis B infection can develop immune complex glomerulonephritis with cryoglobulins (cryoglobulinemic glomerulonephritis) or without cryoglobulins. Membranous glomerulonephritis is the best-known renal complication in patients with chronic hepatitis B antigenemia. Membranoproliferative pattern of hepatitis B–associated immune complex glomerulonephritis is usually of type I, but cases of type III MPGN (Bruckholder type) have been described.[10] Furthermore, cases of IgA nephropathy and renal vasculitis can be seen as well.[29]

By light microscopy the MPGN pattern is indistinguishable from that of primary MPGN. In cases with cryoglobulins, characteristic intraluminal hyaline thrombi (cryoglobulin deposits) can be seen.

By immunofluorescence (frozen or paraffin sections) or immunohistochemistry (paraffin sections), deposits of IgG, IgM, and C3 are predominantly found. In contrast to hepatitis C, hepatitis B–specific antigens (HBsAg, HBcAg, and HBeAg) may be detected in the glomerular deposits, providing evidence for the immune-complex-mediated pathogenesis of glomerulonephritis.[30]

By electron microscopy, relatively dense deposits are seen in mesangial, subendothelial, and/or subepithelial locations. As a sign of chronic viral infection, tubuloreticular inclusions might be found in the endoplasmic reticulum of glomerular endothelial cells.

Differential Diagnosis in Renal Biopsy

In addition to all three pathologic techniques (light microscopy, electron microscopy, and immunofluorescence/immunohistochemistry), the differential diagnostic workup of biopsies with an MPGN pattern of glomerulonephritis has to include comprehensive clinical information, including serologic findings. Three major categories of differential diagnosis should be considered.

First, MPGN-like variants of other glomerulonephritis have to be excluded. IgA nephropathy and Henoch-Schönlein purpura nephritis can present with an MPGN-like pattern but will be readily distinguished by a predominant mesangial deposition of IgA and C3. In the majority of cases of thrombotic microangiopathy, characteristic changes (thrombi or onion skinning) are found in small, preglomerular arterioles. Furthermore, the material found by electron microscopy in the widened subendothelial space between the double contours of the basement membranes consists of organized products of coagulation and not true deposits. The material has a somewhat electron-lucent, fluffy appearance. In renal allografts the differential diagnosis of MPGN and transplant glomerulopathy can be challenging in patients in whom MPGN was the original disease or chronic viral hepatitis is apparent. However, transplant glomerulopathy is often a segmental process, whereas glomerulonephritis is more commonly diffuse. By electron microscopy in transplant glomerulopathy, an accompanying transplant capillaropathy[31] can frequently be observed, and the subendothelial deposits are more like those in thrombotic microangiopathy and less electron dense than in immune-complex-mediated MPGN. Cases of MPGN-like glomerulopathy in patients with dysproteinemias can be distinguished by the respective clonal light or heavy chain in the glomeruli found by immunofluorescence/immunohistochemistry. Recent variants with organized deposits and MPGN-like glomerular pattern, namely fibrillar and immunotactoid glomerulopathy, can be distinguished by electron microscopy. Both show either randomly oriented fibrillar or highly organized (tactoid) microtubular electron deposits in the mesangium and adjacent basement membranes. Rare cases of MPGN-like glomerulopathy such as in chronic liver cirrhosis, alpha-1-antitrypsin deficiency, and sickle cell disease can show slight differences in the ultrastructural appearance of the deposits but definitely need clinical background information for final diagnosis.

Having excluded all the aforementioned glomerulopathies with a potential MPGN-like appearance, cases traditionally regarded as classical MPGN remain. These now require thorough differentiation of primary MPGN from the numerous secondary forms (Table 17-2). This can be accomplished only by clinical exclusion of possible underlying autoimmune (e.g., SLE, cryoglobulinemia) and infectious diseases (e.g., hepatitis B and hepatitis C, endocarditis, malaria, shunt nephritis, chronic visceral infections). Therefore the diagnosis of primary MPGN is one of exclusion.

Finally, the three subtypes of primary MPGN must be differentiated by careful analysis of morphologic, immunofluorescence/immunohistochemical, and electron microscopic findings.

Many authors believe that MPGN type II/DDD represents a separate entity and should be completely distinguished from type I and III MPGN.[32] The fact that transformation of type I/III MPGN into DDD and vice versa has not yet been described and that differentiation between DDD and type I/III MPGN is usually reliable by electron microscopy supports this point of view. However, large multicentric and prospective trials are needed to clarify whether distinction of MPGN (types I and III) and DDD (type II) as two separate entities is of therapeutic and prognostic relevance.

MPGN TYPE II/DDD AS COMPLEMENT-MEDIATED DISEASE*

Although a key role of the complement system in the pathogenesis of MPGN has been appreciated since the first description,[1] during recent years it has become evident that the alternative complement pathway, specifically dysregulation of the alternative pathway C3 convertase C3bBb, plays a central role in the pathogenesis of MPGN type II/DDD.[33,34]

A key finding in patients with complement-based MPGN type II/DDD is the activation of the alternative complement pathway.[35] The recent observation that animals lacking plasma Factor H, the main soluble regulator of the alternative complement pathway, develop MPGN type II/DDD further supports the observation that the complement system is involved in the pathogenesis of MPGN type II/DDD, and that defective complement control is a major cause for this disease.[36-38] This concept is supported by the presence of C3 nephritic factor (C3NeF)—an IgG autoantibody that stabilizes the alternative C3 convertase C3bBb, thus preventing degradation of this complex—in some MPGN Type II/DDD patients.[39-41] Even though C3NeF not only shows interindividual but also intraindividual variability, the presence of this factor suggests a crucial role of complement dysregulation in the pathogenesis of MPGN type II/DDD. Both the presence of C3NeF and the absence or defective function of Factor H result in unrestricted activity of the alternative C3 convertase C3bBb, leading to complement activation and deposition of activated complement.[34]

*The following section has in part been recently published by us (Licht C, Schlotzer-Schrehardt U, et al: MPGN II—genetically determined by defective complement regulation? *Pediatr Nephrol* 22[1]:2-9, 2007).

Alternative Complement Pathway: Central Role of C3bBb

The complement system is an integral part of innate immunity but also plays a complementary role for acquired (humoral) immunity. It is mainly designed to defend the body against invading microbes such as pyogenic bacteria or fungi. The complement system consists of a large family of soluble and surface-bound proteins that interact in a tightly regulated fashion. Activated complement proteins (e.g., C3b) bind to the surface of microbes or to antibodies within antigen-antibody complexes and induce the activation of the late steps of the complement cascade, consisting of inflammation, opsonization and phagozytosis, and formation of the membrane attack complex (MAC) and cytolysis (Figure 17-10).[42-44]

The complement system can be involved in diseases in two general ways. Deficiencies in any of the complement cascade components may lead to abnormal complement activation, resulting in either deficient or unrestricted activation of the complement system.[42-44] With respect to renal diseases, however, in most cases unrestricted activation of the complement cascade, especially of the alternative pathway, prevails.[45]

Complement can be activated by four different pathways (Figure 17-10): whereas the classical and lectin pathways are induced by antigen-antibody complexes (classical pathway) or repetitive carbohydrate structures (mannose lectin pathway), the alternative pathway, the most ancient of these three, is constantly active and therefore needs to be tightly regulated by inhibitors to avoid fatal self-attack of the body.[42-44] As recently identified, C5—and thereby the terminal complement cascade—can be activated directly by thrombin, a finding that directly links the complement and the coagulation systems.[46]

Within the alternative complement pathway, the central complement protein C3 is spontaneously activated by constant low-rate cleavage (C3 tickover) which—upon binding to and activation of Factor B—cleaves additional C3 molecules (initiation). The newly generated C3b binds to cell surfaces and, together with other soluble factors, forms the alternative pathway C3 convertase C3bBb, which is stabilized by properdin. This "enzyme" rapidly activates more C3 molecules (amplification). If not limited at this stage, the complement cascade proceeds and the actions of the terminal complement cascade (inflammation, opsonization and phagocytosis, and membrane attack and cell lysis) are carried out (Figure 17-10).[42-44]

With few exceptions, mammalian cells are protected by a multilayered system of soluble and membrane-anchored factors, summarized as "regulators of complement activation (RCA)."[†] Functional redundancy of this system ensures that

[†]Soluble factors: C1 inhibitor; C4 binding protein; Factor H and FHL-1 (Factor H–like protein = alternate splice variant of Factor H); FHR 1-5 (Factor H–related protein 1-5); Factor I; clusterin; vitronectin (S-protein). Membrane-anchored factors: MCP (membrane cofactor protein); DAF (decay-accelerating factor); CR1 (complement receptor 1); protectin (CD59).

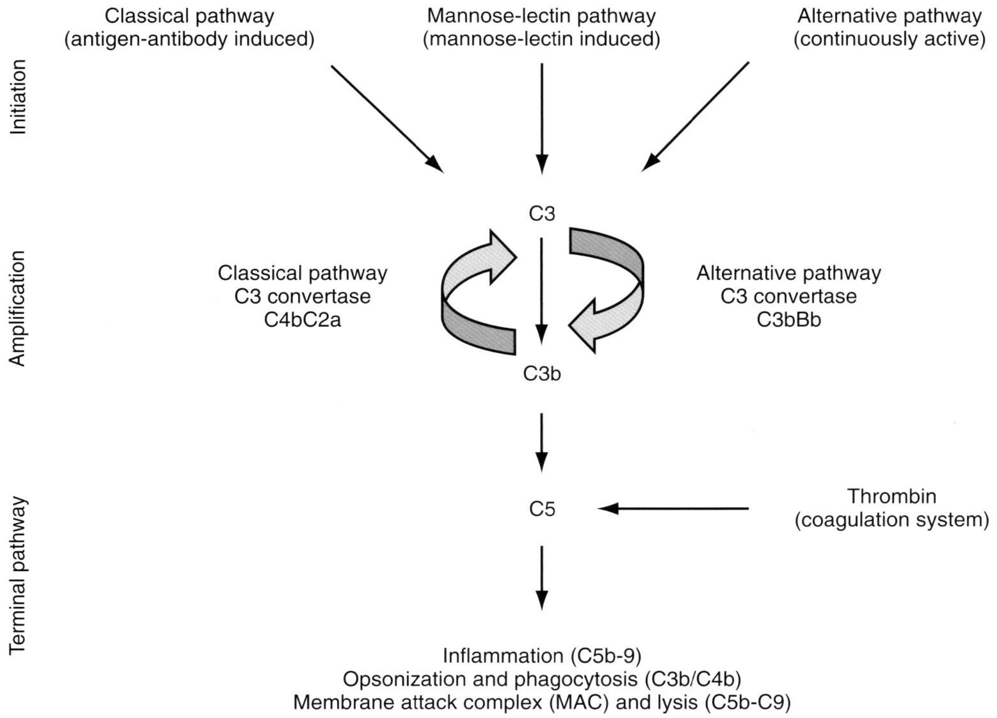

Figure 17-10 The crucial role of the alternative pathway C3 convertase C3bBb within the activation cascade of the complement system.

activation of the complement cascade is site restricted and time restricted. Furthermore, the distribution of the regulators directs the action of the complement system specifically to the surface of target cells. Whereas microbial cells lack surface-anchored regulators, host cells are protected by the presence of such proteins (e.g., MCP, DAF, and CR1). However, in the absence of membrane-anchored regulators, as in the case of the GBM, protection of host surfaces depends solely on the action of soluble factors (e.g., Factor I and Factor H), which are present as circulating plasma proteins and act both in the fluid phase and upon binding to surfaces.[47-48]

Among these complement regulators, plasma Factor H is of significant importance to the homeostasis of the alternative pathway. Factor H consists of 20 sushi domains, also referred to as short consensus repeats (SCR) or complement cofactor proteins (CCP). *N*-terminal SCRs 1 to 4 form the regulatory domain of Factor H (cofactor and decay-accelerating activity, binding to C3b), and C-terminal SCRs 19 and 20 form the recognition domain (heparin and cell binding, binding to C3d).[48] Factor H competes with Factor B for binding to C3b-targeted surfaces.[49,50] Furthermore, Factor H destabilizes C3bBb (decay-accelerating activity) and, as cofactor of Factor I, inactivates C3b (cofactor activity) (Figure 17-11).

Whereas activation of the central complement component C3 is the key step within the activation cascade of the alternative complement pathway, regulation of the alternative pathway C3 convertase C3bBb becomes crucial. Control of C3bBb activity is the key to complement control, and all regulatory mechanisms controlling activation of the alternative complement pathway revolve around this center.[42-44]

Opposing the function of these complement regulators is the IgG autoantibody C3 nephritic factor (C3NeF), which is assumed to stabilize C3bBb. C3NeF is supposed to covalently bind to C3bBb, thereby preventing Factor H–induced dissociation of this complex and thus increasing the half-life of this "enzyme" by approximately 10-fold.[51,52]

In summary, each defect—quantitative or qualitative—of one or more of the complement regulator proteins or the presence of C3NeF unavoidably leads to unrestricted complement activation.

MPGN Type II/DDD Caused by Dysregulation of C3bBb

The complement system has been linked to MPGN type II/DDD, and with the detection of C3NeF in MPGN type II/DDD patients a central pathophysiologic role of the alternative C3 convertase C3bBb has been identified for more than 30 years. However, this insight has not resulted in further progress in the understanding of the pathogenesis of MPGN type II/DDD, nor has it helped develop specific treatment strategies. Only recent research that has identified Factor H as the most potent soluble regulator of the alternative complement pathway and has linked Factor H deficiency to the development of MPGN type II/DDD in different animal models and in humans has led to a conclusive pathogenetic concept for MPGN type II/DDD based on the dysregulation of the alternative C3 convertase C3bBb.

A number of different scenarios, all of which result in unrestricted activation of the alternative pathway C3 convertase C3bBb, are known to cause MPGN type II/DDD. In order of frequency they include (a) presence of C3NeF, (b) missing

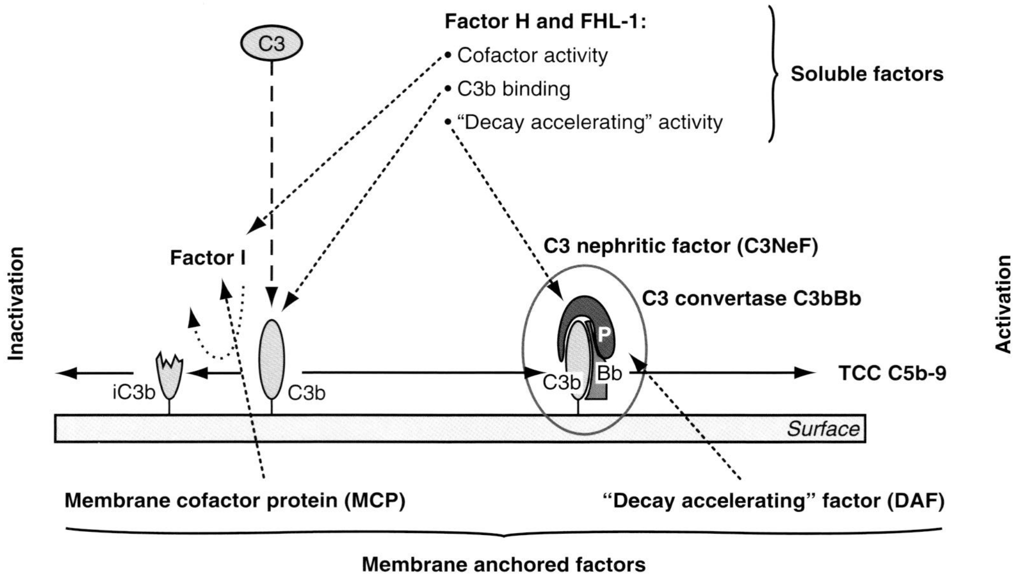

Figure 17-11 Regulation of complement activation on surfaces. A multilayered system of soluble (Factor I, Factor H, FHL-1), as well as membrane-anchored regulators (membrane cofactor protein: MCP, CD46; decay-accelerating factor: DAF, CD55; complement receptor 1: CR1, CD35—not shown) prevents progression of the complement cascade by (1) prevention of C3b from binding to surfaces (Factor H and FHL-1), (2) degradation of C3b (Factor I together with Factor H and/or MCP), (3) interference with assembly of and degradation of assembled alternative pathway C3 convertase C3bBb (Factor H and/or DAF). By contrast, C3 nephritic factor (C3NeF), an IgG autoantibody against C3Bb, binds to and stabilizes C3bBb, thus preventing its degradation and prolonging its half-life. (Modified from Peter F. Zipfel, with permission.)

TABLE 17-3 MPGN Type II/DDD Caused by Dysregulation of C3bBb

Deficiency/Defect	Pathophysiologic Consequence
Factor H	
Deficiency	Missing cofactor activity for Factor I
Functional defect	Missing cofactor activity (but intact binding activity)
Autoantibodies	
C3NeF	Increased half-life of C3bBb
Factor H	Inactivation of Factor H—missing cofactor activity
Rare Causes	
Marder's disease	Factor H unable to bind to C3
C3 autoantibodies	Increased half-life of C3 and C3bBb

or impaired Factor H activity (Factor H deficiency, defective Factor H function, inhibitory Factor H autoantibodies), and (c) rare causes (mutant Factor H binding site of C3 [Marder's disease], C3 autoantibodies)[34] (Table 17-3).

C3 Nephritic Factor

It is well known that the IgG autoantibody C3NeF is linked to MPGN type II/DDD[39-41]: about 55% of the adult and 80% of the pediatric MPGN type II/DDD patients are positive for C3NeF.[8] However, C3Nef is observed not only in patients with MPGN type II/DDD but also in patients with MPGN type I and MPGN type III (MPGN type II > MPGN type I > MPGN type III), partial lipodystrophy, retinal alterations, meningococcal meningitis, and even in healthy individuals.[33] Moreover, it is possible that the same patient may initially test C3NeF positive but become negative during the course of disease (or vice versa).[8]

As already outlined, both C3NeF and Factor H control the same "enzyme," the alternative pathway C3 convertase C3bBb. Factor H dissociates the C3bBb complex (decay-accelerating activity), C3NeF stabilizes the convertase and increases its half-life.[51,52] Thus the presence of C3NeF, absence or defective function of Factor H, and inhibition of Factor H function by antibodies result in an impaired control of C3bBb activity, which eventually results in unrestricted activation of the complement cascade.

Absent or Impaired Factor H Activity

A multilayered system composed of soluble and membrane-anchored regulators normally prevents unrestricted complement activation on host cells. Certain tissue surfaces, however, lack membrane-anchored regulators. Consequently, these structures exclusively depend on attached soluble regulators such as Factor H. Although several renal cell types (endothelial, mesenchymal, epithelial) express membrane-inserted regulators such as CR1 (CD35), MCP (CD46), DAF (CD55), or protectin (CD59),[53] the GBM lacks such proteins.[33,54] Supporting a crucial role of Factor H for protection of the GBM is the fact that it colocalizes with collagen IVα3 (COLIVα3) (Figure 17-12), and, in addition, a transmembrane gradient of Factor H across the GBM is found with maximum Factor H concentration on the blood side and minimum Factor H concentration on the urine side of the GBM (Figure 17-13).

Lack or inactivity of Factor H results in continuous C3 deposition within the lamina densa of the GBM, which is the layer in which under physiologic conditions Factor H is detected in the highest concentration (Figure 17-13).

Factor H Deficiency Absence of Factor H in plasma as a cause of MPGN type II/DDD has been observed in humans, in naturally mutant Factor H–deficient pigs, and in genetically engineered Factor H knockout mice.[33]

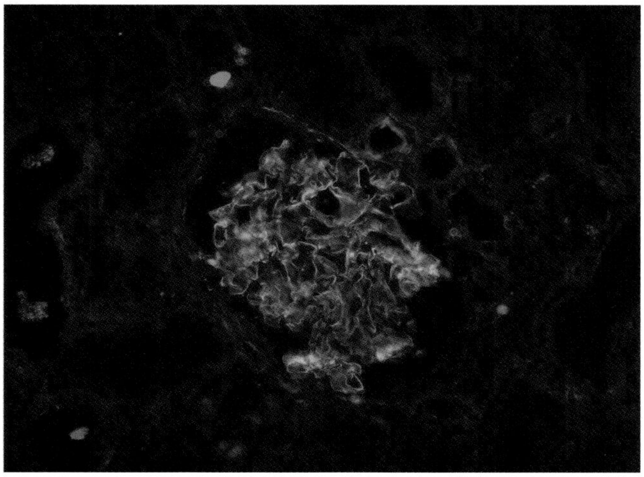

Figure 17-12 Light microscopic immunofluorescence double labeling of Factor H (green fluorescence) and collagen type IVα3 (red fluorescence) in a normal human kidney specimen; colocalization in glomeruli is indicated by yellow fluorescence (merge). For indirect immunofluorescence, cryostat-cut sections were fixed in cold acetone, blocked with 10% normal goat serum, and incubated in primary antibodies overnight at 4°C using a rabbit polyclonal antibody against Factor H (*N*-terminal domain; dilution 1 : 500) and a rat monoclonal antibody against collagen type IVα3 (dilution 1 : 5; gift of Dr. Y. Sado, Kumamoto, Japan). Antibody binding was detected by Alexa 488-conjugated and Alexa 555-conjugated secondary antibodies (molecular probes). (IF by Ursula Schlotzer-Schrehardt, Erlangen, Germany.)

Analysis of the genetic defects leading to complete deficiency of Factor H in plasma of patients revealed homozygous or compound heterozygous Factor H gene mutations in SCRs 2, 4, 9, 11, and 16, which result in nonframework amino acid exchanges or in mutations of framework Cys residues affecting disulphide bond formation within the Factor H molecule.[55,56]

Factor H–deficient pigs represent natural mutants[36,37] and Factor H knock-out mice have been genetically designed.[38] Deficient pigs display amino acid mutations located within SCRs 9 and 20.[47]

All these mutations result in a block of protein secretion: the mutant protein is expressed in hepatocytes but is retained in the endoplasmic reticulum, thereby accumulating in the cytoplasm. As a consequence, absence of Factor H in plasma causes sustained activation of the alternative complement pathway reflected by consumption of C3 and accumulation of the C3 degradation product C3d in plasma.[47]

Defective Factor H Function Different from the absence of Factor H in plasma, we recently described a novel pathomechanism for MPGN type II/DDD: two siblings with MPGN type II/DDD and complement activation expressed normal plasma levels of a mutant and functionally defective Factor H protein; in addition, they were both positive for C3NeF. Genetic analysis revealed several mutations within the Factor H gene. One—considered relevant for disease—causes deletion of three nucleotides (genomic DNA: 57967-57969; cDNA: 743-745) and results in homozygous deletion of a Lys residue in position 224 (K224) located within the complement regulatory domain of Factor H protein in SCR 4. Functional studies of the mutant Factor H protein isolated from the patients revealed normal C-terminal activity

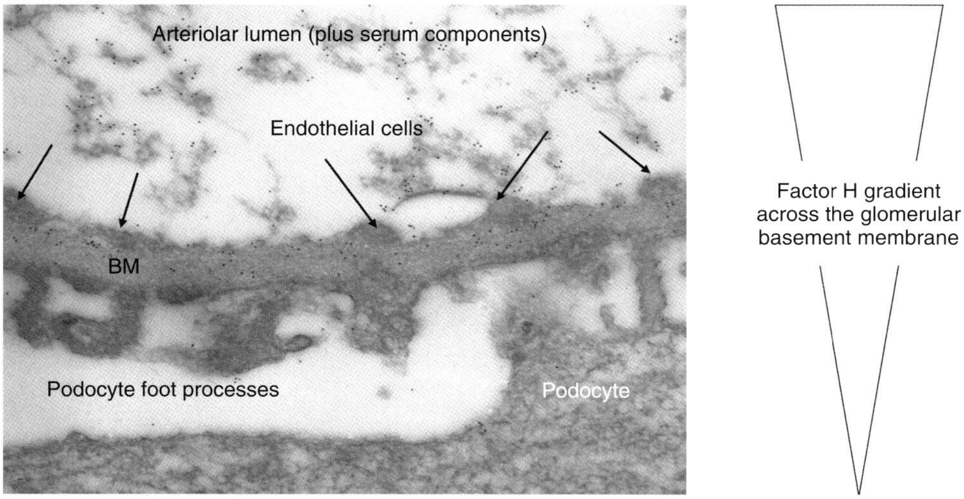

Figure 17-13 Electron microscopic immunogold localization of Factor H along the GBM of a normal human kidney specimen revealing a transmembrane gradient of Factor H across the GBM with maximum Factor H concentration on the blood side and minimum Factor H concentration on the urine side of the GBM. For postembedding immunogold labeling, tissue specimens were fixed in 4% paraformaldehyde and 0.1% glutaraldehyde in 0.1M cacodylate buffer for 5 hours at 4°C and embedded in resin (LR White). Ultrathin sections were blocked with 0.5% ovalbumin and 0.5% fish gelatin, incubated in primary antibody (Factor H, *N*-terminal domain; dilution 1 : 200) overnight at 4°C and in 10 nm gold-conjugated secondary antibody (BioCell) for 1 hour, followed by staining with uranyl acetate. (EM by Ursula Schloetzer-Schrehardt, Erlangen, Germany.)

(binding to heparin, cell surfaces, and C3d), whereas *N*-terminal functions (cofactor and decay-accelerating activity, as well as binding to C3b) were severely reduced. Both parents carried the mutation heterozygously, but normal Factor H function was observed in plasma and the complement system was not activated.

Both siblings and also their healthy mother were positive for C3NeF, indicating that defective control of the alternative pathway by both C3NeF and Factor H dysfunction supports the development of MPGN type II/DDD in the two patients, whereas in this study C3NeF alone in the absence of mutant and functionally defective Factor H did not cause disease in the mother per se.[57]

In a recently performed genotype-phenotype study, potential cosegregation of specific allele variants of the genes encoding for Factor H (CFH) and Factor H–related protein 5 (CFHR-5) with MPGN type II/DDD was reported. However, further functional tests are required to evaluate pathophysiologic relevance of these findings.[58]

Factor H Inhibiting Autoantibodies Meri et al. isolated a factor associated with dysfunction of the alternative complement pathway from serum and urine of a patient with hypocomplementemic MPGN type II/DDD (atypical histology with additional subendothelial deposits: intermediate type between MPGN type I and MPGN type II/DDD). When mixed with fresh normal serum, the patient's serum induced almost complete conversion of C3. This activity was due to a circulating factor different from C3NeF that interacted directly with Factor H and could therefore be considered as Factor H autoantibody. The binding site of this antibody was located in SCR 3 within the regulatory domain of Factor H, which explains impairment of the complement regulatory function of Factor H upon antibody binding.[59,60]

Rare Causes

Mutant Factor H Binding Site of C3 (Marder's Disease) Marder et al. described a C3 mutation that alters the Factor H binding site of C3. This mutation renders the C3b molecule unable to bind Factor H, thus preventing Factor H–mediated dissociation of the alternative pathway convertase C3bBb. Consequently, this defect, called Marder's disease, which has so far been found in only a small group of patients, also prevents control of C3bBb activity and thereby causes unrestricted complement activation.[61,62]

C3 Autoantibodies Normal human IgG contains naturally occurring anti-C3 antibodies (anti-C3 NAbs) that have been proposed to regulate complement amplification. Anti-C3 NAb preparations exhibited nephritic factor activity that was up to 60 times stronger than that of total IgG from a patient with MPGN type II/DDD. Anti-C3 NAbs associated with framework-specific antiidiotypic NAbs stabilize C3 convertase and promote its generation, but their activity is compensated for in whole IgG.[63]

Extrarenal Manifestations in MPGN Type II/DDD

MPGN type II/DDD can be associated with extrarenal manifestations. Besides the renal phenotype MPGN type II/DDD, patients may develop acquired partial lipodystrophy (APL) and ocular lesions similar to soft drusen seen in age-related macular degeneration (AMD).[14]

APL becomes manifest in the loss of subcutaneous fat tissue, which typically occurs in the upper half of the body and precedes the onset of renal disease by several years. Median interval between the onset of APL and MPGN type II/DDD is about 8 years.[64] The majority of APL patients display low C3 levels and in addition are C3NeF positive, which leads to enhanced alternative complement pathway activation. Patients with combined disease are more likely to show decreased C3 levels and develop APL earlier in life (about 12.5 years of age).[64] A common pathophysiologic cause—unrestricted activation of the alternative complement pathway—for both APL and MPGN II/DDD is suggested, and complement-mediated destruction of adipocytes has been shown.[65,66]

Patients with MPGN II/DDD can also develop ocular lesions in the form of drusen. Drusen are retinal changes seen as crystalline yellow or white dots that lie between the retinal pigment epithelium and Bruch's membrane.[67] Drusen can develop in the second decade of life and are responsible for visual disturbances in up to 10% of patients with MPGN type II/DDD.[14] The drusen seen in patients with MPGN type II/DDD are similar to those seen in AMD, which represents the major cause of blindness in the Western aging population. In the early phase of AMD, drusen can develop without any visual problems (i.e., soft drusen) but can progress to visual loss after 65 years of age (Figure 17-14).[68,69] Genome scan studies have linked AMD to the regulators of complement activation RCA gene cluster on chromosome 1q32. Moreover, recently a single-nucleotide polymorphism (Y402H) of the Factor H gene (CFH) was found to play a crucial role in the development of AMD.[70-73] Studies of the composition of drusen support this link by confirming the presence of Factor H in drusen of AMD patients (Figure 17-15).[67,71] However, functional relevance of the Y402H mutation for the development of AMD remains to be established.

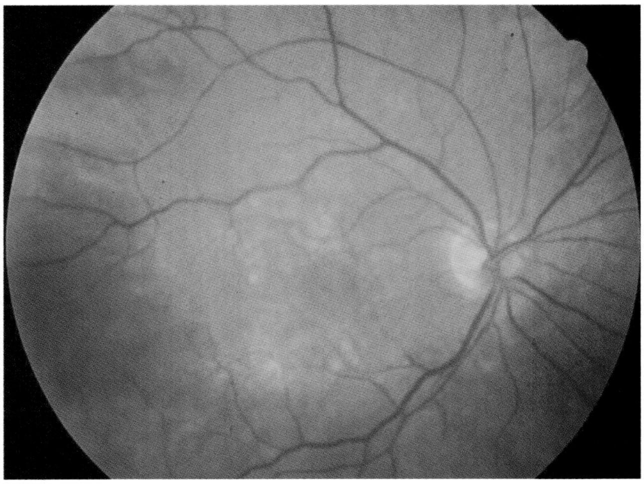

Figure 17-14 Fundoscopic picture of MPGN type II/DDD–associated retinal changes with scattered clumps of hyperpigmentation throughout the macular region (drusen).

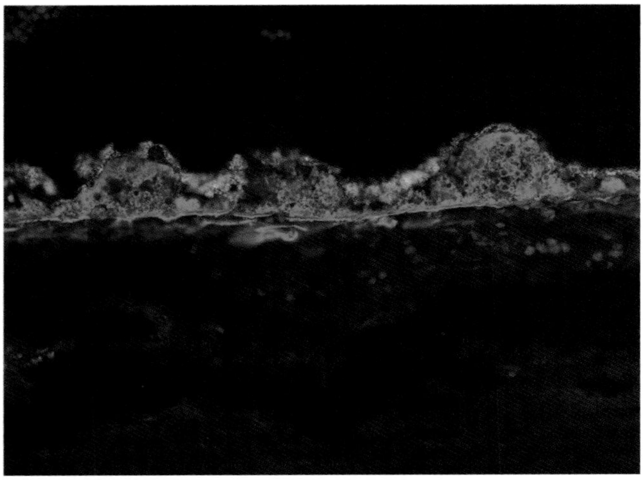

Figure 17-15 Immunofluorescence labeling of Factor H (C-terminal domain; dilution 1 : 500; green fluorescence) in drusen located underneath the retinal pigment epithelium (red autofluorescence) of a human donor eye (age 79 years) with age-related macular degeneration (nuclear counterstain: propidium iodide). (IF by Ursula Schloetzer-Schrehardt, Erlangen, Germany.)

In further support of a crucial role of the alternative complement pathway for AMD, recently certain polymorphisms of Factor B[74]—a protein involved in the assembly of the alternative C3 convertase C3bBb—and Factor H–related proteins 1 and 3 (CFHR1 and CFHR3)[75]—proteins assumed to exert complement regulatory functions similar to Factor H—were also linked to AMD and, surprisingly, were found to reduce the risk of AMD development.

EXPANDED CONCEPT OF MPGN AS COMPLEMENT-MEDIATED DISEASE

Currently three paradigms are in place to explain the amplification of renal injury initiated by the deposition of immune complexes in the glomerulus.[76]

The first paradigm explains the activation of the complement cascade via the classical pathway, resulting in inflammation and cell and tissue injury through binding of complement component C1 to the deposited immune complexes.[76]

The second, and recently established, paradigm recognizes the crucial role of the alternative complement pathway for the pathogenesis of MPGN. As discussed previously, quite distinct abnormalities can cause dysregulation of the alternative complement pathway C3 convertase C3bBb. A multilayered system of soluble and membrane-anchored RCAs prevents unrestricted activation of the complement cascade. Particular tissue surfaces, however, lack membrane-anchored regulators. These structures consequently depend on soluble regulators such as Factor H. The GBM represents such a sensitive structure, which lacks endogenous, membrane-anchored complement regulators. Given this background, lack or functional inactivation of Factor H causes continued C3 deposition within the lamina densa of the GBM, eventually resulting in DDD with deleterious consequences for glomerular and eventually global renal function.[34]

Although the concept of complement-based pathogenesis with deposition of complement factors in the lamina densa of the GBM for type II MPGN/DDD is now well established, it remains unclear whether MPGN type II/DDD should be considered an independent disease entity, or whether the complement system, specifically defects in the regulation of the alternative complement pathway, contribute to the pathophysiology of MPGN in general. Rennke recently suggested defining MPGN as a "disease pattern" and classifying specific phenotypes based on the underlying pathophysiology.[3] However, a recent study by Servais et al. that examined patients with primary glomerulonephritis with isolated C3 deposits identified a small group of patients with type I MPGN carrying mutations in the Factor H or the MCP (CD46) gene, respectively, suggesting an association between constitutional or acquired dysregulation of the alternative complement pathway and MPGN.[77]

The third paradigm identifies a role of Fc receptors, especially of the Fcγ receptor, for the amplification of inflammatory injury of the glomerulus upon immune complex deposition.[76] Fc receptors are expressed by leukocytes and potentially by intrinsic renal cells, and can exert both activating and inhibiting effects on inflammatory processes depending on the differential activation of intracellular pathways through different receptor subtypes.[78-80] The pathogenetic relevance of these receptors is supported by the finding that mice lacking the inhibitory receptor Fcγ subtype develop MPGN.[81]

Further expanding the concept of an autoimmune system–centered pathogenesis for MPGN with a crucial role for innate immunity, Smith et al. suggested inclusion of the recently detected Toll-like receptors (TLRs).[76]

TLRs are a family of innate immune receptors expressed by macrophages and dendritic cells that help regulate inflammation and ensure immune responses in the kidney. TLRs recognize and become activated by pathogen-associated molecular patterns, which are absent or underrepresented in hosts, and upon activation initiate inflammatory responses but also the repair of tissue injury and the priming of adaptive immune responses. In addition, TLRs can direct the immune response toward T helper type 1 (T_H1) or type 2 (T_H2) immune reponse, which potentially results in the development of immunologic sequelae.[82,83]

TLRs probably contribute to the activation of immune responses in inflammatory glomerular and tubulointerstitial diseases and might thus be involved in renal inflammation in general.[82] The observation that MPGN—like other glomerular diseases (e.g., postinfectious glomerulonephritis, IgA-nephropathy, Henoch-Schönlein purpura)—is associated with preceding infections caused by viruses (e.g., hepatitis C virus)[84,85] or, less frequently, other infections[86] including Lyme disease[87] leads to the hypothesis that an infection-specific immune response eventually results in the deposition of immune complexes or the induction of other immune responses within the glomerulus, and that the type of inducing infection is decisive for the resultant glomerular pathology.[88] An ineffective immune response failing to eradicate the infectious agent results in continuous stimulation of the immune system, causing sustained glomerular immune complex deposition.[76]

In summary, both experimental and clinical observations support a crucial role of the immune system, specifically innate immunity and the alternative complement pathway, for the pathogenesis of MPGN. Although with the detection of C3NeF a link between the alternative complement pathway and MPGN type II/DDD has already been appreciated for several decades, there is now evidence that immune mechanisms—involving the classical and alternative complement pathway and specific leukocyte receptors such as Fcγ and TLRs—are also closely involved in the pathogenesis of MPGN subtypes that were so far exclusively linked to infectious diseases (e.g., MPGN type I in HCV infection).

This progress in the understanding of the pathogenesis of MPGN will potentially reconcile the current traditional classification of MPGN into three subtypes, with the suggested novel nomenclature of an MPGN-like injury pattern, to establish a novel, pathophysiologic classification of MPGN. This novel concept would not only simplify and clarify the classification of MPGN but also provide a rationale for a systematic evaluation of MPGN patients for underlying defects of the immune (complement) system. In addition, it would allow for the development of specific treatment strategies for a disease that has few treatment options and a persistently poor outcome.

MANAGEMENT OF MPGN

A standard therapy for patients with MPGN does not exist, either for adults or for children.[89,90] Treatment options are scarce and choices are usually made empirically.[14] Only an improved understanding of the pathogenesis of MPGN will allow the development of specific treatment strategies in the long term.

The key for successful therapy of a patient with MPGN is the identification of the underlying pathophysiology—in short, the correct diagnosis. Besides renal biopsy with the exact characterization of the histopathologic findings and identification of any concomitant systemic disease, detailed examination of the classical and alternative complement pathway should become part of the routine management of MPGN patients.[34]

Treatment of MPGN Type I

Nonspecific treatment of primary and secondary MPGN type I includes (a) treatment of an underlying infectious disease (e.g., antibiotic treatment of shunt sepsis or antiviral treatment of hepatitis C); (b) angiotensin converting enzyme (ACE) inhibitors and/or angiotensin receptor II type 1 (ARB) inhibitors, both aiming for reduction of proteinuria and delay of inflammatory and fibrotic injury of renal parenchyma; and (c) lipid-lowering agents such as HMG CoA reductase inhibitors aimed at delaying progression of renal disease and decreasing endothelial cell dysfunction.[91]

Specific treatment of primary MPGN type I includes corticosteroids (prednisone), other immunosuppressive and antiplatelet/anticoagulant agents, as well as plasma exchange for selected patients with MPGN type II/DDD.[89,91-93] Current (Table 17-4) and novel (Table 17-5) therapeutic concepts are discussed in the following paragraphs, and a stepwise approach for the treatment of children with primary (idiopathic) MPGN is suggested (Figures 17-16 and 17-17).

In children with all three subtypes of primary MPGN, prednisone (specifically, long-term, low-dose use) was found to have a beneficial effect with respect to the degree of proteinuria and renal survival.[89,90,94,95] Treatment with prednisone 2 mg/kg (maximum 60 mg) every other day for 1 year, followed by a maintenance dosage every other day for up to 10 years, was reported as successful.[89] This observation was confirmed by subsequent studies in which therapy with prolonged alternate-day prednisone delayed deterioration of

TABLE 17-4 **Current Therapeutic Concepts for MPGN Type I**

Diagnosis	Therapy	Regimen
Primary MPGN Type I		
	Alternate-day corticosteroids	1-year alternate-day prednisone (2 mg/kg; max 60 mg) + up to 10 years maintenance alternate-day prednisone (5-10 mg every other day) Methylprednisolone pulses (e.g., 3 × 30 mg/kg) + maintenance alternate-day prednisone (5-10 mg every other day)
	Immunosuppressants	Calcineurin inhibitors (cyclosporin, tacrolimus) Mycophenolate mofetil (MMF)
	Antiplatelet/anticoagulant agents	Acetylsalicylic acid, dipyridamole, heparin
	Plasma exchange	Acute: 10-12 consecutive treatments Chronic: 1 treatment every week/every second week (0.5-1.5 × plasma volume/treatment)
Secondary MPGN Type I		
	Supportive therapy only: Angiotensin converting enzyme (ACE) inhibitors Angiotensin receptor II type 1 (ARB) inhibitors Lipid-lowering agents (e.g., HMG CoA reductase inhibitors) Antihypertensives	

TABLE 17-5 Therapeutic Concepts for MPGN Type II/DDD

Abnormality	Mode	Measures
Deficiency of complement factor	Replacement	Plasma infusion: 10-20 ml/kg body weight/every 1-2 weeks Plasma exchange: Acute: 10-12 consecutive treatments Chronic: 1 treatment every week/every second week (0.5-1.5 × plasma volume/treatment) Purified complement factor (in development)
	Inhibition of complement cascade	C5 antibody (eculizumab)*
Functional defect of complement factor	Replacement	Plasma infusion Plasma exchange Purified complement factor
	Inhibition of complement cascade	C5 antibody (eculizumab)*
Autoantibodies against complement factor	Removal	Plasma exchange
	Suppression	Steroids (prednisone 0.5-2 mg/kg)
	Removal	i.v. IgG (400-500 mg/kg i.v. ×1-2) +/− combination with steroids

*From: Hillmen P, Hall C et al: Effect of eculizumab on hemolysis and transfusion requirements in patients with paroxysmal nocturnal hemoglobinuria, *N Engl J Med* 350(6):552-59, 2004; and Hillmen P, Young NS, et al: The complement inhibitor eculizumab in paroxysmal nocturnal hemoglobinuria, *N Engl J Med* 355(12):1233-43, 2006.

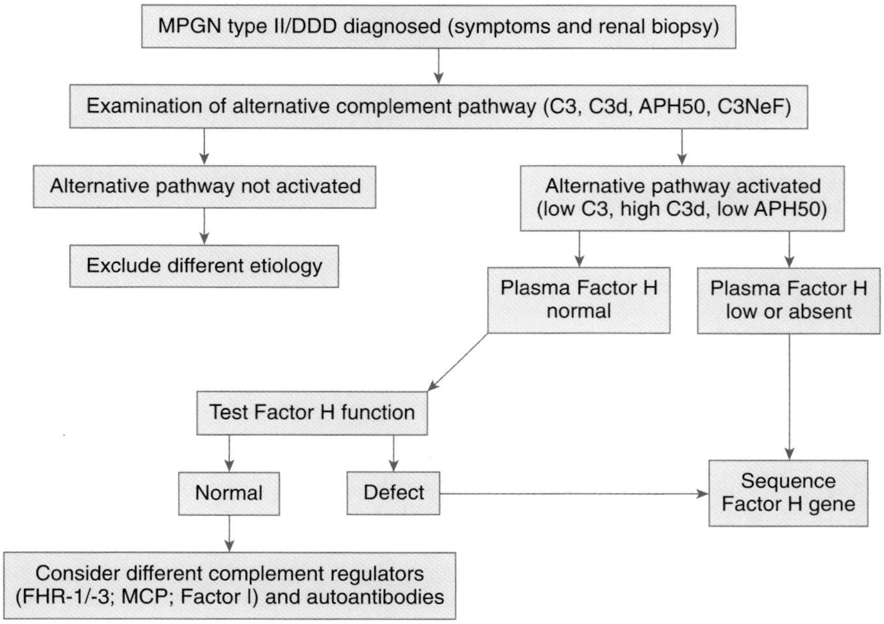

Figure 17-16 Diagnostic algorithm for MPGN type II/DDD. In-depth analysis of the complement system and examination of complement regulatory proteins—especially functional analysis—are available only in specialized laboratories. (From Licht C, Schlotzer-Schrehardt U et al: MPGN II—genetically determined by defective complement regulation? *Pediatr Nephrol* 22[1]:2-9, 2007.)

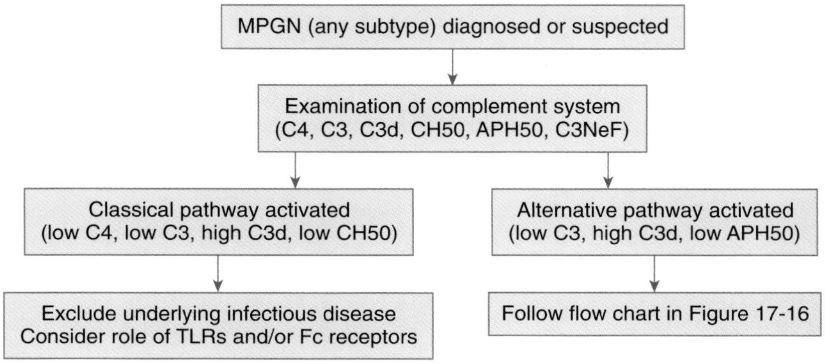

Figure 17-17 General algorithm for MPGN.

renal function.[90,96] Different authors reported individualized treatment strategies using intravenous pulse methylprednisolone (30 mg/kg per day for 3 consecutive days), or prednisone 2 mg/kg (maximum 60 mg) every day, or prednisone 2 mg/kg (maximum 60 mg) every other day depending on the severity of disease. Prednisone was then individually tapered to a maintenance dosage after treatment response (but after an 8-week maximum of daily prednisone). The corticosteroid therapy was accompanied by a concomitant treatment of hypertension. The reported success of this regimen suggests a beneficial effect of early and aggressive treatment of MPGN, including blood pressure control.[95] Finally, in a recent study of idiopathic disease unrelated to hepatitis C, MPGN remission was sustained after steroid withdrawal.[97]

Response of MPGN patients to corticosteroids is not homogeneous. An MPGN subtype–specific analysis of the effect of corticosteroid treatment revealed a lack of efficacy in patients with MPGN type II/DDD despite a beneficial effect in all MPGN patients regardless of the MPGN subtype.[90] In a different study comparing corticosteroid response of MPGN type I and type III patients, decreases in renal function and relapse rate were significantly higher in MPGN type III patients.[98]

Despite a few reports about the use of mycophenolate mofetil (MMF) and the CD20 antibody rituximab in patients with primary or secondary MPGN type I, reports about the treatment of patients with MPGN type II/DDD are so far not available.[14] In MPGN type I patients, MMF was administered alone or in combination with corticosteroids and generated encouraging results in early, short-term use.[92]

In accordance with the observation that thromboembolic-type alterations of the glomeruli are part of the spectrum of pathohistologic findings of the MPGN pattern of injury,[3] a potential rationale for the use of antiplatelet/anticoagulant agents in the treatment of MPGN seems evident, since these agents might be able to reduce platelet consumption in the glomeruli involved in the disease. Accordingly, Donadio et al. found a beneficial effect of a 1-year treatment of MPGN type I patients with the combination of acetylsalicylic acid and dipyridamole with respect to decline in GFR and progression to ESRD.[99] Necessity of prolonged treatment (1 vs. 3 years) is suggested by a different study.[100] The use of warfarin in combination with dipyridamole[101] or in combination with dipyridamole and cyclophosphamide[102] in the treatment of patients with MPGN type I and type II/DDD showed conflicting results and was accompanied by bleeding complications, which strongly contradicts clinical use in children.

Recent progress in the understanding of the role of platelets in the pathogenesis of atypical hemolytic uremic syndrome (aHUS) has provided a link between platelets and the alternative complement pathway. Platelets are carriers of complement regulators (e.g., Factor H), which are required to control complement activation on the surface of activated platelets.[103,104] In addition, platelets might deliver complement regulators to sites of complement activation, thus acting within the multilayered system of complement control.[104] The potential beneficial effect of antiplatelet agents in the treatment of MPGN as just discussed might in the future be explainable in this context.

In secondary MPGN, however, prognosis is considered to be good and mainly depends on the spontaneous remission or successful treatment of an underlying infection.[91] Supportive therapy consists of ACE inhibitors and ARB inhibitors, lipid-lowering agents (e.g., HMG CoA reductase inhibitors), and antihypertensives (Table 17-4). The use of immunosuppressive agents in secondary MPGN can even be harmful, such as in a patient with MPGN secondary to HBV-infection treatment with MMF-stimulated virus replication.[105]

Treatment of MPGN Type II/DDD

Besides corticosteroids (see "Treatment of MPGN Type I"), calcineurin inhibitors (i.e., cyclosporine and tacrolimus) are also used in the treatment of MPGN, but contradictory results have been published about their efficacy in the treatment of patients with MPGN type II/DDD. Although Kiyomasu et al. reported the successful treatment of a patient with MPGN type II/DDD resulting in the recovery from nephrotic syndrome using a combination of alternate-day, low-dose prednisone and cyclosporine,[106] a beneficial effect of calcineurin inhibitors was not seen in other patients.[14]

Whereas an important role of immune mechanisms for the pathogenesis of all subtypes of MPGN is becoming more evident, a crucial role of the alternative complement pathway especially for the pathogenesis of MPGN type II/DDD has been confirmed.[34] We therefore suggest a standardized stepwise diagnostic workup of a patient with MPGN II/DDD, which may reveal specific treatment options (Figure 17-16).

The suggested workup includes the analysis of complement components C3 and C4, as well as of the C3 breakdown product C3d. In addition, analysis of CH50 (test of classical pathway activation) and of APH50 (test of alternative pathway activation) is suggested. If the results are normal, a complement-based etiology can most likely be ruled out. However, if the alternative complement pathway is activated (i.e., low C3, high C3d, low APH50), known complement regulators such as Factor H, Factor I, and possibly in the future Factor H–related proteins 1 and 3 (FHR-1/FHR-3), MCP, DAF, CR-1, and protectin (CD59) should be analyzed by Western blot, examination of protein function, and gene sequencing. If the classical pathway is activated (i.e., low C4 and low C3, high C3d, low CH50), an infection-triggered antigen-antibody complex-mediated pathogenesis is suggested and pathways involving TLRs or Fc receptors might play a role (Figure 17-17). In-depth analysis, especially functional analysis, of the complement system and examination of complement regulatory proteins are available only in specialized laboratories.

With the observation of a crucial role for the complement system in the pathogenesis of MPGN, replacement of potentially missing or dysfunctional complement factors or blockade of the complement cascade by antibodies targeting key activation steps offers a specific therapeutic tool for MPGN.[14,56,107]

The complement system can be compromised in three different ways, each of which can affect one or more complement factors and can occur alone or in combination (Table 17-3). They include (1) deficiency of one or more complement factors, (2) functional defect of one or more complement factors, and (3) presence of inhibiting autoantibodies.

In all three scenarios, replacement of such factor or factors by either plasma infusion or plasma exchange is the appropriate therapeutic approach.[34] Similar to the treatment of aHUS, also recently identified as a complement-based disease,[108] plasma volumes of 10-45 (typically 20-25 ml)ml/kg/treatment (fresh frozen or cryosupernatant) and treatment intervals of 14 days based on the measured Factor H half-life of about 6 days[109] seem to be adequate or appropriate for MPGN.[57,93,110]

This approach is supported by the observation of a beneficial effect of the infusion of porcine plasma in piglets lacking expression of Factor H that developed MPGN type II/DDD.[36,37,47]

Furthermore, in accordance with this concept, we recently described the treatment of two siblings with MPGN type II/DDD showing mild hematuria and proteinuria caused by a functional defect of Factor H protein. In these patients complement activation (low C3, high C3d, low APH50) was present despite low normal plasma Factor H levels. Patients were treated with regular plasma infusions (20 ml/kg/14 days) in order to substitute functionally intact Factor H. Acutely, plasma infusion reduced complement activation both under normal conditions and under biologic stress caused by infections when the complement system was strongly activated. Chronically, plasma infusion prevented disease progression and development of ESRD.[57,93]

Plasma exchange allows administration of an increased volume of plasma. In addition, plasma exchange allows removal of either dysfunctional endogenous complement factors, which—in addition to their functional impairment—might also compete for potential binding partners/receptors, thus possibly weakening the efficacy of plasma replacement therapy. Furthermore, plasma exchange removes antibodies such as the IgG autoantibody C3NeF or Factor H autoantibodies, thus optimizing therapy. Plasmapheresis/plasma exchange is reported to be beneficial in MPGN type I[111] and in MPGN type II/DDD.[112,113] In addition, Kurtz et al. reported a child with rapidly progressive recurrent MPGN type II/DDD on the background of the presence of C3NeF. In this patient, disease progression toward chronic renal failure was delayed by periodic plasmapheresis.[114]

It is likely that in the near future pure Factor H (or other deficient or dysfunctional complement regulators in pure form) will be available either isolated from donor plasma or in recombinant form and may replace whole plasma in the treatment of complement-based MPGN. The use of such a compound would not only offer a specific therapeutic tool that could be administered more frequently and in higher doses if required, but would also reduce the infection risk and facilitate treatment of patients by offering the possibility of subcutaneous or intramuscular administration as compared with the current routine of clinic visits not exceeding every 14 days for plasma infusions.

Finally, antibodies targeting key components of the complement cascade (i.e., complement factor C3 or C5) are under development, and the C5 antibody eculizumab has already been successfully used in adults in the treatment of paroxysmal nocturnal hemoglobinuria, a complement-mediated hemolytic disease.[115-117] However, it is currently unclear whether such antibodies will become a therapeutic option for the treatment of MPGN in children. A potential beneficial effect of complement inhibition in the treatment of complement-based diseases needs to be balanced against the detrimental effect of complement inhibition in situations where complement activation is required as part of the immune defense of the host, and thorough clinical trials are required before the use of these novel substances in children can be recommended.

RECURRENCE OF MPGN AFTER TRANSPLANTATION

All subtypes of MPGN can recur with variable risk after renal transplantation in children.[118,119] Specific risk factors of disease recurrence have not yet been identified. However, a recent study found an association between donor HLA type and risk of recurrent glomerular diseases, including MPGN, after renal transplantation.[120]

For MPGN type I, recurrence risk is reported to be at least 20% to 30%.[119,121] The risk of allograft loss at 10 years posttransplantation due to recurrent MPGN type I was found to be 14.4% in one study.[122] A different study found an impact of the allograft source on the recurrence rate. In patients with deceased donor kidneys, recurrence risk was 33% but was 60% in patients with living-related donor kidneys.[123]

Although recurrence of MPGN type I in a renal allograft can remain asymptomatic, patients with disease recurrence usually display with hematuria, proteinuria, and hypertension, and hypocomplementemia may or may not be present.[124] An association between cytomegalovirus (CMV) infection and renal allograft glomerulopathy has been postulated for a long time,[125] and recent reports support a triggering role of certain virus infections (i.e., CMV, EBV) for disease recurrence in renal allografts. However, whereas recurrent MPGN type I was described in a patient with CMV infection without identifiable virus in the renal allograft,[126] de novo EBV infection in a different patient with recurrent MPGN type I was associated with the presence of the virus in the transplant kidney.[127]

For MPGN type II/DDD patients, recurrence risk is much higher than for MPGN type I patients and is reported to be as high as 50% to 100%.[113,121,128-133] In a recent study the risk of allograft loss at 5 years posttransplantation was about 50% and, in contrast to the finding in MPGN type I living-related donor kidneys, had a significantly better 5 years' survival (about 66%) compared with deceased-donor kidneys (about 34%).[113] In other studies the risk of graft loss was found to be significantly lower, ranging from 0% to 25%.[122,133,134]

The degree of proteinuria was strongly associated with disease recurrence, and the presence of glomerular crescents in biopsies of renal allografts had a significant negative correlation with graft survival.[113] A correlation between the severity of hypocomplementemia either at initial presentation or at the time of disease recurrence in the renal allograft was not found.[113]

Reports about recurrence of MPGN type III in renal allografts are scarce. Only two case reports exist and do not permit a firm statement about the risk of recurrence or allograft loss in this MPGN subtype.[135,136]

As for primary MPGN, there is no proven beneficial therapy for recurrent MPGN in the renal allograft. Therapeutic approaches are similar to those used in primary MPGN and are therefore not discussed in detail here. Reported treatment of recurrent MPGN type I beyond conservative medications such as ACE inhibitors and/or ARB inhibitors to control proteinuria and hypertension includes antiplatelet/anticoagulant agents,[137] corticosteroids,[138] cyclosporine,[139] cyclophosphamide,[140] and plasmapheresis.[138,141] Reported treatment of recurrent MPGN type II/DDD includes dose reduction, discontinuation or switch (cyclosporine to tacrolimus) of the calcineurin inhibitors used as part of the post-transplant immunosuppression regimen, modification of the prednisone dose (increase; switch from daily to alternate day), pulse methylprednisolone, or plasmapheresis/plasma exchange.[112,113] Reports about treatment of recurrent MPGN type III are scarce. In a small case series of recurrent glomerulopathies in renal allografts, however, one patient with MPGN type III was reported to have responded well to high-dose MMF, whereas a previous attempt with steroid pulses had failed to induce remission.[142]

SUMMARY AND PERSPECTIVES

We have presented a novel concept for MPGN that integrates the traditional three MPGN subtypes (MPGN type I, MPGN type II/DDD, and MPGN type III) as complement-based diseases and extends the traditional morphologic classification to include pathophysiologic mechanisms. The current concept highlights the key roles of both the classical (MPGN type I) and the alternative (MPGN type II/DDD) complement pathways, which was first suggested some 30 years ago for both primary MPGN and MPGN recurrence in renal allograft rejection.[143] Mutations of the key complement regulator Factor H resulting in deficiency or functional defect, and presence of inhibiting Factor H autoantibodies are now linked with MPGN type II/DDD (alternative complement pathway), and TLRs and Fc receptors have been associated with MPGN type I (classical pathway). In the future even more complement factors may be identified as important for the pathogenesis of MPGN. Besides Factor H, the family of Factor H–related proteins, Factor I, and Factor B (all soluble factors), and membrane cofactor protein (MCP, CD46), decay-accelerating factor (DAF, CD55), complement receptor 1 (CR1, CD35), and protectin (CD59) (all membrane-bound factors) might also be identified as disease causing when deficient or defective.

Our concept is supported by two different lines of argument that have developed independently over the past few years. One evolves from recent progress in the interpretation of the morphologic findings in MPGN, resulting in the recommendation of the term *membranoproliferative pattern of injury*,[3] which has also been recently adopted by other pathologists,[11] and the other evolves from the rapid progress in understanding the impact of the complement system on the pathogenesis of MPGN.[33,44]

Additional support for an integrative concept of complement-based glomerular diseases has been provided by Mathieson et al., who described development of aHUS in infancy and MPGN (subtype not specified) in adulthood in one patient with sustained alternative complement pathway activation.[144] Also, Jha et al. reported a child who clinically presented with symptoms of HUS but showed MPGN on renal biopsy, and who recovered completely with resolution of both diseases upon institution of plasma exchange.[145]

The concept we have described needs to be further evaluated. Because patient numbers are small in individual centers, multicenter patient registries* are required to provide in-depth analysis of the underlying pathogenetic mechanisms and to establish a conclusive classification system of MPGN, as well as to develop successful treatment strategies for both primary disease and recurrent disease in renal allografts.

REFERENCES

1. West CD, McAdams AJ, et al: Hypocomplemententemic and normocomplemententemic persistent (chronic) glomerulonephritis: clinical and pathologic characteristics, *J Pediatr* 67:1089-112, 1965.
2. Habib R, Kleinknecht C, et al: Idiopathic membranoproliferative glomerulonephritis in children. Report of 105 cases, *Clin Nephrol* 1(4):194-214, 1973.
3. Rennke HG: Secondary membranoproliferative glomerulonephritis, *Kidney Int* 47(2):643-56, 1995.
4. Johnson RJ, AC, Schena FP (2003). Membranoproliferative glomerulonephritis and cryoglobulinemic glomerulonephritis. Comprehensive clinical nephrology. FJ Johnson RJ Edinburgh, Mosby: 25.1-25.10.
5. The primary nephrotic syndrome in children. Identification of patients with minimal change nephrotic syndrome from initial response to prednisone. A report of the International Study of Kidney Disease in Children, *J Pediatr* 98:561-64, 1981.
6. Iitaka K, Nakamura S, et al: Hypocomplementemia and membranoproliferative glomeruloneophritis in children, *Clin Exp Nephrol* 9(1):31-33, 2005.
7. Schwertz R, de Jong R, et al: Outcome of idiopathic membranoproliferative glomerulonephritis in children. Arbeitsgemeinschaft Padiatrische Nephrologie, *Acta Paediatr* 85(3):308-12, 1996.
8. Schwertz R, Rother U, et al: Complement analysis in children with idiopathic membranoproliferative glomerulonephritis: a long-term follow-up, *Pediatr Allergy Immunol* 12(3):166-72, 2001.
9. D'Agati V, Jennette JC, et al: Membranoproliferative glomerulonephritis. In D'Agati V, Jennette JC, Silva FG, editors: *Non-Neoplastic Kidney Diseases*, vol 1, Silver Spring, MD, 2005, ARP Press.
10. Silva FG: Menbranoproliferative glomerulonephritis. In Jennette JC, Olson JL, Schwartz MM, Silva FG, editors: *Heptinstall's Pathology of the Kidney*, vol 1, Philadelphia, 1998, Lippincott-Raven.
11. Gokden N, Rossini M, et al: Membranoproliferative injury pattern in a renal allograft, *Am J Kidney Dis* 46(3):573-76, 2005.
12. Nakopoulou L: Membranoproliferative glomerulonephritis, *Nephrol Dial Transplant* 16 (suppl 6):71-73, 2001.
13. Ferrario F, Rastaldi MP: Histopathological atlas of renal diseases. Membranoproliferative glomerulonephritis, *J Nephrol* 17(4):483-86, 2004.
14. Appel GB, Cook HT, et al: Membranoproliferative glomerulonephritis type II (dense deposit disease): an update, *J Am Soc Nephrol* 16(5):1392-403, 2005.
15. Burkholder PM: Ultrastructural demonstration of injury and perforation of glomerular capillary basement membrane in acute proliferative glomerulonephritis, *Am J Pathol* 56(2):251-65, 1969.
16. Burkholder PM, Bradford WD: Proliferative glomerulonephritis in children. A correlation of varied clinical and pathologic patterns

*Europe or Canada: www.mpgn-registry.de / USA: www.nursing.uiowa.edu/MPGNDatabase/

utilizing light, immunofluorescence, and electron microscopy, *Am J Pathol* 56(3):423-67, 1969.
17. Burkholder PM, Marchand A, et al: Mixed membranous and proliferative glomerulonephritis. A correlative light, immunofluorescence, and electron microscopic study, *Lab Invest* 23(5):459-79, 1970, and in *Complement and kidney disease,* Zipfel PF (editor), Birkhäuser Company, Basel, Switzerland, pp. 165-97.
18. Anders D, Agricola B, et al: Basement membrane changes in membranoproliferative glomerulonephritis. II. Characterization of a third type by silver impregnation of ultra thin sections, *Virchows Arch A Pathol Anat Histol* 376(1):1-19, 1977.
19. Strife CF, Jackson EC, et al: Type III membranoproliferative glomerulonephritis: long-term clinical and morphologic evaluation, *Clin Nephrol* 21(6):323-34, 1984.
20. Iitaka K, Nakamura S, et al: Long-term follow-up of type II membranoproliferative glomerulonephritis in two children, *Clin Exp Nephrol* 7(1):58-62, 2003.
21. Habib R, Gubler MC, et al: Dense deposit disease: a variant of membranoproliferative glomerulonephritis, *Kidney Int* 7(4):204-15, 1975.
22. Cameron JS, Turner DR, et al: Idiopathic mesangiocapillary glomerulonephritis. Comparison of types I and II in children and adults and long-term prognosis, *Am J Med* 74(2):175-92, 1983.
23. Anders D, Thoenes W: Basement membrane-changes in membranoproliferative glomerulonephritis: a light and electron microscopic study, *Virchows Arch A Pathol Anat Histol* 369(2):87-109, 1975.
24. Anders D, Blaker F, et al: [Membranoproliferative glomerulonephritis. Variability of a morphologically definable disease], *Klin Padiatr* 194(3):173-81, 1982.
25. Strife CF, McAdams AJ, et al: Membranoproliferative glomerulonephritis characterized by focal, segmental proliferative lesions, *Clin Nephrol* 18(1):9-16, 1982.
26. Meyers KE, Finn L, et al: Membranoproliferative glomerulonephritis type III, *Pediatr Nephrol* 12(6):512-22, 1998.
27. Johnson RJ, Gretch DR, et al: Membranoproliferative glomerulonephritis associated with hepatitis C virus infection, *N Engl J Med* 328(7):465-70, 1993.
28. Martin M, Sole M: Membranoproliferative glomerulonephritis associated with hepatitis C infection, *J Hepatol* 41(5):881, 2004.
29. Johnson RJ, Couser WG: Hepatitis B infection and renal disease: clinical, immunopathogenetic and therapeutic considerations, *Kidney Int* 37(2):663-76, 1990.
30. Venkataseshan VS, Lieberman K, et al: Hepatitis-B-associated glomerulonephritis: pathology, pathogenesis, and clinical course, *Medicine (Baltimore)* 69(4):200-16, 1990.
31. Ivanyi B: Transplant capillaropathy and transplant glomerulopathy: ultrastructural markers of chronic renal allograft rejection, *Nephrol Dial Transplant* 18(4):655-60, 2003.
32. Mazzucco G, Barbiano di Belgiojoso G, et al: Glomerulonephritis with dense deposits: a variant of membranoproliferative glomerulonephritis or a separate morphological entity? Light, electron microscopic and immunohistochemical study of eleven cases, *Virchows Arch A Pathol Anat Histol* 387(1):17-29, 1980.
33. Zipfel PF, Heinen S, et al: Complement and diseases: defective alternative pathway control results in kidney and eye diseases, *Mol Immunol* 43(1-2):97-106, 2006.
34. Licht C, Schlotzer-Schrehardt U, et al: MPGN II—genetically determined by defective complement regulation?, *Pediatr Nephrol* 22(1):2-9, 2007.
35. Ault BH: Factor H and the pathogenesis of renal diseases, *Pediatr Nephrol* 14(10-11):1045-53, 2002.
36. Hogasen K, Jansen JH, et al: Hereditary porcine membranoproliferative glomerulonephritis type II is caused by factor H deficiency, *J Clin Invest* 95(3):1054-61, 1995.
37. Jansen JH, Hogasen K, et al: Porcine membranoproliferative glomerulonephritis type II: an autosomal recessive deficiency of factor H, *Vet Rec* 137(10):240-44, 1995.
38. Pickering MC, Cook HT, et al: Uncontrolled C3 activation causes membranoproliferative glomerulonephritis in mice deficient in complement factor H, *Nat Genet* 31(4):424-28, 2002.
39. Daha MR, Fearon DT, et al: C3 nephritic factor (C3NeF): stabilization of fluid phase and cell-bound alternative pathway convertase, *J Immunol* 116(1):1-7, 1976.
40. West CD: Nephritic factors predispose to chronic glomerulonephritis, *Am J Kidney Dis* 24(6):956-63, 1994.
41. West CD, McAdams AJ: The alternative pathway C3 convertase and glomerular deposits, *Pediatr Nephrol* 13(5):448-53, 1999.
42. Walport MJ: Complement. First of two parts, *N Engl J Med* 344(14):1058-66, 2001.
43. Walport MJ: Complement. Second of two parts, *N Engl J Med* 344(15):1140-44, 2001.
44. Thurman JM, Holers V: The central role of the alternative complement pathway in human disease, *J Immunol* 176(3):1305-10, 2006.
45. Quigg RJ: Complement and the kidney, *J Immunol* 171(7):3319-24, 2003.
46. Huber-Lang M, Sarma JV, et al: Generation of C5a in the absence of C3: a new complement activation pathway, *Nat Med* 12(6):682-87, 2006.
47. Hegasy GA, Manuelian T, et al: The molecular basis for hereditary porcine membranoproliferative glomerulonephritis type II: point mutations in the factor H coding sequence block protein secretion, *Am J Pathol* 161(6):2027-34, 2002.
48. Jozsi M, Manuelian T, et al: Attachment of the soluble complement regulator factor H to cell and tissue surfaces: relevance for pathology, *Histol Histopathol* 19(1):251-58, 2004.
49. Fearon DT: Regulation by membrane sialic acid of beta1H-dependent decay-dissociation of amplification C3 convertase of the alternative complement pathway, *Proc Natl Acad Sci U S A* 75(4):1971-75, 1978.
50. Pangburn MK, Pangburn KL, et al: Molecular mechanisms of target recognition in an innate immune system: interactions among factor H, C3b, and target in the alternative pathway of human complement, *J Immunol* 164(9):4742-51, 2000.
51. Weiler JM, Daha MR, et al: Control of the amplification convertase of complement by the plasma protein beta1H, *Proc Natl Acad Sci U S A* 73(9):3268-72, 1976.
52. Daha MR, Van Es LA: Stabilization of homologous and heterologous cell-bound amplification convertases, C3bBb, by C3 nephritic factor, *Immunology* 43(1):33-38, 1981.
53. Timmerman JJ, van der Woude FJ, et al: Differential expression of complement components in human fetal and adult kidneys, *Kidney Int* 49(3):730-40, 1996.
54. Pavenstadt H, Kriz W, et al: Cell biology of the glomerular podocyte, *Physiol Rev* 83(1):253-307, 2003.
55. Ault BH, Schmidt BZ, et al: Human factor H deficiency. Mutations in framework cysteine residues and block in H protein secretion and intracellular catabolism, *J Biol Chem* 272(40):25168-75, 1997.
56. Cunningham PN, Quigg RJ: Contrasting roles of complement activation and its regulation in membranous nephropathy, *J Am Soc Nephrol* 16(5):1214-22, 2005.
57. Licht C, Heinen S, et al: Deletion of Lys224 in regulatory domain 4 of factor H reveals a novel pathomechanism for dense deposit disease (MPGN II), *Kidney Int* 70(1):42-50, 2006.
58. Abrera-Abeleda MA, Nishimura C, et al: Variations in the complement regulatory genes factor H (CFH) and factor H related 5 (CFHR5) are associated with membranoproliferative glomerulonephritis type II (dense deposit disease), *J Med Genet* 43(7):582-89, 2006.
59. Meri S, Koistinen V, et al: Activation of the alternative pathway of complement by monoclonal lambda light chains in membranoproliferative glomerulonephritis, *J Exp Med* 175(4):939-50, 1992.
60. Jokiranta TS, Solomon A, et al: Nephritogenic lambda light chain dimer: a unique human miniautoantibody against complement factor H, *J Immunol* 163(8):4590-96, 1999.
61. Marder HK, Coleman TH, et al: An inherited defect in the C3 convertase, C3b,Bb, associated with glomerulonephritis, *Kidney Int* 23(5):749-58, 1983.
62. Linshaw MA, Stapleton FB, et al: Hypocomplementemic glomerulonephritis in an infant and mother. Evidence for an abnormal form of C3, *Am J Nephrol* 7(6):470-77, 1987.
63. Jelezarova E, Lutz HU: IgG naturally occurring antibodies stabilize and promote the generation of the alternative complement pathway C3 convertase, *Mol Immunol* 42(11):1393-403, 2005.

64. Misra A, Peethambaram A, et al: Clinical features and metabolic and autoimmune derangements in acquired partial lipodystrophy: report of 35 cases and review of the literature, *Medicine (Baltimore)* 83(1):18-34, 2004.
65. Mathieson PW, Wurzner R, et al: Complement-mediated adipocyte lysis by nephritic factor sera, *J Exp Med* 177(6):1827-31, 1993.
66. Mathieson PW, Peters DK: Lipodystrophy in MCGN type II: the clue to links between the adipocyte and the complement system, *Nephrol Dial Transplant* 12(9):1804-06, 1997.
67. De Jong PT: Age-related macular degeneration, *N Engl J Med* 355(14):1474-85, 2006.
68. Hogg RE, Chakravarthy U: Visual function and dysfunction in early and late age-related maculopathy, *Prog Retin Eye Res* 25(3):249-76, 2006.
69. Magnusson KP, Duan S, et al: CFH Y402H confers similar risk of soft drusen and both forms of advanced AMD, *PLoS Med* 3(1):e5, 2006.
70. Edwards AO, Ritter R III, et al: Complement factor H polymorphism and age-related macular degeneration, *Science* 308(5720):421-24, 2005.
71. Hageman GS, Anderson DH, et al: A common haplotype in the complement regulatory gene factor H (HF1/CFH) predisposes individuals to age-related macular degeneration, *Proc Natl Acad Sci U S A* 102(20):7227-32, 2005.
72. Haines JL, Hauser MA, et al: Complement factor H variant increases the risk of age-related macular degeneration, *Science* 308(5720):419-21, 2005.
73. Klein RJ, Zeiss C, et al: Complement factor H polymorphism in age-related macular degeneration, *Science* 308(5720):385-89, 2005.
74. Gold B, Merriam JE, et al: Variation in factor B (BF) and complement component 2 (C2) genes is associated with age-related macular degeneration, *Nat Genet* 38(4):458-62, 2006.
75. Hughes AE, Orr N, et al: A common CFH haplotype, with deletion of CFHR1 and CFHR3, is associated with lower risk of age-related macular degeneration, *Nat Genet* 38(10):1173-77, 2006.
76. Smith KD, Alpers CE: Pathogenic mechanisms in membranoproliferative glomerulonephritis, *Curr Opin Nephrol Hypertens* 14(4):396-403, 2005.
77. Servais A, Fremeaux-Bacchi V, et al: Primary glomerulonephritis with isolated C3 deposits: a new entity which shares common genetic risk factors with hemolytic uremic syndrome, *J Med Genet* 44(3):193-99, 2006.
78. Ravetch JV, Lanier LL: Immune inhibitory receptors, *Science* 290(5489):84-89, 2000.
79. Ravetch JV, Bolland S: IgG Fc receptors, *Annu Rev Immunol* 19:275-90, 2001.
80. Tarzi RM, Cook HT: Role of Fcgamma receptors in glomerulonephritis, *Nephron Exp_Nephrol* 95(1):e7-12, 2003.
81. Muhlfeld AS, Segerer S, et al: Deletion of the Fcgamma receptor IIb in thymic stromal lymphopoietin transgenic mice aggravates membranoproliferative glomerulonephritis, *Am J Pathol* 163(3): 1127-36, 2003.
82. Anders HJ, Banas B, et al: Signaling danger: toll-like receptors and their potential roles in kidney disease, *J Am Soc Nephrol* 15(4):854-67, 2004.
83. Pulendran B: Variegation of the immune response with dendritic cells and pathogen recognition receptors, *J Immunol* 174(5):2457-65, 2005.
84. Meyers CM, Seeff LB, et al: Hepatitis C and renal disease: an update, *Am J Kidney Dis* 42(4):631-57, 2003.
85. Wornle M, Schmid H, et al: Novel role of toll-like receptor 3 in hepatitis C-associated glomerulonephritis, *Am J Pathol* 168(2): 370-85, 2006.
86. Anders HJ, Banas B, et al: Bacterial CpG-DNA aggravates immune complex glomerulonephritis: role of TLR9-mediated expression of chemokines and chemokine receptors, *J Am Soc Nephrol* 14(2):317-26, 2003.
87. Kirmizis D, Efstratiadis G, et al: MPGN secondary to Lyme disease, *Am J Kidney Dis* 43(3):544-51, 2004.
88. Pasare C, Medzhitov R: Toll-like receptors: linking innate and adaptive immunity, *Microbes Infect* 6(15):1382-87, 2004.
89. West, CD: Childhood membranoproliferative glomerulonephritis: an approach to management, *Kidney Int* 29(5):1077-93, 1986.
90. Tarshish P, Bernstein J, et al: Treatment of mesangiocapillary glomerulonephritis with alternate-day prednisone—a report of the International Study of Kidney Disease in Children, *Pediatr Nephrol* 6(2):123-30, 1992.
91. Levin A: Management of membranoproliferative glomerulonephritis: evidence-based recommendations, *Kidney Int Suppl* 70:S41-46, 1999.
92. Jones G, Juszczak M, et al: Treatment of idiopathic membranoproliferative glomerulonephritis with mycophenolate mofetil and steroids, *Nephrol Dial Transplant* 19(12):3160-64, 2004.
93. Habbig S, Kirschfink M, et al: Long-term treatment of MPGN II tue to functional factor H defect via FFP infusion, *J Am Soc Nephrol* 17(abstracts issue):575A, 2006.
94. McEnery PT: Membranoproliferative glomerulonephritis: the Cincinnati experience—cumulative renal survival from 1957 to 1989, *J Pediatr* 116(5):S109-14, 1990.
95. Ford DM, Briscoe DM, et al: Childhood membranoproliferative glomerulonephritis type I: limited steroid therapy, *Kidney Int* 41(6):1606-12, 1992.
96. Yanagihara T, Hayakawa M, et al: Long-term follow-up of diffuse membranoproliferative glomerulonephritis type I, *Pediatr Nephrol* 20(5):585-90, 2005.
97. Kazama I, Matsubara M, et al: Steroid resistance in prolonged type I membranoproliferative glomerulonephritis and accelerated disease remission after steroid withdrawal, *Clin Exp Nephrol* 9(1):62-68, 2005.
98. Braun MC, West CD, et al: Differences between membranoproliferative glomerulonephritis types I and III in long-term response to an alternate-day prednisone regimen, *Am J Kidney Dis* 34(6):1022-32, 1999.
99. Donadio JV Jr, Anderson CF, et al: Membranoproliferative glomerulonephritis. A prospective clinical trial of platelet-inhibitor therapy, *N Engl J Med* 310(22):1421-26, 1984.
100. Zauner I, Bohler J, et al: Effect of aspirin and dipyridamole on proteinuria in idiopathic membranoproliferative glomerulonephritis: a multicentre prospective clinical trial. Collaborative Glomerulonephritis Therapy Study Group (CGTS), *Nephrol Dial Transplant* 9(6):619-22, 1994.
101. Zimmerman SW, Moorthy AV, et al: Prospective trial of warfarin and dipyridamole in patients with membranoproliferative glomerulonephritis, *Am J Med* 75(6):920-27, 1983.
102. Cattran DC, Cardella CJ, et al: Results of a controlled drug trial in membranoproliferative glomerulonephritis, *Kidney Int* 27(2):436-41, 1985.
103. Vaziri-Sani F, Hellwage J, et al: Factor H binds to washed human platelets, *J Thromb Haemost* 3(1):154-62, 2005.
104. Karpman D, Manea M, et al: Platelet activation in hemolytic uremic syndrome, *Semin Thromb Hemost* 32(2):128-45, 2006.
105. Sayarlioglu H, Erkoc R, et al: Mycophenolate mofetil use in hepatitis B associated-membranous and membranoproliferative glomerulonephritis induces viral replication, *Ann Pharmacother* 39(3):573, 2005.
106. Kiyomasu T, Shibata M, et al: Cyclosporin A treatment for membranoproliferative glomerulonephritis type II, *Nephron* 91(3):509-11, 2002.
107. Licht C, Hoppe B: Complement defects in children which result in kidney diseases: diagnosis and therapy, *Progress in Inflammation Research*, Parnham MJ (series editor), Springer, 2006.
108. Noris M, Remuzzi G: Hemolytic uremic syndrome, *J Am Soc Nephrol* 16(4):1035-50, 2005.
109. Licht C, Weyersberg A, et al: Successful plasma therapy for atypical hemolytic uremic syndrome caused by factor H deficiency owing to a novel mutation in the complement cofactor protein domain 15, *Am J Kidney Dis* 45(2):415-21, 2005.
110. Filler G, Radhakrishnan S, et al: Challenges in the management of infantile factor H associated hemolytic uremic syndrome, *Pediatr Nephrol* 19(8):908-11, 2004.
111. McGinley E, Watkins R, et al: Plasma exchange in the treatment of mesangiocapillary glomerulonephritis, *Nephron* 40(4):385-90, 1985.

112. Oberkircher OR, Enama M, et al: Regression of recurrent membranoproliferative glomerulonephritis type II in a transplanted kidney after plasmapheresis therapy, *Transplant Proc* 20(suppl 1):418-23, 1988.
113. Braun MC, Stablein DM, et al: Recurrence of membranoproliferative glomerulonephritis type II in renal allografts: The North American Pediatric Renal Transplant Cooperative Study experience, *J Am Soc Nephrol* 16(7):2225-33, 2005.
114. Kurtz KA, Schlueter AJ: Management of membranoproliferative glomerulonephritis type II with plasmapheresis, *J Clin Apher* 17(3):135-37, 2002.
115. Hillmen P, Hall C, et al: Effect of eculizumab on hemolysis and transfusion requirements in patients with paroxysmal nocturnal hemoglobinuria, *N Engl J Med* 350(6):552-59, 2004.
116. Appel GB, Waldman M, et al: New approaches to the treatment of glomerular diseases, *Kidney Int Suppl*(104):S45-50, 2006.
117. Hillmen P, Young NS, et al: The complement inhibitor eculizumab in paroxysmal nocturnal hemoglobinuria, *N Engl J Med* 355(12): 1233-43, 2006.
118. Denton MD, Singh AK: Recurrent and de novo glomerulonephritis in the renal allograft, *Semin Nephrol* 20(2):164-75, 2000.
119. Floege J: Recurrent glomerulonephritis following renal transplantation: an update, *Nephrol Dial Transplant* 18(7):1260-65, 2003.
120. Karakayali FY, Ozdemir H, et al: Recurrent glomerular diseases after renal transplantation, *Transplant Proc* 38(2):470-72, 2006.
121. Habib R, Antignac C, et al: Glomerular lesions in the transplanted kidney in children, *Am J Kidney Dis* 10(3):198-207, 1987.
122. Briganti EM, Russ GR, et al: Risk of renal allograft loss from recurrent glomerulonephritis, *N Engl J Med* 347(2):103-09, 2002.
123. Andresdottir MB, Assmann KJ, et al: Recurrence of type I membranoproliferative glomerulonephritis after renal transplantation: analysis of the incidence, risk factors, and impact on graft survival, *Transplantation* 63(11):1628-33, 1997.
124. McLean RH, Geiger H, et al: Recurrence of membranoproliferative glomerulonephritis following kidney transplantation. Serum complement component studies, *Am J Med* 60(1):60-72, 1976.
125. Richardson WP, Colvin RB, et al: Glomerulopathy associated with cytomegalovirus viremia in renal allografts, *N Engl J Med* 305(2):57-63, 1981.
126. Andresdottir MB, Assmann KJ, et al: Type I membranoproliferative glomerulonephritis in a renal allograft: A recurrence induced by a cytomegalovirus infection? *Am J Kidney Dis* 35(2):E6, 2000.
127. Andresdottir MB, Assmann KJ, et al: Primary Epstein-Barr virus infection and recurrent type I membranoproliferative glomerulonephritis after renal transplantation, *Nephrol Dial Transplant* 15(8):1235-37, 2000.
128. Droz D, Nabarra B, et al: Recurrence of dense deposits in transplanted kidneys: I. Sequential survey of the lesions, *Kidney Int* 15(4): 386-95,1979.
129. Briner J: Glomerular lesions in renal allografts, *Ergeb Inn Med Kinderheilkd* 49:1-76, 1982.
130. Cameron JS: Glomerulonephritis in renal transplants, *Transplantation* 34(5):237-45, 1982.
131. Mathew TH: Recurrence of disease following renal transplantation, *Am J Kidney Dis* 12(2):85-96, 1988.
132. Kotanko P, Pusey CD, et al: Recurrent glomerulonephritis following renal transplantation, *Transplantation* 63(8):1045-52, 1997.
133. Andresdottir MB, Assmann KJ, et al: Renal transplantation in patients with dense deposit disease: morphological characteristics of recurrent disease and clinical outcome, *Nephrol Dial Transplant* 14(7):1723-31, 1999.
134. Eddy A, Sibley R, et al: Renal allograft failure due to recurrent dense intramembranous deposit disease, *Clin Nephrol* 21(6):305-13, 1984.
135. Morales JM, Martinez MA, et al: Recurrent type III membranoproliferative glomerulonephritis after kidney transplantation, *Transplantation* 63(8):1186-88, 1997.
136. Ramesh Prasad GV, Shamy F, et al: Recurrence of type III membranoproliferative glomerulonephritis after renal transplantation, *Clin Nephrol* 61(1):80-81, 2004.
137. Glicklich D, Matas AJ, et al: Recurrent membranoproliferative glomerulonephritis type 1 in successive renal transplants, *Am J Nephrol* 7(2):143-49, 1987.
138. Saxena R, Frankel WL, et al: Recurrent type I membranoproliferative glomerulonephritis in a renal allograft: successful treatment with plasmapheresis, *Am J Kidney Dis* 35(4):749-52, 2000.
139. Tomlanovich S, Vincenti F, et al: Is cyclosporine effective in preventing recurrence of immune-mediated glomerular disease after renal transplantation? *Transplant Proc* 20(3 suppl 4):285-88, 1988.
140. Lien Y, Scott K: Long-term cyclophosphamide treatment for recurrent type I membranoproliferative glomerulonephritis after transplantation, *Am J Kidney Dis* 35(3):539-43, 2002.
141. Muczynski KA: Plasmapheresis maintained renal function in an allograft with recurrent membranoproliferative glomerulonephritis type I, *Am J Nephrol* 15(5):446-49, 1995.
142. Wu J, Jaar BG, et al: High-dose mycophenolate mofetil in the treatment of posttransplant glomerular disease in the allograft: a case series, *Nephron Clin Pract* 98(3):c61-66, 2004.
143. Fearon DT, Daha MR, et al: Pathways of complement activation in membranoproliferative glomerulonephritis and allograft rejection, *Transplant Proc* 9(1):729-39, 1997.
144. Mathieson P: Complement factor H and haemolytic uraemic syndrome, *Lancet* 359(9308):801-02, 2002.
145. Jha V, Murthy MS, et al: Secondary membranoproliferative glomerulonephritis due to hemolytic uremic syndrome: an unusual presentation, *Ren Fail* 20(6):845-50, 1998.

CHAPTER

18 IgA Nephropathy

Rosanna Coppo and Alessandro Amore

DEFINITION AND EPIDEMIOLOGY

IgA nephropathy (IgAN) is a glomerular disease characterized by the presence of IgA deposits prevalent over other classes of immunoglobulins.[1,2] This histologic picture can be observed in association with features of systemic vasculitis in Henoch-Schönlein purpura[2,3] or can be renal limited, as described by Berger (primary IgAN).[1,3,4] These two entities are the most common glomerular diseases characterized by predominant IgA deposits in the pediatric age group[5]; rarely is this associated with dermatitis herpetiformis or celiac disease.

Primary IgAN is more frequent in males than in females.[6] It is common in children and adolescents with isolated microscopic hematuria (up to 35%) or hematuria associated with non-nephrotic proteinuria (30%).[7,8]

Its prevalence varies in different areas based on ethnic and environmental factors, being particularly common in the Mediterranean and northern Europe, Asia, and Australia.[6,9] Most of these discrepancies are likely due to screening examination of urine for microscopic hematuria in some countries,[7,9,10,11,12] which increases the detection of IgAN, and the variable criteria for renal biopsy,[7,11,13] which is often not performed in cases of isolated microscopic hematuria.

PATHOGENESIS

The hallmark of these forms of nephritis is IgA deposition[1,14] (Figure 18-1) together with high serum levels of IgA, mainly IgA1 in polymeric form,[15,16] in more than 50% of patients; increased number of IgA-bearing B lymphocytes,[17] with prevalence of Th2 subset[18] and activated Tα helper cells. Considering these abnormalities, it is likely that systemic as well as mucosal immunity are involved in the pathogenesis of the disease.

The accumulation of IgA containing immune material along with complement fractions within glomeruli was initially ascribed to deposition of IgA immune complexes (IgAIC) due to a mucosal immune response with predominant synthesis of polymeric IgA.[19,20] This hypothesis offered a unifying explanation of the relationship between mucosal infections and gross hematuria. High levels of IgAIC are detectable in 30% to 70% of patients, mostly of IgA1 subclass of bone marrow origin.[21,22] However, no specific viral or alimentary antigens have been found in renal mesangial deposits, instead suggesting a role for a dysregulated IgA immune response.

Recent attention has been focused on the character of the IgA produced by IgAN patients,[20,23] and particularly on the IgA1 subclass (Figure 18-2), which is most predominant in glomerular deposits of this disease.The presence of an insertion of 18 amino acids in the hinge region between CH1 and CH2 domains in IgA1 represents the major structural difference between IgA1 and IgA2.[20] The amino acid sequence shows three threonine and three serine residues bound to five short O-linked oligosaccharide chains. The O-glycosylation consists of a core of N-acetyl galactosamine (GalNAc), which occurs alone or extended with β1,3-linked galactose (Gal) or further with sialic acid in α2,3 and/or α2,6 linkage.[20] Thus each glycan may consist of one of four different forms, including the desialylated T (Thomsen-Friedenreich) antigen and the agalactosyl GalNAc moiety (Tn antigen). The IgA1 O-glycans are short, mucin-type carbohydrate chains, which are unusual in serum proteins. In healthy subjects, serum IgA1 consists of a mixture of molecules with different O-glycoforms, whereas an abnormal IgA1 O-glycoform pattern has been detected in IgAN by using different techniques such as lectin-binding assay, matrix-assisted laser desorption spectroscopy,[24] gas-liquid chromatography, and more recently fluorophore-assisted carbohydrate electrophoresis, which demonstrates a high frequency of O-glycans consisting of GalNAc alone.[25]

Such aberrantly glycosylated IgA1 can circulate in monomeric form or participate in the formation of self-aggregates IgA1/IgA; they can bind to IgG forming IgG/IgA1IC or react with antigens and form true IgAIC. After a report of experimental IgAN in mice deficient in uteroglobulin (UG), a similar defect was sought in human IgAN, but initial observations do not support a role for a primary defect of UG in these patients.[26] IgAIC constituted by aberrantly glycosylated IgA1 likely escapes clearance by hepatic receptors and is preferentially deposited in the kidneys by virtue of enhanced lectinic reactivity with fibronectin, laminin, and collagen within the mesangial matrix.[23]

The possibility of DNA point mutations or deletions in the nucleotide sequence that codifies the core amino acid sequence of IgA1 in IgAN patients was investigated. However, there was no difference found in the nucleotide sequence of the α1 hinge region between IgAN patients and controls.

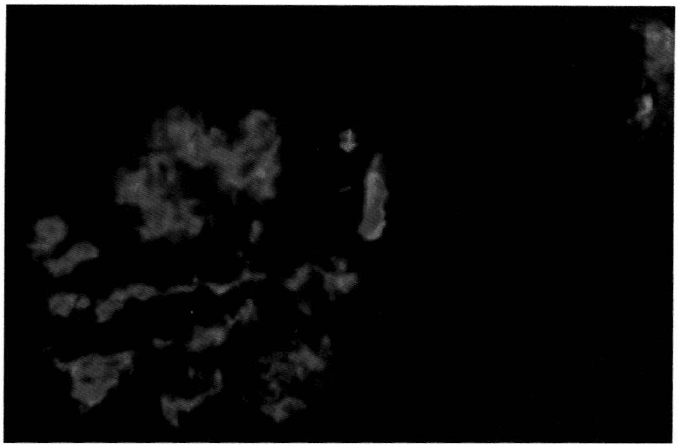

Figure 18-1 Immunofluorescent deposits of IgA in IgA nephropathy. Magnification ×250.

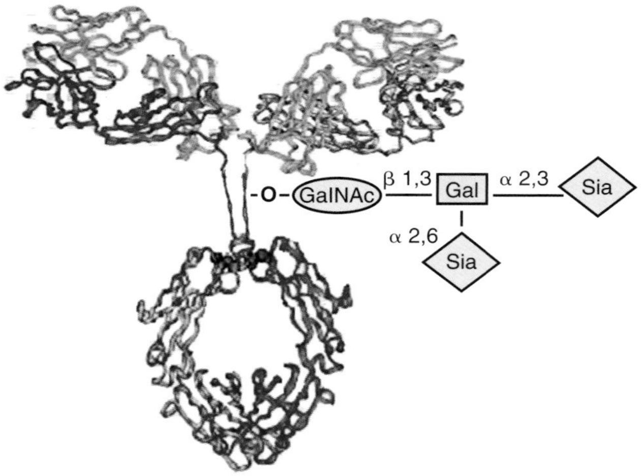

Figure 18-2 The IgA1 molecule with particular magnification of the hinge region. *Gal*, galactose; *GalNAc*, N-acetyl galactosamine; *Sia*, sialic acid.

The addition of Gal to GalNAc is modulated by glycosyltransferases. The activity of β1,3 galactosyltransferase (β1,3 GT) responsible for galactosylation of O-linked sugars, initially seen to be reduced in B cells from IgAN patients in phases of clinical activity,[27] was finally found to be unmodified in IgAN patients. Also from genetic analysis of the *B3GALT1* gene, no data on polymorphism studies have provided evidence of a genetic conditioning.

Increased production of IL-4 and IL-5 by Th2 subset lymphocytes in IgAN may explain the production of abnormally glycosylated IgA1 molecules that deposit in the glomeruli. A relatively or absolutely increased production of Th2 cytokines in response to mucosal infections may be the pathogenic factor responsible for reduced terminal galactosylation and sialylation.[28]

The interaction with Fcα receptors on mesangial cells results in cellular activation and phlogistic mediator synthesis, including a variety of cytokines (IL6, PDGF, IL1, TNF-α, TGFβ), vasoactive factors (prostaglandins, thromboxane, leukotrienes, endothelin, PAF, NO), or chemokines (MCP-1, IL-8, MIP-1, RANTES) (reviewed in Davin et al.[3]). The influx of monocytes and lymphocytes into the mesangium is enhanced by the C3 present in deposited IgA.

The activation of mesangial cells leads to cell contraction, hemodynamic modifications, and activation of the renin-angiotensin system (RAS).[29] Angiotensin II enhances the activation of cytokines and chemokines and potentiates the actions of PDGF and TGFβ as growth factors for mesangial cells, favoring proliferation and accumulation of extracellular matrix and ultimately promoting sclerosis.

GENETICS

Reports of familial cases of IgAN suggest a role for genetic factors. The candidate genes investigated have included those coding for the major histocompatibility proteins and the genes regulating immunoglobulin heavy chain rearrangement. The results, initially encouraging, have not been conclusive to date.

A multicenter study in which 30 IgAN families (from Italy and the United States) were analyzed by whole-genome scanning revealed, by linkage analysis, a close association with the trait 6q 22-23 in 60% of familial IgAN.[30] These findings support the hypothesis that familial IgAN is a multifactorial or "complex" disease in which one or more genes, probably in combination with environmental factors, may be responsible for the onset of the disease.

Particular attention has recently been devoted to genes possibly involved in IgAN progression, such as the polymorphism of RAS genes, because of a correlation between angiotensin II levels in tissue and the activity of the gene encoding angiotensin converting enzymes (ACEs). In IgAN, there is no clear evidence of a significant alteration in the ACE genotype frequency, but several reports, only partially confirmed, associate one genotype (DD) with a greater rate of progression in IgAN and a better response to treatment with ACE inhibitors (ACEIs).[31] Several genes have been found to influence the evolution of IgAN, including genes encoding cytoskeletal proteins such as adducin, or genes encoding for cytokines such as IL6, IL2R, PDGF, TNFα, and TGFβ, which could modulate the mesangial cell response (reviewed in Davin et al.[3]). Recently an association between uteroglobin (UG) polymorphism and rate of progression of IgAN has been observed,[32] but this report has not been confirmed.

CLINICAL PRESENTATION

Primary IgAN, or Berger's disease, is mostly characterized by recurrent episodes of gross hematuria concomitant with upper respiratory tract infections or other mucosal inflammatory processes; it rarely occurs after vaccination or heavy physical exercise. In other patients microscopic hematuria and/or proteinuria are the only signs.[6] The diagnosis is made in the absence of any recognizable systemic disease (lupus erythematosus, Henoch-Schönlein purpura, cryoglobulinemia), liver disease, or lower urinary tract diseases.

The first episode of macroscopic hematuria generally occurs between 15 and 30 years of age, which is often 7 to 10 years earlier than a biopsy diagnosis is made.[6] Since it is conceivable that the pathogenetic process leading to IgA deposit formation and clinical symptoms lasts several years, the true onset of primary IgAN is thus usually in the teens or even earlier. Affected children do not present symptoms or urinary signs before the age of 3; thereafter the frequency increases with age. Gross hematuria affects 30% to 40% of children with IgAN.[7,8,11,12] The interval between the precipitating event and the appearance of macrohematuria is very short (12 to 72 hours) compared with 1 to 3 weeks in postinfectious acute glomerulonephritis. The macrohematuria persists for less than 3 days and is sometimes accompanied by flank and loin pain and occasionally fever. The urine is red or brown (cola colored); blood casts are common but blood clots can rarely be found. These episodes can recur, and microscopic hematuria of various degree, isolated or associated with low degree of proteinuria, can be residual in between. Several other children (30% to 50% of cases)[12] are biopsied because of persistent microscopic hematuria with or without proteinuria (Figures 18-3 and 18-4). They often have isolated microscopic hematuria for several years before the manifestation of proteinuria.

In asymptomatic patients, such as those detected at routine medical examination, proteinuria may be found in 3% to 13% of cases.[7,8,10,11] A transient increase in proteinuria occurs coinciding with episodes of gross hematuria. In some children (6%) the clinical onset can be with a classic nephrotic syndrome, and only the renal biopsy allows a correct diagnosis of IgAN. In some cases primary IgAN is superimposed upon a preceding, undiagnosed minimal change disease.[7,8,11,12]

In a few cases there is an acute nephritic syndrome, similar to poststreptococcal glomerulonephritis, at the onset of disease. In these children macrohematuria is associated with increased serum creatinine and urea, and also hypertension.[7,8,11,12] In rare cases the onset may be a severe nephritic syndrome progressing to chronic renal failure due to crescentic lesions.[5]

Furthermore, in a few patients, acute oliguric failure, usually spontaneously reversible, accompanies the episodes of macrohematuria and is attributed to tubular obstruction by red blood cells. Hypertension usually develops during follow-up over several years or in severe cases.[7,8]

NATURAL HISTORY AND CLINICAL RISK FACTORS FOR PROGRESSION

The prognosis was initially considered to be benign in children compared with adults, but long-term studies have failed

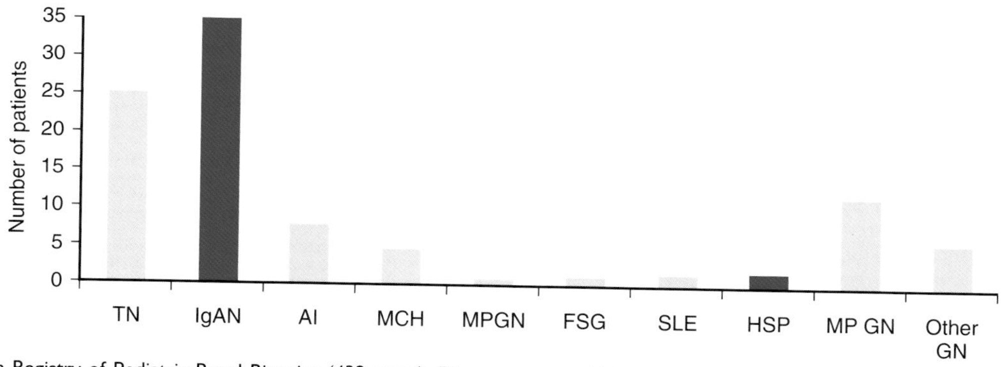

Figure 18-3 Italian Registry of Pediatric Renal Biopsies (432 cases). Diagnosis at renal biopsy in children with isolated microscopic hematuria (83 cases). (From Coppo et al: *Nephrol Dial Transplant* 13:293-97, 1998.)

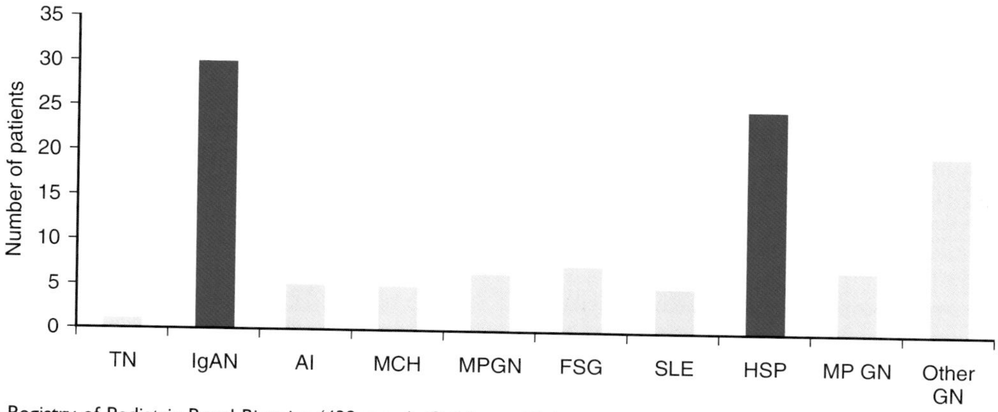

Figure 18-4 Italian Registry of Pediatric Renal Biopsies (432 cases). Children with hematuria and proteinuria (135 cases). (From Coppo et al: *Nephrol Dial Transplant* 13:293-97, 1998.)

TABLE 18-1 Ten Years' Renal Survival in Adults and Children with IgAN Diagnosis

		Adults 10 Years' Survival	Children 10 Years' Survival
Kusumoto (1987)[11]	All patients	80%	95%
	Hypertension and/or nephrotic range proteinuria	31%	24%
Wyatt (1984, 1995)[7,65]	All patients	78%	87%
	Hypertension and/or nephrotic range proteinuria	18%	15%

to confirm this assessment. The European Renal Association-European Dialysis and Transplant Association (ERA-EDTA) registry reports that 67% of IgAN patients between the ages of 24 and 54 enter a chronic dialysis program and that 22% of these patients are less than 30 years of age.[33] Since the decline of renal function is slow (25% of cases need dialysis in 20 years), it is clear that several progressive IgANs begin in childhood.

With few exceptions, the natural history of IgAN in children represents the early phase of the overall natural history of the disease. Severe clinical signs usually develop after 5 to 15 years, indicating the need for long-term follow-up to define the history and the progression of IgAN in children. In short-term follow-up studies in both adults and children, a better prognosis is observed in children; however, the 20-year survival shows that IgAN in children is as progressive as in adults[7,8,9,11,34,35] (Table 18-1).

Some children, usually those showing moderate microscopic hematuria without proteinuria and displaying the mildest lesions, do not, over decades of observation, progress to end-stage renal failure. In children with progressive IgAN, the clinical course is often slow and indolent. Among the factors that determine progression over the years, the most relevant, such as reduced renal function at onset and persistent hypertension, are uncommon in children with IgAN. Conversely, proteinuria is a relevant risk factor for progression that can be detected in early phases of IgAN and frequently in children.[36]

Significantly different actuarial survivals are reported for IgAN patients according to levels of proteinuria greater or less than 1 g per day. More significant than proteinuria at onset, follow-up proteinuria (percent duration of massive proteinuria), or proteinuria at 1 year, duration and amount of proteinuria over years of follow-up were the only independent predictors of end-stage renal failure by stepwise multiple regression analysis.

In general, most studies consider proteinuria greater than 1 g/1.73 m^2 per day as a risk factor for progression. However, an increasing number of reports indicate that patients showing clinical features at onset that are generally not thought to be related to progression can experience decline in renal function over long-term follow-up. A study from China investigated 72 adult patients with normal renal function and proteinuria of less than 0.4 g per day. After a 7-year follow-up, an increase in proteinuria of more than 1 g per day was observed in one third of cases, development of hypertension in 26% of patients, and decline in renal function in 7% of the patients.[37] These data were confirmed by another report on a large cohort of 400 adult patients with a median follow-up of 6.7 years; it showed that creatinine levels above the upper limits developed in 20% of the cases and that 5% of patients required dialysis.[38]

Not only quantity but also composition of proteinuria has been correlated with clinical outcome. In particular, an elevated tubular proteinuria, as increased urinary excretion of low molecular weight proteins and particularly α_1-microglobulin, has been found to be a negative prognostic index. Similarly, an increased excretion of cytokines and chemokines of tubular origin, such as interleukin 6 (IL-6) or chemokines (monocyte chemoattractant protein MCP-1),[39] with reduced excretion of tubular epithelial growth protein (EGF) were found to be significant risk factors. Data from our group indicated, in both adults and children, the prognostic value of tubular proteinuria and increased urinary excretion of IL-6, MCP-1, and EGF in proteinuric IgAN.[40]

The search for a possible role of hematuria in predicting the progression of IgAN is particularly appropriate in that this nephropathy is characterized by microscopic and gross hematuria. Because the most typical clinical feature of IgAN is recurrent bouts of macroscopic hematuria, the first risk factor evaluated for outcome was the meaning of *recurrent gross hematuria*. Two apparently conflicting positions were proposed by D'Amico, who pointed out the benign nature of recurrent gross hematuria when the urinary sediment was inactive between bouts,[41] and Kincaid-Smith, who, having found segmental necrosis and small, florid, noncircumferential crescents in renal biopsies during gross hematuria episodes, suggested a less-favorable prognosis for patients exposed to repeated episodes of clinical and histologic activity.[42,43] What can unify these two apparently conflicting positions is represented by the regression potential, with disappearance of urinary abnormalities in the periods between episodes of gross hematuria. Patients with recurrent macroscopic hematuria who experience total regression with an almost-normal urinary sediment between episodes of gross hematuria are clinically very different from those showing persistent heavy microscopic hematuria, often accompanied by significant proteinuria. Glomerular hematuria in IgAN is an expression, per se, of an acute inflammatory process that likely involves release of free radicals produced by the oxidative stress and cytokines originating from mesangial or infiltrating cells. Hematuria might follow parcellar endothelial necrosis and metalloproteinase activation leading to collagen degradation. Levels and severity of the damage induced by these products depend on the duration of the pathogenetic event and the capacity for healing and damage regression. The process can be rapidly followed by repair, or it can activate the formation of more or less extensive crescents. Segmental necrotizing lesions of the capillary wall, indicating a limited vasculitic lesion, are often observed. These patients experience a clinical course characterized by repeated bouts of activity and accelerated progression toward renal failure.[43] Some peculiar deposits characterized by the parietal extension of glomerular deposits, or qualitative properties, are likely to activate the mediators of renal damage, leading to focal necrotizing lesions that give rise to floccular-capsular adhesions. These pathogenetic events clinically manifest with increase in hematuria and intermittent bouts of activity, leading to worsening of the clinical course and progression to renal fibrosis.

When evaluating the natural history of IgAN in children, long-term analysis including adult life should be considered. Since the first report by Levy et al.[5] in which a follow-up of 13 years in 91 children demonstrated that only 8 children (9%) developed renal failure, other studies from different areas of the world have been performed. In Europe, Linné et al.[34] found the persistence of clinical signs of disease in 47% of patients who were followed for a mean period of 10 years. Urine abnormalities were present in all patients, proteinuria in 35%, hypertension in 9%, and decreased glomerular filtration rate (GFR) in 3%. The more common histologic lesions in these patients consisted of focal segmental glomerular changes.

A multicenter US study reviewed clinical and pathologic features in 80 children with primary IgAN who were followed for at least 4 years. Seven markers were found to be predictive of end-stage kidney disease in children: presence of glomerular sclerotic changes, especially when these were associated with proliferation or when sclerosis affected 20% or more of the glomeruli; African American race; hypertension at biopsy; proteinuria at biopsy; age at presentation; crescents; and male gender[36] (Table 18-2).

From a cohort of 103 pediatric patients, Wyatt et al.[44] reported normal renal function in 87% after 10 years from the time of apparent onset of IgAN. In Japan, Yoshikawa et al.[45] found urinary abnormalities in 38% of patients, persistent heavy proteinuria in 10%, and progression to chronic renal failure in 5% of 200 children less than 15 years of age who were followed for a mean period of 5 years. The poor outcome was characterized by heavy proteinuria at biopsy; diffuse mesangial proliferation; a high proportion of glomeruli showing sclerosis, crescents, or capsular adhesions in more than 30% of glomeruli; the presence of tubulointerstitial infiltrates; subepithelial electron-dense deposits; and lysis of the glomerular basement membrane.

In the 89 cases of pediatric IgAN detected and followed in the Turin Center over the last 15 years (Table 18-3), significant proteinuria developed in 39% of the children and hypertension in 3%, whereas progression to dialysis, over a median follow-up of 6 years, was not frequent (only one child on dialysis and two with impaired renal function). A complete remission was found in 7% of the cases. This probably does not represent the true natural history of IgAN in children, since 39% were treated with steroids in various protocols and 46% received angiotensin antagonists. In studies from centers following the children over decades, the 10-year survival of IgAN initiated in childhood was calculated to be around 87% to 93%, with complete clinical remission in one third of the cases.

TABLE 18-2 Factors Affecting Progression of IgAN in Children

Factor	Significance
Age (<9 years) at presentation	n.s.
Sex (male)	n.s.
Race (African American)	<0.005
Gross hematuria	n.s.
GFR reduced at biopsy	n.s.
Proteinuria at biopsy	<0.0001
Hypertension at biopsy	<0.003
Mesangial proliferation with mesangial sclerosis	<0.0001
Sclerosis in >20% of glomeruli	<0.0001
Focal global sclerosis	<0.01
Crescents/synechiae	<0.03
Tubulointerstitial disease	<0.03
Peripheral capillary wall deposits (EM)	n.s.
Other GBM changes (EM)	n.s.

n.s., Not significant.
From Hogg RJ, Silva FG, Wyatt RJ, Reisch JS, et al: Prognostic indicators in children with IgA nephropathy—Report of the Southwest Pediatric Nephrology Study Group, *Pediatr Nephrol* 8:15-20, 1994.

TABLE 18-3 Follow-up of 89 Children with IgAN in the Turin Center

NATURAL HISTORY DURING A MEDIAN FOLLOW-UP OF 6 YEARS (0.5-19 YEARS)	
Percentage of Cases	**Feature or Therapeutic Intervention during Follow-Up**
39	Increase in proteinuria >1 g/day/1.73 m^2
3	Hypertension
7	Complete clinical remission (proteinuira <0.160 mg/day/1.73 m^2, no hematuria, normal GFR)
2	Decrease in GFR <70 ml/min/1.73 m^2 at the end of FU
1	Progression to end-stage renal disease
39	Steroids in various protocols
45	ACEI for >6 months

In conclusion, pediatric patients often have an earlier diagnosis than adults due to the more frequent onset with gross hematuria or because of population screening. Hence the medium-term prognosis is better than that usually found in adult patients since less-severe clinical signs (hypertension, proteinuria, impaired renal function) and histologic lesions (extent of sclerosis and tubulointerstitial damage) are present at the time of renal biopsy. However, the disease is progres-

TABLE 18-4 Histologic Classification of IgA Nephropathy

I:	Minimal or no mesangial hypercellularity without glomerular sclerosis
II:	Focal and segmental glomerular sclerosis without active cellular proliferation
III:	Focal proliferative GN
IV:	Diffuse proliferative GN
V:	Any biopsy showing > or = 40% globally sclerotic glomeruli and/or > or = 40% estimated cortical tubular atrophy or loss

(From Haas M: Histologic subclassification of IgA nephropathy: a clinicopathologic study of 244 cases, *Am J Kidney Dis* 29:829-42, 1997.)

sive over decades, and the long-term prognosis becomes similar to patients with clinical onset in adult age. Lifelong follow-up is needed in these children in order to detect the manifestations of signs of progressive disease and the need to initiate a therapy.

HISTOLOGY AND HISTOLOGIC RISK FACTORS FOR PROGRESSION

Primary IgAN presents with focal or diffuse mesangial hypercellularity and expansion of the extracellular matrix. Other glomerular lesions include focal or diffuse endocapillary proliferation, extracapillary proliferation with crescent formation, glomerular hyalinosis, and segmental or global sclerosis. Limited areas of tuft necrosis, indistinguishable from those seen in association with small vessel vasculitis, have been described, most often in IgAN with particularly acute disease. The histologic features in children are usually moderate and crescentic rapidly progressive forms are exceptional. Interstitial and arteriolar changes are infrequently found. The extent of interstitial cellular infiltration and fibrosis is an important negative prognostic marker.

On the basis of these features, IgAN has been stratified into five histologic classes (Haas classification)[14] in order of increasing severity of renal damage (Table 18-4). A new classification is under evaluation by a Consensus of Pathologists and Nephrologists.

The changes observed by light microscopy are not specific and IgAN is identified by the predominance of IgA deposits in mesangial areas, mostly of the IgA1 subclass. The extension of IgA into the capillary walls has been considered a marker for poor prognosis, as has codeposition of IgG and C3.

Analysis of the most relevant reports from the literature reveal that the strongest independent predictors of progression by Cox multivariate analysis are the severity of glomerulosclerosis and interstitial fibrosis (widespread global and/or segmental glomerulosclerosis, marked tubulointerstitial lesions or elevated glomerular and/or tubulointerstitial score of lesions, or in general classes of highest severity of overall damage).[6,46] The presence of crescents, which are generally not circumferential, is a risk factor in almost all studies by univariate analysis. However, by multivariate analysis, only when crescents were analyzed together with tuft adhesions, which possibly result from previous segmental necrosis, did they maintain statistical significance as a risk factor.[47]

The extent of mesangial proliferation and parietal expansion of deposits were significantly associated with an unfavorable prognosis in a few studies only, and never by multivariate analysis. Also, vascular lesions were only occasionally significant when analyzed by multivariate analysis.[6,46]

It is clear that the only histologic and immunohistologic factors predictive of progression are those indicating that renal disease has already progressed to sclerosis. Therefore it is unfortunately not possible to predict progression from early changes on renal biopsy before development of irreversible damage, because neither the extension of glomerular deposits nor the mesangial cellularity are predictors of long-term outcome. Hopefully the new classification will offer additional and more sentitive risk factors.

LABORATORY INVESTIGATION AND GUIDELINES FOR DIAGNOSIS

High levels of IgA are found in 35% to 50% of patients.[48] This marker may suggest possible presence of the disease, but the diagnosis is made on a histologic basis only. High levels of macromolecular IgA (IgAIC, mixed IgA/IgGIC, IgA/fibronectin aggregates) are frequently found, particularly during the phases of clinical activity.[23]

Complement values are generally within the normal limits when C3 or C4 are measured, whereas signs of subclinical complement activation can be detected by measuring the C3d breakdown product.

In about half of the cases, serial measurement of 24-hour proteinuria or urinary protein/creatinine ratio is highly recommended as the most useful parameter to follow over the years.

Urinary excretion of cytokines, mostly MCP-1 and IL6, is increased in patients with proteinuric disease and in those with severe interstitial changes.[39,40]

THERAPY

Attempts to intervene in the pathogenic events leading to IgAN should take into account a reduction in antigen challenge; because tonsils are a frequent source of infections, interest has focused on tonsillectomy for many years. Abandoned as a routine approach in Europe, tonsillectomy is still favored in some regions of the world, notably in Japan.[49] This procedure may be of some value in preventing episodic gross hematuria in the short term, whereas long-term effects are still being debated. Tonsillectomy is supported by two large retrospective studies from Japan, which reported that the benefit on renal functional decline is demonstrated after a follow-up exceeding 10 years.[50,51] Tonsillectomy has a clear indication when tonsils are a true infectious focus; otherwise the efficacy of the procedure is often proposed in association with other therapies and the benefit is unclear.[52] Other attempts to reduce antigen exposure include long-term antibiotics and a gluten-free diet, which are not effective in preventing functional decline even though the latter significantly reduces IgA immunologic abnormalities.[53] Similar conclusions can be drawn from other previously suggested therapies, including dapsone, which solubilizes IgA aggregates; diphenylhydantoin, which reduces polymeric IgA; and disodium cromoglycate, which impairs absorption of food antigens.

Current therapeutic strategies for IgAN have been directed toward modulating the glomerular response to immune deposits in order to decrease the resultant tissue damage and progression toward sclerosis.

It is important to identify patients at risk for progressive renal injury. Therapeutic intervention should be attempted in rapidly progressive IgAN (i.e., with florid crescent formation involving more than 50% of glomeruli, hypertension, and/or severe proteinuria). The protocols include a cycle of 10 plasmaphereses, cyclophosphamide 3 mg/kg/day, and prednisone 1 mg/kg/day for 8 weeks or a course of high-dose methylprednisolone pulses alone or in association with 3 mg/kg/day cyclophosphamide for 8 weeks.[54] In a cohort of children with severe IgAN and slowly progressive course, treatment with prednisone and azathioprine for 1 year was reported to produce a favorable outcome.[55] A similar protocol in association with heparin-warfarin and dipyridamole may be used for children with histologic signs of diffuse mesangial proliferation.[56]

Children with IgAN and high levels of proteinuria are at risk for progressive disease. Patients with severe proteinuria (>3.5 g/day/1.73 m^2) who even still have normal renal function should be treated, according to recently published, evidence-based recommendations. Treatment with prednisone 2 mg/kg/day for 4 weeks, with a progressive reduction over the following 8 weeks and then small doses for a total period of 1 to 3 years is indicated for patients with nephrotic-range proteinuria,[57] and eicosapentanoic acid (fish oil) for 2 years in those with high or moderate proteinuria (>1 <2 g/day) with initial GFR reduction.[58] It was recently found that 3 pulses of methylprednisolone at 1, 3, and 5 months followed by low doses of prednisone provided a significant protective effect on functional decline in adults.[59] Interestingly, the benefit of this therapy lasted for several years after pulse treatment, protecting the patients from proteinuria and even more from loss of renal function.[60] No data are available for children, but our personal experience is fairly good.

Cyclosporin A is ineffective in that it does not provide protection from recurrence of IgAN in transplanted kidneys, indirectly indicating that any benefit on the original disease would be moderate.

ACEIs have a strong basis for use in the treatment of IgAN not only because they improve two principal progression factors (hypertension and proteinuria), but because their use may inhibit the long series of potentially negative angiotensin II effects. However, a metaanalysis of ACEI results in adult IgAN patients failed to find significant conclusions and suggested the need for prospective controlled studies.[61]

In 1995 we designed a double-blind placebo RCT, because the effect of ACEIs had just been proven on progression of chronic nephropathies at that time but not on IgAN. This trial was supported by the European Community Concerted Action of Biomedicine and Health. It included children and young patients (3 to 35 years old) with a constant level of moderate proteinuria (>1 <3.5 g/day/1.73 m^2 over the 3 months before enrollment) and normal or moderately reduced renal function. Fifty-seven patients, randomized to receive benazepril 0.2 mg/kg/day or placebo, completed the trial (median follow-up 42 months). The primary outcome of renal disease progression, defined as a decrease greater than 30% in baseline CrCl and/or worsening of proteinuria to nephrotic range, was significantly different between the two groups. A stable remission of proteinuria (<0.5 g/day/1.73 m^2) was observed in 56.5% of ACEI patients versus 8% of placebo patients. The multivariate Cox analysis showed that treatment with ACEI was the independent predictor of prognosis, whereas no influence on the progression of renal damage was found for gender, age, baseline CrCl, systolic or diastolic blood pressure, mean arterial pressure, or proteinuria.[37]

A new, ongoing trial is testing whether angiotensin inhibition by both ACEI and angiotensin receptor blockers (ARB) may decrease the risk of progression in patients with IgAN so far considered benign (proteinuria <0.5 g/day). Such inhibition will first be achieved with a unique pharmacologic class (ACEI or ARB), then shifting to the combination of the two classes as soon as the inhibition with one drug becomes ineffective.[62]

Results of a randomized, placebo-controlled, double-blind trial in the United States using prednisone (60 mg/m^2 every other day for 3 months, then 40 mg/m^2 every other day for 9 months, then 30 mg/m^2 every other day for 12 month) or fish oil (4 g/day for 2 years) or placebo has recently been reported by Hogg et al.[63] The authors demonstrated the three groups comparable at baseline except that the O3FA (fish oil) group had higher urine protein to creatinine (UP/C) ratios than the placebo group ($p = 0.003$). Neither treatment group showed benefit over the placebo group regarding time to failure, with 14 patient failures overall (2 in the prednisone group, 8 in the O3FA group, and 4 in the placebo group). The primary factor associated with time to failure was higher baseline UP/C ratios ($p = 0.009$). Superiority of prednisone or O3FA over placebo in slowing progression of renal disease was not demonstrated in this study. However, the relatively short follow-up period, inequality of baseline UP/C ratios, and the small numbers of patients precludes any definitive conclusion.

IgAN benefits from treatment of potentially progressive cases: there is indication for prednisone in children with very active histologic lesions (sometimes using pulses of methylprednisolone in association with alkylating agents, according to data in adults[64]), and cases with proteinuria also have to be treated. Prednisone or ACEIs are the treatment of choice.

The effectiveness of new drugs such as mycophenolate mofetil is still debated in adults: an RCT using this drug in children and young subjects is ongoing in the United States.[64]

The present treatment recommendations derived from the literature data mentioned here can be administered as depicted in Table 18-5.

TABLE 18-5 **Treatment Recommendations for IgAN According to Clinical Features**	
Clinical Presentation	**Recommended Treatment**
Recurrent macroscopic hematuria with normal renal function; no proteinuria and no microscopic hematuria between episodes	No specific treatment, no present indications
Proteinuria <0.5 g/1.73 m^2/day ± microscopic hematuria	No specific treatment
Proteinuria between 0.5 and 1 g/1.73 m^2/day ± microscopic hematuria	ACEI or ARB might be useful (RCT in progress)
Proteinuria between 1 and 3 g/1.73 m^2/day ± microscopic hematuria	ACEI beneficial (RCT evidence) Combined RAS blockade with ACEI and ARB in cases of inadequate proteinuric response If no effect, 3 pulses of methylprednisolone 10 mg/kg for 3 days on alternate months (3 courses)
Proteinuria >3.5 g/1.73 m^2/day	Oral prednisone 2 mg/kg/day for 2 months, followed by reduced doses. Alternatively, 3 courses of 3 pulses of methylprednisolone (10 mg/kg), for 3 days on alternate months
Nephrotic syndrome with minimal change on light microscopy	Prednisolone 2 mg/kg/day for up to 8 weeks, followed by reduced doses
Acute Renal Failure	
Acute tubular necrosis	Supportive measures
Crescentic IgAN (with little or no chronic damage)	Methylprednisolone 3 pulses 10 mg/kg Induction (8 weeks) Prednisone 1 mg/kg/day Cyclophosphamide 2 mg/kg/day *Maintenance* Prednisone tapering; azathioprine 2.5 mg/kg/day

REFERENCES

1. Berger J, Hinglais N: Les depots intercapillaires d'IgAIgG, *Journal d'Urologie et Nephrologie* 74:694-95, 1998.
2. Coppo R, Amore A, Hogg R, Emancipator S: Idiopathic nephropathy with IgA deposits, *Pediatr Nephrol* 15:139-50, 2002.
3. Davin JC, Ten Berge IJ, Weening JJ: What is the difference between IgA nephropathy and Henoch-Schönlein purpura nephritis? *Kidney Int* 59:823-34, 2001.
4. Schena FP, Coppo R: IgA nephropathies. In Davison AM, editor: *Oxford Textbook of Clinical Nephrology*, ed 3, Oxford, 2005, Oxford University Press.
5. Levy M, Gonzalez-Burchard G, Broyer M, et al: Berger's disease in children. Natural history and outcome, *Medicine* 64:157-80, 1985.
6. D'Amico G et al: Idiopathic IgA mesangial nephropathy. Clinical and histological study of 374 patients, *Medicine* 64:49-60, 1985.
7. Wyatt RJ, Julian BA, Bhathena DB, et al: IgA nephropathy: Presentation, clinical course, and prognosis in children and adults, *Am J Kidney Dis* 4:192-200, 1984.
8. Yagucki Y et al: Comparative studies of clinicalpathologic changes in patients with adult and juvenile-onset of IgA nephropathy, *J Nephrol* 7:182-85, 1994.
9. Schena FP: A retrospective analysis of the natural history of primary IgA nephropathy worldwide, *Am J Med* 89:209-15, 1990.
10. Koyama A, Igarashi M, Kobayashi M, Members and Coworkers of the Research Group on Progressive Renal Disease: Natural history and risk factors for immunoglobulin A nephropathy in Japan, *Am J Kidney Dis* 29:526-32, 1997.
11. Kusumoto Y, Takebayashi S, Taguchi T, Harada T, et al: Long-term prognosis and prognostic indices of IgA nephropathy in juvenile and in adult Japanese, *Clin Nephrol* 28:118-24, 1987.
12. Yoshikawa N, Iijima K, Ito H: IgA nephropathy in children, *Nephron* 83:1-12, 1999.
13. Coppo R, Gianoglio B, Porcellini MG, Maringhini S (for the group of Renal Immunopathology of the Italian Society of Pediatric Nephrology and group of Renal Immunopathology of the Italian Society of Nephrology): Frequency of renal diseases and clinical indications for renal biopsy in children, *Nephrol Dial Transplant* 13:293-97, 1998.
14. Haas M: Histologic subclassification of IgA nephropathy: a clinicopathologic study of 244 cases, *Am J Kidney Dis* 29:829-42, 1997.
15. Harper SJ, Allen AC, Layward L, Hattersley J, et al: Increased immunoglobulin A and immunoglobulin A1 cells in bone marrow trephine biopsy specimens in immunoglobulin A nephropathy, *Am J Kidney Dis* 24:888-92, 1994.
16. Schena FP, Pastore A, Ludovico N, et al: Increased serum levels of IgA1–IgG immune complexes and anti-F(ab′) 2 antibodies in patients with primary IgA nephropathy, *Clin Exp Immunol* 77:15-20, 1989.
17. Harper SJ, Allen AC, Bene MC, Pringle JH, et al: Increased dimeric IgA-producing B cells in tonsils in IgA nephropathy determined by in situ hybridization for J chain mRNA, *Clin Exp Immunol* 101:442-48, 1995.
18. Lim CS, Zheng S, Kim YS, Ahn C, et al: Th1/Th2 predominance and proinflammatory cytokines determine the clinicopathological severity of IgA nephropathy, *Nephrol Dial Transplant* 16:269-75, 2001.
19. Emancipator SN: Aspects of the pathogenesis of IgA nephropathy, *Clinical Immunological News* 12:149-56, 1992.
20. Coppo R, Amore A, Hogg R, Emancipator S: Idiopathic nephropathy with IgA deposits, *Pediatr Nephrol* 15:139-50, 2000.
21. Coppo R, Basolo B, Martina G, Rollino C, De Marchi M, et al: Circulating immune complexes containing IgA, IgG and IgM in patients with primary IgA nephropathy and with Henoch-Schönlein nephritis. Correlation with clinic and histologic signs of activity, *Clin Nephrol* 18:230-39, 1982.
22. Valentijn RM, Kauffmann RH, De la Reveliere GB, Daha MR, Van Es LA: Presence of circulating macromolecular IgA in patients with hematuria due to primary IgA nephropathy. *Am J Med* 74:375-81, 1983.
23. Coppo R, Amore A, Gianoglio B, Porcellini MG, et al: Macromolecular IgA and abnormal IgA reactivity in sera from children with IgA nephropathy. Italian Collaborative Paediatric IgA Nephropathy Study, *Clin Nephrol* 43:1-13, 1995.
24. Hiki Y, Tanaka A, Kokubo T, Iwase H, et al: Analyses of IgA1 hinge glycopeptides in IgA nephropathy by matrix-assisted laser desorp-

tion/ionization time-of-flight mass spectrometry, *J Am Soc Nephrol* 9:577-82, 1998.

25. Allen AC, Bailey EM, Barratt J, Buck KS, et al: Analysis of IgA1 O-glycans in IgA nephropathy by fluorophore-assisted carbohydrate electrophoresis, *J Am Soc Nephrol* 10:1763-71, 1999.
26. Coppo R, Chiesa M, Cirina P, Peruzzi L, et al: In human IgA nephropathy uteroglobin does not play the role inferred from transgenic mice, *Am J Kid Dis* 40(3):495-503, 2002.
27. Allen AC, Topham PS, Harper SJ, Feehally J: Leucocyte beta 1,3 galactosyltransferase activity in IgA nephropathy, *Nephrol Dial Transplant* 12:701-06, 1997.
28. Chintalacharuvu SR, Nagy NU, Sigmund N, Nedrud JG, et al: T cell cytokines determine the severity of experimental IgA nephropathy by regulating IgA glycosylation, *Clin Exp Immunol* 126:326-33, 2001.
29. Coppo R, Amore A, Gianoglio B, Cacace G, et al: Angiotensin II local hyperreactivity in the progression of IgA nephropathy, *Am J Kid Dis* 21(6):593-602, 1993.
30. Gharavi AG, Yan Y, Scolari F, Schena FP, et al: IgA nephropathy, the most common cause of glomerulonephritis, is linked to 6q22-23, *Nat Genet* 26:354-57, 2000.
31. Schena FP, D'Altri C, Cerullo G, Manno C, et al: ACE gene polymorphism and IgA nephropathy. An ethically homogeneous study and a meta-analysis review, *Kidney Int* 60:732-40, 2001.
32. Szelestei T, Bahring S, Kovacs T, Vas T, et al: Association of a uteroglobin polymorphism with rate of progression in patients with IgA nephropathy, *Am J Kid Dis* 36(3):468-73, 2000.
33. Fassbinder W, Brunner FP, Brynger H, Ehrich JH, Geerlings W, et al: Combined report on regular dialysis and transplantation in Europe, XX, 1989, *Nephrol Dial Transplant* 6(1):5-35, 1991.
34. Linné T, Berg U, Bohman SO, Sigstrom L: Course and long-term outcome of idiopathic IgA nephropathy in children, *Pediatr Nephrol* 5:383-86, 1991.
35. Mina SM, Murphy WM: IgA nephropathy: A comparative study of the clinicopathologic features in children and adults, *Am J Clin Path* 83(6):669-75, 1985.
36. Hogg RJ, Silva FG, Wyatt RJ, Reisch JS, et al: Prognostic indicators in children with IgA nephropathy—Report of the Southwest Pediatric Nephrology Study Group, *Pediatr Nephrol* 8:15-20, 1994.
37. Coppo R, Peruzzi L, Amore A, Piccoli A, Cochat P, et al: 2006 IgACE: first prospective double-blind randomized placebo-controlled multicenter trial of ACE-inhibitors (ACE-I) in moderately proteinuric IgA nephropathy in the young, *J Am Soc Nephrol*, in press.
38. Szeto CC, Lai FM, To KF, Wong TY, et al: The natural history of immunoglobulin a nephropathy among patients with hematuria and minimal proteinuria, *Am J Med* 15:110, 434-37, 2001.
39. Ranieri E, Gesualdo L, Petrarulo F, Schena FP: Urinary IL-6/EGF ratio: a useful prognostic marker for the progression of renal damage in IgA nephropathy, *Kidney Int* 50:1990-2001, 1996.
40. Roasio L, Balegno S, Camilla R, Magnetti F, Dotti G, et al: Urinary IL-6/EGF and MCP-1/EGF ratio in patients with IgA nephropathy during a prospective, double blind, placebo controlled trial of ACE-inhibitors, *J Am Soc Nephrol* 16:553A, 2005.
41. D'Amico G: Clinical features and natural history in adults with IgA nephropathy, *Am J Kid Dis* 12(5):353-57, 1998.
42. Nicholls KM, Fairley KF, Dowling JP, Kincaid-Smith P: The clinical course of mesangial IgA associated nephropathy in adults, *Quarterly Journal of Medicine* 53:22-50, 1984.
43. Bennett WM, Kincaid-Smith P: Macroscopic hematuria in mesangial IgA nephropathy: correlation with glomerular crescents and renal dysfunction, *Kidney Int* 23:393-400, 1993.
44. Wyatt RJ, Julian BA, Weinstein A, Rothfield NF, et al: Partial H (beta 1H) deficiency and glomerulonephritis in two families. *J Clin Immunol* 2:110-17, 1982.
45. Yoshikawa N, Ito H, Nakamura H: Prognostic indicators in childhood IgA nephropathy, *Nephron* 60:60-67, 1992.
46. D'Amico G, et al: Prognostic indicators in idiopathic IgA mesangial nephropathy, *Quarterly Journal of Medicine* (59):363-78, 1986.
47. Roodnat JI, van Stiphout WAHJ, Rosendaal FR, van Es LA, et al: What do we really know about the long-term prognosis of IgA-nephropathy? *J Nephrol* 3:145-51, 1991.
48. Coppo R, D'Amico G: Factors predicting progression of IgA nephropathies, *J Nephrol* 18(5):503-12, 2005.
49. Kosaka M: Long-term prognosis for tonsillectomy patients with IgA nephropathy, *Nippon Jibiinkoka Gakkai Kaiho* 101:916-23, 1998.
50. Akagi H, Kosaka M, Hattori K, Doi A, Fukushima K, et al: Long-term results of tonsillectomy as a treatment for IgA nephropathy, *Acta Otolaryngol Suppl* 555:38-42, 2004.
51. Sato M, Hotta O, Tomioka S, Horigome I, Chiba S, et al: Cohort study of advanced IgA nephropathy: efficacy and limitations of corticosteroids with tonsillectomy, *Nephron Clin Pract* 93(4):c137-45, 2003.
52. Akagi H, Kosaka M, Hattori K, Doi A, Fukushima K, et al: Long-term results of tonsillectomy as a treatment for IgA nephropathy, *Acta Otolaryngol Suppl* 555:38-42, 2004.
53. Coppo R, Roccatello D, Amore A, Quattrocchio G, Molino A, et al: Effects of a gluten-free diet in primary IgA nephropathy, *Clin Nephrol* 33(2):72-86, 1990.
54. Roccatello D, Ferro M, Coppo R, Giraudo G, et al: Report on intensive treatment of extracapillary glomerulonephritis with focus on crescentic IgA nephropathy, *Nephrol Dial Transplant* 10:2054-59, 1995.
55. Andreoli SP, Bergstein JM: Treatment of severe IgA nephropathy in children, *Pediatr Nephrol* 3:248-53, 1989.
56. Yoshikawa N, Ito H, Sakai T, Takekoshi Y, Honda M, et al: A controlled trial of combined therapy for newly diagnosed severe childhood IgA nephropathy. The Japanese Pediatric IgA Nephropathy Treatment Study Group, *J Am Nephrol* 10(1):101-09, 1999.
57. Kobayashi Y, Hiki Y, Kokubo T, Horii A, Tateno S: Steroid therapy during the early stage of IgA nephropathy, *Nephron* 72:237-42, 1996.
58. Donadio JV Jr, Begstralh EJ, Offord KP, Spencer DC: A controlled trial of fish oil in IgA nephropathy. Mayo Nephrology Collaborative Group, *N Engl J Med* 331:1194-9, 1994.
59. Pozzi C, Bolasco PG, Fogazzi GB, Andrulli S, et al: Corticosteroids in IgA nephropathy: a randomised controlled trial, *Lancet* 353:883-87, 1999.
60. Pozzi C, Andrulli S, Del Vecchio L, Melis P, Fogazzi GB, et al: Corticosteroid effectiveness in IgA nephropathy: long-term results of a randomized, controlled trial, *J Am Soc Nephrol* 15(1):157-63, 2004.
61. Dillon JJ: Treating IgA nephropathy, *J Am Soc Nephrol* 12:846-47, 2001.
62. Pozzi C, Del Vecchio L, Casartelli D, Pozzoni P, Andrulli S, et al: ACE inhibitors and angiotensin II receptor blockers in IgA nephropathy with mild proteinuria: the ACEARB study. *J Nephrol* 19:508-14, 2006.
63. Hogg RJ, Lee J, Nardelli N, Julian BJ, Cattran D, et al: Clinical trial evaluate omega-3 fatty acids and alternate day prednisone in patients with IgA nephropathy: Report from the Southwest Pediatric Nephrology Study Group, *Clin J Am Soc Nephrol* 1:467-74, 2006.
64. Hogg RJ, Wyatt RJ (for Scientific Planning Committee of the North American IgA Nephropathy Study): A randomized controlled trial of mycophenolate mofetil in patients with IgA nephropathy, *BMC Nephrol* 5:3, 2004.
65. Wyatt RJ, Krichevsky SB, Woodford SY, Miller PM, Roy S 3rd, et al: IgA nephropathy: long-term prognosis for pediatric patients, *J Pediatr* 127(6):913-19, 1995.

CHAPTER

19 Membranous Nephropathy

Sanjeev Gulati and Alok Kumar

Nephrotic syndrome is one of the most common renal problems encountered in day-to-day nephrology practice. In children it has a reported incidence of 2 per 100,000 per year and a cumulative prevalence of 16 per 100,000 children.[1] Membranous nephropathy (MN) is an uncommon cause of nephrotic syndrome in children.[2,3] This is in contrast to adults, in whom MN is one of the more common forms of nephrotic syndrome and a leading cause of end-stage renal disease (ESRD).[4] It can be idiopathic or secondary, which can be distinguished by clinical, laboratory, and histologic features.

PATHOPHYSIOLOGY

MN is an immunologically mediated disease that occurs in genetically predisposed individuals and is precipitated by some endogenous or exogenous insults.

Genetic Factors

Genetic factors appear important in MN. There is a strong link to the major histocompatibility antigens in humans. Many studies have shown association of HLA-DR3 with MN in Caucasians.[5] A strong association with HLA-DQA1 allelle has also been reported in two HLA-identical brothers.[6] In patients with MN, there is an extra Bss HII restriction enzyme cutting site in the vicinity of the HLA-DP genes.[7] This structural heterogeneity in the area containing genes for antigen peptide processing and transport could have implications for genetic susceptibility for developing MN. A significant increase in HLA-DR2 antigens and relatively low frequency of HLA-DR3 antigens have been found in the Japanese population.

Pathogenesis

The morphologic changes seen on biopsy in MN suggest that the podocyte injury and subepithelial immune deposits are central in the pathogenesis of the disease. The characteristic feature of MN is the presence of immune-complex deposits in the subepithelial space in the glomerulus. In the experimental Heymann nephritis model of MN, the disease can be produced in susceptible rats by active immunization with antigen extracted from the kidney and Freund's adjuvant.[8] The injected antigen stimulates antibody production and these antibodies react with FXIA, a component of the tubular brush border. The histopathologic findings in this model mimic those of MN in humans. Heymann antigen was found to be a 330 kDa cell surface glycoprotein (gp 330), which is expressed in higher concentration in the brush border of tubular epithelial cells and in lesser concentration on glomerular epithelial cells. The gp 330 is synthesized and expressed by podocytes on their surface in clathrin-coated pits only. The circulating antibodies pass through glomerular basement membrane (GBM) and bind to the antigen in the coated pits, forming immune complexes in situ. The immune complexes condense and attach firmly to the GBM at the level of the filtration slit. Then new gp 330 molecules are formed by podocytes that may interact with antibody. Repeated cycles of immune-complex formation and shedding into lamina externa take place and lead to growth of immune deposits.[8] In humans, gp 330 has been found in the brush border of proximal tubules, but it has not been seen in human glomeruli. These findings indicate that antigen targets in humans probably differ from those found in rat models of Heymann nephritis.

In antenatal MN, neutral endopeptidases (NEP) have been identified as the podocyte target antigen of circulating antibodies produced by mother granulocyte expression of NEP. Severity of renal disease was determined by the maternal IgG response to fetal NEP antigens expressed on podocytes.[9] Recently two compound heterozygous or homozygous mutations were identified in five mothers in the metallomembrane endopeptidase gene (*MME*). These mutations are the cause of alloimmunization during pregnancy. Idiopathic renal failure in early adulthood may be caused by immune-mediated fetal nephron loss.[9] NEP deficiency should also be considered in patients developing de novo MN after transplantation. Many of the antigens associated with secondary MN are not known. However, hepatitis B surface antigens (HbsAg) and hepatitis B e antigens (HbeAg) have been identified in immune deposits, as have thyroid antigens in patients with thyroiditis.

Data from various experimental models suggest that the following three mechanisms may be responsible for immune-complex deposition.

1. Acute serum sickness in rabbits (associated with neutralization of some glomerular anionic sites) appears to favor subepithelial deposition of immune complexes formed in circulation.[10] This mechanism may account for some forms of secondary glomerulonephritis.
2. Glomerular subepithelial in situ immune-complex formation by formation of antibodies (reactive with

movable structural antigen) may be responsible for MN with autoimmune disease or penicillamine administration.[11]

3. Immune-complex formation in situ by antibodies reactive with exogenous antigen (planted in subepithelial space) appear responsible for MN by chronic administration of cationized bovine serum albumin.[12]

Once immune deposits are formed, complement activation ensues and results in formation of terminal membrane attack complex (C5b-9). The C5b-9 triggers the biosynthesis of oxygen radical–producing enzymes within the glomerular epithelial cells. The finding of urinary C5b-9 has been suggested as a diagnostic test for following disease activity.[13,14]

Proteinuria is not due to disruption of the plasma membrane but to activation of specific signaling pathways. These include activation of protein kinases, phospholipases, cyclooxygenase, transcription factors, NADPH oxidase, stress protein proteinases, etc. Their impact leads to alteration or disturbances in cell metabolic signalling pathways and in the structure and function of lipids. This also alters various key proteins involved in maintenance of the cytoskeleton and slit diaphagm. Therefore C5b-9 induces partial dissolution of active skeleton, reduces nephrin expression, and F actin-bound reprint and loss of slit diaphragm integrity.[15] Endoplasmic reticulum stress may limit injury. Further evidence of complement-mediated injury comes from the fact that nephritogenic serum contains antibodies to complement regulatory proteins (Crry). On the other hand, overexpression of Crry has a protective effect on immune-complex-mediated MN.[16] The alteration of glomerular extracellular matrix is also seen in MN and it may not be induced by complement-mediated injury. Some studies suggest that thickening of basement membrane seen in MN may be caused at least in part by a reduced fibrinolytic activity due to stabilization of plasminogen activator inhibitor (PAI) and vitronectin in the subepithelial deposits.

INCIDENCE

The peak incidence of idiopathic membranous nephropathy (IMN) is around the fourth and fifth decades of life, although it can occur in any age group, including infants. In the International Study of Kidney Disease in Childhood (ISKDC) study, IMN accounted for only 8 in 521 cases (1.5%) of all children with idiopathic nephrotic syndrome.[17] In our recent series of 600 children with idiopathic nephrotic syndrome, of whom 290 were biopsied, MN was seen on histopathology in 5 of 290 children (1.7%).[18] When we analyzed the subgroup of 136 children with steroid-resistant nephrotic syndrome (SRNS), IMN was observed in 6 children (4.4%).[19] All these children were HbsAg and HCV negative. In contrast, Bhimma et al. have observed that in African Americans, MN accounted for 40% of cases of nephrotic syndrome; 86.2% were associated with hepatitis B virus antigens.[20] Since all children with asymptomatic proteinuria are not referred to pediatric nephrologists and also because renal biopsy examinations are not performed in these patients, it is possible that the frequency of IMN in children may be higher than what has been reported. MN has a predilection for males over females, with a male-to-female ratio of 2 : 1.

ETIOLOGY

MN can be idiopathic or secondary. Often, distinguishing between idiopathic and secondary causes (Table 19-1) on the basis of clinical evidence alone is not possible. In secondary MN, such as with lupus or hepatitis, concomitant mesangial or subendothelial deposits may be present.[21] Children have a higher frequency of secondary MN than adults. The secondary variety has been described in 43% of children compared with 22% in adults.[22,23] The principal causes of the secondary variety in children appear to be infections and autoimmune disease. Drugs and neoplasms are rare causes of membranous glomerulopathy in children.[23] Hepatitis B is an important factor in the etiology of disease in parts of the world where hepatitis B is endemic.[20,24,25] Other infections such as schistosomiasis, filariasis, malaria, and syphilis are also important

TABLE 19-1 Secondary Causes of Membranous Nephropathy

Autoimmune diseases	Systemic lupus erythematosus Enteropathy/diabetes mellitus Pemphigus Ulcerative colitis Ankylosing spondylitis Dermatomyositis Graves disease Hashimoto disease Mixed connective-tissue disease Rheumatoid arthritis Sjögren syndrome Systemic sclerosis
Infectious diseases	Hepatitis B: Occurs in children in endemic areas Hepatitis C Quartan malaria Leprosy Hydatid cyst Schistosomiasis Congenital syphilis Enterococcal endocarditis Filariasis
Drugs and heavy metals	Penicillamine Gold Captopril Nonsteroidal antiinflammatory agents
Neoplastic	Neuroblastoma Ovarian tumors Wilms' tumor Gonadoblastoma
Other conditions	IgA deficiency Kidney transplant (de novo) Fanconi syndrome Sickle cell disease Stem cell transplant Antitubular basement membrane Antialveolar basement membrane antibodies Idiopathic thrombocytopenia Juvenile cirrhosis Familial truncating mutation in metallomembrane endopeptidase

conditions linked to development of MN in the prevalent area.[23,26,27]

CLINICAL FEATURES

The clinical features of MN are similar to those in other children with idiopathic nephrotic syndrome, and children with MN also exhibit anasarca, microhematuria, and hypertension.[18] However, they are almost always nonresponsive to a standard course of prednisone therapy.[19] A finding of acute renal failure is unusual and should direct investigation toward other diagnoses or related conditions, such as bilateral renal vein thrombosis, excessive diuresis, or the use of nephrotoxic medications. Hence the diagnosis is most often made when children with SRNS are biopsied. The clinical manifestations of HBV-associated nephropathy are different. These children either exhibit nephrotic syndrome or the manifestations are detected by routine urine and serologic testing. Microscopic hematuria has rarely been reported. Occasionally microscopic hematuria has been reported without proteinuria. The mean age at presentation for HBV-related MN is 5 to 7 years in cases of horizontal transmission, whereas children who acquire infection vertically display in infancy. The incidence of hypertension is less than 25%.[20,22]

INVESTIGATIONS

To confirm the diagnosis, MN children should be subjected to the standard biochemical investigations used for any child with nephrotic syndrome. These include the following:

- Urine microscopy: Urine sediment is typically nephrotic with oval fat bodies and fatty casts. In mild cases the urinalysis may reveal proteinuria without formed elements in the sediment.
- Serum creatinine
- Blood urea nitrogen
- Serum albumin
- Lipid profile
- Proteinuria (quantitative) with a 24-hour urine collection: A ratio of spot urine protein to creatinine is easier to obtain, and the findings may be sufficient for screening purposes.
- Creatinine clearance
- Ultrasound of the abdomen: An ultrasound is essential before a renal biopsy. It provides information about kidney size and echogenicity of the kidneys, and also information about extrarenal involvement, especially of the liver and splenoportal axis.
- Renal biopsy: Definitive diagnosis is made based on findings from a renal biopsy.

In addition, the following investigations are recommended to find a secondary cause and the underlying etiology:

- Antinuclear antibodies
- Anti-double-stranded DNA if results from antinuclear antibody testing are positive
- Hepatitis B serology (if positive, DNA quantitation)
- Hepatitis C serology (if positive, RNA quantitation)
- Syphilis serology
- Complement levels
- Cryoglobulin, particularly if hepatitis C and/or low levels of complement are found
- Urinary C5b-9
- Urinary β_2-microglobulin (prognosis worse with an increased level)

Membranous Nephropathy and Hepatitis B

Children with HBV-related MN show positivity of HbsAg and usually hepatitis B surface antibody is not detected. The hepatitis B early antigen (HbeAg) can be detected in serum of 90% of patients.[27] Hypocomplementemia is observed at the onset of disease (low C3 and C4), but titers of C3, C4 return to normal in the later part of disease.[27] Circulatory immune complexes are detected in 80% of patients. Serum levels of transaminases may be raised on presentation.[20,24] Liver biopsy shows evidence of chronic persistent hepatitis mainly in children, but chronic active hepatitis is seen in adults.

HISTOLOPATHOLOGY

Pathologic features can be observed using light microscopy, immunofluorescence microscopy, and electron microscopy.

Light Microscopy

All glomeruli are involved. The histologic hallmark under light microscopy is diffuse global capillary wall thickening.[28] The size of the glomerulus appears normal or slightly increased. The cellularity is not increased. The epithelial cells appear normal but occasionally may be enlarged or prominent. Epithelial cell crescents are rarely seen in the clinical setting of rapidly progressive glomerulonephritis. The mesangial matrix is not increased and capillary loops are usually patent. The diffuse capillary wall thickening is best appreciated in the periodic acid methenamine silver-stained sections in which subepithelial deposits are not stained and the GBM is stained black (Figure 19-1). The unstained deposits are surrounded by black-staining, newly synthesized GBM that appears as small black spikes projecting from the GBM toward the urinary space (Figure 19-2). The light microscopic

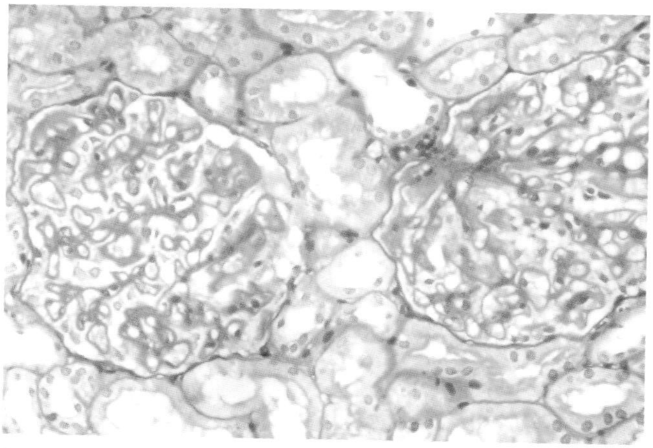

Figure 19-1 Photomicrograph depicting thick refractile PAS-positive glomerular basement membrane. Light microscopy.

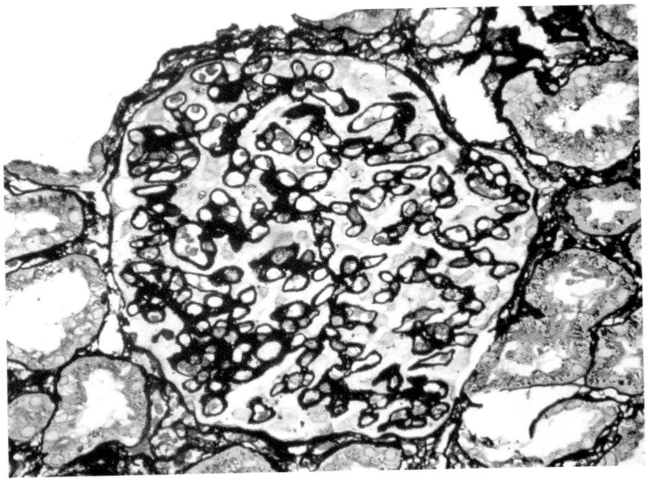

Figure 19-2 Silver stain showing subepithelial argyrophilic spikes along glomerular basement membrane. Light microscopy.

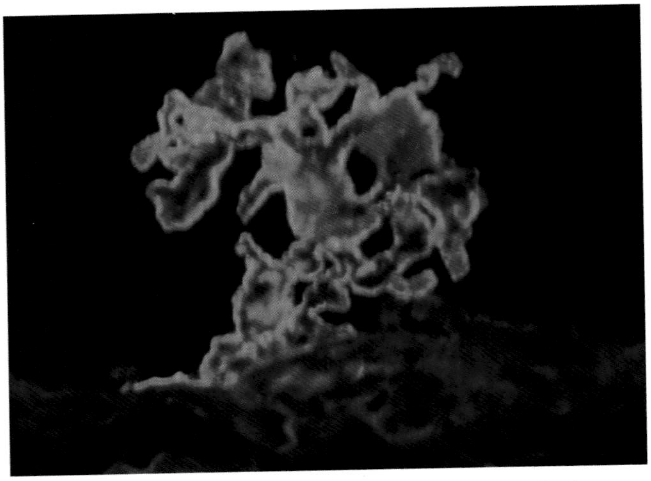

Figure 19-3 Coarse granular IgG deposits along glomerular basement membrane. Immunofluorescent microscopy.

features may vary with the stage of disease. As the disease progresses, progressive tubular atrophy, increasing interstitial fibrosis, and mononuclear cell infiltration take place. Glomeruli become segmentally and globally sclerotic and develop adhesions to Bowman's capsule. Overt mesangial hypercellularity is suggestive of secondary MN. An infiltrate of numerous mononuclear cells in the interstitium may carry higher risk of renal dysfunction.

Immunofluorescence Microscopy

The hallmark of immunofluorescence microscopy is uniform, granular capillary wall staining for IgG and C3.[28,29] The most intense staining is seen for IgG and it is universal. C3 deposition is also found in more than 95% of cases but is weaker in intensity (Figure 19-3). The predominant IgG staining is for IgG4 by using monoclonal antibodies against human IgG subclass. If mesangial deposits of IgG are seen, then a secondary cause, for example, systemic lupus erythematosus (SLE), should be suspected. Staining for C1q and C4 has been

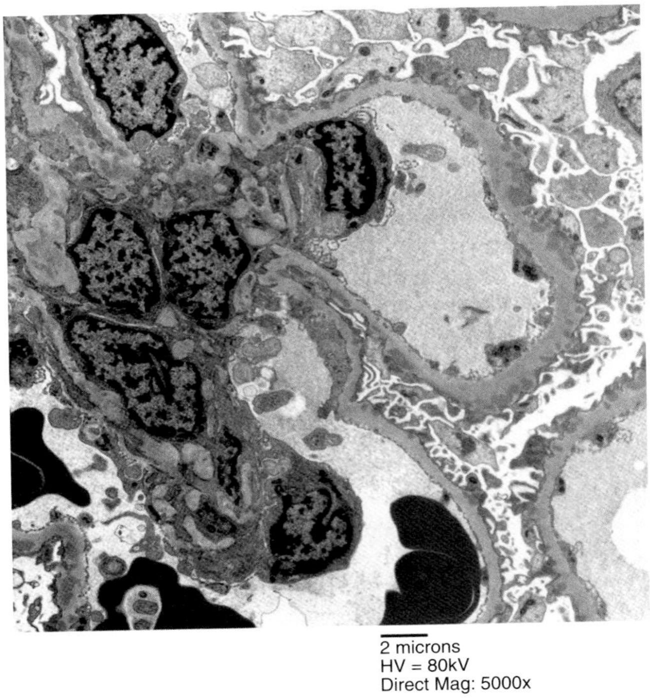

Figure 19-4 Subepithelial electron-dense immune-complex deposits along glomerular basement membrane. Electron microscopy, magnification ×5000.

described, but intense staining for C1q should raise suspicion of SLE. C4d and C4bp have been identified in 92% of cases.[30] IgM and IgA are less often demonstrable. Staining for C5b-9 has been demonstrated in a location similar to IgG. Recently CD20+ve infiltrates have been demonstrated in human membranous glomerulonephritis.[31] In another recent study, the amount of complement deposition has been shown to correlate with the rate of progression of renal dysfunction.[32]

Electron Microscopy

The characteristic electron microscopy finding in MN is the presence of subepithelial electron-dense, immune-complex deposits. These correspond to the granular IgG deposits seen under immunofluorescence microscopy (Figure 19-4). Epithelial foot process effacement and microvillous transformation occur in all stages of MN when there is heavy proteinuria. No electron-dense deposits are observed in the subendothelial space or in the mesangium. The presence of mesangial deposits of complement or immunoglobulin indicates a secondary form of MN such as SLE. The subendothelial deposits are also common in SLE.

Five morphologic stages of MN are recognized.[33] Based on a combination of light and electron microscopic features, the stages are as follows:

Stage I. Light microscopy shows normal GBM in thickness and appearance. The electron-dense deposits are small and flat but discrete. The smaller deposits are located at the site of the slit diaphragm, whereas moderate-size deposits are located adjacent to the fused foot process.

Stage II. In stage II, thickening of the GBM is discernible by light microscopy. The electron-dense deposits are increased in number and size. These deposits are flanked by prominent spikes in almost every capillary loop.

Stage III. The basement membrane material (spikes) completely surrounds the deposits. These are larger and acquire intramembranous position. The capillary wall is irregular and has a moth-eaten appearance. A few synechiae can be seen.

Stage IV. The GBM is severely altered and irregularly thickened. The deposits are few or completely absent. The vacuolated appearance of the GBM is discernible, and loss of deposits is seen as electrolucent areas in the basement membrane.

Stage V. This stage is characterized by return of the GBM to normal. The only residual membrane disturbance is seen in the inner aspect of the basement membrane. The GBM appears very delicate and only partially thickened.

The most common lesion seen in children is stage II, followed by stage III and mixed stage.[34,35] A relationship between histologic stage and clinical outcome has been shown in adults. There is a paucity of data to determine a correlation between the histologic stages and clinical outcome in children.[36]

NATURAL HISTORY

IMN is well characterized in adults and hence it is easier to understand its course by looking at adult data. These patients are at risk of complications such as thrombotic events and progression to ESRD. A review of studies that reported on the long-term outcome of untreated adults showed that 50% of these patients either died or developed ESRD within 10 years of onset.[3,37,38] The risk was increased in patients with interstitial fibrosis on biopsy. On the other hand, about 20% to 40% of patients in most series have been observed to go into spontaneous remission without any therapy within 5 years.[37-40] In children, MN differs from the disease as it is seen in adults in several important respects: an apparent associated cause is more common, macroscopic hematuria is often seen, a relapsing course is more often noted, renal venous thrombosis is rarely found, and evolution to renal failure occurs less often. All the existing data about natural history and treatment of IMN in children is not only uncontrolled, but there is also considerable variability regarding the therapeutic protocols used and the definition of *remission.* Hence it is not possible to recommend any particular drug. However, it is evident from this data that children with asymptomatic proteinuria have a good outcome. On the other hand, about 25% of children with nephrotic syndrome develop chronic renal failure after a variable follow-up of 1 to 17 years.[40]

The natural history of HBV-associated MN is incompletely understood. Approximately 30% to 60% of patients may experience spontaneous regression of nephrotic syndrome. The duration of nephrotic syndrome tends to be 12 months or longer in these patients. The remaining patients continue to have edema and proteinuria.

TREATMENT

MN is an uncommon cause of nephrotic syndrome in children. In the absence of any large series and controlled trials, guidelines for treatment are extrapolated from studies done in adults.

The first and foremost step is to investigate for any secondary causes such as hepatitis B, hepatitis C, and SLE. Successful treatment of the underlying cause may be curative in secondary forms.

Supportive Management

During the first 6 months (after diagnosis), immunosuppressive therapy is generally avoided, as a significant number of the patients may undergo a spontaneous remission. During this period supportive management should be instituted in all these children. This can go a long way in controlling edema and anasarca and preventing complications of a prolonged nephrotic state. These measures include the following:

- A low-salt diet is key in reducing anasarca. Protein should be given as per RDA for age, and restriction is not useful in reducing the rate of progression of chronic kidney disease.
- Diuretics help control edema. Loop diuretics are the most potent. A combination of diuretics can be used in cases of massive anasarca.
- Hypertension should be treated aggressively. Angiotensin converting enzyme (ACE) inhibitors and angiotensin II receptor blockers (ARBs) decrease proteinuria and control hypertension. Both these drugs have been shown to reduce intraglomerular pressure and proteinuria in a variety of nondiabetic renal diseases. Furthermore, there are suggestions that a combination of these may have a synergistic effect. Enalapril or lisinopril is generally initiated in a dosage of 0.08 mg/kg/day and increased at 2 to 4 weekly intervals thereafter. Losartan is used in a dosage of 25 to 100 mg day.
- Hepatic 3-methylglutaryl coenzyme A reductase inhibitors (simvastatin, lovastatin) help treat hypercholesterolemia. There is preliminary evidence in studies from adult patients that these might also help in retarding the progression of renal disease by a mechanism other than the antilipidemic effect.
- NSAIDs help decrease proteinuria. These have been largely supplanted by ACE inhibitors and ARBs. Also, NSAIDs may cause interstitial nephritis.
- Routine anticoagulation is not advisable. However, it is generally recommended in patients with a history of venous thrombosis (renal vein thrombosis and other deep vein thromboses). The clinician must be vigilant in monitoring for signs of venous thrombosis.

Immunosuppressive Therapy

Patients with asymptomatic nonnephrotic proteinuria should be monitored on conservative therapy for at least 6 months. These patients may undergo spontaneous remission, particularly if they have normal renal function and an early lesion.

Therapy with immunosuppressive agents is indicated in patients who have one or more of the following features:[39]

Increased creatinine level at presentation
Progressive decline in renal function
Persistent nephrotic syndrome

Thromboembolism
Elevation of urinary excretion of complement activation products
Tubulointerstitial changes or focal sclerosis

The role of immunosuppressive therapy in children with IMN is controversial.[40] There are only short case series and no good controlled trials. Hence the therapy is extrapolated from management experience in adults with this condition. A recent metaanalysis of randomized trials has shown that protocols based on corticosteroids alone improve neither the probability of remission nor the 5-year survival when compared with symptomatic treatments.[37] Thus monotherapy with steroids has no role in management of patients with IMN. In the landmark trial by Ponticelli et al., a daily combination of three daily high-dose intravenous methylprednisone pulses and alternating oral prednisone with monthly chlorambucil was found to be beneficial.[41] The probability of being alive at 10 years without dialysis was 92% for treated patients and 60% for untreated controls. In a randomized trial by Cattran et al. in adults with nephrotic syndrome, cyclosporin A (CsA) given for 1 year was found to be superior to placebo in patients with nephrotic syndrome and/or renal dysfunction.[42] These results were confirmed in a German multicenter trial where it was observed that 34% of patients treated with CsA alone or CsA plus prednisone achieved complete remission during treatment. In the majority of patients, remission was observed within 6 months of therapy.[43] There are case reports on the beneficial effect of tacrolimus.[44] Because the immunosuppressive potency of tacrolimus is superior to that of cyclosporin, further studies are warranted with this agent. It is prudent to avoid immunosuppressive therapy in patients with advanced renal failure, severe hyperechogenicity of the kidneys on ultrasonography, and/or diffuse glomerular sclerosis/interstitial fibrosis at renal biopsy.

Currently one of the following three protocols can be used[45,46]:

1. The first line of therapy in any child with persistent nephrotic range proteinuria is a combination of three daily high-dose intravenous methylprednisone pulses (600 mg/m^2), each followed by oral prednisone 0.5-1 mg/kg/day for 1 month and alternating with monthly chlorambucil in a dosage of 0.15-0.2 mg/kg/day. It is, however, advisable not to exceed a cumulative dose of chlorambucil of 8-10 mg/kg, especially in boys in view of the risk of azoospermia. A similar regimen using alternate monthly prednisone therapy with oral cyclophosphamide (2.5 mg/kg/day) has been found to be equally effective (not to exceed a cumulative dose of 200-300 mg/kg). The peripheral blood counts should be monitored and the cytotoxic agents discontinued if the TLC is less than 3,000/mm^3 or in the presence of an active infection. The usual duration of therapy is 6 months. In order to minimize the risk of gonadal toxicity, we have used monthly intravenous cyclophosphamide infusions in a dose of 500 mg/m^2/month (along with alternate monthly prednisone) and have observed it to be beneficial in our anecdotal experience with this protocol.
2. CsA in a dosage of 3.5 mg/kg/day for 1 year is usually administered in combination with oral prednisone (2 mg/kg/day), which is gradually tapered off over 3 to 6 months.
3. There are preliminary reports of success with tacrolimus in adults, although so far there is no experience in children.[44] However, tacrolimus has been used in children with SRNS secondary to focal segmental glomerulosclerosis (FSGS) and minimal change disease (MCD) with encouraging results.

Secondary Membranous Nephropathy

In hepatitis-associated MN, the following agents have been used:

Interferon. A metaanalysis showed that α interferon (IFN) therapy had a beneficial effect in adult HbeAg-positive patients with MN who were treated for 3 to 6 months. There is only one prospective trial in children. Lin[47] observed that all 20 patients who were treated with IFN underwent remission, whereas 50% of patients in the control group had persistent nephrotic syndrome and 50% had mild proteinuria.[48] (Patients in both groups were HBV positive.) In the IFN group, 18 patients had HbsAg and HbeAg seroconversion to negative status and 4 patients had HbeAg seroconversion only. There was no seroconversion in patients undergoing conservative treatment.

Lamivudine. This agent has a role in patients who have persistent proteinuria. A recent study compared renal outcome of adults (with chronic HBV infection with MN) taking lamivudine with patients using conservative treatment.[49] The 10 lamivudine-treated patients had a 100% 3-year survival versus 58% of the 12 conservatively treated patients. There are anecdotal reports showing reversal of MN in a child treated with lamivudine.[50] This appears to be a promising therapy for the future.

Of all patients with lupus nephritis, 10% to 20% have MN. Children with pure MN secondary to lupus nephritis are treated with Ponticelli's protocol.[41] In cases of superimposed features of class IV nephritis (diffuse proliferative glomerulonephritis), patients are treated with a combination of intravenous cyclophosphamide and oral prednisone.

MORTALITY/MORBIDITY

The course of IMN is variable, and patients may be divided into three groups of approximately equal size (i.e., rule of thirds).

Spontaneous complete remission. Renal function is normal, with or without subsequent relapse.

Persistent proteinuria of variable degree. Renal function is normal or impaired but stable.

Progressive disease leading to (ESRD). The incidence rate of ESRD in adult series is 14% at 5 years, 35% at 10 years, and 41% at 15 years. There are no similar large series in children because of the uncommon nature of this entity. However, in the series by Habib et al., of 50 children with MN followed for 1 to 10 years, 26 (52%) attained remission, 19 (38%) continued to have active disease, and 5 (10%) developed chronic kidney disease (CKD).[34] In another large series, the Southwest Pediatric Nephrology Study group reported the outcome of 54 children with follow-up of 2 to 14 years. Of these, 13 (25%) attained remission and 10 (18.5%) developed CKD.[36] Children with hypertension had the worst outcome.[34-36] In a review of 163 children who had been followed in different studies, 39% were documented to be in remission, 38% had active disease, and 19% developed CKD. All patients who developed CKD exhibited nephrotic syndrome.[40]

There is general agreement that impaired function at the time of biopsy and hypertension portends a poor prognosis. Biopsy findings may correlate with prognosis, especially the degree of tubulointerstitial damage.

CONCLUSION

MN remains an uncommon cause of nephrotic syndrome in children. The diagnosis is often made when these children are biopsied after being labeled steroid resistant. It is imperative to rule out secondary causes in these children. Initially, IMN children should be managed conservatively. Immunosuppressive therapy should be considered in children who develop nephrotic proteinuria and/or progressive renal dysfunction.

REFERENCES

1. Nash MA, Edelmannn CM Jr, Bernstein J, Barnett JL: The nephrotic syndrome. In Edelmann CM Jr, editor: *Paediatric Kidney Disease,* ed 2, Boston, 1992, Little, Brown and Co.
2. Eddy AA, Symons JM: Nephrotic syndrome in childhood, *Lancet* 362(9384):629-39, 2003.
3. Cameron, JS: Membranous nephropathy in childhood and its treatment, *Pediatr Nephrol* 4(2):193-98, 1990.
4. Honkanen E, Tornroth T, Gronhagen-Riska C: Natural history, clinical course and morphological evolution of membranous nephropathy, *Nephrol Dial Transplant* 7(suppl 1):35-41, 1992.
5. Dyer PA, Short CD, Clarke EA, Mallich NP: HLA antigen and gene polymorphism and haplotypes by family studies in membranous nephropathy, *Nephrol Dial Transplant* 7:42-47, 1992.
6. Vangelista A, Tazzari R, Bonomini V: Idiopathic membranous nephropathy in 2 twin brothers. *Nephron* 50(1):79-80, 1988.
7. Sacks SH, Warner C, Campbell RD, Dunham I: Molecular mapping of the HLA class II region in HLA-DR3 associated idiopathic membranous nephropathy, *Kidney Int Suppl* 39:S13-19, 1993.
8. Kerjaschki D: Molecular pathogenesis of membranous nephropathy (clinical conference), *Kidney Int* 41:1090-105, 1992.
9. Debiec H, Nauta J, Coulet F et al: Role of truncating mutations in MME gene in fetomaternal alloimmunisation and antenatal glomerulopathies, *Lancet* 364(9441):1252-59, Oct 2-8, 2004.
10. Border WA: Experimental membranous nephropathy: the pathogenetic role of cationic proteins. In Davison AM, editor: *Nephrology, Proceedings of the 10th International Congress of Nephrology,* vol 2, London, 1988, Balliere Tindall.
11. Mallick NP, Short CD, Manos J: Clinical membranous nephropathy, *Nephron* 34:209-19, 1983.
12. Adler SG, Wang HJ, Cohen AH, Border WA: Electric charge. Its role in the pathogenesis and prevention of experimental membranous nephropathy in the rabbits, *J Clin Invest* 71:487-89, 1983.
13. Kon SP, Coupes B, Short CD, Solomon LR, Raftery MJ et al: Urinary C5b-9 excretion and clinical course in idiopathic human membranous nephropathy, *Kidney Int* 48:1953-58, 1995.
14. Coupes B, Brenchley PE, Short CD, Mallick NP: Clinical aspects of C3dg and C5b-9 in human membranous nephropathy, *Nephrol Dial Transplant* 7(suppl 1):32-34, 1992.
15. Cubulsky AV, Quigy RJ, Salant DJ: Experimental membranous nephropathy redux, *Am J Physiol Renal Physiol* 289(4):F660-71, 2005.
16. Quigg RJ, Holers VM, Berthiaume D et al: Crry and CD 59 regulate complement in rat glomerular epithelial cells and are inhibited by the nephritogenic antibody of passive Heymann nephritis, *J Immunol* 154:3437-43, 1995.
17. International Study of Kidney Disease in Children: Nephrotic syndrome: prediction of histopathology from clinical and laboratory characteristics at time of diagnosis, *Kidney Int* 13:159-65, 1978.
18. Kumar J, Gulati S, Sharma AP, Sharma RK, Gupta RK: Histopathological spectrum of childhood nephrotic syndrome in Indian children, *Pediatr Nephrol* 18(7):657-60, Jul 2003.
19. Gulati S, Sengupta A, Sharma RK, Gupta RK, Sharma AP, Gupta A: Steroid resistant nephrotic syndrome, *Indian Pediatr* 43(4):373-74, 2006.
20. Bhimma R, Coovadia HM, Adhikari M: Nephrotic syndrome in South African children: changing perspectives over 20 years, *Pediatr Nephrol* 11(4):429-34, Aug 1997.
21. Glassock RJ: Secondary membranous glomerulonephritis, *Nephrol Dial Transplant* 7(suppl 1):64-71, 1992.
22. Kingswood JC, Banks RA, Tribe R, Owes Jones J, Mackenjie J: Renal biopsy in the elderly: clinicopathological correlations in 143 patients, *Clin Nephrol* 22:183-87, 1984.
23. Kleinknecht C, Habib R: Membranous glomerulonephritis. In Holliday MA, Barratt TM, Vernier RL, editors: *Pediatric Nephrology,* Baltimore, 1987, Williams & Wilkins.
24. Lin CY: Hepatitis B virus associated membranous nephropathy: clinical features, immunological profiles and outcome, *Nephron* 55:37-44, 1990.
25. Hu HC, Wu CY, Lin CY et al: Membranous nephropathy in 52 hepatitis B surface antigen (HBsAg) carrier children in Taiwan, *Kidney Int* 36:1103-07, 1989.
26. Hendrickise RG, Adeniyi A: Quartan malarial nephrotic syndrome in children, *Kidney Int* 16:67-74, 1979.
27. Ngu JL, Chatelanet F, Leke R et al: Nephropathy in Cameroon: evidence for filarial derived immune complex pathogenesis in some cases, *Clin Nephrol* 24:128-34, 1985.
28. Schwartz MM: Membranous glomerulonephritis. In Jenette JC, Olson JL, Schwartz MM, Silva FG, editors: *Heptinstall's Pathology of the Kidney,* Philadelphia, 1998, Lippincott-Raven.
29. Jenette JC: Immunohistology of renal disease. In Jenette JC: *Immunohistopathology in diagnostic pathology,* Boca Raton, 1998, CRC Press.
30. Kusonoki Y, Itami N, Tochimarn H, Takekoshi Y, Nagasawa S, Yoshiki T: Glomerular deposition of C4 cleavage fragment (C4d) and C4 binding protein in idiopathic membranous glomerulonephritis, *Nephron* 51:17-19, 1989.
31. Cohen CD, Calvaresi N, Armelloni S, Schmid H, Henger A et al: CD20 positive infiltrates in human membranous glomerulonephritis, *J Nephrol* 18(3):328-33, 2005.
32. Troyanov S, Roasio L, Pandes M, Herzenberg AM, Cattran DC: Renal pathology in idiopathic membranous nephropathy: a new perspective, *Kidney Int* 69(9):1641-48, 2006.
33. Ehrenreich T, Churg J: Pathology of membranous nephropathy. In Scommers SC, editor, *Pathology Annual,* New York, 1968, Appleton-Century-Crofts.
34. Habib R, Kleinknecht C, Gubler MC: Extramembranous glomerulonephritis in children: report of 50 cases, *J Pediatr* 82:754-66, 1973.
35. Latham P, Poucell S, Koresaar A et al: Idiopathic membranous glomerulopathy in Canadian children: a clinicopathologic study, *J Pediatr* 101:682-85, 1992.
36. Southwest Pediatric Nephrology Study Group: Comparison of idiopathic and systemic lupus erythematosus associated membranous glomerulonephritis in children, *Am J Kidney Dis* 7:115-24, 1986.
37. Hogan SL, Muller KE, Jennette JC, Falk RJ: A review of therapeutic studies of idiopathic membranous glomerulopathy, *Am J Kid Dis* 25(6):862-75, 1995.
38. Hunt LP: Statistical aspects of survival in membranous nephropathy, *Nephrol Dial Transplant* 7(suppl 1):53-59, 1992.
39. Reichert LJ, Koene RA, Wetzels JF: Prognostic factors in idiopathic membranous nephropathy, *Am J Kidney Dis* 31(1):1-11, 1998.
40. Makker SP, Treatment of membranous nephropathy in children, *Semin Nephrol* 23(4):379-385, 2003.

41. Ponticelli C, Zucchelli P, Passerini P et al: A 10-year follow-up of a randomized study with methylprednisolone and chlorambucil in membranous nephropathy, *Kidney Int* 48(5):1600-04, 1995.
42. Cattran D, Greenwood C, Ritchie S et al: Management of membranous nephropathy: when and what for treatment, *Kidney Int* 47:1130-35, 1995.
43. Fritsche L, Budde K, Farber L, Charisse G, Kunz R et al: Treatment of membranous glomerulopathy with cyclosporin A: how much patience is required? *Nephrol Dial Transplant* 14:1036-38, 1999.
44. McCauley J, Shapiro R, Ellis D, Igdal H, Tzakis A, Starzl TE: Pilot trial of FK 506 in the management of steroid-resistant nephrotic syndrome, *Nephrol Dial Transplant* 8(11):1286-90, 1993.
45. Cattran D: Management of membranous nephropathy: when and what for treatment, *J Am Soc Nephrol* 16:1188-94, 2005.
46. Muirhead N: Management of idiopathic membranous nephropathy: evidence-based recommendations, *Kidney Int Suppl* 70:S47-55, 1999.
47. Lin CY: Treatment of hepatitis B virus associated membranous nephropathy with recombinant alfa interferon, *Kidney Int* 47:225-30, 1995.
48. Bhimma R, Coovadia HM, Kramvis A, Adhikari M, Kew MC: Treatment of hepatitis B virus associated nephropathy in black children, *Pediatr Nephrol* 17:393-99, 2002.
49. Tang S, Lai FM, Lui YH, Tang CS, Kung NN et al: Lamivudine in hepatitis B associated MN, *Kidney Int* 68:1750-58, 2005.
50. Filler G, Feber J, Weiler G, Le Saux S: Another case of HBV associated membranous glomerulonephritis resolving on lamivudine, *Arch Dis Child* 88(5):460, 2003.

CHAPTER 20

Postinfectious Glomerulonephritis

Velibor Tasic

INTRODUCTION

Acute postinfectious glomerulonephritis (APIG) is the most common renal pathology in underdeveloped countries and may be caused by a wide spectrum of infective agents that may produce acute glomerular injury. The prototype of APIG is acute poststreptococcal glomerulonephritis. The clinical presentation of APIG varies from subclinical disease to acute renal failure, and is usually accompanied by transient hypocomplementemia. Sites of infection may include pneumonia, meningitis (particularly with infected ventriculo-atrial or ventriculo-peritoneal shunts), sepsis, or infected endocarditis (SBE). There is a growing list of infective agents that may cause APIG (bacteria, viruses, fungi, and parasites) (Table 20-1). In the majority of cases the disease has a mild clinical course, although clearly this may be influenced by the course of the underlying infection (e.g., SBE).

Poststreptococcal Glomerulonephritis

Poststreptococcal glomerulonephritis (PSGN) is still the most common glomerulopathy in undeveloped countries. The disease is characterized by sudden onset of nephritic signs, such as hematuria, edema, hypertension, oliguria, and azotemia.[1-8] The disease was recognized as a complication of scarlet fever in the 18th century. Owing to antibiotic therapy and improved social, economic, education, and health care, PSGN is seen in advanced industrialized countries mainly as sporadic cases.[9,10]

EPIDEMIOLOGY

The disease is seen all around the world.[11-16] In the tropics, it is a complication of pyoderma due to hot climate and high humidity. Minor skin injuries, insect bites, and poor hygiene predispose to infection with group A beta hemolytic streptococcus (GABHS).[17] In countries with moderate and cold climates, PSGN is a complication of upper respiratory tract infections (pharyngitis) during the winter months. M types 2, 47, 49, 55, 57, and 60 are associated with PSGN following pyoderma, while M types 1, 2, 3, 4, 12, 25, and 45 are associated with PSGN following pharyngitis. The disease has a seasonal character, although isolated cases may be seen throughout the year. In the past, epidemics of PSGN following impetigo were reported. In some areas (e.g., Trinidad, Maracaibo), epidemics appear cyclically every 5 to 7 years; there is no clear explanation for this phenomenon.[8] Populations at risk were children and soldiers due to intimate contact, overcrowded living conditions, and poor hygiene and sanitation systems. The male : female ratio is up to 2 : 1, but when subclinical cases are included, male predominance disappears. The disease is most common in children aged 3 to 12 years, although PSGN has been reported in infants.[18] The risk for developing PSGN after infection with a nephritogenic strain of GABHS is about 15%; for M type 49, it is 5% after pharyngeal infection and 25% after pyoderma.[19] Rarely, PSGN has been reported as a complication of piercing[20] and circumcision,[21] and in a transplanted kidney.[22] Besides GABHS, streptococci from groups C and G can also cause acute glomerulonephritis; this is due to the common nephritogenic antigen (endostreptosin), which has been isolated from these strains.[23,24]

PATHOGENESIS

It is clear that PSGN is an immune complex disease, but the nephritogenic antigen is still a matter of debate.[25,26] The proposed mechanisms are (1) deposition of circulating immune complexes containing nephritogenic antigen in glomeruli, (2) implantation of the nephritogenic antigen into glomerular structures and in situ formation of immune complexes, (3) molecular mimicry between streptococcal antigens and normal glomerular antigens that react with antibodies against streptococcal antigens, and (4) direct activation of the complement system by implanted streptococcal antigens. Many proteins such as endostreptosin, preabsorbing antigen, nephritis strain–associated protein, streptococcal pyrogenic exotoxin B (SPEB), nephritis-associated plasmin receptor (NaPlr) have been considered as potent nephritogenic antigens in PSGN.[27-35]

To document pathogenicity, nephritogenic antigen in renal biopsy specimens from patients with PSGN should be identified; the same antigen should be extracted from streptococci obtained from PSGN patients, but not from streptococci cultured from patients with rheumatic fever. Finally, sera from PSGN patients in the convalescent phase should contain significant titers of antibodies against the nephritogenic antigen. Lange et al.[29,30] surmised that endostreptosin (ESS) was the ideal nephrotogenic antigen because it fulfilled three of the above-mentioned criteria. Interestingly, ESS was identified in early biopsy specimens, but not in later ones.

TABLE 20-1 Etiological Agents Associated with Acute Postinfectious Glomerulonephritis

Bacterial	Viral	Fungal	Parasites
Streptococcus group A, C, G	Coxsackievirus	Coccidioides immitis	*Plasmodium malariae*
Streptococcus viridans	Echovirus		*Plasmodium falciparum*
Staphylococcus (aureus, albus)	Cytomegalovirus		*Schistosoma mansoni*
Pneumococcus	Epstein-Barr virus		*Toxoplasma gondii*
Neisseria meningitidis	Hepatitis B, C		Filariasis
Mycobacteria	HIV		Trichinosis
Salmonella typhosa	Rubella		Trypanosomes
Klebsiella pneumoniae	Measles		
Escherchia coli	Varicella		
Yersinia enterocolitica	Vaccinia		
Legionella	Parvovirus		
Brucella melitensis	Influenza		
Treponema pallidum	Adenovirus		
Corynebacterium bovis	Rickettsial scrub typhus		
Actinobacilli	Mumps		
Cat-scratch bacillus			

The authors proved in animal experiments that ESS implanted very early in the course of the disease on the glomerular basement membrane was identified with a fluorescent technique using anti-ESS antibodies. In the late course of the disease, the organism produced anti-ESS antibodies that coupled with ESS and thus enabled detection of the ESS. The two main drawbacks to this theory are (1) ESS is an anionic antigen, and its implantation on the GBM is not explained, and (2) injections of ESS have never induced histological changes and clinical features compatible with PSGN.

Vogt et al.[32] pointed out that cationic antigens were responsible for immunopathogenesis of PSGN; they identified cationic antigens in 8 of 18 biopsy specimens from PSGN patients and confirmed that streptococci cultured from PSGN patients produced cationic antigens. Later this antigen was confirmed to be streptococcal pyrogenic exotoxin B (zymogen) (SPEB). Besides SPEB, a plasmin-binding membrane receptor, the glyceraldehyde phosphate dehydrogenase (NAPlr/Plr, GAPDH), has also been considered as a serious candidate for the nephritogenic antigen.[26,] Both these antigens induce long-lasting antibody response, and antibodies against NaPlr can be detected 10 years after an acute episode; this explains why second attacks of PSGN are extremely rare. The common pathway for both antigens is plasmin binding, which activates complement, and promotes chemotaxis and degradation of GBM components. Nephritogenic potential is not limited to GABHS, but also includes groups C and G, as sporadic and epidemic cases of PSGN have also reported after infection with these streptococcal groups.

In a recent study, glomerular deposits and serum antibodies against these two putative antigens have been examined concurrently in biopsies and sera from the same PSGN patients.[35] The results of this study suggested that SPEB is the most likely major antigen involved in pathogenesis of PSGN.

Immune complexes deposited from the circulation or formed in situ activate the complement cascade that leads to production of various cytokines and other cellular immunity factors that initiate an inflammatory response manifested by cellular proliferation and edema of the glomerular tuft.[36,37]

In some PSGN patients rheumatoid factor, cryoglobulins, and antineutrophil cytoplasmic antibodies are present.[38-42] The significance of these autoimmune (epi)phenomena is not defined.

PATHOLOGY

The most typical feature observed via light microscopy is diffuse enlargement of all glomeruli due to hypercellularity (Figure 20-1). There is swelling of the endothelial cells that leads to the obliteration of the capillary loops. The number of mesangial cells is increased. There is recruitment of numerous inflammatory cells in the glomeruli, mainly polymorphonuclear leukocytes and monocytes; thus this pathological picture is termed exudative proliferative glomerulonephritis. If the mesangial proliferation is axial, the glomerulus has a lobular appearance. Capillary walls are not thickened. Arterioles and tubules are not affected, although polymorphonuclear leukocytes may be seen in the tubular lumen. Edema of the interstitium and infiltration with inflammatory cells may be found. Rarely, proliferation of parietal cells of Bowman's capsule may result in the formation of crescents; if the proportion of crescents is high, the disease may run a rapidly progressive course.

With the use of immunofluorescent study, irregular granular deposits of complement and immunoglobulins may be

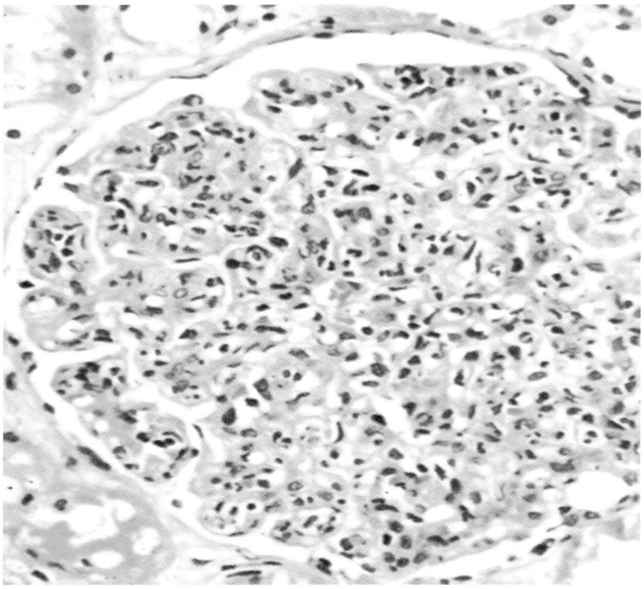

Figure 20-1 Acute poststreptococcal glomerulonephritis. The glomerulus is enlarged and hypercellular, capillary loops are obliterated, and there is infiltration with polymorphonuclear leukocytes (hematoxylin and eosin, ×400).

demonstrated in glomeruli (Figure 20-2). The most common finding is the presence of C3 and IgG, but C4, C1q, IgM, fibrinogen, and factor B may be found. Sorger et al. described three types of immune deposits in PSGN.[43] Starry sky is the fine granular deposition of C3 and IgG along the capillary walls in the first week of the disease (Figure 20-2A). Mesangial pattern is found between the 4th and 6th week after disease onset; the only immune reactant is C3, which is found in mesangial location. Garland type is characterized by dense, confluent deposits along the capillary loops, while mesangial and endocapillary locations are preserved (Figure 20-2B). Subepithelial location of the deposits correlates with the humps seen via electron microscopy. Garland type is associated with massive proteinuria and does not correlate with the time of renal biopsy.[44]

The typical finding in the acute phase of the disease seen via electron microscopy is deposits on the subepithelial side of the GBM (humps) (Figure 20-3). These deposits disappear after the 6th week from disease onset.[45]

With clinical resolution of the disease, there is marked change in the histological picture with resolution of exudative and endocapillary changes; in the convalescent phase, there is still mesangial proliferation (resolving mesangioproliferative glomerulonephritis). As already mentioned, subepithelial deposits disappear or their number significantly diminishes after the 6th week; the same happens with immune deposits. It takes usually 1 year for complete normalization of histological findings.

CLINICAL FEATURES

The latent period is usually 10 to 14 days after pharyngitis/angina or 2 to 3 weeks after pyoderma. One-third of APSGN

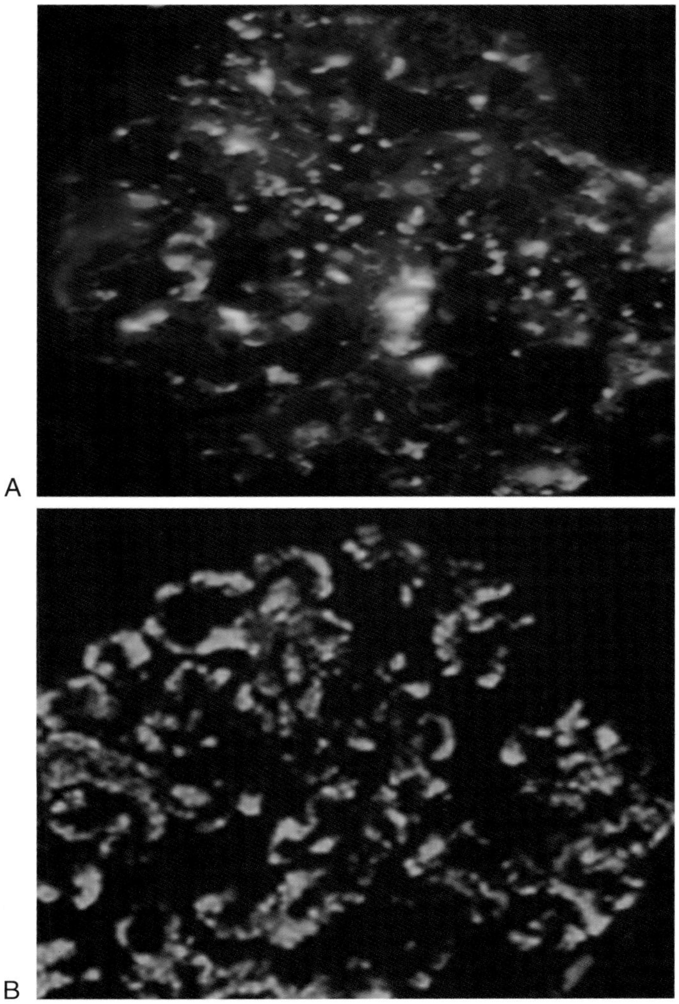

Figure 20-2 Immunofluorescent study in acute poststreptococcal glomerulonephritis showing intensive immune deposition of C3. **A,** Starry-sky pattern (×400). **B,** Garland pattern (×400). (Courtesy of M. Polenakovic, Department of Nephrology, University Clinical Center, Skopje, Macedonia.)

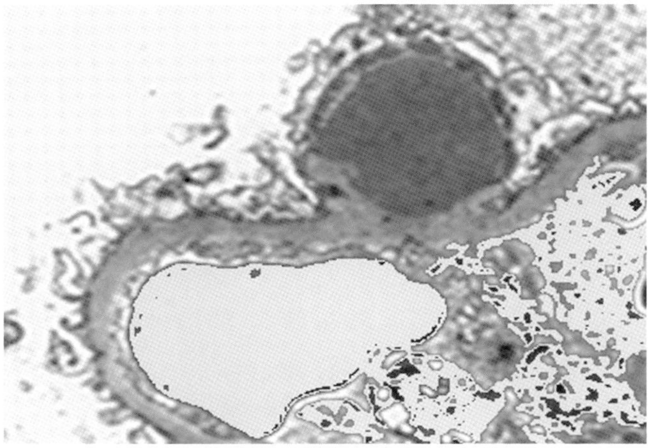

Figure 20-3 Acute poststreptococcal glomerulonephritis. A typical dense deposit (hump) located on the subepithelial side of the glomerular basement membrane (electron micrograph, ×8000).

patients develop discrete microscopic hematuria and/or proteinuria in the latent period. Usually the disease has sudden onset with development of nephritic syndrome (edema, oliguria, azotemia, hematuria, hypertension). At the onset of the disease, initial nonspecific symptoms may be present, such as pallor, malaise, low-grade fever, lethargy, anorexia, and headache.

If a child with upper respiratory tract infection develops nephritic signs after 2 to 3 days, pathology other than PSGN should be suspected (e.g., IgA nephropathy, or Alport syndrome).

Gross hematuria is present in 30% to 70% of patients with PSGN, while microscopic hematuria is present in all patients. Microscopic examination of the urine reveals the presence of dysmorphic red blood cells and casts. The urine is described as being smoky, cola colored, tea colored, or rusty. Gross hematuria may last a few hours during the day. Usually it resolves after 1 to 2 weeks and transforms into microscopic hematuria. Once gross hematuria has resolved, relapses may appear after physical exercise or intercurrent infections. Anecdotally, a few patients had minimal urinary findings (few red blood cells per high-power field), which contrasted with a severe clinical presentation of the disease.[46,47]

Edema in PSGN results from retention of salt and water. Edema is not often recognized by parents, but it becomes obvious that a child had significant edema in the diuretic phase when there is marked weight loss. Most children have mild morning periorbital edema. Also edema may be located in the pretibial area and may be generalized (anasarca) with presence of pleural effusion and ascites. When careful restriction of water and salt is undertaken early, edema as well as circulatory congestion and hypertension may be prevented.

Hypertension is the third cardinal sign in PSGN, and is found in up to 70% of hospitalized children. Hypertension in PSGN is the low-renin type due to retention of water and salt, which leads to expansion of the extracellular fluid volume with consequent suppression of the renin-angiotensin-aldosterone axis. Usually it is mild and has a biphasic character. If hypertension is severe and associated with retinal changes, preexisting renal disease should be suspected. Normalization of the blood pressure correlates with increased diuresis and recovery of renal function. If elevated blood pressure persists 4 weeks after disease onset, rapidly progressive disease or chronic glomerulonephritis should be suspected.

COMPLICATIONS

Circulatory congestion is the most common complication in hospitalized children with PSGN. If severe, it can lead to pulmonary edema which represents an emergency state and requires prompt and appropriate therapy. The signs of circulatory congestions are tachycardia, dyspnea, orthopnea, and cough. On auscultation, pulmonary rales may be audible. Sometimes clinical signs may be subtle, but chest radiograph shows signs of congestion. Since children and youths typically have healthy cardiovascular systems, cardiac failure is rarely seen.

Hypertensive encephalopathy is another serious complication found in 0.5% to 10% of hospitalized patients.[8] The most common clinical signs are nausea, vomiting, headache, and impairment of consciousness that varies from somnolence to coma. The children may manifest seizures, hemiparesis, amaurosis, and aphasia. These symptoms are a consequence of sudden elevation of the blood pressure, which impairs cerebral autoregulation leading to vasogenic edema. EEG recordings show nonspecific changes, which resolve in parallel with resolution of the neurological symptoms. Analysis of the cerebrospinal fluid may reveal increased protein but no cellular elements. Nuclear magnetic resonance imaging shows typical alteration of the posterior white matter, which is termed reversible posterior leukoencephalopathy syndrome.[48] Neurological complication in PSGN cannot be attributed exclusively to hypertensive encephalopathy or abnormal serum biochemistry, particularly in patients with normal blood pressure during the accident (e.g., seizure). With advances in neuroimaging techniques, there is clear evidence that some children develop cerebral vasculitis.[49,50] This has practical implications because of varying treatment modalities.

The third serious complication in PSGN is acute renal failure characterized by oliguria to anuria, severe azotemia, and acid–base and electrolyte disturbances. Hyperkalemia may be a fatal complication due to cardiovascular effects, and requires urgent conservative treatment and dialysis.

CLINICAL VARIANTS

Rodriguez-Iturbe[8] estimates that clinical PSGN represents only 10% of all cases, while 90% of cases develop subclinical disease and thus escape medical attention due to absence of symptoms. Nephrotic syndrome (0.4%) and rapidly progressive disease (0.1%) are rare presentations. The incidence of subclinical disease (expressed as the ratio subclinical to clinical disease) varies from 0.03 to 19.0.[51,52] This difference is most likely due to the applied methodology and the type of population studied—epidemic contacts,[19] family contacts,[51,53,54] or patients with well-documented streptococcal infections.[52,55] The incidence also depends on whether the population at risk was tested for urinary abnormalities and hypocomplementemia once or sequentially; the latter increases the chance of detecting urinary abnormalities and hypocomplementemia, which may be transitory and normalize within a week.

In an excellent study by Sagel et al.,[52] 248 children from various locales in New York State had been followed 4 to 6 weeks after well-documented streptococcal infection.[52] Twenty children displayed abnormal urinalysis and hypocomplementemia and only one of these children had symptomatic disease. The incidence of nephritis after streptococcal infection in this report was 8.08%, and the ratio of subclinical/clinical nephritis was 19.0. Renal biopsy was performed in all 20 children and showed histological lesions varying from mild focal cellular proliferation to classical exudative and proliferative glomerulonephritis. Only one child had normal histology and lack of immune deposits. The authors concluded that in clinical practice only a minority of PSGN cases (clinical) are detected ("the tip of the iceberg").

Yoshizawa et al.[55] performed a similar study in Japan; 12 out of 49 patients with well-documented streptococcal infection developed subclinical nephritis (24%) and all 12 patients had abnormal renal biopsies.

In a study of family contacts in Macedonia, the incidence of nephritis in parents and siblings was 0% and 9.4%, respectively.[54] It seems that parents are "protected" from developing PSGN. The ratio of subclinical to clinical nephritis in contacts was 1.28. Additional family contacts had glomerular-type microhematuria and elevated ASO titer; thus, one may speculate that they also had subclinical PSGN and that their complement levels normalized before the occurrence of nephritis in index cases. Lange et al.[29,56] pointed out that the finding of significant titers of endostreptosin antibodies in patients with chronic glomerulonephritis or on hemodialysis suggested the possibility of previously undetected subclinical PSGN.

Nephrotic syndrome may be seen in 4% to 25% of hospitalized children with PSGN. It usually resolves within 2 to 3 weeks; if the syndrome persists beyond this period it is associated with an unfavorable outcome of the disease. Less than 1% of hospitalized children develop rapidly progressive disease, which is characterized by prolonged oligo-anuria, uremia, hypertension, anemia, and persistent nephrotic syndrome. On renal biopsy, crescentic nephritis is found, and the percentage of crescents correlates with the severity of the disease and final outcome.

As already mentioned a few patient may develop cerebral vasculitis; cutaneous and gastrointestinal vasculitis have also been reported in PSGN patients and may mimic Henoch-Schönlein purpura.[57] In a very few cases, PSGN may be associated with rheumatic fever.[58,59] An unusual or atypical course of the disease is reported in patients with concurrent IgA nephropathy, diabetes mellitus, hemolytic uremic syndrome, reflux nephropathy, and bilateral renal hypoplasia.[60-63] Simultaneous occurrence of acute thrombocytopenic purpura has also been reported in a few PSGN patients.[64,65] The most likely mechanism is production of autoantibodies cross-reactive against GABHS and against platelets.[65]

LABORATORY FINDINGS

Proteinuria and hematuria are found in almost all patients with PSGN. The presence of red blood cell casts and dysmorphic erythrocytes points to a glomerular origin of hematuria. In a few patients, minimal urinary findings contrast with the severe clinical presentation.

A mild dilutional anemia may be seen at the onset of the disease, and is due to expansion of the extracellular fluid volume. Thrombocytopenia is extremely rare and its presence suggests systemic lupus erythematosus or hemolytic uremic syndrome. If there is no significant impairment of glomerular filtration rate (GFR), blood chemistry is almost normal. A severe reduction of renal function leads to hyperkalemia, uremia, and acidosis. Hypoproteinemia, hypoalbuminema, and hyperlipidemia are evident in the event of associated nephrotic syndrome. Evidence for previous streptococcal infection should be sought in all patients.

Cultures from the throat or skin should be obtained depending on the site of the initial infection. Antibodies against streptococcal antigens (antistreptolysin O, antihyaluronidase, antiDNA-se B titer), or a combination of antigens (streptozyme) should be measured serially during the course of the disease. Of note in postpyodermic disease is an insignificant rise in antistreptolysin O titers. Testing with antizymogen titers is very sensitive and specific for diagnosing streptococcal infection in PSGN patients, but this test is not available for routine practice. In addition, high titer of antibodies against glyceraldehydes phosphate dehydrogenase is found in PSGN patients.

Complement Studies

There is marked depression of serum hemolytic component CH50 and C3 due to activation of the alternative pathway. In some patients, there is also depression of C2 and C4 fractions, which suggests activation of both classical and alternative pathways.[66] Typically, complement levels normalize in 6 to 8 weeks. If hypocomplementemia persists more than 3 months, an alternative diagnosis, such as membranoproliferative glomerulonephritis, should be strongly considered.

Recently, Kozyro et al.[67] tested children with PSGN for presence of antibodies against C1q, and found that 8 of 24 were positive for anti-C1q. The anti–C1q-positive children had more a severe clinical presentation with hypertension, proteinuria, and unfavorable resolution of the disease.

RENAL BIOPSY AND DIFFERENTIAL DIAGNOSIS

In the majority of cases of PSGN, the course of the disease is typical with favorable outcome, so that renal biopsy is not necessary. If the clinical presentation is atypical and resolution of the disease delayed, then renal biopsy is mandatory. Indications for renal biopsy are given in Table 20-2.

PSGN should be differentiated from the following diseases: IgA nephritis (short latent period), hereditary nephritis (family history, short latent period), membranoproliferative glomerulonephritis (persistent hypocomplementemia and unresolving nephritic syndrome), lupus nephritis (persistent hypocomplementemia, systemic manifestation), glomerulonephritis in acute and chronic infections (evidence for other nonstreptococcal infection), vasculitides (polyarteritis nodosa, Henoch Schönlein purpura), and hemolytic-uremic syndrome (hemolysis, thrombocytopenia).

TABLE 20-2 **Indications for Renal Biopsy**

Early Stage	Recovery Phase
Short latent period	Depressed GFR >4 weeks
Severe anuria	Hypocomplementemia >12 weeks
Rapid progressive course	Persistent proteinuria >6 months
Hypertension >2 weeks	Persistent microhematuria >18 months
Depressed GFR >2 weeks	
Normal complement levels	
Nonsignificant titres of antistreptococcal antibodies	
Extrarenal manifestation	

TREATMENT

Bed rest and limited activity are indicated in the early stage of the disease, particularly if circulatory overload and hypertension are present. There is no evidence that prolonged bed rest hastens recovery.

In most cases, fluid and salt restriction are sufficient to prevent edema and hypertension. Salt intake should be limited to less than 1.0 g/day. Usually protein intake should be limited to 1.0 g/kg/day. In case of marked azotemia, calories should be provided from carbohydrates and fats. It is essential to individualize the diet according to clinical and biochemical indices. Diuresis and body weight should be monitored every day. Loop diuretics (furosemide 1-2 mg/kg/day) are indicated if there is moderate circulatory congestion. Higher doses up to 5 mg/kg per intravenous (IV) dose are indicated if there is pulmonary edema. Particular caution is necessary for patients with severe azotemia because of potential furosemide ototoxicity.

Moderate hypertension should be treated with diuretics and oral antihypertensive drugs (nifedipine, hydralazine, prazosin). Although short treatment with captopril is promising in controlling hypertension, this may worsen hyperkalemia.[68] In a hypertensive emergency, the drug of choice is labetalol 0.5-1.0 mg/kg/hour IV. An alternative emergency drug is diazoxide 2-3 mg/kg IV slowly over 30 minutes or nitroprusside 0.5-2 mcg/kg/min IV. Short-acting nifedipine (0.25-0.5 mg/kg/dose) administered by the oral/sublingual route was very popular for hypertensive emergencies in patients without encephalopathy. Because serious or fatal adverse effects have been reported in adults, it should be administered in children with great caution.[69]

Hyperkalemia should be prevented by restricting potassium intake. If present, conservative treatment should be started immediately to prevent fatal complications. Severe hyperkalemia, azotemia, acidosis, uncontrolled hypertension, cardiovascular insufficiency, and pulmonary edema are indications for immediate dialysis.

Digoxin is not indicated in patients with cardiovascular insufficiency since it accumulates in renal failure. Children with pre-existing cardiac disease should continue digitalization and adjust the dose according to the level of renal dysfunction.

There is no clear evidence that immunosuppressive therapy has a beneficial effect in children with crescentic PSGN. In those with over 30% crescents may be treated with pulse methylprednisolone 0.5-1.0 g/1.73 m^2 for 3 to 5 days. In a study by Roy et al.,[70] 5 of 10 children with crescentic PSGN were given quintuple therapy (including immunosuppressive drugs) and 5 were given only supportive treatment. At the end of the follow-up, there was no significant advantage to any of the treatment options; a benefit of quintuple treatment was faster normalization of serum creatinine and shortening of the hospital stay. When there is acute renal failure and crescents on biopsy, corticosteroids, methylprednisolone pulses, and cyclophosphamide may be beneficial.[5]

Antibiotic therapy is indicated if there are still signs of streptococcal infection (pharyngitis, pyoderma) or patients have a positive throat or skin culture. Oral penicillin V (or erythromycin for allergic patients) is preferred over parenteral treatment. Antibiotic treatment does not alter the course of the disease, but it is very important in preventing the spread of nephritogenic strains of GABHS to close contacts. Long-term antibiotic prophylaxis is not justified since second attacks of PSGN are very rare.[71]

PROGNOSIS

There is general agreement that the prognosis of PSGN in children in the acute phase is excellent, with mortality of less than 1% due to improved conservative management and availability of dialysis. Concerning the medium- and long-term outcomes, the data are inconsistent, ranging from unfavorable outcomes in the Baldwin et al.[72,73] series to excellent outcomes reported by Potter et al.[74] This is mainly due to different selection criteria for patients included in prognostic studies as elegantly discussed by Cameron.[75] When comparing results, one should bear in mind that only clinical cases (10%) are included in the analysis, while those with subclinical and mild disease may escape clinicians' attention. Of those who go to the doctor, only a minority with severe clinical presentation are referred to the nephrologist for biopsy. The series mentioned above differs vis-a-vis the following parameters: pediatric/adult, sporadic/epidemic, evidence/no evidence for previous streptococcal infection, with/without renal biopsy, and with/without crescents on renal biopsy.

In a study by Vogl et al.,[76] 36 children and 101 adults had biopsy and serological confirmation of PSGN and had been followed for 2 to 13 years. None of these children reached end-stage renal disease, but 10% had elevated serum creatinine between 1 and 2 mg/dl. Clark et al.[77] provided excellent data concerning the long-term outcome of PSGN in children. Although their series was small, it was exclusively pediatric with adequate documentation of streptococcal infection and initial biopsy in all children and re-biopsies in some of them. Thirty children had been followed up from 14.6 to 22 years (mean 19 years). Urinary abnormalities were found in 20% of patients during the follow-up, but none had reduced GFR, as assessed by creatinine clearance. Clark et al.[77] questioned the role of renal biopsy for diagnosis and follow-up of children with typical PSGN.

As already mentioned, Baldwin et al.[72,73] reported unfavorable data on the long-term prognosis of PSGN. In their series, 37 of 126 patients were children; 11 patients progressed to terminal uremia, and 9 of these in the first 6 months. During the follow-up of 2 to 15 years, proteinuria, hypertension, and reduced GFR were documented in half of the patients. A total of 174 renal biopsies were obtained. In the first years after the acute episode, proliferative changes were prevalent, while sclerosing lesions were found in two-thirds of the late biopsies, which Baldwin et al.[72,73] considered to be an indicator of chronicity. The results of this study were criticized because it was a highly selected patient population, 20% of whom presented with nephrotic syndrome. Patients who died or rapidly progressed to uremia had crescentic nephritis on biopsy, and a substantial number of patients were lost during the follow-up, with selection of those who had more severe disease. Furthermore, GFR in this study was not corrected for gender, age, and body surface area. The same group reported six patients with PSGN who progressed to terminal uremia 2 to 12 years after resolution of acute nephritis and normalization of the GFR.[78] Of note, five of these six patients had nephrotic syndrome at the disease onset. In addition, Gallo et al.[79] presented data on the morphologic alteration in renal biopsies from patients who recovered from PSGN and found that the incidence of glomerular and vascular sclerosis increased with time.[79] The clinical consequence of this healing process is reduced renal functional reserve after a protein-loading test.[80,81]

Two studies from Maracaibo, Venezuela, also pointed to the progressive character of PSGN.[82,83] A total of 120 (101 children) who had survived the epidemics in 1968 were evaluated between 1973 and 1975. Proteinuria, microhematuria, hypertension, or reduced GFR were found in 36.7% of adult patients compared with 8.7% of pediatric patients. Renal biopsies showed advanced glomerulosclerosis in all patients with abnormal findings. Mild to moderate mesangial proliferation and glomerulosclerosis were observed even in those patients without functional abnormality. In contrast to these reports, Dodge et al.[84] and Travis et al.[85] reported excellent clinical and histological healing of the disease in their pediatric series. Dodge et al.[84] found that the presence of proteinuria was associated with histological abnormality, and that proteinuria was orthostatic before it finally cleared. In a Macedonian study, 40 postnephritic children were investigated 3 months to 10 years after the acute episode, but no increase in proteinuria was found after moderate to strenuous physical activity.[86] Perlman et al.[87] reevaluated 61 children 10 years after an epidemic in 1963.[87] All children had normal GFR, 3 had proteinuria greater than 100 mg/24 hours, but all had normal morphology on renal biopsy. A total of 16 children had renal biopsies, four of whom had minimal focal proliferation, but no sclerosing lesions were seen.

Three studies from Trinidad evaluated medium- and long-term prognoses of PSGN. These are the largest predominantly pediatric studies as of this writing, and all reported excellent results concerning levels of urinary abnormalities, hypertension, or impaired renal function.[74,88,89] Many studies did not include renal biopsy for diagnosis and follow-up of PSGN in children, but the diagnosis was based on firm clinical and serological documentation of previous streptococcal infection as well as transitory hypocomplementemia. Results of these studies unquestionably confirmed the benign course of PSGN in children with a very low percent of urinary abnormalities, hypertension, or reduced GFR.[90-92] Besides clinical healing, there was complete functional recovery in almost all patients, and Drukker et al.[93] found that natriuretic response was excellent in postnephritic children after IV saline loading.

Unlike the typical PSGN due to GABH streptococci, the prognosis of PSGN caused by group C *Streptococcus zooepidemicus* is not as promising. An average 5.4 years following epidemics in Brazil, a relatively high percent of patients had increased microalbuminuria, hypertension, and reduced GFR.[94] Since only a few children were evaluated in this study, conclusions could not be drawn for this age group.

Based on various studies, the following risk factors for an unfavorable outcome were identified: older age, high serum creatinine at presentation, and nephrotic syndrome and crescents on renal biopsy. Even after initial normalization of renal function, impairment of the GFR may ensue many years after disease onset; thus, children who present with crescents need indefinite follow-up.[95]

REFERENCES

1. Sulyok E: Acute proliferative glomerulonephritis. In Avner ED, Harmon WE, Niaudet P, editors: *Pediatric nephrology*, ed 5, Philadelphia, 2004, Lippincott, Williams and Wilkins, pp. 601-13.
2. Forrest JW, John F, Mills LR, et al: Immune complex glomerulonephritis associated with Klebsiella pneumonia infection, *Clin Nephrol* 7:76-80, 1977.
3. Rainford DJ, Woodrow DF, Sloper JC, et al: Post meningococcal acute glomerulo-nephritis, *Clin Nephrol* 9:249-53, 1978.
4. Doregatti C, Volpi A, Torri Tarelli L, et al: Acute glomerulonephritis in human brucellosis, *Nephron* 41:365-66, 1983.
5. Sadikoglu B, Bilge I, Kilicaslan I, Gokce MG, et al: Crescentic glomerulonephritis in a child with infective endocarditis, *Pediatr Nephrol* 21:867-69, 20.
6. Ferrario F, Kourilsky O, Morel-Maroger L: Acute endocapillary glomerulonephritis: a histologic and clinical comparison between patients with and without acute renal failure, *Clin Nephrol* 19:17-23, 1983.
7. Moroni G, Pozzi C, Quaglini S, et al: Long-term prognosis of diffuse proliferative glomerulonephritis associated with infection in adults, *Nephrol Dial Transplant* 17:1204-11, 2002.
8. Rodriguez-Iturbe B: Acute poststreptococcal glomerulonephritis, In Schrier RW, Gottschalk CW, editors: *Diseases of the kidney*, Boston, 1988, Little, Brown, pp. 1929-47.
9. Meadow SR: Poststreptococcal glomerulonephtis—a rare disease? *Arch Dis Child* 50:379-82, 1975.
10. Yap H, Chia K, Murugasu B, et al: Acute glomerulonephritis-changing patterns in Singapore children, *Pediatr Nephrol* 4:482-84, 1990.
11. Knuffash FA, Sharda DC, Majeed HA: Sporadic pharyngitis-associated acute poststreptococcal glomerulonephritis, *Clin Pediatr* 25:181-84, 1986.
12. Sarkissian A, Papazian M, Azatian G, Arikiants N, et al: An epidemic of acute postinfectious glomerulonephritis in Armenia, *Arch Dis Child* 77:342-44, 1997.
13. Majeed HA, Khuffash FA, Sharda DC, Farwana SS, et al: Children with acute rheumatic fever and acute poststreptococcal glomerulonephritis and their families in a subtropical zone: a three-year prospective comparative epidemiological study, *Int J Epidemiol* 16:561-68, 1987.
14. Streeton CL, Hanna JN, Messer RD, Merianos A: An epidemic of acute post-streptococcal glomerulonephritis among aboriginal children, *J Paediatr Child Health* 31:245-48, 1995.
15. Leung DTY, Tseng RYM, Go SH, et al: Post-streptococcal glomerulonephritis in Hong Kong, *Arch Dis Child* 198762:1075-76, 1987.
16. Margolis HS, Lum MKW, Bender TR, et al: Acute glomerulonephritis and streptococcal skin lesions in Eskimo children, *Am J Dis Child* 134:681-85, 1980.
17. Svartman M, Potter EV, Poon-King T, Earle DP: Streptococcal infection of scabetic lesions related to acute glomerulonephritis in Trinidad, *J Lab Clin Med* 81:182-93, 1973.
18. Li Volti S, Furnari ML, Garozzo R, et al: Acute poststreptococcal glomerulonephritis in an 8-month old girl, *Pediatr Nephrol* 7:737-39, 1993.
19. Anthony BF, Kaplan EL, Wannamaker LW, et al: Attack rates of acute nephritis after type 49 streptococcal infection of the skin and of the respiratory tract, *J Clin Invest* 48:1697-702, 1969.
20. Ahmed-Jushuf IH, Selby PL, Brownjohn AM: Acute post-streptococcal glomerulonephritis following ear piercing, *Postgrad Med J* 60 (699):73-74, 1984.
21. Tasic V, Polenakovic M. Acute poststreptococcal glomerulonephritis following circumcision, *Pediatr Nephrol* 15:274-75, 2000.

22. Sorof JM, Weidner N, Potter D, Portale AA: Acute poststreptococcal glomerulonephritis in a renal allograft, *Pediatr Nephrol* 9:317-20, 1995.
23. Gnann JW, Gray BM, Griffin FM, Dismukes WE: Acute glomerulonephritis following group G streptococcal infection, *J Infect Dis* 156:411-12, 1987.
24. Barnham M, Thornton T, Lange K: Nephritis caused by streptococcus zooepidemicus (Lancefield group C), *Lancet* I:945-48, 1983.
25. Yoshizawa N: Acute glomerulonephritis, *Intern Med* 39:687-94, 2000.
26. Rodriguez-Iturbe B: Nephritis-associated streptococcal antigens. Where are we now? *J Am Soc Nephrol* 15:1961-62, 2004.
27. Cronin W, Deol H, Azadegan A, Lange K: Endostreptosin: isolation of the probable immunogen of acute poststreptococcal glomerulonephritis (PSGN), *Clin Exp Immunol* 76:198-203, 1989.
28. Cronin WJ, Lange K: Immunologic evidence for the in situ deposition of a cytoplasmatic streptococcal antigen (endostreptosin) on the glomerular basement membrane in rats, *Clin Nephrol* 31:143-46, 1990.
29. Lange K, Selingson G, Cronin W: Evidence for the in situ origin of poststreptococcal glomerulonephritis: glomerular localization of endostreptosin and the clinical significance of the subsequent antibody response, *Clin Nephrol* 19:3-10, 1983.
30. Lange K, Ahmed U, Kleinberger H, Treser G: A hitherto unknown streptococcal antigen and its probable relation to acute poststreptococcal glomerulonephritis, *Clin Nephrol* 5:207-15, 1976.
31. Rodriguez-Iturbe B, Rabideau D, Garcia R, et al: Characterization of the glomerular antibody in acute poststreptococcal glomerulonephritis, *Ann Intern Med* 92:478-81, 1980.
32. Vogt A, Batsford S, Rodriguez-Iturbe B, Garcia R: Cationic antigens in poststreptococcal glomerulonephritis, *Clin Nephrol* 20:271-79, 1983.
33. Parra G, Rodriguez-Iturbe B, Batsford S, Vogt A, et al: Antibody to streptococcal zymogen in the serum of patients with acute glomerulonephritis: a multicentric study, *Kidney Int* 54:509-17, 1998.
34. Yoshizawa N, Yamakami K, Fujino M, Oda T, et al: Nephritis-associated plasmin receptor and acute glomerulonephritis: characterization of the antigen and associated immune response, *J Am Soc Nephrol* 15:1785-93, 2004.
35. Batsford SR, Mezzano S, Mihatsch M, Schiltz E, Rodriguez-Iturbe B. Is the nephritogenic antigen in post-streptococcal glomerulonephritis pyrogenic exotoxin B (SPE B) or GAPDH? *Kidney Int* 68:1120-29, 2005.
36. Soto HM, Parra G, Rodriguez-Iturbe B: Circulating levels of cytokines in poststreptococcal glomerulonephritis, *Clin Nephrol* 47:6-12, 1997.
37. Matsell DG, Wayatt RJ, Gaber LW: Terminal complement complexes in acute poststreptococcal glomerulonephritis, *Pediatr Nephrol* 8:671-77, 1994.
38. Garin E, Fenell R, Shulman S, et al: Clinical significance of the presence of cryoglobulins in patients with glomerulonephritis not associated with systemic disease, *Clin Nephrol* 13:5-11, 1980.
39. Mezzano S, Olavarria F, Ardiles L, Lopez MI: Incidence of circulating immune complexes in patients with acute postreptococcal glomerulonephritis and in patients with streptococcal impetigo, *Clin Nephrol* 26:61-65, 1986.
40. Sesso RC, Ramos OL, Pereira AB: Detection of IgG-rheumatoid factor in sera of patients with acute poststreptococcal glomerulonephritis and its relationship with circulating immunocomplexes, *Clin Nephrol* 25:55-60, 1986.
41. Villches AR, Williams DG: Persistent anti-DNA antibodies and DNA-anti-DNA complexes in post-streptococcal glomerulonephritis, *Clin Nephrol* 22:97-101, 1984.
42. Ardiles LG, Valderrama G, Moya P, Mezzano SA: Incidence and studies on antigenic specificities of antineutrophil-cytoplasmic autoantibodies (ANCA) in poststreptococcal glomerulonephritis, *Clin Nephrol* 47:1-5, 1997.
43. Sorger K, Gessler U, Hubner FK, et al: Subtypes of acute postinfectious glomerulo-nephritis. Synopsis of clinical and pathological features, *Clin Nephrol* 17:114-28, 1982.
44. Sorger K, Balun J, Hubner FK, et al: The garland type of acute postinfectious glomerulonephritis: morphological characteristics and follow-up studies, *Clin Nephrol* 20:17-26, 1983.
45. Tornroth T: The fate of subepithelial deposits in acute poststreptococcal glomerulonephritis, *Lab Invest* 35:461-74, 1976.
46. Cohen JA, Levitt MF: Acute glomerulonephritis with few urinary abnormalities. Report of two cases proved by renal biopsy, *N Engl J Med* 268:749-53, 1963.
47. Robson WL, Leung AK: Post-streptococcal glomerulonephritis with minimal abnormalities in the urinary sediment, *J Singapore Paediatr Soc* 34:232-34, 1992.
48. Fux CA, Bianchetti MG, Jakob SM, Remonda L: Reversible encephalopathy complicating post-streptococcal glomerulonephritis, *Pediatr Infect Dis J* 25:85-87, 2006.
49. Kaplan RA, Zwick DL, Hellerstein S, et al: Cerebral vasculitis in acute poststreptococcal glomerulonephritis, *Pediatr Nephrol* 7:194-96, 1993.
50. Rovang RD, Zawada ET Jr, Santella RN, Jaqua RA, et al: Cerebral vasculitis associated with acute post-streptococcal glomerulonephritis, *Am J Nephrol* 17:89-92, 1997.
51. Sharrett AR, Poon-King T, Potter EV, et al: Subclinical nephritis in South Trinidad, *Am J Epidemiol* 91:231-45, 1971.
52. Sagel I, Treser G, Ty A, et al: Occurrence and nature of glomerular lesions after group A streptococci infections in children, *Ann Intern Med* 79:492-99, 1973.
53. Rodriguez-Iturbe B, Rubio L, Garcia R: Attack rate of poststreptococcal glomerulonephritis in families. A prospective study, *Lancet* I:401-405, 1981.
54. Tasic V, Polenakovic M: Occurrence of subclinical post-streptococcal glomerulonephritis in family contacts, *J Paediatr Child Health* 39:177-79, 2003.
55. Yoshizawa N, Suzuki Y, Oshima S, et al: Asymptomatic acute poststreptococcal glomerulonephritis following upper respiratory tract infections caused by Group A streptococci, *Clin Nephrol* 46:296-301, 1996.
56. Lange K, Azadegan AA, Seligson G, Bovie RC, Majeed H: Asymptomatic poststreptococcal glomerulonephritis in relatives of patients with symptomatic glomerulonephritis. Diagnostic value of endostreptosin antibodies, *Child Nephrol Urol* 9:11-15, 1988-89.
57. Goodyer PR, de Chadarevian JP, Kaplan BS: Acute poststreptococcal glomerulonephritis mimicking Henoch-Schönlein purpura, *J Pediatr* 93:412-15, 1978.
58. Said R, Hussein M, Hassan A: Simultaneous occurrence of acute poststreptococcal glomerulonephritis and acute rheumatic fever, *Am J Nephrol* 6:146-48, 1986.
59. Matsell DG, Baldree LA, DiSessa TG, et al: Acute poststreptococcal glomerulonephritis and acute rheumatic fever: occurrence in the same patient, *Child Nephrol Urol* 10:112-14, 1990.
60. Hiki Y, Tamura K, Shigematsu H, Kobayashi Y: Superimposition of poststreptococcal acute glomerulonephritis on the course of IgA nephropathy, *Nephron* 57:358-64, 1991.
61. Chadaverian JP, Goodyer PR, Kaplan BS, et al: Acute glomerulonephritis and hemolytic uremic syndrome, *CMAJ* 123:391-94, 1980.
62. Sheridan RJ, Roy S, Stapleton BF: Reflux nephropathy complicated by acute post-streptococcal glomerulonephritis, *Intern J Pediatr Nephrol* 4:119-21, 1983.
63. Naito Yoshida Y, Hida M, Maruyama Y, Hori N, Awazu M. Post-streptococcal acute glomerulonephritis superimposed on bilateral renal hypoplasia, *Clin Nephrol* 63:477-80, 2005.
64. Kaplan BS, Esseltine D: Thrombocytopenia in patients with acute poststreptococcal glomerulonephritis, *J Pediatr* 93:974-76, 1978.
65. Tasic V, Polenakovic M: Thrombocytopenia during the course of acute poststreptococcal glomerulonephritis, *Turk J Pediatr* 45:148-51, 2003.
66. Wayatt RJ, Forristal J, West CD, et al: Complement profiles in acute poststreptococcal glomerulonephritis, *Pediatr Nephrol* 2:219-23, 1988.
67. Kozyro I, Perahud I, Sadallah S, Sukalo A, et al: Clinical value of autoantibodies against C1q in children with glomerulonephritis, *Pediatrics* 117:1663-68, 2006.
68. Parra G, Rodriguez-Iturbe B, Colina-Chourio J, Garcia R: Short term treatment with captopril in hypertension due to acute glomerulonephritis, *Clin Nephrol* 29:58-62, 1988.
69. Yiu V, Orrbine E, Rosychuk RJ, et al: The safety and use of short-acting nifedipine in hospitalized hypertensive children, *Pediatr Nephrol* 19:644-50, 2004.

70. Roy S, Murphy WM, Arant BS: Poststreptococcal crescentic glomerulonephritis in children: comparison of quintuple therapy versus supportive care, *J Pediatr* 98:403-10, 1981.
71. Roy S, Wall HP, Etteldorf JN: Second attacks of acute glomerulonephritis, *J Pediatr* 75:758-67, 1969.
72. Baldwin DS: Poststreptococcal glomerulonephritis. A progressive disease, *Am J Med* 62:1-11, 1977.
73. Baldwin DS, Gluck MC, Schacht RG, Gallo G: The long-term course of poststreptococcal glomerulonephritis, *Ann Intern Med* 80:342-58, 1974.
74. Potter E, Lipschultz SA, Abidh S, et al: Twelve- to seventeen-year follow-up of patients with poststreptococcal acute glomerulonephritis in Trinidad, *N Engl J Med* 307:725-30, 1982.
75. Cameron JS: The long-term outcome of glomerular disease. In Schrier RW, Gottschalk CW, editors: *Diseases of the kidney*, 3 vols, Boston, 1988, Little, Brown, pp. 2127-89.
76. Vogl W, Renke M, Mayer-Eichberger D, et al: Long term prognosis for endocapillary glomerulonephritis of poststreptococcal type in children and adults, *Nephron* 44:58-65, 1986.
77. Clark G, White R, Glasgow EF, et al: Poststreptococcal glomerulonephritis in children: clinicopathological correlations and long term prognosis, *Pediatr Nephrol* 2:381-88, 1988.
78. Schacht RG, Gluck MC, Gallo GR, et al: Progression to uremia after remission of acute poststreptococcal glomerulonephritis, *N Engl J Med* 295:977-81, 1976.
79. Gallo GR, Feiner HD, Steele JM, et al: Role of intrarenal vascular sclerosis in progression of poststreptococcal glomerulonephritis, *Clin Nephrol* 13:49-57, 1980.
80. Rodriguez-Iturbe B, Herrera J, Garcia R: Response to acute protein load in kidney donors and in apparently normal postacute glomerulonephritis patients: evidence for glomerular hyperfiltration, *Lancet* II:461-64, 1985.
81. Cleper R, Davidovitz M, Halevi R, Eisenstein B: Renal functional reserve after acute poststreptococcal glomerulonephritis, *Pediatr Nephrol* 11:473-76, 1997.
82. Rodriguez-Iturbe B, Garcia R, Rubio L, et al: Epidemic glomerulonephritis in Maracaibo. Evidence for progression to chronicity, *Clin Nephrol* 5:197-206, 1976.
83. Garcia R, Rubio L, Rodriguez-Iturbe B: Long-term prognosis of epidemic poststreptococcal glomerulonephritis in Maracaibo: follow-up studies 11-12 years after the acute episode, *Clin Nephrol* 15:291-98, 1981.
84. Dodge WF, Spargo BH, Travis LB, et al: Poststreptococcal glomerulonephritis. A prospective study in children, *N Engl J Med* 286:273-78, 1971.
85. Travis LB, Dodge WF, Beathard GA, et al: Acute glomerulonephritis in children. A review of the natural history with emphasis on prognosis, *Clin Nephrol* 1:169-81, 1973.
86. Tasic V, Korneti P, Gucev Z, Korneti B: Stress tolerance test and SDS-PAGE for the analysis of urinary proteins in children and youths, *Clin Chem Lab Med* 39:478-83, 2001.
87. Perlman LV, Herdman RC, Kleinman H, Vernier RL: Poststreptococcal glomerulo-nephritis. A ten-year follow-up of an epidemic, *JAMA* 194:63-70, 1965.
88. Potter EV, Abidh S, Sharrett AR, et al: Clinical healing two to six years after poststreptococcal glomerulonephritis in Trinidad, *N Engl J Med* 298:767-72, 1978.
89. Nissenson AR, Mayon-White R, Potter EV, et al: Continued abscence of clinical renal disease seven to twelve years after poststreptococcal acute glomerulonephritis in Trinidad, *Am J Med* 67:255-62, 1979.
90. Popovic-Rolovic M, Kostic M, Antic-Peco A, et al: Medium- and long-term prognosis of patients with acute poststreptococcal glomerulonephritis, *Nephron* 58:393-99, 1991.
91. Tasic V, Polenakovic M, Kuzmanovska D, Sahpazova E, Ristoska N: Prognosis of poststreptococcal glomerulonephritis five to fifteen years after an acute episode, *Pediatr Nephrol* 12:C167, 1998.
92. Kasahara T, Hayakawa H, Okubo S, et al: Prognosis of acute poststreptococcal glomerulonephritis (APSGN) is excellent in children, when adequately diagnosed, *Pediatr Int* 43:364-67, 2001.
93. Drukker A, Pomeranz A, Reichenberg J, Mor J, Stankiewicz H: Natriuretic response to i.v. saline loading after acute poststreptococcal glomerulonephritis, *Isr J Med Sci* 22:779-82, 1986.
94. Sesso R, Wyton S, Pinto L: Epidemic glomerulonephritis due to *Streptococcus zooepidemicus* in Nova Serrana, Brazil, *Kidney Int* Suppl 97:S132-36, 2005.
95. Tasic V, Polenakovic M, Cakalarovski K, Kuzmanovska D: Progression of crescentic poststreptococcal glomerulonephritis to terminal uremia twelve years after recovery from an acute episode, *Nephron* 79:496 (letter), 1988.

CHAPTER

21 Rapidly Progressive Glomerulonephritis

Arvind Bagga and Shina Menon

Rapidly progressive glomerulonephritis (RPGN) is a rare syndrome in children, characterized by clinical features of glomerulonephritis (GN) and rapid loss of renal function. Renal histology shows crescentic extracapillary proliferation in Bowman's space affecting the majority of glomeruli. This clinical course may be seen in any form of GN including poststreptococcal GN, renal vasculitis, IgA nephropathy, systemic lupus erythematosus (SLE), and membranoproliferative GN. RPGN is a medical emergency, which if untreated might rapidly progress to irreversible loss of renal function. Prompt evaluation and specific therapy are necessary to ensure satisfactory outcome in most cases.

DEFINITION

RPGN is a clinical syndrome characterized by an acute nephritic illness accompanied by a rapid loss of renal function (>50% decrease in GFR) over days to weeks.[1] The histopathological correlate is the presence of crescents (crescentic GN) involving 50% or more glomeruli. The presence of crescents is a histologic marker of severe glomerular injury, which may occur in a number of conditions including postinfectious GN, IgA nephropathy, SLE, renal vasculitis, and membranoproliferative GN.[1,2] The severity of clinical features correlates with the proportion of glomeruli that shows crescents. While patients with circumferential crescents involving more than 80% of glomeruli present with advanced renal failure, those with crescents in less than 50% of glomeruli, particularly if the crescents are noncircumferential, often have an indolent course.

While the terms RPGN and crescentic GN are used interchangeably, similar clinical presentation might occur in conditions without crescents, including hemolytic uremic syndrome (HUS), diffuse proliferative GN, and acute interstitial nephritis.

Table 21-1 lists common conditions that present with RPGN in children.

PATHOGENESIS OF CRESCENT FORMATION

Crescents are defined as the presence of two or more layers of cells in Bowman's space. The chief participants in formation of crescents are coagulation proteins, macrophages, T cells, fibroblasts, and parietal and visceral epithelial cells.[1,3] Perturbations of humoral immunity as well as the Th1 cellular immune response contribute to the pathogenesis.[1,2]

Initiating Events

The initial event in formation of crescents is the occurrence of a physical gap in the glomerular capillary wall and glomerular basement membrane (GBM), mediated by macrophages and T lymphocytes. Breaks in the integrity of the capillary wall lead to passage of inflammatory mediators and plasma proteins into the Bowman's space with fibrin formation, influx of macrophages and T cells, and release of proinflammatory cytokines, such as interleukin-1 (IL-1) and tumor necrosis factor-α (TNF-α). Similar breaks in the Bowman's capsule allow cells and mediators from the interstitium to enter Bowman's space and for contents of the latter to enter the interstitium, resulting in periglomerular inflammation.

Formation

The development of a crescent results from the participation of coagulation factors and various proliferating cells, chiefly macrophages, parietal glomerular epithelial cells, and interstitial fibroblasts. The presence of coagulation factors in the Bowman's space results in formation of a fibrin clot and recruitment of circulating macrophages. Activated neutrophils and mononuclear cells release procoagulant tissue factor, IL-1, TNF-α, serine proteinases (elastase, PR3), and matrix metalloproteinases. The proteases cause lysis of the GBM proteins and facilitate the entry of other mediators in the Bowman's space. Release of IL-1 and TNF-α results in upregulated expression of adhesion molecules, leading to macrophage recruitment and proliferation. Apart from macrophages, the other major cellular components of the crescents are proliferating parietal and visceral epithelial cells.[4]

Resolution of Crescents

The stage of inflammation is followed by the development of fibrocellular and fibrous crescents. The expression of fibroblast growth factors and transforming growth factor (TGF-β) is important for fibroblast proliferation and production of type I collagen, which is responsible for the transition from cellular to fibrocellular and fibrous crescents. The transition from cellular to fibrous crescents, which occurs over days, is clinically important since the latter is not likely to resolve following immunosuppressive therapy. The plasminogen-plasmin system is responsible for fibrinolysis and resolution of crescents.

TABLE 21-1 Causes of RPGN
Immune Complex GN
Postinfectious GN. Poststreptococcal nephritis, infective endocarditis, shunt nephritis, *Staphylococcus aureus* sepsis, other infections (e.g., HIV, hepatitis B and C, syphilis)
Systemic disease. Systemic lupus erythematosus, Henoch-Schönlein purpura, cryoglobulinemia, mixed connective tissue disorder, juvenile rheumatoid arthritis
Primary GN. IgA nephropathy, MPGN, membranous nephropathy, C1q nephropathy
Pauci-Immune Crescentic GN
Microscopic polyangiitis, Wegener's granulomatosis, renal limited vasculitis, Churg-Strauss syndrome
Idiopathic crescentic GN
Medications: penicillamine, hydralazine, hydrocarbons, propylthiouracil
Anti-GBM GN
Anti-GBM nephritis, Goodpasture's syndrome, Post Renal transplantation in Alport syndrome
Postrenal Transplantation
Recurrence of IgA nephropathy, Henoch-Schönlein purpura, MPGN, systemic lupus
RPGN without Crescents
Hemolytic uremic syndrome
Acute interstitial nephritis
Diffuse proliferative GN

GBM, Glomerular basement membrane; *GN,* glomerulonephritis; *HIV,* human immunodeficiency virus; *MPGN,* membranoproliferative GN.

CAUSES AND IMMUNOPATHOLOGIC CATEGORIES

Based on pathology and immunofluorescence-staining patterns, crescentic GN is classified into three categories that reflect various mechanisms of glomerular injury.[1]

Immune-complex GN with granular deposits of immune complexes along capillary wall and mesangium
Pauci-immune GN with scant or no immune deposits, and associated with systemic vasculitis
Anti-GBM GN with linear deposition of anti-GBM antibodies

Immune Complex Crescentic GN

These patients form a heterogeneous group in which multiple stimuli lead to proliferative GN with crescents. Immunohistology shows granular deposits of immunoglobulin and complement along capillary walls and in the mesangium. The causes include infections, systemic diseases, and pre-existing primary GN.

Systemic Infections

Poststreptococcal GN can rarely present with crescentic histology. While most patients recover completely, the presence of nephrotic-range proteinuria, sustained hypertension, and crescents is associated with an unsatisfactory outcome.[5,6] Other infectious illnesses associated with crescentic GN include infective endocarditis, infected atrioventricular shunts, and visceral abscesses. Crescentic GN associated with other infectious agents including methicillin-resistant *Staphylococcus aureus,* hepatitis B and C virus, leprosy, and syphilis are reported anecdotally.

Systemic Immune Complex Disease

Rapidly progressive glomerulonephritis with glomerular crescents might be seen in patients with class IV and, less commonly, class III lupus nephritis. Extensive crescent formation is associated with an unsatisfactory outcome in Henoch Schönlein purpura and rheumatoid arthritis.

Primary GN

Patients with IgA nephropathy, membranoproliferative GN, and rarely membranous nephropathy may present with rapid deterioration of renal function and crescentic GN.[5,7]

Pauci-Immune Crescentic GN

Microscopic polyangiitis, Wegener's granulomatosis, and renal limited vasculitis are characterized by small-vessel vasculitis; when involving glomerular capillaries, the vasculitis results in necrotizing crescentic GN with few or no immune deposits on immunofluorescence microscopy.[2,8] Most (80%) show antineutrophil cytoplasmic autoantibodies (ANCA) in blood.

The majority of patients with pauci-immune crescentic GN have or will develop clinical features of vasculitis. This variety of RPGN is considered a part of the Wegener's granulomatosis/microscopic polyangiitis spectrum, since the histological features are similar and some patients who present with renal-limited vasculitis might later show systemic vasculitis.[2] Some cases of ANCA-positive disease might be induced by drugs, including penicillamine, propylthiouracil, and hydralazine. Patients with ANCA-negative, pauci-immune RPGN should be considered part of this spectrum, since they show similar clinical and histological features and outcomes.[9]

Anti-GBM Crescentic GN

This condition is uncommon in childhood, accounting for less than 10% of cases in children.[1,5,10-12] The nephritogenic autoantibody is directed against a 28-kDa monomer located on the $\alpha 3$ chain of type IV collagen (Goodpasture antigen). Pulmonary involvement (Goodpasture syndrome) is uncommon.

Approximately 5% of patients with Alport syndrome who receive a renal allograft show anti-GBM autoantibodies and anti-GBM nephritis within the first year of the transplant.[13] Unlike de novo anti-GBM nephritis, pulmonary hemorrhage is not observed in post-transplant anti-GBM nephritis because the patient's lung tissue does not contain the putative antigen. The risk of post-transplantation anti-GBM nephritis is low in subjects with normal hearing, late-progression to end-stage renal disease, or females with X-linked Alport syndrome.

Idiopathic RPGN

This term denotes patients with immune complex crescentic GN who do not fit into any identifiable category, and those with pauci-immune disease that is ANCA-negative. The former is rare, while the latter accounts for less than 5% of cases of crescentic GN in children.

EPIDEMIOLOGY

The incidence of RPGN in children is not known. Crescentic GN comprises approximately 5% of unselected renal biopsies in children. While there are no population-based studies in children, a recent report from Romania suggested an annual incidence of 3.3 per million adult population.[14] The 2006 North American Pediatric Renal Trials and Collaborative Studies database shows that idiopathic crescentic GN contributes to 1.8% of all transplanted patients.[15] This figure is an underestimate since other conditions in the database, including membranoproliferative GN (2.7%), SLE (1.6%), systemic immune disorders (0.4%), Wegener's granulomatosis (0.5%), chronic glomerulonephritis (3.4%), and IgA nephropathy and Henoch Schönlein purpura (2.5%), might present as RPGN.

Table 21-2 outlines the underlying conditions in four large series of crescentic GN reported from India,[5] United States,[10] United Kingdom,[11] and France.[12] Immune complex GN is the most common pattern of crescentic GN in children accounting for over 75% to 80% of cases in most reports. Pauci-immune crescentic GN, while common in adults, is infrequent in children, accounting for 15% to 20% of cases. The decline in the incidence of postinfectious GN has resulted in a change in the etiological profile of crescentic GN, and a recent survey of 73 patients aged 1 to 20 years showed similar frequencies of immune complex (45%) and pauci-immune crescentic GN (42%).[1]

The severity of clinical, laboratory, and histological features at presentation varies with the underlying cause, the most severe being anti-GBM disease, followed by pauci-immune GN and finally immune complex crescentic GN.[1,16]

CLINICAL FEATURES

The presenting complaints in RPGN are similar to severe postinfectious GN with the course extending over several days. The spectrum of presenting features is variable, and includes macroscopic hematuria (in 60%-90% patients), oliguria (60%-100%), hypertension (60%-80%), and edema (60%-90%).[5,8,10] The illness may be complicated by the occurrence of hypertensive emergencies, pulmonary edema, and cardiac failure. Occasionally, RPGN has an insidious onset with the initial symptoms being fatigue or edema. Nephrotic syndrome is rare and seen in patients with less severe renal insufficiency.

Systemic complaints, involving the upper respiratory tract (cough, sinusitis), skin (vasculitic rash over lower limbs), musculoskeletal (joint pain, swelling), and/or the nervous system (seizures, altered sensorium) are common in patients with pauci-immune RPGN, with or without ANCA positivity. Relapses of systemic and renal symptoms occur in one-third of patients with vasculitis.[2,8]

Patients with anti-GBM antibody disease may present with hemoptysis and, less often, pulmonary hemorrhage. Similar complications may be found in Wegener's granulomatosis, SLE, Henoch-Schönlein purpura, and severe GN with pulmonary edema.

INVESTIGATIONS

Hematuria, characterized by dysmorphic red cells and red cell casts, is seen in all patients; most also have gross hematuria. A variable degree of nonselective proteinuria (2+ to 4+) is present in more than 65% of patients. Urinalysis also shows leukocyte, granular, and tubular epithelial cell casts.

Renal insufficiency is present at diagnosis in almost all cases, with the plasma creatinine concentration often exceeding 3 mg/dl (264 μmol/L). The degree of renal failure is usually more than that estimated by the serum creatinine. Anemia, if present, is mild; peripheral smear shows normocytic normochromic red cells. Microangiopathic hemolytic anemia with reticulocytosis, thrombocytopenia, and elevated blood levels of LDH are characteristic of HUS. Similar features may be seen in SLE with superimposed throm-

TABLE 21-2 Causes of Crescentic Glomerulonephritis in Children (%)

	SPNSG[10] (*n* = 50)	Srivastava et al.[5] (*n* = 43)	Niaudet, Levy[12] (*n* = 41)	Jardim et al.[11] (*n* = 30)
Immune complex disease				
Unspecified	26	—	4.8	—
Systemic lupus erythematosus	18	2.3	2.4	3.3
Poststreptococcal GN	12	25.5	12.1	6.6
Henoch-Schönlein purpura, IgA nephropathy	14	6.9	34.1	30
Membranoproliferative GN	4	—	21.9	23.3
Vasculitis	6	—	7.3	16.6
Idiopathic crescentic GN	14	60.4	7.3	13.3
Antiglomerular basement disease	6	2.3	7.3	6.6
Others	—	2.3	2.4	—

GN, Glomerulonephritis; *SPNSG*, Southwest Pediatric Nephrology Study Group.

botic microangiopathy. Nonspecific markers of inflammation including CRP and ESR may be elevated.

Serology

Serological investigations assist in evaluation of the cause and monitoring disease activity (Table 21-3) (Figure 21-1). Low levels of total hemolytic complement (CH50) and complement 3 (C3) are seen in postinfectious GN, SLE, and membranoproliferative GN, and inversely correlate with disease activity. Patients with SLE and type 1 membranoproliferative GN additionally show reduced levels of C1 and C4 due to activation of the classic complement pathway. Positive antistreptolysin O titers and anti–deoxyribonuclease B suggest streptococcal infection in the past 3 months. Patients with SLE show antinuclear (ANA) and anti–double-stranded DNA autoantibodies.

Elevated levels of ANCA suggest an underlying vasculitic cause, and are present in most patients with pauci-immune crescentic GN. Most ANCA have specificity for myeloperoxidase (MPO) or proteinase-3 (PR3). ANCA should be screened by indirect immunofluorescence and positive tests confirmed by both PR3-ELISA and MPO-ELISA. In patients with pauci-immune crescentic GN, negative results from indirect immunofluorescence should be tested by ELISA, because 5% of serum samples are positive only by the latter. Wegener's granulomatosis is usually associated with PR3 ANCA, which produces a cytoplasmic staining pattern on indirect immunofluorescence (c-ANCA). Renal limited vasculitis and drug induced pauci-immune crescentic GN are typically associated with MPO ANCA that shows perinuclear staining on indirect immunofluorescence (p-ANCA). Patients with microscopic polyangiitis have almost equal distribution of MPO ANCA/p-ANCA and PR3 ANCA/c-ANCA. Approximately 10% of patients with Wegener's granulomatosis or microscopic polyangiitis have negative assays for ANCA. The autoantibodies (usually p-ANCA) are also found in 20% to 30% patients with anti-GBM GN, and occasionally in idio-

TABLE 21-3 Diagnostic Evaluation of Patients with RPGN
Complete blood counts, peripheral smear for type of anemia, reticulocyte count
Blood levels of urea, creatinine, electrolytes, calcium, phosphate
Urinalysis: proteinuria, microscopy for erythrocytes and leukocytes, casts
Complement (C3, C4, CH50)
Antistreptolysin O, antinuclear antibody, anti–double-stranded DNA antibodies
Antinuclear cytoplasmic antibodies (ANCA)
Renal biopsy (light microscopy, immunofluorescence, electron microscopy)
Required in Specific Instances
Anti-GBM IgG antibodies
Blood levels of cryoglobulin, hepatitis serology
Chest: radiograph, CT (patients with Goodpasture's syndrome and vasculitides)
Sinuses: radiograph, CT (patients with Wegener's granulomatosis)

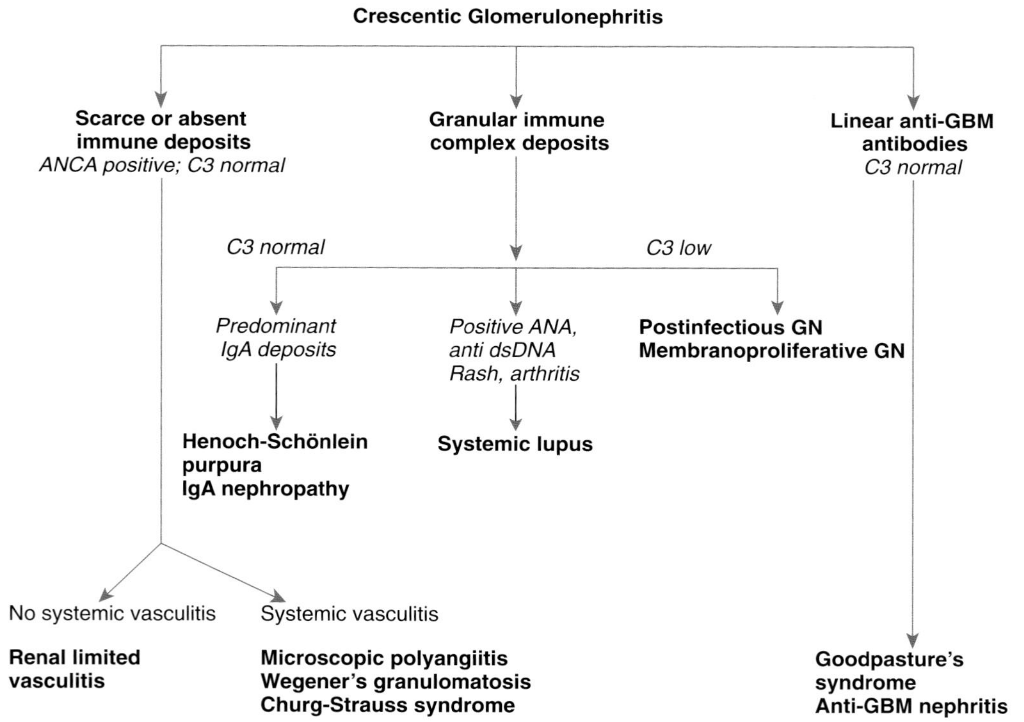

Figure 21-1 Diagnostic evaluation of crescentic glomerulonephritis, based on renal histology and serological findings.

pathic immune-complex RPGN, inflammatory bowel disease, rheumatoid arthritis, and SLE.[17]

Apart from diagnosis, ANCA titers have also been used for monitoring activity of systemic vasculitis. Persistent or reappearing ANCA positivity in patients in remission may be associated with disease relapse in ANCA-associated vasculitides. Similarly, the risk of relapse in patients who show persistently negative ANCA titers is low. However, it is proposed that an isolated rise in ANCA titers not be used for modifying treatment in patients with systemic vasculitis.[18] Patients with ANCA-associated crescentic GN in remission, with persistent or reappearing ANCA positivity or rise in its titer, should be closely followed up and diagnostic efforts intensified to detect and treat relapses.

High titers of anti-GBM IgG antibodies, demonstrated by immunofluorescence or ELISA, are seen in anti-GBM nephritis or Goodpasture's syndrome and correlate with disease activity. About 5% of ANCA positive samples are also anti-GBM positive and approximately 20% to 30% of anti–GBM-positive samples are ANCA positive. Serology for ANCA is therefore recommended in all patients with either anti-GBM antibodies in blood or linear IgG deposition along the GBM. The initial clinical outcome for these patients is similar to that of anti-GBM disease, although relapses may occur as in systemic vasculitis.[1]

Renal Histology

Light Microscopy

Renal histological findings in various forms of crescentic GN are similar. A glomerular crescent is an accumulation of two or more layers of cells that partially or completely fill the Bowman's space. The crescent size varies from circumferential to segmental depending on the plane of the tissue section and the underlying disease. Crescents in anti-GBM nephritis or ANCA-associated disease are usually circumferential, while they are often segmental in immune-complex GN. Interstitial changes range from acute inflammatory infiltrate to chronic interstitial scarring and tubular atrophy. Once the glomerular capillary loop is compressed by the crescent, tubules that derive their blood flow from that efferent arteriole show ischemic changes.

Crescents may be completely cellular or show variable scarring and fibrosis. Cellular crescents are characterized by proliferation of macrophages, epithelial cells, and neutrophils (Figure 21-2). Fibrocellular crescents show admixture of collagen fibers and membrane proteins among the cells (Figure 21-3). In fibrous crescents, the cells are completely replaced by collagen (Figure 21-4).

Renal biopsies from patients with vasculitis often show crescents in various stages of progression indicating episodic inflammation. Early lesions have segmental fibrinoid necrosis with or without an adjacent small crescent. Severe acute lesions show focal or diffuse necrosis in association with circumferential crescents. Features of small vessel vasculitis affecting interlobular arteries (Figure 21-5) and rarely angiitis involving the vasa recta might be seen.

Immunohistology and Electron Microscopy

These investigations assist in determining the cause of crescentic GN, based on presence, location, and nature of immune

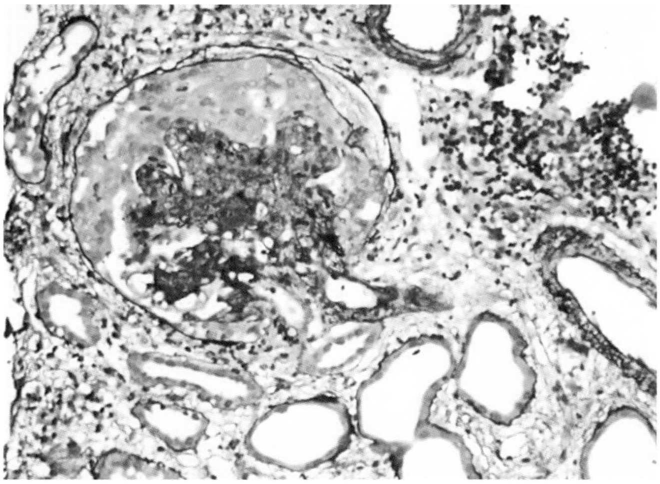

Figure 21-2 Cellular crescent compressing the glomerular tuft. Silver methanamine stain (×800).

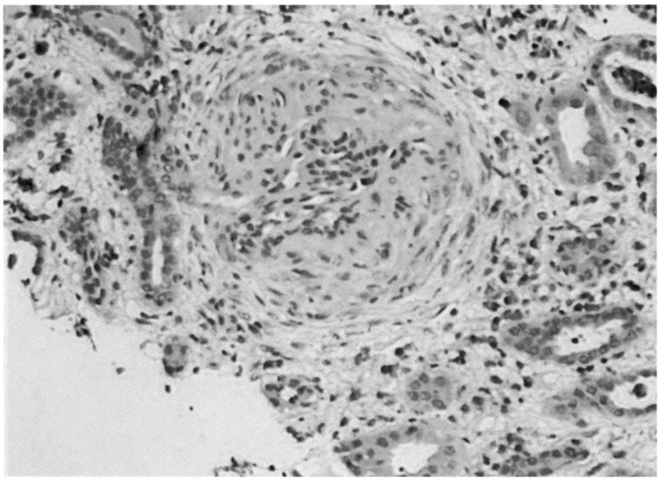

Figure 21-3 Fibrocellular crescent with compression of glomerular tuft and partial sclerosis. There is chronic interstitial inflammation, tubular atrophy, and interstitial fibrosis in surrounding area (H&E ×800).

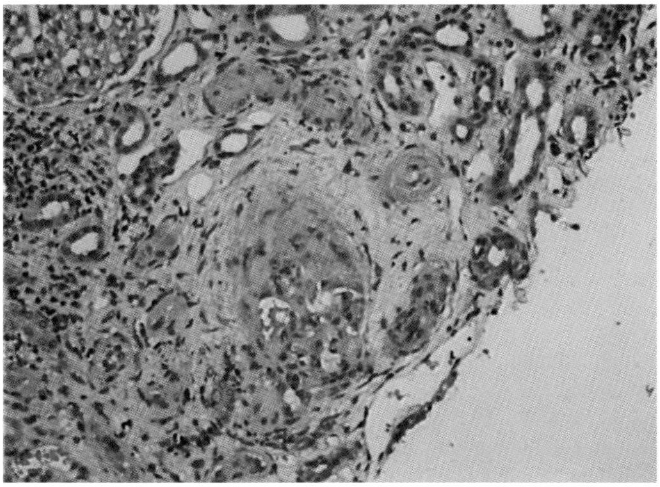

Figure 21-4 Fibrous crescent compressing glomerular tuft (H&E ×800).

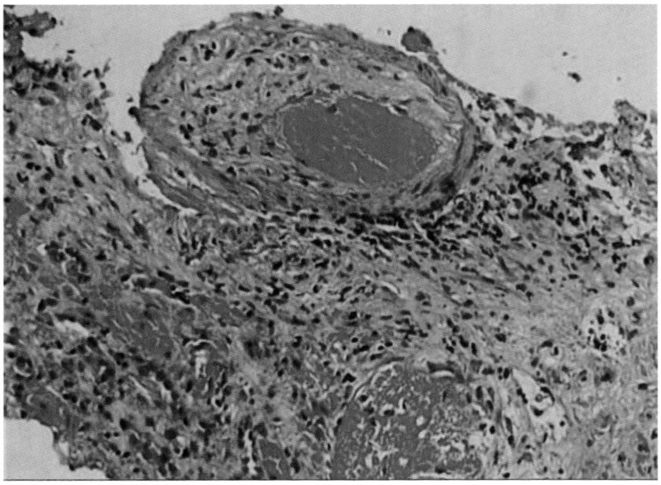

Figure 21-5 A patient with pauci-immune crescentic glomerulonephritis. A small artery shows features of active vasculitis; its wall shows neutrophil infiltration, fibrin deposition, and lumen occluded by a thrombus. Perivascular area shows interstitial hemorrhage and inflammation (H&E ×600).

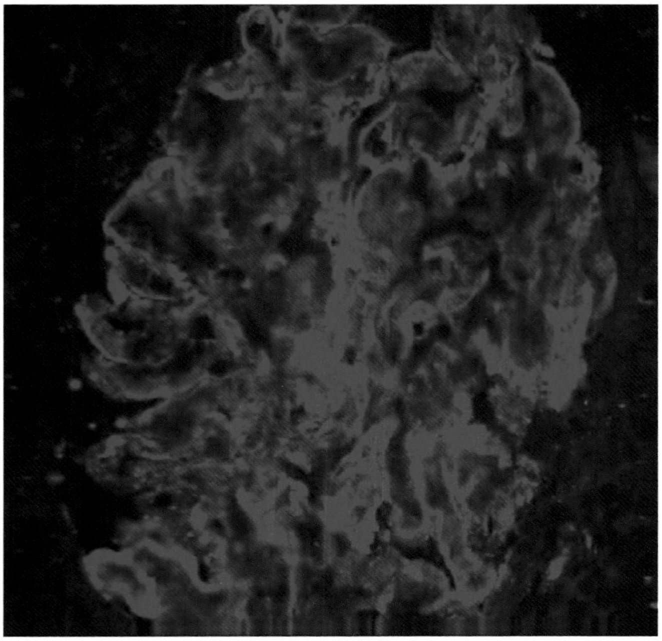

Figure 21-6 Immunofluorescence microscopy (×1200) in a patient with crescentic glomerulonephritis secondary to systemic lupus erythematosus showing granular deposition of IgG on the capillary wall.

deposits. The crescents stain strongly for fibrin on immunofluorescence. Mesangial deposits of IgA are found in IgA nephropathy and Henoch-Schönlein purpura; granular, subepithelial deposits of IgG and C3 in postinfectious GN; mesangial, subendothelial, and intramembranous deposits of IgG and C3 in MPGN; and "full house" capillary wall and mesangial deposits of granular IgG, IgA, IgM, C3, C4, and C1q in SLE (Figure 21-6). Glomeruli of patients with vasculitis, both with and without ANCA positivity, have few or no immune deposits. Anti-GBM disease is characterized by linear staining of the GBM with IgG (rarely IgM and IgA) and C3.

EVALUATION AND DIAGNOSIS

It is necessary to make an accurate and rapid diagnosis in RPGN, as treatment strategies vary and delay in instituting treatment results in risk of irreversible disease. All patients should immediately undergo a kidney biopsy. While the majority shows the presence of crescentic GN, the detection of thrombotic microangiopathy (affecting interlobular arteries and arterioles) or diffuse proliferative GN is not unusual.

The diagnosis of the etiology of crescentic GN depends on integration of clinical data and findings on serology and renal histology (Table 21-3) (Figure 21-1). In this way, anti-GBM disease or ANCA-associated RPGN can be distinguished from other causes of crescentic GN. Timely and appropriate therapy is indicated in view of the widely recognized unsatisfactory outcome in untreated patients.

TREATMENT

The heterogeneity and unsatisfactory outcome of RPGN have led to the use of multiple treatments. Evidence-based data are limited and specific treatment guidelines for children are based on data from case series and prospective studies in adults.[16] Besides specific therapy, supportive management for RPGN includes maintenance of fluid and electrolyte balance, providing adequate nutrition, and control of infections and hypertension.

The specific treatment of RPGN broadly comprises two phases: *induction* of remission and its *maintenance* (Table 21-4). The first phase aims at control of inflammation and the associated immune response. Once remission is induced, the maintenance phase attempts to prevent further renal damage and relapses.

Combination therapy with high-dose corticosteroids and cyclophosphamide is the current standard for *induction* treatment, with additional therapy for those with life- or organ-threatening disease. Treatment includes IV pulses of methylprednisolone (15-20 mg/kg, maximum 1 g/day) for 3 to 6 days, followed by high-dose oral prednisone (1.5-2 mg/kg daily) for 4 weeks, with tapering to 0.5 mg/kg daily by 3 months and alternate-day prednisone for 6 to 12 months. Cyclophosphamide is an important part of the induction regimen, though there is debate on benefits of oral versus IV treatment. Oral and IV administration of cyclophosphamide were compared in the CYCLOPS trial of the European Vasculitis Study Group (EUVAS). Analysis of data from this trial shows that IV pulse cyclophosphamide is equally effective as daily oral treatment for induction of remission, but with significantly reduced dose and thereby lower toxicity.[19] A meta-analysis of nonrandomized studies showed that pulse cyclophosphamide was significantly more likely to induce remission (odds ratio 0.29, 95% confidence interval 0.12-0.73) and had a lower risk of infection and leukopenia. Pulse cyclophosphamide dosing may, however, be associated

TABLE 21-4 Treatment of Crescentic Glomerulonephritis

Induction
Methylprednisolone 15-20 mg/kg (maximum 1 g) IV daily for 3-6 doses
Prednisone 1.5-2 mg/kg/day PO for 4 weeks; taper to 0.5 mg/kg daily by 3 months; 0.5-1 mg/kg on alternate days for 3 months
Cyclophosphamide 500-750 mg/m^2 IV every 3-4 weeks for 6 pulses[a]
Plasmapheresis (double volume) on alternate days for 2 weeks[b]
Maintenance
Azathioprine 1.5-2 mg/kg/d for 12-18 months
Alternate-day low-dose prednisolone
Consider mycophenolate mofetil (1000-1200 mg/m^2/day) or cyclosporin if disease activity is not controlled with azathioprine
Agents for Refractory Disease
Intravenous immunoglobulin, TNF-α antibody (infliximab), anti-CD20 (rituximab)

[a] The dose of cyclophosphamide is increased to 750 mg/m^2 if no leukopenia before the next dose. Dose reduction is necessary in patients showing impaired renal function. Alternatively, the medication is given orally at a dose of 2 mg/kg daily for 12 weeks.
[b] Plasmapheresis should begin early, especially if patient is dialysis dependent at presentation or if biopsy shows severe histological changes (>50% crescents). Plasma exchange is particularly useful in anti-GBM nephritis and ANCA-associated vasculitis. It should be considered in patients with immune complex RPGN if there is unsatisfactory renal recovery after steroid pulses.

with a greater risk of relapses, exposing patients to further immunosuppression.[20] Cyclophosphamide is administered at an oral dose of 2 mg/kg/day, or intravenously starting at 500 mg/m^2 and increased monthly by 125 mg/m^2 to a maximum of 750 mg/m^2. The dose should be adjusted to maintain a nadir leukocyte count, 2 weeks post-treatment, of 3000 to 4000/mm^3.

The requirement for *maintenance* therapy in crescentic GN depends on the underlying disease. Most patients with ANCA-associated disease need long-term maintenance immunosuppression due to the risk of relapses. Extended treatment with cyclophosphamide has been used in adults, but carries significant risks and is currently not preferred for children. While azathioprine does not appear to be effective at inducing remission, it is useful for long-term prevention of relapses. The timing of the switch from cyclophosphamide to azathioprine was clarified by the CYCAZAREM trial, which compared switching from cyclophosphamide to maintenance azathioprine at 3 versus 12 months.[21] Those converted to azathioprine at 3 months had similar remission rates, renal function,[2] and patient survival compared to those continuing on cyclophosphamide at 18 months. The duration of maintenance treatment is debatable, with most patients of pauci-immune crescentic GN treated for 2 or more years.

Plasmapheresis

Plasmapheresis or plasma exchange (PE) has been used for the treatment of crescentic GN with variable success. The mechanism of action is not clear, but is believed to involve removal of pathogenic autoantibodies, coagulation factors, and cytokines. PE has been shown in randomized controlled trials in adults to have therapeutic benefit in patients with anti-GBM disease with clearance of anti-GBM antibodies, lower serum creatinine, and improved patient and renal survival.[22] The benefits were limited in adults who were anuric with severe azotemia, dialysis dependent, or having more than 85% crescents on renal biopsy.

Evidence regarding the use of PE in other categories of crescentic GN is outlined below. Retrospective data in children with RPGN show benefits of PE if commenced within 1 month of disease onset.[23] Prospective studies in pauci-immune crescentic GN suggest that discontinuation of dialysis and renal recovery were better when patients received PE along with immunosuppression (91% with PE and immunosuppression vs. 38% in the group without PE).[24] The role of intensive PE versus IV methylprednisolone, in addition to oral steroids and cyclophosphamide, was examined by the EUVAS MEPEX trial on 151 patients with renal vasculitis.[25] Interim analysis showed that after 3 months, 69% of the PE group were alive and dialysis independent compared to 49% of those given methylprednisolone (p = 0.02). This benefit was sustained at the 1-year follow-up. Anecdotal reports also confirm the effectiveness of plasmapheresis in patients with RPGN due to SLE, Henoch-Schönlein purpura, severe proliferative GN, and in life-threatening pulmonary hemorrhage.

Immune-Complex Crescentic GN

There are no evidence-based recommendations on treatment for these patients. Therapy for immune-complex GN largely depends on the underlying disease. The treatment of IgA nephropathy and lupus nephritis presenting with RPGN is discussed in respective chapters in this volume.

Poststreptococcal RPGN

Poststreptococcal GN presenting with extensive crescents is rare and the benefits of intensive immunosuppressive therapy are unclear, since most patients recover spontaneously. Nevertheless, immunosuppressive therapy with corticosteroids and alkylating agents has been used in patients with renal failure and extensive glomerular crescents.[10,26] Despite the lack of evidence-based data, we recommend that patients with poststreptococcal RPGN and crescents involving 50% or more glomeruli be treated with 3 to 6 IV pulses of methylprednisolone, followed by tapering doses of oral steroids for 6 months. Therapy is usually combined with cyclophosphamide, and administered orally (for 3 months) or by IV (monthly for 6 months).

Eradication of the infection and removal of infected prostheses are necessary for resolution of immune-complex GN associated with active infections. Patients with idiopathic immune-complex crescentic GN should be treated similarly to those with pauci-immune crescentic GN.

Pauci-Immune Crescentic GN

Induction therapy comprises of treatment with IV pulses of methylprednisolone (administered daily for 3-6 days) followed by oral prednisone and cyclophosphamide (given either orally for 3 months or by the IV route every 3-4 weeks for 6 months).[2,16] Intensive PE for 2 weeks has been recommended for children who are dialysis dependent, have pulmonary hemorrhage, or are not responding satisfactorily to induction treatment. Based on data from recent multicenter studies, patients with severe renal failure are likely to benefit from early and intensive PE instituted in combination with steroids and cyclophosphamide.[25]

Therapy is continued during the maintenance phase with tapering doses of oral prednisolone and azathioprine. Steroid and immunosuppressive therapy is required for 18 to 24 months in most cases. A longer duration of therapy, extended to 3 to 5 years, is required in patients showing relapses, elevated ANCA titers and those with PR3-ANCA.[2] Approximately one-third of patients with pauci-immune crescentic GN have one or more relapses. Reinstitution of induction therapy with cyclophosphamide is often necessary. Less-intensive treatment with mycophenolate mofetil has been proposed for relapses that are mild and diagnosed early.

Intensive immunosuppression is associated with a significant risk of infection. Prophylactic antimicrobials especially against *Pneumocystis carinii* and *Candida* may be required during induction. Patients are also at risk of other complications of prolonged therapy with corticosteroids and alkylating agents.

Anti-GBM Crescentic GN

Prompt institution of PE is necessary in subjects with anti-GBM nephritis. Double-volume PE is implemented daily, and subsequently on alternate days until anti-GBM antibodies are no longer detectable (usually 2-3 weeks).[1,16]

The patients are also treated with IV methylprednisolone (described above) followed by high-dose oral prednisolone, with subsequent tapering over several months. Co-administration of cyclophosphamide (2 mg/kg daily for 3 months) is effective in suppressing further antibody production. Pulmonary hemorrhage responds to therapy with three doses of methylprednisolone (20 mg/kg on alternate days) with oral prednisone thereafter. PE is also beneficial in these patients.

As anti-GBM disease does not usually have a relapsing course, long-term maintenance therapy is not required and steroids are withdrawn slowly over the next 6 to 9 months. Patients treated early in the course of their illness respond satisfactorily. In patients who develop end-stage renal disease, transplantation should be deferred until anti-GBM antibodies are undetectable for 12 months, at which point disease recurrence is unlikely.

A proportion of patients with anti-GBM nephritis also show positive ANCA, most often p-ANCA. While the precise significance of the dual positivity is unclear, the initial clinical outcome for these patients is similar to that for classical anti-GBM disease. In view of a higher risk of relapse, these patients require a longer course of maintenance immunosuppressive therapy (as for ANCA-associated GN).

Newer Agents

A number of studies have examined the efficacy of intravenous immunoglobulin in subjects with ANCA positive systemic vasculitis and RPGN, with benefit lasting for up to 3 months.[27] The EUVAS NORAM study compared the effectiveness of orally administered methotrexate and cyclophosphamide in adult patients with early systemic vasculitis and mild renal involvement. Induction of remission was similar in the two groups at 6 months (90% vs. 94%, respectively), but relapses were significantly more frequent after treatment withdrawal in the methotrexate-treated patients.[28] Methotrexate, however, accumulates in renal impairment, and is therefore not recommended for patients with moderate or severe renal dysfunction.

The efficacy of other agents, including mycophenolate mofetil,[29] cyclosporin, leflunomide, deoxyspergualin, and mizoribine is being examined prospectively. Rituximab, a monoclonal antibody directed against CD20 antigen on B cells, has been used successfully in therapy-resistant lupus nephritis and Wegener's granulomatosis.[30] Case series in patients with refractory Wegener's granulomatosis found satisfactory results following treatment with antithymocyte globulin, anti–T-cell antibodies (e.g., anti-CD52 antibodies) and infliximab (anti-TNF monoclonal antibody).[31] Although potentially useful for treatment of individual patients, there is currently insufficient evidence to recommend general use of these agents.

OUTCOME

The outcome for patients has improved in recent decades, such that almost 60% to 70% of patients recover renal function, which is maintained in the long term. The outcome is largely determined by the severity of renal failure at presentation and the promptness of intervention, renal histology, and the underlying diagnosis.[1,2,16] Patients with poststreptococcal crescentic GN have a better prognosis, with most showing spontaneous improvement after supportive management. The outcome in patients with pauci-immune crescentic GN, MPGN, and idiopathic RPGN is less favorable than Henoch-Schönlein purpura or SLE.

The potential for recovery corresponds with the relative proportion of cellular or fibrous components in the crescents, and the extent of tubulointerstitial scarring and fibrosis. Histological changes that are not reversible with treatment and suggest unsatisfactory outcome include fibrous crescents, tubular atrophy, interstitial fibrosis, and glomerulosclerosis. The prognosis is better in patients with poststreptococcal crescentic GN with subepithelial rather than subendothelial or intramembranous deposits.

Post-Transplant Recurrence

The immunosuppression following transplantation and different antigenic characteristics of the graft compared to the native kidney prevent severe recurrence in most patients. Increasing graft survival has, however, increased the likelihood of disease recurrence in the allografts. Nonetheless, graft losses are uncommon and occur in less than 5% of cases. Conditions associated with a high risk of histological recurrence include MPGN type II, IgA nephropathy, Henoch-Schönlein purpura, and SLE. A positive ANCA titer at the time of transplantation does not increase the risk of recurrence in the allograft.

REFERENCES

1. Jennette JC: Rapidly progressive crescentic glomerulonephritis, *Kidney Int* 63 (3):1164-77.
2. Morgan MD, Harper L, Williams J, Savage C: Anti-neutrophil cytoplasm–associated glomerulonephritis, *J Am Soc Nephrol* 17 (5):1224-34, 2006.
3. Atkins RC, Nikolic-Paterson DJ, Song Q, Lan HY: Modulators of crescentic glomerulonephritis, *J Am Soc Nephrol* 7:2271-78, 1996.
4. Bariety J, Bruneval P, Meyrier A, Mandet C, et al: Podocyte involvement in human immune crescentic glomerulonephritis, *Kidney Int* 68 (3):1109-19, 2005.
5. Srivastava RN, Moudgil A, Bagga A, Vasudev AS, et al: Crescentic glomerulonephritis in children: a review of 43 cases, *Am J Nephrol* 12 (3):155-61, 1992.
6. El-Husseini AA, Sheashaa HA, Sabry AA, Moustafa FE, Sobh MA: Acute postinfectious crescentic glomerulonephritis: clinicopathologic presentation and risk factors, *Int Urol Nephrol* 37 (3):603-09, 2005.
7. Hoschek JC, Dreyer P, Dahal S, Walker PD: Rapidly progressive renal failure in childhood, *Am J Kidney Dis* 40 (6):1342-47, 2002.
8. Hattori M, Kurayama H, Koitabashi Y, Japanese Society for Pediatric Nephrology: Antineutrophil cytoplasmic autoantibody-associated glomerulonephritis in children, *J Am Soc Nephrol* 12 (7):1493-500, 2001.
9. Eisenberger U, Fakhouri F, Vanhille P, et al: ANCA-negative pauci-immune renal vasculitis: histology and outcome, *Nephrol Dial Transplant* 20 (7):1392-99, 2005.
10. Southwest Pediatric Nephrology Study Group: A clinico-pathologic study of crescentic glomerulonephritis in 50 children, *Kidney Int* 27 (2):450-58, 1985.
11. Jardim HM, Leake J, Risdon RA, Barratt TM, Dillon MJ: Crescentic glomerulonephritis in children, *Pediatr Nephrol* 6 (3):231-35, 1992.
12. Niaudet P, Levy M: Glomerulonephritis a croissants diffuse. In: Royer P, Habib R, Mathieu H, Broyer M, editors: *Nephrologie pediatrique*, ed 3, Paris, 1983, Flammarion, pp. 381-94.
13. Kashtan CE: Renal transplantation in patients with Alport syndrome, *Pediatr Transplant* 10 (6):651-57, 2006.
14. Covic A, Schiller A, Volovat C, et al: Epidemiology of renal disease in Romania: a 10 year review of two regional renal biopsy databases, *Nephrol Dial Transplant* 21 (2):419-24, 2006.
15. North American Pediatric Renal Trials and Collaborative Studies: NAPRTCS 2006 annual report. https://web.emmes.com/study/ped/annlrept/annlrept2006.
16. Jindal KK: Management of idiopathic crescentic and diffuse proliferative glomerulonephritis: evidence-based recommendations, *Kidney Int Suppl* 70:S33-40, 1999.
17. Bosch X, Guilabert A, Font J: Antineutrophil cytoplasmic antibodies, *Lancet* 368:404-18, 2006.
18. Schmitt WH, van der Woude FJ: Clinical applications of antineutrophil cytoplasmic antibody testing, *Curr Opin Rheumatol* 16:9-17, 2004.
19. de Groot K, Jayne D, Tesar V, Savage C; EUVAS Investigators: Randomised controlled trial of daily oral versus pulse cyclophosphamide for induction of remission in ANCA-associated systemic vasculitis, *Kidney Blood Press Res* 28:103, 2005.
20. de Groot K, Adu D, Savage CO: The value of pulse cyclophosphamide in ANCA-associated vasculitis: meta-analysis and critical review, *Nephrol Dial Transplant* 16:2018-27, 2001.
21. Jayne D, Rasmussen N, Andrassy K, et al: A randomized trial of maintenance therapy for vasculitis associated with antineutrophil cytoplasmic autoantibodies, *N Engl J Med* 349 (1):36-44, 2003.
22. Gianviti A, Trompeter RS, Barratt TM, Lythgoe MF, Dillon MJ: Retrospective study of plasma exchange in patients with idiopathic rapidly progressive glomerulonephritis and vasculitis, *Arch Dis Child* 75 (3):186-90, 1996.
23. Levy JB, Turner AN, Rees AJ, Pusey CD: Long-term outcome of anti-glomerular basement membrane antibody disease treated with plasma exchange and immunosuppression, *Ann Intern Med* 134 (11):1033-42, 2001.
24. Pusey CD, Rees AJ, Evans DJ, Peters DK, Lockwood CM: Plasma exchange in focal necrotizing glomerulonephritis without anti-GBM antibodies, *Kidney Int* 40:757-63, 1991.
25. Gaskin G, Jayne D, Group EVS: Adjunctive plasma exchange is superior to methylprednisolone in acute renal failure due to ANCA-associated glomerulonephritis, *J Am Soc Nephrol* 13:2A, 2002.
26. Raff A, Hebert T, Pullman J, Coco M: Crescentic post-streptococcal glomerulonephritis with nephrotic syndrome in the adult: is aggressive therapy warranted? *Clin Nephrol* 63 (5):375-80, 2005.
27. Ito-Ihara T, Ono T, Nogaki F, et al: Clinical efficacy of intravenous immunoglobulin for patients with MPO-ANCA-associated rapidly progressive glomerulonephritis, *Nephron Clin Pract* 102 (1):c35-42, 2006.
28. de Groot K, Rasmussen N, Bacon PA, et al: Randomized trial of cyclophosphamide versus methotrexate for induction of remission in early systemic antineutrophil cytoplasmic antibody-associated vasculitis, *Arthritis Rheum* 52:2461-69, 2005.
29. Koukoulaki M, Jayne DR: Mycophenolate mofetil in anti-neutrophil cytoplasm antibodies-associated systemic vasculitis, *Nephron Clin Pract* 102 (3-4):c100-07, 2006.
30. Keogh KA, Ytterberg SR, Fervenza FC, Carlson KA, et al: Rituximab for refractory Wegener's granulomatosis: report of a prospective, open-label pilot trial, *Am J Respir Crit Care Med* 173:180-87, 2006.
31. Booth A, Harper L, Hammad T, et al: Prospective study of TNF-alpha blockade with infliximab in anti-neutrophil cytoplasmic antibody-associated systemic vasculitis, *J Am Soc Nephrol* 15:717-21, 2004.

CHAPTER 22

Lupus Nephritis

Stephen D. Marks and Kjell Tullus

INTRODUCTION

Systemic lupus erythematosus (SLE) is an unpredictable, multisystemic, autoimmune disorder, which is episodic in nature with a broad spectrum of clinical and immunological manifestations. It is characterized by widespread inflammation of blood vessels and connective tissues affecting the skin, joints, kidneys, heart, lungs, and nervous and other systems, with a higher rate and more severe organ involvement than in adults (especially with respect to hematological and renal disease).[1-4] Biopsy-proven lupus nephritis, occurring in up to 80% of all cases of childhood-onset SLE, is a major determinant of the prognosis, which has improved over the last 20 years with an increasing armamentarium of immunosuppressive agents used to treat active disease. However, due to the variable clinical course of childhood-onset SLE, which is often progressive, there is still significant morbidity and mortality for severe disease with considerable physical and psychosocial morbidity. This results from both the sequelae of disease activity and the side effects of medications, including the infectious risks from overimmunosuppression, and longer-term risks with accelerated atherosclerosis.[5] Patients in clinical studies are diagnosed with SLE if they have at least 4 of the 11 American College of Rheumatology criteria for classification of SLE, which gives 95% sensitivity and 96% specificity in clinical practice[6,7] (Table 22-1).

EPIDEMIOLOGY

SLE presenting in childhood accounts for up to 20% of all cases, with epidemiological studies demonstrating its unpredictable natural history and sometimes progressive clinical course resulting in significant morbidity and mortality.

From the literature, there is a minimum incidence in a pediatric population of 0.28 per 100,000 children at risk per year[8] with a prevalence in children and adults of between 12.0 and 50.8 per 100,000.[9-16] However, SLE has been reported to be common and more severe in children in China, Hong Kong, and Taiwan, and three times more frequent in Afro-Caribbean than Caucasian children, although it is surprisingly rare in black African children.[17,18] In addition, the prevalence and severity of renal and neuropsychiatric lupus are increased in Afro-Caribbean children.[19] In the United Kingdom, Asian and Afro-Caribbean children are over six times more likely to be affected when compared to Caucasian children.[20] SLE is more prevalent in females of childbearing age due to hormonal influences, and in pediatric practice is more common over the age of 10 years.[21,22]

PATHOGENESIS

Despite the etiology of SLE being elusive, recent studies have made progress in our understanding of the pathogenic mechanisms via abnormal regulation of cell-mediated and humoral immunity that lead to tissue damage. The developing immune system is immature compared to that of adults and the heterogeneity of the clinical manifestations probably reflects the complexity of the disease pathogenesis. SLE is a multifactorial disorder with multigenic inheritance and various environmental factors implicated in its etiopathogenesis.

The immune system in SLE is characterized by a complex interplay among overactive B cells, abnormally activated T cells, and antigen-presenting cells, which lead to the production of an array of inflammatory cytokines, apoptotic cells, and diverse autoantibodies and immune complexes that in turn activate effector cells and the complement system, leading to tissue injury and damage, which are the hallmarks of the clinical manifestations.[23] Moreover, several autoantibodies against cell wall components or circulating proteins can produce specific disease manifestations, although 88% of SLE patients have presence of autoantibodies (including ANA, anti-dsDNA, and anti-Smith) up to 9.4 years before SLE is ever diagnosed.[24] It is generally assumed that anti-dsDNA antibodies play an important role in the pathogenesis of LN, as an increase in anti-dsDNA titer often precedes onset of renal disease, immune deposits are present in glomeruli and eluates of glomeruli are enriched for anti-dsDNA. However, the classical concept of deposition of DNA–anti-DNA complexes inciting glomerular inflammation is questionable, as free, naked, DNA is not present in the circulation, and injection of these complexes hardly leads to glomerular localization. The pathogenicity of anti-DNA has been proven with circulating immune complexes, in situ immune complexes, direct binding to renal and nonrenal antigens, penetration into cells, and stimulation of cytokines in the form of immune complexes. However, there are pathogenic and nonpathogenic anti-DNA, and current assays do not distinguish these classes.

Genomic and gene expression studies in patients with SLE have revealed novel gene mutations and cytokine alterations

TABLE 22-1 American College of Rheumatology Criteria for Classification of Systemic Lupus Erythematosus

Malar rash
Discoid rash
Photosensitivity
Oral ulcers
Arthritis
Serositis
Pleuritis
Pericarditis
Renal disorder
Proteinuria (>0.5 g/day or persistently ≥+++)
Red blood cell casts
Neurological disorder
Seizures
Psychosis (after excluding other causes)
Hematological disorder
Hemolytic anemia
Leukopenia (<4 × 10^9/L on two occasions)
Lymphopenia (<1.5 × 10^9/L on two occasions)
Thrombocytopenia (<100 × 10^9/L)
Immunological disorder
Elevated anti–double-stranded DNA
Elevated anti-Smith antibodies
Positive antiphospholipid antibodies (previously lupus erythematosus cell tests or false-positive *Treponema pallidum* immobilization/Venereal Disease Reference Laboratory)
Elevated antinuclear antibodies (after exclusion of drug-induced lupus)

that may explain many of the features of the disease as well as genetic susceptibility. There is a familial incidence of SLE in 12% to 15% of cases with a tenfold to twentyfold increased risk of developing the disease if a sibling is affected compared to the general population (prevalence increases from 0.4% of populations up to 3.5% if there is a first-degree relative with SLE).[10] The concordance rate of SLE in monozygous twins is 24% compared with 2% in heterozygous pairs, highlighting the importance of genetic (including HLA haplotypes, complement components, and Fcγ receptor polymorphisms) and environmental factors in the etiology of SLE.[25-28] The genetics of SLE is not fully understood; with many susceptible loci, there is a complex multifactorial inheritance with associated environmental factors. Genetic linkage studies using microsatellite markers and single nucleotide polymorphisms have identified at least seven loci displaying significant linkage to SLE, including 1q23 (FcγRIIA, FcγRIIB, FcγRIIIA), 1q25-31, 1q41-42, 2q35-37, 4p16-15.2, 6p11-21 (MHC haplotypes), and 16q12.

Although complement activation is involved in tissue damage, from initial murine lupus models and later human studies, homozygous deficiencies of the components of the classical complement pathway (C1q, C1r, C1s, C2, and C4) predispose to the development of SLE. The complement system is protective against the development of SLE, which occurs in 75% and 90% of patients with complete deficiencies of C4 and C1q, respectively.[29] Although initially anti-C1q was neither specific nor sensitive for SLE, in vitro testing has shown that anti-C1q is pathogenic in conjunction with complement-fixing antibodies and immune complexes with an increased prevalence of LN. Anti-C1q autoantibodies are strongly associated with renal involvement in SLE and deposit in glomeruli together with C1q.[30] Anti-C1q antibodies are especially pathogenic in patients with SLE, as they induce overt renal disease in the context of glomerular immune complex disease.[31]

Children and adult SLE patients exhibit profound alterations in B-cell compartments[32,33] with characteristic hypergammaglobulinemia and increased serum autoantibody titers, explaining why B-cell depletion may be an effective therapy.[34,35]

As well as autoantibodies and immune complexes, autoreactive T cells cause tissue damage in SLE with evidence of alterations in human SLE T-cell signaling molecules and loss of self-tolerance.[36] Compared to healthy T cells, there is increased and accelerated signaling responses in T cells from patients with SLE with hyperreactivity to antigenic triggers, which may be due to genetic influences.[37,38]

Many cytokines including interferon and interleukins (IL-6, IL10, IL12 (p40), and IL-18), which are elevated in the serum of SLE patients correlate with disease activity.[39]

In SLE, the increase in autoantigens may be due to impaired immune complex clearance and apoptosis. There is evidence of defective clearance of apoptotic cells in some SLE patients, due to the genetic deficiency of molecules, including complement deficiencies with autoantigens undergoing structural modifications during the process of apoptosis that may induce immunogenicity.[40]

Myeloid and plasmacytoid dendritic cells, which are key regulators of the immune system by acting as antigen-presenting cells, are significantly decreased in the blood of children with SLE, although they are present in high number on biopsies of active skin lesions.[41]

Although the influences for the development of SLE may be attributable to genetic susceptibility with changes in the hormonal milieu, environmental, pharmaceutical, and toxic agents (including crystalline silica, solvents, and pesticides),[42] there is also an association with infectious factors on the developing immune system of children who develop SLE, including Epstein–Barr virus.[43,44]

CLINICAL PRESENTATION

The presentation of SLE in childhood is varied, although typically there are nonspecific symptoms of being generally unwell with lethargy, aches, pains, episodic fever, anorexia, nausea, and weight loss with a typical butterfly rash over a period of a few weeks or months. Most organ systems can be involved[45] (Table 22-2), although unusual presentations are sometimes encountered, which is why SLE has been called one of the great mimickers.[46]

TABLE 22-2 Presenting Symptoms of Systemic Lupus Erythematosus (% of cases)

Malaise, weight loss, growth retardation	96%
Cutaneous abnormalities	96%
Hematological abnormalities	91%
Fever	84%
Lupus nephritis	84%
Musculoskeletal complaints	82%
Pleural/pulmonary disease	67%
Hepatosplenomegaly and/or lymphadenopathy	58%
Neurological disease	49%
Other disease manifestations (including cardiac, ocular, gastrointestinal, Raynaud's phenomenon)	13%-38%

From Cameron JS: Lupus nephritis in childhood and adolescence, *Pediatr Nephrol* 8 (2):230-49, 1994.

TABLE 22-3 Presenting Features of Lupus Nephritis (% of cases)

Nephrotic syndrome (>3 g/day)	55%
Proteinuria (<3 g/day)	43%
Macroscopic hematuria	1.4%
Microscopic hematuria	79%
Hypertension	40%
Reduced GFR (<80 ml/min/1.73m^2)	50%
Acute renal failure	1.4%

From Cameron JS: Lupus nephritis in childhood and adolescence, *Pediatr Nephrol* 8 (2):230-49, 1994.

Disease onset for 20% of all SLE patients occurs during childhood, with most children presenting in adolescence. From one of the largest cohorts of 201 children with SLE from Toronto, Canada, six children (3%) presented before the age of six years, 41 (20%) between 6 and 10 years, 62 (31%) between 11 and 13 years, and 92 (46%) between 14 and 18 years.[47] There was a female predominance of 80% with a slightly higher proportion of male patients compared to later in adulthood.

Lupus Nephritis

As many as 60% to 80% of children have some renal involvement close to the onset of the disease.[45] In a 1994 review of the presentation of lupus nephritis from different studies involving 208 children, 55% presented with nephrotic syndrome and 43% with proteinuria of lesser degrees (Table 22-3). Most children have microscopic hematuria while relatively few (1.4%) presented with macroscopic hematuria. Fifty percent of the children have impaired renal function at onset, while only 1.4% had acute renal failure requiring renal replacement therapy. A small proportion will present with a rapidly progressive glomerulonephritis with biopsy-proven crescentic glomerulonephritis. Hypertension was found in 40% of children.

Other Organ Systems

Dermatological

The classic rash of SLE is the butterfly rash over the cheeks and nose with photosensitivity to sunlight. Other kinds of rashes can be present including maculopapular or purpuric rashes, livedo reticularis, and urticaria. Hair loss and brown discoloration of the nails are rather common findings.

Cerebral

Neuropsychiatric symptoms are among the most severe found in SLE. They include headache, seizures, and mood disorders. The psychiatric symptoms can range from fatigue and depression to frank psychotic symptoms with hallucinations. Poor academic achievement is a common problem of multifactorial origin that is important to address in these children.

Hematological

Coombs' positive hemolytic anemia, leucopenia, and thrombocytopenia are very common findings in children with SLE. Erythrocyte sedimentation rate (ESR) is markedly raised in most children with SLE, while high C-reactive protein (CRP) is found in only a small minority. Therefore, CRP can be helpful in differentiating between flares of disease activity of SLE or an infectious complication, such as septicemia due to the disease itself and/or treatment.

Rheumatological

Generalized pain involving the musculoskeletal system is a very common finding in SLE patients, with severe arthritis less common than a milder arthritis or arthralgia. Bone pain can also occur, in particular as a complication of steroid treatment.

Other Organs

All serous membranes including pleura and pericardium are frequently affected. Hepatosplenomegaly and lymphadenopathy are commonly found in some children. Growth delay is often seen in children, partly related to pubertal delay. Primary and secondary amenorrhea are manifestations of SLE and lupus nephritis, but are also complications of high doses of cyclophosphamide treatment.

Antiphospholipid Syndrome

Antiphospholipid syndrome (APS) with anticardiolipin antibodies and/or lupus anticoagulant are found in 65% of children with SLE.[48] Patients with APS are prone to developing both venous and arterial thrombosis. APS is an independent risk factor for more severe renal disease due to microangiopathy in the kidneys and may require treatment as outlined below.

American College of Rheumatology Criteria

These diagnostic criteria are listed in Table 22-1. The diagnosis of SLE is made in typical cases with classical organ involvement, elevated autoantibodies, and hypocomplementemia. However, in many cases, the initial diagnosis is more difficult due to the evolution of disease, and these cases may not initially fulfill the criteria developed by the American College of Rheumatology (ACR), which have been refined for children.[6,7] They consist of 11 criteria, of which four should be fulfilled for the diagnosis of SLE, although meeting these criteria is not enough for a diagnosis of SLE because many children with other diseases can also formally match a number of them.

Disease Activity Scoring Systems

Various disease activity and damage scoring systems are very helpful in monitoring disease activity and damage in children and adolescents with SLE with respect to both clinical long-term follow-up and scientific studies. Scales of indices of disease activity continue to evolve and include SLEDAI (Systemic Lupus Erythematosus Disease Activity Index), SLAM (Systemic Lupus Activity Measure), and ECLAM (European Consensus Lupus Activity Measure). The British Isles Lupus Activity Assessment Group (BILAG) index is another scoring system that can be used and has been evaluated in children.[49] The BILAG index is based on the principle of the physician's intention to treat, and is a clinical measure of disease activity in SLE patients that has been validated to be reliable, comprehensive, and sensitive to change. It was developed to report disease activity in eight different systems (general, mucocutaneous, neurological, musculoskeletal, cardiorespiratory, vasculitis, renal, and hematological), which differentiates it from other lupus activity indices.

INVESTIGATIONS

The initial investigations of a child with suspected SLE include hematological, biochemical, and immunological investigations. Further investigations are warranted depending on organ involvement, so a percutaneous renal biopsy and imaging of relevant organ systems are often required.

Blood Investigations

The initial blood test should include a full blood count with a blood film, ESR, and reticulocyte count. Anemia, leukopenia, and thrombocytopenia are common findings during active disease that normally improve when the disease is brought under control. The leukocyte count, in particular the neutrophil count, should be monitored during active immunosuppressive treatment, as the presence of neutropenia influences the doses of immunosuppressive therapies. However, lymphopenia is often seen with treatment, and is mostly regarded as a "desired" side effect, which can sometimes be a marker of the effectiveness of treatment. ESR is a marker of disease activity, which can be clinically useful, although it is not uncommon for it to be markedly elevated even during clinical and serological remission. A coagulation screen and a direct Coombs' test should be performed to look for evidence of hemolysis.

The biochemistry profile should include estimation of renal function with plasma creatinine and urea, serum electrolytes, bone, thyroid and liver function tests (including serum albumin), pancreatic enzymes, and C-reactive protein (where sepsis is clinically suspected). It is useful to calculate the estimated glomerular filtration rate using the Schwartz formula.

TABLE 22-4 Auto-Antibodies in Patients with Lupus Nephritis

	Frequency	Specificity	Association with Disease Activity
Anti-dsDNA	40%-90%	High	Yes
Anti-SSA/Ro	35%	Low	No
Anti-SSB/La	15%	Low	No
Anti-Sm	5%-30%	High	No
Anti-C1q	80%-100%	High	Yes

Anti-C1q, Anti-complement factor C1q; *Anti-Sm*, Anti-Smith; *Anti-SSA/Ro*, Anti-Sjögren's syndrome A; *Anti-SSB/La*, anti-Sjögren's syndrome B; *dsDNA*, double-stranded DNA.

Immunology Testing

Nearly all children with SLE will have evidence of immune dysregulation with positive immunological tests and antinuclear antibodies (ANA) are the most common. ANA can sometimes be a nonspecific finding but the use of anti–double-stranded DNA (dsDNA), and the extractable nuclear antibodies (ENA) and anti-C1q increases the specificity (Table 22-4). The pathogenic significance of these antibodies is debated, and they can be found in serum sometimes several years before the development of symptoms.[24] However, it is clear that dsDNA and anti-C1q can be used to monitor disease activity as a marker of improvement or a pending flare of disease activity. Anti-C1q antibodies have also been shown to predict more severe renal involvement.[50]

Complement, in particular C3 and C4, are reduced during the active phases of disease. They are also useful markers of disease activity. Anticardiolipin antibodies and lupus anticoagulant should be regularly monitored. Hypergammaglobulinemia is a feature of SLE, and it is useful to monitor serum immunoglobulins. Although it is controversial whether hypogammaglobulinemia should be supplemented, we do not routinely administer substitutive intravenous immunoglobulin in children treated with B-lymphocyte depletion therapies (rituximab) who should have their B-lymphocyte counts monitored (by measuring the number of CD19 positive cells).

Urine Investigations

Urine should be regularly monitored in all children with SLE with urinalysis by dipstick performed for hematuria and proteinuria or albuminuria. Urine microscopy is also helpful in looking for red blood cells and casts during the acute phase of lupus nephritis. Some standardized measurement of proteinuria or albuminuria should be regularly followed, which in most centers is carried out by analyzing an early morning spot urine sample relating the urine excretion of protein or albumin to the urine levels of creatinine. Evidence of tubular dysfunction may help to identify lupus nephritis prior to the onset of albuminuria by measuring NAG (N-acetyl-beta-D-glucosaminidase):creatinine ratio, RBP (retinol binding protein):creatinine ratio or other tubular markers.[51]

Other Investigations

It is important to base treatment decisions on the histopathology of percutaneous renal biopsies, as it has been shown that the severity of the renal involvement sometimes is difficult to predict from clinical symptoms and signs. Formal measurements of glomerular filtration rate should be performed on all children with a clinical suspicion of impaired renal function. Pulmonary function tests, electrocardiography, echocardiography, and chest x-rays are important investigations in selected children.

Follow-Up

Each child should at every clinic visit have a full clinical evaluation including weight, height, and a disease activity score (as above). Blood pressure should be monitored and urine tested for proteinuria and hematuria. Regular blood tests should include full blood count, ESR and CRP, renal and liver function tests, electrolytes, complement C3 and C4, and autoantibodies including dsDNA. Fasting blood lipids including cholesterol, triglycerides, HDL, LDL, and VLDL should be monitored at least once a year. Bone density should be measured on an annual basis, in particular in children with long-term corticosteroid therapy.

HISTOLOGICAL CLASSIFICATION OF LUPUS NEPHRITIS

The histological classification of lupus nephritis (LN) was initially formatted in 1975 by the World Health Organization (WHO) and modified in 1982 and 1995. It describes the spectrum of LN as the type and extent of renal lesion and provides information on the immunosuppression required and prognosis. This classification was revised by the International Society of Nephrology (ISN) and Renal Pathology Society (RPS) Working Group after a consensus conference in 2002 in order to standardize definitions, emphasize clinically relevant lesions, and encourage uniform and reproducible reporting among centers[52,53] (Table 22-5). This new classification facilitates clinical management by increased comprehension of the etiopathogenesis of SLE and guides the clinician with treatment decisions, protocols, and clinical research. However, there is widespread variation of the timing, type, and distribution of histological lesions, including immune-complex–mediated vasculitis, fibrinoid necrosis, inflammatory cell infiltrate, and collagen sclerosis. Although some data suggest that tubular dysfunction may be evident prior to glomerular dysfunction in children with SLE, the emphasis is on glomerular compared to tubulo-interstitial or vascular lesions.[51]

Classes I and II denote purely mesangial involvement (I, mesangial immune deposits without mesangial hypercellularity; II, mesangial immune deposits with mesangial expansion and hypercellularity), III for focal glomerulonephritis (involving <50% of total number of glomeruli) with subdivisions for active and chronic lesions; IV for diffuse glomerulonephritis (involving ≥50% of total number of glomeruli with examples in Figures 22-1, 22-2, and 22-3) either with segmental (class IV-S) or global (class IV-G) involvement, and also with subdivisions for active and chronic lesions; V for membranous lupus nephritis (combinations of membranous and prolifera-

TABLE 22-5 **International Society of Nephrology and Renal Pathology Society Working Group (ISN/RPS) Revised Histopathological Classification of LN**

I. Minimal mesangial LN	Normal glomeruli by LM, but mesangial immune deposits by IF
II. Mesangial proliferative LN	Purely mesangial hypercellularity of any degree or mesangial matrix expansion by LM with mesangial immune deposits, with none or few isolated subepithelial or subendothelial deposits by IF or EM, not visible by LM
III. Focal LN	Active or inactive focal (<50% involved glomeruli), segmental, or global endo- or extra-capillary GN, typically with focal, subendothelial immune deposits, with or without focal or diffuse mesangial alterations*,†
III (A)	Active focal proliferative LN
III (A/C)	Active and sclerotic focal proliferative LN
III (C)	Inactive sclerotic focal LN
IV. Diffuse segmental (IV-S) or global (IV-G) LN	Active or inactive diffuse (≥50% involved glomeruli), segmental, or global endo- or extra-capillary GN with diffuse subendothelial immune deposits, with or without mesangial alterations. This class is divided into diffuse segmental (IV-S) when ≥50% of the involved glomeruli have segmental lesions, and diffuse global (IV-G) when ≥50% of the involved glomeruli have global lesions*,†
IV (A)	Active diffuse segmental or global proliferative LN
IV (A/C)	Diffuse segmental or global proliferative and sclerotic LN
IV (C)	Diffuse segmental or global sclerotic LN
V. Membranous LN	Numerous global or segmental subepithelial immune deposits or their morphologic sequelae by LM and IF or EM with or without mesangial alterations. May occur in combination with III or IV in which case both will be diagnosed. May show advanced sclerosis.
VI. Advanced sclerotic LN	90% or more glomeruli globally sclerosed without residual activity

* Indicate the proportion of glomeruli with active and with sclerotic lesions.
† Indicate the proportion of glomeruli with fibrinoid necrosis and/or cellular crescents.
EM, Electron microscopy; *IF*, immunoflourescence; *GN*, glomerulonephritis; *LN*, lupus nephritis; *LM*, light microscopy.

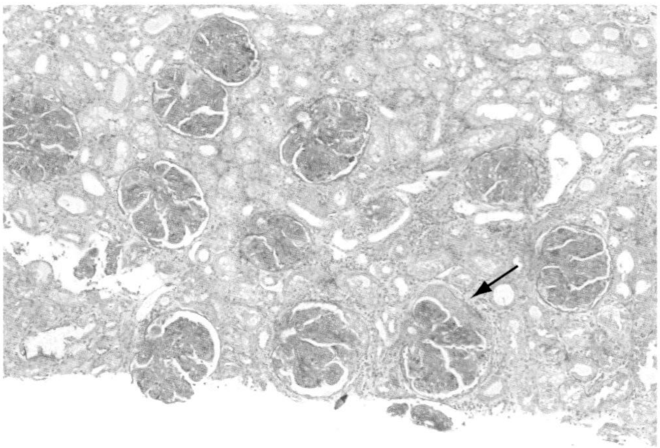

Figure 22-1 Photomicrograph of a case of lupus nephritis demonstrating predominant diffuse endocapillary proliferative change with scattered superimposed extracapillary proliferative lesions *(arrow)*. Lupus nephritis class IV-G (A/C) (PAS, original magnification ×100). (From Marks SD, Tullus K, Sebire NJ: Current issues in pediatric lupus nephritis: role of revised histopathological classification, *Fetal Pediatr Pathol* 25(6):297-309, 2006.)

TABLE 22-6 **Activity and Chronicity Indices of Lupus Nephritis**

Activity Index	Chronicity Index
Glomerular	
Endocapillary hypercellularity	
Fibrinoid necrosis	
Karyorrhexis	Glomerular sclerosis
Cellular crescents	Fibrous crescents
Hyaline thrombi	Fibrous adhesions
Wire loops (subendothelial deposits)	Extramembranous deposits
Hematoxylic bodies	
Leukocyte infiltration	
Tubulointerstitial	
Mononuclear cell infiltration	Interstitial fibrosis
Tubular necrosis	Tubular atrophy

tive glomerulonephritis, that is, classes III and V or classes IV and V) should be reported individually in the diagnostic line), and VI for advanced sclerosing lesions (which now for the first time categorically states that ≥90% of glomeruli need to be globally sclerosed without residual activity). In addition, the new ISN/RPS classification includes overlap cases (see Figure 22-4 for an example of mixed class IV and class V lupus nephritis).

The histopathological features of LN include the delineation of active and chronic histological lesions, which has been extensively investigated[54] (Table 22-6). The active glomerular and tubulointerstitial lesions, which are potentially reversible and are scored up to 24 (with 12 denoting poor renal prognosis), include endocapillary hypercellularity, fibrinoid necrosis, karyorrhexis, cellular crescents, hyaline thrombi, wire loops (subendothelial deposits), hematoxylin bodies, leukocyte infiltration, and tubulo-interstitial disease with tubular atrophy and mononuclear cell infiltration. The chronic lesions are irreversible and include glomerular sclerosis, fibrous crescents, fibrous adhesions, extramembranous deposits, and tubulo-interstitial disease with interstitial fibrosis and tubular atrophy.

The clinicopathological correlation of LN has been evaluated in both adults and children according to different histopathological classifications. The largest adult series investigating the clinicopathological outcomes according to the new ISN/RPS classification of LN followed 60 Japanese subjects for 1 to 366 (mean 187) months[55] (Figure 22-5). The primary outcome was defined as developing end-stage renal failure (ESRF) with secondary outcome as death and/or ESRF. The primary and secondary outcomes of all subjects were 82% and 78% at 10 years, and 80% and 73% at 20 years, respectively. The primary outcome of subjects with nephrotic syndrome ($n = 21$) was statistically poorer ($p = 0.0007$), with the mean time of 50% renal survival of 200 (standard deviation 29) months as compared to that of subjects without nephrotic syndrome ($n = 39$).

In comparison with adult-onset SLE, there are usually fewer patients in the series of childhood cases of LN. There have been larger series investigating clinicopathological outcomes of 39 to 67 children according to the WHO classification[56] and the new ISN/RPS classification of LN,[57] which provide evidence that up to half of children with LN will have the most severe class (class IV or diffuse LN). The new ISN/RPS classification demonstrates that the subgroup of diffuse global sclerosing (IV-G(C)) LN is associated with the worst clinical outcome.[57]

TREATMENT

The optimal treatment of children and adolescents with SLE is with a multidisciplinary team of health professionals, including a pediatric rheumatologist and pediatric nephrologist, with a dedicated specialist nurse and members of a psychosocial team.

Drug Treatment

Treatment of lupus with or without nephritis is based on evaluation of the severity of the disease. The treatment should be individually tailored depending on the presenting symptoms and severity of renal involvement, with emphasis on renal dysfunction and the degree of proteinuria. In all cases with suspected renal involvement, the histopathological grading of the renal biopsy is very helpful in deciding further treatment. Other potentially life-threatening symptoms, such as cerebral lupus, should also be taken into consideration when deciding on the initial treatment. Most treatments have common or potential side effects that need to be considered when deciding on the treatment for an individual child.

The treatment of childhood-onset SLE is not based on large randomized controlled trials comparing various therapies head to head, but on some studies in adult patients and clinical experience. Therefore, a rather wide variation among

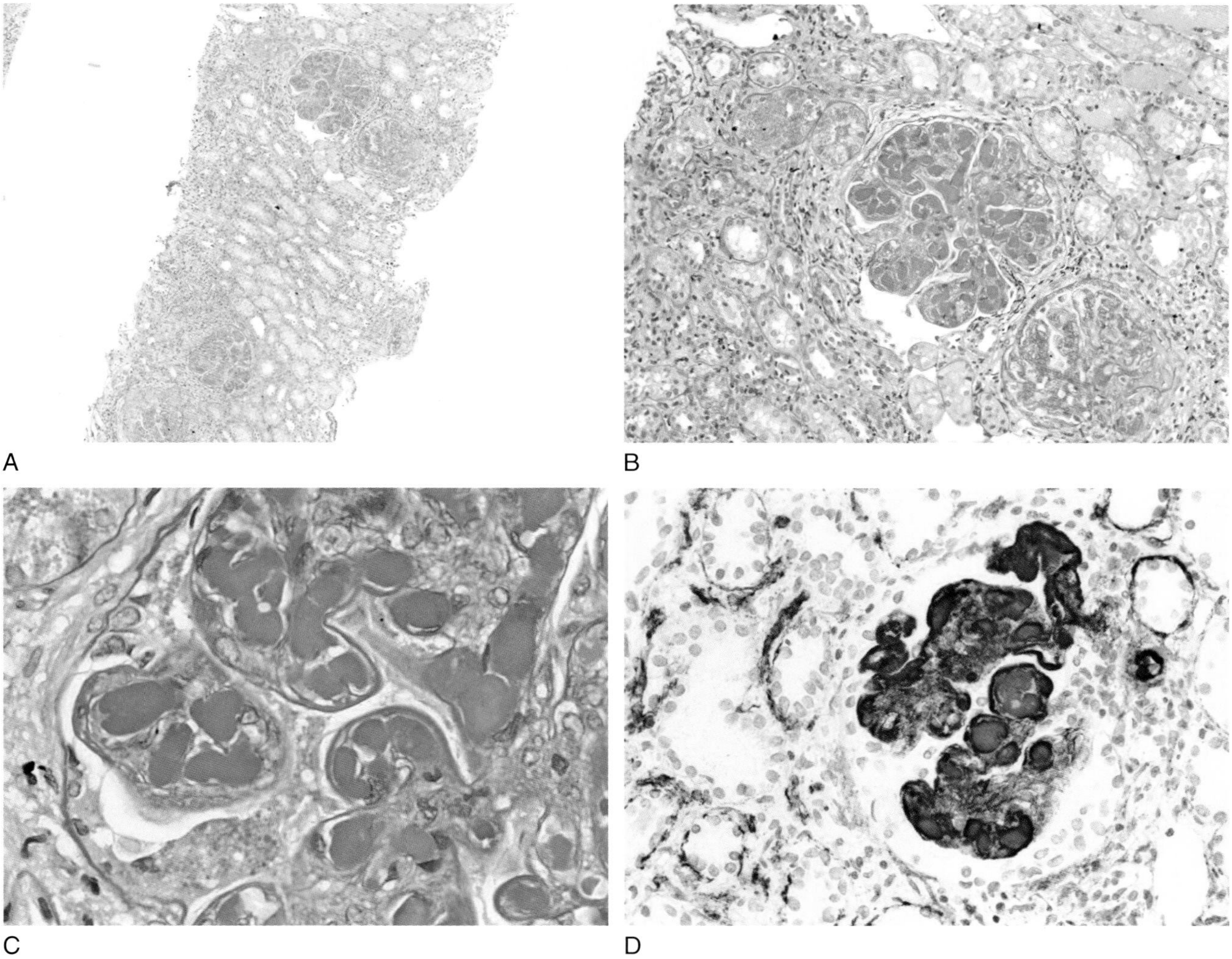

Figure 22-2 Photomicrographs of a case of lupus nephritis presenting as apparent acute renal failure, demonstrating diffuse endocapillary proliferative change with scattered crescent formation **(A, B)** and extensive subendothelial deposits visualized as wire-loop and hyaline drop lesions **(B, C).** Immunostaining revealed a characteristic "full-house" pattern of immunoglobulin and complement deposition **(D).** Lupus nephritis class IV-G **(A).** (PAS and immunostain, original magnifications ×40-400.) (From Marks SD, Tullus K, Sebire NJ: Current issues in pediatric lupus nephritis: role of revised histopathological classification, *Fetal Pediatr Pathol* 25(6):297-309, 2006.)

centers exists. The guidelines below describe our current protocol for treating children with SLE; other regimens may be equally appropriate. The armamentarium of immunosuppressive agents is presently developing quickly, so guidelines may change substantially in the near future.

Traditionally, treatment has been divided into induction therapy to gain control of acute disease, and maintenance therapy to maintain control over the disease. This is a helpful approach, but a difficult-to-define flare of disease activity is not uncommon.

Severe Multisystem Disease with or without Nephritis (ISN/RPG Classes III-V)

Induction Therapy

A common presentation to the nephrologist is a child who has developed generalized symptoms over a few weeks or months and at assessment by his or her local medical team is found to have an acute nephritic and/or nephrotic syndrome with a suspicion of SLE that is later confirmed by serology. It is important in cases with significant renal disease to commence treatment early without unnecessary delay to protect the kidneys from developing chronic damage.

The mainstay of treatment at the present time is based on corticosteroids and cyclophosphamide (Table 22-7). For children with the worst disease spectrum, incorporating severe renal dysfunction and crescentic glomerulonephritis, we have added plasma exchange to the treatment, and more recently, B-lymphocyte depletion therapy with intravenous rituximab.[35,58] There are large international centers that have used azathioprine as induction therapy with seemingly similar outcome results.[47,56] In adult patients, data are emerging that mycophenolate mofetil (MMF) is at least equally effective as cyclophosphamide.[59-61]

Corticosteroids Intravenous pulses of methylprednisolone should be given during 3 consecutive days (600-1000 mg/m^2)

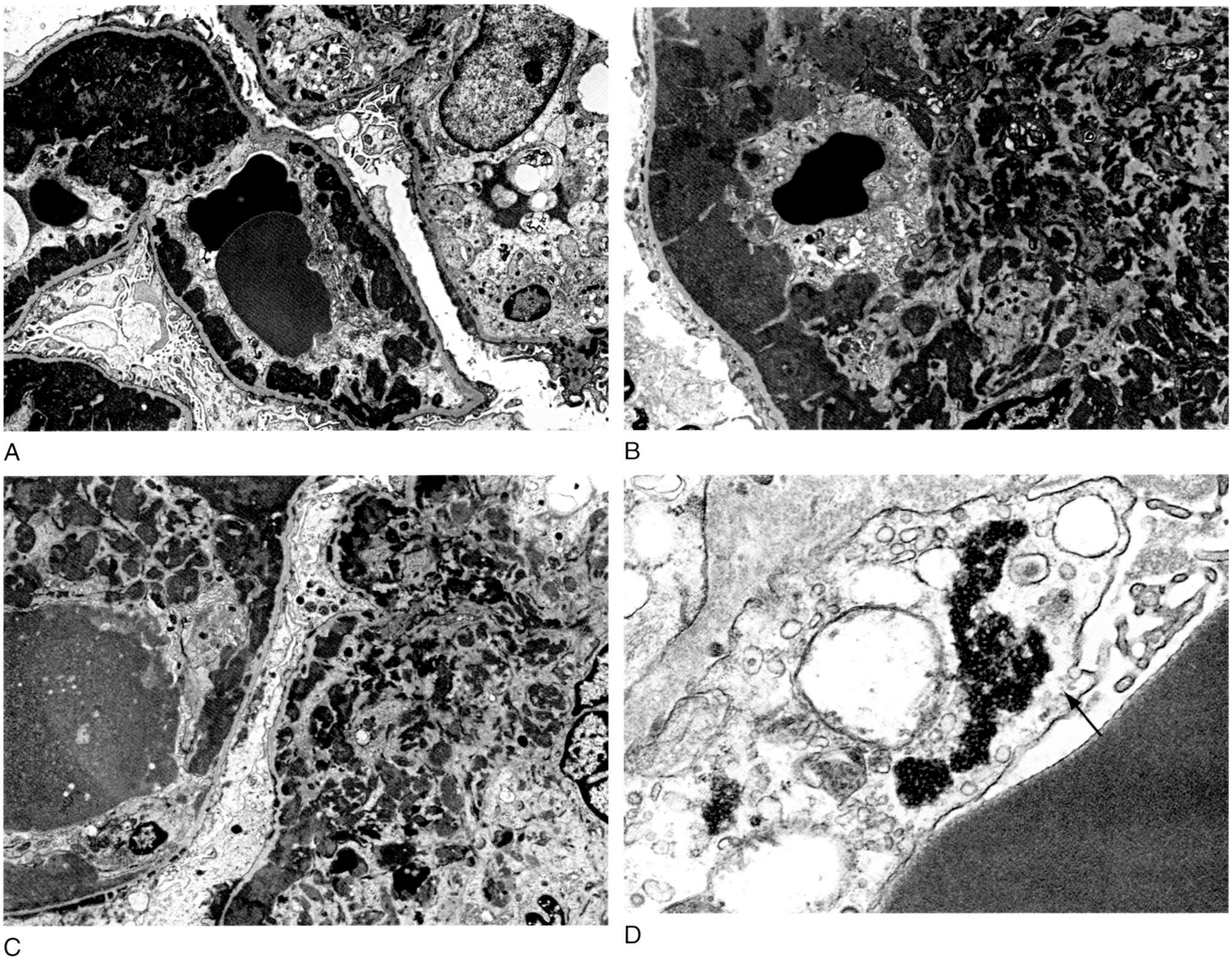

Figure 22-3 Electron micrographs of lupus nephritis demonstrating extensive mesangial and paramesangial electron-dense deposits in association with massive subendothelial deposits. **A** corresponds to the case in Figure 22-1, and **B** and **C** correspond to the case in Figure 22-2. In addition, some cases may demonstrate the presence of tubuloreticular inclusions **(D).** (From Marks SD, Tullus K, Sebire NJ: Current issues in pediatric lupus nephritis: role of revised histopathological classification, *Fetal Pediatr Pathol* 25(6):297-309, 2006.)

TABLE 22-7 Induction Therapy of ISN/RPS Class III, IV, and V Lupus Nephritis

Methylprednisolone (intravenous) pulses ×3	600-1000 mg/m^2 (maximum 1 g)
Prednisolone (oral)	1-2 mg/kg/day (maximum 60-80 mg/day with rapid weaning)
Cyclophosphamide (intravenous)[a]	Monthly pulses for 6 months, 500-1000 mg/m^2
In Very Severe Cases or When Not Responding to the Above:	
Plasma exchange	Daily for 5-10 days
Rituximab	See protocol in text

[a] Induction therapy with oral mycophenolate mofetil or azathioprine is an alternative in less severe cases.

with a maximum of 1 g, infused over at least 30 minutes. In severe cases, these pulses may need to be repeated.

The methylprednisolone pulses will be followed by high doses of oral prednisolone (1-2 mg/kg/day to a maximum dose 60-80 mg/day). This high dose is dictated by the severity of the clinical situation, but should be weaned down to a dose of 0.5 mg/kg/day within 6 to 8 weeks. This treatment will inevitably result in Cushingoid side effects, which can be debilitating for adolescents (such as fluid and water retention with increased appetite and weight gain, rounded facies, striae, and growth delay). Other important side effects include mood changes, hypertension, steroid-induced diabetes mellitus, osteoporosis, and osteopenia. Therefore, for long-term adherence to therapy, it is very important to reduce the corticosteroid dose as quickly as the clinical situation allows to try to minimize these side effects.

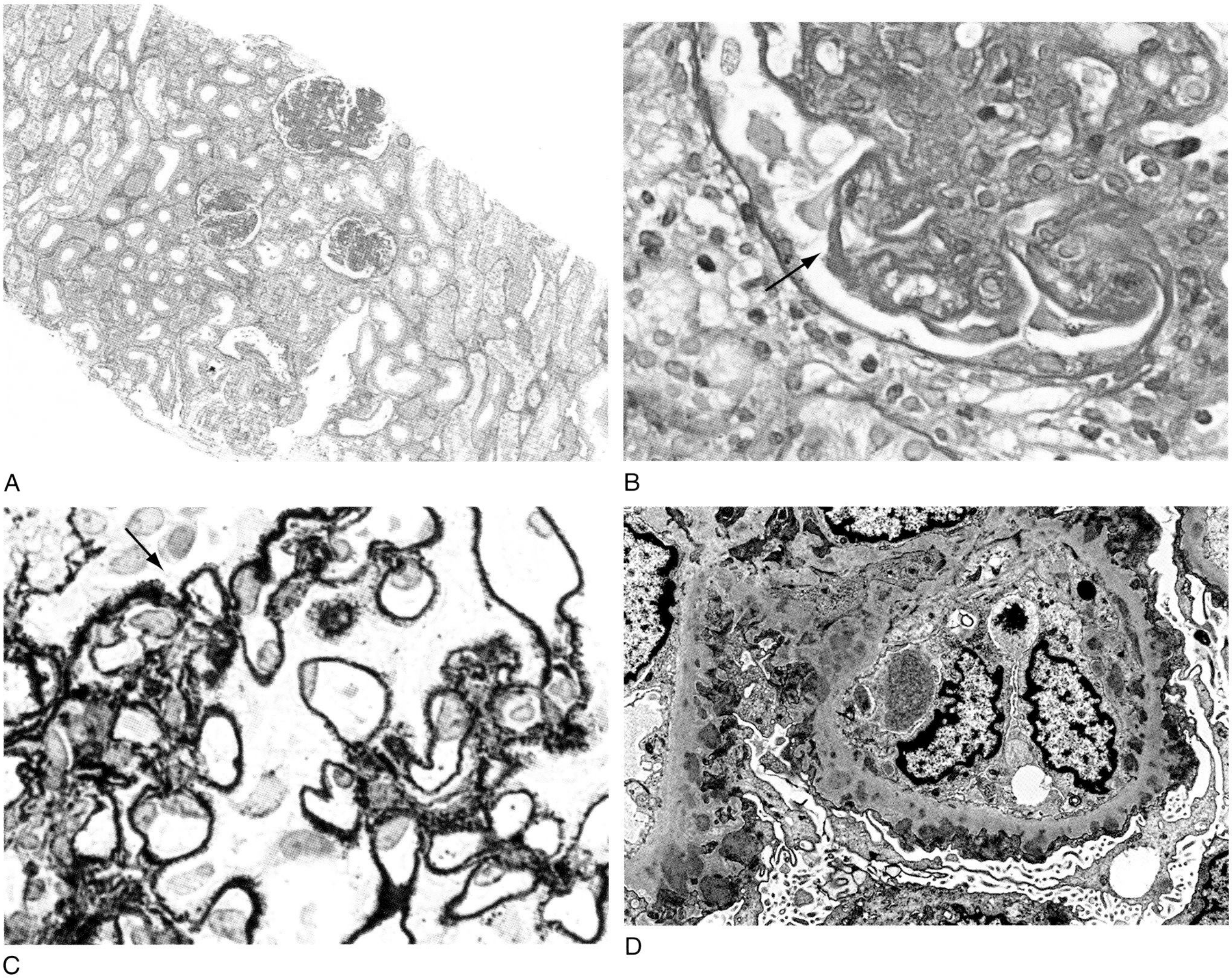

Figure 22-4 Photomicrographs of a case of lupus nephritis presenting with nephrotic syndrome demonstrating diffuse endocapillary proliferative change with subendothelial deposits. **A, B:** PAS, original magnifications ×40 and 400, respectively). In addition, some glomeruli show florid "spike" formation on silver staining (**C;** PAMS, original magnification ×400), with mesangial, subendothelial, and subepithelial deposits on ultrastructural examination **(D).** Lupus nephritis, mixed class IV and class V changes. (From Marks SD, Tullus K, Sebire NJ: Current issues in pediatric lupus nephritis: role of revised histopathological classification, *Fetal Pediatr Pathol* 25(6):297-309, 2006.)

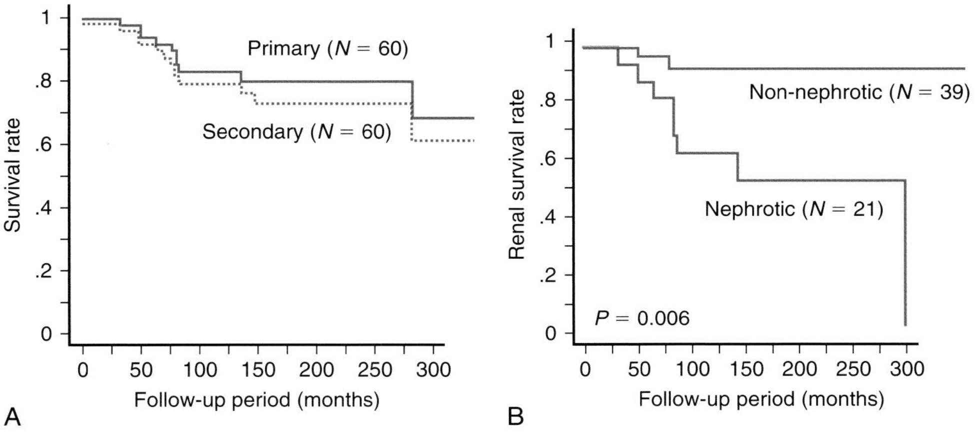

Figure 22-5 The primary (end-stage renal failure [ESRF]) and secondary (patients' death and/or ESRF) outcomes of 60 Japanese adult lupus-nephritis subjects with and without nephrotic syndrome at mean follow-up of 187 months. (From Yokoyama H, Wada T, Hara A, et al: The outcome and a new ISN/RPS 2003 classification of lupus nephritis in Japanese, *Kidney Int* 66:2382-88, 2004.)

Cyclophosphamide Intravenous pulses of cyclophosphamide are presently the most important steroid-sparing agent in achieving remission in severe SLE and lupus nephritis. However, this treatment has substantial short- and long-term side effects, including nausea (which can be alleviated with routine use of ondansetron), alopecia, hemorrhagic cystitis, and infectious risks of septicemia due to neutropenia. Many girls develop amenorrhea, and with high doses, there is a risk for infertility. The modified National Institute of Health protocol of intravenous cyclophosphamide (500-1000 mg/m^2 with dose reduction in renal failure) can be administered as monthly pulses for 6 months. It is important to keep the child well hydrated and to administer MESNA to protect the child from developing hemorrhagic cystitis.

Controlled studies in adult patients show that intravenous cyclophosphamide results in significantly more side effects, including severe infections compared to oral azathioprine or mycophenolate mofetil (MMF).[59-62] Therefore, it is important to closely monitor the total white-cell, neutrophil, and lymphocyte counts, with the nadir usually occurring around 7 to 10 days after the infusion. Subsequent doses may need to be reduced based on hematological side effects.

Cyclophosphamide also causes significantly more amenorrhea.[63] There is a long-term increased risk for developing malignancies and for infertility. Up to 14% of cyclophosphamide-treated patients younger than 41 years have premature ovarian failure, which is a common consequence of cyclophosphamide treatment. The PREGO Study (Prospective Randomized Study On Protection Against Gonadal Toxicity), which compares randomized monthly injection versus no injection of gonadotropin-releasing hormone analog, will investigate whether temporary induction of a prepubertal hormonal milieu during cyclophosphamide therapy significantly decreases the risk of premature ovarian failure.[64]

Plasma Exchange We advocate the use of plasmapheresis in very severe and refractory cases of SLE with cerebral lupus and/or crescentic glomerulonephritis in which 5 to 10 plasma exchanges seem to be useful in acutely improving some patients.[58] However, this is a controversial area, and a controlled trial in adult patients with severe lupus nephritis could not confirm any benefits from adding plasma exchange to the standard treatment of methylprednisolone and cyclophosphamide,[65] which was recently confirmed in a meta-analysis.[66]

Rituximab Rituximab is a humanized anti-CD20 antibody that was designed for treatment of B-cell lymphoma, and in adults has been increasingly used for B-cell depletion therapy in autoimmune diseases such as rheumatoid arthritis or SLE.[34] We have used intravenous rituximab in over 20 children with SLE or vasculitis, and have published the results of our first seven children.[35,67] All our patients have shown very good response to the treatment and have not experienced any severe side effects.

The experience in other centers has also been very favorable but there are no published randomized controlled trials. The indications for rituximab therapy in children include severe life threatening disease and those patients with active disease despite standard treatment. Different protocols have been used and our protocol involves administration of intravenous rituximab as an infusion of 750 mg/m^2 (rounded up to the nearest 100 mg with a maximum dose of 1 g) on days 1 and 15, and intravenous cyclophosphamide as an infusion of 375 mg/m^2 on days 2 and 16. In addition, an intravenous dose of 100 mg methylprednisolone is given immediately prior to the rituximab infusion.

Mycophenolate Mofetil (MMF) and Azathioprine There is evolving evidence from recent studies in some centers that suggests MMF and possibly also azathioprine in adult patients may be equally good for induction therapy as cyclophosphamide. In a cohort of 42 adult patients from Hong Kong treated with 12 months of oral MMF therapy or 6 months of intravenous cyclophosphamide followed by 6 months of azathioprine, both groups responded equally well to the treatment, but there were significantly more side effects in the cyclophosphamide group.[59] The follow-up of these patients for a median of 63 months was recently published with similar long-term treatment results with 6.3% and 10.0%, respectively, of the patients in each group showing doubling of their plasma creatinine.[60] MMF treatment was associated with fewer infections than cyclophosphamide, and four patients in the cyclophosphamide group and none in the MMF group reached the composite end-point of end-stage renal failure or death. A 24-week trial in 140 adult patients showed significantly more patients entering remission after MMF compared to cyclophosphamide, and again with fewer severe side effects in the MMF group.[61] However, the patients on MMF had increased gastrointestinal side effects with more diarrhea.

Intravenous Immunoglobulin Intravenous immunoglobulin (at a dose of 2 g/kg to a maximum of 70 g) can be useful, particularly in children with severe hematological disease. Some children benefit from regular infusions, which can be administered repeatedly (such as every 6 weeks).

Maintenance Therapy

All cases of severe lupus require maintenance therapy for a long period of time, although the length of treatment is not well defined. We advocate maintenance therapy for at least 2 to 3 years and possibly indefinitely in many cases.

Corticosteroids After the initial rather rapid reduction of the oral corticosteroid, the prednisolone dose should be continuously weaned down more slowly. The clinical response will decide how quickly the dose can be reduced. Long-term treatment with steroids for several years is likely to be needed, although there are different approaches on preferred maintenance dose. One goal is to aim for an alternate-day treatment at a dose on the order of 10 to 15 mg every other day (Table 22-8), and another to aim for a low once-daily dose of 5 to 10 mg. These doses of prednisolone should allow the child to grow normally.[68]

Azathioprine Azathioprine at a dose of 2 to 2.5 mg/kg/day is presently the first-line maintenance therapy with its generally favorable side-effect profile. In a recent study of aza-

TABLE 22-8 Maintenance Therapy of Lupus Nephritis

Prednisolone (oral)	10-15 mg alternate or every day
Azathioprine (oral)	2.0-2.5 mg/kg once daily
Alternatively:	
Mycophenolate mofetil (oral)	Start dose of 500 mg/day to a maximum of 30 mg/kg/day (or 2 g/day) in two divided doses
Hydroxychloroquine (oral)	4-6 mg/kg/day; normal dose 200 mg once daily

thioprine or mycophenolate mofetil used as maintenance therapy in adult patients after 6 months of intravenous cyclophosphamide, the outcomes were similar with significantly better patient and event-free survival compared to continuation of cyclophosphamide every 3rd month.[62] MMF and azathioprine treated patients had significantly less hospitalization, amenorrhea, infections, nausea, and vomiting compared to cyclophosphamide. The mortality rate was 8.5% (5 out of 59 patients in the study) due to infectious complications (four in the cyclophosphamide group and one in the MMF group).

Mycophenolate Mofetil Mycophenolate mofetil (MMF) is another good choice for long-term maintenance therapy.[62] By slowly increasing the dose, the main side effect of abdominal pain and diarrhea can mostly be avoided. A normal starting dose is 500 mg/day in two divided doses up to a final dose of 2 g/day (maximum dose of 15 mg/kg twice daily). If gastrointestinal side effects are a continuing problem, then the daily dose may be divided up and given three or four times a day.

Hydroxychloroquine The use of antimalarial drugs (such as hydroxychloroquine at a dose of 4 to 6 mg/kg/day) should be considered for all lupus patients. It is especially helpful in children with marked skin disease, lethargy, and arthritis. Hydroxychloroquine also seems to reduce blood lipids and possibly the risk for later atherosclerosis. A high dose of 10 mg/kg has been used in lung disease up to a total maximum dose of 400 mg/day. Patients should have annual optician reviews to check color vision.

Treatment of Antiphospholipid Syndrome

Treatment for APS includes reducing lupus disease activity and appropriate anticoagulation treatment (such as aspirin or life-long warfarin for severe thromboembolic disease).

General Renal Management

As outlined in other parts of this book general renal care is important in all children with renal impairment. This includes monitoring and treatment of hypertension and proteinuria. It is important to continuously evaluate renal function of these children with estimated GFR, and if appropriate a formal GFR measurement. Supportive treatment of chronic renal failure is needed in some of these children.

General Management

Sun Protection

All children with SLE and especially those with active skin disease should be advised to always use appropriate sunscreen and protect themselves from the sun.

Immunizations

Children with SLE, treated with immunosuppressive drugs, should avoid immunization with live vaccines. Vaccination with killed vaccines should be carefully considered as they might induce a flare of the disease and also might not be as effective as they normally would be. In the United Kingdom and other countries, pneumococcal vaccinations are recommended for all patients likely to be on steroids for more than a month.

Management of Infection

Children on immunosuppressive treatment are more susceptible to severe infections than other children and it should be emphasized to the parents and the children that they should seek medical advice early in the case of fever or symptoms of an infection.

PROGNOSIS

In the era before treatment became available, the prognosis of patients with SLE was very poor; very few patients with a severe nephritis survived more than 2 years.[69] The introduction of corticosteroids and immunosuppressive treatment with cyclophosphamide and azathioprine has made a huge impact on the long-term prognosis. In a long-term follow-up study (mean of 11 years) of 67 patients with lupus nephritis from a single center, 4 (6%)[4] of children died and 6 (9%)[6] developed ESRF.[56] From the same center with a follow-up (mean 9 years), there was a 97% survival of 201 children with SLE.[47]

The acute and short- to medium-term mortality from SLE is now caused both by active disease and complications to the treatment. In recent years, it has also become evident that patients with SLE face another important threat to their long-term survival due to increased atherosclerosis.

Disease Related Complications and Mortality

Data compiled by Cameron from various studies showed that some 40% of the mortality in children with lupus nephritis was due to renal failure and infections, respectively, while the remaining 20% were caused by active disease in other organs (mainly the brain but also the lungs and heart).[45] The proportion of children dying from renal failure is now most likely lower with increasing use of effective therapies, although the prognostic factors for developing renal failure remain the same (male gender, non-Caucasian race, and severity of disease on renal biopsy).[56]

Treatment-Related Complications and Mortality

In recent studies, infections have been the main cause of death, therefore suggesting that the most important short-term goal is to find therapies that are as good as current treatments but with fewer side effects. Recent comparative studies in adults showed that cyclophosphamide treatment was associated with significantly more severe infections compared to treatment with azathioprine or MMF.[59-62] This emphasizes the importance of monitoring white cell and neutrophil counts during therapy and early treatment of infectious complications. However, infections can sometimes be difficult to differentiate from a flare of disease activity, especially in children who are in ESRF on renal replacement therapy. CRP can be used as a helpful tool in these situations, as very few patients even with active lupus have raised CRP levels[45] while most children with septicemia do.

Severe viral infections, in particular varicella zoster virus, are seen, and children exposed to the virus or with early symptoms of varicella (or more often herpes zoster virus) should be treated with acyclovir therapy to reduce the risk of generalized infection.

Growth failure is a major problem in children with lupus, which can be related to the inflammatory disease or a complication of corticosteroid treatment. Sometimes it can be difficult to differentiate between them; this is a controversial area, but it is our opinion that ongoing inflammation more often causes the growth failure than the treatment with low corticosteroid doses. Therefore, increasing immunosuppression rather than reducing treatment is often more beneficial for the growth of these children.

SLE patients have an increased risk of osteoporosis partly caused by their long-term treatment with steroids.[70] Treatment with calcium and vitamin D is advocated from some centers, but unfortunately it seems as if the beneficial effects from that treatment only persist during the treatment itself.[71] However, an increased nutritional calcium intake does seem to be able to improve bone accretion over a longer period.[72] It is recommended that children with SLE should be monitored with regular bone density scans.

Children on long-term immunosuppressive treatment are considered to have an increased risk for developing malignancies, in particular skin cancers and lymphoma, and should be advised to use sun protection. Bladder cancer has been reported to be associated with the use of cyclophosphamide in children with SLE.[73] A 10-year follow-up of a very large cohort of 1000 adult lupus patients found that 23 developed malignancies with breast and uterine cancers being the most common.[74] Therefore, the risk of malignancy does not seem to be excessive.

Active lupus often causes amenorrhea and delayed puberty, whereas treatment with cyclophosphamide can also reduce fertility. A study of 39 women younger than 40 years showed that 12.5% (2 out of 16) receiving seven intravenous doses of cyclophosphamide developed sustained amenorrhea compared to 39% (9 out of 23) receiving 15 or more doses (with a higher risk in women older than 25).[63]

Thrombosis

In the aforementioned 10-year follow-up of 1000 adult patients, 9.2% (92) developed thrombosis and of the 68 patients who died, 26.5% had a thrombotic event. This is more commonly occurring in children with antiphospholipid syndrome. A ten-year follow-up of 149 children with SLE from Toronto showed that 24 were positive for lupus anticoagulant and that 13 of them experienced 21 thromboembolic events.[75] The authors emphasized the need for life-long anticoagulation treatment for this subgroup of children.

Cardiovascular Disease

A recent Swedish register study on 4737 patients with SLE from 1964 to 1994 showed a 16-fold increased risk of death from cardiovascular diseases.[76] Therefore, our new challenge is to try to prevent atherosclerosis and to improve patients' long-term survival. The increased risk for cardiovascular death is multifactorial and includes classical risk factors, such as hypertension, hyperlipidemia, and corticosteroid treatment, but also proteinuria, vasculitis, low-grade systemic inflammation, antiphospholipid syndrome, and elevated levels of homocysteine.[77]

Carotid plaque and coronary artery calcifications are significantly increased in lupus patients.[78,79] Therefore, prevention of this increased atherosclerosis includes good control of inflammation, aggressive treatment of any hypertension and proteinuria, and efforts to prevent steroid-induced obesity. Treatment of hyperlipidemia with statins is not yet established in most pediatric centers but should be considered for the future. Hydroxycholoroquine has been shown to have a beneficial influence on the cardiovascular risk profile.[80]

Adherence to Treatment

One important prognostic factor in children with lupus nephritis, as in all our children with chronic kidney disease, is adherence with treatment, especially during puberty. Nonadherence in adolescents is a common reason for relapse of symptoms and sometimes an acute presentation with renal failure after initially successful treatment. In such serious clinical situations, we would advocate the use of intravenous therapies (with cyclophosphamide or rituximab treatment reserved for children who have already had large cumulative doses of cyclophosphamide) instead of oral treatments to ensure adherence and disease control.

Renal Transplantation

Patients with ESRF due to lupus nephritis seem to do as well as matched controls after renal transplantation with less than 10% recurrence of lupus nephritis and similar long-term patient and graft survival.[81] However, the risk for thromboembolic complications was higher in the SLE group.

CONCLUSION

In recent decades, the prognosis for children with SLE has improved in a major way with most children now able to look forward to long lives without debilitating symptoms. However, the first important challenge for the future is to find ways to minimize treatment-related mortality and morbidity. This will most likely include reduced use of cyclophosphamide due to replacement by other less toxic drugs such as azathioprine and most likely MMF and rituximab. The other important challenge is to find ways to reduce the burden of future premature cardiovascular disease in these children.

REFERENCES

1. Brunner HI, Silverman ED, To T, Bombardier C, Feldman BM: Risk factors for damage in childhood-onset systemic lupus erythematosus: cumulative disease activity and medication use predict disease damage, *Arthritis Rheum* 46 (2):436-44, 2002.
2. Jimenez S, Cervera R, Font J, Ingelmo M: The epidemiology of systemic lupus erythematosus, *Clin Rev Allergy Immunol* 25 (1): 3-12, 2003.
3. Rood MJ, ten Cate R, Suijlekom-Smit LW, den Ouden EJ, et al: Childhood-onset systemic lupus erythematosus: clinical presentation and prognosis in 31 patients, *Scand J Rheumatol* 28 (4):222-26, 1999.
4. Tucker LB, Menon S, Schaller JG, Isenberg DA: Adult- and childhood-onset systemic lupus erythematosus: a comparison of onset, clinical features, serology, and outcome, *Br J Rheumatol* 34 (9): 866-72, 1995.
5. Schanberg LE, Sandborg C: Dyslipoproteinemia and premature atherosclerosis in pediatric systemic lupus erythematosus, *Curr Rheumatol Rep* 6 (6):425-33, 2004.
6. Hochberg MC: Updating the American College of Rheumatology revised criteria for the classification of systemic lupus erythematosus, *Arthritis Rheum* 40 (9):1725, 1997.
7. Tan EM, Cohen AS, Fries JF, Masi AT, et al: The 1982 revised criteria for the classification of systemic lupus erythematosus, *Arthritis Rheum* 25 (11):1271-77, 1982.
8. Malleson PN, Fung MY, Rosenberg AM: The incidence of pediatric rheumatic diseases: results from the Canadian Pediatric Rheumatology Association Disease Registry, *J Rheumatol* 23 (11):1981-87, 1996.
9. Fessel WJ: Systemic lupus erythematosus in the community. Incidence, prevalence, outcome, and first symptoms: The high prevalence in black women, *Arch Intern Med* 134 (6):1027-35, 1974.
10. Hochberg MC: Prevalence of systemic lupus erythematosus in England and Wales, 1981-2, *Ann Rheum Dis* 46 (9):664-66, 1987.
11. Hochberg MC: Systemic lupus erythematosus, *Rheum Dis Clin North Am* 16 (3):617-39, 1990.
12. Hopkinson ND, Doherty M, Powell RJ: The prevalence and incidence of systemic lupus erythematosus in Nottingham, UK, 1989-1990, *Br J Rheumatol* 32 (2):110-15, 1993.
13. Hopkinson ND, Doherty M, Powell RJ: Clinical features and race-specific incidence/prevalence rates of systemic lupus erythematosus in a geographically complete cohort of patients, *Ann Rheum Dis* 53 (10):675-80, 1994.
14. Johnson AE, Gordon C, Palmer RG, Bacon PA: The prevalence and incidence of systemic lupus erythematosus in Birmingham, England. Relationship to ethnicity and country of birth, *Arthritis Rheum* 38 (4):551-58, 1995.
15. Nived O, Sturfelt G, Wollheim F: Systemic lupus erythematosus in an adult population in southern Sweden: incidence, prevalence and validity of ARA revised classification criteria, *Br J Rheumatol* 24 (2):147-54, 1985.
16. Siegel M, Lee SL: The epidemiology of systemic lupus erythematosus, *Semin Arthritis Rheum* 3 (1):1-54, 1973.
17. Citera G, Wilson WA: Ethnic and geographic perspectives in SLE, *Lupus* 2 (6):351-53, 1993.
18. Symmons DP: Frequency of lupus in people of African origin, *Lupus* 4 (3):176-78, 1995.
19. Vyas S, Hidalgo G, Baqi N, Von Gizyki H, Singh A: Outcome in African-American children of neuropsychiatric lupus and lupus nephritis, *Pediatr Nephrol* 17 (1):45-49, 2002.
20. Gardner-Medwin JM, Dolezalova P, Cummins C, Southwood TR: Incidence of Henoch-Schönlein purpura, Kawasaki disease, and rare vasculitides in children of different ethnic origins, *Lancet* 360 (9341):1197-202, 2002.
21. Lahita RG: Sex hormones and systemic lupus erythematosus, *Rheum Dis Clin North Am* 26 (4):951-68, 2000.
22. McMurray RW: Sex hormones in the pathogenesis of systemic lupus erythematosus, *Front Biosci* 6:E193-206, 2001.
23. Kyttaris VC, Katsiari CG, Juang YT, Tsokos GC: New insights into the pathogenesis of systemic lupus erythematosus, *Curr Rheumatol Rep* 7 (6):469-75, 2005.
24. Arbuckle MR, McClain MT, Rubertone MV, Scofield RH, et al: Development of autoantibodies before the clinical onset of systemic lupus erythematosus, *N Engl J Med* 349 (16):1526-33, 2003.
25. Deapen D, Escalante A, Weinrib L, Horwitz D, et al: A revised estimate of twin concordance in systemic lupus erythematosus, *Arthritis Rheum* 1992 35 (3):311-18, 1992.
26. Kelly JA, Moser KL, Harley JB: The genetics of systemic lupus erythematosus: putting the pieces together, *Genes Immun* 3 (Suppl 1):S71-85, 2002.
27. Manderson AP, Botto M, Walport MJ: The role of complement in the development of systemic lupus erythematosus, *Annu Rev Immunol* 22:431-56, 2004.
28. Tsao BP: The genetics of human systemic lupus erythematosus, *Trends Immunol* 24 (11):595-602, 2003.
29. Pickering MC, Botto M, Taylor PR, Lachmann PJ, Walport MJ: Systemic lupus erythematosus, complement deficiency, and apoptosis, *Adv Immunol* 76:227-324, 2000.
30. Seelen MA, Trouw LA, Daha MR: Diagnostic and prognostic significance of anti-C1q antibodies in systemic lupus erythematosus, *Curr Opin Nephrol Hypertens* 12 (6):619-24, 2003.
31. Trouw LA, Groeneveld TW, Seelen MA, Duijs JM, et al: Anti-C1q autoantibodies deposit in glomeruli but are only pathogenic in combination with glomerular C1q-containing immune complexes, *J Clin Invest* 114 (5):679-88, 2004.
32. Odendahl M, Jacobi A, Hansen A, Feist E, et al: Disturbed peripheral B lymphocyte homeostasis in systemic lupus erythematosus, *J Immunol* 165 (10):5970-79, 2000.
33. Tangye SG, Liu YJ, Aversa G, Phillips JH, de Vries JE. Identification of functional human splenic memory B cells by expression of CD148 and CD27, *J Exp Med* 188 (9):1691-703, 1998.
34. Leandro MJ, Cambridge G, Edwards JC, Ehrenstein MR, Isenberg DA: B-cell depletion in the treatment of patients with systemic lupus erythematosus: a longitudinal analysis of 24 patients, *Rheumatology (Oxford)* 44 (12):1542-45, 2005.
35. Marks SD, Patey S, Brogan PA, Hasson N, et al: B lymphocyte depletion therapy in children with refractory systemic lupus erythematosus, *Arthritis Rheum* 52 (10):3168-74, 2005.
36. Shlomchik MJ, Craft JE, Mamula MJ: From T to B and back again: positive feedback in systemic autoimmune disease, *Nat Rev Immunol* 1 (2):147-53, 2001.
37. Tsokos GC, Nambiar MP, Tenbrock K, Juang YT: Rewiring the T-cell: signaling defects and novel prospects for the treatment of SLE, *Trends Immunol* 24 (5):259-63, 2003.
38. Tsokos GC, Mitchell JP, Juang YT: T cell abnormalities in human and mouse lupus: intrinsic and extrinsic, *Curr Opin Rheumatol* 15 (5):542-47, 2003.
39. Grondal G, Gunnarsson I, Ronnelid J, Rogberg S, et al: Cytokine production, serum levels and disease activity in systemic lupus erythematosus, *Clin Exp Rheumatol* 18 (5):565-70, 2000.
40. Casciola-Rosen L, Andrade F, Ulanet D, Wong WB, Rosen A: Cleavage by granzyme B is strongly predictive of autoantigen status: implications for initiation of autoimmunity, *J Exp Med* 190 (6):815-26, 1999.
41. Farkas L, Beiske K, Lund-Johansen F, Brandtzaeg P, Jahnsen FL: Plasmacytoid dendritic cells (natural interferon-alpha/beta-producing cells) accumulate in cutaneous lupus erythematosus lesions, *Am J Pathol* 159 (1):237-43, 2001.
42. Cooper GS, Parks CG: Occupational and environmental exposures as risk factors for systemic lupus erythematosus, *Curr Rheumatol Rep* 6 (5):367-74, 2004.
43. Incaprera M, Rindi L, Bazzichi A, Garzelli C: Potential role of the Epstein-Barr virus in systemic lupus erythematosus autoimmunity, *Clin Exp Rheumatol* 16 (3):289-94, 1998.
44. Moon UY, Park SJ, Oh ST, Kim WU, et al: Patients with systemic lupus erythematosus have abnormally elevated Epstein-Barr virus load in blood, *Arthritis Res Ther* 6 (4):R295-302, 2006.
45. Cameron JS: Lupus nephritis in childhood and adolescence, *Pediatr Nephrol* 8 (2):230-49, 1994.

46. Iqbal S, Sher MR, Good RA, Cawkwell GD: Diversity in presenting manifestations of systemic lupus erythematosus in children, *J Pediatr* 135 (4):500-505, 1999.
47. Marks SD, Hiraki L, Hagelberg S, Silverman ED, Hebert D: Age-related renal prognosis of childhood-onset SLE, *Pediatr Nephrol* 17 (9):C107, 2002.
48. Lee T, von Scheven E, Sandborg C: Systemic lupus erythematosus and antiphospholipid syndrome in children and adolescents, *Curr Opin Rheumatol* 13 (5):415-21, 2001.
49. Marks SD, Pilkington C, Woo P, Dillon MJ: The use of the British Isles Lupus Assessment Group (BILAG) index as a valid tool in assessing disease activity in childhood-onset systemic lupus erythematosus, *Rheumatology (Oxford)* 43 (9):1186-89, 2004.
50. Marto N, Bertolaccini ML, Calabuig E, Hughes GR, Khamashta MA: Anti-C1q antibodies in nephritis: correlation between titres and renal disease activity and positive predictive value in systemic lupus erythematosus, *Ann Rheum Dis* 64 (3):444-48, 2005.
51. Marks SD, Shah V, Pilkington C, Woo P, Dillon MJ: Renal tubular dysfunction in children with systemic lupus erythematosus, *Pediatr Nephrol* 20 (2):141-48, 2005.
52. Weening JJ, D'Agati VD, Schwartz MM, Seshan SV, et al: The classification of glomerulonephritis in systemic lupus erythematosus revisited, *Kidney Int* 65 (2):521-30, 2004.
53. Weening JJ, D'Agati VD, Schwartz MM, Seshan SV, et al: The classification of glomerulonephritis in systemic lupus erythematosus revisited, *J Am Soc Nephrol* 15 (2):241-50, 2004.
54. Austin HA III, Muenz LR, Joyce KM, Antonovych TA, et al: Prognostic factors in lupus nephritis. Contribution of renal histologic data, *Am J Med* 75 (3):382-91, 1983.
55. Yokoyama H, Wada T, Hara A, Yamahana J, et al: The outcome and a new ISN/RPS 2003 classification of lupus nephritis in Japanese, *Kidney Int* 66 (6):2382-88, 2004.
56. Hagelberg S, Lee Y, Bargman J, Mah G, et al: Long-term follow-up of childhood lupus nephritis, *J Rheumatol* 29 (12):2635-42, 2002.
57. Marks SD, Sebire NJ, Pilkington C, Tullus K: Clinicopathological correlations of pediatric lupus nephritis, *Pediatr Nephrol* 22 (1): 77-83, 2007.
58. Wright EC, Tullus K, Dillon MJ: Retrospective study of plasma exchange in children with systemic lupus erythematosus, *Pediatr Nephrol* 19 (10):1108-14, 2004.
59. Chan TM, Li FK, Tang CS, Wong RW, et al: Efficacy of mycophenolate mofetil in patients with diffuse proliferative lupus nephritis. Hong Kong-Guangzhou Nephrology Study Group, *N Engl J Med* 343 (16):1156-62, 2000.
60. Chan TM, Tse KC, Tang CS, Mok MY, Li FK: Long-term study of mycophenolate mofetil as continuous induction and maintenance treatment for diffuse proliferative lupus nephritis, *J Am Soc Nephrol* 16 (4):1076-84, 2005.
61. Ginzler EM, Dooley MA, Aranow C, Kim MY, et al: Mycophenolate mofetil or intravenous cyclophosphamide for lupus nephritis, *N Engl J Med* 353 (21):2219-28, 2005.
62. Contreras G, Pardo V, Leclercq B, Lenz O, et al: Sequential therapies for proliferative lupus nephritis, *N Engl J Med* 350 (10):971-80, 2004.
63. Langevitz P, Klein L, Pras M, Many A: The effect of cyclophosphamide pulses on fertility in patients with lupus nephritis, *Am J Reprod Immunol* 28 (3-4):157-58, 1992.
64. Manger K, Wildt L, Kalden JR, Manger B: Prevention of gonadal toxicity and preservation of gonadal function and fertility in young women with systemic lupus erythematosus treated by cyclophosphamide: the PREGO-Study, *Autoimmun Rev* 2006 5 (4):269-72, 2006.
65. Lewis EJ, Hunsicker LG, Lan SP, Rohde RD, Lachin JM: A controlled trial of plasmapheresis therapy in severe lupus nephritis. The Lupus Nephritis Collaborative Study Group, *N Engl J Med* 326 (21):1373-79, 1992.
66. Flanc RS, Roberts MA, Strippoli GF, Chadban SJ, et al: Treatment for lupus nephritis, *Cochrane Database Syst Rev* (1):CD002922, 2004.
67. Marks SD, Tullus K: Successful outcomes with rituximab therapy for refractory childhood systemic lupus erythematosus, *Pediatr Nephrol* 21 (4):598-99, 2006.
68. Simmonds J, Trompeter R, Calvert T, Tullus K: Does long-term steroid use influence long-term growth? *Pediatr Nephrol* 20:C107, 2005.
69. Zetterstrom R, Berglund G: Systemic lupus erythematosus in childhood; a clinical study, *Acta Paediatr* 45 (2):189-204, 1956.
70. Lee C, Ramsey-Goldman R: Bone health and systemic lupus erythematosus, *Curr Rheumatol Rep* 7 (6):482-89, 2005.
71. Lee WT, Leung SS, Leung DM, Cheng JC: A follow-up study on the effects of calcium-supplement withdrawal and puberty on bone acquisition of children, *Am J Clin Nutr* 64 (1):71-77, 1996.
72. Stark LJ, Davis AM, Janicke DM, Mackner LM, et al: A randomized clinical trial of dietary calcium to improve bone accretion in children with juvenile rheumatoid arthritis, *J Pediatr* 148 (4):501-07, 2006.
73. Alivizatos G, Dimopoulou I, Mitropoulos D, Dimopoulos AM, et al: Bladder cancer in a young girl with systemic lupus erythematosus treated with cyclophosphamide, *Acta Urol Belg* 59 (1):133-37, 1991.
74. Cervera R, Khamashta MA, Font J, Sebastiani GD, et al: Morbidity and mortality in systemic lupus erythematosus during a 10-year period: a comparison of early and late manifestations in a cohort of 1,000 patients, *Medicine (Baltimore)* 82 (5):299-308, 2003.
75. Levy DM, Massicotte MP, Harvey E, Hebert D, Silverman ED: Thromboembolism in pediatric lupus patients, *Lupus* 12 (10): 741-46, 2003.
76. Bjornadal L, Baecklund E, Yin L, Granath F, et al: Decreasing mortality in patients with rheumatoid arthritis: results from a large population based cohort in Sweden, 1964-95, *J Rheumatol* 29 (5):906-12, 2002.
77. Stichweh D, Arce E, Pascual V: Update on pediatric systemic lupus erythematosus, *Curr Opin Rheumatol* 16 (5):577-87, 2004.
78. Asanuma Y, Oeser A, Shintani AK, Turner E, et al: Premature coronary-artery atherosclerosis in systemic lupus erythematosus, *N Engl J Med* 349 (25):2407-15, 2003.
79. Roman MJ, Shanker BA, Davis A, Lockshin MD, et al: Prevalence and correlates of accelerated atherosclerosis in systemic lupus erythematosus, *N Engl J Med* 349 (25):2399-406, 2003.
80. Wallace DJ, Metzger AL, Stecher VJ, Turnbull BA, et al: Cholesterol-lowering effect of hydroxychloroquine in patients with rheumatic disease: reversal of deleterious effects of steroids on lipids, *Am J Med* 89 (3):322-26, 1990.
81. Moroni G, Tantardini F, Gallelli B, Quaglini S, et al: The long-term prognosis of renal transplantation in patients with lupus nephritis, *Am J Kidney Dis* 45 (5):903-11, 2005.

CHAPTER

23 Henoch-Schönlein Nephritis

Yukihiko Kawasaki and Hitoshi Suzuki

INTRODUCTION

Henoch-Schönlein purpura (HSP) was first recognized by Heberden in 1801 and first described as an association between purpura and arthritis by Schönlein in 1837. Henoch added descriptions of gastrointestinal involvement in 1874 and renal involvement in 1899. HSP is a small-vessel vasculitis whose major manifestations include arthritis, nonthrombocytopenic purpura, abdominal pain, and renal disease. In 1990, the American College of Rheumatology published diagnostic criteria for HSP, which include (1) palpable purpura, with slightly raised "palpable" hemorrhagic skin lesions, not related to thrombocytopenia; (2) age less than 20 at disease onset, with patients 20 years or younger at onset of first symptoms; (3) bowel angina, with diffuse abdominal pain, worse after meals, or the diagnosis of bowel ischemia, usually including bloody diarrhea; and (4) wall granulocytes on biopsy, with histological changes including granulocytes in the walls of arterioles or venules.[1] The classification further states that for purposes of classification, a patient shall be said to have HSP if at least two of these four criteria are present. HSP is one of the most common vasculitides of childhood and is considered to be self-limiting. One manifestation of HSP that can continue to cause lifelong problems is renal involvement.[2]

INCIDENCE OF DISEASE

Gardner-Medwin et al.[3] examined the frequency and ethnic variation of childhood vasculitides in the West Midlands region of the United Kingdom. Their survey was completed using monthly questionnaires sent to consultants and a single questionnaire sent to family doctors along with review of case notes with diagnostic codes for vasculitis. The annual incidence of HSP in the study was 22.1 per 100,000, and higher than previous estimates of 13.5 to 18.0 per 100,000. The authors postulated that a higher incidence of HSP may lead to increased incidence of renal disease and need for renal medical treatment.

CLINICAL AND LABORATORY FINDINGS

Skin

The characteristic rash is purpuric and is symmetrically distributed over the extensor surfaces of the lower legs and arms and over the sides of the buttocks. It is nearly always present in the area of the lateral malleolus and at times is present only there. It usually begins as a red maculopapular rash that then becomes purpuric and eventually takes on a fawn color as it fades. The patches of purpura may be tiny or very large. Sometimes the rash does not have a purpuric stage. It does not itch. In children under 5 years of age, the illness may start with a generalized urticarial rash, which may later become purpuric. Edema of the scalp and face and of the dorsa of the hands and feet is common. Subcutaneous bleeding may occur anywhere and is often seen in the scrotum, eyelids, and conjunctivae.

Joints

Pain, with or without swelling and tenderness, predominantly affects the ankles and knees. Other joints of the hands and feet may be affected. There is periarticular edema of short duration. There is no residual injury of the joints.

Gastrointestinal Tract

Gastrointestinal involvement occurs in approximately two-thirds of cases of HSP, is usually manifested by abdominal pain, and symptoms precede the rash in 14% to 36% of patients. Vomiting, diarrhea, periumbilical pain mimicking appendicitis, and bloody stool are the main abdominal symptoms. Major gastrointestinal complications develop in about 5% of patients, with intussusception the most common. Bowel ischemia and infarction, necrosis, intestinal perforation, fistula formation, late ileal stricture, acute appendicitis, massive upper gastrointestinal hemorrhage, pancreatitis, hydrops of the gallbladder, and pseudomembranous colitis are seen infrequently. Ultrasonography has in recent years proved useful for diagnosing intra-abdominal pathology in these patients, and is sensitive in distinguishing bowel wall edema, bowel dilatation, ascites, ileus, and intussusception. Serial ultrasonography and/or computed tomography scanning has permitted a more conservative approach, with the avoidance of unnecessary surgery. Color Doppler ultrasonography may be a useful adjunct to grayscale examination in demonstrating blood flow signals in diseased bowel wall. The most common indications for surgical intervention include intussusception, perforation, necrosis, and massive gastrointestinal bleeding.

Blood

The peripheral blood count may reveal a neutrophilic leukocytosis at onset. The erythrocyte sedimentation rate is variable and may be elevated. Platelet count, bleeding time, and clotting time are normal (the purpura is of vascular, not thrombocytopenic, origin). Fibrin-stabilizing factor, factor 13, is a clotting factor that is significantly decreased in children with HSP.[4] It has been suggested that measurement of factor 13 is useful in determining the prognosis and in management of patients, since those who have a particularly low level early in the course of the disease are more likely to have serious renal complications. However, even after fibrin-stabilizing factor has returned to a normal level, nephritis may progress.[5]

Elevated titers of ASO, anti-DNase B, and anti-NADase are present in a third of children, but titers do not differ significantly from those of matched normal control subjects.[6] Serum IgG, IgM, and IgD are usually normal. Serum IgA is increased in a significant number of children, particularly at onset.[7] A marked increase in IgA-bearing lymphocytes in the peripheral blood has been found during the acute phase of the disease. The level returned to normal after the acute symptoms had disappeared, but remained high for more than 12 months in those with marked nephritis.[8] Increased levels of IgA immune complexes were found in 13 of 18 children with HSP whether or not they developed nephritis.[9] It is known that IgA complexes may be dissolved by complement and that they may activate the alternative complement pathway.[10] Serum C3 level is normal. Although rheumatoid factor of IgG or IgM isotype is usually negative in HSP, IgA rheumatoid factor was found in 13 of 24 children with HSP. Although concentration of it tended to be highest during the acute phase of illness, there was no correlation between the level of it and the severity or duration of illness.[11] Although increased numbers of dimeric IgA-secreting cells have been found in the tonsils of patients with HSP, and those with primary IgA nephropathy, there is no evidence of increased production of IgA1 in the jejunal mucosa of patients with either of these two conditions.[12]

Significant cryoglobulinemia has been found in children with recent HSP and also in those with current glomerular disease resulting from the syndrome.[13] Analysis of cryoglobulins revealed IgA and properidin, suggesting activation of complement through the alternative pathway, but isolated cryoglobulins capable of splitting C3 in vitro did so through the classical pathway. One group of 23 children studied in the first month of illness included a third who had low serum CH50 and low serum properidin; C1q, C4, and C3 levels were not depressed.[14]

Because HSP is the most commonly encountered vasculitis in childhood, there has been speculation concerning the possibility of abnormal vascular prostaglandin metabolism in its pathophysiology. There are limited findings supporting the existence of this abnormality.[15] Plasma from 13 of 17 children with recent HSP exhibited diminished ability to support prostacyclin-like activity in vitro, and six of the children exhibited evidence of inhibitory activity. Most of the children had decreased concentrations of plasma prostacyclin metabolites, but there was no significant change in serum thromboxane A2 metabolite concentrations. It has been suggested that decreased prostaglandin I2 (PGI2) synthesis may play a role in the pathogenesis of HSPN, even though reduced levels of prostaglandin precursors do not explain everything.[16] Low-density lipoprotein components of plasma phospholipids may have an inhibitory effect, and high-density lipoproteins a protective effect, on PGI2 synthesis. It was reported that leukotriene (LT) E4 levels in patients with HSP were higher at onset than those in healthy children, and that cysteinyl LTs may play a role in the pathophysiology of purpura in HSP.[17]

Other Extrarenal Manifestations

A large variety of problems may occur in association with HSP. Nose-bleeding may be severe, and bleeding into the calf may occur, simulating deep-vein thrombosis. Convulsions, encephalopathy, facial palsy, and chorea occasionally occur. Anterior uveitis has been recorded. The liver may be enlarged. The peripheral blood exhibits a normal hemoglobin level and platelet count and no clotting defects. The white cell count and erythrocyte sedimentation rate may be moderately increased.

Kawasaki et al.[18] reported that interleukin-5 and eosinophil activation may be involved in the onset mechanism of nephritis.

Renal Manifestations

Incidence of Renal Involvement

The proportion of patients reported to have renal involvement varies between 20% and 80%.[2,8,9,19-21] Part of this variation can be accounted for by the differences in criteria used to define "renal involvement," as well as by the differences in methods used to detect microscopic hematuria. Urinary abnormalities may be transient, and unless repeated checks are performed, may be missed. Study of the surveys referred to above suggests that 20% to 30% of children have macroscopic hematuria, whereas 30% to 70% have albuminuria, or microscopic hematuria, or both, persisting for more than a week. However, increased rates of red cell excretion in urine have been found in all children with HSPN.[19]

Renal Presentation

Just as skin, joint, and gut symptoms may occur in any order at any time over a period of several days or weeks, so too may renal manifestations occur at any time. In general, the first urinary abnormality is noted after other symptoms, but hematuria may occasionally be the initial feature. In 80% of children with a urinary abnormality, the first abnormality is detected within 4 weeks of onset of the illness. In most of the remainder, urinary abnormality develops within the next 8 weeks, and a small minority of affected children are found to have urinary abnormalities several months later.[20]

The nonrenal manifestations of illness fluctuate over a period of days or weeks before disappearing. Recurrences are common and appear to be particularly common in those in whom severe renal damage has occurred. Meadow et al.[19] found that 25% of 88 children with HSPN had suffered a late relapse of the syndrome 2 months or more after the initial episode. Relapses may occur at the time of an upper respiratory tract infection.[19]

The most common urinary abnormalities are albuminuria and microscopic hematuria. A smaller number of patients have macroscopic hematuria. Acute nephritic syndrome occurs in the more severe cases and may lead to nephrotic syndrome or to renal insufficiency. Both of these may develop independently and insidiously, but they are much more likely to develop in the child who has had an acute nephritic stage in the course of illness.

PATHOLOGIC CHANGES

Light Microscopy

The basic pattern of glomerular involvement is that of mesangial injury or mesangial proliferative glomerulonephritis with varying degrees of hypercellularity, similar to the lesions in IgA nephropathy. Segmental capillary thrombosis, possibly related to the development of necrosis and crescents, is often present.[22] For classification of the degree of involvement and correlation of it with clinical manifestations and prognostic indices, the following categories have been established. Glomerular changes were graded according to a classification devised by pathologists of the International Study of Kidney Disease in Children (ISKDC), shown in Table 23-1. In general, nephrotic syndrome is present in only about 25% of patients of groups I, II, and III, and hematuria is present in all groups. Patients with group II and IIIa histologic findings tend to have better outcomes, with return of normal renal function or persistent microscopic hematuria and proteinuria, whereas patients in groups IIIb, IV, and V have persistent proteinuria and hematuria or progress to terminal renal failure.[19,22] Occasionally patients develop rapidly progressive renal failure accompanied by exuberant crescent formation.

Glomeruli

The model of histological expression of HSPN incorporates mesangial proliferative glomerulonephritis in the tufts. Probably 30% to 35% of all patients have mesangial proliferation (Figure 23-1), characterized by increased numbers of cells confined to mesangial areas and associated expansion of mesangial matrix, but without conspicuous crescents. Considerable interglomerular and segmental variation is regularly observed in biopsies, as in those of IgA nephropathy patients.[23] One-half of biopsies with proliferation confined to the mesangium also reveal foci of necrosis (Figure 23-2), segmental splitting of capillary walls, areas of parietal epithelial hyper-

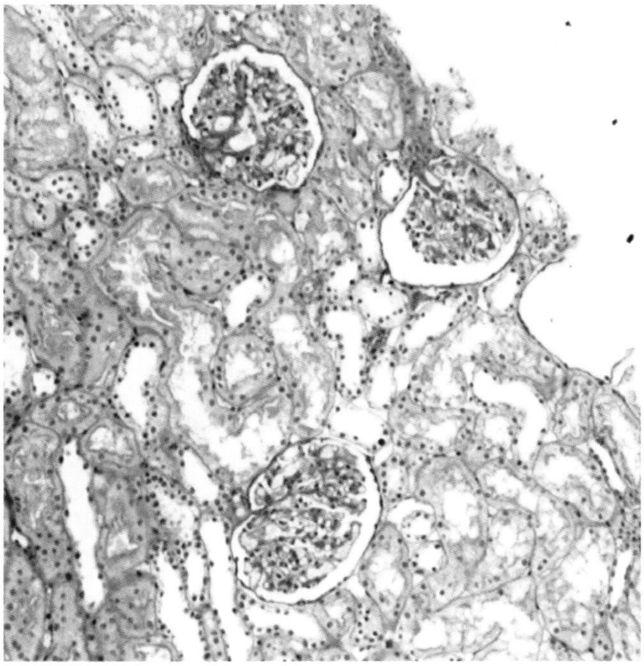

Figure 23-1 The glomerulus shows mild segmental mesangial proliferation (PAS, ×400).

TABLE 23-1 Henoch-Schönlein Purpura Nephritis Pathology Classification of International Study of Kidney Disease in Children

Group I	Minimal changes
Group II	Pure mesangial proliferation without crescents
Group III	Mesangial proliferative glomerulonephritis with <50% crescents IIIa. Focal IIIb. Diffuse
Group IV	Mesangial proliferative glomerulonephritis with 50%-75% crescents IVa. Focal IVb. Diffuse
Group V	Mesangial proliferative glomerulonephritis with >75% crescents Va. Focal Vb. Diffuse
Group VI	Membranoproliferative (mesangiocapillary) glomerulonephritis

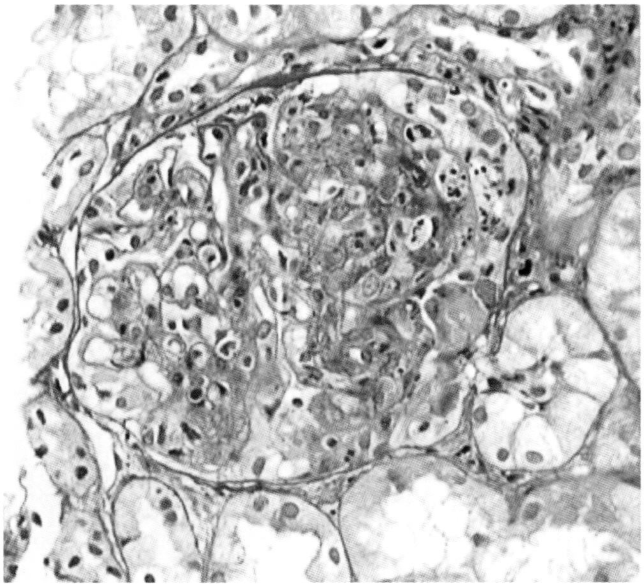

Figure 23-2 The glomerulus shows a localized area of cellular proliferation and an area of necrosis in the lobule (PAS, ×400).

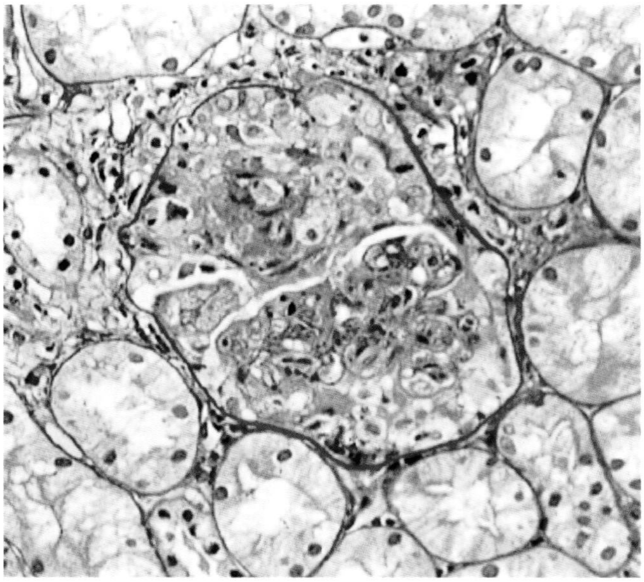

Figure 23-3 The glomerulus shows a cellular crescent (PAS, ×400).

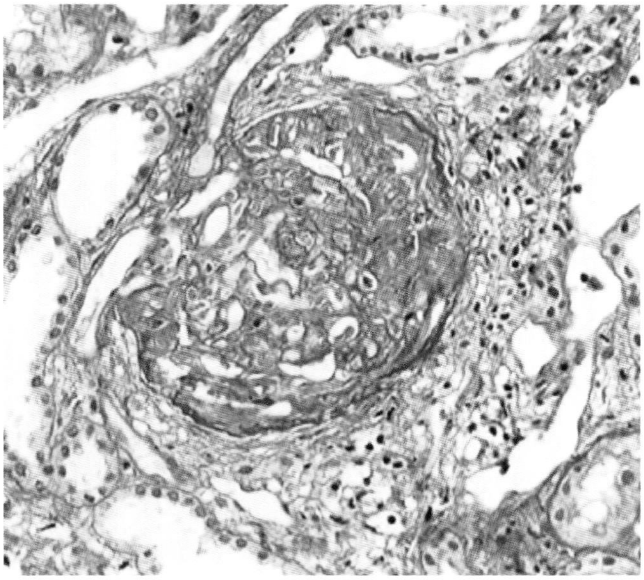

Figure 23-4 The glomerulus shows a fibrous crescent (PAS, ×400).

plasia, and small and scattered foci of segmental capillary collapse.

Another 20% of patients exhibit a true segmental endocapillary proliferation superimposed on mesangial proliferation without crescents; 13% of patients exhibit diffuse but segmentally variable endocapillary proliferative glomerulonephritis without conspicuous crescents.[23-25] Neutrophils and monocytes infiltrate many glomeruli in approximately one-half of these patients. In 2%, a pattern closely resembling membranoproliferative glomerulonephritis type I can be seen.[23]

Crescents are a conspicuous component of the appearance of glomeruli in 40% of patients with HSPN (Figures 23-3 to 23-5). Most of those patients (32% overall) have crescents in fewer than 50% of the glomeruli, and nearly all of the remainder (6%-7%) have 50% to 75% of glomeruli involved.[23,26-28]

Of biopsies with crescents, proliferation is confined to the mesangium in 25%, is distributed in the mesangium and in capillaries in a focal segmental pattern in 30%, and shows diffuse endocapillary involvement in 45%.[23] Proliferation within the tufts is distributed similarly in glomeruli with and without crescents. In many affected glomeruli, the segments with proliferation exhibit adhesion of the tuft to Bowman's capsule.

Interstitium

The interstitium is affected to a degree consonant with the severity of the glomerular injury. A patchy leukocytic infiltrate consisting mainly of lymphocytes, macrophages, and plasma cells is seen, with a minor degree of edema, in 15% to 20% of patients.[24,28] There is often a periglomerular or perivascular accentuation of the infiltrates, which generally occupy less than 25% of the cortex. Tubular casts and atrophy are also encountered focally in most biopsies, and in most

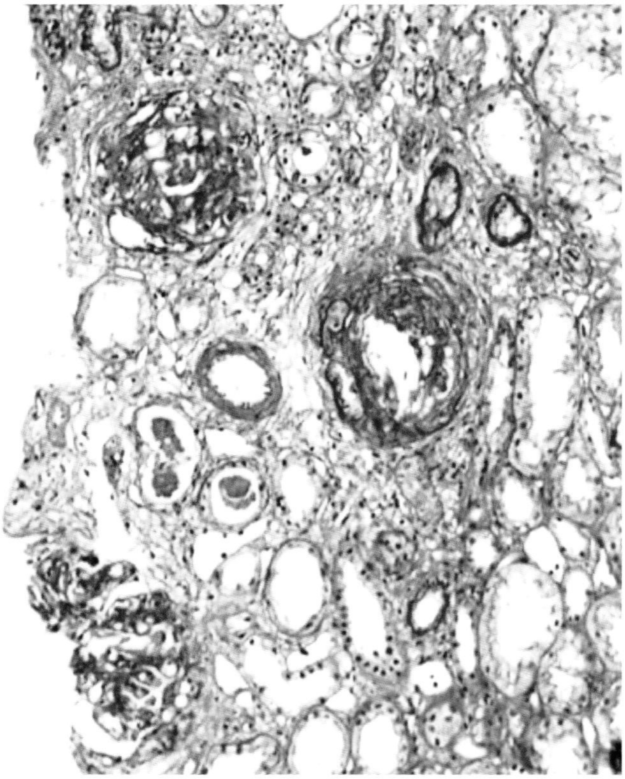

Figure 23-5 Circumferential crescents are evident in most glomeruli in this florid case of HSPN. The tubular degeneration is extensive (PAS, ×200).

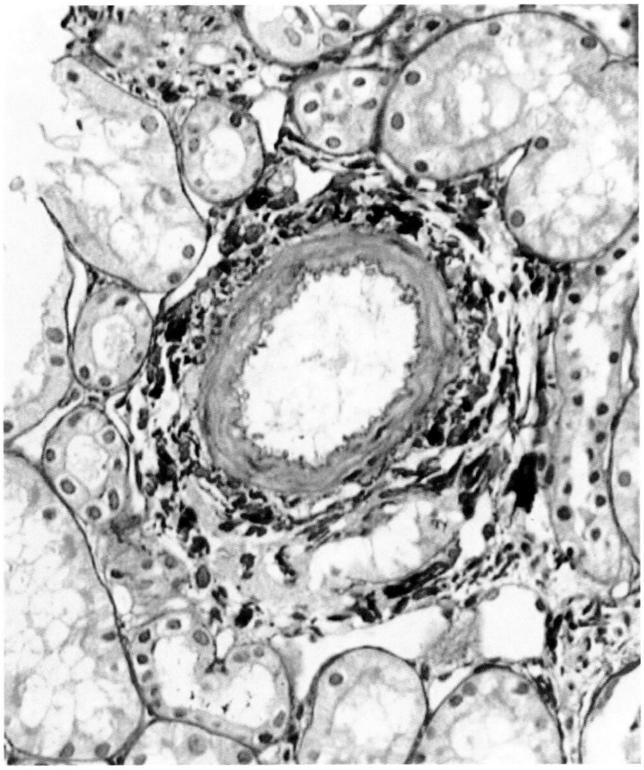

Figure 23-6 A small, intralobular renal artery shows necrotizing vasculitis with intense leukocytic infiltration (PAS, ×400).

cases erythrocytes and red cell casts are seen in some tubular lumens. Tubular degeneration is extensive in only 10% of patients.

Blood Vessels

Medial hypertrophy and intimal fibrotic thickening are present in biopsies from some patients, although in most reported series details are scanty, and the incidence of vascular sclerosis cannot be reliably estimated. Hyaline change and accumulation of fibrinoid material or frank necrotizing vasculitis (Figure 23-6) may be present, but the latter is rare, even in association with the more florid lesions.

Electron Microscopy

On electron microscopy, the principal abnormalities are found in the mesangium. Focal proliferation, increase in mesangial matrix, and electron-dense deposits may be seen. Similar electron-dense deposits may be found scattered in the subendothelial areas adjacent to the mesangium. These deposits have been shown to contain IgA by immunoelectron microscopy.[29] The findings are similar to those of IgA nephropathy. The capillary lumen may contain platelets and fibrin. Although not described in earlier reports, subepithelial deposits were noted by Urizar et al.[30] in 6 of 25 biopsy specimens studied; in 3 specimens, these deposits were virtually identical to the humps classically described in acute poststreptococcal glomerulonephritis. Similar deposits have been described in several other reports. In any location, the deposits are easier to identify in thick sections embedded in plastic and stained with toluidine blue than in the material prepared for electron microscopic study. Basement membrane lysis or dissolution, especially in association with subepithelial deposits and neutrophils in capillary lumens, is found in more than half of biopsies. These changes correlate well with more severe glomerular damage as assessed by light microscopy and by heavy proteinuria.

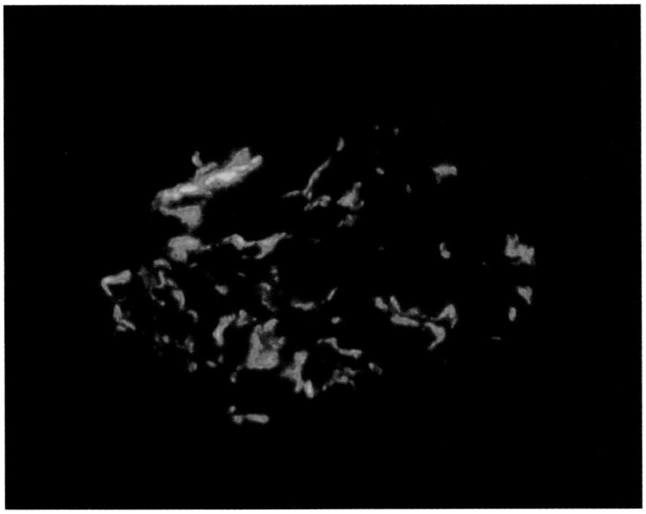

Figure 23-7 The immunofluorescence micrograph reveals the mesangial distribution of IgA in a child with HSPN (PAS, ×400).

Immunofluorescence

In contrast to the frequently focal and segmental nature of the glomerular lesions observed on light microscopy, one of the striking features on immunofluorescence study is the widespread involvement of glomeruli. These abnormalities are granular deposits of IgA (Figure 23-7) and, to a lesser extent, IgG or IgM.[22-25] Secretory pieces are absent but J chains may be detected, indicating the polymeric nature of the IgA deposits. The later-acting components of the complement sequence, C3 and properdin, are more frequently found than C1q or C4. The deposits are largely mesangial in distribution, with an occasional segmental paramesangial capillary deposit. Fibrin-related antigens are frequently deposited in the mesangial areas.

PATHOGENESIS

The pathogenesis of HSP remains unknown; however, HSP is generally believed to be an immune complex–mediated disease characterized by the presence of polymeric IgA1 (pIgA1)–containing immune complexes predominantly in dermal gastrointestinal and glomerular capillaries.[31] The pathognomonic granular IgA and C3 deposits in the mesangium are indistinguishable from those seen in IgA nephropathy. Similar immunohistologic findings have been observed in the kidneys of patients with liver cirrhosis, dermatitis herpetiformis, celiac disease, and chronic inflammatory disease of the lung.

Biology of IgA

In healthy subjects, IgA is found abundantly in mucosal fluids, but its concentration in the serum is relatively low. The IgA in primates occurs as two isotypes, IgA1 and IgA2, which are distinguished by the presence in IgA1 of a hinge region containing five O-linked oligosaccharide side chains composed of serine-linked N-acetylgalactosamine (GalNAc) and galactose, the latter of which may be sialylated. Sixty percent of IgA in secretions is of the IgA2 subclass, is primarily polymeric, and has a secretory component synthesized by glandular epithelial cells. Serum IgA is mostly IgA1 and is 90% monomeric. In HSPN, mesangial deposits contain predominantly pIgA1, with bridging J protein absent in the secretory component.[25]

Site of pIgA Production and Roles of Impaired IgA Synthesis and Clearance

Both increased IgA synthesis and diminished clearance have been implicated in the pathogenesis of IgA immune complex deposition. Increased pIgA production by the mucosal immune system in response to a mucosally presented antigen has been hypothesized as a potential mechanism for the development of HSP.[32] Hyper-reactivity of both B and T cells in response to specific antigenic stimuli in vitro has been reported in patients with HSP. Clinical observations in vivo have implicated infectious antigens as immunomodulators, and clinical associations have been observed between mucosal infections and HSP (Table 23-2). Other antigens, including dietary proteins (gliadin) and extracellular matrix components (collagen and fibronectin), have also been implicated. No exogenous antigen has been consistently identified either in circulating immune complexes (CIC) or in the mesangial deposits.[23] Some studies have demonstrated increased pIgA production in mucosal and tonsillar cells, whereas others have unexpectedly revealed down-regulation of pIgA production in the mucosa and upregulation in the bone marrow.[33] Alteration of mucosal pIgA production allowing increased antigen penetration to stimulate an exaggerated marrow response has been suggested to occur.[32] Total serum levels of IgA are increased in 40% to 50% of patients with HSP, with elevations of both monomeric IgA and pIgA.[34,35]

TABLE 23-2 Antigens Implicated in Precipitation of Henoch-Schönlein Purpura

Infections	Upper respiratory tract infections, measles, rubella, human parvovirus B19, mycoplasma, Coxsackie virus, toxocara, amebiasis, *Salmonella hirschfeldii, Clostridium difficile*, morganella morganii, streptococcus, mumps, tuberculosis, *Legionella longbeachae, Helicobacter pylori*, adenovirus
Medications	Vancomycin, ranitidine, streptokinase, cefuroxime, diclofenac, enalapril, captopril
Miscellaneous	Leukemias and lymphomas, breast cancer, small-cell lung cancer, myelodysplastic syndrome, autosomal-recessive chronic granulomatous disease, exposure to cold, food hypersensitivity

Mechanism of Mesangial IgA Deposition

Capillary IgA immune complexes are likely the result of either CIC deposition or in situ complex formation. There is reasonable clinical evidence to suggest that CIC deposition is unlikely to be the sole explanation. Serum IgA1 has been shown to be abnormally O-glycosylated in patients with HSP and IgA nephropathy.[28] Circulating IgA1 has reduced terminal galactose on 0-linked sugars, and a B cell defect in β-1,3-galactosyltransferase has been implicated.[25] Altered hinge-region glycosylation may change IgA1 structure, modifying interaction with matrix proteins, IgA receptors, and complement, causing mesangial deposition and subsequent injury.[23] A study demonstrating abnormal IgA glycosylation restricted to those HSP patients with clinical nephritis lends support to a role for altered IgA1 O-glycosylation in the pathogenesis of IgA-associated glomerular disease. The presence and potential pathogenetic role of circulating IgA-antineutrophil cytoplasmic antibodies (ANCA) and IgA rheumatoid factor observed in patients with HSP have also been reported.

Pathogenesis of Glomerular Injury

Traditional mediators of inflammation have been implicated in the glomerular injury that occurs in HSP. Deposition of C3 and properdin without C1q and C4 is typical, suggesting alternate pathway activation. Despite the demonstration of complement components in skin and renal biopsies, controversy remains regarding the role of complement in the pathogenesis of HSP. Some authors believe that IgG co-Ig deposition may induce complement activation and modulate disease activity.[9] The roles of cytokines, growth factors, chemokines, and adhesion molecules in mesangial proliferation are under investigation. Interleukin-1 (IL-1), IL-6, platelet-derived growth factor, tumor necrosis factor, free oxygen radicals, prostanoids, leukotrienes, vascular cell adhesion molecule-1, membrane attack complex (C5b-9), and a circulating immunostimulatory protein have all been implicated.

Diagnostic Investigation

There is no specific serologic test available to diagnose HSP. Elevated levels of IgA, IgA-rheumatoid factor, and IgA-containing immune complexes have been detected in patients with HSP,[34,35] and although a correlation between serum IgA level and clinical features has been suggested, it has not been consistently demonstrated. The diagnosis is made on the basis of clinical suspicion, and laboratory tests are mainly directed toward excluding other diagnostic possibilities and assessing the extent of renal involvement. Renal biopsy is especially useful in distinguishing HSP from other disorders and, for patients with renal disease, in assessing prognosis and suggesting the need for treatment.

COURSE AND CLINICOPATHOLOGICAL CORRELATIONS

Although HSP is generally a benign, self-limited disorder, there may be episodic and recurrent bouts of rash, arthralgia, gastrointestinal symptoms, and hematuria for several months or even years after the initial onset.

In patients with focal and segmental proliferative glomerular lesions, the overall mortality is less than 10% at 5 and 10 years after onset.[19,36,37] In a large series of patients seen by Meadow et al.[19] 2 years or more after diagnosis, 55% were entirely normal, 22% had residual urinary abnormalities but normal GFR, 10% had both abnormal urine sediment and reduced GFR, and 8% had severe reduction in GFR, were receiving dialysis, or had died of renal failure. The occurrence of acute nephritic syndrome at onset, persistent nephrotic syndrome, and older age were indicators of a poor prognosis. All renal deaths occurred in patients with clinical and histological pictures of crescentic glomerulonephritis. In a group of patients who recovered or improved clinically, repeated biopsies also revealed lessening of severe glomerular alterations. Hypercellularity diminished or disappeared, and focal lesions decreased in number and extent of glomerular involvement. Furthermore, IgA deposits diminished to a considerable extent or even disappeared in a few patients. Capillary wall deposits also disappeared with clinical improvement.[37]

In long-term follow-up of 78 patients, averaging 23 years, Goldstein et al.[36] noted that 44% of patients who presented with nephrotic syndrome or acute nephritis had persisting hypertension or progressive decline in GFR, while 82% of those who presented with hematuria alone were normal. More than one-third of pregnancies in these patients were complicated. Subsequent deterioration in clinical status after initial, apparently full recovery occurred in approximately 20% to 25% of patients, indicating the need for long-term follow-up of patients with HSP.

TREATMENT

The extrarenal manifestations of HSPN are managed by appropriate symptomatic measures. Severe skin lesions may require oral corticosteroids,[22,23] which may also improve abdominal pain and protein-losing enteropathy.[38] Severe gastrointestinal complications may occasionally require surgical intervention.[39] The treatment of HSPN is controversial, and recommendations are based on small, often uncontrolled series.

Steroids

The majority of patients with HSPN have no clinical renal involvement or microhematuria, mild proteinuria, and normal renal function. These patients do not require steroid therapy, and the disease is usually managed symptomatically. An uncontrolled prospective study of 38 children with severe forms of HSPN suggested improvement in activity and chronicity indices on renal biopsy after the administration of methylprednisolone pulse therapy.[40] Another study appeared to verify that early administration of prednisone can be useful in preventing the development of HSPN.[41,42] One group suggested treating patients with risk factors for renal involvement with corticosteroids at the onset of disease. In an uncontrolled study, Kawasaki et al.[41] reported that methylprednisolone and urokinase pulse therapy are effective for those patients with risk of progression of HSPN, especially if they were started early during the course of disease before crescents became fibrous.

Multiple-Drug Therapy

A prospective study of 12 patients with HSP who presented with rapidly progressive glomerulonephritis suggested benefit from intensive multiple-drug therapy.[42,43] Clinical improvement with combined corticosteroid and azathioprine therapy was suggested by another study of 21 children with severe HSPN. Kawasaki et al.[44] reported that methylprednisolone and urokinase pulse therapy combined with cyclophosphamide significantly reduced urinary protein excretion and prevented any increase in crescentic and sclerosed glomeruli in HSPN patients with at least type IV, compared with methylprednisolone and urokinase pulse therapy alone. At most recent follow-up, there were no patients with persistent nephropathy or renal insufficiency among those treated with methylprednisolone and urokinase pulse therapy combined with cyclophosphamide.

Plasmapheresis

The clinical courses of nine children with a rapidly progressive type of HSPN demonstrated that early use of plasmapheresis may have been effective in improving prognosis.[45] In another case series study without controls, multiple-drug therapy combined with plasmapheresis may have been of benefit to children with the rapidly progressive type of HSPN.[46]

Other Types of Treatment

The use of intravenous immunoglobulin (IVIg) for the treatment of HSP is anecdotal. It has been advocated as effective for abdominal pain and other gastrointestinal symptoms.[47]

Some studies have reported that tonsillectomy was effective for patients with severe HSPN.[48]

Transplantation

After transplantation HSPN may recur, and rates of recurrence are increased in recipients of living-related transplantations.[49,50] Meulders et al.[49] reported the actuarial risks for renal recurrence and for graft loss due to recurrence were 35% and 11%, respectively, at 5 years after transplantation. Recurrence appeared to be associated with shorter duration of the original episode of disease, occurred despite delay of more than 1 year between disappearance of purpura and transplantation, and was not prevented by a triple immunosuppressive regimen that included cyclosporin.

Finally, our recommendations for treatment of HSPN in our hospital are shown in Table 23-3. We try to perform renal biopsy soon after onset of HSPN and give aggressive therapy according to the severity of pathological lesions. We believe these treatments of HSPN effectively improve the prognosis for HSPN.

TABLE 23-3 Treatment of Henoch-Schönlein Purpura Nephritis in Our Hospital	
Severity	**Treatment**
International Study of Kidney Disease in Children (ISKDC) Classification	
I or II	Antiplatelet agents*
IIIa	Steroid + antiplatelet agents + anticoagulant*
IIIb	Methylprednisolone + urokinase pulse + steroid + antiplatelet agents + anticoagulant (MUT)†
IVa, IVb	MUT with cyclophosphamide (MUCT)‡
Va, Vb	MUCT
VI	MUCT
Other	
Patients with rapidly progressive Henoch-Schönlein purpura nephritis	MUCT with plasmapheresis§
Patients with ISKDC IIIa presenting as nephrotic syndrome	MUT

* From Kawasaki Y, Suzuki J, Suzuki H, et al: Clinical and pathological features of children with Henoch-Schönlein purpura nephritis: risk factors associated with poor prognosis. *Clin Nephrol* 60:153-60, 2003.
† From Kawasaki Y, Suzuki J, Suzuki H, et al: Efficacy of methylprednisolone and urokinase pulse therapy for severe Henoch-Schönlein nephritis. *Pediatrics* 111:785-89, 2003.
‡ From Kawasaki Y, Suzuki J, Suzuki H: Efficacy of methylprednisolone and urokinase pulse therapy combined with or without cyclophosphamide in severe Henoch-Schönlein nephritis: a clinical and histological study. *Nephrol Dial Transplant* 19:858-64, 2004.
§ From Kawasaki Y, Suzuki J, Suzuki H, et al: Plasmapheresis therapy for rapidly progressive Henoch-Schönlein nephritis. *Pediatr Nephrol* 19:920-23, 2004.

REFERENCES

1. Mills JA, Michel BA, Bloch DA, et al: The American College of Rheumatology 1990 criteria for the classification of Henoch-Schönlein purpura, *Arthritis Rheum* 33:1114-21, 1990.
2. Saulsbury FT: Epidemiology of Henoch-Schönlein purpura, *Cleve Clin J Med* 69:S187-89, 2002.
3. Gardner-Medwin JM, Dolezalova P, Cummins C, et al: Incidence of Henoch-Schönlein purpura, Kawasaki disease, and rare vasculitides in children of different ethnic origins, *Lancet* 360:1197-202, 2002.
4. Henriksson P, Hedner U, Nilsson IM: Factor III (fibrin stabilising factor) in Henoch-Schönlein's purpura, *Acuta Paediatr Scand* 66:273-76, 1977.
5. Dalens B, Travade P, Labbe A, et al: Diagnostic and prognostic value of fibrin stabilising factor in Schönlein-Henoch syndrome, *Arch Dis Child* 58:12-14, 1983.
6. Ayoub EM, Hoyer J: Anaphylactoid purpura: Streptococcal antibody titers and beta1c-globulin levels, *J Pediatr* 75:193-201, 1969.
7. Trygstad CW, Stiehm ER: Elevated serum IgA globulin in anaphylactoid purpura, *Pediatrics* 47:1023-28, 1971.
8. Kuno-Saki H, Sakai H, Nomoto Y, et al: Increase of IgA-bearing peripheral blood lymphocytes in children with Henoch-Schönlein purpura, *Pediatrics* 64:1979-84, 1979.
9. Levinsky RJ, Barratt TM: IgA immune complexes in Henoch-Schönlein purpura, *Lancet* 2:1100-103, 1979.
10. Gotze O, Muller-Ererhard HG: The C3 activator system: An alternate pathway of complement activation, *J Exp Med* 134:90-95, 1971.
11. Rogers PW, Bunn SM, Kurtzman NA, et al: Schönlein-Henoch syndrome associated with exposure to cold, *Arch Intern Med* 128:782-86, 1971.
12. Hene RJ, Schuurman H, Kater L: Immunoglobulin A subclass-containing plasma cells in the jejunum in primary IgA nephropathy and in Henoch-Schönlein purpura, *Nephron* 48:4-7, 1988.
13. Garcia-Fuentes M, Chantler C, Williams DG: Cryoglobulinaemia in Henoch-Schönlein purpura, *BMJ* 2:163-65, 1977.
14. Garcia-Fuentes M, Martin A, Chantler C, et al: Serum complement components in Henoch-Schönlein purpura, *Arch Dis Child* 53: 417-19, 1978.
15. Turi S, Belch JJF, Beattie TJ, et al: Abnormalities of vascular prostaglandins in Henoch-Schönlein purpura, *Arch Dis Child* 61:173-77, 1986.
16. Turi S, Nagy J, Haszon I, et al: Plasma factors influencing PGI2-like activity in patients with IgA nephropathy and Henoch-Schönlein purpura, *Pediatr Nephrol* 3:61-67, 1989.
17. Tsuji Y, Abe Y, Hisano M, et al: Urinary leukotriene E4 in Henoch-Schönlein purpura, *Clin Exp Allergy* 34:1259-61, 2004.
18. Kawasaki Y, Hosoya M, Suzuki H: Possible pathologenic role of interleukin-5 and eosino cationic protein in Henoch-Schönlein purpura nephritis, *Pediatr Int* 47:512-17, 2005.
19. Meadow SR, Glasgow EF, White RHR, et al: Schönlein-Henoch nephritis, *Q J Med* 41:241-45, 1972.
20. Hurly RM, Drummond KN: Anaphylactoid purpura nephritis. Clinicopathological correlations, *J Pediatr* 81:904-11, 1972.
21. Kawasaki Y, Suzuki J, Suzuki H, et al: Clinical and pathological features of children with Henoch-Schönlein purpura nephritis: risk factors associated with poor prognosis, *Clin Nephrol* 60:153-60, 2003.
22. Glassock RJ, Cohen AH, Adler SG, et al: Secondary glomerular disease. In Brenner BM, Rector FC Jr, editors: *The kidney*, ed 4, Philadelphia, 1991, WB Saunders, pp. 1280-302.
23. Silva FG: IgA nephropathy and Henoch-Schönlein syndrome. In Jennette JC, Olson JL, Schwartz MM, Silva FG, editors: *Heptinstall's pathology of the kidney*, ed 15, Philadelphia, 1998, Lippincott Raven, pp. 479-540.
24. Coppo R, Mazzucco G, Cagnoli L, et al: Henoch-Schönlein purpura in adult and children: renal features and prognostic factors, *Nephrol Dial Transplant* 12:2277-83, 1997.
25. Kobayashi O, Wada H, Okawa K, et al: Schönlein-Henoch's syndrome in children, *Contrib Nephrol* 4:48-71, 1977.
26. Counahan R, Winterborn MH, White RHR, et al: Prognosis of Henoch-Schönlein nephritis in children, *BMJ* 2:11-18, 1977.
27. Farine M, Poucell S, Geary DL, et al: Prognostic significance of urinary findings and renal biopsies in children with Henoch-Schönlein nephritis, *Clin Pediatr* 25:257-59, 1986.
28. Niaudet P, Habib R: Schönlein-Henoch purpura nephritis: prognostic factors and therapy, *Ann Med Intern* 145:577-80, 1994.

29. Yoshiara S, Yoshikawa N, Matsuo T: Immunoelectron microscopic study of childhood IgA nephropathy and Henoch-Schönlein nephritis, *Virchows Arch A* 412:95-102, 1987.
30. Urizar EE, Singh JK, Muhammad T, et al: Henoch-Schönlein anaphylactoid purpura nephropathy: electron microscopic lesions mimicking acute poststreptococcal nephritis, *Hum Pathol* 9:223-28, 1978.
31. Vogler C, Eliason SC, Wood EG: Glomerular membranopathy in children with IgA nephropathy and Henoch-Schönlein purpura, *Pediatr Dev Pathol* 2:227-35, 1999.
32. Allen A, Harper S, Feehally J: Origin and structure of pathogenic IgA in IgA nephropathy, *Biochem Soc Transac* 25:486-90, 1997.
33. Moja P, Quesnel A, Resseguier V, et al: Is there IgA from gut mucosal origin in the serum of children with Henoch-Schönlein purpura? *Clin Immunol Immunopathol* 86:290-97, 1998.
34. Jones CL, Powell HR, Kincaid-Smith P et al: Polymeric IgA and immune complex concentrations in IgA-related renal disease, *Kidney Int* 38:323-31, 1990.
35. Allen AC, Willis FR, Beattie TJ, et al: Abnormal IgA glycosylation in Henoch-Schönlein purpura restricted to patients with clinical nephritis, *Nephrol Dial Transplant* 13:930-34, 1998.
36. Goldstein AR, White RH, Akuse R, et al: Long-term follow-up of childhood Henoch-Schönlein nephritis, *Lancet* 339:280-82, 1992.
37. Mollica F, LiVolti S, Garozzo R, et al: Effectiveness of early prednisone treatment in preventing the development of nephropathy in anaphylactoid purpura, *Eur J Pediatr* 151:40-43, 1992.
38. Reif S, Jain A, Santiago J, et al: Protein-losing enteropathy as a manifestation of Henoch-Schönlein purpura, *Acuta Paediatr Scand* 80:482-85, 1991.
39. Cull DL, Rosario V, Lally KP, et al: Surgical implications of Henoch-Schönlein purpura, *J Pediatr Surg* 25:741-43, 1990.
40. Niaudet P, Habib R: Methylprednisolone pulse therapy in the treatment of severe forms of Schönlein-Henoch purpura nephritis, *Pediatr Nephrol* 1998,12:238-43, 1998.
41. Kawasaki Y, Suzuki J, Suzuki H, et al: Efficacy of methylprednisolone and urokinase pulse therapy for severe Henoch-Schönlein nephritis, *Pediatrics* 111:785-89, 2003.
42. Iijima K, Nakamura H, Yoshikawa N, et al: Multiple combined therapy for severe Henoch-Schönlein nephritis in children, *Pediatr Nephrol* 12:244-48, 1998.
43. Oner A, Tinaztepe K, Erdogan O: The effect of triple therapy on rapidly progressive type of Henoch-Schönlein purpura nephritis to corticosteroid and azathioprine therapy, *Clin Nephrol* 49:9-14, 1998.
44. Kawasaki Y, Suzuki J, Suzuki H: Efficacy of methylprednisolone and urokinase pulse therapy combined with or without cyclophosphamide in severe Henoch-Schönlein nephritis: a clinical and histological study, *Nephrol Dial Transplant* 19:858-64, 2004.
45. Hattori M, Ito K, Konomoto T, Kawaguchi H, et al: Plasmapheresis as the sole therapy for rapidly progressive Henoch-Schönlein purpura nephritis in children, *Am J Kidney Dis* 33:427-33, 1999.
46. Kawasaki Y, Suzuki J, Suzuki H, et al: Plasmapheresis therapy for rapidly progressive Henoch-Schönlein nephritis, *Pediatr Nephrol* 19:920-23, 2004.
47. Heldrich FJ, Minkin S, Gatdula CI: Intravenous immunoglobulin in Henoch-Schönlein purpura: a case study, *Md Med J* 42:577-79, 1993.
48. Suguyama H, Watanabe N, Onoda T, et al: Successful treatment of progressive Henoch-Schönlein purpura nephritis with tonsillectomy and steroid pulse therapy, *Intern Med* 44:611-15, 2005.
49. Meulders Q, Pirson Y, Cosyns JP, et al: Course of Henoch-Schönlein nephritis after renal transplantation: report on ten patients and review of the literature, *Transplantation* 58:1179-86, 1994.
50. Ramos EL: Recurrent diseases in the renal allograft, *J Am Soc Nephrol* 2:109-21, 1991.

CHAPTER

24 Wegener's Granulomatosis, Microscopic Polyangiitis, and Childhood Polyarteritis Nodosa

Aysin Bakkaloglu and Seza Ozen

Vasculitis is an inflammation of blood vessels. Systemic vasculitides often affect the kidney as well. Renal disease is a major cause of morbidity and mortality. Vasculitis may affect vessels of various sizes, including the renal artery, renal arterioles, or glomerular capillaries.

This chapter will focus on the systemic vasculitides that commonly affect the kidney: Wegener's granulomatosis (WG), microscopic polyangiitis (MPA), and childhood polyarteritis nodosa (PAN).

WEGENER'S GRANULOMATOSIS

Wegener's granulomatosis is a granulomatous inflammation involving the respiratory tract and necrotizing vasculitis affecting small- to medium-sized vessels.[1,2] The etiology of WG, like other primary systemic vasculitides, remains unknown.

The disease is rare in children. According to the 1999 U.S. Renal Data System annual data report, WG was the underlying cause of end-stage renal disease (ESRD) in 40 pediatric patients.[3] Environmental factors appear to be necessary for the development of WG. These factors may explain the epidemiological distribution of WG. Watts and Scott[4] have reported the disease to be more frequent in Northern Europe compared to microscopic polyarteritis, which seems to be more common in southern Europe. On the other hand, in a recent report from New Zealand the prevalence of the disease was found to be 152 per million which is equivalent to northern European figures.[5] Among exogenous factors, *Staphylococci* as well as heavy metals have been implicated in the pathogenesis.[6]

Pathogenesis

Wegener's granulomatosis is among the heterogeneous group of anti-neutrophil cytoplasmic antibodies (ANCA)—associated systemic vasculitides. As a multifactorial disease, WG is characterized by the presence of specific ANCA subtypes that are often directed against proteinase 3 (PR3).[7] Recent studies have shown that ANCA interact with primed neutrophils that express PR3 on their surface.[8] This interaction depends on adherence mediated by factors such as Fc gamma receptor IIa and integrins at the endothelial surface.[9] ANCA induce stable adherence of rolling neutrophils to affirm integrin-mediated adhesion to the endothelial surface.[6,8] Neutrophils and monocytes activated by ANCA undergo a respiratory burst as well as showing expression and secretion of prostimulatory cytokines such as TNF and IL8, and these primed neutrophils and monocytes are cytotoxic to the endothelial cell.[6,8]

The genetics of WG is quite complex. The disease has been associated with a region on chromosome 6p21.3.[7] The polymorphisms of the natural inhibitor of PR3, alpha-1-antitrypsin, was also studied as a susceptibility factor for the disease: heterozygosity for alpha-1-antitrypsin deficiency has been associated with an increased risk and morbidity of WG.[10] Polymorphisms for Fc gamma receptor and PR3 also seemed to be involved in the predisposition to WG.[6,7]

Among the environmental factors that are effective in disease pathogenesis, *Staphylococcus aureus* has been frequently implicated, especially because of its association with disease relapses.

Clinical Manifestations

The disease mostly affects the respiratory system and kidneys but may affect almost any organ. There are only a few rather small published childhood series, and mainly case reports.

Disease onset in these reports varies from infancy to adolescence. Most features are similar to those in adults. However, subglottic stenosis and nasal deformity are more common in children.[11-13] The most affected organs are the upper airways, lungs, and kidneys in the three largest childhood series.

The kidneys are involved in 10% to 100% of childhood cases.[6] Necrotizing glomerulonephritis is one of the most serious disease manifestations in WG. Hematuria, proteinuria, and renal insufficiency are common, whereas hypertension and gross hematuria are unusual. Fifty-seven percent of children with WG developed renal insufficiency and 14% required dialysis.[3]

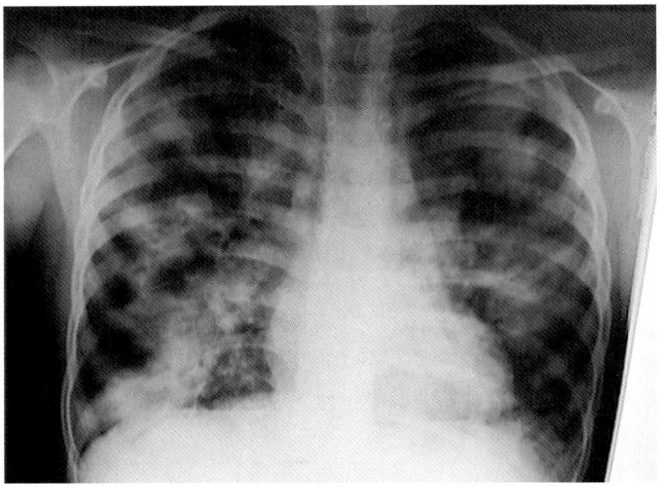

Figure 24-1 Chest x-ray of a patient revealing nodular infiltrates.

Lower respiratory tract involvement may present as cough, dyspnea, and hemoptysis.[14] A chest x-ray may show nodular infiltrates and nodules (Figure 24-1).

Other clinical findings may include blurred vision, eye pain, conjunctivitis, episcleritis of the eye, and persistent otitis media. Arthralgia may occur in 30% to 78% of patients, and myalgia may also occur.[11-13] Skin lesions may be in the form of leukocytoclastic vasculitis or may be nodular, vesicular, or papular in nature, and central nervous system involvement (CNS) may also occur as cranial nerve palsies, seizures, or neuropathies.[14] Cardiac involvement is very rare.

Laboratory Features and ANCA

The complete blood count usually reveals anemia, normal white blood cell count, and thrombocytosis. Acute-phase reactants are elevated. Urinalysis is essential and will show hematuria, proteinuria, and casts when there is kidney involvement. Chest x-ray and pulmonary function tests are indicated for the assessment of lung disease,[14] and computerized tomography of the lung provides more detailed evaluation for pulmonary involvement.

ANCA is highly associated with WG and is included in the new classification of the disease.[2] A cytoplasmic pattern on immunofluorescent staining of ANCA (c-ANCA) is present in 70% to 90% of active WG patients.[6,8] The target antigen is PR-3. ELISA tests against PR3-ANCA will confirm this specificity in a large proportion of patients. However, a positive c-ANCA should not routinely replace a biopsy for establishing the diagnosis.[6]

Kidney biopsy is indicated especially in children with kidney involvement. Characteristically, it shows focal necrotizing crescentic glomerulonephritis.[15] In about half of these patients, renal vasculitis can also be seen. Unlike the biopsy of lung or sinuses, the renal biopsy rarely shows a granuloma. The kidney disease is characteristically pauci-immune.[6,11] Few if any electron-dense deposits are present on electron microscopy.[15]

If kidney involvement is minimal, lung or sinus biopsies are indicated, and involved areas will show patchy necrosis, granulomatous inflammation, and vasculitis.

Diagnosis and Differential Diagnosis

A definite diagnosis of WG would be based on characteristic changes on biopsies of the lung, kidney, or skin. A typical clinical presentation together with presence of antibodies to PR3 antigen is strongly suggestive of the diagnosis.

Recently a group of pediatricians has suggested that the presence of "PR3-ANCA or c-ANCA staining" and "subglottic, tracheal or endobronchial stenosis" be added as new criteria to classify the disease in addition to four items previously suggested by the American College of Rheumatology (ACR).[2]

Differential diagnosis includes infectious processes that lead to sino-pulmonary symptoms alone, other ANCA-associated vasculitides such as microscopic polyarteritis (MPA), and Churg-Strauss syndrome, pulmonary-renal syndromes, such as Goodpasture disease, anti-glomerular basement membrane disease, systemic lupus erythematosus (SLE), Henoch-Schönlein purpura (HSP), and other granulomatous diseases such as sarcoidosis, lymphomatoid granulomatosis, and tuberculosis.

Treatment and Prognosis

Treatment of all ANCA-associated diseases is similar. Steroids and cyclophosphamide are mainstays. In severe patients with kidney involvement, intravenous methylprednisolone for 1 to 3 days (15-30 mg/kg/day, maximum 1 g), followed by daily oral corticosteroids (1.5 mg/kg/day, maximum 60 mg/day) and cyclophosphamide (2 mg/kg/day or monthly intravenous pulses at 0.75 g/m^2) may be initiated as induction therapy.

For maintenance treatment, again there are many different regimens for oral corticosteroids. However, we suggest a starting dose of 1.5 mg/kg/day after three pulses. The dose is tapered according to clinical and laboratory response, not before 2 weeks, to 1 mg/kg/day, and the dose is then decreased by 10 mg every 2 weeks to reach a minimum dose of 10 mg/day, and then subsequently every other day. This dose is continued for a year after clinical remission.

For the maintenance regimen, there are a number of protocols suggesting continuation of cyclophosphamide. Some have suggested continuing oral cyclophosphamide for a year after remission at varying doses.[14] The CYCAZAREM study has shown that the replacement of cyclophosphamide with azathioprine at 3 months and continuation for a year in remission is also effective for disease control.[16] Methotrexate has also been shown to be an alternative for maintenance treatment.[17] In a study of limited ANCA-associated vasculitis in adults, methotrexate was administered at a dose of 15 mg/week, and escalated to 25 mg/week by 6 weeks and continued for 12 months.[17] In children, the drug can be administered orally, subcutaneously, or intramuscularly.

In the setting of life-threatening disease, and especially for severe kidney disease, plasmapheresis in addition to immunosuppressive treatment may be used. Plasmapheresis can be performed on alternate days, with duration varying according to the response of the patient. The effect of biologic treatments is not yet conclusive. Etanercept, which is a TNF receptor blocker, has not been shown to be effective in WG in a prospective and randomized trial.[18] Rituximab, which is an anti-CD20 molecule, has been shown to be effective in small series.[19] It is too early to make recommendations in children for anti-CD20 treatment, and this should be reserved for patients who do not respond to the more standard treatment outlined above. Autologous hematopoietic stem cell transplantation is also being evaluated.[6]

Several reports suggest the benefit of the use of trimethoprim sulphamethaxasole in WG prophylaxis; however, whether it reduces relapses is controversial. Although 5-year survival is now more than 80%, relapses are frequent.[20] Rottem et al.[12] have reported that 53% of childhood patients had at least one relapse requiring treatment. Therefore, the rates of remission and relapse are similar to those of adults. Stegmayr et al.[20] have found that relapses occurred after a median of 28 (4-120) months.[20] Treatment-related morbidity also becomes an important concern in patients with WG.

Relapses may occur after renal transplantation in ANCA-associated vasculitis (WG and microscopic polyangiitis).[21,22] Nachman et al.[21] performed a pool analysis where they showed that 17.3% of the patients had a relapse. However, the outcome of renal transplant is not different from other causes of renal disease, and thus transplantation is recommended.[22]

MICROSCOPIC POLYARTERITIS/ POLYANGIITIS

Microscopic polyarteritis/polyangiitis is a nongranulomatous, multisystem, pauci-immune vasculitis without upper airway involvement. The EULAR/PRES Consensus Conference has defined the disease as a necrotizing pauci-immune vasculitis affecting predominantly small vessels, and is often associated with a high titer of myeloperoxidase antineutrophil cytoplasmic antibodies (MPO)-ANCA or positive perinuclear-ANCA (p-ANCA) staining by immunofluorescence.[2] Necrotizing glomerulonephritis is very common. Pulmonary capillaritis often occurs in the absence of granulomatous lesions of the respiratory tract.[1] The only modification of the Chapel Hill Consensus Conference report is that ANCA was added to the description of microscopic polyangiitis.[2] MPA can often mimic classic polyarteritis nodusa (PAN) histologically, as both diseases produce a necrotizing arteritis. The key distinction is in the involved vessel size since MPA is predominantly a small vessel vasculitis, whereas according to the Chapel Hill consensus criteria, classic PAN is confined to mid-size artery involvement.[1]

Watts and Scott[4] have described PAN to be more common in Southern Europe. In accordance with this, two childhood series, albeit small, come from Turkey and Serbia.[23,24]

Pathogenesis

Infections may have an initiating role although a specific antigen has not been indicated. MPO-ANCA is implicated in the pathogenesis of this vasculitis similar to the role of PR3-ANCA in WG.[8] A recent report showed strong support for a direct pathogenic role for ANCA IgG in human glomerulonephritis and vasculitis in an elegant mouse model.[25] Mice that received anti-MPO IgG developed focal necrotizing and crescentic glomerulonephritis with a paucity of glomerular immunoglobulin deposition.[25] Together with the chemokines and cytokines, MPO-ANCA cause adherence of leukocytes to the walls of small vessels with subsequent injury to the glomerular capillaries and arterioles.

Clinical and Laboratory Manifestations

Patients often present with progressive glomerulonephritis with or without pulmonary symptoms.[26] Urinalysis will reveal an active urine sediment, and renal function is often impaired. Thrombocytosis is frequent and acute-phase reactants are elevated.

In a childhood series including 10 patients, median age 9.5,[23] six developed renal failure and three of the 10 had pulmonary-renal syndrome. All had high MPO-ANCA levels. Six (60%) had renal biopsies showing pauci-immune, necrotizing crescentic glomerulonephritis. Four of them (40%) progressed to chronic renal insufficiency.

In the seven patients reported from Serbia, all had hematuria/proteinuria, 57% had pulmonary-renal syndrome, and two had acute renal failure progressing to ESRD.[24] Another developed chronic renal failure (42.8%). In another series of six pediatric patients from India, 50% presented with pulmonary renal syndrome.[27]

Hattori et al.[28] have reviewed 34 ANCA-seropositive Japanese pediatric patients with biopsy-proven pauci-immune necrotizing crescentic glomerulonephritis, and 21 were classified as microscopic polyangiitis. The authors concluded that the disease was similar to that of adults except for female dominance. Patients who subsequently developed end-stage renal disease ($n = 9$) had significantly higher average peak serum creatinine levels and more chronic pathologic lesions at diagnosis compared with patients with favorable renal outcome.[28] A series on adults has reviewed 107 MPA patients followed for 2.5 years.[26] Indirect immunofluorescence (IIF) revealed 65% p-ANCA and 35% c-ANCA staining. Twelve disease-related deaths occurred and 46 progressed to ESRD. Pulmonary disease was present in 36% and skin involvement in 12% of these patients. Pulmonary hemorrhage and increased serum creatinine levels were associated with increased mortality.[26]

Diagnosis and Differential Diagnosis

Diagnosis depends on characteristic biopsy findings in the typical clinical setting and a positive MPO-ANCA by ELISA or p-ANCA staining with IIF. The renal biopsy will show necrotizing crescentic glomerulonephritis (Figure 24-2). Immunofluorescence shows pauci-immune staining with no significant immune deposits.

Differential diagnosis includes childhood PAN, HSP, other ANCA-associated vasculitides including WG and Churg-Strauss syndrome (CSS), and pulmonary renal syndromes such as SLE.

Treatment and Outcome

Treatment is similar to that of WG. Weidner et al.[29] have reported that patients with MPO-ANCA had a better outcome compared to patients with PR3-ANCA. Overall, relapses seem to be less frequent as compared to WG in MPA patients. In the two small childhood series, about 40% have progressed to ESRD.[24] Two of our MPA patients have been

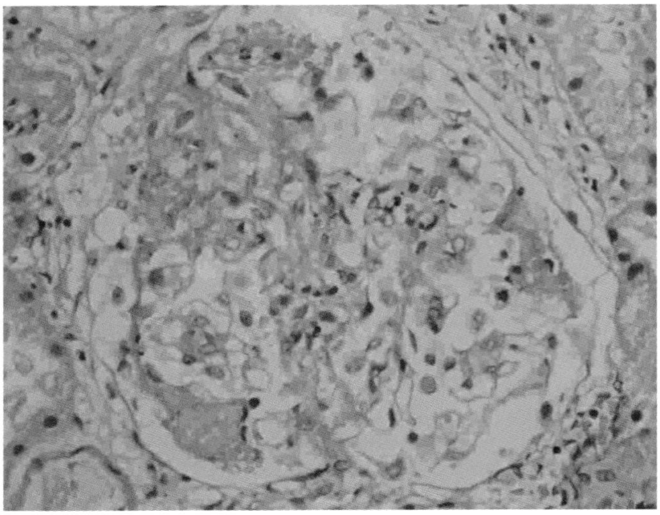

Figure 24-2 Renal biopsy of a patient with MPA shows fibrinoid necrosis and crescent formation (H&E stain).

TABLE 24-1 Classification Criteria for Childhood Polyarteritis Nodosa

A systemic illness characterized by the presence of at least 2 of the following 7 criteria: 1. Skin involvement (livedo reticularis, tender subcutaneous nodules, other vasculitic lesions) 2. Myalgia or muscle tenderness 3. Systemic hypertension, relative to childhood normative data 4. Mononeuropathy or polyneuropathy 5. Abnormal urine analysis and/or impaired renal function 6. Testicular pain or tenderness 7. Signs or symptoms suggesting vasculitis of any other major organ system (gastrointestinal, cardiac, pulmonary, or central nervous system)
In the presence of (one of the below as a mandatory criterion):
Biopsy showing small and mid-size artery necrotizing vasculitis *OR*
Angiographic abnormalities (aneurysms or occlusions)

From Ozen S, Ruperto N, Dillon MJ, Bagga A, et al: EULAR/PRES endorsed consensus criteria for the classification of childhood vasculitides, *Ann Rheum Dis* 65:936-41, 2006.

successfully transplanted and followed without complications through 4 to 5 years.[30]

CHILDHOOD POLYARTERITIS NODOSA

Polyarteritis nodosa is a necrotizing vasculitis of medium- and/or small-sized arteries. Childhood PAN is typically a multisystem disease resulting from vascular inflammation predominantly in skin, abdominal viscera, kidneys, CNS, and muscles.[14] The ACR requires the presence of three of the following 10 criteria for classification of a patient with PAN: weight loss, livedo reticularis, testicular pain, myalgia, mono- and poly-neuropathy, elevated diastolic blood pressure, increased serum BUN or creatinine, presence of Hepatitis B virus, arteriographic changes, and characteristic biopsy.[31] Jennette et al.[1] have divided PAN into classic and microscopic polyarteritis/polyangiitis: they have defined classic PAN as a necrotizing inflammation of small- or medium-sized arteries without glomerulonephritis or vasculitis in arterioles, capillaries, or venules. Pediatric patients are often not limited to this description, and the disease has certain characteristic features in children. Thus, an attempt has been made to classify childhood PAN patients with the recently developed EULAR/PRES criteria for the classification of childhood PAN[2] (Table 24-1).

PAN is rare in childhood, especially in North America. In children it occurs with equal frequency in girls and boys. The peak age at onset is 9 to 11, but may occur in very young children.[32,33] The largest and most recent reports come from Turkey and Japan.[32,33]

Pathogenesis

The cause of PAN is not known but infectious processes are implicated.[14] A number of reports have suggested that the disease is associated with streptococcal infections; however, the matter is still controversial.[33] PAN occurring after hepatitis C, parvovirus B19, and cytomegalovirus have also been described.[14] The most classical association with infection is HBV-associated PAN patients. The pathogenesis of HBV-PAN, the most typical form of classic PAN, is not well known, and initial reports suggested that the deposition of circulating immune complexes in vessel walls was responsible for the disease.[34] Guillevin et al.[34] have suggested that their therapeutic strategies in this disease confirm this pathogenic hypothesis. In animals, polyarteritis-like vascular lesions have been induced by infectious agents.[35]

Familial occurrence is rare. A report from Turkey has suggested that PAN is more frequent in familial Mediterranean fever (FMF) and that this may be associated with the increased inflammatory milieu in these patients.[36,37]

Clinical Manifestations

Childhood PAN often starts with an insidious onset of constitutional symptoms (fever, weight loss), abdominal and musculoskeletal pain, as well as maculopapular or nodular or necrotic skin lesions.[14] The nodules of childhood PAN are subcutaneous, painful, and are especially common in the calf and foot. Cutaneous involvement may also include livedo reticularis, digital ischemia, and peripheral gangrene. Musculoskeletal involvement may be in the form of myalgia or arthritis. Other system involvement types include neurological, cardiac, and pulmonary diseases, reflecting the vasculitis in these organ systems.[33] Abdominal pain is quite frequent due to ischemia of the intra-abdominal arteries and/or infarction. CNS findings are present in 14.5% to 70% of the patients. This may present as an organic brain syndrome, focal neurologic defects, blindness, seizures, hemiparesis, or ptosis.[38]

The patients may present with signs suggesting primary renal disease or renovascular hypertension. Renal symptoms at presentation may be in the form of isolated proteinuria, nephritic, and/or nephrotic syndrome or renal failure.[39] Most of the patients reported as classic PAN in childhood series would better be classified as childhood PAN since some have

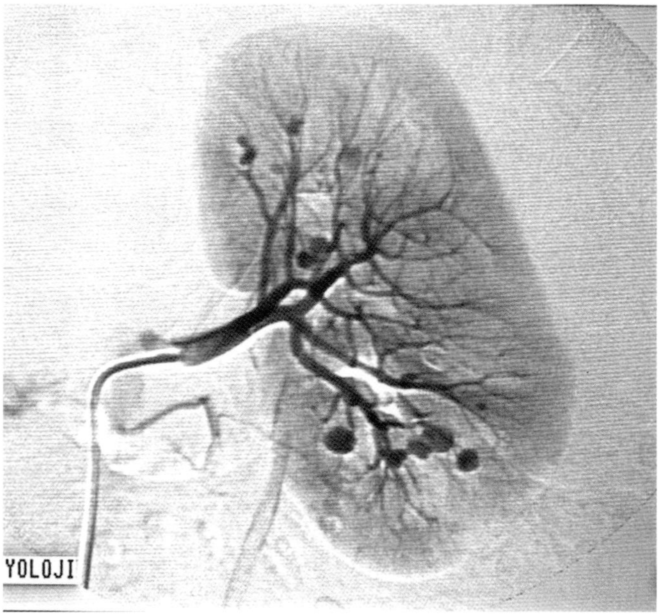

Figure 24-3 Renal angiogram of a childhood PAN patient who presented with hypertension. Multiple typical aneurysms are seen.

small vessel involvement, although this is an exclusion criteria for classic PAN. In a multicenter study of 110 patients hypertension was the presenting symptom in 14.5% of the patients.[33] Renovascular hypertension is due to vasculitis of the renal artery, which can be documented by a renal angiography.[40]

Laboratory Findings

Complete blood count may reveal anemia, leukocytosis, and thrombocytosis. Acute-phase reactants and especially C-reactive protein are elevated.

If there is renal involvement, urinalysis may show an active urinary sediment with casts, erythrocytes, and proteinuria of varying degrees. End-stage renal disease is rare. If renal involvement is present, a kidney biopsy or renal angiogram is indicated. A typical finding is renal aneurysms (Figure 24-3). However, Brogan et al.[40] retrospectively reviewed the angiograms of 25 children with PAN; only 40% of these children had aneurysms demonstrated on selective renal angiography. In this study, nonaneurysmal changes were detected more commonly on renal angiography than aneurysms in the PAN group. The most reliable nonaneurysmal signs were perfusion defects, the presence of collateral arteries, lack of crossing of peripheral renal arteries, and delayed emptying of small renal arteries.[40]

Serology is not typical. Antineutrophil cytoplasmic antibodies, ANA, RF, and immune complexes may be rarely present. Factor VIII–related antigen may reflect vascular inflammation.[41]

Diagnosis and Differential Diagnosis

There are no pathognomonic laboratory features. The diagnosis depends on the multisystem involvement along with the characteristic biopsy and/or angiogram changes cited above. A biopsy of the affected tissue will reveal necrotizing arteritis of small- and/or mid-size arteries. Recent childhood series show that the disease is not confined to medium- and small-size arteries in pediatric patients.[2]

Childhood PAN needs to be differentiated from other childhood vasculitides, including HSP, Kawasaki disease, and WG, as well as systemic infections. Tissue infarcts caused by mid-size artery involvement may need to be differentiated from thrombophilia and primary central nervous system vasculitis.

Treatment and Outcome

Treatment of the systemic disease is similar to that of ANCA-related vasculitides. Corticosteroids remain the mainstay of treatment. In patients with limited disease, the use of immunosuppressives may not be necessary. However, long-term, multicenter studies are required to reach evidence-based conclusions. For severe organ involvement, in the pediatric literature cyclophosphamide is the first choice for treatment in addition to steroids.[14]

In older series, the prognosis of pediatric patients with PAN was guarded. However, with the judicious use of immunosuppressives the prognosis is better than in adults in recent series.[33]

In conclusion, the kidney is an important target organ for the aforementioned diseases. A judicious evaluation for diagnosis and careful management are required for renal and patient survival.

REFERENCES

1. Jennette JC, Falk RJ, Andrassy K, et al: Nomenclature of systemic vasculitides. Proposal of an international consensus conference, *Arthritis Rheum* 37(2):187-92, 1994.
2. Ozen S, Ruperto N, Dillon MJ, Bagga A, et al: EULAR/PRES endorsed consensus criteria for the classification of childhood vasculitides, *Ann Rheum Dis* 65:936-41, 2006 (Epub ahead of print December 2005).
3. U.S. Department of Health and Human Services: Pediatric end-stage renal disease. USRDS 1999 annual data report, Bethesda MD, 1999, United States Renal Data System.
4. Watts RA, Scott DG: Epidemiology of the vasculitides, *Semin Respir Crit Care Med* 25(5):455-64, 2004.
5. Gibson A, Stamp LK, Chapman PT, O'Donnell JL: The epidemiology of Wegener's granulomatosis and microscopic polyangiitis in a Southern Hemisphere region, *Rheumatology* 45(5):624-28, 2006.
6. Frosch M, Foell D: Wegener granulomatosis in childhood and adolescence, *Eur J Pediatr* 163(8):425-34, 2004.
7. Jagiello P, Gross WL, Epplen JT: Complex genetics of Wegener granulomatosis, *Autoimmun Rev* 4(1):42-47, 2005.
8. Pankhurst T, Savage CO: Pathogenic role of anti-neutrophil cytoplasmic antibodies in vasculitis, *Curr Opin Pharmacol* 6(2):190-96, 2006.
9. Reumaux D, Kuijpers TW, Hordijk PL, Duthilleul P, Roos D: Involvement of Fcgamma receptors and beta2 integrins in neutrophil activation by anti-proteinase-3 or anti-myeloperoxidase antibodies, *Clin Exp Immunol* 134(2):344-50, 2003.
10. Segelmark M, Elzouki AN, Wieslander J, Eriksson S: The PiZ gene of alpha 1—antitrypsin as a determinant of outcome in PR3-ANCA-positive vasculitis, *Kidney Int* 48(3):844-50, 1994.

11. Belostotsky VM, Shah V, Dillon MJ: Clinical features in 17 paediatric patients with Wegener granulomatosis, *Pediatr Nephrol* 17(9):754-61, 2002.
12. Rottem M, Fauci AS, Hallahan CW, Kerr GS, et al: Wegener granulomatosis in children and adolescents: clinical presentation and outcome, *J Pediatr* 122(1):26-31, 1993.
13. Hoffman GS, Kerr GS, Leavitt RY, Hallahan CW, et al: Wegener granulomatosis: an analysis of 158 patients, *Ann Intern Med* 116(6):488-98, 1992.
14. Cassidy JT, Petty RE: Polyarteritis nodosa and related vasculitides. In Cassidy JT, Petty RE, editors: *Textbook of pediatric rheumatology*, ed 5, Philadelphia, 2005, Elsevier Saunders, pp. 512-20.
15. Valentini RP, Smoyer WE: Renal vasculitis. In Avner ED, Harmon WE, Niaudet P, editors: *Pediatric Nephrology*, ed 5, Philadelphia, 2004, Lippincott Williams & Wilkins, 835-50.
16. Jayne D: Update on the European Vasculitis Study Group trials, *Curr Opin Rheumatol* 13(1):48-55, 2001.
17. de Groot K, Jayne D: What is new in the therapy of ANCA-associated vasculitides? Take home messages from the 12th workshop on ANCA and systemic vasculitides, *Clin Nephrol* 64(6): 480-84, 2005.
18. Wegener's Granulomatosis Etanercept Trial (WGET) Research Group. Etanercept plus standard therapy for Wegener's granulomatosis, *N Engl J Med* 352(4):351-61, 2005.
19. Hellmich B, Lamprecht P, Gross WL: Advances in the therapy of Wegener's granulomatosis, *Curr Opin Rheumatol* 18(1):25-32, 2006.
20. Stegmayr BG, Gothefors L, Malmer B, Muller Wiefel DE, et al: Wegener granulomatosis in children and young adults. A case study of ten patients, *Pediatr Nephrol* 14(3):208-13, 2000.
21. Nachman PH, Segelmark M, Westman K, Hogan SL, et al: Recurrent ANCA-associated small vessel vasculitis after transplantation: a pooled analysis, *Kidney Int* 56(4):1544-50, 1999.
22. Elmedhem A, Adu D, Savage CO: Relapse rate and outcome of ANCA-associated small vessel vasculitis after transplantation, *Nephrol Dial Transplant* 18(5): 1001-04, 2003.
23. Bakkaloglu A, Ozen S, Baskin E, Besbas N, et al: The significance of antineutrophil cytoplasmic antibody in microscopic polyangitis and classic polyarteritis nodosa, *Arch Dis Child* 85(5):427-30, 2001.
24. Peco-Antic A, Bonaci-Nikolic B, Basta-Jovanovic G, Kostic M, et al: Childhood microscopic polyangiitis associated with MPO-ANCA, *Pediatr Nephrol* 21(1):46-53, 2006.
25. Xiao H, Heeringa P, Liu Z, Huugen D, et al. The role of neutrophils in the induction of glomerulonephritis by anti-MPO antibodies, *Am J Pathol* 167(1):39-45, 2005.
26. Guillevin L, Lhote F, Cohen P, Jarrousse B, et al: Corticosteroids plus pulse cyclophosphamide and plasma exchanges versus corticosteroids plus pulse cyclophosphamide alone in the treatment of polyarteritis nodosa and Churg-Strauss syndrome patients with factors predicting poor prognosis. A prospective, randomized trial in sixty-two patients, *Arthritis Rheum* 38(11):1638-45, 1995.
27. Handa R, Wali JP, Gupta SD, Dinda AK, et al: Classical polyarteritis nodosa and microscopic polyangiitis—a clinicopathologic study, *J Assoc Physicians India* 49:314-49, 2001.
28. Hattori M, Kurayama H, Koitabashi Y, Japanese Society for Pediatric Nephrology: Antineutrophil cytoplasmic autoantibody-associated glomerulonephritis in children, *J Am Soc Nephrol* 12(7):1493-500, 2001.
29. Weidner S, Geuss S, Hafezi-Rachti S, Wonka A, Rupprecht HD: ANCA-associated vasculitis with renal involvement: an outcome analysis, *Nephrol Dial Transplant* 19(6):1403-11, 2004.
30. Besbas N, Ozaltin F, Tinaztepe K, Gucer S, et al: Successful renal transplantation in a child with ANCA-associated microscopic polyangiitis, *Pediatr Nephrol* 18(7):696-99, 2003.
31. Lightfoot RW Jr, Michel BA, Bloch DA, Hunder GG, et al: The American College of Rheumatology 1990 criteria for the classification of polyarteritis nodosa, *Arthritis Rheum* 33(8):1088-93, 1993.
32. Maeda M, Kobayashi M, Okamoto S, Fuse T, et al: Clinical observation of 14 cases of childhood polyarteritis nodosa in Japan, *Acta Paediatr Jpn* 39(2):277-79, 1997.
33. Ozen S, Anton J, Arisoy N, Bakkaloglu A, et al: Juvenile polyarteritis: results of a multicenter survey of 110 children, *J Pediatr* 145(4):517-22, 2004.
34. Guillevin L, Mahr A, Callard P, Godmer P, et al: Hepatitis B virus—associated polyarteritis nodosa: clinical characteristics, outcome, and impact of treatment in 115 patients, (*Medicine (Baltimore)* 84(5):313-22, 2005.
35. Thibault S, Drolet R, Germain MC, D'Allaire S, et al: Cutaneous and systemic necrotizing vasculitis in swine, *Vet Pathol* 35(2):108-16, 1998.
36. Ozen S, Bakkaloglu A, Yilmaz E, Duzova A, et al: Mutations in the gene for familial Mediterranean fever: do they predispose to inflammation? *J Rheumatol* 30(9):2014-18, 2003.
37. Ozen S: The spectrum of vasculitis in children, *Best Pract Res Clin Rheumatol* 16(3):411-25, 2002.
38. Kirkali P, Topaloglu R, Kansu T, Bakkaloglu A: Third nerve palsy and internuclear ophthalmoplegia in periarteritis nodosa, *J Pediatr Ophthalmol Strabismus* 21:45-46, 1991.
39. Besbas N, Ozen S, Saatci U, Topaloglu R, et al: Renal involvement in polyarteritis nodosa: evaluation of 26 Turkish children, *Pediatr Nephrol* 14(4):325-27, 2000.
40. Brogan PA, Davies R, Gordon I, Dillon MJ: Renal angiography in children with polyarteritis nodosa, *Pediatr Nephrol* 17(4):277-83, 2002.
41. Ates E, Bakkaloglu A, Saatci U, Soylemezoglu O: von Willebrand factor antigen compared with other factors in vasculitic syndromes, *Arch Dis Child* 70(1):40-43, 1994.

CHAPTER 25

Hemolytic Uremic Syndrome

Sharon Phillips Andreoli and Lothar Bernd Zimmerhackl

DEFINITION OF HEMOLYTIC UREMIC SYNDROME

In the literature, the acronyms HUS[1] and TTP[2] have often been used interchangeably for similar diseases. This has caused confusion in many discussions. Historically, hemolytic uremic syndrome (HUS) and thrombotic thrombocytopenic purpura (TTP) were based on the clinical criteria of the original reports.[3,4] HUS is the clinical triad of acute renal failure, microangiopathic hemolytic anemia and thrombocytopenia; TTP has the added features of fever and neurological signs. However, in many patients with HUS fever and neurological signs are often obvious. Both share the pathological finding of thrombotic microangiopathy, an arteriolar-capillary occlusive lesion consisting of platelet-fibrin thrombus and/or intimal vascular damage.[5,6] However, there is great overlap of the two definitions. A major difference is age. In general, patients with clinical features of HUS are younger (1 to 5 years), while TTP patients tend to be adults aged 20 to 40 years.

New concepts of the etiology and pathogenesis of some of the disorders that comprise HUS and TTP challenge previous attempts to classify the syndrome according to clinical description. Although it is self-evident that in each case of HUS or TTP the individual etiology and pathogenesis to a large extent determine the clinical course, a growing literature that confirms this. For example, the childhood form of HUS immediately preceded by diarrhea (so-called diarrhea-positive HUS [D+HUS]) is closely linked to verocytotoxin (synonyms are Shiga toxin [Stx] or Shiga-like toxin [Slx])-producing *Escherichia coli* (VTEC, STEC, or enterohemorrhagic *E. coli* [EHEC]) infection. This is usually a short-lived event that has a comparatively benign early outcome and there is no relapse. By contrast, HUS associated with mutations in the complement regulator factor H has a poor prognosis, and a high risk of relapse and graft loss after transplantation. Subgroups of HUS and TTP defined by etiology require subgroup-specific therapies.

In clinical practice, beyond a few well-defined subgroups, the etiology and pathogenesis often remain unexplained. This is partly because the etiology has not been fully considered, or the necessary investigations proved unavailable outside a research setting. The European Paediatric Research Study Group for HUS operates a disease registry for childhood cases of HUS, and encourages comprehensive investigation upon which to make valid clinico-pathological and etiological correlations. In order to clarify these issues we use a new classification as shown in Table 25-1 based on accepted published pathophysiological grounds.[7] This chapter is based in part on original work of the authors.

HEMOLYTIC UREMIC SYNDROME CAUSED BY INFECTIONS: INTRODUCTORY COMMENTS

HUS caused by infectious agents is a common cause of acute renal failure in children and leads to significant morbidity and mortality during the acute phase of the disease. In addition to acute morbidity and mortality, long-term renal and extrarenal complications can occur in a substantial number of children years after the acute episode of HUS. While the most common infectious agent causing HUS is enterohemorrhagic *E. coli* that produce Shiga toxin (STEC), *Shigella* can also be associated with HUS and as described below HUS following infections by *Streptococcus pneumoniae* can be particularly severe and has a higher acute mortality and higher long-term morbidity compared to HUS caused by STEC. D+HUS or typical HUS was linked to infection with Shiga toxin–producing *E. coli* in the early 1980s by Karmali et al.,[3] and much has been learned about the pathophysiology of HUS since that seminal observation. While the pathophysiology of HUS is beginning to be understood, more research needs to be performed to understand the precise mechanisms of cell injury in HUS so that specific therapies can be developed. Importantly, strategies to prevent EHEC infection and HUS also need to be developed.

HUS ASSOCIATED WITH SHIGA TOXIN–PRODUCING *ESCHERICHIA COLI*

Epidemiology

The classic clinical features of HUS include the triad of microangiopathic hemolytic anemia, thrombocytopenia, and acute renal failure.[3-9] However, epidemiologic studies in outbreaks of hemorrhagic colitis and D+HUS have clearly shown that some patients develop hemolytic anemia and/or thrombocytopenia with little evidence of renal involvement while other children develop substantial renal disease with a normal platelet count and/or minimal hemolysis.[4-8] Similarly, Shiga toxin–producing *E. coli* has been isolated from children with

TABLE 25-1 Classification of HUS, TTP, and Related Disorders

Part 1. Recognized Etiology or Pathogenesis
1. Infection induced Shiga and verocytotoxin (Shiga-like toxin)–producing bacteria; enterohemorrhagic *Escherichia coli*, *Shigella dysenteriae* type 1, *Citrobacter* *Streptococcus pneumoniae*, neuraminidase, and T-antigen exposure Human immunodeficiency virus
2. Disorders of complement regulation Genetic disorders of complement regulation Acquired disorders of complement regulation, such as anti–Factor H antibody
3. von Willebrand proteinase deficiency, ADAMTS13 Genetic disorders of ADAMTS13 Acquired von Willebrand proteinase deficiency; autoimmune, drug induced
4. Defective cobalamin metabolism
5. Drug induced Mitomycin C Ticlopidine clopidogrel Quinine Calcineurin antagonists
Part 2. Unknown Etiology and Pathogenesis
1. Associated with pregnancy, HELLP syndrome, and oral contraception
2. Superimposed on preexisting disorders Systemic lupus erythematosus and antiphospholipid antibody syndrome Glomerulopathy Malignancy Bone marrow transplantation Ionizing radiation
3. Genetic Familial, not included in Part 1, no. 2 above
4. Unclassified

HUS without prodromal diarrhea, making the distinction of D+HUS related to infection with EHEC and diarrhea-negative HUS (D-HUS) due to other etiologies less clear.[10]

Well-publicized outbreaks of hemorrhagic colitis and HUS have highlighted the morbidity and mortality of infection with Shiga toxin–producing *E. coli*. In 1993, an outbreak in the western United States resulted in several cases of severe HUS with substantial extrarenal complications.[11] In 1996, over 5,000 Japanese schoolchildren were infected with verocytotoxin-producing *E. coli*, an outbreak in Scotland resulted in 20 deaths, and an outbreak in the United States was traced to contaminated apple juice.[12,13] In case–control studies, consumption of a hamburger and/or consumption of cold, precooked sliced meat was associated with Shiga toxin–producing *E. coli* infection.[14] Although undercooked hamburger has been the most common vector for transmission of EHEC infection in the past, apple juice, radish sprouts, and sausages, as well as other food sources have also been implicated in the spread of verocytotoxin-producing *E. coli* infections. While epidemics are notable, the majority of cases of HUS from Shiga toxin–producing *E. coli* are sporadic without identification of a specific source for the Shiga toxin–producing *E. coli*.[15]

In a prospective surveillance of Canadian children, in a total of 136 cases over 2 years, 121 were endemic while 15 were epidemic.[16] The annual incidence in that study was 1.11 cases per 100,000 children under age 16. In a well-documented prospective multicenter surveillance study in Germany and Austria involving 394 children, the incidence of HUS was 0.7 per 100,000 and 0.4 per 100,000 children under 15 years of age, respectively.[17,18] The reason for variable incidence in different regions is unclear, but may be related to exposure to STEC and potential genetic susceptibilities of specific populations.[19]

While consumption of contaminated food products is the most common mechanism of exposure to Shiga toxin–producing *E. coli*, person-to-person transmission is also an important mode of transmission; in people exposed to STEC, synchronous onset of symptoms suggests a common exposure, while onset of symptoms several days apart suggests person-to-person transmission in the people developing symptoms at a later time.[1-6] Recently, mother-to-child transmission was described in a 7-day-old child who presented with bloody diarrhea; she subsequently developed severe HUS with long-term neurological sequelae.[20]

The O157 : H7 serotype is most commonly implicated in Shiga toxin–producing infection in the United States and Europe, but in Europe and other areas of the world non-O157 : H7 strains are emerging as important pathogens.[17,18,21-23] *E. coli* O111 : H^- caused a large outbreak of hemorrhagic colitis and HUS in Australia, and other serotypes have been associated with hemorrhagic colitis and HUS as well.[14,15,18-20] In the prospective European study of 394 children described above, serotypes other than O157 : H7 was detected in 43% of the stool samples from patients with HUS; O26 was detected in 15%, sorbitol-fermenting O157 : H^- was detected in 10%, O145 in 9%, O103 in 3%, and O111 was detected in 43%.[17]

Once a person is infected with Shiga toxin–producing *E. coli*, the percentage of patients who progress to HUS ranges from approximately 5% to 15%. In children under 5 years of age, the percentage who develop hemolytic anemia or HUS was 12.9% compared to 6.8% and 8% for children aged 5 to 9.9 years and over 10 years of age, respectively.[8] In another study, children with a white blood cell count greater than 13,000/mm^3 during the initial 3 days of illness with Shiga toxin–producing *E. coli* infection had a seven-fold increase in the risk of developing HUS compared to age-matched children with a white blood cell count less than 13,000/mm^3.[24] The use of antimotility agents was also associated with a higher risk for the development of HUS.[24] A recent study demonstrated that children with hemorrhagic colitis associated with Shiga toxin–producing *E. coli* who received antibiotic therapy were more likely to progress to HUS.[25] However, a subsequent meta-analysis did not support this conclusion.[26] A study of 29 children who developed HUS found that children who received intravenous hydration and volume expansion have less severe HUS and were more likely to have nonoliguanuric renal failure.[27] Environmental or genetic factors that might predispose to the progression of hemorrhagic colitis associated with Shiga toxin–producing

E. coli to HUS are currently unknown. It has been suggested that alterations in the gene for factor H recently described in patients with atypical HUS may also be relevant to epidemic D+HUS.[19]

Clinical Manifestations

Once a person is exposed to Shiga toxin–producing *E. coli*, symptoms of diarrhea typically occur 3 to 7 days after exposure and the diarrhea becomes bloody in the majority of children. Other symptoms include crampy abdominal pain that can be quite severe. In children who develop HUS, the diarrhea begins to subside at the time the child begins to appear pale and decreased urine output may be noted. The major manifestations of HUS include the triad of thrombocytopenia, microangiopathic hemolytic anemia, and acute renal insufficiency. The hemolytic anemia is Coombs negative and schizocytes are prominent.[3,4,15] While the kidney and gastrointestinal tract are the organs most commonly affected in HUS, evidence of central nervous system (CNS), pancreatic, skeletal, and myocardial involvement may also be present.[3-11,28-33] Gastrointestinal involvement with severe colitis can result in transmural necrosis with perforation and/or the later development of colonic stricture.[15,32,33] Brisk hemolysis has been associated with the development of bilirubin gallstones that may become apparent after the acute phase of HUS has subsided.[34,35] Elevation of pancreatic enzymes is common, and edema of the pancreas indicative of pancreatitis can be detected by ultrasound or CT scan.[36] Glucose intolerance and frank insulin-dependent diabetes mellitus (IDDM) occurs in a minority of children with HUS, and severe pancreatic involvement is nearly always associated with severe renal disease and other extrarenal manifestations.[28,34,35] Glucose intolerance and IDDM may be transient with recovery of pancreatic islet cell function, but such children are at risk for the later development of insulin insufficiency[37,38] (Figure 25-1). As described below, extrarenal disease is associated with microthrombi in multiple extrarenal organs and can lead to ischemic injury.

Central nervous system involvement in typical HUS is common, and frequently presents as lethargy, irritability, seizures. In more severe cases, CNS disease may present with paresis, coma, and cerebral edema.[4-6,8,15,17] Isolated abducens nerve palsy that resolved spontaneously has been described in a 20-month-old child with HUS.[39] Skeletal muscle involvement manifesting as rhabdomyolysis occurs in rare cases, and fortunately myocardial involvement is rare as well[29-32] (Figure 25-2). When myocardial involvement occurs, elevated troponin I level may reflect the degree of myocardial ischemia.[40] The mortality of HUS is reported to be between 3% and 5%, and death due to HUS is nearly always associated with severe extrarenal disease including severe CNS disease.[4-6,8,15]

During the acute phase of HUS, pathologic specimens of the kidney reveal microvascular injury characterized by microthrombi deposition in association with swollen and detached glomerular endothelial cells and infiltration of inflammatory cells[40] (Figure 25-3A). Similar pathologic changes have been described in other organs including the colon, CNS, pancreas, skeletal and myocardial muscle, and red blood cells[32,34] (Figure 25-3B). These findings demonstrate that HUS is a systemic disease characterized by endothelial cell injury. The precise mechanisms of this microvascular injury are unknown, but evidence points to a role for Shiga toxin in mediating endothelial cell injury with a resultant change in the normal anticoagulant profile of the endothelial cell to a procoagulant state as described below.

Long-Term Complications

Technical advances in dialysis therapy and improved care of the critically ill child has resulted in a significant reduction of the acute mortality of HUS such that chronic complications in long-term survivors are becoming more apparent. Some children never recover renal function and require long-term renal replacement therapy, while those who recover are

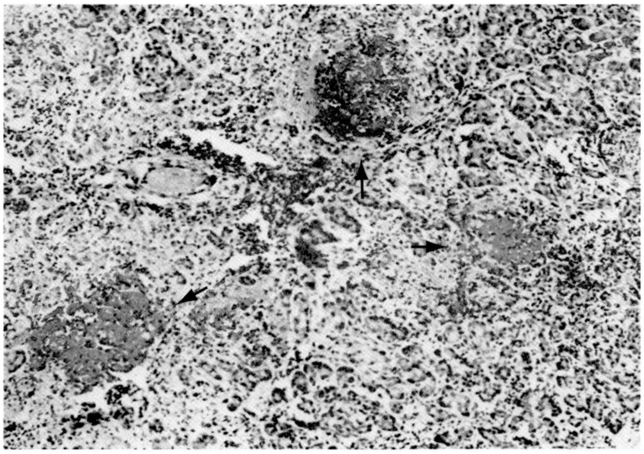

Figure 25-1 Hematoxylin and eosin light microscopy of pancreas from a patient with insulin dependence during the acute phase of HUS. Three islets (arrows) demonstrate necrosis and are obliterated and replaced by fibrin and hemorrhage. (Reprinted with permission from Burns JC, Berman ER, Fagre J, et al: Pancreatic islet cell necrosis: association with cell necrotic syndrome, *J Pediatr* 100:582-84, 1982.)

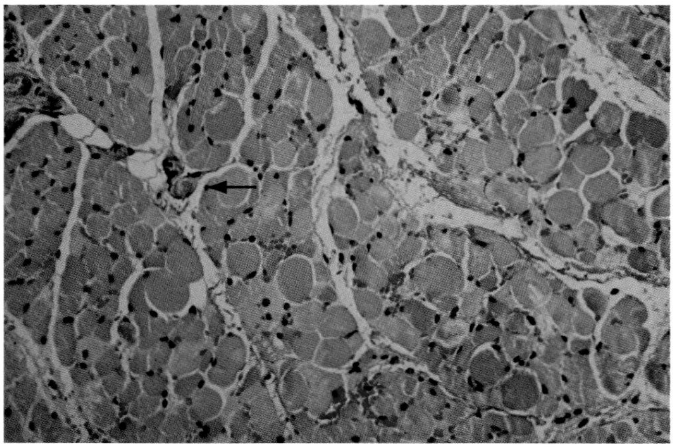

Figure 25-2 Hematoxylin and eosin light microscopy of muscle from a child with rhabdomyolysis during the acute phase of HUS. The arrow demonstrates a microthrombus in the vasculature. (Reprinted with permission from Andreoli SP, Bergstein JM: Acute rhabdomyolysis associated with the hemo-uremic syndrome, *J Pediatr* 103:78-80, 1983.)

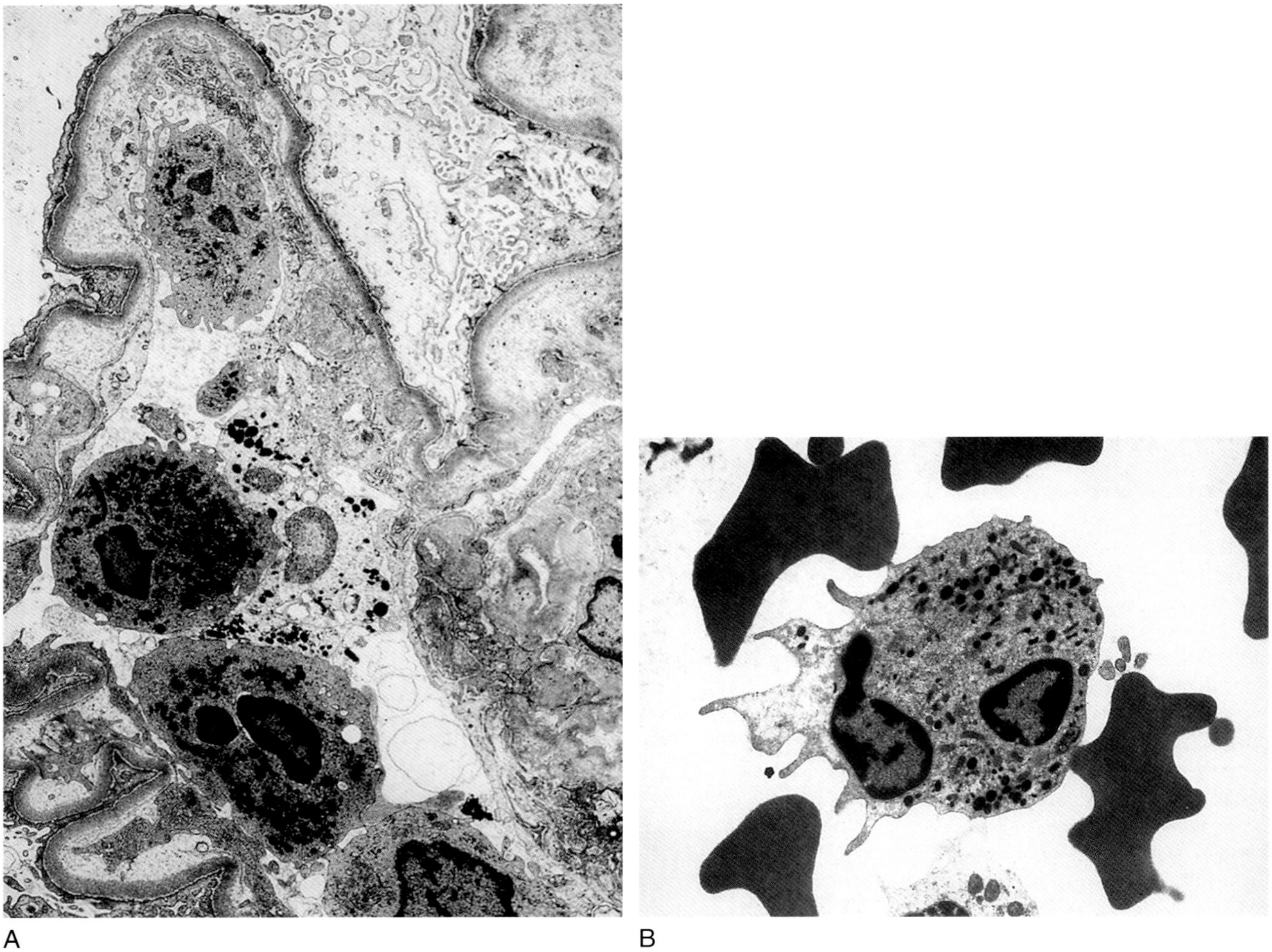

Figure 25-3 **A,** Electron micrograph of a glomerulus from a child during the acute phase of HUS demonstrating swollen endothelial cells with three PMNs adhering to the injured endothelial cells. **B,** Electron micrograph of a red blood cell and PMN from a patient with HUS demonstrating the adherence of the PMN to red blood cells. (**B,** reprinted with permission from Taylor M: Role of oxidants in the pathophysiology of HUS. In Kaplan BS, Trompeter R, Moak J, editors: *The hemolytic uremic syndrome: thrombotic thrombocytopenia purpura,* New York, Marcel Decker, 1992, pp. 355-73.)

at risk for the late development of renal disease.[41-43] In addition, some children have residual extrarenal problems including neurological defects, insulin-dependent diabetes mellitus, pancreatic insufficiency, and/or gastrointestinal complications[4-6,8,15,24-26,37,38] (Figure 25-4). Thus, HUS is a disease with substantial acute and chronic mortality and multisystem morbidity.

Several studies have demonstrated that children who have recovered from the acute episode of HUS are at risk for long-term complications, including hypertension, renal insufficiency, end-stage renal failure (ESRF), and insulin-dependent diabetes mellitus.[42-48] One study found that that 39% of 61 children with a history of HUS demonstrated late complications including hypertension, proteinuria, and renal insufficiency during a mean 9.6 years after the acute episode.[45] The duration of oligo/anuria was found to be the best predictor of late complications. A histopathological study demonstrated that focal and segmental glomerulosclerosis and arteriolar hyalinosis may be found sclerosis and several years following HUS, and in this study, only a quarter of the chil-

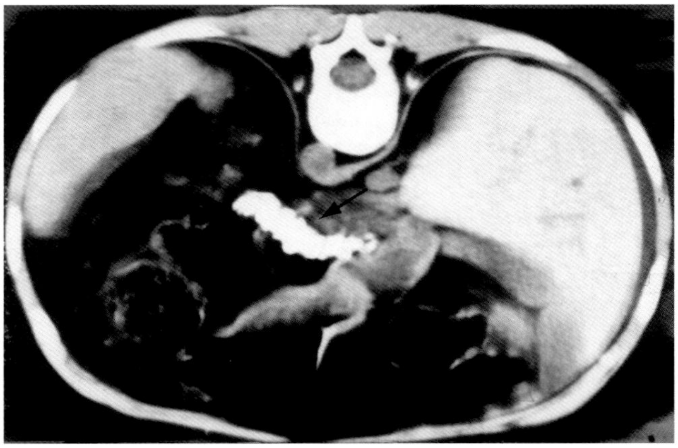

Figure 25-4 CT scan from a patient with permanent insulin-dependent diabetes mellitus and pancreatic insufficiency from HUS. The CT scan was obtained approximately 2 years after the acute episode and demonstrated a calcified pancreas *(arrow).* (Reprinted with permission from Andreoli SP: Pancreatic involvement in the hemolytic uremic syndrome. In Kaplan BS, Trompeter R, Moak J, editors: *The hemolytic uremic syndrome: thrombotic thrombocytopenia purpura,* New York, Marcel Decker, 1992, pp. 131-41.)

dren had normal renal function during long-term follow-up.[42,43] Kidney biopsies performed in children with a history of HUS and residual proteinuria demonstrated that the majority of these children had global and segmental sclerosis with interstitial fibrosis, suggesting that these children are risk for later development of renal insufficiency.[42] Oral protein loading in 17 children with a past history of HUS who had normal renal function and normal blood pressure demonstrated reduced functional renal reserve compared to normal children, although baseline renal function and blood pressure are normal.[47] In addition, ambulatory blood pressure monitoring was abnormal in children with a history of HUS and normal casual blood pressure.[49]

A meta-analysis demonstrated that death or end-stage renal disease (ESRD) occurred in 12% of children with diarrhea-associated HUS, and 25% of survivors demonstrate long-term renal sequelae.[50] In a study comparing children who had HUS from 1960 to 1980 who received therapy with low-sodium diet, antihypertensive therapy and late dietary protein restriction with children who had HUS from 1988 to 2002 who had received low-sodium diet, antihypertensive therapy with angiotensin-converting enzyme inhibitors, and earlier restriction of protein, the latter group had improved renal function.[51] This suggests that contemporary management of the residual sequelae of HUS with ACEI may help preserve renal function as it does in other diseases.[51]

Children with HUS who were discharged without neurological injury did not have an increased risk of subclinical problems with learning behavior or attention,[52] while some children who had major neurological symptoms had evidence of subtle neurological sequelae including clumsiness, poor fine motor coordination, hyperactivity, and distractibility.[53] Long-term gastrointestinal complications such as colonic stricture and bilirubin gallstones can develop following apparent recovery of HUS.[30-33] Permanent or transient insulin-dependent diabetes mellitus occurs in a small percentage of children with HUS, and children who have transient IDDM are at risk for later return of IDDM (Figure 25-1). Interestingly, these children do not have anti-islet cell antibodies, and the pathogenesis of their IDDM is not related to immunologic injury but rather due to decreased beta cell function.[28,38]

Mechanisms of Shiga Toxin–Mediated Cell Injury

Shiga toxins (also called verotoxins, verocytotoxin [VT], or Shiga-like toxins [ST]) are composed of two subunits—a larger A subunit that inhibits protein synthesis by blocking elongation factor-1–dependent binding of aminoacyl-tRNA to ribosomes, and five of the smaller B subunits that mediate binding of the toxin with a membrane glycolipid, globotriaosylceramide or Gb3.[54,55] Shiga toxin 1 (ST-1) produced by *E. coli* is almost identical to Shiga toxin typically produced by other gram-negative organisms, including *Shigella,* and differs by only one amino acid in the A subunit, while Shiga toxin 2 (ST-2) varies considerably, demonstrating approximately 55% to 60% homology.[54,55] *E. coli* O157 : H7 strains and other STEC that are isolated from patients with HUS usually produce both ST-1 and ST-2 or only ST-2 and strains that produce only ST-1 are unusual.[17,54,55] A recent epidemic of Shiga toxin 1–producing *E. coli* led to the development of hemorrhagic colitis in 526 children and 35 adults, but was not associated with the development of HUS.[23] While mild abnormalities in the urinalysis were detected in some patients, none of the patients developed typical symptoms of HUS.[23] This epidemiologic study emphasizes the probable important role of ST-2 in the development of HUS compared to the role of ST-1. Although free Shiga toxin has not been demonstrated in the circulation of children with HUS, Shiga toxin has been shown to traverse polarized gastrointestinal epithelial cells probably via transcellular pathways.[56] Immunohistochemical studies have also demonstrated ST-1 and ST-2 binding to renal tubular epithelial cells in a fatal case of typical D+HUS, suggesting that Shiga toxin is absorbed into the systemic circulation, binds to renal cells, and contributes to cell injury.[57] In a primate model of HUS, a single intravenous dose of purified ST-1 resulted in thrombocytopenia, hemolytic anemia, and renal microangiopathy, while animals that received the same amount of Shiga toxin divided into four doses did not develop clinical or histological features of HUS.[58] This suggests that the rate of absorption of Shiga toxin from the gastrointestinal tract plays a role in the development of HUS.

The association of Shiga toxin–producing *E. coli* and HUS is very strong but the mechanism(s) of Shiga toxin–mediated cell injury in HUS is uncertain. Studies with ST-1 and human umbilical vein endothelial cells (HUVEC) demonstrated that Shiga toxin was directly toxic to nonconfluent, growing endothelial cells, but Shiga toxin was much less toxic to confluent, quiescent endothelial cells. When quiescent Shiga toxin–resistant human umbilical vein endothelial cells were pre-treated with tumor necrosis factor-α (TNF-α) or interleukin-1 (IL-1), the endothelial cells became susceptible to the toxicity of Shiga toxin.[54,55] The sensitivity of specific cell lines and tissues to Shiga toxin was shown to be related to membrane expression of the Gb3 receptor, and maneuvers to increase expression of the Gb3 receptor increase sensitivity to the cytotoxic effects of Shiga toxin.[54,55] The Gb3 plasma membrane receptor mediates binding and internalization of the Shiga toxin by receptor-mediated endocytosis.

Studies in human glomerular endothelial cells documented that renal glomerular endothelial cells are sensitive to the cytotoxic effects of Shiga toxin. In highly confluent glomerular microvascular cells, Shiga toxin–mediated cytotoxicity required pre-treatment of the cells with TNF-α, which induced an increase in the number of Gb3 receptors on the glomerular endothelial cells.[59] Interestingly, ST-1 and ST-2 induced similar cytotoxic effects on glomerular microvascular endothelial cells. Thus, the strong association of HUS with ST-2–producing *E. coli* infections may not be related to a higher sensitivity of endothelial cells to toxicity mediated by ST-2 as compared to toxicity mediated by ST-1. Other studies have shown that Shiga toxin–induced programmed cell death in a dose- and time-dependent manner in microvascular endothelial cells.[60]

Other very interesting studies have demonstrated that the sensitivity of some cells to the cytotoxic effects of Shiga toxin can be greatly influenced without a significant change in Gb3 receptor expression. In a series of studies, Lingwood and others have demonstrated that in addition to receptor concentration, the fatty acid composition of Gb3 and the phospholipid chain length within the phospholipid bilayer play an important role in internal sorting of the toxin and subsequent cytotoxic effects of the toxin.[61-63] When cells were sensitized to Shiga toxin by sodium butyrate, the intracellular retrograde transport to the receptor-bound internalized toxin was to the endoplasmic reticulum/nuclear envelope rather than the Golgi, and this correlated with a marked increase in the cell sensitivity to Shiga toxin. The increased sensitivity was not related to increased Gb3 expression but appeared to be related to Gb3 receptors containing shorter chain fatty acid species, which directed the intracellular sorting of the toxin to the nuclear envelope. This may explain why some cells are resistant to the cytotoxic effects of the toxin despite expression of the Gb3 receptor on the plasma membrane.[63] The investigators speculated that genetic differences in Gb3 receptor fatty acid composition could play a role in the susceptibility of individuals to HUS when exposed to Shiga toxin.

In many of these studies, inhibition of protein synthesis and cell death were the determinants of Shiga toxin–mediated cell injury. While some cells respond to Shiga toxin by progressing to cell death, other cells do not die and these cells are likely to demonstrate sublethal effects of Shiga toxin. In bovine aortic endothelial cells, ST-1 and ST-2 each induced a concentration-dependent increase in preproendothelin-1 mRNA transcript levels.[64] In contrast, endothelin converting enzyme-1 and constitutive nitric oxide synthase activity was not altered by ST-1 or ST-2, suggesting that Shiga toxin–mediated alterations in endothelial-derived vasomediators may play a pathophysiologic role in the microvascular injury characteristic of HUS and hemorrhagic colitis. In addition, sublethally injured endothelial cells exposed to Shiga toxin are more susceptible to injury mediated by activated polymorphonuclear leukocytes compared to endothelial cells not exposed to Shiga toxin.[65] It is likely that VT-1 and VT-2 induce multiple sublethal changes in cells that will recover from injury.

While the endothelial cell has been considered to be the major target of Shiga toxin–mediated injury, recent studies have demonstrated that mesangial cells, renal tubular epithelial cells, monocytes, and monocyte-derived cell lines are targets of Shiga toxin–mediated biological effects and/or cytotoxicity as well. Mesangial cells have been shown to express Gb3 receptors and when exposed to ST-1 mesangial cells demonstrated inhibition of protein synthesis that was potentiated by preincubation with IL-1a or TNF-α. In addition, ST-1 induced dose- and time-dependent increases in MCP-1 mRNA levels.[66] Prolonged incubation with ST-1 resulted in substantial cytotoxicity in mesangial cells. In other studies, human mesangial cells exposed to ST-1 demonstrated decreased protein synthesis and no induction of cytokines or chemokines.[67]

Renal tubular epithelial cells have been shown to demonstrate diverse biologic responses when exposed to Shiga toxin. Cultured human proximal tubules were sensitive to the cytotoxic effects of ST-1 and the cytotoxic effect was increased when the cells were preexposed to IL-1, lipopolysaccharide, and butyrate, but not when preincubated with TNF-α.[68] Sublethal concentrations of ST-1 induced increased release of TNF-α and IL-1, and increased expression of TNF-α and IL-1 mRNA.[69] In other studies, Shiga toxin was found to induce cell death and apoptosis in a human renal tubular epithelial–derived cell line.[70,71] Interestingly, apoptosis of renal tubular cells has been observed in pathologic specimens from patients with HUS, and Shiga toxin was demonstrated to be bound to distal tubule cells in HUS.[57,72] As described below, Shiga toxins have also been demonstrated to elicit multiple biological responses from monocytes and macrophages. Taken together, these studies suggest that mesangial cells, renal tubular epithelial cells, monocytes, and macrophages are important targets of Shiga toxin–mediated cell injury in HUS.

While Shiga toxins have direct effects on endothelial cells, mesangial, and epithelial cells, it is very likely that inflammatory mediators are important in the pathogenesis of endothelial cell injury as well[34,73-76] (Figure 25-5). Animal studies have shown that macrophages are important in mediating Shiga toxin–induced cell injury and that Shiga toxin induces TNF

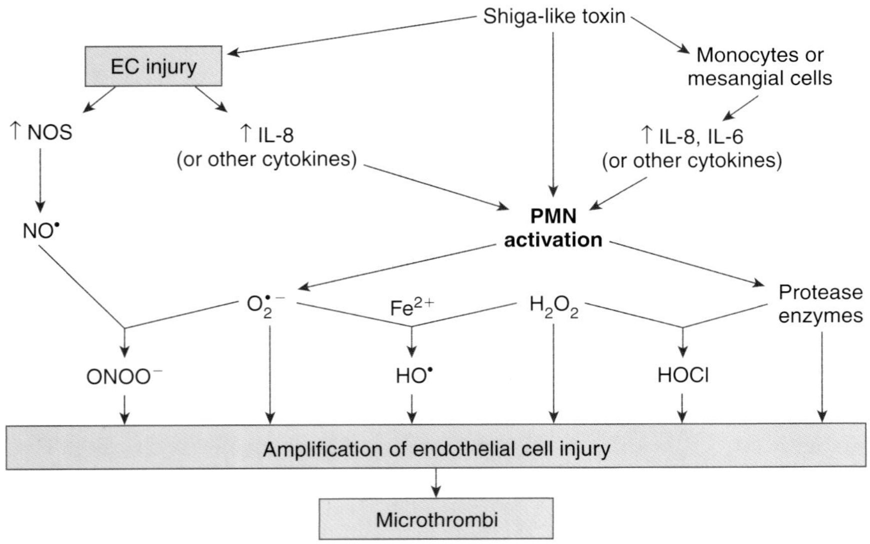

Figure 25-5 Potential mechanisms of cell injury in HUS. Shiga-like toxins can cause direct cytotoxicity as well as amplification of injury with activation of inflammatory cytokines and PMNs. (Reprinted with permission from Andreoli SP: The pathophysiology of the hemolytic uremic syndrome, *Curr Opin Nephrol Hypertens* 8:459-64, 1999.)

expression in mice, while other animal studies have also demonstrated that nitric oxide production was increased in mouse macrophages exposed to Shiga toxin.[77,78] Human monocytes and monocyte-derived cell lines respond to Shiga toxin with increased secretion of inflammatory cytokines, including TNF-α, IL-1, and IL-6.[73,79] Increased expression of TNF-α mRNA was preceded by the nuclear translocation of the transcriptional activators NF-κB and AP-1.[80]

Elevated levels of IL-8 and TNF and signs of oxidant stress have been described in children with HUS, suggesting that the inflammatory response and PMNs in particular are very important in mediating microvascular injury in HUS.[34,73-76] In addition, urinary levels of MCP-1 and IL-8 levels were recently found to be significantly elevated in children during the acute phase of HUS.[73] Several studies support a role for oxidant injury in the pathogenesis of HUS. A high PMN count is typical of the disease and a high WBC is associated with more severe disease and a worse outcome.[17,75] In addition, blood levels of interleukin-8, a cytokine that stimulates PMNs to degranulate and generate oxidants, are elevated in children with HUS, and the PMN degranulation enzyme, elastase (in complex with alpha-1-antitrypsin), is elevated in children during the acute phase of HUS and in animal models of HUS[34,74-76] (Figure 25-6). PMNs isolated from patients with HUS were found to be functionally impaired and demonstrated features of previous degranulation, indicating a previous activation with release of oxidants and protease enzymes.[81] A recent study also demonstrated that urinary neutrophil gelatinase-associated lipocalcin was significantly higher in children with more severe HUS and in children with HUS who required dialysis.[82]

In in vitro studies, PMNs were more adherent to HUVEC exposed to Shiga toxin (VT-1).[83] Human umbilical vein endothelial cells and human glomerular endothelial cells exposed to TNF and Shiga toxin are more susceptible to PMN-mediated cell injury compared to endothelial cells not exposed to Shiga toxin.[65] Studies have also demonstrated that Shiga toxin is rapidly bound to PMNs, and Shiga toxin bound to PMNs can be transferred to the Shiga toxin receptors on glomerular microvascular endothelial cells to induce cell injury.[83] Taken together, these studies suggest an important role for oxidants and protease enzymes derived from activated PMNs in the pathogenesis of HUS (Figure 25-6). However, this view is not yet widely accepted.[84]

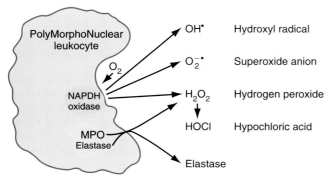

Figure 25-6 Activated PMNs produce oxidants including superoxide anion, hydrogen peroxide, hydroxyl radical, hypochlorus acid, and release elastase and myeloperoxidase, which generates hypochlorus acid from hydrogen peroxide.

The resulting injured endothelial cell then alters its normal thromboresistant characteristics and becomes thrombogenic. Indeed, decreased thrombomodulin expression has been demonstrated in human glomerular endothelial cells exposed to ST-2, and increased circulating levels of tissue factor have been demonstrated in children with HUS.[85,86]

Management and Therapy of Shiga Toxin–Mediated HUS

The majority of children with HUS develop some degree of renal insufficiency and approximately two-thirds of children with HUS will require dialysis therapy, while about one-third will have milder renal involvement without the need for dialysis therapy. Thus, the management of HUS encompasses the usual management of children with acute renal failure with additional management issues specific to HUS. General management of acute renal failure includes appropriate fluid and electrolyte management, antihypertensive therapy if the child demonstrates hypertension, and the initiation of renal replacement therapy when appropriate.

Specific management issues in HUS include management of the hematological complications of HUS, monitoring for extrarenal involvement in HUS, avoiding antidiarrheal drugs, and possibly avoiding antibiotic therapy. Management of the hematological complications of HUS, including hemolytic anemia and thrombocytopenia, should involve frequent laboratory studies as children may become quietly anemic due to rapid hemolysis. In addition, jaundice may develop due to the hemolytic process, and is characterized by an increase in indirect bilirubin. Transfusion of packed red blood cells is needed when the hemoglobin is falling rapidly and/or when the hemoglobin reaches 6 to 7 g/dl (unpublished data). Children should be transfused over a 2 to 4 hour interval, with diuretic therapy in case of volume overload. Careful monitoring of blood pressure, urine output, and respiratory status is important to ensure that the child does not develop pulmonary edema.

Thrombocytopenia can be profound, but platelet transfusions are usually limited to the child in need of a surgical procedure or the child with active bleeding. The rationale for limited platelet transfusions is that platelet transfusions can contribute to the development of microthrombi formation and promote tissue ischemia. Since microthrombi form during the course of HUS in multiple organs, including the kidney, CNS, colon, pancreas, skeletal muscle, and myocardium, as well as other organs, accelerated deposition of microthrombi may occur following platelet transfusions and promote tissue injury.

The kidney and the gastrointestinal tract are the organs most commonly affected in HUS, but other organs are also affected in a substantial number of children. CNS involvement may manifest as irritability, seizures, obtundation, and/or coma. In some patients, pancreatitis with or without glucose intolerance will develop during the acute phase of the disease, while skeletal and myocardial involvement may also be present. It is very important to evaluate the presence and extent of extrarenal involvement, as these extrarenal complications contribute to the mortality of HUS. Neurological examination will screen for CNS involvement and radiographic imaging will be needed in symptomatic patients, including those with combativeness, irritability, seizures, and decreased level of consciousness. In addition to monitoring the level of renal function, hemoglobin, hemolytic parameters (LDH, haptoglobin), hematocrit, and platelet count as described above, amylase, lipase, glucose, and liver function studies should be performed during the acute phase of the disease.

In children with hemorrhagic colitis due to Shiga toxin–producing *E. coli* infection, the use of antimotility agents has been associated with a greater risk for the development of HUS. Thus, antidiarrhea agents are usually avoided in children with HUS, as it is thought that this contributes to retention of Shiga toxin within the colon, which could enhance absorption of the toxin.[87]

Antibiotic Treatment and Potential Preventive Agents

Some studies have demonstrated harmful effects of antibiotic therapy in hemorrhagic colitis. Children with hemorrhagic colitis associated with Shiga toxin–producing *E. coli* who received antibiotic therapy were more likely to develop HUS compared to children who did not receive antibiotic therapy.[25] Other studies have not demonstrated such an association, and a recent metaanalysis concluded that administration of antibiotics in people infected with Shiga toxin–producing *E. coli* was not associated with the development of HUS.[26,88] In vitro studies have shown that some antibiotics promote production and release of Shiga toxin from *E. coli*.[82,89] Currently there is no consensus on the use of antibiotic therapy in children with hemorrhagic colitis or HUS; however, antibiotics are not usually prescribed unless there are specific indications for antibiotic therapy.[90] While clearly indicated in some children with atypical HUS, therapy with plasmapheresis and/or plasma exchange has not been proven beneficial in Shiga toxin–associated HUS.[91]

A diatomaceous silicon-diamide compound linked to an oligosaccharide chain (Synsorb Pk) has been shown to avidly bind and neutralize Shiga toxin. A clinical trial has recently been completed to determine if oral administration of Synsorb Pk can decrease the rate of progression of hemorrhagic colitis to HUS, or if it can reduce the need for dialysis or extrarenal complications in children with established HUS.[92,93] Unfortunately, the Synsorb Pk was not found to be beneficial in preventing extrarenal complications or in reducing dialysis duration in children with new-onset HUS. Starfish is a new compound that has recently been developed which binds to Shiga toxin 1000 times more efficiently than Synsorb Pk. Starfish is a pentamer and has the potential to be administered intravenously.[94] Starfish has been shown to protect mice against a lethal dose of ST-1, but not ST-2, while a modified version of Starfish called Daisy protected mice against lethal doses of ST-1 and ST-2.[95] Very interesting studies have also demonstrated that monoclonal antibodies specific for the A subunit of ST-2 prevented lethal complications in mice when administered after the onset of diarrhea.[96,97] The authors suggested that treatment of children with this antibody after the onset of bloody diarrhea may be protective against the development of HUS.[97,98] Other recent studies demonstrated that vaccination with a plant-based oral vaccine protected mice against a lethal systemic intoxication with ST-2.[98] An improved understanding of the mechanisms of Shiga toxin infections and the pathophysiology of cell injury in HUS will hopefully lead to new therapeutic strategies for children with HUS to prevent acute mortality and long-term morbidity of HUS.

HUS ASSOCIATED WITH *S. PNEUMONIAE*, NEURAMINIDASE, AND T-ANTIGEN

A rare but unique form of HUS may occur following an invasive infection of *S. pneumoniae*. The preceding infection is usually severe and invasive, and children may present with septicemia, meningitis, and/or pneumonia with empyema.[94-103] The incidence of *S. pneumoniae*–associated HUS in the Canadian surveillance program was one definitive and three probable cases among 140 cases of HUS from April 2000 to March 2002.[101] When compared with children with STEC-associated HUS, children with *S. pneumoniae*–associated HUS were generally younger, had more severe renal and hematological disease, and were more likely to require dialysis.[102] The mortality of SP-associated HUS is 30% to 50% (much higher than STEC-associated HUS), and the incidence of cortical necrosis and long-term renal and extrarenal complications is also higher in SP-associated HUS compared to STEC-associated HUS.[94-103] The mechanism of cellular injury in SP-associated HUS is thought to be related to exposure of the normally hidden Thomsen-Freidenreich T-antigen, by circulating neuraminidase produced by the *Streptococcus pneumoniae* organism. The neuraminidase removes the N-acetylneuraminic acid, and normally circulating anti–T-antigen antibodies react with the newly exposed T-antigen on red blood cells, platelets, and endothelial cells, which precipitates hemolytic anemia, thrombocytopenia, and microvascular injury characteristic of HUS.[103] In children with SP-associated HUS, all blood products should be washed and plasma infusion should be avoided so as to prevent administration of additional anti–T-antigen antibodies.[103]

HUS ASSOCIATED WITH *SHIGELLA DYSENTERIAE* TYPE I AND OTHER INFECTIONS

HUS associated with *Shigella dysenteriae* occurs in India and in Africa. It is usually complicated by severe dysentery, intravascular volume depletion, and cardiovascular collapse, and has a higher morbidity and mortality rate than HUS associated with *E. coli*.[104,105] A large severe outbreak of HUS following *Shigella* dysentery occurred in Kwazulu/Natal from 1994 to 1996; this outbreak resulted in impaired renal function and chronic renal failure in over 40% of the cases and the death rate was 17.3%.[106] Severe HUS following *Shigella* infection was also observed in 11 children from two families in France, including the index case, who had recently returned from Senegal.[107]

HUS has also been reported following *Entamoeba histolytica* intestinal infection and also in association with HIV infection and HTLV-1 infection.[108-110] The endothelial cell is a target of injury in chronic states of HIV infection, and the basic fibroblast growth factor is an angiogenic growth factor produced by injured endothelial cells. Studies have shown that basic fibroblast growth factor was elevated in children with HUS associated with HIV infection, and that fibroblast growth factor is upregulated in the kidney of such children.[111-113] Since the introduction of effective retroviral medications, the incidence of HUS-associated HIV infection seems to have decreased.

ATYPICAL-RECURRENT HUS

"Atypical HUS," often used by pediatricians to indicate a presentation of HUS without preceding diarrhea, is clearly a misnomer if it is used to refer to a *typical* example of a known but rare subgroup of HUS, such as HUS induced by pneumococcal sepsis with T-antigen exposure.

This may be a semantic issue, but atypical HUS in this chapter refers to the term "diarrhea negative/VTEC negative" to separate this heterogeneous group from the more common VTEC-induced form that mostly affects young children.

In all cases of HUS/TTP, the history and the clinical pattern are important and may be sufficient by themselves to point towards an appropriate subgroup and appropriate therapy.[114-135] Nevertheless, with the exception of a first episode of VTEC-positive, diarrhea-associated HUS in a child with no family history of HUS or TTP, it should be emphasized that there should be a comprehensive investigation. For example, a woman with HUS/TTP associated with pregnancy should have investigation of vWF protease activity and complement regulatory pathways. The clinical implications of finding an abnormality in any of these would be considerable, and override the descriptive diagnosis of "pregnancy-associated HUS." Similarly, all infants presenting at less than 3 months of age should be fully investigated for congenital risk factors. Clinicians should resist the temptation to drop further exploration once a seemingly satisfactory diagnosis has been reached as dual causation may be missed.[1,2,114-137]

It is increasingly clear that patients with atypical or recurrent forms have what we call "susceptibility genes" that may influence the clinical course and outcome of the disease. It is at present unclear whether atypical HUS is a monogenic disease. Recent results from several laboratories indicate that patients may have two genetic defects in different complement genes, or rearrangements in an area on chromosome 1 where the RCA cluster is located, that is, a cluster of genes associated with the complement system.[138]

Genetic Disorders of Complement Regulation

Almost all patients with atypical-recurrent HUS have a defect in the alternative pathway. Since defects in the classical pathway are common, an association with HUS is unclear. It is not known whether patients have an abnormal lectin pathway. Therefore, we focus in this chapter on defects or alterations in the alternative complement pathway.

Mutations in the genes for complement Factor H (FH), Factor I (FI), and membrane co-factor protein (MCP) (CD46) are associated with HUS. Mutations in the FH gene are described more often.

FH, the most abundant complement regulator in plasma, is composed of 20 complement control protein (CCP) motifs in a single glycopeptide of 155 kDa, and is mostly made in the liver. FH accelerates the decay of C3bBb, the C3 convertase of the alternative pathway. With factor I as a co-factor, C3b is cleaved, interrupting the complement cascade before the generation of the effector pathways, anaphylatoxin C5a, and the membrane attack complex (C5b-C9) (see Figure 25-7 for details). Complement C5a and the membrane attack complex are essential in certain laboratory models of HUS.[139,140] FH operates both in the soluble phase and on host cells, protecting them from complement-induced injury.[141] FH is known to bind to vascular endothelium, erythrocytes, and platelets[142-144] (Figure 25-8A and B).

FH mutations have been found in about a fifth of families with HUS where the onset of the disease is nonsynchronous, and in about 8% in sporadic cases not associated with other known causes such as VTEC infection.[19,145] Most mutations are heterozygous and affect the C-terminal domain of the FH molecule. This part of the molecule is important for C3b binding. The loss of that part of the gene causes a loss of function with reduced[140] binding affinity to C3b, heparin and endothelial cells in vitro (using either synthesized muta-ted FH proteins or FH purified from the plasma of affected patients).[143,146-149] The role of FH polymorphisms in the susceptibility to HUS from other causes has not been fully understood, but an association of three frequent single nucleotide polymorphisms with HUS has been suggested.[150,151]

Not all patients with proven FH mutations show C3 reduction. Generally, those with homozygous FH deficiency are more likely to have persistently low C3, manifest HUS in early life (the neonatal period in some families),[150,152] or exhibit mesangioproliferative (mesangiocapillary) glomerulonephritis (MPGN).[153] Heterozygotes have a variable phenotype. This is best described in investigations of families.[150] The plasma concentration of C3 may be normal and HUS may present at any age. The fact that some individuals do not manifest HUS until adulthood has been used to argue that a separate trigger event may be necessary to initiate microvascular damage.

A typical feature of HUS associated with FH mutations is the poor prognosis, with over 50% of cases progressing to ESRF, sometimes during the first episode. In the Innsbruck recHUS study, 60% of patients developed ESRD within 12 months. Others have fluctuating renal function and a high risk of relapse. Hypertension is frequent and severe. The risk of graft loss soon after transplantation approaches 80%, mostly reflecting disease recurrence.[154-156]

Mutations have also been found in the genes encoding for complement FI[154,157] and the membrane-bound regulator MCP (CD46).[158,159] FI circulates in plasma and, using FH as a co-factor, cleaves C3b to iC3b. The patients thus far described with HUS are heterozygous for stop codons that abolish the synthesis of full-length protein, and plasma concentrations of FI are reduced. MCP, a membrane-bound regulator expressed in glomerular endothelium, which comprises four extracellular CCPs and a transmembranous and cytoplasmic domain, also acts as a co-factor for the cleavage

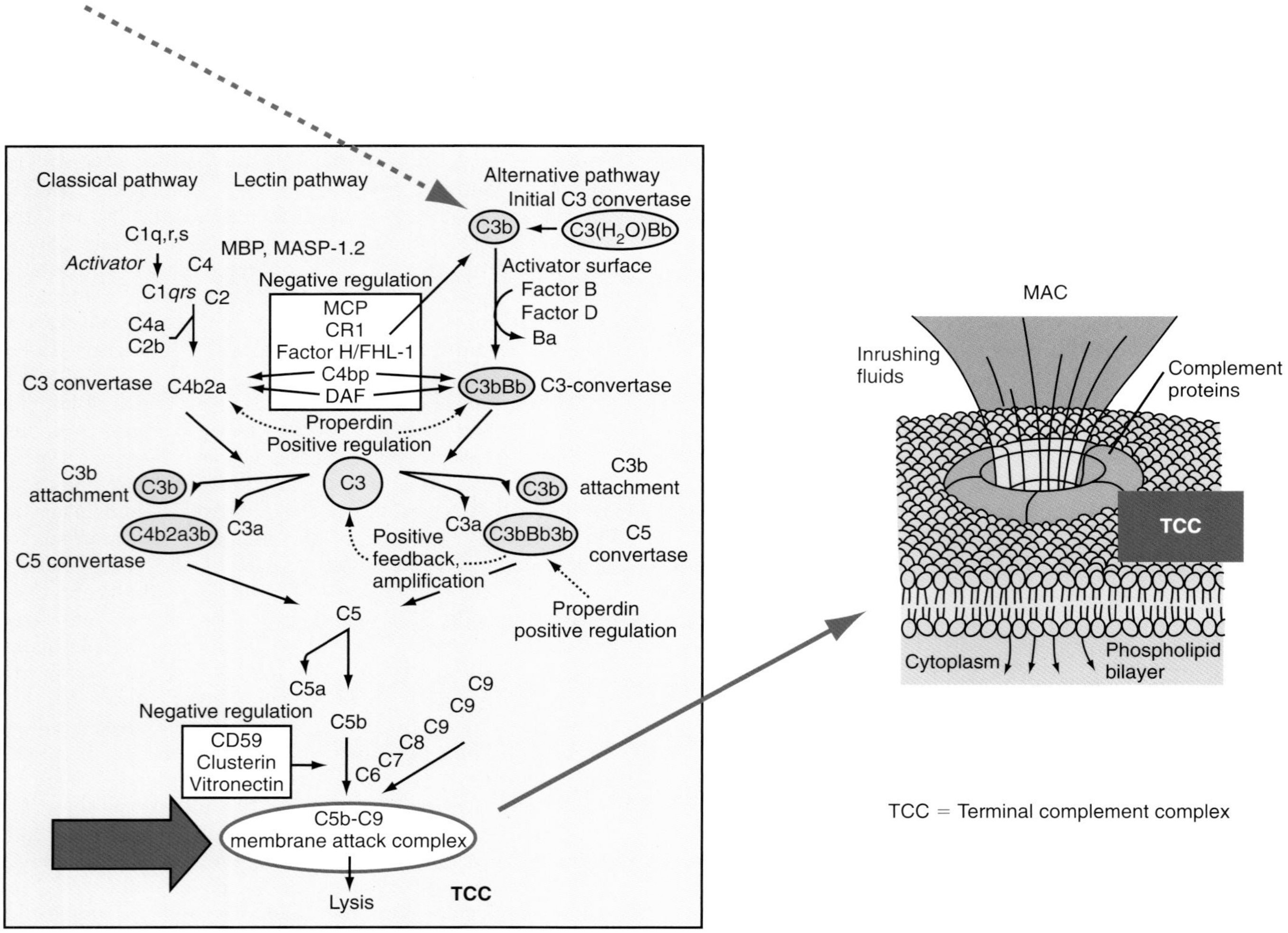

Figure 25-7 Complement system scheme. Formation of C3b from C3 is an initial path of the alternative pathway. C3b and Bb form C3bBb, which is a protease activating C5. Finally, the membrane attack complex (MAC) is formed from C5b-9. The MAC is considered toxic to cells. (Copyright J. Hellwage)

of C3b and C4b by FI. Heterozygous MCP mutations have been identified in more than 15 cases. Mutations are predicted to cause loss of C3b recognition or loss of the C-terminal of the protein, and reduced tissue expression has been shown in some patients. Unlike patients with FH or FI mutations, those with MCP abnormalities should not have disease recurrence after transplantation, because the donor organ retains its expression of normal MCP.[158,159]

The diagnosis of primary complement dysregulation in HUS is difficult without genetic expertise. A low C3 cannot be relied on to indicate deficiency of a membrane-bound complement regulator, nor does a normal plasma concentration of FH or FI exclude the possibility of a functional defect. Conversely, low C3 is a positive indicator, and in families with HUS those with hypocomplementemia are at increased risk of developing the disorder.[153] The fact that at least three regulators have been found to be abnormal in HUS adds to the concept that defective complement control predisposes to HUS, and raises the possibility that other regulatory defects, either individual or compound,[160-163] will be found.

Histology

The histological findings of thrombotic microangiopathy (TMA) are described as mesangial cell proliferation with interposition leading to double contours of the capillary loops and a lobulated appearance of the glomerular tuft not unlike MPGN.[87,137,143,159] Complement deposition in glomerular capillaries and arterioles is present but scanty. Arteriolar or arterial lesions are frequently seen. However, it is unclear if there are specific findings in atypical versus typical HUS. Most biopsies were performed in the years before the complement defects were described. At present, biopsies are rarely performed in patients with atypical or relapsing HUS. Therefore, histological interpretation with regard to etiology is not clear.[38,160,164-166]

Clinical Features

Patients with HUS and FH abnormalities have certain clinical peculiarities. The onset of the disease usually occurs without a previous gastrointestinal infection, and is seldom precipitated by diarrhea. However, other types of infections

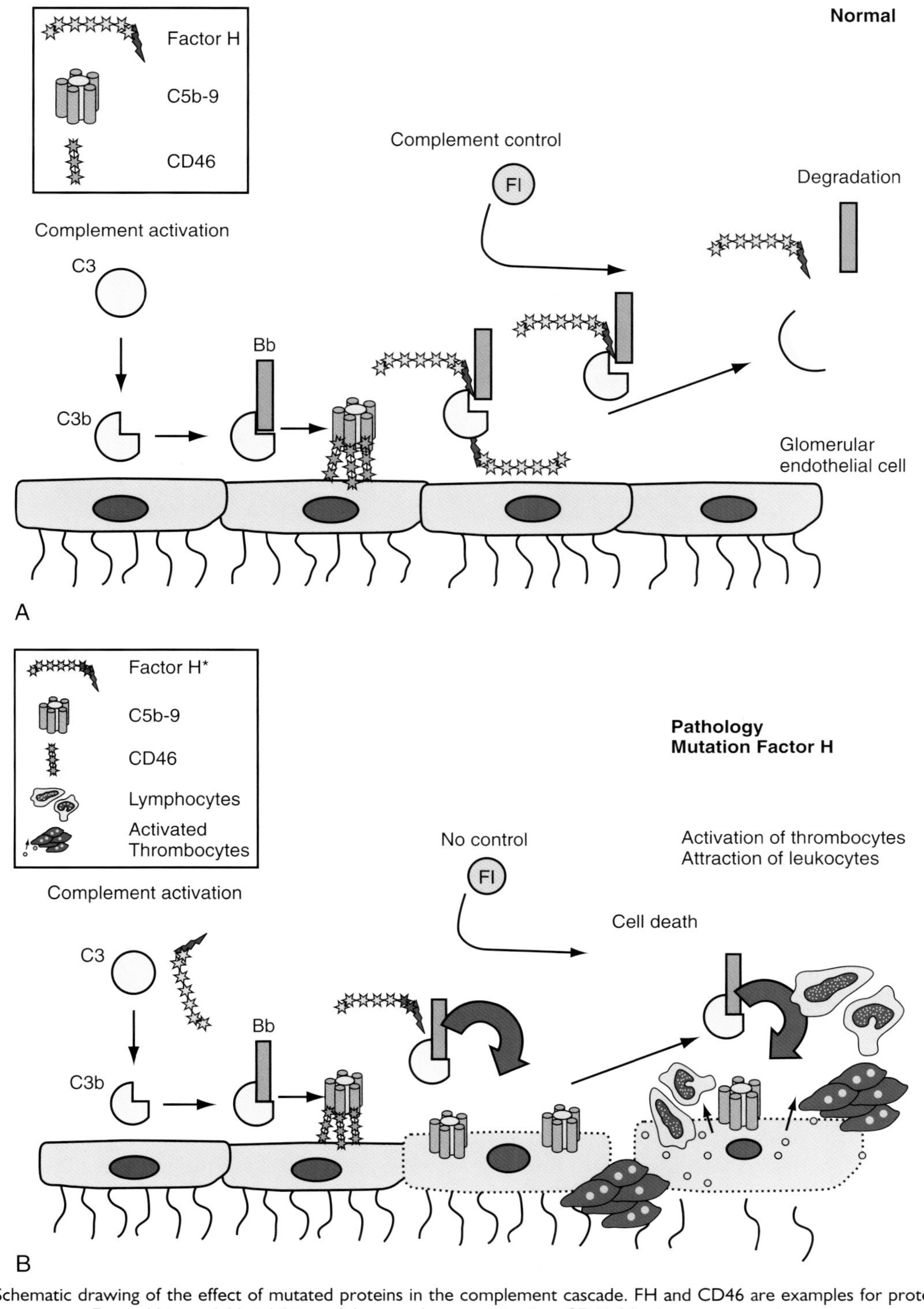

Figure 25-8 **A,** Schematic drawing of the effect of mutated proteins in the complement cascade. FH and CD46 are examples for proteins that inhibit the activated complement system. Factor H is a soluble inhibitor of the complement activation. CD46 (also known as membrane complement protein I [MCP I]) is a membrane-bound complement inhibitor. **B,** Mutation in FH. In atypical and recurrent HUS, mainly the alternative pathway is activated (C3). If activated complement cannot be controlled, cell damage and death occur through the incorporation of the membrane attack complex (C5b-9) into the (glomerular or arteriolar) endothelial cell. This attracts lymphocytes and macrophages. Finally, the damaged cells are replaced by fibroblasts. Renal function decreases and tubular damage follows. Renal replacement therapy is necessary. In this scheme, the mutation of FH causes prolonged activation of complement. Thus, the membrane-bound protection system is not sufficient. C5b-9 attacks the renal cells.

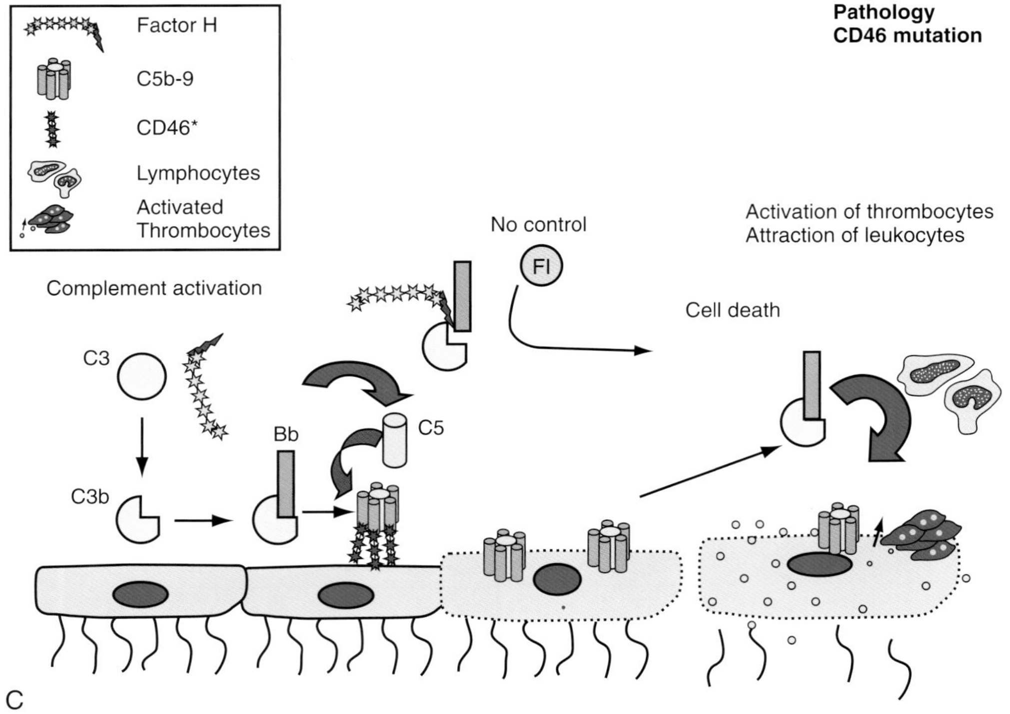

Figure 25-8, cont'd **C,** Mutation in CD46. In atypical and recurrent HUS, mainly the alternative pathway is activated (C3). If activated complement cannot be controlled, cell damage and death occur through the incorporation of the membrane attack complex (C5b-9) into the (glomerular or arteriolar) endothelial cell. This attracts lymphocytes and macrophages. Finally, the damaged cells are replaced by fibroblasts. Renal function decreases and tubular damage follows. Renal replacement therapy is necessary. Mutation in CD46 is associated with decreased protection on the cellular membrane. Even normal complement activation may be associated with cellular damage.

including upper respiratory tract infections with flulike symptoms may precede HUS.[156,162]

Occasionally, women develop HUS during pregnancy or while using the contraceptive pill. The onset is often insidious with pallor, malaise, nausea, and vomiting. A wide age range is seen.

In cases of onset in infancy, there is likely to be marked hypocomplementemia and homozygous or compound heterozygous FH deficiency. Adult onset is more in keeping with heterozygosity, although there are exceptions. Where the disease is familial, individual families tend to have distinctive patterns of presentation and outcome. Hypertension is frequent and severe. Proteinuria is common and renal function tends to fluctuate.[94,164,166] This is different from the abrupt oliguric renal failure of STEC-induced HUS. However, the clinical picture does not differ from patients with EHEC-associated disease in many cases (Figure 25-9).

Pathogenesis

FH, the most abundant complement regulator in plasma, is a 155 kDa protein made in the liver. FH accelerates the decay of C3bBb, the C3 convertase of the alternative pathway, and with FI as a co-factor it cleaves and inactivates C3b. It therefore interrupts the complement cascade before the generation of the effector pathways, anaphylatoxin C5a, and the membrane attack complex C5b-C9. The FH molecule has binding sites for sialic acid by which it attaches to host cell surfaces. It operates both in the soluble phase and on host cells including vascular endothelium.[137,142,143,164]

The pathogenesis has not been fully elucidated yet, but it seems likely that the FH defect might allow unrestrained complement activation against microvascular endothelium. Clearly this is unlikely to be the whole explanation. Some individuals do not develop HUS before adulthood and yet will have had the complement regulatory problem for many years without incident. It is therefore proposed that an unknown trigger event occurs to initiate microvascular injury that, once started, involves complement activation that cannot be switched off (Figure 25-8A, B, and C). Similar pathogenesis is likely for other regulators of complement activation localized on chromosome 1 (Figure 25-9).

Treatment

In addition to the obligatory supportive treatment and tight control of hypertension, plasma therapy may induce remission and in some cases maintain it. Fresh-frozen plasma contains FH at physiological concentrations. The dosage required to regulate complement is unclear (see below). It is certainly greater than that needed to replace missing vWF protease in TTP, and therefore plasma exchange is at present the treatment of choice initially.[150] The evidence is unclear as to how long therapy should be maintained. Plasma treatment may have to be continued for life (Table 25-2). These recommendations should be considered expert advice rather than

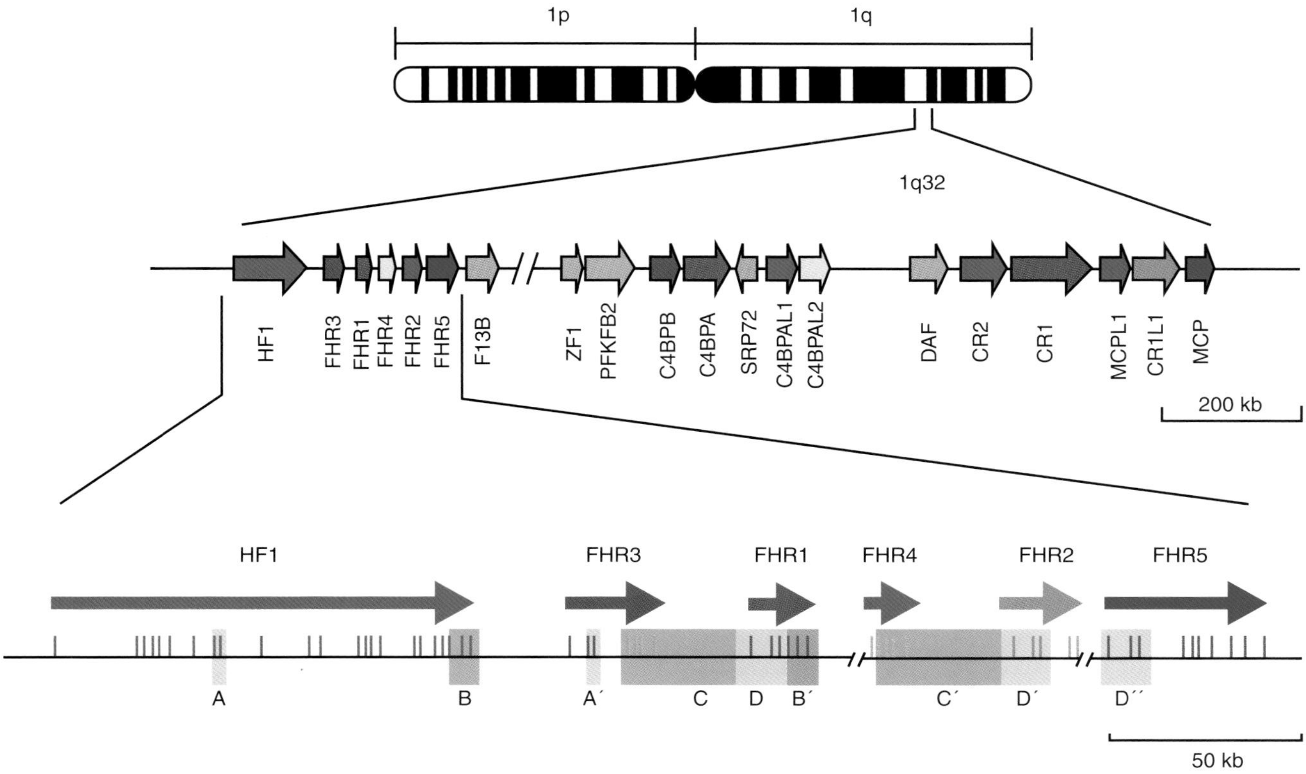

Figure 25-9 Regulators of complement activation (RCA). A cluster of complement inhibitors is located on chromosome 1. This RCA cluster is schematically drawn. Note that similar colors represent similar genetic areas. (With permission, from Rodríguez de Córdoba S, Esparza-Gordillo J, Goicoechea de Jorge E, Lopez-Trascasa M, Sánchez-Corral P: The human complement factor H: functional roles, genetic variations and disease associations, *Mol Immunol* 41:355-67, 2004.)

TABLE 25-2 Recommendations for Treatment in Patients with Atypical or Recurrent HUS (Not Evidence Based)

1.	Plasma exchange if infusion with fresh frozen plasma not sufficient or not tolerated.
2.	Pathogen-reduced FFP (Octaplas®) preferred, as mentioned in text.[167a]
3.0.	If complement is activated, intensive plasma exchange is warranted. In the first 2 weeks, 10-14 sessions with 40-60 ml/kg should be initiated. If not sufficient, increase to plasma volume of up to 420 ml/kg for 7 days.
3.1.	After the first 2 weeks (5-10 sessions), FFP volume 60-65 ml/kg per treatment.
4.	FFP volume during maintenance 20-25 ml/kg per week. This can be given as an infusion.
5.	Delay/avoid transplantation in patients with soluble complement disorders.
5.1.	Combined transplantations of liver and kidney may be an option in the future.
6.	Immunization program (including hepatitis A and B, varicella, influenza, and meningococci).

evidence-based measures. Plasma therapy should be performed with reduced pathogen content (Octaplas).[167,167a]

Steroids[168] should be avoided, and anticoagulant therapy was not proven beneficial in HUS.

New Therapeutic Strategies

Given the previous discussion, it is obvious that new treatment strategies are needed. These will include production of single complement proteins such as FH for substitutions, but also new inhibitors of complement activation such as anti-C5 antibodies. Both strategies are underway.[156]

TRANSPLANTATION

Risk of Recurrence

In 2003, Loirat and Niaudet[3] published a study on the risk of HUS recurrence after renal transplantation in children. They compared the outcomes and recurrence risks between D+HUS and D-HUS, and found that renal transplantation in children with D+HUS is not associated with an increased risk of graft failure compared with non-HUS patients. In addition, HUS has never recurred post-transplant in patients with proven verotoxin-producing *E. coli*–induced HUS.

On the other hand, they showed the incidence of HUS recurrence in 63 children who received 77 kidney transplants after D-HUS of unknown etiology. Of these 63 children, 13

(21%) had recurrence of HUS in one or several grafts. The time between initial HUS and renal transplantation varied from 4 months to 17.6 years. Therefore, it appears that a prolonged interval between initial HUS and transplantation does not reduce the risk of recurrence.

Eleven patients with HUS associated with Factor H deficiency received 11 kidneys. Five (45%) of them developed recurrence in their graft. Another seven patients with HUS associated with normal FH plasma concentration but FH gene mutation received seven kidneys, and recurrence occurred in two (28%) of them. In three patients with HUS associated with low C3 without identifiable FH deficiency or mutation, three kidneys were transplanted; recurrence developed in all (100%) of them. Eleven patients (adults) with autosomal recessive HUS of unknown etiology received 14 kidneys. Recurrence occurred in seven (36%) patients and 9 (64%) grafts.

Since 2001, we have evaluated 43 patients with recurrent HUS in a multicenter study including Germany, Austria, Switzerland, Hungary, and the Czech Republic.[156,157,162] In 44.8% of the patients, complement analysis demonstrated low C3. FH abnormalities were found in 15.4%.

In 10 of the 43 patients with recHUS (24%), 20 kidneys were transplanted. Only three patients were successfully transplanted. Five patients (50%) were retransplanted because of recurrence in the graft, and two patients developed thrombosis in the graft. One patient was transplanted four times because of recurrences in the transplanted kidney.

At present combined transplantation of liver and kidney is still considered experimental. In any case, a complete genetic workup should be performed to help the clinician to evaluate the risk. May be indicated in patients with abnormalities of circulating complement regulators (FH, cofactor I), but not in patients with CD46 mutations.

Prognosis

The outcome after recurrence is poor. In the French series, 3 of 30 patients with recurrence died, one each from hypertension, cerebral infarct, and disseminated intravascular coagulation. Twenty-five patients (83%) lost their graft because of recurrence. Three patients returned to dialysis after recurrence and only two patients had a functioning graft despite recurrence.[154]

Recurrent HUS causes terminal renal insufficiency in over 60% of patients. The problem of this disease is the high rate of recurrence after transplantation.[9,10] In addition, the chance for successful re-transplantation is low. These patients demonstrate a high rate of thrombosis and rejection.

The therapy of patients with D-HUS is difficult. They often progress to ESRD despite continuous plasma therapy, which only has a transient effect.[7,9] Complications in other organs, including heart failure, are high.

Conclusion

Identification of the specific genetic defect in patients with atypical HUS should improve diagnostic precision and help to predict clinical outcomes. Knowledge of the exact pathomechanisms will hopefully translate into improved management of the disease.

Since the soluble complement inhibitors like FH or FHR are plasma proteins produced mainly by the liver, kidney transplantation in patients with atypical HUS with FH mutations who have progressed to ESRD is associated with graft loss in 80% due to disease recurrence.[12] Therefore, the underlying pathogenesis should be known before transplantation in order to avoid high risk of transplant failure. Furthermore, patients with abnormalities in soluble complement inhibitors might benefit from specific replacement therapies with plasma fractions enriched in these proteins.[7,162]

ACQUIRED DISORDERS OF COMPLEMENT REGULATION

Evidence of IgG autoantibodies to complement FH has been reported in some patients with atypical HUS.[163,169] In these patients, the plasma concentration of FH, and the FH gene mutation analysis were normal. The antibody to purified FH was identified by ELISA, and functional experiments indicated that the antibody probably interfered with FH binding to the C3bBb convertase. The plasma concentration of C3 was mildly reduced in two cases and factor B reduced in two cases, which indicated alternative pathway activation. It seems that autoantibodies are more often involved but not recognized. Most centers are not able to identify these specific antibodies yet. However, substantial research activity is ongoing. Furthermore, treatment strategies are numerous. Vigorous plasmapheresis is helpful in some patients. However, immunosuppression with anti–B-lymphocyte strategies (i.e., steroids, cyclophosphamide, azathioprin, or rituximab) is probably needed to ensure long-term remission.

GENETIC DISORDERS OF VON WILLEBRAND FACTOR–CLEAVING PROTEASE (ADAMTS13)

The finding of unusually large multimeric forms of von Willebrand factor (vWF) in the plasma of patients with HUS/TTP and chronic relapsing TTP was first reported by Moake et al.[170,171] These large multimers are able to cause agglutination of platelets under high shear stress conditions. In 1997, Furlan et al.[171] identified severe deficiency (<7% of normal plasma activity) of a specific protease that cleaves multimeric vWF protein in patients with chronic relapsing TTP. Later, two groups confirmed decreased plasma activity of von Willebrand factor–cleaving protease (vWFCP) in a large group of patients with familial and nonfamilial TTP.[172-174] The decreased activity was shown to be due to either constitutional deficiency of vWF-CP or to the presence of autoantibodies against it.

In healthy adults, the vWFCP plasma activity ranges from 50% to 178% of normal control. Low activity can be found in patients with liver disease, disseminated cancers, and chronic inflammatory and metabolic conditions, and in pregnant patients and newborns. These low levels do not correspond to the extremely low levels associated with "TTP."[164,174]

Normally, vWF-CP prevents the emergence and persistence of unusually large multimers of vWF in the circulation by cleaving multimeric vWF released from the endothelium and platelets into monomeric subunits at position 842-843. The protease has recently been purified from plasma and the gene sequenced,[174,175] and shown to be a member of a family of metalloproteases, designated ADAMTS13. ADAMTS is an acronym for "a disintegrin-like and metalloprotease with thrombospondin type I repeats." ADAMTS13 is encoded on chromosome 9q34, and genetic analysis from patients with familial chronic relapsing TTP has demonstrated mutations throughout the gene.[176-179] vWFCP is predominantly produced by stellate cells in the liver,[180-183] and has a plasma half-life of 2 to 3 days.[183]

Chronic relapsing thrombotic thrombocytopenic purpura due to inherited vWFCP deficiency may present in the neonatal period. Often the diagnosis is not made at this time, and the thrombocytopenia, hemolytic anemia, and need for exchange transfusions appear unexplained.[178,184] Later in infancy or early childhood, recurrent episodes of hemolysis and thrombocytopenia recur at intervals, typically every 3rd to 4th week. The clinical presentation varies. About 50% of patients with less than 5% vWFCP activity have their first attack before age 5 years. In the other 50%, the diagnosis is made in adulthood. There are a few cases of vWFCP deficiency reported in patients who have not, or have not yet, developed clinical symptoms, implying that different genetic defects are important or that environmental triggering events are necessary to develop HUS/TTP.[185,186]

Not all patients present with the complete diagnostic criteria of HUS/TTP. The family history and the clinical presentation of recurrent thrombocytopenia and hemolytic anemia as well as unexplained thrombocytopenia and hemolytic anemia are an indication to examine vWFCP activity in blood. Several assays of vWFCP activity and vWFCP inhibiting autoantibodies (see below) have been developed. The tests are labor-intensive and mostly done in specialized hematology laboratories. The assays are based on detection of degraded multimers of vWF by immunoblotting, binding of vWF to collagen, binding of antibodies that detect the vWF cleavage products, ristocetin co-factor activity, and ELISA that detects vWF cleavage at the A2 domain. These assays have typically been found to be reliable and comparable.[187]

Chronic relapsing TTP/HUS due to constitutional deficiency of vWFCP can be reversed or prevented by prophylactic infusion of fresh-frozen plasma or cryoprecipitate-poor plasma (cryosupernatant) at 2- to 3-week intervals without concurrent plasmapheresis. If diagnosed early, chronic relapsing TTP due to congenital deficiency of vWFCP can be adequately treated as above, but long-term follow-up studies are warranted.

ACQUIRED DISORDERS OF VON WILLEBRAND FACTOR–CLEAVING PROTEASE

Severely decreased vWFCP activity in patients with acute acquired, mainly nonfamilial, TTP is mostly due to IgG autoantibodies that inhibit vWFCP in plasma.[172,173] These antibodies are found in 48% to 80% of adult TTP patients, and are transient or intermittent in the majority. In addition, antibodies to vWFCP have been identified in patients with TTP associated with the platelet inhibitory agent ticlopidine (see Figure 25-1). This acquired form of thrombotic microangiopathy can occur at any age, but is mainly seen in adults and is usually a single acute episode, although recurrences have been reported in 11% to 36% of patients.

Patients with vWFCP deficiency due to inhibiting autoantibodies usually respond to intensive plasmapheresis, but may require additional immunosuppression or even splenectomy. Rituximab, the monoclonal antibody against CD20 on B-lymphocytes, has also been effective.[166,188,189] Historically, patients with untreated TTP had mortality approaching 90%. Plasma exchange with replacement by fresh-frozen plasma has reduced the mortality to 20%.[190] Platelet infusions risk exacerbating microvascular thrombosis and should be avoided in these patients unless there are life-threatening hemorrhages or the patient is undergoing a surgical procedure.

DEFECTIVE COBALAMIN METABOLISM

A peculiar form of HUS in infants (age <1 year) was attributed to an inborn error of cobalamin-C (Cbl-C) metabolism by Baumgartner et al. in 1979.[191] It is an autosomal recessive disorder with variable clinical expression. Vitamin B_{12} undergoes intracellular metabolism for full biological action. After uptake by endocytosis, the transcobalamin II–cobalamin complex is cleaved and released from the lysosomes as cobal(III)amin to further undergo reduction to cobal(II)amin and cobal(I)amin. Cobal(I)amin initiates the synthesis of two co-enzymes, adenosylCbl and methylCbl. AdenosylCbl is the co-enzyme of methylmalonoyl-CoA mutase, and methylCbl is the co-enzyme of methionine synthase. Defects in the synthesis of these co-enzymes lead to hyperhomocysteinemia and methylmalonic aciduria, the two biochemical characteristics of Cbl-C deficiency. It is postulated that the high levels of homocysteine may be responsible for the vascular manifestations. Patients with Cbl-C deficiency usually present in the early days and months of life with failure to thrive, poor feeding, and vomiting. Rapid deterioration of the patient's condition is the rule due to metabolic acidosis, gastrointestinal bleeding, hemolytic anemia, thrombocytopenia, severe respiratory and hepatic failure, and renal insufficiency.[191-194] The incidence of the disease is unknown, but it is likely that many patients die undiagnosed. Besides the early fulminant course, the disease can manifest later in childhood with a more protracted course. Labrune et al.[195] described such a patient diagnosed at the age of 18 months and in need of renal replacement therapy at age 13 years. A few adolescent patients have been reported recently. The case of a 16-year-old boy who presented with a chronic illness and died at age 21 years following cerebrovascular bleeding has been published.[196] Van Hove et al.[197] reported a brother and a sister with a chronic illness characterized by hematuria, proteinuria, and arterial hypertension. Renal biopsy showed a chronic thrombotic angiopathy. Serum homocysteine was 10-fold higher than normal values, and urinary methylmalonic acid markedly increased. Both anomalies were corrected by the daily administration of 5 mg of hydroxycobalamin associated with betaine.

DRUG-INDUCED HUS

Chemotherapeutic Agents Mitomycin C and Gemcitabine

Mitomycin is an antibiotic with antimitotic properties, used mainly in gastric and breast cancer. Early reports associated this drug with cases, usually fatal, that displayed histological features of thrombotic microangiopathy (TMA).[197] Survival was obtained in some cases using a combination of steroids and plasma exchanges[198]; however, patients surviving the acute phase often remain on chronic dialysis, or die later from their malignancy. According to a recent report that mentioned 12 cases, gemcitabine, another chemically related anticancer drug used in the treatment of pulmonary, pancreatic, and urothelial carcinomas, is also thought to be the cause of cancer-associated HUS/TTP.[200] Given that HUS has been described in cancer itself, the specific role of these drugs is uncertain. However, Cattell[201] was able to induce renal lesions resembling human HUS by injecting mitomycin into the renal artery of rats, giving credence to a causative role for these agents.

Ticlopidine and Clopidogrel

Ticlopidine and clodipogrel, both thienopyridine derivatives, are antiplatelet agents used in the treatment of patients with cerebrovascular and peripheral diseases and to reduce the risk of thrombosis in patients undergoing coronary artery stenting. In the first 4 years of marketing of ticlopidine, the U.S. Food and Drug Administration received 25 reports of patients developing thrombotic thrombocytopenic purpura. Bennett et al.[202] described the clinical characteristics and outcomes in 60 patients with ticlopidine-associated TTP,[201] and it became clear that the occurrence of TTP was not as rare as previously thought. TTP became one of the most serious hematological side effects of the drug, with a frequency of one case per 1600 to 5000 patients. TTP usually occurred after 2 weeks of treatment, and within 1 month in 80% of cases. Besides the hemolytic anemia and thrombocytopenia, 75% of the 98 investigated cases developed neurological manifestations, and renal insufficiency was observed in almost 30%. The overall mortality rate was estimated at 33%. Plasmapheresis was shown to be the treatment of choice and clearly reduced the mortality rate for patients with ticlopidine-associated TTP in comparison to those who did not undergo plasmapheresis.[202] The mechanism by which ticlopidine induces TTP is unconfirmed, but an immune mechanism may be responsible. In a recent study, a deficiency of ADAMTS13 was found in all of seven patients with ticlopidine-associated TTP/HUS. In five of these patients, antibodies against ADAMTS13 were present.[203]

Clopidogrel differs from ticlopidine by a having an extra carboxymethyl group, and has largely replaced ticlopidine as it has fewer adverse effects, notably neutropenia, and cutaneous and gastrointestinal reactions. In the first clinical trials of 20,000 closely monitored patients, no signs of TTP were mentioned. However, in 2000 the first cases of clopidogrel-associated TTP-HUS were reported.[204] In these, TTP occurred more often in the first 2 weeks after starting clopidogrel. Patients were more prone to recurrence than those with ticlopidine-associated TTP and needed more plasma exchanges before improvement occurred. The incidence of clopidogrel-associated TTP has been estimated to be the same as TTP in the general population (about 3.7 cases per million). This makes a causal relation less certain, although in two patients severe ADAMTS13 deficiency due to antibodies was found in the acute phase. In the 11 cases published by Bennett et al.,[205] almost half of the patients also used cholesterol-lowering agents, and this drug combination deserves further evaluation in relation to TTP.

Quinine

The intake of quinine, whether as a medication or a bitter flavoring in drinks, is associated with TTP/HUS, with predominant renal involvement.[205-207] In a series of HUS/TTP patients, 11% reported taking quinine compared to 6% taking other drugs.[166] In patients sensitized to quinine, the typical clinical pattern is one of abrupt onset of chills, myalgia, vomiting, and oliguria immediately after quinine exposure. The accompanying anemia is often mild. Patients can be shown to have antibodies that recognize various glycoprotein epitopes on platelets, red cells, and leukocytes.[208,209] This interaction is quinine dependent, suggesting that a neoantigen is formed. In platelets, the antibody has been found to cross-react with glycoprotein IIb/IIIa and sometimes Ib/IX. The disorder is comparatively mild, and remits with avoidance of quinine and if plasma exchange is started early enough. ADAMTS13 plasma activity is typically normal.

Calcineurin Inhibitors

HUS/TTP occasionally occurs de novo in recipients of solid organ allografts. The first report was in 1984[211] in a patient treated with cyclosporin (CsA) for liver transplantation. Recovery after CsA withdrawal suggested an etiological role. At the same time, van Buren et al.[212] described three adult patients receiving CsA for renal transplantation, and subsequently it has become clear that this complication occurs in heart, kidney-pancreas, and bone marrow transplantation, and with both CsA and tacrolimus. The vast majority of patients reported are adults. In an overview, Young et al.[213] described 13 of their own patients and summarized the findings in 76 cases published between 1983 and 1993. In their own patients, CsA or tacrolimus was discontinued, and the patients were treated with isradipine (a calcium channel blocker), aspirin, and pentoxifylline. All survived and only three did not regain renal function.

In a review of 188 transplants Zarifian et al.[214] calculated that incidence of CsA-associated TMA was 14%, while for tacrolimus, where the number of patients is smaller, the estimate was between 1% and 5%. Trimarchi et al.[215] reviewed 21 cases of tacrolimus-associated TMA and found that patients might be almost asymptomatic or present with the full-blown clinical picture of HUS/TTP. Trough levels of the drug were not predictive of the development of TMA, but a reduction of the dose was often beneficial in terms of recovery of renal function. The first pediatric case was published in 1999.[203] The 16-year-old girl developed TMA under conventional therapy of methylprednisolone, azathioprine, and CsA. A change to tacrolimus resulted in graft recovery.

The pathophysiology of HUS associated with calcineurin inhibitors is speculative.[215] Plasma activity of ADAMTS13 has not been measured in this setting. These drugs exert both direct and endothelin-1–mediated vasoconstriction that reduces renal plasma flow and glomerular filtration rate, and perhaps this leads to prothrombotic changes in endothelium. An unsolved problem is clinical management. The replacement of CsA with tacrolimus, or by sirolimus or mycophenolate mofetil has benefited some patients.

Calcineurin inhibitors are the mainstay of immunosuppression for kidney transplantation. It is not clear if they should be avoided for those cases of HUS where relapse after transplantation is a known risk. In a recent report on renal transplant outcome in 71 patients with ESRD secondary to non-Stx-HUS, cyclosporine A and FK506 administration were not associated with a higher incidence of HUS recurrence, when compared with regimens excluding these drugs.[216,217] The efficacy of sirolimus in these circumstances is doubtful,[218] as illustrated by the recurrence of HUS in two children whose immunosuppressive regimen was based on sirolimus, without calcineurin inhibitors.[216,218]

HUS ASSOCIATED WITH PREGNANCY, HELLP SYNDROME, AND ORAL CONTRACEPTIVES

Epidemiological studies confirm that TTP is more prevalent in women than in men, and in women occurs more often in childbearing years. An association with the use of the oral contraceptive pill remains speculative, but an association with pregnancy is clear.[219] The syndrome may manifest at any time during pregnancy, but is more common in the last trimester and about the time of delivery. For this reason, it may be difficult initially to distinguish HUS/TTP from pre-eclampsia. Cases have been described in which TTP recurs in subsequent, although not always consecutive, pregnancies. Patients with previous HUS/TTP not associated with pregnancy may or may not relapse when pregnant.

Comprehensive investigation of the cause of pregnancy-associated HUS/TTP has been undertaken in relatively few cases. Von Willebrand protease activity is reduced in the last trimester of normal pregnancy, but not to the very low levels observed in idiopathic TTP.[220] Estrogens cause only a modest reduction in vWFCP. However, in a few cases severely reduced protease activity, with or without an inhibitor, and the presence of ultra-large VWF multimers in plasma have been found.[220-224] There are also cases of pregnancy-associated HUS/TTP in which the protease is clearly normal. Complement activation in this group has not been reported.

HELLP syndrome, consisting of hemolytic anemia, elevated liver enzymes, and low platelets, is also a disorder occurring in the last trimester or at parturition, and patients may have features of pre-eclampsia. The blood film typically has evidence of microangiopathic hemolytic anemia with fragmented red blood cells. Von Willebrand protease activity is reduced in this disorder more than is seen in normal pregnancy, but not to the low levels seen in idiopathic TTP and without ultra-large VWF multimers in plasma.[210] Whether the moderately reduced activity of the protease plays any role in the pathogenesis is unclear. One might predict that pregnancy, and pre-eclampsia in particular, would exacerbate a prothrombotic state and add to the causation of HUS/TTP, perhaps providing a "second hit." Meanwhile the association with pregnancy cannot at present imply causation.[223]

HUS SUPERIMPOSED ON EXISTING DISORDERS: SYSTEMIC LUPUS ERYTHEMATOSUS AND ANTIPHOSPHOLIPID ANTIBODY SYNDROME

The clinical picture of HUS/TTP, systemic lupus erythematosus (SLE), and antiphospholipid antibody syndrome (ALS) may overlap and, if any two of the three conditions coexist in the same patient, the diagnosis may be difficult at the time of initial presentation.

HUS/TTP has been reported in 2% to 3%[225] and 8.4%[226] of SLE patients, with over 50 cases to date. It may manifest at any age, either before or years after SLE has been diagnosed.[225-229] The etiology is unclear. Autoantibodies to ADAMTS13, platelets, and the platelet glycoprotein CD-36 have been described in patients with SLE, and it has been postulated that these antibodies incite endothelial injury and trigger the release of ultra-large von Willebrand factor multimers, culminating in TMA.[225,230] Immunosuppressive and cytotoxic drugs have been used, in conjunction with plasmapheresis, with the objective of suppressing production and increasing clearance of these antibodies, with most patients achieving remission of microangiopathic symptoms. Not all patients need cytotoxics to achieve remission, and some respond very well to plasmapheresis alone.[225,230]

HUS/TTP is a rare complication of ALS. It may be the first clinical manifestation of the syndrome[218] or occur in patients with established primary ALS. The main clinical consequences are systemic hypertension, which is usually severe, variable degrees of proteinuria and renal impairment, and cortical atrophy. Interestingly, in two patients a severe ADAMTS13 deficiency was found due to high titers of autoantibodies.[231] Antiphospholipid antibodies may also have a role in the development of HUS/TTP in patients with SLE, as suggested by findings of anticardiolipin antibodies in four of five patients with coexistent SLE and TTP.

Glomerular capillary thrombosis is the additional renal vascular lesion that occurs mainly among SLE patients with anti-phospholipid antibodies. This causes glomerular sclerosis and leads to renal insufficiency.[232] Steroids and plasma exchange, alone or in combination, are the most common treatment. As shown in a recent meta-analysis,[230] in the cases in which steroids alone were the first treatment used, the clinical status and laboratory abnormalities worsened, whereas recovery occurred in 73% of episodes treated with plasma exchange. Immunosuppressive agents, vincristine, intravenous immunoglobulins, and anticoagulant and antithrombotic agents have also been used, with no clear-cut benefit.[230]

HUS SUPERIMPOSED ON RENAL DISORDERS

A small number of cases appear to develop HUS superimposed on different forms of glomerular diseases. These are often children who are often nephrotic at presentation. De

Chadarevian et al.[232] described a 5-year-old boy with acute glomerulonephritis (AGN) associated with HUS. Renal biopsy displayed features of both disorders, that is, mesangial proliferation and subepithelial humps on the one hand and glomerular thrombi with fibrin deposition on the other hand. A similar patient reported 15 years later was a 14-year-old boy with acute renal failure, severe hypertension, low platelets, and hemolytic anemia with very low haptoglobin levels.[233] Clinical hallmarks of AGN were lacking. Yet, renal biopsy showed marked diffuse glomerular hypercellularity and the presence of immune complexes on either side of the basement membrane without fibrin. Habib et al.[165] reported five patients with severe hypertension who developed a HUS-like picture. The preexisting disorders were idiopathic nephrotic syndrome, reflux nephropathy, Henoch-Schönlein nephritis, congenital nephrotic syndrome, and nail-patella syndrome. All patients were biopsied and severe TMA was found. Further single-case observations include a baby with crescentic membranoproliferative glomerulonephritis,[167] a child with membranous glomerulopathy,[234] and man with IgA nephropathy.[235] HUS and membranoproliferative glomerulonephritis may coincide. Both are associated with alternative pathway complement activation and in a few cases where mutations affecting complement factor H have been identified.

HUS SUPERIMPOSED ON MALIGNANCY

Disseminated metastatic carcinoma, gastric,[236] prostatic,[237] or colon,[238] has been associated with HUS/TTP in adults. No information is currently available for pediatric patients. In a registry established in 1984 at the Lombardi Cancer Research Center, Georgetown University, Washington, D.C., 85 patients met the criteria of hemolysis, thrombocytopenia, and serum creatinine above 1.6 mg/dl.[239] Eighty-nine percent of them had adenocarcinoma, 26% being gastric cancer. HUS/TTP developed before cancer was diagnosed in a third of the patients, giving credence to the primary association. Mortality is high, but several reports ascribe a good outcome from the HUS to the use of plasmapheresis. It should be mentioned that these patients may in addition receive irradiation or drugs associated with HUS/TTP, such as mitomycin, cyclosporin, and others. Infectious complications of cancer may also play a role.[240,241]

HUS SUPERIMPOSED ON BONE MARROW TRANSPLANTATION (STEM CELL TRANSPLANTATION)

HUS and TTP are reported to occur up to several months after bone marrow transplantation. In a review, Moake and Byrnes[242] point out the difficulties in identifying factors that correlate with this complication. For example, total body radiation and cyclophosphamide were used almost universally, making it impossible to determine whether the preconditioning had a pathogenic role. The radiation dose used is less than that associated with radiation nephropathy, but a synergistic effect with cyclophosphamide has been considered. Cyclosporin used in graft versus host disease may independently promote the syndrome. George et al.[243] reviewed data from the Oklahoma registry question on whether the association between BMT and HUS/TTP is causative. They concluded that the association is rare, and that most cases, and all in their series who came to death, had evidence of underlying sepsis. The pathogenesis has not been convincingly shown. VWFcp activity has been found to be decreased in patients undergoing allogeneic BMT, but not to the very low levels associated with idiopathic TTP,[244] and in some the activity is normal. In children, HUS often occurs in patients after allogeneic stem cell transplantation with graft-versus-host disease. Since these patients have a tremendous increase in antibody production against many proteins, it is also possible that in these children, HUS is part of the graft-versus-host reaction. However, information on these patients is scarce. The mortality rate is high despite intensive plasma substitution or plasmapheresis.[245-248]

HUS SUPERIMPOSED ON IONIZING RADIATION

Radiation nephropathy requires radiation doses of more than 2000 rads and presents with hypertension, proteinuria, or renal impairment up to a year after exposure. Cases with superadded microangiopathic hemolytic anemia typical of HUS are rare. Hemolytic anemia, thrombocytopenia, and consumptive disseminated intravascular coagulation are also reported without red cell fragmentation. Some of the cases of apparent radiation-induced HUS also had cancer or received chemotherapy, making it less certain that radiation is the primary cause.

In the kidney, the most sensitive cells to ionizing radiation are those of the glomerular endothelium and tubular epithelium. In radiation nephropathy, electron microscopy shows that glomerular endothelial cells are swollen and separated from the capillary basement membrane by electron-lucent material. The basement membrane becomes split, and some capillaries are denuded of endothelium altogether. A late finding is fibrinoid necrosis and thrombosis of arteries and arterioles. This resembles thrombotic microangiopathy and adds credence to the association. Modern concepts of pathogenesis have not been applied.

FAMILIAL/GENETIC DISORDERS WITH UNKNOWN UNDERLYING DISEASE

It is not surprising that the etiology cannot be identified in most case history reports of familial HUS and TTP where abnormalities of complement regulation or the processing of vWF have not been considered. However, there are also current undiagnosed familial cases extensively investigated for their causes. This suggests that other inherited risk factors will be found in the near future.[84,138,249-260]

UNCLASSIFIABLE HUS

In practice, no obvious clinical associations or causes are found in the majority of childhood patients with HUS presenting without a diarrheal prodrome, or in adults with HUS and TTP. However, in the past these cases were often not fully investigated and even now there are omissions in the diagnostic work-up of patients. As our understanding of HUS improves, this group should decrease.[260-277]

CONCLUSION

In conclusion, HUS is not a benign disease. Even the so-called "classical" D+HUS has substantial long-term morbidity. This is even more true for the atypical forms (Figure 25-10). New strategies are urgently needed for this devastating disease (Figure 25-11). Only interdisciplinary research will allow us to reduce the burden on these children and their parents or caregivers. In addition to the medical support one should not forget the high demand for psychological support for these patients and parent groups. Some international patient groups are devoted to improving conditions of these sick children. However, research is still scarce and surveillance measures for shigatoxin-producing bacteria are not available in many areas of the world. In addition, testing is not carried out according to a standardized procedure. Furthermore, many countries are still struggling with low awareness of this disease. Even in the European Union, research support is inadequate. Consequently, international efforts and financial support should be encouraged for research in this field.

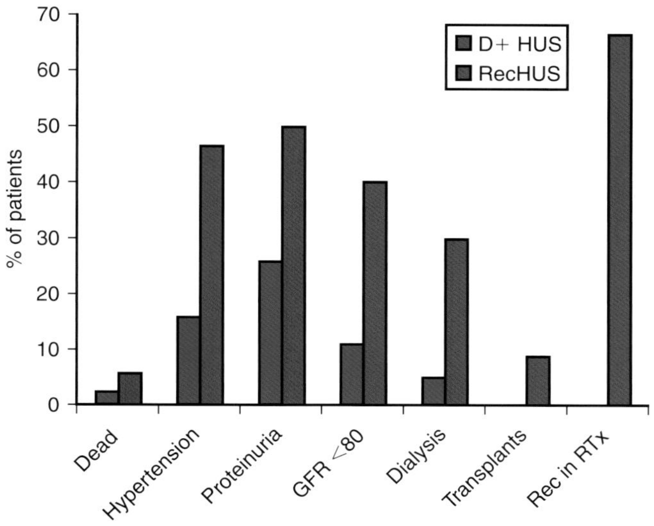

Figure 25-10 Clinical outcome of patients with recurrent form of HUS after 1 year (authors, unpublished data).

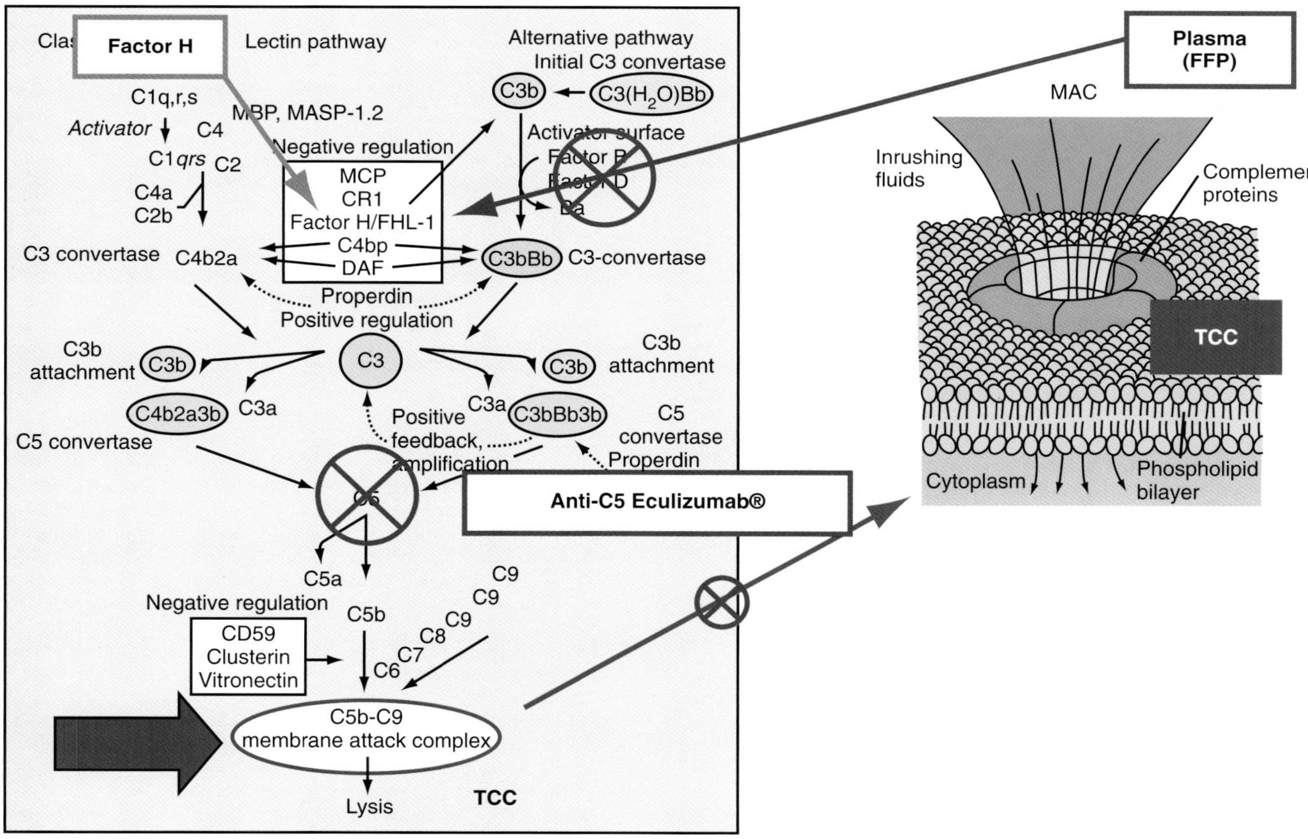

Figure 25-11 Future and present treatment strategies. Schematic drawing of the complement system. Strategies to treat inadequate complement activation. At present only plasma is used to substitute a missing factor. Factor H would substitute the defined missing protein factor H. Eculizumab is an antibody against C5, which inhibits the formation of C5b-9, therefore preventing (theoretically) the damage to renal cells. In addition, inhibition of complement activators like factor B may be beneficial. (Copyright J. Hellwage)

Internet Links

National Institute of Health (NIH): http://kidney.niddk.nih.gov/kudiseases/pubs/childkidneydiseases/hemolytic_uremic_syndrome/

European Society of Paediatric Nephrology: http://espn.cardiff.ac.uk/guidelines.htm: Innsbruck HUS Database: www.hus-net.uki.at

Private homepage on atypical HUS with many links: http://www.atypicalhus.50megs.com/

ACKNOWLEDGMENTS

We wish to thank the European Study Group for Haemolytic Uraemic Syndrome and Related Disorders (HUSNET) for thorough discussion of the subject (present members are C. Loirat, N. von de Kar, C.M. Taylor, N. Besbas, W. Proesmans, D. Karpman, D. Landau, G. Rizzoni, and L.B. Zimmerhackl). Claudia Lenz provided excellent secretarial assistance.

REFERENCES

1. Gasser C, Gautier E, Steck A, et al: Hämolytisch-urämische syndrome: bilaterale nierenrinden nekrosen bei akuten erworbenen hämolytischen anämien, *Schweitz Med Wochenschr* 85:905-909, 1955.
2. Moschcowitz E: An acute febrile pleiochromic anemia with hyalin thrombosis of the terminal arterioles and capillaries. An undescribed disease, *Arch Intern Med* 36:89-93, 1925.
3. Karmali MA, Petric M, Lim C, et al: The association between idiopathic hemolytic uremic syndrome and infection by verotoxin-producing *E. coli*, *J Infect Dis* 151:775-82, 1985.
4. Repetto HA: Epidemic hemolytic uremic syndrome in children, *Kidney Int* 52:1708-119, 1997.
5. Boyce TG, Swerdlow DL, Griffin PM: *Escherichia coli* O157 : H7 and the hemolytic-uremic syndrome, *N Engl J Med* 33:364-68, 1995.
6. Su C, Brandt LJ: *Escherichia coli* 0157 : H7 infection in humans, *Ann Intern Med* 123:698-714, 1995.
7. Besbas N, Karpman D, Landau D, Loirat C, Proesmans C, et al; European Paediatric Working Group for HUS: A classification of hemolytic uremic syndrome and thrombotic thrombocytopenic purpura and related disorders, *Kidney Int* 70:423-31, 2006.
8. Rowe PC, Orrbine E, Wells GA, Yetisir E, et al: Risk of hemolytic uremic syndrome after sporadic *Escherichia coli* O157 : H7 infection: results of a Canadian collaborative study, *J Pediatr* 132:777-82, 1998.
9. BS, Meyers KE, Schulman SL: The pathogenesis and treatment of the hemolytic uremic syndrome, *J Am Soc Nephrol* 9:1126-33, 1998.
10. Gianvita A, Tozzi AE, De Petris, et al: Risk factors for poor prognosis in children with hemolytic uremic syndrome, *Pediatr Nephrol* 18:1229-35, 2003.
11. Brandt JR, Fouser LS, Watkins SL, Zelikovic I, et al: *Escherichia coli* O157 : H7-associated hemolytic-uremic syndrome after ingestion of contaminated hamburgers, *J Pediatr* 125:519-26, 1994.
12. Yamasaki S, Takeda Y: Enterohemorrhagic *Escherichia coli* O157 : H7 episode in Japan with a perspective on vero toxins (Shiga-like toxins), *J Toxicol Toxin Rev* 16:229-40, 1997.
13. Cody SH, Glynn K, Farrar JA, Cairns KL, et al: An outbreak of *Escherichia coli* O157 : H7 infection from unpasteurized commercial apple juice, *Ann Intern Med* 130:202-209, 1999.
14. Parry SM, Salmon RL, Willshaw GA, Cheasty T: Risk factors for and prevention of sporadic infections with verocytotoxin (Shiga toxin) producing *Escherichia coli* O157, *Lancet* 351:1019-22, 1998.
15. Tarr PI, Gordon CA, Chandler WL: Shiga-toxin producing *Escherichia coli* and haemolytic uremic syndrome, *Lancet* 365:1073-86, 2005.
16. Proulz F, Sockett P: Prospective surveillance of Canadian children with the hemolytic uremic syndrome, *Pediatr Nephrol* 20:786-90, 2005.
17. Gerber A, Karch H, Allerberger F, et al: Clinical course and the role of Shiga toxin producing *Escherichia coli* infection in the hemolytic uremic syndrome in pediatric patients, 1997-2000 in Germany and Austria: a prospective study, *J Infect Dis* 186:493-500, 2002.
18. Verweyen HM, Karch H, Allerberger F, Zimmerhackl LB: Enterohemorrhagic *Escherichia coli* (EHEC) in pediatric hemolytic uremic syndrome: a prospective study in Germany and Austria, *Infection* 27:341-47, 1999.
19. Warwicker P, Goodship TJH, Donne RL, Pirson Y, et al: Genetic studies into inherited and sporadic hemolytic syndrome, *Kidney Int* 53:836-44, 1998.
20. Ulinski T, Lervat C, Ranchin, et al: Neonatal hemolytic uremic syndrome after mother to child transmission of *Escherichia coli* O157, *Pediatr Nephrol* 20:1334-35, 2005.
21. Voss E, Paton AW, Manning PA, Paton JC: Molecular analysis of Shiga toxigenic *Escherichia coli* O111:H$^-$ proteins which react with sera from patients with hemolytic uremic syndrome, *Infect Immun* 66:1467-72, 1998.
22. Henning PH, Tham ECB, Martin AA, Beare TH, Jureidinid KF: Hemolytic-uremic syndrome outbreak caused by *Escherichia coli* O111:H$^-$: clinical outcomes, *Med J Aust* 168:552-55, 1998.
23. Hashimoto H, Mizukoshi K, Nishi M, Kawakita T, et al: Epidemic of gastrointestinal tract infection including hemorrhagic colitis attributing to Shiga toxin 1-producing *Escherichia coli* O118:H2 at a junior high school in Japan, *Pediatrics* 103:e2, 1999.
24. Bell BP, Griffin PM, Lozano P, Christie DL, et al: Predictors of hemolytic uremic syndrome in children during a larger outbreak of *Escherichia coli* O157 : H7 infections, *Pediatrics* 100:e12, 1997.
25. Wong CS, Jelacic S, Habeeb RL, Watkins SL, Tarr PI: The risk of hemolytic uremic syndrome after antibiotic treatment of *Escherichia coli* O157 : H7 infections, *N Engl J Med* 342:1930-36, 2000.
26. Safdar N, Said A, Gangnon RE, Maki GD: Risk of hemolytic uremic syndrome after antibiotic treatment of *Escherichia coli* O157 : H7 enteritis: a meta-analysis, *JAMA* 288:996-1001, 2002.
27. Ake JA, Jelacic S, Ciol MA, et al: Relative nephroprotection during *Escherichia coli* O157 : H7 infections: association with intravenous volume expansion, *Pediatrics* 115:673-80, 2005.
28. Andreoli SP, Bergstein JM: Development of insulin-dependent diabetes mellitus during the hemolytic uremic syndrome, *J Pediatr* 100:541-45, 1982.
29. Andreoli SP, Bergstein JM: Acute rhabdomyolysis associated with the hemolytic-uremic syndrome, *J Pediatr* 103:78-80, 1983.
30. Siegler RL: Spectrum of extrarenal involvement in post-diarrhea hemolytic uremic syndrome, *J Pediatr* 125:511-18, 1994.
31. Sebbag H, Lemelle JL, Moller C, Schmitt M: Colonic stenosis after hemolytic uremic syndrome, *Eur J Pediatr Surg* 9:119-20, 1999.
32. Burns JC, Berman ER, Fagre J, et al: Pancreatic islet cell necrosis: association with hemolytic uremic syndrome, *J Pediatr* 100:582-84, 1982.
33. Masumoto K, Nishimoto Y, Taguchi T: Colonic stricture secondary to hemolytic uremic syndrome caused by *Escherichia coli* O-157, *Pediatr Nephrol* 20:1496-99, 2005.
34. Taylor M: Role of oxidants in the pathophysiology of HUS. In Kaplan BS, Trompeter R, Moak J, editors: *The hemolytic uremic syndrome: thrombotic thrombocytopenia purpura*, New York, Marcel Dekker, 1992, pp. 355-73.
35. Brandt JR, Joseph MW, Fouser LS, et al: Cholelithiasis following *Escherichia coli* O157 : H7 associated hemolytic uremic syndrome, *Pediatr Nephrol* 12:222-25, 1998.

36. Grodinsky S, Telmesani A, Robson WLM, et al: Gastrointestinal manifestations of hemolytic uremic syndrome: pancreatitis, *J Pediatr Gastroenterol Nutr* 11:518-24, 1990.
37. Andreoli SP, Bergstein JM: Exocrine and endocrine pancreatic insufficiency and calcinosis following the hemolytic uremic syndrome, *J Pediatr* 110:816-17, 1987.
38. Andreoli SP: Pancreatic involvement in the hemolytic uremic syndrome. In Kaplan BS, Trompeter R, Moake J, editors: *The hemolytic uremic syndrome: thrombotic thrombocytopenia purpura*, New York, 1992, Marcel Dekker, pp. 131-41.
39. Durkan A, Menascu S, Langlois V: Isolated abducens nerve palsy in hemolytic uremic syndrome, *Pediatr Nephrol* 19:915-16, 2004.
40. Askitia V, Hendrickson K, Fish AJ, Braunlin E, Sinaiko AR: Troponin I levels in a hemolytic uremic syndrome patient with severe cardiac failure, *Pediatr Nephrol* 19:345-48, 2004.
41. Inward CD, Howie AJ, Fitzpatrick MM, Rafaat F, et al: Renal histopathology in fatal cases of diarrhea associated hemolytic uremic syndrome, *Pediatr Nephrol* 11:556-59, 1997.
42. Moghal NE, Ferreira MAS, Howie AJ, Milford DV, et al: The late histologic finding in diarrhea associated hemolytic uremic syndrome, *J Pediatr* 133:220-23, 1998.
43. Caletti MG, Gallo G, Gianantonio CA: Development of focal segmental sclerosis and hyalinosis in hemolytic uremic syndrome, *Pediatr Nephrol* 10:687-92, 1996.
44. Turfo A, Arrizurieta EE, Repetto H: Renal functional reserve in children with a previous episode of HUS, *Pediatr Nephrol* 5:184-88, 1991.
45. Siegler RL, Milligan MK, Burningham TH, Christofferson RD, et al: Long-term outcome and prognostic indicator in the hemolytic uremic syndrome, *J Pediatr* 118:195-200, 1991.
46. Gagnadoux MF, Habib R, Gubler MC, Bacri LJ, Broyer M: Long-term (15-25 years) outcome of childhood hemolytic-uremic syndrome, *Clin Nephrol* 46:39-41, 1996.
47. Perelstein EM, Grunfeld BG, Simsolo RB, Gimenez M, Gianantonio CA. Renal functional reserve compared in hemolytic uraemic syndrome and single kidney, *Arch Dis Child* 65:728-31, 1991.
48. Spizzirri FD, Rahman RC, Bibiloni N, Ruscasso JD, Amoreo OR: Childhood hemolytic uremic syndrome in Argentina: long-term follow-up and prognostic features, *Pediatr Nephrol* 11:156-60, 1997.
49. De Petris L, Gianviti A, Giordano U, et al: Blood pressure in the long term follow-up of children with hemolytic uremic syndrome, *Pediatr Nephrol* 19:1241-44, 2004.
50. Garg AX, Suri RS, Barrowman, et al: Long term renal prognosis of diarrhea associated hemolytic uremic syndrome, *JAMA* 290:1360-70, 2003.
51. Caletti MG, Lejarraga H, Kelmansky D, Missoni M: Two different therapeutic regimens in patients with sequelae of hemolytic uremic syndrome, *Pediatr Nephrol* 19:1148-52, 2004.
52. Schlieiper A, Orrbine E, Wells, et al: Neurological sequelae of hemolytic uremic syndrome, *Arch Dis Child* 80:214-20, 1999.
53. Qamar IU, Ohali M, MacGregor DL, et al: Long-term neurological sequelae of hemolytic uremic syndrome: a preliminary report, *Pediatr Nephrol* 10:504-506, 1996.
54. Keusch GT, Acheson DWK: Thrombotic thrombocytopenia purpura associated with Shiga toxins, *Semin Hematol* 34:106-16, 1997.
55. Paton JC, Paton AW: Pathogenesis and diagnosis of Shiga toxin-producing *Escherichia coli* infections, *Clin Microbiol Rev* 11:450-79, 1998.
56. Acheson DWK, Moore R, DeBreuler S: Translocation of Shiga-like toxins across polarized intestinal cells in tissue culture, *Infect Immun* 64:3294-300, 1996.
57. Uchida H, Kiyokawa N, Horie H, Fujimoto J, Takeda T: The detection of Shiga toxins in the kidney of a patient with hemolytic uremic syndrome, *Pediatr Res* 45:133-37, 1999.
58. Siegler RL, Physher TJ, Tesh VL, Taylor FB: Response to single and divided doses of Shiga toxin-1 in a primate model of hemolytic uremic syndrome, *J Am Soc Nephrol* 12:1458-67, 2001.
59. van Setten PA, van Hinsbergh VWM, van der Velden TJAN, van de Kar NCAJ, et al: Effects of TNF-α on verocytotoxin cytotoxicity in purified human glomerular microvascular endothelial cells, *Kidney Int* 51:1245-56, 1997.
60. Pijpers AHJM, Van Setten PA, Van den Heuvel LPWJ, et al: Verocytotoxin induced apoptosis of human microvascular endothelial cells, *J Am Soc Nephrol* 12:767-78, 2001.
61. Kiarash A, Boyd B, Lingwood CA: Glycosphingolipid receptor function is modified by fatty acid content, *J Biol Chem* 269:1138-46, 1994.
62. Sandvig K, Garred O, van Helvoort A, van Meer G, van Deurs B: Importance of glycolipid synthesis for butyric acid induced sensitization to Shiga toxin and intracellular sorting of toxin in A431 cells, *Mol Biol Cell* 7:1391-404, 1996.
63. Arab S, Lingwood CA: Intracellular targeting of the endoplasmic reticulum/nuclear envelope by retrograde transport may determine cell hypersensitivity to verotoxin via globotriosyl ceramide fatty acid isoform traffic, *J Cell Physiol* 117:646-60, 1998.
64. Bitzan MM, Wang Y, Lin J, Marsden PA: Verotoxin and ricin have novel effects on preproendothelin-1 expression but fail to modify nitric oxide synthase (ecNOS) expression and NO production in vascular endothelium, *J Clin Invest* 101:372-82, 1998.
65. Andreoli SP: The pathophysiology of the hemolytic uremic syndrome, *Curr Opin Nephrol Hypertens* 8:459-64, 1999.
66. Simon M, Learly TG, Hernandez JD, Abboud HA. Shiga toxin 1 elicits diverse biological response in mesangial cells, *Kidney Int* 54:1117-27, 1998.
67. Van Setten PA, Van Hinsbergh VWM, Van den Heuvel LPWJ, Van der Velden TJAN, et al: Verocytotoxin inhibits mitogenesis and protein synthesis in purified human glomerular mesangial cells without affecting cell viability: evidence for two distinct mechanisms, *J Am Soc Nephrol* 8:1877-88, 1997.
68. Hughes AK, Sticklett PK, Kohan DE: Cytotoxic effect of Shiga toxin-1 on human proximal tubular epithelial cells, *Kidney Int* 54:426-37, 1998.
69. Hughes AK, Stricklett PK, Kohan DE: Shiga toxin-1 regulation of cytokine production by human proximal tubule cells, *Kidney Int* 54:1093-106, 1998.
70. Taghchi T, Uchida H, Kiyokawa N, Mori T, et al: Verotoxins induce apoptosis in human renal tubular epithelium derived cells, *Kidney Int* 53:1681-88, 1998.
71. Hughes AK, Stricklett PK, Schmid D, Kohan DE: Cytotoxic effect of Shiga-toxin on human glomerular epithelial cells, *Kidney Int* 57:2350-59, 2000.
72. Karpman D, Hakansson A, Perez MT, Isaksson C, et al: Apoptosis of renal cortical cells in the hemolytic uremic syndrome: in vivo and in vitro studies, *Infect Immun* 66:636-44, 1998.
73. Van Setten PA, van Hinsbergh VWM, van den Heuvel LPWJ, Preyers F, et al: Monocytes chemoattractant protein-1 and interleukin-8 levels in urine and serum of patients with hemolytic uremic syndrome, *Pediatr Res* 43:759-67, 1998.
74. Fitzpatrick MM, Shah V, Trompeter RS, Dillon MJ, Barratt TM: Interleukin-8 and polymorphonuclear leukocyte activation in hemolytic uremic syndrome of childhood, *Kidney Int* 42:951-56, 1992.
75. Walters MDS, Matthei IU, Kay R, Dillon MJ, Barratt TM. The polymorphonuclear leukocyte count in childhood hemolytic uraemic syndrome, *Pediatr Nephrol* 3:130-34, 1989.
76. Morigi M, Micheletti G, Figliuzzi M, Imberti B, et al. Verotoxin-1 promotes leukocyte adhesion to cultured endothelial cells under physiologic flow conditions, *Blood* 86:4553-58, 1995.
77. Harel Y, Silva M, Giroir B, Weinberg A, et al: A reporter transgene indicates renal specific induction of tumor necrosis factor (TNF) by Shiga-like toxin, *J Clin Invest* 92:2110-16, 1993.
78. Yuhas H, Kaminsky E, Mor M, Ashkenazi S: Induction of nitric oxide production in mouse macrophages by Shiga toxin, *J Med Microbiol* 45:97-102, 1996.
79. Inward CD, Varagunam M, Milford DV, Taylor CM: Cytokines in hemolytic uremic syndrome associated with verocytotoxin-producing *Escherichia coli* infection, *Arch Dis Child* 77:145-47, 1997.
80. Sakiri R, Ramegowda B, Tesh TL: Shiga toxin type 1 activates tumor necrosis factor-α gene transcription and nuclear translocation of the transcriptional activators nuclear factor κB and activator protein-1, *Blood* 92:558-66, 1998.
81. Fernandez GC, Gómez SA, Rubel CJ, et al: Impaired neutrophils in children with the typical form of hemolytic uremic syndrome, *Pediatr Nephrol* 20:1306-14, 2005.

82. Trachtman H, Christen E, Cnaan A, et al: Urinary neutrophil gelatinase-associated lipocalcin in D+HUS: a novel marker of renal injury, *Pediatr Nephrol* 21:989-94, 2006.
83. Maroeska D, te Loo WM, Monnens LAH, et al: Binding and transfer of veroytotoxin by polymorphonuclear leukocytes in hemolytic uremic syndrome, *Blood* 95:3396-402, 2000.
84. Exeni RA, Fernandes GC, Palermo MS: Role of polymorphonuclear leukocytes in the pathophysiology of typical hemolytic uremic syndrome, *Scientific World J* 7:1155-64, 2007.
85. Kamitsuji H, Nonaami K, Ishikawa N, et al: Elevated tissue factor circulating levels in children with hemolytic uremic syndrome caused by verotoxin producing E. coli, *Clin Nephrol* 53:319-24, 2000.
86. Fernandez GC, Te Loo MW, van der Velden TJA, et al: Decrease of thrombomodulin contributes to the procoagulant state of the endothelium in hemolytic uremic syndrome, *Pediatr Nephrol* 18:1066-68, 2003.
87. Siegler R, Oakes R: Hemolytic uremic syndromepathogenesis, treatment, and outcome, *Curr Opin Pediatr* 17:200-04, 2005.
88. Molbak K, Mead PS, Griffin PM: Antimicrobial therapy in patients with *Escherichia coli* O157 : H7 infection, *JAMA* 288:1014-16, 2002.
89. Grif K, Kierich MP, Karch H, Allerberger F: Strain-specific differences in the amount of Shiga toxin released from enterohemorrhagic *Escherichia coli* O157 following exposure to subinhibitory concentrations of antimicrobial agents, *Eur J Clin Microbiol Infect Dis* 17:761-66, 1998.
90. Zimmerhackl LB: *E. coli*, antibiotics, and the hemolytic-uremic syndrome, *N Engl J Med* 342(26):1990-91, 2000.
91. Rizzoni G, Claris-Appaini A, Edefonti A, et al: Plasma infusion for hemolytic uremic syndrome in children: results of a multicenter controlled trial, *J Pediatr* 112:284-90, 1988.
92. Heerze LD, Kelm MA, Talbot JA, Armstrong GD: Oligosaccharide sequences attached to an inert support (SYNSORB) as potential therapy for antibiotic associated diarrhea and pseudomembranous colitis, *J Infect Dis* 169:1291-96, 1994.
93. Armstrong GD, Fodor E, Vanmaele R: Investigation of Shiga-like toxin binding to chemically synthesized oligosaccharide sequences, *J Infect Dis* 164:1160-70, 1991.
94. Kitov PI, Sadowska JM, George M, Armstrong GD, et al: Shiga like toxins are neutralized by tailored multivalent carbohydrate ligands, *Nature* 403:669-72, 2000.
95. Mulvey GL, Marcato P, Kitov PE, et al: Assessment in mice of the therapeutic potential of tailored, multivalent Shiga toxin carbohydrate ligands, *J Infect Dis* 187:640-49, 2003.
96. Mukherjee J, Chios K, Fishwild D, et al: Human Stx2 specific monoclonal antibodies prevent systemic complications of *Escherichia coli* O157 : H7 infection, *Infect Immun* 70:612-19, 2002.
97. Sheoran AS, Chapman-Bonofiglio S, Harvey BR, et al: Human antibody against Shiga toxin 2 administered to piglets after the onset of diarrhea due to *Escherichia coli* O157 : H7 prevents fatal systemic complications, *Infect Immun* 73:4607-13, 2005.
98. Wen SX, Teel LD, Judge NA, O'Brien AD: A plant based oral vaccine to protect against systemic intoxication by Shiga toxin type 2, *Proc Natl Acad Sci U S A* 103:7082-87, 2006.
99. Cabreba GR, Fortenberry JD, Warshaw BL, et al: Hemolytic-uremic syndrome associated with invasive *Streptococcus pneumoniae* infection, *Pediatrics* 101:699-703, 1998.
100. Nathanson S, Deschenes G: Prognosis of *Streptococcus pneumoniae* induced hemolytic uremic syndrome, *Pediatr Nephrol* 16:362-65, 2001.
101. Proulz F, Liet JM, Michele D, et al: Hemolytic uremic syndrome associated with invasive *Streptococcus* infection, *Pediatrics* 105:462-63, 2000.
102. Brandt J, Wong C, Mihm S, et al: Invasive pneumococcal disease and hemolytic uremic syndrome, *Pediatrics* 110:371-75, 2002.
103. Cochran JB, Panzarino VM, Maes LY, Tecklenburg FW: *Pneumococcus*-induced T-antigen activation in hemolytic uremic syndrome, *Pediatr Nephrol* 19:317-21, 2004.
104. Raghupathy P, Date A, Shastry JCM, et al: Hemolytic uremic syndrome complicating *Shigella* dysentery in south Indiana children, *BMJ* 1:1518-21, 1978.
105. Butler T, Islam MR, Azad MAK, Jones PK: Risk factors for development of hemolytic uremic syndrome during shigellosis, *J Pediatr* 110:894-97, 1987.
106. Bhimma R, Rollins NC, Coovadia HM, Adhikari M: Post-dysenteric hemolytic uremic syndrome in children during an epidemic of *Shigella* dysentery in Kwazulu/Natal, *Pediatr Nephrol* 11:560-64, 1997.
107. Houdouin V, Doit C, Mariana P, et al: A pediatric cluster of *Shigella dysenteriae* serotype 1 diarrhea with hemolytic uremic syndrome in 2 families from France, *Clin Infect Dis* 38:96-99, 2004.
108. Cabagnaro F, Guzman C, Harris P: Hemolytic uremic syndrome associated with *Entamoeba histolytica* intestinal infection, *Pediatr Nephrol* 21:126-28, 2006.
109. Turner ME, Kher K, Rakusan T, et al: Atypical HUS in human immunodeficiency virus 1 infected children. *Pediatr Nephrol* 11:161-63, 1997.
110. Ucar A, Fernandez HF, Byrnes JJ, et al: Thrombotic microangiopathy and retroviral infections: a 13-year experience, *Am J Hematol* 45:304-09, 1994.
111. Ray PE, Liu XH, Xu L, Rakusan T: Basic fibroblast growth factor in HIV associated hemolytic uremic syndrome, *Pediatr Nephrol* 13:586-93, 1999.
112. Liu XHH, Aigner A, Wellstein A, Ray PE: Up-regulation of a fibroblast growth factor binding proteins in children with renal diseases, *Kidney Int* 59:1717-28, 2001.
113. Ray PE, Tassi E, Liu XH, Wellstein A: Role of fibroblast growth factor binding protein in the pathogenesis of HIV associated hemolytic uremic syndrome, *Am J Physiol* 290:R105-13, 2006.
114. Symmers WSTC: Thrombotic microangiopathic haemolytic anaemia (thrombotic microangiopathy), *BMJ* 2:897-903, 1952.
115. Habib R: Pathology of the hemolytic uremic syndrome. In Kaplan B, Trompeter R, Moake J, editors: *Hemolytic uremic syndrome and thrombotic thrombocytopenic purpura*. New York, 1992, Marcel Dekker, pp. 315-53.
116. Tschape H, Prager R, Strekel W,, et al: Verotoxigenic *Citrobacter freundii* associated with severe gastroenteritis and cases of haemolytic uraemic syndrome in a nursery school: green butter as the infection source, *Epidemiol Infect* 114:441-50, 1995.
117. Griffin P, Tauxe R: The epidemiology of infections caused by *Escherichia coli* O157 : H7, other enterohemorrhagic *E. coli*, and the associated hemolytic uremic syndrome, *Epidemiol Rev* 13:60-98, 1991.
118. Rowe PC, Orrbine E, Wells GA, et al: Epidemiology of hemolytic-uremic syndrome in Canadian children from 1986 to 1988. The Canadian Pediatric Kidney Disease Reference Centre, *J Pediatr* 119:218-24, 1991.
119. Milford D, Taylor CM, Guttridge B, et al: Haemolytic uraemic syndromes in the British Isles 1985-8: association with verocytotoxin-producing *Escherichia coli*. Part 1: clinical and epidemiological aspects, *Arch Dis Child* 65:716-21, 1990.
120. Decludt B, Bouvet P, Mariani-Kurkdjian P, et al: Haemolytic uraemic syndrome and Shiga toxin-producing *Escherichia coli* infection in children in France. The Societe de Nephrologie Pediatrique, *Epidemiol Infect* 124:215-20, 2000.
121. Elliot EJ, Robins-Browne RM, O'Loughlin EV, et al: Nationwide study of haemolytic uraemic syndrome: clinical, microbiological and epidemiological features, *Arch Dis Child* 85:125-31, 2001.
122. Friedrich AW, Bielaszewska M, Zhang WL, et al: *Escherichia coli* harboring Shiga toxin 2 gene variants: frequency and association with clinical symptoms, *J Infect Dis* 185:74-84, 2002.
123. Beutin L, Krause G, Zimmerman S, et al: Characterization of Shiga toxin-producing *Escherichia coli* strains isolated from human patients in Germany over a 3-year period, *J Clin Microbiol* 42:1099-108, 2004.
124. Lynn R, O'Brien SJ, Taylor CM, et al: Childhood hemolytic uremic syndrome, United Kingdom and Ireland, *Emerg Infect Dis* 11:590-96, 2005.
125. Lopez EL, Diaz M, Grinstein S, et al: Hemolytic uremic syndrome and diarrhea in Argentine children: role of Shiga-like toxins, *J Infect Dis* 160:469-75, 1989.
126. Chandler W, Jelacic S, Boster D, et al: Prothrombotic coagulation abnormalities preceding the hemolytic-uremic syndrome, *N Engl J Med* 346:23-32, 2002.

127. Richardson S, Karmali M, Becker L, et al: The histopathology of the hemolytic uremic syndrome associated with verocytotoxin-producing *Escherichia coli* infections, *Hum PatholHum Pathol* 19:1102-108, 1988.
128. de Loos F, Huijben KMLC, van der Kar NCAJ, Monnens LAH, et al: Hemolytic uremic syndrome attributable to *Streptococcus pneumoniae* infection: a novel cause of secondary protein N-glycan abnormalities, *Clin Chem* 48:781-85, 2005.
129. Klein PJ, Bulla M, Newman RA, Muller P, Uhlenbruck G, et al: Thomsen-Friedenreich antigen in haemolytic uraemic syndrome, *Lancet* 2:1024-25, 1977.
130. Eder A, Manno C: Does red-cell T activation matter? *Br J Haematol* 114:25-30, 2001.
131. Strauss J, Abitbol C, Zilleruelo G, Montane B: HIV nephropathy. In Barratt TM, Avner ED, Harmon WE, editors: *Pediatric Nephrology*, ed 4, Baltimore, 1999, Lippincott, Williams and Wilkin, pp. 1103-107.
132. Badesha PS, Saklayen MG: Hemolytic uremic syndrome as a presenting form of HIV infection, *Nephron* 72:472-75, 1996.
133. Peraldi MN, Maslo C, Akposso K, Mougenot B, et al: Acute renal failure in the course of HIV infection: a single institution retrospective study of ninety-two patients and sixty renal biopsies, *Nephrol Dial Transplant* 14: 1578-85, 1999.
134. Ray PE, Rakusan T, Loechelt BJ, Selby DM, et al: Human immunodeficiency virus (HIV) associated nephropathy in children from the Washington, DC, area: 12 years' experience, *Semin Nephrol* 18:396-405, 1998.
135. Sahud MA, Claster S, Liu L, Ero M, et al: Von Willebrand factor cleaving protease inhibitor in a patients with human immunodeficiency syndrome associated thrombotic thrombocytopenic purpura, *Br J Haematol* 116:909-11, 2002.
136. Segerer S, Eitner F, Cui Y, Hudkins KL, Alpers CE: Cellular injury associated with renal thrombotic microangiopathy in human immunodeficiency virus-infected macaques, *J Am Soc Nephrol* 13:370-78, 2002.
137. Zipfel PF, Jokiranta TS, Hellwage J, Koistinen V, Meri S: The factor H protein family, *Immunopharmacology* 42:53-60, 1999.
138. Esparza-Gordillo J, Goicoechea de Jorge E, Abarrategui Garrido C, Carreras L, López-Trascasa M, et al: Insights into haemolytic uremic syndrome: segregation of three independent predisposition factors in a large, multiple affected pedigree, *Mol Immunol* 43:1769-75, 2006.
139. Kondo C, Mizuno M, Nishikawa K, Yusawa Y, et al: The role of C5a in the development of thrombotic glomerulonephritis in rats, *Clin Exp Immunol* 124:323-29, 2001.
140. Nangaku M, Alpers CE, Pippin J, Shankland SJ, et al: CD59 protects glomerular endothelial cells from immune-mediated thrombotic microangiopathy in rats, *J Am Soc Nephrol* 9:590-97, 1998.
141. Pangburn MK: Host recognition and target differentiation by factor H, a regulator of the alternative pathway of complement, *Immunopharmacology* 49:149-51, 2000.
142. Hellwage J, Jokiranta TS, Friese MA, Wolk TU, et al: Complement C3b/C3d and cell surface polyanions are recognised by overlapping binding sites on the most carboxyl-terminal domain of complement factor H, *J Immunol* 169:6935-44, 2002.
143. Manuellian T, Hellwage J, Meri S, Caprioli J, et al: Mutations in factor H reduce binding affinity to C3b and heparin and surface attachment to endothelial cells in haemolytic uremic syndrome, *J Immunol* 169:6935-44, 2002.
144. Vaziri-Sani F, Hellwage J, Zipfel PF, Sjoholm AG, et al: Factor H binds to washed human platelets, *J Thromb Haemostas* 2:1-9, 2004.
145. Rougier N, Kazatchkine MD, Rougier J-P, Fremeaux-Bacchi V, et al: Human complement factor H deficiency associated with hemolytic uremic syndrome, *J Am Soc Nephrol* 9:2318-26, 1998.
146. Pangburn MK: Localisation of the host recognition functions of complement factor H at the carboxyl terminal: implications for hemolytic uremic syndrome, *J Immunol* 169:4702-706, 2002.
147. Sanchez-Corral P, Gonzales-Rubio C, Rodrigues de Cordoba S, Lopez-Trascasa M: Functional analysis in serum from atypical hemolytic uremic syndrome patients reveals impaired protection of host cells associated with mutations in factor H, *Mol Immunol* 41:81-84, 2004.
148. Sanchez-Corral P, Perez-Caballero D, Huarte O, Simckes AM, et al: Structural and functional characterization of factor H mutations associated with atypical hemolytic uremic syndrome, *Am J Hum Genet* 71:1285-95, 2002.
149. Ault BH, Schmidt BZ, Fowler NL, et al: Human factor H deficiency. Mutations in framework cysteine residues and block in H protein secretion and intracellular catabolism, *J Biol Chem* 272:25168-75, 1997.
150. Caprioli J, Castelletti F, Bucchioni S, et al: Complement factor H mutations and gene polymorphisms in haemolytic uraemic syndrome: theC-257T, the A2089G and the G2881T polymorphisms are strongly associated with the disease, *Hum Mol Genet* 15:3385-95, 2003.
151. Esparza-Gordillo J, Goicoechea de Jorge E, Buil A, et al: Predisposition to atypical haemolytic uremic syndrome involves the concurrence of different susceptibility alleles in the regulators of complement activation gene cluster in 1q32, *Hum Mol Genet* 14:703-12, 2005.
152. Landau D, Shalev H, Levy-Finer G, et al: Familial haemolytic uremic syndrome associated with complement factor H deficiency, *J Pediatr* 138:12-17, 2001.
153. Ault BH. Factor H and the pathogenesis of renal disease, *Pediatr Nephrol* 14:1045-53, 2000.
154. Loirat C, Niaudet P. The risk of recurrent haemolytic uremic syndrome after renal transplantation in children, *Pediatr Nephrol* 18:1095-101, 2003.
155. Fremeaux-Bacchi V, Dragon-Durey MA, Blouin J, Vigneau C, et al: Complement factor I: the susceptibility gene for atypical haemolytic uraemic syndrome, *J Med Genet* 41:e84, 2004.
156. Zimmerhackl LB, Scheiring J, Prufer F, Taylor CM, Loirat C: Renal transplantation in HUS patients with disorders of complement regulation, *Pediatr Nephrol.* 22:10-16, 2007.
157. Kavanagh DM, Kemp EJ, Mayland E, Winney RJ, et al: Mutations in complement factor I predispose to development of atypical haemolytic uremic syndrome, *J Am Soc Nephrol* 16:2150-55, 2005.
158. Richards A, Kemp EJ, Liszewski MK, Goodship JA, et al. Mutations in human complement regulator, membrane cofactor protein (CD46), predisposes to development of familial hemolytic uremic syndrome, *Proc Natl Acad Sci USA* 100:12966-71, 2003.
159. Noris M, Brioschi S, Caprioli J, Todeschini M, et al: International registry of recurrence and familial HUS/TTP. Familial hemolytic uremic syndrome and an MCP mutation, *Lancet* 362:1542-47, 2003.
160. Noris M, Ruggenenti P, Perna A, Orisio S, et al: Hypocomplementemia discloses genetic predisposition to hemolytic uremic syndrome and thrombotic thrombocytopenic purpura: role of factor H abnormalities, *J Am Soc Nephrol* 10:281-93, 1999.
161. Prufer F, Scheiring J, Sautter S, Jensen DB, et al: Terminal complement complex (C5b-9) in children with recurrent hemolytic uremic syndrome, *Semin Thromb Hemost* 32(2):121-27, 2006.
162. Zimmerhackl LB, Besbas N, Jungraithmayr T, van de Kar N, et al: European Study Group for Haemolytic Uraemic Syndromes and Related Disorders. Epidemiology, clinical presentation, and pathophysiology of atypical and recurrent hemolytic uremic syndrome, *Semin Thromb Hemost* 32(2):113-20, 2006.
163. Fremeaux-Bacchi V, Kemp EJ, Goodship JA, et al: The development of atypical HUS is influenced by susceptibility factors in factor H and membrane cofactor protein—evidence from two independent cohorts, *J Med Genet* 42(11):852-56, 2005.
164. Moake JL: Thrombotic microangiopathies, *N Engl J Med* 347 (8):589-600, 2002.
165. Habib R: Pathology of the hemolytic uremic syndrome. In Kaplan BS, Trompeter R, Moak J, editors: *The hemolytic uremic syndrome: thrombotic thrombocytopenia purpura*, New York, Marcel Dekker, 1992, pp. 341-42.
166. Tsai HM: Advances in the pathogenesis, diagnosis, and treatment of thrombotic thrombocytopenic purpura, *J Am Soc Nephrol* 14:1072-81, 2003.
167. Siegler RL, Brewer ED, Pysher J: Hemolytic uremic syndrome associated with glomerular disease, *Am J Kidney Dis* 13:144-47, 1989.

167a. O'Shaughnessy DF, Atterbury C, Bolton Maggs P, Murphy M, et al: Guidelines for the use of fresh-frozen plasma, cryoprecipitate and cryosupernatant, *Br J Haematol* 126(1):11-28, 2004.
168. Perez N, Spizzirri F, Rahman R, Suarez A, et al: Steroids in the hemolytic uremic syndrome, *Pediatr Nephrol* 12:101-104, 1998.
169. Dragon-Durey M-A, Loirat C, Cloarec S, Macher M-A, et al: Anti-factor H autoantibodies associated with atypical haemolytic uremic syndrome, *J Am Soc Nephrol* 16:555-63, 2005.
170. Moake JL, Byrnes CK, Troll JH, Weinstein MJ, Colannini NM, Azocar J, et al: Unusually large plasma factor VIII:von Willebrand factor multimers in chronic relapsing thrombotic thrombocytopenic purpura, *N Engl J Med* 307:1432-35, 1982.
171. Moake JL, Byrnes JJ, Troll JH, Rudy CK, et al: Abnormal VIII: von Willebrand factor pattern in the plasma of patients with the haemolytic uremic syndrome, *Blood* 64:592-98, 1984.
172. Furlan M, Robles R, Solenthaler M, Wassmer M, et al: Deficient activity of von Willebrand factor-cleaving protease in chronic relapsing thrombotic thrombocytopenic purpura, *Blood* 89:3097-103, 1997.
173. Furlan MF, Robles R, Galbusera M, Remuzzi G, et al: Von Willebrand factor–cleaving protease in thrombotic thrombocytopenic purpura and the hemolytic uremic syndrome, *N Engl J Med* 339:1578-84, 1998.
174. Tsai H-M, Chun-Yet Lain E: Antibodies to von Willebrand factor-cleaving protease in acute thrombotic thrombocytopenic purpura, *N Engl J Med* 338:1585-94, 1998.
175. Mannucci PM, Canciani MT, Forza I, Lussana F, et al: Changes in health and disease of the metalloprotease that cleaves von Willebrand factor, *Blood* 98:2730-35, 2001.
176. Fujikawa K, Suzuki H, McMullen B, Chung D: Purification of human von Willebrand factor-cleaving protease and its identification as a new member of the metalloproteinase family, *Blood* 98:1662-66, 2001.
177. Gerritsen HE, Robles R, Lämmle B, Furlan M: Partial amino acid sequence of purified von Willebrand factor–cleaving protease, *Blood* 98:1654-61, 2001.
178. Levy GC, Nichols WC, Lian EC, Foroud T, et al: Mutations in a member of the *ADAMTS* gene family cause thrombotic thrombocytopenic purpura, *Nature* 413:488-94, 2001.
179. Kokame K, Matsumoto M, Soejima K, Yagi H, et al: Mutations and common polymorphisms in ADAMTS13 gene responsible for von Willebrand factor-cleaving protease activity, *Proc Natl Acad Sci U S A* 99:11902-907, 2002.
180. Assink K, Schiphorst R, Allford S, Karpman D, et al: Mutation analysis and clinical implications of von Willebrand factor-cleaving protease deficiency, *Kidney Int* 63:1995-99, 2003.
181. Schneppenheim R, Budde U, Oyen F, Angerhaus D, et al: Von Willebrand factor cleaving protease and ADAMTS13 mutations in childhood TTP, *Blood* 101:1845-50, 2003.
182. Zheng X, Chung D, Takayama TK, Majerus EM, et al: Structure of von Willebrand factor-cleaving protease (ADAMTS13), a metalloprotease involved in thrombotic thrombocytopenic purpura, *J Biol Chem* 276:41059-63, 2001.
183. Soejima K, Mimura N, Hirashima M, Maeda H, et al: A novel human metalloprotease synthesized in the liver and secreted into the blood: possibly, the von Willebrand factor-cleaving protease? *J Biochem* 130:475-80, 2001.
184. Uemara M, Tatsumi K, Matsumoto M, Fujimoto M, et al: Localization of ADAMTS13 to the stellate cells of human liver, *Blood* 106:922-24, 2005.
185. Furlan M, Robles R, Morselli B, Sandoz P, Lämmle B: Recovery and half life of von Willebrand factor–cleaving-protease after plasmatherapy in patients with thrombotic thrombocytopenic purpura, *Thromb Haemost* 81:8-13, 1999.
186. Jubinsly PT, Moraille R, Tsai HM: Thrombotic thrombocytopenic purpura in a newborn, *J Perinatol* 23(1):85-87, 2003.
187. George JN, Sadler JE, Lämmle B: Platelets: thrombotic thrombocytopenic purpura, *Hematology* 1:315-42, 2002.
188. Tripodi A, Chantarangkul V, Bohm M, Budde U, et al: Measurements of von Willebrand factor cleaving protease (ADAMTS13): results of an international collaborative study involving 11 methods testing the same set of coded plasmas, *J Thromb Haemostas* 2:1601-609, 2004.
189. Zheng X, Pallera AM, Goodnough LT, Sadler JE, Blinder MA: Remission of chronic thrombotic thrombocytopenic purpura after treatment with cyclophosphamide and rituximab, *Ann Intern Med* 138:105-108, 2003.
190. Fakhouri F, Vernant JP, Veyradier A, Wolf M, et al: Efficiency of curative and prophylactic treatment with rituximab in ADAMTS13-deficient thrombotic thrombocytopenic purpura: a study of 11 cases, *Blood* 106:1932-37, 2005.
191. Rock GA, Shumak KH, Buskard NA, Blanchette VS, et al: Comparison of plasma exchange with plasma infusion in the treatment of thrombotic thrombocytopenic purpura. A Canadian apheresis study group, *N Engl J Med* 325:393-97, 1991.
192. Baumgartner ER, Wick H, Maurer R, Egli F, Steinmann B: Congenital defect in intracellular cobalamin metabolism resulting in homocystinuria and methylmalonic aciduria, a case report and histopathology. *Helv Paediatr Acta* 34:465-82, 1979.
193. Russo PA, Doyon J, Sonsino E, Ogier H, Saudubray JM: Thrombotic thrombocytopenic purpura. In Kaplan BS, Trompeter R, Moae J, editors: *The hemolytic uremic syndrome,* New York, Marcel Dekker, 1992, pp. 255-70.
194. Geraghty MT, Perlman EJ, Martin LS, Hayflick SJ, et al: Cobalamin C defect associated with hemolytic-uremic syndrome, *J Pediatr* 120:934-37, 1992.
195. Labrune P, Zittoun J, Duvaltier I, Trioche P, et al: Haemolytic uraemic syndrome and pulmonary hypertension in a patient with methionine synthase deficiency, *Eur J Pediatr* 158:734-39, 1999.
196. Brunelli SM, Meyers KEC, Guttenberg M, Kaplan P, Kaplan BS. Cobalamin C deficiency complicated by an atypical glomerulopathy, *Pediatr Nephrol* 17:800-803, 2002.
197. Van Hove JLK, Van Damme Lombaerts R, Grünewald S, Peters H, et al: Cobalamin disorder Cbl-C presenting with late-onset thrombotic microangiopathy, *Am J Med Genet* 111:195-201, 2002.
198. Crocker J, Jones EL: Haemolytic-uraemic syndrome complicating long-term mitomycin C and 5-fluorouracil therapy for gastric carcinoma, *J Clin Pathol* 36:24-29, 1983.
199. Lyman NW, Michaelson R, Viscuso RL, et al: Successful treatment with corticosteroids and intense plasma exchange, *Arch Intern Med* 143:1617-18, 1983.
200. Teixeira L, Debourdeau P, Zammit C, et al: [Gemcitabine-induced thrombotic microangiopathy], *Presse Méd* 31:740-42, 2002.
201. Cattell V: Mitomycin-induced hemolytic uremic kidney. An experimental model in the rat, *Am J Pathol* 121:88-95, 1985.
202. Bennett CL, Weinberg PD, Rozenberg-Ben-Dror, et al: Thrombotic thrombocytopenic purpura associated with ticlopidine. A review of 60 cases, *Ann Intern Med* 128:541-44, 1998.
203. Bennett CL, Davidson CJ, Raisch DW, et al: Thrombotic thrombocytopenic purpura associated with ticlopidine in the setting of coronary artery stents and stroke prevention, *Ann Intern Med* 159:2524-28, 1999.
204. Tsai HM, Rice L, Sarode R, et al: Antibody inhibitors to von Willebrand factor metalloproteinase and increased binding of von Willebrand factor to platelets in ticlopidine-associated thrombotic thrombocytopenic purpura, *Ann Intern Med* 132:7984-89, 2000.
205. Bennet CL, Connors JM, Carwile JM, et al: Thrombotic thrombocytopenic purpura associated with clopidogrel, *N Engl J Med* 342:1773-77, 2000.
206. Gottschall JL, Neahring B, MacFarland JG, et al: Quinine-induced immune thrombocytopenia with haemolytic uremic syndrome: clinical and serological findings in nine patients and review of literature, *Am J Hematol* 47:283-89, 1994.
207. Aster RH: Quinine sensitivity. A new cause of the haemolytic uremic syndrome, *Ann Intern Med* 119:243-44, 1993.
208. Kojouri K, Vesely SK, George JN: Quinine-associated thrombotic thrombocytopenic purpura-hemolytic uremic syndrome: frequency, clinical features and long-term outcomes, *Ann Intern Med* 135:1047-51, 2001.
209. Stroncek DF, Vercellotti GM, Hammerschmidt DE, et al: Characterization of multiple quinine-dependent antibodies in a patient with episodic haemolytic uremic syndrome and immune agranulocytosis, *Blood* 80:241-48, 1992.
210. Glynne P, Salama A, Chaudhry A, et al: Quinine-induced immune thrombocytopenic purpura followed by hemolytic uremic syndrome, *Am J Kidney Dis* 33:133-37, 1999.

211. Bonser RS, Adu D, Franklin I, McMaster P: Cyclosporin-induced haemolytic uraemic syndrome in liver allograft recipient, *Lancet* 2 (8415):1337, 1984.
212. Van Buren D, Van Buren CT, Flechner SM, et al: De novo hemolytic uremic syndrome in renal transplant recipients immunosuppressed with cyclosporine, *Surgery* 98:54-62, 1985.
213. Young BA, Marsh CL, Alpers CE, Davis CL: Cyclosporine-associated thrombotic microangiopathy/hemolytic uremic syndrome following kidney and kidney-pancreas transplantation, *Am J Kidney Dis* 28:561-71, 1996.
214. Zarifian A, Meleg-Smith S, O'Donovan R, Tesi RJ, Batuman V: Cyclosporine-associated thrombotic microangiopathy in renal allografts, *Kidney Int* 55:2457-66, 1999.
215. Trimarchi HN, Truong LD, Brennan S, Gonzalez JM, Suki WN: FK506-associated thrombotic microangiopathy. Report of two cases and review of the literature, *Transplantation* 67:539-44, 1999.
216. Burke GAA, McGraw ME, MacIver AG: The role of early renal biopsy in cyclosporin induced thrombotic microangiopathy, *Pediatr Nephrol* 13:564-66, 1999.
217. Reynolds JC, Agodoa LY, Yuan CM, Abbott KC: Thrombotic microangiopathy after renal transplantation in the United States, *Am J Kidney Dis* 42:1058-68, 2003.
218. Tarr PI, Gordon CA, Chandler WL: Shiga-toxin-producing *Escherichia coli* and haemolytic uraemic syndrome, *Lancet* 365 (9464):1073-86, 2005.
219. Florman S, Benchimol C, Lieberman K, et al: Fulminant recurrence of atypical haemolytic uremic syndrome during a calcineurin inhibitor-free immunosuppression regimen, *Pediatr Transpl* 6:352-55, 2002.
220. George JN, Vesely SK, Terrell DR: The Oklahoma thrombotic thrombocytopenic purpura-hemolytic uremic syndrome (TTP-HUS) registry: a community perspective of patients with clinically diagnosed TTP-HUS, *Semin Hematol* 41:60-67, 2004.
221. Lattuada A, Rossi E, Calzarossa R, Mannucci PM: Mild to moderate reduction of a von Willebrand factor cleaving protease (ADAMTS-13) in pregnant women with Willebrand microangiopathic syndrome, *Haematologica* 88:1029-34, 2003.
222. Cosmai EM, Puzis L, Tsai H-M, Lian ECY: Thrombocytopenic purpura and cardiomyopathy in pregnanacy reversed by combined plasma exchange and infusion, *Eur J Haematol* 68:239-42, 2002.
223. Ducloy-Bouthors A-S, Caron C Subtil D, et al: Thrombotic thrombocytopenic purpura: medical and biological monitoring of six pregnancies, *Eur J Obstet Gynecol Reprod Biol* 111:146-52, 2003.
224. Veyradier A, Obert B, Houlier A, Meyer D, Girma J-P, et al: Specific von Willebrand factor-cleaving protease in thrombotic microangiopathies: a study of 111 cases, *Blood* 98:1765-71, 2001.
225. Vesely SK, George JN, Lammle B, et al: ADAMTS13 activity in thrombotic thrombocytopenic purpura-hemolytic uremic syndrome: relation to presenting features and clinical outcomes in a prospective cohort of 142 patients, *Blood* 102:60-68, 2003.
226. Vasoo S, Thumboo J, Fong KY: Thrombotic thrombocytopenic purpura in systemic lupus erythematosus: disease activity and the use of cytotoxic drugs, *Lupus* 11:443-50, 2002.
227. Banfi G, Bertani T, Boeri V, et al: Renal vascular lesions as a marker of poor prognosis in patients with lupus nephritis, *Am J Kidney Dis* 18:240-48, 1991.
228. Kawasaki Y, Suzuki J, Nozawa R, et al: A 12-year-old girl with hemolytic uremic syndrome as initial symptom of systemic lupus erythematosus and a literature review, *Am J Nephrol* 22:576-80, 2002.
229. Espinosa G, Bucciarelli S, Cervera R, et al: Thrombotic microangiopathic haemolytic anaemia and antiphospholipid antibodies, *Ann Rheum Dis* 63:730-36, 2004.
230. Amoura Z, Costedoat-Chalumeau N, Veyradier A, et al: Thrombotic thrombocytopenic purpura with severe ADAMTS-13 deficiency in two patients with primary antiphospholipid syndrome, *Arthritis Rheum* 50:3260-64, 2004.
231. Ruggenenti P, Noris M, Remuzzi G: Thrombotic microangiopathy, hemolytic uremic syndrome, and thrombotic thrombocytopenic purpura, *Kidney Int* 60(3):831-46, 2001.
232. De Chadarevian JP, Goodyer PR, Kaplan BS: Acute glomerulonephritis and hemolytic uremic syndrome, *CMAJ* 123:391-94, 1980.
233. Proesmans W, Baten E, Van Damme B: A boy with acute renal failure. A case for diagnosis, *Pediatr Nephrol* 9:389-91, 1995.
234. Dische FE, Culliford EJ, Parsons V: Haemolytic uremic syndrome and idiopathic membranous glomerulonephritis, *BMJ* 1:1112-13, 1978.
235. Morita S, Sakai T, Okamoto N,, et al: Hemolytic uremic syndrome associated with immunoglobulin A nephropathy: a case report and review of cases of haemolytic uremic syndrome with glomerular disease, *Intern Med* 38:495-99, 1999.
236. Carr DJ, Kramer BS, Dragonetti DE: Thrombotic thrombocytopenic purpura associated with metastatic gastric adenocarcinoma: successful management with plasmapheresis, *South Med J* 79:476-79, 1986.
237. Mungall S, Mathieson P: Hemolytic uremic syndrome in metastatic adenocarcinoma of the prostate, *Am J Kidney Dis* 40:1334-36, 2002.
238. Majhail NS, Hix JK, Almahameed A: Carcinoma of the colon in a patient presenting with thrombotic thrombocytopenic purpura-hemolytic uremic syndrome, *Mayo Clin Proc* 77:873, 2002.
239. Lesesne JB, Rothschild N, Erickson B, et al: Cancer-associated hemolytic-uremic syndrome: analysis of 85 cases from a national registry, *J Clin Oncol* 7:781-89, 1989.
240. Cavagnaro F, Barriga F: Hemolytic uremic syndrome in a child with leukemia and CMV infection, *Pediatr Nephrol* 14:1118-20, 2000.
241. Matsuda Y, Hara J, Miyoshi H, et al: Thrombotic microangiopathy associated with reactivation of human herpesvirus-6 following high-dose chemotherapy with autologous bone marrow transplantation in young children, *Bone Marrow Transpl* 254:919-23, 1999.
242. Moake JL, Byrnes JJ: Thrombotic microangiopathies associated with drugs and bone marrow transplantation, *Hematol Oncol Clin North Am* 10(2):485-97, 1996.
243. George JN, Li X, McMinn JR, et al: Thrombotic thrombocytopenic purpura—haemolytic uremic syndrome following allogenic hematopoetic stem cell transplantation: a diagnostic dilemma, *Transfusion* 44:294-304, 2004.
244. Melnyk AM, Solez K, Kjellstrand CM: Adult hemolytic-uremic syndrome. A review of 37 cases, *Arch Intern Med* 155:2077-84, 1995.
245. Remuzzi G, Galbusera, M, Mannucci PM: ADAMTS13 in microangiopathies, *Blood* 100:3842, 2002.
246. Hunt BJ, Lammle B, Nevard CHF, Haycock GB: Von Willebrand factor–cleaving protease in childhood diarrhoea-associated haemolytic uraemic syndrome, *Thromb Haemost* 85:975-78, 2001.
247. Noris M, Bucchioni S, Galbusera M, Donadelli R, et al: Complement factor H mutation in familial thrombotic thrombocytopenic purpura with ADAMTS13 deficiency and renal involvement, *J Am Soc Nephrol* 16:1177-83, 2005.
248. Allford SL, HuntBJ, Rose P, Machin SJ, et al: Guidelines on the diagnosis and management of the thrombotic microangiopathic haemolytic anaemias, *J Haematol Br J Haematol* 120:556-73, 2003.
249. Cochran JB, Panzarino VM, Maes LY, Tecklenburg FW: Pneumococcus-induced T-antigen activation in haemolytic uremic syndrome and anemia, *Pediatr Nephrol* 19:317-21, 2004.
250. Hilmen P, Young NS, Schubert J, Brodsky RA, et al: The complement inhibitor eculizumab in paroxysmal nocturnal hemoglobinuria, *N Engl J Med* 355:1233-43, 2006.
251. Caprioli J, Noris M, Brioschi S, Pianetti G, et al: Genetics of HUS: the impact of MCP, CFH and IF mutations of clinical presentation, response to treatment and outcome, *Blood* 108(4):1267-79, 2006.
252. Zakarija A, Benett C: Drug-induced thrombotic microangiopathy, *Semin Thromb Hemost* 31 (6):681-90, 2005.
253. Liszewski MK, Kemper C, Price JD, Atkinson JP: Emerging roles and new functions of CD 46, *Springer Semin Immun* 27:345-58, 2005.
254. Repetto HA: Long-term course and mechanisms of progression of renal disease in haemolytic uremic syndrome, *Kidney Int* 68 (Suppl 97):S102-106, 2005.
255. Ahmed A, Li J, Shiloach Y, Robbins JB, Szu SC: Safety and immunogenicity of *Escherichia coli* O157 O-specific polysaccharide con-

jugate vaccine in 2-5 year-old children, *J Infect Dis* 193:515-21, 2006.
256. Manz Rudolf: Regulation of plasma cell homeostasis in protective and autoreactive immunity, PhD diss: Free University (FU) Berlin, 2004.
257. Yassa SK, Blessios G, MarinidesG, Venuto RC: Anti-CD 20 monoclonal antibody (rituximab) for life-threatening haemolytic-uremic syndrome, *Clin Transplant* 19:423-26, 2005.
258. Dragon-Durey MA, Frémeaux-Bacchi V: Atypical haemolytic uraemic syndrome and mutations in complement regulator genes, *Springer Semin Immun* 27:359-74, 2005.
259. Zipfel PF, Misselwitz J, Licht C, Skerka C: The role of defective complement control in haemolytic uremic syndrome, *Semin Thromb Hemost* 32(2):146-54, 2006.
260. Choy BY, Chan TM, Lai KN: Recurrent glomerulonephritis after kidney transplantation, *Am J Transpl* 6 (11):2535-42, 2006.
261. Bresin E, Daina E, Noris M, Castelletti F, et al: Outcome of renal transplantation in patients with non-Shiga-toxin-associated haemolytic uremic syndrome: prognostic significance of genetic background, *Clin J Am Soc Nephrol* 1:88-99, 2006.
262. Garg AX, Clark WF, Salvadori M, Thiessen-Philbrook HR, Matsell D: Absence of renal sequelae after childhood *Escherichia coli* O157 : H7 gastroenteritis, *Kidney Int* 70:807-12, 2006.
263. Trachtman A: Does parenteral volume expansion improve outcomes in children infected with *Escherichia coli* O157 : H7? *Nat Clin Pract Nephrol* 1:14-15, 2005.
264. George JN: Thrombotic thrombocytopenic purpura, *N Engl J Med* 354:1927-35, 2006.
265. Lämmle B, Kremer Hovinga JA, Alberio L: Thrombotic thrombocytopenic purpura, *J Thromb Haemostasis* 3:1663-75, 2005.
266. Wyllie BF, Garg AX, Macnab J, Rock GA, Clark WF: Thrombotic thrombocytopenic purpura/haemolytic uraemic syndrome: a new index predicting response to plasma exchange, *Br J Haematol* 132:204-209, 2006.
267. Lowe EJ, Werner EJ: Thrombotic thrombocytopenic purpura and haemolytic uremic syndrome in children and adolescents, *Semin Thromb Hemost* 31(6):717, 2005.
268. Chandler WL, Jelacic S, Boster DR, Ciol MA, et al: Prothrombotic coagulation abnormalities preceding the haemolytic-uremic syndrome, *N Engl J Med* 346(1):23-32, 2002.
269. Galbusera M, Noris M, Remuzzi G: Thrombotic thrombocytopenic purpura—then and now, *Semin Thromb Hemost* 32(2):81-89, 2006.
270. Rodríguez de Córdoba S, Esparza-Gordillo J, Goicoechea de Jorge E, Lopez-Trascasa M, Sánchez-Corral P: The human complement factor H: functional roles, genetic variations and disease associations, *Mol Immunol* 41:355-67, 2004.
271. Rougier N, Kazatchkine MD, Rougier JP, Fremebaux-Bacchi V, et al: Human complement factor H deficiency associated with haemolytic uremic syndrome, *J Am Soc Nephrol* 9:2318-26, 1998.
272. Jokiranta TS, Jaakola VP, Lehtinen MJ, Pärepalo M, et al: Structure of complement factor H carboxyl-terminus reveals molecular basis of atypical haemolytic uremic syndrome, *EMBO J* 25:1784-94, 2006.
273. Sánchez-Corral P, Pérez-Caballero D, Huarte O, Simckes AM, et al: Structural and functional characterization of factor H mutations associated with atypical haemolytic uremic syndrome, *Am J Hum Genet* 71:1285-95, 2002.
274. Vaziri-Sani F, Holmber L, Sjöholm AG, Kristoffersson AC, et al: Phenotypic expression of factor H mutations in patients with atypical haemolytic uremic syndrome, *Kidney Int* 69:981-88, 2006.
275. Sethi S, Iida S, Sigmund C, Heistad D: Renal thrombotic microangiopathy in a genetic model of hypertension in mice, *Exp Biol Med* 231:196-203, 2006.
276. Goodship THJ: Factor H genotype–phenotype correlations: lessons from aHUS, MPGN II and AMD, *Kidney Int* 70:12-13, 2006.
277. Tsai HM: The molecular biology of thrombotic microangiopathy, *Kidney Int* 70:16-23, 2006.

CHAPTER 26

Disordered Hemostasis and Renal Disorders

Mary Bauman, M. Patricia Massicotte, and Verna Yiu

Hemostasis, the balance between bleeding and clotting in the body, differs in normal children compared to adults. In children with renal disease, disturbances in the balance of hemostasis can occur resulting in either bleeding or thrombosis. Bleeding often occurs as a result of platelet function disturbance in uremia. Thrombosis occurs as a result of acquired thrombophilia due to decreased inhibitor levels in nephrotic syndrome, the presence of antiphospholipid antibodies in primary or secondary antiphospholipid antibody syndrome or damaged endothelium due to central line placement (arterial or venous), and postrenal transplant at the anastomotic vasculature site or in hemolytic uremic syndrome (HUS).

HEMOSTASIS

Normal Hemostasis

The coagulation system consists of a series of inactive proteins that circulate in the blood. Normal hemostasis is the controlled activation of both clot formation and clot lysis that stops bleeding without permitting inappropriate clotting (thrombosis). Understanding normal hemostasis is critical to managing disordered hemostasis, presenting as either bleeding or thrombosis in the child with renal disease.

Normal hemostasis occurs when a stimulus causes tissue factor (TF) to be released from the endothelium, which activates the coagulation proteins. TF activates factors XII and VII. FVIIa binds to TF on the surface of endothelial cells and the monocytes situated at the surface of vascular injury (Figure 26-1). This complex then activates factor X to Xa, and then factor IX to IXa. Factor Xa in the presence of factor Va activates prothrombin to thrombin, and a clot is formed.

Thrombin, or factor IIa, is the most important protein in the coagulation pathway (Figure 26-1). Thrombin (IIa) initiates a number of major reactions in coagulation (thrombus formation with platelet participation), fibrinolysis (thrombus degradation), anticoagulation, and inflammation. Uncontrolled thrombin generation results in significant abnormalities including disseminated intravascular coagulation (DIC) and overwhelming inflammation such as occurs in HUS. Thrombin generation is controlled by inhibitor proteins of coagulation as follows:

- Tissue factor pathway inhibitor (TFPI) inactivates tissue factor-FVIIa complex.
- Antithrombin inactivates thrombin, factors IX, X, and XI.
- Activated protein C in combination with protein S inactivates factors Va and VIIIa.
- Factor Xa is inactivated by protein Z, a vitamin K–dependent protein.

Platelets

Normal platelets, when activated, change shape from discoid to round with stellate formation.[1] Upon activation, a number of internal reactions occur that result in the release of adenosine diphosphate (ADP), thromboxane A2 (TxA2), prostaglandins, and multiple proteins stored in platelet granules. Thromboxane A2 increases the number of transmembrane glycoproteins (GP Ib/V/IX) that join together on the platelet surface to form a heterodimer glycoprotein (GP IIb/IIIa). GP IIb/IIIa in turn binds to fibrinogen. Serotonin and ADP, released by platelet granules when activated, act as platelet attractants to the injured endothelium. ADP stimulates further platelet activation, while serotonin increases fibrinogen and thrombospondin, resulting in a procoagulant state.

Platelet interaction with damaged endothelium is an important contributor to hemostasis.[1] Platelet adhesion at sites of vessel wall injury is mediated by von Willebrand factor (vWF). This is a large multimeric protein which binds with the platelet transmembrane adhesion glycoproteins (GP Ib/V/IX). By doing so, this leads to the cascade of events previously described with activation of GP IIb/IIIa that binds to fibrinogen and thus results in a procoagulant state.

Platelets require adequate numbers of red blood cells to facilitate their movement toward sites of injured endothelium. Red blood cells also enhance platelet function by releasing ADP and inactivating PGI2. Erythropoietin increases the number of GP IIb/IIIa receptors on platelets and enhances its function by promoting thrombin activation.[2]

Measurement of Hemostasis

Hemostasis can be measured using laboratory testing. Overall hemostasis including platelet involvement can be measured using an activated clotting time (ACT) and the thromboelastogram. Tests measuring different parts of the coagulation pathway (excluding platelets) include the international normalized ratio (INR), partial thromboplastin time (PTT), and the fibrinogen level.

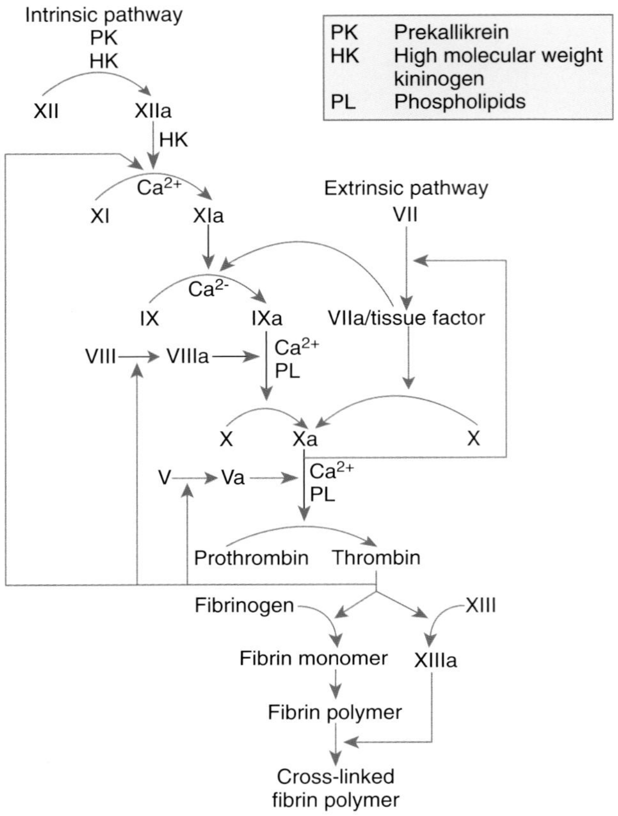

Figure 26-1 Coagulation pathway.

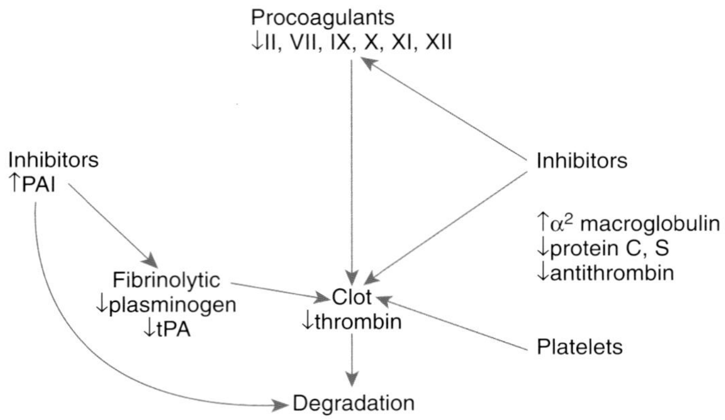

Figure 26-2 Coagulation/fibrinolytic system: the differences in children.

There are no reliable screening tests to assess platelet function.[3] The two tests that are the most utilized and readily available are the bleeding time (BT) and platelet function analyzer (PFA100), and will be discussed below.

Bleeding time, first introduced in 1910 by Duke, is an in vivo test of primary hemostasis that assesses the formation of a platelet plug in a skin wound.[4] It is found to be abnormal in patients with quantitative and/or qualitative platelet disorders or in those with vessel wall integrity abnormalities. In states of uremia, the BT has been found to be elevated. Older studies have suggested a correlation with an elevated BT and bleeding risk, and BT was considered a standard in preoperative assessment in uremic patients. Recent studies have failed to show the usefulness of BT as a predictor for clinically significant bleeding with invasive procedures or renal biopsies. A recent review of two large studies led to the conclusion that BT is not informative in predicting the risk of bleeding. Due to the lack of clinical correlation, in a position paper the College of American Pathologists and American Society of Clinical Pathologists have recommended that in the absence of a clinical history of a bleeding disorder, the BT is not a useful predictor of bleeding risk with invasive surgical procedures, and conversely, that a normal BT does not rule out the risk of excessive bleeding.[4]

There are a number of ongoing studies that evaluate the use of platelet function analyzers, and the PFA-100 to estimate platelet adhesion and aggregation.[3] These tests can be influenced by the degree of anemia resulting in false positives due to low sensitivity and specificity (30% and 84%, respectively).

The best and most reliable screen for concerns of a bleeding risk is to take a careful bleeding history.[3] It is considered to be significant if there is greater or equal to two distinct sites of spontaneous or provoked bleeding (skin, gums, nose, gastrointestinal, or genitourinary), or a single episode of bleeding requiring transfusion, or single episodes of bleeding on three separate occasions.

Activation of Coagulation

Activation of hemostasis resulting in thrombus formation results in the production of a protein, called the d-dimer. The d-dimer can be measured and increased levels compared to age-matched normals indicate activation of the coagulation system. Caution is necessary when interpreting the results of the d-dimer test as any activation of the clotting system (surgery, line insertion, injury, trauma, malignancy, and so on) will be reflected in an elevated d-dimer.

Developmental Hemostasis

Developmental hemostasis describes the evolving nature of the coagulation system of infants and children. An understanding of developmental hemostasis is necessary to avoid misdiagnosing what may appear to be disordered coagulation or thrombophilia. Normal infants and children have major differences in hemostasis compared to adults. These differences—coagulation factors, fibrinolytic proteins, inhibitor levels, amount of thrombin generation, and composition of thrombus formed—are collectively known as developmental hemostasis[5-7] (Figure 26-2).

Thrombophilia

The contribution of congenital thrombophilia to thrombosis in children with renal disease remains unknown. The need to screen for prothrombotic disorders in children with renal disease undergoing an invasive procedure or with a history of confirmed thrombosis remains uncertain. In normal children, congenital prothrombotic disorders are relatively rare, but include factor V Leiden; prothrombin gene G20210A; dysfibrinogenemia; deficiencies of protein C, protein S, and antithrombin; and increased FVIII. Most children with factor V

Leiden or prothrombin gene G20210A do not develop thrombosis in childhood. Excessive plasma levels of homocysteine resulting from homozygous deficiencies of enzymes, such as cystathione β synthase or methylenetetrahydrofolate reductase (MTHFR), may be associated with severe venous thrombosis in children. In addition, there is an association between lipoprotein A, antiphospholipid antibody syndrome, and thrombosis in children. Thrombosis in children usually results from at least two risk factors including immobility, malignancy, placement of a central line, and thrombophilia.[8]

BLEEDING IN RENAL DISEASE

Uremic Coagulopathy

The association between uremia and bleeding was first described in 1764 by Morgagni. In 1836, Bright published a report on 100 cases of patients with albuminous urine and again noted the connection between purpura and uremia. The observation that bleeding in uremic patients occurs despite having normal clotting factors led to the supposition that the primary abnormality must be within the platelet system.[9]

Clinical Manifestations

Bleeding in uremia has been reported in many locales.[10] This includes potential bleeding in the areas of the skin and mucosa, the gastrointestinal tract, the retroperitoneum, ocular tissues, genitourinary system, and intracranium. There are potential risks of bleeding during surgery or postoperatively from venipuncture sites and renal biopsy sites. Pleural and pericardial hemorrhagic effusions have also been described. Most of these reports have been in the adult population with only a few scattered reports of bleeding risks in uremic children.[9] Whether the adult risks of bleeding can be extrapolated to children is still unknown.

Pathogenesis

Studies have measured the levels and function of coagulation factors in chronic renal failure, and results have been found to be normal.[10] From these data, it is assumed that platelets in the uremic state are primarily responsible for the bleeding risk in chronic renal failure. When placed into normal plasma, uremic platelets demonstrate normal function, implying that causative factors are present in the surrounding uremic plasma. However, researchers have found both intrinsic and extrinsic platelet abnormalities that result in the uremic coagulopathy.

Intrinsic Platelet Abnormalities

In chronic kidney disease (CKD) and uremia, the content of ADP and serotonin is reduced in the platelet granules. This is felt to be either an acquired storage pool defect or a defect in secretory mechanisms.[1] Cyclic adenosine monophosphate (cAMP) has been reported to be increased in CKD, which can affect the mobilization of calcium in response to stimulus and ultimately, platelet activation. It may be through an imbalance between ADP, serotonin, and cAMP that results in platelet activation defects. Other defects include low levels of GP Ib/V/IX in association with elevated levels of glycocalicin, a proteolytic byproduct released by GP Ib/V/IX when damaged on the platelet surface.[11] Thromboxane A2 levels, generated from free arachidonic acid, have also been found to be low in uremia and result in poor platelet adhesion and aggregation.[12]

Platelet contractility defects may be another factor contributing to platelet dysfunction by reducing its mobility and secretory capacity.[13] In uremic states, platelets have deficient cytoskeletal proteins, such as α-actin and tropomyosin, with the abnormalities becoming more pronounced after activation by thrombin.

Platelet–Vessel Wall Abnormalities

Levels of vWF and fibrinogen have been documented to be normal in uremic states.[10] There is also normal binding of vWF to the platelet receptor GP Ib/V/IX as well as normal surface expression of GP Ib/V/IX, although as previously mentioned, the total levels of GP Ib/V/IX have been found to be suboptimal.[11] Another noted abnormality is reduced binding capacity of vWF and fibrinogen to GP IIb/IIIa resulting in reduced platelet adhesion to injured endothelium. This may be secondary to receptor blockade by fibrinogen, or through substances that are dialyzable as dialysis improves this anomaly.

Other extrinsic factors that might come into play include prostaglandins.[10] Prostaglandin I2 (PGI2) is a vasodilator released by endothelial cells and inhibits platelet function through its action on adenylyl cyclase through its modulating effects on cAMP and calcium mobilization within platelets. Although several studies have shown increased production of PGI2 in endothelium of uremic models, blockage of PGI2 production does not result in improved coagulation, thereby suggesting that there are other factors that are involved in platelet dysfunction in renal failure. Patients with chronic kidney disease often present with anemia, which may also influence platelet function.[2] Circulating uremic toxins may also play a role in uremic coagulopathy. Substances such as urea, creatinine, phenol, phenolic acids, or guanidinosuccinic acid (GSA) have all been investigated for their potential effects on platelet function.[11] Phenolic acid impairs primary aggregation of platelets to ADP, and GSA has been found to inhibit the second wave of ADP-induced platelet aggregation. This is further supported by the observation that dialysis can improve or partially correct these defects.

Finally, platelet number and volume are both reduced in uremia.[10] Platelet numbers are lower in uremia when compared to healthy controls, although they are rarely less than 80×10^9/L. The reduction in platelet volume can further reduce the amount of circulating platelet mass resulting in ineffectual platelet contact with injured endothelium.

Treatment

Treatment for uremic coagulopathy in the past was based on its ability to correct or normalize the prolonged BT observed in uremic patients. However, as noted in the previous sections, BT has no in vivo correlation with risk of bleeding so that treatment should only be directed toward active cases of bleeding in the setting of uremia. Treatments utilized include desmopressin (DDAVP), estrogens, and cryoprecipitate. Discussion here will focus around the use of DDAVP in settings where there is a significant history of clinical bleeding.

DDAVP was first utilized for its antidiuretic properties when it was discovered in the 1970s to have hemostatic properties.[14] Infusions of DDAVP have been found to increase vWF, factor VIII coagulant activity, ristocetin co-factor, and tissue plasminogen activator. The rise of coagulation factors is rapid, likely related to release of endogenous reserves rather than new synthesis. DDAVP may also promote the glycoprotein transmembrane proteins as both vWF and GP IIb/IIIa.

DDAVP is administered via intravenous, subcutaneous, or intranasal routes. The maximal effects on clotting factor levels occur at 30 minutes, lasting up to 6 hours with an intravenous dose of 0.3 μg/kg. With subcutaneous dosing, the levels peak at 1 to 2 hours. For intranasal administration, a dose of 300 μg is comparable to a 0.2-μg/kg intravenous dose.

Adverse effects of DDAVP include facial flushing, headache, hypotension, tachycardia, water retention, hyponatremia, and seizures (uncommon but higher incidence in children under 5 years of age). Hypotonic solutions should be administered with caution in children who have received DDAVP.

DDAVP should not be used in cases of polydipsia, unstable angina, or severe cases of congestive heart failure because of its antidiuretic effects.

Estrogens have been reported to improve BT in uremia by increasing platelet responsiveness.[10] There have been no reports of its use in children, although adult studies recommend a dosage of 0.6 mg/kg/day given intravenously daily for 4 to 5 days. Effects start within 6 hours and can last for up to 2 weeks after an intravenous course. It can also be given as an oral dose, but the effect is shorter, lasting up to 5 days. Side effects include hypertension, fluid retention, and raised liver transminases.

Cryoprecipitate is rich in factor VIII, vWF, fibrinogen, and fibrinectin, but carries with it the risks of blood-borne infections and anaphylaxis.

CLOTTING IN RENAL DISEASE

Nephrotic Syndrome

Nephrotic syndrome is a hypercoagulable state that leads to an increased predisposition to the development of thromboembolic events.[15-19] Prevalence is highest in the adult population with membranous nephropathy and is estimated at 37%. In pediatrics, where the most common cause of nephrotic syndrome is minimal change lesion, prevalence is much lower with the majority of studies estimating it to be less than 10% (range between 0.8% to as high as 28%). It has been suggested that pediatric cases of thromboembolism in the setting of nephrotic syndrome are more severe, with a poorer prognosis as compared with adult counterparts.

Thrombotic Manifestations of Nephrotic Syndrome

Both venous and arterial thrombosis cases have been reported in the pediatric age group.[15,18] Commonly affected areas for venous thrombosis include: deep leg veins, inferior vena cava, superior vena cava, hepatic veins, sagittal sinus, and sinovenous vessels. Arterial thromboses are also more common in nephrotic children and can involve any artery including femoral, mesenteric, and intracardiac areas. Pulmonary vascular clots can occur both as a spontaneous in situ phenomenon or as a consequence of an embolic event.

Pathogenesis

The prothrombotic tendencies in nephrotic patients have been attributed to a number of factors including state of hydration and hyperviscosity, imbalance between clotting factors and thrombophilic proteins, increase in platelets and platelet activation, abnormalities of the fibrinolytic system, and use of medications.[16,19]

Antithrombin (AT) is an endogenous anticoagulant that has been documented in numerous studies to be low in nephrotic patients.[14-16] In several studies, AT had a strong correlation with plasma albumin levels and a negative correlation with urinary protein excretion, suggesting that one of the mechanisms involved in low AT levels is due to its loss in the urine.[20] Subsequent remission of the nephrotic syndrome results in normalization of AT levels. Data on other in vivo anticoagulants have not been conclusive, although the majority of studies suggest that protein C, protein S, and tissue factor pathway inhibitor are all elevated during acute nephrotic relapses.[16,21,22] This might exert a protective effect against clotting and might explain why, in children, episodes of thromboembolic events are less frequent when compared to adult nephrotic patients.

Platelets have been found to be higher in numbers and more active in nephrotic children. Studies suggested improved platelet availability due to their higher numbers and increased exposure of the normally albumin bound arachidonic acid leading to thromboxane A2 activation and subsequent platelet aggregation.[23] Hyperlipidemia may also promote platelet aggregation, based on the simple observation that treatment with lipid-lowering agents improves platelet hyperaggregability in nephrotics.

Elevated levels of fibrinogen add to the prothrombotic state by providing more substrate for thrombin to produce fibrin.[20] Fibrinogen also enhances platelet aggregation and increases blood viscosity and subsequent red cell aggregation. Elevation in fibrinogen is likely secondary to the nonspecific response to increased synthesis of all proteins to compensate for urinary protein losses. This increase in fibrinogen levels is countered by an overactive fibrinolysis system, which is protective against thrombosis.

Finally, use of corticosteroids for the management of childhood nephritic syndrome has been reported to be associated with hypercoagulability.[24] Mechanisms responsible include increase in coagulation factors and reduction in fibrinolysis.

ANTIPHOSPHOLIPID ANTIBODY SYNDROME

Antiphospholipid antibody syndrome (APS) is a form of acquired autoimmune thrombophilia that has the following clinical manifestations: arterial and venous thrombosis, including renal artery and vein, recurrent fetal loss, thrombocytopenia, and neurologic complications. These autoantibodies have been labeled lupus anticoagulant (LA), anticardiolipin antibody (ACLA), and anti β2 glycoprotein 1, and bind to plasma proteins (β2 glycoprotein 1, prothrombin, protein C, protein S, or annexin V) on negatively charged phospholipids. These proteins have been associated with the development of thrombosis due to a number of different prothrombotic mechanisms.[25]

Primary APS is rare in children; secondary APS occurs in children with systemic lupus erythematosus (SLE) with a prevalence of ACLA of 9% to 87% and LA of 11% to 62%.[26,27] There is a higher prevalence of thrombosis in children with LA. If a patient with APS, with or without SLE, develops a thrombosis, anticoagulant therapy should be initiated in the absence of contraindications. Treatment may include thrombectomy (arterial thrombosis), fibrinolysis (if potential loss of life, organ such as kidney, or limb), and anticoagulation (see "Treatment" section). If the APA continues to be present on laboratory testing separated by 6 weeks, strong consideration should be given to continuing anticoagulation until the APA is negative.[28] Some data suggest that thromboprophylaxis studies in children with APLA and SLE may be warranted.[29] The data are inconclusive; therefore, no definitive recommendations can be made for thromboprophylaxis.

RENAL ARTERY THROMBOSIS

In neonates, renal artery thrombosis occurs as a result of umbilical arterial cannulation with the incidence currently unknown. In older children, renal artery thrombosis is most commonly associated with renal transplant and occurs at the site of vascular anastomosis. The incidence as estimated from the North American Pediatric Renal Transplant Cooperative Study (NAPRTCS) is approximately 3%, with recent estimates due to advanced immunosuppressive therapy being as low as 1%.[30] Previous analyses of the NAPRTCS identified the following risk factors for renal artery thrombosis in a graft: cadaver donor source, peritoneal dialysis, in excess of five pretransplant blood transfusions, cold ischemia time of more than 24 hours, and prior renal transplant.[30-33] There are no studies in the treatment of renal artery thrombosis determining the safety and efficacy of embolectomy, fibrinolysis, or anticoagulation. If renal artery thrombosis associated with renal transplant is diagnosed, embolectomy or fibrinolytic/anticoagulation therapy should be considered in the absence of contraindications (bleeding) to attempt to save the graft.[8]

RENAL VEIN THROMBOSIS

Although renal vein thrombosis is the most common non–catheter-related thrombosis in the newborn period, few long-term outcome studies have been carried out.[8,33-36] Most renal vein thromboses present in the first month, with the majority of these in the first week of life. The clinical features of renal vein thrombosis are variable and include hematuria, oliguria-anuria, hypertension, decreased renal function, palpable flank mass, thrombocytopenia, and abnormal Doppler ultrasound results (decrease in amplitude or absence of venous signal, abnormal flow patterns in a number of renal venous branches, or evidence of venous collateral development). The etiology of renal vein thrombosis in most cases is unknown. Risk factors reported for the development of renal vein thrombosis include maternal diabetes mellitus (either type 1 or gestational), pathologic states associated with thrombosis (e.g., shock, dehydration, perinatal asphyxia, polycythemia, cyanotic heart disease), sepsis, umbilical venous catheterization, and conjoined twins. Inherited prothrombotic abnormalities have been described in case reports of renal vein thrombosis.[35] However, the prevalence of these disorders has not been studied in a cohort of patients with neonatal renal vein thrombosis.

Treatment

The optimal immediate management of renal vein thrombosis is unknown. The use of anticoagulant or fibrinolytic therapy is therefore controversial. There are no data to confirm that active treatment improves the long-term outcome in the absence of acute renal failure.[8] If the renal vein thrombosis on ultrasound has extended in the absence of therapy, then if there are no contraindications (bleeding, high risk of bleeding), anticoagulation should be considered.

The long-term management for renal vein thrombosis includes follow-up to ensure that renal function normalizes. Patients with bilateral renal vein thrombosis should be followed through life because of the high likelihood of chronic renal failure. It should be recognized that some neonates who are labeled as having unilateral renal vein thrombosis may have bilateral disease or damage to the contralateral kidney (e.g., from acute renal failure caused by acute tubular necrosis developing into cortical necrosis) and may need a longer follow-up period. Patients require a clinical examination for manifestations of chronic kidney disease, including hypertension and proteinuria, both of which may aggravate progression of renal failure. Renal function should be monitored by serial plasma creatinine levels and calculation of GFR. Formal measurement of GFR is recommended at 12 months of age to determine whether chronic renal failure is present. Serial Doppler ultrasound screening will demonstrate the change from the acute finding of enlarged, echogenic kidney(s) to the chronic changes with renal atrophy. Nuclear medicine imaging with technetium-99m dimercaptosuccinic acid should be carried out to assess the functional status of the kidney(s).[35]

The sequelae of renal vein thrombosis reported in the literature include glomerular disease (3% to 100%), tubular dysfunction (9% to 47%), hypertension (9% to 100%), and evidence of renal scarring or atrophy (27% to 100).[35-38] Performance of multicenter, randomized clinical trials is urgently required to investigate the safety and efficacy of treatment for renal vein thrombosis and to determine long-term outcomes.

HEMOLYTIC UREMIC SYNDROME AND COAGULATION

Hemolytic uremic syndrome (HUS) is the most common cause of acute renal failure in children. HUS has significant morbidity and mortality with no difference in clinical outcome between typical and atypical forms of HUS.[39,40] The triad of hemolytic anemia, thrombocytopenia, and renal involvement underscore the primary abnormality with this entity, which is related to a procoagulant state initiated by endothelial injury.[41] Plasma taken from patients with HUS will induce aggregation of normal platelets.[42] Similarly, in the presence of shiga toxin, platelets adhered with the formation of thrombin when whole blood was perfused over human microvascular endothelial cells. Shiga toxin has also been found to inhibit prostacyclin production and increase thromboxane A2 release from endothelial cells, thereby favoring platelet aggregation.

The procoagulant state of HUS is evidenced by the clinical manifestations of the formation of microthrombi throughout systemic circulation. Subclinical thrombogenesis occurs even prior to the onset of HUS with elevation of markers of thrombin activation (increase in prothrombin fragments 1 and 2 and thrombin–antithrombin complexes).[41] In the normal state, levels of thrombin activation markers are negligible. TF, expressed on mononuclear and endothelial cells and an initiator of the coagulation cascade leading to thrombin generation, has been found to be upregulated by shiga toxin. Blockade of thrombin activity with lepirudin prevented lethal shiga toxin effects in greyhounds suggesting that shiga toxin may mediate injury via thrombin activation.

The thrombocytopenia in HUS is also intertwined in this process and is due to a consumptive process with platelet deposition in the microthrombi.[42] The platelets are activated with degranulation, as evidenced by reduction in intracellular levels of β-thromboglobulin and impaired aggregation in vitro. Other evidence of platelet activation includes an increase in platelet microparticles and platelet-derived factors including platelet factor-4, β-thromboglobulin, and P-selectin. The resultant effect is the formation of platelet aggregates through binding of fibrinogen leading to thrombus formation.

Fibrinolysis has been suggested to be depressed in the setting of HUS, adding to the prothrombotic state in HUS.[41,42] However, studies are conflicting as to whether indications of this, such as elevated levels of plasminogen activator inhibitor type 1 (PAI-1), support this finding.[43]

Finally, other evidence of vascular activation includes increases in circulating levels of the following: Fas-ligand and soluble Fas, interleukin-1 receptor antagonist, transforming growth factor, platelet activating factor, degraded vWF multimers, and numerous plasma factors as previously noted.[44]

DIAGNOSIS OF THROMBOSIS

The diagnosis of thrombosis in children is challenging due to a number of factors. Many children with a clinical suspicion of thrombosis are critically ill and unable to be transported to a radiology suite for testing. Most radiographic testing used in children has not been properly studied to determine sensitivity and specificity; however, clinical studies have determined the most sensitive diagnostic methods for diagnosing upper system venous thrombosis in children[45] to be ultrasound for jugular venous thrombosis, and venography for intrathoracic vessels.

Ultrasound may be used to assess for upper or lower system venous or arterial thrombosis but it is important to understand its limitations. If clinical suspicion is high for thrombosis, and the ultrasound is negative, magnetic resonance imaging with venography (MRI/V), venogram, or computed tomography (CT) of the vessels should be performed to rule out thrombosis. All tests have limitations, including ultrasound. Due to its noninvasive nature, ultrasound is still the first test that patients will undergo to diagnose thrombosis. However, there is a high false-negative rate. If clinical suspicion is high despite a negative result, further investigation is warranted using the studies previously listed.

Pulmonary Embolism

The gold standard test for pulmonary embolism, pulmonary angiography, is invasive and thus rarely performed in infants and children. The sensitivity and specificity of ventilation perfusion scans, MRI/A, and spiral CT have not been determined in infants and children. Due to the lack of data in children, it is difficult to make specific recommendations. In adults, VQ scans have a significant false-negative rate. In these cases, spiral CT may have a higher sensitivity and specificity. When clinical suspicion is high, consideration should be given to the possibility of false negatives and more than one imaging test may be warranted to ensure accurate diagnosis.

Renal Vein and/or Artery Thrombosis

Renal function compromise or unexplained hypertension warrants ultrasound investigation to rule out arterial and/or venous thrombosis. If ultrasound is inconclusive and clinical suspicion of thrombosis exists, MRI/V/A should be performed. The sensitivity and specificity of MRI/V/A has not been determined in infants and children.

ANTITHROMBOTIC THERAPY IN INFANTS AND CHILDREN

Influence of Developmental Hemostasis on Antithrombotic Therapy

Developmental hemostasis has significant implications on current recommendations for the use of antithrombotic therapy. In children, the dosing and intensity of antithrombotic therapy is based on adult guidelines. The use of unfractionated heparin in infants may require antithrombin replacement (antithrombin concentrate or fresh frozen plasma) to achieve an effect due to developmentally low antithrombin levels.

Treatment of Venous or Arterial Thrombosis

With confirmed symptomatic and asymptomatic proximal venous thromboembolism (VTE), in the absence of contraindications, anticoagulation should be strongly considered. Therapy can be initiated with either unfractionated heparin (UFH) or low-molecular-weight heparin (LMWH), for a minimum of 5 to 7 days. Therapy is increased to 10 to 14 days in extensive deep venous thrombosis or pulmonary embolism, followed by warfarin or LMWH for the duration of therapy. (Use with caution in children with renal disease; see LMWH section below.)

For a deep venous thrombosis (DVT) secondary to an acquired insult, 3 months of therapy is usually sufficient. In cases of idiopathic VTE, a minimum of 6 months should be considered. Objective imaging of the thrombosis is recommended prior to discontinuation of anticoagulant therapy.

TABLE 26-1 Heparin Dosing Nomogram

aPTT (seconds)	Antifactor Xa (units/ml)	Hold (minutes)	Rate Change	Repeat aPTT
<50	<0.1	0	Increase 20%	4 hours
50-70	0.1-0.34	0	Increase 10%	4 hours
70-120	0.35-0.70	0	0	24 hours
121-135	0.71-0.89	0	Decrease 10%	4 hours
135-160	0.90-1.20	30	Decrease 10%	4 hours
>160	>1.20	60	Decrease 15%	4 hours

aPTT, Activated partial thromboplastin time.

Practical Guidelines for Anticoagulant Use in Children

Prior to the initiation of therapy, obtain the patient's weight and blood for hemoglobin, platelets, and INR; if LMWH is being considered, obtain activated partial thromboplastin time (aPTT), urea, and creatinine as well. Dosing nomograms for each anticoagulant are available.[8,46,47]

Where possible, avoid intramuscular injections and arterial punctures during anticoagulation therapy. If necessary, appropriate precautions should be taken, including the use of extended periods (5 minutes) of firm external pressure.

Avoid concomitant antiplatelet drugs. Acetaminophen (paracetamol) is recommended for analgesia.

For patients on long-term vitamin K antagonist therapy (warfarin or acenocoumoral for more than 6 months), consider bone densitometry studies at baseline and then every 12 months to assess for possible reduced bone mineral density.[48]

TABLE 26-2 Reversal of Heparin Therapy

Time Since End of Infusion, or Last Heparin Dose	Protamine per 100 Units Unfractionated Heparin Dosed (maximum 50 mg/dose)
<30 min	1 mg
30-60 min	0.5-0.75 mg
61-120 min	0.375-0.5 mg
>120 min	0.25-0.375 mg

From Kuhle S, Massicotte P, Chan A, Mitchell L: A case series of 72 neonates with renal vein thrombosis. Data from the 1-800-NO-CLOTS Registry, *Thromb Haemost* 92(4):729-33, 2004.

Unfractionated Heparin Therapy

Unfractionated heparin therapy is the anticoagulant of choice for children with a high risk of bleeding and those requiring invasive procedures, because it has a short half-life allowing for quick reversal of anticoagulation by simply discontinuing the infusion, and rapid reversal with the use of protamine sulfate.

Age-related dosing is required in children. Initiation of therapy follows: infants of 28 weeks gestational age up to 12 months of age require 28 IU/kg/hour, and children over 12 months of age require 20 IU/kg/hour. The dosage is then titrated based on laboratory results.[8,47,49]

A bolus should be considered in cases of extensive thrombosis or acute pulmonary embolus. The recommended bolus is UFH 75 units/kg administered over 10 minutes, followed by an age-appropriate infusion.

Dosing and Monitoring

Monitoring of therapy is necessary as a result of the poor bioavailability of UFH. It has been shown that aPTT and anti-factor Xa levels only correspond in approximately 70% of children and rarely in children less than 12 months of age.

In all age groups, if possible, an anti-factor Xa and an aPTT should be drawn within 24 hours of initiating therapy to ensure that the aPTT is accurately reflecting the UFH concentration. In children where the aPTT and the anti-factor Xa level do not correspond, UFH therapy should be monitored using anti-factor Xa level. Blood sampling should be performed (aPTT or anti-factor Xa level) 4 to 6 hours after initiation of therapy.

The UFH must be adjusted to maintain an anti-factor Xa at 0.35 to 0.7 IU/ml or an aPTT that corresponds to the therapeutic anti-factor Xa range (Table 26-1).

If anticoagulation with UFH needs to be discontinued for clinical reasons, termination of the infusion will usually suffice because of the rapid clearance of UFH. If an immediate effect is required, consider administering protamine sulfate. Following IV administration, neutralization occurs within 5 minutes. The dose of protamine sulfate required to neutralize UFH is based on the dosage of UFH received in the previous 2 hours as shown in Table 26-2.

The maximum dose of protamine sulfate—regardless of the amount of UFH received—is 50 mg, and should be administered in a concentration of 10 mg/ml at a rate not exceeding 5 mg/min. When administered too quickly, protamine sulfate may result in cardiovascular collapse.

An aPTT performed 15 minutes after administration will demonstrate if reversal has been partial or complete.

Heparin-induced thrombocytopenia is relatively rare in children. There have been a number of case reports of pediatric heparin-induced thrombocytopenia (HIT) in the literature, ranging in age from 3 months to 15 years.[50,51]

If an abrupt drop in platelets by more than 50% from baseline occurs, with no other etiology, then a HIT screen should be performed.

TABLE 26-3 Enoxaparin Dosing Nomogram: Dose Adjustment

Anti-Factor Xa Level	Hold Next Dose?	Change Dose?	Next Anti-Factor Xa Level?
<0.35 units/ml	No	Increase by 25%	4 hours post next morning dose
0.35-0.49 units/ml	No	Increase by 10%	4 hours post next morning dose
0.5-1 units/ml	No	0	1× per week at 4 hours post morning dose
<1.20 units/ml	No	Decrease by 20%	4 hours post next morning dose. Hold dose. Do a trough level. If trough is <0.5 at 10 hours post dose, administer scheduled dose at 20% of previous dose.

Note: The above nomogram assumes that there is no bleeding or renal compromise. Dose adjustments ordered in 1.0-mg increments for doses greater than 5 mg are sufficient to achieve targeted anti-factor Xa level.
From Massicotte P: Improving warfarin therapy in children: anticoagulation clinics are just the beginning, *Thromb Res* 114(1):1-3, 2004.

Low-Molecular-Weight Heparin in Infants and Children

The use of LMWH (enoxaparin) should be considered in most patients with normal renal function who require anticoagulation for therapy or prophylaxis. The potential advantages of LMWH are directly related to its high bioavailability. For children, these advantages include the following:

The need for minimal monitoring (important in pediatric patients with poor venous access).
Lack of interference by other drugs or diet, such as exists for warfarin.
Reduced risk of HIT.
Probable reduced risk of osteoporosis.[8,47,52]

The following dosage guidelines apply to enoxaparin only and cannot be directly extrapolated to other LMWHs: at 3 months and older, 1.5 mg/kg dose given at 12-hour intervals; and at less than 3 months, 1.0 mg/kg dose given every 12 hours.

In Children with Renal Dysfunction

Modifications are strongly recommended in children with renal compromise or failure, use with caution, start at 80% of recommended dose and monitor levels frequently. The guidelines for therapeutic LMWH suggest maintaining an anti-Xa level of 0.50 to 1.0 IU/ml in a sample taken 4 to 6 hours following a subcutaneous injection.

Monitor the creatinine level prior to initiating LMWH therapy and throughout the treatment period. Accumulation of LMWH may occur if renal clearance is impeded. Dosing nomograms are available, but should be adjusted for children with renal compromise (Table 26-3).

If anticoagulation with LWMH needs to be terminated for clinical reasons, discontinuation of LMWH injections will usually suffice. If an immediate reversal of effect is required, protamine sulfate reverses 80% of the anti-factor Xa activity of LMWHs.

Tips for Therapy Administration in Infants and Children

LMWH may be administered using an insulin syringe with a short ultrafine needle. An Insuflon catheter may be used to avoid pain associated with needle pokes. Close monitoring of the site for bruising and bleeding is necessary.

TABLE 26-4 Warfarin Dosing Nomogram: Loading Phase, after Initial Dose

If INR Is	Then
1.1-1.4	Repeat initial dose.
1.5-2.9	Use 50% of initial dose.
>3.0	Hold until <2.5, and then restart at 50% less than the previous dose.

INR, International normalized ratio.

Warfarin Therapy

Monitoring oral anticoagulant therapy in children is difficult and requires close supervision with frequent dosage adjustments. Reasons contributing to the need for frequent monitoring include variations in daily intake, medications, primary medical problems and concomitant childhood illnesses. For these reasons, warfarin is not recommended in children under 1 year of age.

The usual loading dose is 0.2 mg/kg as a single daily oral dose, with a maximum of 5 mg. Full diet should be tolerated prior to initiating warfarin therapy in children. It is helpful to use LMWH until the child is adequately tolerating feeds, as this will result in achieving the maintenance phase safely and efficiently.

Dosing nomograms are available for loading warfarin (Table 26-4) and for maintenance dose adjustments (Table 26-5).[8,47,52]

Control of warfarin is improved when patients are managed through dedicated anticoagulation clinics.[53-55] Referral to a dedicated clinic should be considered.

The antidote for warfarin is dependent on whether urgent or nonurgent reversal is necessary. *For non-urgent reversal,* vitamin K1 is administered in a dose of 0.5 to 2 mg orally, depending on the patient's size. The administration of vitamin K either subcutaneously or intramuscularly has been shown to be less efficacious than orally, providing that gut absorption is not severely compromised. *For urgent reversal* (major bleeding or interventional procedure), prothrombin complex concentrate or fresh frozen plasma (20 ml/kg) is administered.

TABLE 26-5 **Warfarin Dosing Nomogram: Maintenance Phase for Target INR 2.5**

INR	Action
1.1-1.4	Check for adherence; if adherent, increase dose by 20%.
1.5-1.9	Increase dose by 10%.
2.0-3.0	No change.
3.1-3.5	Decrease dose by 10%.
>3.5-4.0	Administer one dose at 50% less than maintenance dose. Then restart at 20% less than maintenance dose.
4.1-5.0	Hold one dose, and then restart at 20% less than maintenance dose.
>5.0	Consider reversal with Vitamin K.

INR, International normalized ratio.

Patients discharged on warfarin therapy may be given an ampoule of vitamin K dispensed as 10 mg/ml ampoules. Vitamin K may be self-administered on the advice of the treating physician[56] as follows (based on adult [60 kg] recommendations): INR of 6 to 10, administer 1.0 mg orally; and INR of more than 10, administer 2.0 mg orally. INR must be repeated within 24 hours.

Home INR Monitors

Whole-blood monitors provide an effective way for monitoring INRs in children on long-term anticoagulant therapy, with needle phobias or poor venous access. The INR is measured using a capillary blood sample. Point-of-care INR monitors have been evaluated in children and were shown to be acceptable and reliable for use in the outpatient laboratory and in home settings.

Thrombolytic Therapy

Systemic thrombolytic therapy is indicated for arterial occlusions, massive pulmonary embolism, and pulmonary embolism not responding to heparin therapy. It may also be indicated for acute extensive DVT, and should be limited to situations where there is a risk for loss of life, organ, or limb, as there exists a high incidence of hemorrhage. Contraindications include acute bleeding or the potential for local bleeding such as general surgery within the previous 10 days, neurosurgery within the previous 3 weeks, hypertension, AV malformations, and severe recent trauma.

Alteplase therapy has been reported in the literature at doses from 0.01 to 0.6 mg/kg/hour intravenously for 6 hours. The thrombus should be reevaluated prior to reinitiating alteplase infusion. During alteplase infusion, UFH at 10 units/kg/hour should be administered simultaneously, and precautions must be taken to minimize the risk for bleeding (such as maintaining fibrinogen over 1.0 g/L, platelets more than 100×10^9/L, and minimal manipulation of the patient during the infusion). In a neonate or a child with arterial thrombosis where the decision has been made to use thrombolysis, plasminogen supplementation (fresh frozen plasma) may be prudent to achieve a high enough plasminogen level to result in a lytic effect.

CONCLUSION

Children with renal disease may have disordered hemostasis, resulting in a risk of either bleeding or clotting. Normal hemostasis in children must be understood by the clinician in order to determine whether, in a child with renal disease, therapeutic intervention to prevent abnormal bleeding or clotting is prudent. Unfortunately, there are few properly designed studies in children with renal disease providing guidelines for best practice relating to diagnosis and treatment of disordered hemostasis. These studies are urgently required to optimize care for this complicated group of children.

REFERENCES

1. Jurk K, Kelvrel BE: Platelet physiology, *Biochem Semin Thromb Hemost* 4:381-92, 2005.
2. Boccardo P, Remuzzi G, Galbusera M: Platelet dysfunction in renal failure, *Semin Thromb Hemost* 5:579-89, 2004.
3. Hassan AA, Kroll MH: Acquired disorders of platelet function, *Hematology* 403-8, 2005.
4. Peterson P, Hayes TE, Arkin CF, Bovill EG, et al: The preoperative bleeding time test lacks clinical effectiveness, *Arch Surg* 133:134-39, 1998.
5. Andrew M, Paes B, Milner R, et al: Development of the human coagulation system in the healthy premature infant, *Blood* 72 (5):1651-57, 1988.
6. Andrew M, Paes B, Milner R, et al: Development of the human coagulation system in the full-term infant, *Blood* 198770(1):165-72, 1987.
7. Andrew M, Vegh P, Johnston M, Bowker J, et al: Maturation of the hemostatic system during childhood, *Blood* 80(8):1998-2005, 1992.
8. Monagle P, Chan A, Massicotte P, Chalmers E, Michelson AD: Antithrombotic therapy in children: the Seventh ACCP Conference on Antithrombotic and Thrombolytic Therapy, *Chest* 126(Suppl 3):645S-87S, 2004.
9. Davidovich E, Schwarz Z, Davidovitch E, Eidelman E, Bimstein E: Oral findings and periodontal status in children, adolescents and young adults suffering from renal failure, *J Clin Periodontol* 32:1076-82, 2005.
10. Kaw D, Malhotra D: Platelet dysfunction and end-stage renal disease, *Semin Dialysis* 19:317-22, 2006.
11. Mezzano D, Tagle R, Panes D, Perez M, et al: Hemostatic disorder of uremia: the platelet defect, main determinant of prolonged bleeding time, is correlated with indices of activation of coagulation and fibrinolysis, *Thromb Haemost* 76:312-21, 1996.
12. DiMinno G, Martinez J, McKean ML, DeLaRosa J, et al: Platelet dysfunction in uremia: multifaceted defect partially corrected by dialysis, *Am J Med* 79:552-59, 1985.
13. Escolar G, Diaz-Ricart M, Cases A: Uremic platelet dysfunction: past and present, *Curr Hematol Rep* 4:359-67, 2005.
14. Lethagen S: Desmopressin and hemostasis, *Ann Hematol* 69:173-80, 1994.
15. Singhal R, Brimble KS: Thromboembolic complications in the nephrotic syndrome: pathophysiology and clinical management, *Thromb Res* 118:397-407, 2006.
16. Mehls O, Andrassy K, Koderisch J, Herzog U, Ritz E: Hemostasis and thromboembolism in children with NS: differences from adults, *J Pediatr* 1987110:862-67, 1987.
17. Hoyer PF, Gonda S, Barthels M, Krohn HP, Brodehl J: Thromboembolic complications in children with nephrotic syndrome: risk and incidence, *Acta Paediatr Scand* 75:804-10, 1986.

18. Citak A, Emre S, Sirin A, Bilge I, Nayr A: Hemostatic problems and thromboembolic complications in nephrotic children, *Pediatr Nephrol* 14:138-42, 2000.
19. Lilova MI, Velkovski IG, Topalov IB: Thromboembolic complications in children with nephrotic syndrome in Bulgaria (1974-1996), *Pediatr NephrolPediatr Nephrol* 15:74-78, 2000.
20. Elidrissy ATH, Abdurrahman MB, Bahakim HM, Jones MD, Gader AMA: Haemostatic measurements in childhood nephrotic syndrome, *Eur J Pediatr* 150:378, 1991.
21. al-Mugeiren MM, Gader AM, al-Rasheed SA, Bahakim HM, et al: Coagulopathy of childhood nephrotic syndrome—a reappraisal of the role of natural anticoagulants and fibrinolysis, *Haemostasis* 26:304-10, 1996.
22. Yermiaku T, Shalev H, Landau D. Dvilansky A: Protein C and protein S in pediatric nephrotic patients, *Sangre (Barc)* 41:155-57, 1996.
23. Anand NK, Chand G, Talib VH, Chellani H, Pande J: Hemostatic profile in nephrotic syndrome, *Indian Pediatr* 33:1005-12, 1996.
24. Patrassi GM, Sartori MT, Livi U, et al: Impairment of fibrinolytic potential in long-term steroid treatment after heart transplantion, *Transplantation* 64:1610-13, 1997.
25. Robertson B, Greaves M: Antiphospholipid syndrome: an evolving story, *Blood Rev* 20(4):201-12, 2006.
26. Falcini F: Vascular and connective tissue diseases in the paediatric world, *Lupus* 13(2):77-84, 2004.
27. Lee T, von Scheven E, Sandborg C: Systemic lupus erythematosus and antiphospholipid syndrome in children and adolescents, *Curr Opin Rheumatol* 13(5):415-21, 2001.
28. Levine JS, Branch DW, Rauch J: The antiphospholipid syndrome, *N Engl J Med* 346(10):752-63, 2002 (see comment).
29. Berube C, Mitchell L, Silverman E, et al: The relationship of antiphospholipid antibodies to thromboembolic events in pediatric patients with systemic lupus erythematosus: a cross-sectional study, *Pediatr Res* 44(3):351-56, 1998.
30. Smith JM, Stablein D, Singh A, Harmon W, McDonald RA: Decreased risk of renal allograft thrombosis associated with interleukin-2 receptor antagonists: a report of the NAPRTCS, *Am J Transplant* 6(3):585-88, 2006.
31. Harmon WE, Stablein D, Alexander SR, Tejani A: Graft thrombosis in pediatric renal transplant recipients. A report of the North American Pediatric Renal Transplant Cooperative Study, *Transplantation* 51(2):406-12, 1991.
32. Massicotte-Nolan P, Glofcheski DJ, Kruuv J, Lepock JR: Relationship between hyperthermic cell killing and protein denaturation by alcohols, *Radiation Res* 87(2):284-99, 1981.
33. Proesmans W, van de Wijdeven P, Van Geet C: Thrombophilia in neonatal renal venous and arterial thrombosis, *Pediatr Nephrol* 20(2):241-42, 2005.
34. Goldenberg NA: Long-term outcomes of venous thrombosis in children, *Curr Opin Hematol* 12(5):370-76, 2005.
35. Marks SD, Massicotte MP, Steele BT, et al: Neonatal renal venous thrombosis: clinical outcomes and prevalence of prothrombotic disorders, *J Pediatr* 146(6):811-16, 2005.
36. Winyard PJD, Bharucha T, De Bruyn R, et al: Perinatal renal venous thrombosis: presenting renal length predicts outcome, *Arch Dis Child Fetal Neonatal Ed* 91(4):F273-78, 2006.
37. Kosch A, Kuwertz-Broking E, Heller C, Kurnik K, et al: Renal venous thrombosis in neonates: prothrombotic risk factors and long-term follow-up, *Blood* 104(5):1356-60, 2004.
38. Kuhle S, Massicotte P, Chan A, Mitchell L: A case series of 72 neonates with renal vein thrombosis. Data from the 1-800-NO-CLOTS Registry, *Thromb Haemost* 92(4):729-33, 2004.
39. Siegler RL: Spectrum of extrarenal involvement in postdiarrheal hemolytic uremic syndrome, *J Pediatr* 125:511-18, 1994.
40. Verweyen HM, Karch H, Allerberger F, Zimmerhackl LB: Enterohemorrhagic *E. coli* in pediatric hemolytic uremic syndrome: a prospective study in Germany and Austria, *Infection* 27:341-47, 1999.
41. Chandler WL, Jolacic S, Boster DR, Ciol MA, et al: Prothrombotic coagulation abnormalities preceding hemolytic uremic syndrome, *N Engl J Med* 346:23-32, 2002.
42. Karpman D, Papadopoulou D, Nilssen K, Sjogren AC, et al: Platelet activation by Shiga toxin and circulating factors as a pathogenetic mechanism in hemolytic uremic syndrome, *Blood* 97:3100-108, 2001.
43. VanGeet C, Proesmans W, Arnout J, Vermylen J, Dederck PJ: Activation of both coagulation and fibrinolysis in childhood hemolytic uremic syndrome, *Kidney Int* 54:1324-30, 1998.
44. Tarr PI: Basic fibroblast growth factor and shiga toxin-0157 : H7-associated hemolytic uremic syndrome, *J Am Soc Nephrol* 13:817-20, 2003.
45. Male C, Chait P, Ginsberg JS, et al: Comparison of venography and ultrasound for the diagnosis of asymptomatic deep vein thrombosis in the upper body in children: results of the PARKAA study. Prophylactic Antithrombin Replacement in Kids with ALL treated with Asparaginase, *Thromb Haemost* 87(4):593-98, 2002.
46. Monagle P, Chan A, deVeber G, Massiccotte M: *Pediatric thromboembolism and stroke,* ed 3, Hamilton, 2006, BC Decker Inc.
47. O'Shaughnessy D, Makris M, Lillicrap D: *Practical hemostasis and thrombosis,* Malden, 2005, Blackwell Publishing Ltd.
48. Barnes C, Newall F, Ignjatovic V, et al: Reduced bone density in children on long-term warfarin. *Pediatr Res* 57(4):578-81, 2005.
49. Monagle P, Chan A, deVeber G, Massicotte M: *Pediatric thromboembolism and stroke,* ed 3, Hamilton, 2006, BC Decker Inc.
50. Schmugge M, Revel-Vilk S, Hiraki L, Rand ML, et al: Thrombocytopenia and thromboembolism in pediatric systemic lupus erythematosus, *J Pediatr* 143(5):666-69, 2003.
51. Klenner AF, Lubenow N, Raschke R, Greinacher A: Heparin-induced thrombocytopenia in children: 12 new cases and review of the literature, *Thromb Haemost* 91(4):719-24, 2004.
52. Monagle P, Chan AKC: Pediatric edition thrombosis research, *Thromb Res* 118(1):1-2, 2006.
53. Newall F, Savoia H, Campbell J, Monagle P: Anticoagulation clinics for children achieve improved warfarin management, *Thromb Res* 114(1):5-9, 2004.
54. Massicotte P: Improving warfarin therapy in children: anticoagulation clinics are just the beginning, *Thromb Res* 114(1):1-3, 2004.
55. Errichetti AM, Holden A, Ansell J: Management of oral anticoagulant therapy. Experience with an anticoagulation clinic, *Arch Intern Med* 144(10):1966-68, 1984.
56. Crowther MA, Donovan D, Harrison L, McGinnis J, Ginsberg J: Low-dose oral vitamin K reliably reverses over-anticoagulation due to warfarin, *Thromb Haemost* 79(6):1116-18, 1998.

CHAPTER 27

Differential Diagnosis and Management of Fluid, Electrolyte, and Acid–Base Disorders

Mario G. Bianchetti and Alberto Bettinelli

INTRODUCTION

In this chapter the various disturbances involving fluid, electrolyte, and acid–base balance will be addressed in sections focused on water, salt, potassium, acid–base, calcium, magnesium, and phosphate. This traditional presentation is didactically relevant. It is worthy of mention, however, that more than one disturbance in fluid, electrolyte, and acid–base homeostasis often concurrently occur in the same patient. For example, hypokalemia rarely occurs in isolation but is often associated with metabolic alkalosis, hypomagnesemia, and reduced urinary calcium excretion. More importantly, the diagnostic approach of the aforementioned constellation of hypokalemia associated with alkalosis is strongly influenced by the concurrent demonstration of arterial hypertension, a marker of expanded effective circulating volume.

Some years ago a boy was admitted to three different hospitals because of a tendency towards renal hypokalemia. Renal biopsy was found to be normal and medical treatment failed to correct the biochemical abnormality. Two years later, a diuretic screen was found to be positive for frusemide, and the child improved after separation from his mother, indicating the diagnosis of nonaccidental poisoning by the parents or someone in loco parentis.[1] This impressive case suggests that the ideal interpreter of some unexplained electrolyte disturbances would be Sherlock Holmes.[2] Hence, the diagnostic approach to initially unexplained "isolated" disturbances involving the fluid, electrolyte, and the acid–base balance (e.g., hypokalemia in a child with muscle weakness) should include both very careful history and examination as well the concurrent assessment of an extended "electrolyte spectrum." In the setting of initially unclassifiable and apparently "isolated" disturbances involving the fluid, electrolyte, and acid–base balance, concomitant determination in blood of pH, pCO_2, HCO_3^-, Na^+, K^+, Cl^-, Ca^{++} (either total or ionized), Mg^{++}, inorganic phosphate, alkaline phosphatase, total protein level (or albumin), uric acid, urea, and creatinine is advised.

WATER AND SALT

Body Fluid Compartments

Water accounts for 50% to 75% of body weight. The most important determinants of the wide range in water content are age and gender. The water content of a newborn, an adolescent, and an elderly man is approximately 75%, 60%, and 50%, respectively. After puberty, water content in females is generally 2% to 10% lower than in males. The intracellular fluid contains approximately two-thirds of total body water, and the remainder is held in the extracellular fluid. The solute composition of the intracellular and extracellular fluid differs considerably because the sodium pump (Na^+-K^+-ATPase) maintains sodium in a primarily extracellular and potassium in a primarily intracellular location. Consequently, sodium largely determines extracellular fluid volume, and potassium determines intracellular fluid volume.[3-6]

The extracellular fluid compartment is further subdivided into the interstitial and the intravascular compartments (blood volume), which contain two-thirds and one-third of the extracellular fluid, respectively. Finally, the transcellular compartment comprises the digestive, cerebrospinal, intraocular, pleural, peritoneal, and synovial fluids.

The size of the intravascular compartment is determined by the overall size of the extracellular fluid compartment and by the Starling forces, that is, the forces controlling partition of fluids between intravascular and interstitial compartments across the capillary membrane, which is crossed by salts like sodium chloride and by glucose but not by blood proteins (especially albumin). Three major forces control the distribution of fluids across the capillary membrane (Figure 27-1).

First, the hydrostatic pressure causes fluids to leave the vascular space. Second, the higher concentration of proteins in the intravascular compartment as compared with that in interstitial fluid, causes fluids to enter the vascular space. This force, which is called oncotic pressure, is due both to the concentration gradient of albumin (blood proteins other than albumin account for 50% of the weight of proteins in blood but only 25% of the oncotic pressure) as well to the fact that

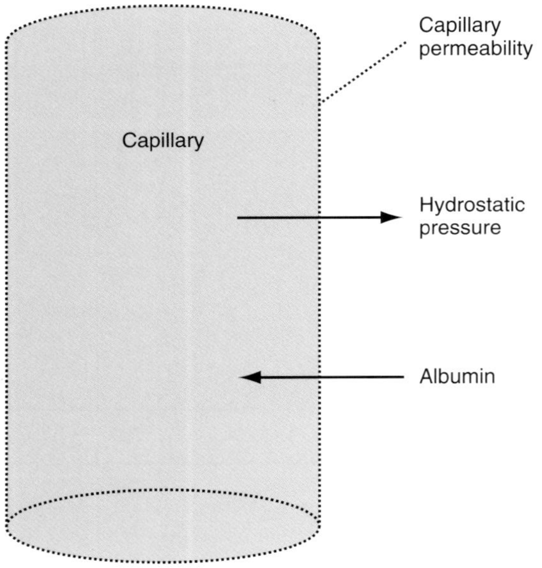

Figure 27-1 Distribution of ultrafiltrate across the capillary membrane. The barrel-shaped structure represents a capillary. A high hydrostatic pressure or increased capillary permeability causes fluid to leave the vascular space. By contrast, increased intravascular albumin concentration and, therefore, increased oncotic pressure causes fluid to enter the vascular space.

albumin is anionic and therefore attracts cations (largely sodium) into the vascular compartment (Gibbs-Donnan effect; Figure 27-2). Third, altered capillary permeability is another major mechanism that modulates the distribution of fluids across the capillary membrane.

Effective Circulating Volume

Effective circulating volume is a clinically relevant but unmeasured entity, which denotes the part of the intravascular compartment that is in the arterial system and is effectively perfusing the tissues. The effective circulating volume (which is biologically more important than the intravascular compartment) usually varies directly with the extracellular fluid volume. As a result, the regulation of extracellular fluid balance (by alterations in urinary sodium excretion) and the maintenance of the effective circulating volume are intimately related. Sodium loading will tend to produce volume expansion, whereas sodium loss (e.g., due to vomiting, diarrhea, or diuretic therapy) will lead to volume depletion. The body responds to changes in effective circulating volume in two steps: (1) the change is sensed by the volume receptors, which are located in the cardiopulmonary circulation, the carotid sinuses and aortic arch, and in the kidney; and (2) these receptors activate effectors that restore normovolemia by varying vascular resistance, cardiac output, and renal water and salt excretion. Briefly, the extrarenal receptors primarily govern the activity of the sympathetic nervous system and natriuretic peptides. On the other side the renal receptors affect volume balance by modulating the renin-angiotensin II-aldosterone system.

In some settings, the effective circulating volume is independent of the extracellular fluid volume. Among patients with heart failure, the extracellular fluid volume is increased but the patient is effectively volume depleted due to low

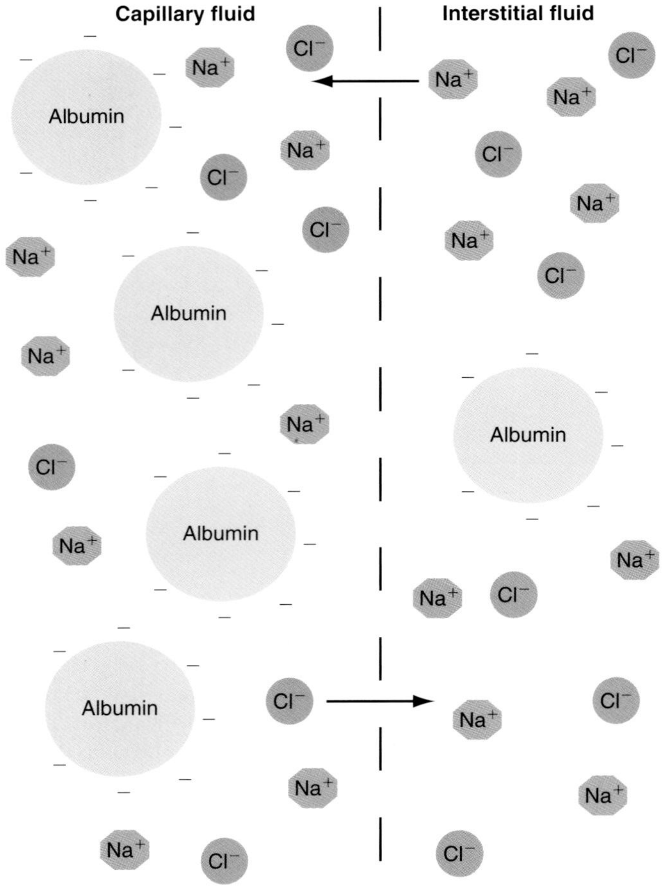

Figure 27-2 The Gibbs-Donnan effect. There is a difference in the concentration of anionic albumin, which is impermeant, between the vascular (albumin approximately 40 g/L) and the interstitial (albumin approximately 10 g/L) compartments. The negative charges of albumin "attract" cations (largely Na^+) into the vascular compartment and "repel" anions (Cl^- and HCO_3^-) out. Because the concentration of Na^+ exceeds that of Cl^- and HCO_3^-, "attraction" outweighs "repulsion." Consequently, the Gibbs-Donnan effect increases the vascular compartment. The capillary bed separating the intravascular and interstitial spaces (represented by dashed line) is freely permeable to Na^+, K^+, Cl^-, and glucose.

cardiac output. Among patients with advanced cirrhosis and ascites, the extracellular fluid volume is expanded because of the ascites, the circulatory volume is increased due in part to fluid accretion in the markedly dilated, but slowly circulating splanchnic venous circulation, and the cardiac output is often elevated because of multiple arteriovenous fistulas throughout the body (such as the spider angiomas on the skin) which bypass the capillary circulation.

Blood Osmolality: Measurement of Sodium

Since osmolality is the concentration of all of the solutes in a given weight of water, blood osmolality is equal to the sum of the osmolalities of the individual solutes in blood. Most of the osmoles in blood are sodium salts, with lesser contributions from other ions, glucose, and urea. Under normal circumstances, the osmotic effect of the ions in blood can usually be estimated from two times the sodium concentration. Total (or true) blood osmolality (in milliosmoles per kilogram of H_2O) can be measured directly (via determination of freezing point depression) or estimated from circulating sodium, glucose, and urea (in millimoles per/l) as

Sodium × 2 + Glucose + Urea.[3-9]

To obtain urea and glucose in millimoles per liter divide blood urea nitrogen (in milligrams per deciliter) by 2.8 and glucose (in milligrams per deciliter) by 18.

The effective blood osmolality, known colloquially as blood tonicity, is another clinically significant entity that denotes the concentration of solutes impermeable to cell membranes (sodium, glucose, mannitol) that are therefore restricted to the extracellular compartment (osmoreceptors sense effective blood osmolality rather than the total blood osmolality). Glucose is a unique solute because, at normal physiological concentrations in blood, it is actively taken up by cells and therefore acts as an ineffective solute, but under conditions of impaired cellular uptake (like diabetes mellitus) it becomes an effective extracellular solute.

Solutes, which are impermeable to cell membranes, are effective because they create osmotic pressure gradients across cell membranes leading to movement of water from the intracellular to the extracellular compartment. Solutes that are permeable to cell membranes (urea, ethanol, methanol) are ineffective solutes because they do not create osmotic pressure gradients across cell membranes, and therefore are not associated with such water shifts. Since no direct measurement of effective blood osmolality (which is biologically more important than the total or true blood osmolality) is possible, the following equations are used to calculate this entity:

Sodium × 2 + Glucose

Measured total blood osmolality − Urea

Flame photometry, the traditional assay for circulating sodium, measures the concentration of sodium per unit volume of solution, with a normal range between 135 and 145 mmol/L. In fact, sodium is dissolved in plasma water, which normally accounts for 93% of the total volume of plasma, the remaining 7% consisting of protein and lipid. The average activity of sodium in plasma water is 150 mmol/L (range 145 to 155 mmol/L), and it is this which is determined by direct ion-selective electrodes that are now used in most laboratories. For convenience, laboratories routinely apply a correction factor so that the reported values still correspond to the traditional normal range of 135 to 145 mmol/L. A kind of "pseudohyponatremia" caused by expansion of the nonaqueous phase of plasma—for example, due to hyperlipidemia or paraproteinemia—is no longer seen because determination by ion-selective electrodes in undiluted samples is unaffected by this. Although, strictly speaking, a sodium concentration outside the range of 135 to 145 mmol/L denotes dysnatremia, clinically relevant hypo- or hypernatremia is mostly defined as a sodium concentration outside the extended normal range of 130 to 150 mmol/L.

Dehydration and Extracellular Fluid Volume Depletion

The terms "dehydration" and "extracellular fluid volume depletion" are mostly used interchangeably. However, these terms denote conditions resulting from different types of fluid losses. Volume depletion refers to any condition in which the effective circulating volume is reduced. It is produced by salt and water loss (as with vomiting, diarrhea, diuretics, bleeding, or third space sequestration). In the strict sense, dehydration refers to water loss alone. The clinical manifestation of dehydration is often hypernatremia. The elevation in blood sodium concentration, and therefore effective blood osmolality, pulls water out of the cells into the extracellular fluid.

However, much of the literature does not distinguish between dehydration and volume depletion, and in medicine the word dehydration means both a loss of water and salt. Depending on the type of pathophysiologic process, water and salts (primarily sodium chloride) may be lost in physiologic proportion or lost disparately, with each type producing a somewhat different clinical picture, designated as normotonic (mostly isonatremic), hypertonic (mostly hypernatremic), or hypotonic (always hyponatremic) dehydration. Dehydration develops when fluids are lost from the extracellular space at a rate exceeding intake. The most common sites for extracellular fluid loss are the intestinal tract (diarrhea, vomiting, or bleeding), skin (fever or burns), and urine (osmotic diuresis, diuretic therapy, or diabetes insipidus). More rarely, dehydration results from prolonged inadequate intake without excessive losses.[3-6,9]

The risk for dehydration is high in childhood for the following causes: higher frequency of diarrhea and vomiting in children compared to adults; children, especially very young children, have a higher surface area-to-volume ratio with proportionally higher insensible losses that are accentuated in disease states like fever or burns; and young children do not communicate their need for fluids or do not independently access fluids to replenish volume losses.

Dehydration reduces the effective circulating volume, thereby impairing tissue perfusion. If not corrected, ischemic end-organ damage occurs, leading to serious morbidity.[3-6,9]

Three groups of symptoms and signs occur in dehydration[3-6,9,10]: those related to the manner in which fluids loss occurs (including diarrhea, vomiting, or polyuria); those related to the electrolyte and acid–base imbalances that sometimes accompany dehydration; and those directly due to dehydration. The following discussion will focus on the third group. When assessing a child with a tendency towards dehydration, the clinician needs to address the degree of extracellular fluid volume depletion. More rarely the clinician will address the laboratory testing and the type of fluid lost (extracellular or intracellular fluid).

Degree of Dehydration

Accurate assessment of the degree of dehydration is imperative since severe extracellular fluid volume depletion calls for rapid isotonic fluid resuscitation.[3-6,9] Dehydration is most objectively measured as a change in weight from baseline (acute loss of body weight reflects the loss of fluid, not lean body mass; thus, a 1.5-kg weight loss should reflect the loss of 1.5 liters of fluid). In most cases, however, a recent weight measurement is unavailable. As a result, a number of findings on physical examination as well as pertinent history are used to assess the severity of dehydration.

Minimal dehydration (absent or less than 3% to 5% volume loss): There is a history of fluid losses but clinical signs are absent.

Mild dehydration (3% to 5% volume loss): There are minimal signs of dehydration including either tachycardia or dry mucous membranes (sometimes the child does not produce tears well while crying). Such patients may have a reduction in urine output.

Moderate dehydration (6% to 9% volume loss): These children have apparent signs of dehydration including tachycardia, dry mucous membranes, irritability, decreased peripheral perfusion with a delay in capillary refill between 2 and 3 seconds, or deep respirations with or without an increase in respiratory rate. There is a history of reduction in urine output, decreased tearing, and an open fontanel will be sunken on physical examination. In childhood, blood pressure may be maintained until relatively late in dehydration (arterial hypotension is a late sign in hypovolemia and is rapidly followed by cardiac arrest).

Severe dehydration (10% volume loss or more): Such patients typically have a near-shock presentation as manifested by decreased peripheral perfusion with a pathologic capillary refill (more than 3 seconds), cool and mottled extremities, deep respirations with an increase in rate, tachycardia, and perhaps even arterial hypotension. Skin turgor, sometimes referred to as skin elasticity, is a sign commonly used to assess the degree of hydration. The skin on the back of the hand, lower arm, or abdomen is grasped between two fingers, is held for a few seconds then released. Skin with normal turgor snaps rapidly back to its normal position. Skin with decreased turgor remains elevated and returns slowly to its normal position. Decreased skin turgor is a late sign in dehydration, which is associated with moderate or, more frequently, severe dehydration.

Laboratory Testing and Type of Fluid Lost

Laboratory testing can confirm the presence of dehydration. The fractional clearance of sodium,

$$\frac{\text{Urinary sodium} \times \text{Circulating creatinine}}{\text{Circulating sodium} \times \text{Urinary creatinine}}$$

is less than 0.5×10^{-2} and the urine spot sodium concentration less than 30 mmol/L (unless the source of dehydration is renal). (The fractional clearance of Na^+ (like that of Cl^-, K^+, Ca^{++}, Mg^{++}, or inorganic phosphate) is the amount of Na^+ actually excreted by the body relative to the amount filtered by the kidney. In a healthy child with a plasma Na^+ level of 140 mmol/L, a plasma creatinine level of 40 µmol/L (0.45 mg/dl), and urinary Na^+ of 131 mmol/L and creatinine of 2860 µmol/L (32 mg/dl) the calculated fractional clearance of Na^+ is 0.014 or 1.49×10^{-2}.)

Furthermore, in dehydration, the urine is concentrated with an osmolality exceeding 450 mosm/kg of H_2O. The urinary concentration can be measured with an osmometer or fairly estimated, in the absence of proteinuria and glucosuria, from the specific gravity, as determined by refractometry (dipstick measurement of specific gravity is rather inaccurate), as follows:

$$(\text{Specific gravity} - 1000) \times 40$$

Furthermore, laboratory testing can detect associated electrolyte and acid–base abnormalities, but determination of circulating electrolytes and acid–base balance is typically limited to children requiring intravenous fluids. These children are more severely volume depleted, and are therefore at greater risk for dyselectrolytemias. Laboratory testing is less useful for assessing the degree of volume depletion.

Circulating HCO_3^- 17.0 mmol/L or less might be the most useful laboratory test to assess dehydration. (In children with diarrhea metabolic acidosis almost always results from the loss of bicarbonate in the stool. Other causes of acidosis associated with diarrhea are type A L-lactate acidosis and fasting ketosis.) The blood urea level reflects the severity of dehydration, the decreased glomerular filtration rate and the increased sodium and water reabsorption. Unfortunately the clinical usefulness of this test is limited, since this blood parameter can be increased by other factors such as bleeding or tissue breakdown (on the other side the rise can be minimized by a concurrent decrease in protein intake).

The sodium concentration varies with the relative loss of solute to water. Changes in sodium concentration play a pivotal role in deciding the type of fluid depletion (Figure 27-3).

Hyponatremic and hypotonic dehydration: The development of hyponatremia reflects net solute loss in excess of water loss. This does not occur directly, as fluid losses such as diarrhea are not hypertonic. Usually solute and water are lost in proportion, but water is taken in and retained in the context of hypovolemia-induced secretion of antidiuretic hormone. Since body water shifts from extracellular fluid to cells under these circumstances, signs of dehydration easily become profound.

Normonatremic and isotonic dehydration: In this setting, solute is lost in proportion to water loss.

Hypernatremic and hypertonic dehydration: This setting reflects water loss in excess of solute loss. Since body water shifts from intracellular to extracellular fluid under these circumstances, these children have less signs of dehydration for any given amount of fluid loss than do children with normonatremic (or normotonic) dehydration and especially those with hyponatremic dehydration.

DYSNATREMIA

Consequences, Symptoms, and Diagnostic Workup

Under normal conditions, blood sodium concentrations are maintained within the narrow range of 135 to 145 mmol/L despite great variations in water and salt intake. Sodium and its accompanying anions, principally chloride and bicarbonate, account for 90% of the extracellular effective osmolality. The main determinant of the sodium concentration is the plasma water content, itself determined by water intake (thirst or habit), "insensible" losses (such as metabolic water and sweat), and urinary dilution. The last of these is under most circumstances crucial and predominantly determined by antidiuretic hormone. In response to this hormone, concentrated urine is produced by water reabsorption across the renal collecting tubules.[3-9] Dysnatremias produce signs and

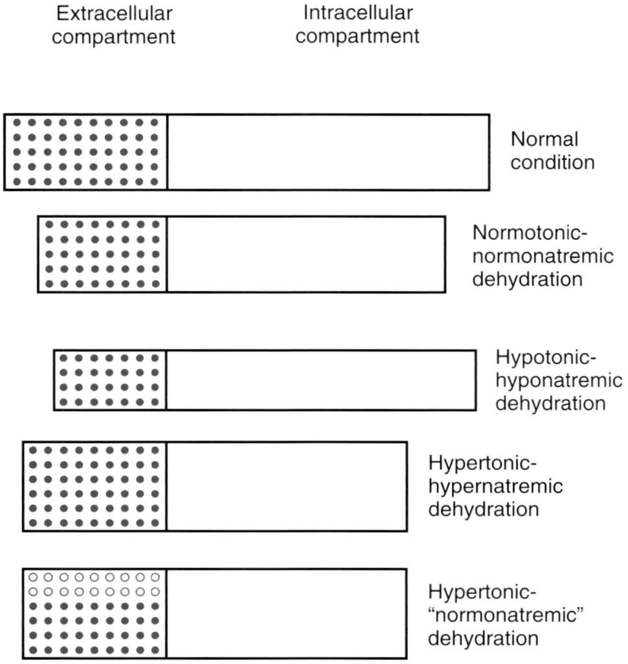

Figure 27-3 Extracellular and intracellular compartments in children with dehydration. Normally the extracellular compartment makes up approximately 20% and the intracellular 40% of body weight (upper panel). The second, third, and fourth panels depict the relationship between extracellular and intracellular compartment in three children with dehydration in the context of an acute diarrheal disease: dehydration is normotonic-normonatremic in the first, hypotonic-hyponatremic (mainly extracellular fluid losses) in the second, and hypernatremic (mainly intracellular fluid losses) in the third. The lower panel depicts the relationship between the extracellular and intracellular compartment (mainly intracellular fluid losses) in a child with dehydration in the context of diabetic ketoacidosis (hypertonic means "normonatremic" dehydration; the brackets indicate that in the context of diabetic ketoacidosis, the concentration of circulating sodium is normal or even reduced). In each panel, the solid circles denote sodium and open circles impermeable solutes that do not move freely across cell membranes (glucose in the present example). For reasons of simplicity, no symbols are given for potassium, the main intracellular cation.

symptoms secondary to central nervous system dysfunction. While hyponatremia may induce brain swelling, hypernatremia may induce brain shrinkage, yet the clinical features elicited by opposite changes in tonicity are remarkably similar.

Hyponatremia

Determining the cause of hyponatremia may be straightforward if an obvious precipitating cause is present, such as in the setting of vomiting or diarrhea.[3,4,6,8,9] In hospital practice, diagnosing the cause is often less evident. The clinical classification of hyponatremia according to the patient's extracellular fluid volume status, as hypovolemic, normovolemic, or hypervolemic, is useful to help with the diagnosis. In practice, however, distinguishing normovolemic and hypovolemic hyponatremia may not be straightforward.

A decrease in sodium concentration and effective blood osmolality causes movement of water into brain cells and results in cellular swelling and raised intracranial pressure. Nausea and malaise are typically seen when sodium level falls below 125 to 130 mmol/L. Headache, lethargy, restlessness, and disorientation follow, as the sodium concentration falls below 115 to 120 mmol/L. With severe and rapidly evolving hyponatremia, seizure, coma, permanent brain damage, respiratory arrest, brain stem herniation, and death may occur. In more gradually evolving hyponatremia, the brain self-regulates to prevent swelling over hours to days by transport of, firstly, sodium, chloride, and potassium and, later, solutes like glutamate, taurine, myoinositol, and glutamine from intracellular to extracellular compartments. This induces water loss and ameliorates brain swelling, and hence leads to few symptoms in chronic hyponatremia.

An accurate history may reveal a clue to the cause of the hyponatremia and establish the rapidity of the symptoms. The key diagnostic factors are the hydration status of the child, the spot urine sodium concentration, and the fractional clearance of sodium, which allows the distinction in hypovolemic hyponatremia between extrarenal (sodium <30 mmol/L, fractional clearance of sodium $<0.50 \times 10^{-2}$) and renal (sodium >30 mmol/L; fractional clearance of sodium $>0.5 \times 10^{-2}$) salt loss. Urinary sodium is similarly helpful in patients whose volume status is difficult to assess, as patients with dilutional hyponatremia have a urinary sodium above 30 mmol/L (fractional clearance of sodium $>0.5 \times 10^{-2}$), whereas those with extracellular fluid depletion (unless the source is renal) will have a urinary sodium less than 30 mmol/L (fractional clearance of sodium $<0.5 \times 10^{-2}$). Effective blood osmolality is almost always low in hyponatremia, and urine is less than maximally dilute (inappropriately concentrated). Thus, although usually measured, blood and urine osmolalities are rarely discriminant.

Hypernatremia

Hypernatremia reflects a net water loss or a hypertonic sodium gain, with inevitable hypertonicity.[3-5,7,9] Severe symptoms are usually evident only with acute and large increases in sodium concentrations to above 160 mmol/L. Importantly, the protecting sensation of thirst is absent or reduced in patients with altered mental status or with hypothalamic lesions and in infancy. Nonspecific symptoms such as anorexia, muscle weakness, restlessness, nausea, and vomiting tend to occur early. More serious signs follow, with altered mental status, lethargy, irritability, stupor, or coma. Acute brain shrinkage can induce vascular rupture, with cerebral bleeding and subarachnoid hemorrhage.

The cause of hypernatremia is almost always evident from the history. Determination of urine osmolality in relation to effective blood osmolality and urine sodium concentration helps if the cause is unclear. Patients with diabetes insipidus present with polyuria and polydipsia (and not hypernatremia unless thirst sensation is impaired). Central diabetes insipidus and nephrogenic diabetes insipidus may be differentiated by the response to water deprivation (failure to concentrate urine) followed by desmopressin, causing concentration of urine in patients with central diabetes insipidus.

Evaluating the Causes of Dysnatremias

Dysnatremias are common in both the inpatient and outpatient settings.

Hyponatremia

The primary defense against developing hyponatremia is the ability to dilute urine and excrete free water. Rarely is excess ingestion of free water alone the cause of hyponatremia. It is also rare to develop hyponatremia from excess urinary sodium losses in the absence of free water ingestion. Development of hyponatremia typically requires a relative excess of free water in conjunction with an underlying condition that impairs the ability to excrete free water.

Renal water handling is primarily under control of antidiuretic hormone, which is released from the posterior pituitary and impairs water diuresis by increasing the permeability to water in the collecting tubule. There are osmotic, hemodynamic, and nonhemodynamic stimuli for release of antidiuretic hormone. In most cases of hyponatremia there is a stimulus for antidiuretic hormone production that results in impaired free water excretion. The body will attempt to preserve the extracellular volume at the expense of the serum sodium; therefore, a hemodynamic stimulus for vasopressin production will override any inhibitory effect of hyponatremia. There are numerous stimuli for production of antidiuretic hormone in hospitalized children that make virtually any hospitalized patient at risk for hyponatremia (Table 27-1).

Hospital-acquired hyponatremia is most often seen in the postoperative period or in association with a reduced effective circulating volume.[6,8,9,11] Very rarely, hospital-acquired hyponatremia is seen in association with the syndrome of inappropriate antidiuretic hormone activity, which is caused by elevated activity of this hormone, independently of increased effective blood osmolality and hemodynamic stimulus (i.e., reduced effective circulating volume). The syndrome of inappropriate antidiuretic hormone secretion should be suspected in any child with hyponatremic hypotonicity, a urine osmolality above 100 mosmol/kg H_2O, a fractional clearance of sodium more than 0.5×10^{-2}, hypouricemia, low blood urea level, and normal acid–base and potassium balance.

Postoperative hyponatremia is a serious problem in children.[11] Postoperative hyponatremia sometimes is caused by a combination of nonosmotic stimuli for release of antidiuretic hormone, such as pain, nausea, stress, narcotics, and edema-forming conditions. However, subclinical depletion of the effective circulating volume and administration of hypotonic fluids are the most important causes of postoperative hyponatremia.

Hyponatremia is also a concern in the outpatient setting.[12] It is primarily attributable to antidiuretic hormone secretion in children with diarrhea, vomiting, or poor fluid intake.

Desmopressin, a synthetic analogue of the natural antidiuretic hormone, is used in central diabetes insipidus, in some bleeding disorders, in diagnostic urine concentration testing, and especially in primary nocturnal enuresis with nocturnal polyuria. Desmopressin is generally regarded as a safe drug and adverse effects due to treatment are uncommon. Nonetheless, hyponatremic water intoxication leading to seizures has been reported as a rare but potentially life-threatening side effect of desmopressin therapy in enuretic children with high fluid intake during the day.[6,13]

Boys have been recently described with hyponatremia and laboratory features consistent with inappropriate antidiuretic hormone release but without detectable circulating antidiuretic hormone. Genetic testing revealed gain-of-function mutations of the X-linked receptor gene that mediates the renal response to antidiuretic hormone, resulting in persistent activation of the receptor.[14] This disease is a kind of mirror image of the X-linked nephrogenic diabetes insipidus, which results from loss-of-function genetic defects in the aforementioned renal receptor.

A syndrome sometimes occurs in patients with cerebral disease that mimics all of the findings in the syndrome of inappropriate antidiuretic hormone activity, except that salt wasting is the primary defect with the ensuing volume depletion leading to a secondary rise in release of antidiuretic hormone. Salt wasting of central origin likely results from

TABLE 27-1 Causes of Hyponatremia in Childhood

Hypovolemic	Normovolemic (or Hypervolemic)
Normotonic hyponatremia (e.g., diabetes mellitus)	**Increased body water**
Intestinal salt loss	Parenteral hypotonic solutions
Diarrheal dehydration	Tap water enemas
Vomiting, gastric suction	Compulsive water drinking
Fistulae	**Nonosmolar release of antidiuretic hormone**[a]
Laxative abuse	Cardiac failure
Transcutaneous salt loss	Severe liver disease (mostly cirrhosis)
Cystic fibrosis	Nephrotic syndrome
Endurance sport	Glucocorticoid deficiency
Renal sodium loss	Drugs causing renal water retention
Mineralocorticoid deficiency (or resistance)	(Hypothyroidism)
Diuretics	**Syndrome of inappropriate antidiuresis**
Salt-wasting renal failure	Classic syndrome of inappropriate secretion of antidiuretic hormone
Salt-wasting tubulopathies (including Bartter syndrome, Gitelman syndrome, and de Toni-Debré-Fanconi syndrome)	Hereditary nephrogenic syndrome of inappropriate antidiuresis
Cerebral salt wasting	**Reduced renal water loss**
Perioperative (e.g., preoperative fasting, vomiting, third space losses)	Chronic renal failure
Third space losses (e.g., burns, major septic shock, surgery)	Oliguric acute renal failure

[a] Effective circulating volume mostly reduced.

increased secretion of brain natriuretic peptide with subsequent suppression of aldosterone synthesis. The distinction between cerebral salt wasting and inappropriate activity of antidiuretic hormone is not always simple to make since the true volume status of the patient is sometimes difficult to ascertain.[15]

Endurance athletes, soldiers during military operations, and desert hikers sometimes replace their dilute, but sodium-containing sweat losses with excessive amounts of hypotonic solutions, with the net effect being a reduction in the circulating sodium level (the effect is likely compounded by a reduced renal blood flow and glomerular filtration rate during exercise). Such individuals may also be taking nonsteroidal anti-inflammatory drugs, which can impair the excretion of free water.[16]

Drugs sometimes cause renal retention of fluids,[6] as given in Table 27-2.

Textbooks indicate that hypothyroidism may cause hyponatremia but the evidence supporting this association is extremely poor.[6,8] Other causes of low sodium concentration should be sought, when hypothyroidism and hyponatremia co-exist.

Hypernatremia

Two mechanisms protect against developing hypernatremia (sodium 145 mmol/L or more) or increased effective blood osmolality: the ability to release antidiuretic hormone and concentrate urine and a powerful thirst mechanism. Release of antidiuretic hormone occurs when the effective blood osmolality exceeds 275 to 280 mosmol/kg H_2O and results in maximally concentrated urine when the effective blood osmolality exceeds 290 to 295 mosmol/kg H_2O. Thirst, the second line of defense, provides additional protection against hypernatremia and increased effective osmolality. If the thirst mechanism is intact and there is unrestricted access to free water, it is rare to develop sustained hypernatremia from either excess sodium ingestion or a renal concentrating defect (Table 27-3).

Hypernatremia is primarily a hospital-acquired condition occurring in children who have restricted access to fluids. Most children with hypernatremia are debilitated by an acute or chronic disease, have neurological impairment, are critically ill, or are born premature. Hypernatremia in the intensive care setting is a particularly common problem, as these children are typically either intubated or moribund, and often are fluid restricted, receive large amounts of sodium as blood products, or have renal concentrating defects from diuretics or renal dysfunction. The majority of hypernatremia results from the failure to administer sufficient free water to children who are unable to care for themselves and have restricted access to fluids.

A frequent cause of hypernatremia in the outpatient setting is breast-feeding–associated hypernatremia, which should more properly be labeled "not-enough-breast-feeding–associated hypernatremia."[17] This condition mostly occurs between days 7 and 15 in otherwise healthy term or near-term (≥35 weeks of gestation) newborns of first-time mothers who are exclusively breast-fed. In all cases, feeding had been difficult to establish and the volume of milk ingested was likely to have been low. The underlying problem is one of water deficiency: sodium concentration rises predominantly as a result of low volume intake and a loss of water, demonstrating that inadequate feeding is the cause of hypernatremic dehydration. In addition, increased breast-milk sodium concentration (which normally may exceed 60 mmol/L in antenatal and postnatal colostrum, falling dramatically by day 3) has been sometimes measured in the milk of mothers whose infant develops hypernatremic dehydration. Monitoring postnatal weight loss provides an objective assessment of the adequacy of nutritional intake, allowing targeted support to those infants who fail to thrive or demonstrate excessive weight loss (10% or more of birth weight).

TABLE 27-2 Antidiuretic Drugs

↑ Water permeability of the renal collecting tubule: arginine vasopressin, vasopressin analogues like desmopressin, oxytocin
↑ Antidiuretic hormone release, ↑ antidiuretic hormone action: carbamazepine, barbiturates, chlorpropamide, clofibrate, colchicine, nicotine, vincristine, cyclophosphamide
↓ Synthesis of prostaglandins: nonsteroidal anti-inflammatory drugs including salicylates, paracetamol
Mechanism unknown: haloperidol, amitriptyline, selective serotonin-reuptake inhibitors like fluoxetine (narcotics like morphine[a])

[a] Evidence supporting the association between narcotics and antidiuresis is rather poor.

Modified from Haycock GB: Hyponatraemia: diagnosis and management, *Arch Dis Child Educ Pract Ed* 91:37-41, 2006.

TABLE 27-3 Cause of Hypernatremia in Childhood

Hypovolemic	Normovolemic	Hypervolemic
Inadequate intake Breast-feeding hypernatremia Poor access to water Altered thirst perception (unconsciousness, mental impairment)	Renal water loss (diabetes insipidus, medullary renal damage) Hypodipsia Fever, hyperventilation	Inappropriate intravenous fluids (e.g., hypertonic saline, $NaHCO_3$) Salt poisoning (accidental, deliberate) Primary aldosteronism (and related conditions)[a]
Intestinal salt loss (diarrheal dehydration)		
Renal water and salt loss (postobstructive polyuria)		

[a] See Table 27-6 (hypernatremia is often mild or even absent in these conditions).

Diarrhea and vomiting are additional reasons for hypernatremia in the outpatient setting, but are much less common than previously reported, presumably because of the advent of low solute infant formulas and the increased use and availability of oral rehydration solutions.[3-5]

Management

The discussion will exclusively focus on some features of parenteral hydration, and the management of hyponatremia with V2 antidiuretic hormone receptor antagonists.

Parenteral Hydration

Intravenous maintenance fluids are designed to provide water and electrolyte requirements in a fasting patient. The prescription for intravenous maintenance fluids was originally described by Holliday,[18] who rationalized a daily H_2O requirement of 1700 to 1800 ml/m^2 body surface area and the addition of 3 and 2 mmol/kg of body weight of Na^+ and K^+, respectively (as it approximates the electrolyte requirements and urinary excretion in healthy infants). This is the basis for the traditional recommendation that hypotonic intravenous maintenance solutions are ideal for children. In clinical practice, the daily parenteral H_2O requirements are mostly calculated as a quantity of milliliters per kilogram of body weight as follows: 100 ml/kg of body weight for a child weighing less than 10 kg plus 50 ml/kg for each additional kilogram up to 20 kg plus 20 ml/kg for each kilogram in excess of 20 kg. In children weighing 5 kg or less, the daily parenteral H_2O requirement is 120 ml/kg of body weight.[18] This approach has been recently questioned because of the potential for these hypotonic solutions to cause hyponatremia and subsequently severe neurological sequelae.[4,19] Surgical patients appear to be the subgroup of children with the highest risk of developing severe hyponatremia with the use of hypotonic intravenous solutions, likely because they tend to be hypovolemic. Furthermore, traditional maintenance fluid recommendations may be much greater than actual water needs in children at risk of hyponatremia.

We suggest that hyponatremia should be prevented by using isotonic (usually normal saline, which contains NaCl at 9 g/L) or near isotonic (usually Ringer lactate) solutions and perhaps also reducing the volume of maintenance fluid (approximately by 20%). Considering the potential for hypoglycemia in infancy, isotonic saline in 5% glucose in water (which contains glucose 50 g/L) seems to be the safest fluid composition for most children. On the other hand, we recommend that this new standard for intravenous fluids be evaluated in rigorous clinical trials.

Dehydration

Oral rehydration therapy is currently the treatment of choice for children with mild to moderate dehydration due to diarrheal diseases.[4,19] Considering the potential of life-threatening hyponatremia in dehydrated children rehydrated parenterally using hypotonic saline solutions, the accelerated intravenous administration of isotonic (or near isotonic) solutions is advised in children with mild to moderate dehydration resistant to initial oral rehydration therapy or with severe dehydration. Children with hypernatremic dehydration are also initially parenterally hydrated with isotonic solutions, followed by slightly hypotonic solution (e.g., half-saline) in order to slowly correct circulating sodium levels (rapidly correcting hypernatremia using a sodium-free glucose solution creates an increased risk for the development of brain edema).

Chronic Hyponatremia

Chronic normovolemic (or hypervolemic) hyponatremia has been traditionally managed either by restricting water intake or by giving salt. An alternative may be the use of nonpeptide antidiuretic hormone receptor antagonists.[20] There are multiple receptors for antidiuretic hormone: the V1a receptor that mediates vasoconstriction, the V1b receptor that mediates adrenocorticotropin release, and especially the V2 receptor that mediates the antidiuretic response. A number of oral V2 receptor antagonists have been approved for the management of normovolemic and hypervolemic hyponatremia: these agents produce a selective water diuresis (without affecting sodium and potassium excretion) that raises the circulating sodium level. No information is currently available for oral V2 receptor antagonists in childhood.

POTASSIUM

Balance

Most (98%) of the potassium in the body (40 to 50 mmol/kg) is in cells. The maintenance of distribution of potassium across cells is largely dependent on the activity of the sodium pump (Na^+-K^+-ATPase). In healthy humans the extracellular potassium concentration is maintained between 3.5 and 5.0 mmol/L. Potassium balance, like that of other ions, is a function of intake and urinary excretion. In adults, the daily potassium intake averages 0.5 to 2.0 mmol/kg of body weight (Figure 27-4). The homeostasis goal of the adult is to remain in zero potassium balance. Thus, approximately 90% to 95% of the typical daily intake of 1 mmol/kg is ultimately eliminated from the body in the urine (the residual 5% to 10% of the daily potassium load is lost through the stool). Infants maintain a state of positive potassium balance (the requirements for growth are estimated to be 1.2 mmol/day during the first 3 months of life, 0.8 mmol/day up to 1 year, and 0.4 mmol/day thereafter). The net accretion of potassium is to ensure the availability of adequate substrate for incorporation into cells newly formed during periods of somatic growth. Postnatal growth is associated with an increase in total body potassium from approximately 8 mmol/cm of body height at birth to more than 14 mmol/cm of body height by 18 years of age. The rate of accretion of body potassium per kg of body weight in the infant is more rapid than in the older child, reflecting both an increase in cell number and potassium concentration, at least in skeletal muscle, with advancing age.[21-23]

Regulation of Circulating Potassium

Circulating potassium concentration is regulated by the total body potassium content, which depends on the external balance—that is, the difference between intake and excretion in the urine, feces, and sweat—and by the internal balance, which represents the relative distribution of potassium between the intracellular and the extracellular space.[21-23]

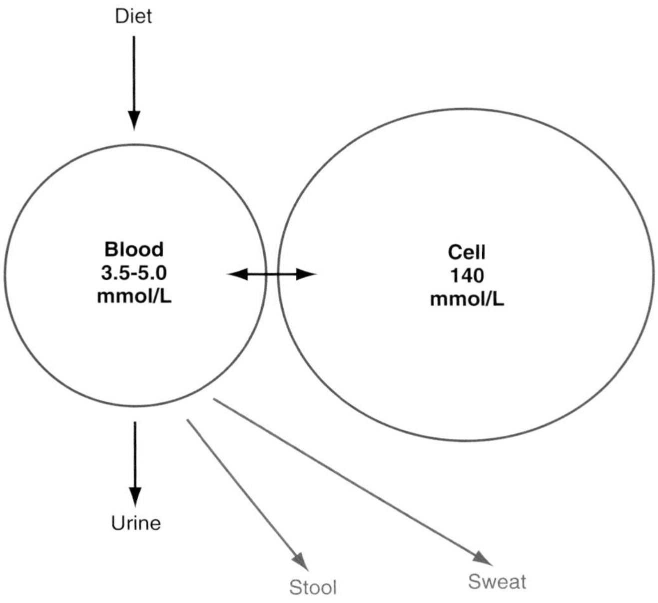

Figure 27-4 Major factors governing the homeostasis of potassium. Most of the potassium in the body is in cells. The maintenance of distribution of potassium across cells is largely dependent on the activity of the sodium pump. Potassium balance, like that of other ions, is a function of intake and urinary excretion. Since only small amounts of potassium are normally lost in the sweat and the stool each day, these factors governing the potassium homeostasis were given a different color. However, substantial intestinal potassium, and therefore potassium depletion, can be seen with vomiting, diarrhea, or other intestinal disease conditions or when sweat production is chronically increased.

TABLE 27-4 **Body Functions Impaired by Hypokalemia**
Cardiovascular Abnormalities
Cardiac arrhythmias (premature atrial and ventricular beats, sinus bradycardia, paroxysmal atrial or junctional tachycardia, atrioventricular block, and ventricular tachycardia or fibrillation)
↑ Systemic vascular resistance
Neuromuscular Disturbances
Skeletal muscle weakness (usually beginning with lower extremities and progressing to trunk and upper extremities; sometimes involvement of respiratory muscles)
Muscle cramps, rhabdomyolysis[a]
Smooth muscle dysfunction (intestinal and urinary system)
Renal Effects
↓ Urinary concentrating ability (decreased expression of the antidiuretic hormone-sensitive water channel aquaporin-2)
↓ Sodium excretion
↑ Renal ammonium production (and therefore ↑ generation of HCO_3)
Hypokalemic nephropathy[b] (interstitial fibrosis, tubular atrophy, cyst formation in the renal medulla)
Endocrine and Metabolic Effects
Negative nitrogen balance (causing growth retardation)
Glucose intolerance (with tendency towards diabetes mellitus)
↓ Aldosterone release (direct adrenal action), ↑ renin secretion
Hepatic encephalopathy (in susceptible individuals)

[a] In rhabdomyolysis hypokalemia may be masked by the release of potassium from the injured muscle.
[b] Following prolonged hypokalemia.

External (Renal) Potassium Homeostasis

Although small amounts of potassium are lost each day in stool and sweat, virtually all regulation of urinary potassium excretion and therefore of external potassium homeostasis occurs in the renal cortical collecting tubule. Indeed, almost all of the filtered potassium is reabsorbed in the proximal tubule and the loop of Henle, so that less than 10% of the filtered load is delivered to the cortical collecting tubule. This tubular segment adjusts the external homeostasis of potassium by modulating its secretion. Little or no potassium secretion or reabsorption takes place in the most distal tubular portions, that is, in the medullary collecting tubule.

The major physiologic regulators of potassium secretion within the cortical collecting tubule are "hyperkalemia" and aldosterone, which act in concert to promote the tubular secretion and therefore the urinary excretion of potassium. Increasing the flow rate traversing the cortical collecting tubule is another factor that may increase the potassium excretion. This response is most prominent in the presence of hyperkalemia, since the concurrent elevations in aldosterone and circulating potassium concentration produce a high level of potassium secretion within the cortical collecting tubule.

Internal Potassium Homeostasis

The main modulators of the distribution of potassium between the intracellular and the extracellular space are insulin, the sympathetic nervous system (via β2-adrenergic receptors), and the acid–base balance (the influence of acid–base balance on potassium homeostasis is discussed in the "Systemic Effects of Acid–Base Abnormalities" section).

Prenatal and Neonatal Potassium Balance

During fetal life, potassium is actively transported across the placenta from the mother to the fetus (indeed, the fetal potassium concentration is maintained at levels exceeding 5.0 mmol/L even in the face of maternal potassium deficiency). The tendency to retain potassium early in postnatal life is reflected by the observation that infants, especially premature newborns, tend to have higher circulating potassium levels than children.[23] Furthermore, in infancy the ability to increase urinary potassium excretion is blunted.

Symptoms, Signs, and Consequences of Hypokalemia and Hyperkalemia

Surplus or deficit of potassium in the extracellular space impairs cardiovascular, neuromuscular, renal, and endocrine-metabolic body functions. The main clinical consequence of these dyselectrolytemias is the predisposition to dangerous cardiac arrhythmias.[21,22] The manifestations of hypokalemia are outlined in Table 27-4, and those of hyperkalemia in Table 27-5.

TABLE 27-5 Body Functions Impaired by Hyperkalemia

Cardiovascular Abnormalities
Cardiac arrhythmias (ventricular fibrillation and standstill are the most severe consequences)
↓ Systemic vascular resistance
Neuromuscular Disturbances
Skeletal muscle weakness (usually beginning with the lower extremities and progressing to trunk and upper extremities; rarely involvement of respiratory muscles)
Smooth muscle dysfunction (intestinal and urinary system)
Renal Effects
↑ Sodium excretion
↓ Renal ammonium production (and therefore ↓ generation of HCO_3)
Endocrine and Metabolic Effects
↑ Aldosterone release (direct adrenal action), ↓ renin secretion

The severity of hypokalemic manifestations is proportionate to the degree and duration of hypokalemia, and symptoms generally do not become manifest until the potassium concentration is below 2.5 or 3.0 mmol/L. Hypokalemia produces characteristic electrocardiographic changes, including depression of the ST segment, decrease in the amplitude of the T wave, and an increase in the amplitude of U waves, which occur at the end of the T wave.

There are very few symptoms or signs of hyperkalemia, and these tend to occur only with very high levels. Symptoms generally do not become manifest until the potassium concentration exceeds 7.0 mmol/L, unless the rise in concentration has been very rapid. Hyperkalemia produces the following electrocardiographic changes: peaked T wave with shortened QT interval is the first change, followed by progressive lengthening of the PR interval and QRS duration. The severity of hyperkalemia is classified as follows: mild, potassium between 5.1 and 6.0 mmol/L and absent or equivocal electrocardiographic changes; moderate, potassium between 6.1 and 7.0 mmol/L and definite electrocardiographic changes in repolarization ("peaked" T waves); and severe, potassium 7.1 mmol/L or more and severe definite eletrocardiographic changes including atrial standstill, advanced atrioventricular heart block, QRS widening, or ventricular arrhythmia (usually associated with weakness of skeletal muscle).

Evaluating the Causes of Hypokalemia and Hyperkalemia (Diagnostic Tests)

The following tests have been developed to evaluate and distinguish the various causes of hypo- or hyperkalemia in childhood.[22,24-26]

The transtubular potassium concentration gradient, which is sometimes colloquially referred as TTKG, measures the potassium secretion within the cortical collecting tubule and represents an estimate of the aldosterone activity. This parameter can be easily calculated, assuming that the urine osmolality at the end of the cortical collecting tubule is similar to that of blood, and that no potassium secretion or reabsorption takes place in the medullary collecting tubule. If these assumptions are accurate, then the potassium concentration in the final urine will rise above that in the cortical collecting tubule due to reabsorption of water in the medullary collecting duct. This effect can be accounted for by dividing the urine potassium concentration by the ratio of the urine to blood osmolality. If, for example, this ratio is 2, then 50% of the water leaving the cortical collecting tubule has been reabsorbed in the medulla, thereby doubling the luminal potassium concentration. This parameter is calculated as follows:

$$\frac{\dfrac{\text{Urinary potassium}}{\text{Urinary osmolality}}}{\dfrac{\text{Blood osmolality}}{\text{Circulating potassium}}}$$

Blood osmolality (in milliosmoles per kilogram) can be measured with an osmometer or very reasonably estimated[26] from circulating sodium, glucose, and urea (in millimoles per liter) as follows: ($Na^+ \times 2$) + glucose + urea. On the other hand, urinary osmolality (in millimoles per/kg H_2O) can be measured with an osmometer or estimated,[26] in the absence of proteinuria and glucosuria, from the specific gravity as determined by refractometry as follows: (specific gravity − 1000) × 40.

Another two frequently used tests, the fractional clearance of potassium (which measures the amount of filtered potassium that is excreted in the urine),

$$\frac{\text{Urinary potassium} \times \text{circulating creatine}}{\text{Circulating potassium} \times \text{urinary creatine}}$$

and the urinary potassium/creatinine ratio (mol/mol),

$$\frac{\text{Urinary potassium}}{\text{Urinary creatinine}}$$

are strongly correlated.

Also suggested are the following closely correlated tests—the fractional clearance of chloride (which measures the amount of filtered chloride that is excreted in the urine),

$$\frac{\text{Urinary chloride} \times \text{circulating creatinine}}{\text{Circulating chloride} \times \text{urinary creatinine}}$$

and especially the urinary chloride/creatinine ratio (moles per mole and millimoles per milligram, respectively)

$$\frac{\text{Urinary chloride}}{\text{Urinary creatinine}}$$

The urinary potassium/creatinine and the urinary chloride/creatinine indices are based on a near-constant creatinine excretion rate, and consequently might have a limited significance in patients with a very low body mass index.

The 24-hour excretion of potassium is another useful diagnostic test. The use of this traditional diagnostic test is not generally advised, considering that 24-hour urine collections are troublesome and difficult to obtain (and often imprecise) in children who are not hospitalized, are not practical in a medical emergency, and almost impossible without invasive techniques such as bladder catheterization in infants.

In our opinion, the following "urinary tests" are useful to distinguish the various causes of hypokalemia and hyperkalemia. In normotensive children with hypokalemia, the transtubular potassium gradient and the urinary potassium/creatinine ratio (and perhaps the fractional clearance of potassium) easily help distinguish hypokalemia due to a short-term shift of the ion into cells (transtubular potassium gradient <2.5, urinary potassium/creatinine <2.5 mol/mol, respectively, or <0.022 mmol/mg) from hypokalemia resulting from a deficit of this ion, including renal potassium-losing conditions and hypokalemia complicating intestinal diseases. (In patients experiencing diarrhea, secondary hyperaldosteronism caused by circulating volume depletion leads to an increased urine potassium excretion. See Table 27-15.)

In normotensive children with hypokalemia and metabolic alkalosis, the urinary excretion of chloride helps distinguish renal (urinary chloride/creatinine ratio largely higher than 10 mol/mol, respectively, or 0.09 mmol/mg) from extrarenal (urinary chloride/creatinine ratio less than 10 mol/mol) causes, as stated in the section on metabolic alkalosis.

Note: Physicians sometimes incorrectly assume that when hypokalemia occurs in the context of extrarenal conditions, the fractional clearance of potassium, the urinary potassium/creatinine ratio, and the 24-hour excretion of potassium are very low, therefore discriminating between extrarenal and renal conditions. However, in most children with extrarenal hypokalemia, extracellular volume depletion is present also, leading to secondary activation of the renin-angiotensin II-aldosterone system, and therefore to increased urinary potassium excretion. As a consequence, urinary potassium excretion sometimes does not discriminate between the extrarenal and renal conditions associated with hypokalemia.

In hyperkalemia, the urinary potassium/creatinine ratio and the transtubular potassium gradient help distinguish impaired from unimpaired urinary potassium excretion. In subjects with unimpaired urinary potassium excretion, the urinary potassium/creatinine ratio is expected to be more than 20 mol/mol (0.18 mmol/mg), the transtubular potassium gradient is greater than 7.0.

Hypokalemia

The clinician evaluating a child with hypokalemia (<3.5 mmol/L) should consider five groups of causes[21,22,27]: spurious hypokalemia; redistribution; true potassium depletion due to extrarenal (mostly intestinal) conditions; potassium depletion due to renal conditions; and hypokalemia associated with an expanded "effective" circulating volume, and therefore with systemic hypertension due to enhanced mineralocorticoid activity (Table 27-6).

The total potassium stores are reduced only in subjects with hypokalemia due to extrarenal or renal conditions. However, the body potassium content is normal in children with spurious hypokalemia, in those with an increased shift of potassium into cells, and in those with hypokalemia associated with an expanded "effective" circulating volume.

Occasionally, metabolically active cells take up potassium after blood has been drawn and before it has been tested in the laboratory. This condition, which has been called spurious hypokalemia, has been noted in patients with acute myeloid leukemia associated with a very high, white blood cell count and in hot weather. The problem of spurious hypokalemia, which is much more rare than spurious hyperkalemia, can be avoided if plasma (or serum) is rapidly separated from the cells or if the blood is stored at 4°C. A useful clue is that there are no characteristic electrocardiogram changes.

Normal total body potassium content with hypokalemia results from an increased shift of this ion into cells. Metabolic alkalosis, increased endogenous secretion or exogenous administration of insulin, sympathetic activation, and exogenous administration of β_2-adrenergic receptors are the main causes of hypokalemia caused by cellular uptake of potassium. Hypokalemic periodic paralysis is an uncommon form of hypokalemia resulting from an increased shift of potassium into cells, which is characterized by recurrent episodes of hypokalemia (associated with hypophosphatemia and mild hypomagnesemia) and muscular weakness or paralysis that occurs primarily in males of Asian descent. The hypokalemic episodes are precipitated by rest after exercise, a carbohydrate meal, or the administration of insulin or β_2-adrenergic agonists (e.g., epinephrine).

The potassium stores may be depleted when dietary potassium is very low and therefore fails to counterbalance the obligatory potassium losses and, in infancy and childhood, the required potassium accretion. Since the kidney is able to lower potassium excretion to very low figures in the presence of potassium depletion, decreased intake alone will cause hypokalemia only in rare cases. However, it contributes to the severity of potassium depletion when another problem is superimposed. Under normal circumstances the net fluid loss from the skin and the gastrointestinal tract is small, therefore preventing the development of potassium depletion. Sometimes, in cases such as prolonged exertion in a hot, dry environment, in cystic fibrosis (in these patients sweat contains a large amount of sodium, potassium, and chloride), and especially in the context of various gastrointestinal conditions (Table 27-6) potassium loss occurs. In most of these cases extracellular volume depletion is present also, leading to secondary activation of the renin-angiotensin II-aldosterone system, and further worsening the potassium deficiency. It has been also suggested that in some patients with diarrheal states an increased urinary potassium excretion plays a more important role than intestinal losses in the development of potassium deficiency. Hypokalemia is mostly associated with metabolic alkalosis after poor dietary potassium intake, in the context of "upper" gastrointestinal conditions or in conditions associated with increased sweating and with acidosis in "lower" gastrointestinal conditions. Finally, renal potassium losses occur either associated with acidosis or, more frequently, with alkalosis.

Excessive mineralocorticoid activity is the main cause of hypokalemia associated with metabolic alkalosis and arterial hypertension. The underlying mechanism will be discussed elsewhere.

Clinical Workup

The clue to the diagnosis of spurious hypokalemia is a normal electrocardiogram without the characteristic changes. Con-

TABLE 27-6 **Causes of Hypokalemia**

Spurious Hypokalemia (cells take up potassium after blood has been drawn)

Hypokalemia Associated with Normal or Low Blood Pressure

- Increased shift of potassium into cells (total body K^+ content normal)
  - Activation of β_2-adrenergic receptors
    - Endogenous: stress, hypothermia
    - Exogenous: β_2-adrenergic agonists (e.g., albuterol), xanthines
  - Hormones
    - Insulin
      - Endogenous: anabolism (e.g., refeeding syndrome)
      - Exogenous: treatment of diabetic ketoacidosis
    - Possibly aldosterone
  - Alkalosis (metabolic)
  - Rare causes
    - Hypokalemic periodic paralysis
      - Congenital (autosomal dominant inheritance)
      - Complicating thyreotoxicosis (particularly in Chinese males)
    - Barium-induced hypokalemia, acute chloroquine intoxication
    - Maturation of red cell precursors after treatment of megaloblastic anemia with vitamin B_{12} or folic acid
    - Paraneoplastic hypokalemia secondary to increased cell synthesis in acute myeloid leukemia[a]

- True potassium depletion (total body K^+ content reduced)
  - Extrarenal "conditions"
    - Prolonged poor potassium intake, protein-energy malnutrition
    - Gastrointestinal conditions
      - Gastric (associated with alkalosis): vomiting, nasogastric suction
      - Small bowel
        - Associated with acidosis: biliary drainage, intestinal fistula, malabsorption, diarrhea (including diarrhea associated with AIDS), radiation enteropathy
        - Associated with alkalosis: congenital chloride diarrhea
      - Large bowel
        - Associated with acidosis: ureterosigmoidostomy
        - Acid–base balance unpredictable: bowel cleansing agents, laxatives, clay ingestion, potassium-binding resin ingestion
    - Sweating, full thickness burns
    - Dialysis
  - Renal "conditions"
    - Interstitial nephritis, postobstructive diuresis, recovery from acute renal failure
    - With metabolic acidosis: renal tubular acidosis (type I or II), carbonic anhydrase inhibitors (e.g., acetazolamide), amphotericin B, outdated tetracyclines
    - With metabolic alkalosis
    - Inherited conditions: Bartter syndrome, Gitelman syndrome, and related syndromes
      - Acquired conditions: normotensive primary aldosteronism, loop and thiazide diuretics, high-dose antibiotics (penicillin, naficillin, ampicillin, carbenicillin, ticarcillin), magnesium depletion
      - Acid–base balance unpredictable: cetuximab[b]

Hypokalemia Associated with High Blood Pressure (often linked with metabolic alkalosis; total K^+ body content normal)

↓ Renin: primary aldosteronism (either hyperplasia or adenoma), apparent mineralocorticoid excess (defect in 11-β-hydroxysteroid-dehydrogenase), Liddle syndrome (congenitally increased function of the collecting tubule sodium channels), dexamethasone-responsive aldosteronism (synthesis of aldosterone promoted not only by renin but also by adrenocorticotropin), congenital adrenal hyperplasia (11-β-hydroxylase or 17-α-hydroxylase deficiency), Cushing disease, exogenous mineralocorticoids, licorice ingestion (11-β-hydroxysteroid-dehydrogenase blockade)

→ or ↑ renin: renal artery stenosis, malignant hypertension, renin-producing tumor

[a] The pathogenic mechanism includes also hyperkaluresis due to activation of the renin-angiotensin II system.
[b] A monoclonal antibody that binds to the epidermal growth factor receptor and thereby inhibits cell proliferation, metastasis, and angiogenesis.

sidering that the great majority of children with true hypokalemia have either a gastrointestinal condition or take drugs associated with renal potassium wasting, the causes of hypokalemia can almost always be discerned clinically. When the data obtained from the clinical history fail to establish a presumptive diagnosis, the following simple steps are suggested:[21,22,24,28]

Repeated measurement of blood pressure.

Concurrent determination of the acid–base balance, Na^+, Cl^-, Ca^{++}, Mg^{++}, inorganic phosphate, alkaline phosphatase, uric acid, and especially urea and creatinine.

In normotensive subjects, the urinary potassium/creatinine ratio distinguishes hypokalemia due to a short-term shift of the ion into cells (ratio <2.5 mol/mol, respectively, or 0.022 mg/mmol) from hypokalemia resulting due to a deficit of the ion.

In normotensive subjects with hypokalemia and metabolic alkalosis, the urinary chloride/creatinine ratio discriminates renal from extrarenal (ratio <10 mol/mol, respectively, 0.09 mmol/mg) causes.

Management

Considering the numerous origins of hypokalemia, this section will focus only on the urgency and the mode of substitution in patients with normotensive hypokalemia.[27]

The urgency for substitution is dictated by the following factors: conditions that increase the likelihood of dangerous cardiac arrhythmias, the possibility that potassium will shift into cells (e.g., during recovery from diabetic ketoacidosis), severe muscle weakness in a child who must intensively hyperventilate because of metabolic acidosis, magnitude of the ongoing potassium losses (e.g., during severe diarrhea), and degree of hypokalemia.

Potassium Preparations

- Potassium chloride: preferred among patients with metabolic alkalosis due to diuretic therapy, or vomiting
- Potassium citrate or potassium bicarbonate: prescribed in patients with hypokalemia and metabolic acidosis (this most often occurs in renal tubular acidosis)
- Potassium phosphate: administered in recovery from diabetic ketoacidosis, in subjects at risk of refeeding syndrome and during total parenteral nutrition

The concurrent intravenous administration of potassium chloride with glucose or bicarbonate is not advised in patients with severe hypokalemia, because they cause a shift of potassium into cells and transiently reduce circulating potassium concentration.

The safest way to administer potassium is by mouth. Intestinal conditions that limit intake or absorption of potassium, severe hypokalemia (<2.5 mmol/L), characteristic electrocardiogram abnormalities (with or without cardiac arrhythmias), or respiratory muscle weakness and an anticipated shift of potassium into cells mandate intravenous substitution.

Intravenous Potassium Chloride

In a child with a very severe degree of hypokalemia and an abnormal electrocardiogram, the aim will be to raise potassium to a theoretical value of 3.0 mmol/L in 1 to 2 minutes. The amount of intravenous potassium (in millimoles) will be chosen from measured potassium (in millimoles/L) and body weight (in kilograms) using the formula:

$$(3.0 - \text{Measured } K^{+}) \times \text{Body weight} \times 0.04$$

The basis for this decision is as follows: the total blood volume approximates 7% of body weight (this volume circulates each minute, cardiac output being at least 70 ml/min/kg of body weight) and plasma volume 60% of blood volume, that is, approximately 4% of body weight. Consequently, a 50.0-kg adolescent with a very severe hypokalemia of 1.5 mmol/L will be given $(3.0 - 1.5) \times 50 \times 0.04 = 3.0$ mmol of potassium chloride in 1 to 2 minutes. Considering that infused potassium will mix with interstitial fluid (approximately three to four times the plasma volume) before reaching the cell membrane, there will be a much smaller increase in potassium concentration near the cell membranes. Following this bolus, the rate of infusion of potassium should be reduced to 0.015 mmol/kg of body weight per minute, and measurement of potassium concentration should be repeated every 5 to 10 minutes.

Note: The potassium supplementation should be minimal if hypokalemia is due exclusively to an abnormal distribution of the total potassium stores (e.g., exogenous administration of β_2-adrenergic receptors or hypokalemic periodic paralysis).

In conditions demanding intravenous potassium but without acute emergency, the rate of infused potassium should not exceed 0.5 to 1.0 mmol/kg of body weight hourly. Furthermore, the potassium concentration in intravenous solutions should be less than 60 mmol/L for use in peripheral veins because higher concentrations lead to local discomfort, venous spasm, and sclerosis.

Parenteral supplemental potassium administration is a common cause of severe hyperkalemia. Consequently, the safest route to give potassium is by mouth. A traditional approach to minimizing hypokalemia is to ensure adequate dietary potassium intake (unfortunately, the potassium contained in foods that have a high potassium content is almost entirely coupled with phosphate rather than with chloride, and therefore is not effective in repairing potassium loss associated with chloride depletion, including use of diuretics, vomiting, or nasogastric drainage). In most circumstances, oral replacement with potassium chloride (1 to 3 mmol/kg of body weight daily in divided doses) is effective in correcting hypokalemia.

Hyperkalemia

The clinician evaluating a child with hyperkalemia (>5.5 mmol/L) will initially consider the possible diagnosis of spurious hyperkalemia (Table 27-7). The term refers to conditions in which the elevation in the measured potassium is due to potassium movement out of the cells during or after the blood specimen has been drawn.[21,22,25,27,29] The major cause of this problem is mechanical trauma during venipuncture, resulting in the release of potassium from red cells and a characteristic reddish tint of the serum (or plasma) due to the release of hemoglobin. In very rare instances, however, red serum (or red plasma) represents severe intravascular hemolysis rather than a hemolyzed specimen. Furthermore, spurious hyperkalemia can also occur in hereditary spherocytosis and in familial pseudohyperkalemia, a rare autosomal dominant disorder recognized as a laboratory artifact. In the circulation, the sodium and potassium content of red cells is normal in familial pseudohyperkalemia. However, the plasma or serum potassium concentration is elevated in the laboratory measurement because of an abnormally high rate of efflux of potassium from the red cells when the temperature is lowered below 22°C. The in vitro potassium efflux can be reversed by incubation at 37°C. Potassium also moves out of white cells and platelets after clotting has occurred. Thus, serum potassium concentration normally exceeds the true value in the plasma by 0.1 to 0.5 mmol/L. Although in normals this difference is clinically insignificant, the measured serum potassium concentration may be as high as 9 mmol/L in patients with marked leukocytosis or thrombocytosis. Spurious hyperkalemia is suspected whenever there is no apparent cause for the elevation in the serum potassium concentration in an asymptomatic patient.

TABLE 27-7 Causes of Hyperkalemia
Spurious Hyperkalemia (potassium movement out of cells during or after blood has been drawn)
Mechanical trauma during venipuncture
Hereditary spherocytosis
Familial pseudohyperkalemia
True Hyperkalemia
Increased potassium load[a]
Increased shift of potassium out of cells Normal anion gap metabolic acidosis Insulin deficiency Extracellular hypertonicity Increased tissue catabolism (severe hemolysis, rhabdomyolysis, tumor lysis syndrome, immediately after cardiac surgery) Severe exercise Familial hyperkalemic periodic paralysis (Gamstorp disease) Hyperkalemia of premature infant
Impaired renal potassium excretion Global renal failure: acute or chronic Hyperreninemic hypoaldosteronism: adrenal insufficiency (Addison disease), salt-losing congenital adrenal hyperplasia (21-hydroxylase deficiency) Hyporeninemic hypoaldosteronism: idiopathic, complicating acute glomerulonephritis or mild-to-moderate renal failure) Pseudohypoaldosteronism Type 1 (cortical collecting tubule) Primary Autosomal recessive[b]: reduced sodium channel activity Autosomal dominant: mutations in gene for mineralocorticoid receptor, phenotype mild and transient Secondary: complicating obstructive uropathy, systemic lupus erythematosus, sickle cell disease, renal transplantation, or renal amyloidosis Type 2 (familial hyperkalemic hypertension or Gordon syndrome[c])

Note: Drugs associated with hyperkalemia appear in Table 27-8.
[a] Not a cause of hyperkalemia, unless very acute (and important) or occurring in subjects with impaired potassium excretion (due, for example, to underlying kidney disease).
[b] Autosomal recessive pseudohypoaldosteronism type 1 is opposite to Liddle syndrome.
[c] The clinical phenotype of Gordon syndrome is opposite to Gitelman syndrome.

True hyperkalemia (Table 27-7) occurs rarely in normal subjects, because cellular and urinary adaptations prevent substantial extracellular potassium accumulation. Furthermore, the efficiency of potassium handling is increased if potassium intake is enhanced, thereby tolerating what might be a fatal potassium load. These observations lead to three conclusions concerning the development of hyperkalemia.

First, increasing potassium load is not a cause of chronic hyperkalemia, unless very acute or occurring in a patient with impaired urinary potassium excretion. In special conditions, acute hyperkalemia can be induced (primarily in infants because of their small size) by the intravenous administration of unusual large doses of potassium or the use of stored blood for transfusions.

Second, the net release of potassium from the cells can cause a transient elevation in the serum potassium concentration (in the presence of normal or even low total body potassium stores). Four causes of true hyperkalemia resulting from release of the ion from cells will be discussed: (1) extracellular hypertonicity, (2) tumor lysis syndrome, (3) hyperkalemic familial periodic paralysis, and (4) nonoliguric hyperkalemia of the premature infant.

Elevated extracellular tonicity results in water movement from the cells into the extracellular fluid. This is linked with potassium movement out of the cells by two mechanisms. The loss of water raises the intracellular potassium level, creating a gradient for passive potassium exit, and second, the friction forces between water and solute result in potassium being carried along with water. Hypertonicity-induced hyperkalemia occurs in hyperglycemia, in hypernatremia, and following administration of mannitol.

The phenotype of acute tumor lysis syndrome is opposite to refeeding syndrome. The term denotes the metabolic abnormalities that occur either spontaneously or immediately after initiation of cytotoxic therapy in neoplastic disorders.[30] The findings include hyperuricemia, hyperkalemia, hyperphosphatemia, hypocalcemia (due to precipitation of calcium phosphate), and acute renal failure. The syndrome has been noted in children with a tumor characterized by rapid cell turnover such as lymphomas (particularly non-Hodgkin's lymphoma) and some leukemias. The distinction between spontaneous tumor lysis syndrome and that noted during therapy is the lack of hyperphosphatemia in the spontaneous form. It has been suggested that rapidly growing tumors with high cell turnover rates lead to high uric acid levels through rapid nucleoprotein turnover, but the tumors reutilize released phosphorus for synthesis of new tumor cells. In contrast, the acute increase in uric acid levels associated with chemotherapy is due to cell destruction; in this setting, there are no new cancer cells to reutilize the released phosphate.

Hyperkalemic familial periodic paralysis, or Gamstorp disease, is a rare inherited autosomal dominant disease that causes patients to experience episodes of flaccid weakness associated with increased potassium levels (please note that the most common cause of hyperkalemic skeletal muscle paralysis results from hyperkalemia of any cause). In this syndrome, hyperkalemia occurs with increased potassium intake, cold weather, exercise, or at rest. The attacks of paralysis, however, are not always linked with hyperkalemia.

Nonoliguric hyperkalemia (>6.5 mmol/L) of the premature infant is a common and serious condition. The features are a rapid rise of potassium concentration to excessively high values at 24 hours after birth, a tendency towards cardiac arrhythmia, and occurrence only within 72 hours after birth exclusively in premature infants. This peculiar condition mainly results from a potassium loss from the intra- into the extra-cellular space. Moreover, renal potassium excretion that is dependent on both glomerular filtration rate and urinary output is slightly decreased in this setting. Finally aldosterone unresponsiveness, rather than a decreased concentration of aldosterone, also contributes to the degree of hyperkalemia. However, since there is no significant potassium intake during the first days of life of premature infants, even total absence of renal potassium excretion cannot increase potassium concentration, if there is no intra- to extra-cellular potassium shift.[25,31]

Third, persistent hyperkalemia requires an impaired urinary potassium excretion (the total body potassium stores are increased in this condition). Two factors modulate renal potassium homeostasis in the cortical collecting tubule: "hyperkalemia" and aldosterone, which act in concert to promote the tubular secretion and therefore the excretion of potassium, and the flow rate traversing the cortical collecting tubule. Consequently, a decreased aldosterone release, a decreased aldosterone effect, or a decreased renal tubular flow rate are the major conditions impairing urinary potassium excretion.

Any cause of decreased aldosterone release or effect can diminish the efficiency of potassium secretion and lead to hyperkalemia. The ensuing tendency towards hyperkalemia directly stimulates potassium secretion, partially overcoming the relative absence of aldosterone. The net effect is that the rise in the serum potassium concentration is generally small in patients with normal renal function, but can be clinically important in the presence of underlying renal insufficiency or with multiple insults.

The ability to maintain potassium excretion at near normal levels is habitually preserved in advanced renal disease as long as both aldosterone secretion and distal flow are maintained. Thus, hyperkalemia generally develops in oliguria or in the presence of an additional problem including high potassium diet, increased tissue breakdown, or reduced aldosterone bioactivity. Impaired cell uptake of potassium also contributes to the development of hyperkalemia in advanced renal failure. Decreased distal tubular flow rate due to marked effective volume depletion, as in heart failure or a salt-wasting nephropathy can also induce hyperkalemia.

Acute and chronic renal failure, the most recognized causes of impaired urinary potassium excretion, will be discussed elsewhere. Hyperkalemia and a tendency towards hyponatremia and metabolic acidosis characteristically occur in children with hyperreninemic hypoaldosteronism (including classic congenital adrenal hyperplasia), hyporeninemic hypoaldosteronism, and end-organ resistance to aldosterone, mostly referred to as pseudohypoaldosteronism. In the United States, Japan, and most European countries, neonatal screening (measurement of 17-hydroxy-hydroxyprogesterone in filter paper blood) identifies children affected by classic congenital adrenal hyperplasia due to 21-hydroxylase deficiency before salt-wasting crises with hyperkalemia develop. Consequently, in these countries classic congenital adrenal hyperplasia is nowadays an uncommon cause of hyperkalemia. In our experience, secondary type 1 pseudohypoaldosteronism is, together with advanced renal failure, a common cause of true hyperkalemia, at least in infancy. Secondary type 1 psedudohypoaldosteronism develops in infants with urinary tract infections, in infants with urinary tract anomalies (either obstructive or vesicoureteral reflux), and especially in infants with both urinary tract infections and urinary tract anomalies. On the contrary, secondary type 1 pseudohypoaldosteronism does not occur in older children with urinary tract infections or urinary tract anomalies.[25,32]

Finally, the syndrome of (acquired) hyporeninemic hypoaldosteronism, which is characterized by mild hyperkalemia and metabolic acidosis, is due to diminished renin release and, subsequently, decreased angiotensin II and aldosterone production. The syndrome, which mostly occurs in subjects with mild renal failure, has been first reported in subjects with overt diabetic kidney disease, has been occasionally noted in children with acute glomerulonephritis and mild-to-moderate chronic renal failure.[25,33]

Prescribed medications, over-the-counter drugs, and nutritional supplements that are used by many people may disrupt potassium balance and promote the development of hyperkalemia, as shown in Table 27-8. Although most of these products are well tolerated, drug-induced hyperkalemia may develop in subjects with underlying renal impairment or other abnormalities in potassium handling. However, their hyperkalemic action is less evident in children than in elderly subjects.

Clinical Workup

The clue to the diagnosis of spurious hyperkalemia, the most common cause of elevated potassium levels in clinically asymptomatic infants and children, is a normal electrocardiogram without the characteristic changes.

Considering that the great majority of children with true hyperkalemia have renal failure (either acute or chronic), secondary type 1 pseudohypoaldosteronism or take drugs that can cause hyperkalemia, the causes of hyperkalemia, a common clinical problem, can almost always be discerned clinically. When the data obtained from the clinical history fail to establish a presumptive diagnosis, the following simple steps are suggested:[21,33,25,26,29]

Repeated measurement of blood pressure.

Concurrent determination of the acid–base balance, Na^+, Cl^-, Ca^{++}, Mg^{++}, inorganic phosphate, alkaline phosphatase, uric acid, and especially urea and creatinine.

In subjects with true hyperkalemia, unrelated to an impaired urinary potassium excretion the expected urinary potassium/creatinine ratio is greater than 20 mol/mol (>0.18 mmol/mg) and the transtubular potassium gradient more than 10.

TABLE 27-8 **Drugs Associated with Hyperkalemia**

Medication	Mechanism of Action
Increased K^+ Input	K^+ ingestion or infusion
K^+ supplements (and salt substitutes)	
Nutritional and herbal supplements	
Stored packed red blood cells	
Potassium-containing penicillins	
Transcellular K^+ Shifts	
β-adrenergic receptor antagonists	↓ β_2-driven K^+ uptake
Intravenous amino acids (lysine, arginine, aminocaproic acid)	↑ K^+ release from cells
Succinylcholine	Depolarized cell membranes
Digoxin intoxication	↓ Na^+ pump
Impaired Renal Excretion	
Potassium-sparing diuretics	
Spironolactone, eplerenone	Aldosterone antagonism
Triamterene, amiloride	Na^+ channels blocked (collecting tubule)
Trimethoprim[a], pentamidine	Na^+ channels blocked (collecting tubule)
Nonsteroidal anti-inflammatory drugs	↓ Aldosterone synthesis, ↓ glomerular filtration rate, ↓ renal blood flow
Blockers of the renin-angiotensin II-aldosterone system (converting enzyme inhibitors, angiotensin II-antagonists, renin inhibitors)	↓ Aldosterone synthesis
Heparins (both unfractionated and low-molecular-weight heparins)	↓ Aldosterone synthesis
Calcineurin inhibitors (e.g., cyclosporine and tacrolimus)	↓ Aldosterone synthesis, ↓ Na^+-pump, ↓ K^+-channels

[a] Including cotrimoxazole, the fixed combination of trimethoprim with sulfomethoxazole.
Modified from Alfonzo AV, Isles C, Geddes C, Deighan C: Potassium disorders—clinical spectrum and emergency management, *Resuscitation* 70:10-25, 2006; and Hollander-Rodríguez JC, Calvert JF Jr: Hyperkalemia, *Am Fam Physician* 73:283-90, 2006.

Management

Because many conditions account for true hyperkalemia, there is no universal therapy for this dyselectrolytemia. The following measures deserve consideration upon recognition of hyperkalemia with increased total body potassium stores[27,29]:

- Interruption of excessive dietary potassium intake.
- Discontinuation of drugs that may cause hyperkalemia.
- Increasing renal potassium excretion (for this purpose children without end-stage renal failure or physical signs of fluid overload must have substantial salt intake via oral or parenteral routes. The use of a loop diuretic, less frequently a thiazide diuretic, also increases renal potassium excretion). (A low salt intake and extracellular fluid volume depletion are the most commonly observed contributing factor in the development of hyperkalemia in children with renal failure. In patients with a salt-retaining disease proper management is achieved by avoiding severe restriction of dietary salt while concurrently administering diuretics.)
- Increasing gastrointestinal potassium excretion using cation exchange resins.
- Institution of dialysis in children with end-stage renal failure.

Emergencies

Because of the deleterious cardiac effects, severe hyperkalemia (potassium at 7.1 mmol/L or more with electrocardiographic abnormalities) requires emergency intervention. The following measures, which are listed according to rapidity of action, have been recommended:

- Intravenous calcium, which directly antagonizes the membrane actions of hyperkalemia.
- Intravenous insulin (and glucose), which lowers extracellular potassium levels by driving potassium into cells.
- Intravenous or nebulized β_2-adrenergic agonists, which, like insulin, drive potassium into cells (the reduction in potassium concentration is more pronounced in adult patients given nebulized β_2-adrenergic agonists than in those given intravenous albuterol but these data likely do not apply for small children who do not inhale correctly).
- Intravenous $NaHCO_3$ results in H^+-ion release from cells (as part of the buffering reaction) is accompanied by potassium movement into cells to preserve electroneutrality.

Available data[27,29] indicate that intravenous (or nebulized) albuterol, a β_2-adrenergic agonist, or intravenous insulin (and glucose) are the best supported recommendations. Their combination may be more effective than either alone, and although there are no properly conducted studies assessing the efficacy of calcium, little doubt remains of its effectiveness in treating arrhythmias. Evidence for the use of intravenous $NaHCO_3$ is equivocal. For practical purposes, the emergency interventions given in Table 27-9 are advised.

ACID–BASE BALANCE

Blood pH, one of the most crucial physiological variables, is maintained within narrow limits, as given in Table 27-10. Inspection of the (simplified) Henderson-Hasselbalch equation,[34,35]

$$pH = pK + \frac{HCO_3}{pCO_2}$$

TABLE 27-9 Currently Recommended Emergency Intervention for Severe Hyperkalemia (≥7.1 mmol/L) with Electrocardiogram Abnormalities

Medication	Dosage	Onset (minutes)	Duration of Effect (hours)	Comments/Cautions
Nebulized albuterol	10-20 mg (diluted in 4 ml of saline) over 10 minutes	15-30	4-6	May increase heart rate
Intravenous albuterol	10 μg/kg body weight over 15 minutes	15-30	4-6	May increase heart rate
Glucose and insulin	Glucose 0.5-1.0 g/kg body weight and insulin 0.1 U/kg body weight intravenously over 15 minutes	15-30	4-6	Tendency towards hypoglycemia (monitor blood glucose level)
Intravenous calcium	4.5-9.0 mg/kg body weight over 1-3 minutes	Immediate	0.5-1	Does not lower potassium level

Notes: Albuterol and intravenous glucose (with insulin) lower extracellular potassium level by driving potassium into the cell, while calcium directly antagonizes the membrane actions of hyperkalemia but does not modify extracellular potassium concentration. None of the recommended emergency interventions modifies total body potassium content.

TABLE 27-10 Acid–Base Balance in Healthy Infants and Children (Reference Values)

Age	pH	pCO_2 (mmHg)[a]	Bicarbonate (mmol/L)
Preterm (1 week)[b]	7.22-7.46	25-37	14.8-19.6
Preterm (6 weeks)[b]	7.34-7.42	23-47	13.1-30.7
Term (birth)[c]	7.14-7.34	29-69	14.4-25.6
Term (1 hour)[c]	7.27-7.47	25-43	14.4-21.6
3-6 months[b]	7.33-7.45	30-42	18.2-25.8
21-24 months[b]	7.36-7.44	29-41	18.8-25.0
2.1-5.4 years[d]	7.31-7.48	29-45	19.9-25.1
5.5-12 years[d]	7.34-7.46	32-44	20.7-25.5
>12 years[d]	7.32-7.44	35-45	22.0-26.5

[a] To obtain SI units (kPa), divide by 7.5.
[b] Arterialized capillary blood.
[c] Umbilical artery blood.
[d] Arterial blood.

makes clear that abnormalities of blood pH result either from a deviation in circulating bicarbonate (millimoles per liter of HCO_3^-) or partial pressure of carbon dioxide (pCO_2, mmHg).

There are four primary disturbances of acid–base balance. Since alveolar ventilation regulates pCO_2, any disturbance in pH that results from a primary change in pCO_2 is called respiratory acid–base disorder. Retention of CO_2 leads to a reduction in pH (<7.35) called respiratory acidosis, a fall in pCO_2 leads to a rise in pH (>7.45) called respiratory alkalosis. On the other side, primary changes in the concentration of HCO_3^- are called metabolic acid–base disorders. A primary reduction in HCO_3^- is termed metabolic acidosis and a primary increase in HCO_3^- is called metabolic alkalosis.

The Henderson-Hasselbalch equation shows that blood pH is determined by the ratio between HCO_3^- and pCO_2, not either compound alone. Thus, primary respiratory disturbances (primary changes in pCO_2) invoke compensatory metabolic responses (secondary changes in HCO_3^-), and primary metabolic disturbances (primary changes in HCO_3^-) elicit compensatory respiratory responses (secondary changes in pCO_2). For instance, metabolic acidosis due to an increase in endogenous acids (e.g., ketoacidosis) lowers extracellular fluid HCO_3^- and decreases extracellular pH. This stimulates the medullary chemoreceptors to increase ventilation and to return the ratio of HCO_3^- to pCO_2, and thus pH, toward normal.[34,35]

The physiologic metabolic and respiratory compensations to simple primary acid–base disturbances can be predicted from the relationships[35] displayed in Table 27-11. In a child with simple metabolic acidosis, the pCO_2 is expected to decrease by 1.3 mmHg for each millimole per liter decrease in HCO_3^-. Thus, a patient with metabolic acidosis and HCO_3^- of 12.0 mmol/L would be expected to have a pCO_2 of approximately 23 mmHg, that is, between 20 and 26 mmHg. Values for pCO_2 below 20 or greater than 26 mmHg define a mixed disturbance (metabolic acidosis and respiratory alkalosis or metabolic acidosis and respiratory acidosis, respectively).

In childhood, arterial blood is often unavailable. As a consequence, in this age group pH and pCO_2 are assessed in venous or arterialized blood samples, whose pH is on the average lower by 0.05 and pCO_2 higher by 6 mmHg. Automated blood gas analyzers measure pH and pCO_2, while the HCO_3^- concentration is calculated from the (unsimplified) Henderson-Hasselbalch equation. Most currently available blood gas analyzers determine circulating L-lactate as well (the assay will not detect D-lactate).

"Base excess" and "standard HCO_3^-" are in vitro generated parameters of the acid–base balance that are of little value and often even misleading. Most authoritative bodies argue against the use of standard HCO_3^- and base excess in clinical practice and recommend the use of the traditional parameters HCO_3^-, pCO_2, and pH.[34,35]

The following sections focus mainly on the systemic effects of acid–base abnormalities and various causes of metabolic acid–base disorders.

Systemic Effects of Acid–Base Abnormalities

The systemic effects of acid–base abnormalities on the cardiovascular system, central nervous system, potassium and

TABLE 27-11 Predicted Metabolic and Respiratory Compensations to Simple Primary Acid–Base Disturbances

Disorder	Primary Change	Compensatory Response
Metabolic acidosis	↓ HCO_3^-	↓ pCO_2 by 1.3[a] mmHg for ↓ 1.0 mmol/L[b] in HCO_3^-
Metabolic alkalosis	↑ HCO_3^-	↑ pCO_2 by 0.6[a] mmHg for ↑ 1.0 mmol/L[b] in HCO_3^-
Respiratory acidosis	↑ pCO_2	
Acute		↑ 1.0 mmol/L[c] in HCO_3 for ↑ 10 mmHg[d] in pCO_2
Chronic		↑ 3.5 mmol/L[c] in HCO_3 for ↑ 10 mmHg[d] in pCO_2
Respiratory alkalosis	↓ pCO_2	
Acute		↓ 2.0 mmol/L[c] in HCO_3 for ↓ 10 mmHg[d] in pCO_2
Chronic		↓ 5.0 mmol/L[c] in HCO_3 for ↓ 10 mmHg[d] in pCO_2

[a] Range approximately ±3 mmHg.
[b] From 25 mmol/L.
[c] Range approximately ±2.0 mmol/L.
[d] From 40 mmHg.
Modified from Laski ME, Kurtzman NA: Acid–base disorders in medicine, *Dis Mon* 42:51-125, 1996; and Whittier WL, Rutecki GW: Primer on clinical acid–base problem solving, *Dis Mon* 50:122-62, 2004.

calcium balance, and metabolism are briefly addressed below.[34]

Cardiovascular System

Acidemia impairs cardiovascular function in four ways:

- Depresses vascular tone
- Alters the release of, and the response to, catecholamines
- Depresses myocardial contractility inducing diastolic dysfunction
- Induces arrhythmias. In mild to moderate acidemia, increased catecholamines produce sinus tachycardia; when acidemia is severe, vagal activity increases and bradycardia ensues; there is also an increased risk of ventricular fibrillation.

Alkalemia exerts fewer effects on the cardiovascular system. The predominant clinical problem is an increase in myocardial irritability. Alkalemia reduces the free calcium inside the cell and out, and most alkalemic patients are also hypokalemic. Changes in both ions contribute to the increased potential for arrhythmias.

Alkalemia has significant effects on vascular tone in the cerebral circulation: hypocarbia constricts the cerebral vasculature as indicated by the fact that subjects with respiratory alkalosis develop lightheadedness and lack of mental acuity, but coma does not occur.

Central Nervous System

Acidosis and alkalosis impair central and peripheral nervous system function. Alkalemia increases seizure activity. If pH is 7.60 or more, seizures may occur in the absence of an underlying epileptic diathesis. Acidosis depresses the central nervous system (this most frequently occurs in respiratory acidosis). Early signs of impairment include tremors, myoclonic jerks, and clonic movement disorders. At pH of 7.10 or less, there is generalized depression of neuronal excitability. Central effects of severe hypercarbia include lethargy and stupor at pCO_2 of 60 mmHg or more, coma occurs at pCO_2 of 90 mmHg or more. Metabolic acidosis causes central nervous system depression less commonly. Fewer than 10% of diabetics with ketoacidosis develop coma (hyperosmolarity and the presence of acetoacetate may be more important than acidosis per se).

Blood pH alters hemoglobin oxygen binding and tissue oxygen delivery. Acidemia decreases hemoglobin oxygen affinity, shifts the oxygen dissociation curve "to the right," and increases tissue delivery of oxygen. On the contrary, alkalemia shifts the curve to the left, increasing the oxygen binding to hemoglobin and tending to decrease tissue delivery.

Potassium Balance

There are major interactions between the internal potassium balance and acute metabolic acid–base changes. In patients with normal anion gap metabolic acidosis, the excess hydrogen ions are buffered in the cell and electroneutrality is maintained by movements of intracellular potassium into the extracellular fluid. Interestingly, metabolic acidosis is much less likely to raise the extracellular potassium concentration in patients with high anion gap acidosis like L-lactate acidosis or ketoacidosis. The underlying mechanisms are briefly explained in Figure 27-5. For similar reasons some tendency towards hypokalemia is noted in metabolic alkalosis (Figure 27-5). Respiratory acidosis and alkalosis do not significantly change potassium balance.

Calcium Balance

Acid–base disorders affect circulating calcium, inorganic phosphate, and potassium. Acidemia increases calcium phosphate dissociation, increasing free (ionized) calcium. Acidemia also permits greater dissociation of calcium from plasma protein. The effect of acidosis on calcium salt dissociation extends to bone. Alkalemia might increase calcium phosphate precipitation and lowers ionized calcium.

Metabolism

A final aspect of acid–base pathophysiology is the effect of pH on metabolism. The most often-cited example of pH control of enzyme activity is the pH regulation of phosphofructokinase, which catalyzes a rate-controlling step in carbo-

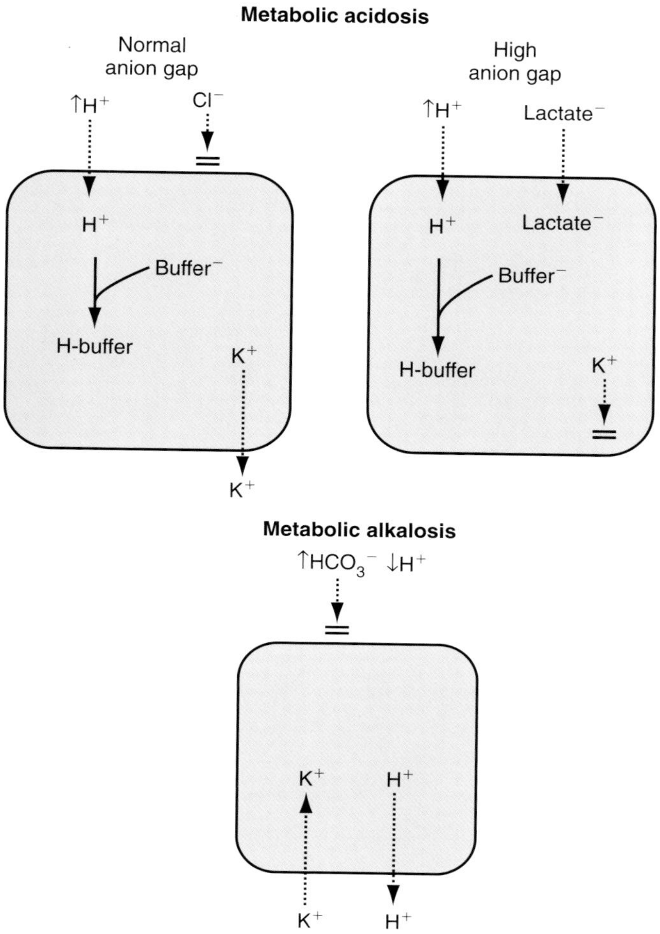

Figure 27-5 Effect of metabolic acidosis or alkalosis on circulating potassium level. Both in normal (hyperchloremic) and in high (normochloremic) anion-gap metabolic acidosis, some extracellular H^+ shifts into the intracellular fluid volume (the squares denote the cell membrane). In normal anion-gap (left panel) metabolic acidosis, Cl^- remains largely in the extracellular fluid volume. On the contrary, in high anion-gap (right panel) metabolic acidosis (e.g., L-lactate acidosis), some organic anions enter the intracellular fluid. Hence, a tendency towards hyperkalemia, the consequence of a shift of K^+ from the intracellular to the extracellular fluid volume, occurs in normal anion gap acidosis only. Please note that hyperkalemia is followed by a stimulated aldosterone release and results in the urinary excretion of the extra K^+. No tendency towards hyperkalemia occurs in respiratory acidosis. In metabolic alkalosis some intracellular H^+ shifts into the extracellular fluid volume. Hence, a tendency towards hypokalemia, the consequence of a shift of K^+ from the extracellular to the intracellular fluid volume, occurs. No tendency towards hypokalemia occurs in respiratory alkalosis.

hydrate metabolism. Glycolysis terminates in lactic and pyruvic acid, and accumulation of these acids reduces pH. This is but one example of pH feedback. Most enzymes operate most effectively at a specific optimum pH. As pH varies from the optimum, enzyme activity changes. The integrated response of the individual enzyme alterations may serve to maintain or restore normal pH.

Metabolic Acidosis

Primary hypobicarbonatemia and, therefore, metabolic acidosis mostly occur when endogenous acids are produced faster than they can be excreted, when HCO_3^- is lost from the body, or when exogenous acids are administered.[34-36]

The main laboratory tool in metabolic acidosis is the calculation of the blood anion gap, the difference between the major measured cations (sodium and potassium; mmol/L) and the major measured anion (bicarbonate and chloride, millimoles per liter) by means of the equation:

$$(\text{Sodium} + \text{Potassium}) - (\text{Chloride} + \text{Bicarbonate})$$

Because electroneutrality must be maintained, the anion gap results from the difference between the unmeasured anions (primarily albumin, which is largely responsible for the normal anion gap, but also phosphate, sulfate, and organic anions such as lactate) and the remaining cations (calcium and magnesium).

Calculation of the blood anion gap (upper reference: 18 mmol/L) allows separation of the two major types of metabolic alkalosis: one type has an increased anion gap (higher than 18 mmol/L; high anion gap metabolic acidosis) and the other does not (normal anion gap metabolic acidosis or hyperchloremic metabolic acidosis), as shown in Table 27-12. (The blood anion gap sometimes does not include the blood concentration of potassium: sodium − [bicarbonate + chloride]. The approximate upper value of this anion gap is lower by 4 mmol/L: 14 mmol/L.)

High Anion Gap Metabolic Acidosis ("Normochloremic")

The HCO_3^- deficit observed in high anion gap metabolic acidosis results from retention of fixed acids, which deplete HCO_3^- stores by releasing their protons. Two mechanisms lead to this form of metabolic acidosis: excessive acid load (endogenous or exogenous) overwhelming the normal capacity to decompose or excrete the acid, and diminished capacity to excrete the normal load of fixed acids in the context of renal failure.

Note: In healthy patients, the blood anion gap is predominantly due to the net negative charge of albumin. Abnormally low albumin levels in blood significantly influence acid–base interpretation through calculation of the anion gap. Imagine a patient with increased production of endogenous acids and therefore a tendency towards high anion gap. Unfortunately, this tendency may be masked by concurrent hypoalbuminemia.[37] In this condition, the anion gap corrected for albumin may be calculated by means of the following formula (albumin in grams per liter):

$$(Na^+ + K^+) - (Cl^- + HCO_3^-) + 0.25 \times (40 - \text{Albumin})$$

Considering that most currently available blood gas analyzers determine circulating L-lactate,[38] the determination of the albumin and lactate corrected anion gap has been recently advised (upper reference: 15 mmol/L):

$$(Na^+ + K^+) - (Cl^- + HCO_3^- + \text{Lactate}) + 0.25 \times (40 - \text{Albumin})$$

Normal Anion Gap Metabolic Acidosis ("Hyperchloremic")

This form of metabolic acidosis develops from a primary loss of HCO_3^-, from the failure to replenish HCO_3^- stores

TABLE 27-12 Causes of Metabolic Acidosis

Metabolic Acidosis with Increased Anion Gap

Excessive acid load
  Endogenous sources of acid (due to abnormal metabolism of substrates)
    Ketoacidosis (largely β-hydroxybutyric acid)
    Congenital organic acidemias (e.g., methylmalonic acidemia and propionic acidemia)
    L-lactate acidosis
      Type A (impaired tissue oxygenation; e.g., sepsis, hypovolemia, cardiac failure)
      Type B (altered metabolism of L-lactate with normal tissue oxygenation in context of mitochondrial impairment)
        Inherited metabolic diseases: either altered production of glucose from lactate or altered degradation of pyruvate derived from pyruvate
        Thiamine deficiency
        Drugs (e.g., biguanides, antiretroviral agents)
        Toxins (e.g., ethanol)
        Chronic diseases (mostly hepatic)
  Overproduction of organic acids in gastrointestinal tract (D-lactate)
  Conversion of alcohols (methanol, ethylene glycol) to acids and poisonous aldehydes

Defective renal excretion of acids due to generalized renal failure ("uremic acidosis")
Metabolic Acidosis with Normal Anion Gap

Losses of bicarbonate HCO_3^-
  Intestinal: diarrhea, surgical drainage of the intestinal tract, gastrointestinal fistulas resulting in losses of fluid rich in HCO_3^-, patients whose ureters have been attached to the intestinal tract (alkali of intestinal secretion is lost by titration with acid urine)
  Urinary: carbonic anhydrase inhibitors (e.g., acetazolamide), proximal renal tubular acidosis (type 2)

Failure to replenish HCO_3 stores depleted by daily production of fixed acids
  Distal renal tubular acidosis (classic, also called type 1 or type 4)
  Diminished mineralocorticoid (or glucocorticoid) activity (adrenal insufficiency, selective hypoaldosteronism, aldosterone resistance)
  Administration of potassium-sparing diuretics (spironolactone, eplerenone, amiloride, triamterene)

Exogenous infusions
  Amino acids like L-arginine and L-lysine (during parenteral nutrition)
  HCl or NH_4Cl
  Rapid administration of normal saline (NaCl 9 g/L) solution ("dilutional" metabolic acidosis)

depleted by the daily production of fixed acids (H^+: 1 to 3 mmol/kg of body weight) in subjects with normal glomerular filtration rate, or from the administration of exogenous acids (including the rapid administration of large volumes of normal saline solution and other chloride-rich fluids).

The following factors account for the metabolic acidosis that is observed after administration of normal saline solution, which is called "dilutional" acidosis: (1) volume expansion, which results from infusion of normal saline, reduces the renal threshold for HCO_3^- leading to bicarbonaturia; and (2) the infusion of normal saline with a Na^+ level almost identical to that of blood results in a relatively stable Na^+ level in blood. By contrast, the concentration of Cl^- in the infused solution, which is much higher than that of normal blood, leads to progressive hyperchloremia and hypobicarbonatemia.

Urine Net Charge

The kidney prevents the development of metabolic acidosis by modulating the HCO_3^- concentration in blood. This is done by preventing loss of large amounts of filtered HCO_3^- (primarily a task of the proximal tubule, which may reclaim the filtered HCO_3^-), and generating HCO_3^- (primarily a task of the distal tubule). The main mechanism by which the distal tubule generates HCO_3^- is the conversion of glutamine to NH_4^+, which is excreted in the urine, plus HCO_3^-, which is added to the blood. As a consequence, the urinary NH_4^+ excretion reflects the renal HCO_3^- generation, and the renal NH_4^+ excretion can be equated with HCO_3^- regeneration on a 1 : 1 basis. In a child with normal anion gap metabolic acidosis and normal renal mechanisms of acidification, a very low urinary concentration of HCO_3^- and, more importantly, a large concentration of NH_4^+ will result. The measurement of urinary NH_4^+, which is complicated by the need to avoid changes in urine composition after voiding (the changes are due to bacterial overgrowth, especially at room temperature, as well as to open exposure to the atmosphere, which produces gas loss), is usually unavailable in clinical practice.[35,36] In the context of metabolic acidosis, a urinary pH significantly less than 6.2 indicates a very low urinary concentration of HCO_3^-, and argues against an altered renal mechanism of acidification. Furthermore, and more importantly, the crucial concept of urinary net charge or urine anion gap (which results from urinary Na^+, K^+, and Cl^-) was developed as an indirect assessment of urinary NH_4^+ concentration. (The term urine anion gap is a misnomer for what should have been named urine cation gap.) Usually, because ammonium (an unmeasured cation) accompanies chloride, in the context of metabolic acidosis the concentration of chloride should be greater than the sum of sodium and potassium, and the net charge negative ($Na^+ + K^+ < Cl^-$). A positive net charge ($Na^+ + K^+ > Cl^-$) indicates impaired ammonium secretion and, therefore, impaired distal acidification of the renal tubule. For instance, in the aforementioned context of metabolic acidosis with normal renal mechanisms of acidification (e.g., a child with normal anion gap metabolic acidosis due to mild

TABLE 27-13 Indirect Assessment of Urinary Excretion of NH_4^+ by Means of Urinary Net Charge in Subjects with Normal Anion Gap Metabolic Acidosis

Distal Acidification of Renal Tubule	Urinary NH_4^+	Urinary Net Charge
Normal	↑ NH_4^+	$Na^+ + K^+ < Cl^-$
Impaired	↓ NH_4^+	$Na^+ + K^+ > Cl^{-a}$

[a] The urine osmolal charge is a more precise estimate of the urinary NH_4^+ concentration in this setting:

$$\frac{\text{Measured osmolality} - [2 \times (\text{Na} + \text{K}) + \text{Urea} + \text{Glucose}]}{2}$$

diarrhea), the enhanced urinary NH_4^+ excretion will result in a large urinary level of urinary NH_4Cl, and consequently the measured urinary cations ($Na^+ + K^+$) will have a concentration lower than the measured anion Cl^-: $Na^+ + K^+ < Cl^-$. On the contrary, in a child with impaired renal acidification due to classic distal renal tubular acidosis, the urine net charge will be as follows: $Na^+ + K^+ > Cl^-$ (Table 27-13).

When the urine net charge is positive ($Na^+ + K^+ > Cl^-$) and it is unclear whether increased excretion of unmeasured anions is responsible, the urinary NH_4^+ concentration can be estimated from calculation of the urine osmolal gap.[36] This calculation requires measurement of urine osmolality (in milliosmoles per kilogram) and urine sodium, potassium, and urea, and, if the dipstick is positive, glucose concentrations (in millimoles per liter):

$$NH_4^+ = \frac{\text{Measured osmolality} - [2 \times (\text{Na} + \text{K}) + \text{Urea} + \text{Glucose}]}{2}$$

In the context of metabolic acidosis, an estimated urinary NH_4^+ concentration of less than 20 mmol/L indicates impaired NH_4^+ excretion.

Metabolic Acidosis during First Months of Life

During the first months of life, bicarbonatemia is lower by 2 to 4 mmol/L than in older children (Table 27-10), and is even lower in preterm infants (ranging from 16 to 19 mmol/L) and during the first 3 weeks of life. This is the consequence of a lower renal threshold for bicarbonate. In addition, in preterm infants and in growing children the daily production of H^+ is higher by 50% to 100% than that noted in adults (this is mainly explained by the fact that the growing skeleton releases 20 mmol of H^+ for each gram of calcium that is incorporated). The clinical implications of these data are that, as compared with older children, newborns and infants have a relatively limited capacity to compensate for hypobicarbonatemia. In this age, the tendency towards metabolic acidosis is compensated for by the large intake of milk, whose alkali content is high. Infants are therefore more prone to develop metabolic acidosis in conditions associated with decreased milk intake.

Symptoms, Signs, and Consequences

The signs and symptoms of acute metabolic acidosis include:

High respiratory rate. In young children and infants, the increase in depth of respiration, as observed in classic Kussmaul-type deep breathing, may not be as apparent as in adults, and the response to metabolic acidosis may be tachypnea alone.
Abdominal pain and vomiting.
Irritability and lethargy.

The gastrointestinal absorption and excretion of dietary base play a major role in acid–base homeostasis in infants in whom the predominantly milk-based diet contributes a considerable amount of alkali. Infants are therefore more vulnerable to developing metabolic acidosis in illnesses associated with decreased milk intake.

Since an excessive chronic acid burden interferes with calcium deposition in the bone and calcium intestinal absorption, metabolic acidosis of any form can impair growth in children. Other signs and symptoms are abdominal pain, vomiting, irritability, lethargy, seizures, and coma. However, the latter manifestations are primarily due to the underlying disease (e.g., organic acidemias or hyperosmolality in diabetic ketoacidosis), not the acidosis itself.

Clinical Workup

The causes of metabolic acidosis, which appear in Table 27-12, can often be discerned clinically. A careful history and physical examination and the determination of the blood anion gap direct an accurate evaluation. For the initial diagnostic approach to metabolic acidosis of unknown origin, the following initial steps are taken[35,36]:

Confirm the diagnosis of metabolic acidosis.
Confirm that the respiratory response is appropriate.
Distinguish high from normal anion gap metabolic acidosis.
  If normal anion gap, consider intestinal loss of HCO_3^-.
  If high anion gap, assess urinary ketones, blood glucose, and blood L-lactate.

The major causes of high anion-gap acidosis are L-lactate acidosis, which results from impaired tissue oxygenation (type A L-lactate acidosis) or from altered metabolism of L-lactate with normal tissue oxygenation in the context of a mitochondrial impairment (type B L-lactate acidosis); diabetic ketoacidosis, which mainly results from the accumulation of β-hydroxybutyrate; and "uremic" metabolic acidosis, which is characterized by the accumulation of phosphate, sulfate, and organic anions.

In children, normal anion gap metabolic acidosis mostly results from intestinal bicarbonate losses due to diarrhea. Renal bicarbonate wasting is much less common. In children with normal anion gap acidosis, but without history of diarrhea, the concurrent determination of urinary Na^+, K^+, and Cl^- will provide information on the renal mechanisms of acidification.

Sometimes there is overlap between the causes of a normal and high anion gap metabolic acidosis. Diarrhea, for example, is most often associated with a normal anion gap. However, severe diarrhea and hypovolemia can result in an increase in the anion gap due hypoperfusion-induced lactic acidosis and starvation ketosis.

Management

Emergency Measures Avoid further production of H^+, including measures to ensure a proper airway, adequate peripheral perfusion and O_2 delivery. For example, in a child with type A L-lactate acidosis in the context of severe dehydration, delivery of O_2 and the rapid administration of normal saline will regenerate adenosine triphosphate. On the other hand, in a child with accidental methanol intoxication the administration of ethanol might stop the production of toxins leading to acidosis.

Increase pH Level The pH level is increased by lowering the pCO_2 to ensure an adequate degree of hyperventilation, if necessary by mechanical ventilation.

Correct Underlying Condition For example, in diabetic ketoacidosis, insulin is administered in addition to normal saline.

Administration of $NaHCO_3$ The use of $NaHCO_3$ is controversial,[39] considering the possible benefits (metabolic advantage of faster glycolysis with better availability of adenosine triphosphate in vital organs, and improved cardiac action) and the risks (extracellular fluid volume expansion, tendency towards hypernatremia, and development of hypokalemia and hypocalcemia). The following guidelines have been suggested for administration of $NaHCO_3$:

Diabetic ketoacidosis: $NaHCO_3$ should be considered when hyperkalemia persists despite insulin therapy, when acidemia worsens despite insulin therapy (suggesting insulin resistance as a result of acidemia), and perhaps when HCO_3^- is 5.0 mmol/L or less. We are very reluctant to use bicarbonate in diabetic ketoacidosis because a large body of evidence indicates that the administration of $NaHCO_3$ is a risk factor for cerebral edema in childhood diabetic ketoacidosis.

Type A L-lactate metabolic acidosis: In this form of acidosis, the primary effort should be directed at improving delivery of O_2. $NaHCO_3$ should be given when HCO_3^- is 5.0 mmol/L or less.

Because the "HCO_3^- space" is approximately 0.5 l/kg of body weight the dose of $NaHCO_3$ in severe metabolic acidosis may be calculated from body weight (kilograms), current blood HCO_3^-, and desired blood HCO_3^- (both in millimoles per liter) using the following equation[34,35,39,40]:

$$\text{Body weight} \times 0.5\ (\text{Desired } HCO_3 - \text{Current } HCO_3)$$

Hence, a child weighing 20.0 kg with a severe hypobicarbonatemia of 3.5 mmol/L will be given 40 mmol of $NaHCO_3$ over several minutes (i.e., 2.0 mmol/kg of body weight) if the "desired" blood HCO_3^- level is 7.5 mmol/l. In most cases, however, the initial dosage of $NaHCO_3$ is 1.0 mmol/kg of body weight, a dosage that is expected to increase blood HCO_3^- by 2.0 mmol/L.

Because correction of metabolic acidosis tends to decrease circulating K^+ levels, one must avoid a severe degree of hypokalemia when $NaHCO_3$ is given.

K^+ depletion and metabolic acidosis are associated in three settings: classic distal renal tubular acidosis, acute diarrheal disease, and diabetic ketoacidosis (Table 27-14).

TABLE 27-14 Conditions Associating Metabolic Acidosis and Potassium Depletion

Condition	Basis of Potassium Depletion
Classic distal renal tubular acidosis	Renal loss
Diarrhea	Renal and intestinal loss
Diabetic ketoacidosis	Renal loss (osmotic diuresis)[a]

[a] Circulating potassium is often initially normal in diabetic ketoacidosis.

The management of renal tubular acidosis will be discussed in Chapter 31, and that of uremic acidosis in the sections on renal replacement therapy.

Metabolic Alkalosis

Primary hyperbicarbonatemia and, therefore, alkalemia, are the hallmarks of metabolic alkalosis.[41] In this peculiar acid–base disorder, hyperbicarbonatemia, alkalemia, and the compensatory hypoventilation (resulting in a rise of the pCO_2) are almost always associated with hypokalemia (see "Systemic Effects of Acid–Base Abnormalities" section).

Within the constraints of electroneutrality, the ways to add HCO_3^- to extracellular space are loss of the anion Cl^- or retention of Na^+. Hence, an increase in circulating HCO_3^- may be associated with a contracted "effective" circulating volume (blood pressure normal) or with an expanded "effective" circulating volume (blood pressure increased).

In metabolic alkalosis associated with a contracted "effective" circulating volume ("unaccompanied" Cl^- deficiency syndrome or normotensive hypokalemic metabolic alkalosis), Cl^- is lost from the extracellular space "not accompanied" by the major cations Na^+ and K^+ but "accompanied" by H^+ or NH_4^+. Since a loss of H^+ or NH_4^+ is equivalent to a gain of HCO_3^-, the final effect is a swap with loss of Cl^- and gain of HCO_3^-. Two further steps complete the development of metabolic alkalosis:

"Extra" HCO_3^-, which is filtered by the kidney, is mostly reabsorbed and only a little HCO_3^- is excreted.

Contraction of the circulating volume activates the renin-angiotensin II-aldosterone system resulting in urinary K^+ excretion, which further aggravates hyperbicarbonatemia.

Secondary hyperaldosteronism resulting in urinary K^+ excretion is the main cause of hypokalemia that accompanies this form of metabolic alkalosis. During the first months of life, metabolic alkalosis is often not associated with hypokalemia (alternatively it is associated with mild hypokalemia). This is likely due to the reduced ability of the kidney to excrete potassium early in life.

Maternal chloride deficiency, deficient chloride intake, gastrointestinal chloride losses, cutaneous chloride losses in the setting of cystic fibrosis, diuretics, and renal tubular disturbances are the most important causes of normotensive hypokalemic metabolic alkalosis (Table 27-15). The urinary excretion of chloride[28,41] is low in patients with extrarenal causes, and normal or high in subjects with renal causes of this peculiar form of metabolic alkalosis. In our experience,

TABLE 27-15 Causes of Metabolic Alkalosis (Linked with Hypokalemia)

Associated with Contracted "Effective" Circulating Volume (and therefore with normal or even low blood pressure)
A. Nonrenal causes (low urine chloride excretion: chloride/creatinine <10 mol/mol) Intestinal causes Low dietary chloride intake (e.g., soybean formula with low chloride content in infancy, "tea and toast diet") Loss of gastric secretions (vomiting, nasogastric suction) Posthypercapnia Congenital chloridodiarrhea (uncommon), villous adenoma (uncommon) Cutaneous cause Cystic fibrosis Excessive sweating (uncommon, associated with low dietary chloride intake) "Posthypercapnia" (posthypercapnic alkalosis) Refeeding syndrome Transient neonatal metabolic alkalosis in infants of mothers affected by chloride deficiency (eating disorders associated with chloride deficiency, Bartter syndrome, Gitelman syndrome)
B. Renal causes (high urine chloride excretion: chloride/creatinine >>10 mol/mol) Primary chloride losing tubulopathies (Bartter syndrome, Gitelman syndrome) Secondary chloride losing tubulopathies (some cases of chronic cisplatin tubulopathy) Current diuretic use (including surreptitious use)[a]
Associated with Expanded "Effective" Circulating Volume (and therefore with high blood pressure)
A. Enhanced mineralocorticoid activity Primary aldosteronism (either hyperplasia or adenoma) Apparent mineralocorticoid excess (defect in 11-β-hydroxysteroid-dehydrogenase), Liddle syndrome (congenitally increased function of the collecting tubule sodium channels), dexamethasone-responsive aldosteronism (synthesis of aldosterone promoted not only by renin but also by adrenocorticotropin), congenital adrenal hyperplasia (11-β-hydroxylase or 17-α-hydroxylase deficiency), Cushing disease Secondary hyperaldosteronism (including renal artery stenosis, malignant hypertension, and renin-producing tumor) Exogenous mineralocorticoids, licorice ingestion (11-β-hydroxysteroid-dehydrogenase blockade)
B. Reduced renal function plus source of HCO_3^+: alkali ingestion, ingestion of ion-exchange resin plus nonreabsorbable alkali

[a] Urinary chloride excretion is low in subjects with remote use of diuretics.

the determination of the urinary chloride/creatinine ratio in spot urine samples from patients with normotensive metabolic alkalosis distinguishes between renal (urinary chloride/creatinine ratio largely higher than 10 mol/mol, respectively, or 0.09 mmol/mg) and extrarenal causes (urinary chloride/creatinine ratio less than 10 mol/mol, respectively, or 0.09 mmol/mg). In clinical practice, this simple parameter is useful in patients in whom the etiology of metabolic alkalosis with normal or low normal blood pressure is not obtainable from the history. Please note that the urinary chloride/creatinine ratio is also usually higher than 10 mol/mol in patients with metabolic alkalosis associated with expanded effective circulating volume (see below).

Posthypercapnic Alkalosis ("Posthypercapnia")

Chronic respiratory acidosis is associated with a compensatory hyperbicarbonatemia. In patients with a tendency towards a contracted circulating volume when pCO_2 falls to normal, there will be a stimulus for persistently increased HCO_3^- levels and hypokalemia. In addition, a rapid correction of chronic respiratory acidosis (e.g., mechanical ventilation) results in an acute rise in cerebral pH that can produce serious neurologic sequelae or even death. Consequently, pCO_2 should be lowered slowly and carefully in chronic hypercapnia.

Metabolic Alkalosis Associated with Expanded "Effective" Circulating Volume (Hypertensive Metabolic Alkalosis)

The second way to add HCO_3^- to the circulating volume while preserving electroneutrality is to retain HCO_3^- along with Na^+, thereby expanding the extracellular fluid volume and increasing blood pressure. Obviously, to retain extra Na^+ (along with HCO_3^-) "permission" of the kidney will be required.

The mechanisms for renal retention of Na^+ and HCO_3^- includes either an enhanced reabsorption of filtered HCO_3^-, or a reduced glomerular filtration rate plus a source of HCO_3^- (e.g., the ingestion of large amounts of milk and the absorbable antacid $CaCO_3$).

Excessive mineralocorticoid activity is the main cause of metabolic alkalosis associated with hypokalemia and expanded circulating volume. The corresponding causes appear in Table 27-15.

Symptoms, Signs, Consequences

There are no specific diagnostic symptoms or signs of metabolic alkalosis. Physical examination may reveal neuromuscular irritability, such as tetany or hyperactive reflexes. These signs will be more pronounced if hypocalcemia is an accompanying feature. The symptoms and signs of accompanying hypokalemia will be discussed elsewhere.

It is recognized that in children with both contracted and expanded circulating volume and metabolic alkalosis, the assessment of the fluid volume status by physical examination and history may be quite inaccurate. This assumption is supported by the experience in infantile hypertrophic pyloric stenosis where the clinical assessment of the fluid volume stated may be quite inaccurate, and the severity of metabolic alkalosis helps to define the amount of fluid replacement required.

Management

The most frequent causes of hypokalemic metabolic alkalosis associated with a contracted "effective" circulating volume include intestinal (mostly gastric) or cutaneous fluid losses, and excessive diuretic therapy. These forms of metabolic alkalosis are termed "chloride responsive," because they are reversed by the oral intravenous administration of NaCl, KCl, and water.[41,42] At our institutions, for example, infants with hypertrophic pyloric stenosis[42] are hydrated parenterally with a "near isotonic" solution containing glucose 5% (50 g/l), sodium chloride 80 to 90 mmol/L and potassium chloride 20 to 30 mmol/L until correction of the acid–base and potassium balance. In "chloride responsive" metabolic alkalosis, the oral administration of K^+ with any anion other the Cl^- (e.g., citrate) prevents the correction of alkalosis.

Occasionally, severe metabolic alkalosis is additionally treated with the carbonic anhydrase inhibitor acetazolamide, which blocks the proximal tubular HCO_3^- reabsorption (inducing bicarbonaturia accompanied by Na^+ and K^+ losses), with NH_4Cl, or with HCl (through a central venous line). Finally, hemodialysis with a low dialysate HCO_3^- (or hemofiltration) in association with saline infusion has been advised for the treatment of severe metabolic alkalosis in advanced kidney disease.

The management of the remaining causes of hypokalemic metabolic alkalosis will be discussed in the chapters on arterial hypertension and renal tubular disorders.

Respiratory Acid–Base Disturbances

These acid–base disorders will not be discussed in this textbook of clinical nephrology, with the exception of Table 27-16, which depicts the main causes.

TABLE 27-16 Causes of Respiratory Acidosis (Hypoventilation) and Alkalosis (Hyperventilation)

Respiratory Acidosis (hypoventilation)
Central nervous system (patient will not breathe!)
Cerebral
Posthypoxic brain damage
Cerebral trauma
Intracranial disease
Psychotropic drugs
Brain stem
Brain stem herniation
Encephalitis
Central sleep apnea
Severe metabolic alkalosis
Sedative or narcotic drugs
Upper airway reflexes
Bulbar palsy
Anterior horn cell lesion (including Guillain-Barré and poliomyelitis)
Disruption of airway
Peripheral disorders (patient cannot breathe)
Respiratory muscle disease
Myasthenia, Guillain-Barré syndrome, poliomyelitis
Myopathy, muscular dystrophy
Muscle fatigue or paralysis (including hypokalemic paralysis)
Airway and pulmonary disease
Interstitial lung disease (including lung fibrosis)
Obstructive disease (including upper airway obstruction, asthma, bronchiolitis, cystic fibrosis)
Obstructive sleep apnea
Obesity, kyphoscoliosis
Respiratory Alkalosis (hyperventilation)
Hypoxia: intrinsic pulmonary disease, high altitude, congestive heart failure, cyanotic congenital heart disease
Pulmonary receptor stimulation: pneumonia, asthma, interstitial lung disease, pulmonary edema, pulmonary thromboembolism
Drugs: salicylates, niketamide, catecholamines, theophylline, progesterone
Central nervous disorders: subarachnoidal hemorrhage, Cheyne-Stokes respiration, primary hyperventilation syndrome
Miscellaneous: psychogenic hyperventilation (rare before puberty), fever, sepsis, recovery from metabolic acidosis

CALCIUM

Balance

A 70-kg man contains one kg of calcium (25 mol), 99% of which resides in the skeleton in the form of hydroxyapatite and 1% of which is found in soft tissues and the extracellular space. Since calcium plays a crucial role in neuromuscular function, blood coagulation, and intracellular signaling, circulating calcium concentrations are maintained within a tight physiologic range. The calcium (and phosphate) homeostasis involves intestinal, bone, and renal function. Regulation of intestinal function is important because, in contrast to the complete absorption of dietary sodium, potassium, and chloride, that of calcium (like magnesium and phosphate) is incomplete. This limitation is due both to the requirement for vitamin D and to the formation of insoluble salts in the intestinal lumen, such as calcium phosphate, calcium oxalate, and magnesium phosphate.

A normal adult may ingest approximately 1000 mg (25 mmol) of calcium per day, of which roughly 40% to 50% may be absorbed. However, 300 mg (approximately 8 mmol) of calcium from digestive secretions are lost in the stool, resulting in the net absorption of no more than 10% to 20%. In the steady state, this amount of calcium is excreted in the urine. Within the blood calcium, roughly 40% is bound to albumin, 15% is complexed with citrate, sulfate, or phosphate, and 45% exists as the physiologically important ionized form.[43]

Considering that a large proportion of circulating calcium is bound to albumin, the determination of albumin (or the direct measurement of ionized calcium) is essential to the diagnosis of true hypocalcemia or hypercalcemia. The following simple formula[44] may be used for total calcium (mmol/L) to account for albumin (g/L) binding:

$$\text{Corrected total Ca} = \text{Measured Ca} + 0.025\ (40 - \text{albumin})$$

(Circulating calcium levels can be reported in either millimoles per liter, metabolic equivalents per liter, milligrams per decaliter, or milligrams per liter. The valence of magnesium is 2 and its molecular mass is 40.1; therefore, 2.5 mmol/L is equivalent to 5.0 meq/L, 10.0 mg/dl, and 100 mg/L.)

Although only a small fraction of the total body calcium is located in the plasma, the blood level of ionized calcium is under control of calciotropic hormones and calcium-sensing receptor: The calcium sensing receptor, which is found on the cell surface of tissues such as the parathyroid gland, kidney, and bone, detects hypocalcemia and leads to enhanced secretion of parathyroid hormone. Summarizing the process briefly, a fall in circulating calcium in normal subjects leads to a compensatory increase in parathyroid hormone secretion, which returns the calcium level to normal by two major actions: increased calcium release from bone and stimulated production of calcitriol (1,25-dihydroxyvitamin D_3), the active metabolite of vitamin D_3, resulting in an increase in intestinal calcium absorption.[44,45]

Parathyroid hormone–related peptide is another calciotropic hormone with the following identified actions:

- During pregnancy, calcium is transferred from the maternal circulation to the fetus by a pump regulated by this hormone.
- Parathyroid hormone–related peptide levels are elevated during lactation and contribute substantially to the movement of calcium from the maternal skeleton to the mammary glands.
- Finally, this peptide is involved in the pathogenesis of hypercalcemia of malignancies.

Non-Neonatal Hypocalcemia

Symptoms and Signs

Symptoms and signs of hypocalcemia, which is often asymptomatic, result from neuromuscular, ocular, ectodermal, dental, gastrointestinal, cardiovascular, skeletal, or endocrine dysfunctions, and are related to the severity and chronicity of the hypocalcemia (Table 27-17). However, some signs and symptoms are unique to chronic hypoparathyroidism and not hypocalcemia, including candidiasis and dysmorphic changes in **a**utoimmune **p**oly**e**ndocrinopathy-**c**andidiasis-**e**ctodermal **d**ystrophy (APECED association). Among the symptoms of hypocalcemia tetany, papilledema and seizures may occur in patients who develop acute hypocalcemia. By comparison, ectodermal and dental changes, cataracts, basal ganglia calcification, and extrapyramidal disorders are features of chronic hypocalcemia, and are common in hypoparathyroidism.[46,47]

Causes

Deficiency or impaired function of parathyroid hormone, calcitriol, or the calcium-sensing receptor are major causes of reduced blood level of ionized calcium. Because bone calcium stores are so large, the major reason for hypocalcemia is decreased bone resorption. Sometimes acute events such as hyperphosphatemia can produce hypocalcemia, even though the regulatory systems are intact. The main causes of hypocalcemia include vitamin D deficiency, calcium deficiency, impaired vitamin D metabolism, impaired parathyroid hormone action (secondary to end-organ resistance), reduced production of parathyroid hormone, and abnormal calcium-sensing receptor or impaired renal function (Table 27-18).

Diagnostic Workup

Hypocalcemia is a rather common clinical problem, the cause of which can very often be determined from the history (as with a breast-fed infant not receiving any supplementation of vitamin D_3 presenting with nonfebrile generalized convulsions, enlargement of the costochondral junction along the anterolateral aspects of the chest, and enlargement of the wrist). In some cases, however, the underlying condition is not readily apparent. A detailed history documenting diet, lifestyle, family, and drug history, as well as development and hearing is important. The examination should include an assessment of skin, nails, teeth, and the skeleton, as well as the cardiovascular system. A comprehensive range of investigations should be performed at baseline, which have been divided into first and second line (Table 27-19). The objective of assessing urine calcium excretion is to establish whether the urine calcium/creatinine (units: mole per mole or milligram per milligram) is inappropriately high in the presence of hypocalcemia. Reference values for urine calcium/creatinine ratio in young children are not well defined and will vary according to factors such as diet. The upper limits of normal urine calcium excretion in healthy children appear in the footnote of Table 27-19. Renal phosphate handling may be abnormal despite a blood phosphate within the quoted laboratory normal range, and should be assessed in more detail by determining the tubular maximum reabsorption threshold of phosphate (see phosphate).

Checking biochemistry of the parents and possibly siblings is crucial when inherited diseases such as hypocalcemic hypercalciuria and hypophosphatemic rickets are suspected. It is also important to measure maternal calcium and vitamin D levels in the case of hypocalcemia in infancy because of the link with maternal vitamin D deficiency and hyperparathyroidism. Maternal hyperparathyroidism is linked with adverse pregnancy outcome and causes transient hypocalcemia in the newborn because the fetal parathyroids are suppressed following exposure to high calcium levels in utero. An autoantibody screen including adrenal, parathyroid, smooth muscle, and microsomal antibodies is useful in cases of isolated hypoparathyroidism and where APECED association is suspected. Renal ultrasound scan is often used to look for evidence of nephrocalcinosis or renal dysplasia.

The biochemical picture of hypocalcemia can be categorized according to the presence of undetectable, normal, or high levels of circulating intact parathyroid hormone, an approach that reflects the underlying pathophysiology.

Undetectable or low levels of this hormone in the hypocalcemic child suggest hypoparathyroidism (Table 27-18). Aplasia or hypoplasia of the parathyroids is most commonly due to the DiGeorge syndrome associated with deletion of chromosome 22q11. A similar phenotype, including hypoparathyroidism has also been associated with deletions of chromosome 10p and, recently, the HDR-association (**h**ypoparathyroidism, **d**eafness, and **r**enal dysplasia) was found to be due to defects in the GATA3 gene. Defects in the parathyroid hormone gene are rare. Diseases such as APECED can present with hypoparathyroidism in the absence of the two other major manifestations, which are candidiasis and adrenal failure. There should be a high index of suspicion for this disease in all cases of hypoparathyroidism presenting in children older than 4 years. Children with APECED may have other "minor" features such as malabsorption, gallstones, hepatitis, and dysplastic nails and teeth. Screening should be considered in the siblings of affected individuals.

TABLE 27-17 **Clinical Signs and Symptoms of Hypocalcemia**
Neuromuscular
Tetany Sensory dysfunction: circumoral and acral paresthesias Muscular dysfunctions Stiffness, myalgia, muscle spasms, and cramps Forced adduction of thumb, flexion of metacarpophalangeal joints and wrists, and extension of fingers Laryngismus stridulus (spasm of respiratory muscles and of glottis causing dyspnea) Autonomic dysfunction: diaphoresis, bronchospasm, biliary colic Trousseau sign: inflation of a sphygmomanometer above systolic blood pressure for 3-4 minutes induces carpal spasm (sign also may be induced by voluntary hyperventilation for 1-2 minutes after release of cuff) Chvostek sign: ipsilateral tapping of the facial nerve just anterior to the ear followed by contraction of the facial muscles (complete sign is contraction of corner of the mouth, nose, and eye; contraction of corner of the mouth alone often occurs in normal subjects)
Myopathy: generalized muscle weakness and wasting with normal creatine kinase (myopathy represents more a feature of vitamin D deficiency than hypocalcemia per se; elevated parathyroid hormone level or hypophosphatemia may contribute to myopathy)
Extrapyramidal disorders: bradykinetic movement disorders, sometimes dystonia, hemiballismus, choreoathetosis, oculogyric crises
Convulsions (generalized or partial)
Mental retardation, psychosis
Ocular
Cataract (rarely keratoconjunctivitis)
Papilledema (often associated with benign intracranial hypertension; rarely optic neuritis is present)
Ectodermal (especially in the context of severe, chronic hypocalcemia)
Dry scaly skin
Hyperpigmentation, dermatitis, eczema, and psoriasis
Coarse, brittle, and sparse hair with patchy alopecia
Brittle nails, with characteristic transverse grooves
Candidiasis: usually as a component of autoimmune polyendocrinopathy-candidiasis-ectodermal dystrophy (APECED association)
Dental (dental hypoplasia, failure of tooth eruption, defective enamel and root formation, and abraded carious teeth)
Gastrointestinal
Loose stools (steatorrhea due to impaired pancreatic secretion)
Gastric achlorhydria
Cardiovascular
Systemic hypotension, decreased myocardial function, congestive heart failure
Prolonged QT interval on standard electrocardiogram with tendency towards cardiac arrhythmias (clinically relevant if hypocalcemia is associated with hypokalemia and hypomagnesemia)
Skeletal
Rachitic findings Delayed closure of the fontanelles Parietal and frontal bossing Craniotabes Rachitic rosary: enlargement of the costochondral junction visible as beading along anterolateral aspects of the chest Harrison sulcus caused by muscular pull of diaphragmatic attachments to lower ribs Enlargement and bowing of distal radius, ulna, tibia, and fibula Progressive lateral bowing of femur and tibia
Children with hypoparathyroidism: increased bone mineral density, osteosclerosis, and thickening of calvarium
Children with pseudohypoparathyroidism: Albright's hereditary osteodystrophy, osteitis fibrosa cystica (due to normal skeletal responsiveness to parathyroid hormone)
Endocrine Manifestations
Impaired insulin release
Hypothyroidism, prolactin deficiency, and ovarian failure associated with polyglandular autoimmune syndromes

TABLE 27-18 Causes of Hypocalcemia in Infants and Children

Intact Parathyroid Hormone Level Low
Abnormal production of parathyroid hormone
Magnesium deficiency[a]
Following neck surgery
Hypoparathyroidism (autosomal recessive, autosomal dominant, or X linked)
Di George anomaly (22q11 deletions), 10p13 deletion, Hall-Hittner or CHARGE association (= coloboma, heart anomaly, choanal atresia, mental retardation, genital hypoplasia, and ear anomalies), HDR association (hypoparathyroidism, deafness, renal dysplasia)
Autoimmune polyendocrinopathy-candidiasis-ectodermal dystrophy (APECED association)
Infiltrative lesions such as Wilson's disease and thalassemia
Mitochondrial diseases (e.g., Kearns-Sayre syndrome)
Altered "set point" (calcium-sensing receptor activating mutations)
Intact Parathyroid Hormone Level High
Hypovitaminosis D, calcium deficiency, impaired vitamin D metabolism
Hypovitaminosis D
Reduced vitamin D intake or production in skin
Decreased intestinal absorption (e.g., celiac disease and cystic fibrosis)
Calcium deficiency
Impaired vitamin D "metabolism"
Severe liver disease
Drugs that "inactivate" vitamin D: anticonvulsants (e.g., carbamazepine, phenobarbital, phenytoin, isoniazid, theophylline, rifampicin)
Enzyme deficiency: defects of the 1-α-hydroxylase gene (vitamin D–dependent rickets type I)
End-organ resistance to vitamin D (vitamin D–dependent rickets type II)
Signaling defects: pseudohypoparathyroidisms
Renal failure, osteopetrosis, excessive fluoride intake

[a] Severe chronic magnesium deficiency (0.45 mmol/L or less) causes hypocalcemia by impairing parathyroid hormone secretion as well as parathyroid hormone action.

Modified from Carmeliet G, Van Cromphaut S, Daci E, Maes C, Bouillon R: Disorders of calcium homeostasis, *Best Pract Res Clin Endocrinol Metab* 17:529-46, 2003; and Singh J, Moghal N, Pearce SH, Cheetham T: The investigation of hypocalcaemia and rickets, *Arch Dis Child* 88:403-07, 2003.

Mitochondrial disease is a rare cause of hypoparathyroidism but is not usually an isolated finding.

Detectable parathyroid hormone values (low-normal or normal) in an asymptomatic individual raise the possibility of hypocalcemic hypercalciuria, an abnormality of the calcium-sensing receptor that can be assessed in more detail by determining urinary calcium excretion. Urine calcium excretion is typically low in longstanding hypoparathyroidism, and a relatively high urine calcium excretion (calcium/creatinine ratio 0.30 mol/mol or more, respectively, or 0.11 mg/mg or more) suggests hypocalcemic hypercalciuria. This abnormality is due to activating mutations of the calcium-sensing receptor with downshift of the set point for calcium responsive parathyroid hormone release. Magnesium levels are low in this disorder because the calcium-sensing receptor also detects this cation. Interestingly, the biochemical picture of hypocalcemic hypercalciuria sometimes resembles Bartter syndromes and includes hypokalemia and hyperbicarbonatemia.

If blood creatinine is normal, thereby excluding renal insufficiency, then increased parathyroid hormone levels point towards a diagnosis of rickets (in hypophosphatemic rickets circulating parathyroid hormone and calcium are usually normal) or pseudohypoparathyroidism. Vitamin D deficiency is still prevalent in the Western world. High-risk groups include families in which the maternal and child diet may be low in calcium and vitamin D and where exposure to sunlight can be limited. The diagnosis of Fanconi-de Toni-Debré syndrome should be considered in any hypocalcemic child with persistent glycosuria, phosphaturia, and acidosis. Pseudohypoparathyroidism is a heterogeneous disorder that results from signaling defects of the cell surface receptors. Patients may become hypocalcemic despite a compensatory increase in parathyroid hormone concentration, and may have other endocrine problems, such as primary hypothyroidism and hypogonadism that are also manifestations of an abnormal signaling mechanism. Some patients are overweight and mentally retarded.[6,7]

Neonatal Hypocalcemia

Hypocalcemia is a common metabolic problem in newborns. During pregnancy, calcium is transferred from the maternal circulation to the fetus by a pump regulated by parathyroid hormone–related peptide, the majority of fetal calcium accretion occurring in the third trimester. This process results in higher blood calcium levels in the fetus than in the mother and leads to fetal hypercalcemia, with total calcium concentration of 2.50 to 2.75 mmol/L in umbilical cord blood.

The cessation of placental transfer of calcium at birth is followed by a fall in total blood calcium concentration to 2.00 to 2.25 mmol/L and ionized calcium to as low as 1.1 to 1.35 mmol/L at 24 hours. Calcium levels subsequently rise, reaching levels seen in older children and adults by 2 weeks of age.

The definition of hypocalcemia depends on birth weight: in term infants or premature infants greater than 1.5 kg at birth, hypocalcemia is defined as a total concentration less than 2.00 mmol/L or an ionized fraction of less than 1.10 mmol/L; and premature infants with birth weight of less than 1.5 kg are hypocalcemic if they have a total calcium

TABLE 27-19 First- and Second-Line Investigations in Childhood Hypocalcemia When Cause Cannot Be Determined from History and Clinical Examination

First-Line Investigations	Second-Line Investigations
Blood Values	
Phosphate,[a] magnesium	Autoantibody screen
Alkaline phosphatase	Parental (and siblings) biochemistry
Sodium, potassium, bicarbonate, creatinine	Maternal vitamin D_3 status
Intact parathyroid hormone	1,25-hydroxy vitamin D_3, genetic studies (e.g., 22q11 deletion)
25-Hydroxyvitamin D_3 (calcidiol)	
Urinary Values	
Urinalysis (for glucose, protein, and pH)	
Calcium,[b] phosphate,[a] creatinine	
Imaging	
Hand and wrist radiograph	Renal ultrasound Skull radiograph

[a] Calculate the fractional excretion of phosphate and the maximal tubular reabsorption of phosphate as indicated in the section on phosphate.
[b] The upper limit of normal for urine calcium/creatinine in healthy children is 2.20 mol/mol (or 0.81 mg/mg) in infants aged 6-12 months, 1.50 mol/mol (or 0.56 mg/mg) in infants aged 13-24 months, 1.40 mol/mol (or 0.50 mg/mg) in infants aged 25-36 months, 1.10 mol/mol (or 0.41 mg/mg) in children aged 3-5 years, 0.80 mol/mol (or 0.30 mg/mg) in children aged 5-7 years, and 0.70 mol/mol (or 0.25 mg/mg) in older children.
Modified from Singh J, Moghal N, Pearce SH, Cheetham T: The investigation of hypocalcaemia and rickets, *Arch Dis Child* 88:403-07, 2003.

concentration less than 1.75 mmol/L or an ionized fraction of less than 1.0 mmol/L.[48]

Symptoms and Signs

Neonatal hypocalcemia is usually asymptomatic. Among those who become symptomatic, the characteristic sign is increased neuromuscular irritability. Such infants are jittery and often have muscle jerking. Generalized or partial clonic seizures can occur. Rare presentations include inspiratory stridor caused by laryngospasm, wheezing caused by bronchospasm, or vomiting, possibly resulting from pylorospasm.[48]

Causes

The causes of neonatal hypocalcemia are classified by the timing of onset. Hypocalcemia is considered to be early when it occurs in the first 2 to 3 days after birth.[48]

Early Neonatal Hypocalcemia Early hypocalcemia is an exaggeration of the normal decline in calcium concentration after birth. It occurs commonly in premature infants, in infants of diabetic mothers, and after perinatal asphyxia or intrauterine growth restriction.

Prematurity One-third of premature infants and the majority of very-low-birth-weight infants develop hypocalcemia during the first 2 days after birth. Multiple factors contribute to the fall and include hypoalbuminemia, and factors that lower both total and ionized calcium such as reduced intake of calcium because of low intake of milk, possible impaired response to parathyroid hormone, increased calcitonin levels, and increased urinary calcium losses.

Infants of Diabetic Mothers Hypocalcemia occurs in 10% to 20% of infants of diabetic mothers. The lowest concentration typically occurs between 24 to 72 hours after birth and often is associated with hyperphosphatemia. Hypocalcemia is caused by lower parathyroid hormone concentrations after birth in this condition compared to normal infants. Hypoparathyroidism is likely related to intrauterine hypercalcemia suppressing the fetal parathyroid glands. Concurrent hypomagnesemia is another contributing factor.

Birth Asphyxia Infants with birth asphyxia frequently have hypocalcemia and hyperphosphatemia. Possible mechanisms include increased phosphate load caused by tissue catabolism, decreased intake due to delayed initiation of feedings, renal insufficiency, acidosis, and increased serum calcitonin concentration.

Intrauterine Growth Restriction Hypocalcemia occurs with increased frequency in infants with intrauterine growth restriction. The mechanism is thought to involve decreased transfer of calcium across the placenta.

Late Neonatal Hypocalcemia Late hypocalcemia develops after the second or third day after birth. It typically occurs at the end of the first week.

Hypoparathyroidism: Hypoparathyroidism associated with excess phosphorus intake is the most common cause of late neonatal hypocalcemia. Hypoparathyroidism often occurs as part of a syndrome, including DiGeorge syndrome, or, more rarely, mitochondrial cytopathies.

Maternal Hyperparathyroidism: Infants born to mothers with hyperparathyroidism frequently have hypocalcemia. The mechanism is related to increased transplacental calcium transport caused by maternal hypercalcemia, which results in excessive fetal hypercalcemia that inhibits fetal and neonatal parathyroid secretion. Affected infants typically develop increased neuromuscular irritability in the first 3 weeks after birth, but they can present later.

Hypomagnesemia: Hypomagnesemia causes resistance to parathyroid hormone and impairs its secretion, both of which can result in hypocalcemia. The most common etiology in newborns is transient hypomagnesemia, although rare disorders of intestinal or renal tubular magnesium transport can occur.

High Phosphate Intake: Intake of excess phosphate is a historically important cause of late hypocalcemia that was seen in term infants fed bovine milk or a formula with a high phosphorus concentration. It has been postulated but the high phosphorus levels antagonize parathyroid hormone or may produce increased calcium and phosphorus deposition in bones. Symptomatic infants typically present with tetany or seizures at 5 to 10 days of age. Severe hyperphosphatemia and hypocalcemia also can be caused by phosphate enemas.

Other Causes: Critically ill or premature infants are exposed to many therapeutic interventions that may cause transient hypocalcemia including bicarbonate infusion resulting in metabolic alkalosis, transfusion with citrated blood or infusion of lipids leading to formation of calcium complexes and decreased ionized calcium level. Finally, mild hypocalcemia has been associated with phototherapy. Other rare causes include acute renal failure of any cause, usually associated with hyperphosphatemia, any disorder of vitamin D metabolism, and rotavirus infections.

Hypercalcemia

Signs and Symptoms

Hypercalcemia is more difficult to diagnose than hypocalcemia because of the nonspecific nature of symptoms and signs (Table 27-20). Major symptoms may include skeletal pain, fatigue, anorexia, nausea, and vomiting, and particularly important are polyuria and polydipsia. Changes in behavior and frank psychiatric disorders may also be a result of hypercalcemia. The extent of symptoms and signs is a function of both the degree of hypercalcemia and the rate of onset of the elevation in the serum calcium concentration. Thus, a rather severe hypercalcemia of 3.50 mmol/L is asymptomatic chronically while an acute rise to these values may cause marked changes in sensorium. It is worthy of mention, however, that symptoms and signs associated with hypercalcemia may be due to the elevation in the calcium concentration or to the underlying disease.[49,50]

TABLE 27-20 Symptoms and Signs of Hypercalcemia

General Weakness Depression Anorexia
Central nervous system Impaired concentration Increased sleep requirement Altered state of consciousness Mental retardation Polydipsia (and polyuria)
Muscular: weakness
Ocular Palpebral calcification Band keratopathy Conjunctival calcification
Dermal: pruritus and skin calcifications
Gastrointestinal Constipation Anorexia, nausea, vomiting Pancreatitis Peptic ulcer
Cardiovascular Shortened QT interval on standard electrocardiogram[a] Arterial hypertension
Skeletal: joint pains (pseudogout)
Renal dysfunction Altered urinary concentration ability with polyuria and polydipsia Nephrolithiasis, nephrocalcinosis, renal failure Distal renal tubular acidosis

[a] Without any major tendency towards cardiac arrhythmias.

Causes

Hypercalcemia results when the entry of calcium into the circulation exceeds the excretion of calcium into the urine or deposition in bone. Since the major sources of calcium are bones and the intestinal tract, hypercalcemia mostly results from increased bone resorption or from increased intestinal absorption. In some cases, however, multiple sites are involved in the development of hypercalcemia. Major textbooks or reviews correctly point out that the great majority of adult patients with elevated calcium concentration will be found to have either primary hyperparathyroidism or malignancy (this form of hypercalcemia is thought in many instances to be caused by secretion of parathyroid hormone–related peptide), although the differential diagnosis is much longer. For these other causes of hypercalcemia, which include vitamin D (or A) intoxication, sarcoidosis, tuberculosis, some fungal infections, thyreotoxicosis, Addison's disease, milk-alkali syndrome related to the prescription of calcium and absorbable alkali, treatment with thiazides or lithium carbonate, familial hypocalciuric hypercalcemia, prolonged immobilization in subjects with high skeletal turnover (including adolescents), and the recovery phase of rhabdomyolysis, the use of the mnemonic VITAMINS TRAPS (Table 27-21) has been suggested.[51] Children present with hypercalcemia less frequently than adults, but the causes that are common in adults are also common in children. Young children and infants, however, present with hypercalcemia in association with a number of rather rare conditions seen almost exclusively in that population.[51,52] The reported causes of hypercalcemia are given in Table 27-21.

Diagnostic Workup

The cause of hypercalcemia can usually be discerned clinically. It is estimated, for example, that clinical history, physical examination, and simple laboratory data (circulating phosphate and creatinine; urinary calcium, phosphate, and creatinine) and chest x-ray (looking for sarcoidosis), provide the correct diagnosis with an accuracy of 80% to 90%. Addition of an assay for intact parathyroid hormone further increases accuracy.[49,50]

Step 1: Assess Clinical and Simple Laboratory Data Clinical history and physical examination are useful in establishing the diagnosis of hypercalcemia induced by immobilization medication or thyreotoxicosis, and the diagnosis of "syndromic" hypercalcemia, including Williams-Beuren syndrome, Down syndrome, and Jansen's metaphyseal chondrodysplasia. Measurement of serum phosphate concentration and urinary calcium excretion also may be helpful in selected cases: hyperparathyroidism and the humoral hypercalcemia of malignancy induced by secretion of parathyroid hormone–related peptide often present with hypophosphatemia resulting from inhibition of renal proximal tubular phosphate

TABLE 27-21 Causes of Hypercalcemia

Classical causes (mnemonic VITAMINS TRAP) *V*itamins D (and A) *I*mmobilization *T*hyrotoxicosis *A*ddison's disease *M*ilk-alkali syndrome *I*nflammatory disorders (granulomatous diseases with excessive production of calcitriol) *N*eoplastic-related disease[a] *S*arcoidosis *T*hiazides[b] and other drugs *R*habdomyolysis (recovery phase) *A*IDS *P*arathyroid disease[a] (including familial hypocalciuric hypercalcemia), parenteral nutrition
Hypercalcemia associated with elevated calcitriol (1,25-dihydroxyvitamin D_3) Sarcoidosis Acute granulomatous pneumonia, lipoid pneumonia Tuberculosis (and other mycobacterial infections) Wegener's granulomatosis Crohn's disease Hepatic granulomatosis Talc and silicone granulomatosis Cat scratch disease Neonatal subcutaneous fat necrosis
Hypercalcemia associated with elevated parathyroid hormone-related peptide Hypercalcemia of malignancy Some benign tumors (ovary, kidney, pheochromocytoma) Systemic lupus erythematosus HIV-associated lymphadenopathy Massive mammary hyperplasia During late pregnancy and lactation in hypoparathyroidism
Drugs associated with the development of hypercalcemia Common: calcium, vitamin D, vitamin A, lithium, thiazides[b] (e.g., hydrochlorothiazide, chlortalidone) Less common: omeprazole, theophyllin (toxic doses), recombinant growth hormone, foscarnet, hepatitis B vaccination, manganese toxicity
Rare causes of hypercalcemia with unknown underlying mechanism Infections: nocardiosis, brucellosis, cytomegaloviric infection (in AIDS), berylliosis Juvenile idiopathic arthritis Advanced chronic liver disease
Rare causes of hypercalcemia in infancy and young children Reduced function of calcium-sensing receptor Deactivating mutations Heterozygous: familial hypocalciuric hypercalcemia Homozygous: severe neonatal hyperparathyroidism Autoantibodies directed at calcium-sensing receptor Congenital hypoparathyroidism Idiopathic infantile hypercalcemia Jansen's metaphyseal chondrodysplasia[c] Williams-Beuren syndrome Down syndrome Hypophosphatasia Congenital lactase deficiency Phosphate depletion in severe prematurity Renal tubular acidosis Primary hyperoxaluria Neonatal subcutaneous fat necrosis

Note: Some causes of hypercalcemia are given twice.
[a] Malignancy and primary hyperparathyroidism account for 80%-90% of cases of hypercalcemia in adulthood.
[b] Although thiazides are frequently cited as a cause of hypercalcemia, it is more common that they bring mild pre-existing hypercalcemia to light.
[c] Consequence of a constitutive activation of the parathyroid hormone receptor.

reabsorption. In comparison, the serum phosphate concentration is normal or elevated in granulomatous diseases, vitamin D intoxication, immobilization, and thyrotoxicosis and metastatic bone disease. Urinary calcium excretion is usually raised or high-normal in hyperparathyroidism and hypercalcemia of malignancy. Two conditions lead to relative hypocalciuria: thiazides, which directly enhance active calcium reabsorption in the distal tubule, and familial hypocalciuric hypercalcemia in which the fractional excretion of calcium is often less than 1.0%. (Two other clues to the possible presence of this disorder are a family history of hypercalcemia and few if any hypercalcemic symptoms.)

Step 2: Analyze Intact Parathyroid Hormone Level An elevated intact parathyroid hormone concentration indicates the presence of primary hyperparathyroidism or a patient taking lithium. Ten percent to 20% of patients with primary hyperparathyroidism have a parathyroid hormone concentration in the upper end of the normal range: such a "normal" level, which indicates that the secretion is not suppressed, is virtually diagnostic of primary hyperparathyroidism, since it is still inappropriately high considering the presence of hypercalcemia. A low or low-normal parathyroid hormone level is consistent with all other non-parathyroid hormone-induced causes of hypercalcemia.

Step 3: Analyze Vitamin D Metabolites The levels of vitamin D metabolites calcidiol and calcitriol should be measured if there is no obvious malignancy, and parathyroid hormone levels are not elevated. An elevated serum concentration of calcidiol is indicative of vitamin D intoxication. On the other hand, increased levels of calcitriol may be induced by direct intake of this metabolite or extrarenal production in granulomatous diseases or lymphoma.

MAGNESIUM

Balance

A 70-kg man contains approximately 1 mole (25 g) of magnesium. About half of it is present in bone tissue, and the other half in soft tissue, whereas no more than 1% to 2% of the total body magnesium is present in extracellular fluids. Intracellular magnesium serves as a cofactor for many enzymes that produce and store energy via hydrolysis of adenosine triphosphate.[53]

In healthy humans the total circulating magnesium concentration is maintained within narrow limits and ranges between 0.75 and 1.0 mmol/L. (Circulating magnesium levels can be reported in millimoles per liter, metabolic equivalents per liter, milligrams per deciliter, or milligrams per liter. The valence of magnesium is 2 and its molecular mass 24.3; therefore, 0.50 mmol/L is equivalent to 1.00 meq/L, 1.21 mg/dl, and 12.1 mg/L.) Approximately one-quarter of the magnesium is bound to albumin. For the remaining three-quarters of the circulating magnesium approximately 10% is complexed to inorganic phosphate, citrate, and other compounds, while 90% (two-thirds of the total circulating magnesium) is in the form of free ion.

Magnesium balance, like that of other ions, is a function of intake and urinary excretion. In adults, daily magnesium intake averages 0.23 to 0.28 mmol/kg of body weight (5.6 to 6.8 mg/kg of body weight). About one-third of this magnesium is absorbed. In healthy adults, there is no net gain or loss of magnesium from bone so that balance is achieved by the urinary excretion of the 0.06 to 0.08 mmol/kg of body weight (1.5 to 1.9 mg/kg of body weight.)

Only 15% to 25% of the filtered magnesium is reabsorbed in the proximal tubule and 5% to 10% in the distal tubule. The major site of magnesium transport is the thick ascending limb of the loop of Henle where 60% to 70% of the filtered load is reabsorbed.[54,55]

With negative magnesium balance, the initial loss comes primarily from the extracellular fluid (equilibration with bone stores begins after several weeks). Thus, circulating magnesium falls rapidly with negative magnesium balance, leading to a conspicuous decrease in magnesium excretion unless urinary magnesium wasting is present. The fractional clearance of magnesium, which is 3.0 to 5.0×10^{-2} in healthy subjects ingesting a normal diet, can fall to below 0.5% with magnesium depletion due to extrarenal losses. This parameter is calculated from the following equation:

$$\frac{\text{Urinary magnesium} \times \text{Circulating creatinine}}{\text{Circulating magnesium} \times \text{Urinary creatinine}}$$

There is no protection against hypermagnesemia with loss of renal function. In this setting, high intake leads to extracellular magnesium retention.

Hypomagnesemia

Hypomagnesemia is not rare (Table 27-21). There are two mechanisms by which hypomagnesemia can be induced: intestinal (including dietary insufficiency) or renal losses. In the presence of hypomagnesemia, the healthy kidney lowers magnesium excretion to very low values. Hence the diagnosis of hypomagnesemia caused by intestinal magnesium losses (or low dietary magnesium intake) is easily established by the demonstration of low urinary magnesium excretion. Conversely, the diagnosis of hypomagnesemia caused by renal losses is established by the demonstration of inappropriately high ("normal") urinary magnesium excretion. If the cause of hypomagnesemia is not apparent from the history, the distinction between intestinal and renal losses can be made by measuring the fractional clearance of magnesium on a random urine specimen.[16]

Decreased Intake, Poor Intestinal Absorption, or Intestinal Loss

Intestinal secretory losses, which contain some magnesium, are continuous and not regulated. Although the obligatory losses are not large, marked dietary deprivation can lead to progressive magnesium depletion. Magnesium loss will also occur when the intestinal secretions are incompletely reabsorbed as with most disorders of the small bowel, including acute or chronic diarrhea, malabsorption and steatorrhea, and small-bowel bypass surgery.

Hypomagnesemia can also be seen in acute pancreatitis. The mechanism is probably similar to that responsible for the associated hypocalcemia: saponification of magnesium and calcium in necrotic fat.

Paunier disease or hypomagnesemia with secondary hypocalcemia is a very rare defect of intestinal magnesium (usually combined with impaired renal magnesium conservation), which presents early in infancy with hypocalcemia responsive to magnesium administration. The disease is caused by a loss of function mutation in an ion channel of the transient receptor potential gene family called TRPM6.[56,57]

Renal Losses

Urinary magnesium losses can be induced by various mechanisms.

Primary renal magnesium wasting: various primary renal magnesium wasting disorders have been recognized, as discussed in Chapter 30.

Loop and thiazide-type diuretics: Both loop and thiazide diuretics can inhibit net magnesium reabsorption, while the potassium-sparing diuretics may lower magnesium excretion. The degree of hypomagnesemia induced by the loop and thiazide diuretics is generally mild, in part because the associated volume contraction will tend to increase proximal sodium, water, and magnesium reabsorption.

Drugs other than diuretics: Many drugs can produce urinary magnesium wasting, as shown in Table 27-22.

Volume expansion: Expansion of the extracellular fluid volume can decrease passive magnesium transport. Mild hypomagnesemia may ensue if this is sustained.

Hypercalcemia: Calcium and magnesium seem to compete for transport in the thick ascending limb of the loop of Henle. The increased filtered calcium load in hypercalcemic states will deliver more calcium to the loop; the ensuing rise in calcium reabsorption will diminish that of magnesium.

Miscellaneous: Magnesium wasting can be seen as part of the tubular dysfunction seen with recovery from acute tubular necrosis, following renal transplantation and during postobstructive diuresis.

Alcohol: Excessive urinary excretion of magnesium is common in alcoholic patients. Dietary deficiency, acute pancreatitis, diarrhea, and refeeding also contribute to hypomagnesemia in these patients.

Additional Causes

Hypomagnesemia, together with hypophosphatemia, hypokalemia, and increasing extracellular fluid volume, occurs in the context of refeeding syndrome (see the Hypophosphatemia section).

Hypomagnesemia sometimes occurs in diabetes mellitus and is related in part to the degree of hyperglycemia.

Hypomagnesemia can be seen following surgery, at least in part due to chelation by circulating free fatty acids.

Hypomagnesemia can occur as part of the "hungry bone" syndrome in which there is increased magnesium uptake by renewing bone following parathyroidectomy (for hyperparathyroidism).

TABLE 27-22 Causes of Hypomagnesemia

Decreased Magnesium Intake and Intestinal Losses
Dietary deprivation
Small bowel disorders, including acute or chronic diarrhea, malabsorption and steatorrhea, and small bowel bypass surgery
Acute pancreatitis
Paunier disease[a] (hypomagnesemia with secondary hypocalcemia)
Renal Losses
Primary renal magnesium-wasting diseases
Drugs Loop and thiazide-type diuretics Drugs other than diuretics (aminoglycoside antibiotics, amphotericin B, cisplatin, pentamidine, cyclosporine, tacrolimus, foscarnet, cetuximab[b]) Volume expansion
Hypercalcemia
Miscellaneous: recovery from acute tubular necrosis following renal transplantation and during a postobstructive diuresis
Further Causes
Alcohol
Refeeding syndrome
Diabetes mellitus
Following surgery
"Hungry bone syndrome" following parathyroidectomy for hyperparathyroidism
Neonatal hypomagnesemia
Maternal hypomagnesemia
Intrauterine growth retardation

[a] Often combined with impaired renal magnesium conservation.
[b] A monoclonal antibody against epithelial growth factor receptor.

Neonatal Hypomagnesemia

Like in older children, in newborns hypomagnesemia may result from decreased magnesium intake, intestinal losses, or renal losses.[55] However, two peculiar causes of neonatal hypomagnesemia deserve consideration: maternal hypomagnesemia and intrauterine growth retardation.

Neonatal hypomagnesemia secondary to maternal hypomagnesemia is a recognized feature of maternal diabetes mellitus. However, maternal hypomagnesemia from any cause has been associated with neonatal hypomagnesemia.

Decreased magnesium levels sometimes occur in infants whose birth weight is small in relation to their gestational age. Circulating magnesium is normally low for the first 3 to 5 days of life.

Symptoms, Signs, Consequences

Magnesium depletion is often associated with two biochemical abnormalities: hypokalemia and hypocalcemia. As a result, it is often difficult to ascribe specific clinical manifestations solely to hypomagnesemia. The typical signs and symptoms of magnesium depletion include tetany, positive Chvostek, Trousseau and Lust signs, or generalized convulsions. Generalized weakness and anorexia sometimes also occur. In addition magnesium depletion can induce ventricular arrhythmias, particularly during myocardial ischemia or cardiopulmonary bypass.[53,56]

Hypokalemia

Hypokalemia, mostly accompanied by metabolic alkalosis, is common in hypomagnesemia. This association is in part due to underlying disorders that cause both magnesium and potassium loss, such as diuretic therapy and diarrhea.

There is also evidence of renal potassium wasting in hypomagnesemia. The following mechanism explains this tendency. Potassium secretion from the cell into the lumen of the loop of Henle is mediated by a potassium channel that is inhibitable by adenosine triphosphate. Hypomagnesemia and the associated reduction in cell magnesium concentration lead to an increase in the number of open potassium channels. Given the high cell potassium level, this change promotes potassium secretion from the cell into the lumen and enhances urinary losses.

Hypocalcemia

Hypocalcemia is the most classical sign of severe hypomagnesemia (0.50 mmol/L or less). The following three factors account for this tendency:

- Inappropriately low circulating parathyroid hormone secretion.
- Inappropriately low calcitriol (1,25-dihydroxyvitamin D, the active metabolite of vitamin D).
- Bone resistance to parathyroid hormone. Hypomagnesemia interferes with G protein activation in response to parathyroid hormone, thereby minimizing the stimulation of adenylate cyclase.

Repletion

Magnesium repletion is controversial in asymptomatic (mostly mild) hypomagnesemia. Oral repletion using lactate, oxide, pidolate, or chloride salts is usually preferred. Because of the laxative effect of oral magnesium, the amounts administered must be tailored to the individual patient (0.30 mmol/kg of body weight of magnesium per day in divided doses results in diarrhea in approximately 10% of patients). The parenteral route is preferred in critically ill patients, but the exact dosage is poorly understood. For true emergencies (e.g., generalized convulsions or ventricular arrhythmias), magnesium is administered (either as sulphate or as chloride) intravenously over 1 to 2 minutes in a dosage of 0.15 to 0.20 mmol/kg of body weight (approximately 3.5 to 4.7 mg of elemental magnesium per kilogram of body weight) (repeated if no response 5 to 10 minutes later). In subjects with moderate to severe but rather oligosymptomatic magnesium deficiency, the mentioned dose is given over 4 to 6 hours until circulating magnesium is returned to normal.

INORGANIC PHOSPHATE

Balance

In a 70-kg man, the phosphate content of the body amounts to approximately 1% of the body weight, or 700 g (23 mol). Of this, 85% is contained in the bone tissue and teeth, 14% in the soft tissues, and the remaining 1% in extracellular fluids.[58-60]

In the blood, phosphate is found both as organic as well as inorganic salt, but clinical laboratories measure the inorganic form. Of the circulating inorganic phosphate, roughly 10% is bound to protein; 5% is complexed with calcium, magnesium, or sodium; and 85% exists as ionized phosphate. The normal blood concentration of inorganic phosphate is highest during the neonatal period and early childhood and declines thereafter (Table 27-23) because infants and children avidly retain phosphate. There is a mean diurnal variation in concentration of phosphate of approximately 0.2 mmol/L (0.6 mg/dl) with a nadir at 11.0, subsequently rising to a plateau at 16.0 hours and peaking in the early night.

The average diet of a 70-kg man provides 800 to 1500 mg (25 to 50 mmol) of phosphate daily. As much as two-thirds of the dietary phosphate is absorbed in the gut, but intestinal secretion, mainly in saliva and bile acids, adds 200 mg (6 mmol) of phosphate into the intestinal lumen daily. Under steady-state conditions, the kidney is the most important modulator of the blood phosphate level, ensuring that urinary phosphate output is equivalent to the net phosphate absorption from the intestine. Phosphate is freely filtered across the glomerulus, and 80% to 90% of the phosphate is reabsorbed by the renal tubules (mostly in the proximal tubule) in subjects aged 6 months or more (Table 27-23). The renal tubular handling of phosphate is best expressed as fractional excretion of phosphate or, more precisely, as maximal tubular reabsorption of phosphate, which clarify the relationship between circulating phosphate and urinary phosphate excretion. The fractional clearance of phosphate, the tubular phosphate reabsorption and the maximal tubular phosphate reabsorption are easily calculated following an overnight fast from plasma (P_{Ph}), urinary (U_{Ph}) phosphate, plasma (P_{Cr}), and urinary (U_{Cr}) creatinine as follows[61,62]:

$$\text{Fractional excretion} = \frac{U_{Ph} \times P_{Cr}}{P_{Ph} \times U_{Cr}}$$

$$\text{Tubular phosphate reabsorption} = 1 - \frac{U_{Ph} \times P_{Cr}}{P_{Ph} \times U_{Cr}}$$

$$\text{Maximal reabsorption} = P_{Ph} - \left(\frac{U_{Ph} \times P_{Cr}}{U_{Cr}}\right)$$

The maximal tubular phosphate reabsorption calculated using this equation and that obtained using the normogram described by Walton and Bijvoet are almost identical. The reference values[62] for the fractional excretion of phosphate and the maximal tubular reabsorption of phosphate are age dependent and appear in Table 27-23.

Three groups of hormonal factors regulate phosphate homeostasis[58-60,63]:

Calcitriol (1,25-dihydroxyvitamin D_3) stimulates the intestinal phosphate reabsorption.

Parathyroid hormone decreases the renal tubular reabsorption and causes phosphaturia.

"Phosphatonins" are phosphaturic factors other than parathyroid hormone. They include fibroblast growth factor 23, frizzled-related protein 4, and matrix extracellular phosphoglycoprotein.

Hypophosphatemia

Hypophosphatemia does not necessarily mean phosphate depletion since it can occur in the presence of low, normal, or high total body phosphate, because in some instances the relationship between extracellular and intracellular phosphate is altered. On the other hand, phosphate depletion may exist with normal, low, or elevated levels of blood phosphate.[58-60]

The normal phosphate level in adolescents and adults ranges between 0.97 and 1.8 mmol/L (2.9 to 5.4 mg/dl). In this age group hypophosphatemia is arbitrarily divided into moderate cases (phosphate 0.32 to 0.65 mmol/L or 0.96 to 1.95 mg/dl) and severe cases (phosphate <0.32 mmol/L or <0.96 mg/dl). There are three major mechanisms by which

TABLE 27-23 Fasting Values for Circulating Inorganic Phosphate, Fractional Phosphate Excretion, and Maximal Tubular Phosphate Reabsorption in Infancy and Childhood

Age	Blood Inorganic Phosphate mmol/L[a]	Fractional Phosphate Excretion 10^{-2}	Maximal Tubular Reabsorption of Phosphate mmol/L[a]
0-3 months	1.62 2.40	11.9-38.7	1.02-2.00
4-6 months	1.78-2.21	3.50-34.9	1.27-1.88
6-12 months	1.38-2.15	10.3-20.0	1.13-1.86
1-2 years	1.32-1.93	5.50-23.3	1.05-1.74
3-4 years	1.02-1.92	≤18.4	0.90-1.78
5-6 years	1.13-1.73	0.60-15.0	1.02-1.62
7-8 years	1.06-1.80	≤16.8	0.98-1.64
9-10 years	1.13-1.70	1.80-14.1	1.00-1.58
11-12 years	1.04-1.79	1.80-12.1	0.97-1.65
13-15 years	0.97-1.80	≤12.6	0.91-1.68

[a] To obtain traditional units (mg/dl), multiply by 3.1.

Modified from Brodehl J: Assessment and interpretation of the tubular threshold for phosphate in infants and children, *Pediatr Nephrol* 8:645, 1994.

TABLE 27-24 **Causes of Hypophosphatemia**
With Normal Fractional Excretion of Phosphate and Maximal Tubular Phosphate Reabsorption
Low dietary intake or poor intestinal absorption Low dietary intake: severe malnutrition, very-low-birthweight infants Poor absorption: steatorrhea, chronic diarrhea, use of phosphate binders
Internal redistribution Refeeding syndrome in malnutrition (including diabetic ketoacidosis treated with insulin) Respiratory alkalosis Hungry bone syndrome after parathyroidectomy
With Increased Fractional Excretion of Phosphate and Reduced Maximal Tubular Phosphate Reabsorption
Hyperparathyroidism
de Toni-Debré-Fanconi syndrome (general impairment of proximal tubule)[a]
Hypophosphatemic rickets[b]
After kidney transplant (post-transplant hypophosphatemia)

[a] Various drugs may cause an incomplete or, more rarely, a complete form of de Toni-Debré-Fanconi syndrome with hypophosphatemia, including paracetamol poisoning, and treatment with ifosfamide, valproic acid, or β_2-adrenoreceptors (e.g., albuterol).
[b] At least in part explained by increased activity of the phosphatonin fibroblast growth factor 23.

hypophosphatemia can occur: (1) low dietary intake or poor intestinal absorption, (2) internal redistribution, and (3) increased urinary loss. In patients with hypophosphatemia caused by decreased intestinal absorption or internal redistribution, the fractional excretion of phosphate and the maximal tubular reabsorption of phosphate are normal (Table 27-24). On the contrary, these parameters are inappropriately altered in patients with increased urinary loss.

Low Dietary Intake or Poor Intestinal Absorption

Given the fact that phosphate is ubiquitous in foods, the development of deficiency would be anticipated only in severe cases of malnutrition or in very-low-birth-weight infants at the time of rapid postnatal growth. If phosphate restriction is severe and prolonged, or if intestinal absorption is reduced by the chronic use of phosphate binders, then the constant intestinal loss may induce phosphate depletion.

Internal Redistribution

In the majority of cases, an acute shift in phosphate from the extracellular to the intracellular compartment is primarily responsible for lowering of serum phosphate. The most frequent cause is refeeding syndrome, a recognized but underdiagnosed and potentially fatal condition that occurs when previously malnourished patients are fed. The fluid and electrolyte abnormalities noted in the refeeding syndrome and those noted in severe diabetic ketoacidosis following the administration of insulin therapy are similar.

Patients who are malnourished develop a total body depletion of phosphate, magnesium, and potassium. Nonetheless, their blood levels are maintained by redistribution from the intracellular space. The delivery of glucose as part of a feeding strategy causes a huge increase in the circulating insulin level that induces a rapid uptake of glucose, potassium, phosphate, and magnesium into cells. The blood concentration of these metabolites falls dramatically. In addition, the body begins to retain fluid, and the extracellular space expands. Although hypophosphatemia is the predominant feature of the syndrome, rapid falls in potassium and magnesium levels, together with some tendency towards metabolic alkalosis, predispose to cardiac arrhythmias, while extracellular space expansion can precipitate acute heart failure in patients with cardiovascular disease. The most effective way to treat refeeding syndrome is to be aware of it. One should start feeds slowly and aggressively supplement and monitor phosphate, potassium, and magnesium for 4 days after feeding is started.

Another cause of hypophosphatemia in hospitalized patients is respiratory alkalosis. Severe hyperventilation can be seen in patients with anxiety, pain, and sepsis, and in patients during mechanical ventilation. The fall in carbon dioxide will result in a similar change in the cell because carbon dioxide readily diffuses across cell membranes. The elevated pH stimulates the glycolysis, leading to an accelerated production of phosphorylated metabolites and a rapid shift of phosphate into the cells.

The hungry bone syndrome, characterized by massive deposition of calcium and phosphate in the bone, can occur after parathyroidectomy for long-standing hyperparathyroidism (both primary and secondary).

Urinary Loss

In hyperparathyroidism, both primary and secondary, there is an increased urinary loss of phosphate. Fanconi-de Toni-Debré syndrome is characterized by a general impairment of the proximal tubule leading to urinary loss of compounds normally reabsorbed by the proximal tubule. It results in hypophosphatemia, glucosuria, hyperaminoaciduria, uricosuria, and hyperbicarbonaturia (causing renal tubular acidosis). The urinary phosphate excretion is also increased in patients with hereditary hypophosphatemic rickets and tumor-induced osteomalacia and rickets, as discussed in Chapter 28. In patients with a kidney transplant, hypophosphatemia has been described in the absence of both hyperparathyroidism and other evidence of proximal tubule dysfunction.

Combined Factors

A combination of factors is often responsible for hypophosphatemia found in patients.

Symptoms, Signs, Consequences

Phosphate depletion can cause a variety of symptoms and signs. Two major mechanisms are responsible for these symptoms: decreases in intracellular adenosine triphosphate and in diphosphoglycerate. In adults, hypophosphatemia is symptomatic when the phosphate level is lower than 0.35 mmol/L. Hypophosphatemia may be asymptomatic under certain clinical situations: patients recovering from diabetic ketoacidosis and patients with prolonged hyperventilation are usually asymptomatic because often there is not real phosphate depletion. The clinical features of phosphate depletion appear in Table 27-25.

TABLE 27-25 Symptoms, Signs, and Consequences of Phosphate Depletion

Skeletal muscle and bone: proximal myopathy, rhabdomyolysis[a]
Cardiovascular system: impaired myocardial contractility
Respiratory system: respiratory failure (and failed weaning)
Neurological system: paresthesias, tremors, seizures, features resembling Guillain-Barré syndrome or Wernicke encephalopathy
Hematological system: hemolysis, impaired granulocyte chemotaxis and phagocytosis causing Gram-negative sepsis, altered platelet function, and thrombocytopenia

[a] In patients with rhabdomyolysis, hypophosphatemia can be masked by the release of phosphate from the injured muscle.

Management

Hypophosphatemia does not automatically mean that replacement therapy with phosphate is indicated. To determine whether treatment is indicated it is necessary to establish the cause of the hypophosphatemia, in which the history and clinical setting are important. The identification and treatment of the primary cause usually lead to normalization of the circulating phosphate level. As an example, the hypophosphatemia found in patients with diabetic ketoacidosis will usually correct spontaneously with normal dietary intake. However, replacement therapy is needed in patients with hypophosphatemia in combination with evidence of renal or gastrointestinal phosphate loss, the presence of underlying risk factors, and particularly if there are the clinical manifestations described above.[58-60]

The safest mode of therapy is oral. Cow's milk is a good source. It contains 1 g (32 mmol) of elemental phosphate per liter. Alternatively, oral preparations in the form of sodium phosphate or potassium phosphate can be used. The average adult patient requires 1 to 2 g (32 to 64 mmol) of phosphate per day for 7 to 10 days to replenish body stores. An important side effect of oral supplementation is diarrhea.

Intravenous phosphate, usually 2.5 to 5.0 mg/kg (0.08 to 0.16 mmol/kg) over 6 hours, is given in patients with symptomatic phosphate deficiency who cannot take milk or tablets. More aggressive repletion with phosphate has been advocated but the magnitude of the response is unpredictable (close monitoring of phosphate level is crucial). Side effects of intravenous phosphate repletion are hypocalcemia, metastatic calcification, hyperkalemia associated with potassium-containing supplements, volume excess, hypernatremia, metabolic acidosis, and hyperphosphatemia.

Hyperphosphatemia

Phosphatemia may be artifactually increased if hemolysis occurs during the collection or processing of blood samples. Spurious hyperphosphatemia due to interference with analytical methods may occur in patients with hyperglobulinemia, hyperlipidemia, and hyperbilirubinemia (among these conditions, the most common is hyperglobulinemia due to Waldenstrom's macroglobulinemia, multiple myeloma, or monoclonal gammopathy, three conditions that do not occur in childhood). True hyperphosphatemia indicates either an increased phosphate load or a decreased renal phosphate excretion, as shown in Table 27-26. High dietary ingestion of phosphate alone rarely causes hyperphosphatemia with the exception of newborns and infants fed cow's milk, whose phosphate content is six times greater than human milk.

TABLE 27-26 Causes of Hyperphosphatemia

Artifactual or Spurious
Increased Phosphate Load (with normal fractional excretion of phosphate and normal maximal tubular phosphate reabsorption)
High dietary intake or increased intestinal absorption Newborns and infants fed cow's milk (rather than breast milk or adapted formula milk) Parenteral administration of phosphate salts Large amounts of phosphate-containing laxatives, phosphate enemas[a] Vitamin D intoxication
Internal redistribution Tumor lysis syndrome (before treatment and after initiation of cytotoxic therapy) Rhabdomyolysis Lactic and ketoacidosis (or severe hyperglycemia alone),[b] including severe dehydration in context of acute diarrhea
Decreased Renal Phosphate Excretion
Reduced renal function (either acute or chronic)
Increased renal tubular phosphate reabsorption (decreased fractional phosphate excretion and increased maximal tubular phosphate reabsorption) Hypoparathyroidism (and pseudohypoparathyroidism) Acromegaly Drugs: growth hormone, biphosphonates, dipyridamole Idiopathic childhood nephrotic syndrome Familial tumoral calcinosis

[a] The danger of hyperphosphatemia secondary to phosphate enema is especially high in children under age 2 years.
[b] Metabolic acidosis blunts glycolysis, and therefore cellular phosphate utilization. In addition, tissue hypoxia or insulin deficiency also plays a crucial role.

Acutely or chronically impaired renal function plays at least a partial role in most instances of hyperphosphatemia, including physiologically low glomerular filtration rate to explain the inability of the neonate to eliminate excess phosphate, mild renal insufficiency (due to volume contraction secondary to diarrhea) in subjects ingesting large amounts of phosphate-containing laxatives, or mild to moderate tubulointerstitial injury secondary to intrarenal accumulation of uric acid in tumor lysis syndrome (see section on hyperkalemia).

Familial tumoral calcinosis is a rare autosomal recessive disorder characterized by hyperphosphatemia due to increased maximal tubular phosphate reabsorption. Available data suggest that the disease might be secondary to deficient fibroblast growth factor 23. Familial tumoral calcinosis is a kind of mirror image of some forms of hypophosphatemic rickets in which increased activity of the phosphatonin fibroblast growth factor 23 decreases maximal tubular phosphate reabsorption.[63]

ACKNOWLEDGMENT

This work is supported by the Associazione per il Bambino Nefropatico, Milan, Italy.

REFERENCES

1. D'Avanzo M, Santinelli R, Tolone C, Bettinelli A, Bianchetti MG: Concealed administration of frusemide simulating Bartter syndrome in a 4.5-year-old boy, *Pediatr Nephrol* 9:749-50, 1995.
2. Peschel RE, Peschel E: What physicians have in common with Sherlock Holmes, *J R Soc Med* 82:33-36, 1989.
3. Moritz ML, Ayus JC: Disorders of water metabolism in children: hyponatremia and hypernatremia, *Pediatr Rev* 23:371-80, 2002.
4. Moritz ML, Ayus JC: Preventing neurological complications from dysnatremias in children, *Pediatr Nephrol* 20:1687-700, 2005.
5. Haycock GB: Hypernatraemia: diagnosis and management, *Arch Dis Child Educ Pract Ed* 91:8-13, 2006.
6. Haycock GB: Hyponatraemia: diagnosis and management, *Arch Dis Child Educ Pract Ed* 91:37-41, 2006.
7. Adrogué HJ, Madias NE: Hypernatremia, *N Engl J Med* 342:1493-99, 2000.
8. Adrogué HJ, Madias NE: Hyponatremia, *N Engl J Med* 342:1581-89, 2000.
9. Gouyon JB: Mouvements d'eau transmembranaires: de l'osmolalité à la tonicité, *Arch Pédiatr* 8:1367-69, 2001.
10. Steiner MJ, DeWalt DA, Byerley JS: Is this child dehydrated? *JAMA* 291:2746-54, 2004.
11. Paut O, Lacroix F: Recent developments in the perioperative fluid management for the paediatric patient, *Curr Opin Anaesthesiol* 19:268-77, 2006.
12. Halberthal M, Halperin ML, Bohn D: Lesson of the week: Acute hyponatraemia in children admitted to hospital: retrospective analysis of factors contributing to its development and resolution, *BMJ* 322:780-82, 2001.
13. Robson WL, Leung AK: Hyponatremia in children treated with desmopressin, *Arch Pediatr Adolesc Med* 152:930-31, 1998.
14. Gitelman SE, Feldman BJ, Rosenthal SM: Nephrogenic syndrome of inappropriate antidiuresis: a novel disorder in water balance in pediatric patients, *Am J Med* 119 (Suppl 1):S54-58, 2006.
15. Berger TM, Kistler W, Berendes E, Raufhake C, Walter M: Hyponatremia in a pediatric stroke patient: syndrome of inappropriate antidiuretic hormone secretion or cerebral salt wasting? *Crit Care Med* 30:792-95, 2002.
16. Noakes T: Hyponatremia in distance runners: fluid and sodium balance during exercise, *Curr Sports Med Rep* 1:197-207, 2002.
17. Shroff R, Hignett R, Pierce C, Marks S, van't Hoff W: Life-threatening hypernatraemic dehydration in breastfed babies, *Arch Dis Child* 91:1025-56, 2006.
18. Holliday MA, Friedman AL, Wassner SJ: Extracellular fluid restoration in dehydration: a critique of rapid versus slow, *Pediatr Nephrol* 13:292-97, 1999.
19. Choong K, Kho ME, Menon K, Bohn D: Hypotonic versus isotonic saline in hospitalised children: a systematic review, *Arch Dis Child* 91:828-35, 2006.
20. Hays RM: Vasopressin antagonists—progress and promise, *N Engl J Med* 355:2146-48, 2006.
21. Kamel KS, Quaggin S, Scheich A, Halperin ML: Disorders of potassium homeostasis: an approach based on pathophysiology, *Am J Kidney Dis* 24:597-613, 1994.
22. Rodríguez-Soriano J: Potassium homeostasis and its disturbances in children, *Pediatr Nephrol* 9:364-67, 1995.
23. Satlin LM: Maturation of renal potassium transport, *Pediatr Nephrol* 5:260-69, 1991.
24. Lin SH, Lin YF, Chen DT, Chu P, et al: Laboratory tests to determine the cause of hypokalemia and paralysis, *Arch Intern Med* 164:1561-66, 2004.
25. Rodríguez-Soriano J, Vallo A: Renal tubular hyperkalaemia in childhood, *Pediatr Nephrol* 2:498-509, 1988.
26. Truttmann AC, Mullis PE, Bianchetti MG: Simple biochemical screening for aldosterone activity in adrenal insufficiency, *Eur J Pediatr* 157:520, 1998.
27. Alfonzo AV, Isles C, Geddes C, Deighan C: Potassium disorders—clinical spectrum and emergency management, *Resuscitation* 70:10-25, 2006.
28. Mersin SS, Ramelli GP, Laux-End R, Bianchetti MG: Urinary chloride excretion distinguishes between renal and extrarenal metabolic alkalosis, *Eur J Pediatr* 154:979-82, 1995.
29. Hollander-Rodríguez JC, Calvert JF Jr: Hyperkalemia, *Am Fam Physician* 73:283-90, 2006.
30. Rossi R, Kleta R, Ehrich JH: Renal involvement in children with malignancies, *Pediatr Nephrol* 13:153-62, 1999.
31. Mildenberger E, Versmold HT: Pathogenesis and therapy of non-oliguric hyperkalaemia of the premature infant, *Eur J Pediatr* 161:415-22, 2002.
32. Watanabe T: Hyponatremia and hyperkalemia in infants with acute pyelonephritis, *Pediatr Nephrol* 19:361-62, 2004.
33. Rodríguez-Soriano J, Vallo A, Sanjurjo P, Castillo G, Oliveros R: Hyporeninemic hypoaldosteronism in children with chronic renal failure, *J Pediatr* 109:476-82, 1986.
34. Laski ME, Kurtzman NA: Acid–base disorders in medicine, *Dis Mon* 42:51-125, 1996.
35. Whittier WL, Rutecki GW: Primer on clinical acid–base problem solving, *Dis Mon* 50:122-62, 2004.
36. Kamel KS, Halperin ML: An improved approach to the patient with metabolic acidosis: a need for four amendments, *J Nephrol* 19 (Suppl 9):S76-85, 2006.
37. Figge J, Jabor A, Kazda A, Fencl V: Anion gap and hypoalbuminemia, *Crit Care Med* 26:1807-10, 1998.
38. Moviat M, van Haren F, van der Hoeven H: Conventional or physicochemical approach in intensive care unit patients with metabolic acidosis, *Crit Care* 7:R41-45, 2003.
39. Kraut JA, Kurtz I: Use of base in the treatment of severe acidemic states, *Am J Kidney Dis* 38:703-27, 2001.
40. Adrogué HJ: Metabolic acidosis: pathophysiology, diagnosis and management, *J Nephrol* 19 (Suppl 9):S62-69, 2006.
41. Galla JH: Metabolic alkalosis, *J Am Soc Nephrol* 11:369-75, 2000.
42. Miozzari HH, Tönz M, von Vigier RO, Bianchetti MG: Fluid resuscitation in infantile hypertrophic pyloric stenosis, *Acta Paediatr* 90:511-14, 2001.
43. Carmeliet G, Van Cromphaut S, Daci E, Maes C, Bouillon R: Disorders of calcium homeostasis, *Best Pract Res Clin Endocrinol Metab* 17:529-46, 2003.
44. Iqbal SJ, Giles M, Ledger S, Nanji N, Howl T: Need for albumin adjustments of urgent total serum calcium, *Lancet* 332:1477-78, 1988.
45. Goodman WG: Calcium-sensing receptors, *Semin Nephrol* 24:17-24, 2004.
46. Singh J, Moghal N, Pearce SH, Cheetham T: The investigation of hypocalcaemia and rickets, *Arch Dis Child* 88:403-407, 2003.
47. Guise TA, Mundy GR: Clinical review 69: Evaluation of hypocalcemia in children and adults, *J Clin Endocrinol Metab* 80:1473-78, 1995.
48. Hsu SC, Levine MA: Perinatal calcium metabolism: physiology and pathophysiology, *Semin Neonatol* 9:23-36, 2004.
49. Inzucchi SE: Understanding hypercalcemia: its metabolic basis, signs, and symptoms, *Postgrad Med* 115:69-70, 73-76, 2004.
50. Jacobs TP, Bilezikian JP: Clinical review: rare causes of hypercalcemia, *J Clin Endocrinol Metab* 90:6316-22, 2005.
51. Pont A: Unusual causes of hypercalcemia, *Endocrinol Metab Clin North Am* 18:753-64, 1989.
52. Rodríguez-Soriano J: Neonatal hypercalcemia, *J Nephrol* 16:606-608, 2003.
53. Truttmann AC, Bettinelli A, Bianchetti MG: Métabolisme du magnésium pour le clinicien: une mise au point actuelle et simple, *Méd Hyg* 55:551-53, 1997.
54. Ariceta G, Rodríguez-Soriano J, Vallo A: Renal magnesium handling in infants and children, *Acta Paediatr* 85:1019-23, 1996.
55. Ariceta G, Rodríguez-Soriano J, Vallo A: Magnesium homeostasis in premature and full-term neonates, *Pediatr Nephrol* 9:423-27, 1995.
56. Agus ZS: Hypomagnesemia, *J Am Soc Nephrol* 10:1616-22, 1999.
57. Schlingmann KP, Konrad M, Seyberth H: Genetics of hereditary disorders of magnesium homeostasis, *Pediatr Nephrol* 19:13-25, 2004.

58. Gaasbeek A, Meinders AE: Hypophosphatemia: an update on its etiology and treatment, *Am J Med* 118:1094-101, 2005.
59. Amanzadeh J, Reilly RF Jr: Hypophosphatemia: an evidence-based approach to its clinical consequences and management, *Nat Clin Pract Nephrol* 2:136-48, 2006.
60. Ritz E, Haxsen V, Zier M: Disorders of phosphate metabolism—pathomechanisms and management of hypophosphataemic disorders, *Best Pract Res Clin Endocrinol Metab* 17:547-58, 2003.
61. Alon U, Hellerstein S: Assessment and interpretation of the tubular threshold for phosphate in infants and children, *Pediatr Nephrol* 8:250-51, 1994.
62. Brodehl J: Assessment and interpretation of the tubular threshold for phosphate in infants and children, *Pediatr Nephrol* 8:645, 1994.
63. Berndt TJ, Schiavi S, Kumar R: "Phosphatonins" and the regulation of phosphorus homeostasis, *Am J Physiol Renal Physiol* 289:F1170-82, 2005.

CHAPTER 28

Fanconi Syndrome

Detlef Böckenhauer and William G. van't Hoff

INTRODUCTION

Fanconi first described the concept that defective renal proximal tubule reabsorption of solutes might contribute to "non-nephrotic glycosuric dwarfing with hypophosphatemic rickets in early childhood."[1] Rickets and albuminuria secondary to kidney disease were described some 50 years previously but attributed to "a disorder of adolescence."[2] Fanconi's first case presented at 3 months with rickets and recurrent fevers. She had glycosuria and albuminuria, and progressed to terminal renal failure by 5 years of age. At autopsy, the renal tubule cells appeared to have been filled with crystals, which were thought to be cystine. In subsequent reports, Debré, de Toni, and Fanconi all described series of children with rickets, glycosuria, and albuminuria, but the presentation, course, and outcome in these reports were markedly different.[3-5] So the syndrome described by Fanconi refers to multiple defects in proximal tubular function, but early and subsequent descriptions have highlighted the heterogeneity of the syndrome.

Tables 28-1 and 28-2 list a large number of secondary causes, some congenital (Table 28-1) and some acquired (Table 28-2). All of these conditions are characterized by multiple defects in proximal tubular function but they differ in the extent and severity of tubular dysfunction. Severe and generalized proximal tubular dysfunction is seen in cystinosis while many children with Dent's disease and some with Lowe's syndrome may, in early life, have no clinically significant disturbance of phosphate and bicarbonate transport. We use the term Fanconi syndrome (FS) to include disorders with multiple tubular dysfunction, but recognize that not every proximal transport system need be affected. This clinical and biochemical heterogeneity is likely to arise from the multiple mechanisms involved in proximal tubular transport, reflecting not only the bulk of solute and water reabsorption but also the re-uptake of proteins, amino acids, vitamins, cytokines, and many other substances. Fanconi syndromes do not therefore have a common and single pathogenetic basis, but reflect the interplay of a number of different biochemical processes.

BIOCHEMICAL ABNORMALITIES

Excessive urinary levels of a wide range of solutes and substances normally reabsorbed in the proximal tubule are the biochemical hallmarks of FS. The tubular transport dysfunction can include bicarbonaturia leading to hyperchloremic metabolic acidosis, phosphaturia leading to hypophosphatemia, rickets, osteomalacia, and growth retardation, as well as abnormal urinary losses of glucose, proteins, hormones, and a variety of other compounds. Proteinuria is made up of albumin, low-molecular-weight proteins and tubular enzymes, such as retinol binding protein (RBP), α-1 microglobulin, β-2 microglobulin, N-acetylglucosaminidase, and alanine aminopeptidase. The urinary level of these very sensitive markers of proximal tubular dysfunction is markedly elevated in FS.[6,7] Albuminuria precedes glomerular dysfunction in Fanconi syndrome and while elevated, does not reach nephrotic range proteinuria.[8] This reflects the amount of filtered albumin requiring tubular reabsorption, which has been estimated at 0.4 to 1 g of albumin per 1.73 m^2 per day.[9,10] Tubular proteinuria may be seen in some forms of nephrotic syndrome, reflecting associated tubulointerstitial damage.[11,12] The aminoaciduria seen in FS is generalized and its pattern is influenced by plasma values, so that in rare situations of severe protein malnutrition, aminoaciduria, as analyzed on thin-layer chromatography, may be recorded as "normal" or "mild."[7] Quantitative analysis by ion-exchange chromatography should be used to determine the degree of aminoaciduria.

Phosphaturia and glycosuria were key features of the original descriptions of FS, and huge losses are seen in severe cases. However, milder cases may not have clinically evident losses. Renal glycosuria in FS is characterized by a low threshold, and a low maximal glucose reabsorption at saturation glucose concentrations in blood, but normal values of maximal reabsorptive capacity (Tm_G) during excessive glucose loading. Bicarbonaturia reflects a reduced threshold for reabsorption and is again variable in extent, according to the underlying cause of FS. In severe acidosis, filtered bicarbonate is reduced to a level below the threshold for proximal reabsorption and urine pH falls below 5.3. The hyperchloremic metabolic acidosis requires treatment with large doses of alkali and also contributes to loss of skeletal calcium and hypercalciuria. Electrolyte, fluid, and mineral losses can be very severe and lead to volume contraction, which, in turn results in hyperaldosteronism with hypokalemia and a paradoxical alkalosis.[13-15] In addition, sodium wasting contributes to hypercalciuria. Defective urinary concentration and features of nephrogenic diabetes insipidus have been seen in cystinosis and following ifosfamide therapy, likely due to the increased solute delivery overwhelming the countercurrent

TABLE 28-1 Congenital Causes of Fanconi Syndrome by Age of Onset

Onset	Disorder	Associated Features	Diagnostic Test
Neonatal	Galactosemia	Liver dysfunction, jaundice, encephalopathy, sepsis	Red cell galactose 1-phosphate uridyl transferase
	Mitochondrial disorders	Usually multisystem dysfunction (brain, muscle, liver, heart)	Lactate/pyruvate (may be normal plasma lactate due to urinary losses), muscle enzymology
	Tyrosinemia	Poor growth, hepatic enlargement and dysfunction	Plasma amino acids, urine organic acids (succinyl acetone)
Infancy	Fructosemia	Rapid onset after fructose ingestion, vomiting, hypoglycemia, hepatomegaly	Hepatic fructose-1-phosphate aldolase B
	Cystinosis	Poor growth; may be blond/fair hair, rickets ± corneal cystine crystals	Leukocyte cystine concentration, mutation analysis *(CTNS)*
	Fanconi-Bickel syndrome	Failure to thrive, hepatomegaly, hypoglycemia rickets, severe glycosuria, galactosuria	Mutation analysis *(GLUT2)*
	Lowe's syndrome	Males (X-linked), cataracts, hypotonia, developmental delay	Clinical and molecular genetic diagnosis *(OCRL)*
Childhood	Cystinosis	As above	
	Dent's disease	Males (X-linked), hypercalciuria, nephrocalcinosis	Molecular diagnosis *(CLCN5, OCRL)*
	Wilson's disease	Hepatic and neurological disease, Kayser-Fleischer rings	Copper, coeruloplasmin

Adapted from Van't Hoff W. Renal tubular disorders. In *Clinical Paediatric Nephrology*, NJA Webb and RJ Postlethwaite, eds. Oxford University Press, 2003, pp. 103-12.

TABLE 28-2 Acquired Causes of Renal Fanconi Syndrome

Drugs and Toxins
Anticancer drugs Ifosfamide (see text) Streptozocin[262,263]
Antibiotics Aminoglykoside (see text) Expired tetracyclines[264,265]
Antiretrovirals Adefovir/cidofovir/tenofovir[266-269] ddI[270,271]
Heavy metals Lead poisoning[272] Cadmium[273]
Sodium valproate[274]
Aristolochic acid (Chinese herb nephropathy)[275-277]
Toluene/glue sniffing[278]
Fumaric acid[279]
Suramin[280]
Paraquat[281]
L-Lysine[282]
Renal Disorders
Tubulointerstitial nephritis[283]
Membranous nephropathy with anti-tubular basement antibodies[221-228,230]

multiplication system in the loop of Henle.[14,16] Carnitine is normally reabsorbed in the proximal tubule and is therefore lost in excess in FS. Low plasma carnitine concentrations have been reported in children with cystinosis and tyrosinemia,[17,18] leading to plasma and muscle deficiencies of carnitine, which could contribute to the myopathy in these disorders. Losses of vitamins, carrier proteins, and chemokines have all been described in FS.[8,19]

PATHOGENESIS

The variation in etiology, manifestations, and severity of FS make it unlikely that there is a single common pathogenetic mechanism. Most studies of the pathogenesis have, of necessity, focused on one biochemical pathway. However, in vivo, it is more likely that a number of interlinked biochemical processes are disrupted in a variable manner.

Disruption of Energy Production

Sodium uptake in the proximal tubule allows the co-transport of solutes such as glucose, phosphate, and amino acids. Sodium crosses the basolateral membrane by the action of NaK-ATPase, which transfers three sodium ions out of the cell in exchange for the inward movement of two extracellular potassium ions. This creates an electrochemical gradient, which drives sodium-coupled solute co-transport. NaK-ATPase function depends on the supply of ATP generated in mitochondria as a result of oxidative phosphorylation.

There has been extensive investigation of mitochondrial function in animal models of FS. Rats treated with intraperitoneal cystine dimethyl ester (CDME) demonstrate an increase in urine volume and excretion of phosphate, glucose, and amino acids compared to controls.[20] Isolated animal renal tubules loaded with CDME exhibit decreased solute and volume transport, reduced oxygen consumption and oxidation of glucose, lactate, butyrate, and succinate compared to control tubules.[20-23] Cystine-loaded tubules have a reduction in intracellular phosphate and in ATP concentrations and the abnormal solute and volume transport can be attenuated by preincubation of the tubules with exogenous phosphate or ATP.[21,24] Cystine accumulation in this model reduces the consumption of oxygen normally utilized by NaK-ATPase,[25] and mitochondria isolated after cystine loading, show reduced oxidation of glutamate but not of succinate.[26]

Similar studies have been undertaken in models of tyrosinemia, which is associated with excessive accumulation of succinyl acetone (SA). SA reduced sodium-dependent uptake of sugar and amino acids across rat brush-border membranes,[27] and intraperitoneal injection of SA to rats led to development of FS.[28] SA inhibits sodium-dependent phosphate transport by brush-border membrane vesicles, decreases ATP production, and inhibits mitochondrial respiration.[29] Administration of maleic acid, used to create an animal model of FS, causes a reduction in ATP and phosphate concentrations, NaK-ATPase activity, and coenzyme A.[30]

Significantly reduced concentrations of ATP compared to controls have been demonstrated in cystinotic fibroblasts, polymorphonuclear leukocytes, and exfoliated proximal renal tubular cells (PTC) grown under hypoxic stress.[31] In cystinotic fibroblasts and exfoliated PTC, under basal conditions, there was no impairment of activity of any of the components of the mitochondrial electron transport chain under basal conditions.[32] However, when these cells were grown under hypoxic conditions, activities of mitochondrial complexes I and IV were increased.[32] When molecular oxygen is limited, there is normally a compensatory increase in complexes I and IV of the electron transport chain in order to maintain the availability of ATP.[33-36] These data suggest that in cystinotic cells, this protective mechanism may be lost.

More recent studies have emphasized the role of glutathione (GSH) in the pathogenesis of FS. GSH has a number of key cellular roles including post-translational protein modification and xenobiotic detoxification, and it also acts as a major antioxidant. In cystinosis, defective lysosomal transport of cystine might lead to cytosolic deficiency of cysteine, which, together with glutamate and glycine, is required for GSH synthesis utilizing the γ-glutamyl cycle (Figure 28-1). Increased urinary 5-oxoproline (pyroglutamate) has been demonstrated in cystinotic patients, suggesting a perturbation of the γ-glutamyl cycle that could lead to GSH depletion.[37] Urinary 5-oxoproline returned to normal levels when the patients were treated with cysteamine and no abnormality in its excretion was seen in other FS patients, suggesting that the biochemical disturbance was specific to untreated cystinosis.[37] Cystinotic fibroblasts exhibited raised pyroglutamate levels compared to controls, and the difference became more marked after cells were stressed.[38]

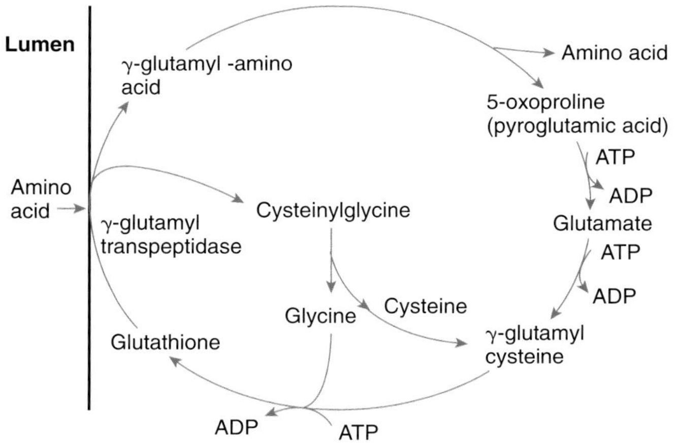

Figure 28-1 The γ-glutamyl cycle.

Data on GSH in cystinosis vary according to the cell types studied and the methods used.[39-41] GSH was unchanged compared to controls in immortalized human cystinotic PTC[42] but significantly depleted in nonimmortalized cystinotic PTC.[32] Inhibition of ATP synthesis in cystinotic fibroblasts caused a marked accumulation of pyroglutamate, reflecting decreased GSH synthesis.[38] Importantly, oxidized GSH (GSSG) is increased in the same cell systems.[39,41,42] There is thus an imbalance in the ratio of total and oxidized GSH in cystinosis cells, which may reflect cytosolic cysteine deficiency and may be implicated in the pathogenesis of FS.

Deficiency of GSH has also been implicated in other forms of the renal FS. Ifosfamide toxicity, which leads to FS, may be mediated by its interaction with γ-glutamyl transpeptidase and by hepatic metabolism to chloroacetaldehyde.[43] Incubation of chloroacetaldehyde with isolated human renal proximal tubules was associated with depletion of GSH, coenzyme A, acetyl-coenzyme A, and ATP.[44] Wistar rats injected with ifosfamide develop renal FS associated with GSH depletion, which is attenuated by treatment with melatonin.[44] Addition of ochratoxin A, the presumed toxin causing FS in Balkan endemic nephropathy, to rat proximal tubular cells causes an elevation of reactive oxygen species and depletion of cellular GSH.[45]

Reduced Activity of Co-Transporters

Increased solute excretion in FS could result from reduced expression or activity of sodium-coupled co-transporters. In the animal maleic acid model of FS, decreased NaPi-2 mRNA expression and consequent reduced NaPi-2 protein were observed.[46] However, phosphaturia preceded these changes, suggesting that other mechanisms (such as energy disruption) accounted for the early phosphate leakage. Cystine dimethyl ester (CDME)–loaded human kidney epithelial cells led to rapid alteration of basal membrane voltage with an initial depolarization followed by a marked hyperpolarization (due to activation of K^+ channels).[47] Prolonged cystine loading (>30 minutes) inhibited the activity of Na^+-alanine co-transporter and the Na^+/H^+ exchanger. The Na^+-phosphate (NaPi2) co-transporter was much more sensitive, with substantial inhibition occurring after very little exposure to CDME (1 to 2 minutes).[47]

Mice lacking hepatocyte nuclear factor 1 alpha (*HNF1α*), a transcription factor expressed in liver, pancreas, kidney, and intestine, develop FS, abnormal bile metabolism, and diabetes.[48] *HNF1α* –/– mice had reduced expression of sodium-coupled transporters for glucose (SGLT-2) and phosphate (NaPi-1 and NaPi-4), but normal levels of NaPi-2, the major phosphate transporter.[49]

Disruption of Endocytic Pathway (Megalin/Cubilin)

An important task of the proximal tubule is to reabsorb filtered proteins, including peptide hormones and small carrier proteins binding fat-soluble vitamins and trace elements. Therefore, by reabsorbing filtered proteins, the proximal tubule actively participates in the homeostasis of hormones,

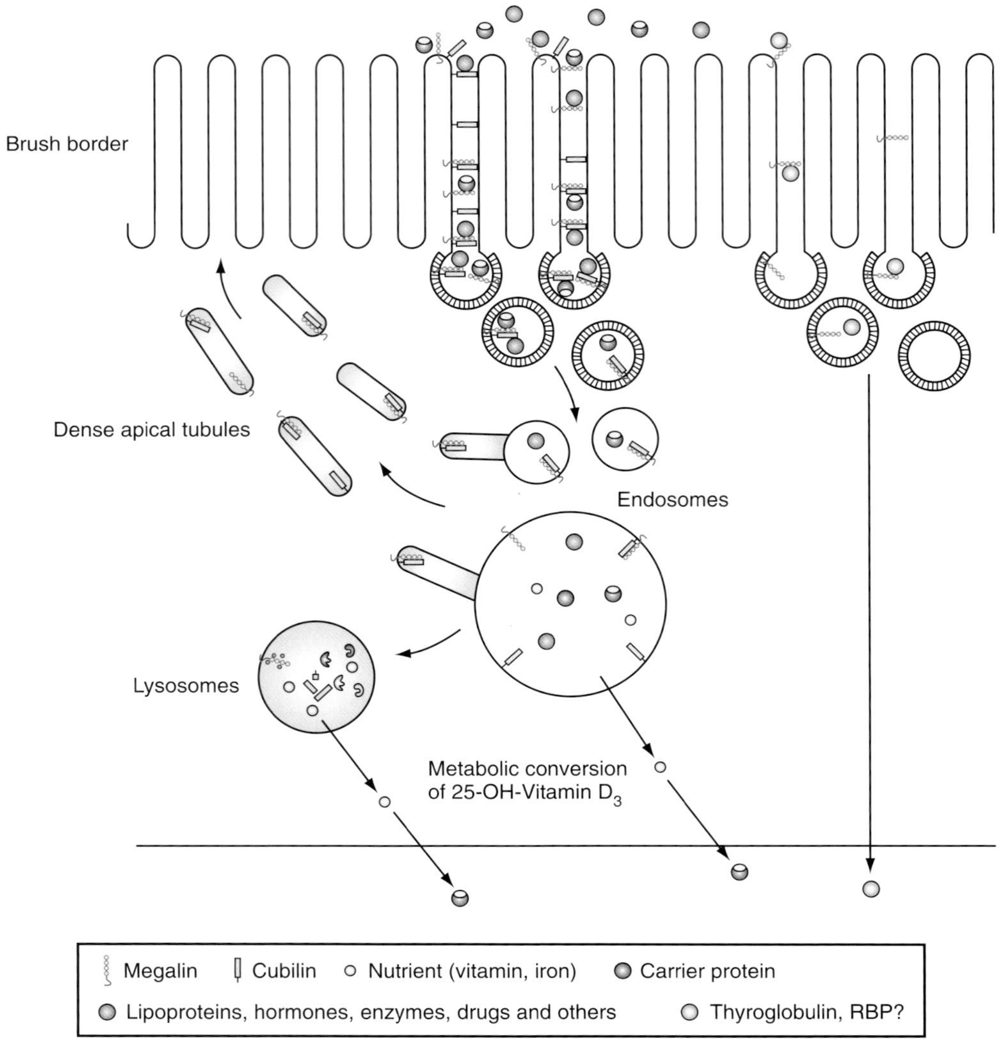

Figure 28-2 Diagram of proximal tubule. (From Christensen EI, Birn H: Megalin and cubilin: multifunctional endocytic receptors, *Nat Rev Mol Cell Biol* 3(4):258-68, 2002.)

trace elements, and vitamins. Reabsorption of the vast majority of filtered proteins is mediated by two endocytotic receptors: megalin and cubilin.[50-52] These receptors contain several protein-binding domains and protrude from the microvilli, which make up the brush border of the proximal tubule, into the tubular lumen. Once a protein is attached, the receptor-ligand complex moves towards the base of the microvilli into clathrin-coated pits, which then bud off into the cytoplasm to form endosomes (Figure 28-2). Subsequently, the receptors are recycled back to the membrane to mediate further uptake. The fate of the protein ligands is different: most are degraded by acid hydrolysis after fusion of the endosome to a lysosome, while others, such as vitamins, are released back into the blood circulation across the basolateral membrane. In this fashion, the megalin/cubilin complex assumes a role in the regulation of several hormonal pathways, the importance of which becomes apparent, when considering, for instance, calcium regulation: megalin competes with the PTH receptor for the binding of filtered PTH and renders it non-functional by endocytosis and subsequent delivery to a lysosome for degradation.[53] In contrast, megalin/cubilin facilitates activation of vitamin D by binding of filtered 25-OH vitamin D–vitamin D binding protein, and thus allowing uptake into the proximal tubule cell and activation by 1-alpha hydroxylase.[54-55]

Megalin is a large transmembrane protein belonging to the family of low-density lipoprotein receptors, and was originally identified as the target of antibodies causing Heymann nephritis in rats.[56] It is expressed in epithelial cells of a variety of other tissues active in endocytosis.[57] Megalin-deficient mice mostly die in utero, but those that survive indeed show Fanconi-type low-molecular-weight proteinuria, confirming the central role of megalin in endocytosis in the proximal tubule.[58]

Cubilin is a peripheral membrane protein, and is dependent on megalin to initiate endocytosis after ligand binding. These two proteins are co-expressed in proximal tubule and along the endocytic pathway and work in tandem to mediate protein uptake.[50,52] Cubilin is otherwise known as the intrinsic factor-vitamin B12 receptor.[59] Loss-of-function mutations are associated with juvenile megaloblastic anemia or Imerslund-Graesbeck disease.[60,61] The anemia is caused by deficient intestinal endocytosis of intrinsic factor-vitamin B12. In addition, some of these patients also have a selective low-molecular-weight proteinuria that identifies those proteins requiring cubilin for endocytosis, such as albumin, transferrin, immunoglobulin light chains, and α1- and β2-microglobulin.[62]

Decreased expression of both megalin and cubilin at the brush border has been described in a mouse model of Dent's disease. Concurrently, decreased levels of megalin have been found in the urine of patients with Dent's disease and Lowe syndrome, suggesting defective trafficking of the receptors as the basis of the low-molecular-weight proteinuria seen in affected patients.[63,64] The loss of vitamins, hormones, and trace elements associated with endocytic dysfunction may explain some of the clinical heterogeneity seen in FS.

Apoptosis

Apoptosis has also been implicated in the pathogenesis of Fanconi syndromes. Mice in whom the genes encoding both fumaryl acetoacetate hydrolase and 4-hydroxyphenylpyruvate dioxygenase have been knocked out, develop a phenotype similar to patients with tyrosinemia when fed homogentisate. There is rapid apoptosis of both hepatocytes and renal tubular cells. Apoptosis (but not the renal tubular dysfunction) can be prevented by co-administration of caspase inhibitors so the role of apoptosis in this model is unclear.[65] Cadmium, which induces a renal Fanconi syndrome, increases apoptotic rates and reactive oxygen species in renal tubular cells. The oxidative damage increases degradation of NaK-ATPase critical to proximal tubular cell transport function.[66]

Increased apoptotic rates have been demonstrated in cultured fibroblasts and exfoliated renal tubular cells from cystinosis patients.[32,67] Protein kinase Cδ (PKCδ) is a pro-apoptotic protein, up-regulated by cysteinylation, which results from lysosomal release of cystine in an in vitro model of cystinosis.[68] An increased susceptibility to apoptosis, associated with lysosomal cystine efflux, is speculated to be implicated in both the renal tubular and multisystem dysfunction characteristic of cystinosis.[68]

CYSTINOSIS

Biochemical and Molecular Basis

Cystinosis is characterized by defective lysosomal transport of cystine, leading to increased intralysosomal cystine accumulation.[69-71] The causative gene, *CTNS*, was isolated using a mapping and positional cloning strategy to the short arm of chromosome 17 (17p13).[72,73] *CTNS* consists of 12 exons and encodes a 367–amino-acid protein, cystinosin, which is predicted to have seven transmembrane domains, eight N-glycosylation sites, and a GY-XX-hydrophobic amino acid motif that acts as a lysosomal targeting signal, characteristic of lysosomal membrane proteins.[73] The lysosomal localization of cystinosin has been confirmed in COS-7 cells expressing either wildtype or mutant cystinosin.[74] A second novel lysosomal targeting motif (YFPQA) located in the fifth inter-transmembrane domain, has subsequently been identified.[75]

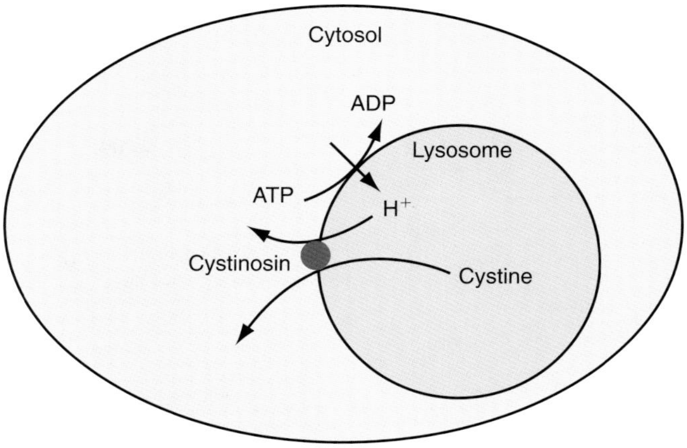

Figure 28-3 Function of cystinosin as the lysosomal cystine transporter. (Adapted from Kalatzis V, Cherqui S, Antignac C, Gasnier B: Cystinosin, the protein defective in cystinosis, is a H(+)-driven lysosomal cystine transporter, *EMBO J* 20(21):5940-49, 2001.)

Cystinosin acts as the lysosomal cystine/H+ symporter, mediating saturable cystine transport out of the lysosome (Figure 28-3).[76]

The most common mutation in cystinosis is a 57-kb deletion, found in 76% of patients of Northern European origin, arising as a founder effect, and enabling a PCR-based rapid diagnostic test for the disorder.[77] A variety of other mutations, mainly causing premature termination of cystinosin, are found in the severe, infantile-onset form of cystinosis.[78] Milder forms are associated with point mutations, often in the intertransmembrane domains or *N*-terminal region that do not affect the open reading frame of cystinosin.[79]

Patients with cystinosis appear normal at birth[70,71] and grow well for the first few months of life. Symptoms usually become prominent in the second half of infancy, with a median age at onset of symptoms of 10 months.[80] Typical symptoms include poor weight gain or weight loss, inadequate and fussy feeding, vomiting, constipation, lethargy, weakness, excessive thirst, and polyuria. Recurrent episodes of fever and dehydration may occur. The weakness may be profound and can lead to an inability to bear weight or walk.

Cystinosis is not associated with dysmorphic features, although most children at presentation are short for their age. Typically, there is frontal bossing, blond hair, and a protuberant abdomen. Most Caucasian patients have a fair complexion and light or blond hair, although the presence of dark hair does not exclude the diagnosis. A cause for the paler skin and hair has yet to be found, although it may be related to impaired melanosome function since melanosomes are the melanocyte counterparts of lysosomes.[70] At the time of diagnosis, hair may be sparse and thin. Children of other racial groups have a complexion identical to their unaffected siblings.

Head circumference is not affected by the growth failure. Frontal bossing secondary to rickets is commonly seen and may persist throughout childhood. Other more marked signs of rickets may be noted, including swelling of the wrists, "rachitic rosary," and genu valgum. The bone age is often delayed with respect to chronological age. One of the authors (WvH) noted a mean bone age delay at diagnosis of 0.76 year (range 0.17 to

1.11 years) in a series of six children aged 0.7 to 1.9 years. Vitamin D metabolism has been studied in a group of 10 cystinosis patients with varying degrees of renal impairment,[81] none of whom were treated with cysteamine. No evidence of 25-hydroxyvitamin D deficiency was found, although levels of 24,25-dihydroxyvitamin D and 1,25-dihydroxyvitamin D were low in some patients, in proportion to their renal parenchymal damage.

Fundoscopy may reveal a patchy depigmentation of the retina with peripheral clumps of pigment. The retinal changes may precede the corneal features and have been observed as early as 5 weeks of age.[82] In addition, the retina may be generally hypopigmented (the "blond fundus"). Demonstration of corneal crystals requires slit lamp examination by an experienced ophthalmologist. Crystals are not present in the neonatal period but can usually be seen by the second year.[82,83] Thus, the inability to see corneal crystals does not exclude the diagnosis of cystinosis in an infant, while their demonstration is virtually pathognomonic. The crystals are fusiform or needle-shaped and are found in the stroma beneath the epithelium. In adults, a similar appearance is seen in patients with myeloma.[82] Slit-lamp examination of the conjunctiva reveals a ground-glass appearance, again due to crystal deposition.

There is often a substantial delay between the onset of symptoms and confirmation of the diagnosis of cystinosis. Data on 129 patients from the UK Cystinosis Registry indicate a fall in delay between onset of symptoms and age of diagnosis from 8.8 months in 1998 to 5.7 months in 2002.[80] Cystine crystals may be seen on slit-lamp examination or in biopsy tissue (bone marrow, lymph node), and sometimes in kidney histology.[84,85] In at-risk fetuses, prenatal diagnosis can be made reliably by either biochemical or molecular methods,[86] and presymptomatic diagnosis of at-risk newborns is possible using either umbilical cord blood or placental samples.[87]

In the absence of cystine-depleting therapy, progressive glomerular damage leads to end-stage renal failure by the end of the first decade, but this can occur as early as 2 to 3 years.[88-90] As the glomerular filtration rate falls, so too do tubular losses of fluid and electrolytes. Less electrolyte supplements are required and the child appears to be "getting better." As chronic renal impairment progresses, salt, water, potassium, and phosphate restriction is required. This relentless course has been dramatically altered by the advent of cysteamine therapy.

Renal biopsy is no longer routinely undertaken in children with cystinosis. There is marked variation in proximal tubule sections, alteration in tubular cell size and shape. The brush border is irregular and may be absent in sections. Glomerular podocytes also vary from relatively normal to multinucleate giant cell.[91] Cystine crystals (which are easily "lost" during processing of the biopsy sample) may be identified in the interstitium, sometimes in podocytes but only very rarely in tubular cells. Spear reported the presence of dark bodies mainly in macrophages but also at other sites.[92] These dark inclusion bodies were further studied and found to contain an elevated content of cystine. They have also been described in biopsies from kidneys transplanted into children with cystinosis.[93] "Dark cells" were not observed in a French review of cystinotic biopsies.[91] Chronic damage is associated with progressive tubulointerstitial, glomerular, and vascular changes.

Renal calcification is common and may contribute to the progressive damage. All 22 children in one UK study had features of nephrocalcinosis on ultrasound.[94] In a series of 46 U.S. patients, only 15 had no evidence of nephrocalcinosis, while the changes were mild in 18, severe in 8, and 5 had renal stones.[95] Gross polyuria can lead to structural abnormalities such as megacystis, megaureters, and hydronephrosis.[96] Rarely, gross albuminuria can lead to hypoalbuminemia and a nephrotic state.

Severe short stature was a universal feature of patients with cystinosis prior to the use of cysteamine. The degree of growth retardation is out of proportion to the extent of renal damage. Poor nutrition, chronic acidosis, loss of electrolytes as a result of the Fanconi syndrome, rickets, and the effects of cystine accumulation in bone and other organs (e.g., thyroid) may all contribute to the poor growth. Historic studies of final height in cystinosis demonstrated that very few reached 150 cm or the third percentile and many are profoundly short.[90,97,98] There are few data on growth hormone (GH) secretion in cystinosis. Spontaneous GH secretion was of normal frequency and maximum peak concentrations, but the mean integrated concentration was slightly lower than normal.[99] Overnight GH concentration profiles in eight patients were not statistically different from controls with chronic renal failure.[100,101] In the thyroid gland, follicular cells atrophy with collapse and condensation of the connective tissue framework.[102] In untreated patients, there is an exaggerated response of TSH to thyrotropin releasing hormone (TRH), suggesting impaired thyroid reserve compared to control children with chronic renal failure.[103] Hypothyroidism is present in 50% of patients without cysteamine aged 10 years and 80% aged 20 years.[97,98,104,105] Children well treated with cysteamine can expect normal thyroid function throughout childhood.[106]

Impaired glucose tolerance occurs in over 50% of patients at 15 years and diabetes mellitus in 50% by 19 years.[107] Impaired insulin production[107,108] is related to beta-cell hyperplasia, demonstrated in postmortem pancreatic tissue from cystinosis patients,[109] which occurs secondary to chronic cystine accumulation. Pubertal development is generally delayed.[110,111] In one study, the mean onset of puberty was 15.5 years (range 12 to 18) in males and 15 years (12 to 18) in females.[111] Bone age at the onset of puberty was delayed by a mean of approximately 4.5 years in both sexes. Females established stable menstrual cycles 2 years after menarche and had appropriate cyclical fluctuations in gonadotrophin and estradiol levels. In males, studies have demonstrated hypergonadotrophic hypogonadism might be due to progressive testicular damage secondary to cystine accumulation.[111] To date, there is no report of males fathering a child, but several cystinosis females have had successful pregnancies.[112,113]

Early neurological development and function appear to be normal in cystinosis. However, in the second and third decades of life, the frequency of neurological manifestations of cystine accumulation increases. Symptoms include bradykinesia, tremor, memory loss, dementia, rigidity, weakness, paresthesia, dysarthria, and dysphagia.[114,115] Neurological examination may be normal or may reveal characteristic distal vacuolar myopathy,[116] tremor, spasticity, and abnormal gait.[114,115] Older patients with severe myopathy are also at risk of respiratory insufficiency with severely reduced lung capacity, FEV (1), and FVC.[117] Several such patients develop conical chests, restricting inflation, but lung imaging indicates normal lung parenchyma.[117] Other manifestations can include stroke-like episodes, and idiopathic intracranial hypertension can occur.[118-120] Imaging or neuropathologic findings often include cerebral atrophy disproportionate to that in other patients with renal disease, dilated ventricles, cystic necrosis of the globus pallidus and lentiform nuclei, patchy demyelination, and calcification in the basal ganglia.[115,120-122] Cystine crystals can be demonstrated in basal ganglia, cortex, thalamus, cerebellum, and pituitary gland.[114,123] Swallowing dysfunction is a common finding in cystinosis, which is evident even in young children and progresses with age.[124,125] Oral, pharangeal, and esophageal phases of swallowing are increasingly affected by disordered neuromuscular activity rather than neurological damage, and the dysfunction is less marked in those with prolonged cysteamine therapy.[125] Longitudinal psychometric testing has shown that children with cystinosis usually have a normal intelligence quotient and can attend normal school.[126] However, detailed psychometric assessment has shown specific deficits in tests of short-term visual memory, spelling, and mathematics that can be negated by adaptation of teaching methods.[127,128]

Although the effects of cystine deposition in the eye can be detected early in life (see above), visual acuity remains good in childhood. However, the long-term prognosis for normal vision is poor.[129] Corneal cystine crystal deposition leads to haziness or clouding, worsening photophobia, corneal erosions, band keratopathy, and corneal revascularization.[130] Crystal deposition in the iris may lead to posterior synechia and glaucoma. In older patients, color vision may be defective, the dark-adaptation thresholds are increased, and electro-retinograms become abnormal. A hemorrhagic retinopathy can occur, leading to retinal detachment, scarring, and angle-closure glaucoma.[131]

Vomiting, abdominal pain, and feeding difficulties are extremely common in cystinosis. These may be mediated by gastric acid hypersecretion and exacerbated by cysteamine, but respond to proton-pump inhibition.[132,133] Pancreatic dysfunction may lead to diabetes mellitus (see above) and very occasionally malabsorption.[108] While hepatomegaly may be evident even in young children,[134] disturbance of liver function is uncommon. In adult patients, there are several reports of noncirrhotic portal hypertension.[97,135,136]

An arteriopathy can occur even in childhood with dilated coronary arteries or even dissecting aneurysm.[137,138] Advanced arteriosclerotic changes occur in coronary arteries in young adult cystinosis patients, and fatal restrictive cardiomyopathy with pseudoaneurysm has been reported.[139,140] There has been a single case report of a patient, transplanted on account of cystinosis, who died in respiratory failure from pulmonary fibrosis.[141]

Milder Forms of Cystinosis

While the majority (95% in UK Cystinosis Registry data) of children with cystinosis present in infancy, a small number have a milder phenotype. Presentation may be in adolescence or early adult life with chronic kidney disease (of a tubulointerstitial type) or proteinuria, and in these case, typical Fanconi features are often absent.[142,143] In general, patients with late-onset cystinosis have a slower progression of renal glomerular damage than do infantile-onset patients and growth is better. Biochemically, the untreated leukocyte cystine concentrations are generally lower and fibroblast lysosomal cystine transport generally greater in late-onset patients than in the infantile group.[144] At the molecular level, such patients usually have milder mutations, often in less critical regions of the *CTNS* gene.[79] A non-nephropathic form of cystinosis with only ocular changes affects adults.[70]

DENT'S DISEASE

Dent's disease is an X-linked recessive proximal tubulopathy, characterized by low-molecular-weight proteinuria and hypercalciuria with nephrocalcinosis and nephrolithiasis, as well as progressive renal failure.[145] Patients may also have aminoaciduria, glucosuria, and phosphaturia, consistent with a complete renal Fanconi syndrome. It was first described as hypercalciuric rickets by Dent and Friedman.[146] Clinical manifestations can vary enormously, and once an underlying gene, *CLCN5,* was identified in 1996, it was realized that mutations in the same gene also caused other tubulopathies, previously thought to be distinct, namely X-linked recessive nephrolithiasis and Japanese idiopathic low-molecular-weight proteinuria.[147-153] Patients typically manifest with complications of hypercalciuria, such as hematuria, nephrocalcinosis, or stones. Progression to ESRD is rare in childhood. Women are rarely affected, probably due to skewed X-chromosome inactivation.[154] The diagnosis is made by the presence of hypercalciuria and low-molecular-weight proteinuria (such as retinol-binding protein or β-2 microglobulin) and typically a family history on the maternal side. Renal histology is nonspecific, showing features of interstitial nephritis and calcium deposits, and is thus not useful in establishing the diagnosis. Treatment is symptomatic and includes a large fluid intake and vitamin D supplementation, if rickets is present. Citrate supplementation has been helpful in a mouse model of the disease.[155] Thiazide diuretics have been shown to reduce calcium excretion, and thus reduce the stone-forming risk in Dent's disease,[156] but are sometimes poorly tolerated. This is interesting, as thiazides are thought to enhance calcium reabsorption in the proximal tubule, the segment affected in these patients.[157] Apparently, *CLCN5* dysfunction does not affect proximal calcium reabsorption directly.

Despite the identification of *CLCN5* as an underlying gene, the pathogenesis of Dent's disease is only incompletely understood. *CLCN5* clearly plays an important part in endocytosis in the proximal tubule (see above). It is highly expressed in endosomes and lysosomes, where it co-localizes with endocytosed proteins.[158] *CLCN5* is likely to provide an electric shunt neutralizing the electrical gradient otherwise created by the H^+-ATPase, to allow its efficient operation. Loss of function of *CLCN5* has been shown to impair lysosomal acidification, and initially this was assumed to be the basis of the low-molecular-weight proteinuria (LMWP).[158] However, *CLCN5* is not only a voltage-gated chloride channel, as initially described, but also a Cl^-/H^+ antiporter.[159,160] Moreover, experiments in *CLCN5*-deleted mice have shown that it is also expressed at the apical surface of proximal tubule cells, where it is important in the assembly of the endocytic complex containing megalin and cubilin (see above).[64,161-163] Indeed, megalin and cubilin expression at the brush border is dramatically reduced in these mice, as is the excretion of megalin in the urine in Dent's patients and the mouse model.[63,64] Therefore, the proteinuria seen in this disease may well be due to altered trafficking of megalin and cubilin.

The hypercalciuria is even less understood. One hypothesis is based on altered endocytosis of PTH and vitamin D–binding protein and a subsequently altered balance of calciotropic hormones.[164] Others propose a more direct role of *CLCN5* in calcium handling by the kidney and bone.[165,166] This discrepancy may in part be due to the fact that there are two different mouse strains with deleted *CLCN5* function, one of which has LMWP but no hypercalciuria.[158] Even more challenging to our understanding of Dent's disease was the discovery of another underlying gene: *OCRL1*.[167] Mutations in *OCRL1*, which encodes a phosphatidylinositol 4,5-bisphosphate (PIP_2) 5-phosphatase, lead to Lowe syndrome, which besides renal proximal tubular dysfunction includes cataracts and developmental delay (see below). Some overlap in the renal phenotype of Dent's disease and Lowe syndrome has been noted, including a very similar pattern on urinary proteomic analysis, suggesting that *CLCN5* and *OCRL* may participate in similar endocytic pathways.[168] Indeed, the renal manifestation in some patients with Lowe syndrome appears to be restricted to a Dent's-like phenotype, while in others it extends beyond the hypercalciuria and LMWP to a more generalized proximal tubular dysfunction. Potentially, in patients with *OCRL1*-based Dent's disease, other PIP_2 5-phosphatases can compensate for the loss of *OCRL1* except with respect to endocytosis and hypercalciuria. Redundancy in PIP_2 5-phosphatases is suggested by the fact that *OCRL*-deleted mice do not show any clinical phenotype.[169] Interestingly, children with *OCRL1*-based Dent's disease appear to have some extrarenal manifestations in the form of a mildly elevated LDH and CK and slightly poorer growth.[170]

LOWE SYNDROME

Lowe syndrome (oculocerebrorenal syndrome) was first described in 1952 as a clinical entity comprising "organic aciduria, decreased renal ammonia production, hydrophthalmus and mental retardation."[171] Severity of symptoms varies, but in its complete form, patients are profoundly hypotonic with absent reflexes, have severe mental retardation, congenital cataracts, glaucoma, and a renal Fanconi syndrome.[172,173] There is often a delay in establishing the diagnosis, and the renal manifestations can be minimal in early years but gross LMWP is characteristic.[7] Renal histology is nonspecific, showing some distortion of proximal tubular architecture and later also glomerular changes.[174] There is slow progression of renal insufficiency with end-stage renal failure typically reported during the fourth and fifth decades of life.[175,176] Treatment is symptomatic and includes supplementation of electrolytes, alkali, and vitamin D, if needed. Nutritional support with tube feeding is often helpful in the more severely affected patients. Occasionally affected females have been reported, probably related to skewed X inactivation.[177,178] The presence of lens opacities has been suggested to identify female mutation carriers, although the reported sensitivity is variable.[7,179-183] In contrast, analysis of the *OCRL1* gene is reported to reveal mutations in virtually all patients.[184-186]

OCRL1 encodes a PIP_2 5-phosphatase, and was cloned as the gene underlying Lowe syndrome in 1992.[187] Our understanding of the pathogenesis, however, has only slowly evolved since. *OCRL1* is expressed in the trans-Golgi network, specifically in clathrin-coated vesicles, and appears to regulate traffic between endosomes and the trans-Golgi network (Figure 28-4).[188-191] Thus, both OCRL1 and CLCN5 appear

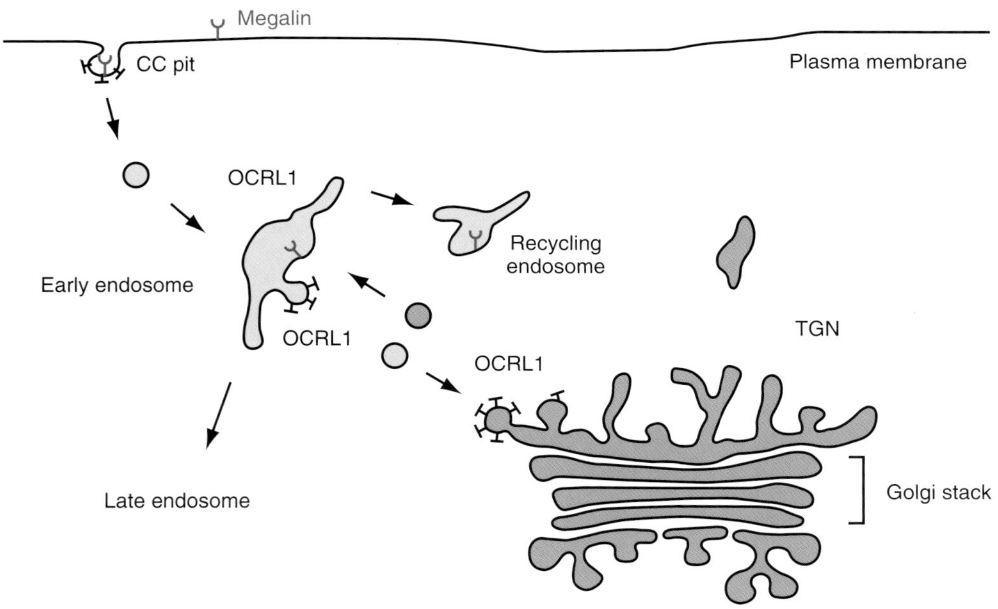

Figure 28-4 Role of OCRL1 in regulation of traffic between apical membrane, endosomes, and the trans-Golgi network (TGN). OCRL is present in clathrin-coated (CC) pits, early endosomes, and the trans-Golgi network. (Adapted from Lowe M: Structure and function of the Lowe syndrome protein OCRL1, *Traffic* 6:711-19, 2005.

to play important parts in intracellular trafficking of clathrin-coated vesicles. Lowe patients, like Dent's, have a reduced excretion of megalin in the urine, suggesting that *OCRL1*, like *CLCN5*, may play a role in the trafficking of megalin.[63] PIP_2 is an important second messenger involved in many cellular processes, including the organization of the cytoskeleton and its interaction with the cell membrane, as well as cell signaling.[192,193] Deficient breakdown of PIP_2 by *OCRL1* has been shown to lead to accumulation of PIP_2 in Lowe cells.[194] Accordingly, an abnormal structure of the cytoskeleton has been observed in fibroblasts from Lowe patients.[195] To what extent these different mechanisms contribute to the development of Lowe syndrome remains to be determined.

TYROSINEMIA

The tyrosinemias are a group of disorders affecting the metabolism of tyrosine. The most severe one is tyrosinemia type 1, which results from a defect in the enzyme fumarylacetoacetate hydrolase. Severity of clinical symptoms is variable, but typically includes hepatic dysfunction with progression to cirrhosis and risk of hepatic cancer, as well as a porphyria-like neuropathy. In addition, patients develop a severe Fanconi syndrome and chronic renal impairment can eventually ensue. The enzymatic defect in tyrosinemia leads to an accumulation of succinylacetone, which is thought to cause the symptoms. In experimental models, succinylacetone inhibits transport in the proximal tubule, potentially by inhibition of mitochondrial function.[27-29] In addition, it inhibits porphobilinogen synthetase, which may explain the porphyria-like neuropathy.[196] Further evidence for the pathogenic role of succinylacetone comes from the discovery that blockade of tyrosine metabolism further upstream effectively remedies the symptoms of tyrosinemia: mice deleted for the gene encoding fumarylacetoacetate hydrolase die in the neonatal period, but are rescued by the additional deletion of the 4-OH-phenylpyruvate dioxygenase (HPD) gene (the basis for tyrosinemia type 3) which prevents the accumulation of succinylacetone.[65] Similarly, administration of nitisinone, a blocker of HPD effectively prevents and even reverses the symptoms of tyrosinemia in the vast majority of patients.[197] Consequently, nitisinone is now the first line therapy for tyrosinemia together with a tyrosine- and phenylalanine-restricted diet.[198] In the roughly 10% of patients where this fails, liver transplantation is an option. However, even though transplantation corrects the enzymatic defect in the liver, elevated levels of succinylacetone are still found in the urine of these patients and some have persisting tubular defects.[199,200]

MITOCHONDRIAL CYTOPATHIES

The proximal tubule has a high energy requirement in order to reabsorb the bulk of filtered solutes. Cellular energy is provided in the form of ATP, produced by the respiratory chain in mitochondria. Therefore, proximal tubular cells are rich in mitochondria and it is not surprising that the proximal tubule is particularly susceptible to mitochondrial dysfunction. Indeed, Fanconi syndrome is the most common renal manifestation of mitochondrial cytopathies. The clinical manifestations of mitochondrial disorders are highly variable, but those with Fanconi syndrome typically have severe multiorgan involvement and present during infancy.[201] Neuromuscular manifestations usually predominate and the prognosis is often poor. Mitochondrial DNA mutations are inherited through the maternal line, as mitochondria derive from the maternal egg. An egg contains several mitochondria, each carrying its own DNA. Mutations in mitochondrial DNA can therefore be present in some mitochondria, but not in others within the same cell, a state termed *heteroplasmy*. Depending on the number of mitochondria with mutations passed on during cell division the ratio of mutated to healthy mitochondria can be highly variable within different tissues and cells, which may explain some of the clinical variability. However, the majority of genes encoding the respiratory chain enzymes are encoded in the nuclear genome, and mutations in these genes are typically inherited in autosomal-recessive fashion and affect all mitochondria uniformly.

An initial investigation in suspected mitochondrial cytopathies is typically to determine the ratio of lactate to pyruvate in the serum. However, in patients with Fanconi syndrome, this ratio is often normal, due to the grossly increased loss of organic acids in the urine.[201] Therefore, measurement of activity of respiratory chain enzymes should be performed in patients with high suspicion of a mitochondrial cytopathy. Renal histology is typically nonspecific, showing tubular damage, but may show giant mitochondria.[202] While some forms of mitochondrial cytopathies can be improved by supplementation with certain vitamins, no definitive treatment exists and is only supportive for the renal manifestations.

FANCONI-BICKEL SYNDROME

Fanconi-Bickel syndrome is a rare autosomal recessive glycogen-storage disease, caused by mutations in the gene *SLC2A2* encoding the glucose transporter GLUT2.[203] Patients typically present in infancy with hepatomegaly, failure to thrive, and renal Fanconi syndrome with excessive glucosuria.[204] GLUT2 is expressed in liver, intestine, pancreatic β cells, and proximal tubule cells. In hepatocytes, the transporter facilitates glucose uptake, as well as release. The impaired release leads to hepatomegaly and hypoglycemia during fasting, while the defective uptake causes postprandial hyperglycemia. In the pancreas, it leads to impaired glucose sensing and insulin release.[204,205] In the kidney, GLUT2 localizes to the basolateral membrane of the proximal tubule, easily explaining the excessive glucosuria, which has been reported to exceed 300 g/day.[206] The renal Fanconi syndrome is less well understood, but may be due to impaired mitochondrial function.[207] Interestingly, GLUT2 knockout mice reproduce the hepatic and pancreatic phenotype and also have glucosuria, but a Fanconi syndrome has not been reported.[205] The mouse model is therefore not helpful in understanding the mechanism for the Fanconi syndrome.

Mutations in *SLC2A2* associated with Fanconi-Bickel are typically severe, and thus are expected to completely abrogate GLUT2 function. Interestingly, some heterozygote missense mutations in *SLC2A2* can cause isolated renal glucosuria.[208-211] Treatment consists of frequent feedings of slowly absorbed carbohydrates, as well as replacement of renal losses of water and solutes.[212]

FRUCTOSE INTOLERANCE

Fructose intolerance is due to a deficiency in the enzyme fructose-1-phosphate aldolase B, also simply called aldolase. Affected infants typically become symptomatic at weaning, with the introduction of fructose-containing food, such as fruits and vegetables. Patients develop nausea, vomiting, and diarrhea, and can progress to hypoglycemia, convulsions, and shock. Proximal tubule dysfunction develops, and is most obvious in the form of a renal tubular acidosis, which is compounded by accumulation of lactic acid in the blood. The mechanism of cellular dysfunction is thought to be intracellular phosphate depletion due to phosphorylation of accumulating fructose. Phosphate is required for the generation of the cellular fuel ATP.[213] Moreover, a direct association between aldolase and the vacuolar proton pump V-H^+-ATPase has been shown.[214] This pump is involved in bicarbonate reabsorption in the proximal tubule, as well as acid secretion in the distal tubule and an inhibition by defective aldolase may explain the pronounced acidosis seen in patients. Treatment consists of a fructose-free diet, which completely reverses the renal symptoms.

GALACTOSEMIA

A reversible and incomplete form of Fanconi syndrome can be seen in infants with classical galactosemia, an autosomal recessive disorder due to loss of function of the enzyme galactose-1-phosphate uridyl transferase. This is a key enzyme for the conversion of galactose to glucose. Affected infants typically present with failure to thrive, and develop vomiting, diarrhea, and jaundice after ingestion of galactose-containing feeds. Untreated hepatomegaly progresses to cirrhosis, cataracts, and mental retardation. Renal manifestations, are aminoaciduria, albuminuria, acidosis, and galactosuria, the latter due to the elevated blood galactose levels.[215] The mechanism of tubular dysfunction is unclear, but may be related to intracellular depletion of free phosphate, due to phosphorylation of the accumulating galactose.

The diagnosis is made by increased blood galactose levels, and confirmed by demonstration of enzyme deficiency. Importantly, the Fanconi syndrome is completely reversible with treatment, which is the elimination of galactose from the diet.

ARC SYNDROME

The combination of arthrogryposis, renal dysfunction, and cholestasis is a rare autosomal recessive disorder, due to mutations in a gene called *VPS33B*, encoding a vacuolar sorting protein involved in intracellular transport.[216] Affected neonates are identified by their contractures, conjugated hyperbilirubinemia, and severe failure to thrive. In addition, giant platelets with a bleeding diathesis are observed. Renal manifestations include severe proximal tubular dysfunction, but nephrocalcinosis, nephrogenic diabetes insipidus, and dysplasia have also been described.[217] No specific treatment exists and the prognosis is poor, with patients typically dying in their first year of life.[216-220]

MEMBRANOUS NEPHROPATHY WITH ANTIPROXIMAL TUBULE BASEMENT-MEMBRANE ANTIBODIES

Several reports exist about an association between membranous nephropathy and Fanconi syndrome.[221-230] In most cases, antibodies have been found directed against the basement membrane of the proximal tubule. In some cases, pulmonary symptoms associated with antialveolar basement membrane antibodies are also present.[221] Most likely the antibodies are directed against an antigen expressed in the glomerulus as well, explaining the combination of glomerular and proximal tubular dysfunction. In two families, the syndrome has been linked to a region on the X chromosome, but no gene has yet been identified.[228]

ACQUIRED FANCONI SYNDROMES

Many exogenous causes of Fanconi syndrome have been reported and are listed in Table 28-2. The mechanism of tubular damage is often unclear, but the treatment, aside from supportive measures, is always the removal of the offending agent, which typically reverses the symptoms. Except for those compounds, where blood levels can be measured (such as lead or aminoglycosides), no specific diagnostic tests exist. Thus, the diagnosis is typically made through suspicion of an exogenous cause and its subsequent removal.

CHEMOTHERAPEUTIC AGENTS

Ifosfamide is the chemotherapeutic agent most commonly associated with Fanconi syndrome, which is seen in up to 10% of patients. Risk factors include total dose, reduced renal mass, young age, or the combination with other nephrotoxic agents, such as cisplatin.[231-235] Symptoms typically reverse within weeks after cessation of the drug, but in some cases persist for several years and chronic impaired kidney function is possible.[236,237]

ANTIBIOTICS

Aminoglycosides are well known for their nephrotoxic side effects. In a small percentage of patients, they can also induce Fanconi syndrome. In fact, aminoaciduria has been proposed as a highly sensitive marker for aminoglycoside-induced renal injury, at least in the rat model.[238] The mechanism of damage is unclear, but the risk appears to be related to the dosage and length of treatment, and symptoms typically reverse after cessation of the drug.[239]

PRIMARY FANCONI SYNDROME

Sometimes, Fanconi syndrome appears in patients without an identified cause. The majority of these primary or idiopathic cases occur in adulthood, but some have also been reported in children.[240] A small number of cases occur in families and different modes of inheritance have been reported.[241-246] In families with autosomal dominant inheritance, two distinct forms are recognized: Fanconi syndrome with early renal failure and one form with preserved GFR into advanced age. No underlying genetic defect has yet been reported, but identification will hopefully provide further insight into the pathophysiology of the proximal tubule. Treatment is symptomatic, and in those with kidney failure, transplantation is an option.

TREATMENT

Treatment of Fanconi syndromes is mainly supportive, although there is a specific cystine-depleting therapy for cystinosis (see below). In severe cases, rehydration initially with 0.9% saline and careful electrolyte correction is necessary and can be hazardous. Historically, fatalities occurred during rehydration with glucose-containing solutions, which exacerbated the profound hypokalemia. Rapid correction of acidosis can precipitate hypocalcemic seizures, the "hungry bone" phenomenon.[247] Once stabilized, many patients require large doses of alkali (3 to 20 mmol/kg/day), to be prescribed in the form of sodium or potassium bicarbonate or citrate, or as a compound preparation (e.g., Polycitra). We favor citrate, as a large proportion of patients are prone to hypercalciuria and subsequent development of nephrocalcinosis. Supplements of sodium chloride may also be needed. For some children, provision of all the above supplements fails to correct the biochemical disturbances and growth failure persists. Indomethacin or an alternative nonsteroidal anti-inflammatory agent is favored by many European pediatric nephrologists.[248] A double-blind trial in children with Fanconi syndrome due to cystinosis failed to show a significant advantage of indomethacin.[249] Chronic administration of thiazide diuretics may also provide symptomatic improvement by contracting extracellular volume.[250] Carnitine supplements have been used to correct the plasma and muscle carnitine deficiencies that occur in cystinosis. Hypophosphatemic rickets requires treatment with phosphate supplementation and 1α-calcidol or calcitriol. In some, provision of all the above supplements fails to correct the biochemical disturbances and growth suffers as a result.

Specific therapy of Fanconi syndrome depends on the underlying cause. The renal features of galactosemia and hereditary fructose intolerance are reversed by appropriate dietary therapy. Removal of the causative toxin or drug usually ameliorates the tubulopathy, although some drugs (e.g., ifosfamide) can cause long-term dysfunction. Niti-sinone (NTBC (2-(2-nitro-4-trifluoromethylbenzoyl)-1,3-cyclohexanedione), reverses the Fanconi syndrome in tyrosinemia (see above).

Cysteamine, used as a cystine-depleting agent in cystinosis, has a beneficial but not curative effect on proximal tubular function. Cysteamine acts by converting cystine into a mixed disulphide that exits the lysosome on the lysine transporter.[251] A multicenter study of cysteamine in 93 children treated for up to 73 months, demonstrated that, compared to historical controls, cysteamine-treated patients had a significantly better creatinine clearance.[252] Compelling evidence of the efficacy of cysteamine in retarding progression of renal damage came from a single-center review of 32 years of experience with cystinosis. In this group, those who started cysteamine under 2 years, and sustained a median leukocyte cystine less than 2 nmol of half-cystine per milligram of protein, had a mean creatinine clearance of 57 compared to a nontreatment group in which (at a similar age), clearance was 8.0 ml/min/1.73m^2.[253] Patients who can be treated early and with sustained compliance have a significantly better outcome compared to historic controls without cysteamine.[90,254] Patients should also be treated with cysteamine after renal transplantation because although cystinosis does not recur in the graft, cystine accumulation continues in nonrenal tissues manifesting multisystem damage (see above). Adequate cysteamine therapy has been shown to reduce thyroid damage, ameliorate swallowing problems, reduce cystine accumulation in muscle and liver and, in some cases, to improve neurological function and imaging.[106,119,125] Growth is also improved in cysteamine-treated patients, although a proportion with severe growth retardation may require growth hormone supplementation.[101,255,256] Topical cysteamine eye drops can reverse the corneal cystine deposition although oral therapy is needed to affect the posterior eye changes.[257-259]

Cysteamine should be started as soon as the diagnosis is confirmed and should be given in 4 divided doses throughout the 24 hours. Cystine depletion is better on a strict 6-hourly cysteamine regimen, but this can be challenging for some families.[260,261] The recommended dose is 1.3 g/m^2/day (maximum 1.95 g/m^2/day), but new patients should be commenced at lower doses (e.g., one-half the maintenance dose) with increases every week. For patients over 12 years or over 50 kg, the recommended dose is 2 g/day. The effective cysteamine dose for each patient will vary according to the leukocyte cystine level they achieve and may vary from the above recommendations. Levels should be taken 4 to 6 hours after the last dose, and therapy should be adjusted to maintain cystine levels less than 1 nmol of half-cystine per milligram of protein.[70] However, it is important to discuss cystine measurements with a specialist metabolic laboratory, as difficulties with the assay tend to cause artificially low results, which may lead to inadequate dosing.[90] Frequent side effects are malodorous breath, nausea, and vomiting, but tolerance can develop. A proton pump inhibitor can reduce the gastrointestinal effects.[132,133] A small number of European patients (mostly on high doses) have experienced an Ehlers-Danlos–like skin reaction, and in one case with fatal complications. Families should be asked to report immediately to their physician any unexpected circumscribed hemorrhagic/bruising rash.

Conflict of Interest:
One author (WvH) has declared a non-personal conflict of interest as a medical consultant to Orphan Europe, distributor of Cystagon (mercaptamine or cysteamine). Payment for this work has been made to a research fund for cystinosis, held at the Institute of Child Health, University College London, for cystinosis research.

REFERENCES

1. Fanconi G: Die nicht diabetischen Glykosurien und Hyperglyklaemien des aelteren Kindes, *Jahrbuch fuer Kinderheilkunde* 133:257-300, 1931.
2. Lucas RC: On a form of late rickets associated with albuminuria, rickets of adolescence, *Lancet* 993-94, 1883.
3. de Toni G: Remarks on the relationship between renal rickets (renal dwarfism) and renal diabetes, *Acta Pediatr* 16:479-84, 1933.
4. Debre R, Marie J, et al: Rachitisme tardif coexistant avec une Nephrite chronique et une Glycosurie, *Arch Med Enfants* 37:597-606, 1934.
5. Fanconi G: Der nephrotisch-glykosurische Zwergwuchs mit hypophosphataemischer Rachitis, *Deutsche Medizinische Wochenschrift* 62:1169-71, 1936.
6. Norden AG, Scheinman SJ, et al: Tubular proteinuria defined by a study of Dent's (CLCN5 mutation) and other tubular diseases, *Kidney Int* 57(1):240-49, 2000.
7. Laube GH, Russell-Eggitt IM, et al: Early proximal tubular dysfunction in Lowe's syndrome, *Arch Dis Child* 89(5):479-80, 2004.
8. Norden AG, Lapsley M, et al: Glomerular protein sieving and implications for renal failure in Fanconi syndrome, *Kidney Int* 60(5):1885-92, 2001.
9. Mogensen CE, Solling K: Studies on renal tubular protein reabsorption: partial and near complete inhibition by certain amino acids, *Scand J Clin Lab Invest* 37(6):477-86, 1977.
10. Birn H, Christensen EI: Renal albumin absorption in physiology and pathology, *Kidney Int* 69(3):440-49, 2006.
11. Bazzi C, Petrini C, et al: A modern approach to selectivity of proteinuria and tubulointerstitial damage in nephrotic syndrome, *Kidney Int* 58(4):1732-41, 2000.
12. VallesP, Peralta M, et al: Follow-up of steroid-resistant nephrotic syndrome: tubular proteinuria and enzymuria, *Pediatr Nephrol* 15(3-4):252-58, 2000.
13. Houston IB, Boichis H, et al: Fanconi syndrome with renal sodium wasting and metabolic alkalosis, *Am J Med* 44(4):638-46, 1968.
14. Lemire J, Kaplan BS: The various renal manifestations of the nephropathic form of cystinosis, *Am J Nephrol* 4(2):81-85, 1984.
15. Yildiz B, Durmus-Aydogdu S, et al: A patient with cystinosis presenting transient features of Bartter syndrome, *Turk J Pediatr* 48(3):260-62, 2006.
16. Rossi R, Godde A, et al: Concentrating capacity in ifosfamide-induced severe renal dysfunction, *Ren Fail* 17(5):551-57, 1995.
17. Gahl WA, Bernardini IM, et al: Muscle carnitine repletion by long-term carnitine supplementation in nephropathic cystinosis, *Pediatr Res* 34(2):115-19, 1993.
18. Nissenkorn A, Korman SH, et al: Carnitine-deficient myopathy as a presentation of tyrosinemia type I, *J Child Neurol* 16(9):642-44, 2001.
19. Moestrup SK, Verroust PJ: Megalin- and cubilin-mediated endocytosis of protein-bound vitamins, lipids, and hormones in polarized epithelia, *Annu Rev Nutr* 21:407-28, 2001.
20. Foreman JW, Bowring MA, et al: Effect of cystine dimethylester on renal solute handling and isolated renal tubule transport in the rat: a new model of the Fanconi syndrome, *Metabolism* 36(12):1185-91, 1987.
21. Foreman JW, Benson L: Effect of cystine loading and cystine dimethylester on renal brushborder membrane transport, *Biosci Rep* 10(5):455-59, 1990.
22. Salmon RF, Baum M: Intracellular cystine loading inhibits transport in the rabbit proximal convoluted tubule, *J Clin Invest* 85(2):340-44, 1990.
23. Coor C, Salmon RF, et al: Role of adenosine triphosphate (ATP) and NaK ATPase in the inhibition of proximal tubule transport with intracellular cystine loading, *J Clin Invest* 87(3):955-61, 1991.
24. Bajaj G, Baum M: Proximal tubule dysfunction in cystine-loaded tubules: effect of phosphate and metabolic substrates, *Am J Physiol* 271(3 Pt 2):F717-22, 1996.
25. Sakarcan A, Aricheta R, et al: Intracellular cystine loading causes proximal tubule respiratory dysfunction: effect of glycine, *Pediatr Res* 32(6):710-13, 1992.
26. Foreman JW, Benson LL, et al: Metabolic studies of rat renal tubule cells loaded with cystine: the cystine dimethylester model of cystinosis, *J Am Soc Nephrol* 6(2):269-72, 1995.
27. Spencer PD, Medow MS, et al: Effects of succinylacetone on the uptake of sugars and amino acids by brush border vesicles, *Kidney Int* 34(5):671-77, 1988.
28. Wyss PA, Boynton SB, et al: Physiological basis for an animal model of the renal Fanconi syndrome: use of succinylacetone in the rat, *Clin Sci (Lond)* 83(1):81-87, 1992.
29. Roth KS, Carter GE, et al: Succinylacetone effects on renal tubular phosphate metabolism: a model for experimental renal Fanconi syndrome, *Proc Soc Exp Biol Med* 196(4):428-31, 1991.
30. Eiam-ong S, Spohn M, et al: Insights into the biochemical mechanism of maleic acid-induced Fanconi syndrome, *Kidney Int* 48(5):1542-48, 1995.
31. Levtchenko EN, Wilmer MJ, et al: Decreased intracellular ATP content and intact mitochondrial energy generating capacity in human cystinotic fibroblasts, *Pediatr Res* 59(2):287-92, 2006.
32. Laube GF, Shah V, et al: Glutathione depletion and increased apoptosis rate in human cystinotic proximal tubular cells, *Pediatr Nephrol* 21(4):503-509, 2006.
33. Lehrer-Graiwer JE, Firestein BL, et al: Nitric oxide mediated induction of cytochrome c oxidase mRNA and protein in a mouse macrophage cell line, *Neurosci Lett* 288(2):107-10, 2000.
34. Vasquez OL, Almeida A, et al: Depletion of glutathione up-regulates mitochondrial complex I expression in glial cells, *J Neurochem* 76(5):1593-96, 2001.
35. Brealey D, Brand M, et al: Association between mitochondrial dysfunction and severity and outcome of septic shock, *Lancet* 360(9328):219-23, 2002.
36. Gegg ME, Beltran B, et al: Differential effect of nitric oxide on glutathione metabolism and mitochondrial function in astrocytes and neurones: implications for neuroprotection/neurodegeneration? *J Neurochem* 86(1):228-37, 2003.
37. Rizzo C, Ribes A, et al: Pyroglutamic aciduria and nephropathic cystinosis, *J Inherit Metab Dis* 22(3):224-26, 1999.
38. Mannucci L, Pastore A, et al: Impaired activity of the gamma-glutamyl cycle in nephropathic cystinosis fibroblasts, *Pediatr Res* 59(2):332-35, 2006.
39. Chol M, Nevo N, et al: Glutathione precursors replenish decreased glutathione pool in cystinotic cell lines, *Biochem Biophys Res Commun* 324(1):231-35, 2004.
40. Butler JD, Key JD, et al: Glutathione metabolism in normal and cystinotic fibroblasts, *Exp Cell Res* 172(1):158-67, 1987.
41. Levtchenko E, de Graaf-Hess A, et al: Altered status of glutathione and its metabolites in cystinotic cells, *Nephrol Dial Transplant* 20(9):1828-32, 2005.
42. Wilmer MJ, de Graaf-Hess A, et al: Elevated oxidized glutathione in cystinotic proximal tubular epithelial cells, *Biochem Biophys Res Commun* 337(2):610-14, 2005.
43. Rossi R, Kleta R, et al: Renal involvement in children with malignancies, *Pediatr Nephrol* 13(2):153-62, 1999.
44. Sener G, Sehirli O, et al: Melatonin attenuates ifosfamide-induced Fanconi syndrome in rats, *J Pineal Res* 37(1):17-25, 2004.
45. Schwerdt G, Freudinger R, et al: The nephrotoxin ochratoxin A induces apoptosis in cultured human proximal tubule cells, *Cell Biol Toxicol* 15(6):405-15, 1999.
46. Haviv YS, Wald H, et al: Late-onset downregulation of NaPi-2 in experimental Fanconi syndrome, *Pediatr Nephrol* 16(5):412-16, 2001.
47. Cetinkaya I, Schlatter E, et al: Inhibition of Na(+)-dependent transporters in cystine-loaded human renal cells: electrophysiological studies on the Fanconi syndrome of cystinosis, *J Am Soc Nephrol* 13(8):2085-93, 2002.
48. Pontoglio M, Barra J, et al: Hepatocyte nuclear factor 1 inactivation results in hepatic dysfunction, phenylketonuria, and renal Fanconi syndrome, *Cell* 84(4):575-85, 1996.
49. Cheret C, Doyen A, et al: Hepatocyte nuclear factor 1 alpha controls renal expression of the Npt1-Npt4 anionic transporter locus, *J Mol Biol* 322(5):929-41, 2002.

50. Verroust PJ, Birn H, et al: The tandem endocytic receptors megalin and cubilin are important proteins in renal pathology, *Kidney Int* 62(3):745-56, 2002.
51. Vormann J: Magnesium: nutrition and metabolism, *Mol Aspects Med* 24(1-3):27-37, 2003.
52. Christensen EI, Gburek J: Protein reabsorption in renal proximal tubule-function and dysfunction in kidney pathophysiology, *Pediatr Nephrol* 19(7):714-21, 2004.
53. Hilpert J, Nykjaer A, et al: Megalin antagonizes activation of the parathyroid hormone receptor, *J Biol Chem* 274(9):5620-25, 1999.
54. Nykjaer A, Dragun D, et al: An endocytic pathway essential for renal uptake and activation of the steroid 25-(OH) vitamin D3, *Cell* 96(4):507-15, 1999.
55. Nykjaer A, Fyfe JC, et al: Cubilin dysfunction causes abnormal metabolism of the steroid hormone 25(OH) vitamin D(3), *Proc Natl Acad Sci U S A* 98(24):13895-900, 2001.
56. Raychowdhury R, Niles JL, et al: Autoimmune target in Heymann nephritis is a glycoprotein with homology to the LDL receptor, *Science* 244(4909):1163-65, 1989.
57. Christensen EI, Birn H: Megalin and cubilin: multifunctional endocytic receptors, *Nat Rev Mol Cell Biol* 3(4):256-66, 2002.
58. Leheste JR, Rolinski B, et al: Megalin knockout mice as an animal model of low molecular weight proteinuria, *Am J Pathol* 155(4): 1361-70, 1999.
59. Moestrup SK, Kozyraki R, et al: The intrinsic factor-vitamin B12 receptor and target of teratogenic antibodies is a megalin-binding peripheral membrane protein with homology to developmental proteins, *J Biol Chem* 273(9):5235-42, 1998.
60. Grasbeck R, Gordin R, et al: Selective vitamin B12 malabsorption and proteinuria in young people. A syndrome, *Acta Med Scand* 167:289-96, 1960.
61. Imerslund O: Idiopathic chronic megaloblastic anemia in children, *Acta Paediatr Suppl* 49 (Suppl 119):1-115, 1960.
62. Wahlstedt-Froberg V, Pettersson T, et al: Proteinuria in cubilin-deficient patients with selective vitamin B12 malabsorption, *Pediatr Nephrol* 18(5):417-21, 2003.
63. Norden AG, Lapsley M, et al: Urinary megalin deficiency implicates abnormal tubular endocytic function in Fanconi syndrome, *J Am Soc Nephrol* 13(1):125-33, 2002.
64. Christensen EI, Devuyst O, et al: Loss of chloride channel ClC-5 impairs endocytosis by defective trafficking of megalin and cubilin in kidney proximal tubules, *Proc Natl Acad Sci U S A* 100(14):8472-77, 2003.
65. Endo F, Sun MS: Tyrosinaemia type I and apoptosis of hepatocytes and renal tubular cells, *J Inherit Metab Dis* 25(3):227-34, 2002.
66. Thevenod F, Friedmann JM: Cadmium-mediated oxidative stress in kidney proximal tubule cells induces degradation of Na+/K (+)-ATPase through proteasomal and endo-/lysosomal proteolytic pathways, *FASEB J* 13(13):1751-61, 1999.
67. Park MA, Thoene JG: Potential role of apoptosis in development of the cystinotic phenotype, *Pediatr Nephrol* 20(4):441-46, 2005.
68. Park MA, Pejovic V, et al: Increased apoptosis in cystinotic fibroblasts and renal proximal tubule epithelial cells results from cysteinylation of protein kinase Cdelta, *J Am Soc Nephrol* 17(11): 3167-75, 2006.
69. Gahl WA, Bashan N, et al: Cystine transport is defective in isolated leukocyte lysosomes from patients with cystinosis, *Science* 217(4566):1263-65, 1982.
70. Gahl W, Thoene J, et al: Cystinosis: a disorder of lysosomal membrane transport. In Scriver CR, Beaudet A, Valle D, Sly W, editors: *The metabolic and molecular basis of inherited disease*, New York, 2001, McGraw-Hill, pp. 5085-108.
71. Gahl WA, Theone JG, et al: Cystinosis, *N Engl J Med* 347(2):111-21, 2002.
72. The Cystinosis Collaborative Research Group: Linkage of the gene for cystinosis to markers on the short arm of chromosome 17, *Nat Genet* 10(2):246-48, 1995.
73. Town M, Jean G, et al: A novel gene encoding an integral membrane protein is mutated in nephropathic cystinosis, *Nat Genet* 18(4):319-24, 1998.
74. Haq MR, Kalatzis V, et al: Immunolocalization of cystinosin, the protein defective in cystinosis, *J Am Soc Nephrol* 13(8):2046-51, 2002.
75. Cherqui S, Kalatzis V, et al: The targeting of cystinosin to the lysosomal membrane requires a tyrosine-based signal and a novel sorting motif, *J Biol Chem* 276(16):13314-21, 2001.
76. Kalatzis V, Cherqui S, et al: Cystinosin, the protein defective in cystinosis, is a H (+)-driven lysosomal cystine transporter, *EMBO J* 20(21):5940-49, 2001.
77. Forestier L, Jean G, et al: Molecular characterization of CTNS deletions in nephropathic cystinosis: development of a PCR-based detection assay, *Am J Hum Genet* 65(2):353-59, 1999.
78. Kalatzis V, Antignac C: New aspects of the pathogenesis of cystinosis, *Pediatr Nephrol* 18(3):207-15, 2003.
79. Attard M, Jean G, et al: Severity of phenotype in cystinosis varies with mutations in the CTNS gene: predicted effect on the model of cystinosin, *Hum Mol Genet* 8(13):2507-14, 1999.
80. Collin S, van't Hoff W: UK Cystinosis Registry (in Abstracts of the 3rd International Cystinosis Conference), *J Inherit Metab Dis* 28:1211-12, 2005.
81. Steinherz R, Chesney RW, et al: Circulating vitamin D metabolites in nephropathic cystinosis, *J Pediatr* 102(4):592-94, 1983.
82. Wong V: The eye and cystinosis. In Schulman JD, editor: *Cystinosis*, Washington, DC, 1972, U.S. Department of Health, Education and Welfare (NIH 72-249), pp. 23-35.
83. Gahl WA, Kuehl EM, et al: Corneal crystals in nephropathic cystinosis: natural history and treatment with cysteamine eyedrops, *Mol Genet Metab* 71(1-2):100-20, 2000.
84. Patrick AD, Lake BD: Cystinosis: electron microscopic evidence of lysosomal storage of cystine in lymph node, *J Clin Pathol* 21(5):571-75, 1968.
85. Schneider JA, Wong V, et al: The early diagnosis of cystinosis, *J Pediatr* 74(1):114-16, 1969.
86. Jackson M, Young E: Prenatal diagnosis of cystinosis by quantitative measurement of cystine in chorionic villi and cultured cells, *Prenat Diagn* 25(11):1045-47, 2005.
87. Smith ML, Clark KF, et al: Diagnosis of cystinosis with use of placenta, *N Engl J Med* 321(6):397-98, 1989.
88. Gretz N, Manz F, et al: Survival time in cystinosis. A collaborative study, *Proceedings of the European Dialysis and Transplant Association* 19:582-89, 1982.
89. Schnaper HW, Cottel J, et al: Early occurrence of end-stage renal disease in a patient with infantile nephropathic cystinosis, *J Pediatr* 120(4 Pt 1):575-78, 1992.
90. van't Hoff WG, Gretz N: The treatment of cystinosis with cysteamine and phosphocysteamine in the United Kingdom and Eire, *Pediatr Nephrol* 9(6):685-89, 1995.
91. Gubler MC, Lacoste M, et al: The pathology of the kidney in cystinosis. In Broyer M, editor: *Cystinosis*, Paris, 1999, Elsevier, pp. 42-48.
92. Spear GS: The pathology of the kidney. In Schulman JD, editor: *Cystinosis*, Washington, DC, 1972, U.S. Department of Health, Education and Welfare (NIH 72-249), pp. 37-53.
93. Spear GS, Gubler MC, et al: Dark cells of cystinosis: occurrence in renal allografts, *Hum Pathol* 20(5):472-76, 1989.
94. Saleem MA, Milford DV, et al: Hypercalciuria and ultrasound abnormalities in children with cystinosis, *Pediatr Nephrol* 9(1):45-47, 1995.
95. Theodoropoulos DS, Shawker TH, et al: Medullary nephrocalcinosis in nephropathic cystinosis, *Pediatr Nephrol* 9(4):412-18, 1995.
96. Strife CF, Strife JL, et al: Acquired structural genitourinary abnormalities contributing to deterioration of renal function in older patients with nephropathic cystinosis, *Pediatrics* 88(6):1238-41, 1991.
97. Broyer M, Tete MJ, et al: Late symptoms in infantile cystinosis, *Pediatr Nephrol* 1(3):519-24, 1987.
98. Ehrich JH, Loirat C, et al: Report on management of renal failure in children in Europe, XXII, 1991, *Nephrol Dial Transplant* 7 (Suppl 2):36-48, 1992.
99. Wilson DP, Jelley D, et al: Nephropathic cystinosis: improved linear growth after treatment with recombinant human growth hormone, *J Pediatr* 115(5 Pt 1):758-61, 1989.
100. Wuhl E, Haffner D, et al: Treatment with recombinant human growth hormone in short children with nephropathic cystinosis: no evidence for increased deterioration rate of renal function. The

European Study Group on Growth Hormone Treatment in Short Children with Nephropathic Cystinosis, *Pediatr Res* 43(4 Pt 1):484-88, 1998.
101. Wuhl E, Haffner D, et al: Long-term treatment with growth hormone in short children with nephropathic cystinosis, *J Pediatr* 138(6):880-87, 2001.
102. Chan AM, Lynch MJ, et al: Hypothyroidism in cystinosis. A clinical, endocrinologic and histologic study involving sixteen patients with cystinosis, *Am J Med* 48(6):678-92, 1970.
103. Burke JR, El-Bishti MM, et al: Hypothyroidism in children with cystinosis, *Arch Dis Child* 53(12):947-51, 1978.
104. Broyer M, Guillot M, et al: Infantile cystinosis: a reappraisal of early and late symptoms, *Adv Nephrol Necker Hosp* 10:137-66, 1981.
105. Gahl WA, Schneider JA, et al: Course of nephropathic cystinosis after age 10 years, *J Pediatr* 109(4):605-608, 1986.
106. Kimonis VE, Troendle J, et al: Effects of early cysteamine therapy on thyroid function and growth in nephropathic cystinosis, *J Clin Endocrinol Metab* 80(11):3257-61, 1995.
107. Robert JJ, Tete MJ, et al: Impaired insulin tolerance and insulin-dependent diabetes mellitus in infantile nephropathic cystinosis. In Broyer M, editor: *Cystinosis*, Paris, 1999, Elsevier, pp. 56-62.
108. Fivush B, Green OC, et al: Pancreatic endocrine insufficiency in posttransplant cystinosis, *Am J Dis Child* 141(10):1087-89, 1987.
109. Milner RD, Wirdnam PK: The pancreatic beta cell fraction in children with errors of amino acid metabolism, *Pediatr Res* 16(3):213-16, 1982.
110. Gahl WA, Kaiser-Kupfer MI: Complications of nephropathic cystinosis after renal failure, *Pediatr Nephrol* 1(3):260-68, 1987.
111. Winkler L, Offner G, et al: Growth and pubertal development in nephropathic cystinosis, *Eur J Pediatr* 152(3):244-49, 1993.
112. Reiss RE, Kuwabara T, et al: Successful pregnancy despite placental cystine crystals in a woman with nephropathic cystinosis, *N Engl J Med* 319(4):223-26, 1988.
113. Andrews PA, Sacks SH, et al: Successful pregnancy in cystinosis, *JAMA* 272(17):1327-28, 1994.
114. Fink JK, Brouwers P, et al: Neurologic complications in long-standing nephropathic cystinosis, *Arch Neurol* 46(5):543-48, 1989.
115. Vogel DG, Malekzadeh MH, et al: Central nervous system involvement in nephropathic cystinosis, *J Neuropathol Exp Neurol* 49(6):591-99, 1990.
116. Gahl WA, Dalakas MC, et al: Myopathy and cystine storage in muscles in a patient with nephropathic cystinosis, *N Engl J Med* 319(22):1461-64, 1988.
117. Anikster Y, Lacbawan F, et al: Pulmonary dysfunction in adults with nephropathic cystinosis, *Chest* 119(2):394-401, 2001.
118. Van Lierde A, Colombo D, et al: Hemiparesis in a girl with cystinosis and renal transplant, *Eur J Pediatr* 153(9):702-703, 1994.
119. Broyer M, Tete MJ: Central nervous system complications in cystinosis. In Broyer M, editor: *Cystinosis*, Paris, 1999, Elsevier, pp. 75-80.
120. Dogulu CF, Tsilou E, et al: Idiopathic intracranial hypertension in cystinosis, *J Pediatr* 145(5):673-78, 2004.
121. Van Damme BJ, Fleuren GJ, et al: Experimental glomerulonephritis in the rat induced by antibodies directed against tubular antigens. V. Fixed glomerular antigens in the pathogenesis of heterologous immune complex glomerulonephritis, *Lab Invest* 38(4):502-10, 1978.
122. Cochat P, Drachman PR, et al: Cerebral atrophy and nephropathic cystinosis, *Arch Dis Child* 61(4):401-403, 1986.
123. Fushimi K, Uchida S, et al: Cloning and expression of apical membrane water channel of rat kidney collecting tubule, *Nature* 361(6412):549-52, 1996.
124. Sonies BC, Ekman EF, et al: Swallowing dysfunction in nephropathic cystinosis, *N Engl J Med* 323(9):565-70, 1990.
125. Sonies BC, Almajid P, et al: Swallowing dysfunction in 101 patients with nephropathic cystinosis: benefit of long-term cysteamine therapy, (*Medicine (Baltimore)* 84(3):137-46, 2005.
126. Wolff G, Ehrich JH, Offner G, Brodehl J: Psychosocial and intellectual development in 12 patients with infantile nephropathic cystinosis, *Acta Scan Paediatr* 71:1007-11, 1982.
127. Trauner DA, Chase C, et al: Neurologic and cognitive deficits in children with cystinosis, *J Pediatr* 112(6):912-14, 1988.
128. Ballantyne AO, Trauner DA: Neurobehavioral consequences of a genetic metabolic disorder: visual processing deficits in infantile nephropathic cystinosis, *Neuropsychiatry Neuropsychol Behav Neurol* 13(4):254-63, 2000.
129. Kaiser-Kupfer MI, Caruso RC, et al: Long-term ocular manifestations in nephropathic cystinosis, *Arch Ophthalmol* 104(5):706-11, 1986.
130. Tsilou ET, Rubin BI, et al: Age-related prevalence of anterior segment complications in patients with infantile nephropathic cystinosis, *Cornea* 21(2):173-76, 2002.
131. Schneider JA, Katz B, et al: Update on nephropathic cystinosis, *Pediatr Nephrol* 4(6):645-53, 1990.
132. Dohil R, Newbury RO, et al: The evaluation and treatment of gastrointestinal disease in children with cystinosis receiving cysteamine, *J Pediatr* 143(2):224-30, 2003.
133. Dohil R, Fidler M, et al: Esomeprazole therapy for gastric acid hypersecretion in children with cystinosis, *Pediatr Nephrol* 20(12):1786-93, 2005.
134. Gahl WA: Cystinosis coming of age, *Adv Pediatr* 33:95-126, 1986.
135. Rossi S, Herrine SK, et al: Cystinosis as a cause of noncirrhotic portal hypertension, *Dig Dis Sci* 50(7):1372-75, 2005.
136. O'Brien K, Hussain N, et al: Nodular regenerative hyperplasia and severe portal hypertension in cystinosis, *Clin Gastroenterol Hepatol* 4(3):387-94, 2006.
137. Strayer DS: Cystinosis and dissecting aortic aneurysm in a 7-year-old boy, *Am J Dis Child* 133(4):436-38, 1979.
138. Olgar S, Nisli K, et al: Can cystinosis cause coronary artery dilatation? *Pediatr Cardiol* 27(2):263-68, 2006.
139. Dixit MP, Greifer I: Nephropathic cystinosis associated with cardiomyopathy: a 27-year clinical follow-up, *BMC Nephrol* 3:8, 2002.
140. Ueda M, O'Brien K, et al: Coronary artery and other vascular calcifications in patients with cystinosis after kidney transplantation, *Clin J Am Soc Nephrol* 1:555-62, 2006.
141. Almond PS, Matas AJ, et al: Renal transplantation for infantile cystinosis: long-term follow-up, *J Pediatr Surg* 28(2):232-38, 1993.
142. Goldman H, Scriver CR, et al: Adolescent cystinosis: comparisons with infantile and adult forms, *Pediatrics* 47(6):979-88, 1971.
143. Langman CB, Moore ES, et al: Renal failure in a sibship with late-onset cystinosis, *J Pediatr* 107(5):755-56, 1985.
144. Gahl WM, Renlund M, et al: Disorders of lysosomal transport: cystinosis and sialic acid storage disorders. In Scriver CR, Beaudet A, Sly W, editors: *The metabolic basis of inherited disease*, New York, 1989, McGraw-Hill, pp. 2619-47.
145. Wrong OM, Norden AG, et al: Dent's disease: a familial proximal renal tubular syndrome with low-molecular-weight proteinuria, hypercalciuria, nephrocalcinosis, metabolic bone disease, progressive renal failure and a marked male predominance, *Q J Med* 87(8):473-93, 1994.
146. Dent CE, Friedman M: Hypercalcuric rickets associated with renal tubular damage, *Arch Dis Child* 39:240-49, 1964.
147. Lloyd SE, Pearce SH, et al: A common molecular basis for three inherited kidney stone diseases, *Nature* 379(6564):445-49, 1996.
148. Akuta N, Lloyd SE, et al: Mutations of CLCN5 in Japanese children with idiopathic low molecular weight proteinuria, hypercalciuria and nephrocalcinosis, *Kidney Int* 52(4):911-16, 1997.
149. Lloyd SE, Pearce SH, et al: Idiopathic low molecular weight proteinuria associated with hypercalciuric nephrocalcinosis in Japanese children is due to mutations of the renal chloride channel (CLCN5), *J Clin Invest* 99(5):967-74, 1997.
150. Langlois V, Bernard C, et al: Clinical features of X-linked nephrolithiasis in childhood, *Pediatr Nephrol* 12(8):625-29, 1998.
151. Igarashi T, Inatomi J, et al: Clinical and genetic studies of CLCN5 mutations in Japanese families with Dent's disease, *Kidney Int* 58(2):520-27, 2000.
152. Scheinman SJ, Cox JP, et al: Isolated hypercalciuria with mutation in CLCN5: relevance to idiopathic hypercalciuria, *Kidney Int* 57(1):232-39, 2000.

153. Thakker RV: Pathogenesis of Dent's disease and related syndromes of X-linked nephrolithiasis, *Kidney Int* 57(3):787-93, 2000.
154. Hoopes RR Jr, Hueber PA, et al: CLCN5 chloride-channel mutations in six new North American families with X-linked nephrolithiasis, *Kidney Int* 54(3):698-705, 1998.
155. Cebotaru V, Kaul S, et al: High citrate diet delays progression of renal insufficiency in the ClC-5 knockout mouse model of Dent's disease, *Kidney Int* 68(2):642-52, 2005.
156. Raja KA, Schurman S, et al: Responsiveness of hypercalciuria to thiazide in Dent's disease, *J Am Soc Nephrol* 13(12):2938-44, 2002.
157. Nijenhuis T, Vallon V, et al: Enhanced passive Ca2+ reabsorption and reduced Mg2+ channel abundance explains thiazide-induced hypocalciuria and hypomagnesemia, *J Clin Invest* 115(6):1651-58, 2005.
158. Piwon N, Gunther W, et al: ClC-5 Cl-channel disruption impairs endocytosis in a mouse model for Dent's disease, *Nature* 408(6810):369-73, 2000.
159. Accardi A, Miller C: Secondary active transport mediated by a prokaryotic homologue of ClC Cl-channels, *Nature* 427(6977):803-807, 2004.
160. Scheel OA, Zdebik AA, et al: Voltage-dependent electrogenic chloride/proton exchange by endosomal CLC proteins, *Nature* 436(7049):424-27, 2005.
161. Wang Y, Cai H, et al: ClC-5: role in endocytosis in the proximal tubule, *Am J Physiol Renal Physiol* 289(4):F850-62, 2005.
162. Hryciw DH, Ekberg J, et al: Regulation of albumin endocytosis by PSD95/Dlg/ZO-1 (PDZ) scaffolds. Interaction of Na+-H+ exchange regulatory factor-2 with ClC-5, *J Biol Chem* 281(23): 16068-77, 2006.
163. Hryciw DH, Ekberg J, et al: ClC-5: a chloride channel with multiple roles in renal tubular albumin uptake, *Int J Biochem Cell Biol* 38(7):1036-42.
164. Gunther W, Piwon N, et al: The ClC-5 chloride channel knock-out mouse—an animal model for Dent's disease, *Pflugers Arch* 445(4):456-62, 2003.
165. Silva IV, Cebotaru V, et al: The ClC-5 knockout mouse model of Dent's disease has renal hypercalciuria and increased bone turnover, *J Bone Miner Res* 18(4):615-23.
166. Devuyst O, Jouret F, et al: Chloride channels and endocytosis: new insights from Dent's disease and ClC-5 knockout mice, *Nephron Physiol* 99(3):69-73, 2005.
167. Hoopes RR Jr, Shrimpton AE, et al: Dent disease with mutations in OCRL1, *Am J Hum Genet* 76(2):260-67, 2005.
168. Norden AG, Sharratt P, et al: Quantitative amino acid and proteomic analysis: very low excretion of polypeptides >750 Da in normal urine, *Kidney Int* 66(5):1994-2003, 2004.
169. Janne PA, Suchy SF, et al: Functional overlap between murine Inpp5b and Ocrl1 may explain why deficiency of the murine ortholog for OCRL1 does not cause Lowe syndrome in mice, *J Clin Invest* 101(10):2042-53, 1998.
170. Utsch B, Bokenkamp A, Benz MR, Besbas N, et al: Novel OCRL1 mutations in patients with the phenotype of Dent disease, *Am J Kidney Dis* 48(6):942-56, 2006.
171. Lowe CU, Terrey M, et al: Organic-aciduria, decreased renal ammonia production, hydrophthalmos, and mental retardation: a clinical entity, *AMA Am J Dis Child* 83(2):164-84, 1952.
172. Abbassi V, Lowe CU, et al: Oculo-cerebro-renal syndrome. A review, *Am J Dis Child* 115(2):145-68, 1968.
173. Charnas LR, Bernardini I, et al: Clinical and laboratory findings in the oculocerebrorenal syndrome of Lowe, with special reference to growth and renal function, *N Engl J Med* 324(19):1318-25, 1991.
174. Witzleben CL, Schoen EJ, et al: Progressive morphologic renal changes in the oculo-cerebro-renal syndrome of Lowe, *Am J Med* 44(2):319-24, 1968.
175. Tricot L, Yahiaoui Y, et al: End-stage renal failure in Lowe syndrome, *Nephrol Dial Transplant* 18(9):1923-25, 2003.
176. Schramm L, Gal A, et al: Advanced renal insufficiency in a 34-year-old man with Lowe syndrome, *Am J Kidney Dis* 43(3):538-43, 2004.
177. Scholten HG: Een meisje met Lowe-syndrome, *Maandschrift voor Kindergeneeskunde* 28:251-55, 1960.
178. Reilly DS, Lewis RA, et al: Tightly linked flanking markers for the Lowe oculocerebrorenal syndrome, with application to carrier assessment, *Am J Hum Genet* 42(5):748-55, 1988.
179. Brown N, Gardner RJ: Lowe syndrome: identification of the carrier state, *Birth Defects* 12(3):579-95, 1976.
180. Delleman JW, Bleeker-Wagemakers EM, et al: Opacities of the lens indicating carrier status in the oculo-cerebro-renal (Lowe) syndrome, *J Pediatr Ophthalmol* 14(4):205-12, 1977.
181. Cibis GW, Waeltermann JM, et al: Lenticular opacities in carriers of Lowe's syndrome, *Ophthalmology* 93(8):1041-45, 1986.
182. Lin T, Lewis RA, et al: Molecular confirmation of carriers for Lowe syndrome, *Ophthalmology* 106(1):119-22, 1999.
183. Roschinger W, Muntau AC, et al: Carrier assessment in families with lowe oculocerebrorenal syndrome: novel mutations in the OCRL1 gene and correlation of direct DNA diagnosis with ocular examination, *Mol Genet Metab* 69(3):213-22, 2000.
184. Lin T, Orrison BM, et al: Spectrum of mutations in the OCRL1 gene in the Lowe oculocerebrorenal syndrome, *Am J Hum Genet* 60(6):1384-88, 1997.
185. Lin T, Orrison BM, et al: Mutations are not uniformly distributed throughout the OCRL1 gene in Lowe syndrome patients, *Mol Genet Metab* 64(1):58-61, 1998.
186. Monnier N, Satre V, et al: OCRL1 mutation analysis in French Lowe syndrome patients: implications for molecular diagnosis strategy and genetic counseling, *Hum Mutat* 16(2):157-65, 2000.
187. Attree O, Olivos IM, et al: The Lowe's oculocerebrorenal syndrome gene encodes a protein highly homologous to inositol polyphosphate-5-phosphatase, *Nature* 358(6383):239-42, 1992.
188. Olivos-Glander IM, Janne PA, et al: The oculocerebrorenal syndrome gene product is a 105-kD protein localized to the Golgi complex, *Am J Hum Genet* 57(4):817-23, 1995.
189. Dressman MA, Olivos-Glander IM, et al: Ocrl1, a PtdIns(4,5)P(2) 5-phosphatase, is localized to the trans-Golgi network of fibroblasts and epithelial cells, *J Histochem Cytochem* 48(2):179-90, 2000.
190. Ungewickell A, Ward ME, et al: The inositol polyphosphate 5-phosphatase Ocrl associates with endosomes that are partially coated with clathrin, *Proc Natl Acad Sci U S A* 101(37):13501-506, 2004.
191. Choudhury R, Diao A, et al: Lowe syndrome protein OCRL1 interacts with clathrin and regulates protein trafficking between endosomes and the trans-Golgi network, *Mol Biol Cell* 16(8):3467-79, 2005.
192. Toker A: The synthesis and cellular roles of phosphatidylinositol 4,5-bisphosphate, *Curr Opin Cell Biol* 10(2):254-61, 1998.
193. Raucher D, Stauffer T, et al: Phosphatidylinositol 4,5-bisphosphate functions as a second messenger that regulates cytoskeleton-plasma membrane adhesion, *Cell* 100(2):221-28, 2000.
194. Zhang X, Hartz PA, et al: Cell lines from kidney proximal tubules of a patient with Lowe syndrome lack OCRL inositol polyphosphate 5-phosphatase and accumulate phosphatidylinositol 4,5-bisphosphate, *J Biol Chem* 273(3):1574-82, 1998.
195. Suchy SF, Nussbaum RL: The deficiency of PIP2 5-phosphatase in Lowe syndrome affects actin polymerization, *Am J Hum Genet* 71(6):1420-27, 2002.
196. Sassa S, Kappas A: Hereditary tyrosinemia and the heme biosynthetic pathway. Profound inhibition of delta-aminolevulinic acid dehydratase activity by succinylacetone, *J Clin Invest* 71(3):625-34.
197. Holme E, Lindstedt S: Tyrosinaemia type I and NTBC(2-(2-nitro-4-trifluoromethylbenzoyl)-1,3-cyclohexanedione), *J Inherit Metab Dis* 21(5):507-17, 1998.
198. McKiernan PJ: Nitisinone in the treatment of hereditary tyrosinaemia type 1, *Drugs* 66(6):743-50, 2006.
199. Tuchman M, Freese DK, et al: Contribution of extrahepatic tissues to biochemical abnormalities in hereditary tyrosinemia type I: study of three patients after liver transplantation, *J Pediatr* 110(3):399-403, 1987.
200. Pierik LJ, van Spronsen FJ, et al: Renal function in tyrosinaemia type I after liver transplantation: a long-term follow-up, *J Inherit Metab Dis* 28(6):871-76, 2005.
201. Niaudet P, Rotig A: Renal involvement in mitochondrial cytopathies, *Pediatr Nephrol* 10(3):368-73, 1996.

202. Thorner PS, Balfe JW, et al: Abnormal mitochondria on a renal biopsy from a case of mitochondrial myopathy, *Pediatr Pathol* 4(1-2):25-35, 1985.
203. Santer R, Schneppenheim, R, et al: Mutations in GLUT2, the gene for the liver-type glucose transporter, in patients with Fanconi-Bickel syndrome, *Nat Genet* 17(3):324-26, 1997.
204. Santer R, Schneppenheim R, et al: Fanconi-Bickel syndrome—the original patient and his natural history, historical steps leading to the primary defect, and a review of the literature, *Eur J Pediatr* 157(10):783-97, 1998.
205. Guillam MT, Hummler E, et al: Early diabetes and abnormal postnatal pancreatic islet development in mice lacking Glut-2, *Nat Genet* 17(3):327-30, 1997.
206. Brivet M, Moatti N, et al: Defective galactose oxidation in a patient with glycogen storage disease and Fanconi syndrome, *Pediatr Res* 17(2):157-61, 1983.
207. Odievre MH, Lombes A, et al: A secondary respiratory chain defect in a patient with Fanconi-Bickel syndrome, *J Inherit Metab Dis* 25(5):379-84, 2002.
208. Sakamoto O, Ogawa E, et al: Mutation analysis of the GLUT2 gene in patients with Fanconi-Bickel syndrome, *Pediatr Res* 48(5):586-89, 2000.
209. Santer R, Steinmann B, et al: Fanconi-Bickel syndrome—a congenital defect of facilitative glucose transport, *Curr Mol Med* 2(2):213-27, 2002.
210. Santer R, Kinner M, et al: Molecular analysis of the SGLT2 gene in patients with renal glucosuria, *J Am Soc Nephrol* 14(11):2873-82, 2003.
211. Francis J, Zhang J, et al: A novel SGLT2 mutation in a patient with autosomal recessive renal glucosuria, *Nephrol Dial Transplant* 19(11):2893-95, 2004.
212. Lee PJ, van't Hoff WG, et al: Catch-up growth in Fanconi-Bickel syndrome with uncooked cornstarch, *J Inherit Metab Dis* 18(2):153-56, 1995.
213. Morris RC Jr, Nigon K, et al: Evidence that the severity of depletion of inorganic phosphate determines the severity of the disturbance of adenine nucleotide metabolism in the liver and renal cortex of the fructose-loaded rat, *J Clin Invest* 61(1):209-20, 1978.
214. Lu M, Holliday LS, et al: Interaction between aldolase and vacuolar H+-ATPase: evidence for direct coupling of glycolysis to the ATP-hydrolyzing proton pump, *J Biol Chem* 276(32):30407-13, 2001.
215. Goldberg L, Holzel A, et al: A clinical and biochemical study of galactosaemiaa possible explanation of the nature of the biochemical lesion, *Arch Dis Child* 31(158):254-64.
216. Gissen P, Johnson CA, et al: Mutations in VPS33B, encoding a regulator of SNARE-dependent membrane fusion, cause arthrogryposis-renal dysfunction-cholestasis (ARC) syndrome, *Nat Genet* 36(4):400-404, 2004.
217. Eastham KM, McKiernan PJ, et al: ARC syndrome: an expanding range of phenotypes, *Arch Dis Child* 85(5):415-20, 2001.
218. Horslen SP, Quarrell OW, et al: Liver histology in the arthrogryposis multiplex congenita, renal dysfunction, and cholestasis (ARC) syndrome: report of three new cases and review, *J Med Genet* 31(1):62-64, 1994.
219. Di Rocco M, Callea F, et al: Arthrogryposis, renal dysfunction and cholestasis syndrome: report of five patients from three Italian families, *Eur J Pediatr* 154(10):835-39, 1995.
220. Gissen P, Tee L, et al: Clinical and molecular genetic features of ARC syndrome, *Hum Genet* 120(3):396-409, 2006.
221. Levy M, Gagnadoux MF, et al: Membranous glomerulonephritis associated with anti-tubular and anti-alveolar basement membrane antibodies, *Clin Nephrol* 10(4):158-65, 1978.
222. Dumas R, Dumas ML, et al: [Membranous glomerulonephritis in two brothers associated in one with tubulo-interstitial disease, Fanconi syndrome and anti-TBM antibodies], *Arch Fr Pediatr* 39(2):75-78, 1982.
223. Wood EG, Brouhard BH, et al: Membranous glomerulonephropathy with tubular dysfunction and linear tubular basement membrane IgG deposition, *J Pediatr* 101(3):414-17, 1982.
224. Yagame M, Tomino Y, et al: An adult case of Fanconi's syndrome associated with membranous nephropathy, *Tokai J Exp Clin Med* 11(2):101-106, 1986.
225. Katz A, Fish AJ, et al: Role of antibodies to tubulointerstitial nephritis antigen in human anti-tubular basement membrane nephritis associated with membranous nephropathy, *Am J Med* 93(6):691-98, 1992.
226. Makker SP, Widstrom R, et al: Membranous nephropathy, interstitial nephritis, and Fanconi syndrome—glomerular antigen, *Pediatr Nephrol* 10(1):7-13, 1996.
227. Griswold WR, Krous HF, et al: The syndrome of autoimmune interstitial nephritis and membranous nephropathy, *Pediatr Nephrol* 11(6):699-702, 1997.
228. Tay AH, Ren EC, et al: Membranous nephropathy with anti-tubular basement membrane antibody may be X-linked, *Pediatr Nephrol* 14(8-9):747-53, 2000.
229. Kazama I, Matsubara M, et al: Adult onset Fanconi syndrome: extensive tubulo-interstitial lesions and glomerulopathy in the early stage of Chinese herbs nephropathy, *Clin Exp Nephrol* 8(3):283-87, 2004.
230. Shenoy M, Krishnan R, et al: Childhood membranous nephropathy in association with interstitial nephritis and Fanconi syndrome, *Pediatr Nephrol* 21(3):441, 2006.
231. Rossi R, Ehrich JH: Partial and complete de Toni-Debre-Fanconi syndrome after ifosfamide chemotherapy of childhood malignancy, *Eur J Clin Pharmacol* 44 (Suppl 1):S43-45, 1993.
232. Skinner R, Pearson AD, et al: Risk factors for ifosfamide nephrotoxicity in children, *Lancet* 348(9027):578-80, 1996.
233. Loebstein R, Koren G: Ifosfamide-induced nephrotoxicity in children: critical review of predictive risk factors, *Pediatrics* 101(6): E8, 1998.
234. Skinner R, Pearson AD, et al: Cisplatin dose rate as a risk factor for nephrotoxicity in children, *Br J Cancer* 77(10):1677-82, 1998.
235. Rossi R, Pleyer J, et al: Development of ifosfamide-induced nephrotoxicity: prospective follow-up in 75 patients, *Med Pediatr Oncol* 32(3):177-82, 1999.
236. Loebstein R, Atanackovic G, et al: Risk factors for long-term outcome of ifosfamide-induced nephrotoxicity in children, *J Clin Pharmacol* 39(5):454-61, 1999.
237. Skinner R, Cotterill SJ, et al: Risk factors for nephrotoxicity after ifosfamide treatment in children: a UKCCSG Late Effects Group study. United Kingdom Children's Cancer Study Group, *Br J Cancer* 82(10):1636-45, 2000.
238. Macpherson NA, Moscarello MA, et al: Aminoaciduria is an earlier index of renal tubular damage than conventional renal disease markers in the gentamicin-rat model of acute renal failure, *Clin Invest Med* 14(2):101-10, 1991.
239. Izzedine H, Launay-Vacher V, et al: Drug-induced Fanconi's syndrome, *Am J Kidney Dis* 41(2):292-309, 2003.
240. Haffner D, Weinfurth A, et al: Body growth in primary de Toni-Debre-Fanconi syndrome, *Pediatr Nephrol* 11(1):40-45, 1997.
241. Neimann N, Pierson M, et al: [Familial glomerulo-tubular nephropathy with the de Toni-Debre-Fanconi syndrome], *Arch Fr Pediatr* 25(1):43-69, 1968.
242. Friedman AL, Trygstad CW, et al: Autosomal dominant Fanconi syndrome with early renal failure, *Am J Med Genet* 2(3):225-32, 1978.
243. Patrick A, Cameron JS, et al: A family with a dominant form of idiopathic Fanconi syndrome leading to renal failure in adult life, *Clin Nephrol* 16(6):289-92, 1981.
244. Tieder M, Arie R, et al: Elevated serum 1,25-dihydroxyvitamin D concentrations in siblings with primary Fanconi's syndrome, *N Engl J Med* 319(13):845-49, 1988.
245. Wen SF, Friedman AL, et al: Two case studies from a family with primary Fanconi syndrome, *Am J Kidney Dis* 13(3):240-46, 1989.
246. Tolaymat A, Sakarcan A, et al: Idiopathic Fanconi syndrome in a family. Part I. Clinical aspects, *J Am Soc Nephrol* 2(8):1310-17, 1992.
247. Frisch LS, Mimouni F: Hypomagnesemia following correction of metabolic acidosis: a case of hungry bones, *J Am Coll Nutr* 12(6):710-13, 1993.
248. Haycock GB, Al-Dahhan J, et al: Effect of indomethacin on clinical progress and renal function in cystinosis, *Arch Dis Child* 57(12):934-39, 1982.

249. Clark KF: A comparative study of indomethacin for the treatment of the Fanconi syndrome in cystinosis. *J Rare Dis* 11:5-12, 1996.
250. Callis L, Castello F, et al: Studies on the site of renal sodium loss in two patients with cystinosis. Effects of hydrochlorothiazide on tubular sodium reabsorptive mechanisms, *Nephron* 18(1):35-40, 1977.
251. Pisoni RL, Thoene JG, et al: Detection and characterization of carrier-mediated cationic amino acid transport in lysosomes of normal and cystinotic human fibroblasts. Role in therapeutic cystine removal? *J Biol Chem* 260(8):4791-98, 1985.
252. Gahl WA, Reed GF, et al: Cysteamine therapy for children with nephropathic cystinosis, *N Engl J Med* 316(16):971-77, 1987.
253. Markello TC, Bernardini IM, et al: Improved renal function in children with cystinosis treated with cysteamine, *N Engl J Med* 328(16):1157-62, 1993.
254. Kleta R, Bernardini I, et al: Long-term follow-up of well-treated nephropathic cystinosis patients, *J Pediatr* 145(4):555-60, 2004.
255. Broyer M: [Cystinosis from childhood to adulthood], *Nephrologie* 21(1):13-8, 2000.
256. Gahl WA: Early oral cysteamine therapy for nephropathic cystinosis, *Eur J Pediatr* 162(Suppl 1):S38-41, 2003.
257. Kaiser-Kupfer MI, Gazzo MA, et al: A randomized placebo-controlled trial of cysteamine eye drops in nephropathic cystinosis, *Arch Ophthalmol* 108(5):689-93, 1990.
258. Iwata F, Kuehl EM, et al: A randomized clinical trial of topical cysteamine disulfide (cystamine) versus free thiol (cysteamine) in the treatment of corneal cystine crystals in cystinosis, *Mol Genet Metab* 64(4):237-42, 1998.
259. Tsilou ET, Thompson D, et al: A multicentre randomised double masked clinical trial of a new formulation of topical cysteamine for the treatment of corneal cystine crystals in cystinosis, *Br J Ophthalmol* 87(1):28-31, 2003.
260. Belldina EB, Huang MY, et al: Steady-state pharmacokinetics and pharmacodynamics of cysteamine bitartrate in paediatric nephropathic cystinosis patients, *Br J Clin Pharmacol* 56(5):520-25.
261. Levtchenko EN, van Dael CM, et al: Strict cysteamine dose regimen is required to prevent nocturnal cystine accumulation in cystinosis, *Pediatr Nephrol* 21(1):110-13, 2006.
262. Sadoff L: Nephrotoxicity of streptozotocin (NSC-85998), *Cancer Chemother Rep* 54(6):457-59, 1970.
263. Kintzel PE: Anticancer drug-induced kidney disorders, *Drug Saf* 24(1):19-38, 2001.
264. Montoliu, J, Carrera M, et al: Lactic acidosis and Fanconi's syndrome due to degraded tetracycline, *BMJ (Clin Res Ed)* 283(6306):1576-77, 1981.
265. Cleveland WW, Adams WC, et al: Acquired Fanconi syndrome following degraded tetracycline, *J Pediatr* 66:333-42, 1965.
266. Vittecoq D, Dumitrescu L, et al: Fanconi syndrome associated with cidofovir therapy, *Antimicrob Agents Chemother* 41(8):1846, 1997.
267. Verhelst D, Monge M, et al: Fanconi syndrome and renal failure induced by tenofovir: a first case report, *Am J Kidney Dis* 40(6):1331-33, 2002.
268. Earle KE, Seneviratne T, et al: Fanconi's syndrome in HIV+ adults: report of three cases and literature review, *J Bone Miner Res* 19(5):714-21, 2004.
269. Izzedine H, Hulot JS, et al: Association between ABCC2 gene haplotypes and tenofovir-induced proximal tubulopathy, *J Infect Dis* 194(11):1481-91, 2006.
270. Crowther MA, Callaghan W, et al: Dideoxyinosine-associated nephrotoxicity, *AIDS* 7(1):131-32, 1993.
271. Izzedine H, Launay-Vacher V, et al: Fanconi syndrome associated with didanosine therapy, *AIDS* 19(8):844-45, 2005.
272. Chisolm JJ Jr, Harrison HC, et al: Amino-aciduria, hypophosphatemia, and rickets in lead poisoning: study of a case, *AMA Am J Dis Child* 89(2):159-68, 1955.
273. Kazantzis G, Flynn FV, et al: Renal tubular malfunction and pulmonary emphysema in cadmium pigment workers, *Q J Med* 32:165-92, 1963.
274. Lande MB, Kim MS, et al: Reversible Fanconi syndrome associated with valproate therapy, *J Pediatr* 123(2):320-22, 1993.
275. Yang SS, Chu P, et al: Aristolochic acid-induced Fanconi's syndrome and nephropathy presenting as hypokalemic paralysis, *Am J Kidney Dis* 39(3):E14, 2002.
276. Lee S, Lee T, et al: Fanconi's syndrome and subsequent progressive renal failure caused by a Chinese herb containing aristolochic acid, *Nephrology (Carlton)* 9(3):126-29, 2004.
277. Hong YT, Fu LS, et al: Fanconi's syndrome, interstitial fibrosis and renal failure by aristolochic acid in Chinese herbs, *Pediatr Nephrol* 21(4):577-79, 2006.
278. Moss AH, Gabow PA, et al: Fanconi's syndrome and distal renal tubular acidosis after glue sniffing, *Ann Intern Med* 92(1):69-70, 1980.
279. Raschka C, Koch HJ: Long-term treatment of psoriasis using fumaric acid preparations can be associated with severe proximal tubular damage, *Hum Exp Toxicol* 18(12):738-39, 1999.
280. Rago RP, Miles JM, et al: Suramin-induced weakness from hypophosphatemia and mitochondrial myopathy. Association of suramin with mitochondrial toxicity in humans, *Cancer* 73(7):1954-59, 1994.
281. Gil HW, Yang JO, et al: Paraquat-induced Fanconi syndrome, *Nephrology (Carlton)* 10(5):430-32, 2005.
282. Lo JC, Chertow GM, et al: Fanconi's syndrome and tubulointerstitial nephritis in association with L-lysine ingestion, *Am J Kidney Dis* 28(4):614-17, 1996.
283. Igarashi T, Kawato H, et al: Acute tubulointerstitial nephritis with uveitis syndrome presenting as multiple tubular dysfunction including Fanconi's syndrome, *Pediatr Nephrol* 6(6):547-49, 1992.

CHAPTER

29 Bartter, Gitelman, and Related Syndromes

Siegfried Waldegger

INTRODUCTION

The focus of this chapter is various forms of renal salt wasting caused by inherited dysfunction of ion-transporting proteins expressed along the thick ascending limb (TAL) of Henle's loop and the early distal convoluted tubule (DCT1). Renal salt wasting due to impaired sodium reabsorption along the aldosterone-sensitive distal nephron (ASDN) composed of the late distal convoluted tubule (DCT2), the connecting tubule (CNT), and the cortical and medullary portions of the collecting duct (CCD and MCD), is accompanied by hyperkalemia and is discussed elsewhere.

BASIC PRINCIPLES OF ION TRANSPORT IN THE TAL AND DCT1

The TAL and DCT1 form a functional unit in that they separate tubular sodium chloride from water. Compared to sodium absorption in the other nephron segments, which occurs via sodium hydrogen exchange or by sodium channels in the proximal nephron and in the ASDN, respectively, TAL and DCT1 sodium transport is accomplished primarily by the active reabsorption of sodium together with chloride from the tubular fluid. These nephron segments in addition are relatively water-tight, and thus prevent osmotically driven absorptive water flow. About 30% of the total sodium load provided by glomerular filtration is absorbed along the TAL and—via counter-current multiplication—contribute to medullary interstitial hypertonicity. TAL sodium absorption thus not only accounts for the—in quantitative terms—most important mechanism of sodium retention (apart from the proximal nephron, which absorbs about 60% of the filtered sodium load), but also generates the osmotic driving force for water absorption along the collecting ducts. For this reason, disturbances in TAL salt absorption result in both salt wasting and severely reduced urinary concentrating capacity (i.e., water wasting). In contrast, DCT-mediated salt absorption accounts for only about 5% of the filtered sodium load and does not contribute to the urinary concentrating mechanisms. Impaired DCT salt absorption therefore does not interfere with urinary concentrating capability, although the accompanying saluresis indirectly increases renal water excretion even with normal urine osmolalities.

Transepithelial NaCl absorption in both nephron segments is driven by secondary active transport processes that depend on a low intracellular sodium concentration maintained by active extrusion of sodium by the basolateral sodium-potassium-ATPase (sodium pump). By far the majority of TAL sodium absorption depends on the operation of the furosemide-sensitive NKCC2 sodium-potassium-chloride co-transporter with about half of the sodium taking the transcellular route and half taking a paracellular route by cationselective intercellular pathways. Potassium that enters the TAL cell by sodium-potassium-chloride co-transport (one potassium-ion being transported with one sodium and two chloride ions) recycles back to the tubular urine through renal outer medullary potassium (ROMK) channels. This guarantees proper activity of NKCC2-mediated transport along the entire length of the TAL by replenishment of urinary potassium that otherwise would rapidly decrease along the TAL through absorption by NKCC2. Even more importantly, luminal potassium secretion in addition establishes a lumen-positive transepithelial voltage gradient that provides—in terms of energy recovery—a low-cost driving force for paracellular transport of cations like sodium, calcium, and magnesium. The essential functions of the TAL thus not only include the reabsorption of sodium chloride, but also that of magnesium and calcium. It is noteworthy that all TAL chloride reabsorption occurs by the transcellular route. Overall parity of sodium (with ~50% transcellular and ~50% paracellular) and chloride (100% transcellular) reabsorption is due to the stoichiometry of the apical NKCC2 transporter that transports two chloride ions for each sodium ion (Figure 29-1).

Taken together, the initial step of transcellular sodium chloride and paracellular sodium transport across the TAL epithelium critically depends on the proper activity of NKCC2 and ROMK.

In contrast to the TAL, sodium chloride absorption in the DCT1 occurs almost exclusively by the transcellular route. Luminal sodium chloride uptake is mediated by the electroneutral thiazide-sensitive sodium chloride co-transporter NCCT that is structurally related to the NKCC2 protein, but transports one sodium ion together with one chloride ion without potassium. A relevant apical potassium conductance seems not to exist in DCT1 cells, which instead express TRPM6 cation channels that permit apical magnesium entry.

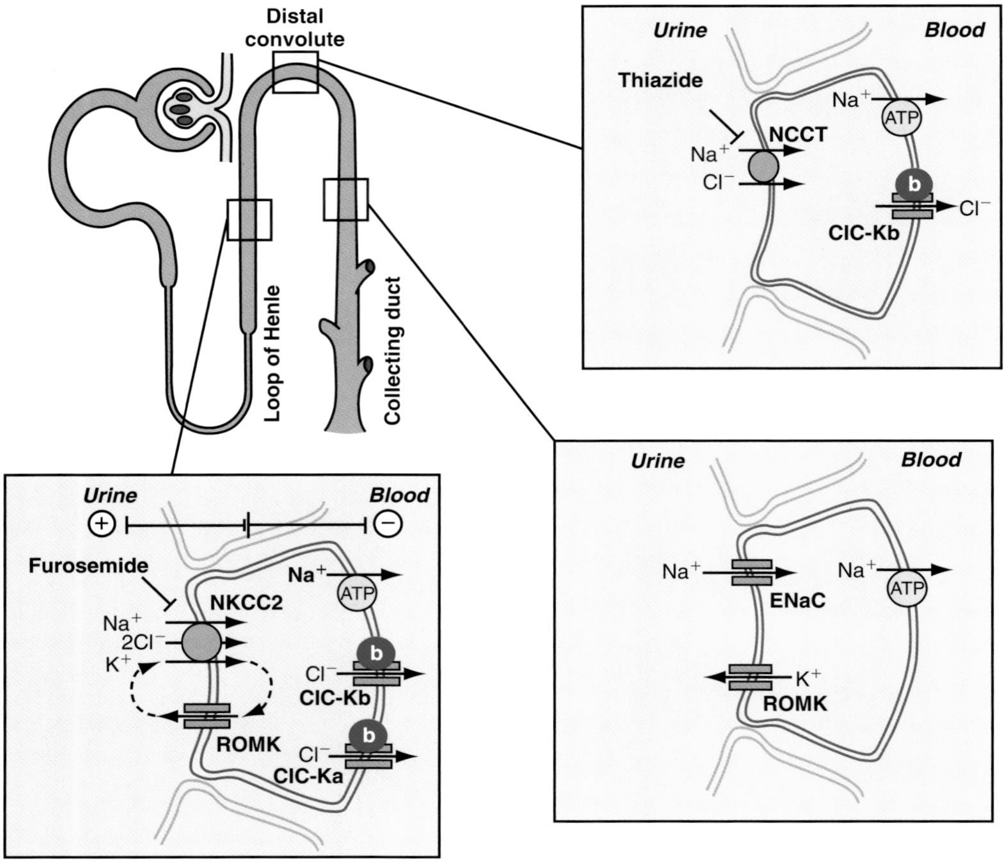

Figure 29-1 Mechanisms of sodium reabsorption along the distal nephron. The key transport proteins and ion channels are shown for TAL, DCT1, and CCD. b, ClC-K chloride channel beta-subunit Barttin.

Inhibition of NCCT transport by long-term administration of thiazides or by genetic ablation in animal models has been shown to reduce the number of DCT1 cells, which might explain impaired renal magnesium reabsorption with consequent hypomagnesemia observed in human diseases caused by impaired NCCT-mediated transport.

DCT1 and TAL cells differ with respect to the apical entry step for sodium chloride. However, as mentioned above, basolateral sodium release in both cell types is accounted for by the sodium pump. Moreover, TAL and DCT1 cells share similar pathways for basolateral chloride exit. In both cell types, two highly homologous ClC-K-type chloride channel proteins (ClC-Ka and ClC-Kb) associate with their beta-subunit barttin to form a basolateral chloride conductance, which accounts for releasing the great majority of reabsorbed chloride ions (Figure 29-1).

Taken together, NCCT mediates DCT1 cell sodium chloride uptake and ClC-K-type chloride channels in association with barttin account for basolateral chloride release in TAL and DCT1 cells.

In the transition zone between the TAL and DCT1, a plaque of closely packed epithelial cells morphologically different from TAL and DCT1 cells forms the macula densa. Together with closely adjacent extraglomerular mesangial cells and granular cells of the afferent arterioles appendant to the same nephron, these specialized tubular cells assemble the juxtaglomerular apparatus. Macula densa cells serve an important function in coupling renal hemodynamics with tubular reabsorption in that they monitor the sodium chloride concentration of the tubular fluid and via paracrine signaling molecules like prostaglandin E_2 (PGE_2), ATP, adenosine, and NO provide a feedback mechanism that adapts glomerular filtration to tubular reabsorption (tubuloglomerular feedback [TGF]). In case of an increased sodium chloride concentration at the macula densa, the TGF induces afferent arteriole vasoconstriction and decreases renin release, whereas a decreased macula densa NaCl concentration dilates the afferent arteriole and increases renin release. To sense the tubular sodium chloride concentration, the macula densa cells seem to take advantage of essentially the same repertoire of transport proteins as found in salt-reabsorbing TAL cells. Via apical sodium chloride uptake (NKCC2 and ROMK) and basolateral chloride release (ClC-K and barttin) changes in luminal sodium chloride concentration are translated in alterations of basolateral transmembrane voltage. This again results from recycling of potassium into the tubular lumen, which guarantees an asymmetric—hence electrogenic—transcellular transport of sodium chloride with one sodium ion being reabsorbed together with two chloride ions, which results in basolateral membrane depolarization by transcellular net movement of one negative charge. This in turn regulates, among other processes, voltage-sensitive calcium entry, which triggers a series of intracellular signaling events, eventually resulting in the release of the above mentioned paracrine signals. Owing to these combined functions in transepithelial transport and sensing of tubular sodium chloride, impaired activity of one of the participating proteins not only results in salt wasting due to reduced TAL salt-reabsorbing capacity, but also abrogates the TGF as an important safety valve, which otherwise would reduce the filtered sodium chloride load by decreasing glomerular filtration. In fact, blinding of the macula densa for the tubular sodium chloride concentration with resultant disinhibition of glomerular filtration might constitute the single most important mechanism underlying the severe salt wasting observed in impaired TAL salt transport. This notion is consistent with findings from NHE3-deficient mice (lacking the sodium/proton exchanger type 3, the dominating sodium reabsorbing protein of the proximal tubule), which surprisingly do not display renal salt wasting. An intact TGF, admittedly together with intact TAL function, thus obviously suffices to compensate for a sodium reabsorption defect exceeding more than 60% of the filtered sodium load.

Taken together, NKCC2, ROMK, the ClC-K type chloride channels, and barttin participate in the salt-sensing mechanism of the macula densa. Impaired function of one of these proteins affects the TGF and prevents adjustment of glomerular filtration with tubular salt-reabsorbing capacity, which further aggravates renal salt wasting.[1]

HYPOKALEMIC SALT-WASTING KIDNEY DISORDERS

With the exception of the MCD that is primarily responsible for the absorption of water, re-absorption of sodium chloride from the glomerular filtrate at least in quantitative terms constitutes the key function of all nephron segments. Given the normal daily amount of 170 liters of glomerular filtrate produced by adult kidneys, at a normal plasma sodium concentration of 140 mmol/L and plasma chloride concentration of 105 mmol/L, the filtered load of sodium and chloride per 24 hours amounts to 23.8 mol (about 550 g) and 17.9 mol (about 630 g), respectively. Healthy kidneys manage the reabsorption of more than 99% of the filtered load, with about 60% by the proximal tubule, 30% by the TAL, 5% by the DCT1, and the remainder by the aldosterone-sensitive distal nephron (ASDN). Impairment of sodium transport in any of these nephron segments causes a permanent reduction in extracellular fluid volume, which in turn causes compensatory activation of sodium-conserving mechanisms, that is, stimulation of renin secretion and aldosterone synthesis. Accordingly, with intact ASDN function, the primary symptoms of renal salt wasting like hypovolemia with tendency for reduced arterial blood pressure, mix with those of secondary hyperaldosteronism, which increases ASDN sodium retention at the expense of an increased potassium excretion that eventually results in hypokalemia. In case of renal salt wasting, hypokalemia thus indicates proper function of the ASDN and points to the involvement of nephron segments more proximal to the ASDN.

As mentioned above, sodium reabsorption along the TAL and DCT1 is coupled to the reabsorption of chloride. Sodium wasting caused by defects in these nephron segments hence is accompanied by decreased reabsorption of chloride. Unlike sodium, which at least partially may be recovered by compensatory increased reabsorption along the ASDN, chloride irretrievably gets lost with the urine. Accordingly, the urinary chloride loss exceeds that of sodium, and for the sake of electroneutrality has to be balanced by other cations like ammonium or potassium. Loss of ammonium, the main carrier of protons in the urine, results in metabolic alkalosis; potassium loss in addition aggravates hypokalemia caused by secondary hyperaldosteronism. For this reason, hypochloremia with metabolic alkalosis, in addition to severe hypokalemia, characterizes salt wasting due to defects along the TAL and DCT1.

Finally, sodium reabsorption along the proximal tubule via the sodium proton exchanger and carboanhydrase is indirectly coupled to the reabsorption of bicarbonate. Proximal tubular salt wasting thus—in addition to hypokalemia—is accompanied by urinary loss of bicarbonate resulting in hyperchloremic metabolic acidosis.

Taken together, in the state of renal salt-wasting determination of plasma potassium, chloride, and bicarbonate concentrations allows for the rapid assessment of the affected nephron segment. Of note, in this context the determination of the plasma sodium concentration is not very helpful, since changes in plasma sodium—the more or less exclusive extracellular cation accounting for plasma osmolality—reflects disturbances in the osmoregulation (i.e., water balance) rather than in the regulation of sodium balance.

Apart from more general disturbances of proximal tubular function, which among other transport processes affect proximal tubular sodium reabsorption (the Fanconi renotubular syndromes), no hereditary defects specifically affecting the proximal tubular sodium proton exchanger have been described in humans. By contrast, several genetic defects affect sodium chloride transport along the TAL and DCT1, and are the focus of the following section.

RENAL SALT WASTING WITH HYPOKALEMIA AND HYPOCHLOREMIC METABOLIC ALKALOSIS

Historical Overview and Nomenclature

In 1957, two pediatricians described an infant with congenital hypokalemic alkalosis, failure to thrive, dehydration, and hyposthenuria, who died at the age of 7.5 months.[2] Some years later, two patients with normotensive hyperaldosteronism, hyperplasia of the juxtaglomerular apparatus, metabolic alkalosis, and severe renal potassium wasting were characterized by the endocrinologist Frederic Bartter.[3] Other features of this syndrome were increased activity of the renin-angiotensin system and a relative vascular resistance to the pressor effect of exogenously applied angiotensin II. Following these original reports, hundreds of such Bartter syndrome (BS) cases have been described. While all shared the findings of hypokalemia and hypochloremic alkalosis, patients differed with respect to age of onset, severity of symptoms, degree of growth retardation, urinary concentration capacity, magnitude of urinary potassium and prostaglandin excretion, presence of hypomagnesemia, and extent of urinary calcium excretion.

Gitelman and colleagues pointed to the susceptibility to carpopedal spasms and tetany in three BS cases.[4] Tetany was attributed to low plasma magnesium levels secondary to impaired renal conservation of magnesium. Further examination of these patients revealed low urinary calcium excretion.[5] Consequently, the association of hypocalciuria with renal magnesium wasting was regarded as a hallmark to separate the then-defined Gitelman syndrome (GS) from other forms of BS.[6] Interestingly, both patients in Bartter's original report displayed positive Chvostek's sign and carpopedal spasms. Indeed, in a recent review of the original observations described by Bartter et al.,[7] one of the coauthors conceded that the majority of patients seen by both endocrinologists perfectly matched the later description of Gitelman.

Phenotypic homogeneity of BS was challenged even more seriously when the pediatricians Fanconi and McCredie described high urinary calcium excretion and medullary nephrocalcinosis in preterm infants initially suspected of having BS.[8,9] Descriptions of this variant in the literature became more frequent in the 1980s, most likely because advances in neonatal medicine resulted in higher survival rates of extremely preterm babies. The neonatologist Ohlsson finally described the antenatal history with maternal polyhydramnios, which likely predisposed to premature birth.[10] Immediately after birth, profound polyuria puts these types of patients at great risk for life-threatening dehydration. Contraction of the extracellular fluid (ECF) volume is accompanied by markedly elevated renal and extrarenal prostaglandin E_2 (PGE_2) production. Treatment with prostaglandin synthesis inhibitors effectively reduced polyuria, ameliorated hypokalemia, and improved growth. To emphasize the obviously critical role of PGE_2 in the pathogenesis of this distinct tubular disorder, Seyberth coined the term hyperprostaglandin E syndrome (HPS).[11,12] Another variant of this severe, prenatal-onset salt-wasting disorder was first described in a Bedouin family. It differs from the above-mentioned hyperprostaglandin E syndrome by the presence of sensorineural deafness, absence of medullary nephrocalcinosis, and slowly deteriorating renal function.[13]

Taken together, renal salt-wasting syndromes associated with hypokalemia and hypochloremic metabolic alkalosis (frequently subsumed as "Bartter syndrome" in a broader sense) present with marked clinical variability. Severe, early onset forms (the "antenatal Bartter syndrome" or "hyperprostaglandin E syndrome") with symptoms directly arising from profound salt wasting with extracellular volume depletion contrast with mild late-onset forms primarily characterized by the features of secondary hyperaldosteronism (the "Gitelman syndrome"). Between these two extremes, the Bartter syndrome *sensu stricto* ("classic Bartter syndrome") presents as a disorder with intermediate severity. Variable extents of extracellular volume depletion and secondary electrolyte disturbances contribute to a rather variable disease phenotype, which in its extremes may mimic antenatal Bartter syndrome or Gitelman syndrome.

This classification based on clinical criteria was enriched by clarification of the underlying genetic defects. As disclosed by molecular genetic analyses, antenatal Bartter syndrome results from disturbed salt reabsorption along the TAL due to defects either in NKCC2,[14] ROMK,[15] barttin,[16] or both ClC-Ka and ClC-Kb.[17] The classic Bartter syndrome is caused by dysfunction of ClC-Kb,[18] which impairs salt transport to some extent along the TAL and in particular along the DCT1. A pure defect of salt reabsorption along the DCT1 due to dysfunction of NCCT finally results in the Gitelman syndrome. Unfortunately, a frequently used classification merely based on molecular genetic criteria, which simply follows the chronology of the identification of the genetic defects, does not accommodate a more easily understood functional classification. According to this molecular genetic classification, Bartter syndrome type I (BS I) refers to a defect of NKKC2 (gene name *SLC12A1*), BS II of ROMK *(KCNJ1)*, BS III of ClC-Kb *(CLCNKB)*, and BS IV of barttin *(BSND)*. Gitelman syndrome, owing to disturbed NCCT *(SLC12A3)* function despite its apparent relatedness to this group of disorders, was not included in this classification. Instead, Bartter syndrome type V (BS V) was suggested for some gain-of-function mutations of the calcium-sensing receptor (CaSR), which, however, in the first instance cause autosomal-dominant hypocalcemia with variable degrees of renal salt wasting explained by the inhibitory effect of CaSR activation on salt transport along the TAL.[19,20] The autosomal-dominant mode of inheritance and the clinically more relevant hypocalcemia are features not compatible with Bartter syndrome and make the designation BS V rather impractical. Consequently, BS V is not considered in the following sections.

Taken together, renal salt wasting with hypokalemia and hypochloremic metabolic alkalosis becomes manifest in three clinically defined syndromes: antenatal Bartter syndrome, classic Bartter syndrome, and Gitelman syndrome. From a functional point of view, antenatal Bartter syndrome arises from sodium chloride transport defects of the TAL. Classic Bartter syndrome combines features of weak TAL defects with disturbed DCT1 function, whereas Gitelman syndrome reflects pure DCT1 dysfunction. Accordingly, genetic defects associated with antenatal Bartter syndrome affect NKCC2, ROMK, barttin, and both ClC-K isoforms. Classic Bartter syndrome results from isolated ClC-Kb dysfunction, whereas Gitelman syndrome typically is caused by mutations of NCCT but may be mimicked by impaired ClC-Kb function.

Genetic Disorders of TAL: Antenatal Bartter Syndrome

Furosemide-Sensitive Na-K-2Cl-Co-Transporter (NKCC2)

Disruption of sodium chloride reabsorption in the TAL due to inactivating mutations in NKCC2 causes a severe disorder with antenatal onset. Within the second trimester, fetal polyuria leads to increasing maternal polyhydramnios. Chloride concentration in the amniotic fluid is elevated up to 118 mmol/L.[21,22] Untreated, premature delivery occurs around 32 weeks of gestation. The most striking abnormality of the newborns is profound polyuria. With adequate fluid replacement, daily urinary outputs can easily exceed half of the newborn's body weight (>20 ml/kg/h). Despite both ECF volume contraction and presence of high AVP levels, urine osmolality hardly approaches that of plasma, indicating a severe renal concentrating defect. Salt reabsorption along the TAL segment is also critical for urine dilution, which explains that urine osmolality, on the other hand, typically does not fall below 160 mosmol/kg. Some preserved ability to dilute urine might be explained by an adaptive increase of DCT1 salt reabsorption, which functions as the most distal portion of the diluting segment. This moderate hyposthenuria clearly separates NKCC2-deficient patients from polyuric patients with nephrogenic diabetes insipidus, who typically display urine osmolalities below 100 mosmol/kg.

Within the first months of life, nearly all patients develop medullary nephrocalcinosis in parallel with persistently high urinary calcium excretion. Amazingly, conservation of magnesium is not affected to a similar extent and NKCC2-deficient patients usually do not develop hypomagnesemia. This is even more surprising given that loss-of-function mutations in paracellin-1, which mediates paracellular transport of divalent cations along the TAL, invariably cause both hypercalciuria and hypermagnesuria, leading to severe hypomagnesemia in paracellin-1-deficient patients.[23] With respect to magnesium transport, the difference between the disorders might be explained by an up-regulation of magnesium reabsorption parallel to a compensatorily increased sodium chloride reabsorption in DCT1 cells in case of an NKCC2 defect.[24]

Renal Outer Medullary Potassium Channel

Renal outer medullary potassium–deficient patients similarly show a history of maternal polyhydramnios, prematurity with median age of gestation of 33 weeks, vasopressin-insensitive polyuria, isosthenuria, and hypercalciuria with secondary nephrocalcinosis. As in the case of NKCC2 dysfunction, the severity of the symptoms argues for a complete defect of sodium chloride reabsorption along the TAL. The mechanism of RAAS activation is virtually identical to that proposed for NKCC2-deficient patients. However, despite the presence of high plasma aldosterone levels, ROMK-deficient patients exhibit transient hyperkalemia in the first days of life.[25] The simultaneous appearance of hyperkalemia and hyponatremia resembles the clinical picture of mineralocorticoid deficiency (which, however, shows low aldosterone levels) or that of pseudohypoaldosteronism type I (PHA-I) (high aldosterone levels). Indeed, several published cases of PHA-I turned out to be misdiagnosed, and subsequent genetic analysis revealed ROMK mutations as the underlying defect.[26] The severity of initial hyperkalemia decreases with gestational age.[27] Hyperkalemia may be attributed to the additional role of ROMK in the cortical collecting duct (CCD) where it participates in the process of potassium secretion (Figure 29-1). Although less pronounced as compared to NKCC2 deficiency, the majority of ROMK-deficient patients develop hypokalemia in the later course of the disease. The transient nature of hyperkalemia may be explained by the upregulation of alternative pathways for potassium secretion in the CCD. An attractive candidate for this alternative route would be a large-conductance potassium channel identified in the apical membrane of CCD principal cells.[28] Because of its low open probability, this potassium channel provides no significant apical potassium release under normal conditions. Experimental data, however, suggest that its activity increases with enhanced fluid and solute delivery to the CCD.[29]

Chloride Channel Beta-Subunit Barttin

Only recently a new player in the process of salt reabsorption along the TAL and DCT1 was identified—the ClC-K channel beta-subunit barttin. Discovery of barttin was initiated by chromosomal linkage of a very rare variant of tubular salt wasting associated with sensorineural deafness. By a positional cloning strategy, a novel gene, *BSND*, was identified and inactivating mutations were found in affected individuals.[16] Because the gene product, barttin, had no homology to any known protein, its physiologic function remained unclear until two groups independently described the role of barttin as an essential beta-subunit of the ClC-K channels.[30,31]

Two ClC-K isoforms of the CLC family of chloride channels are highly expressed along the distal nephron, with ClC-Ka being exclusively expressed in the thin ascending limb and decreasing expression levels along the adjacent distal nephron. Its homologue ClC-Kb is predominantly expressed in the DCT1. Along the TAL, both channel isoforms are equally expressed. Barttin, which is found in all ClC-K-expressing nephron segments, is essential for proper ClC-K channel function in that it facilitates the transport of ClC-K channels to the cell surface and modulates biophysical properties of the assembled channel complex.

In affected individuals, the barttin defect seems to completely disrupt chloride exit across the basolateral membrane in TAL as well as DCT1 cells. Accordingly, patients display the severest salt-wasting kidney disorder described so far. As with defects of NKCC2 and ROMK, the first symptom of a barttin defect is maternal polyhydramnios due to fetal polyuria beginning at approximately 22 weeks of gestation. Again, polyhydramnios accounts for preterm labor and extreme prematurity. Postnatally, patients are at high risk of volume depletion. Plasma chloride levels fall to approximately 80 mmol/L; a further decrease usually can be avoided by close laboratory monitoring and rapid intervention on neonatal intensive care units. Polyuria again is resistant to vasopressin and urine osmolalities range between 200 and 400 mosmol/kg.

Unlike patients with loss-of-function mutations of ROMK and NKCC2, barttin-deficient patients exhibit only transitory hypercalciuria.[32] Medullary nephrocalcinosis is absent, yet progressive renal failure is common, with histologic signs of pronounced tissue damage like glomerular sclerosis, tubular atrophy, and mononuclear infiltration. The mechanisms underlying the deterioration of renal function are not yet understood. The lack of hypercalciuria, however, may be explained by disturbed sodium chloride reabsorption along the DCT1. Isolated DCT1 dysfunction like in Gitelman syndrome (see below) or after long-term inhibition of NCCT-mediated transport by thiazides is known to induce hypocalciuria. This effect might counterbalance the hypercalciuric effect of TAL dysfunction in case of a combined impairment of salt reabsorption along the TAL and DCT1. In contrast to calcium, the renal conservation of magnesium is severely impaired, leading to pronounced hypomagnesemia. This might be explained by the disruption of both magnesium reabsorption pathways—the paracellular one in the TAL and the transcellular one in the DCT1.

The barttin defect is invariably associated with sensorineural deafness. Clarification of the pathogenesis of this rare disorder has provided a deeper insight into the mechanisms of potassium-rich endolymph secretion in the inner ear: Marginal cells of the *stria vascularis* contribute to the endolymph formation by apical potassium secretion. Transcellular potassium transport is mediated by the furosemide-sensitive Na-K-2Cl-co-transporter type 1 (NKCC1), ensuring basolateral potassium entry into the marginal cells. Voltage-dependent potassium channels mediate apical potassium secretion into the endolymph. Proper function of NKCC1 requires basolateral recycling of chloride. Deafness associated with barttin deficiency suggests that this recycling is enabled by the ClC-K/barttin channel complex.

Digenic Disorder: ClC-Ka/b Phenotype

The concept of the physiologic role of barttin as a common beta-subunit of ClC-K channels was substantiated by the recent description of an individual harboring inactivating mutations in both the ClC-Ka and ClC-Kb chloride channels, respectively.[17] The clinical symptoms resulting from this digenic disease are indistinguishable from those of barttin-deficient patients. This observation not only proves the concept of the functional interaction of barttin with both ClC-K isoforms, but also excludes important other functions of barttin not related to ClC-K channel interaction.

Disorders of DCT1: Classic Bartter Syndrome and Gitelman Syndrome

Basolateral Chloride Channel ClC-Kb

In the context of normal ClC-Ka function, an isolated defect of the ClC-Kb gene leads to a more variable phenotype. Several studies have indicated that the clinical variability is not related to a certain type of mutation.[33,34] Even the most deleterious mutation, which implies the absence of the complete coding region of the ClC-Kb gene, and which affects nearly 50% of this patient cohort, can cause varying degrees of disease severity. Features of tubular dysfunction distal from the TAL predominate, suggesting a major role of ClC-Kb along the DCT1. Although TAL salt transport can be impaired to a variable extent, its function is never completely perturbed. Obviously, alternative routes of basolateral chloride exit can be recruited in the TAL segment, most likely via ClC-Ka.

With respect to renal function, the neonatal period in ClC-Kb-deficient patients usually passes without major problems. Maternal polyhydramnios is observed in only one-fourth of the patients and usually is mild. Accordingly, duration of pregnancy is not substantially decreased. More than half of the patients are diagnosed within the first year of life. Symptoms at initial presentation include failure to thrive, dehydration, muscular hypotonia, and lethargy. Laboratory examination typically reveals low plasma chloride concentrations (down to 60 mmol/L), decreased plasma sodium concentration, and severe hypokalemic alkalosis. At first presentation, electrolyte derangement is usually more pronounced as compared to the other groups. However, because renal salt wasting progresses slowly and polyuria may be absent, medical consultation may be delayed. Plasma renin activity is greatly increased, whereas plasma aldosterone concentration is only slightly elevated. This discrepancy might be attributed to negative feedback regulation of aldosterone incretion by hypokalemia and alkalosis. Therefore, normal or slightly elevated aldosterone levels under conditions of profound hypokalemic alkalosis are in fact inappropriately low.

Urinary concentrating ability is preserved at least to a certain extent and a number of patients achieve urinary osmolalities above 700 mosmol/kg in morning urine samples. Because renal medullary interstitial hypertonicity is critically dependent on sodium chloride reabsorption in the TAL, the ability to concentrate urine above 700 mosmol/kg indicates nearly intact TAL function despite ClC-Kb deficiency. Moreover, the integrity of TAL function is also reflected by the finding that hypercalciuria is not a typical feature of ClC-Kb dysfunction and—if present—occurs only temporarily. The majority of patients exhibit normal or even low urinary calcium excretion. Accordingly, medullary nephrocalcinosis—a hallmark of pure TAL dysfunction—is rare. The plasma magnesium concentration gradually decreases over time owing to impaired renal magnesium conservation, as is observed in other forms of abnormal DCT1 function. Accordingly, several ClC-Kb-deficient patients exhibit both hypomagnesemia and hypocalciuria, a constellation that usually is thought to be highly indicative for an NCCT defect. ClC-Kb deficiency thus may mimic Gitelman syndrome.

The symptoms associated with malfunction of ClC-Kb largely parallel the features of Bartter's original description. The ethnic origin of Bartter's first patients supports this idea. Both were African Americans, and among this racial group only ClC-Kb mutations have been identified to date. It has also been suggested that African Americans are affected by BS more frequently and suffer from a more severe course of the disease. In a recent study in five African American patients with ClC-Kb mutations, two of them had a history of polyhydramnios that elicited extreme prematurity.[35] Postnatal polyuria and electrolyte derangement led to diagnosis in the early neonatal period. The incidence of chronic renal failure tends to be higher among African American BS patients as compared to other ethnic groups.

Thiazide-Sensitive NaCl-Co-Transporter

DCT epithelia contain two cell types: DCT1 cells, which express the NCCT as its predominant apical sodium entry pathway, and further distal residing DCT2 cells, which express the epithelial Na-channel (ENaC) as the main pathway for apical sodium reabsorption (Figure 29-2). Both sodium entry pathways are inducible by aldosterone. DCT1 and DCT2 cells probably also differ with respect to their function in divalent cation transport.

NCCT deficiency results in only mild renal salt wasting. Initial presentation frequently occurs at school age or later with the characteristic symptoms being muscular weakness, cramps, fatigue, and dwarfism. Not uncommonly, patients are diagnosed accidentally while seeking medical consultation because of growth retardation, constipation, or enuresis. A history of salt craving is common. Urinary concentrating ability typically is not affected. Laboratory examination

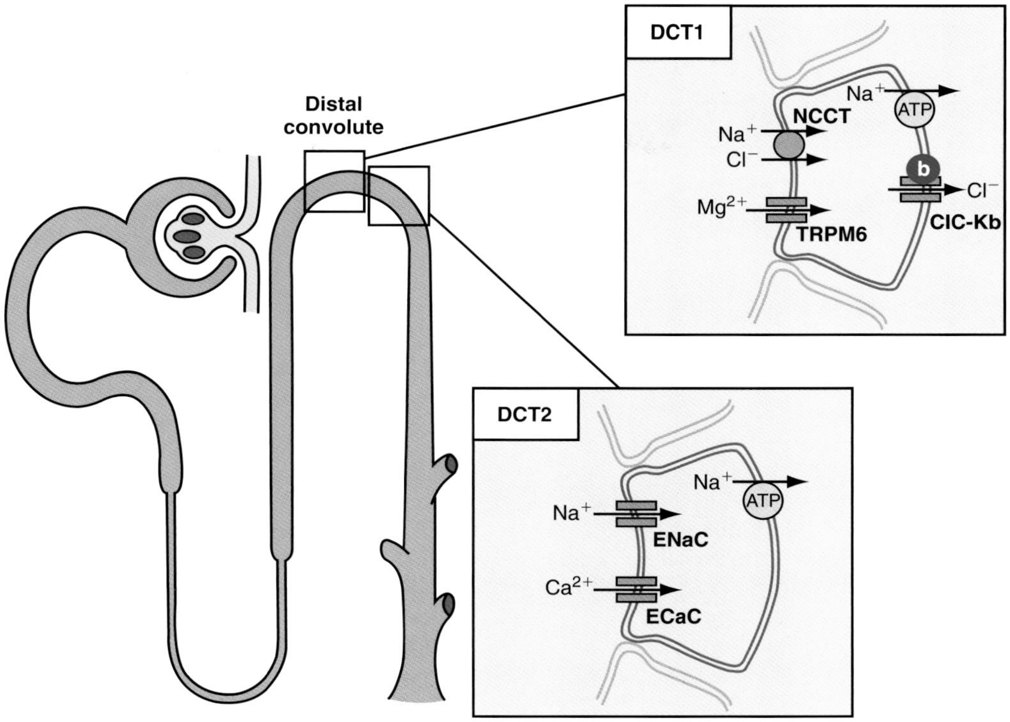

Figure 29-2 Divalent cation reabsorption along the distal convoluted tubule. DCT1 cells express an apical magnesium conductance (TRPM6), whereas DCT2 cells provide an apical calcium conductance formed by ECaC (TRPV5). Impairment of DCT1 cell function by mutations of NCCT or ClC-Kb might shift the DCT1/DCT2 cell ratio in favor of DCT 2 cells, resulting in increased magnesium and decreased calcium excretion.

shows a typical constellation of metabolic alkalosis, low normal chloride levels, hypokalemia, and hypomagnesemia; urine analysis shows hypocalciuria. Family studies revealed that electrolyte imbalances are present from infancy, although the affected infants displayed no obvious clinical signs. Of note, the combination of hypokalemia and hypomagnesemia exerts an exceptionally unfavorable effect on cardiac excitability, which puts these patients at high risk for cardiac arrhythmias.

The pathognomonic feature of Gitelman syndrome is the dissociation of renal calcium and magnesium handling, with low urinary calcium and high urinary magnesium levels. Subsequent hypomagnesemia causes neuromuscular irritability and tetany. Decreased renal calcium elimination together with magnesium deficiency favors deposition of mineral calcium as demonstrated by increased bone density as well as chondrocalcinosis. Although the combination of hypomagnesemia and hypocalciuria is typical for NCCT deficiency, it is neither a specific nor universal finding. Clinical observations in NCCT-deficient patients disclosed intra- and interindividual variations in urinary calcium concentrations that can be attributed to gender, age-related conditions of bone metabolism, intake of magnesium supplements, and changes in diuresis and urinary osmolality. Likewise, hypomagnesemia might not be present from the beginning. Because less than 1% of total body magnesium is circulating in the blood, renal magnesium loss can be balanced temporarily by magnesium release from bone and muscle stores as well as by an increase of intestinal magnesium reabsorption. Accordingly, the strict definition of hypomagnesemia with coincident hypocalciuria in order to separate Gitelman (NCCT) syndrome from classic Bartter (ClC-Kb) syndrome appears arbitrary.

The mechanisms compromising distal magnesium reabsorption and favoring reabsorption of calcium are not yet completely understood. The occasional coexistence of hypomagnesemia and hypocalciuria in ClC-Kb-deficient patients indicates that this phenomenon is not restricted to NCCT defects, but is rather a consequence of impaired transcellular sodium chloride reabsorption along the DCT1. It is tempting to speculate that with a functional defect of DCT1 cells, which in addition to sodium chloride normally reabsorb magnesium by apical TRPM6 magnesium channels, these cells are replaced by DCT2 cells, which reabsorb sodium via ENaC channels and calcium via epithelial calcium channels (ECaC or TRPV5). Accordingly, reabsorption of magnesium would decrease and that of calcium increase. Moreover, other phenomena such as the redistribution of renal tubular sodium chloride reabsorption to more proximal nephron segments (proximal tubule and TAL) might contribute to alterations in renal calcium and magnesium handling.

A summary of the most important clinical features and the ordinary age of disease manifestation is given in Table 29-1.

TREATMENT

As with other hereditary diseases, the desirable correction of the primary genetic defects is not yet feasible. In the case of

TABLE 29-1 Age at Manifestation and Leading Symptoms of Genetically Defined Salt-Wasting Kidney Disorders

	NKCC2	ROMK	Barttin	ClC-Kb	NCCT
Polyhydramnios	+++	+++	+++	+	–
Age at first manifestation	Perinatal	Perinatal	Perinatal	0-5 years	>5 years
Leading symptoms	Polyuria Hypochloremia Alkalosis Hypokalemia Nephrocalcinosis	Polyuria Hypochloremia Alkalosis Initially hyperkalemia, later hypokalemia Nephrocalcinosis	Polyuria Hypochloremia Alkalosis Hypokalemia Deafness	Hypokalemia Hypochloremia Alkalosis Failure to thrive	Hypokalemia Hypomagnesemia Alkalosis Hypocalciuria Growth retardation

salt-wasting kidney disorders, however, the correction of secondary phenomena such as increased renal prostaglandin synthesis or disturbed electrolyte homeostasis have been part of treatment virtually from the first description of the diseases. To the present, the cornerstones in treating renal salt wasting are nonsteroidal anti-inflammatory drugs (NSAID) and long-term electrolyte substitution.

In the case of antenatal Bartter syndrome, inhibition of renal and systemic prostaglandin synthesis leads to reduced urinary prostaglandin E_2 (PGE_2) excretion, dramatically decreases polyuria, converts hyposthenuria to isosthenuria, reduces hypercalciuria, and stimulates catch-up growth. Maintenance of euvolemia in the immediate postnatal period by meticulous replacement of renal fluid and salt loss is of central importance before starting NSAID therapy, which might precipitate acute renal failure if extracellular volume is depleted. There is long-standing experience with the unselective cyclooxygenase (COX) inhibitor indomethacin, which is started at 0.05 mg/kg per day and may be gradually increased to 1.5 mg/kg per day according to its effects on urinary output, renal PGE_2-synthesis, and blood aldosterone levels. Gastrointestinal side effects like gastritis and peptic ulcers are the main drawbacks of prolonged indomethacin therapy. These might be reduced by the use of COX-2–specific inhibitors like rofecoxib, which show a comparable effect on renal salt wasting but adversely affect blood pressure. A convincing explanation for these unsurpassed effects of NSAIDs is still missing, although a reduction of glomerular filtration and blockage of aberrant tubuloglomerular feedback certainly are important contributors. Despite these beneficial effects of NSAIDs, lifelong substitution of potassium chloride usually is required to prevent life-threatening episodes of hypokalemia.

Consistent with the combined defect of the TAL and DCT1, NSAID treatment of antenatal Bartter syndrome with deafness proved clearly less effective. In addition to high NSAID doses, these patients need ample amounts of extra fluid and electrolytes (sodium chloride, potassium chloride, magnesium) to prevent ECV contraction and electrolyte derangements.

In contrast to TAL defects, disturbed salt reabsorption along the DCT1 does not affect tubuloglomerular feedback, and thus is not associated with increased renal prostaglandin synthesis.[36] Accordingly, NSAIDs are of little benefit in Gitelman syndrome. Substitution of potassium chloride and magnesium is therefore central in the treatment of this disorder. As pointed out above, avoidance of factors that, in addition to hypokalemia and hypomagnesemia might affect cardiac excitability (in particular QT-time prolonging drugs), is mandatory to prevent life-threatening cardiac arrhythmias.

CONCLUSION

Parallel loss of sodium and chloride from disturbed renal tubular function is the basis of several distinct diseases that differ with respect to the degree of ECV contraction and secondary electrolyte derangements. Common features of all combined sodium chloride transport defects are ECV contraction, hypokalemia, hypochloremia, and metabolic alkalosis. Clarification of the underlying genetic defects has contributed greatly to understanding the contribution of the affected proteins to renal salt transport.

REFERENCES

1. Jeck N, Schlingmann KP, Reinalter SC, Komhoff M, et al: Salt handling in the distal nephron: lessons learned from inherited human disorders, *Am J Physiol Regul Integr Comp Physiol* 288:R782-95, 2005.
2. Rosenbaum P, Hughes M: Persistent, probably congenital, hypokalemic metabolic alkalosis with hyaline degeneration of renal tubules and normal urinary aldosterone, *Am J Dis Child* 94:560, 1957.
3. Bartter FC, Pronove P, Gill JR Jr, Maccardle RC: Hyperplasia of the juxtaglomerular complex with hyperaldosteronism and hypokalemic alkalosis. A new syndrome, *Am J Med* 33:811-28, 1962.
4. Gitelman HJ, Graham JB, Welt LG: A new familial disorder characterized by hypokalemia and hypomagnesemia, *Trans Assoc Am Physicians* 79:221-35, 1966.
5. Rodriguez-Soriano J, Vallo A, Garcia-Fuentes M: Hypomagnesaemia of hereditary renal origin, *Pediatr Nephrol* 1:465-72, 1987.
6. Bettinelli A, Bianchetti MG, Girardin E, Caringella A, et al: Use of calcium excretion values to distinguish two forms of primary renal tubular hypokalemic alkalosis: Bartter and Gitelman syndromes, *J Pediatr* 120:38-43, 1992.
7. Bartter FC, Pronove P, Gill JR Jr, MacCardle RC: Hyperplasia of the juxtaglomerular complex with hyperaldosteronism and hypokalemic alkalosis. A new syndrome 1962, *J Am Soc Nephrol* 9:516-28, 1998.
8. Fanconi A, Schachenmann G, Nussli R, Prader A: Chronic hypokalaemia with growth retardation, normotensive hyperrenin-hyperaldosteronism ("Bartter's syndrome"), and hypercalciuria.

Report of two cases with emphasis on natural history and on catch-up growth during treatment, *Helv Paediatr Acta* 26:144-63, 1971.
9. McCredie DA, Blair-West JR, Scoggins BA, Shipman R: Potassium-losing nephropathy of childhood, *Med J Aust* 1:129-35, 1971.
10. Ohlsson A, Sieck U, Cumming W, Akhtar M, Serenius F: A variant of Bartter's syndrome. Bartter's syndrome associated with hydramnios, prematurity, hypercalciuria and nephrocalcinosis, *Acta Paediatr Scand* 73:868-74, 1984.
11. Seyberth HW, Koniger SJ, Rascher W, Kuhl PG, Schweer H: Role of prostaglandins in hyperprostaglandin E syndrome and in selected renal tubular disorders, *Pediatr Nephrol* 1:491-7, 1987.
12. Seyberth HW, Rascher W, Schweer H, Kuhl PG, et al: Congenital hypokalemia with hypercalciuria in preterm infants: a hyperprostaglandinuric tubular syndrome different from Bartter syndrome, *J Pediatr* 107:694-701, 1985.
13. Landau D, Shalev H, Ohaly M, Carmi R: Infantile variant of Bartter syndrome and sensorineural deafness: a new autosomal recessive disorder, *Am J Med Genet* 59:454-59, 1995.
14. Simon DB, Karet FE, Hamdan JM, DiPietro A, et al: Bartter's syndrome, hypokalaemic alkalosis with hypercalciuria, is caused by mutations in the Na-K-2Cl cotransporter NKCC2, *Nat Genet* 13:183-88, 1996.
15. Simon DB, Karet FE, Rodriguez-Soriano J, Hamdan JH, et al: Genetic heterogeneity of Bartter's syndrome revealed by mutations in the K+ channel, ROMK, *Nat Genet* 14:152-56, 1996.
16. Birkenhager R, Otto E, Schurmann MJ, Vollmer M, et al: Mutation of BSND causes Bartter syndrome with sensorineural deafness and kidney failure, *Nat Genet* 29:310-14, 2001.
17. Schlingmann KP, Konrad M, Jeck N, Waldegger P, et al: Salt wasting and deafness resulting from mutations in two chloride channels, *N Engl J Med* 350:1314-19, 2004.
18. Simon DB, Bindra RS, Mansfield TA, Nelson-Williams C, et al: Mutations in the chloride channel gene, CLCNKB, cause Bartter's syndrome type III. *Nat Genet* 17:171-78, 1997.
19. Hebert SC: Bartter syndrome, *Curr Opin Nephrol Hypertens* 12:527-32, 2003.
20. Watanabe S, Fukumoto S, Chang H, Takeuchi Y, et al: Association between activating mutations of calcium-sensing receptor and Bartter's syndrome, *Lancet* 360:692-94, 2002.
21. Massa G, Proesmans W, Devlieger H, Vandenberghe K, et al: Electrolyte composition of the amniotic fluid in Bartter syndrome, *Eur J Obstet Gynecol Reprod Biol* 24:335-40, 1987.
22. Proesmans W, Massa G, Vandenberghe K, Van Assche A: Prenatal diagnosis of Bartter syndrome, *Lancet* 1:394, 1987.
23. Simon DB, Lu Y, Choate KA, Velazquez H, et al: Paracellin-1, a renal tight junction protein required for paracellular Mg2+ resorption, *Science* 285:103-106, 1999.
24. Kamel KS, Oh MS, Halperin ML: Bartter's, Gitelman's, and Gordon's syndromes. From physiology to molecular biology and back, yet still some unanswered questions, *Nephron* 92(Suppl 1):18-27, 2002.
25. Jeck N, Derst C, Wischmeyer E, Ott H, et al: Functional heterogeneity of ROMK mutations linked to hyperprostaglandin E syndrome, *Kidney Int* 59:1803-11, 2001.
26. Finer G, Shalev H, Birk OS, Galron D, et al: Transient neonatal hyperkalemia in the antenatal (ROMK defective) Bartter syndrome, *J Pediatr* 142:318-23, 2003.
27. Peters M, Jeck N, Reinalter S, Leonhardt A, et al: Clinical presentation of genetically defined patients with hypokalemic salt-losing tubulopathies, *Am J Med* 112:183-90, 2002.
28. Schlatter E, Frobe U, Greger R: Ion conductances of isolated cortical collecting duct cells, *Pflugers Arch* 421:381-87, 1992.
29. Taniguchi J, Imai M: Flow-dependent activation of maxi K+ channels in apical membrane of rabbit connecting tubule, *J Membr Biol* 164:35-45, 1998.
30. Estevez R, Boettger T, Stein V, Birkenhager R, et al: Barttin is a Cl-channel beta-subunit crucial for renal Cl-reabsorption and inner ear K+ secretion, *Nature* 414:558-61, 2001.
31. Waldegger S, Jeck N, Barth P, Peters M, et al: Barttin increases surface expression and changes current properties of ClC-K channels. *Pflugers Arch* 444:411-18, 2002.
32. Jeck N, Reinalter SC, Henne T, Marg W, et al: Hypokalemic salt-losing tubulopathy with chronic renal failure and sensorineural deafness, *Pediatrics* 108:E5, 2001.
33. Konrad M, Vollmer M, Lemmink HH, van den Heuvel LP, et al: Mutations in the chloride channel gene CLCNKB as a cause of classic Bartter syndrome, *J Am Soc Nephrol* 11:1449-59, 2000.
34. Zelikovic I, Szargel R, Hawash A, Labay V, et al: A novel mutation in the chloride channel gene, CLCNKB, as a cause of Gitelman and Bartter syndromes, *Kidney Int* 63:24-32, 2003.
35. Schurman SJ, Perlman SA, Sutphen R, Campos A, et al: Genotype/phenotype observations in African Americans with Bartter syndrome, *J Pediatr* 139:105-10, 2001.
36. Luthy C, Bettinelli A, Iselin S, Metta MG, et al: Normal prostaglandinuria E2 in Gitelman's syndrome, the hypocalciuric variant of Bartter's syndrome, *Am J Kidney Dis* 25:824-28, 1995.

CHAPTER

30 Disorders of Magnesium Metabolism

Martin Konrad

MAGNESIUM PHYSIOLOGY

Magnesium (Mg^{2+}) is the second most abundant intracellular cation in the body. As a cofactor for many enzymes, it is involved in energy metabolism and protein and nucleic acid synthesis. It also plays a critical role in the modulation of membrane transporters and in signal transduction. Under physiologic conditions, serum Mg^{2+} levels are maintained at almost constant values. Homeostasis depends on the balance between intestinal absorption and renal excretion. Mg^{2+} deficiency can result from reduced dietary intake, intestinal malabsorption, or renal loss. The control of body Mg^{2+} homeostasis primarily resides in the kidney tubules.

The daily dietary intake of Mg^{2+} varies substantially. Within physiologic ranges, diminished Mg^{2+} intake is balanced by enhanced Mg^{2+} absorption in the intestine and reduced renal excretion. These transport processes are regulated by metabolic and hormonal influences.[1,2] The principal site of Mg^{2+} absorption is the small intestine, with smaller amounts being absorbed in the colon. Intestinal Mg^{2+} absorption occurs via two different pathways: a saturable active transcellular transport and a nonsaturable paracellular passive transport[1,3] (Figure 30-1*A*). Saturation kinetics of the transcellular transport system are explained by the limited transport capacity of active transport. At low intraluminal concentrations, Mg^{2+} is absorbed primarily via the active transcellular route, and, with rising concentrations, it is absorbed via the paracellular pathway, thereby yielding a curvilinear function for total absorption (Figure 30-1*B*).

In the kidney, approximately 80% of the total serum Mg^{2+} is filtered in the glomeruli, of which more than 95% is reabsorbed along the nephron. Mg^{2+} reabsorption differs in quantity and kinetics, depending on the different nephron segments, and approximately 15% to 20% is reabsorbed in the proximal tubule of the adult kidney. Interestingly, the premature kidney of the newborn is able to reabsorb up to 70% of the filtered Mg^{2+} in this nephron segment.[4]

From early childhood on, the majority of Mg^{2+} (around 70%) is reabsorbed in the loop of Henle, especially in the cortical thick ascending limb (TAL). Transport in this segment is passive and paracellular, driven by the lumen-positive transepithelial voltage (Figure 30-2*A*). Although only 5% to 10% of the filtered Mg^{2+} is reabsorbed in the distal convoluted tubule (DCT), this is the part of the nephron where the fine adjustment of renal excretion is accomplished. The reabsorption rate in the DCT defines the final urinary Mg^{2+} excretion, because there is no significant uptake of Mg^{2+} in the collecting duct. Mg^{2+} transport in this part of the nephron is an active transcellular process (Figure 30-2*B*). Physiologic studies indicate that apical entry into DCT cells is mediated by a specific and regulated Mg^{2+} channel that is driven by a favorable transmembrane voltage.[5] The mechanism of basolateral transport into the interstitium is unknown. Here, Mg^{2+} has to be extruded against an unfavorable electrochemical gradient. Most physiologic studies favor a sodium (Na^+)-dependent exchange mechanism.[6] Mg^{2+} entry into DCT cells appears to be the rate-limiting step and the site of regulation. Mg^{2+} transport in the distal tubule has been recently reviewed in detail by Dai and colleagues.[5] Finally, 3% to 5% of the filtered Mg^{2+} is excreted in the urine.

MAGNESIUM DEPLETION

Mg^{2+} depletion is usually the result of another disease process or of a therapeutic agent. Some disorders that can be associated with Mg^{2+} depletion are summarized in Table 30-1.[7] Mg^{2+} may be lost via the gastrointestinal tract, either by the excessive loss of secreted fluids or by the impaired absorption of both dietary and endogenous Mg^{2+}. The Mg^{2+} content of the upper intestinal tract fluids is approximately 0.5 mmol/L, and vomiting or nasogastric suction may contribute to Mg^{2+} depletion from the loss of these fluids. The Mg^{2+} content of diarrheal fluids and fistulous drainage is much higher (up to 7.5 mmol/L), and, consequently, Mg^{2+} depletion is common among patients with acute or chronic diarrhea. Malabsorption syndromes such as celiac disease may also result in Mg^{2+} deficiency. In addition, acute severe pancreatitis may be associated with hypomagnesemia.

Excessive excretion of Mg^{2+} into the urine is another cause of Mg^{2+} depletion. Renal Mg^{2+} excretion is proportional to tubular fluid flow as well as to Na^+ and calcium (Ca^{2+}) excretion. Therefore, both chronic intravenous fluid therapy with Na^+-containing fluids and disorders in which there is extracellular volume expansion may result in Mg^{2+} depletion. An osmotic diuresis will result in increased renal Mg^{2+} excretion as a result of excessive urinary volume. Osmotic diuresis caused by glucosuria can therefore result in hypomagnesemia. The degree of Mg^{2+} depletion in patients with diabetes mellitus has been related to the amount of glucose excreted into the urine and, hence, with the degree of osmotic diuresis.

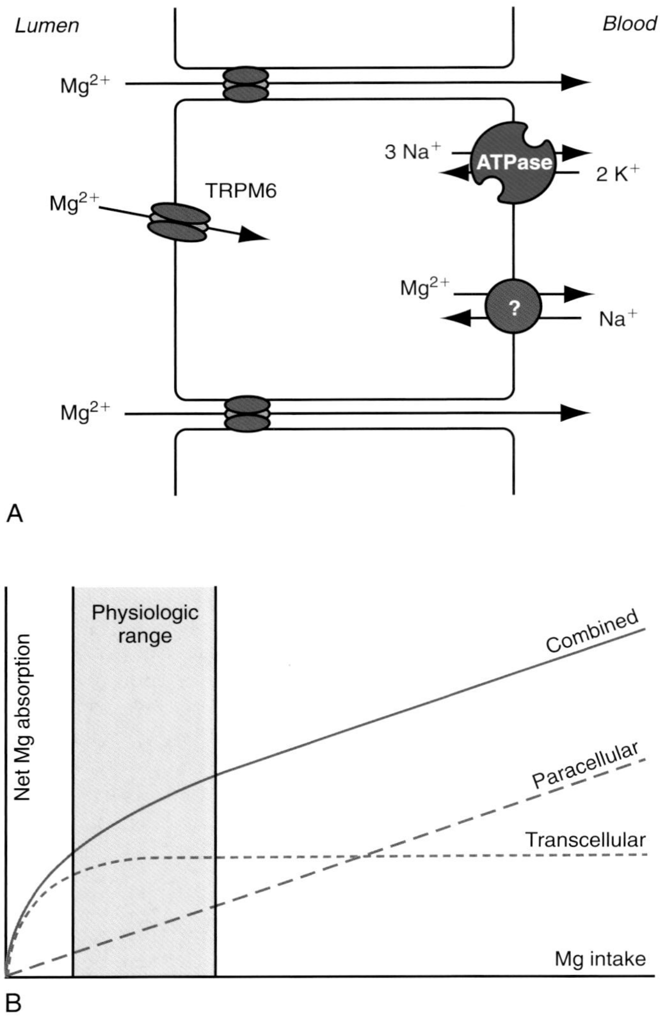

Figure 30-1 Intestinal Mg^{2+} reabsorption. **A,** A model of intestinal Mg^{2+} absorption via two independent pathways: passive absorption via the paracellular pathway and active transcellular transport that consists of an apical entry through a putative Mg^{2+} channel and a basolateral exit mediated by a putative Na^{+}-coupled exchange. **B,** The kinetics of intestinal Mg^{2+} absorption in humans. Paracellular transport linearly rising with intraluminal concentrations *(dotted line)* and saturable active transcellular transport *(dashed line)* together yield a curvilinear function for net Mg^{2+} absorption *(solid line)*.

TABLE 30-1 Major Causes of Magnesium Deficiency

Gastrointestinal Disorders
Prolonged nasogastric suction/vomiting
Acute and chronic diarrhea
Malabsorption syndromes (e.g., celiac disease)
Extensive bowel resection
Intestinal and biliary fistulas
Acute hemorrhagic pancreatitis
Renal Loss
Chronic parenteral fluid therapy
Osmotic diuresis (e.g., as a result of the presence of glucose in a patient with diabetes mellitus)
Hypercalcemia
Drugs (e.g., diuretics, aminoglycosides, calcineurin inhibitors)
Alcohol
Metabolic acidosis
Renal diseases
• Chronic pyelonephritis, interstitial nephritis, and glomerulonephritis
• Diuretic phase of acute tubular necrosis
• Postobstructive nephropathy
• Renal tubular acidosis
• Postrenal transplantation
• Inherited tubular diseases
Endocrine Disorders
Hyperparathyroidism
Hyperthyroidism
Hyperaldosteronism
Syndrome of inappropriate secretion of antidiuretic hormone (SIADH)

Hypercalcemia and hypercalciuria have been shown to decrease renal Mg^{2+} reabsorption, and they are probably the cause of the excessive renal Mg^{2+} excretion and hypomagnesemia observed in many hypercalcemic states. A number of drugs can also cause renal Mg^{2+} wasting and Mg^{2+} depletion; these are described later in this chapter. Various renal diseases (e.g., chronic pyelonephritis, postobstructive nephropathy) may also be accompanied by Mg^{2+} losses.

During infancy and childhood, a substantial proportion of patients receiving medical attention for signs of hypomagnesemia are affected by inherited renal disorders associated with Mg^{2+} wasting. In patients with these disorders, hypomagnesemia may either be a leading symptom or part of a complex phenotype that results from tubular dysfunction, which is described in detail later in this chapter.

Finally, Mg^{2+} wasting may be caused by endocrine disorders (e.g., from hyperparathyroidism as a result of hypercalcemia), or it may occur within the context of the syndrome of inappropriate antidiuretic hormone secretion. Among patients with this syndrome, Mg^{2+} losses are explained by the volume expansion.

MANIFESTATIONS OF HYPOMAGNESEMIA

Mg^{2+} deficiency and hypomagnesemia often remain asymptomatic. Clinical symptoms are usually not very specific, and Mg^{2+} deficiency is frequently associated with other electrolyte abnormalities. The biochemical and physiologic manifestations of severe Mg^{2+} depletion are summarized in Table 30-2.

Hypokalemia

A common feature of Mg^{2+} depletion is hypokalemia.[7] During Mg^{2+} depletion, there is a loss of potassium from the cell with intracellular potassium depletion, which is enhanced as a

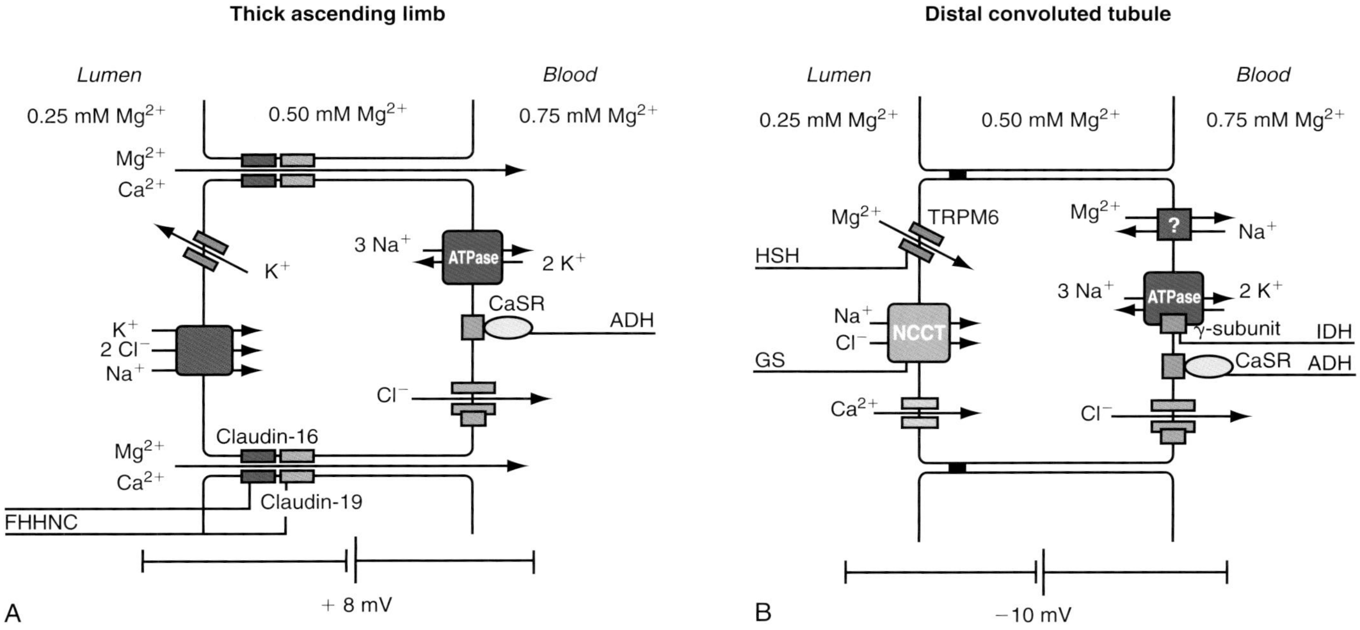

Figure 30-2 Mg^{2+} reabsorption in the loop of Henle and the distal tubule. **A,** Mg^{2+} reabsorption in the thick ascending limb of Henle's loop. Paracellular reabsorption of Mg^{2+} and Ca^{2+} is driven by lumen-positive transcellular voltage generated by the transcellular reabsorption of sodium chloride. **B,** Mg^{2+} reabsorption in the distal convoluted tubule. Mg^{2+} is actively reabsorbed via the transcellular pathway involving an apical entry step through an Mg^{2+}-permeable ion channel (TRPM6) and a basolateral exit, presumably mediated by an Na^+-coupled exchange mechanism. The molecular identity of the basolateral exchange is unknown.

result of the inability of the kidney to conserve potassium. Attempts to replete the potassium deficit with potassium therapy alone are not successful without simultaneous Mg^{2+} therapy. This potassium depletion may be a contributing cause of the electrocardiologic findings and cardiac arrhythmias.

Hypocalcemia

Hypocalcemia is also a common manifestation of moderate to severe Mg^{2+} depletion. The hypocalcemia may be a major contributing factor to the increased neuromuscular excitability that is often present in Mg^{2+}-depleted patients. The pathogenesis of hypocalcemia is multifactorial. Impaired parathyroid hormone (PTH) secretion appears to be a major factor in hypomagnesemia-induced hypocalcemia. Serum PTH concentrations are usually low in these patients, and Mg^{2+} administration will immediately stimulate PTH secretion. Patients with hypocalcemia caused by Mg^{2+} depletion also exhibit both renal and skeletal resistance to exogenously administered PTH as manifested by subnormal urinary cyclic adenosine monophosphate and phosphate excretion and a diminished calcemic response. All of these effects are reversed after several days of Mg^{2+} therapy. The basis for the defect in PTH secretion and PTH end-organ resistance is not known. Because cyclic adenosine monophosphate is an important second messenger in PTH secretion and is required for mediating PTH effects in the kidney and bone, it has been postulated that there may be a defect in the activity of adenylate cyclase. Mg^{2+} is both an essential part of the substrate (magnesium adenosine triphosphate [MgATP]) for adenylate cyclase and important for catalytic activity.

Vitamin D metabolism and action may also be abnormal in hypocalcemic Mg^{2+}-deficient patients. Resistance to vitamin D therapy has been reported in such cases. This resistance may be the result of the impaired metabolism of vitamin D because plasma concentrations of 1,25-dihydroxyvitamin D are low. Because PTH is a major stimulator of the synthesis of 1,25-dihydroxyvitamin D production, the decrease in PTH secretion observed in hypomagnesemia and hypocalcemia may also be a cause of the impaired metabolism of vitamin D.

Neuromuscular Manifestations

Neuromuscular hyperexcitability may be the prominent complaint of patients with Mg^{2+} deficiency. Tetany and muscle cramps may be present, and generalized seizures (convulsions) may also occur. Other neuromuscular signs may include dizziness, disequilibrium, muscular tremor, wasting, and weakness.[7] Although hypocalcemia often contributes to the neurologic signs, hypomagnesemia without hypocalcemia has also been reported to result in neuromuscular hyperexcitability.

Cardiovascular Manifestations

Mg^{2+} depletion may also result in electrocardiographic abnormalities as well as in cardiac arrhythmias,[8] which may be manifested by tachycardia, premature beats, or a totally irregular cardiac rhythm (fibrillation). Cardiac arrhythmias are also known to occur during potassium (K^+) depletion; therefore, the effect of Mg^{2+} deficiency on K^+ loss from the body may be the cause of the arrhythmias.[7] Patients with myocardial infarction also commonly have cardiac arrhythmias. Mg^{2+} administration to patients with acute myocardial infarction has been shown to decrease the mortality rate in some[9] but not all studies.[10]

TABLE 30-2 **Major Manifestations of Magnesium Depletion**
Biochemical
Hypokalemia Excessive renal potassium excretion Decreased intracellular potassium Hypocalcemia Impaired parathyroid hormone (PTH) secretion Renal and skeletal resistance to PTH Resistance to vitamin D
Neuromuscular
Positive Chvostek's and Trousseau's signs Spontaneous carpal–pedal spasm Seizures Vertigo, ataxia, nystagmus, athetoid, and choreiform movements Muscular weakness, tremor, fasciculation, and wasting
Psychiatric
Depression Psychosis
Cardiovascular
Electrocardiographic Abnormalities
Prolonged PR and QT intervals U waves
Cardiac Arrhythmias
Atrial tachycardia, fibrillations Torsades de pointes
Gastrointestinal
Nausea and vomiting Anorexia

CLINICAL ASSESSMENT OF MAGNESIUM DEFICIENCY

Although Mg^{2+} is a relatively abundant cation in the body, more than 99% of it is located either intracellularly or in the skeleton. The less than 1% of total Mg^{2+} present in the body fluids is the most assessable for clinical testing, and the total serum Mg^{2+} concentration is the most widely used measure of Mg^{2+} status, although its limitations for reflecting Mg^{2+} deficiency are well recognized.[11] The reference range for normal total serum Mg^{2+} concentration is a subject of ongoing debate, but concentrations of 0.7 to 1.1 mmol/L are widely accepted. Because the measurement of serum Mg^{2+} concentration does not necessarily reflect the true total body Mg^{2+} content, it has been suggested that the measurement of ionized serum Mg^{2+} or intracellular Mg^{2+} concentrations may provide more precise information about Mg^{2+} status. However, the relevance of such measurements to body Mg^{2+} stores has been questioned, because the ionized serum Mg^{2+} and intracellular Mg^{2+} levels did not correlate with tissue Mg^{2+} levels, and the correlation with the results of Mg^{2+} retention tests was contradictory.[12-14] The use of stable Mg^{2+} isotopes and muscle ^{31}P-nuclear magnetic resonance spectroscopy represent promising new methods for the noninvasive estimation of body and/or tissue Mg^{2+} pools. However, they are not particularly suitable for routine measurements.

Hypomagnesemia develops late during the course of Mg^{2+} deficiency, and intracellular Mg^{2+} depletion may be present despite normal serum Mg^{2+} levels. As a result of the kidney's ability to sensitively adapt its Mg^{2+} transport rate to imminent deficiency, the urinary Mg^{2+} excretion rate is important during the assessment of the Mg^{2+} status. In hypomagnesemic patients, urinary Mg^{2+} excretion rates help to discern renal Mg^{2+} wasting from extrarenal losses. In the presence of hypomagnesemia, the 24-hour Mg^{2+} excretion rate is expected to decrease to less than 1 mmol.[15] Mg^{2+}/creatinine ratios and fractional Mg^{2+} excretion have also been advocated as indicators of evolving Mg^{2+} deficiency.[16,17] However, the interpretation of these results seems to be limited as a result of both intra- and inter-rater variability.[18,19] Normal values for Mg^{2+}/creatinine ratios have been assessed by Matos and colleagues.[20]

Among patients who are at risk for Mg^{2+} deficiency but who have normal serum Mg^{2+} levels, the Mg^{2+} status can be further evaluated by determining the amount of Mg^{2+} excreted in the urine after an intravenous infusion of Mg^{2+}. This procedure has been described as a "parenteral Mg^{2+} loading test," and it is still the gold standard for the evaluation of the body's Mg^{2+} status.[11,12] Normal subjects excrete at least 80% of an intravenous Mg^{2+} load within 24 hours, whereas patients with Mg^{2+} deficiency excrete much less. The Mg^{2+} loading test, however, requires normal renal handling of Mg^{2+}. If excess Mg^{2+} is being excreted by the kidneys as a result of diuresis, the Mg^{2+} load test may yield an inappropriate negative result. Conversely, if renal function is impaired and less blood is being filtered, this test could give a false-positive result.

ACQUIRED HYPOMAGNESEMIA

Cisplatin and Carboplatin

The cytostatic agent cisplatin and the newer antineoplastic drug carboplatin are widely used in various protocols for the therapy of solid tumors. Among their different side effects, nephrotoxicity receives the most attention as the major dose-limiting factor. Carboplatin has been reported to have less severe side effects than cisplatin.[21-23] Hypomagnesemia as a result of renal Mg^{2+} wasting is regularly observed among patients who are treated with cisplatin.[23,24] The incidence of Mg^{2+} deficiency is greater than 30%, but it increases to more than 70% with longer cisplatin usage and greater accumulated doses. Interestingly, cisplatin-induced Mg^{2+} wasting is relatively selective.[23] Hypocalcemia and hypokalemia may be observed, but only with prolonged and severe Mg^{2+} deficiency.[25] The influence of Mg^{2+} deficiency on PTH secretion and end-organ resistance is the likely explanation for enhanced urinary Ca^{2+} excretion and diminished mobilization, which result in low plasma Ca^{2+} concentrations. The effects on potassium balance are more difficult to explain. The hypokalemia observed with Mg^{2+} deficiency is refractory to potassium supplementation. The effects of cisplatin may persist months or even years later, long after the inorganic platinum has disappeared from the renal tissue.[26,27]

Aminoglycosides

Aminoglycosides (e.g., gentamicin) induce renal impairment in up to 35% patients, depending on the dose and duration of administration. In addition, aminoglycosides cause hypermagnesiuria and hypomagnesemia.[28] As many as 25% of patients receiving gentamicin will present with hypomagnesemia.[28] The hypermagnesiuric response occurs soon after the onset of therapy; it is dose-dependent and readily reversible upon withdrawal. Both adults and neonates display an immediate increase of Ca^{2+} and Mg^{2+} excretion after gentamicin infusion.[29,30] Hypokalemia is frequently observed with the Mg^{2+} deficiency. Mg^{2+} wasting is associated with hypercalciuria that may lead to diminished plasma Ca^{2+} concentrations; this would suggest that aminoglycosides affect renal Mg^{2+} and Ca^{2+} transport in the tubular segments where both are reabsorbed (i.e., the TAL and the distal convoluted tubule). The cellular mechanisms are not completely understood, but hypermagnesiuria and hypercalciuria are observed in the absence of histopathologic changes. Because gentamicin is a polyvalent cation, it was postulated that it may exert its effects on the Ca^{2+}-sensing receptor (CaSR).[5,31] The activation of this receptor by polyvalent cations inhibits the passive absorption of Mg^{2+} and Ca^{2+} in the loop of Henle and the active hormone-mediated transport in the distal convoluted tubule that leads to renal Mg^{2+} and Ca^{2+} wasting.

Calcineurin Inhibitors

The calcineurin inhibitors cyclosporine and tacrolimus are widely prescribed as immunosuppressants to organ transplant recipients and for numerous immunologic disorders. With this therapy, patients are at a high risk for developing renal injury and hypertension. Tubular dysfunction with the subsequent disturbance of mineral metabolism is another common side effect. Both drugs commonly lead to renal Mg^{2+} wasting and hypomagnesemia.[32] Unlike the other agents mentioned previously, these drugs also cause modest hypercalcemia with hypercalciuria and hypokalemia.[32] The hypomagnesemic effect is probably attenuated by the fall in the glomerular filtration rate and the reduction in filtered Mg^{2+}, but this defect appears to be specific for Mg^{2+}. Calcineurin inhibitor therapy is associated with an inappropriately high fractional excretion rate of Mg^{2+} (>4% despite hypomagnesemia), which suggests impaired passive reabsorption in the TAL or active Mg^{2+} transport in the DCT.[33] Tacrolimus has been shown to downregulate specific Ca^{2+} and Mg^{2+} transport proteins in the DCT. In an animal study, Nijenhuis and colleagues demonstrated that tacrolimus induces a decrease in TRPV5, calbindin-D28k, and TRPM6 at the mRNA level.[34] There may also be a decrease in TRPV5 and calbindin-D28k at the protein level. These effects appeared to be specific, because no morphologic features of tubular toxicity were observed. With respect to Mg^{2+}, it is interesting to note that TRPM6 expression in the intestine was not changed after tacrolimus administration. It is not known whether these drugs act through calcineurin, which is the intracellular receptor for these agents. It is speculated that tacrolimus-binding proteins, which are known to bind and regulate the Ca^{2+}-permeable transient receptor potential-like cation channels, might be involved, because tacrolimus disrupts this binding.[35] Analogously, one might speculate that certain FK506-binding proteins may also regulate TRPV5 or TRPM6 expression or activity. Hypomagnesemia has been implicated as a contributor to the nephrotoxicity and arterial hypertension associated with calcineurin inhibitors. Mervaala and colleagues demonstrated that the adverse effects of cyclosporine in spontaneously hypertensive rats is directly related to dietary Na^{+} and that these adverse effects can be prevented by Mg^{2+} supplementation.[36] Mg^{2+} supplementation also had a beneficial effect on cyclosporine nephrotoxicity in a rat model used by Miura and colleagues.[37]

Miscellaneous Agents

A number of antibiotics, tuberculostatics, and antiviral drugs may result in renal Mg^{2+} wasting. The cellular basis by which these agents lead to abnormal Mg^{2+} reabsorption are largely unknown. Many are associated with general cytotoxicity. Amphotericin B may lead to an acquired distal tubular acidosis that in turn reduces renal Mg^{2+} reabsorption. Pamidronate, which is used for the treatment of tumor-associated hypercalcemia, has been reported to cause transient hypomagnesemia. The cellular mechanisms are difficult to predict, because this drug is used in patients with hypercalcemia that may aggravate renal Mg^{2+} wasting.

Metabolic Acidosis

It has long been known that systemic acidosis is associated with renal Mg^{2+} wasting. Acute metabolic acidosis produced by the infusion of ammonium chloride or hydrochloride leads to significant increases in urinary Mg^{2+} excretion.[6] Chronic acidosis also leads to urinary Mg^{2+} wasting, which, together with the acidosis itself, may be partially corrected by the administration of bicarbonate.[6] In contrast with metabolic acidosis, acute and chronic metabolic alkalosis consistently leads to a fall in urinary Mg^{2+} excretion. The cellular basis for the acid-base effects on Mg^{2+} transport appears to be multifactorial.

Phosphate Restriction and Phosphate Depletion

One of the hallmarks of hypophosphatemia and cellular phosphate depletion is the striking increase in urinary Ca^{2+} and Mg^{2+} excretion.[5] The hypermagnesiuria may be sufficiently large to lead to overt hypomagnesemia. The increase in divalent ion excretion occurs within hours of dietary phosphate restriction. Three mechanisms have been proposed to account for the increased renal excretion: (1) the mobilization of Ca^{2+} and Mg^{2+} from bone; (2) the suppression of parathyroid hormone secretion; and (3) aberrant tubular transport. It is evident from clearance experiments that the urinary excretion of divalent cations in phosphate-depleted human subjects is inappropriate for the plasma concentration, thus supporting the notion of defective tubular transport.[38]

Cellular Potassium Depletion

Hypokalemia and cellular K^{+} depletion are associated with diminished Mg^{2+} absorption within the TAL and the DCT that may lead to increased Mg^{2+} excretion.[6] This increase in the urinary excretion of divalent cations may be explained by the effects of K^+-depletion on sodium chloride absorption in the TAL. Chloride conservation is impaired in potassium-depleted rats, and this may be related to altered basolateral Na^+-K^+ transport that results in impaired Na^+-K^+-$2Cl^-$-cotransport. To date, there is no direct evidence for changes in Mg^{2+} absorption in the TAL in states of potassium depletion. However, because Mg^{2+} and Ca^{2+} are absorbed by passive mechanisms, it is very likely that impaired sodium chloride transport can lead to diminished divalent cation absorption in this segment. In addition, potassium depletion may have additional important effects on Mg^{2+} transport in the DCT.[39]

THERAPY OF HYPOMAGNESEMIA

The supplementation of Mg^{2+} in patients with hypomagnesemia is primarily aimed at the relief of clinical symptoms. Unfortunately, for patients with renal Mg^{2+} wasting, normal values for total serum Mg^{2+} are difficult to achieve by oral substitution without considerable side effects that mainly result from the cathartic effects of Mg^{2+} salts.

The primary route of administration depends on the severity of the clinical findings. Acute intravenous infusion is usually reserved for patients with symptomatic hypomagnesemia (i.e., those with cerebral convulsions[40]) or those who are unable to tolerate oral administration. Intravenous administration should be preferred to painful intramuscular injections, especially for children.

In neonates and children, the initial treatment usually consists of 35 to 50 mg of Mg^{2+} sulfate (0.1 to 0.2 mmol Mg^{2+}) per kilogram of body weight given slowly (over a period of 20 minutes) and intravenously up to a maximum of 2 g Mg^{2+} sulfate, which is the adult dosage. This dose can be repeated every 6 to 8 hours, or it can be followed by a continuous infusion of 100 to 200 mg of Mg^{2+} sulfate (0.4 to 0.8 mmol Mg^{2+}) per kilogram of body weight given over a period of 24 hours.[41,42]

In the presence of hypocalcemia, this regimen can be continued for 3 to 5 days. When Mg^{2+} is administered intravenously, intravenous calcium gluconate should be available as an antidote. The control of blood pressure, heart rate, and respiration is of special importance, and so is the close monitoring of serum Mg^{2+} levels. Before administration, normal renal function has to be ascertained. Special caution is required in cases of renal insufficiency.

In asymptomatic hypomagnesemic or Mg^{2+}-deficient patients, oral replacement represents the preferred route of administration. The exact dosages required to correct Mg^{2+} deficiency are largely unknown. For the pediatric population, 10 to 20 mg of Mg^{2+} (0.4 to 0.8 mmol) per kg of body weight given three to four times a day has been recommended to correct hypomagnesemia.[43] However, a continuous administration of Mg^{2+} (e.g., dissolved in mineral water) has also been shown to be of advantage, because peak Mg^{2+} blood levels are avoided.

Solubility, intestinal absorption, and side effects differ greatly depending on the Mg^{2+} salt used for oral treatment. The bioavailability and pharmacokinetics of diverse Mg^{2+} salts have been reviewed recently.[44] Considering solubility, intestinal absorption, and bioavailability, organic Mg^{2+} salts such as Mg^{2+} citrate or aspartate appear to be most suitable for oral replacement therapy. In addition, the laxative effect of these preparations seems to be less pronounced as compared with inorganic Mg^{2+} salts.

In addition to replacement therapy, the use of certain diuretics has been proposed for the reduction of renal Mg^{2+} excretion. The aldosterone antagonist spironolactone and K^+-sparing diuretics such as amiloride exert Mg^{2+}-sparing effects.[45,46] Studies in patients with hereditary Mg^{2+} wasting showed a beneficial effect of these diuretics on renal Mg^{2+} excretion, serum Mg^{2+} levels, and clinical manifestations.[47,48]

HEREDITARY DISORDERS OF MAGNESIUM HANDLING

Recent advances in the molecular genetics of hereditary hypomagnesemia substantiated the role of a variety of genes and their encoded proteins in human epithelial Mg^{2+} transport (Table 30-3). The knowledge of underlying genetic defects helps to distinguish different clinical subtypes of hereditary disorders of Mg^{2+} homeostasis. Also, with the use of careful clinical observation and additional biochemical parameters, in most cases, the different disease entities can be distinguished, even when there is a considerable overlap in the phenotypic characteristics (Table 30-4).

Gitelman Syndrome (OMIM #263800)

Gitelman and colleagues pointed to the susceptibility to carpopedal spasms and tetany in three patients with Bartter syndrome.[49] Tetany was attributed to low plasma Mg^{2+} levels as a result of renal Mg^{2+} wasting. The further examination of these patients revealed low urinary Ca^{2+} excretion, which is rarely observed in hypomagnesemic states.[50] Consequently, the association of hypocalciuria with renal Mg^{2+} wasting was regarded as a hallmark to separate the then-defined Gitelman syndrome (GS) from other forms of hypokalemic salt-losing tubular disorders (Bartter-like syndromes).[51] Interestingly, both patients in Bartter's original report displayed positive Chvostek's sign and carpopedal spasms. Indeed, in a recent review of the original observations described by Bartter and colleagues, one of the coauthors conceded that the majority of patients seen by both endocrinologists perfectly matched the later description provided by Gitelman.[52]

The molecular defect in GS was first described by Simon and colleagues in 1996.[53] By a positional cloning approach, GS patients were found to have a loss of function mutations in the apical sodium chloride cotransporter (NCCT) of the DCT. NCCT deficiency results in only mild renal salt wasting. Initial presentation frequently occurs at school age or later, with the characteristic symptoms being muscular weakness, cramps, and fatigue. Affected individuals are frequently diagnosed accidentally while seeking medical advice for growth retardation, constipation, or enuresis; a history of salt craving is common. Urinary concentrating ability is typically not affected. Laboratory examination shows a typical constellation of metabolic alkalosis, low normal chloride levels, hypokalemia, and hypomagnesemia; urine analysis shows

TABLE 30-3 Inherited Disorders of Magnesium Handling

Disorder	OMIM #	Inheritance	Gene Locus	Gene	Protein
Gitelman syndrome	263800	AR	16q13	*SLC12A3*	NCCT, (NaCl cotransporter)
Isolated dominant hypomagnesemia	154020	AD	11q23	*FXYD2*	γ-subunit of the Na^+-K^+-ATPase
Isolated recessive hypomagnesemia	248250	AR	?	?	?
Autosomal dominant hypoparathyroidism	601198	AD	3q21	*CASR*	CaSR (Ca^{2+}/Mg^{2+} sensing receptor)
Familial hypocalciuric hypercalcemia	145980	AD	3q21	*CASR*	CaSR (Ca^{2+}/Mg^{2+} sensing receptor)
Neonatal severe hyperparathyroidism	239200	AR	3q21	*CASR*	CaSR (Ca^{2+}/Mg^{2+} sensing receptor)
Familial hypomagnesemia with hypercalciuria/ nephrocalcinosis	248250	AR	3q28	*CLDN16*	Claudin-16 (paracellin-1), tight junction protein
Familial hypomagnesemia with hypercalciuria/ nephrocalcinosis and severe ocular involvement	248190	AR	1p34	*CLDN19*	Claudin-19, tight junction protein
Hypomagnesemia with secondary hypocalcemia	602014	AR	9q22	*TRPM6*	TRPM6, putative ion channel
Hypomagnesemia/metabolic syndrome	500005	Maternal	mtDNA	*MTTRNA*	Mitochondrial tRNA (isoleucine)

AD, Autosomal dominant; *AR*, autosomal recessive.

hypocalciuria. Family studies reveal that electrolyte imbalances are present from infancy, although the affected infants display no obvious clinical signs. Of note is that the combination of hypokalemia and hypomagnesemia exerts an exceptionally unfavorable effect on cardiac excitability, which puts these patients at high risk for cardiac arrhythmias.

The pathognomonic feature of Gitelman syndrome is the dissociation of renal Ca^{2+} and Mg^{2+} handling, with low urinary Ca^{2+} and high urinary Mg^{2+} levels. Subsequent hypomagnesemia causes neuromuscular irritability and tetany. Decreased renal Ca^{2+} elimination together with Mg^{2+} deficiency favors the deposition of mineral Ca^{2+} as demonstrated by increased bone density as well as chondrocalcinosis. Although the combination of hypomagnesemia and hypocalciuria is typical for NCCT deficiency, it is neither a specific nor universal finding. Clinical observations in NCCT-deficient patients disclosed intra- and interindividual variations in urinary Ca^{2+} concentrations that can be attributed to gender, age-related conditions of bone metabolism, the intake of Mg^{2+} supplements, and changes in diuresis and urinary osmolality. Likewise, hypomagnesemia might not be present from the beginning. Because less than 1% of total body Mg^{2+} is circulating in the blood, renal Mg^{2+} loss can be balanced temporarily by Mg^{2+} release from bone and muscle stores as well as by increased intestinal Mg^{2+} reabsorption. The mechanisms that compromise distal Mg^{2+} reabsorption and favor Ca^{2+} reabsorption are not yet completely understood.

In contrast with TAL defects, disturbed salt reabsorption along the DCT does not affect the tubuloglomerular feedback and thus it is not associated with increased renal prostaglandin synthesis.[54] Accordingly, nonsteroidal anti-inflammatory drugs are of little benefit for patients with GS. Supplementation with potassium chloride and Mg^{2+} is therefore central to the treatment of this disorder. As mentioned previously, the avoidance of factors that, in addition to hypokalemia and hypomagnesemia, may affect cardiac excitability (particularly QT-interval prolonging drugs) is mandatory to prevent life-threatening cardiac arrhythmias.

Isolated Dominant Hypomagnesemia (OMIM #154020)

Isolated dominant hypomagnesemia (IDH) is caused by a mutation in the *FXYD2* gene on chromosome 11q23, which encodes a γ-subunit of the Na^+K^+-ATPase.[55] Only two IDH families have been described so far.[56,57] The two index patients presented with seizures during childhood (at 7 and 13 years). Serum Mg^{2+} levels in the two patients at that time were approximately 0.4 mmol/L. One index patient was treated for seizures of unknown origin with antiepileptic drugs until serum Mg^{2+} levels were evaluated during adolescence. At that time, severe mental retardation was evident. Systematic serum Mg^{2+} measurements performed in members of both families revealed low serum Mg^{2+} levels (approximately 0.5 mmol/L) in numerous apparently healthy individuals. A ^{28}Mg-retention study in one index patient pointed to a primary renal defect.[56] The intestinal absorption of Mg^{2+} was preserved and even stimulated in compensation for the increased renal losses. Urinary Mg^{2+} measurements in affected family members revealed daily Mg^{2+} excretion rates of around 5 mmol per day despite profound hypomagnesemia.[56] In addition, urinary Ca^{2+} excretion rates were low in all hypomagnesemic family members, which is a finding that is reminiscent of patients presenting with GS. However, in contrast with patients with GS, no other associated biochemical abnormalities were reported (especially hypokalemic alkalosis).

Pedigree analysis in the two families pointed to an autosomal-dominant mode of inheritance. A genome-wide linkage study mapped the disease locus on chromosome 11q23.[58] Detailed haplotype analysis demonstrated a common haplotype segregating in the two families that suggested a common ancestor. Indeed, subsequent mutational screening of the *FXYD2* gene demonstrated the identical mutation G41R in all affected individuals of both family branches.

The γ-subunit encoded by *FXYD2* is a member of a family of small single transmembrane proteins that share the common amino acid motif *F-X-Y-D*. Out of the seven members

TABLE 30-4 **Clinical and Biochemical Characteristics of Inherited Hypomagnesemia**

Disorder	Age at Onset	Serum Magnesium Level	Serum Calcium Level	Serum Potassium Level	Blood pH	Urine Magnesium Level	Urine Calcium Level	Nephrocalcinosis	Renal Stones
Gitelman syndrome	Adolescence	↓	Normal	↓	↑	↓	↓	No	No
Isolated dominant hypomagnesemia	Childhood	↓	Normal	Normal	Normal	↑	↓	No	No
Isolated recessive hypomagnesemia	Childhood	↓	Normal	Normal	Normal	↑	Normal	No	No
Autosomal dominant hypoparathyroidism	Infancy	↓	↓	Normal	Normal or ↓	↑	↑ - ↑↑	Yes*	Yes*
Familial hypocalciuric hypercalcemia	Often asymptomatic	Normal to ↑	↑	Normal	Normal	↓	↓	No	?
Neonatal severe hyperparathyroidism	Infancy	Normal to ↑	↑↑↑	Normal	Normal	↓	↓	No	?
Familial hypomagnesemia with hypercalciuria/nephrocalcinosis	Childhood	↓	Normal	Normal	Normal or ↓	↑↑	↑↑	Yes	Yes
Hypomagnesemia with secondary hypocalcemia	Infancy	↓↓↓	↓	Normal	Normal	↑	Normal	No	No

* Common complication during therapy with calcium and vitamin D.

that differ in their tissue specificity, *FXYD2* and *FXYD4* (also called *channel-inducing factor*) are highly expressed along the nephron displaying an alternating expression pattern.[59] The γ-subunit comprises two isoforms, γ-α and γ-β, that are differentially expressed in the kidney. The γ-α isoform is present predominantly in the proximal tubule, and the expression of the γ-β isoform predominates in the distal nephron, especially in the DCT and connecting tubule.[60] The ubiquitous Na^+K^+-ATPase is a dimeric enzyme that invariably consists of one α and one β subunit. FXYD proteins constitute a third or γ subunit that represents a tissue-specific regulator of Na^+K^+-ATPase. The FXYD2 γ subunit increases the apparent affinity of Na^+K^+-ATPase for adenosine triphosphate while decreasing its Na^+ affinity.[61] Thus, it might provide a mechanism for balancing energy use and maintaining appropriate salt gradients.

Expression studies of the mutant G41R γ subunit in mammalian renal tubule cells revealed a dominant-negative effect of the mutation leading to a retention of the γ-subunit within the cell. Whereas initial data pointed to a retention of the entire Na^+K^+-ATPase complex in intracellular compartments, more recent data demonstrate an isolated trafficking defect of the mutant γ subunit while trafficking of the α/β complex is preserved.[62] The mutant γ subunit is obviously retained in the Golgi complex, thus indicating disturbed posttranslational processing. The assumption of a dominant-negative effect is substantiated by the observation that individuals with a large heterozygous deletion of chromosome 11q (including the *FXYD2* gene) exhibit normal serum Mg^{2+} levels.[63]

Urinary Mg^{2+} wasting together with the expression pattern of the *FXYD2* gene indicate defective transcellular Mg^{2+} reabsorption in the DCT in IDH patients. But how can a defect of Na^+K^+-ATPase modulation lead to impaired renal Mg^{2+} conservation? One possible explanation is based on changes in intracellular Na^+ and K^+ levels. Meij and colleagues have suggested that diminished intracellular K^+ may depolarize the apical membrane, thereby resulting in a decrease in Mg^{2+} uptake.[55] Alternatively, an increase in intracellular Na^+ could impair basolateral Mg^{2+} transport, which is presumably achieved by an Na^+-coupled exchange mechanism. Another explanation is that the γ-subunit is not only involved in Na^+K^+-ATPase function but that it is also an essential component of a yet unidentified adenosine-triphosphate–dependent transport system that is specific for Mg^{2+}. Similar to Ca^{2+}, both a specific Mg^{2+}-ATPase and an Na^+-coupled exchanger might exist. Further studies are needed to clarify this issue.

An interesting feature of IDH is the finding of hypocalciuria, which is primarily observed in cases of GS (described previously). Unfortunately, only one large family with IDH has been described, and an animal model for IDH is still lacking. Mice lacking the γ-subunit do not demonstrate any abnormalities in Mg^{2+} conservation or balance.[64] Therefore, data about the structural integrity of the DCT in patients with IDH do not exist. One could speculate that, as in GS, a defect in Na^+K^+-ATPase function and energy metabolism may lead to an apoptotic breakdown of the early DCT responsible for Mg^{2+} reabsorption, whereas later parts of the distal nephron remain intact. In IDH, there is no evidence for renal salt wasting and no stimulation of the renin–angiotensin–aldosterone system. The finding of hypocalciuria without apparent volume depletion apparently contradicts recent experimental data that favor an increase in proximal tubular Ca^{2+} reabsorption as a result of volume depletion in GS.[65]

Isolated Recessive Hypomagnesemia (OMIM #248250)

Geven and colleagues reported a form of isolated hypomagnesemia in a consanguineous family, thereby indicating autosomal recessive inheritance.[66] Two affected girls presented with generalized seizures during infancy. Unfortunately, late diagnosis resulted in neurodevelopmental deficits in both patients. A thorough clinical and laboratory workup at 4 and 8 years of age, respectively, revealed serum Mg^{2+} levels of approximately 0.5 to 0.6 mmol/L with no other associated electrolyte abnormalities. A ^{28}Mg-retention study in one patient pointed to a primary renal defect, although intestinal Mg^{2+} uptake was preserved.[66] Both patients exhibited renal Mg^{2+} excretions of 3 to 6 mmol per day despite hypomagnesemia confirming renal Mg^{2+} wasting. In contrast with IDH, renal Ca^{2+} excretion rates in isolated recessive hypomagnesemia are within the normal range. Haplotype analysis performed in this family excluded the gene loci involved in IDH, familial hypomagnesemia with hypercalciuria and nephrocalcinosis, and GS, thereby indicating that isolated recessive hypomagnesemia is not allelic with these diseases.[63]

Disorders of the Calcium-Sensing Receptor

The extracellular Ca^{2+}/Mg^{2+}-sensing receptor (CaSR) plays an essential role in Mg^{2+} and Ca^{2+} homeostasis by influencing not only PTH secretion in the parathyroid but also by directly regulating the rate of Mg^{2+} and Ca^{2+} reabsorption in the kidney. It was first cloned by Brown and colleagues in 1993.[67] Along the distal nephron, the CaSR is expressed basolaterally in TAL and DCT as well as at both the apical and basolateral membranes of the collecting duct.[68] Activation of the CaSR leads to coordinated changes in renal Ca^{2+} and Mg^{2+} excretion and in water diuresis.[69] The dilution of the urine by decreasing aquaporin expression in the collecting duct is thought to minimize the risk of stone formation in the face of an increase in Ca^{2+} and Mg^{2+} excretion. Several diseases associated with both activating and inactivating mutations in the *CASR* gene have been described. Because alterations in CaSR activity also affect renal Mg^{2+} handling, they are presented in this chapter with a special focus on Mg^{2+}.

Autosomal-Dominant Hypoparathyroidism (OMIM #601198)

Activating mutations of the *CASR* result in autosomal-dominant hypoparathyroidism. The condition typically manifests during childhood with seizures or carpopedal spasms. Laboratory evaluation reveals the typical combination of hypocalcemia and low PTH levels, but the majority of patients also exhibit moderate hypomagnesemia, with serum levels of approximately 0.5 to 0.6 mmol/L.[70,71] Affected individuals are often given the incorrect diagnosis of primary hypoparathyroidism on the basis of inadequately low PTH levels despite their hypocalcemia. Serum Ca^{2+} levels are typically in a range of 6 to 7 mg/dl. The differentiation from primary hypoparathyroidism is of particular importance, because treatment with vitamin D can result in a dramatic increase in hypercalciuria and the occurrence of nephrocalcinosis and the impairment of renal function in autosomal-dominant hypoparathyroidism patients. Therefore, therapy with vitamin D or Ca^{2+} supplementation should be reserved for symptomatic patients, with the aim of maintaining serum Ca^{2+} levels that are just sufficient for the relief of symptoms.[71]

Activating *CASR* mutations leads to a lower setpoint of the receptor or an increased affinity for extracellular Ca^{2+} and Mg^{2+}. This inadequate activation by physiologic extracellular Ca^{2+} and Mg^{2+} levels then results in diminished PTH secretion and the decreased reabsorption of both divalent cations, mainly in the cortical TAL (cTAL). For Mg^{2+}, the inhibition of PTH-stimulated reabsorption in the DCT may significantly contribute to an increased renal loss in addition to the effects observed in the TAL.[5,72] A pronounced hypomagnesemia is observed in patients with complete activation of the CaSR at physiologic serum Ca^{2+} and Mg^{2+} concentrations who also exhibit a Bartter-like phenotype.[73] In these patients, CaSR activation inhibits TAL-mediated salt and divalent cation reabsorption to an extent that cannot be compensated for in later nephron segments.

Familial Hypocalciuric Hypercalcemia (OMIM #145980) and Neonatal Severe Hyperparathyroidism (OMIM #239200)

Familial hypocalciuric hypercalcemia (FHH) and neonatal severe hyperparathyroidism (NSHPT) result from inactivating mutations that present in either the heterozygous or homozygous (or compound heterozygous) state, respectively.[70,74] FHH patients normally present with mild to moderate hypercalcemia accompanied by few if any symptoms, and they often do not require treatment. Urinary excretion rates for Ca^{2+} and Mg^{2+} are markedly reduced, and serum PTH levels are inappropriately high. In addition, affected individuals also show mild hypermagnesemia.[75] By contrast, NSHPT patients with two mutant CaSR alleles usually present during early infancy with polyuria and dehydration as a result of severe symptomatic hypercalcemia. Unrecognized and untreated, hyperparathyroidism and hypercalcemia result in skeletal deformities, extraosseous calcifications, and a severe neurodevelopmental deficit. Therefore, early treatment with partial to total parathyroidectomy seems to be essential for a positive outcome.[76] Data regarding serum Mg^{2+} levels in NSHPT are sparse. However, elevations to levels of around 50% above normal have been reported.

Familial Hypomagnesemia with Hypercalciuria and Nephrocalcinosis (OMIM #248250)

Familial hypomagnesemia with hypercalciuria and nephrocalcinosis (FHHNC) is an autosomal-recessive tubular disorder. Since its first description, at least 50 different kindreds have been reported, which has allowed for a comprehensive characterization of the clinical spectrum of this disorder and for distinction from other Mg^{2+}-losing tubular diseases.[77-79] As a result of excessive renal Mg^{2+} and Ca^{2+} wasting, patients develop the characteristic triad of hypomagnesemia, hypercalciuria, and nephrocalcinosis that gave the disease its name. FHHNC patients usually present during early childhood with recurrent urinary tract infections, polyuria/polydipsia, nephrolithiasis, and/or failure to thrive. Signs of severe hypomagnesemia, such as cerebral convulsions and muscular tetany, are less common. Extrarenal manifestations, especially ocular involvement (e.g., severe myopia, nystagmus, chorioretinitis) have also been reported.[77-79] Additional laboratory findings include elevated serum PTH levels before the onset of chronic renal failure, incomplete distal tubular acidosis, hypocitraturia, and hyperuricemia, which are present in most patients.[80] The clinical course of FHHNC patients is often complicated by the development of chronic renal failure early in life. A considerable number of patients exhibit a marked decline in glomerular filtration rate (<60 ml/min per 1.73 m^2) before the time of diagnosis, and about one third of patients develop end-stage renal disease during adolescence. Hypomagnesemia may completely disappear with the decline in glomerular filtration rate as a result of a reduction in filtered Mg^{2+} that limits urinary Mg^{2+} excretion.

In addition to continuous Mg^{2+} supplementation, therapy aims to reduce Ca^{2+} excretion by using thiazides to prevent the progression of nephrocalcinosis and stone formation. The degree of renal calcification has been correlated with the progression of chronic renal failure.[77] In a short-term study, thiazides have been demonstrated to effectively reduce urinary calcium excretion in patients with FHHNC.[81] However, these therapeutic strategies have not yet been shown to significantly influence the progression of renal failure. Supportive therapy is important for the protection of kidney function, and it should include the provision of sufficient fluids. As expected, after kidney transplantation recurrence of FHHNC has never been observed, because the primary defect resides in the kidney.

Using a positional cloning approach, Simon and colleagues identified a new gene (*CLDN16*, formerly *PCLN1*) that is mutated in patients with FHHNC.[82] *CLDN16* codes for claudin-16, a member of the claudin family. More than 20 claudins identified so far comprise a family of approximately 22 kD proteins with four transmembrane segments, two extracellular domains, and intracellular N and C termini. Claudins are important components of various sorts of tight junctions. The individual composition of tight junction strands with different claudins confers the characteristic properties of different epithelia for paracellular permeability and/or transepithelial resistance. In this context, a crucial role has been attributed to the first extracellular domain of the claudin protein, which is extremely variable with regard to the number and position of charged amino acid residues.[83] Individual charges have been shown to influence paracellular ion selectivity, thereby suggesting that claudins that are positioned on opposing cells and that form the paracellular pathway provide charge-selective pores within the tight junction barrier.

The majority of mutations reported so far in patients with FHHNC are simple missense mutations that affect the transmembrane domains and the extracellular loops, with a particular clustering in the first extracellular loop, which contains the putative ion selectivity filter. Within this domain, patients originating from Germany and Eastern European countries exhibit a common mutation (L151F) as a result of a founder effect.[80] Because this mutation is present in approximately

50% of mutant alleles, molecular diagnosis is greatly facilitated in patients originating from these countries. Defects in *CLDN16* have also been shown to underlie the development of a chronic interstitial nephritis in Japanese cattle that rapidly develop chronic renal failure shortly after birth.[84] Interestingly, affected animals typically show hypocalcemia but no hypomagnesemia, which may be explained by advanced chronic renal failure being present at the time of examination. The fact that (in contrast with the point mutations identified in human FHHNC) large deletions of *CLDN16* are responsible for the disease in cattle may explain the more severe phenotype with early-onset renal failure. In patients with FHHNC, progressive renal failure is more likely a consequence of massive urinary Ca^{2+} wasting and nephrocalcinosis. Concerning the ocular abnormalities observed in some FHHNC patients, it is interesting to note that *cldn16* expression has been identified in bovine cornea and retinal pigment epithelia.[85] Further examination of the eyes of affected Japanese cattle and of *Cldn16* knockout mice will hopefully provide an answer to the question of whether myopia, nystagmus, and chorioretinitis observed in patients with FHHNC are directly linked to *CLDN16* mutations. Furthermore, there is evidence from family analyses that carriers of heterozygous *CLDN16* mutations may also present with clinical symptoms. Two independent studies describe a high incidence of hypercalciuria, nephrolithiasis, and/or nephrocalcinosis among first-degree relatives of FHHNC patients.[77,80] A subsequent study also reported a tendency toward mild hypomagnesemia in family members with heterozygous *CLDN16* mutations.[86] Thus, one might speculate that *CLDN16* mutations could be involved in idiopathic hypercalciuric stone formation.

A homozygous *CLDN16* mutation (T303R) affecting the C-terminal PDZ domain has been identified in two families with isolated hypercalciuria and nephrocalcinosis without disturbances in renal Mg^{2+} handling.[87] Interestingly, the hypercalciuria disappeared during follow up, and urinary Ca^{2+} levels reached normal values beyond puberty. Transient transfection of Madine-Darby canine kidney cells with the *CLDN16* (T303R) mutant revealed a mistargeting into lysosomes, whereas wild-type claudin-16 was correctly localized to tight junctions. It still remains to be determined why this type of misrouting is associated with transient isolated hypercalciuria without increased Mg^{2+} excretion.

The exact physiologic role of claudin-16 is still not fully understood. From the FHHNC disease phenotype, it was concluded that claudin-16 may regulate the paracellular transport of Mg^{2+} and Ca^{2+} ions by contributing to a selective paracellular conductance. Claudin-16 might be involved in the formation of a pore permitting paracellular fluxes of Mg^{2+} and Ca^{2+} down their electrochemical gradients.[82,88] However, recent functional studies in porcine renal tubule epithelial kidney cells (LLC-PK1) demonstrated that the expression of claudin-16 selectively and significantly increased the permeability of Na^+ with a far less pronounced change of Mg^{2+} flux. From these observations, it was hypothesized that, in the TAL, claudin-16 probably contributes to the generation of the lumen-positive potential (thus allowing for the passive reabsorption of divalent cations) rather than to the formation of a paracellular channel that is selective for Ca^{2+} and Mg^{2+}.[89]

As mentioned previously, many FHHNC patients develop chronic renal failure that is associated with progressive tubulointerstitial nephritis. The pathophysiology of this phenomenon, which is not usually observed in other tubular disorders, is unclear. Traditionally, renal failure in FHHNC has been attributed to the concomitant hypercalciuria and nephrocalcinosis, but a true correlation has not been established. Therefore, it has been speculated that claudin-16 is not only involved in paracellular electrolyte reabsorption but also in tubular cell proliferation and differentiation.[90] This hypothesis is supported by the bovine *cldn16* knockout phenotype observed among Japanese Black cattle, which exhibit early-onset renal failure as a result of interstitial nephritis with diffuse zonal fibrosis.[84,91] Tubular epithelial cells were reported as "immature," with loss of polarization and attachment to the basement membrane. A close association between fibrosis and abnormal tubules was noted, and the term *renal tubular dysplasia* was used to emphasize that the lesions develop first in the epithelial cells of the renal tubules.[92] These cattle have large homozygous deletions, whereas human FHHNC mutations are mainly missense mutations that affect the extracellular loops of claudin-16. From these observations, it appears that the site and extent of the mutation determine the phenotypic manifestations, which range from isolated alterations in channel conductance to an alteration in cell proliferation and differentiation.

FHHNC is a genetically heterogenous disease; mutations in another tight junction gene encoding claudin-19 have also been demonstrated to cause this disease.[93] In addition, the identification of *CLDN19* mutations could explain the variable ocular phenotype, because *CLDN19* defects seem to be invariably associated with severe ocular abnormalities as previously described (including severe myopia, nystagmus, or macular coloboma).[77-79] By contrast, only a small subset of FHHNC patients with *CLDN16* defects display severe myopia, whereas nystagmus or colobomata have not been described in a large cohort of patients.[80] The renal phenotype is very similar between these two FHHNC subtypes. Expression studies revealed that claudin-16 and claudin-19 perfectly colocalize at tight junctions of the TAL.[93] It remains to be determined whether both proteins are part of the same molecular structure, thus enabling the paracellular reabsorption of divalent cations.

Hypomagnesemia with Secondary Hypocalcemia (OMIM #602014)

Hypomagnesemia with secondary hypocalcemia (HSH) is a rare autosomal-recessive disorder that manifests during early infancy with generalized seizures or other symptoms of increased neuromuscular excitability as first described in 1968.[94] Delayed diagnosis or noncompliance with treatment can be fatal or result in permanent neurologic damage.

Biochemical abnormalities include extremely low serum Mg^{2+} (about 0.2 mmol/L) and low serum Ca^{2+} levels. The mechanism leading to hypocalcemia is still not completely understood. Severe hypomagnesemia results in an impaired synthesis and/or release of PTH.[95] PTH levels in HSH patients were consistently found to be inappropriately low. The hypocalcemia observed in HSH is resistant to treatment with Ca^{2+} or vitamin D. The relief of clinical symptoms, normocalcemia, and normalization of PTH levels can only be achieved by the administration of high doses of Mg^{2+}.[96]

Transport studies of patients with HSH point to a primary defect in intestinal Mg^{2+} absorption.[97,98] However, in some patients, an additional renal leak for Mg^{2+} is suspected.[99]

By linkage analysis, a gene locus (*HOMG1*) for HSH was mapped to chromosome 9q22 in 1997.[100] Later, two independent groups identified *TRPM6* at this locus and reported loss-of-function mutations (mainly truncating mutations) as the underlying cause of HSH.[101,102] Mutations in *TRPM6* have been identified in more than 20 families affected by HSH to date.[103,104] *TRPM6* encodes a member of the transient receptor potential (TRP) family of cation channels. The TRPM6 protein is homologous to TRPM7, a Ca^{2+}- and Mg^{2+}-permeable ion channel that is regulated by MgATP.[105] TRPM6 is expressed along the entire small intestine and colon but also in the kidney in the distal tubule cells. Immunofluorescence studies with an antibody generated against murine TRPM6 localized TRPM6 to the apical membrane of the DCT.[106] The detection of TRPM6 expression in the DCT confirms the hypothesis of an additional role of renal Mg^{2+} wasting in the pathogenesis of HSH.[107] This was also supported by intravenous Mg^{2+} loading tests in HSH patients, which disclosed a considerable renal Mg^{2+} leak (albeit with the patient still being hypomagnesemic).[102]

The observation that, in patients with HSH, the substitution of high oral doses of Mg^{2+} achieves at least subnormal serum Mg^{2+} levels supports the theory of two independent intestinal transport systems for Mg^{2+}. TRPM6 probably represents a molecular component of active transcellular Mg^{2+} transport. An increased intraluminal Mg^{2+} concentration (by increased oral intake) enables compensation for the defect in active transcellular transport by increasing absorption via the passive paracellular pathway (see Figure 30-1).

TRPM6 is closely related to TRPM7, and it represents the second TRP protein being fused to a C-terminal α-kinase domain. The *TRPM6* gene is composed of 39 exons that code for a total of 2022 amino acid residues. *TRPM6*-mRNA shows a more restricted expression pattern than TRPM7, with the highest levels found along the intestine (duodenum, jejunum, ileum, colon) and the DCT of the kidney.[101] Immunohistochemistry shows a complete colocalization with the Na^+-Cl^--cotransporter NCCT (also serving as a DCT marker) but also with parvalbumin and calbindin-D_{28K}, which are two cytosolic proteins that putatively act as intracellular (Ca^{2+}) and Mg^{2+} buffers.[106]

The biophysical characterization of TRPM6 is controversial. Voets and colleagues demonstrated striking parallels between TRPM6 and TRPM7 with respect to gating mechanisms and ion selectivity profiles (because TRPM6 was shown to be regulated by intracellular Mg^{2+} levels), and both were shown to be permeable for Mg^{2+} and Ca^{2+}.[106] Permeation characteristics with currents almost exclusively carried by divalent cations with a higher affinity for Mg^{2+} than Ca^{2+} support the role of TRPM6 as the apical Mg^{2+} influx pathway. Furthermore, TRPM6-analogous to TRPM7-exhibits a marked sensitivity to intracellular Mg^{2+}. Thus, one may speculate about an inhibition of TRPM6-mediated Mg^{2+} uptake by rising intracellular Mg^{2+} concentrations as a possible mechanism for the regulation of intestinal and renal Mg^{2+} (re-)absorption. This inhibition may in part be mediated by intracellular MgATP, as has been shown for TRPM7.[105]

Using a similar expression model (but a different expression vector), Chubanov and colleagues reported that TRPM6 is only present at the cell surface when it is associating with TRPM7.[108] Furthermore, fluorescence resonance energy transfer analyses showed a specific and direct protein–protein interaction between both proteins. Electrophysiologic data in a *Xenopus* oocyte expression system indicated that the coexpression of TRPM6 results in a significant amplification of TRPM7-induced currents.[108] The idea of the heteromultimerization of TRPM7 with TRPM6 was confirmed by Schmitz and colleagues.[109] The authors further demonstrated that TRPM6 and TRPM7 are not functionally redundant but that there is evidence that both proteins can influence each other's biologic activity. It has also been shown that TRPM6 can phosphorylate TRPM7 and that TRPM6 may modulate TRPM7 function in an Mg^{2+}-dependent manner.[109]

Mitochondrial Hypomagnesemia (OMIM #500005)

Recently, a mutation in the mitochondrial-coded isoleucine tRNA gene $tRNA^{Ile}$ (or MTTI) was discovered in a large Caucasian kindred.[110] An extensive clinical evaluation of this family was prompted after the discovery of hypomagnesemia in the index patient. Pedigree analysis was compatible with mitochondrial inheritance, because the phenotype was exclusively transmitted by affected females. The phenotype includes hypomagnesemia, hypercholesterolemia, and hypertension. Of the adults on the maternal lineage, the majority of offspring exhibited at least one of the mentioned symptoms, approximately half of the individuals showed a combination of two or more symptoms, and around 1 in 6 had all three features. Serum Mg^{2+} levels of family members on the maternal lineage varied greatly, ranging from ~0.8 to ~2.5 mg/dl (equivalent to ~0.3 to ~1.0 mmol/L), with approximately 50% of individuals being hypomagnesemic.

The hypomagnesemic individuals (serum Mg^{2+} <0.9 mmol/L) showed higher fractional excretions (median, approximately 7.5%) than their normomagnesemic relatives on the maternal lineage (median, approximately 3%), which clearly pointed to renal Mg^{2+} wasting as being causative for hypomagnesemia. Interestingly, hypomagnesemia was accompanied by decreased urinary Ca^{2+} levels; this finding points to the DCT as the affected tubular segment.

The mitochondrial mutation observed in the affected family involves the $tRNA^{Ile}$ gene (MTTI). The observed nucleotide exchange occurs at the T nucleotide directly adjacent to the anticodon triplet. This position is highly conserved among species, and it is critical for codon–anticodon recognition. The functional consequences of the tRNA defect for mitochondrial function remain to be elucidated in detail. Because adenosine triphosphate consumption along the tubule is highest in the DCT, the authors speculate about an impaired energy metabolism of DCT cells as a consequence of the mitochondrial defect that could, in turn, lead to disturbed transcellular Mg^{2+} reabsorption. Further studies involving these patients may further the understanding of the mechanism of distal tubular Mg^{2+} wasting in this disease.

REFERENCES

1. Kerstan D, Quamme G: Physiology and pathophysiology of intestinal absorption of magnesium. In Massry SG, Morii H, Nishizawa Y, editors: *Calcium in internal medicine,* London, 2002, Springer-Verlag, pp 171-83.
2. Quamme GA, de Rouffignac C: Epithelial magnesium transport and regulation by the kidney, *Front Biosci* 5:D694-711, 2000.
3. Fine KD, Santa Ana CA, Porter JL, Fordtran JS: Intestinal absorption of magnesium from food and supplements, *J Clin Invest* 88:396-402, 1991.
4. de Rouffignac C, Quamme G: Renal magnesium handling and its hormonal control, *Physiol Rev* 74:305-22, 1994.
5. Dai LJ, Ritchie G, Kerstan D, Kang HS, et al: Magnesium transport in the renal distal convoluted tubule, *Physiol Rev* 81:51-84, 2001.
6. Quamme GA: Renal magnesium handling: new insights in understanding old problems, *Kidney Int* 52:1180-95, 1997.
7. Whang R, Hampton EM, Whang DD: Magnesium homeostasis and clinical disorders of magnesium deficiency, *Ann Pharmacother* 28:220-26, 1994.
8. Hollifield JW: Magnesium depletion, diuretics, and arrhythmias, *Am J Med* 82:30-37, 1987.
9. Woods KL, Fletcher S, Roffe C, Haider Y: Intravenous magnesium sulphate in suspected acute myocardial infarction: results of the second Leicester Intravenous Magnesium Intervention Trial (LIMIT-2), *Lancet* 339:1553-58, 1992.
10. ISIS-4: ISIS-4: a randomised factorial trial assessing early oral captopril, oral mononitrate, and intravenous magnesium sulphate in 58,050 patients with suspected acute myocardial infarction. ISIS-4 (Fourth International Study of Infarct Survival) Collaborative Group, *Lancet* 345:669-85, 1995.
11. Elin RJ: Magnesium: the fifth but forgotten electrolyte, *Am J Clin Pathol* 102:616-22, 1994.
12. Hebert P, Mehta N, Wang J, Hindmarsh T, et al: Functional magnesium deficiency in critically ill patients identified using a magnesium-loading test, *Crit Care Med* 25:749-55, 1997.
13. Hashimoto Y, Nishimura Y, Maeda H, Yokoyama M: Assessment of magnesium status in patients with bronchial asthma, *J Asthma* 37:489-96, 2000.
14. Arnold A, Tovey J, Mangat P, Penny W, Jacobs S: Magnesium deficiency in critically ill patients, *Anaesthesia* 50:203-05, 1995.
15. Sutton RA, Domrongkitchaiporn S: Abnormal renal magnesium handling, *Miner Electrolyte Metab* 19:232-40, 1993.
16. Elisaf M, Panteli K, Theodorou J, Siamopoulos KC: Fractional excretion of magnesium in normal subjects and in patients with hypomagnesemia, *Magnes Res* 10:315-20, 1997.
17. Tang NL, Cran YK, Hui E, Woo J: Application of urine magnesium/creatinine ratio as an indicator for insufficient magnesium intake, *Clin Biochem* 33:675-78, 2000.
18. Nicoll GW, Struthers AD, Fraser CG: Biological variation of urinary magnesium, *Clin Chem* 37:1794-95, 1991.
19. Djurhuus MS, Gram J, Petersen PH, Klitgaard NA, et al: Biological variation of serum and urinary magnesium in apparently healthy males, *Scand J Clin Lab Invest* 55:549-58, 1995.
20. Matos V, van Melle G, Boulat O, Markert M, et al: Urinary phosphate/creatinine, calcium/creatinine, and magnesium/creatinine ratios in a healthy pediatric population, *J Pediatr* 131:252-57, 1997.
21. Boulikas T, Vougiouka M: Recent clinical trials using cisplatin, carboplatin and their combination chemotherapy drugs (review), *Oncol Rep* 11:559-95, 2004.
22. English MW, Skinner R, Pearson AD, Price L, et al: Dose-related nephrotoxicity of carboplatin in children, *Br J Cancer* 81:336-41, 1999.
23. Goren MP: Cisplatin nephrotoxicity affects magnesium and calcium metabolism, *Med Pediatr Oncol* 41:186-89, 2003.
24. Lajer H, Daugaard G: Cisplatin and hypomagnesemia, *Cancer Treat Rev* 25:47-58, 1999.
25. Mavichak V, Coppin CM, Wong NL, Dirks JH, et al: Renal magnesium wasting and hypocalciuria in chronic cis-platinum nephropathy in man, *Clin Sci (Lond)* 75:203-07, 1988.
26. Bianchetti MG, Kanaka C, Ridolfi-Luthy A, Hirt A, et al: Persisting renotubular sequelae after cisplatin in children and adolescents, *Am J Nephrol* 11:127-30, 1991.
27. Markmann M, Rothman R, Reichman B, Hakes T, et al: Persistent hypomagnesemia following cisplatin chemotherapy in patients with ovarian cancer, *J Cancer Res Clin Oncol* 117:89-90, 1991.
28. Shah GM, Kirschenbaum MA: Renal magnesium wasting associated with therapeutic agents, *Miner Electrolyte Metab* 17:58-64, 1991.
29. Elliott C, Newman N, Madan A: Gentamicin effects on urinary electrolyte excretion in healthy subjects, *Clin Pharmacol Ther* 67:16-21, 2000.
30. Giapros VI, Cholevas VI, Andronikou SK: Acute effects of gentamicin on urinary electrolyte excretion in neonates, *Pediatr Nephrol* 19:322-25, 2004.
31. Ward DT, McLarnon SJ, Riccardi D: Aminoglycosides increase intracellular calcium levels and ERK activity in proximal tubular OK cells expressing the extracellular calcium-sensing receptor, *J Am Soc Nephrol* 13:1481-89, 2002.
32. Rob PM, Lebeau A, Nobiling R, Schmid H, et al: Magnesium metabolism: basic aspects and implications of ciclosporine toxicity in rats, *Nephron* 72:59-66, 1996.
33. Lote CJ, Thewles A, Wood JA, Zafar T: The hypomagnesaemic action of FK506: urinary excretion of magnesium and calcium and the role of parathyroid hormone, *Clin Sci (Lond)* 99:285-92, 2000.
34. Nijenhuis T, Hoenderop JG, Bindels RJ: Downregulation of Ca(2+) and Mg(2+) transport proteins in the kidney explains tacrolimus (FK506)-induced hypercalciuria and hypomagnesemia, *J Am Soc Nephrol* 15:549-57, 2004.
35. Goel M, Garcia R, Estacion M, Schilling WP: Regulation of Drosophila TRPL channels by immunophilin FKBP59, *J Biol Chem* 276:38762-73, 2001.
36. Mervaala EM, Pere AK, Lindgren L, Laakso J, et al: Effects of dietary sodium and magnesium on cyclosporin A-induced hypertension and nephrotoxicity in spontaneously hypertensive rats, *Hypertension* 29:822-27, 1997.
37. Miura K, Nakatani T, Asai T, Yamanaka S, et al: Role of hypomagnesemia in chronic cyclosporine nephropathy, *Transplantation* 73:340-47, 2002.
38. Coburn JW, Massry SG: Changes in serum and urinary calcium during phosphate depletion: studies on mechanisms, *J Clin Invest* 49:1073-87, 1970.
39. Dai LJ, Friedman PA, Quamme GA: Cellular mechanisms of chlorothiazide and cellular potassium depletion on Mg2+ uptake in mouse distal convoluted tubule cells, *Kidney Int* 51:1008-17, 1997.
40. Agus ZS: Hypomagnesemia, *J Am Soc Nephrol* 10:1616-22, 1999.
41. Koo WWK, Tsang RC: Calcium and magnesium homeostasis. In Avery GB, Fletcher MA, MacDonald MG, editors: *Neonatology—pathophysiology and management of the newborn,* vol 1, ed 5, Philadelphia, Baltimore, New York, 1999, Lippincott Williams & Wilkins, p 730.
42. Cronan K, Norman ME: Renal and electrolyte emergencies. In Fleisher GR, Ludwig S, editors: *Pediatric emergency medicine,* vol 1, ed 4, Philadelphia, Baltimore, New York, 2000, Lippincott Williams & Wilkins, p 827.
43. Gal P, Reed MD: Medications. In Behrman RE, Kliegman R, Jenson HB, editors: *Textbook of pediatrics,* ed 16, Philadelphia, Toronto, London, 2000, WB Saunders.
44. Ranade VV, Somberg JC: Bioavailability and pharmacokinetics of magnesium after administration of magnesium salts to humans, *Am J Ther* 8:345-57, 2001.
45. Ryan MP: Magnesium and potassium-sparing diuretics, *Magnesium* 5:282-92, 1986.
46. Netzer T, Knauf H, Mutschler E: Modulation of electrolyte excretion by potassium retaining diuretics, *Eur Heart J* 13 Suppl G:22-27, 1992.
47. Colussi G, Rombola G, De Ferrari ME, Macaluso M, Minetti L: Correction of hypokalemia with antialdosterone therapy in Gitelman's syndrome, *Am J Nephrol* 14:127-35, 1994.

48. Bundy JT, Connito D, Mahoney MD, Pontier PJ: Treatment of idiopathic renal magnesium wasting with amiloride, *Am J Nephrol* 15:75-77, 1995.
49. Gitelman HJ, Graham JB, Welt LG: A new familial disorder characterized by hypokalemia and hypomagnesemia, *Trans Assoc Am Physicians* 79:221-35, 1966.
50. Rodriguez-Soriano J, Vallo A, Garcia-Fuentes M: Hypomagnesaemia of hereditary renal origin, *Pediatr Nephrol* 1:465-72, 1987.
51. Bettinelli A, Bianchetti MG, Girardin E, Caringella A, et al: Use of calcium excretion values to distinguish two forms of primary renal tubular hypokalemic alkalosis: Bartter and Gitelman syndromes, *J Pediatr* 120:38-43, 1992.
52. Bartter FC, Pronove P, Gill JR Jr, MacCardle RC: Hyperplasia of the juxtaglomerular complex with hyperaldosteronism and hypokalemic alkalosis. A new syndrome. 1962, *J Am Soc Nephrol* 9:516-28, 1998.
53. Simon DB, Nelson-Williams C, Bia MJ, Ellison D, et al: Gitelman's variant of Bartter's syndrome, inherited hypokalaemic alkalosis, is caused by mutations in the thiazide-sensitive Na-Cl cotransporter, *Nat Genet* 12:24-30, 1996.
54. Luthy C, Bettinelli A, Iselin S, Metta MG, et al: Normal prostaglandinuria E2 in Gitelman's syndrome, the hypocalciuric variant of Bartter's syndrome, *Am J Kidney Dis* 25:824-28, 1995.
55. Meij IC, Koenderink JB, van Bokhoven H, Assink KF, et al: Dominant isolated renal magnesium loss is caused by misrouting of the Na(+),K(+)-ATPase gamma-subunit, *Nat Genet* 26:265-66, 2000.
56. Geven WB, Monnens LA, Willems HL, Buijs WC, ter Haar BG: Renal magnesium wasting in two families with autosomal dominant inheritance, *Kidney Int* 31:1140-44, 1987.
57. Meij IC, Koenderink JB, De Jong JC, De Pont JJ, et al: Dominant isolated renal magnesium loss is caused by misrouting of the Na^+,K^+-ATPase gamma-subunit, *Ann N Y Acad Sci* 986:437-43, 2003.
58. Meij IC, Saar K, van den Heuvel LP, Nuernberg G, et al: Hereditary isolated renal magnesium loss maps to chromosome 11q23, *Am J Hum Genet* 64:180-88, 1999.
59. Sweadner KJ, Arystarkhova E, Donnet C, Wetzel RK: FXYD proteins as regulators of the Na,K-ATPase in the kidney, *Ann N Y Acad Sci* 986:382-87, 2003.
60. Arystarkhova E, Wetzel RK, Sweadner KJ: Distribution and oligomeric association of splice forms of Na(+)-K(+)-ATPase regulatory gamma-subunit in rat kidney, *Am J Physiol Renal Physiol* 282:F393-407, 2002.
61. Arystarkhova E, Donnet C, Asinovski NK, Sweadner KJ: Differential regulation of renal Na,K-ATPase by splice variants of the gamma subunit, *J Biol Chem* 277:10162-72, 2002.
62. Blostein R, Pu HX, Scanzano R, Zouzoulas A: Structure/function studies of the gamma subunit of the Na,K-ATPase, *Ann N Y Acad Sci* 986:420-27, 2003.
63. Meij IC, Van Den Heuvel LP, Hemmes S, Van Der Vliet WA, et al: Exclusion of mutations in FXYD2, CLDN16 and SLC12A3 in two families with primary renal Mg(2+) loss, *Nephrol Dial Transplant* 18:512-16, 2003.
64. Jones DH, Li TY, Arystarkhova E, Barr KJ, et al: Na,K-ATPase from mice lacking the gamma subunit (FXYD2) exhibits altered Na^+ affinity and decreased thermal stability, *J Biol Chem* 280:19003-11, 2005.
65. Nijenhuis T, Vallon V, van der Kemp AW, Loffing J, et al: Enhanced passive Ca2+ reabsorption and reduced Mg2+ channel abundance explains thiazide-induced hypocalciuria and hypomagnesemia, *J Clin Invest* 115:1651-58, 2005.
66. Geven WB, Monnens LA, Willems JL, Buijs W, Hamel CJ: Isolated autosomal recessive renal magnesium loss in two sisters, *Clin Genet* 32:398-402, 1987.
67. Brown EM, Gamba G, Riccardi D, Lombardi M, et al: Cloning and characterization of an extracellular Ca(2+)-sensing receptor from bovine parathyroid, *Nature* 366:575-80, 1993.
68. Riccardi D, Lee WS, Lee K, Segre GV, et al: Localization of the extracellular Ca(2+)-sensing receptor and PTH/PTHrP receptor in rat kidney, *Am J Physiol* 271:F951-56, 1996.
69. Hebert SC: Extracellular calcium-sensing receptor: implications for calcium and magnesium handling in the kidney, *Kidney Int* 50:2129-39, 1996.
70. Pollak MR, Brown EM, Estep HL, McLaine PN, et al: Autosomal dominant hypocalcaemia caused by a Ca(2+)-sensing receptor gene mutation, *Nat Genet* 8:303-07, 1994.
71. Pearce SH, Williamson C, Kifor O, Bai M, et al: A familial syndrome of hypocalcemia with hypercalciuria due to mutations in the calcium-sensing receptor [see comments], *N Engl J Med* 335:1115-22, 1996.
72. Vargas-Poussou R, Huang C, Hulin P, Houillier P, et al: Functional characterization of a calcium-sensing receptor mutation in severe autosomal dominant hypocalcemia with a Bartter-like syndrome, *J Am Soc Nephrol* 13:2259-66, 2002.
73. Watanabe S, Fukumoto S, Chang H, Takeuchi Y, et al: Association between activating mutations of calcium-sensing receptor and Bartter's syndrome, *Lancet* 360:692-94, 2002.
74. Pollak MR, Brown EM, Chou YH, Hebert SC, et al: Mutations in the human Ca(2+)-sensing receptor gene cause familial hypocalciuric hypercalcemia and neonatal severe hyperparathyroidism, *Cell* 75:1297-303, 1993.
75. Marx SJ, Attie MF, Levine MA, Spiegel AM, et al: The hypocalciuric or benign variant of familial hypercalcemia: clinical and biochemical features in fifteen kindreds, *Medicine (Baltimore)* 60:397-412, 1981.
76. Cole DE, Janicic N, Salisbury SR, Hendy GN: Neonatal severe hyperparathyroidism, secondary hyperparathyroidism, and familial hypocalciuric hypercalcemia: multiple different phenotypes associated with an inactivating Alu insertion mutation of the calcium-sensing receptor gene, *Am J Med Genet* 71:202-10, 1997.
77. Praga M, Vara J, Gonzalez-Parra E, Andres A, et al: Familial hypomagnesemia with hypercalciuria and nephrocalcinosis, *Kidney Int* 47:1419-25, 1995.
78. Rodriguez-Soriano J, Vallo A: Pathophysiology of the renal acidification defect present in the syndrome of familial hypomagnesaemia-hypercalciuria, *Pediatr Nephrol* 8:431-35, 1994.
79. Benigno V, Canonica CS, Bettinelli A, von Vigier RO, et al: Hypomagnesaemia-hypercalciuria-nephrocalcinosis: a report of nine cases and a review, *Nephrol Dial Transplant* 15:605-10, 2000.
80. Weber S, Schneider L, Peters M, Misselwitz J, et al: Novel paracellin-1 mutations in 25 families with familial hypomagnesemia with hypercalciuria and nephrocalcinosis, *J Am Soc Nephrol* 12:1872-81, 2001.
81. Zimmermann B, Plank C, Konrad M, Stohr W, et al: Hydrochlorothiazide in CLDN16 mutation. *Nephrol Dial Transplant* 21:2127-32, 2006.
82. Simon DB, Lu Y, Choate KA, Velazquez H, et al: Paracellin-1, a renal tight junction protein required for paracellular Mg2+ resorption, *Science* 285:103-06, 1999.
83. Colegio OR, Van Itallie C, Rahner C, Anderson JM: Claudin extracellular domains determine paracellular charge selectivity and resistance but not tight junction fibril architecture, *Am J Physiol Cell Physiol* 284:C1346-54, 2003.
84. Ohba Y, Kitagawa H, Kitoh K, Sasaki Y, et al: A deletion of the paracellin-1 gene is responsible for renal tubular dysplasia in cattle, *Genomics* 68:229-36, 2000.
85. Meij IC, van den Heuvel LP, Knoers NV: Genetic disorders of magnesium homeostasis, *Biometals* 15:297-307, 2002.
86. Blanchard A, Jeunemaitre X, Coudol P, Dechaux M, et al: Paracellin-1 is critical for magnesium and calcium reabsorption in the human thick ascending limb of Henle, *Kidney Int* 59:2206-15, 2001.
87. Muller D, Kausalya PJ, Claverie-Martin F, Meij IC, et al: A novel claudin 16 mutation associated with childhood hypercalciuria abolishes binding to ZO-1 and results in lysosomal mistargeting, *Am J Hum Genet* 73:1293-301, 2003.
88. Wong V, Goodenough DA: Paracellular channels!, *Science* 285:62, 1999.
89. Hou J, Paul DL, Goodenough DA: Paracellin-1 and the modulation of ion selectivity of tight junctions, *J Cell Sci* 118:5109-18, 2005.
90. Lee DB, Huang E, Ward HJ: Tight junction biology and kidney dysfunction, *Am J Physiol Renal Physiol* 290:F20-34, 2006.
91. Hirano T, Kobayashi N, Itoh T, Takasuga A, et al: Null mutation of PCLN-1/Claudin-16 results in bovine chronic interstitial nephritis, *Genome Res* 10:659-63, 2000.

92. Sasaki Y, Kitagawa H, Kitoh K, Okura Y, et al: Pathological changes of renal tubular dysplasia in Japanese black cattle, *Vet Rec* 150:628-32, 2002.
93. Konrad M, Schaller A, Seelow D, Pandey AV, et al: Mutations in the tight-junction gene claudin 19 (CLDN19) are associated with renal magnesium wasting, renal failure, and severe ocular involvement, *Am J Hum Genet* 79:949-57, 2006.
94. Paunier L, Radde IC, Kooh SW, Conen PE, Fraser D: Primary hypomagnesemia with secondary hypocalcemia in an infant, *Pediatrics* 41:385-402, 1968.
95. Anast CS, Mohs JM, Kaplan SL, Burns TW: Evidence for parathyroid failure in magnesium deficiency, *Science* 177:606-08, 1972.
96. Shalev H, Phillip M, Galil A, Carmi R, Landau D: Clinical presentation and outcome in primary familial hypomagnesaemia, *Arch Dis Child* 78:127-30, 1998.
97. Lombeck I, Ritzl F, Schnippering HG, Michael H, et al: Primary hypomagnesemia. I. Absorption studies, *Z Kinderheilkd* 118:249-58, 1975.
98. Milla PJ, Aggett PJ, Wolff OH, Harries JT: Studies in primary hypomagnesaemia: evidence for defective carrier-mediated small intestinal transport of magnesium, *Gut* 20:1028-33, 1979.
99. Matzkin H, Lotan D, Boichis H: Primary hypomagnesemia with a probable double magnesium transport defect, *Nephron* 52:83-86, 1989.
100. Walder RY, Shalev H, Brennan TM, Carmi R, et al: Familial hypomagnesemia maps to chromosome 9q, not to the X chromosome: genetic linkage mapping and analysis of a balanced translocation breakpoint, *Hum Mol Genet* 6:1491-97, 1997.
101. Schlingmann KP, Weber S, Peters M, Niemann Nejsum L, et al: Hypomagnesemia with secondary hypocalcemia is caused by mutations in TRPM6, a new member of the TRPM gene family, *Nat Genet* 31:166-70, 2002.
102. Walder RY, Landau D, Meyer P, Shalev H, et al: Mutation of TRPM6 causes familial hypomagnesemia with secondary hypocalcemia, *Nat Genet* 31:171-74, 2002.
103. Schlingmann KP, Sassen MC, Weber S, Pechmann U, et al: Novel TRPM6 mutations in 21 families with primary hypomagnesemia and secondary hypocalcemia, *J Am Soc Nephrol* 16:3061-69, 2005.
104. Jalkanen R, Pronicka E, Tyynismaa H, Hanauer A, et al: Genetic background of HSH in three Polish families and a patient with an X;9 translocation, *Eur J Hum Genet* 14:55-62, 2006.
105. Nadler MJ, Hermosura MC, Inabe K, Perraud AL, et al: LTRPC7 is a Mg.ATP-regulated divalent cation channel required for cell viability, *Nature* 411:590-95, 2001.
106. Voets T, Nilius B, Hoefs S, van der Kemp AW, et al: TRPM6 forms the Mg2+ influx channel involved in intestinal and renal Mg2+ absorption, *J Biol Chem* 279:19-25, 2003.
107. Cole DE, Quamme GA: Inherited disorders of renal magnesium handling, *J Am Soc Nephrol* 11:1937-47, 2000.
108. Chubanov V, Waldegger S, Mederos y Schnitzler M, Vitzthum H, et al: Disruption of TRPM6/TRPM7 complex formation by a mutation in the TRPM6 gene causes hypomagnesemia with secondary hypocalcemia, *Proc Natl Acad Sci U S A* 101:2894-99, 2004.
109. Schmitz C, Dorovkov MV, Zhao X, Davenport BJ, et al: The channel kinases TRPM6 and TRPM7 are functionally nonredundant, *J Biol Chem* 280:37763-71, 2005.
110. Wilson FH, Hariri A, Farhi A, Zhao H, et al: A cluster of metabolic defects caused by mutation in a mitochondrial tRNA, *Science* 306:1190-94, 2004.

CHAPTER 31

Renal Tubular Acidosis

Manjula Gowrishankar and Maury Pinsk

INTRODUCTION

Under normal physiologic conditions, an individual consuming a typical Western diet will generate approximately 1 mmol/kg/day of hydrogen ion (H^+) from metabolism and food.[1] These H^+ are buffered by intracellular and extracellular buffers to maintain homeostasis. This process will progressively deplete these buffers, including bicarbonate (HCO_3^-), and the individual will develop metabolic acidosis unless the buffers are returned to previous levels. The kidney returns the body buffers to normal with the use of two processes:

1. *Reclaiming all of the filtered* HCO_3^-. This will not allow for further loss of HCO_3^-; however, it will not replenish the quantity of HCO_3^- that went to buffer the added H^+.
2. *Excreting the added* H^+ *as ammonium (major contributor [approximately 80%]) or with filtered buffers such as phosphate and creatinine (minor contributors)*. This will result in the regeneration of HCO_3^-, which was used to buffer the added H^+.

Thus, both processes together will return the body HCO_3^- level back to normal, and the individual will maintain his or her acid-base homeostasis.

When either of the two mechanisms is impaired, there is a renal cause for the metabolic acidosis, and it is called *renal tubular acidosis* (RTA). RTA is characterized by the presence of hyperchloremic metabolic acidosis with a normal anion gap. The majority of the children will have a normal glomerular filtration rate. Complications of RTA include failure to thrive, growth retardation, osteopenia, rickets, nephrocalcinosis, nephrolithiasis, and renal failure.

This chapter is divided into three sections: the physiology of renal HCO_3^- reabsorption and H^+ secretion; the classification of RTA, which includes diagnostic testing; and case illustrations.

PHYSIOLOGY WITH MOLECULAR INSIGHTS

The daily filtered load of HCO_3^- is approximately 4500 mmol (glomerular filtration rate, 180 L/day; plasma [HCO_3^-], 25 mmol/L). Of this, approximately 80% to 90% (3600 to 4050 mmol) is reabsorbed by the proximal tubule, 10% to 15% (450 to 675 mmol) by the loop of Henle, and 3% to 5% (135 to 225 mmol) by the distal tubule, including the cortical collecting duct (CCD). The excretion of added H^+ as ammonium and phosphate resulting in the addition of HCO_3^- (1 mmol/kg/day) to the body occurs in the collecting tubules. Thus, the proximal tubule functions as the bulk reabsorber, whereas the distal nephron's function is to fine-tune acid-base homeostasis.

Mechanism of Bicarbonate Reabsorption in the Proximal Tubule and the Loop of Henle

Figure 31-1 illustrates the mechanism of and the transporters involved in HCO_3^- reabsorption in the proximal tubule. This is an indirect process via H^+ secretion. H^+ and HCO_3^- are generated inside the cell from carbon dioxide (CO_2) and water (H_2O). This is facilitated by carbonic anhydrase type II. Approximately two thirds of the H^+ exit the cell into the lumen via the sodium (Na^+)/H^+ exchanger (NHE-3), whereas the remainder do so via the H^+-ATPase pump.[2,3] The energy for NHE-3 is provided by Na^+/K^+-ATPase, which is a pump in the basolateral membrane. This pump maintains a low Na^+ concentration and a negative potential within the cell, both of which favor Na^+ entry into the cell via NHE-3. This passive Na^+ entry drives H^+ secretion against a concentration gradient. Angiotensin II is a potent stimulator of NHE-3.

After H^+ enters the lumen, it binds to the filtered HCO_3^-, forming carbonic acid (H_2CO_3), which is rapidly dehydrated to CO_2 and H_2O by the luminal carbonic anhydrase type IV. The H_2O and CO_2 diffuse back into the cell to keep this whole process active. By the end of the proximal tubule, the fluid pH has only fallen by approximately 0.6 units from 7.40 in the filtrate.[4] This is achieved by the presence of carbonic anhydrase type IV, which enhances the secretion of H^+ into the lumen. When a carbonic anhydrase inhibitor is used, this effect is inhibited; the patient then has bicarbonaturia and may develop metabolic acidosis with a normal anion gap.

The HCO_3^- that is formed within the cell exits via the basolateral Na^+-HCO_3^- cotransporter and, to a minor extent, via the chlorine (Cl^-)-HCO_3^- exchanger.[5]

The net result of H^+ secretion is the removal of filtered HCO_3^-; the process is neutral, without a net gain or loss of HCO_3^-. For example, if 5 mmol/L of HCO_3^- went to buffer the H^+ added to the body (thereby resulting in a fall in the plasma HCO_3^- concentration to 20 from 25 mmol/L), even if all of the HCO_3^- filtered is reabsorbed, the HCO_3^- concentration in the plasma will still only be 20 mmol/L rather than 25 mmol/L.

Proximal H^+ secretion is enhanced by increased extracellular pH, hypokalemia, decreased effective circulating

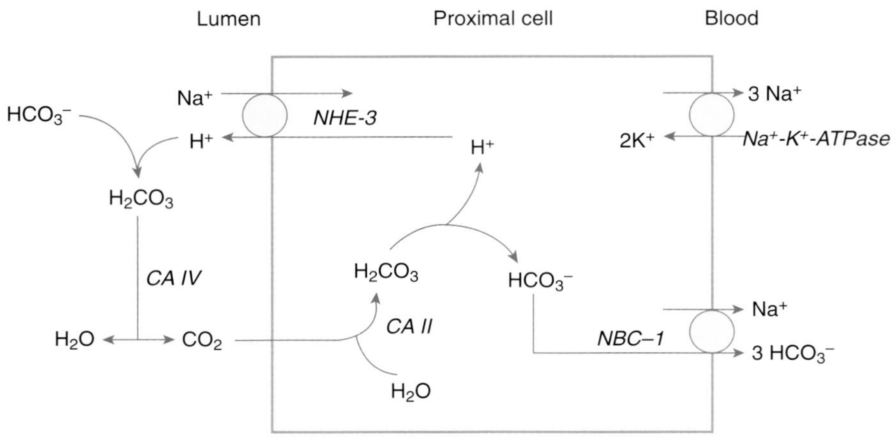

Figure 31-1 Model of proximal tubular bicarbonate reabsorption.

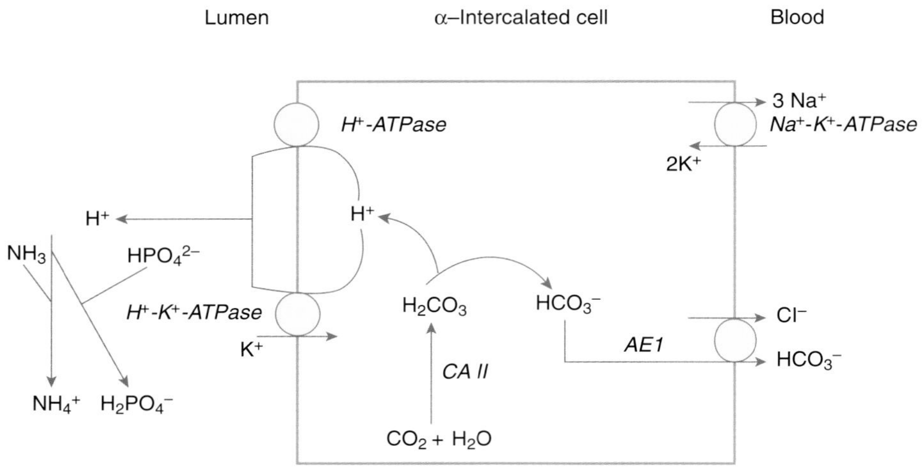

Figure 31-2 Model of cortical collecting duct hydrogen ion secretion.

volume, angiotensin II, increased peritubular partial pressure of carbon dioxide (pCO_2), and several other factors.[6] NHE-3 appears to be the major transport protein for the reabsorption of HCO_3^- in the thick ascending limb of the loop of Henle by a similar mechanism.[7]

Mechanism of Hydrogen Ion Secretion in the Distal Nephron

The vast majority of H^+ secretion occurs in the collecting duct.[8] The CCD is the main segment involved, although the medullary collecting duct also contributes. The CCD has principal cells and intercalated cells. The principal cells are responsible for Na^+ reabsorption and K^+ secretion; α intercalated cells are responsible for H^+ secretion, and β intercalated cells are responsible for HCO_3^- secretion. β intercalated cells are almost the mirror image of α intercalated cells. Experimental studies in animal CCDs have shown that metabolic acidosis causes a reduction in the number of β intercalated cells as well as a reversal of their polarity such that HCO_3^- secretion occurs through the basolateral membrane, thus adding more HCO_3^- to the blood.[9]

Figure 31-2 illustrates the mechanism and transporters involved in H^+ secretion in the CCD. Just like in the proximal tubule, H^+ and HCO_3^- are generated inside the cell from CO_2 and H_2O. This is facilitated by carbonic anhydrase type II. Most of the H^+ is secreted into the lumen via H^+-ATPase.[8] This secretion is enhanced and the back diffusion of H^+ lowered by the electronegativity of the lumen, because H^+ is a positive ion. The electronegative potential of the lumen is created as a result of electrogenic Na^+ reabsorption by the adjacent principal cells. Thus, if for some reason the electronegative potential in the lumen is reduced such that it is relatively more positive, H^+ secretion will be impaired. In low effective circulating volume states, the amount of Na^+ delivered to the principal cell is so low that, even if most of it is reabsorbed, the electronegative potential generated is not adequate to facilitate H^+ secretion. H^+K^+-ATPase is another pump that is involved in H^+ secretion into the lumen and that exchanges H^+ for K^+. This appears to play an active role in K^+ homeostasis (i.e., in hypokalemic states) but not in acid–base homeostasis.[10]

After H^+ enters the lumen, it is very quickly buffered by ammonia (NH_3) and monohydrogen phosphate (HPO_4^{2-}) to form ammonium (NH_4^+) and titratable acid ($H_2PO_4^-$). Net acid excretion is the sum of NH_4^+ and $H_2PO_4^-$, which results in the removal of H^+, thereby promoting further H^+ secretion into the lumen. Some of the secreted H^+ binds to the small fraction of filtered HCO_3^- (<5%) that was not reabsorbed by the upstream nephron segments. The HCO_3^- formed within the cell exits via the Cl^--HCO_3^- exchanger.[2,8,11]

Thus, H^+ secretion in this segment results in the following two changes:

1. The reabsorption of the final quantity of the filtered HCO_3^-, which, in body terms, is neutral in that there is no net addition or loss of HCO_3^-
2. The excretion of H^+ in the form of NH_4^+ and $H_2PO_4^-$, which results in a net gain of HCO_3^- so that the HCO_3^- concentration in the body is returned to its baseline

H^+ secretion is enhanced by systemic acidosis, increased peritubular pCO_2, higher transepithelial potential difference (TEPD; which depends on distal Na delivery and aldosterone activity), aldosterone, and hypokalemia.

Ammonium Excretion

The major urinary buffer that maintains the acid–base balance is NH_3, because buffering by HPO_4^{2-} is limited. Therefore, the kidney is able to adapt to an acid load mainly by increasing NH_4^+ excretion. With an acid load, NH_4^+ excretion starts to increase within 2 hours as a result of increased NH_3 transfer in the interstitium due to a higher H^+ secretion in the CCD and the medullary collecting duct. In chronic acidosis, the NH_4^+ excretion rate can increase by five- to sixfold, and maximum excretion is achieved at 5 to 6 days as a result of increased NH_4^+ production.[12] The mechanisms involved in achieving this include the production, secretion, reabsorption, and recycling of NH_4^+; this allows for a high concentration of NH_3 in the cortical and medullary interstitium, which will promote the easy diffusion of NH_3 into the lumen of the CCD and the medullary collecting duct to bind the secreted H^+ to form NH_4^+ and be excreted in the final urine. NH_4^+ excretion will be discussed later in this chapter, and the mechanism is illustrated in Figure 31-3.

Production and Secretion

NH_4^+ is produced within the proximal cell from the metabolism of primarily glutamine. The net result is that one HCO_3^- is generated and added to the body when one NH_4^+ is produced and excreted. NH_4^+ exits via the luminal NHE-3,[13] whereas HCO_3^- exits via the basolateral Na^+-HCO_3^- cotransporter. NH_4^+ production is tied to adenosine triphosphate production. Most of the adenosine triphosphate produced within the proximal cell is used during Na^+ reabsorption. Thus, when there is a decreased glomerular filtration rate that results in a reduction in the amount of filtered load of Na^+ and therefore a reduction in the amount of Na^+ reabsorbed by the cell, NH_4^+ production is also reduced. In addition, because glutamine is the major source of NH_4^+ production, if the supply of glutamine is reduced or the supply of fat-derived fuels is increased, such as is the case with total parenteral nutrition, NH_4^+ production is also reduced, which results in total-parenteral-nutrition–associated metabolic acidosis. Glutamine has to enter the mitochondria for the production of NH_4^+. This entry and further metabolism by phosphate-dependent glutaminase appear to be enhanced by chronic metabolic acidosis and hypokalemia but inhibited by hyperkalemia. Aldosterone appears to enhance NH_4^+ production, but whether it is a direct effect or the result of hypokalemia is unknown. A detailed review of these processes is discussed by Halperin and colleagues.[14] One can also appreciate from this physiology the metabolic acidosis with a normal anion gap that may be seen in some mitochondrial diseases.

Medullary Recycling

Both NH_4^+ (by active secretion, because it is lipid insoluble) and NH_3 (by passive diffusion) enter the proximal tubular cell lumen after being produced. There is a potential for NH_3 to be lost via the peritubular capillary, because it can diffuse out through the basolateral membrane. In addition, a high concentration of NH_3 is needed in the medullary interstitium to diffuse into the lumen of the collecting duct to form NH_4^+ when H^+ is secreted. Thus, 75% of the tubular NH_4^+ recycles within the medulla. The NH_4^+ that is produced and secreted by the proximal cell is reabsorbed in the thick ascending limb of loop of Henle via the Na^+-K^+-$2Cl^-$ cotransporter, where

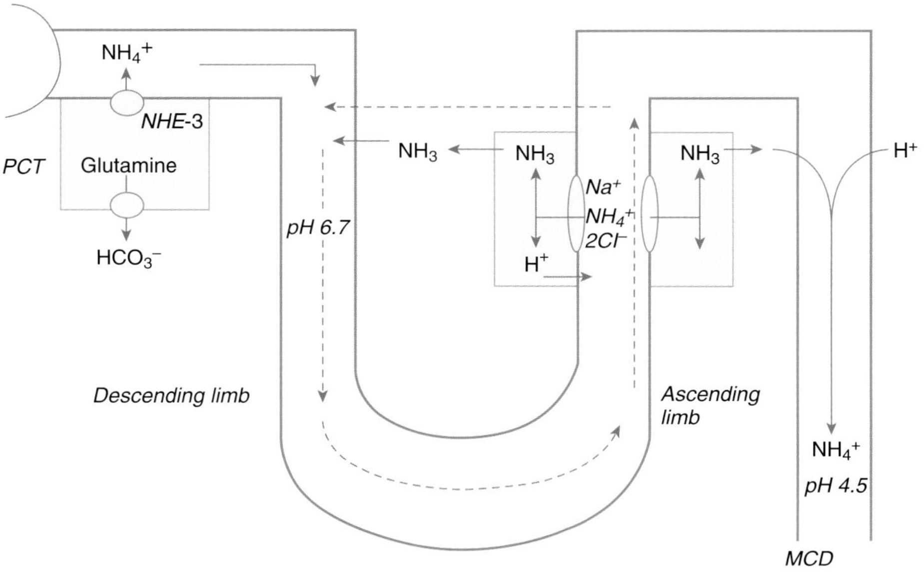

Figure 31-3 Model of NH_4^+ production, secretion, and excretion. The dashed lines show how NH_3 recycles. Refer to the text for details.

NH_4^+ takes the place of K^+.[15] After it is inside the cell, NH_4^+ dissociates to form NH_3 and H^+. The H^+ is secreted back into the lumen via mostly NHE-3, and it reclaims the filtered HCO_3^- that was not reabsorbed by the proximal cell. Because the luminal membrane is not permeable to NH_3, it diffuses out into the medullary interstitium through the basolateral membrane. From here, NH_3 will diffuse into those compartments that have low concentrations of NH_3, namely the S3 segment and the early descending limb of loop of Henle, which results in recycling. Hyperkalemia can lead to reduced NH_4^+ reabsorption in the thick ascending limb, most likely as a result of competition for the site on the Na^+-K^+-$2Cl^-$ cotransporter. In such a situation, correction of the hyperkalemia will lead to normal NH_4^+ excretion as a result of removing the inhibition for NH_4^+ production in the proximal cell as well as recycling. If the interstitium is diseased, a high concentration of NH_3 may not be achieved, thus resulting in low NH_4^+ excretion. An intact medullary interstitium and Na^+-K^+-$2Cl^-$ cotransporter function are important for achieving maximum urinary osmolality. Hence, an important clue in these individuals is that they have low urine osmolality, and they will not be able to attain maximum osmolality when deprived of water.

Secretion into the Cortical Collecting Duct and the Medullary Collecting Duct

The secreted H^+ in these segments is buffered by the luminal NH_3, resulting in low NH_3 concentration within the lumen. This results in a favorable concentration gradient for NH_3 to diffuse from the interstitium into the lumen, and the cycle continues. When there is an insufficient quantity of NH_3 as a result of hyperkalemia, NH_4^+ excretion falls, and the urine pH rises as the secretion of H^+ falls due to a reduction in buffering, which will normally create a favorable concentration gradient for H^+ secretion. That H^+ secretion is intact is confirmed when an acid load results in the maximal acidification of the urine.

Ontogeny of Bicarbonate Reabsorption and Hydrogen Ion Secretion

In newborns, the plasma HCO_3^- concentration is lower than that of adults. However, during the postnatal period, the concentration continues to increase, and, generally by the age of 2 years, the level is the same as that of an adult. This has been shown to be the result of a maturational increase in the expression, distribution, and activity of all of the acid–base transporters discussed previously.[16,17] Corticosteroids accelerate some of these processes.

CLASSIFICATION

Metabolic acidosis is divided into two categories on the basis of a normal or increased anion gap. The anion gap is the difference in the plasma concentration between measured cations and measured anions. This is depicted in the following equation:

$$\text{Anion gap} = [Na^+] + [K^+] - [Cl^-] + [HCO_3^-]$$

Anion gap is the result of unmeasured anions in the plasma, and, under normal physiologic conditions, the majority of these anions are from the negative charge on albumin. The normal anion gap ranges from 8 to 16 mmol/L. However, if the albumin level is low, the anion gap will also be low. Generally, there is a 4 mmol/L decrease in anion gap for every 10 g/L decrease in albumin concentration. Unmeasured anion is the result of an acid being added (endogenous or exogenous) to the body where the anion is not chloride and the anion is not completely excreted so that it remains in the body and raises the anion gap.

RTA is a disorder in which the anion gap is normal because there is no addition of an unmeasured anion. The chloride concentration increases proportionally to the decrease in bicarbonate concentration as a result of the renal tubule reabsorbing more chloride to balance electrical neutrality when it absorbs sodium.

RTA has been traditionally classified into three major types: proximal RTA (type 2); distal RTA (type 1); and RTA with hyperkalemia (type 4). However, as can be appreciated from the previous discussion, classifying RTA on the basis of impaired HCO_3^- reabsorption and impaired NH_4^+ excretion allows for a better understanding of the type of RTA on the basis of the physiology of renal H^+ secretion. This approach will also help to broaden the scope of the diagnosis, because one or more segments of the nephron may be affected when giving rise to HCO_3^- loss or reduced NH_4^+ excretion.

Impaired Hydrogen Ion Secretion in the Proximal Tubule

Because the bulk of HCO_3^- reabsorption occurs in the proximal tubule, when there is bicarbonaturia, the culprits are the proximal cell and the lumen. The proximal cell may only have a disorder of H^+ secretion (isolated), or it may, in addition, have other transport defects, such as aminoaciduria, glycosuria, phosphaturia, and uricaciduria (Fanconi syndrome). Table 31-1 provides a differential diagnosis, but it is by no means complete. In steady state, these patients with chronic metabolic acidosis will have low urine pH (no bicarbonaturia). This is because the filtered load of HCO_3^- in a

TABLE 31-1 Causes of Impaired Hydrogen Ion Secretion in the Proximal Tubule

Proximal hydrogen ion secretion defect
1. Primary isolated
   a. Autosomal dominant
   b. Autosomal recessive with ocular anomaly
   c. Defect in sodium-bicarbonate cotransporter NBC-1
2. Secondary
   a. Fanconi syndrome
   b. Genetic disorders such as cystinosis, galactosemia, tyrosinemia, Lowe's syndrome, Wilson's disease, and fructose intolerance
   c. Toxin- and drug-induced disorders such as heavy metals, aminoglycosides, ifosfamide, mercaptopurine, outdated tetracycline, and multiple myeloma

Carbonic anhydrase II deficiency (combined proximal and distal cell dysfunction)

Carbonic anhydrase inhibitors

Other associated conditions such as vitamin D deficiency and hyperparathyroidism patient with normal glomerular filtration rate and a plasma HCO_3^- concentration of 15 mmol/L (180 L × 15 mmol/L = 2700 mmol/day) is a lot lower than normal (180 L × 25 mmol/L = 4500 mmol/day) and falls within the reabsorptive capacity of the loop of Henle and the distal nephron. The excretion of NH_4^+ is borderline. This may be the result of a defect in the basolateral Na^+-HCO_3^- cotransporter, which causes HCO_3^- to remain within the cell (proximal cell alkalosis) and results in an inhibition of NH_4^+ production or impaired NH_4^+ secretion as a result of a defect in NHE-3 (see Figure 31-1). Filtered citrate is reabsorbed by the proximal cell to produce HCO_3^- when there is acidosis. Thus, citrate level in the urine is very low in other types of RTA. However, in the case of proximal cell dysfunction, citrate is not reabsorbed, and the measurement of citrate in the urine helps to identify whether there is a proximal cell dysfunction. Because citrate is an inhibitor of stone formation, patients with proximal cell dysfunction tend to not have nephrolithiasis unless they also have Fanconi syndrome.

Diagnostic Tests

1. Urine pH is low because there is no distal H^+ secretion problem.
2. Urine NH_4^+ excretion is normal to borderline.
3. Urine citrate excretion is normal or high.
4. Confirmatory test: Administer $NaHCO_3$ 1 mmol/kg either intravenously or orally, and monitor urine pH and plasma HCO_3^- concentration. If, after bicarbonate administration, the urine pH is ≥7 whereas the plasma HCO_3^- is only partially corrected (<22 mmol/L) or if a large quantity of $NaHCO_3$ is required to maintain near-normal serum HCO_3^- concentration while the urine pH increases to 7, there is a proximal defect in H^+ secretion. One can calculate the fractional excretion of HCO_3^- by the formula below, and it will be ≥15%:

$$\text{Fractional excretion} = \frac{\text{Urine}\left[HCO_3^-\right]/\text{Plasma}\left[HCO_3^-\right]}{\text{Urine}\left[\text{creatinine}\right]/\text{Plasma}\left[\text{creatinine}\right]}$$

5. There may be generalized proximal cell dysfunction with aminoaciduria, glycosuria, phosphaturia, and uricaciduria.

Impaired NH_4^+ Excretion

This condition may be as a result of a low NH_3 concentration in the medullary interstitium and/or a low H^+ secretion in the distal nephron.[18] This is traditionally considered to be distal RTA.

Low NH3 Concentration in the Medulla

This may be a result of low NH_4^+ production in the proximal cell as a result of a variety of reasons as can be seen from Table 31-2 and Figure 31-3. These patients have a low urine pH; this indicates a normal H^+ secretion, which can be appreciated by the equation:

$$NH_3 + H^+ \rightarrow NH_4^+$$

Because the NH_4^+ excretion is already known to be low, urine pH will indicate whether this is a low NH_3 problem or a low H^+ secretion problem. If there is no defect in H^+ secretion, the urine pH will be low. If the urine pH is low, there is a defect in either NH_4^+ production by the proximal cell, a defect in the reabsorption of NH_4^+ (recycling), or a combination of the two. The former is seen in patients with low glomerular filtration rates or patients receiving total parenteral nutrition, which is why most patients receiving total parenteral nutrition develop metabolic acidosis if acetate or citrate is not added to the total parenteral nutrition.[19] Recycling can be defective in medullary interstitial diseases such as pyelonephritis and sickle cell disease. A combined defect in the production and recycling of NH_4^+ can be seen in a patient with hyperkalemia.

TABLE 31-2 Causes of Low NH_4^+ Excretion

1. Low NH_3 concentration in the medullary interstitium
    a. Low NH_4^+ production in the proximal convoluted tubule
        i. Low glomerular filtration rate
        ii. Total parenteral nutrition
        iii. Hyperkalemia
        iv. A defect in cotransporter NBC-1 causing the proximal convoluted tubule to be alkaline
    b. Low NH_4^+ recycling
        i. Hyperkalemia
        ii. Tubulointerstitial disease (e.g., pyelonephritis, renal transplant rejection)
        iii. Medullary destruction (e.g., sickle cell disease, medullary sponge kidney)
2. Low hydrogen ion secretion in the distal nephron
    a. Defect in hydrogen ion-ATPase function
        i. Mutation in gene encoding the protein; sporadic or inherited as autosomal-recessive trait with or without deafness
        ii. Inadequate number (e.g., medullary destruction, obstructive uropathy, medullary sponge kidney)
        iii. Inhibition by autoimmune diseases (e.g., Sjögren's syndrome)
        iv. Low transepithelial potential difference with amiloride, trimethoprim, cyclosporine, Gordon syndrome, lithium, and low extracellular fluid volume states
        v. Low aldosterone activity (e.g., congenital adrenal hyperplasia, therapy with angiotensin-converting enzyme inhibitors or angiotensin receptor blockers)
    b. Defect in chloride-bicarbonate exchanger AE-1
        i. Autosomal dominant
    c. Back leak of secreted hydrogen ions
        i. Amphotericin B

Low Hydrogen Ion Secretion in the Distal Nephron

If the urine pH is high (>5.5) when there is systemic acidosis, there is a H^+ secretion problem, or the secreted H^+ leaks out of the lumen and back into the cell. Table 31-2 lists the causes, and Figure 31-2 illustrates the mechanisms.

One of the reasons for impaired H^+ secretion is a defect in H^+-ATPase function. This may be sporadic or inherited (autosomal recessive) and with or without sensorineural deafness. Most sporadic cases and cases of the inherited form without deafness appear to be caused by mutations in the gene that encodes the 116-kD subunit of H^+-ATPase; this is the most common primary distal RTA among children.[20] Where there is deafness, the mutations appear to be in the gene encoding the β1-subunit of H^+-ATPase.[21] These patients will have low urine pCO_2 when given an alkali load (described later).

Secondary or acquired forms of defective function of H^+-ATPase are the result of medullary destruction as seen in tubulointerstitial disease, possible inhibition or deficiency of H^+-ATPase in Sjögren's syndrome, and low TEPD states. Transepithelial potential difference is the difference in the electrical charge within the cell versus that of the lumen. When this difference is high, it means that there is more negative charge in the lumen, thus favoring H^+ (positive charge) secretion. When the difference is low, H^+ secretion is impaired. A low TEPD may be the result of low Na^+ delivery to the principal cell of the CCD or high Na^+ concentration within the lumen of the CCD as a result of the inhibition of Na^+ reabsorption by the epithelial Na^+ channel. When there is a low Na^+ delivery to the principal cell, the amount of Na^+ available for electrogenic reabsorption (which generates the negative voltage in the lumen) is low. Thus, TEPD is low in these states. A low Na^+ delivery may be the result of a low effective circulating volume state (nephrotic syndrome, congestive heart failure, cirrhosis) or of hyperabsorption by the upstream Na-Cl cotransporter in the distal tubule, such as is seen in Gordon syndrome[22] and possibly with the use of cyclosporine (discussed later). Low TEPD may also be the result of defective reabsorption of Na^+ in the CCD resulting in large quantities of Na^+ being present in the lumen (as is seen with obstructive uropathy[23]), of drugs that block epithelial Na^+ channels (amiloride, trimethoprim), or of low aldosterone activity (inherited or congenital, aldosterone receptor blocker, angiotensin-converting enzyme inhibitor, angiotensin receptor blocker) that results in a lack of stimulation of H^+-ATPase as well as a low luminal negative charge as a result of Na^+ wasting. Patients with low TEPD will have hyperkalemia and low transtubular potassium gradient (TTKG) as a result of the concomitant defect in K^+ secretion by the principal cell. This is also considered RTA type 4.

Another reason for low H^+ secretion in the distal nephron is the cell being relatively alkalotic. This appears to be the case with defective Cl^--HCO_3^- exchanger function, which causes HCO_3^- to be retained within the cell. An autosomal-dominant disorder with mutations in the gene SLC4A1, which encodes the Cl^--HCO_3^- exchanger, has been identified in some families.[24] Because this is also expressed in red cells, these patients are expected to have red cell abnormalities; however, this does not appear to be the case. An autosomal-recessive type has been identified in some kindreds from Thailand with both hemolytic anemia (ovalocytosis) and RTA.[25]

A back leak of H^+ is seen with amphotericin therapy.[26] Here, the function of H^+-ATPase is normal as demonstrated by the achievement of a high urine pCO_2 when given an alkali load (described later).

In this form of RTA in which NH_4^+ excretion is impaired (distal RTA), there is hypocitraturia as a result of an acidotic proximal cell reabsorbing the filtered citrate. With relatively high urine pH and low citrate to chelate, these patients develop nephrocalcinosis and or nephrolithiasis, which further destroys the medulla and may result in renal failure. Patients with distal RTA generally have normal or slightly low serum K^+ concentration. However, if the RTA is the result of a defect in TEPD, the patient will have hyperkalemia.

NH_4^+ has to be excreted out of the body to result in the regeneration of HCO_3^-. In some situations, although the renal component is normal, it does not get excreted. For instance, a patient with a bladder diversion procedure such as an ileal pouch/conduit may have a blockage or delayed emptying that causes NH_4^+ to be reabsorbed because the ileal mucosal epithelium is permeable to NH_4^+. Thus, these patients will have metabolic acidosis with hyperchloremia and a normal anion gap, but they do not have RTA. A urine sample will reveal that the NH_4^+ excretion is normal (i.e., a normal osmolal gap, which is described later).

Diagnostic Tests

1. Determine that the NH_4^+ excretion is low. Because NH_4^+ is not measured in regular laboratories, one has to estimate it, which can be done as follows:
   a. *Determine the urine net charge (urine anion gap):*

   $$\text{Urine net charge} = [Na^+] + [K^+] - [Cl^-]$$

   This assumes that all cations of significant quantity (Na^+, K^+, and NH_4^+) are excreted with the anion Cl^-. Thus, if the sum of the concentrations of Na^+ and K^+ is less than that of Cl^-, the difference is the concentration of NH_4^+. Alternatively, if the sum of the concentrations of Na^+ and K^+ is more than or equal to that of Cl^-, one cannot use this method to assess the concentration of NH_4^+ in the urine, because NH_4^+ may be excreted with another anion that is not normally present in the urine, such as ketones, lithium, and hippurate (from toluene).

   b. *Urine osmolal gap.* This assumes that the cations excreted in the urine in substantial quantities are Na^+, K^+, and NH_4^+ and that the solutes that are osmotically active are these cations and their anions, urea, and glucose. The concentrations of Na^+, K^+, and NH_4^+ are multiplied by 2 for the osmolality, because they all have one valence. This removes the uncertainty associated with the type of anion being excreted.[27]

$$\text{Measured urine osmolality} = \text{Urine [urea]} + \text{[glucose]} + 2[Na^+ + K^+ + NH_4^+]$$

(If urea is measured as blood urea nitrogen in mg/dl, divide it by 2.8, and if glucose is measured in mg/dl, divide it by 18 to convert to mmol/L.)

Thus:

$$2[NH_4^+] = \text{Measured urine osmolality} - \{[\text{Urea}] + [\text{Glucose}] + 2[Na^+ + K^+]\}$$

$$[NH_4^+] = \frac{\text{Measured urine osmolality} - \{[\text{Urea}] + [\text{Glucose}] + 2[Na^+ + K^+]\}}{2}$$

Normal daily NH_4^+ excretion is approximately 0.7 to 0.8 mmol/kg of body weight when there is no acidosis. During metabolic acidosis, this value increases to nearly 3 to 5 mmol/kg/day. Because the above calculation only provides the concentration of NH_4^+, this has to be converted into a daily rate. In steady state, creatinine excretion remains unchanged. One can use the expected creatinine excretion rate to convert the concentration of NH_4^+ to its daily rate, as described later.

A child with a body weight of 10 kg is expected to excrete 30 to 50 mmol (mEq) of NH_4^+ per day when acidotic. Because the urinary excretion of creatinine is in the range of 125 to 150 μmol/kg/day (14 to 17 mg/kg/day), the total creatinine excretion is 1.5 mmol/day (170 mg/day). If the random urine sample had a creatinine concentration of 1 mmol/L (11.3 mg/dl) and, by calculation, the concentration of NH_4^+ in that urine was 10 mmol/L, then the child is excreting 15 mmol/day of NH_4^+ ($[10 \div 1] \times 1.5$). This is an inadequate response.

2. Next, look at the urine pH, as discussed previously.
3. Urine citrate excretion will be low.
4. With regard to HCO_3^- loading (similar to proximal RTA testing), if the H^+ secretion is normal, then the urine pCO_2 should be high. This is because, when there is a large amount of HCO_3^- in the lumen of the CCD, the secreted H^+ is buffered by HCO_3^- and forms H_2CO_3. Because there is no carbonic anhydrase in the lumen of the CCD, this H_2CO_3 dehydrates slowly and causes a high pCO_2 in the urine. A urine to plasma pCO_2 U-B pCO_2 gradient of less than 30 mm Hg has been found to be highly sensitive and specific for H^+ secretion defect.[28] If the pCO_2 is high but the fractional excretion of HCO_3^- is low, there is a back leak of secreted H^+ in the distal tubule.
5. Urine osmolality will be low if there is medullary interstitial disease.
6. Serum K will be normal or low.

Combined Proximal Hydrogen Ion Secretion Defect and Distal NH_4^+ Excretion Defect

This condition was previously called *RTA type 3*. Patients with this condition have an inability to reabsorb the filtered HCO_3^- by the proximal cell, and they also have low NH_4^+ excretion as a result of impaired H^+ secretion by the distal nephron. This has been shown to be the result of a mutation in the gene that encodes carbonic anhydrase type II. This is an autosomal-recessive syndrome called *osteopetrosis*, which includes RTA, mental retardation, and cerebral calcification as its syndrome complex.[29,30] There may be autoantibodies against carbonic anhydrase type II in patients with Sjögren's syndrome that result in this form of RTA.[31]

Diagnostic Tests

1. Determine that there is a distal defect:
   a. Low excretion of NH_4^+
   b. High urine pH
   c. Low urine to plasma pCO_2 U-B pCO_2
2. Determine that there is a proximal defect:
   a. High fractional excretion of HCO_3^-
   b. High urinary citrate level

RTA Associated With Hyperkalemia

This condition is also called *RTA type 4*. This disorder is seen in many different disease states that result in hyperkalemia, most notably in states of hypoaldosteronism or pseudohypoaldosteronism types 1 and 2. As a result of decreased aldosterone activity, both K^+ and H^+ secretion (directly via H^+-ATPase and as a result of low TEPD) are impaired. In addition, hyperkalemia impairs ammoniagenesis and recycling. This results in low NH_3 availability in the medullary interstitium. Thus, the secreted H^+ is not buffered adequately, which results in the blunting of H^+ secretion. Distal H^+ secretion can be enhanced by an acid load that results in systemic acidosis such that the concentration gradient for H^+ is high enough to favor its secretion into the lumen. Thus, these patients produce maximally acidic urine when an acid load is given unless the medulla has been destroyed with a disease such as obstructive uropathy. Moreover, NH_4^+ excretion continues to be low despite acidosis as a result of the effect of hyperkalemia.

In pseudohypoaldosteronism type 1, there is resistance to aldosterone action. This results in marked Na^+ wasting with polyuria and elevated plasma renin activity and aldosterone level. The autosomal-dominant form is the result of a mutation in the gene that encodes the mineralocorticoid receptor; the autosomal-recessive form, which involves multiple organs, is the result of a mutation in the gene that encodes the β and γ subunits of the epithelial Na^+ channel in the principal cell.[32,33] In pseudohypoaldosteronism type 2 (Gordon syndrome), there is hyperabsorption of NaCl in the early distal tubule by the Na-Cl cotransporter. This has also been called *chloride-shunt syndrome*. These patients have hypertension as a result of excessive NaCl reabsorption, which results in the suppression of plasma renin activity and the aldosterone level. This is inherited as an autosomal-dominant disorder. The aldosterone level may be reported as normal as a result of two opposing factors: stimulation by hyperkalemia, which increases the level, and expanded extracellular fluid volume, which inhibits the level through the renin-angiotensin pathway. As a result of the low Na^+ delivery to the CCD, the secretion of K^+ by the principal cell and of H^+ by the α-intercalated cell is impaired. Recent genetic studies have identified mutations in WNK1 and WNK4 as the cause of this syndrome.[34] Therapy with a thiazide diuretic that blocks the Na-Cl cotransporter will largely correct the disorder.[35] Patients with pseudohypoaldosteronism types 1 and 2 generally do not develop nephrocalcinosis or nephrolithiasis. This is probably a result of the normal excretion of citrate as well as of the lower urine pH as compared with other low NH_4^+ excretion disorders, although the urine pH is still high for a patient with systemic acidosis. The mechanism of cyclosporine-associated RTA with hyperkalemia may be similar to that of Gordon syndrome.[36] Moreover, cyclosporine has been shown to reduce the reversal in the adaptive polarity change seen in the intercalated cells when there is metabolic acidosis,[37] which probably worsens the degree of acidosis.

Diagnostic Tests

1. Determine that there is hyperkalemia present.
2. Determine that there is low urine K^+ excretion.
   a. *Low TTKG*. TTKG is a measure of the driving force of K^+ secretion in the CCD. Because the K^+ concentration

in the CCD cannot be measured, three major assumptions are made to deduce the value from urinary and plasma measurements of K^+ concentration and osmolality: (1) When antidiuretic hormone is working, the osmolality of the fluid in the CCD is equal to the osmolality of plasma; (2) K^+ is not reabsorbed or secreted in the medullary cortical collecting duct; and (3) Only water is absorbed—no particles (Na^+, K^+, NH_4^+, and urea) are secreted or reabsorbed between the time fluid leaves the lumen of the CCD to the time it arrives in the bladder as final urine. With these assumptions, the urine osmolality (which is measured) is used to calculate the amount of water reabsorbed. For example, if the urine osmolality is 600 mOsm/kg H_2O and the plasma osmolality is 300 mOsm/kg H_2O, then the urine volume in the lumen of the CCD must have been twice as much as that of the final urine (600 ÷ 300). If the final urine K^+ concentration is 20 mmol/L, then the CCD luminal K^+ concentration would have been 10 mmol/L. If the plasma K^+ concentration is 5 mmol/L, then the TTKG is 2 (10 ÷ 2). This is depicted in the following formula and illustrated in Figure 31-4:

$$\text{TTKG} = \text{Urine}[K^+]/(\text{Urine osmolality}/\text{Plasma osmolality})/\text{Plasma }[K^+]$$

If the TTKG is <7 when there is hyperkalemia, then there is a defect in K^+ secretion.

3. Determine that there is a distal defect:
   a. Low excretion of NH_4^+
   b. High urine pH
4. Determine if there is normal or high citrate excretion.
5. Perform the furosemide test. The principle of this test is that, if Na^+ delivery (low TEPD) was the limiting factor for H^+ secretion, then providing a large quantity of Na^+ to this area should enhance H^+ secretion as a result of the reabsorption of Na^+ by the principal cell creating a lumen-negative voltage. This will result in the lowering of urine pH and an increase in NH_4^+ excretion. Administer 1 mg/kg intravenously, monitor the urine pH, and calculate the urine osmolal gap. This can also be achieved with a saline load. If the urine pH does not fall, it does not always mean that there is a permanent defect in H^+ secretion, because this effect is also dependent on increased aldosterone activity to reabsorb the Na^+.
6. Perform the acid loading test. NH_4Cl or sodium sulfate (and several others) can be administered to determine whether the patient is able to maximally acidify the urine if the furosemide test is equivocal. In this case, the administration of any of the previously mentioned agents results in systemic acidosis, which should result in maximally acidic urine with the lowest possible urine pH if H^+ secretion is intact.
7. Treat the hyperkalemia, and the metabolic acidosis disappears.

THERAPY OF RENAL TUBULAR ACIDOSIS

Obviously, therapy will depend on the cause of the RTA. The general principles are to provide adequate amounts of alkali (either in the form of Na HCO_3 or $KHCO_3$) or citrate to achieve optimal growth and bone mineralization and to prevent nephrocalcinosis and progression to renal failure. Because the proximal tubule is the bulk reabsorber, a defect in this segment will require a large amount of alkali therapy (somewhere on the order of 10 to 15 mmol/kg/day). Distal RTA will require approximately 2 to 4 mmol/kg/day. It is important to realize that children with this condition will continue to lose the HCO_3^- given to them and hence the dose should be divided and, whenever possible, given at frequent intervals through the day and night.

CASE ILLUSTRATIONS

Case 1

A 6-month-old male presents to the emergency department with a 2-week history of decreased oral intake, increased fussiness, and weight loss. He was a previously healthy term

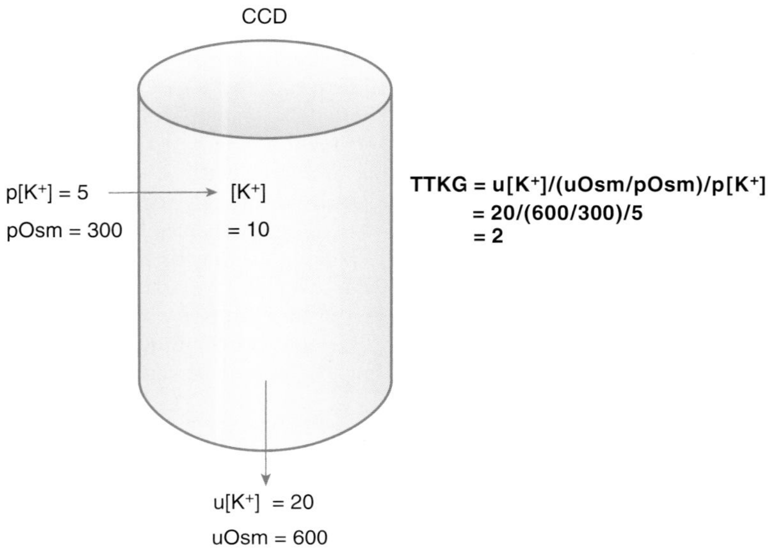

Figure 31-4 Transtubular potassium gradient. Refer to the text for details.

infant who up until that time was growing and developing normally. Despite his poor oral intake, he was described as having normal urine output of 5 to 6 wet diapers per day. There was no history of vomiting or diarrhea. In the emergency department, the infant was presumed to have a viral illness.

Initial Laboratory Values

- Plasma Na^+ — 140 mmol/L
- Plasma K^+ — 2.8 mmol/L
- Plasma Cl^- — 113 mmol/L
- Creatinine — 34 μmol/L (0.4 mg/dl)
- Urea — 1.4 mmol/L (3.9 mg/dl)
- Glucose — 5.2 mmol/L (94 mg/dl)
- HCO_3^- — 15 mmol/L
- Arterial pH — 7.30
- Arterial pCO_2 — 30 mmHg
- Arterial HCO_3^- — 13 mmol/L
- Urine pH — 6.5
- Specific gravity — 1.010
- Protein — 0.3 g/L
- Glucose — 28 mmol/L (504 mg/dl)

Assessment

1. The blood pH of 7.30 indicates acidemia. The low pCO_2 supports the diagnosis of primary metabolic acidosis. The respiratory compensation is appropriate (ΔHCO_3^- of 12, ΔpCO_2 of 10). Because the anion gap is normal (15), this is a nonanion gap metabolic acidosis. The cause of this can be the gastrointestinal or renal loss of HCO_3^- or the inability of the kidney to excrete the dietary or metabolic H^+ load. Because there is no gastrointestinal loss, the possible causes that are left are renal. Glucosuria and low-grade proteinuria suggest a generalized proximal tubular disorder, such as Fanconi syndrome. To prove this theory, the urine is further examined:
   - Na^+ — 54 mmol/L
   - K^+ — 75 mmol/L
   - Cl^- — 34 mmol/L
   - Osmolality — 586 mOsm/L
   - Glucose — 28 mmol/L (504 mg/dl)
   - Urea — 12 mmol/L (33.8 mg/dl)
2. Urine anion gap = 54 + 75 − 34 = **+95**
   Thus, it appears that there is no missing cation (i.e., no NH_4^+) in the urine. This suggests that there is a problem with H^+ secretion or with low NH_4^+ availability in the medullary interstitium rather than proximal tubular dysfunction. Therefore, the urine osmolal gap was determined, because there may be other anions in the urine that could mask the detection of NH_4^+.[4,27]
   - Calculated osmolality: 2(54) + 2(75) + 12 + 28 = 298
   - Measured osmolality: 586 mOsm/L
   - Osmolal gap: 586 − 298 = **288 mOsm/L**

   This suggests that about **144 mmol/L** of an unaccounted osmole (most likely NH_4^+) is present in the urine, thus supporting the hypothesis of a proximal tubular disorder.
3. Generalized proximal tubular dysfunction was confirmed with phosphaturia and aminoaciduria.
4. An elevated white blood cell cystine level of 15 nmol half cystine/mg protein (N < 0.2) confirms the diagnosis of nephropathic cystinosis.[38]

Case 2

A 14-year-old male presents to the outpatient clinic for the assessment of a blood pressure level of 145/95 of 4 weeks' duration. He denies any facial flushing, headache, eye disturbances, or chest pain, and he is physically active with a healthy weight. His family history is not significant for early-onset stroke, renal failure, or hypertension.

Initial Laboratory Values

- Plasma Na^+ — 138 mmol/L
- Plasma K^+ — 6.5 mmol/L
- Plasma Cl^- — 113 mmol/L
- Plasma HCO_3^- — 19 mmol/L
- Creatinine — 45 μmol/L (0.5 mg/dl)
- Urea — 4.5 mmol/L (12.7 mg/dl)
- Arterial pH — 7.32
- pCO_2 — 34 mmHg
- HCO_3^- — 18 mmol/L
- Urine pH — 8.0
- Specific gravity — 1.020

Assessment

1. The pH of 7.30 indicates acidemia. The low serum HCO_3^- and low pCO_2 support the diagnosis of a primary metabolic acidosis. The respiratory compensation is appropriate (ΔHCO_3^- of 7, ΔpCO_2 of 6). Because the anion gap is normal (12.5), this is a nonanion gap metabolic acidosis. As in the previous case, the absence of diarrhea indicates a renal cause of the acidosis. Hyperkalemia suggests decreased NH_4^+ excretion as a result of the decreased production and transfer in the medulla. The urine anion and osmolal gaps confirm this:
   - Na^+ — 169 mmol/L
   - K^+ — 17.1 mmol/L
   - Cl^- — 117 mmol/L
   - Osmolality — 640 mOsm/L
   - Glucose — 0 mmol/L
   - Urea — 263 mmol/L (741 mg/dl)

   Urine anion gap: 169 + 17.1 − 117 = **+69.1**
   Calculated osmolality: 2(169) + 2(17.1) + 0 + 263 = 635 mOsm/L
   Measured osmolality: 640 mOsm/L
   Osmolal gap: 635 − 640 = **−5**
   Both the urine anion gap and the urine osmolal gap confirm that there is no NH_4^+ in the urine.
2. Low NH_4^+ excretion is a result of the following: (a) low NH_4^+ production and recycling as a result of hyperkalemia; and (b) low H^+ secretion as evidenced by high urine pH.
3. A urine pH of 8 indicates that there is a significant impairment in H^+ secretion. Because there is hyperkalemia, the most likely cause for the impaired H^+ secretion is low TEPD, because the elevated K^+ can also be caused by low TEPD. This may arise from defects in the epithelial Na^+ channel and aldosterone activity (synthesis or signaling) or as a result of low distal Na^+ delivery (as seen in activating mutations of NaCl cotransporter [NaCC] [Gordon syndrome]). Of these possibilities, only Gordon syndrome is associated with hypertension.
4. Gordon syndrome is characterized by metabolic acidosis presenting with hyperkalemia as a result of mutations in

either of the WNK1 or WNK4 kinases. These are phosphokinase regulators of the sodium-chloride transporter in the distal tubule. Mutations in either of these proteins result in a gain of function of the Na-Cl transporter, thereby causing increased sodium and chloride uptake and hypertension.[8,34,39] This suppresses the renin-angiotensin-aldosterone system. However, hyperkalemia may induce aldosterone release, with the net effect of having inappropriately normal aldosterone levels.

5. Undetectable plasma renin activity and normal serum aldosterone levels confirm the diagnosis. Genetic analysis confirms a WNK4 kinase D564H mutation.

Case 3

A 10-year-old male presents with a 2-year history of urinary dribbling, a weak urine stream, and short stature. He is developmentally normal, and he has no history of urine infections. His physical examination is notable for height in less than the fifth percentile, easily palpable kidneys, and a blood pressure that is at the ninetieth percentile for height.

Laboratory Investigations

• Plasma Na^+	135 mmol/L
• Plasma K^+	5.2 mmol/L
• Plasma Cl^-	114 mmol/L
• Plasma HCO_3^-	16 mmol/L
• Creatinine	115 μmol/L (1.3 mg/dl)
• Urea	7.2 mmol/L (20.3 mg/dl)
• Osmolality	300 mOsm/L
• Arterial pH	7.33
• Arterial pCO_2	32 mmHg

Assessment

1. The low plasma HCO_3^- in combination with a low pCO_2 indicates a primary metabolic acidosis. The change in pCO_2 (8 mm Hg) and the change in HCO_3^- (9 mmol/L) indicate an appropriate respiratory compensation. The plasma anion gap is normal and, in the absence of diarrhea, suggests a renal cause for the acidosis. Urine studies were done:

• Na^+	137 mmol/L
• K^+	15 mmol/L
• Cl^-	128 mmol/L
• Osmolality	355 mOsm/L
• pH	6.5
• Glucose	0 mmol/L
• Urea	50 mmol/L (141 mg/dl)
• Creatinine	0.4 mmol/L (4.5 mg/dl)

   Anion gap: 137 + 15 − 128 = **+24**
   Calculated osmolality: 2(137) + 2(15) + 0 + 50 = 354 mOsm/L
   Measured osmolality: 355 mOsm/L
   Osmolal gap: 355 − 354 = **+1**

2. The urine anion gap and the urine osmolal gap confirm the absence of NH_4^+. Low NH_4^+ with high urine pH indicates an H^+ secretion problem. However, hyperkalemia is also likely inhibiting NH_4^+ production and recycling so that NH_3 concentration is reduced in the medullary interstitium. Assessing tubular function with respect to Na^+ and K^+ suggests a cause:
   a. Fractional excretion of Na =
      (Plasma sodium/Plasma creatinine) × 100 =
      (137/400)/(135/115) = **29%** (N < 1%)
   b. Transtubular K gradient =
      (Urine K/Urine osmolality)/
      (Plasma K/Plasma osmolality) =
      (15/355)/(5.2/300) = **2.5** (>7 is expected in the setting of hyperkalemia)
3. The high urine Na^+ and low K^+ excretion suggest that there is a problem with aldosterone activity or epithelial Na^+ channel.
4. The plasma aldosterone was elevated, thus supporting the idea of a defect in renal response to aldosterone. A renal ultrasound is done and reveals bilateral obstructive uropathy, which is further clarified as being the result of posterior urethral valves on a voiding cystourethrogram. Obstructive uropathy may cause insensitivity to aldosterone with the development of tubular interstitial disease and fibrosis.[23]
5. Although it was not performed, a water deprivation test would have confirmed that there was medullary interstitial damage by exhibiting the patient's inability to maximally concentrate the urine.

Case 4

A 6-year-old female is admitted to the pediatric intensive care unit with sepsis during chemotherapy for neuroblastoma. She is started on piperacillin and tobramycin for broad-spectrum antibiotic coverage. A chest x-ray shows the presence of coin-shaped lesions throughout both lung fields, and an ultrasound shows echogenic foci in the liver. The kidneys appear normal. Blood cultures are negative for bacteria, but fungal cultures grow *Aspergillus nigricans*. Liposomal amphotericin is initiated. Three days later, the patient has clinical improvement, but she is noted to have a new-onset acidosis.

Laboratory Values

• Plasma Na^+	145 mmol/L
• Plasma K^+	3.4 mmol/L
• Plasma Cl^-	116 mmol/L
• Plasma HCO_3^-	18 mmol/L
• Creatinine	130 μmol/L (1.5 mg/dl)
• Urea	7.2 mmol/L (20.3 mg/dl)
• Osmolality	300 mOsm/L
• Arterial pH	7.32
• pCO_2	34 mm Hg

Assessment

1. The low HCO_3^- and the low pCO_2 indicate a primary metabolic acidosis. The change in pCO_2 (6 mm Hg) and the change in HCO_3^- (7 mmol/L) show an appropriate respiratory compensation. The plasma anion gap is calculated to be 14.4, thus confirming a nonanion gap metabolic acidosis. In the absence of gastrointestinal symptoms, a renal cause is sought, and urine studies are done:

• Na^+	76 mmol/L K^+ 65 mmol/L
• Cl^-	116 mmol/L
• Osmolality	348 mOsm/L
• pH	6.0
• Glucose	0 mmol/L

- Urea 65 mmol/L (183.3 mg/dl)
- Creatinine 0.5 mmol/L (5.6 mg/dl)

Anion gap: 76 + 65 − 116 = **+25**
Calculated osmolality: 2(76) + 2(65) + 0 + 65 = 347 mOsm/L
Measured osmolality: 348 mOsm/L
Osmolal gap: 348 − 347 = **+1**

2. The urine studies confirm the absence of NH_4^+. Urine pH is high in a patient who is in a state of acidosis; thus, there must be an H^+ secretion problem. The patient was given an HCO_3^- load, and the urine to plasma pCO_2 was assessed. The plasma HCO_3^- was 27 when the urine pH was 7.5, and the urine pCO_2 was 46 mmol/L higher than the plasma. This indicates that both HCO_3^- reabsorption and H^+ excretion are intact. This appears to be contradictory, because both proximal and distal function appear good, despite the presence of a renal tubular acidosis.
3. One explanation for this phenomenon is an H^+ back leak. Amphotericin disrupts the luminal membrane and increases the permeability to H^+, thus allowing a back leak of H^+ to occur at a lower lumen H^+ concentration.[26] The presence or absence of ammonium in the urine is therefore determined by the kinetics of the H^+ back leak: a large increase in H^+ membrane permeability allows for the rapid reentry of H^+ into the cell before the sequestration of H^+ by titratable acids can occur. Similarly, a small increase in H^+ permeability will allow some degree of titratable acid protonation and net acid excretion but not under situations in which a large acid load is given. To test this theory, the patient was given a large acid load (NH_4Cl) to see if the urine pH would drop below 5.5. The urine pH was measured at 5.8, which suggests that a mild back leak may be preventing efficient H^+ excretion.

REFERENCES

1. Halperin ML, Jungas RL: Metabolic production and renal disposal of hydrogen ions, *Kidney Int* 24:709-13, 1983.
2. Preisig PA, Ives HE, Cragoe EJ Jr, Alpern RJ, Rector FC Jr: Role of the Na+/H+ antiporter in rat proximal tubule bicarbonate absorption, *J Clin Invest* 80:970-78, 1987.
3. Wang T, Yang CL, Abbiati T, Schultheis PJ, et al: Mechanism of proximal tubule bicarbonate absorption in NHE3 null mice, *Am J Physiol* 277:F298-302, 1999.
4. Gottschalk CW, Lassiter WE, Mylle M: Localization of urine acidification in the mammalian kidney, *Am J Physiol* 198:581-85, 1960.
5. Kurtz I: Basolateral membrane Na+/H+ antiport, Na+/base cotransport, and Na+-independent Cl-/base exchange in the rabbit S3 proximal tubule, *J Clin Invest* 83:616-22, 1989.
6. Maddox DA, Deen WM, Gennari FJ: Control of bicarbonate and fluid reabsorption in the proximal convoluted tubule, *Semin Nephrol* 7:72-81, 1987.
7. Good DW: Regulation of bicarbonate and ammonium absorption in the thick ascending limb of the rat, *Kidney Int Suppl* 33:S36-42, 1991.
8. Wagner CA, Geibel JP: Acid-base transport in the collecting duct, *J Nephrol* 15 Suppl 5:S112-27, 2002.
9. Schwartz GJ, Al-Awqati Q: Role of hensin in mediating the adaptation of the cortical collecting duct to metabolic acidosis, *Curr Opin Nephrol Hypertens* 14:383-88, 2005.
10. Garg LC: Respective roles of H-ATPase and H-K-ATPase in ion transport in the kidney, *J Am Soc Nephrol* 2:949-60, 1991.
11. Star RA: Basolateral membrane sodium-independent Cl-/HCO3-exchanger in rat inner medullary collecting duct cell, *J Clin Invest* 85:1959-66, 1990.
12. Owen OE, Licht JH, Sapir DG: Renal function and effects of partial rehydration during diabetic ketoacidosis, *Diabetes* 30:510-18, 1981.
13. Preisig PA, Alpern RJ: Pathways for apical and basolateral membrane NH3 and NH4+ movement in rat proximal tubule, *Am J Physiol* 259:F587-93, 1990.
14. Haperin ML, Kamel KS, Ethier JH, Stinebaugh BJ, Jungas RL: Biochemistry and physiology of ammonium excretion. In Seldin DW and Giebisch G, editers: *The kidney: physiology and pathophysiology*, New York, 1992, Raven Press, pp. 2645-79.
15. Garvin JL, Burg MB, Knepper MA: Active NH4+ absorption by the thick ascending limb, *Am J Physiol* 255:F57-65, 1988.
16. Shah M, Gupta N, Dwarakanath V, Moe OW, Baum M: Ontogeny of Na+/H+ antiporter activity in rat proximal convoluted tubules, *Pediatr Res* 48:206-10, 2000.
17. Bonnici B, Wagner CA: Postnatal expression of transport proteins involved in acid-base transport in mouse kidney, *Pflugers Arch* 448:16-28, 2004.
18. Halperin ML, Lin S-H, Gowrishankar M, Kamel KS: Disorders of acid-base balance. In Malluche HH, Sawaya BP, Hakim RM, and Sayegh MH, editors: *Clinical nephrology, dialysis, and transplantation*, Munich, Germany, 1999, Dustri-Verlag, pp. 1-54.
19. Kushner RF: Total parenteral nutrition-associated metabolic acidosis, *JPEN J Parenter Enteral Nutr* 10:306-10, 1986.
20. Karet FE, Finberg KE, Nayir A, Bakkaloglu A, et al: Localization of a gene for autosomal recessive distal renal tubular acidosis with normal hearing (rdRTA2) to 7q33-34, *Am J Hum Genet* 65:1656-65, 1999.
21. Karet FE, Finberg KE, Nelson RD, Nayir A, et al: Mutations in the gene encoding B1 subunit of H+-ATPase cause renal tubular acidosis with sensorineural deafness, *Nat Genet* 21:84-90, 1999.
22. Gordon RD: Syndrome of hypertension and hyperkalemia with normal glomerular filtration rate, *Hypertension* 8:93-102, 1986.
23. Chandar J, Abitbol C, Zilleruelo G, Gosalbez R, et al: Renal tubular abnormalities in infants with hydronephrosis, *J Urol* 155:660-63, 1996.
24. Bruce LJ, Cope DL, Jones GK, Schofield AE, et al: Familial distal renal tubular acidosis is associated with mutations in the red cell anion exchanger (Band 3, AE1) gene, *J Clin Invest* 100:1693-707, 1997.
25. Vasuvattakul S, Yenchitsomanus PT, Vachuanichsanong P, Thuwajit P, et al: Autosomal recessive distal renal tubular acidosis associated with Southeast Asian ovalocytosis, *Kidney Int* 56:1674-82, 1999.
26. Steinmetz PR, Lawson LR: Defect in urinary acidification induced in vitro by amphotericin B, *J Clin Invest* 49:596-601, 1970.
27. Kamel KS, Ethier JH, Richardson RM, Bear RA, Halperin ML: Urine electrolytes and osmolality: when and how to use them, *Am J Nephrol* 10:89-102, 1990.
28. Kim S, Lee JW, Park J, Na KY, et al: The urine-blood PCO2 gradient as a diagnostic index of H(+)-ATPase defect distal renal tubular acidosis, *Kidney Int* 66:761-67, 2004.
29. Nagai R, Kooh SW, Balfe JW, Fenton T, Halperin ML: Renal tubular acidosis and osteopetrosis with carbonic anhydrase II deficiency: pathogenesis of impaired acidification, *Pediatr Nephrol* 11:633-36, 1997.
30. Sly WS, Whyte MP, Sundaram V, Tashian RE, et al: Carbonic anhydrase II deficiency in 12 families with the autosomal recessive syndrome of osteopetrosis with renal tubular acidosis and cerebral calcification, *N Engl J Med* 313:139-45, 1985.
31. Takemoto F, Hoshino J, Sawa N, Tamura Y, et al: Autoantibodies against carbonic anhydrase II are increased in renal tubular acidosis associated with Sjogren syndrome, *Am J Med* 118:181-84, 2005.
32. Chang SS, Grunder S, Hanukoglu A, Rosler A, et al: Mutations in subunits of the epithelial sodium channel cause salt wasting with hyperkalaemic acidosis, pseudohypoaldosteronism type 1, *Nat Genet* 12:248-53, 1996.
33. Geller DS, Rodriguez-Soriano J, Vallo Boado A, Schifter S, et al: Mutations in the mineralocorticoid receptor gene cause autosomal dominant pseudohypoaldosteronism type I, *Nat Genet* 19:279-81, 1998.

34. Kahle KT, Wilson FH, Lalioti M, Toka H, et al: WNK kinases: molecular regulators of integrated epithelial ion transport, *Curr Opin Nephrol Hypertens* 13:557-62, 2004.
35. Gordon RD, Hodsman GP: The syndrome of hypertension and hyperkalaemia without renal failure: long term correction by thiazide diuretic, *Scott Med J* 31:43-44, 1986.
36. Ling BN, Eaton DC: Cyclosporin A inhibits apical secretory K+ channels in rabbit cortical collecting tubule principal cells, *Kidney Int* 44:974-84, 1993.
37. Watanabe S, Tsuruoka S, Vijayakumar S, Fischer G, et al: Cyclosporin A produces distal renal tubular acidosis by blocking peptidyl prolyl cis-trans isomerase activity of cyclophilin, *Am J Physiol Renal Physiol* 288:F40-47, 2005.
38. Kleta R, Kaskel F, Dohil R, Goodyer P, et al: First NIH/Office of Rare Diseases Conference on Cystinosis: past, present, and future, *Pediatr Nephrol* 20:452-54, 2005.
39. Farfel Z, Mayan H, Yaacov Y, Mouallem M, et al: WNK4 regulates airway Na+ transport: study of familial hyperkalaemia and hypertension, *Eur J Clin Invest* 35:410-15, 2005.

CHAPTER 32

Diabetes Insipidus

Detlef Böckenhauer

HISTORY

Diabetes insipidus (DI) derives from the Greek word *diabinein* for "flow through" and the Latin word *insapere* for "non–sweet-tasting"; this separates it from another polyuric disorder, diabetes mellitus ("like honey"). A familial form affecting "chiefly males on the female side of the house" was first described by McIlraith in 1892.[1] In 1935, De Lange reported a family with DI and no male-to-male transmission that was unresponsive to injections of posterior lobe extracts.[2] In 1945, Forssman[3] and Waring[4] recognized the disorder in these families as a renal problem. In 1947, Williams and Henry[5] established the unresponsiveness to arginine–vasopressin (AVP) in these patients and coined the term *nephrogenic DI* (NDI). In 1969, the "Hopewell Hypothesis" was suggested by Bode and Crawford, who proposed that most cases of NDI in the United States and Canada could be traced to descendants of Ulster Scots, who arrived on the ship *Hopewell* in Nova Scotia in 1761.[6] Bichet[7] later refuted this by molecular analysis. In 1992, the *AVPR2* gene encoding the AVP2 receptor was cloned and mutations identified in patients with X-linked NDI.[8-11] Shortly thereafter, the *AQP2* gene encoding the vasopressin-regulated water channel aquaporin-2 (*AQP2*) was cloned,[12,13] and, in 1994, mutations in *AQP2* were found to underlie autosomal recessive DI.[14]

CLINIC

Presentation During Infancy

Patients with congenital NDI typically present during the first weeks of life with dehydration. Sometimes patients receive repeated investigations for sepsis, because the dehydration can be associated with low-grade temperatures; this may be suspected until a set of serum electrolytes is obtained, which will reveal hypernatremia. Failure to thrive and irritability are additional symptoms. Patients often suck vigorously but develop vomiting shortly after they start to feed. Vomiting may be the result of reflux exacerbated by the large volumes of fluid that are necessary to compensate for the renal losses. Interestingly, breast-fed infants with NDI typically thrive better than formula-fed infants, because breast milk presents a lower osmolar load than most standard formulas (described later). Of note is that pregnancies resulting in babies with NDI are not complicated by polyhydramnios, because the AVP-dependent mechanisms for urinary concentration are not fully developed until after birth, and the osmolar load is cleared by the placenta.[15]

Symptoms During Childhood and Infancy

Symptoms typically improve with advancing age, especially after food intake has changed to solids and the child has free access to water, which allows for the self-regulation of serum osmolality. Patients remain polyuric, however, and typical problems include constipation and nocturnal enuresis. The frequency of voiding and drinking, especially during the night, is useful information when assessing the severity of the problem. Parents also often report problems with concentration and attention span in their children, and, in one study, almost half of the patients were diagnosed with attention-deficit/hyperactivity disorder.[16] The reason for this is unclear, but it may partly be a result of the constant need to drink and void.

With treatment, patients with NDI can function well.[16] Untreated, patients typically have persistent failure to thrive, probably because the constant intake of fluids limits their appetite. In addition, mental retardation used to be an almost invariable feature, likely as a result of the repeated episodes of hypernatremic dehydration.[17-19] Some patients develop dilatation of the urinary tract from the high urinary flow, especially if they have poor voiding habits.[17,20,21]

PHYSIOLOGIC PRINCIPLES

Tubular Concentration/Dilution Mechanism (Countercurrent Mechanism with Figure)

The kidney creates a concentration gradient via a so-called countercurrent multiplication system.[22,23] The tonicity (osmolality) of urine as it proceeds along the nephron is depicted in Figure 32-1. In the proximal tubule, the urine remains isotonic to plasma because of the high water permeability of this segment, which is mediated by aquaporin 1.[24-26] Urine then enters the tubular segment that is most important for countercurrent multiplication: the loop of Henle. The thin descending limb also expresses aquaporin 1 and is thus permeable for water.[27] However, it is impermeable for sodium.[28] Because water exits the tubular lumen following the interstitial concentration gradient, urine is concentrated as it descends the thin descending limb. Conversely, the thick ascending limb is impermeable for water, but it actively transports sodium chloride via the cotransporter NKCC2.[29]

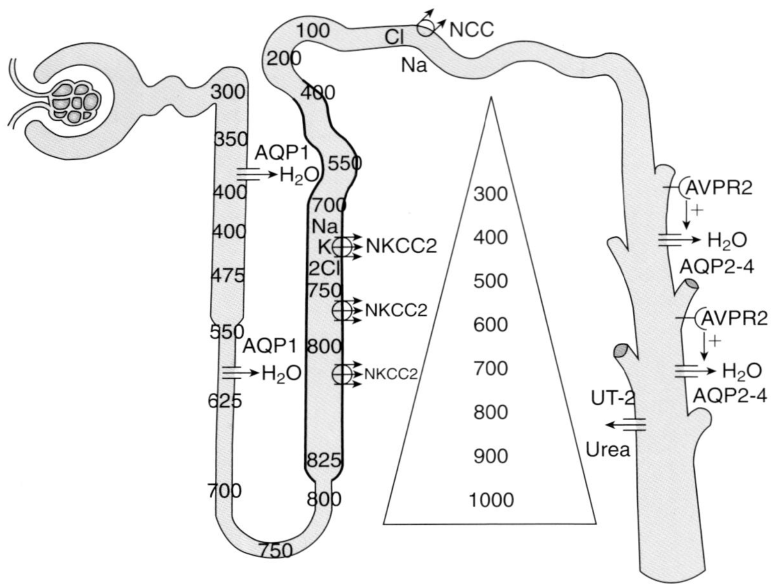

Figure 32-1 Diagram of the renal concentration and dilution mechanism. The numbers indicate the osmolalities of the tubular and interstitial fluids. The names of relevant transport proteins are indicated, and the gradient is generated by the active reabsorption of solutes in the thick ascending limb by the transporter NKCC2. Note that urine entering the collecting duct is hypotonic. Final urine concentration is then dependent on water permeability in the collecting duct, which is mediated by AVP via the AVP receptor and the water channel AQP2. For further details, see the text.

Thus, urine is diluted on its way up the thick ascending limb by the active removal of solutes. The accumulation of solutes in the interstitium in turn generates the driving force for the removal of water from the thin descending limb (described previously), thereby completing the countercurrent multiplier.

There is a further removal of sodium chloride in the distal convoluted tubule via the thiazide-sensitive cotransporter NCC; at its entry into the collecting duct, urinary osmolality is typically around 50 to 100 mOsm/kg. The final osmolality of the urine is now solely dependent on the water permeability of the collecting duct and thus the availability of water channels. If water channels are present, water will exit the tubule following the interstitial concentration gradient and the urine will be concentrated. If no water channels are present, dilute urine will be excreted.

Arginine–Vasopressin Effects in the Kidney

The availability of water channels in the collecting duct is under the control of AVP. The final regulated step is the insertion of AQP2 into the apical (urine-facing) side of the membrane of the principal cells of the collecting duct.[30] Figure 32-2 shows a model of a principal cell. AVP binds to the vasopressin receptor (AVPR2) on the basolateral (blood-facing) side. AVPR2 is a G-protein–coupled receptor that, upon activation, stimulates adenylate cyclase, thus raising cyclic adenosine monophosphate production.[31-34] Protein kinase A is stimulated by cyclic adenosine monophosphate and phosphorylates AQP2 at a consensus site in the cytoplasmic carboxy-terminal tail of the protein, serine 256.[12,35,36] Unphosphorylated AQP2 is present in intracellular vesicles that, upon phosphorylation at serine 256, are fused in the apical membrane.[37] Of note is that AQP2 water channels are homotetramers that consist of four subunits. In vitro evidence suggests that, minimally, three subunits need to be phosphorylated for the channel to be fused in the plasma membrane.[38]

After the insertion of AQP2 in the apical membrane, water can enter from the tubular lumen into the cell and exit via the basolateral water channels AQP3 and AQP4. Although AQP4 appears to be constitutively expressed in the collecting duct, there is some evidence that AVP may also regulate the expression of AQP3.[39-41]

Extrarenal Effects of Arginine–Vasopressin

The vasopressive and glycogenolytic effects of AVP are mediated through AVP1 receptors expressed in the vasculature and the liver, whereas the renal effects (especially the increase in the water permeability of the collecting duct) are mediated by AVPR2.[42] Interestingly, the administration of the AVPR2-specific agonist DDAVP results not only in an increase in urine osmolality, but it also has extrarenal effects, including the following:

- a small depression of blood pressure with a concomitant increase in heart rate and an increase in plasma renin activity[43,44]; and
- an increase in factor VIIIc and von Willebrand factor with a decrease in bleeding time.[43,45,46]

These extrarenal effects are abolished in patients with X-linked NDI, which suggests that AVPR2 is expressed beyond the kidney. Clinically, this can be used to differentiate between X-linked and autosomal-recessive NDI (described later).

DIAGNOSIS

The presence of inappropriately dilute urine in the face of an elevated serum osmolality defines DI. Dehydration in a child with good urine output should always prompt the consideration of a urinary concentrating defect. The diagnosis is easily made by obtaining serum and urine biochemistries. Maximal urinary concentrating ability increases with age, but a urine osmolality below 500 mOsm/kg in a dehydrated child establishes a diagnosis of DI.[47] In classic NDI, the urine osmolality is always below 200 mOsm/kg.

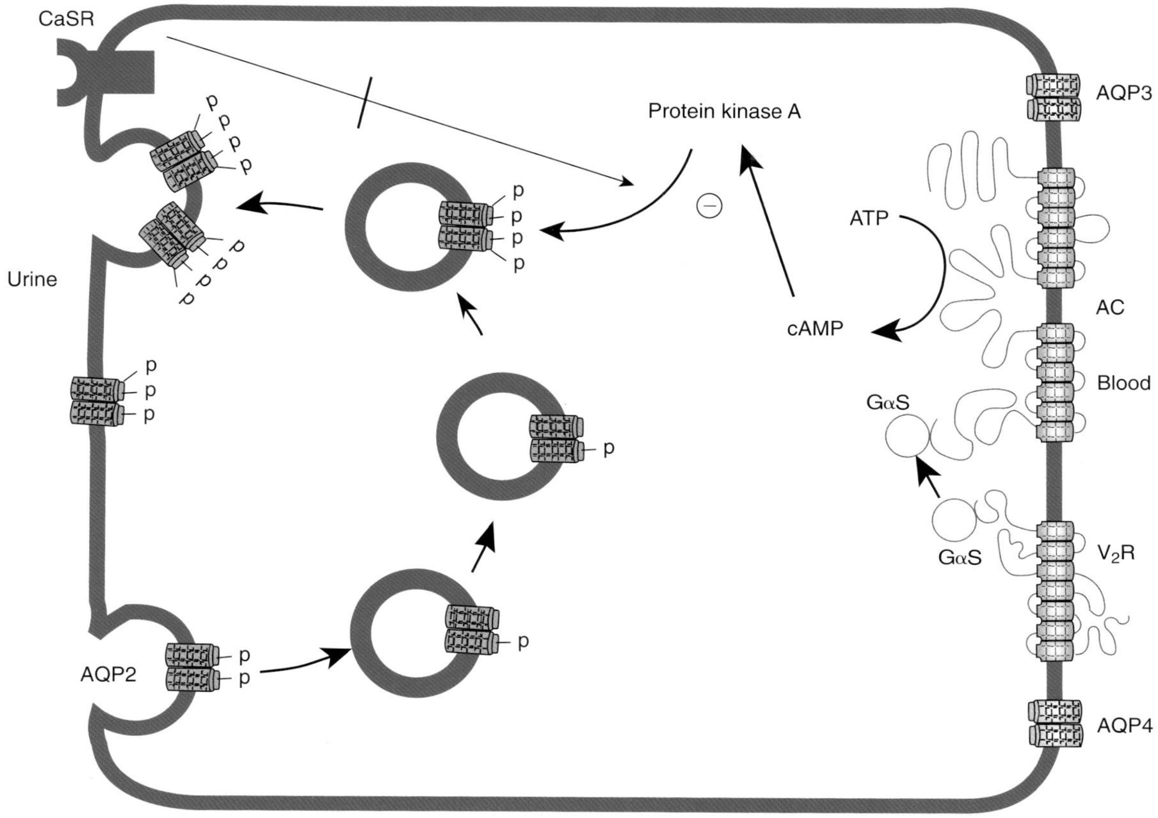

Figure 32-2 Diagram of a principal cell. Depicted is a principal cell with the relevant proteins for water transport. AVP binds to its receptor AVPR2 (expressed on the basolateral side), which in turn stimulates adenylcyclase. The increased production of cyclic adenosine monophosphate leads to the phosphorylation of the water channel AQP2 subunits, which in turn are inserted into the apical membrane. Note that the calcium-sensing receptor (expressed at the apical membrane) and the prostaglandins can inhibit cyclic adenosine monophosphate formation and thus impair urinary concentration. Water entering the cell through AQP2 can exit on the basolateral side via AQP3 and AQP4. For further details, see the text. (Adapted from Nielsen S, Frokiaer J, Marples D, Kwon TH, Agre P, and Knepper MA: Aquaporins in the kidney: from molecules to medicine, *Physiol Rev* 82(1):205-44, 2002.

Diagnostic Procedures

DDAVP Test

The kidney concentrates the urine in response to the pituitary hormone AVP. Failure to concentrate can, therefore, be the result of a deficiency in AVP (central DI or CDI) or an inability of the kidney to respond to it (NDI). AVP effects are mediated via two different receptors: (1) the vasoconstriction ("vasopressin") is mediated by AVP receptor 1 (AVPR1), whereas the antidiuretic response is mediated by the AVP receptor type 2 (AVPR2). The AVP analog 1-desamino-8-D-arginine vasopressin (DDAVP) has a high specificity for AVPR2, and it can therefore be used to assess the renal response while avoiding the systemic effects mediated by AVPR1. Different protocols exist in the literature with respect to the dosage and route of administration of DDAVP. Some authors use intranasal DDAVP, whereas others use oral, subcutaneous, intramuscular, or intravenous administration (0.3 mcg/kg).[43,48,49] Although oral or intranasal DDAVP is less invasive, absorption is less reliable. Thus, if the result of the test is inconclusive, it may need to be repeated using injected DDAVP. DDAVP given intravenously requires a shorter observation period (2 hours) than other modes of administration (4 to 6 hours) with which absorption is more protracted. Interestingly, DDAVP at high doses induces some systemic side effects in the form of a mild decrease in blood pressure and a concomitant increase in the heart rate via AVPR2.[43] Consequently, patients with mutated AVPR2 (X-linked DI) do not experience these hemodynamic changes, whereas patients with intact AVPR2 but mutated AQP2 (autosomal DI) do. The DDAVP test can therefore help differentiate between these two forms. A typical protocol (modified from reference 43) is given in Table 32-1. A commonly feared but actually rare complication of the DDAVP test is hyponatremia. Patients with an intact thirst mechanism who respond to DDAVP will stop drinking water as a result of their stable serum osmolality. Only patients with psychogenic polydipsia, who will keep on drinking despite lowered serum osmolality, and infants, who continue to be fed by their caregivers throughout the test, are at risk for hyponatremia. Thus, close observation and a limitation of fluid intake to a volume equal to the amount of urine excreted during the test period are critical to the prevention of this complication.

A urine osmolality after DDAVP below 200 mOsm/kg is consistent with a diagnosis of NDI, whereas patients with intact urinary concentrating ability typically achieve urine osmolalities of more than 800 mOsm/kg (>500 in infants).[47] Patients with intermediate values should be assessed for inaccurate test results (especially when DDAVP was admin-

TABLE 32-1 DDAVP Test

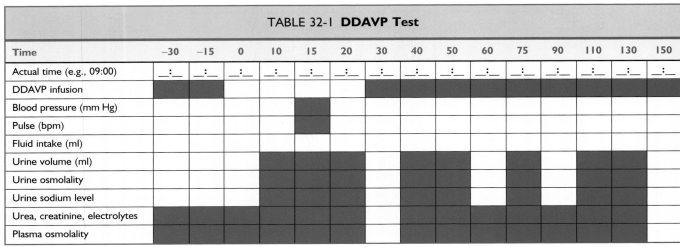

Time	−30	−15	0	10	15	20	30	40	50	60	75	90	110	130	150
Actual time (e.g., 09:00)	__:__	__:__	__:__	__:__	__:__	__:__	__:__	__:__	__:__	__:__	__:__	__:__	__:__	__:__	__:__
DDAVP infusion															
Blood pressure (mm Hg)															
Pulse (bpm)															
Fluid intake (ml)															
Urine volume (ml)															
Urine osmolality															
Urine sodium level															
Urea, creatinine, electrolytes															
Plasma osmolality															

Duration 2 hours after intravenous DDAVP administration; otherwise 4 to 6 hours. Limit fluid intake to urine output during test. See the text for more information about the interpretation of the results.

istered intranasally) or intrinsic renal disease limiting the urinary concentrating capacity (including chronic renal failure and obstructive uropathy, which are described later).

Water-Deprivation Test

The aim of the water-deprivation test is to induce mild dehydration and thus challenge the kidney to preserve water. Water is withheld until the serum osmolality is just above the upper limit of normal (>295 mOsm/kg). Obviously, no child presenting with hypernatremia needs to undergo this test, because the challenge had already presented naturally. A water-deprivation test carries the risk of severe hypernatremic dehydration, especially in infants, because there may be delays in obtaining and reacting to laboratory results. It is useful to distinguish psychogenic polydipsia from central DI in patients with a good response to DDAVP, and thus usually reserved for those particular patients. However, a simple and informal water-deprivation test is to ask the parents to obtain the first morning urine from their child and to note the last time that the child has drunk (however, water should not be withheld from the child). This can be used as a simple screening test in some polyuric patients, because a concentrated urine excludes a diagnosis of DI.

DIFFERENTIAL DIAGNOSIS

Central Diabetes Insipidus

A urinary concentrating defect can be the result of a lack of AVP (central DI) or the inability of the kidney to respond to it (NDI). A DDAVP test helps to differentiate between the two (described previously). Central DI is most commonly the consequence of head trauma or other diseases that affect the hypothalamus or pituitary, but there are some rare cases of hereditary DI that result from mutations in the gene that encodes AVP.[50,51]

X-Linked and Autosomal Nephrogenic Diabetes Insipidus

A careful family history and the assessment of systemic effects in the DDAVP test can discriminate the common X-linked NDI (90% of patients) from the rare autosomal NDI (10%). Because patients with mutations in *AQP2* (autosomal) have intact AVPR2 receptors, they demonstrate normal extrarenal responses to DDAVP, such as a decrease in blood pressure with an increased heart rate and increases in von Willebrand factor and factor VIIIc, whereas patients with mutations in *AVPR2* (X-linked) do not have these characteristics.[43] Genetic testing can be helpful to confirm the affected gene (described later).

Partial Nephrogenic Diabetes Insipidus

An intermediate urine osmolality that is between 200 and 800 mOsm/kg after the administration of DDAVP is referred to as *partial NDI*. As discussed previously, children who are less than 3 years of age may not be able to maximally concentrate their urine yet, and a value between 500 and 800 mOsm/kg can be physiologic.[47] In addition, technical problems with the DDAVP test should be excluded (especially if administration was done intranasally) before a diagnosis of partial NDI is considered. Obviously, because these patients have a partially retained ability to concentrate their urine, their clinical symptoms are milder.

Inherited forms of partial DI are typically the result of mutations in the AVPR2 gene, which allows for the proper expression of the receptor at the cell membrane but decreases the affinity to AVP, thus shifting the dose-response curve and requiring higher amounts of AVP to increase urinary concentration.[52] However, mutations in AQP2 with some retained urinary concentrating ability have also been identified.[53]

Acquired Nephrogenic Diabetes Insipidus

Obstructive Uropathy

Polyuria after the release of urinary tract obstruction is a well-recognized phenomenon (postobstructive diuresis). However, if obstruction is incomplete, it is often associated with polyuria as well. Animal studies show a decreased level of AQP2 expression with bilateral ureteric obstruction.[54] Experiments with unilateral obstruction show a marked decrease in AQP2 in the obstructed kidney, which is consistent with the view that local factors, such as increased pressure, affect AQP2 expression.[55] Supporting this view is also the fact that other signs of distal tubular dysfunction are usually present in obstructive uropathies, like hyperkalemia and acidosis. The downregulation of AQP2 persists for up to 30 days after the release of the obstruction, thus explaining the postobstructive diuresis.[30]

Renal Failure

Polyuria is frequently seen in renal failure, especially if the underlying cause primarily affects the renal tubule, such as nephronophthisis (see Chapter 8) or tubulointerstitial nephritis (see Chapter 34). It is also commonly seen after ischemic renal failure.[56,57] Because urinary concentration and dilution are active tasks, patients with a generalized impairment of tubular function will present with polyuria and isosthenuria.

Lithium

Although it is rarely used in children, lithium therapy is a common treatment for manic-depressive disease in adults, and roughly a fifth of patients receiving it develop polyuria.[58] Animal studies have shown a decreased expression of AQP2 in principal cells, probably as a result of the inhibition of cyclic adenosine monophosphate formation in the collecting duct.[59-61]

Hypercalcemia

Hypercalcemia is associated with polyuria. Two mechanisms have been proposed to explain the AVP-resistant concentrating defect, both of which likely involve the calcium-sensing receptor. This receptor is expressed on the basolateral (blood) side of the thick ascending limb cells, and it indirectly inhibits the NKCC2 cotransporter, thus impairing the generation of a medullary concentration gradient.[62-64] Secondly, this receptor is also expressed on the luminal (urine) side of the collecting duct cells, and it is thought to affect AQP2 trafficking.[65,66] The latter mechanism would thus be mediated by hypercalciuria, and it may constitute a protective measure against the formation of calcium-containing stones.[67]

Hypokalemia

Hypokalemia causes an AVP-resistant concentration defect. As in the other forms of acquired NDI, the reduced expression of AQP2 has been demonstrated.[68] Thus, the downregulation of AQP2 seems to be a common feature of acquired NDI.[30] However, the mechanism by which hypokalemia affects this remains to be elucidated.

Disorders Impairing the Generation of a Medullary Concentration Gradient

Bartter Syndrome

As discussed previously, the loop of Henle and active salt reabsorption in thick ascending limb are necessary for the generation of a medullary concentration gradient. Therefore, factors that impair salt reabsorption in the thick ascending limb will lead to a urinary concentration defect (hypo- or isosthenuria). Patients with Bartter syndrome have inherited defects in thick ascending limb salt transport; symptoms include polyuria and episodes of hypernatremic dehydration (see Chapter 29: Bartter, Gitelman, and Related Syndromes), which are similar to those of patients with NDI. However, the presence of a hypokalemic alkalosis and elevated urinary electrolytes (particularly chloride) help differentiate it from NDI, although the former may be absent in young infants.[69] A history of polyhydramnios further helps to exclude a diagnosis of NDI.

Fanconi Syndrome

Polyuria and hyposthenuria are observed in patients with Fanconi syndrome (see Chapter 28: Fanconi Syndrome), likely as a result of the increased distal delivery of water and solutes as well as of the hypercalciuria resulting from decreased proximal sodium reabsorption.[70]

Urea Transporter

Urea is an important constituent of the medullary interstitial concentration gradient. Urea is a bipolar molecule, and, thus, it can only diffuse slowly through membranes.[71] Diffusion is facilitated by urea transporters, and two genes that encode these transporters have been identified in humans.[72] A mild urinary concentrating defect has been described in patients who do not express the minor blood group antigen Kidd (Jk).[73] Later, this antigen was identified to be identical with the urea transporter UT-1, which is encoded by *SLC14A1*, and several mutations in this gene have been identified in Kidd-negative individuals.[74-76] Interestingly, no mutations have been found so far in the gene that encodes the urea transporter expressed in renal tubule UT-2 (*SLC14A2*). Recent evidence suggests that UT-1 is also expressed in the endothelium of the vasa recta and that the combined defect in red cell and vascular urea diffusion impairs countercurrent concentration.[77,78]

GENETICS

AVPR2

The majority of cases of NDI (90%) are the result of mutations in the AVPR2 gene.[79,80] The gene is located on chromosome region Xq28, and the mode of inheritance is X-linked recessive. Therefore, the majority of patients with NDI are male, but, as a result of skewed X-inactivation (lionization), females can be affected with variable degrees of polyuria and polydipsia.[17,81-83] Indeed, in some families, X-inactivation is strongly biased, and this leads to a pseudodominant inheritance pattern.[84] X-inactivation may be strongly biased as a result of chance, a coexistent mutation on the affected X-chromosome that affects cell survival, or a coexisting mutation in a gene that regulates X-inactivation.[85]

So far, more than 180 distinct putative disease-causing mutations have been described in more than 280 families.[79] When investigated in vitro, these mutations can be classified according to their effect[86-103]:

1. Class 1 mutations result in frame shifts, premature stop codons, and aberrant splicing, and they prevent the translation of the receptor protein.
2. Class 2 mutations are missense mutations that allow for the translation of the protein but that lead to aberrant trafficking. Typically, these mutations induce improper folding with subsequent trapping in the endoplasmic reticulum.

3. Class 3 mutations allow the mutated protein to reach the cell surface, but they impair the receptor's signaling, typically by affecting the binding of AVP.

The majority of mutations identified in X-linked NDI belong to class 2.[104] Conversely, mutations identified in inherited partial NDI fall into class 3: these mutated receptors reach the cell membrane, but they have a decreased affinity for AVP.[48,52]

Interestingly, another class 3 mutation was recently identified in the *AVPR2* gene that led to gain of function with constitutive activation of the receptor and thus to a "nephrogenic syndrome of inappropriate antidiuresis."[105]

AQP2

The analysis of a pedigree with affected females and the presence of intact extrarenal responses to DDAVP in some patients with NDI lead to the postulation of an autosomal inherited "post-receptor" defect in these individuals.[106-108] The molecular basis for this distinct form of NDI was identified in 1994 to be the water channel aquaporin-2, which is expressed in the collecting duct.[14] Approximately 10% of all patients with NDI carry mutations in *AQP2*. As expected for a loss-of-function defect, inheritance is usually recessive and, similar to AVPR2, the majority of mutations fall into class 2, with retention in the endoplasmic reticulum.[104,109] Interestingly, there are some families with autosomal-dominant inheritance of NDI. Molecular analysis has shown that affected members carry mutations in the c-terminus of AQP2.[38,110-112] So why does this lead to a dominant inheritance? The final water channel is a homotetramer, which means that it consists of four AQP2 subunits (see Figure 32-2). Dominant mutations in the c-terminus lead to aberrant trafficking (class 2), but they are able to oligomerize with wild-type protein to form the tetramer. Because tetramerization takes place before export to the plasma membrane, these mutations exert a dominant-negative effect on AQP2 function by misguiding the trafficking of the assembled tetramer. Interestingly, specific mutations direct AQP2 trafficking to distinct cellular compartments, such as the Golgi complex,[38] late endosomes/lysosomes,[110] or the basolateral membrane.[112]

TREATMENT

General Aspects of Treatment

The importance of the prompt treatment of NDI is highlighted by the fact that mental retardation used to be an invariable feature, but nowadays can be completely prevented by proper treatment. Caring for a patient with NDI is most difficult during infancy, when the babies are dependent on their caregivers for access to fluids. Fluids should be offered at 2-hour intervals, which places a considerable burden on the caregivers, particularly at night. Feeding per nasogastric tube is often helpful during this period. A continuous overnight feed delivered by a pump will provide fluid and calories to the baby and much needed rest to the parents. Families also need to be instructed to bring the child for immediate medical attention when there are increased extrarenal fluid losses, such as when diarrhea, vomiting, or fever are present. It is often helpful for the parents to have a letter detailing the condition of their child and the need for prompt physical and biochemical assessment that they can present in these instances to avoid being sent home by medical personnel with no experience with this condition. There should be a low threshold for admission and intravenous hydration in these instances to prevent dehydration. When in hospital, hypotonic fluids (e.g., 0.22% normal saline) are usually appropriate for intravenous hydration as a result of the obligate water losses in the urine. Replacement fluids with a higher osmolality than urine osmolality will exacerbate hypernatremia. For instance, 0.45% saline has an osmolality of 154 mOsm/kg (77 mOsm sodium and 77 mOsm chlorine). A patient with a maximal urine osmolality of 100 mOsm/kg will need to excrete 1.54 L of urine for each liter of 0.45% saline received to excrete the osmotic load presented by the replacement fluid (described later). Thus, in patients with NDI, the administration of fluids that are hypertonic as compared with urine can lead to hypernatremic dehydration, even though the fluid may be hypotonic to plasma. However, if there are increased salt losses (as can occur with diarrhea) or if hypotonic fluids are administered at a rate that is higher than the urine losses, hyponatremia could ensue. Close monitoring of the patient with respect to weight, fluid balance, clinical symptoms, and biochemistries is therefore imperative to prevent complications.

Osmotic Load Reduction

The most important part of the treatment of patients with NDI is a reduction of their osmotic load (also called the *renal solute load*), which determines urine volume. Therefore, the close involvement of a dietician with experience in the management of children with kidney problems is necessary. The osmotic load consists of proteins (they are metabolized to urea) and salts, both of which need to be excreted by the kidney. A typical Western diet contains an osmotic load of about 800 mOsm per day. Thus, an individual with a urine osmolality of 800 mOsm/kg only needs 1 L of water to excrete that load. However, a patient with NDI and a maximal urine osmolality of 100 mOsm/kg needs at least 8 L of water for excretion, and, if the urine osmolality is 50 mOsm/kg, then 16 L of water are required. One gram of table salt is equivalent to about 18 mmol of sodium chloride, thus providing an osmolar load of 36 mOsm (18 mOsm sodium and 18 mOsm chlorine). Consequently, for a patient with a urine osmolality of 100 mOsm/kg, each gram of salt ingested increases obligatory urine output by 360 ml. The osmolar load of a diet can be roughly estimated by the following formula: twice the millimolar amount of sodium and potassium (to account for the accompanying anions) plus protein (g) times 4.[113] Because lipids and sugars are metabolized without byproducts requiring renal excretion, only protein intake needs to be limited, but it should still meet the recommended daily allowance. A reasonable goal is a diet that contains about 15 mOsm/kg/d. A child with a urine osmolality of 100 mOsm will need a fluid intake of 150 ml/kg/d to be able to excrete that load, which is achievable. Enriching the fluid with carbohydrates will provide additional calories without increasing the osmolar load.

Diuretics

The use of a diuretic by a patient with a polyuric disorder appears at first glance to be counterintuitive, but it does make physiologic sense. The successful use of thiazides in patients with NDI with a subsequent increase in urine osmolality and a concomitant decrease in urine output was first reported in 1959.[114,115] Thiazides inhibit the reabsorption of sodium and chloride in the distal convoluted tubule (part of the urinary dilution mechanism, described previously) and thus increase the salt concentration and osmolality of the urine. The increased salt losses decrease the intravascular volume with a subsequent upregulation of the proximal tubular reabsorption of salt and water. Consequently, less volume is delivered to the collecting duct and lost in the urine. Typically used is hydrochlorothiazide at 2 mg/kg/d in two divided doses. The more long-acting bendroflumethiazide (50 to 100 mcg/kg/d) can be given as a single daily dose. Hypokalemia is a common complication of thiazide administration, but supplementation with potassium salts increases the osmolar load. Therefore, the combination of the thiazide with a potassium-sparing diuretic (e.g., amiloride, 0.1 to 0.3 mg/kg/d) is advantageous, but the latter can cause gastrointestinal side effects, especially nausea.

Prostaglandin Synthesis Inhibitors

As with many other tubular disorders, prostaglandin synthesis inhibitors are used in NDI with the aim of reducing the glomerular filtration rate and thus providing a "partial chemical nephrectomy" to minimize losses. However, experiments in animals and humans suggest that prostaglandin synthesis inhibitors can increase urine osmolality without decreasing the glomerular filtration rate. The exact mechanism remains to be elucidated, but it appears to be independent of antidiuretic hormone.[116-118] Some evidence suggests that the activation of basolateral prostaglandin receptors by prostaglandin E2 inhibits adenylcyclase and/or the shuttling of AQP2 to the apical membrane.[119-121]

Typically used is indomethacin (1 to 3 mg/kg/d in three to four divided doses). The long-term use of this drug is associated with the deterioration of renal function and with hematologic and gastrointestinal side effects, including life-threatening hemorrhage.[122,123] The latter may be avoided by using a selective COX-2 inhibitor, and the successful use of these in patients with NDI has been reported.[124,125] However, there are concerns about the cardiotoxic side effects of these drugs, as evidenced by the removal of rofecoxib from the marketplace.[126] In our experience, the combination of hydrochlorothiazide with indomethacin is useful during the first years of life, with a subsequent switch to bendroflumethiazide with or without amiloride. The key is the close observation of the individual patient for side effects and for changes in urine output or growth percentiles.

The use of anti-gastrointestinal reflux medications such as a histamine H2-antagonist (e.g., ranitidine, 2 to 4 mg/kg/dose twice daily) and a prokinetic (e.g., domperidone, 250 to 500 mcg/kg three to four times daily) can help with the vomiting that is often seen in infants with NDI and help prevent the gastrointestinal side effects of indomethacin.

Future Perspectives: Molecular Chaperones

The vast majority of mutations identified in the *AVPR2* gene lead to the improper folding of the resultant protein with entrapment in the endoplasmic reticulum (described previously). Retention is dependent on specialized endoplasmic reticulum proteins, many of which require calcium for optimal function. Therefore, the depletion of endoplasmic reticulum calcium stores by inhibiting the sarcoplasmatic calcium pump may be useful for overcoming entrapment.[127] Indeed, this approach has been successfully used in vitro to induce the surface expression of an AVPR2 mutant.[128] Even more promising—and more specific—is the idea of using small pharmacologic chaperones that can enter the cell, bind to the mutant receptor, and thus induce proper folding with subsequent release from the endoplasmic reticulum.[129,130] With the development of small membrane-permeable AVPR2-receptor antagonists that are designed to fit neatly into the binding fold of the receptor, this approach has become feasible and indeed successful in vitro.[131-133] More importantly, a recent trial of an AVP antagonist in five patients with NDI who bore either the mutation del62-64, R137H, or W164S (all of which lead to endoplasmic reticulum retention), demonstrated a significant decrease in urine output with a concomitant increase in urine osmolality.[134] Total 24-hour urine volume decreased from a mean of 11.9 to 8.2 L, and mean urine osmolality rose from 98 to 170 mOsm/kg; thus the observed effect was modest. Nevertheless, these results hold the promise of a targeted, mutation-specific therapy for patients with NDI.

REFERENCES

1. McIlraith CH: Notes on some cases of diabetes insipidus with marked family and hereditary tendencies, *Lancet* 2:767, 1892.
2. de Lange C: Ueber erblichen diabetes insipidus. *Jahrbuch fuer Kinderheilkunde* 145(1):135, 1935.
3. Forssman HH: On hereditary diabetes insipidus, *Acta Medica Scandinavica* 121(supplement 159):9, 1945.
4. Waring AJ, Kajdi L, Tappan V: A congenital defect of water metabolism, *Am J Dis Child* 69:323-24, 1945.
5. Williams RH, Henry C: Nephrogenic diabetes insipidus: transmitted by females and appearing during infancy in males, *Ann Intern Med* 27:84-95, 1947.
6. Bode HH, Crawford JD: Nephrogenic diabetes insipidus in North America—the Hopewell hypothesis, *N Engl J Med* 280:750-54, 1967.
7. Bichet DG, Arthus MF, Lonergan M, Hendy GN, et al: X-linked nephrogenic diabetes insipidus mutations in North America and the Hopewell hypothesis, *J Clin Invest* 92(3):1262-68, 1993.
8. Lolait SJ, O'Carroll AM, McBride OW, Konig M, et al: Cloning and characterization of a vasopressin V2 receptor and possible link to nephrogenic diabetes insipidus, *Nature* 357(6376):336-39, 1992.
9. Rosenthal W, Seibold A, Antaramian A, Lonergan M, et al: Molecular identification of the gene responsible for congenital nephrogenic diabetes insipidus, *Nature* 359(6392):233-35, 1992.
10. van den Ouweland AM, Dreesen JC, Verdijk M, Knoers NV, et al: Mutations in the vasopressin type 2 receptor gene (AVPR2) associated with nephrogenic diabetes insipidus, *Nat Genet* 2(2):99-102, 1992.
11. Pan Y, Metzenberg A, Das S, Jing B, Gitschier J: Mutations in the V2 vasopressin receptor gene are associated with X-linked nephrogenic diabetes insipidus, *Nat Genet* 2(2):103-06, 1992.
12. Fushimi K, Uchida S, Hara Y, Hirata Y, et al: Cloning and expression of apical membrane water channel of rat kidney collecting tubule, *Nature* 361(6412):549-52, 1993.

13. Sasaki S, Fushimi K, Saito H, Saito F, et al: Cloning, characterization, and chromosomal mapping of human aquaporin of collecting duct, *J Clin Invest* 93(3):1250-56, 1994.
14. Deen PM, Verdijk MA, Knoers NV, Wieringa B, et al: Requirement of human renal water channel aquaporin-2 for vasopressin-dependent concentration of urine, *Science* 264(5155):92-95, 1994.
15. Bonilla-Felix M: Development of water transport in the collecting duct, *Am J Physiol Renal Physiol* 287(6):F1093-101, 2004.
16. Hoekstra JA, van Lieburg AF, Monnens LA, Hulstijn-Dirkmaat GM, Knoers VV: Cognitive and psychosocial functioning of patients with congenital nephrogenic diabetes insipidus, *Am J Med Genet* 61(1):81-88, 1996.
17. van Lieburg AF, Knoers NV, Monnens LA: Clinical presentation and follow-up of 30 patients with congenital nephrogenic diabetes insipidus, *J Am Soc Nephrol* 10(9):1958-64, 1999.
18. Hillman DA, Neyzi O, Porter P, Cushman A, Talbot NB: Renal (vasopressin-resistant) diabetes insipidus; definition of the effects of a homeostatic limitation in capacity to conserve water on the physical, intellectual and emotional development of a child, *Pediatrics* 21(3):430-35, 1958.
19. Vest M, Talbot NB, Crawford JD: Hypocaloric dwarfism and hydronephrosis in diabetes insipidus, *Am J Dis Child* 105:175-81, 1963.
20. Yoo TH, Ryu DR, Song YS, Lee SC, et al: Congenital nephrogenic diabetes insipidus presented with bilateral hydronephrosis: genetic analysis of V2R gene mutations, *Yonsei Med J* 47(1):126-30, 2006.
21. Stevens S, Brown BD, McGahan JP: Nephrogenic diabetes insipidus: a cause of severe nonobstructive urinary tract dilatation, *J Ultrasound Med* 14(7):543-45, 1995.
22. Stephenson JL: Concentration of urine in a central core model of the renal counterflow system, *Kidney Int* 2(2):85-94, 1972.
23. Kokko JP, Rector FC Jr: Countercurrent multiplication system without active transport in inner medulla, *Kidney Int* 2(4):214-23, 1972.
24. Zhang R, Skach W, Hasegawa H, van Hoek AN, Verkman AS: Cloning, functional analysis and cell localization of a kidney proximal tubule water transporter homologous to CHIP28, *J Cell Biol* 120(2):359-69, 1993.
25. Sabolic I, Valenti G, Verbavatz JM, Van Hoek AN, et al: Localization of the CHIP28 water channel in rat kidney, *Am J Physiol* 263(6 Pt 1):C1225-33, 1992.
26. Nielsen S, Smith BL, Christensen EI, Knepper MA, Agre P: CHIP28 water channels are localized in constitutively water-permeable segments of the nephron, *J Cell Biol* 120(2):371-83, 1993.
27. Nielsen S, Pallone T, Smith BL, Christensen EI, et al: Aquaporin-1 water channels in short and long loop descending thin limbs and in descending vasa recta in rat kidney, *Am J Physiol* 268(6 Pt 2): F1023-37, 1995.
28. Imaï M, Kokko JP: Sodium chloride, urea, and water transport in the thin ascending limb of Henle. Generation of osmotic gradients by passive diffusion of solutes, *J Clin Invest* 53(2):393-402, 1974.
29. Obermuller N, Kunchaparty S, Ellison DH, Bachmann S: Expression of the Na-K-2Cl cotransporter by macula densa and thick ascending limb cells of rat and rabbit nephron, *J Clin Invest* 98(3):635-40, 1996.
30. Nielsen S, Frokiaer J, Marples D, Kwon TH, et al: Aquaporins in the kidney: from molecules to medicine, *Physiol Rev* 82(1):205-44, 2002.
31. Eggena P, Christakis J, Deppisch L: Effect of hypotonicity on cyclic adenosine monophosphate formation and action in vasopressin target cells, *Kidney Int* 7(3):161-69, 1975.
32. Edwards RM, Jackson BA, Dousa TP: ADH-sensitive cAMP system in papillary collecting duct: effect of osmolality and PGE2, *Am J Physiol* 240(4):F311-18, 1981.
33. Nielsen S, Chou CL, Marples D, Christensen EI, et al: Vasopressin increases water permeability of kidney collecting duct by inducing translocation of aquaporin-CD water channels to plasma membrane. *Proc Natl Acad Sci U S A* 92(4):1013-17, 1995.
34. Knepper MA, Nielsen S, Chou CL, DiGiovanni SR: Mechanism of vasopressin action in the renal collecting duct, *Semin Nephrol* 14(4):302-21, 1994.
35. Katsura T, Gustafson CE, Ausiello DA, Brown D: Protein kinase A phosphorylation is involved in regulated exocytosis of aquaporin-2 in transfected LLC-PK1 cells, *Am J Physiol* 272(6 Pt 2):F817-22, 1997.
36. Fushimi K, Sasaki S, Marumo F: Phosphorylation of serine 256 is required for cAMP-dependent regulatory exocytosis of the aquaporin-2 water channel, *J Biol Chem* 272(23):14800-04, 1997.
37. Christensen BM, Zelenina M, Aperia A, Nielsen S: Localization and regulation of PKA-phosphorylated AQP2 in response to V(2)-receptor agonist/antagonist treatment, *Am J Physiol Renal Physiol* 278(1):F29-42, 2000.
38. Mulders SM, Bichet DG, Rijss JP, Kamsteeg EJ, et al: An aquaporin-2 water channel mutant which causes autosomal dominant nephrogenic diabetes insipidus is retained in the Golgi complex, *J Clin Invest* 102(1):57-66, 1998.
39. Ecelbarger CA, Terris J, Frindt G, Echevarria M, et al: Aquaporin-3 water channel localization and regulation in rat kidney, *Am J Physiol* 269(5 Pt 2):F663-F672, 1995.
40. Terris J, Ecelbarger CA, Nielsen S, Knepper MA: Long-term regulation of four renal aquaporins in rats, *Am J Physiol* 271(2 Pt 2): F414-22, 1996.
41. Terris J, Ecelbarger CA, Marples D, Knepper MA, Nielsen S: Distribution of aquaporin-4 water channel expression within rat kidney, *Am J Physiol* 269(6 Pt 2):F775-85, 1995.
42. Holmes CL, Landry DW, Granton JT: Science review: Vasopressin and the cardiovascular system part 1—receptor physiology, *Crit Care* 7(6):427-34, 2003.
43. Bichet DG, Razi M, Lonergan M, Arthus MF, et al: Hemodynamic and coagulation responses to 1-desamino[8-D-arginine] vasopressin in patients with congenital nephrogenic diabetes insipidus, *N Engl J Med* 318(14):881-87, 1988.
44. Williams TD, Lightman SL, Leadbeater MJ: Hormonal and cardiovascular responses to DDAVP in man, *Clin Endocrinol (Oxf)* 24(1):89-96, 1986.
45. Mannucci PM, Canciani MT, Rota L, Donovan BS: Response of factor VIII/von Willebrand factor to DDAVP in healthy subjects and patients with haemophilia A and von Willebrand's disease, *Br J Haematol* 47(2):283-93, 1981.
46. Mannucci PM, Aberg M, Nilsson IM, Robertson B: Mechanism of plasminogen activator and factor VIII increase after vasoactive drugs, *Br J Haematol* 30(1):81-93, 1975.
47. Winberg J: Determination of renal concentration capacity in infants and children without renal disease. *Acta Paediatrica* 48:318-28, 1958.
48. Vargas-Poussou R, Forestier L, Dautzenberg MD, Niaudet P, et al: Mutations in the vasopressin V2 receptor and aquaporin-2 genes in 12 families with congenital nephrogenic diabetes insipidus, *J Am Soc Nephrol* 8(12):1855-62, 1997.
49. Monnens L, Smulders Y, van Lier H, de Boo T: DDAVP test for assessment of renal concentrating capacity in infants and children, *Nephron* 29(3-4):151-54, 1981.
50. Ito M, Mori Y, Oiso Y, Saito H: A single base substitution in the coding region for neurophysin II associated with familial central diabetes insipidus, *J Clin Invest* 87(2):725-28, 1991.
51. Ghirardello S, Malattia C, Scagnelli P, Maghnie M: Current perspective on the pathogenesis of central diabetes insipidus, *J Pediatr Endocrinol Metab* 18(7):631-45, 2005.
52. Sadeghi H, Robertson GL, Bichet DG, Innamorati G, Birnbaumer M: Biochemical basis of partial nephrogenic diabetes insipidus phenotypes, *Mol Endocrinol* 11(12):1806-13, 1997.
53. Canfield MC, Tamarappoo BK, Moses AM, Verkman AS, Holtzman EJ: Identification and characterization of aquaporin-2 water channel mutations causing nephrogenic diabetes insipidus with partial vasopressin response, *Hum Mol Genet* 6(11):1865-71, 1997.
54. Frokiaer J, Marples D, Knepper MA, Nielsen S: Bilateral ureteral obstruction downregulates expression of vasopressin-sensitive AQP-2 water channel in rat kidney, *Am J Physiol* 270(4 Pt 2): F657-68, 1996.
55. Frokiaer J, Christensen BM, Marples D, Djurhuus JC, et al: Downregulation of aquaporin-2 parallels changes in renal water excretion

in unilateral ureteral obstruction, *Am J Physiol* 273(2 Pt 2):F213-23, 1997.
56. Kwon TH, Frokiaer J, Fernandez-Llama P, Knepper MA, Nielsen S: Reduced abundance of aquaporins in rats with bilateral ischemia-induced acute renal failure: prevention by alpha-MSH, *Am J Physiol* 277(3 Pt 2):F413-27, 1999.
57. Johnston PA, Rennke H, Levinsky NG: Recovery of proximal tubular function from ischemic injury, *Am J Physiol* 246(2 Pt 2): F159-66, 1984.
58. Boton R, Gaviria M, Batlle DC: Prevalence, pathogenesis, and treatment of renal dysfunction associated with chronic lithium therapy, *Am J Kidney Dis* 10(5):329-45, 1987.
59. Carney SL, Ray C, Gillies AH: Mechanism of lithium-induced polyuria in the rat, *Kidney Int* 50(2):377-83, 1996.
60. Christensen S, Kusano E, Yusufi AN, Murayama N, Dousa TP: Pathogenesis of nephrogenic diabetes insipidus due to chronic administration of lithium in rats, *J Clin Invest* 75(6):1869-79, 1985.
61. Marples D, Christensen S, Christensen EI, Ottosen PD, Nielsen S: Lithium-induced downregulation of aquaporin-2 water channel expression in rat kidney medulla, *J Clin Invest* 95(4):1838-45, 1995.
62. Watanabe S, Fukumoto S, Chang H, Takeuchi Y, et al: Association between activating mutations of calcium-sensing receptor and Bartter's syndrome, *Lancet* 360(9334):692-94, 2002.
63. Hebert SC: Bartter syndrome, *Curr Opin Nephrol Hypertens* 12(5):527-32, 2003.
64. Wang W, Kwon TH, Li C, Frokiaer J, et al: Reduced expression of Na-K-2Cl cotransporter in medullary TAL in vitamin D-induced hypercalcemia in rats, *Am J Physiol Renal Physiol* 282(1):F34-44, 2002.
65. Sands JM, Naruse M, Baum M, Jo I, et al: Apical extracellular calcium/polyvalent cation-sensing receptor regulates vasopressin-elicited water permeability in rat kidney inner medullary collecting duct, *J Clin Invest* 99(6):1399-405, 1997.
66. Earm JH, Christensen BM, Frokiaer J, Marples D, et al: Decreased aquaporin-2 expression and apical plasma membrane delivery in kidney collecting ducts of polyuric hypercalcemic rats, *J Am Soc Nephrol* 9(12):2181-93, 1998.
67. Hebert SC, Brown EM, Harris HW: Role of the Ca(2+)-sensing receptor in divalent mineral ion homeostasis, *J Exp Biol* 200(Pt 2):295-302, 1997.
68. Marples D, Frokiaer J, Dorup J, Knepper MA, Nielsen S: Hypokalemia-induced downregulation of aquaporin-2 water channel expression in rat kidney medulla and cortex, *J Clin Invest* 97(8):1960-68, 1996.
69. Bettinelli A, Ciarmatori S, Cesareo L, Tedeschi S, et al: Phenotypic variability in Bartter syndrome type I, *Pediatr Nephrol* 14(10-11):940-45, 2000.
70. Nijenhuis T, Vallon V, van der Kemp AW, Loffing J, et al: Enhanced passive Ca2+ reabsorption and reduced Mg2+ channel abundance explains thiazide-induced hypocalciuria and hypomagnesemia, *J Clin Invest* 115(6):1651-58, 2005.
71. Gallucci E, Micelli S, Lippe C: Non-electrolyte permeability across thin lipid membranes, *Arch Int Physiol Biochim* 79(5):881-87, 1971.
72. Sands JM: Renal urea transporters, *Curr Opin Nephrol Hypertens* 13(5):525-32, 2004.
73. Gillin AG, Sands JM: Urea transport in the kidney, *Semin Nephrol* 13(2):146-54, 1993.
74. Sidoux-Walter F, Lucien N, Nissinen R, Sistonen P, et al: Molecular heterogeneity of the Jk(null) phenotype: expression analysis of the Jk(S291P) mutation found in Finns, *Blood* 96(4):1566-73, 2000.
75. Lucien N, Sidoux-Walter F, Olives B, Moulds J, et al: Characterization of the gene encoding the human Kidd blood group/urea transporter protein. Evidence for splice site mutations in Jknull individuals, *J Biol Chem* 273(21):12973-80, 1998.
76. Olives B, Mattei MG, Huet M, Neau P, et al: Kidd blood group and urea transport function of human erythrocytes are carried by the same protein, *J Biol Chem* 270(26):15607-10, 1995.
77. Pallone TL, Turner MR, Edwards A, Jamison RL: Countercurrent exchange in the renal medulla, *Am J Physiol Regul Integr Comp Physiol* 284(5):R1153-75, 2003.
78. Promeneur D, Rousselet G, Bankir L, Bailly P, et al: Evidence for distinct vascular and tubular urea transporters in the rat kidney, *J Am Soc Nephrol* 7(6):852-60, 1996.
79. Sands JM, Bichet DG: Nephrogenic diabetes insipidus, *Ann Intern Med* 144(3):186-94, 2006.
80. Bichet DG, Oksche A, Rosenthal W: Congenital nephrogenic diabetes insipidus. *J Am Soc Nephrol* 8(12):1951-58, 1997.
81. Sato K, Fukuno H, Taniguchi T, Sawada S, et al: A novel mutation in the vasopressin V2 receptor gene in a woman with congenital nephrogenic diabetes insipidus, *Intern Med* 38(10):808-12, 1999.
82. Arthus MF, Lonergan M, Crumley MJ, Naumova AK, et al: Report of 33 novel AVPR2 mutations and analysis of 117 families with X-linked nephrogenic diabetes insipidus, *J Am Soc Nephrol* 11(6):1044-54, 2000.
83. Kinoshita K, Miura Y, Nagasaki H, Murase T, et al: A novel deletion mutation in the arginine vasopressin receptor 2 gene and skewed X chromosome inactivation in a female patient with congenital nephrogenic diabetes insipidus, *J Endocrinol Invest* 27(2):167-70, 2004.
84. Friedman E, Bale AE, Carson E, Boson WL, et al: Nephrogenic diabetes insipidus: an X chromosome-linked dominant inheritance pattern with a vasopressin type 2 receptor gene that is structurally normal, *Proc Natl Acad Sci U S A* 91(18):8457-61, 1994.
85. Puck JM, Willard HF: X inactivation in females with X-linked disease, *N Engl J Med* 338(5):325-28, 1998.
86. Holtzman EJ, Kolakowski LF Jr, Geifman-Holtzman O, O'Brien DG, et al: Mutations in the vasopressin V2 receptor gene in two families with nephrogenic diabetes insipidus, *J Am Soc Nephrol* 5(2):169-76, 1994.
87. Pan Y, Wilson P, Gitschier J: The effect of eight V2 vasopressin receptor mutations on stimulation of adenylyl cyclase and binding to vasopressin, *J Biol Chem* 269(50):31933-37, 1994.
88. Tsukaguchi H, Matsubara H, Mori Y, Yoshimasa Y, et al: Two vasopressin type 2 receptor gene mutations R143P and delta V278 in patients with nephrogenic diabetes insipidus impair ligand binding of the receptor, *Biochem Biophys Res Commun* 211(3):967-77, 1995.
89. Tsukaguchi H, Matsubara H, Inada M: Expression studies of two vasopressin V2 receptor gene mutations, R202C and 804insG, in nephrogenic diabetes insipidus, *Kidney Int* 48(2):554-62, 1995.
90. Tsukaguchi H, Matsubara H, Taketani S, Mori Y, et al: Binding-, intracellular transport-, and biosynthesis-defective mutants of vasopressin type 2 receptor in patients with X-linked nephrogenic diabetes insipidus, *J Clin Invest* 96(4):2043-50, 1995.
91. Yokoyama K, Yamauchi A, Izumi M, Itoh T, et al: A low-affinity vasopressin V2-receptor gene in a kindred with X-linked nephrogenic diabetes insipidus, *J Am Soc Nephrol* 7(3):410-14, 1996.
92. Oksche A, Schulein R, Rutz C, Liebenhoff U, et al: Vasopressin V2 receptor mutants that cause X-linked nephrogenic diabetes insipidus: analysis of expression, processing, and function, *Mol Pharmacol* 50(4):820-28, 1996.
93. Wenkert D, Schoneberg T, Merendino JJ Jr, Rodriguez Pena MS, et al: Functional characterization of five V2 vasopressin receptor gene mutations, *Mol Cell Endocrinol* 124(1-2):43-50, 1996.
94. Sadeghi HM, Innamorati G, Birnbaumer M: An X-linked NDI mutation reveals a requirement for cell surface V2R expression, *Mol Endocrinol* 11(6):706-13, 1997.
95. Schoneberg T, Schulz A, Biebermann H, Gruters A, et al: V2 vasopressin receptor dysfunction in nephrogenic diabetes insipidus caused by different molecular mechanisms, *Hum Mutat* 12(3):196-205, 1998.
96. Ala Y, Morin D, Mouillac B, Sabatier N, et al: Functional studies of twelve mutant V2 vasopressin receptors related to nephrogenic diabetes insipidus: molecular basis of a mild clinical phenotype, *J Am Soc Nephrol* 9(10):1861-72, 1998.
97. Wildin RS, Cogdell DE, Valadez V: AVPR2 variants and V2 vasopressin receptor function in nephrogenic diabetes insipidus, *Kidney Int* 54(6):1909-22, 1998.
98. Pasel K, Schulz A, Timmermann K, Linnemann K, et al: Functional characterization of the molecular defects causing nephrogenic diabetes insipidus in eight families, *J Clin Endocrinol Metab* 85(4):1703-10, 2000.

99. Albertazzi E, Zanchetta D, Barbier P, Faranda S, et al: Nephrogenic diabetes insipidus: functional analysis of new AVPR2 mutations identified in Italian families, *J Am Soc Nephrol* 11(6):1033-43, 2000.
100. Postina R, Ufer E, Pfeiffer R, Knoers NV, Fahrenholz F: Misfolded vasopressin V2 receptors caused by extracellular point mutations entail congenital nephrogenic diabetes insipidus, *Mol Cell Endocrinol* 164(1-2):31-39, 2000.
101. Knoers NV, Deen PM: Molecular and cellular defects in nephrogenic diabetes insipidus, *Pediatr Nephrol* 16(12):1146-52, 2001.
102. Hermosilla R, Oueslati M, Donalies U, Schonenberger E, et al: Disease-causing V(2) vasopressin receptors are retained in different compartments of the early secretory pathway, *Traffic* 5(12):993-1005, 2004.
103. Robben JH, Knoers NV, Deen PM: Characterization of vasopressin V2 receptor mutants in nephrogenic diabetes insipidus in a polarized cell model, *Am J Physiol Renal Physiol* 289(2):F265-72, 2005.
104. Fujiwara TM, Bichet DG: Molecular biology of hereditary diabetes insipidus, *J Am Soc Nephrol* 16(10):2836-46, 2005.
105. Feldman BJ, Rosenthal SM, Vargas GA, Fenwick RG, et al: Nephrogenic syndrome of inappropriate antidiuresis, *N Engl J Med* 352(18):1884-90, 2005.
106. Brenner B, Seligsohn U, Hochberg Z: Normal response of factor VIII and von Willebrand factor to 1-deamino-8D-arginine vasopressin in nephrogenic diabetes insipidus, *J Clin Endocrinol Metab* 67(1):191-93, 1988.
107. Knoers N, Monnens LA: A variant of nephrogenic diabetes insipidus: V2 receptor abnormality restricted to the kidney, *Eur J Pediatr* 150(5):370-73, 1991.
108. Langley JM, Balfe JW, Selander T, Ray PN, Clarke JT: Autosomal recessive inheritance of vasopressin-resistant diabetes insipidus, *Am J Med Genet* 38(1):90-94, 1991.
109. Marr N, Bichet DG, Hoefs S, Savelkoul PJ, et al: Cell-biologic and functional analyses of five new Aquaporin-2 missense mutations that cause recessive nephrogenic diabetes insipidus, *J Am Soc Nephrol* 13(9):2267-77, 2002.
110. Marr N, Bichet DG, Lonergan M, Arthus MF, et al: Heteroligomerization of an Aquaporin-2 mutant with wild-type aquaporin-2 and their misrouting to late endosomes/lysosomes explains dominant nephrogenic diabetes insipidus, *Hum Mol Genet* 11(7):779-89, 2002.
111. Kuwahara M, Iwai K, Ooeda T, Igarashi T, et al: Three families with autosomal dominant nephrogenic diabetes insipidus caused by aquaporin-2 mutations in the C-terminus, *Am J Hum Genet* 69(4):738-48, 2001.
112. Kamsteeg EJ, Bichet DG, Konings IB, Nivet H, et al: Reversed polarized delivery of an aquaporin-2 mutant causes dominant nephrogenic diabetes insipidus, *J Cell Biol* 163(5):1099-109, 2003.
113. Coleman J: Diseases of organ system: the kidney. In Shaw V, Lawson M, editors: *Clinical paediatric dietetics*, ed 2, Oxford, 2001, Blackwell Science.
114. Kennedy GC, Crawford JD: Treatment of diabetes insipidus with hydrochlorothiazide, *Lancet* 1(7078):866-67, 1959.
115. Crawford JD, Kennedy GC: Chlorothiazide in diabetes insipidus, *Nature* 183(4665):891-92, 1959.
116. Stoff JS, Rosa RM, Silva P, Epstein FH: Indomethacin impairs water diuresis in the DI rat: role of prostaglandins independent of ADH, *Am J Physiol* 241(3):F231-37, 1981.
117. Walker RM, Brown RS, Stoff JS: Role of renal prostaglandins during antidiuresis and water diuresis in man, *Kidney Int* 21(2):365-70, 1982.
118. Usberti M, Pecoraro C, Federico S, Cianciaruso B, et al: Mechanism of action of indomethacin in tubular defects, *Pediatrics* 75(3):501-07, 1985.
119. Tamma G, Wiesner B, Furkert J, Hahm D, et al: The prostaglandin E2 analogue sulprostone antagonizes vasopressin-induced antidiuresis through activation of Rho, *J Cell Sci* 116(Pt 16):3285-94, 2003.
120. Huber TB, Simons M, Hartleben B, Sernetz L, et al: Molecular basis of the functional podocin-nephrin complex: mutations in the NPHS2 gene disrupt nephrin targeting to lipid raft microdomains, *Hum Mol Genet* 12(24):3397-405, 2003.
121. Hebert RL, Breyer RM, Jacobson HR, Breyer MD: Functional and molecular aspects of prostaglandin E receptors in the cortical collecting duct, *Can J Physiol Pharmacol* 73(2):172-79, 1995.
122. Langman MJ, Weil J, Wainwright P, Lawson DH, et al: Risks of bleeding peptic ulcer associated with individual non-steroidal anti-inflammatory drugs, *Lancet* 343(8905):1075-78, 1994.
123. Garcia Rodriguez LA, Jick H: Risk of upper gastrointestinal bleeding and perforation associated with individual non-steroidal anti-inflammatory drugs, *Lancet* 343(8900):769-72, 1994.
124. Soylu A, Kasap B, Ogun N, Ozturk Y, et al: Efficacy of COX-2 inhibitors in a case of congenital nephrogenic diabetes insipidus, *Pediatr Nephrol* 20(12):1814-17, 2005.
125. Pattaragarn A, Alon US: Treatment of congenital nephrogenic diabetes insipidus by hydrochlorothiazide and cyclooxygenase-2 inhibitor, *Pediatr Nephrol* 18(10):1073-76, 2003.
126. Dogne JM, Hanson J, Supuran C, Pratico D: Coxibs and cardiovascular side-effects: from light to shadow, *Curr Pharm Des* 12(8):971-75, 2006.
127. Egan ME, Glockner-Pagel J, Ambrose C, Cahill PA, et al: Calcium-pump inhibitors induce functional surface expression of Delta F508-CFTR protein in cystic fibrosis epithelial cells, *Nat Med* 8(5):485-92, 2002.
128. Robben JH, Sze M, Knoers NV, Deen PM: Rescue of vasopressin V2 receptor mutants by chemical chaperones: specificity and mechanism, *Mol Biol Cell* 17(1):379-86, 2006.
129. Romisch K: A cure for traffic jams: small molecule chaperones in the endoplasmic reticulum, *Traffic* 5(11):815-20, 2004.
130. Ulloa-Aguirre A, Janovick JA, Brothers SP, Conn PM: Pharmacologic rescue of conformationally-defective proteins: implications for the treatment of human disease, *Traffic* 5(11):821-37, 2004.
131. Morello JP, Salahpour A, Laperriere A, Bernier V, et al: Pharmacological chaperones rescue cell-surface expression and function of misfolded V2 vasopressin receptor mutants, *J Clin Invest* 105(7):887-95, 2000,
132. Tan CM, Nickols HH, Limbird LE: Appropriate polarization following pharmacological rescue of V2 vasopressin receptors encoded by X-linked nephrogenic diabetes insipidus alleles involves a conformation of the receptor that also attains mature glycosylation, *J Biol Chem* 278(37):35678-86, 2003.
133. Wuller S, Wiesner B, Loffler A, Furkert J, et al: Pharmacochaperones post-translationally enhance cell surface expression by increasing conformational stability of wild-type and mutant vasopressin V2 receptors, *J Biol Chem* 279(45):47254-63, 2004.
134. Bernier V, Morello JP, Zarruk A, Debrand N, et al: Pharmacologic chaperones as a potential treatment for X-linked nephrogenic diabetes insipidus, *J Am Soc Nephrol* 17(1):232-43, 2006.

CHAPTER 33

Urolithiasis and Nephrocalcinosis in Childhood

Bernd Hoppe, Ernst Leumann, and Dawn S. Milliner

INTRODUCTION

Urolithiasis in the pediatric age group plays an important role not only in parts of the world with a high incidence of stone disease such as the Near and Far East but also in industrialized countries. Pediatric urolithiasis should not be underestimated, because it is associated with significant morbidity, particularly because stones tend to recur. Although great progress has been made during the last few decades with regard to a better understanding of the cause, pathophysiology, therapy, and prevention of stone disease, many aspects still remain controversial or unsolved.

As compared with the adult population, a far higher proportion of pediatric patients have a well-defined underlying condition that favors stone formation (e.g., metabolic disorders, infections, urinary tract anomalies). For these reasons, it is imperative to evaluate carefully all pediatric stone patients as soon as stone disease is recognized and to pay great attention to the prevention of further stone formation.[1]

An interdisciplinary approach is important, and it should involve pediatricians, pediatric surgeons and urologists, experts in diagnostic imaging and metabolic diseases, and even biochemists. However, the pediatric nephrologist is best situated to correctly interpret all incoming information and to coordinate the diagnostic evaluation and treatment.

History of Urolithiasis

Kidney stone disease has been known since ancient times as documented by different archaeologic findings as well as writings about painful stone colic and attempts at stone treatment, including removal. In earlier centuries, urolithiasis was often a disastrous disease, all too often leading to the patient's death.

The examination of Egyptian mummies revealed kidney and bladder stone disease, such as a 5000-year-old bladder stone in the funeral site of El Amrah. Regimens for treatment were found in the papyrus Ebers (1500 BC), which is the main source of information about traditional Egyptian medicine. Saltpeter and turpentine oil were known to increase urine production, and pulverized eggshell (mainly from ostrich eggs) with a high content of calcium carbonate was ingested to intestinally bind lithogenic substances.

Sushruta, who was the main physician of Kaniska, the king of India (circa 6th century BC), was the first to describe stone removal via the urethra using a splint. Some time later, he recommended the so-called "Steinschnitt" procedure. Although many patients died during this procedure, it was still the only possible intervention. "Stein Schneider," who were people who removed urinary stones, were traveling throughout Europe until the late 18th century. Because most of the patients were boys between the ages of 9 and 14 years, it is assumed that stone disease was most prevalent among this age group.

The prevalence of kidney stone disease increased during the 16th, 17th, and 18th centuries among all ages and social groups. During the late 17th century Frère Jacques Beaulieu was the first to use the lateral approach for a perineal lithotomy; unfortunately, his method was accompanied by severe morbidity and mortality.[2] Thus, all kinds of conservative measures became quite popular. A variety of plant ingredients were used that resulted in increased urinary volume and reduced pain or that had anti-inflammatory properties.

Definitions

The term *urolithiasis* means urinary stones and comprises calculi formed in the kidney (nephrolithiasis) that may be found anywhere in the urinary tract as well as primary bladder stones.

Nephrocalcinosis is the term used for deposits of calcium salts in the tubules, the tubular epithelium, or the interstitial tissue of the kidney. It is usually diagnosed at the macroscopic level by ultrasonography, and, hence, its composition (calcium phosphate or calcium oxalate) is not known. However, pathologists distinguish between nephrocalcinosis (calcium phosphate) and oxalosis (deposits of calcium oxalate). Nephrocalcinosis occurs either alone or in combination with calculi. The latter finding is strongly suggestive of an underlying metabolic disorder such as renal tubular acidosis or primary hyperoxaluria.

Epidemiology

The incidence of urolithiasis in childhood is believed to be approximately 10% of that seen in adults, although a significant proportion of patients remain undiagnosed or misdiagnosed. Incidental discovery occurs in 15% to 40% of patients; therefore, numbers should be interpreted with caution. The incidence of kidney stone disease in adults in the Western hemisphere has increased over the last 20 years from roughly 0.5% during the late 1970s to about 1.5% in 2000, and this is accompanied by an increase of the prevalence rate from 4% to 4.7%.[3] About 5% of all women and 12% of men will develop a kidney stone at least once during their lifetimes.[4] About 40% of children with urolithiasis have a positive family history of kidney stones. Urolithiasis in children appears in all age groups, usually with a male preponderance, which is also observed in the adult population. The occurrence and causes of stone disease vary greatly, both between and within certain countries. For example, young aboriginal children in tropical and desert climates in Australia may develop urate renal stones at an early age,[5] and urolithiasis is endemic in certain parts of the world, like the Near and Far East.[6-8] Nephrolithiasis in North America accounts for 1 in every 1000 to 1 in every 7600 pediatric hospital admissions per year.[6] Surprisingly, the incidence of kidney stones is high in Iceland, with an annual rate of 5.6 to 6.3 per 100,000 children.[9] Primary bladder stones used to be very frequent, but they have almost disappeared in the industrialized countries, which also suggests a cause that differs from that of nephrolithiasis. Nevertheless, bladder calculi still account for up to 5% of urinary calculi worldwide, and they are frequent in endemic areas.[8,10]

DIAGNOSIS

Medical History

Urolithiasis during childhood differs substantially from that seen in the adult population with regard to causes, symptoms, imaging techniques, and treatments. Obtaining a thorough medical history and following it with a careful physical examination is indispensable for early and correct diagnosis. It is important to obtain information from the family about stones, hematuria, renal failure, and metabolic diseases (i.e., draw a pedigree). Particular attention must be paid to nutrition, fluid intake, medications (especially vitamins D and A, steroids, and diuretics), and any mineral supplementation. Children with chronic bowel disease (e.g., Crohn's disease, cystic fibrosis, after a bowel resection), neurologic disorders (e.g., anticonvulsant drugs, low fluid intake), or anomalies of the urinary tract that may predispose them to urine stasis and urinary tract infection (e.g., neurogenic bladder, ileal loops, megaureter) are at special risk for stone formation (Table 33-1).

Clinical Findings

Symptoms of urinary tract stones are often nonspecific, particularly in infants and young children. In addition, stones may remain asymptomatic for long periods of time. The most common symptom of urolithiasis is abdominal pain. In older children, this is clearly identifiable as colicky pain, but in infants and children it is only recognized as nonspecific abdominal pain and thus difficult to differentiate from acute appendicitis and other conditions. Unexplained sterile pyuria or recurrent urinary tract infections should raise the level of suspicion for urolithiasis, especially in the younger child.

TABLE 33-1 Diagnostic Steps in Urolithiasis

History	Family/patient Diet, drugs Chronic diseases? Malabsorption? Immobilization?
Clinical findings	Pain, hematuria Passage of stones, gravel
Stone localization, anatomic anomalies	Ultrasonography, plain film (intravenous urography, spiral computed tomography scanning)
Urine	Density, specific gravity (osmolality), pH, glucose, protein, sediment, culture Spot urine: Ratios of calcium and oxalate (uric acid, citrate) to creatinine Cystine screening 24-hour urine collection: Volume, pH (lithogenic and stone-inhibitory parameters to estimate saturation)
Blood/serum	Electrolytes, calcium, phosphorus, magnesium, creatinine, urea, uric acid, alkaline phosphatase, acid–base status
Stone analysis	Infrared spectroscopy or x-ray diffraction

Gross or microscopic nonglomerular hematuria and, more rarely, flank tenderness and urinary retention are other symptoms that are encountered. Hematuria may be present for some time before urolithiasis or nephrocalcinosis become manifest. Sometimes the gastrointestinal tract is also involved, with vomiting, flatulence, or constipation.

Symptoms differ according to the location of the stone. Stones of the lower urinary tract may manifest with dysuria, voiding problems, or complete urine retention, but enuresis, frequent voiding, hematuria, and fever may also be diagnostic hints. In addition, playing with the genitals in younger children may be a first sign of urolithiasis. Especially in infants, stones may become lodged and therefore palpable in the urethra such that the first symptom of stones is the inability to pass urine.

A missed diagnosis may have serious consequences. For example, the diagnosis of primary hyperoxaluria is often only made after end-stage renal failure has occurred years or decades after the first symptom of urolithiasis had appeared.[11,12]

In contrast with urolithiasis, nephrocalcinosis is mostly asymptomatic, especially during infancy and early childhood. Hence, diagnosis is often only made when nephrocalcinosis is incidentally noted on an imaging study performed for other reasons or when symptoms of reduced renal tubular concentrating capacity are obvious. However, the underlying pathology is not always evident, and finding it requires a detailed history and workup. Renal colic has been reported in some infants with nephrocalcinosis, but, in this situation, it is likely the result of the passage of tiny calculi. It is not unusual for nephrocalcinosis to be diagnosed during systematic renal ultrasound examination in high-risk infants or as part of the diagnostic evaluation of urinary tract infection. The first clinical symptoms, if any, are gross or microscopic hematuria and/or sterile leukocyturia, which may be misdiagnosed as urinary tract infection.[13]

Diagnostic Imaging

Initial diagnostic testing is designed to systematically uncover obstruction, stasis, infection, and metabolic abnormalities (see Table 33-1), and it relies heavily on imaging of the urinary tract. Indeed, with the availability of minimally invasive imaging modalities such as ultrasound and computed tomography (CT) scanning, stones are increasingly detected incidentally during the evaluation of nonspecific symptoms or unrelated problems. Imaging of the urinary tract should be sufficiently thorough at baseline to confidently rule out stasis or obstruction, which may be related either to a stone or to congenital or acquired abnormalities of the urinary tract (Figure 33-1).

The appearance of a stone on imaging studies depends on its composition (Table 33-2). Those comprised of calcium oxalate or calcium phosphate are very dense on conventional radiographs and with CT scanning. Struvite (magnesium ammonium phosphate) and cystine stones are of intermediate density, and small stones that are comprised of either can be difficult to appreciate by conventional radiography. Uric acid stones are radiolucent on radiographs, requiring the administration of contrast agents for adequate visualization.

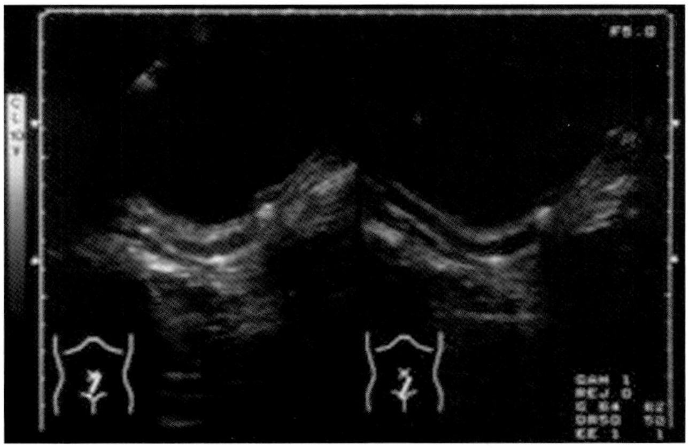

Figure 33-1 Obstructive prevesical urolithiasis in a 5-year-old patient with primary hyperoxaluria and recurrent stone passages. Secondary stenosis of the ureter made reimplantation procedure necessary during follow-up.

They are of low density on CT scans. Stones that are comprised of indinavir or matrix (both infrequent) are of variable density, and they may be difficult to differentiate from surrounding soft tissue by any modality, including ultrasound.

Stones of all composition, with the exception of indinavir and matrix, have distinguishing characteristics of echogenicity and shadowing on ultrasonography. Ultrasonography has the additional advantages of wide availability, the avoidance of ionizing radiation, the ready detection of hydronephrosis, and the ability to define some aspects of the anatomy of the urinary tract. However, ultrasonography is not as sensitive as CT scanning for the detection of small stones or stones in the ureter. Indeed, small stones may not be detectable by routine ultrasound examination, even when they are strongly suspected (Figure 33-2). The measurement of stone size is less reproducible by ultrasound than with conventional radiographs or CT imaging, thus reducing its utility for the monitoring of metabolic stone-forming activity over time.

Most stone imaging can be performed without the use of contrast agents. However, when obstruction is a concern, when radiolucent or low-density stones require careful delineation, or when details of urinary tract anatomy are needed (e.g., for confirmation of a duplicated collecting system), contrast agents in the form of CT urography, intravenous pyelography, or retrograde ureteroscopy or pyelography are usually employed.

Individual clinical characteristics, the type of stone, and questions to be addressed should be considered when making decisions regarding the best imaging modality. Ultrasonography is almost always a good initial choice, and, in uncomplicated situations, it may be all that is needed.

The typical stone location is within the renal pelvis and/or the renal calyces or the ureter and, less often, within the bladder. The most common ureteral calcification is a stone that has migrated down from the kidney. These stones typically become impacted at anatomic sites of narrowing, and they are especially difficult to detect when they overlie bony structures such as the sacrum. The detection of a ureteral stone via ultrasonography is difficult, but the stone may lead to obstruction (hydroureter or hydronephrosis) and may thus be suspected, even if it is not directly visualized. Stones are

TABLE 33-2 Radiodensity of Specific Stones and Frequency of Stone Composition in Large Cohorts of Adult and Pediatric Patients[3,4,18,76,87,91]

Radiodensity	Stone Composition	Frequency (%)
Opaque	Calcium oxalate	70% to 75%
	• Whewellite (calcium oxalate monohydrate)	80%
	• Weddelite (calcium oxalate dihydrate)	20%
	Carbonate apatite (carbonate containing calcium phosphate, Dahllite)	4% to 6%
	Brushite (calcium hydrogen phosphate dihydrate)	0.5% to 1%
Intermediate	Cystine	1% to 5%
	Struvite (magnesium ammonium phosphate hexahydrate)	5% to 7%
Radiolucent	Uric acid (Uricite)	10% to 15% in adults Less frequent in children
	Uric acid dihydrate	~1%
	Ammonium acid urate	~0.5%
	2,8-Dihydroxyadenine	Rare
	Xanthine	Rare

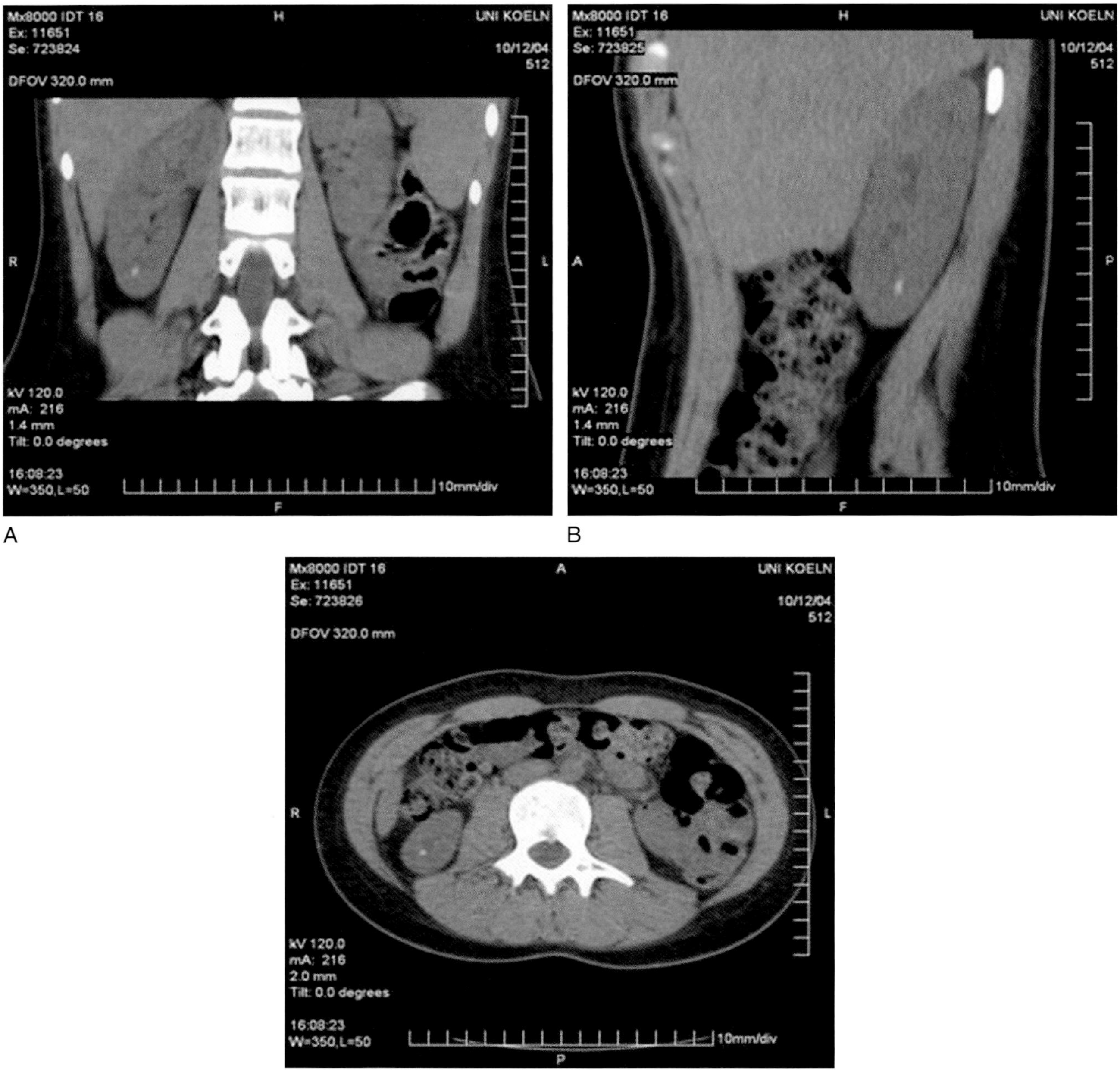

Figure 33-2 **A,** Axial, **B,** sagittal, and **C,** transversal documentation of a kidney stone in the lower pole of the right kidney in a 15-year-old girl with recurrent colicky abdominal pain and a negative ultrasound examination.

rarely found in the urethra, but they may be lodged there. In a boy with penile pain, urethral palpation should be performed.

Studies in adult patients showed that non–contrast-enhanced CT scanning is more effective than intravenous urography for identifying and localizing ureteral stones and that virtually all urinary calculi are now visible with the appropriate selection of imaging techniques, no matter where they reside in the urinary tract.[14,15] However, in infants and young children particularly, the minimization of exposure to ionizing radiation and the occasional need for sedation with CT imaging favors the use of ultrasonography or conventional radiography over CT scanning whenever they provide the necessary visualization.

For detecting and monitoring nephrocalcinosis, high-resolution ultrasonography is the optimal imaging method. Nephrocalcinosis is classified according to the anatomic area involved. Medullary nephrocalcinosis is differentiated from either cortical (e.g., in acute cortical necrosis, chronic glomerulonephritis, and chronic graft rejection) or diffuse nephrocalcinosis, and it is divided into three subtypes according to the degree of echogenicity (Table 33-3 and Figure 33-3). Common causes of nephrocalcinosis and its differential diag-

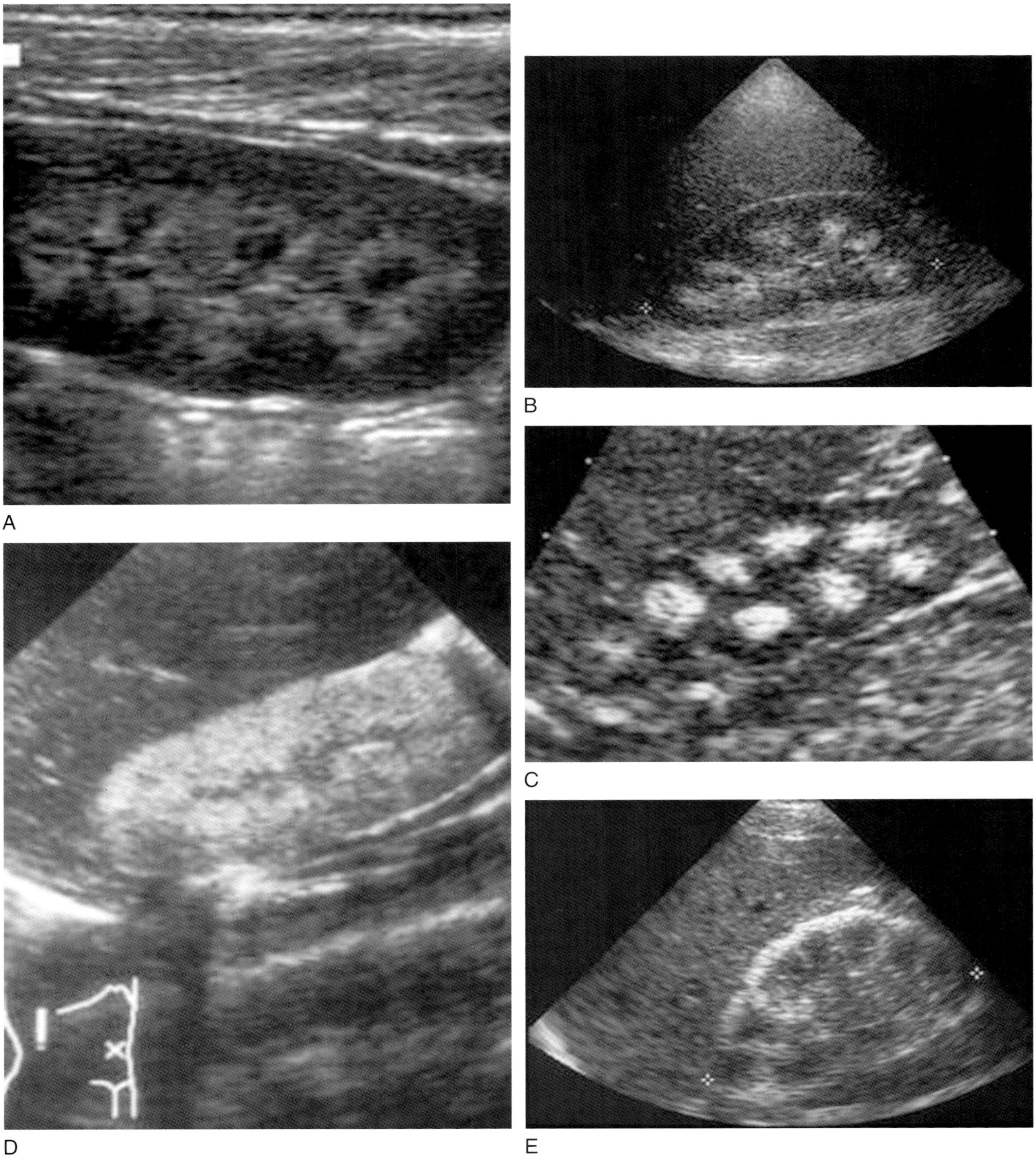

Figure 33-3 **A,** Grade 1, **B,** grade 2, **C,** grade 3 medullary, **D,** corticomedullary, and **E,** cortical nephrocalcinosis.

nosis are listed in Table 33-4. Thanks to the routine use of ultrasonography in premature infants and in children who are at risk, a large number of conditions are now recognized to be associated with nephrocalcinosis (see Table 33-4).[16]

Some peculiarities of renal ultrasonography in neonates and especially in preterm infants need to be recognized: Tamm-Horsfall protein deposits within the renal calyces may look like nephrocalcinosis (Figure 33-4). This deposition, however, disappears within 1 to 2 weeks, and follow-up will show completely normal kidneys. Furthermore, the echogenicity of the renal cortex in neonates is physiologically increased, hence the detection of cortical nephrocalcinosis

TABLE 33-3 **Grading Scale for Medullary Nephrocalcinosis**[131]

Grade I	Mild increase in the echogenicity around the border of the medullary pyramids
Grade II	Mild diffuse increase in the echogenicity of the entire medullary pyramid
Grade III	Greater, more homogeneous increase in the echogenicity of the entire medullary pyramid

TABLE 33-4 **Common Causes of Nephrocalcinosis and Differential Diagnosis**

Nephrocalcinosis	Causes
Medullary	• Adrenal insufficiency • Adrenocorticotropic hormone therapy • Bartter syndrome • Bone metastases • Cushing syndrome • Distal renal tubular acidosis • Hyperoxaluria • Hyperparathyroidism • Hyperthyroidism and hypothyroidism • Idiopathic hypercalcemia • Lipoid necrosis • Lesch-Nyhan syndrome • Lowe syndrome • Malignant neoplasm • Medication: furosemide, dexamethasone • Medullary sponge kidney • Nutrition: long-term parenteral nutrition, ascorbic acid supplementation • Tyrosinemia • Sarcoidosis and other granulomatous diseases • Sickle cell disease • Vitamin D or A intoxication • William syndrome • Wilson disease
Cortical	• Chronic hypercalcemia • Ethylene glycol intoxication • Primary hyperoxaluria • Sickle cell disease
Differential diagnosis	• Acute cortical necrosis • Chronic glomerulonephritis • Kidney transplant rejection • Pyelonephritis • Renal tuberculosis • Renal vein thrombosis • Tamm-Horsfall deposits

can be difficult, and it may become evident only some weeks later, when a rim of cortical calcification appears visible. However, diffuse cortical nephrocalcinosis may already be detectable shortly after birth in patients with suspected primary hyperoxaluria, and it is directly visible both by ultrasonography and x-ray. Medullary nephrocalcinosis can only be sonographically diagnosed when an increased echogenicity appears in the area of the renal medulla. Normally the renal pyramids are hypoechoic in relation to the cortex.

A plain film of the abdomen is less helpful, because only the association of hyperechoic pyramids with a posterior acoustic shadow is a clear sign of nephrocalcinosis. Gross

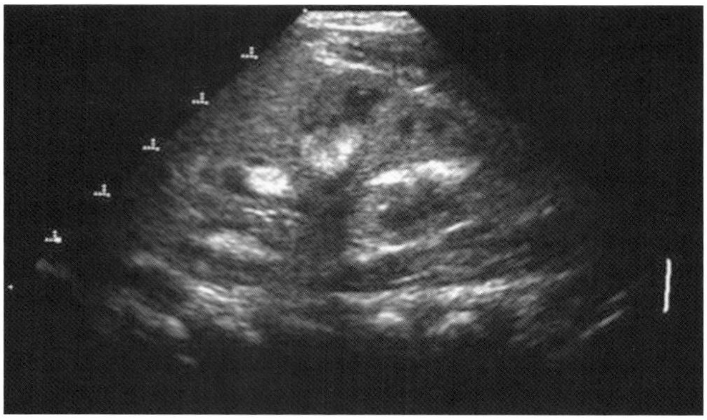

Figure 33-4 Tamm Horsfall protein deposition within the calyces of the kidney in a preterm infant. The resolution of such deposition normally occurs within 10 to 14 days.

calcifications are thus required before nephrocalcinosis can be diagnosed by conventional radiographs.

A comparison of ultrasonography and CT scanning for experimental nephrocalcinosis in rabbits demonstrated a higher sensitivity for ultrasonography (96% versus 64%) but a better specificity for CT scanning (96% versus 85%).[17] Still, renal ultrasound examination is the first diagnostic imaging option for infants and children with suspected stones or nephrocalcinosis.

Examination of Urine and Blood

The complete urinalysis of a randomly voided urine specimen is a necessary diagnostic evaluation for every acute stone episode. Hematuria, white blood cell count, pathogens (nitrite testing), and urinary protein excretion can easily be determined. Microscopic examination of the urine is important not only for the differentiation between glomerular and nonglomerular hematuria (see Chapter 10) but also for the white blood cell count and the detection of certain crystals, such as hexagonal cystine crystals (Figure 33-5), 2,8-dihydroxyadenine, and crystals formed from medications or their metabolites in the urine. Because the pH of the urine is a major factor in the formation of many stones, its measurement (preferably by glass electrode or, if a pH electrode is not available, by special pH paper) is of utmost importance. Sometimes it is advisable to determine a daily profile of both the urinary pH and the density (specific gravity or osmolality) of the urine. This may also be used for follow-up (e.g., to assess the effect of the administration of alkali or to check the patient's compliance regarding a sufficient fluid intake). The presence or absence of infection can be addressed by a urine culture. Chemical analysis of the urine includes (apart from creatinine) calcium, uric acid, oxalic acid, phosphate, magnesium, and citrate. Cystine is screened by cyanide-nitroprusside testing or by chromatography for amino acids. In all patients, the analysis of serum calcium, phosphorus, magnesium, uric acid, alkaline phosphatase, bicarbonate, and creatinine should be performed (see Table 33-1).

Identification of Predisposing Causes

Predisposing causes for urolithiasis can be recognized in more than 75% of children and adolescents who are found to have

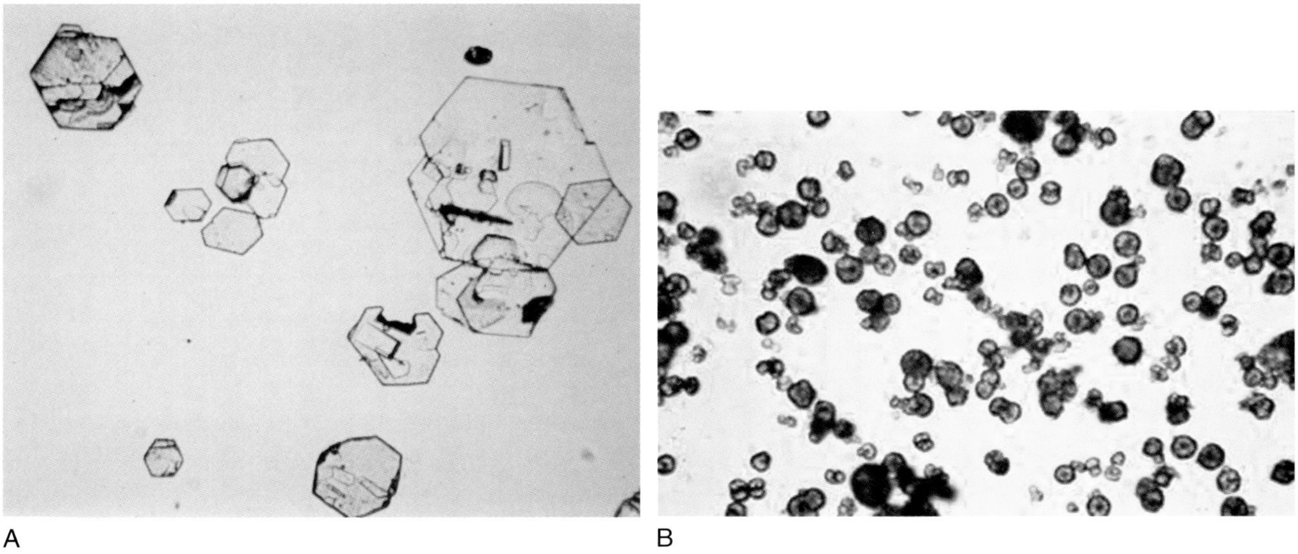

Figure 33-5 Urine sediment with **A,** hexagonal cystine crystals or **B,** typical 2,8-dihydroxyadenine crystals.

urinary tract stones.[7,8,18,19] Accordingly, every young patient with urolithiasis deserves a comprehensive evaluation. Infection, obstruction, or stasis will be identified by the diagnostic evaluation outlined previously. However, the systematic detection of predisposing metabolic factors requires further testing.

Metabolic factors—among which hypercalciuria and hyperoxaluria are the most common—are determined by urine measurements of relevant solutes and naturally occurring inhibitors of crystal and stone formation, such as citrate. Blood levels of calcium and other analytes are also of importance, because they are determinants of urine composition or indicators of underlying disorders relevant to stone formation (e.g., metabolic acidosis). Because many of the urine components are influenced by dietary intake, 24-hour urine collections (excluding diurnal fluctuations related to the intake of food and beverages) provide the best information, and they also provide an objective assessment of the child's daily intake of fluid. For infants or young children or for situations in which a 24-hour urine collection is difficult, random urine measurements using the ratio of the concentration of each analyte to that of urine creatinine provide valuable information. Best results are obtained if urine is collected while patients are receiving their usual diets and fluid intake. Misleading results may be obtained if obstruction or infection is present or when stone fragments are being passed in the urine after a recent stone fragmentation procedure. Analysis should be deferred until infection has been treated and until at least 1 month has passed after lithotripsy or the resolution of obstruction.

Normal values for the excretion rates of the solutes that are most often implicated in stone formation are shown in Table 33-5. Specific abnormalities may dictate more directed testing. It is important to keep in mind that the excretion rates of solutes influence stone risk as continuous (rather than discrete) variables. For example, the child whose urine calcium excretion is in the upper quartile of normal and who has a low urine volume is at risk for stone formation and may benefit from a reduction in urine calcium. Many children and adolescents with stones have more than one predisposing factor (Table 33-6). With this in mind, it is important to complete a systematic evaluation, even when the cause seems obvious. For example, patients with congenital ureteropelvic junction obstruction and stones may have hypercalciuria as a second predisposing cause. When an inherited metabolic disorder is suspected, urine samples from family members can be of help for the primary diagnosis, and they are also valuable for the detection of affected family members.

Among patients with multiple stones at the onset or for those in whom there is active stone formation and no abnormalities have been identified, additional testing can be helpful. This testing should include a timed (preferably 24-hour) urine collection for a full supersaturation profile.[20,21] As a result of day-to-day variations in diet and fluid intake, three separate determinations on different days have been demonstrated to provide the best information.[22]

Stone Analysis

The qualitative analysis of the stone obtained after spontaneous stone passage or intervention is one of the most important diagnostic measures. Only one third of all stones are composed of a single substance. All components exceeding 5% should be determined. The methods of choice are infrared spectroscopy and x-ray diffraction. Even amounts of less than 1 mg can be analyzed. Chemical stone analysis is inappropriate, because it is prone to errors and thus is now obsolete. With infrared spectroscopy, the loss of energy in the infrared spectrum as a result of the circulation of the activated chemical molecules is determined. The analytic principle of x-ray diffraction is based on the crystal structure of the stone substances. The diagrams of either method (their so-called fingerprints) provide an exact analysis (Figure 33-6).

Recurrent stones should be analyzed again, because the stone composition may change. After lithotripsy, only stone

TABLE 33-5 Normal Values for Molar Creatinine Ratios, Upper Limits of Normal for Specific Urinary Lithogenic Substances, and Lower Limits of Normal for Stone Inhibitory Substances

Parameter and Age Range	Ratio solute ÷ Creatinine		Urinary Excretion
Calcium			<0.1 mmol/kg body weight
	mol/mol	g/g	(<4 mg/kg body weight)
<12 months	<2.2	0.8	
1 to 3 years	<1.5	0.53	
3 to 5 years	<1.1	0.4	
5 to 7 years	<0.8	0.3	
>7 years	<0.6	0.21	
Oxalate			<0.5 mmol/1.73 m^2/24 hours
	mmol/mol	mg/g	(<45 mg/1.73 m^2/24 hours)
0 to 6 months	<325 to 360	288 to 260	
7 to 24 months	<132 to 174	110 to 139	
2 to 5 years	<98 to 101	80	
5 to 14 years	<70 to 82	60 to 65	
>16 years	<40	32	
Cystine			<10 years: <55 µmol/1.73 m^2/24 hours (13 mg)
	mmol/mol	mg/g	>10 years: <200 µmol/1.73 m^2/24 hours (48 mg)
<1 month	<85	180	Adults: <250 µmol/1.73 m^2/24 hours (60 mg)
1 to 6 months	<53	112	
>6 months	<18	38	
Uric acid			Excretion substantially higher throughout childhood than in adults
	mol/mol	g/g	>1 year: <815 mg/1.73 m^2/24 hours
<1 J	1.5	2.2	Mmol/L GFR / mg/dl GFR
1 to 3 J	1.3	1.9	<2 years: <0.18 / <3.3
3 to 5 J	1.0	1.5	>2 years: <0.035 / <0.53
5 to 10 J	0.6	0.9	(Ratio × Plasma creatinine)
>10 J	0.4	0.6	
Citrate			>0.8 mmol/1.73 m^2/24 hours
	mol/mol	g/g	(>0.14 g/1.73 m^2/24 hours)
0 to 5 years	>0.12 to 0.25	0.20 to 0.42	
>5 years	>0.08 to 0.15	0.14 to 0.25	

GFR, Glomerular filtration rate.
Normal values may show regional variations. Values given were derived from different studies that were mostly performed in industrialized countries. This is especially the case with regard to urinary calcium/creatinine ratios. For citrate, there are relatively few normal values studies in children; hence, a range for normal molar ratios is given. In addition, differences in analysis have to be kept in mind when comparing normal levels. Therefore, we recommend using these normal values as a guideline but to also look for regional reference values.[13,38,132,133]

fragments are available, and these can be recovered by straining the urine. All fragments should be sent for analysis to allow additional tests, if needed.

With regard to treatment regimens, all stone components are of importance (Table 33-7). Apart from the main stone components, several other substances may be found, such as the salts of uric acid (urate), rare calcium phosphate compositions, protein matrix stones, stones that are comprised of medications or their metabolites (e.g., indinavir), and artifacts, like gypsum or seeds.

PATHOGENESIS OF NEPHROCALCINOSIS AND UROLITHIASIS

Pathophysiology of Nephrocalcinosis

Nephrocalcinosis is related to calcium oxalate or calcium phosphate deposits in the tubulointerstitial regions of the kidney. Medullary nephrocalcinosis is the typical pattern that is seen in 98% of cases.[23] Nephrocalcinosis does not necessarily lead to stone formation, and renal calculi may occur in the apparent absence of macroscopic nephrocalcinosis, although the two are often seen together in the same patient. The two pathologies are distinct, but they are intimately related, and they share many of the same risk factors.[23] Nephrocalcinosis appears, more often than urolithiasis, to be associated with a loss of renal function.[23] In one series of 152 German patients with nephrocalcinosis, glomerular filtration rate and maximal urinary osmolality were related to the stage of nephrocalcinosis.[24]

Nephrocalcinosis is commonly related to tubulopathies such as Dent disease, Bartter syndrome, and Lowe syndrome, and it is also observed in patients with primary hyperoxaluria and distal renal tubular acidosis[23] (see Table 33-4). It is well described in patients with a history of hypercalcemia or vitamin D excess.[24] Hypercalciuria is common to many of these conditions.[23,24]

The most frequently encountered clinical setting in which nephrocalcinosis occurs is in premature infants. The risk of nephrocalcinosis appears to be related to the degree of prematurity and the birth weight, and it has been reported in 7% to 65% of infants born at less than 32 weeks' gestation.[25] Infants who receive furosemide or corticosteroids, who receive longer periods of parenteral nutrition, who are of white race, or who have a family history of urolithiasis appear

TABLE 33-6 Metabolic Background of Urolithiasis During Childhood

Condition	Metabolic Background
Normocalcemic hypercalciuria	• Idiopathic hypercalciuria • Distal renal tubular acidosis • Diuretic induced • Dent disease • Bartter syndrome • Familial hypomagnesemia and hypercalciuria syndrome
Hypercalcemic hypercalciuria	• Primary hyperparathyroidism • Immobilization • Cushing syndrome • Adrenal insufficiency • Metastatic bone disease
Intestinal hyperabsorption of calcium	• Hypervitaminosis D or A • Idiopathic hypercalcemia of childhood • Sarcoidosis
Hyperoxaluria	• Primary hyperoxaluria • Secondary hyperoxaluria as a result of malabsorption syndromes like cystic fibrosis, inflammatory bowel diseases, short bowel syndrome, and/or lack of intestinal oxalate-degrading bacteria
Hyperuricosuria	• Inborn errors of metabolism • Lesch-Nyhan syndrome • Gout • Glycogen storage disease types I, III, V, and VII • Overproduction in leukemia or tumor lysis syndrome • Protein-rich diet
Hypocitraturia	• Distal renal tubular acidosis • Idiopathic or treatment induced
Cystinuria	• Different types
Xanthinuria	• Primary or secondary xanthinuria

to be at greater risk. In addition, hypocitraturia during the first 8 weeks of life was found to be one of the main risk factors for the development of nephrocalcinosis in preterm infants.[25,26] Over time, the nephrocalcinosis will frequently resolve ultrasonographically.[27] However, even after the resolution of nephrocalcinosis, there may be renal compromise. Downing and colleagues[27] studied a small group of 1- to 2-year-old patients who were born prematurely and who had nephrocalcinosis. Although the nephrocalcinosis of six of the seven patients had resolved, they demonstrated both glomerular and tubular dysfunction as compared with a group of infants who had not developed nephrocalcinosis despite a similar degree of prematurity. In a separate study, children who were born prematurely who had renal calcification during infancy were studied when they were 4 to 12 years old. Sixty-four percent of those with a history of renal calcifications had hypercalciuria, hypocitraturia, and reduced ammonium excretion in response to furosemide.[28] Nephrolithiasis associated with nephrocalcinosis, particularly when it is seen in older children or adolescents, suggests a metabolic disorder such as distal renal tubular acidosis or hyperoxaluria.[29]

Scattered calcium oxalate crystals are not infrequently seen in renal tubule cells in patients undergoing allograft biopsies after transplantation.[30,31] The significance of these crystals remains to be established, but it likely reflects renal cell injury from acute tubular necrosis, medications, or other factors. Low citrate excretion, which is often seen in this setting, may also play a role.[31]

Pathophysiology of Urolithiasis

The initial event in the process of stone development is the formation of a crystal of calcium phosphate, calcium oxalate, sodium urate, or another of the elements of which urinary tract stones are comprised. For this to occur, concentrations of relevant solutes in the urine must exceed the saturation threshold. High urine concentrations can result from either

TABLE 33-7 Possible Causes According to the Composition of Renal Stones

Stone Composition	Possible Causes
Calcium oxalate (monohydrate and dihydrate, pure or mixed)	Hypercalciuria, hyperoxaluria, low citrate
Calcium oxalate (pure monohydrate)	Primary hyperoxaluria
Calcium phosphate	
Carbonate apatite	pH > 7.0 (infection, distal renal tubular acidosis, immobilization)
Brushite	pH between 6.5 and 6.8, severe hypercalciuria
Struvite	Infection
Ammonium urate	Infection or endemic; in anorexia
Cystine	Cystinuria (different types)
Uric acid	Fixed acid urine (pH around 5.4); endemic Hyperuricosuria (primary or secondary)
Uric acid dihydrate	Occasional component of uric acid, suggesting very acid urine (pH always <5.5)
2,8-Dihydroxyadenine	Adenine phosphoribosyltransferase deficiency
Xanthine	Primary xanthinuria (xanthinoxidase deficiency) Secondary xanthinuria (side effect of allopurinol treatment)

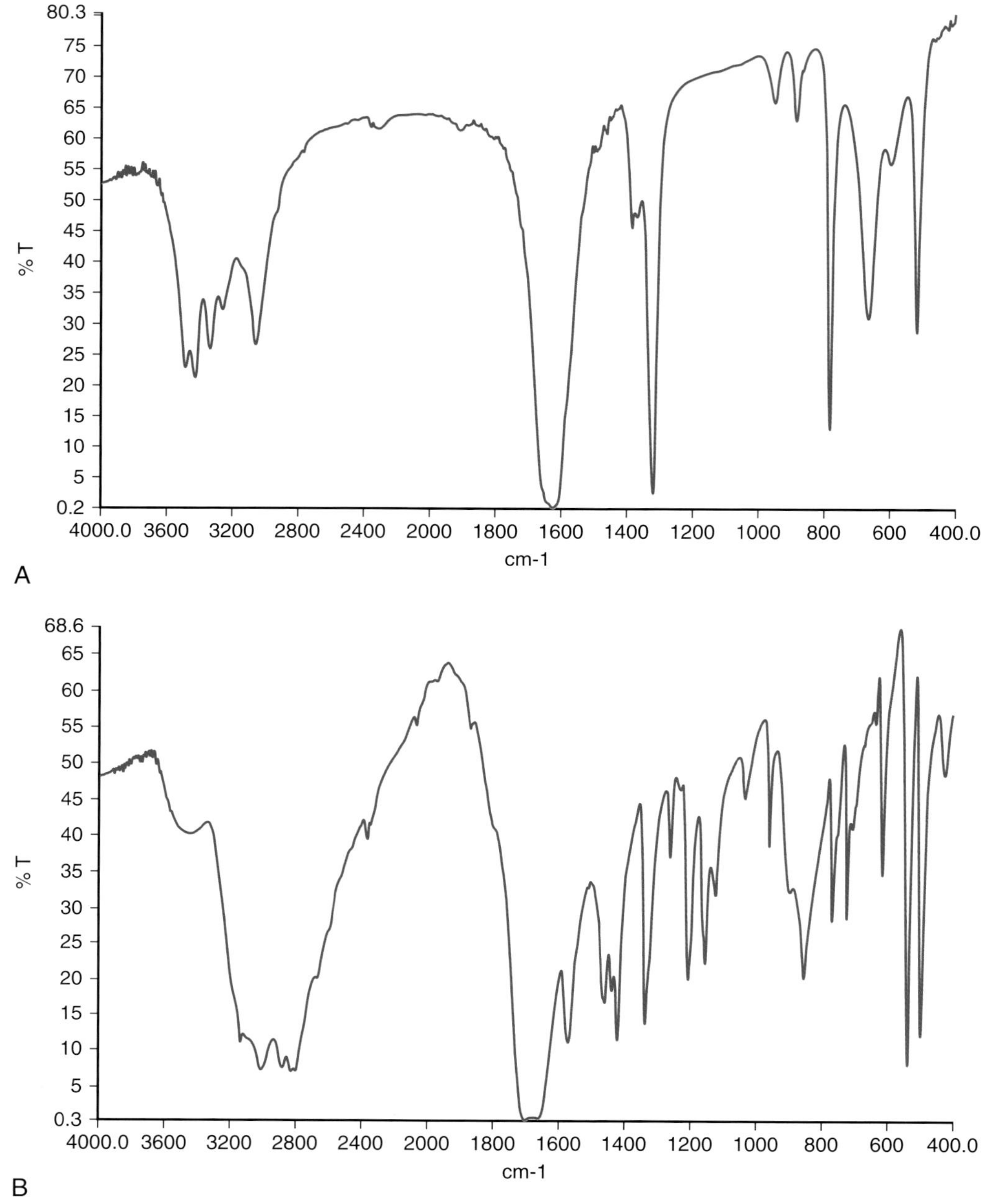

Figure 33-6 Infrared-spectroscopy analysis of **A,** a pure whewellite stone and **B,** a pure xanthine stone.

increased excretion rates or a low urine volume. Diet, physiologic or pathophysiologic processes that influence renal handling of solutes, and medications can all influence excretion rates. Oral fluid intake is the primary determinant of urine volume. Other factors that influence crystallization and aggregation are urinary pH and naturally occurring constituents of the urine that inhibit this process, including citrate, pyrophosphate, sulfate, and magnesium. For example, cystine and uric acid are much more soluble at a pH of 7 than at a pH of 5, whereas calcium phosphate precipitates more readily at an alkaline pH.

These factors are important for understanding the causes of stone formation in a given patient, and they also can be used to advantage during treatment. Dehydration is an obvious source of low urine volume, and repeated episodes are a risk for stone formation. More commonly, low urine volumes result from habitually low fluid intake. A daily fluid volume that is adequate for one child may constitute an important added risk factor for stone formation in a child or adolescent with elevated or even high-normal excretion rates of one or more minerals.

Urine is supersaturated for calcium oxalate in most healthy individuals at some times, thus raising the question of why urinary tract stones are not seen in everyone. After a crystal has formed, aggregation with other crystals and adherence to the renal tubule cell are important next steps. Were it not for attachment, the crystals formed would be expected to be washed readily out of the tubule into the renal pelvis and eliminated by urination. The washout of aggregates of crystals and of small stones is impaired when there is stasis of the urinary tract. It is in part for this reason that children with congenital urinary tract anomalies or other causes of urinary stasis are predisposed to stone formation. Infection is also more likely when there is urinary stasis. A number of common urinary tract pathogens produce urease, which predisposes an individual to the development of stones by virtue of high local concentrations of magnesium ammonium phosphate and alkaline pH (see the discussion of infection stones later in this chapter).

Crystals attach more readily to injured renal tubules than to healthy ones.[32] Thus, factors that cause renal injury (e.g., infection) and medications that damage the renal tubule epithelium (e.g., gentamicin, calcineurin inhibitors [cyclosporine A, tacrolimus]) may predispose individuals to the early stages of stone formation. It is not unusual to see crystals attached to renal tubules in the renal biopsies of patients with acute tubular necrosis or other tubular injury. Immature and rapidly proliferating renal tubular cells also appear to be more susceptible to crystal attachment. This mechanism has been among those proposed for the nephrocalcinosis and stone formation that is observed in premature infants.[25]

Valuable insights into the early stages of stone formation have been provided by the work of Evan and colleagues.[33] Calcium oxalate is the sole or principal constituent of the majority of stones (≥75%). Calcium phosphate had been thought to play a role in a lesser percentage of stones. However, recent work suggests a central role for calcium phosphate crystallization in idiopathic calcium oxalate stone formers.[34] Initial calcium phosphate crystals appear to form in the thin limb of the loop of Henle, resulting in interstitial suburothelial particles that become an apatite plaque. Calcium oxalate crystals form on the surface of this plaque, which is exposed to the urinary space. After it is attached to the apatite plaque, the growth of the calcium oxalate crystal aggregate gradually leads to stone formation, with the growing stone typically attached to the papillary tip of the kidney. The growing stone may remain attached, or it may at any time detach to float free in the renal pelvis or wash down the ureter.

Most of the steps in the process of stone formation can be exploited to minimize stone-forming activity. Such interventions form the basis of effective treatment and should be employed to advantage (see Therapeutic and Preventive Measures later in this chapter).

In contrast with the situation in adult stone formers, metabolic disorders can be found in a large proportion of pediatric patients. Metabolic abnormalities account for 25% to 96% of cases in recent pediatric nephrolithiasis series from Western countries,[18,19] having surpassed primary infection stones. Monogenic disorders leading to inborn errors of metabolism play a major role (Table 33-8). Polygenic disorders likewise appear to play a significant role in urolithiasis, although they are less well understood. Candidate polygenic traits include idiopathic calcium nephrolithiasis and idiopathic hypercalciuria.[34] Molecular genetics has an increasingly important role in diagnosis of urolithiasis, it has stimulated the investigation of specific pathophysiologic mechanisms,[4] and it has contributed to an understanding of the underlying causes of many stone diseases.

STONES AND UNDERLYING CONDITIONS

Calcium-Containing Stones

Calcium and oxalate are the main stone components (≥75%) in the Western hemisphere in both adult and pediatric patients.[3] Urinary tract stones mainly consist of calcium oxalate and, less frequently, of calcium phosphate. Calcium oxalate stones appear either in the monohydrate (whewellite, ~80%) or the dihydrate (weddelite, ~20%) form. As outlined previously, many lithogenic and inhibitory factors are involved in calcium-containing stone formation, apart from fluid intake and dietary factors. Urinary calcium is the best known promoting substance, but oxalate and low citrate also play important roles, in addition to the high excretion of uric acid and a high protein load.

Hypercalciuria

Hypercalciuria is said to be the most common form of metabolic stone formation, with an occurrence rate that varies greatly from 37% to 74%.[35,36] This large range is caused not only by differences in ethnic background and nutrition but also by great discrepancies in the definition of hypercalciuria, which may be overdiagnosed. In fact, for practical reasons, calcium is determined far more often than, for example, oxalate and citrate.

Definition of Hypercalciuria One difficulty is that no sharp limit exists between normal and abnormal urinary calcium excretion. More by convention than by hard data, the upper limit of normal calcium excretion has been set at 4 mg (0.1 mmol)/kg of body weight per day. However, it is actually the urinary concentration of calcium (and of the other constituents) that determines the risk of stone formation. Furthermore, 24-hour urine collections for measuring the excretion of calcium are often unreliable and impractical for younger children; hence, urinary ratios of calcium over creatinine are preferred in this situation. The ratio of individual analytes to osmolality is an alternative to creatinine.[37] The calcium-to-creatinine ratios are strongly age dependent, and they decrease considerably during the first 7 years of life[38] (see Table 33-5). Conventionally, values exceeding the 95th percentile are considered as abnormal. However, to obtain reliable reference values, large series are required.

To complicate matters even further, ratios indicating abnormal values vary considerably from one study to another, presumably because of differences in nutrition, methodology, and the genetic background of the individuals involved. Before classifying a child as hypercalciuric, it is thus necessary to have repeated urinary samples or urine collections from different days that show values that consistently and clearly exceed the upper limits of "normal." Whether hypercalciuric children will ultimately form stones or develop nephrocalcinosis depends on additional factors (e.g., urine volume, pH) and the concentration of the other urinary constituents, primarily of oxalate and citrate.

Idiopathic Hypercalciuria Idiopathic (primary) hypercalciuria is considered to be the most common cause of calcium-

TABLE 33-8 Monogenic Disorders That Cause Stones

	Mendelian Inheritance in Man	Gene, Locus	Inheritance	Gene Product	Phenotype
Hypercalciuric Stone-Forming Diseases					
Autosomal dominant hypocalcemic hypercalciuria	146200 601199	*3q 13.3-q 21* *CASR*	Autosomal dominant	Calcium-sensing receptor	Hypercalciuria, hypocalcemia, chronic renal failure
Familial hypomagnesemia with hypercalciuria and nephrocalcinosis	248250 603959	*3q 27, 1p34.2* *CLDN16, 19*	Autosomal recessive	Paracellin 1 (claudin 16, 19) Tight junction protein	Hypercalciuria, hypercalcemia, hypomagnesemia, distal renal tubular acidosis, chronic renal failure, hypermagnesiuria, polyuria, tetany seizures
Dent disease	300009 310468 300008	*Xp11.22* *CLCN5*	X-linked recessive	ClC-5 chloride channel	Hypercalciuria, renal phosphate leak (variable), low-molecular-weight proteinuria, hypophosphatemia (variable)
Nephrolithiasis and osteoporosis associated with hypophosphatemia resulting from a mutation in the type II sodium phosphate cotransporter	182309	*5q35*	Unknown	NPTZa	Renal phosphate leak, hypercalciuria, osteoporosis, increased 1,25-dihydroxy vitamin D
Lowe syndrome	309000	*Xq25-26* *OCRL1*	X-linked recessive	OCRL1 protein	Hypercalciuria, megalin deficiency, phosphate leak, Fanconi syndrome
Hyperoxaluric Stone-Forming Diseases					
Primary hyperoxaluria type I	259900 604285	*2q37.3* *AGXT*	Autosomal recessive	AGT	Hyperoxaluria, hyperglycolic aciduria, chronic renal failure, systemic oxalosis
Primary hyperoxaluria type II	260000 604296	*9q11* *GRHPR*	Autosomal recessive	GR/HPR	Hyperoxaluria, hyperglycolic aciduria, chronic renal failure
Cystinuric Stone-Forming Diseases					
Cystinuria type A	104614	*2p q16.3* *SLC 3A1*	Autosomal recessive	r BAT	Cystinuria
Cystinuria type B	604144	*19 q13.1* *SLC7A9*	Autosomal recessive	$B^{\alpha+}$ AT	Cystinuria
Purine/Pyrimidine Stone-Forming Diseases					
Lesch-Nyhan syndrome	300322	*Xq26* *HPRT*	X-linked recessive	Hypoxanthine phosphoribosyltransferase	Hyperuricosuria
Partial hypoxanthine phosphoribosyltransferase deficiency	308000	*Xq26-27.2* *HPRT*	X-linked recessive	Hypoxanthine phosphoribosyltransferase	Hyperuricosuria
Glycogenosis type Ia	232200	*17q21* *G6PC*	Autosomal recessive	Glucose-6-phosphatase	Hyperuricosuria
Glycogenosis type Ib	232220	*11q23* *SLC37A4*	Autosomal recessive	Transporter	Hyperuricosuria
Phosphoribosylphosphate synthetase I superactivity	311850	*Xq21* *PRPS1*	X-linked		Hyperuricosuria
Adenine phosphoribosyltransferase deficiency	102600	*16q24.3* *APRT*	Autosomal recessive	Adenine phosphoribosyltransferase	Dihydroxyadeninuria
Xanthinuria (classical)	278300	*2p22* *XDH*	Autosomal recessive	Xanthine oxidoreductase or dehydrogenase	Xanthinuria, hypouricemia
Distal Renal Tubular Acidosis					
Autosomal dominant renal tubular acidosis	179800 109270	*17q21-q22* *SLC 4A1, AE1*	Autosomal dominant	AE1 chloride-bicarbonate exchange	Hypocitric aciduria, hypercalciuria, hypokalemia, osteomalacia
Autosomal recessive distal renal tubular acidosis with hearing loss	267300 192132	*2cen-q13* *ATP6B1*	Autosomal recessive	B1 subunit vacuolar ATPase	Hypercalciuria, hypocitric aciduria, hypokalemia, rickets, hearing loss
Autosomal recessive distal renal tubular acidosis	602722 605239	*7q33-34* *SLC4A1*	Autosomal recessive	A4 subunit of vacuolar ATPase	Hypercalciuria, hypocitric aciduria, hypokalemia

containing stones. Traditionally, attempts have been made to distinguish between defects of the kidney (renal leak), the gut (absorptive), and the bones (resorptive). Theoretically, urinary calcium excretion in the fasting state is elevated in the renal form but normal in the absorptive one. However, many pediatric patients cannot be reliably classified, because they may appear to have the renal subtype at one examination and the absorptive subtype the next time.[39] Furthermore, a primary defect in one organ can lead to secondary changes in others. For these reasons, such a distinction has limited value in pediatric patients. Primary hypercalciuria has a complex genetic background: monozygotic twins show concordance for hypercalciuria in 32% as compared with dizygotic twins (17%).[40] From these data, the authors estimated that more than 52% of hypercalciuria is related to heritability. Successive inbreeding in rats has resulted in a strain of rats with urinary calcium excretion rates that are eight to ten times higher than those seen in control rats that spontaneously form kidney stones.[41]

Clinical symptoms of idiopathic hypercalciuria are obviously those of urolithiasis, but idiopathic hypercalciuria is also incriminated in isolated microscopic hematuria and urinary tract infections. It is therefore recommended to look for hypercalciuria in children with nonglomerular hematuria, although the relationship is not always obvious. More doubtful is the postulated relationship between idiopathic hypercalciuria and urinary tract infection, because small calculi may also cause (sterile) leukocyturia. Given the frequency of both hypercalciuria and urinary tract infection, there is considerable chance of a mere coincidence of both conditions.

Secondary Forms of Hypercalciuria Distal renal tubular acidosis (d-RTA) almost invariably leads to medullary nephrocalcinosis and/or calcium phosphate lithiasis (see Chapter 31). Three factors contribute to these complications: (1) a high urinary pH; (2) hypercalciuria (as a result of systemic acidosis); and (3) hypocitraturia (as a result of a tubular defect and the acidosis).[42] In the complete form of d-RTA, the urine pH cannot be lowered to less than 6.1 after an ammonium-chloride acid-loading test. In addition to the alkaline urine and the hypocitraturia, another risk factor in patients with d-RTA is overt and persistent hyperoxaluria, which may be the result of a primary or secondary defect of tubular oxalate transporters in patients with tubular acidosis (e.g., SLC26A6).[43] Hypercalciuria is also observed in a number of other disorders that are characterized by renal tubule dysfunction, such as Dent disease and Lowe syndrome (see Tables 33-4, 33-6, and 33-8; see Disorders with Abnormalities of Renal Tubule Function later in this chapter).

There are a number of diseases that lead to hypercalcemia with resulting hypercalciuria. Hypervitaminosis D caused by the use of multivitamin preparations, including vitamin D, or of vitamin D added to milk preparations is another example. An excessive daily amount of vitamin A (>10,000 units) may also lead to hypercalcemia and secondary hypercalciuria. Immobilization in growing children, even for a relatively short period, will lead to a reduction of bone calcium and bone mass of about 15% to 20% accompanied by hypercalciuria.[44]

The long-term administration of either furosemide or dexamethasone can lead to hypercalciuria and nephrocalcinosis or stone disease. Hypercalciuria is also found in several syndromes, and it is either linked to the pathogenesis (Bartter and Williams syndrome, Dent disease) or caused by renal tubular damage (Wilson and Lowe syndrome.)[13] Primary hyperparathyroidism, which is the most frequent cause of hypercalcemic hypercalciuria in adults, is very rarely seen in children, and it is practically excluded if the serum calcium level is normal.

Further conditions that lead to hypercalciuria include both hyper- and hypothyroidism, Cushing syndrome, adrenal insufficiency, metastatic malignant bone disease,[34] long-term assisted ventilation (acid–base changes), and parenteral nutrition.[45]

Hyperoxaluria

Primary Hyperoxaluria Under physiologic conditions, more than half of the oxalate excreted by the kidneys is derived from hepatic synthesis and, to a small extent, from the breakdown of ascorbic acid.[46] The primary hyperoxalurias are inborn errors of metabolism, which result in a marked increase in the synthesis of oxalate by the liver, and in primary hyperoxaluria type II, which is also caused by other body cells. The excess oxalate produced is eliminated primarily by the kidneys. As a result of the nature of the metabolic defect, hyperoxaluria is present at birth. High concentrations of oxalate excreted in the urine combine with calcium to cause nephrocalcinosis or to form stones. In addition, calcium oxalate crystals induce renal injury. Stone formation typically begins early during life, although patients may be asymptomatic for many years. The first sign or symptom is usually blood in the urine, pain, the passage of a stone, or urinary tract infection related to a kidney stone. Some patients present with kidney failure as the first symptom, which can occur as early as infancy. Patients with renal failure caused by infantile oxalosis present with the triad of failure to thrive, anemia, and acidosis, and the majority of patients are symptomatic before 10 years of age.[11] In some cases, however, the disease may go unrecognized, either as a result of the absence of symptoms or of the incorrect diagnosis, until patients reach 30 to 50 years of age.[11,47-49]

Calcium oxalate crystals are directly injurious to renal cells and incite a granulomatous reaction in the renal interstitium.[50] Over time, the effects of such injury, often in combination with obstruction or infection related to stones, lead to kidney failure. Earlier literature showed that about 50% of patients developed kidney failure by 15 years of age and that about 80% developed kidney failure by 30 years of age. With improved diagnosis and management, more recent information suggests that the median age at renal failure is 33 years.[11,49,51]

After renal function declines to a glomerular filtration rate of less than 30 to 40 ml/min/1.73 m^2, renal excretion of oxalate is reduced. Plasma oxalate concentration rises and can exceed the supersaturation threshold for calcium oxalate as soon as it reaches a level above 30 μmol/L (the normal level depending on the method used is less than 6 μmol/L).[52] Calcium oxalate then begins to deposit in the eyes, bones, muscles, blood vessels, heart, and other major organs (systemic oxalosis). Serious morbidity and death can result from oxalosis. Because of these problems, renal replacement with dialysis or transplantation should be initiated earlier in patients with primary hyperoxaluria than in patients with other causes of progressive renal insufficiency.[53]

The early diagnosis of primary hyperoxaluria is of vital importance so that treatment can be initiated as soon as possible. However, as a result of the lack of familiarity with the disease, delays of many years from the onset of symptoms to diagnosis are common.[49,54] The onset of calcium oxalate stone formation during childhood or adolescence or of calcium oxalate stones or nephrocalcinosis in patients with renal failure of any age are important clues to the diagnosis and warrant specific diagnostic testing for this disease.[55]

Primary Hyperoxaluria Type I Type I primary hyperoxaluria, which is caused by mutations of the *AGXT* gene (see Table 33-8), accounts for a majority of patients with the primary hyperoxalurias. To date, nearly 100 mutations have been described. This autosomal recessive disease has an estimated prevalence in central Europe of 1 to 2.9 persons per million population.[48,56] However, this rate underestimates the true prevalence because of early death and undiagnosed cases. No reliable estimates of prevalence are available for the United States. In both Europe and the United States, primary hyperoxaluria is the cause of renal failure in less than 1% of children and adolescents who reach end-stage renal disease.[48] The disease is seen with higher frequency in certain parts of the world, including Tunisia and the Canary Islands. The increased hepatic production of both glycolate and oxalate is the result of the deficient activity of liver-specific peroxisomal alanine : glyoxylate aminotransferase (AGT). Reduced enzyme activity may occur as a result of inactive, partially active, or mistargeted enzyme. AGT must be present within the peroxisome for the effective disposition of glyoxylate. In a subset of patients with type I primary hyperoxaluria, AGT is mistargeted to the mitochondria, where it is metabolically ineffective. A deficiency of AGT caused by any of these mechanisms results in the marked overproduction of oxalate.

The diagnosis is strongly suggested by marked hyperoxaluria (usually greater than 1.0 mmol/1.73 m^2/24 hours) and hyperglycolic aciduria, although the latter is not consistently present. Confirmation of the diagnosis can often be obtained by screening DNA for common mutations,[57] particularly when there is a known high regional prevalence of specific mutations. However, even in selected populations, this approach is complicated by the number of mutations responsible and the frequency of compound heterozygosity. In some patients, liver biopsy for the measurement of AGT enzyme activity is needed. As a result of the autosomal recessive nature of primary hyperoxaluria type I and the importance of early diagnosis, siblings of affected patients should always be screened. An algorithm to assist with diagnosis has been published.[55]

In patients whose findings are highly suggestive of primary hyperoxaluria, treatment should be initiated as soon as accurate and reproducible baseline measurements of urine oxalate excretion have been obtained (see Specific Therapeutic and Preventive Measures for Hyperoxaluria later in this chapter). Approximately 30% to 50% of patients respond favorably to treatment with pharmacologic doses of pyridoxine (vitamin B6). The reason for the effectiveness of pyridoxine is unknown, but it may be related to its role as a cofactor for the AGT enzyme. Patients with certain AGT mutations are likely to respond to pyridoxine, sometimes even with the normalization of urinary oxalate.[47,58] The only other currently available means for a reduction in oxalate production is by liver transplantation.

With optimal medical management and prompt attention to stones that pose a risk of obstruction, infection, or other problems, patients with primary hyperoxaluria often maintain adequate renal function for many years.

When reduction in renal function to a glomerular filtration rate of less than 30 ml/min/1.73 m^2 occurs, the concentration of oxalate in the blood rises and can exceed the supersaturation for calcium oxalate in plasma. In this situation, renal replacement with transplantation or dialysis is needed promptly to avoid the systemic deposition of calcium oxalate (oxalosis) with its attendant morbidity and mortality. If dialysis is needed as a bridge to transplantation, intensive dialysis is necessary to remove as much oxalate as possible. Transplantation should be performed as soon as possible to minimize systemic oxalosis. Most patients with type I primary hyperoxaluria will require combined liver and kidney transplantation to correct the metabolic defect and restore kidney function. Otherwise, the transplanted kidney remains at risk as a result of ongoing high oxalate production. Patients who are known to have a normalization of urine oxalate during pharmacologic treatment with pyridoxine may be an exception in that a number of such patients have done well with kidney transplantation alone.

Primary Hyperoxaluria Type II and Other Primary Hyperoxalurias Primary hyperoxaluria type II occurs as a result of deficient glyoxylate reductase/hydroxypyruvate reductase enzyme activity (see Table 33-8). Most glyoxylate reductase/hydroxypyruvate reductase resides in the liver, although it is present in other tissues as well.[57] As a result of the reduced enzyme activity, both oxalate and L-glyceric acid production are increased and are excreted by the kidney. Diagnosis is strongly suggested by marked hyperoxaluria and the elevation of urine L-glyceric acid. Confirmation can often be obtained by the screening of DNA for known mutations. Some patients require liver biopsy for the measurement of glyoxylate reductase/hydroxypyruvate reductase activity. Primary hyperoxaluria type II is encountered much less often than type I, and it appears to account for less than 10% of patients with primary hyperoxaluria overall.[49] However, its general prevalence may be underestimated.

Patients with type II primary hyperoxaluria do not benefit from pyridoxine. Although the clinical course is similar, patients with type II primary hyperoxaluria appear to have less active stone formation and better preservation of renal function as compared with patients with type I disease.[59] The potential for renal failure followed by systemic oxalosis remains, however, regardless of whether the patient has type I or type II disease. Because liver transplantation has not been demonstrated to correct the metabolic defect in patients with type II disease and because such patients may do well with kidney transplant alone, distinguishing between type I and type II primary hyperoxaluria is especially important when managing primary hyperoxaluria patients who have renal failure. The clinical and analytic similarities between primary hyperoxaluria I and II make differentiating the two types difficult. In most patients, molecular genetic testing or liver enzyme measurement is required. Without careful testing, patients may be misclassified.

Patients with hyperoxaluria and clinical features similar to primary hyperoxaluria types I and II but who have normal hepatic AGT and glyoxylate reductase/hydroxypyruvate reductase levels have been described.[60] These patients have marked sustained hyperoxaluria, early-onset urolithiasis, and no apparent secondary causes of hyperoxaluria. In several such patients, the enteric absorption of oxalate has been demonstrated to be normal.[60] Only a small number of patients with nontype I/nontype II primary hyperoxaluria have been identified, and further studies will be required to identify the underlying cause(s).

Secondary Hyperoxalurias Dietary sources of oxalate have historically been believed to account for approximately 10% to 20% of urinary excretion, but more recent information suggests a much higher 25% to 50%.[46] The absorption of oxalate occurs in the stomach, the duodenum, and the colon, and this is influenced by the types of foods consumed and other dietary constituents as well as by the intestinal flora of oxalate-degrading bacteria. The fraction of ingested oxalate that is absorbed is particularly affected by the amount of calcium,[46] because calcium in the diet binds with oxalate in the lumen of the intestine, thus reducing oxalate absorption. Low-calcium, high-oxalate diets are particularly problematic. The influence of dietary calcium on oxalate absorption may account for the epidemiologic observations of Curhan and colleagues,[61] which were that individuals with the lowest quartile of diet calcium had the highest stone incidence.

Another major contributor to urinary excretion is oxalate produced by the liver as an end product of normal metabolism. Oxalate cannot be degraded by humans. Thus, the maintenance of physiologic balance requires the excretion of the amount of oxalate absorbed from the gastrointestinal tract plus that produced by body metabolism. Under physiologic conditions, oxalate is excreted primarily (>90%) by the kidneys, with a small amount excreted by the intestinal tract.[62]

The role of the gastrointestinal tract in oxalate physiology is becoming better understood and appears to play a greater role in the elimination of oxalate when renal function is compromised. Colonic secretion and the absorption of oxalate are regulated by physiologic stimuli, including the renin-angiotensin system.[63] Recently, the function of the ion exchanger SLC26A6 has been shown to be important in gastrointestinal and renal oxalate excretion.[43] Certain microorganisms in the colon, such as *Oxalobacter formigenes*, contain enzymes that can metabolize oxalate, thereby reducing luminal concentrations and thus oxalate absorption. The organisms also appear to be capable of stimulating the colonic secretion of oxalate.[62] Thus, these microorganisms or their enzymes have promise as therapeutic agents for patients with primary as well as secondary hyperoxaluria.[64]

Abnormalities of the intestinal tract that are associated with the malabsorption of fat can result in the enhanced enteric absorption of oxalate. *Enteric hyperoxaluria*, as it is called, has been reported in association with such diverse conditions affecting the gastrointestinal tract as inflammatory bowel disease, cystic fibrosis, short bowel syndrome after intestinal resection, and after gastric bypass surgery.[64] Mechanisms include the binding of calcium by fatty acids. This leaves less calcium in the lumen to bind oxalate so that the oxalate is absorbed more readily. In addition, bile salts cause injury to the colonic epithelium, thus promoting enhanced absorption. The degree of hyperoxaluria in this situation is highly dietary dependent and varies from day to day, but it can be severe. In addition to urolithiasis, enteric hyperoxaluria is a cause of renal failure. Management includes a low-oxalate, low-fat diet; calcium administered with meals to bind oxalate in the lumen of the intestine; and a high fluid intake to the degree tolerable in a patient with fat malabsorption. In some patients, bile acid sequestrants are helpful. The therapeutic use of *Oxalobacter* or its enzymes seems to be a promising avenue for the future.

Dietary and idiopathic hyperoxaluria can result from a very high intake of oxalate in the diet, especially in combination with a low level of dietary calcium. Thus, a careful diet history is important during the evaluation of any patient with hyperoxaluria. In addition, approximately 15% to 20% of patients with idiopathic calcium stone disease have hyperoxaluria. In this situation, the hyperoxaluria does not appear to result from dietary oxalate excess, and it is often associated with hypercalciuria.

Urinary oxalate excretion rates in combination with clinical findings help to distinguish secondary and idiopathic forms of hyperoxaluria from primary hyperoxaluria. Dietary and idiopathic hyperoxaluria are associated with mild increases in urine oxalate excretion, typically in the range of 0.46 to 0.7 mmol/1.73 m^2/24 hours (reference values, <0.45 mmol). Enteric hyperoxaluria is characterized by moderate to marked increases in urinary oxalate, most often ranging from 0.7 to 1.0 mmol/1.73 m^2/24 hours; these levels are usually associated with a history of diarrhea and other signs of malabsorption. By contrast, most patients with primary hyperoxaluria have urine oxalate excretion rates of greater than 1.0 mmol/1.73m^2/24 hours, with values of 1.5 to 3.0 mmol/1.73 m^2/24 hours being frequently observed.

Hypocitraturia

A low citrate excretion is not always adequately recognized as a risk factor in the pathogenesis of calcium-containing stones.[65] Hypocitraturia, possibly of dietary origin, may be more important than hypercalciuria in certain regions of the world (e.g., Turkey).[66] Citric acid, which is a tricarbonic acid, is a very potent inhibitor of calcium oxalate and calcium phosphate crystallization. Some 10% to 35% of the citrate filtered in the glomerulus is excreted in the urine. More citrate is excreted during alkalosis as a result of diminished proximal tubular reabsorption.[42] As citrate forms stable complexes with calcium, less (ionized) calcium remains available in the urine for binding to oxalate. The solubility product of calcium oxalate will therefore improve. Whereas only 16% of calcium is bound to citrate in an acid urine, more than 45% will be bound to citrate at a pH of 8.[67]

Low urinary citrate excretion is characteristic of the complete form of d-RTA.[68] Hypocitraturia is also observed in patients with metabolic acidosis, including mild or latent forms, in patients with hypokalemia, and in patients with malabsorption syndromes.[69] Idiopathic hypocitraturia may be the result of low intestinal alkali absorption.[70]

Phosphate Stones

Phosphate is a component of a number of stones, depending on the cause (see Tables 33-2 and 33-7). Thus, the term *phosphate stones* is not particularly informative. Calcium-phosphate stones (carbonate apatite and brushite) are seen in d-RTA and hypercalciuria, and carbonate-apatite forms are seen with infections. For struvite and carbonate apatite, see Infection Stones later in this chapter.

Brushite stones ($CaHPO_4 \cdot 2H_2O$) grow at a pH of approximately 6.5 and when urinary calcium and phosphate concentrations are elevated, often on a nidus of calcium oxalate.[71] With extremely high urinary calcium concentrations (e.g., approximately 10 mmol/L), pure brushite can precipitate. If the urinary pH increases above 6.8, carbonate apatite instead of brushite is formed. Brushite stones grow very rapidly and often recur. They are very hard as a result of their compact and crystalline structure, which makes them poorly suited for extracorporeal shock wave lithotripsy treatment.[72] In patients with brushite stones, urine is often supersaturated as a result of either severe hypercalciuria or extreme hypocitraturia. Patients with brushite stones may have primary hyperparathyroidism or any other form of renal calcium loss, incomplete renal tubular acidosis, or, rarely, the complete form of renal tubular acidosis. When a urinary tract infection is present in a patient with brushite stones, it is usually a result of stone formation.

Cystine

Cystinuria accounts for approximately 1% to 5% of urolithiasis in children and adolescents. Under normal circumstances, 99% of cystine in the glomerular filtrate is reabsorbed by transporters located along the luminal brush border of the proximal renal tubule cells. Mutations of these transporters interfere with reabsorption, resulting in high concentrations of dibasic amino acids in the urine. High urinary concentrations of the acids ornithine, arginine, and lysine pose no problems. Cystine is much less soluble, particularly at low urine pH levels, and it forms stones. The *SLC3A1* gene encodes a subunit glycoprotein rBAT, which is responsible for cystine and dibasic amino acid transport. Mutations of the *SLC3A1* gene appear to be responsible for most cases of type I disease (also referred to as type A) or “classic” cystinuria, which is inherited as an autosomal recessive trait[73] (see Table 33-8). Heterozygotes have normal urine dibasic amino acids. A second component of the cystine transporter is encoded by the gene *SLC7A9*, and mutations of this appear to be responsible for most type II and type III disease (also referred to as type B). Heterozygotes for mutations of *SLC7A9* exhibit the elevated excretion of cystine and dibasic amino acids demonstrating autosomal dominant inheritance with incomplete penetrance.

The genetics of cystinuria is further complicated by frequent compound heterozygosity,[74] a report of mutations of *SLC7A9* associated with fully recessive cystinuria,[74] and indications that other, as yet unidentified, genes are involved. The genetic subtypes do not appear to correlate with the severity of the disease nor with the response to treatment.[75] Thus, genetic subtyping at present offers little clinical advantage.

The diagnosis of cystinuria is strongly suggested by stones that are comprised of cystine and by characteristic hexagonal cystine crystals that are visible in 17% to 25% of urine samples from patients with this diagnosis (see Figure 33-5). Confirmation is obtained by the measurement of urine cystine, which typically exceeds 1000 μmoL/g creatinine and which may be as high as 8000 μmoL/g creatinine.[76] The renal expression of dibasic amino acid transporters is incomplete at birth and appears to mature only by 3 to 4 years of age. Thus, the degree of cystinuria in heterozygotes is exaggerated, particularly during the first 2 years of life, and it may lead to an erroneous diagnosis of the disease: so-called *transient neonatal cystinuria.*[77] For this reason, diagnosis before 3 to 4 years of age should be made with caution.

Stone formation is clinically evident during childhood in 25% of patients with cystinuria,[78] and, in 224 patients in a multinational database, 83% had their first stone identified during the first two decades of life.[79] In patients in this database, stones were more likely to occur among males than females, and males produced a larger number of stones. A small proportion of patients appear not to form stones.[79] Most stones are composed of cystine, although stones of mixed composition containing calcium are observed. Large staghorn calculi are often seen. Cystine stones are of intermediate density as seen by conventional radiography such that smaller stones may be difficult to see in the absence of contrast agents. Ultrasonography and CT imaging provide better visualization.

Cystine stones are difficult to fragment with extracorporeal lithotripsy. Larger stones usually require percutaneous nephrostomy placement and removal. Episodic stone symptoms and the need for repeated procedures to remove stones are typical. Dello Strologo and colleagues[79] found that renal function was impaired in 17% of their patients, with a trend toward higher serum creatinine levels starting at 20 years of age. Only 1 of 224 patients, however, reached end-stage renal failure.[79] Despite these concerns, most patients do well over time.

Purine Stones

Uric Acid

Uric acid stones are more often found in adults as compared with pediatric patients, both in the Western world and in developing countries. Uric acid as an end product of purine metabolism has to be excreted via the kidneys. The solubility of uric acid is strongly pH dependent, and a low urine pH (<6.0) is the main risk factor for the development of uric acid stones. Food rich in purine or protein favors the precipitation of uric acid, and the metabolic end products of the amino acids methionine and cysteine provide acid valences (protons) that are excreted via the kidneys, thus leading to an acid urine. Most uric acid stones are, therefore, induced by the diet. Uric acid production is increased, even during the fasting state, in patients with myeloproliferative disorders, the tumor lysis syndrome (all as a result of cell destruction), or enzyme defects. Hence, a high fluid intake and the alkalinization of the urine are two of the most important therapeutic measures.

Patients with gout also have an increased risk of forming uric acid stones, and the increased renal clearance of uric acid has been observed in patients with diabetes mellitus. The so-called *metabolic syndrome* is an increasingly frequent problem as obesity has become more prevalent, even among children and adolescents during recent years. A deficiency of renal acid production associated with insulin resistance in this syndrome predisposes an individual to the development of uric acid stones. Hyperuricosuria can also be induced by medications (e.g., uricosurics, analgesics, diuretics). In addition to their role in uric acid stone formation, uric acid crystals in the urine are of importance as a nidus for the formation of calcium oxalate stones.

Primary purine overproduction occurs in rare inherited deficiencies of the purine salvage enzymes hypoxanthine phosphoribosyltransferase and adenine PRT (see Table 33-8). A complete deficiency of hypoxanthine phosphoribosyltransferase leads to the X-linked Lesch-Nyhan syndrome, which is characterized by mental retardation, automutilation, choreoathetosis, gout, and uric acid stones. A partial deficiency of hypoxanthine phosphoribosyltransferase results in urolithiasis and renal failure. Gout and urolithiasis have also been reported in glycogen storage disease type I.[80]

Uric acid dihydrate is a marker of an extremely acid urine ($pH < 5.5$), and it is rarely seen in its pure form. However, in 6% of all kidney stones, this uric acid variant can be found as a stone component.

Urate Stones

All urate stones are composed of salts of uric acid, which means that one or two hydrogen ions are replaced by other cations like $NH4^+$, potassium, sodium, or calcium. In contrast with uric acid, the formation of urate stones mostly starts at physiologic pH levels of greater than 6.5. Nevertheless, no urate stone develops without elevated urinary uric acid excretion. The only urate stone of clinical relevance is the ammonium urate stone, which is known to develop in patients with recurrent urinary tract infections or endemically (see Infection Stones later in this chapter).

2,8-Dihydroxyadenine

A deficiency of adenine phosphoribosyltransferase (see Table 33-8), which is inherited as an autosomal recessive trait, results in increased adenine, which is then oxidized by xanthine oxidase to 2,8-dihydroxyadenine. The diagnosis is suggested by yellow-brown, round dihydroxyadenine crystals in the urine (see Figure 33-5); brown spots on the diaper; or crystals in the renal tubules and parenchyma of patients undergoing biopsy for the evaluation of increased creatinine. The confirmation of the diagnosis is by determination of the adenine phosphoribosyltransferase activity in red blood cells or from the measurement of urinary hydroxyadenine excretion. Serum and urine uric acid levels are normal.

2,8-dihydroxyadenine stones are easily confused with uric acid stones, because dihydroxyadenine is an analog of uric acid. There is a wide spectrum of clinical expression, with 15% of affected patients free of clinical symptoms and others with renal failure as their initial manifestation of the disease. Renal failure may occur in the absence of stones, and the diagnosis may remain unrecognized until renal function is significantly compromised or even until there is a recurrence of crystal deposition or stones in a transplanted kidney.[81]

Most affected patients reported to date are Caucasian, although the abnormality has been reported in African-American, Arab, and Asian families (particularly in Japan). The frequency of heterozygosity in Caucasian populations has been estimated at 0.4% to 1.1%.[82] That observation, in combination with the frequency of compound heterozygosity in affected patients, suggests that the disease may be more frequent than is appreciated. This discrepancy could be related to mild manifestations of the disease in the majority of patients or to underdiagnosis.

Xanthine

Xanthinuria is a rare autosomal recessive disorder of purine metabolism that leads to urolithiasis.[83] A deficiency of xanthine oxidoreductase or dehydrogenase that catalyzes the last two steps of the purine degradation pathway results in the production of large amounts of xanthine and hypoxanthine associated with the reduced production of uric acid. Xanthine stones can form at any age, even in infants, as a result of the poor solubility of xanthine. However, there is a large clinical variability that is not explained by the genetic defect; only about half of all patients have urolithiasis.[83] Acute renal failure caused by crystal nephropathy is a rare complication.[84] Most patients are of Middle Eastern or Mediterranean origin.[83] Xanthinuria is rare in other parts of the world.

The diagnosis is made from stone analysis or from the presence of excessive xanthine excretion in the urine. A hint is the finding of an orange-brown urinary sediment, orange-stained diapers,[85] or profound hypouricemia that is often discovered incidentally.

Two types of classical xanthinuria are known. In type I, the conversion of allopurinol to oxypurinol is not impaired, whereas in type II the additional deficiency of aldehyde oxidase blocks the conversion of allopurinol to oxypurinol. Both types are clinically identical, and they are presumably caused by different mutations of the same *XDH* gene.

In contrast with both types of classical xanthinuria, xanthinuria resulting from the congenital absence of a molybdenum cofactor with combined xanthine dehydrogenase/sulfite oxidase deficiency is a complex disease. Such patients usually present with neonatal seizures, severe neurologic symptoms, and dysmorphic features, and they excrete sulfocysteic acid in the urine.[83]

Secondary xanthine stones and even xanthine nephropathy may develop as a result of the treatment with allopurinol of severe hyperuricemia associated with the gross overproduction of uric acid, as seen in the Lesch-Nyhan syndrome and in myeloproliferative disorders. However, such stones often contain additional constituents apart from xanthine.[83]

Infection Stones

A distinction must be made between stones that are induced by infection and those that are merely associated with urinary tract infection. The latter situation is not so rare, because calculi act as foreign bodies that favor infection, and they may lead to obstruction and thus aggravate infection. Differentiation between stones induced by infection and stones associated with infection is not always easy, but it is important for proper management; hence, stone analysis is essential. Occasionally, stones associated with infection have a mixed composition: for example, the core may contain cystine or calcium oxalate, and the surface may be made of struvite.

The typical primary infection stone consists of struvite ($MgNH_4PO_4 \cdot 6H_2O$, magnesium ammonium phosphate) and is referred to as a *triple-phosphate stone*. This term refers to the presence of the three different cations (NH_4^+, Mg^{2+}, and Ca^{2+}) found together with a single anion (PO_4^{3-}). These stones often also contain carbonate apatite ($Ca_{10}[PO_4]_6 \cdot CO_3$), the crystallization of which is favored by a high urinary pH (>7.0) of any cause. Both constituents look similar to the naked eye and have a friable structure and a white or grey appearance. The amorphous material easily molds into the renal calyces, thereby resulting in a staghorn calculus, which is so named because of its resemblance to the antlers of a male deer (i.e., a stag).

A third component that is less frequently found is ammonium urate (NH_4^+ urate). High concentrations of ammonium ions and uric acid and a high pH of the urine promote its crystallization. Such stones are compact and look, as a result of their reddish-brown color, like uric acid stones; however, they have very different chemical properties and remain insoluble, even at a low pH.

Urease-producing bacteria are responsible for the formation of struvite calculi:

$$\text{Urea} \rightarrow NH_3 + H_2O \rightarrow NH_4^+ + OH^-$$

This results in high concentrations of ammonium ions and in a high urinary pH. The high pH also promotes the formation of carbonate ions (CO_3^{2-}) and the production of trivalent phosphate ions, both of which are components of struvite calculi. Many gram-positive and gram-negative bacteria produce urease; however, *Proteus* species are the predominant organisms. Other urease-producing bacteria include *Haemophilus influenzae*, *Staphylococcus aureus*, *Pseudomonas aeruginosa*, *Klebsiella pneumoniae*, *Serratia marcescens*, and *Citrobacter* and *Morganella* species.[86] *Escherichia coli*, however, does not produce urease. *Ureaplasma urealyticum* is an organism to be specifically considered when standard urine cultures are negative in patients with struvite stones, because it requires specific culture techniques.

Struvite stones cause serious morbidity. In addition, they are hard to treat, and they tend to recur. They have become rare in the industrialized countries, but they are still frequent elsewhere, and they affect mainly boys under the age of 5 years. In a third of patients, there is a primary anomaly of the urinary tract, most often a ureteropelvic junction obstruction or a primary megaureter and more rarely a ureterocele, urethral valves, augmentation cystoplasty, or a urinary diversion (Figure 33-7). Patients with neurogenic bladder (especially those with a meningomyelocele) are particularly prone to developing struvite stones, but metabolic stones are increasingly being found in such patients.[87]

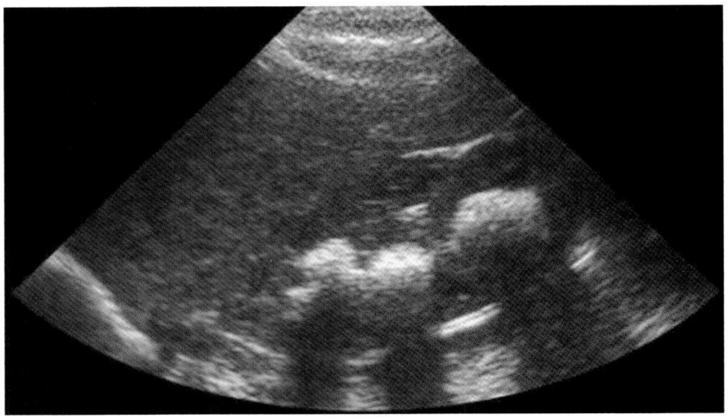

Figure 33-7 Multiple struvite stones in a 9-month-old male patient with recurrent urinary tract infections and vesicoureteral reflux. The stones were removed surgically, and an antireflux operation was performed.

Urinary Stasis

Urinary stasis increases the potential for stone formation. Stones found in patients with ureteropelvic obstruction or primary megaureter are therefore not necessarily of infectious origin. The conditions that most often lead to calculus formation are primary megaureter and polymegacalicosis. Polymegacalicosis is a congenital anomaly with calices that are too numerous (up to 25 instead of <12) and too large. Urolithiasis in such a kidney may be misinterpreted as a primary pelvic stone with secondary obstruction and hydronephrosis. Polymegacalicosis may occur unilaterally, or it may even be found on both sides, and it may accompany other malformation syndromes (e.g., the Schinzel-Giedion syndrome).

In patients with autosomal dominant polycystic kidney disease, uric acid kidney stones are frequently observed to lead to severe pain episodes that are often misinterpreted as cyst rupture.[88] Small calculi may also develop in medullary sponge kidney, a condition that is rarely diagnosed in the pediatric age group. The French name *ectasie tubulaire précalicielle* well describes the major underlying pathology, which is the considerable dilatation of the distal collecting ducts within the pyramids. Although it is a congenital anomaly, the clinical symptoms (urolithiasis, hematuria, urinary tract infections) are usually seen only in adults. Medullary sponge kidneys (not to be confused with medullary cystic disease, which is the term now used for the dominant form of nephronophthisis) may occur either as an isolated finding or as a part of a syndrome (e.g., hemihypertrophy).

Endemic Stones

The term *endemic stones* is used to describe certain renal stones and primary bladder stones. Endemic renal stones are seen in children in developing countries, and they are mainly the result of an unbalanced diet. The early administration of white rice to infants (as early as the first weeks of life) and continuing this form of nutrition during the first year of life seems to constitute a specific risk factor.[89] A slightly elevated uric acid excretion in certain populations, (e.g., in Israeli Arabs) may also play a role.[90] Endemic renal stones mostly consist of uric acid, a constituent that is rarely seen in children (in contrast with adults) in Western countries, and of ammonium acid urate, a constituent that is otherwise associated with infection.[8,91]

Primary bladder stones still account for up to 5% of urinary calculi worldwide,[10] but they have disappeared in industrialized countries. They constitute an important group in endemic areas, accounting for one fourth to one third of all pediatric stones in Tunisia and Turkey and for more than half in Cameroon and India. The main bladder stone components are calcium oxalate, uric acid, and ammonium acid urate, often arranged in concentric layers.[8] Specific dietary habits also seem to play an important role.

Primary (nonendemic) bladder stones may develop as a result of bladder outlet obstruction, neurogenic bladder, infection, or foreign bodies (e.g., suture material).

Medications and Intoxications Causing Nephrocalcinosis or Stones

Medication-Induced Urolithiasis

A number of medications are known to induce nephrolithiasis, and as many as 1% to 2% of all kidney stones may be drug related.[92] Certain drugs, especially those excreted by the kidneys and those with poor solubility, either provide the nidus for stone formation (e.g., triamterene, sulfadiazine, indinavir) or increase the excretion of lithogenic substances (e.g., loop diuretics, topiramate, calcium/vitamin D supplementation, carbonic-anhydrase inhibitors; Table 33-9). The hypercalciuria induced by furosemide has been implicated in the nephrocalcinosis and stones observed in premature infants.[93] Carbonic anhydrase inhibitors result not only in hypercalciuria but also in hypocitraturia as a result of metabolic acidosis and an alkaline urine pH, which together predispose individuals to calcium phosphate precipitation in the urinary tract. Not infrequently, patients with drug-induced nephrolithiasis have additional metabolic abnormalities (e.g., hypercalciuria, low urinary pH levels) as risk factors for stone formation.

Indinavir is a protease inhibitor that is used for the treatment of human immunodeficiency virus infection. It is excreted unchanged in the urine, and it is poorly soluble at a pH of greater than 5. Stones have been observed in 2% to 28% of patients who receive this agent, including children.[94] The stones may be comprised of indinavir alone, or they may be of mixed composition as a result of indinavir crystals acting as a nidus for calcium oxalate or calcium phosphate precipitation. Stones comprised solely of indinavir are radiolucent and difficult to see on CT scanning as a result of the similarity of their density to that of soft tissue. Discontinuation of the medication, urine acidification, and increased fluid administration can successfully dissolve indinavir stones.

TABLE 33-9 **Medications and Intoxications That Cause Urinary Tract Stones**

Medications	Ingestions and Intoxications
• Furosemide	• Ethylene glycol
• Carbonic anhydrase inhibitors	• Paracetamol elixirs containing diethylene glycol
• Methoxyflurane	• Xylitol
• Ceftriaxone	• Rhubarb
• Ampicillin	• Sorrel
• Triamterene	• Ascorbic acid
• Guaifenesin	• Naftidrofuryl
• Phenazopyridine	• Carambola (star fruit)
• Oxypurinol	
• Sulfonamides	
• Topiramate, acetazolamide,	
• Zonisamide, dorzolamide	
• Indinavir	
• Pancreatic enzymes	
• Pyridoxilate	
• Nimesulide	
• Calcineurin inhibitors	
• Orlistat	

The precipitation of other medications in the urinary tract causing stones or the obstruction of tubules from crystals is rare,[92] but it has been reported with ceftriaxone, sulfonamides, ampicillin, amoxicillin, triamterene, acyclovir, guaifenesin, phenazopyridine, and oxypurinol. Patients receiving triamterene (e.g., patients with Liddle syndrome) will have stones that mostly contain triamterene itself or its main metabolite, hydroxytriamterene (see Table 33-9).

Medications and Intoxications Associated with Hyperoxaluria

Certain medications and intoxications associated with marked hyperoxaluria deserve particular mention, because they often have severe clinical consequences, including renal failure.

Intoxication with ethylene glycol, which is usually observed after the accidental ingestion of antifreeze or after suicide attempts with that substance, results in severe hyperoxaluria.[95] Ethylene glycol per se is not toxic, but toxicity is based on its conversion to glycolic acid, formalin, and oxalic acid via alcohol dehydrogenase. These and other acids lead to severe metabolic acidosis. The concurrent overproduction of oxalic acid results in acute renal failure as a result of calcium-oxalate crystal agglomeration in the renal parenchyma.[95,96] Diagnostic hints are an extreme anion gap and abundant calcium-oxalate crystals in the urine.

Treatment consists of the administration of ethanol or 4-methylpyrazole, which both block the alcohol dehydrogenase. Bicarbonate is administered to treat the metabolic acidosis, and hemodialysis is performed to remove both ethylene glycol and its metabolites.[95] The overall prognosis is guarded, with approximately 20% morbidity.[95,96] The highest toll (76 victims) was reported in the United States after the ingestion of a sulfazide-containing medication that was dissolved in ethylene glycol. Decades later, 47 children died in Nigeria after ingesting a paracetamol syrup sweetened with ethylene glycol.[97]

Other Agents

Xylitol, which is sometimes infused as a constituent of parenteral nutrition, is metabolized to oxalate. Renal failure has been reported after its administration,[96] although, unless a large amount is administered, the resulting oxalate can usually be eliminated without serious consequences. One of the components of the medication piridoxilate is metabolized to oxalate and has been reported to cause renal failure from calcium oxalate crystal deposition in the kidney.[98] Methoxyflurane can have similar effects after its administration as an anesthetic agent. Ascorbic acid is also metabolized to oxalate, although very large doses are needed to cause clinically significant hyperoxaluria.[99] The chronic use of ascorbic acid at usual doses does not appear to be associated with stones.

Oxalate poisoning from foods is rare,[100] but it has been reported with carambola (star fruit), sorrel, and rhubarb.[101,102] The absorption of oxalate from the gastrointestinal tract is low (approximately 3% to 18%), particularly when a food high in oxalate is ingested with other foods. For this reason, a very large or highly concentrated amount of the offending agent must be eaten before blood or urinary concentrations of oxalate reach toxic levels.

Other Disorders Complicated by Urolithiasis and/or Nephrocalcinosis

Cystic Fibrosis and Other Malabsorption Syndromes

Urolithiasis and nephrocalcinosis are frequently found in patients with malabsorption syndromes, with prevalence rates ranging from 12% in patients with cystic fibrosis up to 26% in male patients with Crohn disease.[69] This is not confined to adult patients, because stone disease develops early during the course of the diseases. The increased risk in cystic fibrosis is primarily the result of hyperoxaluria[69] (see Secondary Hyperoxalurias earlier in this chapter). Oxalate is increased not only as a result of the malabsorption typically seen in cystic fibrosis but also as a result of the absence of intestinal oxalate-degrading bacteria like *Oxalobacter formigenes,* which is a side effect of long-term antibiotic treatment.[69] The combination of hyperoxaluria and hypocitraturia (found in one third of patients with cystic fibrosis) leads to a significantly increased urinary saturation for calcium oxalate.[69]

The same pathophysiologic background exists in patients with Crohn disease, ulcerative colitis, enteric sprue, A-β-lipoproteinemia, exudative enteropathy, and short bowel syndrome.[64] Patients with malabsorption often have low urine volumes and acid urine as a result of diarrhea, and they are also prone to the development of uric acid stones[103] (Figure 33-8). In addition, they are often volume depleted as a result of chronic diarrhea; hence, their urine volume is low, and the urine is supersaturated, particularly with respect to uric acid and/or calcium oxalate.

A ketogenic diet is used for childhood epilepsy, and it can be associated with uric acid stones (because of an acidic urine and a low fluid intake) or with calcium oxalate stones as a result of hypercalciuria and hypocitraturia.[104]

Disorders with Abnormalities of Renal Tubule Function

A number of hereditary and acquired causes of renal tubule dysfunction result in nephrocalcinosis and/or nephrolithiasis (see Tables 33-4 and 33-6). Both primary and secondary forms of d-RTA, such as those that occur with Wilson disease, Sjögren syndrome, type Ia glycogen storage disease,[80] and cerebrotendinous xanthomatosis, are associated with stones and nephrocalcinosis. Urolithiasis is not usually seen with proximal or type IV renal tubular acidosis. With proximal renal tubular acidosis, the high urine citrate level that accompanies the hypercalciuria may protect against stone formation. With type IV renal tubular acidosis, reductions in urinary calcium appear to balance reductions in urine citrate such that the urinary saturation of calcium oxalate remains normal.

In disorders with generalized proximal renal tubule dysfunction (e.g., Fanconi syndrome), hypercalciuria appears to be an important contributor to stone formation. There may be other contributing factors that have not yet been defined. Medullary nephrocalcinosis and urolithiasis are seen in Dent disease, in Lowe syndrome, and in some patients with cystinosis, and they have occasionally been documented in the absence of hypercalciuria.

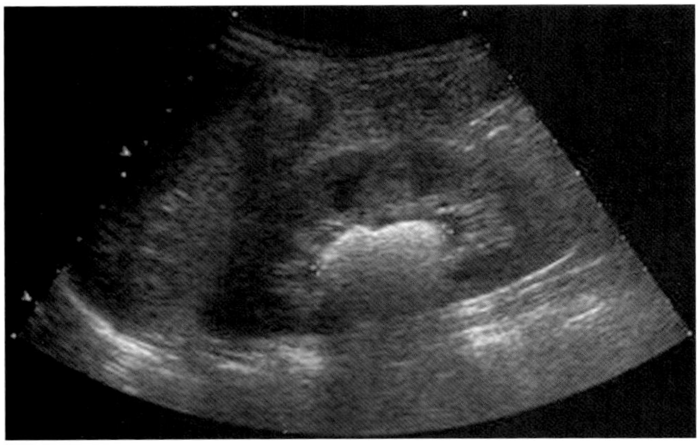

Figure 33-8 Staghorn calculus (100% uric acid) in a 7-year-old patient with ulcerative colitis after total colectomy and a continuously acid urine. The stone was removed by percutaneous nephrolithotomy, and further stone production was prevented with alkaline citrate treatment.

Dent Disease

Dent disease, which is an X-linked disorder of renal tubular epithelial function, is characterized by hypercalciuria, low-molecular-weight proteinuria, glycosuria, aminoaciduria, and phosphaturia, but without the typical proximal renal tubular acidosis of Fanconi syndrome[105] (see Table 33-8). Nephrocalcinosis and urolithiasis are often found, but, more importantly, Dent disease usually leads to early renal failure. Rickets has been reported in a minority of patients, and it is probably the result of excessive phosphaturia[105] (see Chapter 29).

Lowe Syndrome

The oculocerebral syndrome of Lowe is an X-linked recessive disorder characterized by congenital cataracts, hypotonia, developmental delay, impaired growth, and renal tubule dysfunction[106] (see Table 33-8). The disorder is the result of a defect in the inositol phosphate signaling pathway that results from mutations of the gene that encodes the OCRL1 protein. Tubular proteinuria and aminoaciduria are evident in infancy, with the subsequent development of Fanconi syndrome. Associated problems in childhood include polyuria, metabolic acidosis, hypophosphatemia, and rickets. Hypercalciuria, nephrocalcinosis, and stones are well described.[107] Hypercalciuria has been observed in the absence of vitamin D therapy and in the face of normal serum calcium and phosphorus levels, and it can persist after the correction of acidosis.[107] There have been anecdotal reports of improvement in hypercalciuria during treatment with thiazides.[107] Later in life, progressive renal failure is typical, with end-stage renal disease occurring by the fourth decade.[106] The cause of the renal failure and its relationship to hypercalciuria and nephrocalcinosis is unclear.

Familial Hypercalciuria and Hypomagnesemia

The syndrome of familial hypercalciuria and hypomagnesemia with renal magnesium wasting (see Table 33-8) leads to progressive nephrocalcinosis with renal failure.[108] It is caused by *CLDN 16* (paracellin-1) gene mutations, and it is often missed unless magnesium is measured in serum and urine (see Table 33-4). No effective therapy is currently available.

Treatment consists mostly of hydrochlorothiazide and oral magnesium supplementation. However, the treatment does not normalize the serum magnesium levels nor does it appear to prevent early end-stage renal failure.[109]

Therapeutic and Preventive Measures

As a result of the progress made regarding the urologic management of urolithiasis by less-invasive measures, there is now a tendency to pay less attention to the proper diagnostic evaluation that is essential for adequate preventive treatment. This not only results in increased morbidity and occasionally even in progressive renal damage, but it has also adverse socioeconomic effects and leads to additional costs that could easily be avoided.

Acute Management

Attacks of colicky pain are treated with analgesic agents parenterally or orally, as indicated. Recent approaches using calcium channel blocking agents and corticosteroids to facilitate stone passage have been quite successful.[110] If there is no significant obstruction, a large fluid administration is advocated, because many pelvic or ureteral stones pass spontaneously. The urine is filtered (a paper coffee filter may be used) to catch any spontaneously passed stone. If obstruction is suspected from ultrasonographic examination, it is imperative to assess whether the kidney involved is actually functioning and excreting urine. A hint is the demonstration of a urinary jet from the ureter into the bladder. Otherwise, renal scintigraphy (MAG-3) may be performed, or, if scintigraphy is unavailable, an intravenous urogram may be needed. Physical activity is recommended. Further intervention is needed if the colicky pain or significant obstruction persists. If the latter is the case, the prompt removal of the obstructing stone ureteroscopically or by extracorporeal lithotripsy or urine drainage (e.g., by placing a nephrostomy tube) may be necessary to avoid kidney damage.

Surgical and Endoscopic Interventions and Extracorporeal Lithotripsy

Stones that are small (<5 mm) or that do not cause any symptoms can be left in situ, but patients need to be followed. Only two kinds of stones can be dissolved chemically: cystine stones, by chelating agents, and uric acid stones, by alkalinization and the administration of allopurinol.[6,111,112]

Although open surgical intervention is now required for only a small minority of adult patients with stones, this is not fully true for pediatric patients, particularly those with additional urinary tract anomalies that need correction and in countries with limited resources. The newer generations of extracorporeal shockwave lithotripters allow for precise focusing and intervention, even in young children. Alternatively, new lithotripters are more powerful than the earlier generations and may lead to additional injury of the renal tissue. Less-aggressive lithotripsy (i.e., not more than 1500 to 2000 shock waves per session) is therefore advocated, and frequently more than one intervention is needed. General anesthesia is usually required for pediatric patients.[113]

Minimally invasive techniques have recently been developed for pediatric use, most notably percutaneous nephrolithotomy or nephrolithotripsy and retrograde (endoscopic) lithotripsy.[114] However, the method preferred for intervention is determined not only by the clinical situation but also by the equipment available and the experience of the pediatric surgeon or urologist.

The classical domain of extracorporeal shockwave lithotripsy is the patient with symptomatic nephrolithiasis without obstruction or dilatation. The minimal stone size is 5 mm. The administration of large quantities of fluid is needed after extracorporeal shockwave lithotripsy, and the urine is filtered to collect the fragments for analysis. A ureteral stent may have to be placed to allow for the free drainage of urine. Episodes of colicky pain may occur after intervention. Often one or more sessions are needed, and a stone-free state is achieved in about 80% of patients.[114] The success rate of extracorporeal shockwave lithotripsy is clearly less in stones with diameters of more than 2 cm. Large or complex upper tract stones are the domain of percutaneous nephrolithotomy. Open surgery may still occasionally be required for pelvic stones with obstruction or for staghorn calculi. Cystine stones and uric acid stones are less amenable to extracorporeal shockwave lithotripsy alone because of their physicochemical properties, and they may require a combination of other methods (e.g., chemical litholysis).[112]

Great care is needed for patients with nephrocalcinosis, particularly in primary hyperoxaluria because of a serious risk of irreversible renal damage by lithotripsy. Such patients require cautious intervention and very generous hydration.

Proximal ureteral stones may also be amenable to extracorporeal shockwave lithotripsy if no spontaneous passage occurs and the calculus is not encrusted. Retrograde ureteroscopic lithotripsy with a holmium : YAG laser is ideally suited for the removal or fragmentation of distal ureteral stones.[114]

Primary bladder stones are often very large, and they are removed by open surgery, which remains the main treatment in children. After they have been removed endemic bladder stones do not tend to recur.[10] Adult patients are usually treated by endoscopic transurethral disintegration with mechanical cystolithotripsy. All of these procedures require anesthesia and hospitalization.

Specific Therapeutic and Preventive Measures

Most of the steps in the process of stone formation can be exploited to reduce stone-forming activity. Concentrations of solutes can be reduced by addressing dietary or other sources of solute excess, by pharmacologic means (e.g., thiazides to reduce urinary calcium excretion), and by increasing urine volume. High fluid intake is beneficial in almost all types of stone formation and should be a mainstay of therapy. Urine pH can also be modified to advantage. For example, in patients with cystinuria or uric acid stones, alkalinization of the urine will enhance the solubility of cystine or uric acid crystals. Naturally occurring inhibitors of crystal formation are found in the urine and include pyrophosphate, citrate, and magnesium. Enhancing inhibitor activity by the oral administration of these agents can be a valuable component of the treatment program.

Treatment that is specifically directed to the causes identified in each child provides the most effective prevention of further stone formation. The simplest effective measure is a regular large fluid intake (>2 L per 1.73 m^2 of body surface area daily) at all times, but this is not easy to achieve in children and even less so in adolescents. Neutral beverages (i.e., water, fruit tea, mineral water with low calcium content) are preferred. For patients who are clearly unable to drink the recommended daily fluid amount, the placement of a percutaneous gastrostomy may be an option. Without an adequate fluid intake, other preventive measures will be of limited effectiveness.

Hypercalciuria (Primary/Secondary)

Nutrition A low-sodium diet can reduce the urinary calcium excretion, and the renal handling of sodium and calcium is closely linked. However, rigorous salt restriction is almost impossible to achieve for a long period of time. A high-protein diet (animal protein) should be avoided, because metabolic acidosis resulting from the increased metabolism of sulfuric-acid–containing amino acids enhances urinary calcium excretion.[34] Although marked dietary excess of calcium should be avoided, dietary calcium restriction does more harm than good: a daily calcium intake of less than 400 to 600 mg will result in a negative calcium balance.[115] Furthermore, low-calcium diets are accompanied by higher urinary oxalate excretion, because intestinal oxalate is no longer bound to calcium.[116] As a result, more unbound (soluble) oxalate will be available for intestinal absorption and will result in a higher level of urinary oxalate excretion. Because oxalate is 10 times more potent than calcium for increasing the urinary calcium oxalate saturation, the propensity for calcium oxalate stone formation will be increased.[116] Nutrition that is rich in fiber to bind intestinal calcium but that is low in oxalate to avoid the enteric hyperabsorption of oxalate is recommended.[64] When high fluid intake and dietary measures are not sufficient to control stone formation, pharmacologic approaches may be needed.

Thiazide Diuretics Thiazides reduce renal calcium excretion by increasing calcium reabsorption in the distal tubules and by stimulating proximal tubular reabsorption via volume control. The hypocalciuric effect of hydrochlorothiazide may result in improved bone density.[44] Hypokalemia is a troublesome side effect that can lead to hypocitraturia and an inadvertent increase of the urinary saturation (e.g., for calcium oxalate).[42] In addition, hydrochlorothiazide medications may also lead to a lower blood pressure.

Citrate Potassium citrate (0.2 to 0.3 g/kg corresponding with 2 to 3 mEq/kg/day of alkali) is given in patients with d-RTA and leads to a reduction of calcium excretion and an increase of urinary citrate and serum potassium by the correction of the acidosis.[68]

Primary Hyperoxaluria

Nutrition Next to a large daily fluid intake (>3 L per 1.73 m^2 per day for the primary hyperoxalurias), special dietary recommendations are not particularly important for patients with primary hyperoxaluria, other than the avoidance of extremely oxalate-rich foods like spinach or rhubarb.

Pyridoxine (Vitamin B6) Pyridoxal phosphate is an essential cofactor of alanine: glyoxylate aminotransferase (AGT), and pharmacologic doses of pyridoxine may significantly reduce hyperoxaluria in patients with type I primary hyperoxaluria. Approximately 30% to 50% of patients with primary hyperoxaluria type I have some degree of sensitivity to pyridoxine.[47,48,58] Certain mutations of *AGXT* appear to be associated with pyridoxine sensitivity, and they can be useful for guiding initial therapy.[58] This is particularly the case for patients with reduced renal function in whom the clinical assessment of the pyridoxine response can be difficult. Pyridoxine is started with 5 mg/kg body weight per day to exclude or demonstrate pyridoxine responsiveness (>30% reduction of urinary oxalate excretion). Recent data suggests that the maximum benefit is likely to be achieved at less than 10 mg/kg/day,[58] although higher doses may occasionally be considered on a trial basis. Occasionally a much smaller daily dose (10 to 20 mg) is also effective.[58] A trial of at least 3 to 6 months is warranted in all primary hyperoxaluria type I patients. Pyridoxine does not appear to be beneficial for patients with type II primary hyperoxaluria, and there is very limited information available regarding its use in idiopathic hyperoxaluria stone disease.

Crystallization Inhibitors Citrate predominantly binds to calcium, thus forming a soluble complex and reducing the precipitation of calcium with other substances like oxalate. Hence, the urinary saturation index decreases significantly.[48,117] The daily dosage of alkali citrate is 0.1 to 0.15 g/kg body weight (0.3 to 0.5 mmol/kg) of a sodium or sodium/potassium citrate preparation. Citrate is metabolized in the liver to bicarbonate, the alkali load leads to the reduction of the intratubular reabsorption of citrate, and, hence, more citrate is later excreted via the urine.[42] The binding of calcium and citrate complexes is even increased at a higher urinary pH, thus less calcium is available to bind with oxalate. Alkali citrate preparations lead to decreased stone production or the lesser expression of nephrocalcinosis.[48] The effect of alkali therapy and the patient's compliance are checked repeatedly by measuring urinary pH and citrate excretion.

Magnesium and Phosphate Preparations The therapeutic effect of neutral phosphate is comparable to that of alkali citrate medication, and magnesium administration is quite often also recommended for patients with recurrent kidney stones.[19,51] Both substances lead to a potent inhibition of calcium oxalate or calcium phosphate crystallization, and, especially in patients with recurrent urolithiasis, a beneficial effect of magnesium treatment has been reported.[4] The dose of neutral phosphate in children and adolescents with good renal function is 25 to 30 mg/kg day of elemental phosphate divided into three or four doses, with the daily dose not to exceed a total of 1600 mg. Phosphate therapy should be avoided in patients with moderate or advanced renal insufficiency. Long-term follow-up reports of neutral phosphate treatment suggest efficacy for patients with primary hyperoxaluria,[51] but they are sparse for other forms of calcium oxalate stone disease.[4]

Renal Replacement Therapy Patients with dietary or idiopathic hyperoxaluria are not at risk for renal failure. However, as a result of the degree of hyperoxaluria seen in both enteric and primary hyperoxaluria, renal failure frequently ensues. Renal replacement therapy is a specific concern only for patients with primary hyperoxaluria as a result of the marked hepatic production of oxalate. With the reduced renal clearance of the excess oxalate, hyperoxalemia ensues, with a risk of systemic oxalosis (see Primary Hyperoxaluria earlier in this chapter). Specific strategies are required.

Dialysis When a reduction in renal function to a glomerular filtration rate of less than 30 ml/min/1.73 m^2 occurs, renal replacement with transplantation or dialysis is needed promptly. In most patients with primary hyperoxaluria, no type of dialysis therapy is able to remove sufficient oxalate to keep pace with daily production.[53] Not even the combination of hemodialysis and peritoneal dialysis, the use of high flux dialyzers, or hemo(dia)filtration is able to prevent oxalate retention,[121] except in those patients who are sensitive to pyridoxine. Therefore, early transplantation is necessary.[48,56,122-124]

Transplantation Except for those patients who respond well to pyridoxine, prompt disease recurrence is a significant risk in isolated kidney transplantation. Transplantation should be performed as soon as possible to minimize systemic oxalosis. Although reasonable outcomes of kidney-only transplantation (including mostly living donors) were observed in North America,[122] this approach has largely been replaced by combined liver and kidney transplantation in patients with type I primary hyperoxaluria who are not fully responsive to pyridoxine.[123,124] With the metabolic defect in the liver and the problem being the overproduction of oxalate without other avenues for its disposition, it is clearly necessary to perform total hepatectomy before transplantation, although the liver is normal in every other aspect. Actuarial patient survival is 80%, with a liver graft survival rate of 72% at 5 years.[123] Specific risk factors for graft failure or the early recurrence of kidney disease are young age (<5 years) and a long period on dialysis (>2 years).[48,123] The administration of generous amounts of fluids and of alkali citrate or neutral phosphate during the first months or even years is essential because of the slow mobilization of the accumulated body calcium oxalate stores and thus persistent hyperoxaluria.[124]

The rationale of preemptive liver transplantation (instead of waiting until end-stage renal failure occurs) appears attractive at first look, and more than a dozen primary hyperoxaluria type I patients have been treated with this approach, with reasonable results.[56,125] However, the risk of losing a graft or even a patient who might have lived many years longer without transplantation and the long-term adverse effects of immunosuppressive medications raise serious ethical questions.

Secondary Hyperoxaluria

Nutrition Next to a large daily fluid intake (>2 L per 1.73 m^2 per day), special dietary recommendations are particularly important for patients with secondary (including enteric) hyperoxaluria.[64] The aim is to keep the urinary oxalate concentration below 0.5 mmol/L. Oxalate-rich nutrients (e.g., spinach, rhubarb) and an excessive intake of ascorbic acid, which is a precursor of oxalate, should be avoided. Calcium supplementation may be beneficial, because calcium binds to oxalate in the intestine, and such complexes are not absorbed but rather excreted in the feces. However, this form of treatment has to be followed with caution. Most of the calcium supplements contain vitamin D. Also, calcium administration that is independent from the main meals may lead to an increase in urinary calcium excretion.

The management of enteric hyperoxaluria includes a low-oxalate, low-fat diet and the avoidance of a low-calcium diet (but the intake of the daily recommended allowance of calcium so that oxalate is intestinally bound). Calcium supplements with meals can be helpful for some patients. In addition, a high fluid intake to the degree tolerable in a patient with fat malabsorption is necessary. In some patients, bile acid sequestrants are helpful.

Crystallization Inhibitors Crystallization inhibitors like potassium citrate, sodium-potassium citrate, and magnesium as well as neutral phosphate preparations may be of help to decrease the urinary saturation index (see Primary Hyperoxaluria earlier in this chapter).

Newer Preventive Concepts A promising potential treatment that is currently awaiting clinical confirmation is the intestinal elimination of endogenous oxalate using the two oxalate-degrading enzymes of *Oxalobacter formigenes*, an anaerobic microbe that normally inhabits the intestinal tract. Lending credence to the importance of such bacteria, secondary hyperoxaluria has been observed in patients with a lack or absence of intestinal *Oxalobacter formigenes*.[64]

Oxalate secretory pathways for intestinal oxalate elimination have also been identified in the large intestine.[118] A physiologic interaction of *O. formigenes* with rat colonic mucosa to modulate the handling of oxalate in colonized animals leading to the induction of enteric secretion/excretion has also been described.[118] This has led to the hypothesis that this organism may be helpful for the treatment not only of patients with secondary hyperoxaluria but also of those with primary hyperoxaluria.[119] The use of chemical chaperones that stabilize the enzyme AGT in patients with primary hyperoxaluria type I may become another option.[120]

Cystinuria The prevention of stone formation can be quite effective. High fluid intake to keep the urine cystine concentration within the soluble range (<1250 μmol/L at a pH of 7) and the alkalinization of the urine are the most valuable options.[112,126] The solubility of cystine strongly depends on the pH, and it gradually increases to a pH of 7.5 with a rapid increase with pH values above 7.5. However, to raise the urine pH to 7.0 or even 7.5 for prolonged periods is difficult. Because dietary sodium may increase cystine excretion, potassium citrate instead of sodium bicarbonate is preferred as alkali therapy. Limiting dietary sodium intake can also be a useful strategy. For patients who continue to form stones despite these measures, α-mercaptopropionylglycine (Thiola) forms a soluble dimer with cystine and can be administered orally (dosage: 10 to 15 mg/kg body weight per day). The medication must be taken multiple times daily, and it has side effects—a few of which are serious—such as severe nephrosis that limit its use in some patients.[112] D-penicillamine and captopril also form soluble dimers with cystine. The former has a higher incidence of side effects than α-mercaptopropionylglycine, and the latter has not been effective for all patients. The direct measurement of urine cystine excretion or even saturation using the EQUIL program can be helpful for guiding therapy.[127] Bucillamine, which is a dithiol compound, is a promising alternative.[126] Because these medications have an antipyridoxine effect, supplemental vitamin B6 should be provided when they are used.

Purine Stones (Uric Acid, 2,8-Dihydroxyadenine, Xanthine) Because of the greater solubility of uric acid at an alkaline urine pH, therapy aims to keep the urine pH above 6.5 by the administration of alkali citrate. This and a high fluid intake may be sufficient to dissolve small stones.[128] In patients with hyperuricosuria, purine-rich meat (e.g., liver, kidney) and protein excess have to be avoided. Allopurinol, which is an inhibitor of xanthine oxidase, is given in hyperuricosuria that is not amenable to dietary restrictions, particularly in partial or complete hypoxanthine-phosphoribosyltransferase deficiency (Lesch-Nyhan syndrome). However, in complete or partial hypoxanthine-phosphoribosyltransferase deficiency, there is a small risk of xanthine stone formation with such treatment. In contrast with uric acid, the solubility of xanthine is not improved by alkalization.[83] A regular high fluid intake is the only effective measure. The lack of a pH effect is also true for 2,8-dihydroxyadenine; therapy includes high fluid intake and the administration of allopurinol.[82] The restriction of dietary adenine and purine intake is also helpful. Acute renal failure as a result of 2,8-dihydroxyadenine can be reversible if treatment is initiated promptly.[129]

Infection Stones Appropriate antibiotic therapy is the most important thing, but infection will not be eradicated unless all calculous material is removed, because it may still harbor organisms.[130] This is not easily achieved, because struvite stones are often crumbly and difficult to remove. Acidification of the urine would be desirable, but it is difficult to achieve: ascorbic acid is not effective, and L-methionine, which is metabolized to sulfate, has only a very weak effect. Ammonium chloride is poorly tolerated and may lead to systemic acidosis in patients in whom prevention is most needed (i.e., those with impaired renal function and neurogenic bladder). Other therapies, such as urease inhibitors and phosphate depletion, have been abandoned as a result of their adverse side effects.

Conclusions

Urolithiasis and nephrocalcinosis are regularly encountered by nephrologists who care for children and adolescents. Every sign of ongoing stone disease or nephrocalcinosis should lead to further evaluation. Predisposing causes are identifiable in a large proportion of such patients and should be systematically sought. Early diagnosis is mandatory in the child with stones, because therapeutic measures may be able to prevent kidney damage and even early renal failure (e.g., in patients with a metabolic disorder like primary hyperoxaluria). The 24-hour urine collection for detecting abnormalities in urinary lithogenic or stone inhibitory substances is the most valuable approach. Two or three such collections are recommended during the initial diagnostic assessment as a result of day-to-day variations in diet and fluid intake. In addition (or whenever possible), stone analysis can provide further evidence of the pathophysiology of recurrent stone formation.

Commonly, ultrasound examination is the imaging method of choice, but, for detecting urolithiasis (especially ureteral stones), spiral CT scanning is the better method. In children, however, a combination of high-resolution ultrasonography with abdominal x-ray is often sufficient.

Stones causing obstruction, those that are likely to do so because of their size or location, and infected stones require removal. A number of surgical techniques are now available for even small children and should be tailored to the individual circumstances of the patient. Smaller, nonobstructing stones should be managed medically, with a goal of preventing stone growth and new stone formation. Effective treatment is available for most forms of stone disease. Preventive therapy is cheaper and much better for the patient than repeated attacks of colicky pain and further stone removal procedures. Finally and most importantly, the patient with recurrent stone formation or (progressive) nephrocalcinosis must be convinced that a high daily fluid intake is the most valuable therapeutic option.

REFERENCES

1. Saigal CS, Joyce G, Timilsina AR; Urologic Diseases in America Project: Direct and indirect costs of nephrolithiasis in an employed population: opportunity for disease management? *Kidney Int* 68:1808-14, 2005.
2. Ganem JP, Carson CC: Frere Jacques Beaulieu: from rogue lithotomist to nursery rhyme character, *J Urol* 161:1067-69, 1999.
3. Hesse A: Urinary calculi 1: epidemiology, laboratory diagnosis, genetics and infections, *Urologe A* 41:496-508, 2002.
4. Coe FL, Evan A, Worcester E: Kidney stone disease, *J Clin Invest* 115:2598-608, 2005.
5. Carson PJ, Brewster DR: Unique pattern of urinary tract calculi in Australian Aboriginal children, *J Paediatr Child Health.* 39:325-28, 2003.
6. Bartosh SM: Medical management of pediatric stone disease, *Urol Clin North Am,* 31:575-87, 2004.
7. Sarica K: Pediatric urolithiasis: etiology, specific pathogenesis and medical treatment, *Urol Res* 34:96-101, 2006.
8. Sarkissian A, Babloyan A, Arikyants N, et al: Pediatric urolithiasis in Armenia: a study of 198 patients observed from 1991 to 1999, *Pediatr Nephrol* 16:728-32, 2001.
9. Edvardsson V, Elidottir H, Indridason OS, Palsson R: High incidence of kidney stones in Icelandic children, *Pediatr Nephrol* 20:940-44, 2005.
10. Papatsoris AG, Varkarakis I, Dellis A, Dliveliotis C: Bladder lithiasis: from open surgery to lithotripsy, *Urol Res* 34:163-67, 2006.
11. Van Woerden CS, Groothoff JW, Wanders RJ: Primary hyperoxaluria type 1 in The Netherlands: prevalence and outcome, *Nephrol Dial Transplant* 18:273-79, 2003.
12. Hoppe B, Latta K, von Schnakenburg C, Kemper MJ: Primary hyperoxaluria—the German experience, *Am J Nephrol* 25:276-81, 2005.
13. Leumann E, Hoppe B: Urolithiasis in childhood. In Proesmans W, editor: *Therapeutic strategies in children with renal disease.* London, 1997, Baillière's Clinical Paediatrics, pp 655-74.

14. Smith RC, Rosenfield AT, Choe KA, et al: Acute flank pain: comparison of non-contrast-enhanced CT and intravenous urography, *Radiology* 194:789-94, 1995.
15. Mindell HJ, Cochran ST: Current perspectives in the diagnosis and treatment of urinary stone disease, *Am J Roentgenol* 163:1314-15, 1994.
16. Alon US: Nephrocalcinosis, *Pediatrics* 9:160-65, 1997.
17. Cramer B, Husa L, Pushpanathan C: Nephrocalcinosis in rabbits—correlation of ultrasound, computed tomography, pathology and renal function, *Pediatr Radiol* 28:9-13, 1998.
18. van't Hoff WG: Aetiological factors in paediatric urolithiasis, *Nephron Clin Pract* 98:45-48, 2004.
19. Cameron MA, Sakkhae K, Moe OW: Nephrolithiasis in children, *Pediatr Nephrol* 20:1587-92, 2005.
20. Battino BS, DeFoor W, Coe F, et al: Metabolic evaluation of children with urolithiasis: are adult references for supersaturation appropriate? *J Urol* 168:2568-71, 2002.
21. Defoor W, Asplin J, Jackson E, et al: Results of a prospective trial to compare normal urine supersaturation in children and adults, *J Urol* 174:1708-10, 2005.
22. Parks JH, Goldfisher E, Asplin JR, Coe FL: A single 24-hour urine collection is inadequate for the medical evaluation of nephrolithiasis, *J Urol* 167:1607-12, 2002.
23. Sayer JA, Carr G, Simmons NL: Nephrocalcinosis: molecular insights into calcium precipitation within the kidney, *Clin Sci* 106:549-61, 2004.
24. Ronnefarth G, Misselwitz J: Nephrocalcinosis in children: a retrospective study, *Pediatr Nephrol* 14:1016-21, 2000.
25. Schell-Feith EA, van Holthe KJE, Conneman N, et al: Etiology of nephrocalcinosis in preterm neonates: association of nutritional intake and urinary parameters, *Kidney Int* 58:2102-10, 2000.
26. Sikora P, Roth B, Kribs A, et al: Hypocitraturia is one of the major risk factors for nephrocalcinosis in very low birth weight (VLBW) infants, *Kidney Int* 63:2194-99, 2003.
27. Downing G, Egelhoff JC, Daily DK, et al: Kidney function in very low birth weight infants with furosemide-related renal calcifications at ages 1 to 2 years, *J Pediatr* 120:599-604, 1992.
28. Monge M, Garcia-Nieto VM, Domenech E, et al: Study of renal metabolic disturbances related to renal lithiasis at school age in very-low-birth-weight children, *Nephron* 79:269-73, 1998.
29. Neuhaus TJ, Belzer T, Blau N, et al: Urinary oxalate excretion in urolithiasis and nephrocalcinosis, *Arch Dis Child* 82:322-26, 2000.
30. Gwinner W, Suppa S, Mengel M, et al: Early calcifications of renal allografts detected by protocol biopsies: causes and clinical implications, *Am J Transplant* 5:1934-41, 2005.
31. Stapenhorst L, Sassen R, Beck B, et al: Hypocitraturia as a risk factor for nephrocalcinosis after kidney transplantation, *Pediatr Nephrol* 20:652-56, 2005.
32. Verkoelen CF, van der Boom BG, Houtsmuller AB, et al: Increased calcium oxalate monohydrate crystal binding to injured renal tubular epithelial cells in culture, *Am J Physiol* 274:F958-65, 1998.
33. Evan AP, Coe FK, Lingeman JE, et al: Insights on the pathology of kidney stone formation, *Urol Res* 33:383-89, 2005.
34. Moe OW: Kidney stones: pathophysiology and medical management, *Lancet* 367:333-44, 2006.
35. Amaro CR, Goldberg J, Amaro JL, Padovani CR: Metabolic assessment in patients with urinary lithiasis, *Int Braz J Urol* 31:29-33, 2005.
36. Damasio B, Massarino F, Durand F, et al: Prevalence of fasting hypercalciuria associated with increased citraturia in the ambulatory evaluation of nephrolithiasis, *J Nephrol* 18:262-66, 2005.
37. Mir S, Serdaroglu E: Quantification of hypercalciuria with the urine calcium osmolality ratio in children, *Pediatr Nephrol* 20:1562-65, 2005.
38. Matos V, van Melle G, Boulat O, et al: Urinary phosphate/creatinine, calcium/creatinine, and magnesium/creatinine ratios in a healthy pediatric population, *J Pediatr* 131:252-57, 1997.
39. Aladjem M, Barr J, Lahat E, Bistritzer T: Renal and absorptive hypercalciuria: a metabolic disturbance with varying and interchanging modes of expression, *Pediatrics* 97:216-19, 1996.
40. Goldfarb DS, Fischer ME, Keich Y, Goldberg J: A twin study of genetic and dietary influences on nephrolithiasis: a report from the Vietnam Era Twin (VET) Registry, *Kidney Int* 67:1053-61, 2005.
41. Bushinsky DA, Asplin JR, Grynpas MD, et al: Calcium oxalate stone formation in genetic hypercalciuric stone forming rats, *Kidney Int* 61:975-87, 2002.
42. Hamm LL: Renal handling of citrate, *Kidney Int* 38:728-35, 1990.
43. Jiang Z, Asplin JR, Evan AP, et al: Calcium oxalate urolithiasis in mice lacking anion transporter SLC26A6, *Nat Genet* 38:474-78, 2006.
44. Zanchetta JF, Rodriguez G, Negir AL, et al: Bone mineral density in patients with hypercalciuric nephrolithiasis, *Nephron* 73:557-60, 1996.
45. Campfield T, Braden G: Urinary oxalate excretion by very low birth weight infants receiving parenteral nutrition, *Pediatrics* 84:860-63, 1989.
46. Holmes RP, Goodman HO, Assimos DG: Contribution of dietary oxalate to urinary oxalate excretion, *Kidney Int* 59:270-76, 2001.
47. Van Woerden CS, Groothoff JW, Wijburg FA, et al: Clinical implications of mutation analysis in primary hyperoxaluria type 1, *Kidney Int* 66:746-52, 2004.
48. Leumann E, Hoppe B: The primary hyperoxalurias, *J Am Soc Nephrol* 12:1986-93, 2001.
49. Lieske JC, Monico CG, Holmes WS, et al: International registry for primary hyperoxaluria and Dent's disease, *Am J Nephrol* 25:290-96, 2005.
50. Khan SR: Crystal-induced inflammation of the kidneys: results from human studies, animal models, and tissue-culture studies, *Clin Exp Nephrol* 8:75-88, 2004.
51. Milliner DS, Eickholt JT, Bergstralh EJ, et al: Results of long term treatment with orthophosphate and pyridoxine in patients with primary hyperoxaluria, *N Engl J Med* 331:1553-58, 1994.
52. Hoppe B, Kemper MJ, Bökenkamp A, et al: Plasma calcium-oxalate supersaturation in children with primary hyperoxaluria and end stage renal disease, *Kidney Int* 56:268-74, 1999.
53. Hoppe B, Graf D, Offner G, et al: Oxalic acid elimination in children with chronic renal failure: comparison between hemodialysis and peritoneal dialysis, *Pediatr Nephrol* 10:488-92, 1996.
54. Hoppe B, Langman C: A United States survey on diagnosis, treatment and outcome of patients with primary hyperoxaluria, *Pediatr Nephrol* 18:986-91, 2003.
55. Milliner DS: The primary hyperoxalurias: an algorithm for diagnosis, *Am J Nephrol* 25:154-60, 2005.
56. Cochat P, Liutkus A, Fargue S, et al: Primary hyperoxaluria type 1: still challenging! *Pediatr Nephrol* 21:1075-81, 2006.
57. Rumsby G, Williams E, Coulter-Mackie M: Evaluation of mutation screening as a first line test for the diagnosis of the primary hyperoxalurias, *Kidney Int* 66:959-63, 2004.
58. Monico CG Rossetti S, Olson JB, Milliner DS: Pyridoxine effect in type I primary hyperoxaluria is associated with the most common mutant allele, *Kidney Int* 67:1704-09, 2005.
59. Milliner DS, Wilson DM, Smith LH: Phenotypic expression of primary hyperoxaluria: comparative features of types I and II, *Kidney Int* 59:31-36, 2001.
60. Monico CG, Persson M, Ford GC, et al: Potential mechanisms of marked hyperoxaluria not due to primary hyperoxaluria I or II, *Kidney Int* 62:392-400, 2002.
61. Curhan GC, Willett WC, Rimm EB, et al: A prospective study of dietary calcium and other nutrients and the risk of symptomatic kidney stones, *N Engl J Med* 328:833-38, 1993.
62. Hatch M, Freel RW: Intestinal transport of an obdurate anion: oxalate, *Urol Res* 33:1-16, 2005.
63. Hatch M, Freel RW, Vaziri ND: Regulatory aspects of oxalate secretion in enteric oxalate elimination, *J Am Soc Nephrol* 10:S324-28, 1999.
64. Hoppe B, Leumann E, von Unruh G, et al: Diagnostic and therapeutic approaches in patients with secondary hyperoxaluria, *Front Biosci* 8:e437-43, 2003.
65. Miller LA, Stapleton FB: Urinary citrate excretion in patients with hypercalciuria, *J Pediatr* 107:263-66, 1985.

66. Tekin A, Tekgul S, Atsu N, et al: A study of the etiology of idiopathic calcium urolithiasis in children: hypocitraturia is the most important risk factor, *J Urol* 164:162-65, 2000.
67. Parks JH, Coe FL: A urinary calcium-citrate index for the evaluation on nephrolithiasis, *Kidney Int* 30:85-90, 1986.
68. Preminger GM, Sakhaee K, Skurla C, Pak CYC: Prevention of recurrent calcium stone formation with potassium citrate therapy in patients with distal renal tubular acidosis, *J Urol* 134:20-24, 1985.
69. Hoppe B, von Unruh GE, Blank G, et al: Absorptive hyperoxaluria leads to an increased risk of urolithiasis or nephrocalcinosis in cystic fibrosis, *Am J Kid Dis* 46:440-45, 2005.
70. Sakhaee K, William RH, Oh MS, et al: Alkali absorption and citrate excretion in calcium nephrolithiasis, *J Bone Miner Res* 8:789-94, 1993.
71. Parks JH, Worcester EM, Coe FL, et al: Clinical implications of abundant calcium phosphate in routinely analyzed kidney stones, *Kidney Int* 66:777-85, 2004.
72. Bouropoulos N, Mouzakis DE, Bithelis G, Liatsikos E: Vickers hardness studies of calcium oxalate monohydrate and brushite urinary stones, *J Endourol* 20:59-63, 2006.
73. Saadi I, Chen XZ, Hediger M, et al: Molecular genetics of cystinuria: mutation analysis of SLC3A1 and evidence for another gene in type I (silent) phenotype, *Kidney Int* 54:48-55, 1998.
74. Leclerc D, Boutros M, Suh D, et al: SLC7A9 mutations in all three cystinuria subtypes. *Kidney Int* 62:1550-59, 2002.
75. Font-Llitjos M, Jimenez-Vidal M, Bisceglia L, et al: New insights into cystinuria: 40 new mutations, genotype-phenotype correlation, and digenic inheritance causing partial phenotype, *J Med Genet* 42:58-68, 2005.
76. Goodyer P, Saadi I, Ong P, et al: Cystinuria subtype and the risk of nephrolithiasis, *Kidney Int* 54:56-61, 1998.
77. Boutros M, Vicanek C, Rozen R, Goodyer P: Transient neonatal cystinuria, *Kidney Int* 67:443-48, 2005.
78. Rodriguez LM, Santos F, Malaga S, Martinez V: Effect of a low sodium diet on urinary elimination of cystine in cystinuric children, *Nephron* 71:416-18, 1995.
79. Dello Strologo L, Pras E, Pontesilli C, et al: Comparison between *SLC3A1* and *SLC7A9* cystinuria patients and carriers: a need for a new classification, *J Am Soc Nephrol* 13:2547-53, 2002.
80. Restaino I, Kaplan BS, Stanley C, Baker L: Nephrolithiasis, hypocitraturia, and a distal renal tubular acidification defect in type 1 glycogen storage disease, *J Pediatr* 122:392-96, 1993.
81. Arnodottir M, Laxdal T, Halldorsdottir B: 2,8-dihydroxyadeninuria: are there no cases in Scandinavia? *Scand J Urol Nephrol* 39:82-86, 2005.
82. Sahota AS, Tischfield JA, Katamani N, Simmonds HA: Adenine phosphoribosyltransferase deficiency and 2,8-dihydroxyadenine lithiasis. In Scriver CR, Beaudet AL, Valle D, Sly WS, editors: *The metabolic bases of inherited disease*, New York, 2001, McGraw Hill, pp. 2571-84.
83. Arikyants N, Sarkissian A, Hesse A, et al: Xanthinuria type I—a rare cause of urolithiasis. *Pediatr Nephrol* 22:310-14, 2007.
84. Bradbury MG, Henderson M, Brocklebank JT, Simmonds HA: Acute renal failure due to xanthine stones, *Pediatr Nephrol* 9:476-77, 1995.
85. Badertscher E, Robson WL, Leung AK, Trevenen CL: Xanthine calculi presenting at 1 month of age, *Eur J Pediatr* 152:252-54, 1993.
86. Cohen TD, Preminger GM: Struvite calculi, *Semin Nephrol* 16:425-36, 1996.
87. Matlaga BR, Kim SC, Watkins SL, et al: Changing composition of renal calculi in patients with neurogenic bladder, *J Urol* 175:1716-19, 2006.
88. Bajwa ZH, Gupta S, Warfield CA, Steinman TI: Pain management in polycystic kidney disease, *Kidney Int* 60:1631-44, 2001.
89. Sayasone S, Odermatt P, Khammanivong K, et al: Bladder stones in childhood: a descriptive study in a rural setting in Caravan Province, Lao PDR, *Southeast Asian J Trop Med Public Health* 35(Suppl 2):50-52, 2004.
90. Landau D, Tovbin D, Shalev H: Pediatric urolithiasis in southern Israel: the role of uricosuria, *Pediatr Nephrol* 14:1105-10, 2000.
91. Balla AA, Salah AM, Khattab AH, et al: Mineral composition of renal stones from the Sudan, *Urol Int* 61:154-56, 1998.
92. Daudon M, Estepa L: Drug induced lithiases, *Presse Med* 11:675-83, 1998.
93. Jacinto JS, Modanlou HD, Crade M, et al: Renal calcification incidence in very low birth weight infants, *Pediatrics* 81:31-35, 1988.
94. Zinn HL, Orentlicher RJ, Haller JO, Cohen HL: Radiographically occult ureteral calculi in an HIV-positive child undergoing indinavir therapy, *Emerg Radiol* 7:114-16, 2000.
95. Hylander B, Kjellstrand CM: Prognostic factors and treatment of severe ethylene glycol intoxication, *Intensive Care Med* 22:546-52, 1996.
96. Meier M, Nitschke M, Perras B, Steinhoff J: Ethylene glycol intoxication and xylitol infusion—metabolic steps of oxalate-induced acute renal failure, *Clin Nephrol* 63:225-28, 2005.
97. Okuonghae HO, Ighogboja IS, Lawson JO, Nwana EJ: Diethylene glycol poisoning in Nigerian children, *Ann Trop Paediatr* 12:235-38, 1992.
98. Daudon M, Réveillaud RJ: Piridoxilate-associated calcium oxalate urinary calculi, a new metabolic drug induced nephrolithiasis, *Lancet* 1:1338, 1985.
99. Wong K, Thomson C, Bailey RR, et al: Acute oxalate nephropathy after a massive intravenous dose of vitamin C, *Aust N Z J Med* 24:410-11, 1994.
100. Sanz P, Reig R: Clinical and pathological findings in fatal plant oxalosis, *Am J Forensic Med Pathol* 13:342-45, 1992.
101. Chen CL, Fang HC, Chou KJ, et al: Acute oxalate nephropathy after ingestion of star fruit, *Am J Kid Dis* 37:418-22, 2001.
102. Farre M, Xirgu J, Salgado A, et al: Fatal oxalic acid poisoning from sorrel soup, *Lancet* 2:8678-79, 1989.
103. Worcester EM: Stones from bowel disease, *Endocrinol Metab Clin North Am* 31:979-99, 2002.
104. Furth SL, Casey JC, Pyzik PL, et al: Risk factors for urolithiasis in children on the ketogenic diet, *Pediatr Nephrol* 15:125-28, 2000.
105. Scheinman SJ: X-linked hypercalciuric nephrolithiasis: clinical syndromes and chloride channel mutations, *Kidney Int* 53:3-17, 1998.
106. Charnas LR, Bernardini I, Rader D, et al: Clinical and laboratory findings in the oculocerebrorenal syndrome of Lowe, with special reference to growth and renal function, *N Engl J Med* 324:1318-25, 1991.
107. Sliman GA, Winters WD, Shaw DW, Avner ED: Hypercalciuria and nephrocalcinosis in the oculocerebrorenal syndrome, *J Urol* 153:1244-46, 1995.
108. Weber S, Schneider L, Peters M, et al: Novel paracellin-1 mutations in 25 families with familial hypomagnesemia with hypercalciuria and nephrocalcinosis, *J Am Soc Nephrol* 12:1872-81, 2001.
109. Zimmermann B, Plank C, Konrad M, et al: Hydrochlorothiazide in CLDN16 mutation, *Nephrol Dial Transplant* 21:2127-32, 2006.
110. Hollingsworth JM, Rogers MA, Kaufman SR, et al: Medical therapy to facilitate urinary stone passage: a meta-analysis, *Lancet* 368:1171-79, 2006.
111. Knoll T, Zollner A, Wendt-Nordahl G, et al: Cystinuria in childhood and adolescence: recommendations for diagnosis, treatment, and follow up, *Pediatr Nephrol* 20:19-24, 2005.
112. Joly D, Rieu P, Mejean A, et al: Treatment of cystinuria, Pediatr Nephrol 13:945-50, 1999.
113. Aldrigde RD, Aldridge RC, Aldridge LM: Anesthesia for pediatric lithotripsy, *Paediatr Anaesth* 16:236-41, 2006.
114. Durkee CT, Balcom A: Surgical management of urolithiasis, *Pediatr Clin North Am* 53:465-77, 2006.
115. Curhan GC, Willett WC, Knight EL, Stampfer MJ: Dietary factors and the risk of incident kidney stones in younger women: Nurses Health Study II, *Arch Intern Med* 26:885-91, 2004.
116. Von Unruh GE, Voss S, Sauerbruch T, Hesse A: Dependence of oxalate absorption on the daily calcium intake, *J Am Soc Nephrol* 15:1567-73, 2004.
117. Laube N, Hoppe B, Hesse A: Problems in the investigation of urines from patients suffering from primary hyperoxaluria type I, *Urol Res* 33:394-97, 2005.
118. Hatch M, Cornelius J, Allison M, et al: *Oxalobacter* sp. reduces urinary oxalate excretion promoting enteric oxalate excretion, *Kidney Int* 69:1-8, 2006.

119. Hoppe B, Beck B, Gatter N, et al: *Oxalobacter formigenes:* a potential tool for the treatment of primary hyperoxaluria type I, *Kidney Int* 70:1305-11, 2006.
120. Danpure CJ: Primary hyperoxaluria: from gene defects to designer drugs, *Nephrol Dial Transplant* 20:1525-29, 2005.
121. Bunchman TE, Swartz RD: Oxalate removal in type I hyperoxaluria or acquired oxalosis using HD and equilibration PD, *Perit Dial Int* 14:81-84, 1994.
122. Saborio P, Scheinman JI: Transplantation for primary hyperoxaluria in the United States, *Kidney Int* 56:1094-100, 1999.
123. Jamieson NV; European PHI Transplantation Study Group: A 20-year experience of combined liver/kidney transplantation for primary hyperoxaluria (PH1): the European PH1 transplant registry experience 1984-2004, *Am J Nephrol* 25:282-89, 2005.
124. Nolkemper D, Kemper MJ, Burdelski M, et al: Long-term results of pre-emptive liver transplantation in primary hyperoxaluria type 1, *Pediatr Transplant* 3:177-81, 2000.
125. Hoppe B, Kemper MJ, Bokenkamp A, et al: Plasma calcium oxalate supersaturation in children with primary hyperoxaluria and end-stage renal failure, *Kidney Int* 56:268-74, 1999.
126. Sakhaee K: Pathogenesis and medical management of cystinuria, *Semin Nephrol* 16:435-37, 1996.
127. Werness PG, Brown CM, Smith LH, Finlayson B: EQUIL 2, a BASIC computer program for the calculation of urinary saturation, *J Urol* 134:1242-44, 1985.
128. Sharma SK, Indudhara R: Chemodissolution of urinary uric acid stones by alkali therapy, *Urol Int* 48:81-86, 1992.
129. Hoffmann M, Talaszka A, Bocquet JP, et al: Acute renal failure and 2,8 dihydroxyadeninuria, *Nephrologie* 25:297-300, 2004.
130. Abrahams HM, Stoller ML: Infection and urinary stones, *Curr Opin Urol* 13:63-67, 2003.
131. Dick PT, Shuckett BM, Tang B, et al: Observer reliability in grading nephrocalcinosis on ultrasound examinations in children, *Pediatr Radiol* 29:68-72, 1999.
132. Stapleton FB, Linshaw MA, Hassanein K, Gruskin AB: Uric acid excretion in normal children, *J Pediatr* 92:911-14, 1978.
133. Tefekli A, Esen T, Ziylan O, et al: Metabolic risk factors in pediatric and adult calcium oxalate urinary stone formers: is there any difference? *Urol Int* 70:273-77, 2003.

CHAPTER 34

Interstitial Nephritis

Priya S. Verghese, Kera E. Luckritz, and Allison A. Eddy

INTRODUCTION AND HISTORICAL PERSPECTIVE

Anatomically, more than 95% of the kidney is comprised of tubules and interstitium. It is therefore crucial to understand the importance of the tubulointerstitium in all renal disease processes. Despite the anatomic dominance of the interstitium, current understanding of its role in both primary and secondary disease processes remains incomplete.

The term *acute interstitial nephritis* was coined by Councilman in 1898, when he collected data from the autopsy specimens of patients dying as a result of diphtheria, scarlet fever, and other infectious diseases; he provided the first and now classic description of the histopathologic changes.[1,2] Acute interstitial nephritis can be defined as presumptive, immune-mediated tubulointerstitial inflammation and damage with relative sparing of the glomeruli and vessels that is usually initiated by drugs, infections, or other causes.[3]

During the preantibiotic era, systemic infections were the most common cause of tubulointerstitial disease. Today, a drug hypersensitivity reaction is a more common inciting event. Ironically, many of these drugs were developed to treat the very infectious disorders that had often been implicated as causes of acute interstitial nephritis. Councilman's early description still has merit, although it may be more accurate to categorize the disease process as acute tubulointerstitial nephritis (TIN), because the renal tubules are also involved in all cases, both clinically and histopathologically.

Progressive chronic kidney disease—irrespective of the primary disease process—can be attributed to chronic TIN, and thus it is reasonable to consider TIN as a spectrum of clinical pathology that ranges from acute and reversible nephritis to chronic and irreversible disease with fibrogenesis.[4] For each individual patient, it is critical to try to identify and discontinue the offending toxin or agent before acute injury progresses to the chronic stage.

EPIDEMIOLOGY

Acute injury to the interstitium and the surrounding tubules is an important cause of renal dysfunction, accounting for 5% to 15% of all cases of acute or chronic renal failure. However, reliable data about the incidence and prevalence of interstitial nephritis are lacking, especially in the pediatric population. Often the diagnosis is made clinically without performing a renal biopsy to confirm the diagnosis. Furthermore, it is likely that many cases are self-limited and clinically silent. Thus, the estimated numbers are likely conservative and lower than the true incidence. Data are varied, but reports often state that acute TIN accounts for 7% of acute renal failure in the pediatric setting, whereas the incidence in adults is closer to 10% to 25% of reported cases of acute renal failure.[5]

HISTOLOGY AND PATHOGENESIS

By definition, TIN is characterized by interstitial cellular infiltrates, usually with sparing of the vessels and glomeruli, although it is noted that severe primary glomerular injury rarely occurs without concurrent tubulointerstitial injury (Figure 34-1, *A*). Tubular cell damage may manifest as epithelial proliferation and/or tubular dilatation, and cast formation is often present as well.[6] Chronic interstitial nephritis is typically associated with interstitial fibrosis and tubular atrophy, and it is often accompanied by a persistent mononuclear cell infiltrate.[6,7] The infiltrate is composed predominately of T cells, with some macrophages and plasma cells.[6-9] An impressive number of eosinophils may be present and suggest a drug-induced cause (Figure 34-1, *D* and *E*). Granuloma formation is a feature of biopsies in 6% of the patients, and it can occur in any form of acute interstitial nephritis; granulomas are considered common in drug-induced TIN, infection-associated TIN, and renal vasculitis[10] (Figure 34-1, *B*). The degree of tubulointerstitial inflammation may be predictive of functional outcome, even in primary glomerular diseases.[7,11]

In primary TIN, immunofluorescence staining for antibodies and complement proteins is typically negative. Occasionally linear or granular deposits of immunoglobulin G or M may be present along the tubular basement membranes.[7] Electron microscopy may reveal a loss of continuity of basement membranes as well as thickened and multilayered areas that are indicative of chronic damage.[7]

These histopathologic findings as well as the apparent clinical response to steroid therapy support a role for immune-mediated pathogenetic mechanisms. Although the specific immunopathogenetic mechanisms remain unclear, recent studies suggest an active role of chemokines and inflammatory mediators.[9] An ideal animal model that faithfully mimics human acute drug- or infection-associated TIN is not available to elucidate specific pathways. Current concepts suggest

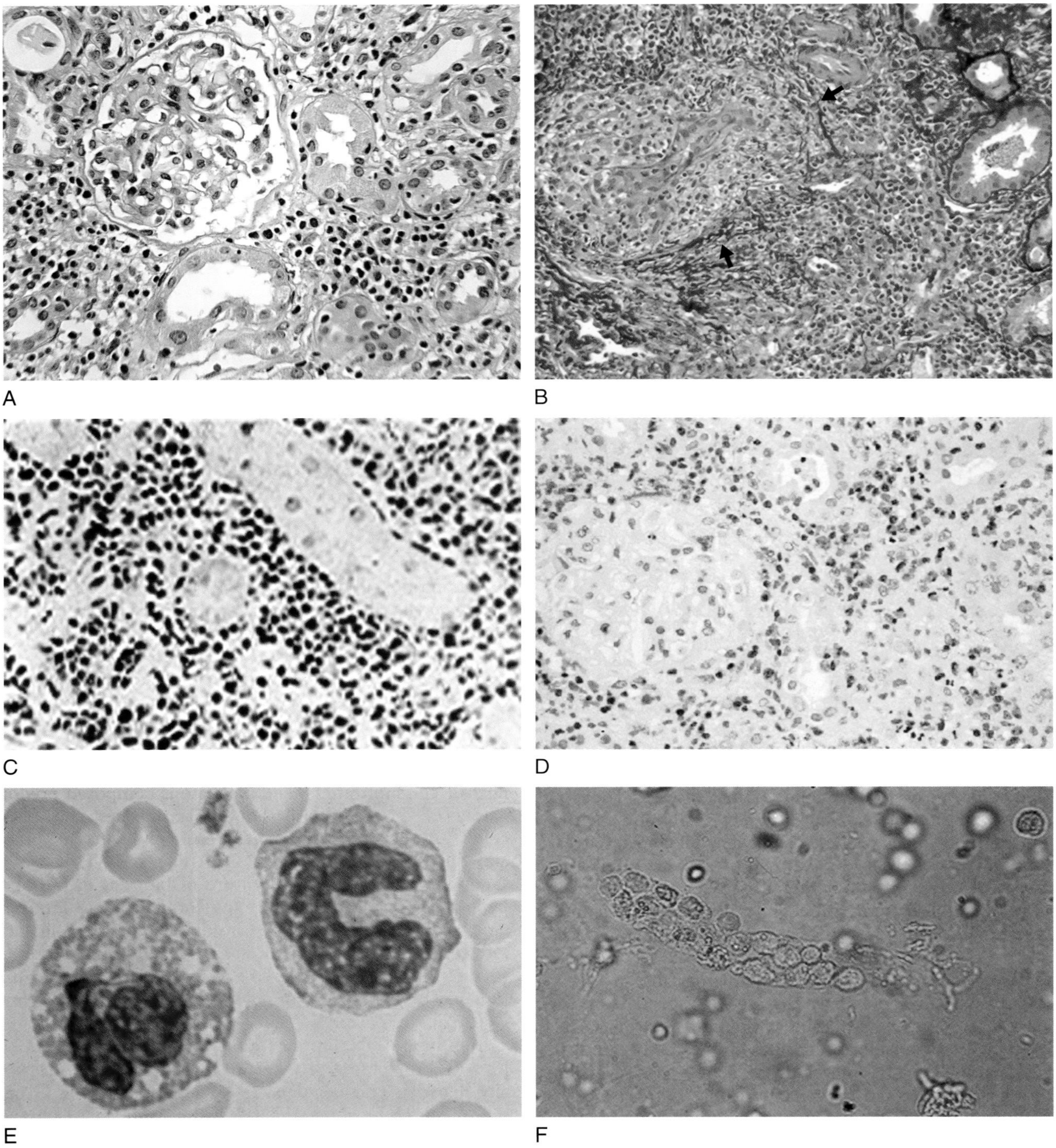

Figure 34-1 Histologic and urinary sediment features of acute interstitial nephritis. Histologic photomicrographs illustrate **A,** an interstitial infiltrate of mononuclear cells, interstitial edema, and tubular dilatation in acute tubulointerstitial nephritis; **B,** acute tubulointerstitial nephritis with granuloma formation *(arrows);* **C,** tubulointerstitial nephritis characterized by an infiltrate of monomorphic interstitial mononuclear cells as a result of lymphoma; and **D,** acute drug-induced tubulointerstitial nephritis with numerous polymorphonuclear eosinophils. Examination of the urinary sediment may show **E,** eosinophils in drug-induced tubulointerstitial nephritis or **F,** white blood cells and while blood cell casts.

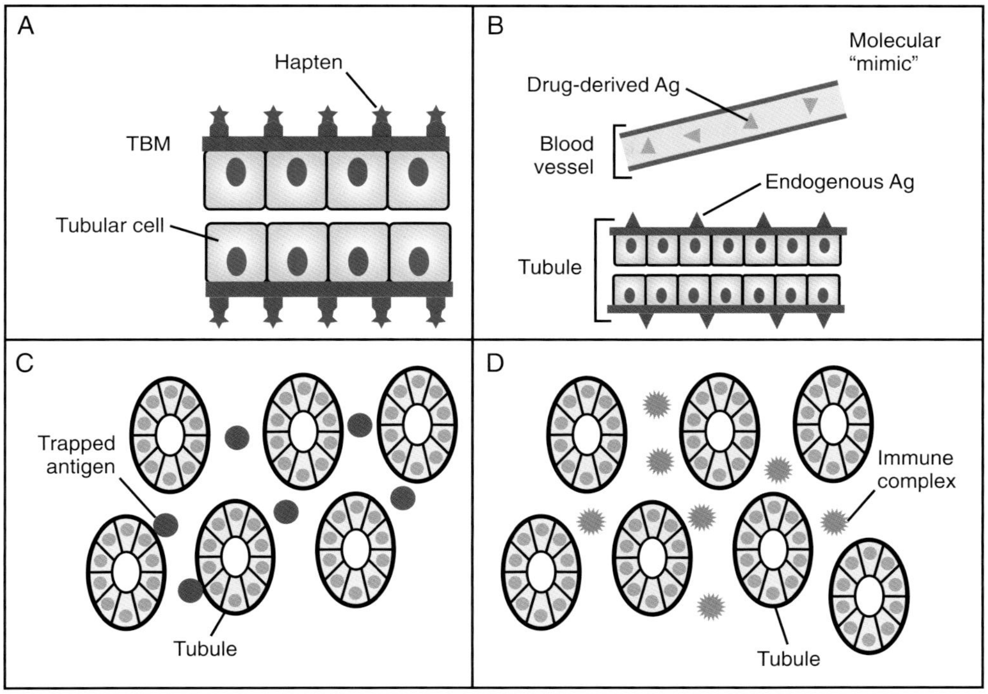

Figure 34-2 Pathogenetic theories of drug-induced acute tubulointerstitial nephritis. **A,** A component of the drug may be trapped along the tubular basement membrane *(TBM)* and act as a hapten, thus becoming the target of immune attack by sensitized T cells or, less commonly, antibody-producing B cells. **B,** A component of the circulating drug may be recognized as a foreign antigen (Ag) that triggers an immune response. The antigen may be structurally similar (molecular "mimic") to a normal component of the tubulointerstitium (endogenous antigen), and, as a consequence, it also becomes a target during the immune attack. **C,** A drug-derived antigen may first be trapped in the tubulointerstitium to which immunologically reactive cells and/or antibodies are recruited (in situ). **D,** Circulating antibodies generated against a drug-derived antigen may form immune complexes within the circulation that are subsequently trapped within the tubulointerstitium and initiate inflammation. Similar theories of pathogenesis have been proposed for reactive acute tubulointerstitial nephritis triggered by an infectious agent. (Redrawn with permission from Rossert J: Drug-induced acute interstitial nephritis, *Kidney Int* 60:804-17, 2001.)

that an antigen—be it a hapten derived from a drug or microbe—is presented to T-helper cells, thereby initiating an immune response and cytokine release. Macrophage and natural killer cell recruitment and activation follow. Evidence of a primary pathogenetic role of T cells is provided by a recent study that demonstrated the presence of drug-specific sensitized T cells in the peripheral blood of patients with acute drug-induced interstitial nephritis.[12] The differentiation of B cells into plasma cells results in the production of specific antibody, although, in most patients with TIN, intrarenal antibody deposition is conspicuously absent. Four non-mutually–exclusive theories of immune pathogenesis have been proposed, and they are summarized in Figure 34-2.[13] There is an animal model of antitubular basement membrane disease that has been well characterized, in which the disease is thought to be caused by an immune response to an endogenous tubular basement membrane antigen.[14] However, human antitubular basement membrane nephritis is distinctly rare; it is most commonly encountered in association with antiglomerular basement membrane disease.

Despite several studies, it is not clear whether the specific cellular phenotyping of the cells within the interstitial infiltrate can differentiate the antigenic trigger. The one exception is interstitial nephritis caused by lymphoma or lymphoproliferative disease, in which a single monomorphic cellular population invades the interstitium (Figure 34-1, C).

CLINICAL FINDINGS

When interstitial nephritis was originally described, it was typically associated with systemic signs of inflammation. A "classic" triad of fever, eosinophilia, and rash was reported in patients with methicillin-induced interstitial nephritis. However, more recent studies suggest that this classic triad is absent in more than 70% of patients,[15] implying that TIN is often clinically silent. When TIN occurs as a manifestation of a multisystem disease process, associated systemic symptoms may be present.

The classic clinical presentation of drug-induced TIN is acute renal failure that begins shortly after ingesting the offending drug. The kinetics of the onset of interstitial nephritis vary depending on the exposure history. Symptoms typically begin 3 to 5 days after reexposure to the inciting drug, although it may take several weeks for the symptoms to develop with first-time drug exposure. The TIN risk is not dependent on the dose, and this observation supports the theory that the pathogenesis of this disease is a hypersensitivity-type immunologic reaction. Extrarenal symptoms and signs of hypersensitivity, such as low-grade fever, a maculopapular rash, and mild arthralgias, may be present. Nonspecific symptoms are often the result of acute renal failure and may include anorexia, nausea, vomiting, and malaise. Interstitial edema may cause renal enlargement and capsular swelling, which are thought to be the cause of the flank pain that is present in some patients with acute interstitial nephritis. Each of these extrarenal manifestations is present in more than 50% of patients, and the concurrent presence of all of these signs and symptoms occurs in less than 5% to 10% of the patients.[8,13] These extrarenal symptoms are more common in patients with TIN that is associated with infectious and autoimmune diseases. Hypersensitivity symptoms may also be present with drug-induced TIN, but their presence does not exclude the possibility of drug-induced nephrotoxicity and/or acute tubular necrosis as the associated renal lesion.

Antimicrobials and nonsteroidal antiinflammatory drugs (NSAIDs) are most commonly implicated as the cause of TIN, but the list of potential offending agents is endless. Fortunately, for almost all drugs, the risk of acute TIN is very low. The hallmark of interstitial nephritis is an acute decline in renal function as evidenced by a rise in the serum creatinine level; this may be the only laboratory abnormality.[7] Acute TIN may also present as one of several more complex clinical scenarios.

Acute Renal Failure

The absence of hypertension, significant proteinuria, and red blood cell casts are clues to a diagnosis of TIN rather than glomerular or vascular disease, although, in a given patient, clinical manifestations may overlap considerably. Recent exposure to a potentially offending agent, significant pyuria in the absence of bacteria, a good urine output, and evidence of tubular dysfunction may favor a diagnosis of TIN. Distinguishing between acute TIN and acute tubular necrosis may be challenging, but the presence of many renal tubular cells and muddy brown casts in the urine sediment is more suggestive of a diagnosis of acute tubular necrosis.

Chronic Renal Failure

When evaluating a new patient, the clinical challenge may be differentiating acute from chronic TIN. Small kidneys with increased echogenicity and anemia suggest a longstanding process. Many of the causes of chronic TIN in the pediatric population are associated with extrarenal manifestations such as cystinosis, certain inborn errors of metabolism, and nephronophthisis.

Tubulopathy

Patients may come to a physician's attention as a result of signs and symptoms of tubular dysfunction such as acidosis, polyuria, hypokalemia, or hypophosphatemia. These are more common in cases of chronic interstitial nephritis.[7] The specific manifestations of tubular cell injury and dysfunction vary, depending on the specific site of injury (Figure 34-3). Proximal tubular injury may cause Fanconi syndrome with glucosuria, proteinuria, and phosphaturia, or it may present as a proximal renal tubular acidosis. Distal tubular cell injury may manifest as acidosis and hyperkalemia (distal renal tubular acidosis), whereas collecting duct damage typically results in a urinary concentrating defect (nephrogenic diabetes insipidus). Tubular cell injury may also manifest as potassium wasting.

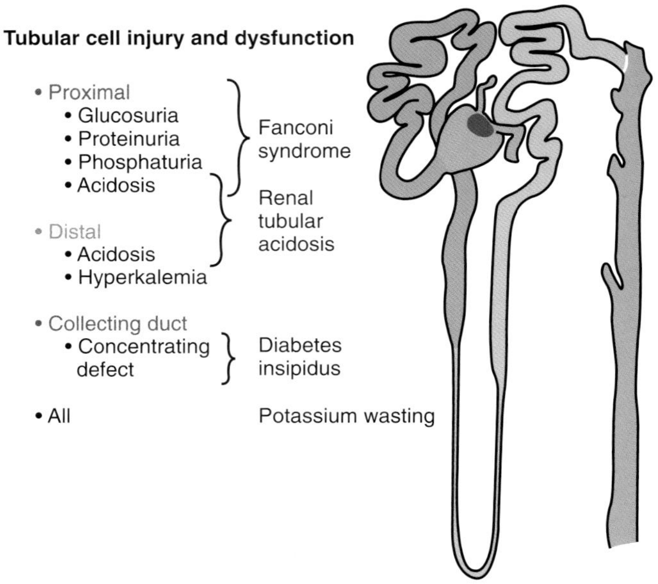

Figure 34-3 Variable patterns of renal functional defects present in patients with tubulointerstitial nephritis depend on which nephron segments (proximal, distal, or collecting ducts) are injured as a consequence of the primary disease process and/or the associated interstitial inflammation.

DIAGNOSIS

There is limited sensitivity and specificity with regard to the various diagnostic studies that can be performed when a diagnosis of TIN is under consideration.

Urinary Sediment

The urinary sediment often shows red cells, white cells, and white cell casts[7] (Figure 34-1, *F*). Sterile pyuria may or may not be associated with eosinophiluria. Urinary eosinophils are thought to be specific although not sensitive for TIN (Figure 34-1, *E*). The identification of urinary eosinophils requires special staining of the urine sediment with Wright or Hansel staining; Hansel staining is thought to be more sensitive. Urinary eosinophilia is said to be present when more than 1% of the urinary white blood cells are positive.[16] Unfortunately, there can be many false positives; eosinophiluria may also occur in acute tubular necrosis, prerenal acute renal failure, schistosomiasis, and atherothromboembolic renal disease. Ruffing and colleages[16] reported a 38% positive predictive value and a 74% negative predictive value for urinary eosinophilia. It is also important to remember that a bland urinary sediment does not exclude the diagnosis of acute TIN.[13]

Proteinuria may be present, but it is typically less than 1 g per 24 hours. Nephrotic range proteinuria is rare except in NSAID-induced TIN, where it is thought to be caused by cytokine-induced glomerular injury.

Radiology

The renal ultrasound usually demonstrates increased echogenicity that is often associated with an increased renal bipolar length, but these findings are nonspecific.[1,7] Gallium scanning has been proposed to differentiate between acute

TIN and acute tubular necrosis, but the findings are often inconclusive.[1] Gallium scanning is very sensitive, but it is not very specific, because numerous other diseases may cause increased gallium uptake (including acute glomerulonephritis and pyelonephritis), and it has occasionally been observed in patients without renal disease.[7]

Biopsy

Because none of the noninvasive studies is both specific and sensitive for TIN, kidney biopsy remains the only definitive diagnostic study for interstitial nephritis. For details regarding biopsy findings, see the previous section of this chapter about histology.

ETIOLOGY

The causes of TIN are numerous, but they can be broadly divided into acute and chronic disorders, although there may be considerable overlap for any single cause. In a recent review of acute TIN cases by Baker and Pusey, 71% were drug related, 16% were infection related, 5% were caused by TIN with uveitis (TINU), 1% were the result of sarcoidosis, and 8% were considered idiopathic[8] (Figure 34-4). The most common causes of TIN are discussed in the following sections; some of the less common disorders are included in Table 34-1.

Drugs

In the current era, drugs clearly surpass infections as the most commonly implicated cause of acute TIN, accounting for more than two-thirds of the cases. Although numerous drugs are suspect, TIN is an infrequent occurrence for most drugs. Antimicrobials and NSAIDs are the most common offenders, but the list of potentially causative agents is extensive and variable with time as drug-prescribing practices change (Table 34-2).

Methicillin was long believed to cause the prototypical drug-induced interstitial nephritis. In fact, as a result of this infamy, the use of this drug has declined worldwide, and it is no longer available in several countries. Methicillin and other β-lactam antibiotics are still more commonly associated with the classic triad of rash, fever, and eosinophilia than any other group of drugs.[3]

Rifampin has been frequently implicated as a cause of acute TIN. Affected patients fall into two groups: (1) patients who receive short-duration therapy with rifampin and (2) patients who have had prior or intermittent exposure to the drug. The first group typically lacks anti-rifampin antibodies, and the onset of clinical symptoms in this group is insidious. The second group may develop antibodies, and clinical symptoms may begin abruptly.[13] Hemolysis or hepatitis may also be present and associated with certain agents, such as rifampin and allopurinol.[13]

NSAID-induced TIN is said to be associated with nephrotic syndrome in 70% of cases.[13] It is reported to occur more frequently among older patients, but it is unclear whether this is the result of underreporting in pediatrics, lower exposure rates, or other factors. In NSAID-induced TIN, hematuria is almost always microscopic, and extrarenal symptoms occur in less than 10% of patients.[13]

The epidemiology of drug-induced TIN appears to be changing. In a study performed between 1995 and 1999 in adult patients, proton pump inhibitors were implicated in 35% of biopsy-confirmed TIN cases.[21] Omeprazole and lan-

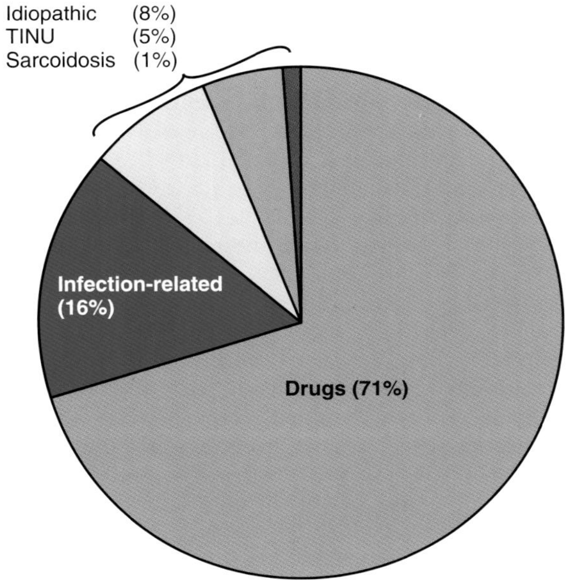

Figure 34-4 Causes of acute tubulointerstitial nephritis based on a review of 128 adults with biopsy-proven disease. (From Baker RJ, Pusey CD: The changing profile of acute tubulointerstitial nephritis, *Nephrol Dial Transplant* 19:8-11, 2004.)

TABLE 34-1 **Other Causes of Tubulointerstitial Nephritis**
Herbs
Aristolochia fangchi (Chinese herb used for weight reduction)
Heavy Metals
Lead
Cadmium
Systemic Disease
Lymphoma/leukemia
Sarcoidosis
Sjögren syndrome
Inflammatory bowel disease
Tubulointerstitial nephritis with uveitis
Hypokalemia[6] (e.g., anorexia nervosa)
Urate nephropathy
Hyperoxaluria
Cystinosis
Radiation nephritis
Other

Adapted with permission from Braden GL, O'Shea MH, Mulhern JG: Tubulointerstitial diseases, *Am J Kidney Dis* 46:560-72, 2005.

TABLE 34-2 Drugs Most Commonly Reported to Cause Acute Tubulointerstitial Nephritis

Antimicrobials	NSAIDs	Diuretics	Others	Potential
Beta-lactams	Almost all agents, including cyclooxygenase-2 inhibitors	Furosemide	Allopurinol[13]	Bisphosphonates
Methicillin		Thiazides	Azathioprine	Ifosfamide
Ampicillin		Triamterenes	Isofosfamide	
Penicillin			Histamine-2 receptor blockers	
Oxacillin			Ranitidine	
Nafcillin			Proton pump inhibitors[21]	
Cephalosporins[17]			Omeprazole	
Sulfonamides			Lansoprazole	
Macrolides			Antihypertensives	
Erythromycin			Amlodipine	
Other antibiotics			Diltiazem	
Colistin[18]			Captopril	
Rifampin			Antiepileptics	
Polymyxin			Carbamazepine	
Ethambutol			Phenytoin	
Tetracycline				
Vancomycin[19,20]				
Ciprofloxacin				
Isoniazid				
Antivirals				
Acyclovir				
Indinavir				
Alpha-interferon				

NSAIDs, Nonsteroidal antiinflammatory drugs.

soprazole were the most common offending agents, and renal function quickly improved after the proton pump inhibitor was discontinued, unless there were confounding factors such as diabetes mellitus. Most patients also had systemic symptoms.[21] As newer therapies and drugs are introduced, one must maintain a high index of suspicion for drugs as a cause of acute renal dysfunction without relying on the presence of the historically "classic" clinical features. Indeed, many recent papers report that the classic clinical triad of rash, fever, and eosinophilia is now distinctly rare.[8,22]

The primary treatment of drug-induced TIN is to discontinue the offending agent. The immunologic trigger must be removed, particularly because persistent tubulointerstitial injury can progress to chronic damage, which may be progressive and/or irreversible. The early removal of the inciting agent alone frequently leads to the complete reversal of renal injury. Additional therapy is not required, particularly if the drug exposure was short term. After drug-induced acute TIN, the mean recovery time to the nadir creatinine level is 1.5 months.[13] A recent retrospective study showed no benefit of the administration of steroids for drug-induced TIN and recommended reserving steroid therapy for patients with delayed recovery.[22]

However, if renal function does not improve shortly after stopping the suspected offending agent, a renal biopsy is recommended to confirm the diagnosis. A biopsy may also be useful for patients with severe or persistent renal insufficiency and before immunosuppressive therapy is considered. In a review of the literature, it is startling to note the complete lack of prospective, randomized, controlled trials of the use of steroids for the treatment of acute TIN. Even consensus guidelines from expert physician panels are not available. A recent study of 42 patients with severe biopsy-proven acute TIN (mean peak serum creatinine level, 7.6 mg/dl; 58% treated with acute dialysis) failed to demonstrate a significant difference in renal function recovery rates between steroid-treated patients and those who were managed conservatively[22] (Figure 34-5, *A*). However, it is not uncommon for patients with severe biopsy-proven acute TIN to be treated with a short course of oral steroids. For patients who show no renal functional improvement despite conservative measures and steroids, immunosuppressive therapy has been recommended, but currently there is a lack of evidence to support its use.

Various studies have analyzed potential prognostic indicators, but none has proved to be useful and reproducible, including the peak serum creatinine level (Figure 34-5, *B*). For example, one study of 30 patients reported that patients with diffuse infiltrates on biopsy had a worse prognosis than those with focal interstitial infiltrates.[23] However, this difference was not confirmed in two subsequent small studies.[24,25] The duration of acute renal failure and of renal dysfunction may prove to be useful predictors of outcome.[13,25]

Infections

Numerous infectious agents have been implicated in the pathogenesis of both acute and chronic TIN (Table 34-3). Interstitial nephritis was first recognized as a unique clinical entity in 1860 in a patient with scarlet fever. However, several decades passed before Councilman introduced the term *interstitial nephritis* and described the histologic lesions. To quote his landmark paper, "Acute interstitial lesions of the kidneys have been considered as common in scarlet fever, and are regarded by some authors as constituting the most frequent pathological alteration of the kidney in this disease. This has also been described in diphtheria and in other infec-

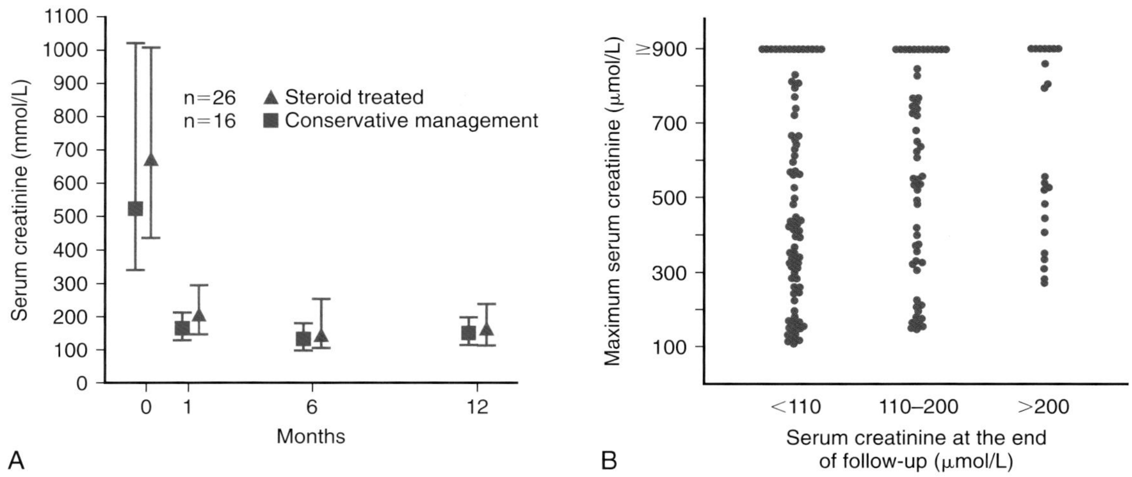

Figure 34-5 Clinical outcomes of patients with acute tubulointerstitial nephritis. **A,** In a review of 42 patients with severe acute renal failure resulting from tubulointerstitial nephritis (92% presumed to be drug-induced cases), the rates and degree of renal functional recovery were similar between those treated with or without steroids for 3 to 6 weeks. **B,** This graph shows that the peak serum creatinine levels of patients with acute tubulointerstitial nephritis do not predict the potential for renal functional recovery. (**A** reproduced from Clarkson MR, Giblin L, O'Connell FP, O'Kelly P, et al: Acute interstitial nephritis: clinical features and response to corticosteroid therapy, *Nephrol Dial Transplant* 19:2778-83, 2004. **B** reproduced from Rossert J: Drug-induced acute interstitial nephritis, *Kidney Int* 60:804-17, 2001.)

tious diseases."[2] The years 1939 through 1945 saw the eradication of serious and fatal streptococcal infections as a result of the introduction of antibiotics. In the current era, the infections implicated as causes of TIN vary from Councilman's time as a result of childhood immunizations together with remarkable progress in the development of newer and more effective antimicrobial agents. In fact, since 1960, antibiotics rather than infections are a more common cause of acute TIN.

The infectious microorganisms may directly invade the renal parenchyma to cause a specific form of interstitial nephritis (pyelonephritis). However, the traditional form of acute TIN is associated with infection at an extrarenal site, and the tubulointerstitial inflammation is thought to represent a secondary or "reactive" immunologic response to the infection. In the latter, the infectious agent is not cultured from the kidney or the urine.

When a renal biopsy is performed in a patient with pyelonephritis (which is not recommended), the interstitial lesion is often localized to a single pyramid, and it is characterized by neutrophil predominance. By contrast, "reactive" TIN that is associated with a systemic infection is characterized histologically as either patchy or diffuse lesions that are associated with interstitial edema and a predominance of mononuclear cells. The pathogenic microbial antigens that initiate the immune response to cause TIN are largely unknown. One exception is leptospirosis, in which an isolated outer membrane protein has been shown to interact in vitro with Toll-like receptor 2 to stimulate the synthesis of inflammatory cytokines, chemokines, and collagen by renal tubules.[28] The primary therapeutic measure is to treat the infection, preferably with non-nephrotoxic antimicrobials.

Granulomatous Interstitial Nephritis

As the name suggests, TIN may be associated with the presence of granulomas on renal biopsy (Figure 34-1, *B*). The differential diagnosis includes drug-induced interstitial nephritis (especially as a result of β-lactam antibiotics or anticonvulsants),[29] which accounts for approximately 25% of cases[10]; infectious causes (tuberculosis, brucellosis, histoplasmosis); Wegener granulomatosis; sarcoidosis; tuberculosis; fungal pyelonephritis; TINU syndrome; multiple myeloma; and other dysproteinemias. In addition, although it is rare in immunocompetent hosts, histoplasmosis has been implicated in case reports.[29]

Tubulointerstitial Nephritis with Uveitis

An association between TIN and anterior uveitis, occasionally in association with bone marrow granulomas, was first reported in 1975, when the term *TINU* was introduced.[30] Although anterior uveitis is more common, posterior uveitis can also occur.[31] When it was first described, there was a female predominance of this syndrome, with a reported female-to-male ratio of 3 : 1. However, the most recent literature suggests that males are now increasingly affected.[32,33] The median age of onset is 15 years (range, 9 to 74 years),[33] and no racial predilection has been identified.

TINU (Figure 34-6) is a syndrome of multiple causes. Although these causes are often idiopathic and presumed to be autoimmune in pathogenesis, it is important to search for evidence of the known causes of TINU, which are summarized in Table 34-4. It is speculated that disease pathogenesis involves an immunologic response that is triggered by a recent drug exposure (often an antimicrobial agent), an infection, or an unknown agent. Some patients have serum autoantibodies, including antinuclear antibodies, rheumatoid factor, antineutrophil cytoplasmic antibodies, and/or anticardiolipin antibodies. Some patients have associated autoimmune diseases such as hyperthyroidism, hyperparathyroidism, and rheumatoid arthritis, or they may have a history of recent insect bites.[33]

Several studies have examined human leukocyte antigens in patients with TINU syndrome, but the numbers are insuf-

TABLE 34-3 **Infectious Causes of Acute Tubulointerstitial Nephritis**

Bacteria
Escherichia coli
Enterococcus
Leptospirosis
Mycobacteria
Legionella
Streptococci
Campylobacter
Brucella[26]
Staphylococci
Corynbacterium diphtheria
Yersinia
Syphilis
Mycoplasma
Viruses
Epstein-Barr virus[27]
BK polyoma virus
Adenovirus
Cytomegalovirus
Hantaan
Hepatitis
Rubeola
Herpes simplex virus
Mumps
Human immunodeficiency virus
Fungi
Histoplasmosis
Parasites
Toxoplasmosis
Leishmaniasis
Rickettsia
Rickettsia diaporica
Rickettsia rickettsii

Adapted with permission from Michel DM, Kelly CJ: Acute interstitial nephritis, *J Am Soc Nephrol* 9:506-15, 1998.

ficient to identify specific human leukocyte antigen associations. The report of TINU in monozygotic male twins separated in onset by 2 years suggests the possibility of a genetic predisposition to the syndrome,[32] as does a report from 1994 of identical female twins with the onset of TINU syndrome being seen 1 year apart.[34] However, the lack of reports of multiple affected family members and the lack of geographic clustering questions the influence of environment and genetic factors.

The nonspecific symptoms of TIN are also manifestations of TINU syndrome. These include fever, weight loss, fatigue, malaise, loss of appetite, weakness, asthenia, abdominal or flank pain, arthralgias, and myalgias. Less commonly, headache, polyuria, lymphadenopathy, edema, pharyngitis, or rash may occur. The ocular manifestations commonly include eye pain and redness (77%), decreased visual acuity (20%), and photophobia (14%).[33] The onset of uveitis varies from several weeks before the onset of renal involvement, concurrent with the interstitial nephritis, or to up to 14 months after the onset of TIN. Both recurrent acute and chronic uveitis are commonly described. The timing of uveitis recurrence has varied from 3 months after steroid tapering to 2 years after the first episode.

TABLE 34-4 **Tubulointerstitial Nephritis with Uveitis Syndrome: Differential Diagnosis**

Sarcoidosis
Sjögren syndrome
Systemic lupus erythematosus
Wegener granulomatosis
Behçet disease
Infections (e.g., tuberculosis, brucellosis, toxoplasmosis, histoplasmosis, Epstein-Barr virus, human immunodeficiency virus, chlamydia, mycoplasma)

Laboratory findings include elevated serum creatinine levels, evidence of tubulopathy, anemia, slightly abnormal liver function tests, eosinophilia, and an elevated erythrocyte sedimentation rate. A variety of serologic markers have been reported without evidence of the associated diseases (i.e., systemic lupus erythematosus, Wegener granuloma, antiphospholipid syndrome, rheumatoid arthritis). However, definitive diagnosis requires a renal biopsy and a formal ophthalmologic slit-lamp examination to identify the uveitis. Bone marrow and lymph node granulomas have been reported, but studies that look for these conditions are rarely performed now that the TINU syndrome has become recognized as a distinct clinical entity.

TINU is self-limited in most patients, although steroid therapy is often administered when renal functional impairment is severe or prolonged.[30,31] There are a few reports of affected individuals requiring long-term renal replacement therapy.[33] The ocular disease often requires treatment with both topical and systemic steroids. Although the acute eye disease usually improves, recurrences, complications, and chronic ocular disease may develop. Most of the long-term complications of TINU have been ocular, and they are estimated to occur in 20% of patients. These include posterior synechiae, optic disc swelling, cystoid macular edema, chorioretinal scar formation, cataracts, and glaucoma.[30,33] Fortunately, the risk of visual loss appears to be low. As a result of the morbidity associated with the ocular manifestations, early detection by slit-lamp examination is essential.

Sjögren Syndrome

Sjögren syndrome is classically described as a sicca syndrome that occurs as a consequence of lymphocytic (mainly by CD4 cells) and plasmacytic infiltrates in the exocrine glands, espe-

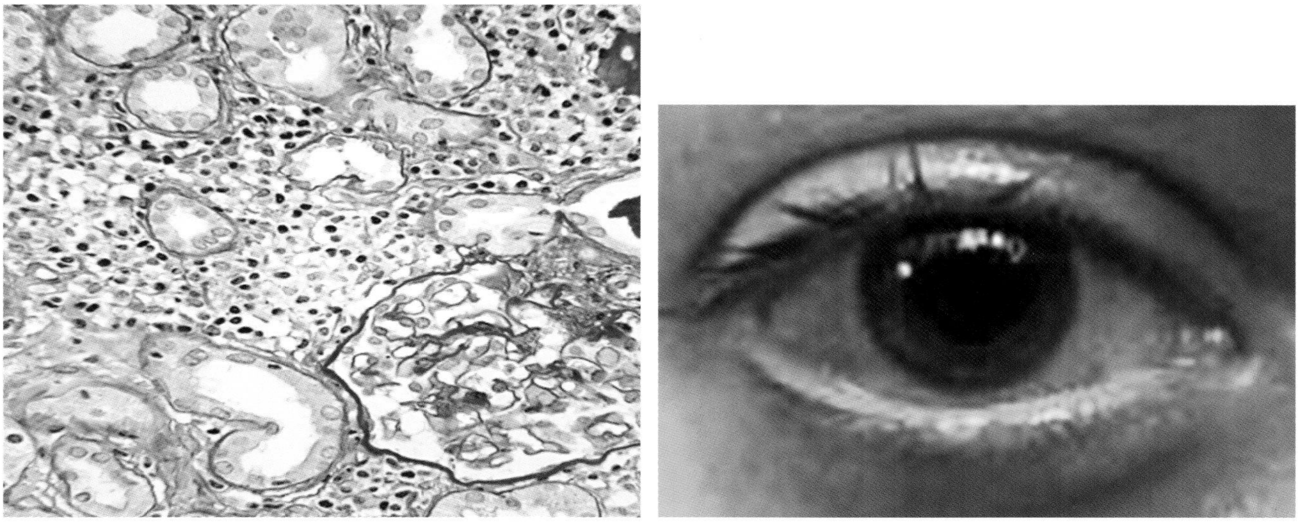

A B

Figure 34-6 Tubulointerstitial nephritis with uveitis syndrome. Although it is often idiopathic, the known secondary causes of this syndrome listed in Table 34-4 should be considered as part of the differential diagnosis, because specific therapy is available for many of them. The eye photomicrograph **(B)**, which was taken from a patient with acute uveitis, serves as a reminder of the importance of performing a slit-lamp examination as part of the evaluation of a patient with suspected acute tubulointerstitial nephritis of unknown cause.

cially the salivary, parotid, and lacrimal glands. This process causes a dry mouth and dry eyes. The pathogenic immune process may also affect nonexocrine organs, including the skin, the lungs, the gastrointestinal tract, the central and peripheral nervous systems, the musculoskeletal system, and the kidneys. The most common renal manifestation is interstitial nephritis with associated tubular dysfunction; glomerular disease has also been reported.[35] Although the presence of renal disease in patients with Sjögren syndrome was first reported during the 1960s, its prevalence and primary pathogenesis remain poorly defined. In the literature, the frequency of renal abnormalities varies widely, from 16% to 67%.[35] The diagnosis of idiopathic Sjögren syndrome is based on clinical and/or histopathologic evidence of ocular, oral, or salivary involvement and the presence of anti-Ro/SSA and/or anti-La/SSB autoantibodies. Although several pharmacologic approaches are available to manage patients with Sjögren syndrome, significant renal disease often requires systemic steroid therapy.[36]

Sarcoidosis

It is well established that sarcoidosis can be associated with significant TIN, but the true incidence remains unknown.[37] Although the histologic evidence of renal involvement is said to be common in sarcoidosis, clinical disease only occurs in 3% to 25% of patients who present with a wide spectrum of clinical manifestations.

Patients with sarcoidosis tend to avidly absorb dietary calcium, and this may lead to hypercalciuria and, less commonly, hypercalcemia. The clinical manifestations of calcium hyperabsorption may be silent, or they may cause nephrolithiasis, nephrocalcinosis, renal insufficiency, or polyuria. Nephrocalcinosis is the most common cause of chronic renal failure in sarcoidosis.[38] Polyuria may be the result of the hypercalcemia and hypercalciuria that decrease tubular responsiveness to antidiuretic hormone, or it may be a manifestation of diabetes insipidus or primary polydipsia that is a consequence of granulomatous infiltration of the hypothalamus. It is important to recognize that the abnormalities in calcium metabolism can occur in other chronic granulomatous diseases as a result of increased calcitriol produced by activated mononuclear cells.[39]

The urinary manifestations of sarcoid granulomatous interstitial nephritis are similar to other forms of chronic TIN, which is often associated with a bland urine sediment, sterile pyuria, and/or mild proteinuria. The serum creatinine level is usually normal, and chronic kidney disease is considered rare. The renal biopsy typically shows normal glomeruli and interstitial nephritis with mononuclear cell infiltration and noncaseating granulomas in the interstitium.[29] Chronic injury is often present with interstitial fibrosis and tubular damage.

Corticosteroids remain the treatment of choice with slowly tapered protocols to prevent disease recurrence. A recent study reported the better preservation of renal function with prolonged steroid therapy, even in patients with advanced disease.[40] Evidence that tumor necrosis factor-α may play a role in the pathogenesis of sarcoidosis suggests that the newer antitumor necrosis factor-α biologic agents may be of benefit, although only anecdotal evidence is currently available.[38] In the rare event that a patient with sarcoidosis progresses to end-stage renal disease (ESRD), it is usually as a result of hypercalcemia and hypercalciuria rather than interstitial nephritis.[38] Renal sarcoidosis does not appear to recur in renal allografts.

Idiopathic Tubulointerstitial Nephritis

Approximately 8% of cases of acute TIN are considered idiopathic.[8] This diagnosis can only be made after all other possible causes have been eliminated by a thorough historical, clinical, and relevant laboratory investigation. In presumed idiopathic TIN, steroid therapy is often prescribed, despite the lack of evidence-based guidelines. A common treatment regimen is prednisone 1 mg/kg/day or 2 mg/kg every other day for 2 to 3 weeks. If renal function fails to improve, a second-line immunosuppressive agent such as cytoxan may be added. Total therapy duration is typically 2 to 3 months, with tapering occurring after serum creatinine normalizes.[41] In the setting of refractory or frequently relapsing disease, other immunosuppressive therapy has occasionally been attempted. Preddie and colleagues[42] recently reported eight patients with steroid-resistant, biopsy-proven TIN in whom renal function improved or stabilized in association with the administration of mycophenolate mofetil over an average of 24 months.

CHRONIC INTERSTITIAL NEPHRITIS

Epidemiology

The exact incidence and prevalence of chronic interstitial nephritis is poorly documented. This topic is somewhat complicated by the fact that chronic interstitial changes typify virtually all chronic renal disorders that eventually progress to ESRD.

Pathology

The early phase of chronic TIN shares histopathologic features with acute TIN, including interstitial inflammation and tubular cell activation. However, as the disease progresses, interstitial fibrosis and chronic tubular injury (dilated tubules with or without cast formation, atrophied tubules, and thickened tubular basement membrane) appear.[6] In the advanced stages, glomerulosclerosis may occur as a consequence of the tubular damage or periglomerular interstitial fibrosis.[6] In almost all chronic kidney diseases, interstitial fibrosis severity is a strong predictor of renal functional loss and risk of progressive renal disease.[43]

Clinical Findings

The clinical findings in chronic TIN are similar to those of acute TIN, but they tend to be more subtle, and they often go undetected until the patient develops signs and symptoms as a result of chronic renal insufficiency. As compared with chronic glomerular disease, in patients with chronic TIN, hypertension is less common, daily protein excretion rates rarely exceed 1.5 g/day, and anemia may be disproportionately worse than the degree of renal functional impairment as a result of the loss of erythropoietin-producing cells in the peritubular interstitium.[6] Bone disease may also be more prominent as a result of chronic phosphate wasting as a result of proximal tubular dysfunction.[6]

Etiology

As in acute TIN, there are numerous causes of chronic TIN (Figure 34-7). In addition to persistent acute TIN as a cause of chronic TIN, several diseases are more typically associated with chronic TIN. The most common pediatric disorders are listed in Table 34-5.

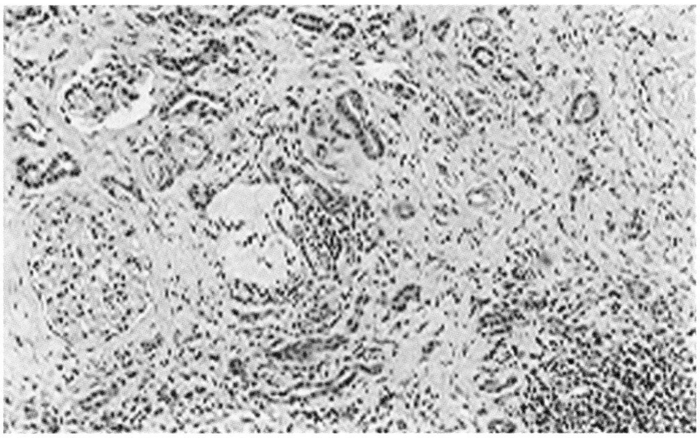

Figure 34-7 Chronic interstitial nephritis. Diseases associated with chronic interstitial nephritis, especially in the pediatric population, are listed in Table 34-5.

TABLE 34-5 Chronic Tubulointerstitial Nephritis: Differential Diagnosis

Persistent acute tubulointerstitial nephritis
Inherited renal disease • Nephronophthisis • Other cystic renal diseases
Inherited disease with renal involvement • Cystinosis • Oxalosis • Methylmalonic acidemia • Mitochondrial diseases
Drugs and toxins • Heavy metals (lead) • Chinese herbs • Drugs (analgesics, lithium, calcineurin inhibitors, cisplatinum)
Metabolic disorders • Calcium (nephrocalcinosis) • Uric acid injury • Potassium deficiency
Structural renal disease • Reflux • Dysplasia • Obstruction

Treatment and Prognosis

The treatment of chronic TIN is based on the treatment of the primary disease process. In addition, there is increasing evidence that the correction of anemia, the reduction of proteinuria, and the suppression of inflammation may also slow the rate of kidney disease progression.[44,45] Angiotensin-converting enzyme inhibitors and angiotensin receptor type I blockers are being used with increasing frequency for a variety of chronic renal diseases, especially when the disease is associated with hypertension and/or proteinuria. It is believed that, in addition to decreasing intraglomerular pressure, these drugs reduce proteinuria, and they may also have an antiinflammatory role in relation to angiotensin II blockade.[43] Other immunosuppressive agents that are under investigation as agents for combating TIN include mycophenolate mofetil, rapamycin, retinoids, and, recently, 1,25-dihydroxyvitamin D.[43]

Erythropoietin therapy not only assists with the management of anemia and the associated renal hypoxia in chronic kidney disease patients, but it may also stimulate vascular endothelial growth factor. In animal models, vascular endothelial growth factor therapy has been associated with renal protection.[44]

Outcomes

Patients with chronic TIN and stage III (glomerular filtration rate, 30 to 59 ml/min/1.73 m^2) or stage IV (glomerular filtration rate, 15 to 29 ml/min/1.73 m^2) chronic kidney disease are destined to progress to ESRD (glomerular filtration rate, <15 ml/min/1.73 m^2). Numerous comorbid factors correlate with a faster rate of renal functional decline, including hypertension, high-grade proteinuria, diabetes, smoking, obesity, dyslipidemia, and anemia.[8,46] Although definitive therapy may not be available for the primary disease process that caused the chronic TIN, many of these comorbidities can be addressed therapeutically to preserve residual nephrons and to slow the rate of chronic kidney disease progression. Further laboratory and clinical studies are needed to identify new evidence-based therapeutic options and to delineate long-term outcomes for patients with chronic TIN.

REFERENCES

1. Kodner CM, Kudrimoti A: Diagnosis and management of acute interstitial nephritis, *Am Fam Physician* 67:2527-34, 2003.
2. Councilman WT: Acute interstitial nephritis, *J Exp Med* 3:393-420, 1898.
3. Behrman RE (Ed.): *Nelson textbook of pediatrics*, ed 17, Philadelphia, 2004, WB Saunders, pp 1764-66.
4. Jones CL, Eddy AA: Tubulointerstitial nephritis, *Pediatr Nephrol* 6:572-86, 1992.
5. Alon US: Tubulointerstitial nephritis. In Avner ED, Harmon WE, Niaudet P, editors: *Pediatric nephrology*, ed 5, Philadelphia, 2004, Lippincott Williams & Wilkins, pp 817-31.
6. Braden GL, O'Shea MH, Mulhern JG: Tubulointerstitial diseases. *Am J Kidney Dis* 46:560-72, 2005.
7. Michel DM, Kelly CJ: Acute interstitial nephritis, *J Am Soc Nephrol* 9:506-15, 1998.
8. Baker RJ, Pusey CD: The changing profile of acute tubulointerstitial nephritis, *Nephrol Dial Transplant* 19:8-11, 2004.
9. Harris DC: Tubulointerstitial renal disease, *Curr Opin Nephrol Hypertens* 10:303-13, 2001.
10. Viero RM, Cavallo T: Granulomatous interstitial nephritis, *Hum Pathol* 26:1347-53, 1995.
11. Cameron JS: Tubular and interstitial factors in the progression of glomerulonephritis, *Pediatr Nephrol* 3:292-303, 1992.
12. Spanou Z, Keller M, Britschgi M, Yawalkar N, et al: Involvement of drug-specific T cells in acute drug-induced interstitial nephritis, *J Am Soc Nephrol* 17:2919-27, 2006.
13. Rossert J: Drug-induced acute interstitial nephritis, *Kidney Int* 60:804-17, 2001.
14. Heeger PS, Smoyer WE, Saad T, Albert S, et al: Molecular analysis of the helper T cell response in murine interstitial nephritis. T cells recognizing an immunodominant epitope use multiple T cell receptor V beta genes with similarities across CDR3, *J Clin Invest* 94: 2084-92, 1994.
15. Eapen SS, Hall PM: Acute tubulointerstitial nephritis, *Cleve Clin J Med* 59:27-32, 1992.
16. Ruffing KA, Hoppes P, Blend D, Cugino A, et al: Eosinophils in urine revisited, *Clin Nephrol* 41:163-66, 1994.
17. Demirkaya E, Atay AA, Musabak U, Sengul A, Gok F: Ceftriaxone-related hemolysis and acute renal failure, *Pediatr Nephrol* 5:733-36, 2006.
18. Kallel H, Hamida CB, Ksibi H, Bahloul M, et al: Suspected acute interstitial nephritis induced by colistin, *J Nephrol* 18:323-26, 2005.
19. Zuliani E, Zwahlen H, Gilliet F, Marone C: Vancomycin-induced hypersensitivity reaction with acute renal failure: resolution following cyclosporine treatment, *Clin Nephrol* 64:155-58, 2005.
20. Hsu SI: Biopsy-proved acute tubulointerstitial nephritis and toxic epidermal necrolysis associated with vancomycin, *Pharmacotherapy* 21:1233-39, 2001.
21. Torpey N, Barker T, Ross C: Drug-induced tubulo-interstitial nephritis secondary to proton pump inhibitors: experience from a single UK renal unit, *Nephrol Dial Transplant* 19:1441-46, 2004.
22. Clarkson MR, Giblin L, O'Connell FP, O'Kelly P, et al: Acute interstitial nephritis: clinical features and response to corticosteroid therapy, *Nephrol Dial Transplant* 19:2778-83, 2004.
23. Laberke HG, Bohle A: Acute interstitial nephritis: correlations between clinical and morphological findings, *Clin Nephrol* 14:263-73, 1980.
24. Buysen JG, Houthoff HJ, Krediet RT, Arisz L: Acute interstitial nephritis: a clinical and morphological study in 27 patients, *Nephrol Dial Transplant* 5:94-99, 1990.
25. Kida H, Abe T, Tomosuqi N, Koshino Y, et al: Prediction of the long term outcome in acute interstitial nephritis, *Clin Nephrol* 22:55-60, 1984.
26. Ustan I, Ozcakar L, Arda N, Duranay M, et al: Brucella glomerulonephritis: case report and review of literature, *South Med J* 98:1216-17, 2005.
27. Becker JL, Miller F, Nuovo GJ, Josepovitz C, et al: Epstein-Barr virus infection of renal proximal tubule cells: possible role in chronic interstitial nephritis, *J Clin Invest* 104:1673-81, 1999.
28. Tian YC, Chen YC, Hung CC, Chang CT, et al: Leptospiral outer membrane protein induces extracellular matrix accumulation through a TGF-β1/Smad-dependent pathway, *J Am Soc Nephrol* 17:2792-98, 2006.
29. Nasr SH, Koscica J, Markowitz GS, D'Agati VD: Granulomatous interstitial nephritis, *Am J Kidney Dis* 41:714-19, 2003.
30. Dobrin RS, Vernier RL, Fish AL: Acute eosinophilic interstitial nephritis and renal failure with bone marrow-lymph node granulomas and anterior uveitis. A new syndrome, *Am J Med* 59:325-33, 1975.
31. Takemura T, Okada M, Hino S, Fukushima K, et al: Course and outcome of tubulointerstitial nephritis and uveitis syndrome, *Am J Kidney Dis* 34:1016-21, 1999.
32. Howarth L, Gilbert RD, Bass P, Deshpande P: Tubulointerstitial nephritis and uveitis in monozygotic twin boys, *Pediatr Nephrol* 19:917-19, 2004.
33. Mandeville JTH, Levinson R, Holland G: The tubulointerstitial nephritis and uveitis syndrome, *Surv Ophthalmol* 46:195-208, 2001.
34. Gianviti A, Greco M, Barsotti P, Rizzoni G: Acute tubulointerstitial nephritis occurring with 1 year lapse in identical twins, *Pediatr Nephrol* 8:427-30, 1994.
35. Bossini N, Savoldi S, Franceschini F, Mombelloni S, et al: Clinical and morphological features of kidney involvement in primary Sjögren's syndrome, *Nephrol Dial Transplant* 16:2328-36, 2001.
36. Kassan SS, Moutsopoulos HM: Clinical manifestations and early diagnosis of Sjogren syndrome, *Arch Intern Med* 164:1275-84, 2004.
37. Bergner R, Hoffman M, Waldherr R, Uppenkamp M: Frequency of kidney disease in chronic sarcoidosis, *Sarcoidosis Vasc Diffuse Lung Dis* 20:126-32, 2003.
38. Thumfart J, Müller D, Rudolph B, Zimmering M, et al: Isolated sarcoid granulomatous interstitial nephritis responding to infliximab therapy, *Am J Kidney Dis* 45:411-14, 2005.
39. Inui N, Muryama A, Sasaki S, Suda T, et al: Correlation between 25-hydroxyvitamin D3 1 alpha-hydroxylase gene expression in alveolar macrophages and the activity of sarcoidosis, *Am J Med* 110:687-93, 2001.
40. Rajakariar R, Sharples EJ, Raftery MJ, Sheaff M, Yaqoob MM: Sarcoid tubulo-interstitial nephritis: long-term outcome and response to corticosteroid therapy, *Kidney Int* 70:165-69, 2006.

41. Neilson EG: Pathogenesis and therapy of interstitial nephritis, *Kidney Int* 35:1257-70, 1989.
42. Preddie DC, Markowitz GS, Radhakrishnan J, Nickolas TL, et al: Mycophenolate mofetil for the treatment of interstitial nephritis, *Clin J Am Soc Nephrol* 1:718-22, 2006.
43. Rodriguez-Iturbe B, Johnson RJ, Herrera-Acosta J: Tubulointerstitial damage and progression of renal failure, *Kidney Int* 68:S82-86, 2005.
44. Nangaku M: Mechanisms of tubulointerstitial injury in the kidney: final common pathways to end-stage renal failure, *Intern Med* 43:9-17, 2004.
45. Remuzzi G, Bertani T: Pathophysiology of progressive nephropathies, *N Engl J Med* 1448-56, 1998.
46. Eddy AA, Neilson EG: Chronic kidney disease progression, *J Am Soc Nephrol* 17:2964-66, 2006.

CHAPTER 35

Diagnosis and Management of Urinary Tract Infections

Gabrielle Williams and Jonathan C. Craig

DEFINITION OF URINARY TRACT INFECTION

The reference standard for urinary tract infection (UTI) is the isolation of a pure growth of bacteria in an uncontaminated sample of urine using semiquantitative culture methods. UTI can be grouped into three clinically distinct presentations: cystitis, acute pyelonephritis, and asymptomatic bacteriuria. Cystitis occurs when infection is limited to the bladder and urethra, and it is most commonly seen among girls who are more than 2 years old. Patients often present with localizing symptoms that can include pain on urination (dysuria), frequency, urgency, cloudy urine, and lower abdominal discomfort.

Acute pyelonephritis is an infection of the kidney, and it is the most severe form of UTI in children. Patients usually present with systemic features such as high fever, vomiting, abdominal pain or tenderness, malaise, poor feeding, or irritability in infants. Diagnosis can be assisted by technetium-99m–labelled dimercaptosuccinic acid (DMSA) scan of the kidneys and inflammatory markers in the blood (e.g., C-reactive protein, erythrocyte sedimentation rate).

A positive urine culture may be found in children without symptoms of illness, such as when urine is collected as part of a routine follow-up or a screening study. Known as asymptomatic, covert, or asymptomatic bacteriuria, some studies suggest that this condition occurs in around 1% of school-aged children.[1] Treatment—and, therefore, detection—is not warranted, because randomized trials have shown that long-term outcomes are no different for treated as compared with untreated patients.[2,3]

DIAGNOSIS

Microbiologic criteria for the diagnosis of UTI are provided in Table 35-1.

The method of collection of a urine sample in children is important for the diagnosis as a result of the problems of contamination and false-positive tests. However, the suprapubic bladder tap, which is the method that is the least likely to be contaminated, may be impractical in some settings. Transurethral catheterization, which is the next best test that uses contamination as a sole criterion, also presents technical challenges, and both of these tests are invasive. Voided samples are more feasible but can be problematic. Pediatric bag collection is used in some settings, but contamination rates are too high to be recommended.[4] The clean-catch method is reasonable, but it requires cooperation and patience from parents. Collection methods thus vary widely across health care settings, because time, skill, the attitudes of parents and clinicians, available facilities, and contamination rates all influence the choice of methods.

Overall, catheterization is the preferred method for urine collection in children who cannot void upon request. The criteria that are taken into consideration are contamination, technical feasibility of obtaining urine, and invasiveness. For children who are more than 2 years old and who are toilet trained, a mid-stream urine sample is recommended.

Diagnostic Tests

Urine culture is the reference standard for the diagnosis of UTI. A commonly used process takes 0.001 ml of urine in a sterile loop and streaks it across a culture plate containing solid media that provides nutrients necessary for bacterial growth. Streaked plates are covered and incubated in a 35°C incubator for a minimum of 18 hours. Plates are viewed for the presence and number of bacterial colonies. At best, such a process is semiquantitative. Colonies are then sampled and streaked on antibiotic selective plates to establish sensitivity.

Because urine culture requires a minimum of 18 hours before a result is known, clinicians often use quicker screening tests in an effort to guide the initial diagnosis and management. Urinalysis (dipsticks) and urine microscopy for white cells or visible bacteria are used routinely in many settings. Dipsticks are fast, simple, and inexpensive, and they can be used anywhere. The microscopic examination of urine requires more specialized equipment and skills, and it is therefore not available as readily; it is also substantially more expensive. A recent systematic review[5] shows that a dipstick with both leukocyte-esterase– and nitrite-positive results is a good indication of UTI (positive test likelihood ratio, 28.2). A dipstick that is negative for both leukocyte esterase and nitrite is also useful for excluding disease (negative test likelihood ratio, 0.2). However, many dipstick results show single positive results, which are less helpful for guiding decisions

TABLE 35-1 Microbiologic Criteria of the Different Urine Sample Collection Methods for the Diagnosis of Urinary Tract Infection in Children

	DEFINITE URINARY TRACT INFECTION*		PROBABLE URINARY TRACT INFECTION†	
Collection Method	Number of Organisms	Colony-Forming Units per Liter	Number of Organisms	Colony-Forming Units per Liter
Suprapubic bladder tap	1	Any	2	Any
Transurethral catheter	1	$\geq 10^7$	1 2	$\geq 10^6$ $\geq 10^7$
Voided samples (clean catch, mid stream, bag)	1	$\geq 10^8$	1 2	$\geq 10^7$ $\geq 10^8$

* Thresholds provided are supported by 52 out of 70 primary studies that evaluated the test performance of urinalysis for the diagnosis of urinary tract infection in children. Given the substantial agreement across the studies, these appear to be well-accepted thresholds.

† Some published studies make use of lower thresholds for the diagnosis of urinary tract infection. These data have been compiled into a "probable" category as a reflection of the uncertainty that may arise with urine culture results.

(leukocyte esterase positive test likelihood ratio, 5.5; nitrite positive test likelihood ratio, 15.9). Combined microscopy findings also perform well for ruling in the diagnosis of UTI in that a positive result for both a high white cell count and bacteria has a likelihood ratio of 37.0. Like the dipstick test, two negative microscopy results also perform reasonably well at excluding UTI (negative test likelihood ratio, 0.21).

Overall, near patient tests such as microscopy and dipstick urinalysis are adjunctive tests only for UTI. In children with suspected UTI, a urine culture should be sent, and a positive urinalysis or microscopy alone should not be relied on for diagnosis. However, clinicians should not wait for a urine culture result (>24 hours) before commencing empiric antibiotics. Children in whom there is a high clinical suspicion of UTI or who have positive urinalysis or microscopy results should be started on antibiotics pending the result of the urine culture.

PATHOGENESIS

Boys are five to ten times as susceptible to UTIs during the neonatal period as compared with girls. After the first year of life, UTI is more common among girls. This increased rate in infant boys is highest among uncircumcised males,[6,7] and it may reflect the presence of the foreskin as a colonizing site[8] in combination with an immature immune system. Higher rates of UTIs among girls are often attributed to a shorter urethra.[9]

It is likely that both human host and bacterial factors contribute to the occurrence of UTI. Bacterial factors that have been well studied in this condition include adherence, growth factors, and features that allow the bacteria to avoid destruction by the human immune response.[10] The importance of human factors in the development of the disease has been demonstrated in a study of healthy volunteers who were inoculated with virulent *Escherichia coli* and who were able to rapidly eradicate the bacteria.[11] Characteristics of the human immune system that are likely to contribute to disease include the types of antimicrobial substances produced (e.g., immunoglobulins), the efficiency of bacterial destruction (e.g., lysozyme, complement), and the responses to antigens (B- and T-cell features). These human defense mechanisms involve many components of the immune system, any of which can vary with genetic background and environmental exposures. Some of these components have been studied in the context of urinary tract infection (e.g., P1 blood type, Lewis blood type), but findings are inconsistent.[12-14] The premise behind many of these studies has been an absolute association between disease and the candidate feature, and, thus, study design was not optimal for the detection of minor influences. It is probable that components convey very slight changes in risk, but this is difficult to examine in any but well-designed genetic epidemiologic studies.

EPIDEMIOLOGY

UTIs are common among children. Precise estimates of rates of UTI are difficult to ascertain, but a large population-based study with a verified diagnosis[15] showed that 8% of girls and 2% of boys had at least one UTI by the age of 7 years. UTI incidence in subgroups of the pediatric population has been studied more frequently. One systematic review of 12 studies of febrile children showed that approximately 5% of febrile infants (0 to 2 months of age) had UTI.[16] Similar rates have been reported among older children with fever (up to 5 years of age).

Recurrence

Between 10 and 30% of children with UTI will have a recurrence of their infection, and most of these recurrences occur within 12 months of the primary infection.[17,18] The risks for recurrence include an age of less than 6 months during the first UTI (odds ratio, 2.9; confidence interval, 1.4-6.2); the presence of a dilating vesicoureteric reflux (odds ratio, 3.6; confidence interval, 1.5-8.3); and renal damage detected during the primary UTI that may be congenital in origin.[17] Other factors, such as dysfunctional voiding, detrusor instability, incomplete bladder emptying, and constipation, are widely believed to be risk factors,[19-21] but supportive epidemiologic data are weak.

Types of Flora

More than 80% of childhood UTIs are caused by *E. coli*. A further 10% to 15% of UTIs are caused by the gram-negative organisms *Klebsiella*, *Enterobacter*, *Proteus*, and *Pseudomonas*. *Staphylococcus* is usually considered a contaminant, but it can cause illness.[22] Signs that suggest contamination include the absence of symptoms, the recent manipulation or catheterization of the urinary tract, the presence of epithelial cells or the absence of leukocytes on urine microscopy, the culture of more than one organism, or a low colony count. Infection with an unusual organism (e.g., *Pseudomonas*) is commonly associated with recurrent infections (with the prolonged use of broad-spectrum antibiotics) or underlying pathology (e.g., neurogenic bladder, obstructive uropathy).[23]

ACUTE TREATMENT

Good-quality evidence on which to base treatment choices for very young children is limited, because such patients are often excluded from randomized, controlled trials. Clinical experience suggests that infants who are 1 month old or younger with UTI require intravenous antibiotics, because there is an approximately 10% risk of concomitant bacteremia[24,25] and a significant chance of finding uropathology (e.g., posterior urethral valves, obstructed duplex systems, high-grade vesicoureteric reflux).[26] The most likely pathogens in this age group are *E. coli* and *Enterococcus faecalis*, which require empiric treatment with a β-lactam antibiotic and an aminoglycoside. Usually intravenous treatment is continued until systemic signs have resolved, at which time an oral antibiotic should be given for 7 to 10 days. In the newborn, empiric combination treatment with ampicillin and gentamicin is the usual treatment. Table 35-2 details suggested antibiotic treatment regimens.

Treatment choices for children who are more than 1 month old with clinical pyelonephritis are based on 18 randomized, controlled trials and summarized in a Cochrane review.[27] Two good trials compared initial intravenous and initial oral antibiotics followed by oral antibiotics, and they showed no difference in time to fever resolution, recurrence of UTI, or renal parenchymal defects (Figure 35-1). Four trials have compared extended intravenous therapy (totaling 10 to 14 days) with initial intravenous therapy followed by oral antibiotic treatment after fever resolution. These trials showed no difference in the recurrence of UTI or renal parenchymal defects. Thus, there is good evidence that oral antibiotics are effective treatment for acute pyelonephritis. Intravenous therapy can be limited to children presenting as seriously unwell or with persistent vomiting. Failure rates of oral antibiotics as first-line treatment for children with acute pyelonephritis are less than 5%. The optimal duration of oral antibiotics for acute pyelonephritis is poorly supported by trial evidence. In clinical practice, between 7 and 14 days of oral antibiotics is usual. Suitable empiric regimens are detailed in Table 35-2, although these depend on local patterns of resistance.

Acute treatment options for children with cystitis are supported by a large evidence base that includes 22 trials and three systematic reviews.[28-30] These data demonstrate that short-duration therapy (3 to 4 days) is as effective as standard therapy (7 to 14 days) for eradicating urinary bacteria[28] (Figure 35-2). Single-dose therapy has been less rigorously explored and thus no recommendation can be made.

PREVENTION OF RECURRENT URINARY TRACT INFECTION

Without a thorough knowledge of causality, it is not possible to reliably prescribe practices that will prevent the recurrence of UTI. Many clinicians advocate treating constipation, ensuring complete bladder emptying and good fluid intake, avoiding local irritation from underclothes or bubble bath, and cleanliness, but there is little or no evidence to support any of these practices.

Prophylaxis and Children with Vesicoureteric Reflux

Vesicoureteric reflux has long been considered a risk factor for the recurrence of UTI, and trials have targeted this group specifically. The use of prophylactic antibiotics for children with vesicoureteric reflux has been standard practice for more than 20 years. A recent systematic review summarizes the existing evidence.[31] Two trials comparing prophylactic antibiotics with no treatment found no difference in the risk of UTI or renal parenchymal abnormality between the groups (Figure 35-3). Six trials have compared ureteric reimplantation surgery plus prophylactic antibiotics with antibiotics alone. These studies show no difference in the risk of UTI at 1 to 2 or 5 years and no difference in the risk of renal paren-

TABLE 35-2 **Antibiotic Treatment Options for Children with Cystitis and Pyelonephritis**

Clinical Features	Antibiotics	Route	Dose	Interval (Hours)	Duration (Days)
Afebrile (cystitis)	Cephalexin Trimethoprim-sulfamethoxazole	Oral Oral	25 mg/kg/dose 4 mg trimethoprim/kg/dose	6 12	3 3
Febrile (pyelonephritis)	Cephalexin Trimethoprim-sulfamethoxazole	Oral Oral	25 mg/kg/dose 4 mg trimethoprim/kg/dose	6 12	7 7
<1 month old or at any age when febrile, extremely unwell, and not able to tolerate oral treatment	Ampicillin and gentamicin	Intravenous	50 mg ampicillin/kg/dose 7.5 mg gentamicin/kg/dose, <10 years of age; 6 mg gentamicin/kg/dose, ≥10 years of age	6 (ampicillin) and 24 (gentamicin)	Until clinically appropriate to switch to oral treatment

Review: Antibiotics for acute pyelonephritis in children
Comparison: 01 Oral (14 days) versus intravenous (3 days) followed by oral (11 days) therapy
Outcome: 01 Time to fever resolution (hours)

Study	Oral therapy N	Oral therapy Mean (SD)	IV then oral therapy N	IV then oral therapy Mean (SD)	Weight (%)	Weighted mean difference (random) 95% CI
Hoberman 1999	153	24.70 (23.20)	153	23.90 (23.30)	38.1	0.80 [−4.41, 6.01]
Montini 2003	185	36.90 (20.20)	202	34.90 (20.80)	61.9	2.00 [−2.09, 6.09]
Total (95% CI)	338		355		100.00	1.54 [−1.67, 4.76]

Test for heterogeneity chi-square = 0.13 df = 1 p = 0.72 I^2 = 0.0%
Test for overall effect: Z = 0.04 p = 0.3

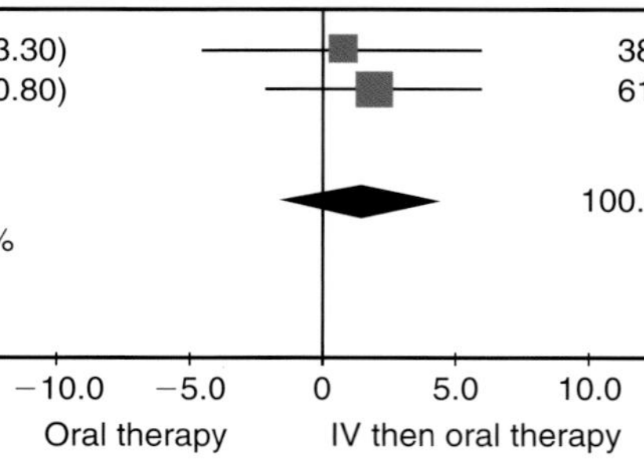

A

Review: Antibiotics for acute pyelonephritis in children
Comparison: 02 Short duration (3–4 days) versus long duration (7–14 days) intravenous therapy
Outcome: 02 Recurrent UTI within 6 months

Study	Oral then IV therapy n/N	IV therapy only n/N	Weight (%)	Relative risk (random) 95% CI
Benador 2001	9/110	6/110	61.5	1.50 [0.55, 4.07]
Francois 1997	0/49	2/53	6.8	0.22 [0.01, 4.39]
Levtchenko 2001	2/44	3/43	20.3	0.65 [0.11, 3.71]
Vilaichone 2001	2/18	1/18	11.5	2.00 [0.20, 20.15]
Total (95% CI)	221	224	100.00	1.15 [0.52, 2.51]

Total events: 13 (Oral then IV therapy), 12 (IV therapy only)
Test for heterogeneity chi-square = 2.11 df = 3 p = 0.55 I^2 = 0.0%
Test for overall effect: Z = 0.35 p = 0.7

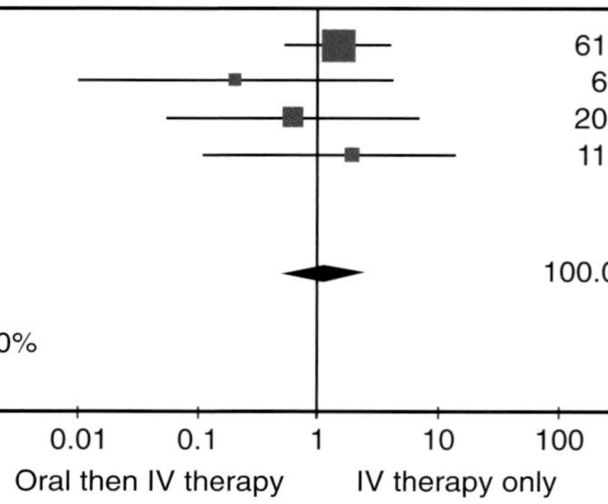

B

Figure 35-1 **A,** Antibiotic treatment for acute pyelonephritis. Initial intravenous versus initial oral antibiotics followed by oral antibiotics. **B,** Antibiotic treatment for acute pyelonephritis. Extended intravenous therapy versus initial intravenous therapy followed by oral antibiotics. (From Bloomfield P, Hodson EM, Craig JC: Antibiotics for acute pyelonephritis in children, *Cochrane Database Syst Rev* (3):CD003772, 2003.)

chymal abnormality between the groups. The only difference was a lower risk of febrile UTI at 5 years in the surgery plus antibiotic group (relative risk, 0.43). Ten-year data is available for one of these trials,[32] and they show that renal growth, UTI recurrence, somatic growth, and renal function were similar between the two groups. The one difference identified was in a higher risk of febrile UTI in the group that only received antibiotics. Two trials and numerous case series of subureteric injection suggest that this treatment "cures" the physical abnormality of vesicoureteric reflux, but the effect on the recurrence of UTI is not known. In summary, the evidence to support surgical treatment, antibiotics, or both for the prevention of recurrent UTI and kidney damage in children with vesicoureteric reflux suggests that the benefit is small at most and that it is limited to reducing febrile infections by a modest amount but without any beneficial effect on overall rates of UTI or kidney outcomes.

Prophylaxis in Children Without Vesicoureteric Reflux

A systematic review of five trials[33] that compared antibiotic prophylaxis with no treatment in children (the majority of whom did not have vesicoureteric reflux) highlights the very poor evidence base for this practice. In only two trials was the outcome symptomatic UTI, and these trials gave conflicting findings (Figure 35-4). To date there is insufficient evidence to support the use of prophylactic antibiotics in children without vesicoureteric reflux.

Cranberries

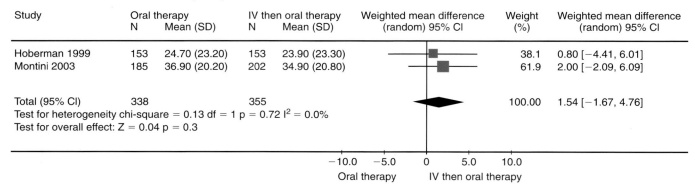

Seven randomized, controlled trials have evaluated the effect of cranberry products on the prevention of recurrent UTIs in adult women; their results are summarized in a systematic review.[34] In two good quality trials, cranberry product significantly reduced the incidence of UTI at 12 months (relative risk, 0.61; 95% confidence interval, 0.4 to 0.91). The dose and the type of product (i.e., tablet or juice) varied across the trials, but no significant differences were found between juice and tablet administration. The remaining five trials were excluded from analyses as a result of methodologic and reporting problems. Thus, there is some evidence to support a beneficial effect of cranberry products on the prevention of UTI in adult women, but evidence for children and dose requirements are lacking. Cranberries do not prevent UTI in children with major predisposing problems like spina bifida. Given that these products are harmless, readily available, and may be beneficial, they should be considered for children.

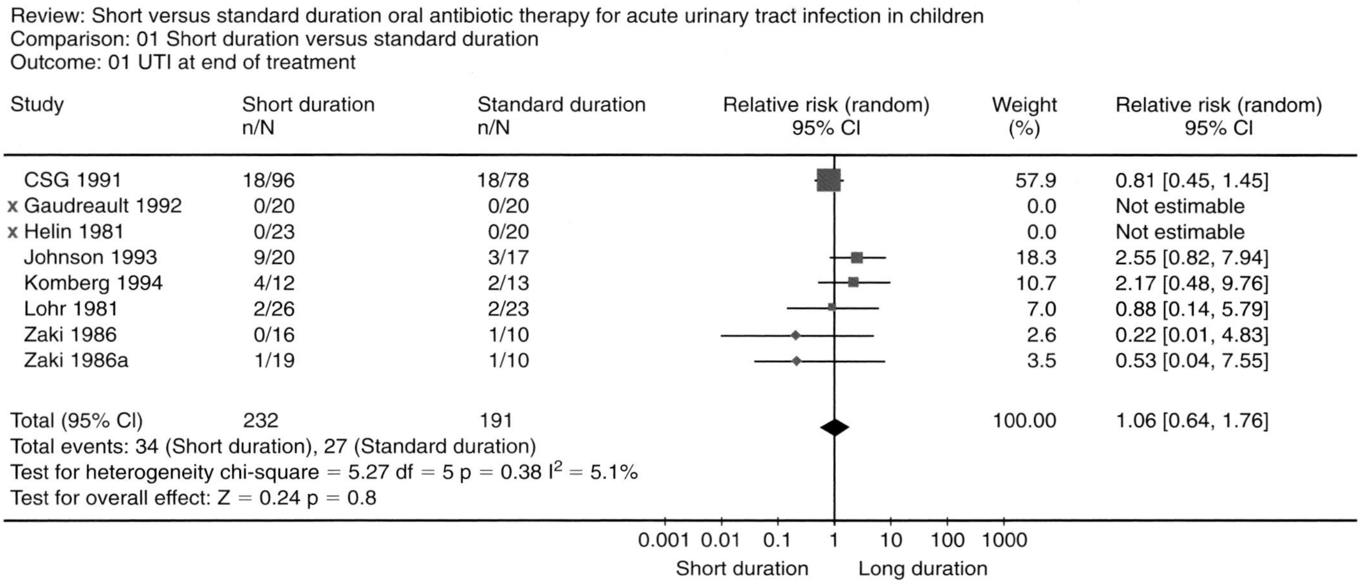
Review: Short versus standard duration oral antibiotic therapy for acute urinary tract infection in children
Comparison: 01 Short duration versus standard duration
Outcome: 01 UTI at end of treatment
Study
Short duration n/N
Standard duration n/N
Relative risk (random) 95% CI
Weight (%)
Relative risk (random) 95% CI
CSG 1991 18/96 18/78 57.9 0.81 [0.45, 1.45]
x Gaudreault 1992 0/20 0/20 0.0 Not estimable
x Helin 1981 0/23 0/20 0.0 Not estimable
Johnson 1993 9/20 3/17 18.3 2.55 [0.82, 7.94]
Komberg 1994 4/12 2/13 10.7 2.17 [0.48, 9.76]
Lohr 1981 2/26 2/23 7.0 0.88 [0.14, 5.79]
Zaki 1986 0/16 1/10 2.6 0.22 [0.01, 4.83]
Zaki 1986a 1/19 1/10 3.5 0.53 [0.04, 7.55]
Total (95% CI) 232 191 100.00 1.06 [0.64, 1.76]
Total events: 34 (Short duration), 27 (Standard duration)
Test for heterogeneity chi-square = 5.27 df = 5 p = 0.38 I² = 5.1%
Test for overall effect: Z = 0.24 p = 0.8
0.001 0.01 0.1 1 10 100 1000
Short duration
Long duration

Figure 35-2 Antibiotic treatment for cystitis, short duration versus standard therapy. (From Michael M, Hodson EM, Craig JC, Martin S, Moyer VA: Short versus standard duration oral antibiotic therapy for acute urinary tract infection in children, *Cochrane Database Syst Rev* (1):CD003966, 2003.)

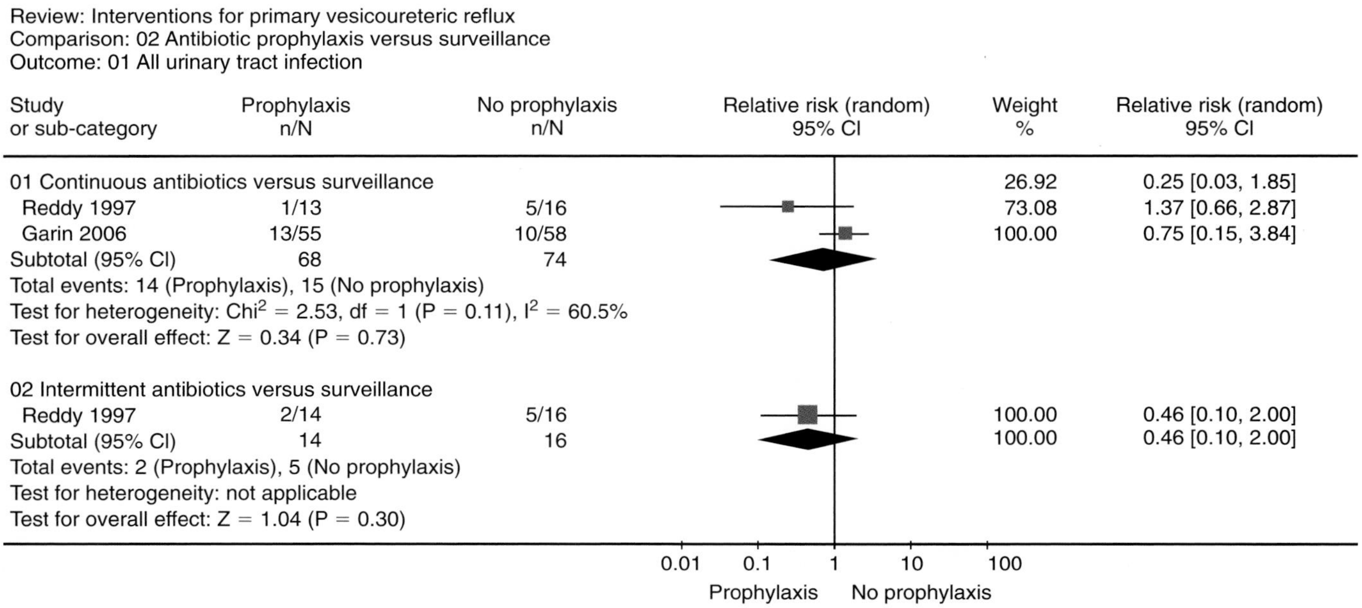
Review: Interventions for primary vesicoureteric reflux
Comparison: 02 Antibiotic prophylaxis versus surveillance
Outcome: 01 All urinary tract infection
Study or sub-category
Prophylaxis n/N
No prophylaxis n/N
Relative risk (random) 95% CI
Weight %
Relative risk (random) 95% CI
01 Continuous antibiotics versus surveillance 26.92 0.25 [0.03, 1.85]
Reddy 1997 1/13 5/16 73.08 1.37 [0.66, 2.87]
Garin 2006 13/55 10/58 100.00 0.75 [0.15, 3.84]
Subtotal (95% CI) 68 74
Total events: 14 (Prophylaxis), 15 (No prophylaxis)
Test for heterogeneity: Chi² = 2.53, df = 1 (P = 0.11), I² = 60.5%
Test for overall effect: Z = 0.34 (P = 0.73)
02 Intermittent antibiotics versus surveillance
Reddy 1997 2/14 5/16 100.00 0.46 [0.10, 2.00]
Subtotal (95% CI) 14 16 100.00 0.46 [0.10, 2.00]
Total events: 2 (Prophylaxis), 5 (No prophylaxis)
Test for heterogeneity: not applicable
Test for overall effect: Z = 1.04 (P = 0.30)
0.01 0.1 1 10 100
Prophylaxis
No prophylaxis

A

Figure 35-3 **A,** Prophylactic treatment of urinary tract infection in children with vesicoureteric reflux. Low-dose prophylactic antibiotics versus surveillance/no treatment.

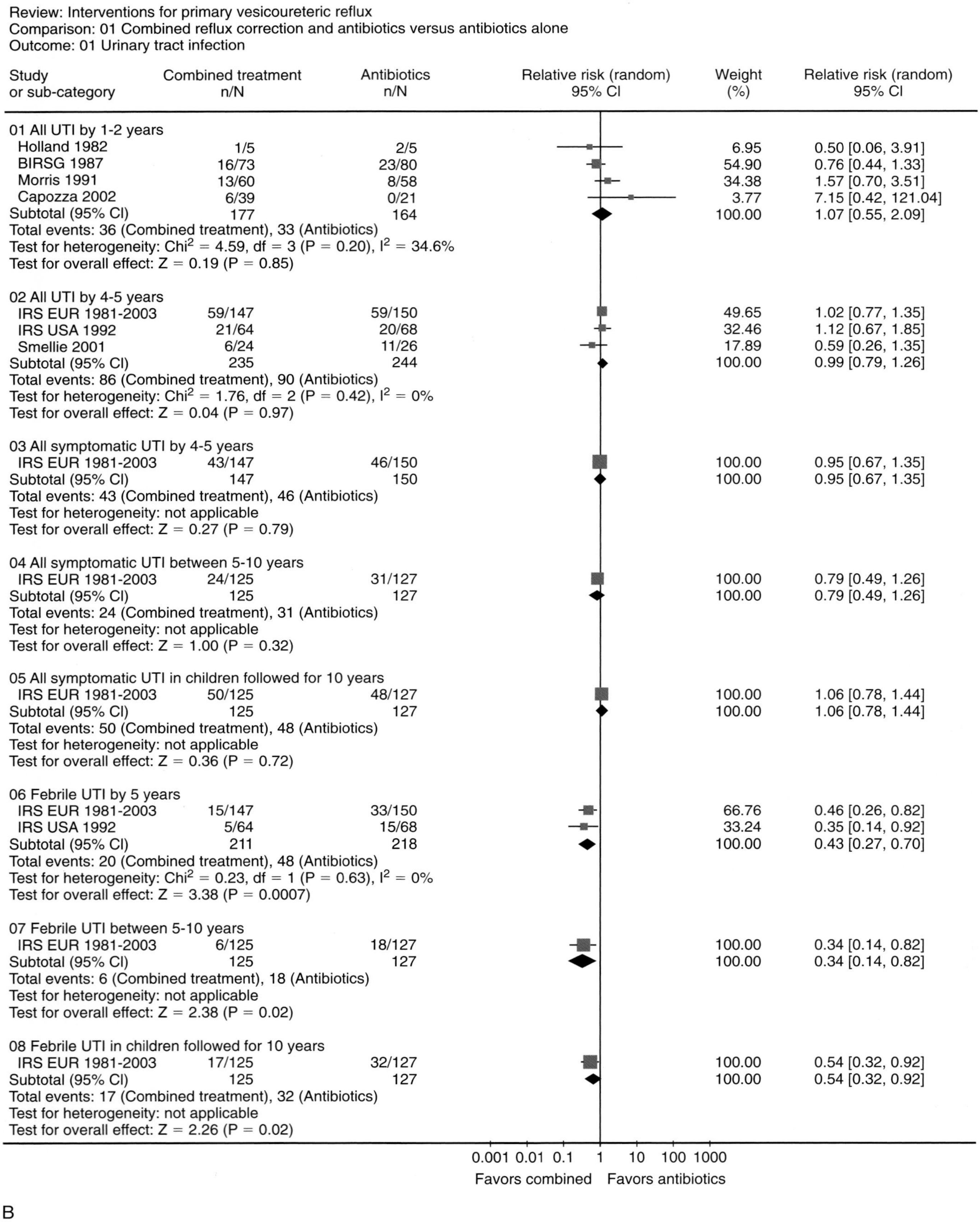

Figure 35-3, cont'd **B,** Prophylactic treatment of urinary tract infection in children with vesicoureteric reflux. Surgery (reimplantation or subureteral injection) and antibiotics versus antibiotics. (From Wheeler DM, Vimalachandra D, Hodson EM, Roy LP, et al: Interventions for primary vesicoureteric reflux, *Cochrane Database Syst Rev* (3):CD001532, 2004.)

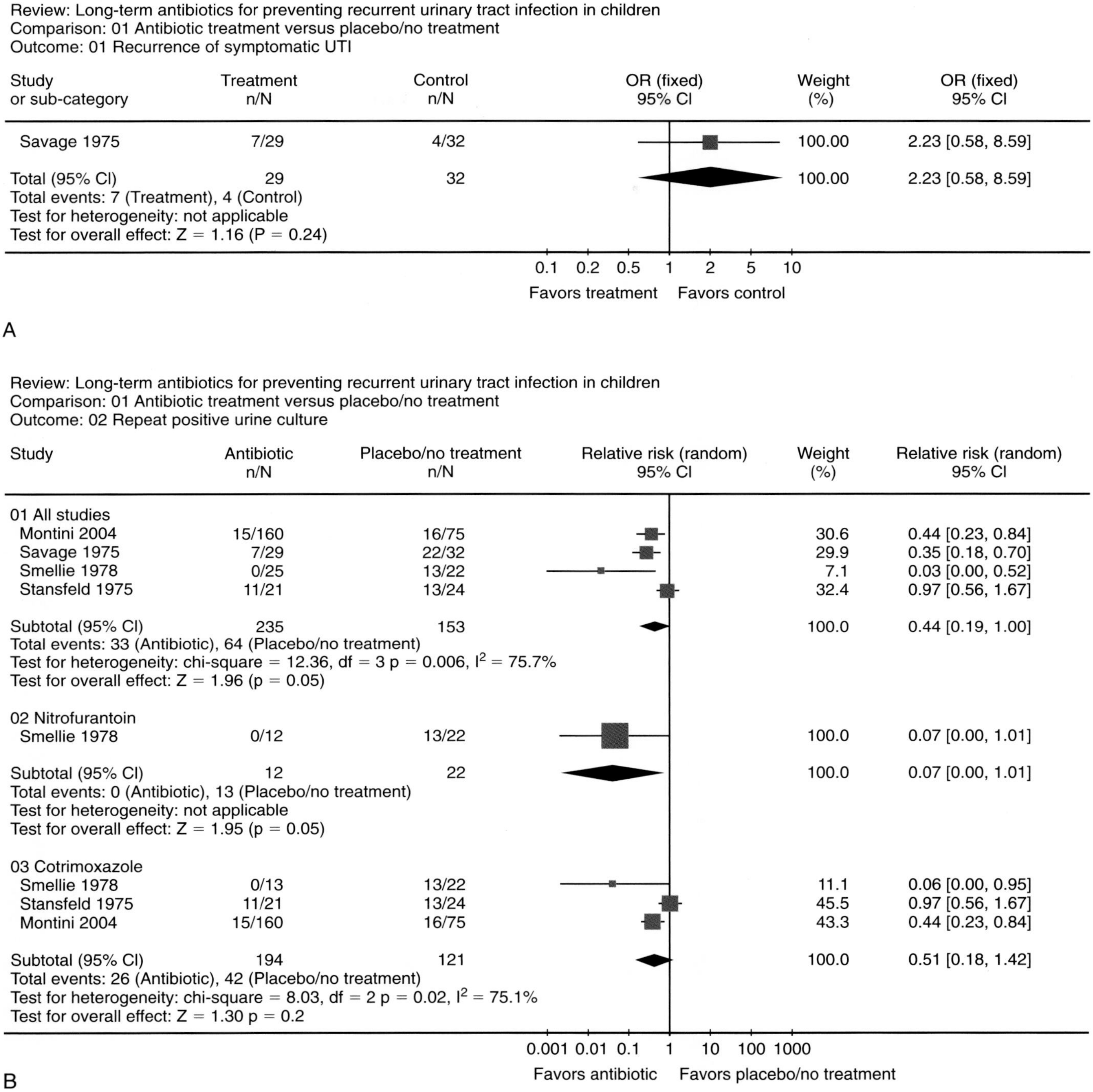
Review: Long-term antibiotics for preventing recurrent urinary tract infection in children
Comparison: 01 Antibiotic treatment versus placebo/no treatment
Outcome: 01 Recurrence of symptomatic UTI
Study or sub-category
Treatment n/N
Control n/N
OR (fixed) 95% CI
Weight (%)
OR (fixed) 95% CI
Savage 1975 7/29 4/32 100.00 2.23 [0.58, 8.59]
Total (95% CI) 29 32 100.00 2.23 [0.58, 8.59]
Total events: 7 (Treatment), 4 (Control)
Test for heterogeneity: not applicable
Test for overall effect: Z = 1.16 (P = 0.24)
0.1 0.2 0.5 1 2 5 10
Favors treatment
Favors control
A
Review: Long-term antibiotics for preventing recurrent urinary tract infection in children
Comparison: 01 Antibiotic treatment versus placebo/no treatment
Outcome: 02 Repeat positive urine culture
Study
Antibiotic n/N
Placebo/no treatment n/N
Relative risk (random) 95% CI
Weight (%)
Relative risk (random) 95% CI
01 All studies
Montini 2004 15/160 16/75 30.6 0.44 [0.23, 0.84]
Savage 1975 7/29 22/32 29.9 0.35 [0.18, 0.70]
Smellie 1978 0/25 13/22 7.1 0.03 [0.00, 0.52]
Stansfeld 1975 11/21 13/24 32.4 0.97 [0.56, 1.67]
Subtotal (95% CI) 235 153 100.0 0.44 [0.19, 1.00]
Total events: 33 (Antibiotic), 64 (Placebo/no treatment)
Test for heterogeneity: chi-square = 12.36, df = 3 p = 0.006, I2 = 75.7%
Test for overall effect: Z = 1.96 (p = 0.05)
02 Nitrofurantoin
Smellie 1978 0/12 13/22 100.0 0.07 [0.00, 1.01]
Subtotal (95% CI) 12 22 100.0 0.07 [0.00, 1.01]
Total events: 0 (Antibiotic), 13 (Placebo/no treatment)
Test for heterogeneity: not applicable
Test for overall effect: Z = 1.95 (p = 0.05)
03 Cotrimoxazole
Smellie 1978 0/13 13/22 11.1 0.06 [0.00, 0.95]
Stansfeld 1975 11/21 13/24 45.5 0.97 [0.56, 1.67]
Montini 2004 15/160 16/75 43.3 0.44 [0.23, 0.84]
Subtotal (95% CI) 194 121 100.0 0.51 [0.18, 1.42]
Total events: 26 (Antibiotic), 42 (Placebo/no treatment)
Test for heterogeneity: chi-square = 8.03, df = 2 p = 0.02, I2 = 75.1%
Test for overall effect: Z = 1.30 p = 0.2
0.001 0.01 0.1 1 10 100 1000
Favors antibiotic
Favors placebo/no treatment
B

Figure 35-4 Antibiotics for the prevention of symptomatic urinary tract infection and repeat positive urine culture in a group of children in which the majority do not have vesicoureteric reflux. (From Williams GJ, Lee A, Craig JC: Long-term antibiotics for preventing recurrent urinary tract infection in children, *Cochrane Database Syst Rev* (3):CD001534, 2006.)

Circumcision

Various studies have attempted to determine the effect of circumcision on the prevention of UTI. A systematic review of existing evidence[35] identified one randomized, controlled trial, four cohort studies, and seven case–control studies that evaluated the effect of circumcision on the risk of UTI in boys. Circumcision reduced the risk of UTI (odds ratio, 0.13; 95% confidence interval, 0.08 to 0.2). However, with regard to clinical relevance, 111 circumcisions would need to be performed to prevent one UTI. Selectively considering boys who are at much greater risk for recurrent UTI improved the benefit–harm balance; for example, for boys with high-grade vesicoureteric reflux, 11 circumcisions would need to be performed to prevent one UTI. Given the potential risks of circumcision (i.e., infection and bleeding), it should probably be reserved for boys with a high risk of UTI (e.g., those with recurrent UTI) rather than used for all boys.

OTHER MANAGEMENT REGIMENS

A systematic review of five trials comparing the immunoactive agent Uro-Vaxom with placebo for the prevention of recurrent UTI claimed a benefit of Uro-Vaxom over placebo.[36] These results should be considered cautiously, because the trial participants were adult women, the follow-up period was only 3 months, and details about key aspects of the design and conduct of this study are unclear.

Probiotics have been studied in the context of the prevention of recurrent urinary tract infection.[37] Most studies have been conducted in women, and results are variable. One randomized, controlled trial in preterm infants[38] found a trend toward a lower rate of UTI but a higher rate of bacterial sepsis in the probiotic group. Although differences were not significant, the possible risk of sepsis outweighs the possible benefit of these products for preterm infants. Until additional data become available, probiotics cannot be recommended for preterm or older children.

Renal Tract Imaging

The American Academy of Pediatrics recommends that children between the ages of 2 months and 2 years undergo renal ultrasound and either voiding cystography or radionuclide cystography after experiencing a UTI.[39] The reported basis of this recommendation is fair, although the authors noted that there are no data that demonstrate that imaging confers improvements in patient outcomes. No recommendations for older children are provided. UK guidelines concur for children who are less than 1 year old and include the addition of a DMSA scan. Children between the ages of 1 and 7 years are reported to require ultrasonography and voiding cystourethrogram, if indicated.[40] Evidence to justify these guidelines is problematic. Two systematic reviews demonstrate an inadequate evidence base to justify the invasive testing of the renal tract after UTI.[41,42]

There are no data that demonstrate that the outcome of children with UTI is improved by the detection and management of renal tract abnormalities found by routine renal tract imaging. Routine imaging has a strong historic basis, but it is not evidence based. Routine imaging by ultrasound can be justified considering the easy access to qualified sonographers, its noninvasive nature, its high sensitivity for renal tract obstruction, and the strong observational evidence base, which demonstrates that the surgical treatment of children with obstructive uropathy improves outcomes. Accordingly, almost all pediatricians report that they recommend ultrasonography for all children with UTI.[43] Considerable variability in the use of DMSA and voiding cystourethrogram reflects the uncertainty about whether these tests do more good than harm in children with UTI.

Renal Ultrasound

Ultrasonography of the renal tract reveals anatomic information about the kidneys and urinary tract, particularly whether there is renal tract dilatation, which may indicate obstructive uropathy. It is noninvasive, readily available, and inexpensive. Only rarely are significant abnormalities detected, and, hence, the subsequent management for the majority of children is not altered after testing. Renal ultrasound detects only a minority of children who have renal parenchymal abnormalities, but this threshold is probably appropriate for the detection of major parenchymal abnormalities, which may be clinically significant for the long term, and for the missing of low-grade abnormalities, which are likely to resolve or to not be of prognostic importance.

Voiding Cystourethrogram

Voiding cystourethrogram is performed to detect vesicoureteric reflux, and it is an invasive and uncomfortable investigation. In the absence of good evidence to support improved outcomes for children who have been diagnosed with and treated for vesicoureteric reflux, this examination is difficult to justify after a first UTI in either sex or at any age, except when renal tract dilatation is detected on ultrasonography and obstructive uropathy therefore requires exclusion.

Dimercaptosuccinic Acid Scan

DMSA scans demonstrate renal focal abnormalities and determine differential renal function. If DMSA is conducted at the time of acute illness, it can be used to differentiate pyelonephritis from cystitis. DMSA is a highly sensitive technique for the detection of renal focal abnormalities. However, it does not distinguish abnormalities that will spontaneously resolve from persisting lesions. The severity of a renal parenchymal abnormality is a reasonable predictor of long-term outcome. One study demonstrated that severe renal scarring identified during the initial UTI was the primary predictor of hypertension in 14 out of 15 cases.[44] However, the ability to discriminate between abnormalities that will resolve and those that will persist and perhaps lead to worse prognoses is not possible. For the majority of children with renal parenchymal abnormalities on DMSA, management is not changed. The threshold of DMSA for detecting renal parenchymal abnormalities is clearly too low for identifying children who have clinically important damage that manifests as hypertension or end-stage kidney disease. Forty percent of children have an abnormal DMSA scan at the time of UTI, which reduces to about 10% by 1 year and 5% at 3 years.

Other Imaging Modes

Intravenous Pyelography

Intravenous pyelography has been generally replaced by renal ultrasound and DMSA for the identification of renal scarring.[45] DMSA has greater sensitivity for the detection of scarring than intravenous pyelography does.[46]

Radionuclide Imaging

Technetium-99m mercaptoacetyltriglycine (MAG-3) and technetium-99m diethylenetriaminepentaacetic acid (DTPA) are both used for the detection of renal obstruction. It is generally a second-stage investigation that is performed after an abnormal ultrasound or DMSA scan.

Further Investigations

Abdominal X-ray

Abdominal X-rays may be used for the management of children with UTI to diagnose renal calculi or to confirm the presence of constipation that may cause bladder dysfunction.

Magnetic Resonance Voiding Cystography

Recent studies suggest magnetic resonance voiding cystography as a replacement for voiding cystourethrogram,[47] but to date there is insufficient evidence to support its use. Ideally evaluation studies should measure whether this technique is a better predictor of clinically relevant outcomes rather than simply comparing detection rates between the two modalities.

REFERENCES

1. Kunin CM, Zacha E, Paquin AJ: Urinary tract infections in school children I. Prevalence of bacteriuria and associated urologic findings, *N Engl J Med* 266:1287-96, 1962.
2. Verrier JK, Asscher AW, Verrier Jones ER, Mattholie K, et al: Glomerular filtration rate in schoolgirls with covert bacteriuria, *Br Med J (Clin Res Ed)* 285:1307-10, 1982.
3. Cardiff-Oxford Bacteriuria Study Group: Sequelae of covert bacteriuria in schoolgirls, *Lancet* 1:889-93, 1978.
4. Al-Orifi F, McGillivray D, Tange S, Kramer MS: Urine culture from bag specimens in young children: are the risks too high? *J Pediatr* 137:221-26, 2000.
5. Whiting P, Westwood M, Watt I, Cooper J, Kleijnen J: Rapid tests and urine sampling techniques for the diagnosis of urinary tract infection (UTI) in children under five years: a systematic review, *BMC Pediatr* 5:4, 2005.
6. Wiswell TE, Roscelli JD: Corroborative evidence for the decreased incidence of urinary tract infections in circumcised male infants, *Pediatrics* 78:96-99, 1986.
7. Wiswell TE, Tencer HL, Welch CA, Chamberlain JL: Circumcision in children beyond the neonatal period, *Pediatrics* 92:791-3, 1993.
8. Fussell EN, Kaack MB, Cherry R, Roberts JA: Adherence of bacteria to human foreskins, *J Urol* 140:997-1001, 1988.
9. Cunningham RJ 3rd: Urinary tract infection in infants and children. Preventing recurrence and renal damage, *Postgrad Med* 75:59-64, 1984.
10. Roberts JA: Factors predisposing to urinary tract infections in children, *Pediatr Nephrol* 10:517-22, 1996.
11. Cox CE, Hinman EJ: Experiments with induced bacteriuria, vesical emptying and bacterial growth on the mechanism of bladder defense to infection, *J Urol* 86:739-48, 1961.
12. Lichodziejewska-Niemierko M, Topley N, Smith C, et al: P1 blood group phenotype, secretor status in patients with urinary tract infections, *Clin Nephrol* 44:376-79, 1995.
13. Jantausch BA, Criss VR, O'Donnell R, Wiedermann BL, et al: Association of Lewis blood group phenotypes with urinary tract infection in children, *J Pediatr* 124:863-68, 1994.
14. Albarus MH, Salzano FM, Goldraich NP: Genetic markers and acute febrile urinary tract infection in the 1st year of life, *Pediatr Nephrol* 11:691-94, 1997.
15. Hellstrom A, Hanson E, Hansson S, Hjalmas K, Jodal U: Association between urinary symptoms at 7 years old and previous urinary tract infection, *Arch Dis Child* 66:232-34, 1991.
16. Slater M, Krug SE: Evaluation of the infant with fever without source: an evidence based approach, *Emerg Med Clin North Am* 17:97-126, 1999.
17. Panaretto K, Craig JC, Knight JF, Howman-Giles R, et al: Risk factors for recurrent urinary tract infection in preschool children, *J Paediatr Child Health* 35:454-59, 1999.
18. Winberg J: What hygiene measures are advisable to prevent recurrent urinary tract infection and what evidence is there to support this advice? *Pediatr Nephrol* 8:652, 1994.
19. Blethyn AJ, Jenkins HR, Roberts R, Verrier Jones K: Radiological evidence of constipation in urinary tract infection, *Arch Dis Child* 73:534-35, 1995.
20. Koff SA, Wagner TT, Jayanthi VR: The relationship among dysfunctional elimination syndromes, primary vesicoureteral reflux and urinary tract infections in children, *J Urol* 160:1019-22, 1998.
21. Lidefelt KJ, Erasmie U, Bollgren I: Residual urine in children with acute cystitis and in healthy children: assessment by sonography, *J Urol* 141:916-17, 1989.
22. Abrahamsson K, Hansson S, Jodal U, Lincoln K: *Staphylococcus saprophyticus* urinary tract infections in children, *Eur J Pediatr* 152:69-71, 1993.
23. Travis LB, Brouhard BH: *Infections of the urinary tract*, Stamford, CT, 1996, Prentice Hall International.
24. Pantell RH, Newman TB, Bernzweig J, Bergman DA, et al: Management and outcomes of care of fever in early infancy, *JAMA* 291:1203-12, 2004.
25. Hsiao AL, Chen L, Baker D: Incidence and predictors of serious bacterial infections among 57- to 180-day-old infants, *Pediatrics* 117:1695-701, 2006.
26. Navarro M, Espinosa L, de las Heras JA, Garcia Meseguer MC, et al: Symptomatic urinary infection in infants less than 4 months old: outcome in 129 cases, *An Esp Pediatr* 21:564-72, 1984.
27. Bloomfield P, Hodson EM, Craig JC: Antibiotics for acute pyelonephritis in children, *Cochrane Database Syst Rev* (3):CD003772, 2003.
28. Michael M, Hodson EM, Craig JC, Martin S, Moyer VA: Short versus standard duration oral antibiotic therapy for acute urinary tract infection in children, *Cochrane Database Syst Rev* (1): CD003966, 2003.
29. Tran D, Muchant DG, Aronoff SC: Short-course versus conventional length antimicrobial therapy for uncomplicated lower urinary tract infections in children: a meta-analysis of 1279 patients, *J Pediatr* 139:93-99, 2001.
30. Keren R, Chan E: A meta-analysis of randomized, controlled trials comparing short- and long-course antibiotic therapy for urinary tract infections in children, *Pediatrics* 109:E70-0, 2002.
31. Wheeler DM, Vimalachandra D, Hodson EM, Roy LP, et al: Interventions for primary vesicoureteric reflux, *Cochrane Database Syst Rev* (3):CD001532, 2004.
32. Jodal U, Smellie J, Lax H, Hoyer PF: Ten year results of randomized treatment of children with severe vesicoureteral reflux. Final report of the international reflux study in children, *Pediatr Nephrol* 21:785-92, 2006.
33. Williams GJ, Lee A, Craig JC: Long-term antibiotics for preventing recurrent urinary tract infection in children, *Cochrane Database Syst Rev* (3):CD001534, 2006.
34. Jepson RG, Mihaljevic L, Craig J: Cranberries for preventing urinary tract infections, *Cochrane Database Syst Rev* (2):CD001321, 2004.
35. Singh-Grewal D, Macdessi J, Craig JC: Circumcision for the prevention of urinary tract infection in boys: a systematic review of randomised trials and observational studies, *Arch Dis Child* 90:853-58, 2005.
36. Bauer HW, Rahlfs VW, Lauener PA, Blessmann GS: Prevention of recurrent urinary tract infections with immuno-active *E. coli* fractions: a meta-analysis of five placebo-controlled double-blind studies, *Int J Antimicrob Agents* 19:451-56, 2002.

37. Reid G, Bruce AW: Could probiotics be an option for treating and preventing urogenital infections? *Medscape Womens Health* 6:9, 2001.
38. Dani C, Biadaioli R, Bertini G, Martelli E, Rubaltelli FF: Probiotics feeding in prevention of urinary tract infection, bacterial sepsis and necrotizing enterocolitis in preterm infants: a prospective double-blind study, *Biol Neonate* 82(2):103-08, 2002.
39. American Academy of Pediatrics, Committee on Quality Improvement, Subcommittee on Urinary Tract Infection: Practice parameter: the diagnosis, treatment, and evaluation of the initial urinary tract infection in febrile infants and young children, *Pediatrics* 103:843-52, 1999.
40. Guidelines for the management of acute urinary tract infection in childhood. Report of a Working Group of the Research Unit, Royal College of Physicians, *J R Coll Physicians Lond* 25:36-42, 1991.
41. Dick PT, Feldman W: Routine diagnostic imaging for childhood urinary tract infections: a systematic overview, *J Pediatr* 128:15-22, 1996.
42. Westwood ME, Whiting PF, Cooper J, Watt IS, Kleijnen J: Further investigation of confirmed urinary tract infection (UTI) in children under five years: a systematic review, *BMC Pediatr* 5:2, 2005.
43. Williams G, Sureshkumar P, Chan S, Macaskill P, Craig JC: Ordering of renal tract imaging by paediatricians after urinary tract infection, *J Paediatr Child Health* 43:271-79, 2007.
44. Goonasekera CD, Gordon I, Dillon MJ: 15-year follow-up of reflux nephropathy by imaging, *Clin Nephrol* 50(4):224-31, 1998.
45. Preston AA: Imaging strategies and discussion of vesicoureteric reflux as a risk factor in the evaluation of urinary tract infection in children, *Curr Opin Pediatr* 6:178-82, 1994.
46. Craig JC, Wheeler D, Williams G, Howman-Giles R, Irwig L: A critical appraisal of the evaluation of children with urinary tract infection (UTI) by diagnostic imaging. 1-57. 2002. A report for the Consultative Committee on Diagnostic Imaging Research Program (CCDIRP). 3-6-2002. Ref Type: Report.
47. Lee SK, Chang Y, Park NH, Kim YH, Woo S: Magnetic resonance voiding cystography in the diagnosis of vesicoureteral reflux: comparative study with voiding cystourethrography, *J Magn Reson Imaging* 21:406-14, 2005.

CHAPTER

36 Vesicoureteral Reflux

Ranjiv Mathews and Tej K. Mattoo

INTRODUCTION

Vesicoureteral reflux (VUR) is the retrograde flow of urine from the bladder to the kidneys. This is considered an abnormal condition in human beings, and it has been implicated in renal injury before birth as well as in the postnatal development of urinary tract infection (UTI) and further renal damage. Although much is known about the diagnosis and the medical and surgical management of VUR, many questions remain regarding the potential of reflux to cause infections and renal injury. This chapter will review the current knowledge and detail the controversies that persist with regard to VUR.

ETIOLOGY

Anatomic Factors

Ureteral development in infants has been studied in an effort to understand the anatomic factors that may lead to VUR. The periureteral sheaths, the intravesical ureteral muscles, and the trigonal muscles have been studied to determine the role of these entities in the development of VUR.[1] On the basis of work done in 11- to 27-week-old fetuses, it was determined that the superficial trigone is derived from the intravesical ureteral muscles and that the deep trigone is derived from the deep periureteral sheath of the ureter. The fixation of the ureters in the appropriate location is very important for the development of a normal trigone and nonrefluxing ureters.

The microscopic evaluation of the ureterovesical junction in children with and without VUR indicated no difference in scarring between these two groups of patients.[2] However, anatomic factors may play a role in the degree of renal injury produced by reflux in that the higher-grade VUR that occurs with lower bladder pressure is associated with an increased risk of nephropathy.[3] The presence of periureteral diverticula also increases the risk of renal damage and the requirement for surgical correction.[4]

Extra-anatomic Factors

The embryologic development of the ureteral bud from the mesonephric duct is dependent on multiple factors. Glial-cell-line–derived neurotrophic factor (GDNF) has been shown in the mouse model to induce the formation of ureteral buds.[5] The misexpression of GDNF has been shown to be associated with the development of multiple ureteral buds. Additionally, GDNF is very focally expressed in the appropriate location of ureteral bud development. If GDNF is expressed in an ectopic location, the ureteral bud will develop in this ectopic location, thereby leading to lateral or medial localization of the ureter in the bladder and predisposing the individual to VUR or obstruction.[5] Additionally, trigonal development is dependent on apoptosis induced by a vitamin A signaling pathway.[6,7] The normal development of the trigone is also necessary to provide appropriate support to the distal ureter. Recent studies have shown that symmetric muscle contractions and unidirectional peristalsis also play a significant role in the competence of the ureterovesical junction.[8] Normal ureters contain greater numbers of interstitial cells of Cajal (a type of pacemaker cell) at the ureterovesical junction.

Associated Conditions

Many anatomic and genetic conditions are associated with the presence of VUR in children. The most commonly noted anatomic conditions are multicystic dysplastic kidney, renal agenesis, and renal or ureteral ectopia.

Multicystic Dysplastic Kidneys

Contralateral VUR is the most common abnormality that is present in children with multicystic dysplastic kidney.[9] VUR has been noted in 12% to 28% of contralateral kidneys in children with this condition.[10] The impact of this contralateral VUR continues to be debated. One study has indicated that contralateral renal growth is compromised in the presence of VUR.[11] However, other studies have revealed that VUR into the contralateral renal unit is usually low grade and does not lead to renal compromise.[12-14] The natural history of VUR in the presence of multicystic dysplastic kidney indicates that most boys and 40% of girls will have a spontaneous resolution.[15]

Renal Agenesis

As with multicystic dysplastic kidney, VUR is the most common abnormality noted in the contralateral kidney in children presenting with unilateral renal agenesis.[16] The management of VUR in the context of a solitary kidney is not different from that seen in patients with two kidneys.[17]

Ectopia

Dilating VUR occurs in up to 26% of children with renal ectopia and hydronephrosis.[18] VUR is the most common associated anomaly in children with renal ectopia.[19] The presence of renal ectopia does not seem to reduce the potential for VUR to resolve spontaneously.[15]

Ureteral duplication is also associated with the presence of VUR, typically into the lower pole of the duplex system. The ureteral orifice is displaced proximally and laterally in children with duplex systems, and it plays a role in the development of VUR into the lower pole moiety. After the endoscopic management of ureteroceles associated with duplex systems, VUR may be unmasked into the lower poles unilaterally or bilaterally, and it may even occur into the upper pole as an iatrogenic entity. The presence of ureteral ectopia does compromise the ability of VUR to subside spontaneously. Many patients with duplex systems will require surgical management of the VUR.[20] Typically surgery in these patients is indicated for the associated conditions that are present (e.g., ureteroceles, ectopic ureters).

Ureteral ectopia may also be noted into the bladder neck and the urethra, thereby leading to VUR during voiding.[21] Bilateral single-system ureteral ectopia is associated with a reduction in bladder growth and capacity, and it requires surgical management with ureteral reimplantation and possible later bladder neck reconstruction to provide continence.[21] Eventual prognosis for this condition is based on the development of adequate bladder capacity.[21]

Syndromes that have been associated with the presence of VUR include VATER/VACTERL syndrome, Townes-Brocks syndrome (SALLI mutation), cat eye syndrome (tetrasomy, chromosome 22), Casamassima-Morton-Nance syndrome, renal-coloboma syndrome (PAX 2 mutation), branchiootorenal syndrome (EYE1 mutation), and Frasier syndrome (WT1 mutation).

INCIDENCE AND PRESENTATION

Antenatal Diagnosis

The widespread use of antenatal ultrasonography has made the early detection of hydronephrosis and subsequent diagnosis of VUR possible before the occurrence of UTI. A fetal pelvic diameter of greater than 5 mm at or beyond 28 weeks of gestation is considered hydronephrosis. About 10% of such patients diagnosed with antenatal ultrasonography will have VUR.[22] Cohorts of infants with VUR diagnosed after the antenatal detection of hydronephrosis include a greater number of boys.[23] Additionally, there are more patients who have low-grade VUR, with a greater propensity for spontaneous resolution.[22,24] Boys with even high grades of VUR (grades IV and V) have a 29% to 37% rate of spontaneous resolution during the first year of life.[24,25] This potential for resolution is attributed to the presence of a mixed pattern of voiding, with coordinated voiding interspersed with high-pressure voiding with increased sphincteric activity.[26]

Urinary Tract Infection

Most children continue to be diagnosed with VUR after an initial UTI. VUR is diagnosed much more frequently in children than in neonates after an initial UTI. Among neonates, although UTI is diagnosed six times more frequently in males, the incidence of VUR is similar between the sexes, with a rate of 15% to 20%.[27,28] Additionally, the incidence of VUR is higher among those neonates who have UTI caused by *Klebsiella* as compared with those whose infections are caused by *Escherichia coli*.[27] In a cohort of patients with UTI (including 68% infants), the overall incidence of VUR was 33%.[29] This incidence was similar to that obtained during a study by Hoberman and colleagues.[30]

Effects of Gender and Race

As noted previously, the relationship of gender and the presence of VUR differs between the patient diagnosed after the identification of hydronephrosis on antenatal ultrasonography and the patient diagnosed after the initial UTI. The incidence of VUR in male infants who are diagnosed after the identification of antenatal hydronephrosis is similar to that found in girls.[31] It has also been noted that the incidence of dysplasia is greater in male infants with VUR.[32] The incidence of the resolution of VUR is greater among male infants.[25] Girls make up a significant majority of patients who present with VUR after a UTI.

African American girls have a lower potential for the development of VUR as compared with Caucasian girls. This difference in incidence was also noted in infants who were diagnosed with VUR after the identification of antenatal hydronephrosis.[33] Additionally, few African American girls presenting with VUR after a UTI have high-grade VUR.[34] The incidence of scarring, however, is reported to be higher among African American girls as compared with their Caucasian counterparts,[35] although the progression of scarring is less among African American girls.[35] Interestingly, the time to spontaneous resolution is shorter in African American girls as compared with Caucasian girls.[35] The incidence of VUR in Hispanic girls is comparable with that of Caucasian girls.[36]

Screening for Vesicoureteral Reflux

The majority of patients with VUR are diagnosed after a febrile UTI, and the number of patients who are found to have VUR at that time ranges from 8% to 50%.[37-39] The current practice guidelines of the American Academy of Pediatrics, which only address children between the ages of 2 and 24 months, recommend performing a voiding cystourethrogram (VCU) after the first febrile UTI for all children in this age group.[40] Screening has also been recommended for other children who are at increased risk for VUR. These include first-degree relatives of children with VUR,[41] the offspring of parents with VUR,[42] children with bladder dysfunction,[43] children with prenatal hydronephrosis/hydroureter,[44,45] and children with unilateral multicystic dysplastic kidney.[10]

ASSOCIATION OF URINARY TRACT INFECTION

VUR is believed to be the primary risk factor for pyelonephritis,[46] although some studies are not very supportive of this association.[47] The International Reflux Study reported recurrent UTI in about 28% of children with medically managed severe VUR.[48] The usual organisms that cause UTI originate from fecal flora that colonize the perineum,[49] and the organisms that cause recurrent UTI can be found on perineal cultures before UTI.[49,50] *E. coli* is the most frequently isolated organism, and it is responsible for approximately 80% of UTIs. The rest are caused by *Klebsiella, Enterobacter, Citrobacter, Proteus, Providencia, Morganella, Serratia,* and *Salmonella* species.[51] There is evidence that a variety of bacterial virulence factors increase the ability of *E. coli* to cause a UTI. The presence of P-antigen-recognizing fimbriae allows *E. coli* to adhere to the epithelial cells of the urinary tract, whereas other virulence factors increase tissue damage and protect the *E. coli* from serum bactericidal activity.[47]

DIAGNOSIS

The gold standard for the diagnosis of VUR is the radiographic VCU.[52] VCU requires urethral catheterization and fluoroscopy. This is also the modality that is used to identify the grade of reflux. Grading has been standardized by the International Reflux Study. Although this is an excellent procedure for identifying the presence or absence of reflux, a discrepancy can be noted between studies and when multiple cycles of filling are used.[52] The performance of VCU within a week of presentation with a UTI is associated with improved compliance, and it does not change the potential for the diagnosis of VUR.[53,54] The discomfort associated with urethral catheterization has led to efforts to identify other modalities for the identification of VUR. Recent studies have shown that sedation can be safely used to improve the tolerance of the procedure,[55] and intermittent radiographic evaluation has been used to reduce the radiation exposure that occurs during VCU.[56]

VCU is also used for the follow-up evaluation of VUR to determine its persistence or improvement. The timing for follow-up VCU remains another area of controversy. An algorithm was developed in an effort to reduce radiation exposure and the numbers of studies based on the grade of reflux.[57] On the basis of this algorithm, VCU can be delayed to every 2 years for mild degrees of reflux (grades I and II) and to every 3 years for those patients with higher grades of reflux. However, most patients continue to have follow-up studies performed every 12 to 18 months.

In an effort to reduce the exposure to radiation that occurs with radiographic VCU, VUR can be diagnosed by using radionuclide agents. Good correlation is noted with the use of nuclear VCU as compared with conventional radiographic VCU.[58] The limitation of this procedure is its inability to grade the VUR in the same manner as the radiographic VCU. By this method, VUR can only be graded as mild, moderate, and severe. However, it can be used for follow-up studies to determine the resolution of VUR. Nuclear VCU has also been used for the determination of the successful surgical correction of reflux. Because this study is very sensitive and because data are collected continuously during the course of the study,[59] it may be used as another modality to identify low-grade reflux in children who have recurrent UTI and negative initial radiographic VCU.[59]

Ultrasonography is the initial test that is performed for most children who present with a UTI.[30] This permits the evaluation of the upper tracts to determine the presence or absence of other anomalies (e.g., duplication, ureteropelvic junction obstruction). The evaluation of the bladder also helps to identify the presence of ureteroceles, diverticulae, or other anomalies that may lead to recurrent UTI. Attempts have been made to use ultrasound for the diagnosis of VUR,[60,61] but the expertise is not widely available, and most patients still require catheterization to detect VUR.[62]

Other imaging modalities have been used in an effort to reduce the radiation exposure that occurs with VCU. Magnetic resonance imaging (MRI) can be used for the detection of reflux.[63] This modality appears to have an accuracy level that is comparable with that of radiographic VCU.[64,65] However, it still requires urethral catheterization, and thus the technique remains limited to a small number of centers.[66] Also, many infants and children require significant sedation and even anesthesia for the performance of MRI.

The major concern with the presence of VUR is the development of infections and subsequent renal scarring. Nuclear renal scanning with 99Tc dimercaptosuccinic acid (DMSA renal scanning) is currently the best modality for evaluating for the presence of scarring in the kidneys.[67-69] The difficulty is in determining whether the scars that are identified are the result of prenatal dysplasia or of recurrent UTI.[70] The technique that has the greatest accuracy for the detection of scarring has not yet been determined.[71] DMSA renal scanning has also been used as an initial study to determine the presence or absence of reflux.[72,73] There is a higher incidence of renal scarring among patients who have higher grades of VUR.[74]

Children who present with recurrent UTI and who have renal scarring but who do not have VUR as determined by standard or nuclear VCU can be evaluated with positional instillation of contrast cystography to determine the presence of low-grade VUR.[75] This procedure is performed with the patient under anesthesia. A cystoscope is placed into the bladder and positioned at the ureteral orifice. Contrast is injected directly at the ureteral orifice and monitored fluoroscopically.[76] When VUR is identified by this modality, correction can be accomplished during the same procedure with the use of a bulking agent. However, experience with this technique remains preliminary, and further studies are required to determine its role in the evaluation of VUR.

GRADING OF VESICOURETERAL REFLUX

The grading of VUR was standardized in 1982[77] using the radiographic VCU. This system of grading divides VUR into five grades (Figure 36-1). The grading of VUR correlates with the degree of renal scarring as well as the potential for spontaneous resolution. Lower grades of VUR have greater potential for spontaneous resolution independent of the age of the patient at diagnosis.[78] Also, the grade of VUR is a consideration when making the appropriate choice regarding the surgical management that is recommended (i.e., endoscopic versus open surgical management).[79,80]

GENETICS OF REFLUX

There is increasing evidence that primary VUR has some genetic basis, and this is best indicated by its familial

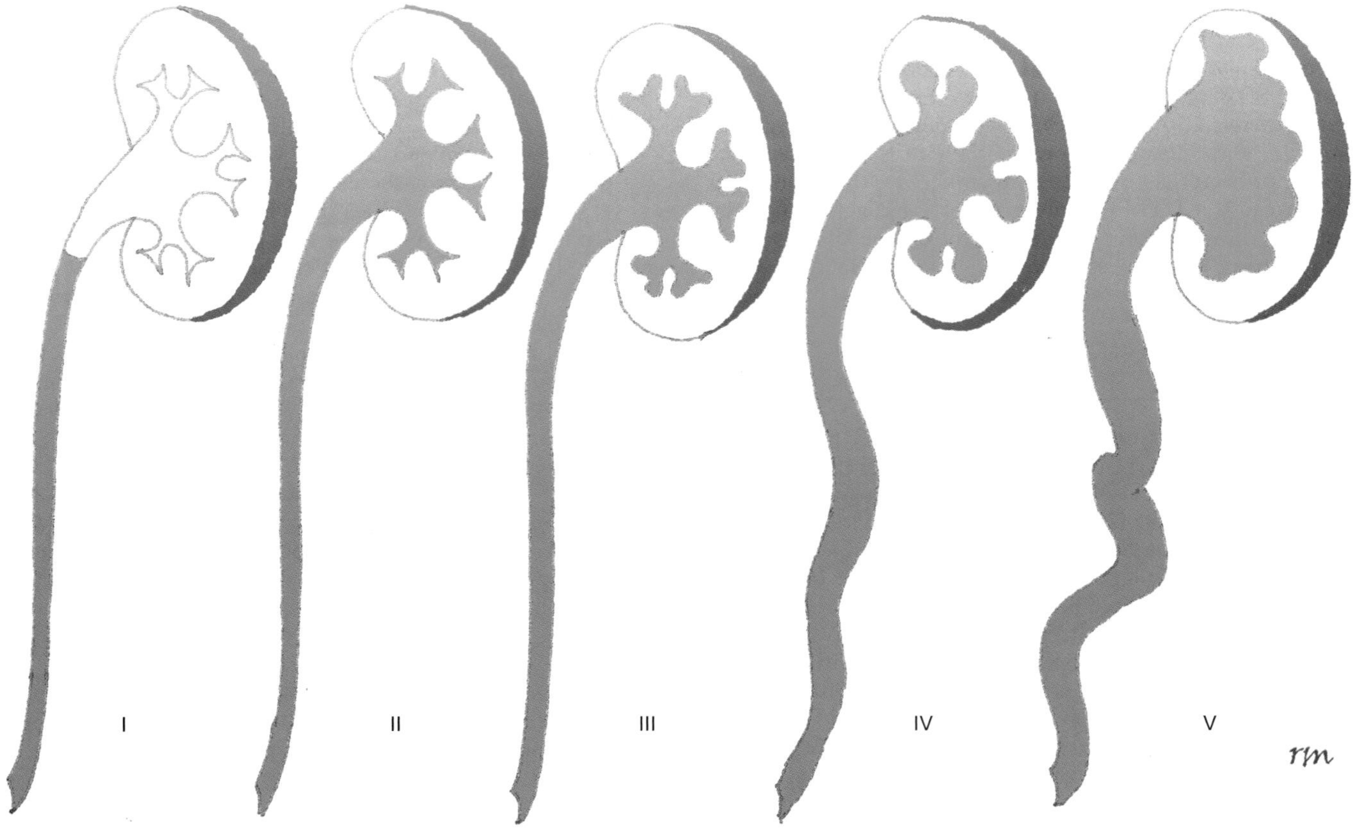

Figure 36-1 International grading system for vesicoureteral reflux. **Grade I,** Contrast in the nondilated ureter. **Grade II,** Contrast in the nondilated ureter and renal pelvis. **Grade III,** Mild dilatation of the ureter and renal pelvis with minimal blunting. **Grade IV,** Moderate tortuosity of the ureter and dilatation of the renal pelvis and calyces. **Grade V,** Gross dilatation of the renal pelvis and calyces with significant ureteral tortuosity. (From International Reflux Study Committee, *Pediatrics* 67:392-400, 1981.)

occurrence. The reported incidence of VUR in the siblings of an affected patient varies from 27% to 45%.[81-83] A higher incidence of VUR has also been reported among children of parents with a history of VUR.[42] The genetics of VUR is not clearly defined, and it is most certainly genetically heterogeneous. Autosomal dominant inheritance with variable expression or multifactorial inheritance has been implicated for VUR and reflux nephropathy. In a study of 88 families with at least one member with primary VUR, the authors concluded that a single major locus was the most important causal factor for this condition.[84] Kaefer and colleagues found 100% concordance among identical twins and 50% concordance among dizygotic twins when only the youngest twins were considered.[85] One gene that is associated with apparent autosomal dominant VUR has been mapped to chromosome 1,[86] although two of the families studies showed negative linkage to this locus, thus further confirming the genetic heterogeneity of VUR.

POTENTIAL FOR VESICOURETERAL REFLUX RESOLUTION

The potential for the spontaneous resolution of VUR is the basis for its conservative nonoperative management. All grades of VUR have the potential for resolution, although the likelihood of resolution is based on the grade and presentation of VUR.[87] Overall, 39% of refluxing ureters will have spontaneous resolution.[88] Even patients with duplex systems have the potential for spontaneous resolution.[89]

Multiple studies have evaluated the rate of resolution of the various grades of VUR. According to one study, the resolution of grade I reflux was noted to be 82%, that of grade II reflux was noted to be 80%, and that of grade III reflux was noted to be 46%.[90] Similar rates of resolution have been noted in other studies that have evaluated the medical management of VUR.[91] The resolution rates for grade IV and V reflux were 30% and 11%, respectively, over 5 years.[87] In patients who were diagnosed with VUR after the evaluation of antenatal hydronephrosis, there is a greater potential for resolution even in the presence of higher grades of VUR.[92]

POTENTIAL FOR RENAL INJURY

Various factors influence the probability of scarring in children with VUR and UTI. The role of VUR, which was initially proven in piglets,[93] has been shown in multiple clinical studies.[94,95] Moreover, children with higher grades of VUR have an increased likelihood of developing renal scarring.[96-99] Renal damage is more common in infants with UTI and VUR because of their unique kidney papillary morphology.[100,101] Children who are less than 2 years old with VUR are more likely to develop scarring,[46,48] although some studies do not show an increased risk of renal damage in younger children after acute pyelonephritis.[102,103] Other factors that affect the probability of renal scarring in children with VUR and UTI include delayed treatment of UTI,[104] recurrent UTI,[105,106] and bacterial virulence.[107,108] Finally, there is evidence that genetic factors predispose patients with VUR to scarring, as demonstrated by studies of angiotensin-converting enzyme (ACE) gene polymorphisms.[109-111]

MANAGEMENT OF VESICOURETERAL REFLUX

The basis for the management of VUR is the prevention of infections of the kidney with the hope that this will lead to the prevention of scarring and the preservation of renal function. The role of intrarenal reflux on the development of renal scars had been noted early in the investigation of VUR.[112] The true causes of reflux nephropathy continue to be elucidated and are described later in this chapter. Additionally, the potential for VUR to resolve spontaneously in many patients has changed the paradigm of management from one of immediate surgical correction to initial medical management with antibiotic prophylaxis to prevent UTI in combination with follow-up.[113] Surgical treatment is typically reserved for those patients in whom spontaneous resolution is in doubt (i.e., those with high-grade reflux), those with recurrent UTI despite appropriate antibiotic prophylaxis, those who cannot comply with antibiotic prophylaxis, and those with a worsening of renal scars during follow-up.

ANTIBIOTIC PROPHYLAXIS

The main objective of treatment in children with VUR is to prevent recurrent UTI and renal parenchymal damage, mostly by long-term antibiotic prophylaxis or surgical correction of the VUR. The concept of antibiotic prophylaxis was introduced in 1975,[114] and controlled trials have demonstrated the effectiveness of low-dose prophylactic trimethoprim-sulfamethoxazole or nitrofurantoin therapy for preventing UTI.[115] Antibiotic prophylaxis is not always effective, with breakthrough rates in children with VUR ranging from 25% to 38%.[116,117] The major concern with long-term antibiotic prophylaxis is antimicrobial drug resistance. In one study, children who received antibiotics for more than 4 weeks during the preceding 6 months had more resistant *E. coli* as compared with those who had not received such treatment (odds ratio, 13.9; 95% confidence interval, 8.2 to 23.5).[118] In another study of childhood UTI, a generalized decrease in bacterial susceptibility to common antibiotics was seen during the year 1999 as compared with that seen in 1991.[119] Other side effects are not uncommon, and these include gastrointestinal disturbances, skin rashes, hepatotoxicity, and hematologic complications.[120]

Numerous multicenter studies have revealed that there is no significant outcome difference between medical and surgical management. The International Reflux Study Group in Europe studied 287 children with severe VUR who were randomly allocated to medical ($N = 147$) or surgical ($N = 140$) groups. Follow-up with DMSA renal scanning over a period of 5 years revealed no difference in outcomes, including renal scarring, between the two groups.[48] In yet another International Reflux Study Group study, which included 306 children, no significant difference in outcome was found between medical or surgical management in terms of the development of new renal lesions or the progression of established renal scars.[121] Similar results were reported by the Birmingham Study.[117] Medical management seems appropriate for VUR grades I, II, and III unless the patient has compliance issues, recurrent UTI, or allergy to prophylactic antibiotics. For grade IV VUR, medical versus surgical treatment is controversial, because the spontaneous resolution rate is less than 40% after 5 years of follow-up.[87,116,122]

SURGICAL MANAGEMENT

Indications

The major indications for surgical intervention in children with VUR include recurrent UTI despite appropriate antibiotic prophylaxis, a worsening of renal scarring during follow-up, and a low chance of resolution (i.e., those patients with grade V VUR). There may be a greater indication for the correction of VUR in those patients who have reflux into a single renal system. However, surgical management decisions should be individualized on the basis of the potential risk to the renal units.

Minimally Invasive Treatment Options

Endoscopy

Multiple attempts have been made to manage VUR with the use of cystoscopy. Endoscopic techniques have typically involved the use of bulking agents to increase resistance at the ureteral orifice to prevent reflux. Polytetrafluoroethylene (Polytef) has been used successfully for the correction of VUR since the early 1980s.[123] The reflux correction achieved with Polytef was comparable to that achieved with open surgical techniques,[124] and this correction was maintained over a long period of follow-up. However, concern about the migration of Polytef particles has prevented the approval of this agent in the United States. As a result of this restriction, other agents have been developed and used. Polydimethylsiloxane has been used in Canada. This agent does not migrate, and it is associated with high success rates[125]; however, it is also not approved for use in the United States. Bovine cross-linked collagen was used successfully,[126] and, although the initial results of collagen seemed very acceptable,[127,128] the long-term results have indicated that recurrence is frequent as a result of the absorption of the collagen over time.[129] Other treatments that have been tried include the use of expanded chondrocytes[130] and the placement of balloons[131]; however, many of these techniques require multiple procedures for completion.[132]

Recently, dextranomer/hyaluronidase (Dx/HA; Deflux) has been used for the bulking of the ureters for the treatment of reflux (Figure 36-2, *A* and *B*). This treatment was initially reported by Stenberg and Lackgren in 1995,[133] and worldwide experience has since grown rapidly. Success rates reported with the use of Dx/HA include overall cure rates

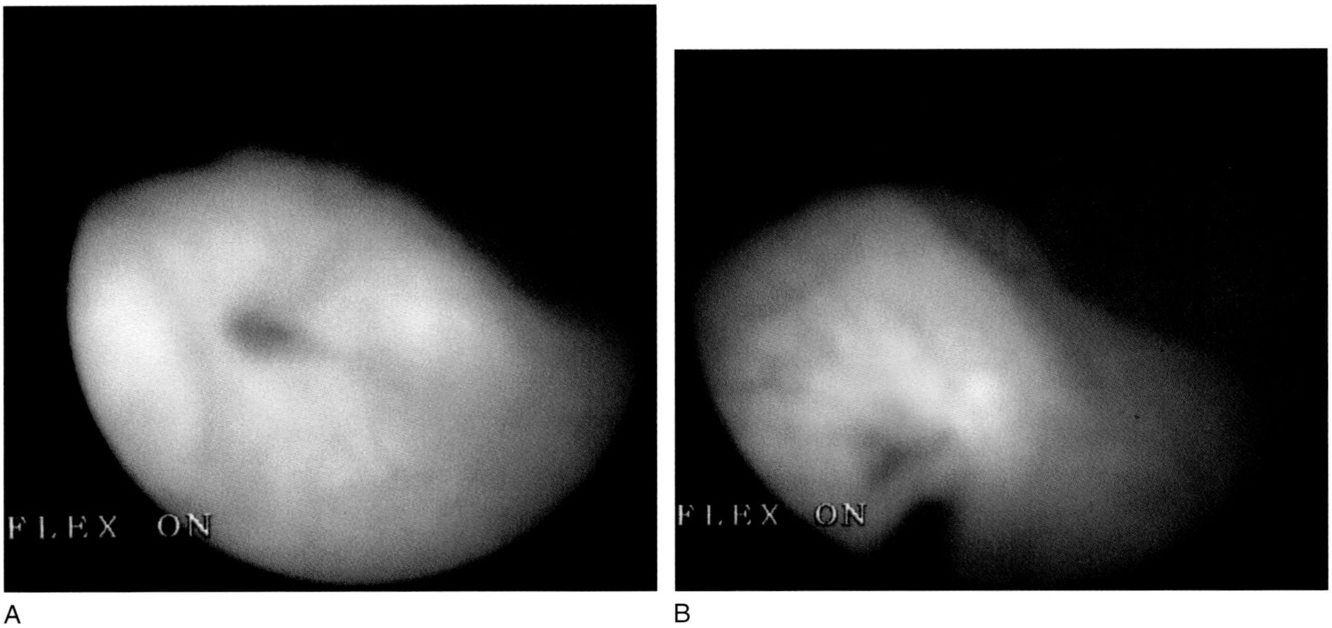

Figure 36-2 **A,** The endoscopic appearance of a right refluxing ureter. **B,** The injection of dextranomer/hyaluronidase for the correction of vesicoureteral reflux.

of 94% for grade I reflux, 85% for grade II reflux, 78% for grade III reflux, and 71% for grade IV reflux.[134] This material has also been shown to be of benefit for those patients for whom prior treatments have failed and for those who have associated urologic anomalies such as ureteroceles and duplex systems.[135] Patients for whom endoscopic management is not effective are still candidates for open surgical reconstruction. The late recurrence of VUR has been noted in patients who have had follow-up evaluations,[102] although the recurrence is of lower grade than what was present before the intervention.

The efficacy and relative simplicity of the use of Dx/HA for the correction of VUR has led some to question the current paradigm of VUR management.[136] It has been suggested that Dx/HA should be used as a first-line treatment for VUR. This procedure does require the use of general anesthesia, and, in infants, this should be a significant consideration.

Laparoscopy

Laparoscopy has been successfully used for the surgical correction of VUR.[137] Laparoscopic techniques allow small incisions to be used, and they have the potential to reduce discomfort and the length of hospital stays. The technique initially involved an extravesical approach for the correction of VUR,[138,139] but intravesical and transvesical techniques have since been reported.[140,141] The presumed benefits of the reduction in hospital stay and smaller incisions have been eclipsed by the advent of improved endoscopic management with Dx/HA. Additionally, there has been a significant reduction in the length of hospital stay with open surgical techniques, and cosmesis is not markedly improved by the use of laparoscopy.

Open Surgical Techniques

Open surgical techniques remain the gold standard for the surgical correction of VUR. The initial technique used was the Leadbetter-Politano approach, which was a combined intra- and extravesical technique.[142] This technique has been supplanted by the two techniques described here. In general, all of the open surgical techniques are associated with a 90% to 95% success rate and a reduction in hospital stay to 1 to 3 days. The success rates are so consistent across multiple studies that the use of routine postoperative VCU has been questioned.[143] Although the techniques are associated with high rates of success for the correction of reflux and for a reduction in the incidence of pyelonephritis,[144] there is no reduction in the incidence of renal scarring noted during follow up.

Intravesical (Cohen Cross-Trigonal) Reimplantation

Since the initial description of the Cohen cross-trigonal technique,[145] it has been rapidly adopted by most pediatric urologists as a result of the consistent rates of the surgical correction of VUR and the low rates of complication.[146] The technique involves the dissection of the ureters within the bladder. The ureters are then placed in submucosal tunnels that are created across the trigone of the bladder. Over time, significant improvements in pain management have permitted a reduction in hospital stays, a reduction in the need for stenting and suprapubic tube placement, and high rates of patient satisfaction.[146] Additionally, the high rates of success have led this technique to be the most frequently performed and taught procedure for the correction of VUR.[147] This technique is routinely used for the correction of bilateral reflux, and it also allows for other bladder abnormalities (e.g., ureteroceles, bladder diverticula) to be corrected at the same time.[148] Potential complications associated with this technique are the development of contralateral reflux (in those patients in whom unilateral correction is performed), ureteral obstruction, and residual reflux.[146,149,150]

Extravesical (Lich-Gregoir) Reimplantation

The Lich-Gregoir technique allows for reimplantation without entry into the bladder.[151] The ureters are dissected before their entry into the bladder, and reimplantation is performed by placing the ureters into troughs created in the bladder wall.[152] This technique has been used most frequently for the management of unilateral reflux, because there is a concern that some patients who have had bilateral reimplantation using this technique have had secondary transient neuropathic bladder dysfunction that requires temporary intermittent catheterization.[153] This technique is also associated with a high degree of success for the correction of reflux. Many patients can be managed with a 24-hour hospitalization, because bladder spasms are less frequently noted.

REFLUX NEPHROPATHY

After acute pyelonephritis, renal scarring takes about 1 to 2 years to develop.[154,155] Shindo and colleagues reported that the mean time from the discovery of VUR to the appearance of a renal scar in their study was 6.1 years.[156] Several studies have shown that scarring develops at the same site as previous infection.[157,158] The exact pathogenesis of renal scarring after acute pyelonephritis is not well understood. The process is an inflammatory response, with chemotaxis, phagocytosis, the release of lysosomal enzymes and superoxides, the production of peroxide and hydroxyl radicals, tubular ischemia, and reperfusion injury.[159-162] The fibrosis that follows is initiated mainly by macrophages.[163] Cytokines that are produced by these cells, which include transforming growth factor-β-1, platelet-derived growth factor, and fibroblast growth factor, attract and stimulate the proliferation of the fibroblasts that are ultimately responsible for collagen production and scarring.[164] Explanations for progressive parenchymal renal injury even after VUR has ceased include autologous tubular antigens, the hyperfiltration of intact nephrons, a reaction to Tamm-Horsfall protein, superoxide production, and persistent hypertension.[165]

In addition to acute complications such as sepsis, drug reactions, and pyonephrosis during acute pyelonephritis, long-term complications and significant morbidity occur with reflux nephropathy. Reflux nephropathy is responsible for 12% to 21% of all children with chronic renal failure.[166,167] Hypertension occurs in 10% to 30% of children and young adults with renal scarring.[168,169] Complications may occur during pregnancy, including significant rises in blood pressure, recurrent UTI, toxemia, and miscarriage.[170-172]

CONTROVERSIES AND FUTURE DIRECTIONS

Renal scars in febrile UTI are known to occur in patients without VUR.[46,98,173-176] Also, up to half of patients with severe VUR exhibit no evidence of renal damage.[177,178] The detection of renal lesions by nuclear scans in as many as 30% of children with prenatal VUR even before the history of UTI has also raised doubts about the role of UTI in causing renal injury in such patients.[179-182] This raises the possibility of reflux-associated, preexisting, congenital renal parenchymal pathology (particularly in boys with VUR), which in the past may have been mistakenly attributed to the inflammatory process.[183] It also raises some doubts about the published literature from the days when antenatal ultrasonography and DMSA scintigraphy were not available. Similarly, serious doubts exist regarding the relevance of long-term antibiotic prophylaxis for VUR. Guidelines from the American Academy of Pediatrics,[40] the American Urological Association,[184] and the Swedish Medical Research Council[185] recommend using long-term antibiotic prophylaxis, but, at the same time, they acknowledge a lack of evidence for this recommendation.

A systematic literature review and meta-analysis of the predictability of renal parenchymal damage by diagnosing VUR in hospitalized children with febrile UTI revealed that VUR is a weak predictor of renal damage in children who are hospitalized with UTI.[186] A recent Cochrane review of the effectiveness of long-term antibiotics for preventing UTI in VUR concluded that most published studies to date have been poorly designed, with biases that are known to overestimate the true treatment effect.[187] Another systematic analysis concluded that it is uncertain whether the identification and treatment of children with VUR confers any clinically important benefit or whether intervention (including anti-biotic prophylaxis or surgery for VUR) is better than no treatment.[188]

The current paradigm for the management of VUR continues to be questioned in light of the concern that VUR may not necessarily lead to renal injury, the presence of scarring of the kidneys at birth in many children with VUR, the lack of compliance with long-term antibiotic prophylaxis, and the inability to categorically demonstrate that the surgical correction of VUR leads to a reduction in UTI or the prevention of renal scarring. Randomized, placebo-controlled trials are currently attempting to answer some of these questions. The most important questions are whether VUR is definitively associated with the development of UTI and renal scarring, and whether prophylaxis with antibiotics has an impact on the prevention of UTI and scarring. The consistency of the diagnosis and grading of VUR among institutions and radiologists, the development of modalities to diagnose reflux without urethral catheterization, and the identification of renal scarring and progression are all being studied. The increasing use of endoscopic techniques is starting to change the surgical algorithm. Parents are being offered endoscopic correction instead of antibiotic prophylaxis as the initial management for VUR. The long-term durability of endoscopic management remains to be determined. If long-term correction is possible with endoscopic techniques, this could offset the problems of antibiotic resistance, side effects, and the lack of compliance that are inherent with long-term antibiotic prophylaxis regimens.

CONCLUSION

The current understanding of the causes, diagnosis, and management of reflux continues to evolve. Questions continue to be raised about the true role of VUR in the predisposition of children to pyelonephritis. Debate also continues regarding the true role of VUR in the worsening of renal scarring over time and the benefit of antibiotic prophylaxis for the prevention of UTI and renal scarring. Carefully planned studies are required to provide answers to these crucial questions and to determine the future of VUR diagnosis and management.

REFERENCES

1. Itatani H, Koide T, Okuyama A, Sonoda T: Development of the ureterovesical junction in human fetus: in consideration of the vesicoureteral reflux, *Invest Urol* 15:232-38, 1977.
2. Hammar E, Helin I: Microanatomy of the intravesical ureter in children with and without reflux, *J Urol* 117:353-54, 1977.
3. Nielsen JB: The clinical significance of the reflux producing intrinsic bladder pressure and bladder volume in reflux and reflux nephropathy, *Scand J Urol Nephrol Suppl* 125:9-13, 1989.
4. Barrett DM, Malek RS, Kelalis PP: Observations on vesical diverticulum in childhood, *J Urol* 116:234-36, 1976.
5. Shakya R, Watanabe T, Costantini F: The role of GDNF/Ret signaling in ureteric bud cell fate and branching morphogenesis, *Dev Cell* 8:65-74, 2005.
6. Batourina E, Tsai S, Lambert S, Sprenkle P, et al: Apoptosis induced by vitamin A signaling is crucial for connecting the ureters to the bladder, *Nat Genet* 37:1082-89, 2005.
7. Batourina E, Choi C, Paragas N, Bello N, et al: Distal ureter morphogenesis depends on epithelial cell remodeling mediated by vitamin A and Ret, *Nat Genet* 32:109-15, 2002.
8. Schwentner C, Oswald J, Lunacek A, Fritsch H, et al: Loss of interstitial cells of Cajal and gap junction protein connexin 43 at the vesicoureteral junction in children with vesicoureteral reflux, *J Urol* 174:1981-86, 2005.
9. Atiyeh B, Husmann D, Baum M: Contralateral renal abnormalities in multicystic-dysplastic kidney disease, *J Pediatr* 121:65-67, 1992.
10. Flack CE, Bellinger MF: The multicystic dysplastic kidney and contralateral vesicoureteral reflux: protection of the solitary kidney, *J Urol* 150:1873-74, 1993.
11. Zerin JM, Leiser J: The impact of vesicoureteral reflux on contralateral renal length in infants with multicystic dysplastic kidney, *Pediatr Radiol* 28:683-86, 1998.
12. Miller DC, Rumohr JA, Dunn RL, Bloom DA, Park JM: What is the fate of the refluxing contralateral kidney in children with multicystic dysplastic kidney? *J Urol* 172:1630-34, 2004.
13. Ismaili K, Avni FE, Alexander M, Schulman C, et al: Routine voiding cystourethrography is of no value in neonates with unilateral multicystic dysplastic kidney, *J Pediatr* 146:759-63, 2005.
14. John U, Rudnik-Schoneborn S, Zerres K, Misselwitz J: Kidney growth and renal function in unilateral multicystic dysplastic kidney disease, *Pediatr Nephrol* 12:567-71, 1998.
15. Guarino N, Casamassima MG, Tadini B, Marras E, et al: Natural history of vesicoureteral reflux associated with kidney anomalies, *Urology* 65:1208-11, 2005.
16. Robson WL, Leung AK, Rogers RC: Unilateral renal agenesis, *Adv Pediatr* 42:575-92, 1995.
17. Palmer LS, Andros GJ, Maizels M, Kaplan WE, Firlit CF: Management considerations for treating vesicoureteral reflux in children with solitary kidneys, *Urology* 49:604-08, 1997.
18. Gleason PE, Kelalis PP, Husmann DA, Kramer SA: Hydronephrosis in renal ectopia: incidence, etiology and significance, *J Urol* 151:1660-61, 1994.
19. Guarino N, Tadini B, Camardi P, Silvestro L, et al: The incidence of associated urological abnormalities in children with renal ectopia, *J Urol* 172:1757-59; discussion 1759, 2004.
20. Jee LD, Rickwood AM, Williams MP, Anderson PA: Experience with duplex system anomalies detected by prenatal ultrasonography, *J Urol* 149:808-10, 1993.
21. Noseworthy J, Persky L: Spectrum of bilateral ureteral ectopia, *Urology* 19:489-94, 1982.
22. Ismaili K, Hall M, Piepsz A, Wissing KM, et al: Primary vesicoureteral reflux detected in neonates with a history of fetal renal pelvis dilatation: a prospective clinical and imaging study, *J Pediatr* 148:222-27, 2006.
23. Penido Silva JM, Oliveira EA, Diniz JS, Bouzada MC, et al: Clinical course of prenatally detected primary vesicoureteral reflux, *Pediatr Nephrol* 21:86-91, 2006.
24. Penido Silva JM, Oliveira EA, Diniz JS, Bouzada MC, et al: Clinical course of prenatally detected primary vesicoureteral reflux. *Pediatr Nephrol* 2005.
25. Sjostrom S, Sillen U, Bachelard M, Hansson S, Stokland E: Spontaneous resolution of high grade infantile vesicoureteral reflux, *J Urol* 172:694-98; discussion 699, 2004.
26. Podesta ML, Castera R, Ruarte AC: Videourodynamic findings in young infants with severe primary reflux, *J Urol* 171:829-33; discussion 833, 2004.
27. Cleper R, Krause I, Eisenstein B, Davidovits M: Prevalence of vesicoureteral reflux in neonatal urinary tract infection, *Clin Pediatr (Phila)* 43:619-25, 2004.
28. Biyikli NK, Alpay H, Ozek E, Akman I, Bilgen H: Neonatal urinary tract infections: analysis of the patients and recurrences, *Pediatr Int* 46:21-25, 2004.
29. Wu CY, Chiu PC, Hsieh KS, Chiu CL, et al: Childhood urinary tract infection: a clinical analysis of 597 cases, *Acta Paediatr Taiwan* 45:328-33, 2004.
30. Hoberman A, Charron M, Hickey RW, Baskin M, et al: Imaging studies after a first febrile urinary tract infection in young children, *N Engl J Med* 348:195-202, 2003.
31. Brophy MM, Austin PF, Yan Y, Coplen DE: Vesicoureteral reflux and clinical outcomes in infants with prenatally detected hydronephrosis, *J Urol* 168:1716-19; discussion 1719, 2002.
32. Arena F, Romeo C, Cruccetti A, Centonze A, et al: Fetal vesicoureteral reflux: neonatal findings and follow-up study, *Pediatr Med Chir* 23:31-34, 2001.
33. Horowitz M, Gershbein AB, Glassberg KI: Vesicoureteral reflux in infants with prenatal hydronephrosis confirmed at birth: racial differences, *J Urol* 161:248-50, 1999.
34. Chand DH, Rhoades T, Poe SA, Kraus S, Strife CF: Incidence and severity of vesicoureteral reflux in children related to age, gender, race and diagnosis, *J Urol* 170:1548-50, 2003.
35. Skoog SJ, Belman AB: Primary vesicoureteral reflux in the black child, *Pediatrics* 87:538-43, 1991.
36. Pinto KJ: Vesicoureteral reflux in the Hispanic child with urinary tract infection, *J Urol* 171:1266-67, 2004.
37. Smellie J, Edwards D, Hunter N, Normand IC, Prescod N: Vesicoureteric reflux and renal scarring, *Kidney Int Suppl* 4:S65-72, 1975.
38. Dick PT, Feldman W: Routine diagnostic imaging for childhood urinary tract infections: a systematic overview, *J Pediatr* 128:15-22, 1996.
39. Wennerstrom M, Hansson S, Jodal U, Stokland E: Disappearance of vesicoureteral reflux in children, *Arch Pediatr Adolesc Med* 152:879-83, 1998.
40. American Academy of Pediatrics. Committee on Quality Improvement. Subcommittee on Urinary Tract Infection: Practice parameter: the diagnosis, treatment, and evaluation of the initial urinary tract infection in febrile infants and young children, *Pediatrics* 103:843-52, 1999.
41. Chertin B, Puri P: Familial vesicoureteral reflux, *J Urol* 169:1804-08, 2003.
42. Noe HN, Wyatt RJ, Peeden JN Jr, Rivas ML: The transmission of vesicoureteral reflux from parent to child, *J Urol* 148:1869-71, 1992.
43. McKenna PH, Herndon CD: Voiding dysfunction associated with incontinence, vesicoureteral reflux and recurrent urinary tract infections, *Curr Opin Urol* 10:599-606, 2000.
44. Phan V, Traubici J, Hershenfield B, Stephens D, et al: Vesicoureteral reflux in infants with isolated antenatal hydronephrosis, *Pediatr Nephrol* 18:1224-28, 2003.

45. Zerin JM: Hydronephrosis in the neonate and young infant: current concepts, *Semin Ultrasound CT MR* 15:306-16, 1994.
46. Ditchfield MR, de Campo JF, Nolan TM, Cook DJ, et al: Risk factors in the development of early renal cortical defects in children with urinary tract infection, *AJR Am J Roentgenol* 162:1393-97, 1994.
47. Majd M, Rushton HG, Jantausch B, Wiedermann BL: Relationship among vesicoureteral reflux, P-fimbriated *Escherichia coli*, and acute pyelonephritis in children with febrile urinary tract infection, *J Pediatr* 119:578-85, 1991.
48. Piepsz A, Tamminen-Mobius T, Reiners C, Heikkila J, et al: Five-year study of medical or surgical treatment in children with severe vesico-ureteral reflux dimercaptosuccinic acid findings. International Reflux Study Group in Europe, *Eur J Pediatr* 157:753-58, 1998.
49. Gruneberg R: Relationship of infecting urinary organism to the faecal flora in patients with symptomatic urinary tract infection, *Lancet* 2:766-68, 1969.
50. Bollgren I, Winberg J: The periurethral aerobic bacterial flora in healthy boys and girls, *Acta Paediatr Scand* 65:74-80, 1976.
51. Rushton HG Jr: Vesicoureteral reflux—new concepts and techniques, *J Urol* 157:1414-15, 1997.
52. Jequier S, Jequier JC: Reliability of voiding cystourethrography to detect reflux, *AJR Am J Roentgenol* 153:807-10, 1989.
53. McDonald A, Scranton M, Gillespie R, Mahajan V, Edwards GA: Voiding cystourethrograms and urinary tract infections: how long to wait?, *Pediatrics* 105:E50, 2000.
54. Mahant S, To T, Friedman J: Timing of voiding cystourethrogram in the investigation of urinary tract infections in children, *J Pediatr* 139:568-71, 2001.
55. Merguerian PA, Corbett ST, Cravero J: Voiding ability using propofol sedation in children undergoing voiding cystourethrograms: a retrospective analysis, *J Urol* 176:299-302, 2006.
56. Ward VL, Barnewolt CE, Strauss KJ, Lebowitz RL, et al: Radiation exposure reduction during voiding cystourethrography in a pediatric porcine model of vesicoureteral reflux, *Radiology* 238:96-106, 2006.
57. Thompson M, Simon SD, Sharma V, Alon US: Timing of follow-up voiding cystourethrogram in children with primary vesicoureteral reflux: development and application of a clinical algorithm, *Pediatrics* 115:426-34, 2005.
58. Gelfand MJ, Strife JL, Hertzberg VS: Low-grade vesicoureteral reflux. Variability in grade on sequential radiographic and nuclear cystograms, *Clin Nucl Med* 16:243-46, 1991.
59. Unver T, Alpay H, Biyikli NK, Ones T: Comparison of direct radionuclide cystography and voiding cystourethrography in detecting vesicoureteral reflux, *Pediatr Int* 48:287-91, 2006.
60. Bosio M, Manzoni GA: Detection of posterior urethral valves with voiding cystourethrosonography with echo contrast, *J Urol* 168:1711-15; discussion 1715, 2002.
61. Piaggio G, Degl'Innocenti ML, Toma P, Calevo MG, Perfumo F: Cystosonography and voiding cystourethrography in the diagnosis of vesicoureteral reflux, *Pediatr Nephrol* 18:18-22, 2003.
62. Uhl M, Kromeier J, Zimmerhackl LB, Darge K: Simultaneous voiding cystourethrography and voiding urosonography, *Acta Radiol* 44:265-68, 2003.
63. Wille S, von Knobloch R, Klose KJ, Heidenreich A, Hofmann R: Magnetic resonance urography in pediatric urology, *Scand J Urol Nephrol* 37:16-21, 2003.
64. Nolte-Ernsting C, Glowinski A, Schaeffter T, Adam G, Gunther RW: Gadolinium-enhanced magnetic resonance fluoroscopy used as micturating cystourethrography: experiences in adult male patients, *Invest Radiol* 38:617-24, 2003.
65. Lee SK, Chang Y, Park NH, Kim YH, Woo S: Magnetic resonance voiding cystography in the diagnosis of vesicoureteral reflux: comparative study with voiding cystourethrography, *J Magn Reson Imaging* 21:406-14, 2005.
66. Kirsch AJ, Grattan-Smith JD, Molitierno JA Jr: The role of magnetic resonance imaging in pediatric urology, *Curr Opin Urol* 16:283-90, 2006.
67. Caione P, Ciofetta G, Collura G, Morano S, Capozza N: Renal damage in vesico-ureteric reflux, *BJU Int* 93:591-95, 2004.
68. Merguerian PA, Jamal MA, Agarwal SK, McLorie GA, et al: Utility of SPECT DMSA renal scanning in the evaluation of children with primary vesicoureteral reflux, *Urology* 53:1024-28, 1999.
69. Ozen HA, Basar I, Erbas B, Ozen S, et al: DMSA renal scanning versus urography for detecting renal scars in vesicoureteral reflux, *Eur Urol* 17:47-50, 1990.
70. Stock JA, Wilson D, Hanna MK: Congenital reflux nephropathy and severe unilateral fetal reflux, *J Urol* 160:1017-18, 1998.
71. Yen TC, Tzen KY, Lin WY, Chen WP, Lin CY: Identification of new renal scarring in repeated episodes of acute pyelonephritis using Tc-99m DMSA renal SPECT, *Clin Nucl Med* 23:828-31, 1998.
72. Ataei N, Madani A, Habibi R, Khorasani M: Evaluation of acute pyelonephritis with DMSA scans in children presenting after the age of 5 years, *Pediatr Nephrol* 20:1439-44, 2005.
73. Hansson S, Dhamey M, Sigstrom O, Sixt R, et al: Dimercapto-succinic acid scintigraphy instead of voiding cystourethrography for infants with urinary tract infection, *J Urol* 172:1071-73; discussion 1073-74, 2004.
74. Ajdinovic B, Jaukovic L, Krstic Z, Dopuda M: Technetium-99m-dimercaptosuccinic acid renal scintigraphy in children with urinary tract infections, *Hell J Nucl Med* 9:27-30, 2006.
75. Tareen BU, Bui D, McMahon DR, Nasrallah PF: Role of positional instillation of contrast cystography in the algorithm for evaluating children with confirmed pyelonephritis, *Urology* 67:1055-57; discussion 1058-59, 2006.
76. Edmondson JD, Maizels M, Alpert SA, Kirsch AJ, et al: Multi-institutional experience with PIC cystography—incidence of occult vesicoureteral reflux in children with febrile urinary tract infections, *Urology* 67:608-11, 2006.
77. Duckett JW, Bellinger MF: A plea for standardized grading of vesicoureteral reflux, *Eur Urol* 8:74-77, 1982.
78. Papachristou F, Printza N, Kavaki D, Koliakos G: The characteristics and outcome of primary vesicoureteric reflux diagnosed in the first year of life, *Int J Clin Pract* 60:829-34, 2006.
79. Routh JC, Vandersteen DR, Pfefferle H, Wolpert JJ, Reinberg Y: Single center experience with endoscopic management of vesicoureteral reflux in children, *J Urol* 175:1889-92; discussion 1892-1883, 2006.
80. Badwan KH, Diamond DA: Vesicoureteral reflux: diagnosis and management, *J Med Liban* 53:61-65, 2005.
81. Wan J, Greenfield SP, Ng M, Zerin M, et al: Sibling reflux: a dual center retrospective study, *J Urol* 156:677-79, 1996.
82. Hollowell JG, Greenfield SP: Screening siblings for vesicoureteral reflux, *J Urol* 168:2138-41, 2002.
83. Ataei N, Madani A, Esfahani ST, Kejbafzadeh A, et al: Screening for vesicoureteral reflux and renal scars in siblings of children with known reflux, *Pediatr Nephrol* 19:1127-31, 2004.
84. Chapman CJ, Bailey RR, Janus ED, Abbott GD, Lynn KL: Vesicoureteral reflux: segregation analysis, *Am J Med Genet* 20:577-84, 1985.
85. Kaefer M, Curran M, Treves ST, Bauer S, et al: Sibling vesicoureteral reflux in multiple gestation births, *Pediatrics* 105:800-04, 2000.
86. Feather SA, Malcolm S, Woolf AS: Primary, nonsyndromic vesicoureteral reflux and its nephropathy is genetically heterogeneous, with locus on chromosome 1, *Am J Hum Genet* 66:1420-25, 2000.
87. McLorie GA, McKenna PH, Jumper BM, Churchill BM, et al: High grade vesicoureteral reflux: analysis of observational therapy, *J Urol* 144:537-40; discussion 545, 1990.
88. Skoog SJ, Belman AB, Majd M: A nonsurgical approach to the management of primary vesicoureteral reflux, *J Urol* 138:941-46, 1987.
89. Husmann DA, Allen TD: Resolution of vesicoureteral reflux in completely duplicated systems: fact or fiction? *J Urol* 145:1022-23, 1991.
90. Arant BS Jr: Medical management of mild and moderate vesicoureteral reflux: followup studies of infants and young children. A preliminary report of the Southwest Pediatric Nephrology Study Group, *J Urol* 148:1683-87, 1992.
91. Huang FY, Tsai TC: Resolution of vesicoureteral reflux during medical management in children, *Pediatr Nephrol* 9:715-17, 1995.

92. Bouachrine H, Lemelle JL, Didier F, Schmitt M: A follow-up study of pre-natally detected primary vesico-ureteric reflux: a review of 61 patients, *Br J Urol* 78:936-39, 1996.
93. Ransley PG, Risdon RA, Godley ML: High pressure sterile vesicoureteral reflux and renal scarring: an experimental study in the pig and minipig, *Contrib Nephrol* 39:320-43, 1984.
94. Smellie JM, Normand IC: Bacteriuria, reflux and renal scarring, *Arch Dis Child* 50:581-85, 1975.
95. Rolleston GL, Shannon FT, Utley WL: Relationship of infantile vesicoureteric reflux to renal damage, *Br Med J* 1:460-63, 1970.
96. Rolleston GL, Shannon FT, Utley WL: Follow-up of vesico-ureteral reflux in the newborn, *Kidney Int Suppl* 4:S59-64, 1975.
97. Bellinger MF, Duckett JW: Vesicoureteral reflux: a comparison of non-surgical and surgical management, *Contrib Nephrol* 39:81-93, 1984.
98. Smellie JM, Ransley PG, Normand IC, Prescod N, Edwards D: Development of new renal scars: a collaborative study, *Br Med J (Clin Res Ed)* 290:1957-60, 1985.
99. Ozen HA, Whitaker JG: Does the severity of presentation in children with vesicoureteric reflux relate to the severity of the disease or the need for operation?, *Br J Urol* 60:110-12, 1987.
100. Ransley PG, Risdon RA: Renal papillary morphology in infants and young children, *Urol Res* 3:111-13, 1975.
101. Verber IG, Meller ST: Serial 99mTc dimercaptosuccinic acid (DMSA) scans after urinary tract infections presenting before the age of 5 years, *Arch Dis Child* 64:1533-37, 1989.
102. Lackgren G, Wahlin N, Skoldenberg E, Stenberg A: Long-term followup of children treated with dextranomer/hyaluronic acid copolymer for vesicoureteral reflux, *J Urol* 166:1887-92, 2001.
103. Stokland E, Hellstrom M, Jacobsson B, Jodal U, Sixt R: Renal damage one year after first urinary tract infection: role of dimercaptosuccinic acid scintigraphy, *J Pediatr* 129:815-20, 1996.
104. Miller T, Phillips S: Pyelonephritis: the relationship between infection, renal scarring and antimicrobial therapy, *Kidney Int* 19:654-62, 1994.
105. Jodal U: The natural history of bacteriuria in childhood, *Infect Dis Clin North Am* 1:713-29, 1987.
106. Jakobsson B, Berg U, Svensson L: Renal scarring after acute pyelonephritis, *Arch Dis Child* 70:111-15, 1994.
107. Lomberg H, Hellstrom M, Jodal U, Leffler H, et al: Virulence-associated traits in *Escherichia coli* causing first and recurrent episodes of urinary tract infection in children with or without vesicoureteral reflux, *J Infect Dis* 150:561-69, 1984.
108. de Man P, Claeson I, Johanson IM, Jodal U, Svanborg Eden C: Bacterial attachment as a predictor of renal abnormalities in boys with urinary tract infection, *J Pediatr* 115:915-22, 1989.
109. Ozen S, Alikasifoglu M, Saatci U: Implications of certain genetic polymorphisms in scarring in vesicoureteric reflux: importance of ACE polymorphism, *Am J Kidney Dis* 34:140-45, 1999.
110. Hohenfellner K, Hunley TE, Brezinska R, Brodhag P, et al: ACE I/D gene polymorphism predicts renal damage in congenital uropathies, *Pediatr Nephrol* 13:514-18, 1999.
111. Ohtomo Y, Nagaoka R, Kaneko K, Fukuda Y, et al: Angiotensin converting enzyme gene polymorphism in primary vesicoureteral reflux, *Pediatr Nephrol* 16:648-52, 2001.
112. Rose JS, Glassberg KI, Waterhouse K: Intrarenal reflux and its relationship to renal scarring, *J Urol* 113:400-03, 1975.
113. Senekjian HO, Suki WN: Vesicoureteral reflux and reflux nephropathy, *Am J Nephrol* 2:245-50, 1982.
114. Gruneberg RN, Leakey A, Bendall MJ, Smellie JM: Bowel flora in urinary tract infection: effect of chemotherapy with special reference to cotrimoxazole, *Kidney Int Suppl* 4:S122-29, 1975.
115. Smellie JM, Katz G, Gruneberg RN: Controlled trial of prophylactic treatment in childhood urinary tract infection, *Lancet* 2:175-78, 1978.
116. Tamminen-Mobius T, Brunier E, Ebel KD, Lebowitz R, et al: Cessation of vesicoureteral reflux for 5 years in infants and children allocated to medical treatment. The International Reflux Study in Children, *J Urol* 148:1662-66, 1992.
117. Birmingham Reflux Study Group: Prospective trial of operative versus non-operative treatment of severe vesicoureteric reflux in children: five years' observation, *Br Med J (Clin Res Ed)* 295:237-41, 1987.
118. Allen UD, MacDonald N, Fuite L, Chan F, Stephens D: Risk factors for resistance to "first-line" antimicrobials among urinary tract isolates of *Escherichia coli* in children, *Can Med Assoc J* 160:1436-40, 1999.
119. Prais D, Straussberg R, Avitzur Y, Nussinovitch M, et al: Bacterial susceptibility to oral antibiotics in community acquired urinary tract infection, *Arch Dis Child* 88:215-18, 2003.
120. Karpman E, Kurzrock EA: Adverse reactions of nitrofurantoin, trimethoprim and sulfamethoxazole in children, *J Urol* 172:448-53, 2004.
121. Smellie JM, Tamminen-Mobius T, Olbing H, Claesson I, et al: Five-year study of medical or surgical treatment in children with severe reflux: radiological renal findings. The International Reflux Study in Children, *Pediatr Nephrol* 6:223-30, 1992.
122. Weiss R, Duckett J, Spitzer A: Results of a randomized clinical trial of medical versus surgical management of infants and children with grades III and IV primary vesicoureteral reflux (United States). The International Reflux Study in Children, *J Urol* 148:1667-73, 1992.
123. O'Donnell B, Puri P: Technical refinements in endoscopic correction of vesicoureteral reflux, *J Urol* 140:1101-02, 1988.
124. Geiss S, Alessandrini P, Allouch G, Aubert D, et al: Multicenter survey of endoscopic treatment of vesicoureteral reflux in children, *Eur Urol* 17:328-29, 1990.
125. Smith DP, Kaplan WE, Oyasu R: Evaluation of polydimethylsiloxane as an alternative in the endoscopic treatment of vesicoureteral reflux, *J Urol* 152:1221-24, 1994.
126. Lipsky H: Endoscopic treatment of vesicoureteric reflux with bovine collagen, *Eur Urol* 18:52-55, 1990.
127. Leonard MP, Canning DA, Peters CA, Gearhart JP, Jeffs RD: Endoscopic injection of glutaraldehyde cross-linked bovine dermal collagen for correction of vesicoureteral reflux, *J Urol* 145:115-19, 1991.
128. Reunanen M: Correction of vesicoureteral reflux in children by endoscopic collagen injection: a prospective study, *J Urol* 154:2156-58, 1995.
129. Frankenschmidt A, Katzenwadel A, Zimmerhackl LB, Sommerkamp H: Endoscopic treatment of reflux by subureteric collagen injection: critical review of 5 years' experience, *J Endourol* 11:343-48, 1997.
130. Atala A, Kim W, Paige KT, Vacanti CA, Retik AB: Endoscopic treatment of vesicoureteral reflux with a chondrocyte-alginate suspension, *J Urol* 152:641-43; discussion 644, 1994.
131. Atala A, Peters CA, Retik AB, Mandell J: Endoscopic treatment of vesicoureteral reflux with a self-detachable balloon system, *J Urol* 148:724-27, 1992.
132. Atala A, Cima LG, Kim W, Paige KT, et al: Injectable alginate seeded with chondrocytes as a potential treatment for vesicoureteral reflux, *J Urol* 150:745-47, 1993.
133. Stenberg A, Lackgren G: A new bioimplant for the endoscopic treatment of vesicoureteral reflux: experimental and short-term clinical results, *J Urol* 154:800-03, 1995.
134. Kirsch AJ, Perez-Brayfield M, Smith EA, Scherz HC: The modified sting procedure to correct vesicoureteral reflux: improved results with submucosal implantation within the intramural ureter, *J Urol* 171:2413-16, 2004.
135. Dean GE, Doumanian LR: The extended use of deflux (dextranomer/hyaluronic acid) in pediatric urology, *Curr Urol Rep* 7:143-48, 2006.
136. Aaronson IA: Does deflux alter the paradigm for the management of children with vesicoureteral reflux? *Curr Urol Rep* 6:152-56, 2005.
137. Atala A, Kavoussi LR, Goldstein DS, Retik AB, Peters CA: Laparoscopic correction of vesicoureteral reflux, *J Urol* 150:748-51, 1993.
138. Kawauchi A, Fujito A, Soh J, Ukimura O, et al: Laparoscopic correction of vesicoureteral reflux using the Lich-Gregoir technique: initial experience and technical aspects, *Int J Urol* 10:90-93, 2003.
139. Janetschek G, Radmayr C, Bartsch G: Laparoscopic ureteral antireflux plasty reimplantation. First clinical experience, *Ann Urol (Paris)* 29:101-05, 1995.

140. Gill IS, Ponsky LE, Desai M, Kay R, Ross JH: Laparoscopic cross-trigonal Cohen ureteroneocystostomy: novel technique, *J Urol* 166:1811-14, 2001.
141. Yeung CK, Sihoe JD, Borzi PA: Endoscopic cross-trigonal ureteral reimplantation under carbon dioxide bladder insufflation: a novel technique, *J Endourol* 19:295-99, 2005.
142. Politano VA, Leadbetter WF: An operative technique for the correction of vesicoureteral reflux, *J Urol* 79:932-41, 1958.
143. Caione P, Capozza N, Asili L, Lais A, Matarazzo E: Is primary obstructive megaureter repair at risk for contralateral reflux? *J Urol* 164:1061-63, 2000.
144. Duckett JW, Walker RD, Weiss R: Surgical results: International Reflux Study in Children—United States branch, *J Urol* 148:1674-75, 1992.
145. Cohen M: The first urinary tract infection in male children, *Am J Dis Child* 130:810-13, 1976.
146. Kennelly MJ, Bloom DA, Ritchey ML, Panzl AC: Outcome analysis of bilateral Cohen cross-trigonal ureteroneocystostomy, *Urology* 46:393-95, 1995.
147. El-Ghoneimi A, Odet E, Lamer S, Baudouin V, et al: Cystography after the Cohen ureterovesical reimplantation: is it necessary at a training center?, *J Urol* 162:1201-02, 1999.
148. Pfister C, Ravasse P, Barret E, Petit T, Mitrofanoff P: The value of endoscopic treatment for ureteroceles during the neonatal period, *J Urol* 159:1006-09, 1998.
149. Hoenig DM, Diamond DA, Rabinowitz R, Caldamone AA: Contralateral reflux after unilateral ureteral reimplantation, *J Urol* 156:196-97, 1996.
150. Diamond DA, Rabinowitz R, Hoenig D, Caldamone AA: The mechanism of new onset contralateral reflux following unilateral ureteroneocystostomy, *J Urol* 156:665-67, 1996.
151. Ringert RH: [Surgical therapy of vesicoureterorenal reflux in children], *Urologe A* 22:410-13, 1983.
152. Linn R, Ginesin Y, Bolkier M, Levin DR: Lich-Gregoir anti-reflux operation: a surgical experience and 5-20 years of follow-up in 149 ureters, *Eur Urol* 16:200-03, 1989.
153. Barrieras D, Lapointe S, Reddy PP, Williot P, et al: Urinary retention after bilateral extravesical ureteral reimplantation: does dissection distal to the ureteral orifice have a role?, *J Urol* 162:1197-1200, 1999.
154. Filly R, Friedland GW, Govan DE, Fair WR: Development and progression of clubbing and scarring in children with recurrent urinary tract infections, *Radiology* 113:145-53, 1974.
155. Goldraich NP, Goldraich IH: Update on dimercaptosuccinic acid renal scanning in children with urinary tract infection, *Pediatr Nephrol* 9:221-26; discussion 227, 1995.
156. Shindo S, Bernstein J, Arant BS Jr: Evolution of renal segmental atrophy (Ask-Upmark kidney) in children with vesicoureteric reflux: radiographic and morphologic studies, *J Pediatr* 102:847-54, 1983.
157. Rushton HG, Majd M, Jantausch B, Wiedermann BL, Belman AB: Renal scarring following reflux and nonreflux pyelonephritis in children: evaluation with 99mtechnetium-dimercaptosuccinic acid scintigraphy, *J Urol* 147:1327-32, 1992.
158. Jakobsson B, Noldstedt L, Svensson L, Soderlundh S, Berg U: 99mTechnetium-dimercaptosuccinic acid scan in the diagnosis of acute pyelonephritis in children: relation to clinical and radiological findings, *Pediatr Nephrol* 6:328-34, 1992.
159. Kaack MB, Dowling KJ, Patterson GM, Roberts JA: Immunology of pyelonephritis. VIII. *E. coli* causes granulocytic aggregation and renal ischemia, *J Urol* 136:1117-22, 1986.
160. Roberts JA: Mechanisms of renal damage in chronic pyelonephritis (reflux nephropathy), *Curr Top Pathol* 88:265-87, 1995.
161. Roberts JA, Domingue GJ, Martin LN, Kim JC: Immunology of pyelonephritis in the primate model: live versus heat-killed bacteria, *Kidney Int* 19:297-305, 1981.
162. McCord JM: Oxygen-derived free radicals in postischemic tissue injury, *N Engl J Med* 312:159-63, 1985.
163. Eddy AA: Interstitial macrophages as mediators of renal fibrosis, *Exp Nephrol* 3:76-79, 1995.
164. Muller GA, Strutz FM: Renal fibroblast heterogeneity, *Kidney Int Suppl* 50:S33-36, 1995.
165. Roberts JA: Pathogenesis of pyelonephritis, *J Urol* 129:1102-06, 1983.
166. Chantler C, Carter JE, Bewick M, Counahan R, et al: 10 years' experience with regular hemodialysis and renal transplantation, *Arch Dis Child* 55:435-45, 1980.
167. Deleau J, Andre JL, Briancon S, Musse JP: Chronic renal failure in children: an epidemiological survey in Lorraine (France) 1975-1990, *Pediatr Nephrol* 8:472-76, 1994.
168. Smellie JM, Prescod NP, Shaw PJ, Risdon RA, Bryant TN: Childhood reflux and urinary infection: a follow-up of 10-41 years in 226 adults, *Pediatr Nephrol* 12:727-36, 1998.
169. Wallace DM, Rothwell DL, Williams DI: The long-term follow-up of surgically treated vesicoureteric reflux, *Br J Urol* 50:479-84, 1978.
170. Jacobson SH, Eklof O, Eriksson CG, Lins LE, et al: Development of hypertension and uraemia after pyelonephritis in childhood: 27 year follow-up, *BMJ* 299:703-06, 1989.
171. Mansfield JT, Snow BW, Cartwright PC, Wadsworth K: Complications of pregnancy in women after childhood reimplantation for vesicoureteral reflux: an update with 25 years of followup, *J Urol* 154:787-90, 1995.
172. Jungers P, Houillier P, Chauveau D, Choukroun G, et al: Pregnancy in women with reflux nephropathy, *Kidney Int* 50:593-99, 1996.
173. Lebowitz RL, Mandell J: Urinary tract infections in children: putting radiology in its place, *Radiology* 165:1-9, 1987.
174. Vandenbossche M, Delhove O, Dumortier P, Deneft F, Schulman CC: Endoscopic treatment of reflux: experimental study and review of Teflon and collagen, *Eur Urol* 23:386-93, 1993.
175. Winberg J, Bollgren I, Kallenius G, Mollby R, Svenson SB: Clinical pyelonephritis and focal renal scarring. A selected review of pathogenesis, prevention and prognosis, *Pediatr Clin North Am* 29:801-14, 1982.
176. Winter AL, Hardy BE, Alton DJ, Arbus GS, Churchill BM: Acquired renal scars in children, *J Urol* 129:1190-94, 1983.
177. Dwoskin JY, Perlmutter AD: Vesicoureteral reflux in children: a computerized review, *J Urol* 109:888-90, 1973.
178. Lenaghan D, Whitaker JG, Jensen F, Stephens FD: The natural history of reflux and long-term effects of reflux on the kidney, *J Urol* 115:728-30, 1976.
179. Anderson PA, Rickwood AM: Features of primary vesicoureteric reflux detected by prenatal sonography, *Br J Urol* 67:267-71, 1991.
180. Crabbe DC, Thomas DF, Gordon AC, Irving HC, et al: Use of 99m technetium-dimercaptosuccinic acid to study patterns of renal damage associated with prenatally detected vesicoureteral reflux, *J Urol* 148:1229-31, 1992.
181. Gordon AC, Thomas DF, Arthur RJ, Irving HC, Smith SE: Prenatally diagnosed reflux: a follow-up study, *Br J Urol* 65:407-12, 1990.
182. Hellerstein S: Long-term consequences of urinary tract infections, *Curr Opin Pediatr* 12:125-28, 2000.
183. Wennerstrom M, Hansson S, Jodal U, Stokland E: Primary and acquired renal scarring in boys and girls with urinary tract infection, *J Pediatr* 136:30-34, 2000.
184. Elder JS, Peters CA, Arant BS Jr, Ewalt DH, et al: Pediatric Vesicoureteral Reflux Guidelines Panel summary report on the management of primary vesicoureteral reflux in children, *J Urol* 157: 1846-51, 1997.
185. Jodal U, Lindberg U: Guidelines for management of children with urinary tract infection and vesicoureteric reflux. Recommendations from a Swedish state-of-the-art conference. Swedish Medical Research Council, *Acta Paediatr Suppl* 88:87-89, 1999.
186. Gordon I, Barkovics M, Pindoria S, Cole TJ, Woolf AS: Primary vesicoureteric reflux as a predictor of renal damage in children hospitalized with urinary tract infection: a systematic review and meta-analysis, *J Am Soc Nephrol* 14:739-44, 2003.
187. Williams G, Lee A, Craig J: Antibiotics for the prevention of urinary tract infection in children: a systematic review of randomized controlled trials, *J Pediatr* 138:868-74, 2001.
188. Wheeler D, Vimalachandra D, Hodson EM, Roy LP, et al: Antibiotics and surgery for vesicoureteric reflux: a meta-analysis of randomized controlled trials, *Arch Dis Child* 88:688-94, 2003.

CHAPTER 37

Obstructive Genitourinary Disorders

Armando J. Lorenzo, Dagmar Csaicsich, Christoph Aufricht, and Antoine E. Khoury

INTRODUCTION

Obstructive uropathy is an all-inclusive term that comprises a heterogeneous group of pathologies. The causes, onset, presentation, and clinical course are quite diverse, thus making generalizations difficult. Nevertheless, to have a working definition, *obstruction* can be thought of as a restriction of urine flow which, if left uncorrected, will lead to progressive renal deterioration[1-3] or hamper normal renal development.[4,5] This concept underscores the fact that, in many cases, we wait for evidence of renal damage before firmly establishing a diagnosis and even acting upon a potentially obstructive process.

The obstructive process can occur at multiple levels of the urinary tract, including the urethra, the bladder outlet, and the ureters. Obstructive uropathy represents one of the largest fractions of identifiable causes of renal failure in the pediatric population.[6] In association with congenital aplasia/hypoplasia/dysplasia, it accounts for almost half of all cases of chronic kidney disease in children.[7] For example, in the ItalKid project (which encompassed a population base of 16.8 million children), hypodysplasia with an identified uropathy affected 43.6% of registered patients and 27.1% of those who reached end-stage renal disease.[8] As shown in Table 37-1, posterior urethral valves are second only to vesicoureteral reflux as the most common underlying diagnosis. However, these figures represent only the tip of the iceberg in that they do not account for the patients with morbidity that is related to borderline renal function or other sequelae (e.g., hypertension).

DEFINITION OF OBSTRUCTION

In the clinical setting, obstruction is usually presumed when dilatation of the urinary tract is detected (i.e., hydronephrosis). Unfortunately, this finding does not necessarily correlate with the presence or degree of antegrade urine flow impediment, because nonobstructive conditions can show similar findings (e.g., vesicoureteral reflux), and great variability in the natural history of different degrees of hydronephrosis has been documented. If anything, hydronephrosis can only be considered a crude marker of obstruction. As a rule of thumb, it can be expected that not every patient with urinary tract dilatation has an obstruction; however, most cases of obstruction will lead to urinary tract dilatation. Importantly, hydronephrosis per se does not allow for any reliable correlation with the affected kidney's function.

In essence, impaired urine flow leads to mechanical distention and elevated intraluminal pressures that, when transmitted to the renal parenchyma, result in a loss of functional mass. How the treating physician reacts is determined by the degree of dilatation, its impact on the renal parenchyma, and the progressive nature of the insult over time (i.e., a progressively worsening pattern is considered more robust evidence than a single set of measurements).

Ultimately, hydronephrosis is a problem when it affects renal function and poses a threat to the child's health. These are the principles that currently guide the management of conditions that are thought to be associated with obstruction, such as antenatal hydronephrosis, primary megaureter, and ureteropelvic junction abnormalities. Some kidneys will have irreversible renal injury at the time of diagnosis, whereas others will have progressive damage if left untreated; however, the largest proportion improves without intervention. Furthermore, other children may present with hydronephrosis caused by a nonobstructive process that leads to progressive renal damage and scarring (i.e., vesicoureteral reflux; Figure 37-1). Identifying and categorizing these groups continue to challenge pediatric nephrologists and urologists.

BIOMECHANICAL PRINCIPLES

From a mechanistic point of view, the urinary tract consists of a series of conduits and reservoirs with the ultimate goal of transporting the urine produced by the kidneys. As such, the static and dynamic properties of this system have to be considered to better understand the consequences of obstruction. Important considerations include structure compliance, the level and degree of flow impairment, urine production and renal function, and the neurohumoral activity (Figure 37-2). Furthermore, the onset and duration of the process appear to correlate with both abnormal renal development and the deterioration of function. These are situations that are difficult to separate at times, because congenital obstruction may affect normal development or renal maturation without necessarily impairing function. It is common to see

TABLE 37-1 Urinary Tract Malformations Associated with Hypodysplasia in Children with Chronic Renal Failure[8]

Urinary Malformation	Number	Percentage
Vesicoureteral reflux	309	59.2%
Posterior urethral valves	124	23.8%
Urethral hypoplasia/atresia	12	2.3%
Ureteropelvic junction stenosis	19	3.6%
Obstructive megaureter	18	3.5%
Ureterocele	9	1.7%
Duplication of collection system	8	1.5%
Other complex uropathies	23	4.4%

TABLE 37-2 Molecules Implicated in Renal Injury after Urinary Tract Obstruction

I. Interstitial inflammation
   a. Angiotensin II
   b. Transforming growth factor β1
   c. Nuclear factor κB
   d. Mutant monocyte chemoatractant protein 1
   e. Activated macrophages
   f. Selectins

II. Tubular apoptosis
   a. Reactive oxygen species
   b. Caspases
   c. Cellular stretch
   d. Epidermal growth factor
   e. Tumor necrosis factor α
   f. Death-associated protein kinase

III. Interstitial fibrosis
   a. CD44
   b. Angiotensin II
   c. Transforming growth factor β1
   d. Smad2 and Smad3
   e. β-catenin
   f. Connective tissue growth factor

(Based on Chevalier RL: Pathogenesis of renal injury in obstructive uropathy, *Curr Opin Pediatr* 18(2):153-60, 2006.)

this clinical variability in patients who are thought to have similar obstructive processes.

The dynamic nature of urinary flow impairment deserves particular attention. Unlike the controlled environment, with the established onset and finite end points found in laboratory experiments, obstruction in vivo changes over time and leads to compensatory processes that condition either better tolerance or the worsening of the functional or morphologic status of the kidney. For example, as obstruction persists or worsens, the system can adapt by means of changes in glomerular filtration that ultimately lead to decreased urine production and lower pressures. Moreover, the renal pelvis or ureter may also change its properties, thus allowing for a higher volume to be accepted without a significant increase in pressure (i.e., improved compliance)[9,10]; this leads to less pressure buildup until a specific threshold is reached. In such specific circumstances, dilatation and increased compliance result in a protective environment with less damage to nephrons over time. This phenomenon helps explain why the grade of hydronephrosis cannot be used as a marker for renal function,[11] why it is important to carefully evaluate the characteristics of the renal parenchyma in contrast with the dilation of the collecting system, and why kidneys may be protected by a large extrarenal pelvis or by the dampening effect of a dilated distal ureter.

PATHOPHYSIOLOGY

Animal Models and Their Limitations

There are multiple animal models that have been used to investigate obstructive uropathy, all with shortcomings that preclude direct extrapolation to humans. Important differences in response to obstruction have been noted among species. One example is the cell-signaling response to epidermal growth factor in unilateral ureteral obstruction, which has opposite apoptotic effects in rats and mice; however, both of these animal models are often used.[12,13] Notwithstanding these limitations, there are many advantages, including the ethical practice of experiments that are not possible in humans. The sheep is commonly used because of the relative ease of performing fetal surgery in these animals. Studies of ureteral ligation and contralateral nephrectomy during early fetal sheep gestation have resulted in severe hydronephrosis and dysplasia[14,15]; this situation contrasts with isolated hydronephrosis when obstruction is created late during gestation.[14] Alternatively, the neonatal rat model is used because only 10% of rat nephrons are present at birth, with the remainder formed during the first 10 postnatal days. Although this development is dramatically different from that of humans, who achieve complete nephron development by 34 weeks' gestation,[16] obstruction of the neonatal rat kidney approximates human fetal obstruction during nephrogenesis. This model has confirmed that the reduction in nephron number is dependent on the duration of obstruction.[17]

Caution should be exercised when extrapolating data from animal models in which the obstructive process is acute and complete rather than partial. Although none of the currently available experimental procedures can accurately recreate spontaneous in utero urine flow impairment, data from models that attempt partial obstruction[18-20] are more likely to be representative of the changes that are expected in the clinical setting of most patients with antenatal hydronephrosis. Some exceptions include the evaluation of multicystic dysplasia and ureteral atresia or situations that could lead to acute postnatal obstruction (e.g., nephrolithiasis).

Mechanical, histopathologic, and humoral effects resulting from obstruction have been described in the different animal models. Reports have shown impaired growth and maturation with a decrease in renal mass, a reduced number of nephrons, hemodynamic changes, tubular atrophy, interstitial fibrosis, and abnormal maturation of the renal vasculature, glomeruli, tubules, and interstitium.[17,21-23] As shown in Table 37-2, molecular analysis has uncovered some of the pathways behind these postobstructive alterations. Reversible models are also beginning to unveil the molecular response to surgical inter-

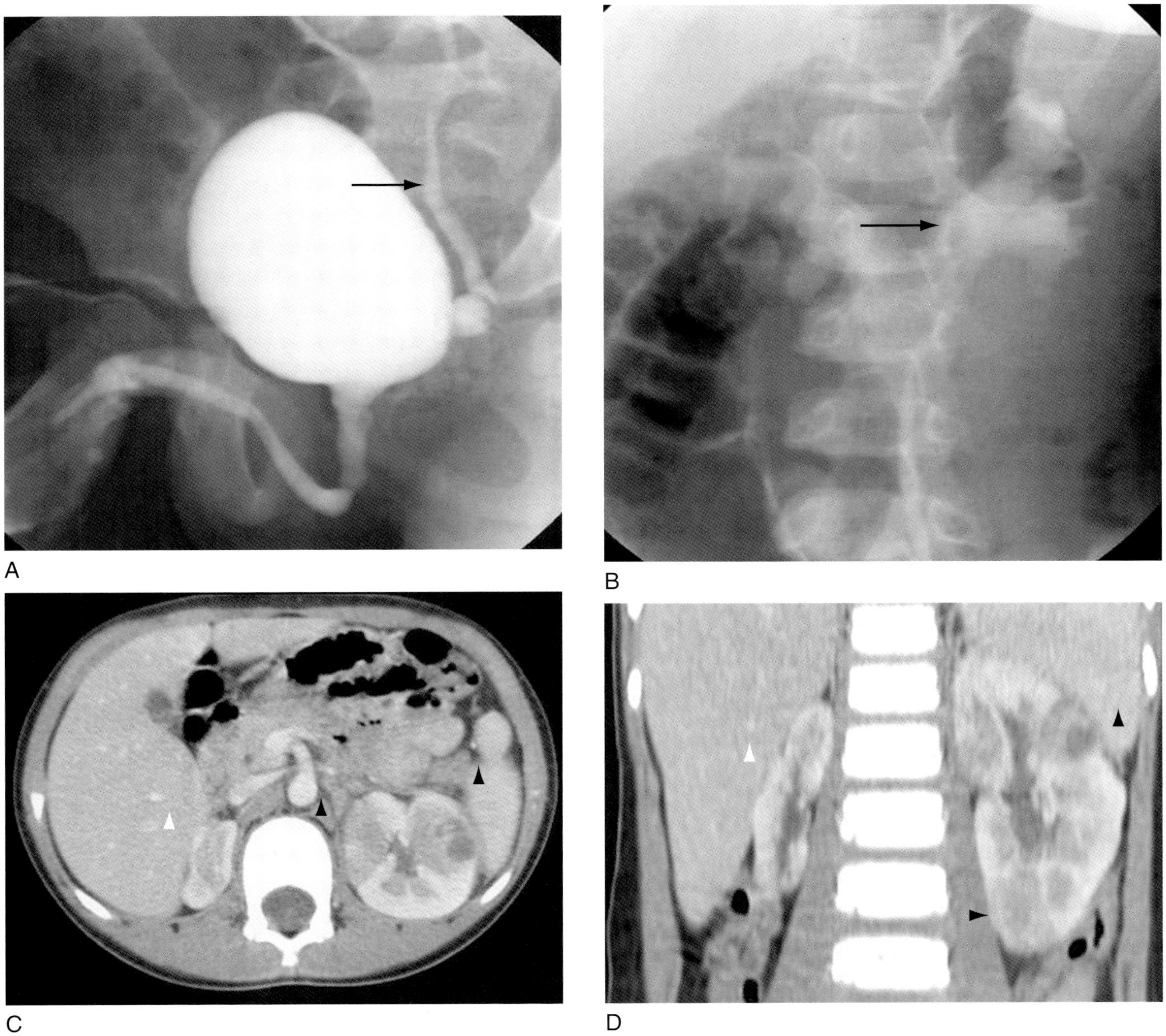

Figure 37-1 **A** and **B,** Vesicoureteral reflux associated with a Hutch diverticulum (*black arrows* point to the ureters). **C,** Atrophic right kidney (adjacent to *white arrowhead*) associated with resolved antenatally detected hydronephrosis. **C** and **D,** Left pyelonephritis *(black arrowhead).*

vention. In fetal sheep, the early relief of unilateral obstruction has resulted in the restoration of nephrogenesis and the renal expression of *PAX2*,[24] whereas similar studies in older rats have shown progressive fibrosis and irreversible changes after obstruction.[25] This latter point is of importance. When the process of interstitial fibrosis involves damage to nephrons and peritubular vasculature, intervention may yield very little recovery. Clinically, fibrosis and irreversible renal damage (i.e., glomerulosclerosis), which are histologically detected in kidneys with poor function, rarely improve after operative correction. Thus, emerging animal data could support the hypothesis that waiting for functional deterioration (as detected by current imaging modalities) may only help prevent or delay further damage after interstitial fibrosis has set in.

Unfortunately, few of the successful animal experiments have resulted in significant changes in clinical practice. For example, although fetal bladder obstruction models showed promising improvement with in utero decompression, human data have been somewhat disappointing.[26-29] Perhaps as a result of the rather simplistic approach to obstruction, researchers have failed to recognize important steps crucial to successful translational work. Therefore, the focus of most modern studies has shifted from hemodynamic and functional analyses to more sophisticated studies of cellular and molecular events.[6] The identification of future biomarkers and molecular therapy is likely to be based on advances in renal function measurement, microscopic anatomy, imaging, and cellular function discovered in experimental models.[30]

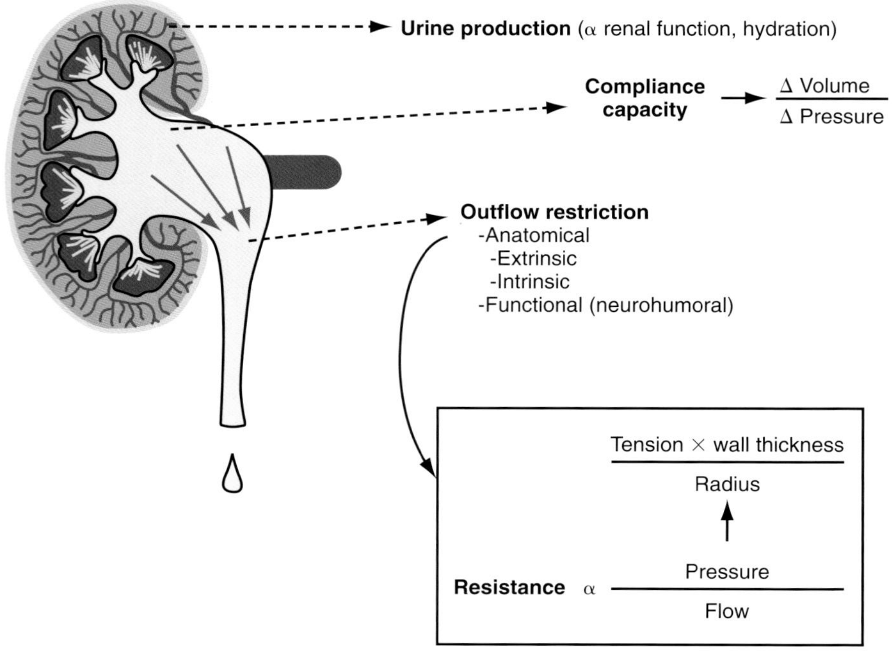

Figure 37-2 Diagram of variables involved in urine flow impairment of the urinary tract. The formulas in the box are based on Laplace's law and the modified Poiseuille-Hagen law.

CLASSIFICATION

As shown in Table 37-3, the differential diagnosis of antenatally detected urinary tract dilatation includes ureteropelvic junction obstruction, ureteral obstruction (ureterovesical obstruction, including ectopic ureteral insertion), posterior urethral valves, prune belly syndrome, urethral atresia or stricture, duplicated collecting system with ureterocele (Figure 37-3), and multicystic renal dysplasia. On the basis of the previously mentioned working definition, many of these patients will improve without intervention or evidence of impaired renal function and thus cannot be classified as obstructed. Hence, many will be considered to have "physiologic" dilatation. In the differential diagnosis, nonobstructive causes of dilatation must also be considered (i.e., vesicoureteral reflux); these may be associated with decreased function as a result of renal dysplasia. At the other end of the spectrum, obstruction may develop as a result of acquired pathologies in an otherwise normally developed urinary tract. In this scenario, the cause can be better understood by dividing the potential causes into extrinsic (i.e., external compression or involvement of the urinary tract), intramural (i.e., pathologic process of the urinary tract wall), and intrinsic (i.e., intraluminal obstructive process). Alternatively, the causes can be divided on the basis of the level of obstruction (i.e., renal/collecting system, ureter, bladder, urethra) and the underlying pathologic process (i.e., neoplastic, inflammatory, traumatic, metabolic). Obviously, congenital and acquired categories may overlap, and patients may present later in life, when it may not be possible to completely differentiate between them.

The level of obstruction is another important consideration. Supravesical lesions are usually unilateral and thus not likely to affect a normal contralateral kidney when present. Conversely, lower abnormalities (bladder, bladder neck, urethra) can put both renal units at risk by affecting the antegrade urine flow of both moieties and/or conditioning a high-pressure/low-compliance reservoir status as seen, for example, in some patients with posterior urethral valves (Figures 37-4 and 37-5). Furthermore, although it is a rela-

TABLE 37-3 **Causes of Prenatal Hydronephrosis Associated with Impaired Antegrade Urine Flow**
Ureteropelvic junction obstruction Extrinsic Intrinsic
Infundibular and infundibulopelvic stenosis
Ureterovesical junction obstruction
Posterior and anterior urethral valves
Ectopic ureteral insertion*
Urethral atresia
Ureteral stricture[105,106]
Retrocaval and retroiliac ureter
Ureterocele*†
Vesicoureteral reflux‡
Prune belly syndrome
Extrinsic compression of urinary tract (pelvic masses, retrocaval ureter, hydrometrocolpos)
Functional pathologies (neurogenic dysfunction, megacystic microcolon intestinal hypoperistalsis syndrome[107])
Complex anatomical abnormalities (cloaca, cloacal exstrophy)

* Commonly seen in association with a duplex system.
† May lead to ipsilateral obstruction or outlet obstruction.
‡ Seen in refluxing obstructive megaureter.

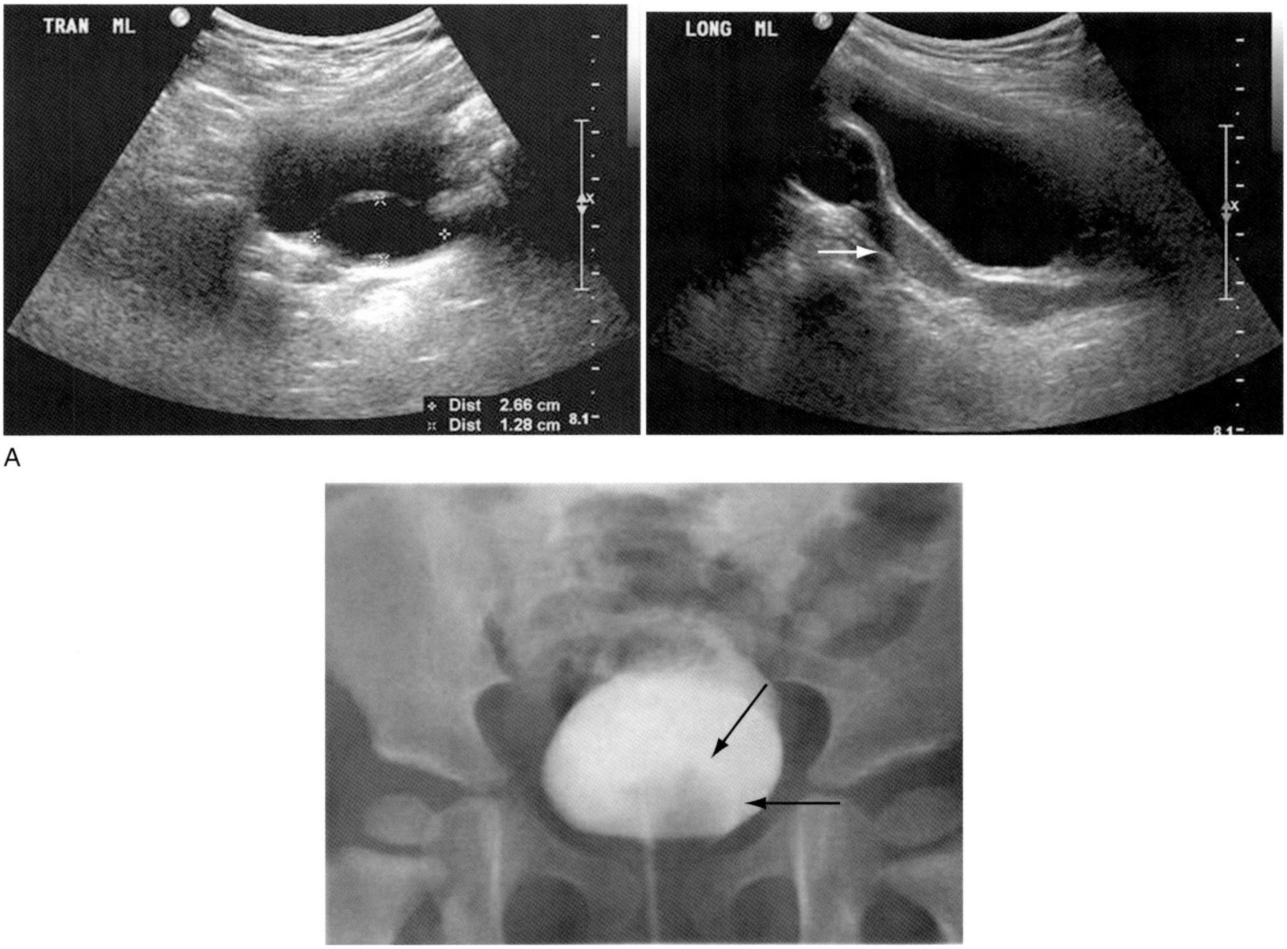

Figure 37-3 Ultrasound images of ureterocele with ipsilateral hydroureter. **A,** Transverse and longitudinal views with a hydroureter *(white arrow)*. **B,** Voiding cystourethrogram, ureterocele defect *(arrows)*.

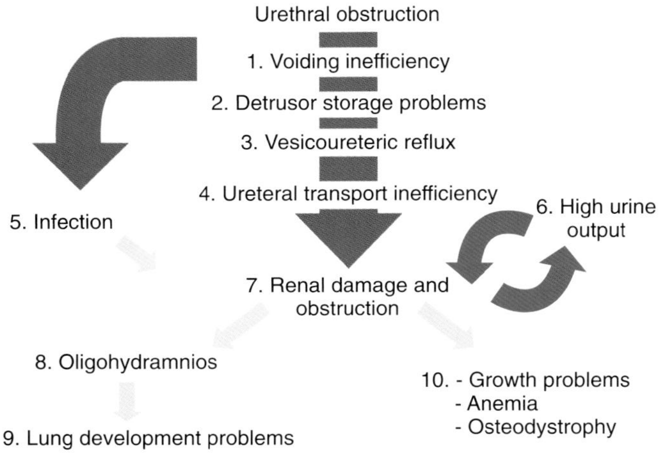

Figure 37-4 Cascade of events associated with congenital urethral obstruction (posterior urethral valves, urethral atresia).

tively rare occurrence, occasionally patients may present with dual abnormalities that complicate the drainage dynamics of the upper tract, such as patients with ureteropelvic junction obstruction and vesicoureteral reflux or children with concurrent hypoperistaltic segments at the ureteropelvic and ureterovesical junctions. Simultaneous abnormalities may not always be readily apparent on imaging studies, and thus they may be difficult to isolate from one another unless more specialized tests are carried out (e.g., percutaneous/retrograde pyelography and/or pressure flow studies).[31-34]

Special situations also arise when patients present with involvement of both renal units (i.e., bilateral ureteropelvic or ureterovesical junction obstruction), when no contralateral kidney is present, or when the contralateral renal unit functions poorly. These patients do not have the benefit of reserve functional parenchyma, thus raising the stakes when a conservative management approach is undertaken.[35,36] Specifically, if the diagnosis of obstruction is based on a loss of function, these situations would be hard to categorize and follow because of the difficulty of interpreting the differential function on a nuclear scan. A decrease of relative function may not only represent a decrease in ipsilateral function but

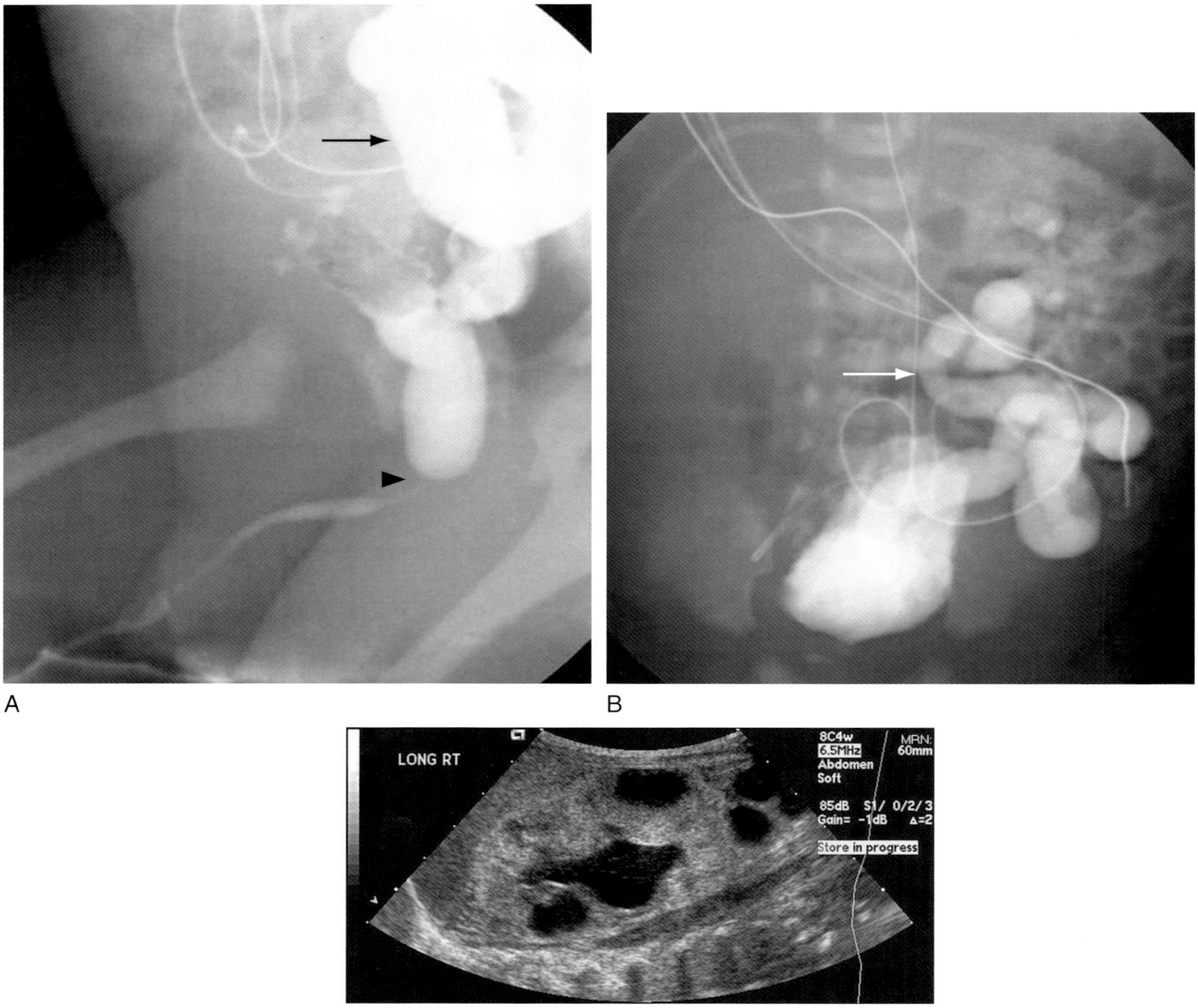

Figure 37-5 Posterior urethral valves. **A** and **B,** Voiding cystourethrogram demonstrating dilated posterior urethra and a change in caliber at the point of obstruction *(black arrowhead)* with high-grade left vesicoureteral reflux *(white arrow)*. The left kidney did not show any residual function on renal scan. **C,** The right kidney appears hyperechoic with multiple cysts and hydronephrosis. As a result of worsening renal function despite valve ablation, the patient had a right pyelostomy (high diversion). He has remained stable with marginal renal function off of dialysis.

also contralateral improvement. Furthermore, stable differential function may represent a parallel worsening of the obstruction in both units. Despite the limitations of ultrasonography, serial evaluations demonstrating a trend toward improvement or worsening may be the best available indicator for intervention in these children. In these circumstances, a low threshold for intervention must be exercised.

Ultimately, obstructive uropathies can also be clinically classified as symptomatic or asymptomatic. With the widespread use of antenatal ultrasonography, symptomatic presentation has become less common. Therefore, the remainder of this section will primarily focus on congenital asymptomatic uropathies that are subclassified by the site of obstruction.

Ureteropelvic junction obstruction is defined as an impediment in urine flow from the renal pelvis to the proximal ureter. There are three basic pathophysiologic processes associated with this common obstruction: extramural, mural, or intramural. Extramural anomalies are extrinsic as a result of aberrant or crossing vessels, kinks, bands, or adhesions. They frequently cause intermittent reductions in urine flow with intermittent dilatation of the pelvicaliceal system. Mural obstructions, which are the most common type, result from a dysfunctional or adynamic ureteral segment that is characterized by an abnormal distribution of smooth muscle and collagen fibers. Intramural anomalies are rare in children, and they are largely the result of a valve-like process (as seen with benign fibroepithelial polyps or stones).

Obstruction of the ureterovesical junction results in a *megaureter*. This anomaly is usually caused by an adynamic distal ureteral segment that results in the so-called *primary megaureter*. Functional continuity of the ureter is disrupted by abnormal collagen deposition, cellular hypoplasia, and/or muscular disarray. In a compensatory response to the distal obstruction, hyperplasia and hypertrophy of smooth muscle cells occur within the walls of the dilated proximal segment. The term *secondary megaureter* is reserved for dilation that results from other processes, such as ureteroceles or infravesical obstruction (i.e., posterior urethral valves, anterior urethral valves, megalourethra, urethral duplications, urethral atresia, cloacal dysgenesis).[37]

Ureteroceles are cystic dilatations of the submucosal or intravesical portion of the ureter that results from the persistence of the embryologic remnant known as *Chwalla's membrane*. They may be solitary, but they are more frequently associated with the upper pole of a duplex system. Approximately 15% are bilateral (Figure 37-6). On the basis of the specific anatomic configuration, size, and location, ureteroceles may not only cause the obstruction of one or both ureters but also of the bladder neck and urethra. As a general rule, bilateral ureteral obstruction caused by ureteroceles does not cause megacystis, whereas the obstruction of the bladder neck and urethra may resemble infravesical obstruction.

Posterior urethral valves are the most common cause of neonatal lower urinary tract obstruction in males. They result from the abnormal development of a valve-like membrane from the verumontanum to the prostatic urethra. This abnormality occurs solely in males; the embryologic female counterpart of the verumontanum, from which the valves originate, is the hymen. Megalourethra, urethral atresia, or urethral agenesis may be sonographically indistinguishable from posterior urethral valves. They are often associated with other severe anomalies, such as the prune belly syndrome, cloacal anomalies, or the VACTERL anomalies (vertebral, anal, cardiac, tracheal, esophageal, renal, and limb). The prognosis of urethral atresia is usually poor unless a fistula develops or prenatal vesicoamniotic drainage is performed.

Anterior urethral valves are a rare anomaly that result from urethral diverticulae, incomplete urethral duplication, or cystic dilation of a periurethral gland. They may represent an attempt at the duplication of the urethra during the first 12 to 14 weeks of gestation. The most common type is cusp-like, and it is most frequently located in the bulbar urethra.[38]

Cloacas results from failure of separation of the urogenital sinus from the hindgut, and they are commonly associated with the obstruction of both the urinary and intestinal tracts.

Prune belly syndrome is characterized by the underdevelopment of the abdominal wall muscles, megacystis, hydroureters, hydronephrosis, and undescended testes. Its nomenclature attempts to describe the wrinkled abdominal appearance that results from mesenchymal maldevelopment and hypoplastic musculature (Figure 37-7). Prenatally, this syndrome presents with bilateral hydronephrosis and hydroureters with a large distended bladder, and it is similar in sonographic appearance to posterior valves. In contrast with posterior urethral valves, both sexes can be affected (although it is rare in females), and the so-called "keyhole" sign, which is characteristic of posterior urethral valves, is typically not detected on ultrasound. Postnatal renal failure may be a result of renal dysplasia, functional impairment to urinary flow (stagnation), scarring from pyelonephritis, or urinary obstruction. In addition to being at risk for genitourinary problems, these children may also have pulmonary problems, which may add significant morbidity and should be considered as part of the anesthetic risk stratification for patients who are scheduled to undergo surgical reconstruction.[39]

Developmental Issues

The above-mentioned pathologies are related to derangements of normal embryologic development. Thus, a good understanding of this process is crucial. Although a thorough description exceeds the scope of this chapter, a brief review is in order. The permanent kidneys (the metanephroi) appear during the fifth week of gestation and start to produce urine about 4 weeks later. The developing ureters are initially solid, and they originate from the wolffian ducts. The abnormal development of the ureteric bud or the failure to meet the mesonephric blastema will lead to renal agenesis or grossly abnormal development (i.e., multicystic dysplastic kidney). Ureteropelvic junction obstruction and megaureters are thought to be caused by the incomplete and/or delayed recanalization of the ureters or the maldevelopment of the ureteral muscle layer. If the ureter is split into a duplex system, the ureter from the upper pole of the kidney inserts into the bladder cranially to the ureter of the lower pole, which is frequently associated with ectopic insertion and/or ureterocele. The urogenital sinus is divided into a cephalad vesical portion, which later becomes most of the bladder, and a caudal pelvic portion, which becomes the bladder neck and the prostatic part of the urethra in males and the entire urethra in the females. The abnormal development of the distal end of the mesonephric duct is thought to be one of the potential causes of the development of posterior urethral valves.

Nephron formation is complete at birth, except in premature infants. After 36 weeks' gestational age, only functional maturation occurs, with the rate of glomerular filtration maximally increasing within the first few weeks after birth. The severity of obstruction is important for determining the renal response to obstruction during early postnatal development. In complete experimental obstruction, the pathologic result is obstructive renal dysplasia. Cysts in the nephrogenic zone disturb nephron induction and tubular development. The abnormal expression of many regulatory molecules results in insufficient nephron numbers and abnormal differentiation not only during the time of initial budding but also during the subsequent ontogenetic processes of the kidney and urinary tract. Incomplete but severe chronic obstruction leads to growth arrest and decreased glomerular filtration rate on the ipsilateral kidney, with compensatory hypertrophy of the contralateral renal unit.[40]

DIAGNOSIS

Clinical Presentation

Prenatal Diagnosis

The widespread use of prenatal ultrasonography, along with improvements in technology, have increased the detection of

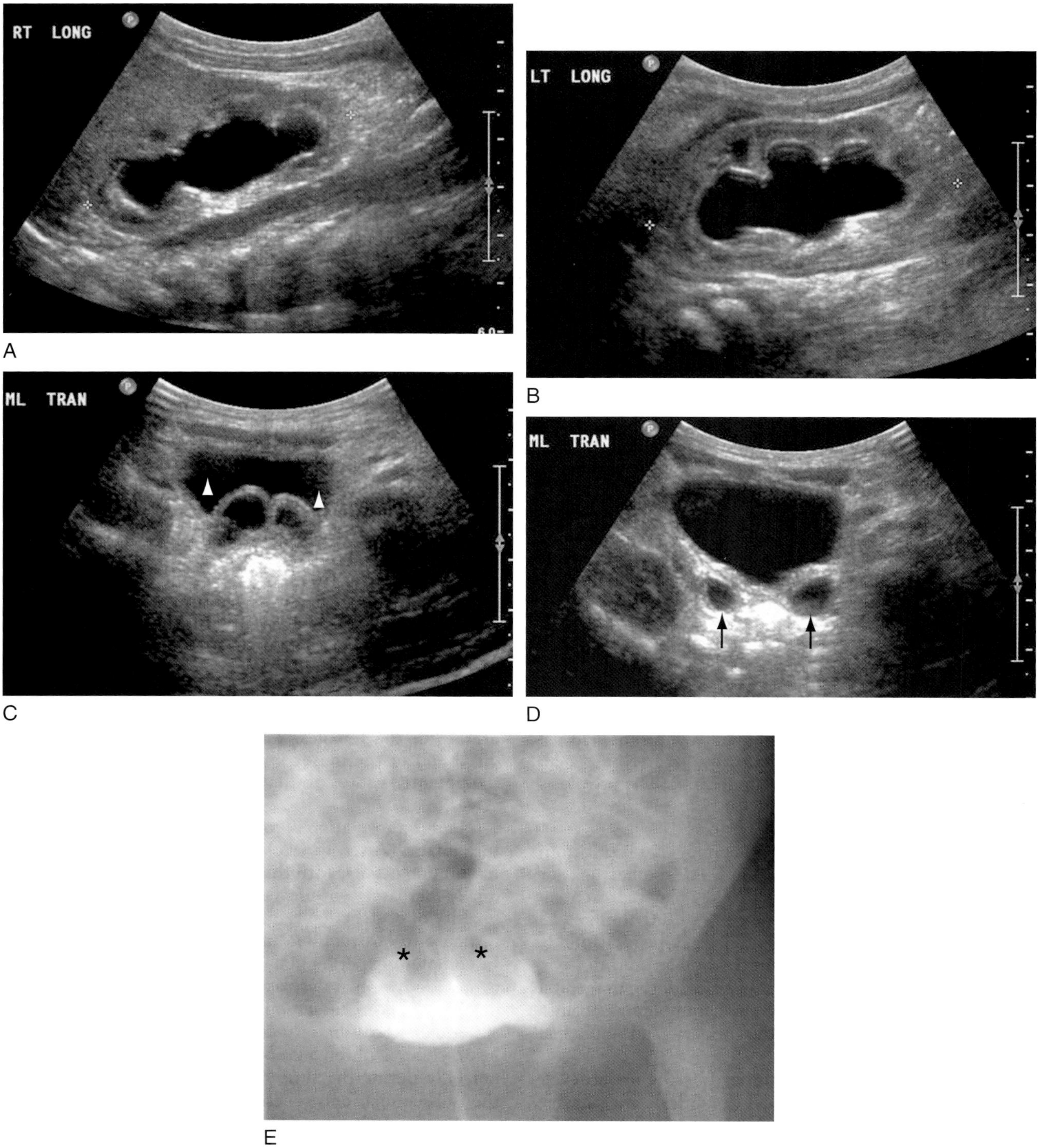

Figure 37-6 Prenatally diagnosed bilateral single system obstructing ureteroceles in a male infant. **A** and **B,** Note grade IV hydronephrosis on both kidneys and **D,** bilateral distal ureteral dilation *(arrows)*. **C** and **E,** Both ureteroceles can be seen in the bladder on ultrasound and voiding cystourethrogram *(arrowheads and sunbursts)*.

urinary structural changes, which are now discovered in up to 1% of pregnancies.[41] Of all prenatal ultrasounds considered to have renal abnormalities, more than 50% demonstrate hydronephrosis with or without dilatation of the ureters[42,43] (see Table 37-3). Unfortunately, no currently available prenatal diagnostic test reliably differentiates obstructive from nonobstructive causes of hydronephrosis or differentiates cases that will have spontaneous resolution as compared with those who may require surgical intervention. Ultrasonography allows for the evaluation of the renal parenchyma for changes that are suggestive of dysplasia (e.g., echogenicity, cysts), amniotic fluid volume (which serves as a proxy for urine output), associated anomalies, and sex determination. Furthermore, it is an invaluable tool for directing diagnostic procedures (amniocentesis) as well as therapeutic interventions (vesicoamniotic shunts). For the rare circumstances in which ultrasound cannot provide sufficient anatomic detail (e.g., maternal obesity, anhydramnios), magnetic resonance imaging appears to be a safe imaging modality.[44,45]

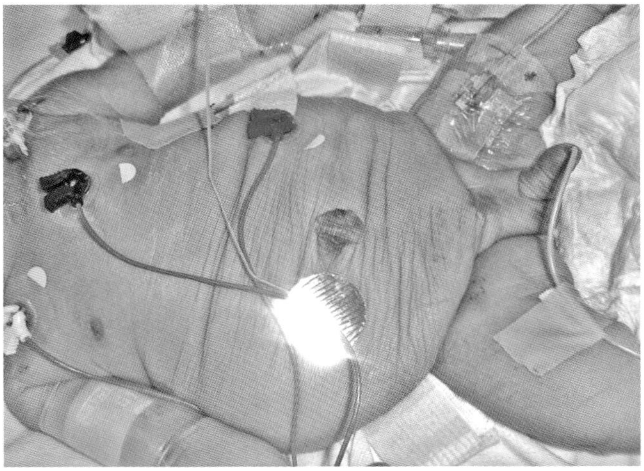

Figure 37-7 A male neonate initially thought to have posterior urethral valves by prenatal ultrasound. Note the appearance of the abdominal wall associated with bilateral undescended testicles and bilateral hydronephrosis, all of which are characteristic of prune belly syndrome.

Postnatal Diagnosis

Upper Urinary Tract Obstruction Patients who escape prenatal diagnosis may develop problems early during the postnatal period. Later on, most older children are diagnosed during the workup of a febrile urinary tract infection, hematuria, a palpable flank mass, or unexplained abdominal or flank pain. Some children may also be diagnosed during the evaluation of hematuria or abdominal pain after abdominal trauma (Figure 37-8). Before the child is able to verbalize complaints, it may be difficult to realize that recurrent episodes of vomiting or discomfort without an apparent cause are related to urinary tract obstruction. These patients often undergo an extensive evaluation for suspected unrelated conditions until the diagnosis is reached. Yet another small group is diagnosed during the workup of associated congenital anomalies (e.g., imperforate anus, VATER association, congenital heart disease) or incidentally on imaging studies that are ordered for a completely unrelated problem.

Lower Urinary Tract Obstruction Early during life, the presence of a palpable bladder and/or delayed voiding may suggest the need for evaluation. Unfortunately, a normal voiding pattern does not rule out obstruction, and an intermittent or irregular flow does not reliably predict it. Bladder outlet obstruction should be suspected in infants with a palpable bladder and urinary ascites and in females with an interlabial cystic mass (prolapsed ureterocele[46]). Later in life, delayed diagnosis is established during the workup of recurrent urinary tract infections, sepsis, renal failure, urinary incontinence, or failure to thrive.

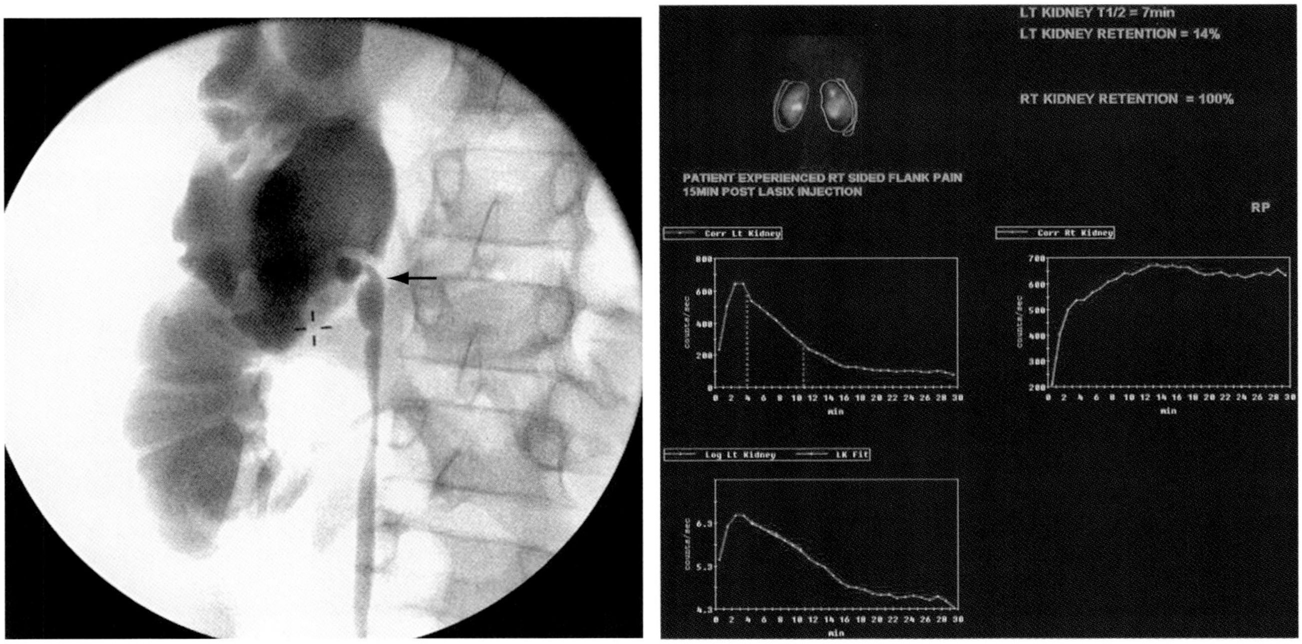

A B

Figure 37-8 A teenager who presented with right flank pain after minor trauma. **A,** A retrograde pyelogram demonstrating an area of stenosis *(arrow)*. Note contrast in the bowel from a previous computed tomography scan. **B,** A nuclear scan after recovery from trauma shows poor drainage with preserved differential function. This patient developed pain after the administration of fluids and furosemide. During surgery, a crossing vessel was encountered at the point of obstruction.

Urinary Tract Infection Urinary tract obstruction and proximal dilatation leads to urinary stasis. Because most infections result from the retrograde migration of bacteria, the same risk factors for bacterial colonization apply to most children, including those with impaired urinary drainage. As a result of the altered drainage mechanism (i.e., decreased or abnormal peristalsis, increased urine transit times), it is conceivable that the child is at higher risk for more severe or difficult-to-treat infection when bacteria reaches above the obstructed segment. One clear example is seen in children with prune belly syndrome in whom the decision to catheterize should be carefully considered, because introduced bacteria may be extremely difficult to eradicate. A similar problem can be seen in patients with associated vesicoureteral reflux in whom catheterization for the diagnostic procedure can lead to colonization of an obstructed system (Figure 37-9). Children who present with pyelonephritis and a potential obstruction should be aggressively treated, with a low threshold for percutaneous or internal drainage of the affected renal units kept in mind.[47]

An important consideration for a child who presents with a febrile urinary tract infection is the presence of associated

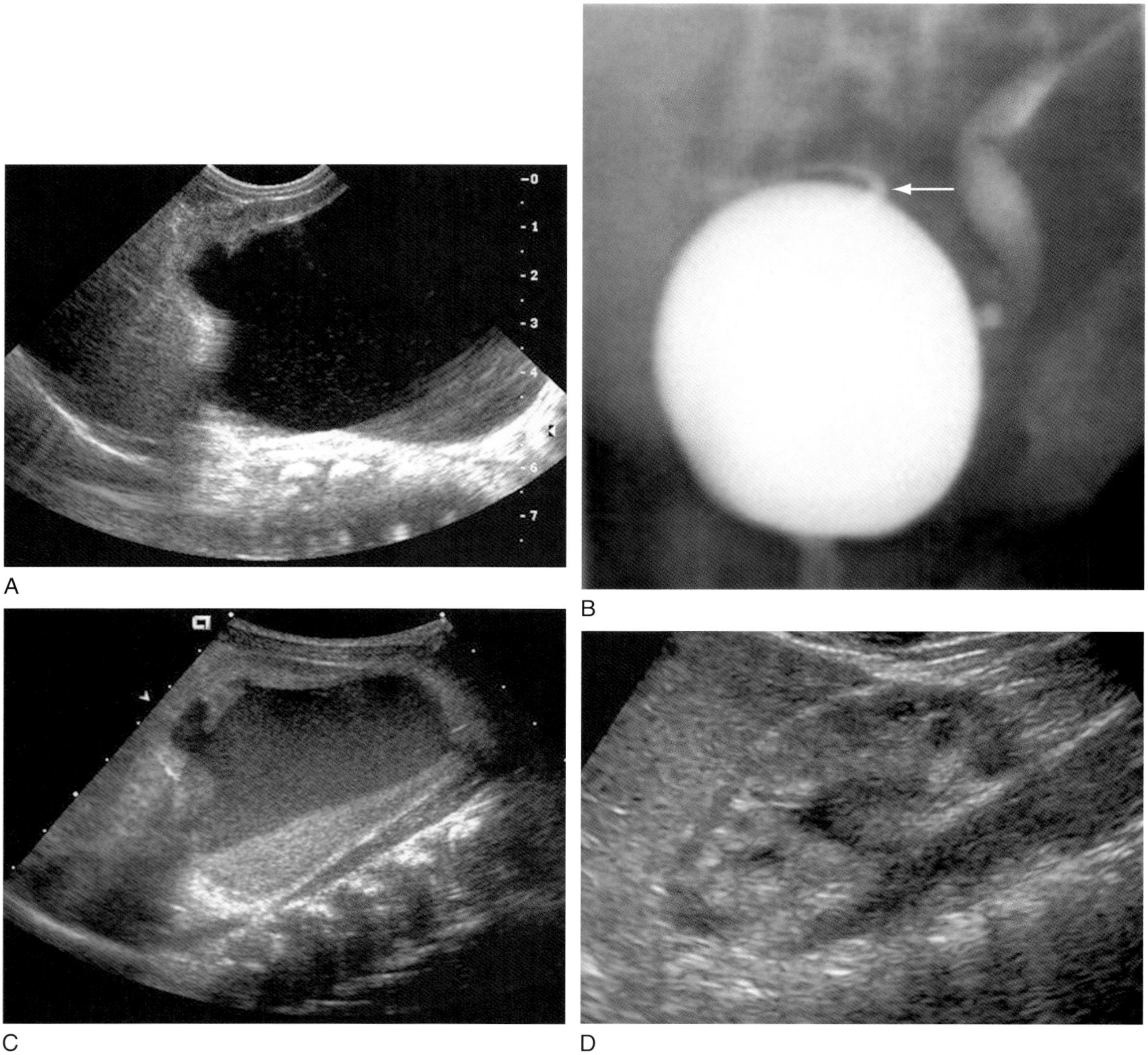

Figure 37-9 A newborn male with a prenatal diagnosis of right hydronephrosis. **A,** Newborn ultrasound documented the massive dilation of the right pelvicaliceal system without ureteral involvement. **B,** A voiding cystogram showed bilateral vesicoureteral reflux. Note that there is a small amount of contrast seen in the right ureter, which is displaced medially by the dilated right kidney *(arrow)*. Twenty-four hours later, the patient presented with fever and lethargy. **C,** An ultrasound was performed upon admission that demonstrated debris and the layering of a fluid-fluid interface. The patient required diversion with a nephrostomy tube. **D,** Note the almost complete resolution of dilation after pyeloplasty.

vesicoureteral reflux. The incidence of reflux in infants and young children who present with pyelonephritis is higher than other structural anomalies, including obstruction.[48] This fact, in combination with the high detection rate as a result of the widespread practice of prenatal ultrasound, has called into question the need for ultrasonography in the workup of young children who present with a febrile urinary tract infection.[49] Despite its relatively low yield, renal ultrasound is quick, it involves little discomfort, it does not require radiation, it detects some cases that ultimately require surgical correction, it provides reassuring information for children with normal studies, and it serves as an excellent baseline study for children who are assigned to conservative management.[50]

Pain In contrast with the asymptomatic presentation early in life, older children with an obstructive process are usually discovered as a result of their symptoms. Pain results from intermittent obstruction at times when the urine flow overwhelms the ability of the urinary tract to drain properly. It is obviously difficult to discern whether younger patients do not complain of pain because they cannot communicate their discomfort or because of the chronic nature of the process (i.e., chronic partial obstruction is painless). Older children with ureteropelvic—and, to a lesser extent, ureterovesical—junction obstruction classically have episodic flank or upper abdominal pain that is associated with nausea and vomiting (Figures 37-10 and 37-11). At their initial presentation, this symptomatology is far more common than febrile urinary tract infections or hematuria.[51] It is important to recognize that patients can have misleadingly unremarkable studies during asymptomatic periods and that they may have a higher rate of extrinsic anatomic abnormalities conditioning the obstructive process (e.g., lower pole crossing vessels[51]). Ultra-

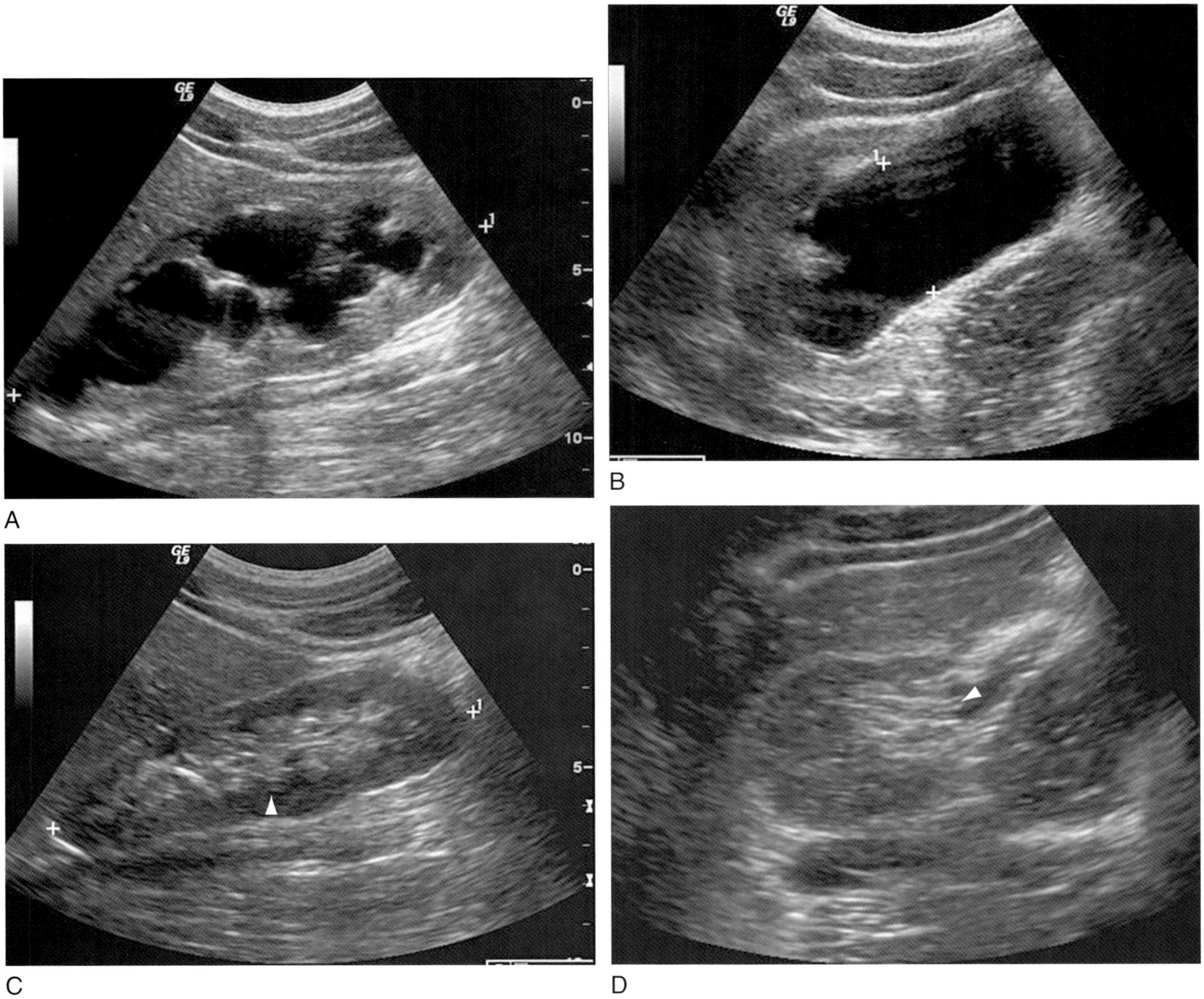

Figure 37-10 Ureteropelvic junction obstruction. This is the case of a teenage boy who presented with intermittent flank pain. **A** and **B,** Preoperative and **C** and **D,** postoperative ultrasound images of the right kidney show a dramatic resolution of the hydronephrosis after pyeloplasty, which was followed by symptom resolution.

sonography while symptomatic can prevent the delay in diagnosis, which is most commonly labeled as a "gastrointestinal disturbance."[52] Pain related to episodes of increased diuresis should also raise the level of suspicion for an obstructive urinary process as can be commonly elicited in children who receive a diuretic challenge during a furosemide renal scan.

Hypertension When a patient demonstrates the now-accepted criteria of an average systolic or diastolic blood pressure at or above the 95th percentile for age and sex measured on at least three separate occasions,[53,54] the diagnosis of secondary hypertension is related to renal parenchymal disease in up to 60% to 80% of cases.[55] Consequences or symptoms of elevated blood pressure are rarely the presenting finding that leads to the diagnosis of obstruction. Conversely, depending on the onset, level, and degree of obstruction as well as the presence of renal parenchymal damage (or dysplasia), hypertension may develop during the

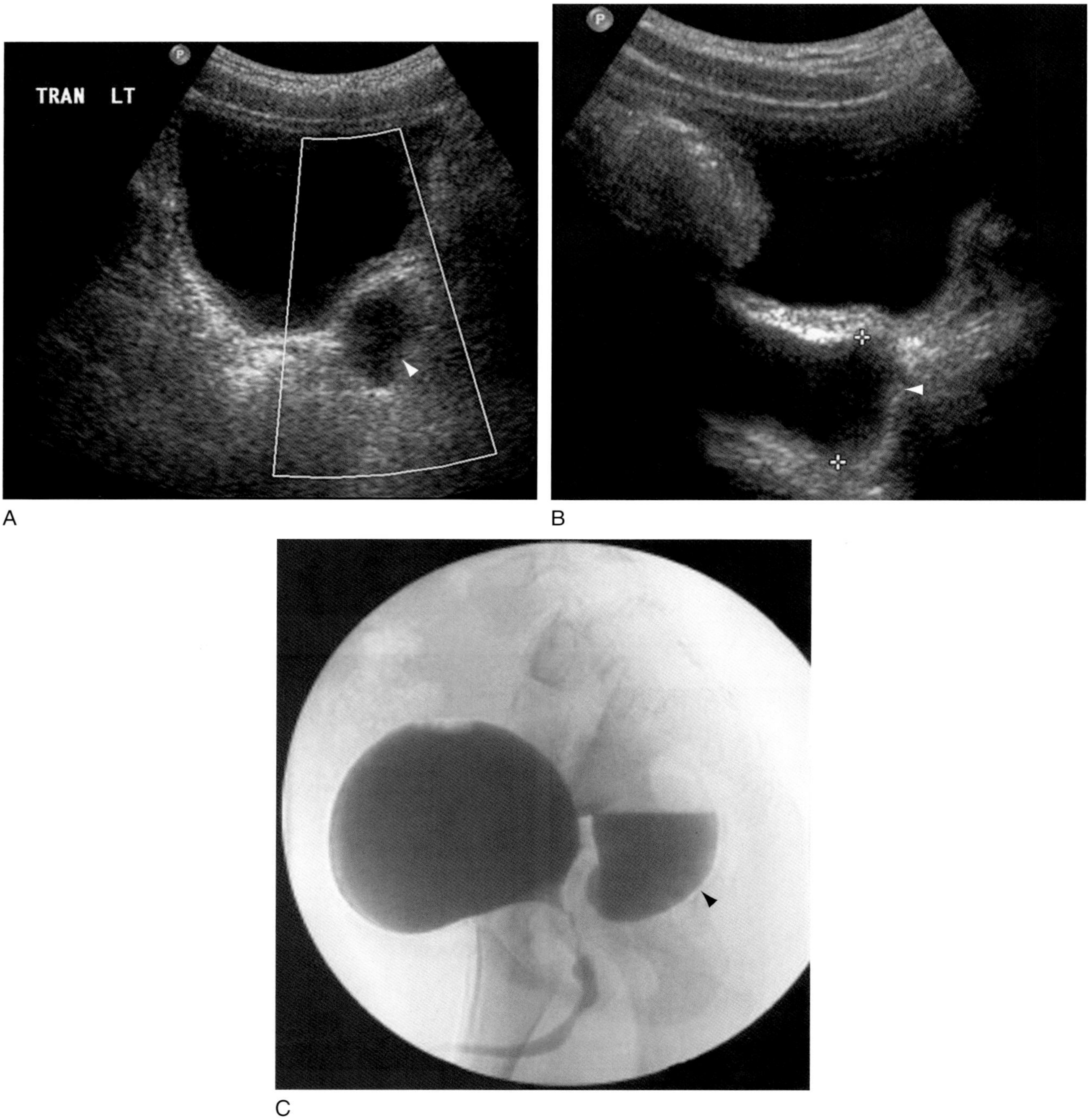

Figure 37-11 Left obstructed refluxing megaureter diagnosed in a child with intermittent flank pain. **A** and **B,** Dilatation of the left ureter to the level of the ureterovesical junction *(arrowhead)*. **C,** Voiding cystourethrogram demonstrates reflux with fluid-fluid layering in the distal left ureter.

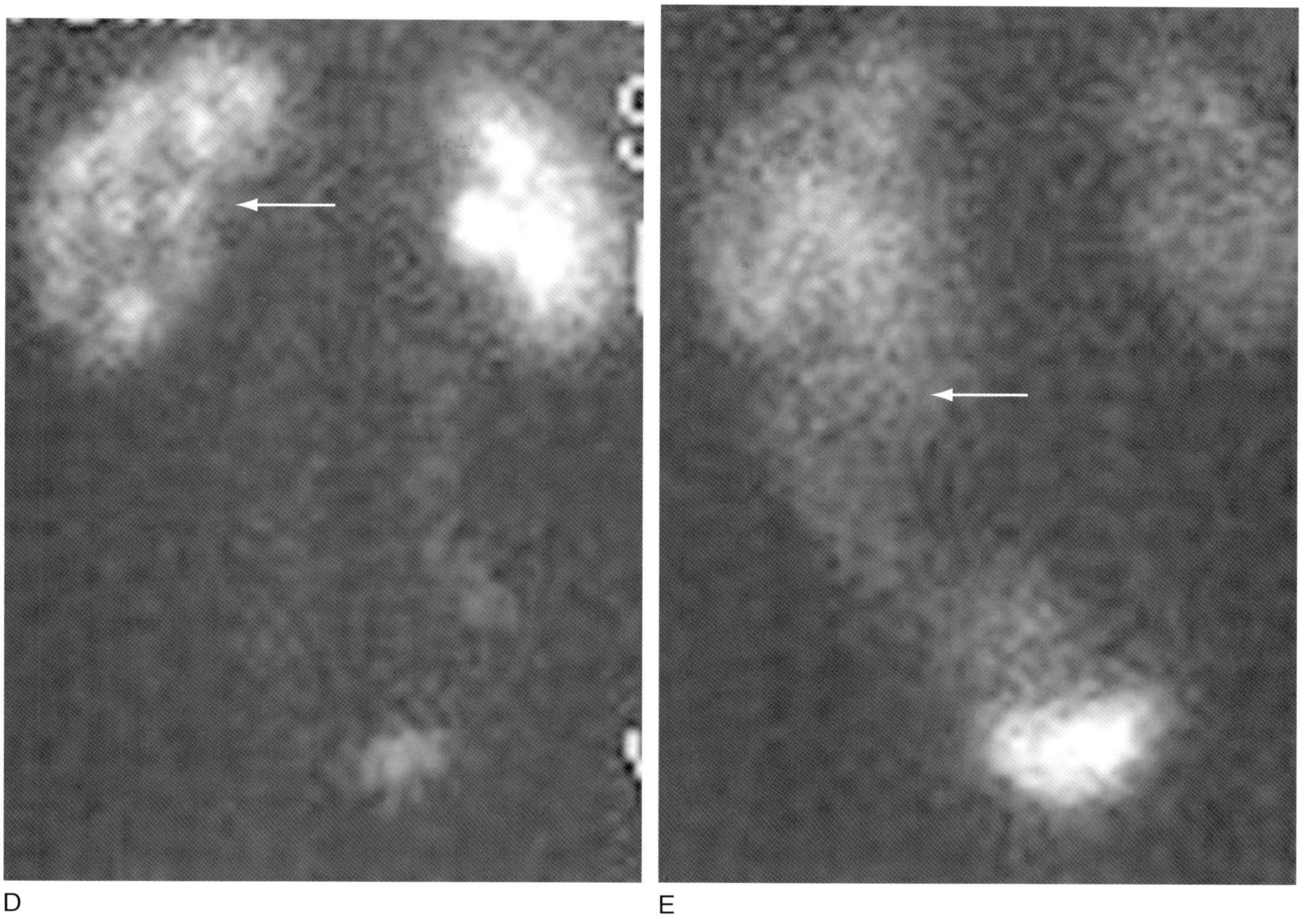

Figure 37-11, cont'd **D** and **E,** Diuretic renal scans showing delayed uptake and excretion of the radiotracer with preserved differential function.

course of conservative management or after surgical intervention.[54] As a result of the widespread use of ultrasonography, most patients are likely to be diagnosed before renal damage has occurred or before it becomes significant enough to lead to elevated blood pressure. When present, investigations should focus on potential interventions that could prevent further renal damage as well as the detection of reversible causes (i.e., renin-mediated hypertension from a poorly functioning/scarred kidney that is amenable to nephrectomy[56,57]).

Imaging Studies

For the most part, currently available diagnostic methods provide complementary information and help establish a diagnosis that is based on trends over time; therefore, they are most significant when combined and repeated during follow up. Of paramount importance is the distinction between detecting morphologic and structural changes (i.e., dilatation of the urinary tract or parenchymal atrophy) as compared with functional changes (i.e., impaired radiotracer excretion or differential renal uptake).

Renal and Pelvic Ultrasound

Ultrasound is a relatively inexpensive, widely available imaging modality that has the added advantage of not requiring ionizing radiation to identify structural changes of the urinary tract. It is the first diagnostic test that is ordered as part of the workup for suspected obstruction, both pre- and postnatally. Ultrasound allows for the excellent morphologic assessment of both the lower and upper urinary tract systems, regardless of renal function. However, it is operator dependent, and it can be difficult to obtain from patients who are not cooperative or who have a challenging body habitus. Because of its perceived nonexistent "toxicity," ultrasound remains the modality of choice for antenatal investigations and for the serial evaluation of patients.

Although renal structures can be visualized as early as gestational weeks 12 to 15, most relevant diagnoses are currently detected during the second trimester.[58] A normal bladder is visible as early as gestational week 13. Bladder detection is facilitated by identifying the umbilical arteries along its sides with the assistance of color Doppler. In healthy babies, the bladder appears as a thin-walled, fluid-filled cavity. Normal ureters are usually not visible on prenatal ultrasound.

Although it is currently believed that longer duration and more severe degrees of antenatal renal dilatation are related to impaired postnatal function, there is no clear agreement about what the upper limit of normal fetal renal pelvis diameter should be. Arbitrarily, pelviectasis can be defined as renal pelvic dilatation of more than 3 mm during the second trimester and of more than 6 mm after 32 weeks' gestation. Although some consider a renal pelvis diameter of more than 5 mm to be abnormal, others define hydronephrosis as a dilatation of the renal pelvis of 10 mm or more (measured at the anteroposterior diameter), regardless of gestational age. Irrespective of the cutoff, postnatal evaluation is currently recommended in most cases, although the benefit of such evaluation in mild cases—especially if they are unilateral—remains to be defined.[59,60]

During the first days after birth, low urinary output may mask hydronephrosis, even when obstruction is present. Therefore, timing appears to be important. When possible, ultrasound should be performed after the third day postdelivery in a stable newborn, and it should be repeated despite normal results immediately after birth, although the significance of missed pathologies has been called into question.[61] The renal pelvis diameter should be examined in the transverse plane and at the anteroposterior diameter (Figure 37-12). In the newborn, an anteroposterior diameter of more than 7 mm is considered abnormal; in an older child, an abnormal diameter is more than 1 cm. As the anteroposterior diameter increases, the likelihood of significant urine flow impairment and the need for intervention increase.[62,63] If possible, ultrasound examination should be performed with both a full and an empty bladder, thus allowing for the better assessment of wall thickening, abnormal filling volume, ureteroceles, incomplete bladder emptying with residual volume, and signs of posterior urethra valves. Also, hydronephrosis may be more obvious or prominent in children with a full bladder; this concept should be kept in mind when comparing studies over time. All measurements should be compared with normal values for age- or size-adjusted nomograms and, when possible, serially assessed to allow for the detection of abnormal renal growth. Hypertrophy of the normal contralateral kidney is a relevant and valuable marker for the decreased function of the hydronephrotic kidney.

Nuclear Medicine Studies

Despite technical advances in other imaging techniques, nuclear medicine studies maintain an important role in the functional assessment of the kidneys. They are relatively noninvasive, although intravenous access is required and sedation is sometimes indicated to reduce motion artefacts. Several imaging agents are available that provide different parameters that are relevant for clinical decision making. Nuclear scans can evaluate relative renal function, estimate absolute renal function (e.g., glomerular filtration rate), portray functional renal parenchyma and renal scars, estimate renal blood flow, and assess excretory function. Because the isotope used (technetium-99m) is a pure gamma emitter and because it has a physical half-life of 6 hours, the radiation burdens to the whole body and to the specific organ are low.

^{99m}Tc-diethylenetriaminepentaacetic acid (DTPA) and ^{99m}Tc-mercaptoacetyltriglycine (MAG-3) are the radionuclides that are most commonly used to evaluate function and clearance. Differences in the mechanism of renal handling, tracer dosing, the timing of the diuretic dose, the patient's level of hydration, and the calculation of the area of interest

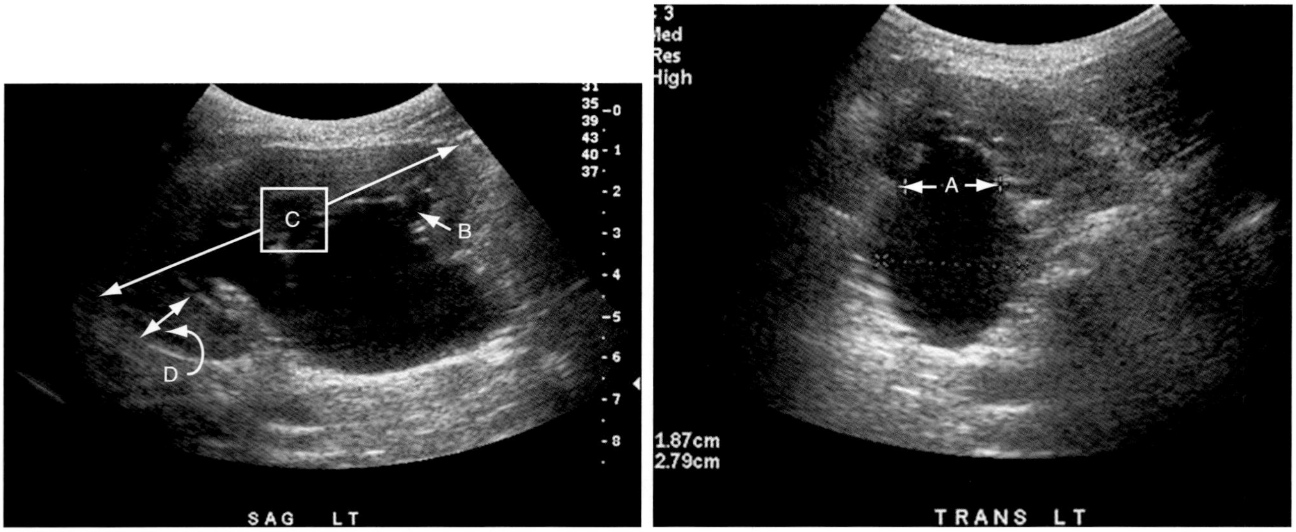

Parameters that should be described on ultrasound:

A. Antero-posterior (AP) diameter of the renal pelvis

B. Degree of caliectasis

C. Renal length

D. Thickness of the renal cortex

E. Echogenicity and cortico-medullary differentiation

F. Grade of hydronephrosis

Figure 37-12 Imaging parameters that should be described on renal ultrasound. Grading is based on the Society of Fetal Urology system.

introduce variability and must be consistent to ensure a valid comparison of test results. Standardized methods for performing diuretic renograms have been developed by the Society for Fetal Urology and the Pediatric Nuclear Medicine Club; these organizations developed the so-called "well-tempered renogram."[64-66] In young children with obstructive uropathies, MAG-3 is the radiopharmaceutical of choice for routine renal imaging as a result of its higher extraction efficiency (which is more apparent when renal function deteriorates) and its widespread availability. Furthermore, MAG-3 scanning allows for the easier estimation of differential renal function as early as the end of the first week of life. Consideration should be given to the fact that the immature nephrons of the newborn kidney demonstrate a blunted response to diuretics. Therefore, whenever possible, it is preferable to defer a diuretic study for at least 4 weeks to allow for renal maturation.

Using computer-generated regions of interest, graphs can be obtained to show the variation of radioactive count by time within organs. What is usually described in reports is the so-called "time-activity curve," which is associated with an individual kidney. Three phases are described: (1) perfusion; (2) parenchymal transit; and (3) excretion. T_{max} (the time it takes to reach the maximum of the curve), relative renal function (using the integral or the Rutland-Patlak method), and transit time (analysis by deconvolution techniques) are computed. The normal time-activity curve is characterized by a steep rising curve that is followed by an early peak and a rapidly descending phase. Dilatation of the collecting system results in a continuously rising curve. The administration of a diuretic (usually furosemide) is used in an attempt to differentiate between obstruction and the "reservoir effect" of nonobstructive dilatation. Theoretically, in a dilated and nonobstructed system, the pharmacologically induced increase in urinary flow leads to a prompt washout, which is a sign of good drainage. In an obstructed system, the drainage curve of the diuretic renogram fails to show a rapid washout curve of the tracer, thereby resulting in a delayed excretion time. Unfortunately, differentiating truly obstructive dilatations of the urinary tract from those that appear to represent no more than nonobstructive variants remains difficult. Drainage curves and transit times as parameters for appropriate urinary flow have been reported to be imprecise. Subjective estimations must be made of the area of interest. Also, the timing of diuretic administration and the time-honored—albeit arbitrary—cutoffs for drainage values (e.g., $t_{1/2}$) remain largely empirical. For example, E_{max}, which is the maximal elimination rate, represents the slope at the turning point of the sigmoidal-shaped washout curve after that administration of furosemide. It is thought to represent complete obstruction if it is lower than 7%, partial obstruction if it is between 7% and 14%, and no functional obstruction if it is more than 14%. Although it is tempting to have clearcut values for labeling obstruction, pressure flow studies have called into question how reliable drainage curves can be[33] (Figure 37-13). In most situations, clinical correlation must be exercised, and management rarely (if ever) relies solely on one value obtained from a diuretic nuclear scan.

Up to the point at which excretion occurs, the relative uptake of the radiopharmaceutical is proportional to the individual renal clearance. The most straightforward method of estimating relative renal function involves summing the counts under the renogram curves between 1 and 3 minutes after the injection of the radiotracer. Relative renal function is given as a percentage of the right and left kidney, with both adding up to 100% global renal function. Under normal conditions, each kidney should contribute equally (~50%). Given a range of normal of two standard deviations, a function of less than 40% is mostly regarded as abnormal for a given renal unit. Decreased function either reflects acquired unilateral renal damage or congenital anomalies (e.g., dysplastic moiety in a duplex kidney). Apparently normal values may also be found with bilaterally damaged kidneys. Poor renal function makes the accurate estimation of differential function harder and limits the interpretation of the drainage curves.

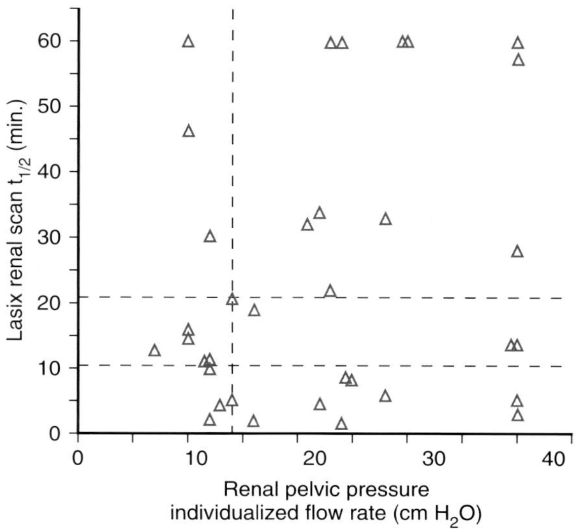

Figure 37-13 Scatter plot of a drainage curve ($t^1/_2$) by diuretic renogram against renal pelvic pressure using individualized flow rate.[33]

Pressure-Flow Studies

The principle underlying these tests is that obstruction produces a restriction to urine flow so that pressures increase to sustain urine flow rates. Whitaker's perfusion test[34] and ureteral opening pressures[9] can be used to evaluate obstruction, but their invasiveness and the requirement of anesthesia or sedation are important drawbacks. In addition, the Whitaker test requires a supraphysiologic flow rate that could potentially overcome the peristaltic flow capacity of a normal child's ureter, and the parameters of obstruction are somewhat empirically defined (i.e., an elevation in renal pressure of more than 22 cm of water over baseline while infusing constantly at 10 cc per minute).[34] The modifications introduced by Fung and colleagues include calculating the infusion rate individually and within a physiologically relevant range, thus identifying obstruction in cases in which the pressure increase within the pelvis is more than 14 cm of water.[9] Although the correlation between perfusion pressures and diuretic nuclear renography is poor, both studies provide valuable information, because the discrepancy is likely the result of measuring different physical parameters (i.e., the rate of radionuclide clearance as a measure of flow across an area of suspected obstruction as compared with the resistance of the collecting system and the ureter to the flow of fluid during a high-flow state). In most situations, management can be planned on the basis of the result of renal nuclear scans and serial ultrasounds, with little additional data obtained by these invasive and somewhat complex tests.[67] Exceptions include renal moieties with extremely poor function and cases in which the diuretic renogram is equivocal or difficult to interpret as a result of a very capacious collecting system.

Voiding Cystourethrogram

This study mainly provides images of the lower urinary tract. In cases of obstructive disease, the voiding cystogram represents the gold standard for delineating the anatomic detail of posterior urethral valves, refluxing/obstructed megaureters, ureteroceles, and bladder diverticulae. It is also used to detect vesicoureteral reflux. Moreover, bladder capacity can be measured. It is an elective test that is commonly ordered to complement the full evaluation of the genitourinary tract. Because of the relatively high incidence of reflux in patients with obstructive uropathies, most physicians keep patients on antibiotic prophylaxis until the study is obtained.

Magnetic Resonance Imaging

This noninvasive, radiation-free imaging modality allows for excellent anatomic imaging. With the administration of a specific non-nephrotoxic, noniodinated intravenous contrast medium and with the use of novel and fast imaging techniques, parenchymal perfusion, glomerular filtration, and the visualization of renal excretory function and urine drainage are possible.

Accepted indications for magnetic resonance urography include preoperative anatomic imaging, the assessment of vascular anatomy, the evaluation of complex abnormalities (e.g., duplex systems, ectopic ureteral insertions), the differential diagnosis of hydronephrosis versus parapelvic cysts, the assessment of complex cystic masses, and the definition of inconclusive findings on ultrasound. Its use is limited by the need for sedation in younger children, its high cost, and its restricted availability. Also, as previously indicated, it can be used in selected cases to clarify findings on a prenatal ultrasound. Examples are shown in Figure 37-14.

Magnetic resonance imaging is based on two main sequences. T2-weighted sequences depict and delineate fluid-filled structures (e.g., the collecting system) without the need for contrast. The T2-weighted sequences employ the prolonged relaxation decay of water; it is very fast and can be performed in less than 10 seconds. This sequence is completely independent of renal function, but it does not allow for enough resolution to identify nondilated ureters (i.e., in ectopically inserted, crossed, or in-duplex systems). The excretory urogram uses T1-weighted sequences with intravenous paramagnetic contrast material (usually gadolinium-DTPA [Gd]) and furosemide for the functional assessment of renal transit and urinary washout. This approach enables an "all-in-one" evaluation of the collecting system and the parenchyma as well as of renal function and drainage. The duration of the investigation varies from about 15 to 20 minutes after furosemide administration to up to 60 minutes with an extensive study (i.e., for baseline T1- and T2-weighted imaging, Gd-enhanced magnetic resonance angiography and Gd-enhanced T1-gradient-recalled-echo (GRE) sequences).[68]

Renal Function Tests

In Utero Function

Because of the invasive nature of the interventions used to obtain fetal blood and urine samples, indirect parameters have been adopted to estimate renal function. After 20 weeks of gestation, some gross correlation between amniotic fluid volume and renal function can be made as a result of the fact that the amount of fluid is progressively determined by fetal urine production as gestation progresses. In normally functioning kidneys, urinary sodium decreases with gestational age; this process is blunted in cases of obstruction, and it could eventually lead to salt wasting. Obstruction also leads to increased concentrations of amniotic microproteins like β_2-microglobulin and α_1-microglobulin, which is an indicator of tubular damage. As discussed later in this chapter, several urinary parameters have been assessed as predictors of renal dysfunction, including sodium, calcium, total protein, microalbumin, phosphate, N-acetyl-β-D-glycosaminidase, and osmolality. These parameters are often used to determine whether intrauterine therapy should be performed.

An important consideration is the relationship between renal and pulmonary function. Severe intrauterine urinary tract obstruction results in oligo-anhydraminos. In these fetuses, the placenta maintains fluid and electrolyte homeostasis as well as other renal functions. Anhydramnios results in the failure of normal pulmonary development as a result of limited lung expansion or a lack of exposure to the soluble growth factors that are important for pulmonary development. Severe pulmonary hypoplasia frequently leads to early neonatal death. Other characteristic associated anomalies include limb and facial anomalies, which are known as Potter's syndrome or sequence.

Postnatal Determination of Renal Function

Exogenous clearance markers (e.g., inulin, radiolabeled compounds) and endogenous markers (e.g., creatinine, cystatin C) may be used to measure glomerular filtration rate as an estimate of global renal function. Methods that are based on exogenous markers are time consuming, labor intensive, and expensive; thus, they are seldom used in clinical practice.

Creatinine, which is the most widely used marker, is endogenously produced at a relatively stable rate from creatine in muscles. To estimate the creatinine clearance, urine must be collected over a period of time (usually 24 hours), and creatinine concentration must be measured in urine and plasma. Alternately, the Schwartz formula[69] is often used to estimate the corrected glomerular filtration rate in infants and children using plasma creatinine, height, age, and sex multiplied by a correction factor. Despite the wide use of creatinine, there are some pitfalls, particularly in infants and small children. In the newborn, the plasma creatinine value is a reflection of the maternal value. Also, in young children, normal values have a wide range, because the mean normal values are close to the methodic standard deviations, especially when nonenzymatic analyzing methods are used.

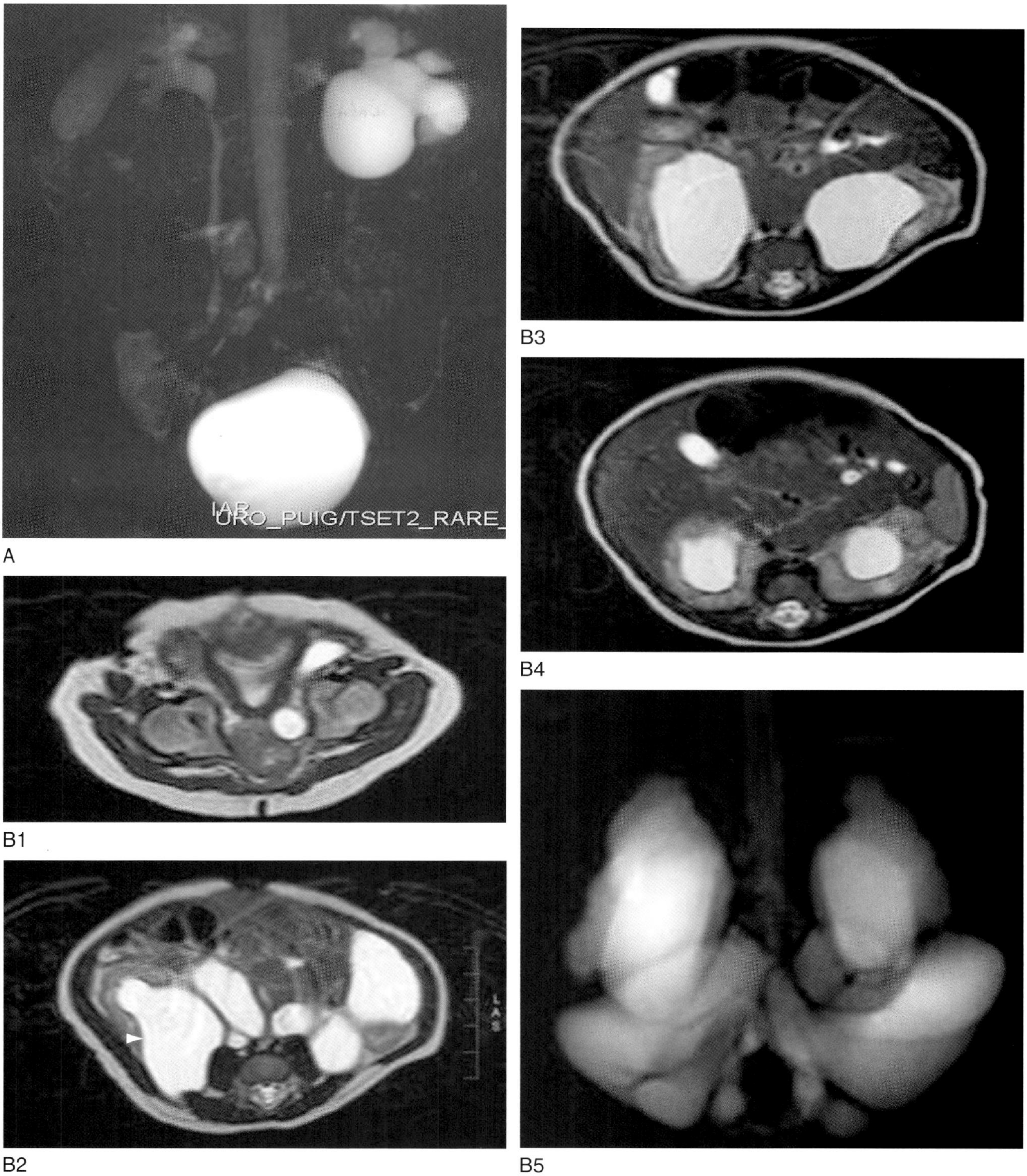

Figure 37-14 Examples of magnetic resonance imaging. **A,** Unilateral ureteropelvic-junction obstruction on the left side. Note that the dilated renal pelvis and bladder are filled, with a lack of enhancement in the ureter. **B1-B8,** A child with prune belly syndrome. Images of the dilated renal pelvises and ureters at 6 weeks of age. **C,** Unilateral ureteropelvic junction and ureterovesical junction obstruction on the left side. Note the contrast in the dilated renal pelvis and ureter on the affected side. **D,** Antenatal imaging in a male fetus with posterior urethral valves demonstrating dilated pelvises and ureters *(arrow)*. Note the oligohydramnios.

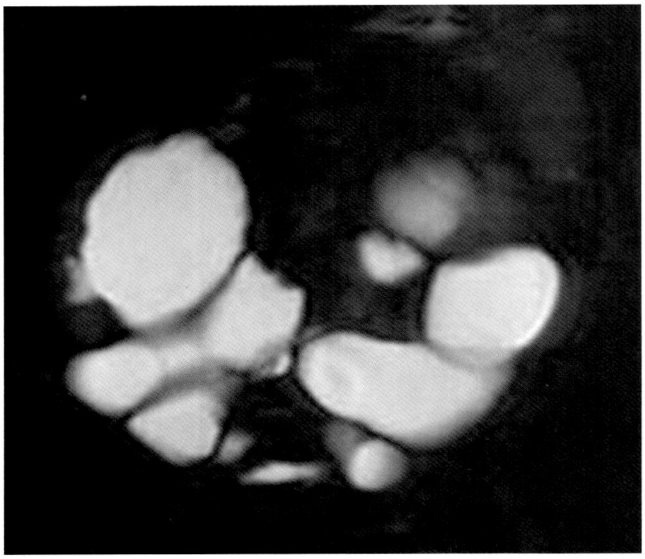

B6

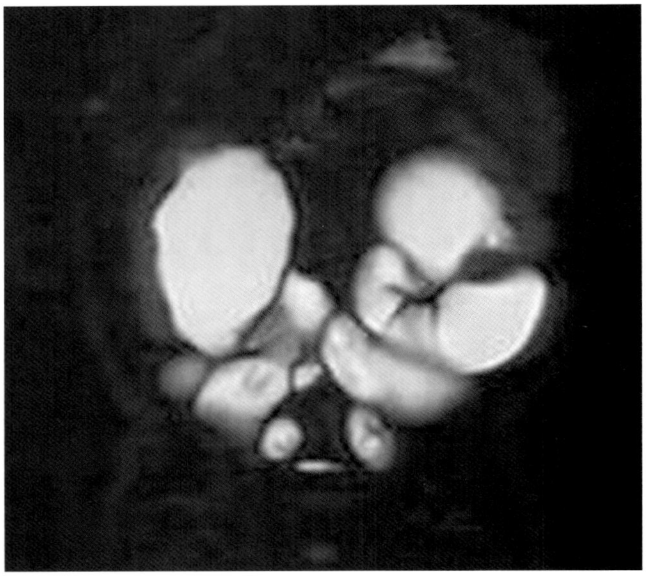

B7

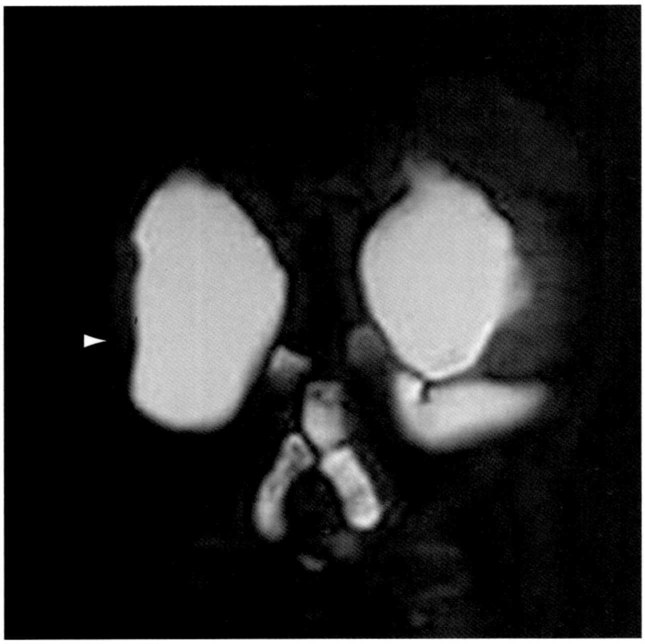

B8

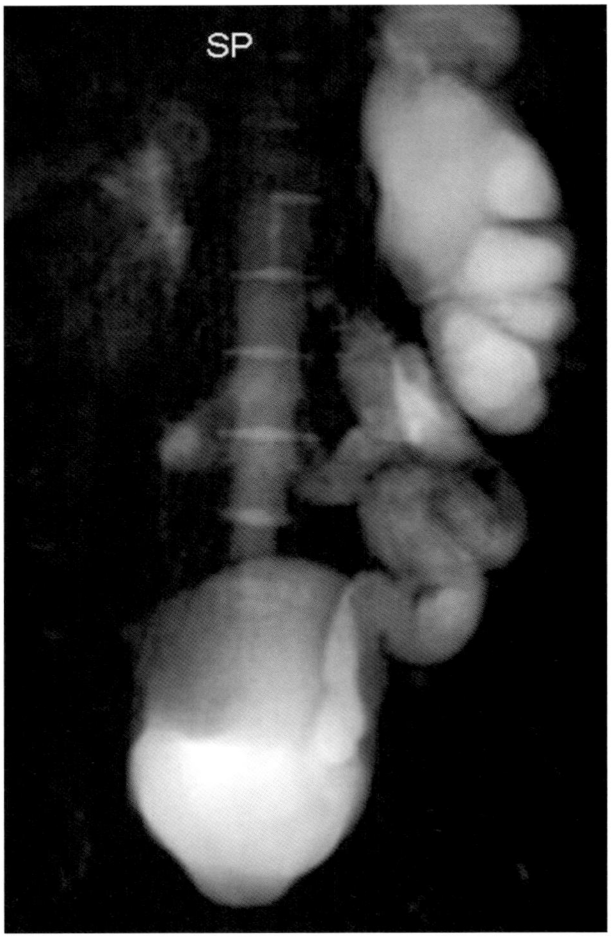

C

Figure 37-14, cont'd

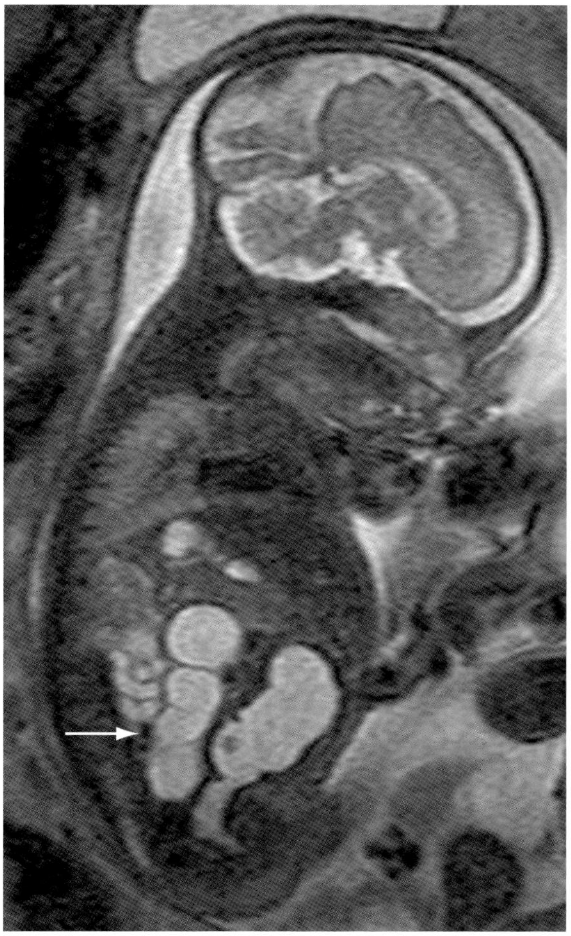

D1

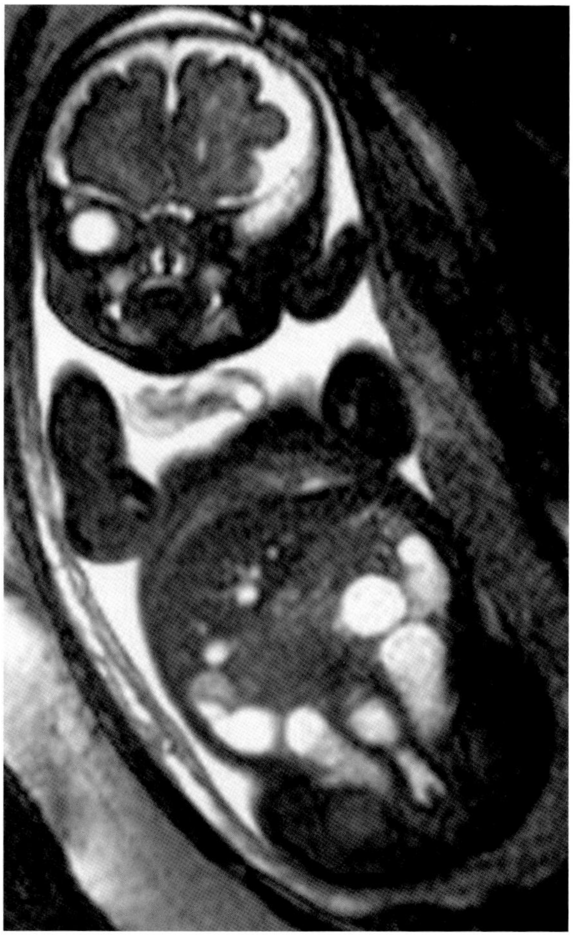

D2

Figure 37-14, cont'd

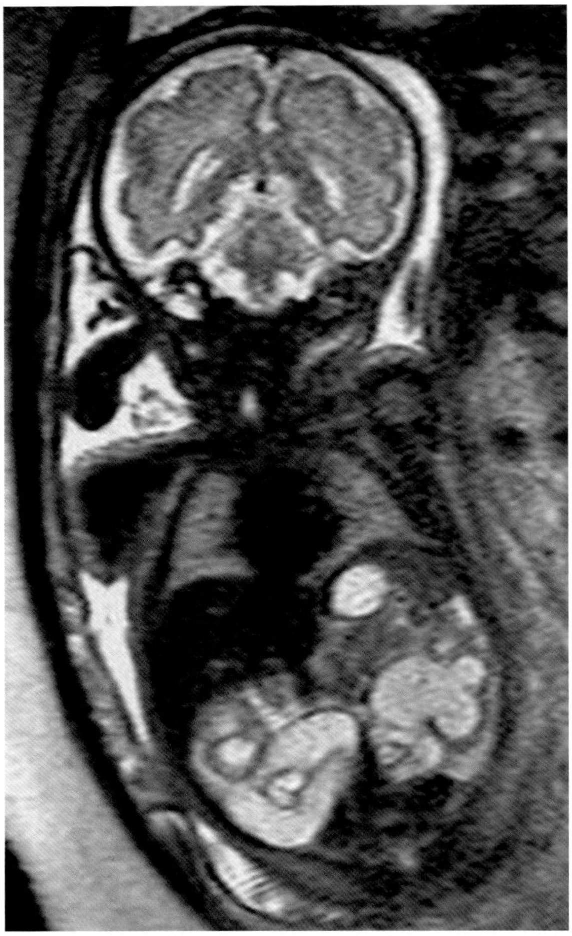

D3

Figure 37-14, cont'd

Moreover, plasma creatinine may be low in patients with low muscle mass (i.e., in patients with meningomyeloceles or malnutrition), thereby masking reduced renal function.

A novel endogenous marker, cystatin C,[70,71] is a low-molecular-weight protein that is produced by all nucleated cells. It is characterized by a stable production rate. Because it is freely filtered by the glomerulus and almost completely reabsorbed and catabolized in the tubules, cystatin C concentration in peripheral blood directly reflects the glomerular filtration rate. In contrast with creatinine, cystatin C seems to be minimally influenced by muscle mass, age, sex, inflammatory states, or nutritional conditions, and, therefore, it does not require any correction for these factors. Furthermore, cystatin C does not cross the placental barrier, and its values after birth directly correlate with the glomerular filtration rate of the neonate.

The above-mentioned methods allow for global renal function assessment, and they may be used to guide therapy when both kidneys are affected. In unilateral disease, global function is mostly normal, and this is reflected by normal creatinine values. In these cases, the unaffected kidney serves as a control, and the contribution of each side to global function can only be compared using nuclear scintigraphy. Isotopic renogram separately assesses renal perfusion and the relative function of each moiety.

MANAGEMENT

Prenatal Management

There are two general points to consider with regard to diagnosis and outcome.[72] First, the likelihood of having a significant postnatal abnormality is proportional to the severity of the antenatal hydronephrosis (94% if the renal pelvis diameter is >20 mm versus 3% if the diameter is <10 mm[73]). Second, the diagnosis may correlate with the degree of hydronephrosis; vesicoureteral reflux is more common if the hydronephrosis is mild, whereas ureteropelvic junction obstruction is more common if the hydronephrosis is marked.[74] Thus, the adoption of a grading system (e.g., the one devised by the Society of Fetal Urology, shown in Table 37-4) and the routine measurement of the renal pelvis diameter can help with the comparison of studies and the evaluation of trends over time. Taking into account the considerations listed in Table 37-5, earlier or more aggressive interventions are offered to patients who are at higher risk, whereas conservative or less-emergent evaluation is reserved for mild cases. The risk/benefit ratio for some interventions has not been fully elucidated (e.g., vesicoamniotic shunts); thus, clinical judgment on a case-by-case basis is warranted.

Most babies can be managed conservatively, with closer monitoring offered to patients who are at higher risk for adverse outcome (e.g., those with bilateral hydronephrosis, megacystis in a male fetus, hydronephrosis in a solitary kidney). Despite the growing experience with prenatal management, currently considered interventions are fairly limited. These include termination of the pregnancy, shunting procedures, and, in rare circumstances, early induction and postnatal care.

The initial enthusiasm for in utero therapy has been tempered as a result of modest outcomes and potentially serious complications. Currently, outside of research protocols, this type of management is usually limited to fetuses with ultrasonographic evidence of bladder outlet obstruction. The challenge remains to determine who benefits from intervention, because some fetuses will reach maturity without problems, whereas some will have a poor outcome despite therapy. Unfortunately, none of the available markers are accurate enough to reliably predict risk before irreversible damage has occurred. Certain ultrasound findings (e.g., renal cysts, hyperechogenicity of the renal parenchyma, hydronephrosis, oligohydramnios) are predictive of renal dysplasia.[75-77] More commonly used in the decision-making process are biochemical markers of fetal renal function, which are measured on single or repeated vesicocentesis samples. Favorable urinary indices include concentrations of sodium of less than 100 mEq/L, chloride of less than 110 mEq/L, calcium of less than 8 mEq/L, β2 microglobulin of less than 10 mg/L, total protein of less than 20 mg/dl, and osmolarity of less than 200 mOsm/L.[77-79] Further considerations before intervention include the presence of associated congenital anomalies (detected in up to 30% of cases), chromosomal abnormalities (seen in up to 23%), and twin pregnancies. Finally, the limited

TABLE 37-4 **Society of Fetal Urology Grading System for Antenatal Hydronephrosis**

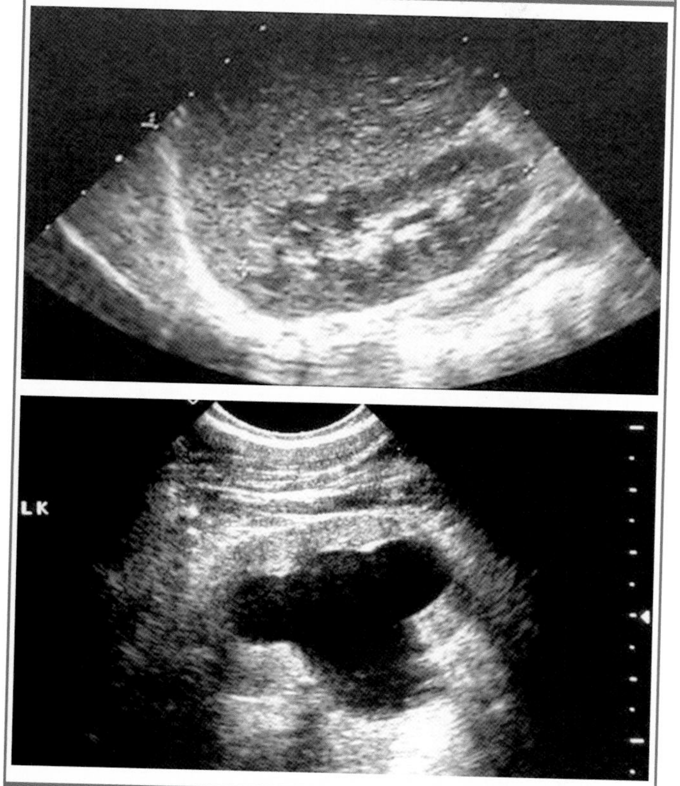

Grade	Renal Pelvis Complex	Renal Parenchymal Thickness
0	Intact	Normal
I (top photo)	Mild splitting*	Normal
II	Moderate splitting (confined to renal border)	Normal
III (bottom photo)	Marked splitting (outside renal border, caliceal dilatation	Normal
IV	Pelvicaliceal dilatation	Thin

* Example of grade I hydronephrosis.
† Example of grade III hydronephrosis.

TABLE 37-5 **Considerations When Evaluating Fetal Hydronephrosis**

1. Is the hydronephrosis unilateral or bilateral?
2. If it is unilateral: a. Is it a solitary kidney? b. Is the contralateral kidney sonographically normal?
3. Is the amniotic fluid volume normal?
4. How dilatation is the renal pelvis?
5. Is the dilatation progressively worsening on serial evaluations?
6. Is there caliceal dilatation? If so, is there cortical thinning?
7. Are there any cystic changes or abnormal echogenic pattern that are suggestive of dysplasia?
8. Are other structures of the genitourinary tract dilated (e.g., bladder, ureters)?
9. Is the bladder visible?
10. Is there evidence of associated urinary tract abnormalities (e.g., duplication, ureterocele)?
11. Are there any other abnormalities outside of the urinary tract?

(Based on Pates JA, Dashe JS: Prenatal diagnosis and management of hydronephrosis, *Early Hum Dev* 82(1):3-8, 2006.)

TABLE 37-6 **Indications for Prenatal Intervention**

Evidence of bladder outlet obstruction
Normal karyotype
No other anomalies
Single male fetus
Oligohydramnios
Noncystic kidneys
Favorable urinary indices

benefit in terms of pulmonary and renal function[29] has to be contrasted with the high rate of vesicoamniotic shunt dysfunction and the risk of urinary ascites, chorioamnionitis, the premature rupture of membranes, premature labor and delivery, and the overall fetal morbidity and mortality. Table 37-6 lists the parameters that are currently used when considering prenatal intervention.

Postnatal Management

Two groups of patients are considered in this category: (1) infants who are managed conservatively after a full workup after birth and (2) children who present at older ages as a result of symptoms or of an incidental finding on studies ordered for unrelated problems.

Indications for Urgent Intervention

Usually, the clinician has time to electively order all of the appropriate tests to evaluate a child with possible urinary tract obstruction (i.e., abdominopelvic ultrasound, voiding cystourethrogram, renal scan). Clear exceptions include patients who present with urosepsis and/or acute renal insufficiency[80,81] in whom emergent intervention may be warranted. Newborn boys with posterior urethral valves should be catheterized and offered valve ablation soon after the diagnosis is established.[82] Similarly, newborns with large ureteroceles obstructing the bladder neck benefit from early catheterization and puncture.[83] Most children with giant hydronephrosis are otherwise asymptomatic and rarely require intervention as a result of the displacement of other structures. Nevertheless, infants with massively dilated

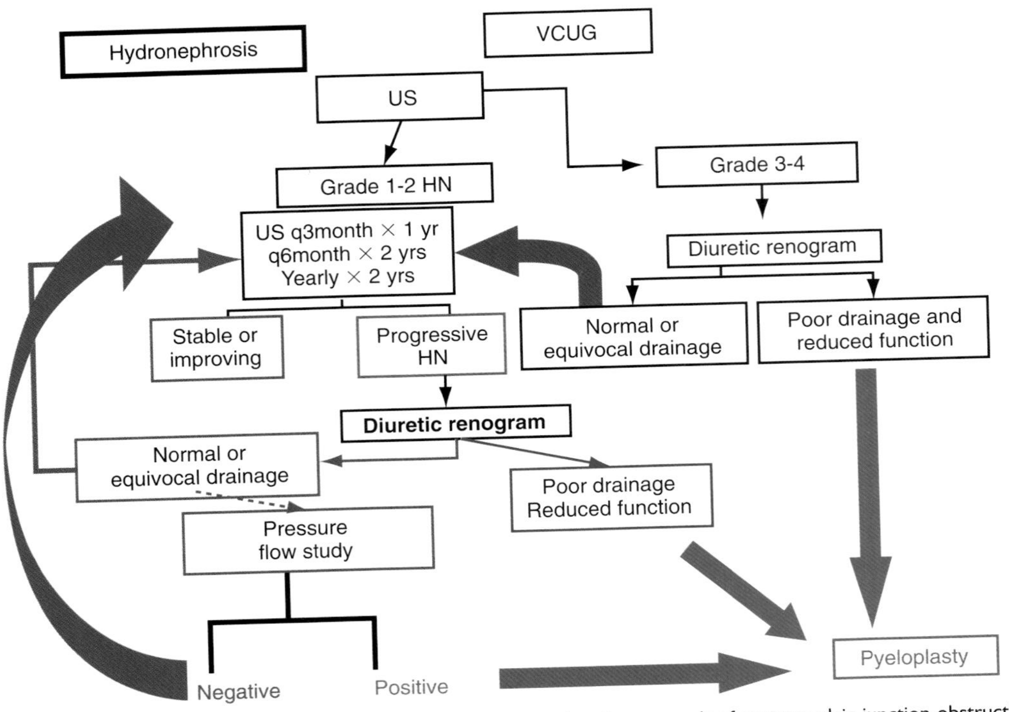

Figure 37-15 Proposed algorithm for the evaluation and management of hydronephrosis as a result of ureteropelvic junction obstruction. *US*, Ultrasound; *VCUG*, voiding cystourethrogram. Grading is based on the Society of Fetal Urology system.

collecting systems rarely improve with conservative management and may benefit from early surgical repair, although most patients—even those with bilateral involvement[35]—are initially observed.

Monitoring

The current basis of conservative management is close monitoring, because no one diagnostic modality can reliably predict spontaneous resolution. In the case of ureteropelvic junction obstruction, after the adoption of selected surgical intervention, the current standard of care has been frequent evaluation to detect worsening renal function or evident progression in dilatation over time[84] (Figure 37-15). The frequency and selection of studies varies among physicians, but a pattern of more aggressive and frequent evaluation is prudent during the first 2 years of life or in cases without a clear trend toward resolution. Keeping in mind that the ultimate goal is the preservation of function, the next issue is the duration of follow up. Although it is reassuring to follow patients, thus avoiding surgical intervention for a long period of time, emerging long-term studies caution about the possibility of late deterioration.[36] A similar policy has been adopted in the management of ureterovesical junction obstruction. Prenatally detected primary megaureters are usually followed expectantly, and only a minority seem to worsen over time. Unfortunately, in the absence of complete resolution, the need for long-term monitoring cannot be overemphasized.[36]

In most cases, early postnatal surgical intervention may prove to be an overtly aggressive approach, because the condition in many children resolves spontaneously. The management approach should balance the cost and risks of surgery with that of close monitoring and renal deterioration, and this must be modulated by other factors such as the level of obstruction, the overall degree of renal function, the likelihood of resolution, and the development of symptoms. For example, in children with presumed ureteropelvic junction obstruction detected by prenatal ultrasound, the ratio favors expectant management, because multiple studies have shown that only about 25% of patients ultimately require surgery. Similarly, primary megaureters are safely monitored in most circumstances.[85] Toward the other end of the spectrum (except for selected cases), many ureteroceles eventually require surgical intervention,[86,87] and most if not all children with posterior urethral valves are treated surgically.[82]

Specific Surgical Interventions

The basic principles behind surgical treatment are to correct the structural defect that is causing the obstructive process and to prevent further renal damage. The specific surgical procedure depends on the level of obstruction. Ureteropelvic junction and proximal ureteral obstructions are commonly managed by performing a pyeloplasty or a ureteroureterostomy. In both circumstances, the abnormal segment is resected, the ureter and pelvis are relocated away from the structures that are causing extrinsic compression, and the system is reconstructed in a watertight fashion. Depending on the patient's age, the surgeon's experience, and the available resources, either an open or a laparoscopic approach may be used.[88,89] Ureterovesical junction obstructions are dealt with in a similar fashion, with the difference being that the distal ureter has to be anastomosed to the bladder;

this process usually requires the creation of an antireflux mechanism. Massively dilated ureters are tailored before reimplantation, and other anatomic abnormalities can be addressed at the same time (e.g., large bladder diverticulum, ureterocele).

Urethral obstructions can be initially managed with temporary diversions above the area of blockage by directly bringing to skin level the bladder (vesicostomy), the ureter (ureterostomy), or the renal pelvis (pyelostomy).[90] As a result of advances in surgical instrumentation, most cases of posterior valves can now be treated endoscopically by transurethral resection.[91] The choice of one approach over others is a matter of surgeon preference, with limited or contradictory reports in the literature supporting one approach over another.[82,92-97] Most newborns undergo transurethral ablation,[98] with urinary cutaneous diversions reserved for selected situations, such as patients with a small urethral lumen (i.e., one that would not allow the resectoscope to be gently advanced to the area of obstruction), those with persistent or worsening hydronephrosis and renal function deterioration despite catheter drainage or transurethral ablation, and those with recurrent infections associated with high-grade vesicoureteral reflux and voiding inefficiency. Children with an obstructing ureterocele can be safely managed by transurethral puncture,[83,99,100] although some cases are better managed by removing the affected renal moiety (if not functioning or poorly functioning) and/or by performing surgical reconstruction of the ureterovesical junction area.[101,102]

Irrespective of the reconstruction performed, infant males at risk for further renal damage as a result of pyelonephritis are likely to be helped by having a circumcision performed during the first year of life.[103] Similarly, in the setting of recurrent or breakthrough febrile infections, consideration should be given to attempting the surgical correction of associated vesicoureteral reflux by either an endoscopic or an open approach.[104,105]

In rare circumstances, lower urinary obstruction is associated with severe and/or progressive structural and functional changes that may worsen already compromised renal function. When high-pressure bladder urine storage fails to improve with anticholinergics and catheterization, the need for a surgical procedure to increase bladder capacity and decrease storage pressures should be considered. It should be highlighted that most children who currently undergo such procedures have underlying neurovesical dysfunction (i.e., neurogenic bladder due to spinal dysraphism), and a minority have an underlying structural obstructive process. For example, most boys with posterior valves do not require augmentation cystoplasty for management, because the natural progression of the "valve bladder" is to go from a small capacity with instability to a large-capacity bladder with a weak detrusor.[106-108]

Bladder capacity may be surgically enhanced with different autologous tissues. Whenever possible, available urothelium-lined structures should be used (i.e., ureterocystoplasty with a dilated ureter associated with a nonfunctioning kidney). Unfortunately, such situations are not common.[109] Therefore, the remaining patients are offered improvement at the expense of using a segment of gastrointestinal tract for augmentation. The benefit has to be counterbalanced with complications that arise from the shortening of the gut, the surgical procedure itself, subsequent urinary tract colonization and recurrent infections, perforation, stones, mucus production, the potential for neoplasia, and metabolic complications from chronic urine exposure.[110] Interestingly, some of these patients may be able to empty their bladders without intermittent catheterization.[111] Those who need clean catheterization may benefit from a catheterizable channel, because the presence of a sensate urethra may not allow for regular instrumentation.[111] Marginal renal function may pose a difficult situation, with worsening azotemia developing as a result of the absorption of solutes through the intestinal epithelium. In those patients who eventually require a renal transplant, previous bladder augmentation does not affect the success of such a procedure or pose an increased risk of complications.[112] Current efforts to devise a bladder replacement with tissue-engineering technology are far from widespread clinical applications, although preliminary human studies are promising.[113]

LONG-TERM ISSUES

In the majority of patients with obstructive urologic disease, the long-term outcomes are remarkably positive. Despite these optimistic outcomes, an important minority have significant sequelae, such as chronic renal failure. Unfortunately, there are relatively few long-term studies that have involved patients with obstructive uropathies. Most of the available data reports are about patients with posterior urethral valves.

In unilateral disease, the development of clinically significant hypertension or proteinuria appears to be very rare. Hypertension may be the result of renal scars from infections or renal dysplasia, and it is renin mediated rather than volume mediated. Perhaps as a result of the early detection and management of prenatally detected cases, later problems appear to be rare. Even with the conservative management of markedly hydronephrotic kidneys, only a small percentage of patients will lose functional renal mass or become symptomatic. Overall, the loss of function resulting in renal insufficiency or failure is not an issue, except in the presence of a solitary kidney.

By contrast, bilateral disease has a more ominous prognosis. In many of these cases, a marked loss of renal mass has already occurred before birth as a result of either maldevelopment or obstructive damage. Adverse prognostic factors in these children include the gestational age at diagnosis, the presence of vesicoureteral reflux or altered renal echogenicity at the time of diagnosis, the level of serum creatinine at one year of age (i.e., <1 mg/dl or ~88 μmol/L in infants born with posterior urethral valves[114]), the occurrence of urinary tract infections, and, later in life, the appearance of proteinuria and/or hypertension. Early-onset hypertension may result from global damage as a result of urinary obstruction and/or scarring from recurrent urinary tract infections. Progressive renal disease, which is frequently seen during adolescence, can be attributed to a combination of factors, including hyperfiltration injury, hypertension, recurrent infections, and persistent obstruction or abnormal bladder dynamics.

Several recent reviews suggest that about a third of patients with posterior urethral valves will go into renal insufficiency before adulthood; many of these patients will ultimately require renal replacement therapy or renal transplantation. Optimal lower urinary tract management is paramount for preserving renal function as long as possible and for protecting the long-term allograft survival if transplantation is required. Therefore, it is crucial to search for and treat abnormal voiding dynamics and to consider urodynamic investigations before transplantation, thus correcting persisting bladder problems early. Further details concerning the management of voiding dysfunction are provided in Chapter 20.

Genetic Counselling

Most urinary tract malformations appear to occur in isolation; only a minority are part of syndromes in which specific mutations have been defined. In the long run, an understanding of the genetic aspects of obstructive uropathies will help unravel the pathogenesis of these disorders, and this may facilitate the design of genetic screening tests with a view toward early diagnosis and appropriate genetic counselling.[115]

Contact Sports

Children with a solitary functioning kidney or a poorly functioning moiety, with or without underlying renal insufficiency, are perceived to be at an increased risk for end-stage renal disease after significant trauma. This is of particular interest for children who want to be involved in collision sports (i.e., those in which athletes purposefully hit each other or inanimate objects with great force) or contact sports (i.e., those in which the collision is less forceful and/or frequent). As compared with adults, children have an increased risk for renal trauma,[116] and, on average, they practice sports more frequently. Interestingly, there are no reports of solitary kidney loss after sports-related trauma. The incidence of posttraumatic end-stage renal disease is low, and more renal injuries occur as a result of other mechanisms (e.g., motor vehicle accidents).[117,118] With these facts taken into account along with the known consequences of inactivity (e.g., childhood obesity, hypertension[119,120]), the child should be allowed to participate in sports if protective gear and adequate supervision are provided and if the patient and family are aware of the risks involved. After all, these sports are practiced all over the world by children who also have other valuable solitary organs, such as the brain, liver, and spleen.

CONCLUSION

The definition and management of obstruction remains a controversial and sometimes difficult clinical problem. The current tendency to observe many patients with presumed obstruction appears to be safe. Although many patients are spared surgical intervention, a smaller group potentially experiences some renal damage before intervention as a result of the fact that the threshold for intervention is based on detecting the effects of such processes (most commonly the loss of renal function). The need for better imaging and molecular markers is evident; this will help physicians to better discriminate "harmful" obstruction from "harmless" dilatation,[5] thereby allowing for earlier detection and treatment with the preservation of function before irreversible damage occurs.

REFERENCES

1. Koff SA: Pathophysiology of ureteropelvic junction obstruction. Clinical and experimental observations, *Urol Clin North Am* 17(2):263-72, 1990.
2. Koff SA, Hayden LJ, Cirulli C, et al: Pathophysiology of ureteropelvic junction obstruction: experimental and clinical observations, *J Urol* 136(1 Pt 2):336-38, 1986.
3. Whitaker RH: Some observations and theories on the wide ureter and hydronephrosis, *Br J Urol* 47(4):377-85, 1975.
4. Chevalier RL, Chung KH, Smith CD, et al: Renal apoptosis and clusterin following ureteral obstruction: the role of maturation, *J Urol* 156(4):1474-79, 1996.
5. Csaicsich D, Greenbaum LA, Aufricht C: Upper urinary tract: when is obstruction obstruction?, *Curr Opin Urol* 14(4):213-17, 2004.
6. Chevalier RL: Pathogenesis of renal injury in obstructive uropathy, *Curr Opin Pediatr* 18(2):153-60, 2006.
7. Chadha V, Warady BA: Epidemiology of pediatric chronic kidney disease, *Adv Chronic Kidney Dis* 12(4):343-52, 2005.
8. Ardissino G, Dacco V, Testa S, et al: Epidemiology of chronic renal failure in children: data from the ItalKid project, *Pediatrics* 111(4 Pt 1):e382-87, 2003.
9. Fung LC, Churchill BM, McLorie GA, et al: Ureteral opening pressure: a novel parameter for the evaluation of pediatric hydronephrosis, *J Urol* 159(4):1326-30, 1998.
10. Koff SA: Pressure volume relationships in human hydronephrosis, *Urology* 25(3):256-58, 1985.
11. Nitzsche EU, Zimmerhackl LB, Hawkins RA, et al: Correlation of ultrasound and renal scintigraphy in children with unilateral hydronephrosis in primary workup, *Pediatr Nephrol* 7(2):138-42, 1993.
12. Kiley SC, Thornhill BA, Belyea BC, et al: Epidermal growth factor potentiates renal cell death in hydronephrotic neonatal mice, but cell survival in rats, *Kidney Int* 68(2):504-14, 2005.
13. Kiley SC, Thornhill BA, Tang SS, et al: Growth factor-mediated phosphorylation of proapoptotic BAD reduces tubule cell death in vitro and in vivo, *Kidney Int* 63(1):33-42, 2003.
14. Beck AD: The effect of intra-uterine urinary obstruction upon the development of the fetal kidney, *J Urol* 105(6):784-89, 1971.
15. Glick PL, Harrison MR, Noall RA, et al: Correction of congenital hydronephrosis in utero III. Early mid-trimester ureteral obstruction produces renal dysplasia, *J Pediatr Surg* 18(6):681-87, 1983.
16. Chevalier RL: Perinatal obstructive nephropathy, *Semin Perinatol* 28(2):124-31, 2004.
17. Chevalier RL, Thornhill BA, Chang AY, et al: Recovery from release of ureteral obstruction in the rat: relationship to nephrogenesis, *Kidney Int* 61(6):2033-43, 2002.
18. Homayoon K, Pippi Salle JL, Agarwal SK, et al: Relative accuracy of renal scan in estimation of renal function during partial ureteral obstruction, *Can J Urol* 5(4):611-19, 1998.
19. Leahy AL, Ryan PC, McEntee GM, et al: Renal injury and recovery in partial ureteric obstruction, *J Urol* 142(1):199-203, 1989.
20. Nguyen HT, Kogan BA: Renal hemodynamic changes after complete and partial unilateral ureteral obstruction in the fetal lamb, *J Urol* 160(3 Pt 2):1063-69, 1998.
21. Chevalier RL, Kim A, Thornhill BA, et al: Recovery following relief of unilateral ureteral obstruction in the neonatal rat, *Kidney Int* 55(3):793-807, 1999.
22. Chung KH, Chevalier RL: Arrested development of the neonatal kidney following chronic ureteral obstruction, *J Urol* 155(3):1139-44, 1996.
23. Thornhill BA, Burt LE, Chen C, et al: Variable chronic partial ureteral obstruction in the neonatal rat: a new model of ureteropelvic junction obstruction, *Kidney Int* 67(1):42-52, 2005.

24. Edouga D, Hugueny B, Gasser B, et al: Recovery after relief of fetal urinary obstruction: morphological, functional and molecular aspects, *Am J Physiol Renal Physiol* 281(1):F26-37, 2001.
25. Ito K, Chen J, El Chaar M, et al: Renal damage progresses despite improvement of renal function after relief of unilateral ureteral obstruction in adult rats, *Am J Physiol Renal Physiol* 287(6):F1283-93, 2004.
26. Freedman AL, Johnson MP, Smith CA, et al: Long-term outcome in children after antenatal intervention for obstructive uropathies, *Lancet* 354(9176):374-77, 1999.
27. Holmes N, Harrison MR, Baskin LS: Fetal surgery for posterior urethral valves: long-term postnatal outcomes, *Pediatrics* 108(1): E7, 2001.
28. Manning FA, Harrison MR, Rodeck C: Catheter shunts for fetal hydronephrosis and hydrocephalus. Report of the International Fetal Surgery Registry, *N Engl J Med* 315(5):336-40, 1986.
29. McLorie G, Farhat W, Khoury A, et al: Outcome analysis of vesicoamniotic shunting in a comprehensive population, *J Urol* 166(3):1036-40, 2001.
30. Chevalier RL: Biomarkers of congenital obstructive nephropathy: past, present and future, *J Urol* 172(3):852-57, 2004.
31. Allen TD, Husmann DA: Ureteropelvic junction obstruction associated with ureteral hypoplasia, *J Urol* 142(2 Pt 1):353-55, 1989.
32. Duel BP, Vates TS, Heiser D, et al: Antegrade pyelography before pyeloplasty via dorsal lumbar incision, *J Urol* 162(1):174-76, 1999.
33. Fung LC, Khoury AE, McLorie GA, et al: Evaluation of pediatric hydronephrosis using individualized pressure flow criteria, *J Urol* 154(2 Pt 2):671-76, 1995.
34. Whitaker RH: Methods of assessing obstruction in dilated ureters, *Br J Urol* 45(1):15-22, 1973.
35. Onen A, Jayanthi VR, Koff SA: Long-term followup of prenatally detected severe bilateral newborn hydronephrosis initially managed nonoperatively, *J Urol* 168(3):1118-20, 2002.
36. Shukla AR, Cooper J, Patel RP, et al: Prenatally detected primary megaureter: a role for extended followup, *J Urol* 173(4):1353-56, 2005.
37. Mouriquand PD, Troisfontaines E, Wilcox DT: Antenatal and perinatal uro-nephrology: current questions and dilemmas, *Pediatr Nephrol* 13(9):938-44, 1999.
38. Van Savage JG, Khoury AE, McLorie GA, et al: An algorithm for the management of anterior urethral valves, *J Urol* 158(3 Pt 2): 1030-32, 1997.
39. Henderson AM, Vallis CJ, Sumner E: Anaesthesia in the prune-belly syndrome. A review of 36 cases, *Anaesthesia* 42(1):54-60, 1987.
40. Balster S, Schiborr M, Brinkmann OA, et al: [Obstructive uropathy in childhood], *Aktuelle Urol* 36(4):317-28, 2005.
41. Grisoni ER, Gauderer MW, Wolfson RN, et al: Antenatal ultrasonography: the experience in a high risk perinatal center, *J Pediatr Surg* 21(4):358-61, 1986.
42. Elder JS: Antenatal hydronephrosis. Fetal and neonatal management, *Pediatr Clin North Am* 44(5):1299-321, 1997.
43. Reddy PP, Mandell J: Prenatal diagnosis. Therapeutic implications. *Urol Clin North Am* 25(2):171-80, 1998.
44. Caire JT, Ramus RM, Magee KP, et al: MRI of fetal genitourinary anomalies, *AJR Am J Roentgenol* 181(5):1381-85, 2003.
45. Zaretsky M, Ramus R, McIntire D, et al: MRI calculation of lung volumes to predict outcome in fetuses with genitourinary abnormalities, *AJR Am J Roentgenol* 185(5):1328-34, 2005.
46. Nussbaum AR, Lebowitz RL: Interlabial masses in little girls: review and imaging recommendations, *AJR Am J Roentgenol* 141(1):65-71, 1983.
47. Riccabona M, Sorantin E, Hausegger K: Imaging guided interventional procedures in paediatric uroradiology—a case based overview, *Eur J Radiol* 43(2):167-79, 2002.
48. Kanellopoulos TA, Salakos C, Spiliopoulou I, et al: First urinary tract infection in neonates, infants and young children: a comparative study, *Pediatr Nephrol* 21(8):1131-37, 2006.
49. Hoberman A, Charron M, Hickey RW, et al: Imaging studies after a first febrile urinary tract infection in young children, *N Engl J Med* 348(3):195-202, 2003.
50. Giorgi LJ Jr, Bratslavsky G, Kogan BA: Febrile urinary tract infections in infants: renal ultrasound remains necessary, *J Urol* 173(2):568-70, 2005.
51. Cain MP, Rink RC, Thomas AC, et al: Symptomatic ureteropelvic junction obstruction in children in the era of prenatal sonography—is there a higher incidence of crossing vessels?, *Urology* 57(2):338-41, 2001.
52. Mergener K, Weinerth JL, Baillie J: Dietl's crisis: a syndrome of episodic abdominal pain of urologic origin that may present to a gastroenterologist, *Am J Gastroenterol* 92(12):2289-91, 1997.
53. Update on the 1987 Task Force Report on High Blood Pressure in Children and Adolescents: a working group report from the National High Blood Pressure Education Program. National High Blood Pressure Education Program Working Group on Hypertension Control in Children and Adolescents, *Pediatrics* 98(4 Pt 1): 649-58, 1996.
54. Farnham SB, Adams MC, Brock JW 3rd, et al: Pediatric urological causes of hypertension, *J Urol* 173(3):697-704, 2005.
55. Bartosh SM, Aronson AJ: Childhood hypertension. An update on etiology, diagnosis, and treatment, *Pediatr Clin North Am* 46(2): 235-52, 1999.
56. Baez-Trinidad LG, Lendvay TS, Broecker BH, et al: Efficacy of nephrectomy for the treatment of nephrogenic hypertension in a pediatric population, *J Urol* 170(4 Pt 2):1655-57; discussion 1658, 2003.
57. Johal NS, Kraklau D, Cuckow PM: The role of unilateral nephrectomy in the treatment of nephrogenic hypertension in children, *BJU Int* 95(1):140-42, 2005.
58. el-Dahr SS, Lewy JE: Urinary tract obstruction and infection in the neonate, *Clin Perinatol* 19(1):213-22, 1992.
59. Lee RS, Cendron M, Kinnamon DD, et al: Antenatal hydronephrosis as a predictor of postnatal outcome: a meta-analysis, *Pediatrics* 118(2):586-93, 2006.
60. Sidhu G, Beyene J, Rosenblum ND: Outcome of isolated antenatal hydronephrosis: a systematic review and meta-analysis, *Pediatr Nephrol* 21(2):218-24, 2006.
61. Docimo SG, Silver RI: Renal ultrasonography in newborns with prenatally detected hydronephrosis: why wait?, *J Urol* 157(4):1387-89, 1997.
62. Dhillon HK: Prenatally diagnosed hydronephrosis: the Great Ormond Street experience, *Br J Urol* 81 Suppl 2:39-44, 1998.
63. Ransley PG, Dhillon HK, Gordon I, et al: The postnatal management of hydronephrosis diagnosed by prenatal ultrasound, *J Urol* 144(2 Pt 2):584-87; discussion 593-94, 1990.
64. Conway JJ: "Well-tempered" diuresis renography: its historical development, physiological and technical pitfalls, and standardized technique protocol, *Semin Nucl Med* 22(2):74-84, 1992.
65. Conway JJ, Maizels M: The "well tempered" diuretic renogram: a standard method to examine the asymptomatic neonate with hydronephrosis or hydroureteronephrosis. A report from combined meetings of The Society for Fetal Urology and members of The Pediatric Nuclear Medicine Council—The Society of Nuclear Medicine, *J Nucl Med* 33(11):2047-51, 1992.
66. Ebel KD: Uroradiology in the fetus and newborn: diagnosis and follow-up of congenital obstruction of the urinary tract, *Pediatr Radiol* 28(8):630-35, 1998.
67. Kass EJ, Majd M, Belman AB: Comparison of the diuretic renogram and the pressure perfusion study in children, *J Urol* 134(1):92-96, 1985.
68. Riccabona M: Pediatric MRU—its potential and its role in the diagnostic work-up of upper urinary tract dilatation in infants and children, *World J Urol* 22(2):79-87, 2004.
69. Schwartz GJ, Haycock GB, Edelmann CM Jr, et al: A simple estimate of glomerular filtration rate in children derived from body length and plasma creatinine, *Pediatrics* 58(2):259-63, 1976.
70. Filler G, Bokenkamp A, Hofmann W, et al: Cystatin C as a marker of GFR—history, indications, and future research, *Clin Biochem* 38(1):1-8, 2005.
71. Zappitelli M, Parvex P, Joseph L, et al: Derivation and validation of cystatin C-based prediction equations for GFR in children, *Am J Kidney Dis* 48(2):221-30, 2006.
72. Woodward M, Frank D: Postnatal management of antenatal hydronephrosis. *BJU Int* 89(2):149-56, 2002.

73. Grignon A, Filion R, Filiatrault D, et al: Urinary tract dilatation in utero: classification and clinical applications, *Radiology* 160(3):645-47, 1986.
74. Podevin G, Mandelbrot L, Vuillard E, et al: Outcome of urological abnormalities prenatally diagnosed by ultrasound, *Fetal Diagn Ther* 11(3):181-90, 1996.
75. Kaefer M, Peters CA, Retik AB, et al: Increased renal echogenicity: a sonographic sign for differentiating between obstructive and non-obstructive etiologies of in utero bladder distension, *J Urol* 158(3 Pt 2):1026-29, 1997.
76. Mahony BS, Filly RA, Callen PW, et al: Fetal renal dysplasia: sonographic evaluation, *Radiology* 152(1):143-46, 1984.
77. Quintero RA: Fetal obstructive uropathy, *Clin Obstet Gynecol* 48(4):923-41, 2005.
78. Freedman AL, Bukowski TP, Smith CA, et al: Use of urinary beta-2-microglobulin to predict severe renal damage in fetal obstructive uropathy, *Fetal Diagn Ther* 12(1):1-6, 1997.
79. Johnson MP, Bukowski TP, Reitleman C, et al: In utero surgical treatment of fetal obstructive uropathy: a new comprehensive approach to identify appropriate candidates for vesicoamniotic shunt therapy, *Am J Obstet Gynecol* 170(6):1770-76; discussion 1776-79, 1994.
80. Filler G: Acute renal failure in children: aetiology and management, *Paediatr Drugs* 3(11):783-92, 2001.
81. Stanley P, Diament MJ: Pediatric percutaneous nephrostomy: experience with 50 patients, *J Urol* 135(6):1223-26, 1986.
82. Yohannes P, Hanna M: Current trends in the management of posterior urethral valves in the pediatric population, *Urology* 60(6):947-53, 2002.
83. Austin PF, Cain MP, Casale AJ, et al: Prenatal bladder outlet obstruction secondary to ureterocele, *Urology* 52(6):1132-35, 1998.
84. Ulman I, Jayanthi VR, Koff SA: The long-term followup of newborns with severe unilateral hydronephrosis initially treated nonoperatively, *J Urol* 164(3 Pt 2):1101-05, 2000.
85. Shokeir AA, Nijman RJ: Primary megaureter: current trends in diagnosis and treatment, *BJU Int* 86(7):861-68, 2000.
86. Direnna T, Leonard MP: Watchful waiting for prenatally detected ureteroceles, *J Urol* 175(4):1493-95; discussion 1495, 2006.
87. Han MY, Gibbons MD, Belman AB, et al: Indications for nonoperative management of ureteroceles, *J Urol* 174(4 Pt 2):1652-55; discussion 1655-56, 2005.
88. Lee RS, Retik AB, Borer JG, et al: Pediatric robot assisted laparoscopic dismembered pyeloplasty: comparison with a cohort of open surgery, *J Urol* 175(2):683-87; discussion 687, 2006.
89. Metzelder ML, Schier F, Petersen C, et al: Laparoscopic transabdominal pyeloplasty in children is feasible irrespective of age, *J Urol* 175(2):688-91, 2006.
90. Jayanthi VR, McLorie GA, Khoury AE, et al: The effect of temporary cutaneous diversion on ultimate bladder function, *J Urol* 154(2 Pt 2):889-92, 1995.
91. Bellinger MF: Optical valvulotomy for urethral valves using a hookblade cold knife, *Urology* 42(4):443-44, 1993.
92. Close CE, Carr MC, Burns MW, et al: Lower urinary tract changes after early valve ablation in neonates and infants: is early diversion warranted?, *J Urol* 157(3):984-88, 1997.
93. Duckett JW: Are "valve bladders" congenital or iatrogenic?, *Br J Urol* 79(2):271-75, 1997.
94. Jaureguizar E, Lopez Pereira P, Martinez Urrutia MJ, et al: Does neonatal pyeloureterostomy worsen bladder function in children with posterior urethral valves?, *J Urol* 164(3 Pt 2):1031-33; discussion 1033-34, 2000.
95. Krueger RP, Hardy BE, Churchill BM: Growth in boys and posterior urethral valves. Primary valve resection vs upper tract diversion, *Urol Clin North Am* 7(2):265-72, 1980.
96. Lopez Pereira P, Martinez Urrutia MJ, Jaureguizar E: Initial and long-term management of posterior ure thral valves, *World J Urol* 22(6):418-24, 2004.
97. Walker RD, Padron M: The management of posterior urethral valves by initial vesicostomy and delayed valve ablation, *J Urol* 144(5):1212-14, 1990.
98. Farhat W, McLorie G, Capolicchio G, et al: Outcomes of primary valve ablation versus urinary tract diversion in patients with posterior urethral valves, *Urology* 56(4):653-57, 2000.
99. Chertin B, Fridmans A, Hadas-Halpren I, et al: Endoscopic puncture of ureterocele as a minimally invasive and effective long-term procedure in children, *Eur Urol* 39(3):332-36, 2001.
100. Jankowski JT, Palmer JS: Holmium: yttrium-aluminum-garnet laser puncture of ureteroceles in neonatal period, *Urology* 68(1):179-81, 2006.
101. Gran CD, Kropp BP, Cheng EY, et al: Primary lower urinary tract reconstruction for nonfunctioning renal moieties associated with obstructing ureteroceles, *J Urol* 173(1):198-201, 2005.
102. Mor Y, Ramon J, Raviv G, et al: A 20-year experience with treatment of ectopic ureteroceles, *J Urol* 147(6):1592-94, 1992.
103. Singh-Grewal D, Macdessi J, Craig J: Circumcision for the prevention of urinary tract infection in boys: a systematic review of randomised trials and observational studies, *Arch Dis Child* 90(8):853-58, 2005.
104. Austin JC, Cooper CS: Vesicoureteral reflux: surgical approaches, *Urol Clin North Am* 31(3):543-57, x, 2004.
105. Elder JS, Diaz M, Caldamone AA, et al: Endoscopic therapy for vesicoureteral reflux: a meta-analysis. I. Reflux resolution and urinary tract infection, *J Urol* 175(2):716-22, 2006.
106. De Gennaro M, Capitanucci ML, Mosiello G, et al: The changing urodynamic pattern from infancy to adolescence in boys with posterior urethral valves, *BJU Int* 85(9):1104-08, 2000.
107. De Gennaro M, Capitanucci ML, Silveri M, et al: Detrusor hypocontractility evolution in boys with posterior urethral valves detected by pressure flow analysis, *J Urol* 165(6 Pt 2):2248-52, 2001.
108. Holmdahl G, Sillen U, Hanson E, et al: Bladder dysfunction in boys with posterior urethral valves before and after puberty, *J Urol* 155(2):694-98, 1996.
109. Husmann DA, Snodgrass WT, Koyle MA, et al: Ureterocystoplasty: indications for a successful augmentation, *J Urol* 171(1):376-80, 2004.
110. Gough DC: Enterocystoplasty, *BJU Int* 88(7):739-43, 2001.
111. Kajbafzadeh AM, Quinn FM, Duffy PG, et al: Augmentation cystoplasty in boys with posterior urethral valves, *J Urol* 154(2 Pt 2):874-77, 1995.
112. DeFoor W, Tackett L, Minevich E, et al: Successful renal transplantation in children with posterior urethral valves, *J Urol* 170(6 Pt 1):2402-04, 2003.
113. Atala A, Bauer SB, Soker S, et al: Tissue-engineered autologous bladders for patients needing cystoplasty, *Lancet* 367(9518):1241-46, 2006.
114. Warshaw BL, Hymes LC, Trulock TS, et al: Prognostic features in infants with obstructive uropathy due to posterior urethral valves, *J Urol* 133(2):240-43, 1985.
115. Woolf AS: A molecular and genetic view of human renal and urinary tract malformations, *Kidney Int* 58(2):500-12, 2000.
116. Brown SL, Elder JS, Spirnak JP: Are pediatric patients more susceptible to major renal injury from blunt trauma? A comparative study, *J Urol* 160(1):138-40, 1998.
117. McAleer IM, Kaplan GW, LoSasso BE: Renal and testis injuries in team sports, *J Urol* 168(4 Pt 2):1805-07, 2002.
118. Psooy K: Sports and the solitary kidney: how to counsel parents, *Can J Urol* 13(3):3120-26, 2006.
119. Mitsnefes MM: Hypertension in children and adolescents, *Pediatr Clin North Am* 53(3):493-512, viii, 2006.
120. Reilly JJ, McDowell ZC: Physical activity interventions in the prevention and treatment of paediatric obesity: systematic review and critical appraisal, *Proc Nutr Soc* 62(3):611-19, 2003.

CHAPTER

38

Voiding Disorders

Jennifer Dart Yin Sihoe, Sik-Nin Wong, and Chung-Kwong Yeung

INTRODUCTION

The lower urinary tract consists of the urinary bladder, the bladder neck/sphincter complex, and the urethra. It has a rich innervation of autonomic and somatic nerves that relay to spinal cord and higher centers. Under normal situation, it works as a coordinated unit, and it achieves the function of storage at low pressure and the intermittent efficient evacuation of urine. Voiding disorders occur when the normal functioning of any of its components is disturbed. This results in urinary incontinence and inadequate emptying or high bladder pressure, with the consequence of urinary tract infection (UTI) and back-pressure damage to the upper urinary tract. In addition to the normal anatomy and developmental physiology of voiding, this chapter will focus on the discussion of neurogenic bladder, functional voiding disorders, and nocturnal enuresis.

NORMAL ANATOMY AND PHYSIOLOGY OF VOIDING

In the human body, the bladder has the dual functions of the storage and the emptying of urine. It is innervated by a complex network of both somatic and autonomic nerves that allow for voluntary and involuntary control of function. The current knowledge of the functional anatomy of the lower urinary tract originates from extensive postmortem studies carried out over the past decades.[1-5]

Anatomy

The bladder is a muscular viscus located in the pelvic cavity; in infants and young children, it is readily palpable as an abdominal organ when full.[6] The bladder wall is lined, from the inside out, by the mucosa, the detrusor muscles, and the adventitia. The detrusor consists of a meshwork of smooth muscle fibers arranged into a single functioning unit with an ability to elicit nearly maximum active tension over a wide range of length. This allows the bladder to fill with urine from the upper tract at low pressures.[7] The ability of the bladder to store urine is determined by the concomitant activity of the detrusor muscle and the bladder outlet. The bladder outlet is made up of the bladder neck and the proximal urethra, and it is supported by the striated muscles of the pelvic floor.[4]

During the storage phase, the bladder continuously receives urine from the ureters. The detrusor relaxes to keep a constant and low intravesical pressure, whereas the sphincter contracts to prevent urine leakage. During the voiding phase, a voluntary relaxation of pelvic floor muscles initiates a reflexive bladder contraction that consists of the funneling of bladder outlet, the relaxation of the sphincter, and the synchronous contraction of the bladder detrusor to effect a coordinated voiding.

The urethral sphincter mechanism plays a major role in urinary continence by closure of the bladder neck and the proximal urethra. It is often thought of as two parts: the internal sphincter and the external sphincter. The external urinary sphincter is situated immediately above the pelvic floor. It extends from the apex of the prostate to include the length of the membranous urethra in males, and it extends from the bladder neck to the mid urethra in females. It consists of an inner layer of smooth muscle and an outer layer of striated muscle arranged into a cylindrical structure, which is accentuated anteriorly and thinned out or actually absent posteriorly, thus giving a characteristic horseshoe or omega shape on cross section. The internal sphincter, however, has not been well delineated anatomically. It has generally been accepted that it consists of smooth muscle fibers that continue from the bladder base and the trigone and that traverse inferiorly through the bladder neck to extend toward the proximal urethra. Its existence has been better delineated on radiologic and urethral pressure measurement studies.

There is limited information about the natural course of development or maturation of the structure and function of the sphincter mechanism. In a postmortem study of the ontogeny of the external urinary sphincter in human fetuses, infants, and young children, Kokoua and colleagues[8] found significant age-related differences in the histologic structure of the sphincter as compared with the adult sphincter. The striated muscle fibers of the sphincter were first shown to appear at around 20 weeks of gestation. They are initially arranged in a concentric pattern as a closed ring that is fused posteriorly to form a tail-like structure that is directed toward the perineal body, with posterior splitting occurring caudally and then progressing in a cephalad manner during the first year of life. Gradual resorption of the "tail" occurs in parallel to eventually form a mature omega-shaped structure.[8] It is postulated that the high intravesical pressures and

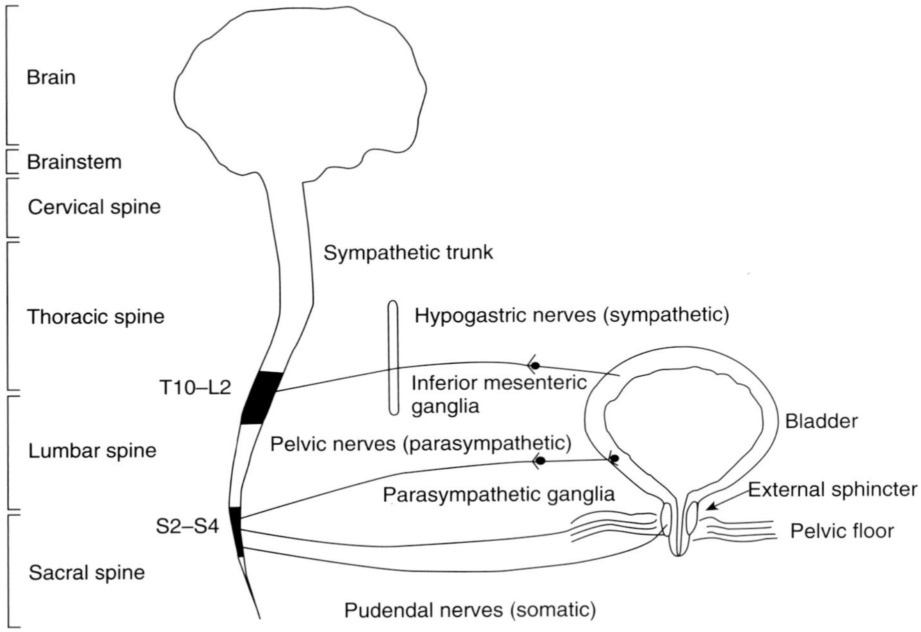

Figure 38-1 Diagram illustrating the innervation of the bladder-sphincter complex.

interrupted voiding commonly observed during urodynamic studies in infants may be the result of the complete closed ring of striated sphincteric muscle that is present in more than 40% of children who are less than 1 year old.[9-11]

Innervation

The nerve supply of the bladder detrusor/sphincter complex consists of sacral parasympathetic, thoracolumbar sympathetic, and sacral somatic nerves[4,7] (Figure 38-1).

The parasympathetic nerve fibers run in the pelvic nerve (S_2 through S_4) to supply the pelvic and vesical plexuses before entering the bladder. Parasympathetic ganglia are found within these plexuses and in the bladder wall.

The sympathetic nerves arise from segments T_{10} through L_2 of the spinal cord and travel through the sympathetic trunk to the inferior mesenteric ganglion and then the pelvic plexus and the bladder as the hypogastric nerves. There are also sympathetic branches that innervate the detrusor and the urethral sphincter.[12]

The somatic nerve fibers run in the pudendal nerve (S_2 through S_4) to supply the periurethral pelvic floor musculature.[7]

The neurologic control of normal micturition occurs at different levels, from the "sacral micturition center" in the spinal cord to the "pontine micturition center" within the brainstem to the cerebellum, the basal ganglia, the limbic system, the thalamus, the hypothalamus, and the cerebral cortex.[4,13-15] Within the spinal cord, information from bladder afferents is integrated with that from other viscera and somatic sources and projected to the brain stem centers that coordinate the micturition cycle.[16]

The parasympathetic and somatic nerves consist of cholinergic fibers. The sympathetic nerves consist of adrenergic fibers that act on beta receptors in the body of the bladder to relax the detrusors and on alpha receptors in the bladder neck to contract the sphincter. In addition, various other neurotransmitters are involved in bladder stimulation. These include prostaglandin substance P, opioid peptides, vasoactive intestinal peptide, and neuropeptide Y.[14] This explains, at least in part, why pharmacologic blockage of the classic neurotransmitters (acetylcholine and norepinephrine) alone may fail to completely abolish the effect of neural stimulation.

DEVELOPMENTAL ASPECTS OF VOIDING

Traditionally, it is believed that micturition in newborns and young infants occurs frequently as a result of a simple spinal cord reflex in response to a full bladder stimulating the afferent limb of the reflex arc, with little or no mediation by the higher neural centers. The voluntary inhibition of the bladder-emptying reflex was thought to be achieved through progressive maturation reached by adulthood. Thus, certain conditions (e.g., primary nocturnal enuresis) were attributed to a delay in this process and hence could improve with age.[17] However, more recent studies have indicated that this is an oversimplification of what actually occurs. Even in full-term fetuses and newborns, it has been shown that micturition is modulated by higher centers. Ohel and colleagues[18] showed that intrauterine micturition almost exclusively occurs while the fetus is awake rather than randomly distributed over various behavioral (sleep/arousal) states. Furthermore, it has been observed that micturition in a full-term fetus can be elicited by vibroacoustic stimulation, all of which indicates that the micturition reflex is probably under higher neural control, even at near gestational term.[19] Further extensive modulation occurs during the postnatal period.

Studies of normal neonates using ambulatory bladder monitoring techniques in conjunction with polysomnographic recordings have shown that, even in newborns, micturition does not occur during sleep.[10] During sleep, the bladder is normally quiescent and stable, with a lack of the facilitation of detrusor contractions. However, during wakefulness, marked detrusor overactivity is observed. Clear electroencephalographic evidence of cortical arousal or actual awakening occurs in response to bladder distension, and sleeping infants are noted to wake up before bladder activity returns and voiding occurs. However, this arousal period may often be transient, with the infant crying or moving for a brief period, micturating, and then going back to sleep without being noticed to have awakened. This wakening response to bladder distension probably involves more complicated neural pathways and higher centers than have been appreciated up until now.

These results also correlate with recent animal studies showing a sophisticated integration of preexisting central and peripheral neural pathways of micturition control at birth, with remodulation occurring during the early postnatal period.[20,21] Extensive studies using experimental animals have indicated that the early postnatal maturation of bladder function probably occurs at different levels: (1) changes in the properties of detrusor muscle; (2) developmental modifications in the peripheral innervation of the bladder; and (3) alterations in the central synaptic circuitry and neuroplasticity in the parasympathetic reflex pathways to the bladder.[22-26] Recordings of spontaneous activity in bladder smooth muscle in neonatal rats showed much larger amplitude and more synchronous rhythmic contractions as compared with those observed in adult rats.[26] This suggests that there is a progressive reduction in intercellular communication between detrusor smooth muscle cells, thereby resulting in less spontaneous activities and hence more efficient urine storage during early postnatal development. In addition, peripheral and central neural mechanisms also change extensively during this period. In cats (and some other species), micturition during the newborn period is dependent on an exteroceptive somatovesical reflex triggered when the mother licks the perineum of the kittens.[22-24] This somatovesical reflex, which is processed in the sacral spinal cord, disappears in older animals but may reappear after spinal cord injury. Further neuroanatomic studies have indicated that spinal bladder reflexes are mediated via interneurons located immediately adjacent to and synapsing with the sacral preganglionic neurons.[25] This interneuron-preganglionic neuron synaptic transmission is very efficient immediately after birth, but it is very abruptly downregulated during the third postnatal week, when the mature supraspinal micturition reflexes start to appear.[24] Transection of the spinal cord prevents this downregulation, thus indicating that the higher neural centers play an important role in this synaptic remodeling, which contributes to the postnatal development of micturition reflexes.

Urodynamic studies of normal infant bladders have also confirmed that bladder function in young children is very different from that in adults. During the first 2 to 3 years of life, there is progressive development from an initially indiscriminate infantile voiding pattern to a more socially conscious and voluntary or adult type of micturition achieved through an active learning process that entails an intact nervous system. This natural evolution of bladder control depends on at least three main events occurring in parallel: (1) a progressive increase in bladder functional storage capacity; (2) a maturation of voluntary control over the urethral striated muscle sphincter; and (3) the development of direct volitional control over the bladder-sphincteric unit so that the child can voluntarily initiate or inhibit the micturition reflex. This process can also be influenced by an awareness of the accepted social norms in families during toilet training.[27]

In addition to changes in bladder storage capacity, the progressive maturation of micturition also involves changes in the following bladder parameters:

1. *Voiding frequency:* During the third trimester of pregnancy, the fetus is voiding at a rate of approximately 30 times every 24 hours.[28] However, immediately after birth, this drops dramatically for the first few days of life only to increase again after the first week to reach a peak by week 2 to 4 of an average of once per hour. Subsequently this rate declines again to about 10 to 15 times per day between 6 to 12 months of age and to about 8 to 10 times per day by 2 to 3 years of age.[28-30] This reduction in voiding frequency observed during the first few years of life appears to be related mainly to an increase in bladder capacity in parallel to body growth, which is proportionately greater than the simultaneous increase in urine volume production.[31,32] By the age of 12 years, the voiding pattern is very similar to that of an adult, and it usually involves 4 to 6 voids per day.
2. *Voided volume:* Several studies have shown that voided volume (also known as *functional bladder capacity*) at a certain age can be accurately estimated and expressed as a function of age with no difference in sex. For young infants, it can be expressed as follows[30]:

   $$\text{Bladder capacity in ml} = 38 + 2.5 \times \text{Age in months}$$

   For older children, one of the most widely accepted formulas is Koff's formula[33]:

   $$\text{Bladder capacity in ml} = (\text{Age in years} + 2) \times 30$$

   Hjalmas' formula is also commonly used[34,35]:

   $$\text{Bladder capacity in ml} = 30 + (\text{Age in years} \times 30)$$

3. *Emptying efficiency:* Urodynamic studies have shown that a significant proportion of infants with incomplete maturation of detrusor-sphincter coordination before the age of 1 year are already able to achieve satisfactory bladder emptying (more than 80% efficacy).[9,10,29,30,36,37]
4. *Detrusor pressure at voiding:* There are limited studies of detrusor pressures at voiding in normal infants as a result of the technical difficulties involved in performing urodynamic studies in young infants and the ethical considerations for justifying doing so. From the data obtained from a natural filling cystometric study of infants with normal lower urinary tracts (as indicated by a normal micturating cystourethrogram) and who had undergone either dismembered pyeloplasty for pelviureteric junction obstruction or nephrectomy for dysplastic kidney, significantly higher maximum detrusor pressures with micturition ($P_{det}max$) have been documented as compared with normal adults. It was also noted that male infants voided with significantly higher pressures than female infants (mean $P_{det}max$, 118 versus 75 cm H_20, respectively; $P < .03$).[9,10,38]

Similar findings were reported in healthy asymptomatic infant siblings of children with vesicoureteral reflux (VUR).[36] Studies have also shown that these high detrusor pressures noted during micturition were mainly observed only during the first year of life and that they decreased progressively with age. Furthermore, an interrupted or "staccato" type of urinary stream was noted in more than half of the patients.[9,10,38] This was demonstrated by fluctuations of the detrusor pressure when it reached maximum during voiding and during the resumption of the urinary stream in conjunction with a sharp fall in the detrusor pressure. The high detrusor pressures during voiding are thought to represent variations among individual infants with regard to the maturation process of detrusor and sphincter coordination during the first 1 to 2 years of life.[9,10,30,35,36] This finding has been further confirmed using video cystometry under fluoroscopy in combination with natural fill urodynamics and perineal electromyography (EMG) in infants with a history of UTI. Periods of increase in perineal or sphincteric EMG activities were noted during voiding and associated with a sudden cessation of urinary flow with a simultaneous isometric rise or high peak of detrusor pressure. By contrast, the resumption of urinary flow was associated with relaxation of the external urinary sphincter and a paradoxic drop in detrusor pressure. Also, the detrusor pressure associated with the initiation of urinary flow was usually significantly lower than the maximal detrusor pressure during micturition (P_{det}max), and the P_{det}max was significantly higher than those recorded in normal adults.

The final steps of maturation of voiding are usually achieved at around the age of 3 to 4 years of age, when most children have developed the adult pattern of urinary control and will be dry both day and night. The child has learned to inhibit a micturition reflex, to postpone voiding, and to voluntarily initiate micturition at socially acceptable and convenient times and places. This development of continence and voluntary micturition is also dependent on behavioral learning, and it can be influenced by toilet training, which in turn depends on the cognitive perception of the maturing urinary tract. It is understandable, therefore, that this series of complex events is highly susceptible to the development of various types of dysfunction.

CLINICAL RECOGNITION OF VOIDING DISORDERS

Voiding disorders should not be viewed rigidly as separate and distinct entities but rather as transitional phases of a complex sequence of events. It must also be emphasized that the use of the term *non-neuropathic* is based purely on the fact that no obvious and identifiable neurologic lesion can be identified. However, certain conditions (e.g., the Ochoa syndrome, the Hinman syndrome) that seem to have no organic underlying neurologic cause but that behave almost identically to the typical neuropathic bladder-sphincter dysfunctions may in fact involve a neuroanatomic lesion that is yet to be identified. Hence, the distinction between neuropathic and non-neuropathic bladder dysfunctions may not be as clear as traditionally thought. In 1997, the International Children's Continence Society put together a standardized set of terminology in an effort to minimize confusion within the profession[39] (Table 38-1).

Transient Detrusor-Sphincter Discoordination in Infancy

It should be noted that, during the assessment of young children with apparent voiding dysfunctions, children may transiently display some degree of abnormal bladder-sphincteric function.[31] Studies have shown that this may be a transient phenomenon in the normal transition from an infantile to an adult pattern of micturition control, and, therefore, investigators should display caution when interpreting intermittent or transient symptoms as pathologic.

During the first 1 to 2 years of life, it has been shown that a significant proportion of normal infants exhibit prominent detrusor-sphincter discoordination and interrupted voiding that may even be brought to a complete stop for 1 to 2 minutes before restarting.[9,10,38] Urodynamic findings show an association with high voiding pressures and the interruption of flow but no impairment of overall bladder emptying. This type of dysfunction usually resolves with a period of successful toilet training; it is only transitory or intermittent and does not persist. However, if voiding dysfunctions persist well beyond the period of toilet training (especially if they are associated with urinary complications like recurrent urosepsis), then the possibility of underlying anatomic and neurologic causes must be considered and duly evaluated.

Overactive Bladder, Urge Syndrome, and Urge Incontinence

Studies using prolonged natural filling bladder monitoring techniques have shown that the normal bladder is quiescent and stable even in newborns.[10] Clinically, the condition of "unstable bladder" is best exhibited by urge syndrome with or without urge incontinence, and it is most prevalent among girls. The syndrome is characterized by frequent attacks of sudden and imperative sensations of urge even with small bladder capacities, which is represented by detrusor overactivity during the filling phase on urodynamics. Clinically, the child or parents may typically describe what is known as the *Vincent's curtsey sign or hold maneuver,* during which the child attempts to voluntarily contract the pelvic floor muscles and externally compress the urethra to counteract the involuntary contractions either by crossing the legs or squatting[40,41] (Figure 38-2). However, despite this move, urge incontinence can still occur, with frequent urine leakage onto the underpants. Urge incontinence occurs most often when the child is preoccupied with play or other activities and has a decreased response to the urge sensation. Children with urge syndrome typically have small bladder capacities for their age, and, behaviorally, they try to overcome this by choosing to drink very infrequently to avoid the social embarrassment of frequent urges to go to the toilet and of urinary incontinence. In addition, habitual voluntary pelvic floor contraction to counteract every urge to void may also lead to inappropriate postponement of defecation, constipation, and fecal soiling.[41,42]

TABLE 38-1 Summary of Functional Voiding Disorders in Children

	Clinical Features	Urodynamic Findings	Management
Transient detrusor-sphincter discoordination	• Age of <2 years • Interrupted voiding • May present with complications such as urinary tract infection	• Detrusor-sphincter discoordination • Interrupted voiding • High voiding pressures • Good bladder emptying	• Transient phenomena • Resolves with toilet training
Detrusor overactivity (overactive bladder)	• Urinary frequency • Urgency • Urge incontinence	• Unstable detrusor contractions during filling	• Anticholinergic drugs • Standard urotherapy • Neuromodulation
Stress incontinence	• Associated with increased intravesical pressure during laughing, running, coughing, and so on	• May be normal • May elicit leakage when the patient is asked to strain or cough during the procedure	• Standard urotherapy • Pelvic floor rehabilitation
Giggle incontinence	• Usually found in girls • Associated with laughing and giggling • May amount to complete bladder emptying	• May be normal • May elicit leakage when the patient is asked to giggle	• Standard urotherapy • Pelvic floor rehabilitation
Postvoid dribbling	• Usually found in toilet-trained girls • Leakage after voiding and on standing	• Usually normal	• Vesicovaginal reflux may be demonstrated with a micturating cystourethrogram • Advise on toilet posture (i.e., sitting with legs apart)
Dysfunctional voiding	• May manifest as daytime urinary symptoms	• Staccato or fractionated voiding • Pelvic floor activity during voiding • Voiding commences with a drop in abdominal pressure	• Standard urotherapy • Biofeedback and pelvic floor rehabilitation
Infrequent voider/ underactive bladder	• Infrequent voiding as a result of diminished urge sensation • Refuses to void when engaged in play • Overflow incontinence • Urinary tract infection	• Poor detrusor contractility • Poor bladder emptying • Increased bladder capacity • Abdominal straining • High compliance	• Standard urotherapy, including timed voiding and scheduled drinking training
Non-neurogenic neurogenic bladder (Hinman syndrome)	• May present as urinary tract infection • Poor bladder emptying • Incontinence • No neurologic pathology identified • May involve bowel dysfunction	• Sphincteric overactivity • Increased pelvic floor activity	• Same as for neurogenic bladders • May require clean intermittent catheterization

Functional Urinary Incontinence

Functional urinary incontinence involves the involuntary loss of urine as a result of a failure of control of the bladder-sphincteric unit. It occurs frequently enough to constitute a social or hygienic problem, and there are no underlying anatomic causes.[39] *Stress incontinence* represents the involuntary leakage of urine occurring at times when the intravesical pressure exceeds the bladder outlet or urethral resistance in the absence of measurable detrusor contraction. Unlike in adults (particularly elderly women), true stress incontinence is extremely uncommon among neurologically normal children, and it is in general not associated with any demonstrable urodynamic abnormalities. Insufficient bladder outlet or urethral resistance is usually not a main factor. Because the amount of urine leakage in most patients is usually small, the incontinence may at times be only scarcely discernible. Therefore, it is possible that the actual incidence of this condition may be underestimated.

Giggle Incontinence

Giggle incontinence is a rare syndrome that is usually described in girls and that is characterized by involuntary and typically unpredictable wetting during or immediately after giggling or laughing. In contrast with stress incontinence, it produces a much larger volume of urine leakage, often amounting to complete bladder emptying. Similar to stress incontinence, however, cystometry is typically normal when the child is not laughing.

Postvoid Dribbling

The term *postvoid dribbling* refers to the involuntary leakage of urine immediately after voiding has finished, and it is applicable to children who have already been toilet trained. Typically this condition is seen in girls who are otherwise normal with no other associated urinary symptoms, where leakage may be a result of vesicovaginal reflux. This occurs when urine gets trapped in the vagina during voiding and

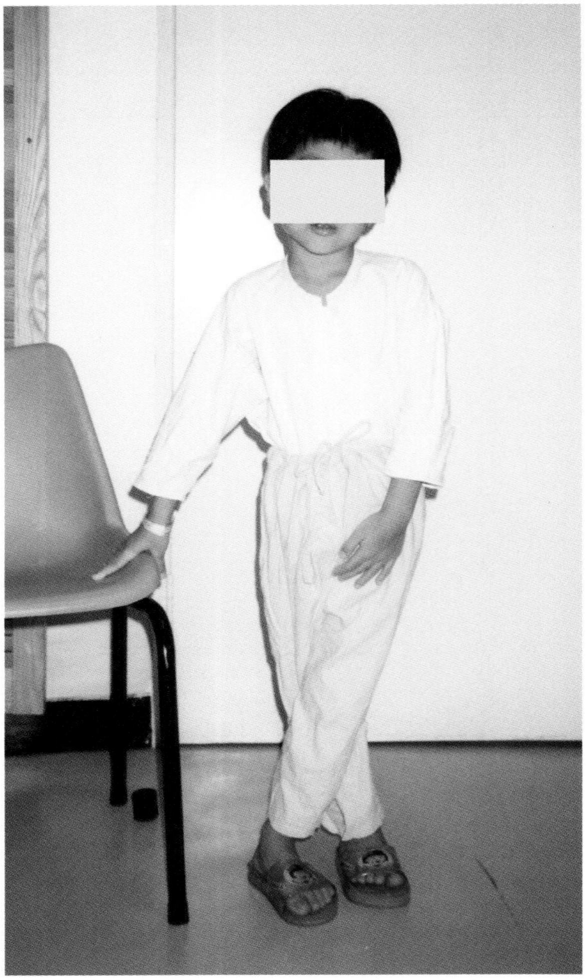

Figure 38-2 Vincent's curtsey sign.

dribbles out after the child stands. It can be confirmed by performing a micturating cystourethrogram or simply by asking the child to void while leaning forward with her legs apart and seeing whether the condition improves. The condition is otherwise harmless, and it tends to resolve with age.

Dysfunctional Voiding

Dysfunctional voiding is actually a urodynamic entity that is characterized by incomplete relaxation or involuntary intermittent contractions of the pelvic floor muscles during voiding in neurologically intact children, typically manifesting as staccato voiding on uroflow. However, it can also manifest in different patterns, depending on the degree of functional outflow obstruction caused as well as the status of the detrusor activity. The term refers to disturbances of the voiding phase alone (Figure 38-3).

Staccato Voiding

Staccato voiding is interrupted voiding that is caused by periodic bursts of pelvic floor muscle activities during voiding. This is seen as characteristic spikes of voiding pressures that coincide with a paradoxic cessation of urinary flow with the delayed passage of urine after the onset of detrusor contraction on urodynamics, which results in a few small squirts of urine that are passed in quick succession. The flow time is usually prolonged, and bladder emptying is often incomplete (Figure 38-4).

Fractionated Voiding

Fractionated voiding involves several small, discontinuous voids that result from poor and unsustained detrusor contractions characterized by infrequent and incomplete emptying. Abdominal straining is usually evident in an effort to improve bladder emptying, but it is often paradoxically counteracted by a reflex increase in activities of the pelvic floor muscles triggered by an increase in intravesical pressure. The bladder capacity is usually large for the child's age.

Infrequent Voiding and the Underactive Bladder (Lazy Bladder Syndrome)

These two conditions represent a spectrum of disease whereby chronic functional bladder outflow obstruction leads to gradual deterioration in detrusor contractility, poor bladder emptying, and a progressive increase in bladder capacity. Because urge sensation is either absent or diminished, voiding is very infrequent. Typically, a child with infrequent voiding syndrome may not void for 8 to 10 hours or even longer if he or she is engaged in activities, and the parents always complain that these children never void unless they are told to do so. This eventually results in a large, floppy bladder with very inefficient emptying: in other words, underactive bladder or lazy bladder syndrome, which is generally regarded as the end point and a fully decompensated system. Urodynamics typically show the recruitment of abdominal straining as the main driving force for bladder emptying with unsustained, low-pressure detrusor contractions that at times may even be completely undetectable (Figure 38-5). Compliance on filling is very high, and electromyography often shows increased activity in the pelvic floor muscle with each abdominal strain. The resultant large volume of postmicturition residual urines predispose patients with this condition to recurrent UTI, and overflow incontinence is usually evident, which may be further associated with constipation and/or fecal soiling.

Hinman Syndrome and Occult Neuropathic Bladder

Hinman, Allen, and Dorfman first used the terms *non-neurogenic neurogenic bladder* and later *Hinman syndrome* to describe the condition of a small group of children with a presumably acquired form of bladder-sphincteric dysfunction characterized by a combination of bladder decompensation with incontinence, poor emptying, and recurrent urinary infections.[43-46] In British literature, the condition is often referred to as *occult neuropathic bladder*.[47] The condition has all the clinical and urodynamic features that are typical of neuropathic bladder dysfunction, but no neurologic pathology can be demonstrated. Most children even have significant bowel dysfunction, including encopresis, constipation, and fecal impaction. Hinman and Baumann initially hypothesized that the condition could be ascribed to acquired psycho-

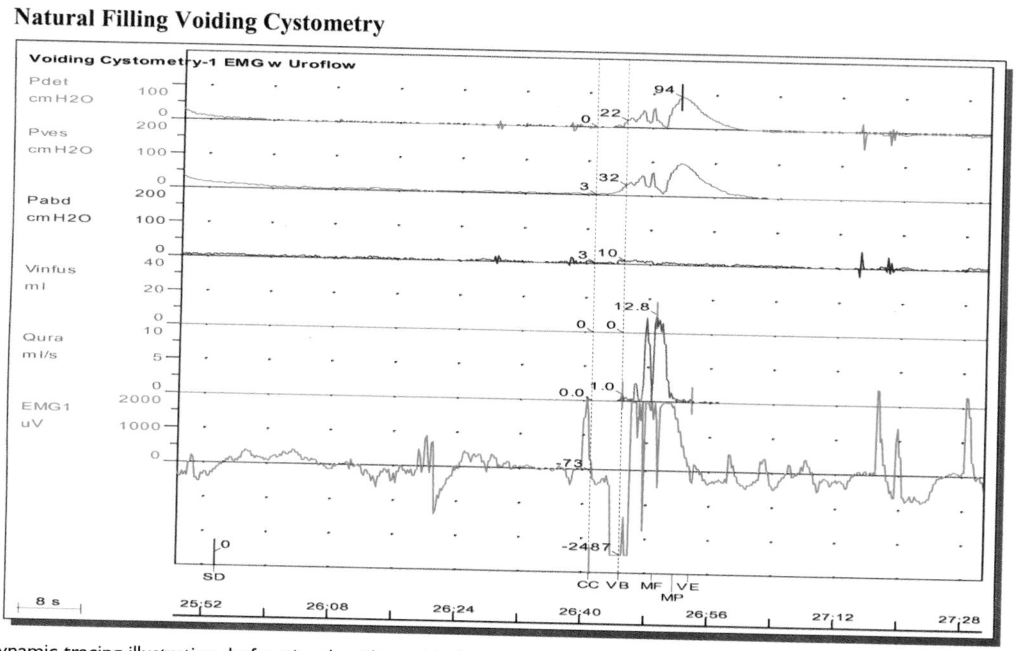

Figure 38-3 Urodynamic tracing illustrating dysfunctional voiding with detrusor-sphincter dyssynergia associated with a marked increase in electromyography activity.

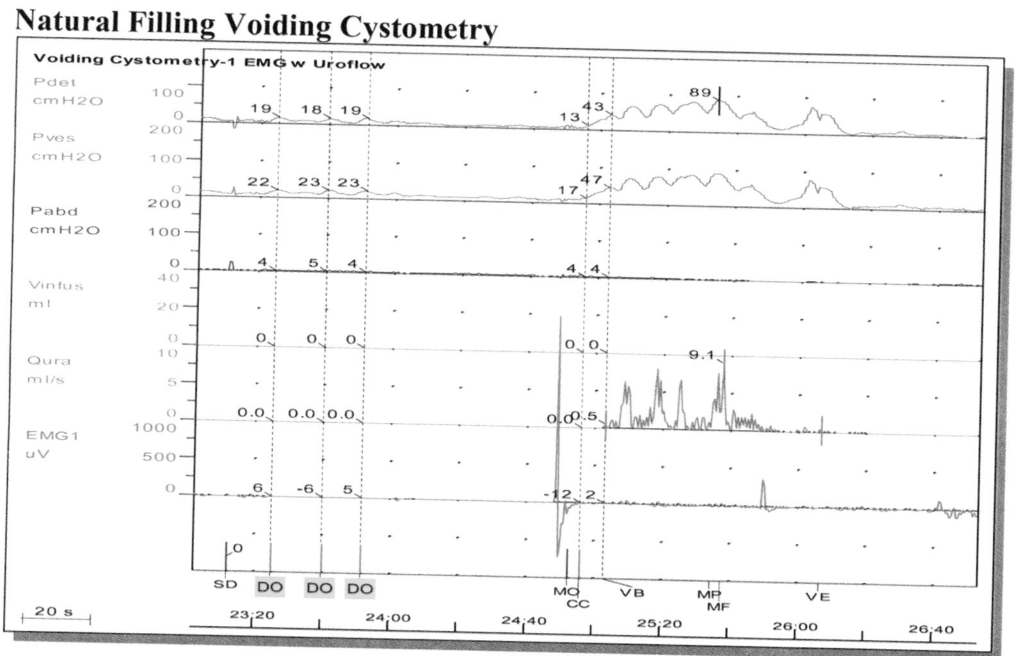

Figure 38-4 Urodynamic tracing illustrating detrusor overactivity and staccato voiding with typical interrupted voids after spikes of voiding pressures. *DO*, Detrusor overactivity.

logically abnormal behavior with voluntary discoordination between the detrusor muscle and the pelvic floor/external urethral sphincter complex during voiding.[43] However, later studies did not support this, and controversies still exist regarding whether a very subtle or occult spinal pathology—although unidentifiable even on magnetic resonance imaging (MRI)—can account for this. Urodynamic studies often show marked sphincteric overactivity and abrupt contractions of the pelvic floor as the child attempts to control incontinence from uninhibited bladder contractions. At the other end of the spectrum, full-blown bladder decompensation can occur with day-and-night wetting, urinary retention, recurrent UTI, upper tract dilatations, and renal scarring.[43-49] Treatment strategies in these children are similar to those for patients

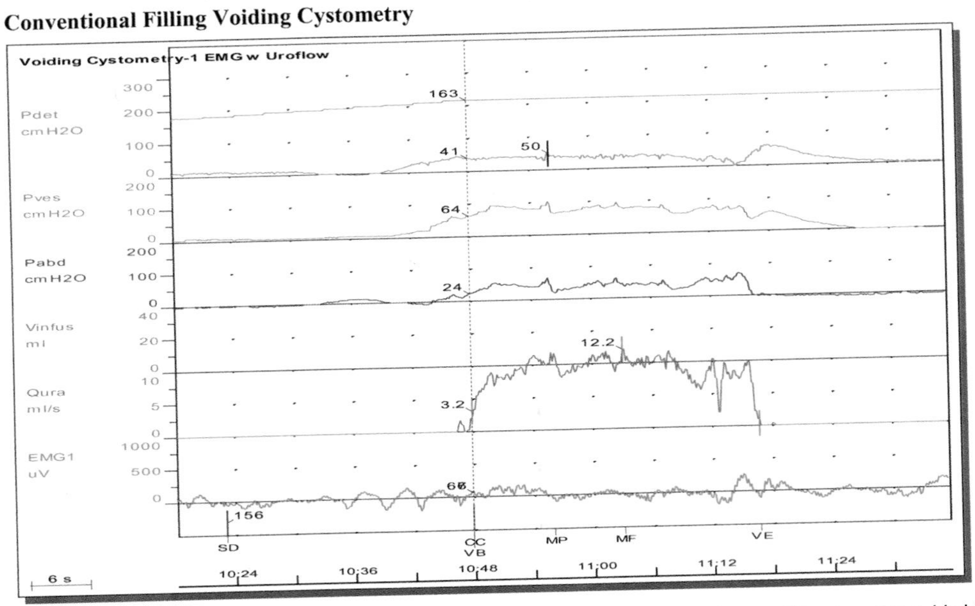

Figure 38-5 Urodynamic tracing illustrating an underactive bladder using abdominal straining throughout voiding to achieve bladder emptying, which is typically incomplete.

with neuropathic bladders and should entail measures to control infection and restore normal bladder storage and emptying function.

The Ochoa (urofacial) syndrome is another described condition of "non-neurogenic neurogenic bladder" among children who are again exhibiting all of the classic features of dysfunctional voiding, including urinary incontinence, recurrent UTI, constipation, reflux, and upper tract damage; in addition, they have a peculiar painful-looking expression that makes it appear that they are crying when they are in fact smiling.[50,51] The condition has an autosomal recessive inheritance, and the gene has been located on chromosome 10. Urodynamic studies characteristically showed a sustained contraction of the external sphincter during voiding, and long-term outcome is usually very dismal. Ochoa[51] reported a series of 66 children of whom 33% had renal functional impairment, 26% had hypertension, and 24% had end stage renal failure, with 5 eventually going on for renal transplantation and 17 dying. It has been speculated that, because the neural ganglia that control the facial muscles are situated very close to the pontine micturition center, a small, genetically predetermined, congenital neurologic lesion in this area may be responsible.

EVALUATION OF VOIDING DISORDERS

History and Clinical Examination

The majority of children with voiding dysfunctions typically present after toilet training with symptoms of either nighttime or daytime urinary incontinence or both. Occasionally they can be recognized at an earlier age, when the child presents for the investigation of UTI or VUR. In any case, it is important to obtain a detailed history from the child (when possible) or the guardian. This should include relevant questions to define the pattern of voiding and wetting. Symptoms of urgency (rushing to the toilet), frequency (eight or more times per day), holding behaviors (squatting or crossing legs), or urge incontinence suggest detrusor overactivity. Symptoms of difficulty with initiating voiding, the need to push or strain during voiding, or a weak urinary stream suggest functional or organic bladder outflow obstruction. Infrequent voiding (three or less times per day) suggests hypocontractile bladder.[52] A detailed bowel history is also important, because bowel dysfunction can coexist in the form of encopresis, constipation, and fecal impaction.

The voiding pattern can be further illustrated with a detailed voiding diary or frequency volume chart. This is used to record daily fluid intake and urine output at home under normal conditions. The number of voidings per day, the time and distribution of voids during the day, and each voided volume is recorded. It can also record any episodes of urgency and leakage, and it is a useful tool for identifying those who may warrant further studies as well as for the follow-up of patients. To get accurate results, the procedure needs to be explained clearly to the child and the family. It is helpful to provide written instructions and a standard urine measuring cup. It has been recommended to do a 2-night, 3-day voiding diary over the weekend.[52] The voiding diary has been found to yield acceptable information for enuresis volume, average voided volume, and functional bladder capacity (taken as the largest voided volume except for the first morning void).

Physical examination is also important to exclude other neurologic and congenital abnormalities in the child. Areas to concentrate on include the spine, the abdomen, and the external genitalia. Abnormalities of the lower spine including asymmetric gluteal folds, hairy patches, dermovascular malformations, and lipomatous abnormalities of the sacral region should prompt further imaging, and the possibility of an occult spinal dysraphism should be excluded. Occasionally, in an otherwise normal child, one may find a palpable bladder on abdominal examination in cases of decompensated bladders. The external genitalia may be examined to exclude any obvious anatomic problems that can explain the urinary symptoms in question. A rectal examination should be performed when the clinical history suggests symptoms of constipation, because this may reveal fecal impaction or a distended rectum in those with chronic constipation; thus dysfunctional elimination syndrome should be excluded.

Laboratory Investigations

Laboratory investigations are not routinely required unless the child has other abnormalities on history or examination, such as history of UTI or short stature. Routine tests may include urinalysis to rule out UTI or bacteriuria and glycosuria, morning urine osmolality to rule out impaired renal concentrating ability, and morning urine calcium-to-creatinine ratio to rule out hypercalciuria.[53]

Imaging Studies

An ultrasonogram is often the first-line investigation in children with voiding dysfunctions, because it is a simple, readily available, and noninvasive tool. When performed by experienced pediatric radiologists, it can be used to illustrate functional problems of the lower urinary tract as well as to provide anatomic information about the lower and upper urinary tracts. Recent studies have shown that the measurement of certain bladder parameters using ultrasonogram can be used to calculate a bladder volume and wall thickness index. This index can be classified as normal, thick, or thin in accordance with measured parameters, and these classifications correspond closely with the urodynamic findings of underlying bladder dysfunction. This suggests that ultrasonogram can be a reliable tool for guiding further invasive investigations.[54]

Other imaging studies may include a plain radiograph of the spine, MRI (if indicated) to exclude the possibility of any neurogenic causes of bladder-sphincter dysfunction, and a micturating cystourethrogram to rule out VUR and outflow obstruction.

Urodynamic Studies

Urodynamic studies, although invasive, are currently still the best means for providing comprehensive detail about the physiologic parameters involved in bladder mechanics during filling and voiding, although one report observed poor interobserver and intraobserver agreement regarding bladder compliance and detrusor activity.[55] Bladder filling and storage are described according to bladder sensation, detrusor activity, bladder compliance, and bladder capacity. Pressure-flow studies are carried out during the voiding phase.

Uroflowmetry

All urodynamics should be preceded by or combined with a uroflow study performed when the child experiences a normal desire to void and does so in the correct sitting or standing position; these studies should be repeated for accuracy. It is also important to note that normal flow rates are different between adults and children. Children usually show a poor correlation between maximal flow rate and outflow resistance, because the detrusor is able to exert much stronger contractions to counteract any increased resistance; thus, it is far more important to study the pattern of the flow curve rather than the flow rates in children. The precise shape of the flow curve is determined by detrusor contractility, by the presence of any abdominal straining, and by the bladder outlet, and it can be described as follows[56]:

- *Bell-shaped:* In normal voiding, a smooth increase and a subsequent decrease in flow rate should be observed.
- *Tower-shaped:* This curve is produced by an explosive voiding contraction that is seen in overactive bladders.
- *Plateau-shaped:* This is representative of an outlet obstruction.
- *Staccato pattern:* This is seen with sphincteric overactivity during voiding, with peaks and troughs throughout voiding.
- *Interrupted flow:* This condition is seen in acontractile or underactive bladders.

Conventional Fill Urodynamic Study

Urodynamic studies combine uroflowmetry with cystometry and perineal EMG studies to provide more comprehensive information about the spectrum of voiding dysfunction and functional bladder outflow obstruction. They also involve more sophisticated instruments and become more invasive to the patient, often requiring a bladder catheter to be introduced transurethrally or suprapubically. Although more invasive, the use of suprapubic catheterization has the advantage of being more physiologic in children, who may find it difficult to void with a catheter in the urethra. Usually a 6-French (6-Fr), double-lumen catheter is placed suprapubically with the patient under sedation and left in situ for 24 hours before the commencement of the urodynamic study to eliminate the effect of any immediate discomfort after placement. The suprapubic catheter is then connected to a computer system and used to measure intravesical pressure. Another catheter is placed in the rectum to measure intra-abdominal pressure surrounding the bladder. By subtracting the latter from the intravesical pressure, the detrusor pressure can be calculated. The study is then commenced, and it is completed when the child successfully micturates after experiencing a normal desire to void. Traditionally, the bladder is filled artificially with water or normal saline to speed up the procedure. The child is asked to indicate his or her desire to void (if old enough to do so) and then to void into a specially designed seat with a uroflowmeter attached. The investigator observing the study should also make note of any events that occur during the study, such as any large movements of the patient, coughing, or, in particular, any urinary dribbling. Sphincteric activity can be measured with simultaneous perineal EMG recordings. All of the measured data are directly fed into a computer for the analysis and display of graphic measurements (Figure 38-6).

Natural Filling Urodynamic Study

More recently, studies have shown that the nonphysiologic filling of the bladder during conventional fill urodynamics, even at low filling rates, can lead to misrepresentations of

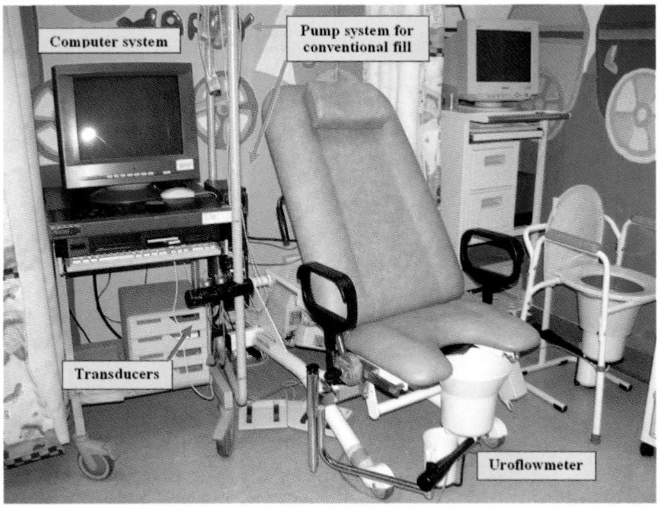

Figure 38-6 Urodynamic setup.

true bladder activity during normal situations. Therefore, natural fill urodynamic studies may be performed in which the child is asked to drink to allow the bladder to fill up at its own rate. Urodynamic studies in children with urge syndrome usually reveal detrusor overactivity associated with a small bladder capacity. However, they may occasionally be normal with only barely perceptible incontinence, particularly if conventional fill cystometry rather than natural filling cystometry is used. It appears that the artificial filling may inhibit the detrusor response and attenuate its maximum contractile potential, thus rendering detrusor instability much less pronounced and undetectable. Therefore, natural fill cystometry is the preferred technique for children. Even better is the combined use of artificial and natural filling urodynamic studies, which are helpful to accurately delineate the underlying bladder dysfunction.[38]

Videourodynamic Study

By combining cystometry with fluoroscopy, videourodynamics can be performed with fluoroscopic images of the bladder, the bladder neck, and the urethra being captured. Conventional fill urodynamics is performed in the usual manner with the child sitting in a specially designed chair with a uroflowmetry device in the fluoroscopy suite. Fluoroscopic images are taken during filling and during voiding. This has the added advantage of allowing for the observation of the shape of the bladder during filling and voiding, of the vesicoureteral reflux, and of the configuration of the urethra and pelvic floor.

Ambulatory Urodynamic Study

The unfamiliar hospital and urodynamic laboratory environment as well as the presence of a urodynamics investigator can sometimes cause significant distress, particularly to young children. To overcome this, an ambulatory urodynamic system was developed. The system consists of an ambulatory urodynamic recorder that converts digital pressure signals into a modulated infrared wave that is strapped to the child. Direct line of sight from the transmitter to the receiver is unnecessary, because the infrared signals reflect from the walls of the room before reaching the receiver. Thus, during the investigation, the child can conduct normal activities, be totally mobile, and be accompanied by one or both of the parents undisturbed in a private cubicle. From an adjoining room, the investigator can observe and record the patient's activities, including urinary dribbling and micturition, through a one-way mirror; real-time online pressure signal displays are monitored continuously on a computer. Only natural fill studies are possible by this means. Overall, it allows for a continuous monitoring of bladder function under near-natural conditions for the child.[57]

More recently, the Bluetooth system has been introduced. This works in much the same way as the infrared system, but it is much less bulky for the patient to carry around. It offers even more freedom of movement, with a much longer transmission range and more reliable reception. If coupled with a camera recorder in the room in which the child is, there is no need for the investigator to sit behind a one-way mirror throughout the procedure. With such advances in technology, it will not be surprising if urodynamics can soon be performed in the setting of one's own home.

CAUSES OF VOIDING DISORDERS

Dysfunction of the lower urinary tract in children can be broadly categorized as disorders that result from the derangement of nervous control, disorders of detrusor and sphincteric muscle function, structural abnormalities, and other unclassified conditions.[39]

Derangement of Nervous Control

Conditions involving the derangement of nervous control include the following:

1. Congenital malformations of the central nervous system, such as myelomeningocele, spina bifida occulta, caudal regression syndrome, and tethered cord syndrome
2. Developmental disturbances, such as mental retardation, dysfunctional voiding, and urge syndrome
3. Acquired conditions, such as cerebral palsy, progressive degenerative diseases of the central nervous system associated with spasticity, transverse myelitis, multiple sclerosis, vascular malformations, and trauma of the spinal cord

Disorders of Detrusor and Sphincteric Muscle Function

These types of disorders include the following:

1. Congenital conditions, such as muscular dystrophy and neuronal dysplasia (megacolon-megacystis syndrome)
2. Acquired conditions, such as chronic bladder distension and fibrosis of the detrusor and the bladder wall

Structural Abnormalities

Structural abnormalities fall into the following two categories:

1. Congenital conditions, such as bladder exstrophy, epispadias, cloacal anomaly, ureteroceles, posterior urethral valves and other urethral anomalies, and prune belly syndrome

2. Acquired conditions, such as traumatic stricture or damage to the sphincter or urethra

Other Unclassified Conditions

Unclassified conditions include the following:

1. Giggle incontinence
2. Hinman syndrome
3. Ochoa syndrome (urofacial syndrome)

Dysfunctional Elimination Syndrome

Since the 1950s, the association of constipation with urologic pathologies has increasingly been described in the literature. Over the last decade, clinicians have recognized the existence of this association with the term *dysfunctional elimination syndrome*, which is used to reflect the broad spectrum of functional disturbances to the urinary tract that result from functional bowel disturbances.

Dysfunctional elimination syndrome can be classified in one of two ways[58]:

1. *Functional disorder of filling:* overactive bladder, overdistension of the bladder, or insensate bladder, which may be associated with fecal impaction or rectal distension with an infrequent call to stool
2. *Functional disorder of emptying:* over-recruitment of pelvic floor activity during voiding, thereby causing interrupted and/or incomplete emptying; also associated with defecation difficulties (as a result of the lack of relaxation of the puborectalis), pain on defecation, or even anismus

NEUROGENIC BLADDER CAUSED BY SPINAL DYSRAPHISMS

The term *spinal dysraphism* refers to both congenital and acquired abnormalities of the spinal cord, including myelomeningocele, myeloschisis, intraspinal lipoma, lipomyelomeningocele, dermoid cyst, diastematomyelia, and tethered conus medullaris. These are the most common causes of neurogenic bladder dysfunction in children. Other common causes include spinal cord injury from trauma, transverse myelitis, and intraspinal neoplasms. Neurogenic bladder has also been reported in children with cerebral palsy,[59] hereditary spinocerebellar ataxia,[60] and adrenoleukodystrophy.[61]

Children with spinal dysraphism are best managed by a multidisciplinary team early in life. The team typically involves neurosurgeons, orthopedic surgeons, pediatric surgeons and urologists, pediatric nephrologists, physiotherapists, continence care nurses, and occupational therapists. Urologic management aims at preserving renal function and improving quality of life through the achievement of urinary and fecal continence as well as independence in self-care. The early involvement of pediatric nephrologists is important, because renal complications are among the most frequent causes of morbidity in these patients.

With the refinements in urodynamic studies, the advent of clean intermittent catheterization (CIC), and the advancements in surgical modalities and techniques, the outcomes and prognoses of these children have been improving during the last two decades. Early functional assessment with urodynamics is now generally advocated, and this is followed by a more proactive management strategy. It has been shown that early intervention has resulted in less need for subsequent bladder augmentation as well as improved outcomes when these children become adults.[62-64]

Assessment

A careful history of urologic symptoms can be obtained from older children and on follow-up evaluations, but it will not be possible for neonates, which is why functional investigations are particularly useful. Physical examination includes blood pressure measurement, inspection of the spine, eliciting perianal and perineal sensation, checking anal tone and reflex, and a neurologic examination of the extremities. A urine culture and a serum creatinine measurement should be performed.

Urodynamics are recommended during the neonatal period before and after the spinal defect is addressed with surgery. However, if the child is considered at high risk for such a procedure, renal ultrasound and postvoid residual urine would be the minimum investigations required at this early stage. If the child cannot empty at least 80% of his or her bladder after a spontaneous void or with a Credé maneuver, then CIC should be commenced even without a urodynamic study.

Other baseline radiologic investigations are required to assess upper and lower tract anatomy and function so that any future deterioration can be determined early. These include a renal ultrasonogram (if one has not already been obtained); a micturating cystourethrogram to assess bladder architecture, urethral obstruction, and the presence of VUR; a MAG3 dynamic radioisotope renogram in cases with hydronephrosis with or without hydroureter; a 99mTc dimercaptosuccinic acid scan to detect renal scarring and to assess differential renal function; and a spinal ultrasonogram or MRI of the spine for the full assessment of spinal cord involvement.

Functional Classification

A combination of dysfunction in bladder contractility and external sphincteric activity may lead to different categories of neurogenic bladder dysfunction, such as synergic, dyssynergic, and complete denervation.[65,66] Synergy is characterized by a silent sphincter during detrusor contraction and at the end of bladder filling with normal detrusor pressures at voiding. Dyssynergy or detrusor-sphincter dyssynergia occurs when the external sphincter fails to relax during a detrusor contraction during both filling and emptying of the bladder, thereby resulting in a high-pressure system. Complete denervation results in the absence of external sphincteric activity throughout filling and emptying, even with sacral stimulation or a Credé maneuver.

Children with a dyssynergic bladder are at the highest risk for urinary tract deterioration. Previous studies have suggested that outlet obstruction is a major contributing factor to such deterioration and that it may be the result of either detrusor-sphincter dyssynergia or poor bladder compliance.[67] Increased intravesical pressure may also lead to dysfunction of the vesicoureteral junction, thereby causing VUR. In addition, the stagnation of urine as a result of a high postvoid residual may lead to recurrent UTI and possible renal scarring and damage.

In a review of urodynamic findings in newborns with myelomeningocele, Snodgrass and Adams[68] reported that 12% to 32% of patients had normal studies. Of the remaining patients, 40% to 76% had detrusor contractility, whereas the rest were areflexic with preserved or diminished compliance. The external sphincter demonstrated normal EMG results in 40%, whereas the others showed evidence of partial or complete denervation. Concerning detrusor-sphincter activity, it was classified as synergic in 16% to 30% and as dyssynergic in 10% to 54%.[68] The findings of high leak point pressure of 40 cm H_2O or more or detrusor-sphincter dyssynergia on initial evaluation predicted a high rate of upper tract deterioration on follow-up.[64,65,69]

Management

Management aims at the early recognition of high-risk systems and early intervention to prevent UTI and pressure damage to the kidneys. Among older children, it is also necessary to consider quality of life in the management plan. This includes continence care and helping the child achieve independence in self-care to be able to lead as normal a life as possible and to improve self-esteem.

CIC has been advocated as a primary treatment for bladder emptying in those children with areflexic detrusors and a high postvoid residual. The advent of CIC during the 1970s changed the whole outlook of the management of neurogenic bladders.[70] The ability to successfully convert a high-pressure system to a low-pressure system has greatly decreased the incidence of urinary tract deterioration and the need for augmentation cystoplasties.[62,63] Campbell and colleagues[71] reported two complications in 137 children during 570 patient-years of follow-up: transient gross hematuria and false passage in the bulbar urethra. Lindehall and colleagues[72] described 28 children on CIC for 438 patient-years. Nineteen patients experienced at least one episode of difficulty inserting the catheter and/or macroscopic hematuria. Other complications were false passages, meatal stenosis, stricture, and epididymitis.

Anticholinergic drugs (typically oxybutynin) may be added in combination with CIC to achieve low bladder pressures and continence, especially in hypercontractile, small bladders[73] (Table 38-2). Newer agents include long-acting oxybutynin,[74] tolterodine,[75] and glycopyrolate,[76] and new routes of administration such as intravesical oxybutynin[77] or resiniferatoxin[78] have also been reported. Alpha-adrenergic blockers have also been tried to relax the urethral sphincter and avoid urine retention, and the use of doxazosin, tamsulosin,[79] alfuzosin,[80] and terazosin[81] in children have been reported although not licensed in many countries. Schurch and Corcos[82] recently reviewed the use of botulinum toxin in children with neurogenic bladders. Multiple injections were given into detrusors to reduce hyperactivity. This substance can also be injected into the urethral sphincter to encourage emptying.[83,84]

Surgery may be considered in different situations. For patients in whom CIC may be difficult (e.g., small neonates) or for whom CIC has failed (i.e., to relieve recurrent UTI or a dilating upper tract system), a *vesicostomy* may be required as a temporizing procedure. Augmentation may be indicated in cases of detrusor hyperreflexia in which anticholinergics fail to achieve low-pressure capacity and continence. Autoaugmentation or enterocystoplasty using sigmoid, colon, small bowel, or stomach have all been advocated, with their associated advantages and disadvantages.[85] Autoaugmentation

TABLE 38-2 **Drugs Used for Neurogenic Bladder and Functional Voiding Disorders**

Medications	Dose	Adverse Events	Comments
Anticholinergics (Relax Detrusor to Reduce Bladder Pressure)			
Oxybutynin hydrochloride (Ditropan)	2.5 to 5 mg two to three times daily (0.2 mg/kg/dose)	Dry mouth, flushing, blurry vision, constipation, heat intolerance	Short-acting preparation; intravesical instillation can be given as 5 mg two to three times daily
Long-acting oxybutynin (Ditropan XL)	5 to 15 mg daily	Same as above	Must be taken without chewing
Tolterodine tartrate	1 to 2 mg two times daily	Same as above; may be less intense than oxybutynin	Use lower dose with cytochrome P450 3A4 inhibitors
Long-acting tolterodine (Detrol LA)	2 to 4 mg daily	Same as above	Same as above; may be sprinkled on food
Long-acting hyoscyamine (Levbid)	0.375 to 0.75 mg two times daily	Same as above; more problems with visual accommodation	May not be chewed; may be halved
Alpha-Adrenergic Blockers (Relax Urethral Sphincter to Encourage Emptying)			
Doxazosin	0.5 to 1 mg/day	Hypotension, dizziness, fatigue, worsened heart failure	Not licensed for children but has been used in clinical trials in children
Tamsulosin	0.4 to 0.8 mg daily	Same as above	Same as above
Alfuzosin	2.5 to 7.5 mg daily	Same as above	Same as above
Terazosin	0.5 to 1 mg daily	Same as above	Same as above

Modified from Schulman SL: Voiding dysfunction in children, *Urol Clin North Am* 31:481-90, 2004.

has the advantage of not requiring any "foreign" material, but its ability to achieve large bladder capacities is limited. Ureterocystoplasty is a good option, but the availability of a nonfunctioning kidney with a dilated megaureter for augmentation is rare, especially with improved recent management. Bowel segments are commonly used to provide the surgical expansion of bladder capacity, but complications such as electrolyte and acid–base derangements can occur.[86,87] Small bowel also has the disadvantage of having intrinsic contractions; thus, demucosalized bowel augmented over the mucosa of the bladder after the detrusor has been stripped off has been advocated. Large bowel has the advantage of having less intrinsic contractions, but it produces more mucus secretions, which may cause repeated UTI, block CIC catheters, and increase the incidence of stone formation. Stomach has less of these problems, but it can cause hyponatremic hypochloremic metabolic alkalosis and hematuria-dysuria syndrome and has therefore lost popularity.[88]

A Mitrofanoff appendicovesicostomy continent catheterizable stoma was introduced during the 1980s to provide a better and more convenient means for CIC in boys with intact urethral sensation and in children who are wheelchair bound or who have severe spinal deformities (e.g., scoliosis, kyphosis). In those without an available appendix, a Monti tube using small bowel can suffice. This has helped improve the quality of life of these children, because it made it easier for them to perform CIC independently.[89] Urinary diversion (e.g., with ileal conduit) is now no longer popular since the introduction of CIC. Bladder neck surgery (or continence surgery) for increasing urethral resistance includes bladder neck reconstruction or bladder neck sling procedures, which are best combined with a continent stoma for CIC. The artificial urinary sphincter has been a viable option for older patients, and it allows them to empty the bladder without CIC. However, it has its complications, such as cuff erosion and device failure. A simpler means is endoscopic bladder neck injection with a bulking agent, but thus far its long-term results have been discouraging. Bladder neck surgery should be performed with caution in patients with poor compliance with treatment, because it can convert low-intravesical-pressure systems to high-pressure systems, thereby leading to upper tract damage.

It is important to not forget the management of the neurogenic bowel as an integral part of patient management. It is also important to be aware that children with spinal dysraphism should be monitored regularly, because changes to their condition can occur throughout childhood and puberty.

FUNCTIONAL VOIDING DISORDERS

It has always been a challenge to define and standardize normal versus abnormal lower urinary tract functions in children, because the development of micturition control over the bladder-sphincter unit in children is age-dependent, variable, and complex. However, with continuous research carried out in this field and with the aid of urodynamic studies, it is now possible to describe various functional disorders of the bladder in children.[90-92] The terminology again follows that set by the International Children's Continence Society in 1997 and updated in 2005 and 2006.[39]

Functional classification is based on the functional state of the bladder-sphincteric complex with respect to detrusor activity, bladder sensation, bladder compliance and capacity, and urethral function both during the filling and the voiding phases of cystometry as follows.

Functional Disorders during Filling

Detrusor Activity

Normal or stable detrusor function allows bladder volume increases during filling without a significant rise in detrusor pressure and without involuntary contractions despite provocation. *Detrusor overactivity,* which replaces the previous term *detrusor instability,* is characterized by phasic involuntary detrusor contractions involving a detrusor pressure rise of more than 15 cm H_2O above baseline and which may occur either spontaneously or on provocation by alterations of posture, coughing, walking, jumping, and other triggering procedures. Detrusor overactivity can be further classified according to cause as either *neurogenic* (replacing the old term *detrusor hyperreflexia*), which occurs when there is objective evidence of a relevant neurologic disorder, or *idiopathic,* which occurs when there is no defined cause.

Bladder Sensation

This can be *normal, increased* (hypersensitive), *reduced* (hyposensitive), or *absent,* and it applies mainly to older children and adolescents, because infants and young children will not be able to indicate differences in bladder sensation, except for possibly a strong desire to void. Both reduced and absent bladder sensations can be observed in underactive detrusors or what was previously known as the "lazy bladder."

Bladder Capacity and Compliance

Bladder capacity and compliance can be described as normal, high, or low. *Bladder compliance* is used to describe the relationship between the change in bladder volume and the change in detrusor pressure as expressed in ml/cm H_2O. During normal bladder filling, little or no pressure change occurs, but there are no standardized reference ranges for compliance in children, because bladder volume varies with age and so it is more important to note the shape of the filling curve rather than to rely on an actual numeric value.

Urethral Function

This can, in general, be described as *normal* when a positive urethral closure pressure is maintained during filling even in the presence of increased abdominal pressure and decreases immediately before micturition to allow flow. *Incompetent urethral function* occurs when a leakage of urine occurs in the absence of detrusor contraction despite urethral closure.

Functional Disorders during Voiding

Detrusor Activity

Normal voiding is achieved by a sustained detrusor contraction that leads to complete bladder emptying within a normal time span in the absence of bladder outlet obstruction. *Detrusor underactivity* is a detrusor contraction of inadequate magnitude and/or duration to effect bladder emptying within a normal time span. An *acontractile detrusor* demonstrates no detrusor contraction at all as a result of an abnormality of nervous control, and it denotes the complete absence of centrally coordinated contractions.

Urethral Function

This can be described as *normal* when a normal urethral opening allows for effective bladder emptying. It is described as *obstructive* when sphincteric overactivity is present, as in dysfunctional voiding or mechanical obstruction resulting from obstructive urethral lesions (e.g., congenital obstructive posterior urethral membrane, syringoceles) that leads to ineffective or prolonged emptying.[93,94]

Clinical Significance of Functional Voiding Disorders

Functional voiding disorders have been reported to be associated with recurrent UTI and VUR. Bachelard and colleagues[95] used videocystometry to study 90 males and 68 females with their first UTI. They found bladder instability (with high voiding detrusor pressure and low bladder capacity) in two thirds of the cases.[95] A survey of 141 Swedish girls between the ages of 3.9 and 18 years with recurrent UTI showed that only 20% did not have functional voiding or defecation abnormalities; infrequent voiding, dysfunctional voiding, and poor fluid intake were the most common.[96] Similar findings were also reported by Wan and colleagues,[97] Hellerstein and Nickell,[98] and Bakker and colleagues.[99] Among infants with congenital VUR, voiding dysfunction was present in about 20%. Patients with 99mTc dimercaptosuccinic acid scan defects have an even higher prevalence of voiding dysfunction (24.3% in girls; 30.4% in boys).[100] Podesta and colleagues[101] also reported that urodynamic studies in 12 children (9 boys and 3 girls) with severe VUR showed reduced bladder capacity during the filling phase but high voiding pressure with concomitant sphincter activity during micturition. Godley and colleagues[102] found a high prevalence of abnormal urodynamic function in children whose VUR did not resolve after a mean of 16 months. In a prospective study of 82 children with grade III or IV VUR who were followed for 2 to 4.8 years, the failure of the resolution of VUR was associated with the presence of abnormal bladder function on initial evaluation.[103] Koff and colleagues[104] also stressed the importance of dysfunctional elimination syndrome in children with VUR. They found that dysfunctional elimination syndrome was associated with a higher incidence of breakthrough UTI despite prophylaxis, a delayed resolution of VUR, persistent UTI recurrence after the resolution of VUR, and more recurrence of VUR after ureteric reimplantation.[104]

Treatment of Functional Voiding Disorders

It is important to exclude anatomic or neuropathic causes by careful history, physical examination, voiding diary, uroflowmetry, and ultrasound scanning. Full urodynamic studies are invasive, and they are generally reserved for children who are unresponsive to conservative treatment. One center reported the use of minimal urodynamic evaluation consisting of standard uroflowmetry and simultaneous perineal electromyograph recordings by cutaneous electrodes. The authors found this to be sufficient to assess children with voiding dysfunction.[105,106]

General Measures

Treatment should be multidisciplinary. It should also be multipronged rather than relying on a single modality. Any concurrent UTI or local perineal irritation such as vulvovaginitis has to be treated first. Constipation is a frequent coexisting and aggravating problem. Fecal retention should be cleared by a series of enemas followed by maintenance laxatives to prevent recurrence. Lactulose and Movicol are stool softeners, but sometimes bowel stimulants such as senna, sodium picosulfate, and high-dose Movicol have to be used to achieve daily bowel movements. Children can be encouraged to keep an elimination diary for monitoring. Dietary advice is important to ensure adequate water and high fiber intake. The American Academy of Pediatrics recommends 0.5 g of dietary fiber per kg of body weight per day up to a maximum of 35 g per day.[107]

For the bladder problem, drugs, behavioral therapy, or a combination should be used, depending on the nature of the functional disorder. In general, children should be encouraged to void every 2 to 3 hours or half hour after a meal. Children can be encouraged to have such a voiding schedule by keeping a voiding diary or using watches to remind them. Caregivers, such as school teachers, should allow adequate toilet time and provide access to a clean and safe toilet. A correct posture during voiding is important, and young children should use age-appropriate toilet seats with their feet supported by a footstool.

Drug Therapy

For children with detrusor overactivity, anticholinergic drugs are helpful to suppress uninhibited contractions during filling. They can increase functional bladder capacity and reduce the severity of VUR. Oxybutynin is most frequently used, but newer alternatives such as long-acting oxybutynin, tolterodine,[108] long-acting hyoscyamine, and darifenacin[109] are better tolerated[73] (see Table 38-2). Children with disturbance during voiding may benefit from alpha-blockers such as doxazosin, terazosin, or tamsulosin, which relax the sphincter.[110-115]

Biofeedback Therapy

Biofeedback programs use modern equipment to give the child an immediate indication of a physiologic process controlled by the central nervous system that is otherwise not perceived clearly or accurately. Through watching urine flow rates, pelvic floor EMG, or detrusor pressures in real time, children can learn to relax the pelvic floor during voiding. Recent reports have demonstrated the efficacy of this process clinically and by pre- and post-treatment urodynamics.[116,117] In general, biofeedback is useful for children who present not only with staccato voiding but also with incontinence. On average, six sessions seem to provide effective treatment. Children as young as 4 years old can be treated effectively. A hyperactive pelvic floor is the most common finding, but some patients have pelvic floor laxity or incontinence as a result of uninhibited bladder contractions. Patients with a low bladder capacity are least likely to respond to a biofeedback program alone; they may respond to anticholinergics followed by biofeedback. A small percentage of patients with low flow but no evidence of pelvic floor hyperactivity (as a result of primary bladder neck dysfunction) may respond to alpha-blockers.[116]

Nonconventional Therapy

Botox (botulinum toxin) has also been used in voiding dysfunction. One study reported 11 children with idiopathic detrusor overactivity who were given Botox A (125 or 250 units) by multiple injections into the bladder wall. There was an increase in functional bladder capacity and a decrease in detrusor contractions and urgency symptoms.[82] Another report described 20 children with urine retention caused by detrusor underactivity. They were given Botox A in 50-unit injections into the urethra. All showed an improvement of reduced mean quality of life score, reduced median voiding pressure, and maximum urethral closure pressure and residual volume.[83]

Neuromodulation has also been tried in refractory cases. The results of acupuncture, posterior tibial nerve stimulation, transurethral electric bladder stimulation, and sacral nerve root stimulation in small case series were summarized in a recent review article.[118]

Rarely children with dysfunctional elimination syndrome or Hinman syndrome with recurrent UTI or upper tract damage may need CIC for effective emptying, just like patients with organic neurogenic bladders.[119]

PRIMARY MONOSYMPTOMATIC NOCTURNAL ENURESIS

Primary nocturnal enuresis (PNE) is a common disorder among children. From published epidemiologic studies, it has been determined that the overall prevalence of PNE remains relatively constant, irrespective of geographic location. It is estimated that 20% to 25% of 4-year-old children and 10% of 7-year-old children have PNE.[52,120] It has been reported that this condition decreases with age, with a resolution rate of 15% per annum.[121,122] According to one study, enuresis persists in 1.5% to 3% of the adult population[123]; another study reported a rate of 0.5%.[124]

Causes and Pathophysiology of Primary Nocturnal Enuresis

Several studies have shown that a large proportion of enuretic children have a deranged circadian rhythm of antidiuretic hormone secretion that results in nocturnal polyuria.[125,126] Hence, desmopressin has been used to treat PNE with a response rate of around 70%.[127,128] However, no satisfactory answer was provided for the remaining 30% of patients who are refractory to treatment. Although some studies tried to explain this mismatch by showing a reduced functional bladder capacity among enuretic patients as compared with age-matched controls,[129-132] other studies had inconsistent findings.[121,133] There is now cumulating evidence that underlying bladder dysfunction may play an important role in the pathophysiology of PNE and that it can further provide reliable predictive clues to the treatment response. Most interestingly, overnight studies in enuretic children with simultaneous sleep electroencephalography and cystometry have revealed marked detrusor instability only after sleep at night but not during wakeful periods in the daytime.[134,135] This per se can result in a marked reduction in the nocturnal functional bladder capacity.[129,130,134,135] The treatment of PNE should therefore include tailored treatment toward the underlying bladder dysfunction rather than solely relying on correcting nocturnal polyuria.

It should be noted that, despite the high prevalence of underlying bladder dysfunction among patients with severe, refractory PNE, many have no identifiable daytime urinary symptoms such as incontinence, frequency, or urgency. A detailed urodynamic study would, however, reveal detrusor instability in 30% to 90% of patients. Many enuretic children with reduced functional bladder capacity have learned—either consciously but more likely subconsciously—to restrict fluid intake during the day in an attempt to avoid the social inconvenience of urinary frequency and urge incontinence. This can often be easily identified by a detailed home-recorded voiding diary of an extraordinarily low fluid intake and infrequent, small-volume voiding. By giving these patients a standard fluid intake and then asking them to repeat a home recording of micturition frequency and urinary volume, one can quite easily obtain a highly reliable estimate of the functional bladder capacity and hence identify those patients with reduced bladder capacities.[134,136]

Whether there is an underlying bladder dysfunction or a mismatch in urine production and storage capacity, there must also be a simultaneous arousal failure in response to bladder fullness before bed wetting can occur. Therefore, more recent studies have looked more closely at the involvement of the central nervous system in the cause of childhood nocturnal enuresis. The region of interest has been hypothesized to lie within a tiny area surrounding the vicinity of the pontine micturition center, the posterior hypothalamus (which is responsible for the secretion of antidiuretic hormone), and the locus coeruleus (which is thought to play an important role in the initiation of cortical arousal and the release of noradrenaline).[9,10,134]

Enuretic boys were shown to be more difficult to arouse than age-matched controls. The arousal inability in patients with nocturnal enuresis may relate to either elevated arousal thresholds or the presence of spontaneous uninhibited bladder contractions.

To further study brainstem involvement, the startle pathway has been examined. A deficiency of the prepulse inhibition of startle has been reported in enuretic children such that a prestimulation at 120 ms before a main stimulus resulted in significantly less inhibition of the blink reflex among enuretic children as compared with healthy controls. This prepulse inhibition is based on an inhibition of the startle pathway by the pedunculopontine tegmental nucleus, which lies in close proximity to the pontine micturition center in the brain stem. Therefore, it has been postulated that a deficient prepulse inhibition and a reduced ability to inhibit micturition during sleep might both originate from a common dysfunction in the pontine tegmentum. This further suggests that a relationship may exist between nocturnal bladder function and brain stem function in humans.[137-139]

Furthermore, it has also been shown that, after the successful treatment of nocturnal enuresis in these children, both the sleep arousal threshold and the prepulse inhibition of startle improved. This suggests that the brain stem dysfunction may be a secondary effect of the underlying bladder dysfunction, thus further supporting the "bladder-brain dialogue" concept whereby there is a bidirectional communication between the bladder and the brain.

Psychologic Consequences of Nocturnal Enuresis

A recent review has found that clinically significant behavioral problems as detected by questionnaire surveys such as Child Behavior Checklist are present in 13.5% to 40.1% of all wetting children and that the relative risk is 1.3 to 4.5 times higher.[52] However, it is possible that such an association with psychiatric problems can be either a consequence of the wetting problem, a precipitating cause, part of a common neurobiologic dysfunction, or mere coincidence. PNE has a low overall comorbidity. In general, PNE has a low overall association with externalizing disorders, and secondary nocturnal enuresis has a high comorbidity of both emotional and externalizing disorders.

One subclinical psychologic symptom of particular concern is low self-esteem among children with PNE. In a recent review, however, there was no conclusive evidence that bed wetting leads to lower self-esteem; however, self-esteem can improve upon attaining dryness.[140] In another study, self-esteem improved with treatment, regardless of any improvement in bed wetting, thereby suggesting that frequent follow-up and emotional support appear to be important for determining the outcome.[141]

Treatment of Nocturnal Enuresis

Initial evaluation includes a careful history, a physical examination, a voiding diary, uroflowmetry, and residual urine volume. This helps not only to exclude other voiding disorders but also to identify the different pathogenetic subtypes of enuresis. Detailed urodynamic evaluation and ultrasound scans should be considered if there is any suspicion of daytime symptoms, multiple wetting episodes per night, or refractory enuresis despite conventional treatment.

General Measures

The International Children's Continence Society presented an evidence-based management strategy in 2004.[52] Before undertaking treatment for enuresis, daytime voiding problems and constipation need to be treated as described previously. Empathetic counseling of the child and the parents ensures that they understand the problem, its natural history, and the effects of treatment. The motivation of the child and family to seek treatment should be assessed, because this is an important determinant of outcome.

General advice for the enuretic child includes adequate duration of sleep for age, restricting fluid intake for several hours before sleep, and voiding before sleep. The parents should be advised not to punish or scold the child for wetting episodes. Generally the child should be 6 to 8 years old before he or she can comply with a treatment such as filling out a "star chart" as a record of dry and wet nights. These simple behavioral measures have been found to be successful.[142] In one study, they achieved dryness in 18% of children.[143]

Behavioral Therapy

Alarm therapy is the most common form of behavioral therapy. It is a learning program with positive reinforcement that includes aversive elements, thus making it an operant type of behavioral approach. It should be offered as first-line treatment for every patient, because four previous systematic reviews all concluded that it is efficacious.[144-148] The recent Cochrane review concluded that about two thirds of children achieved dryness, and it is more effective than no treatment, with a 60% reduction in the risk of failure. As compared with desmopressin (although desmopressin has more immediate effects), alarm therapy is more effective than desmopressin at the end of the program (relative risk for failure, 0.71; 95% confidence interval, 0.50 to 0.99). Alarm therapy probably has a greater long-term effect (relative risk for failure, 0.27 as compared with desmopressin; 95% confidence interval, 0.21 to 0.69).[144] Its efficacy increased with the duration of treatment. Dische and colleagues[149] reported dryness in 25% at 2 months, in 50% at 3 months, and in 90% at 6 months. The motivations of the child and the family and higher wetting frequency were reported to be predictive of success. Children achieved dryness by waking up in 35% of cases or sleeping through the night (hence they developed an increased bladder capacity) in 65% of cases.[150,151] It is recommended that treatment be used until the child is dry for 1 month. Although 29% to 66% of responders relapsed, they often responded to further alarm therapy.

Other behavioral therapies have also been effective if combined with alarm therapy. "Overlearning" involves increasing fluid intake before sleep after achieving dryness with alarm therapy; this has been shown to reduce relapse rates.[152] "Dry bed training" is a complex behavioral program that involves positive practice, cleanliness training, waking schedules, social reinforcement, and increased fluid intake. It is not more effective than alarm therapy alone.[153,154] A reward for correct behavior at the time of wetting promotes alarm therapy efficacy, whereas a penalty for wetting the bed reduces alarm therapy efficacy.[144,155] Combination therapy with both alarms and desmopressin has been shown to be more effective than either alone in several controlled trials.[156-159]

Drug Therapy

Desmopressin is an analog of vasopressin that has increased antidiuretic activity but no vasopressor activity. By correcting the loss of antidiuretic hormone upsurge during sleep, desmopressin reduces nocturnal urine production and prevents enuresis. The Cochrane review of randomized controlled trials has shown that patients on desmopressin were 4.6 times more likely to achieve 14 consecutive dry nights as compared with those receiving placebo. In most trials, 60% to 70% of patients could achieve more than a 50% reduction in wetting frequency. However, in early trials, most patients relapsed when treatment was stopped.[160] Long-term therapy for 6 to 24 months (with a 1-week interruption every 3 months to test lasting cure) has been reported to achieve an annual cure rate of 30% in the Swedish Enuresis Trial (SWEET) trial, which is higher than the usually quoted spontaneous cure rate.[161]

Theoretically, desmopressin is ideal for the patient with nocturnal polyuria. In practice, desmopressin is used when the child has failed to respond to alarm therapy or when alarm therapy is unacceptable. It is also preferred if a rapid response is needed in families that are highly stressed by the bed wetting problem. A short course of desmopressin is also useful to ensure complete dryness when the child is sleeping away from home.

The usual dose of desmopressin is 0.2 to 0.4 mg orally or 20 to 40 mcg nasally at bedtime. It is well tolerated. Parents should be cautioned about the risk of water intoxication.[162] In general, children should be instructed to take one 8-oz glass of water at dinner, to have no more than one 8-oz glass afterward, and to have nothing to drink for 2 hours before sleep.[52]

Anticholinergic drugs have a role in children with both day- and nighttime wetting. Even in children without daytime voiding symptoms, the bladder may be normal during waking hours but overactive during sleep. These drugs are usually used as an adjunct in combination with desmopressin.[163,164] However, constipation may occur, which further aggravates detrusor overactivity and increases residual urine. Tolterodine is better tolerated than oxybutynin.

Tricyclic antidepressants (especially imipramine) were used in the 1960s for treating enuretic children. The Cochrane review found that, as compared with placebo, imipramine was effective during treatment. The mean weighted reduction in wet nights per week was 1.04, and the odds ratio of achieving 14 consecutive dry nights was 7.23. However, after stopping treatment, there was no difference between the treatment group and the placebo group. Another tricyclic antidepressant called viloxazine may be better; it demonstrated a sustained reduction in wet nights on follow-up.[165] The mechanism of beneficial action is unclear, but it is probably a central noradrenergic facilitation effect. However, because of its potentially fatal cardiotoxicity, it should only be used carefully in cases that are refractory to previously described treatment.[52]

SUMMARY

Over the past decades, research has allowed for a better understanding of the anatomy and developmental physiology of the bladder-sphincter complex, especially in infants. Advances of imaging (e.g., ultrasound, MRI) and urodynamic techniques (e.g., natural filling, ambulatory urodynamic studies) have made possible the more accurate assessment of voiding disorders. The early assessment and intervention of newborns with spinal dysraphism have improved the management and outcome of neurogenic bladder in these patients, and urine diversion is no longer indicated. The importance of functional voiding problems is more widely appreciated. There have also been great advances in our knowledge of nocturnal enuresis that have rationalized its treatment.

REFERENCES

1. Gosling JA: The structure of the female lower urinary tract and pelvic floor, *Urol Clin North Am* 12:207-14, 1985.
2. Gosling JA, Dixon JS, Critchley HOD, Thompson SA: A comparative study of the human external sphincter and periurethral levator ani muscle, *Br J Urol* 53:35-41, 1981.
3. DeLancey JOL: Structural aspects of urethrovesical function in the female, *Neurourol Urodyn* 7:509-19, 1988.
4. de Groat WC: Anatomy and physiology of the lower urinary tract, *Urol Clin North Am* 20:383-401, 1993.
5. Zvara P, Carrier S, Kour NW, Tanagho EA: The detailed neuroanatomy of the human striated urethral sphincter, *Br J Urol* 74:182-87, 1994.
6. Wiegel JW: Neurogenic bladder and urinary diversion. In Ashcraft KW, editor: *Pediatric urology*, Philadelphia, 1990, WB Saunders, pp 175-210.
7. Mattiasson A: Bladder and urethral physiology and pathophysiology. In Krane RJ, Siroky MB, Fitzpatrick JM, editors: *Clinical urology*, Philadelphia, 1994, JB Lippincott, pp 536-57.
8. Kokoua A, Homsy Y, Lavigne JF, et al: Maturation of the external urinary sphincter: a comparative histotopographic study in humans, *J Urol* 150:617-22, 1992.
9. Yeung CK, Godley ML, Dhillon HK, Duffy PG, Ransley PG: Urodynamic patterns in infants with normal lower urinary tracts or primary vesico-ureteric reflux, *Br J Urol* 81:461-67, 1998.
10. Yeung CK, Godley ML, Ho CKW, et al: Some new insights into bladder function in infancy, *Br J Urol* 6:235-40, 1995.
11. Sillen U, Hjalmas K, Aili M, Bjure J, et al: Pronounced detrusor hypercontractility in infants with gross bilateral reflux, *J Urol* 148:598-99, 1992.
12. Bradley WE, Timm GW: Innervation of the detrusor muscle and urethra, *Urol Clin North Am* 1:3-27, 1974.
13. Blaivas JG: The neurophysiology of micturition: a clinical study of 550 patients, *J Urol* 127:958-63, 1982.
14. Fernandes ET, Reinberg Y, Vernier R, Gonzalez R: Neurogenic bladder dysfunction in children: review of pathophysiology and current management, *J Pediatr* 124:1-7, 1994.
15. McLorie GA, Husmann DA: Incontinence and enuresis, *Pediatr Clin North Am* 34:1159-74, 1987.
16. Harrison SCW, Abrams P: Bladder function. In Sant GR, editor: *Pathophysiologic principle of urology*, London, 1994, Blackwell Scientific Publications, pp 93-121.
17. Nash DFE: The development of micturition control with special reference to enuresis, *Ann R Coll Surg Engl* 5:318-44, 1949.
18. Ohel G, Haddad S, Samueloff A: Fetal urine production and micturition and fetal behavioral state, *Am J Perinatol* 12:91-92, 1995.
19. Zimmer EZ, Chao CR, Guy GP, Marks F, Fifer WP: Vibroacoustic stimulation evokes human fetal micturition, *Obstet Gynecol* 81:178-80, 1993.
20. Maggi CA, Santicioli P, Meli A: Postnatal development of micturition in rats, *Am J Physiol* 250:R926-31, 1986.
21. Thor KB, Blais DP, de Groat WC: Behavioral analysis of the postnatal development of micturition in kittens, *Dev Brain Res* 46:137-44, 1989.
22. de Groat WC, Booth AM, Yoshimura N: Neurophysiology of micturition and its modification in animal models of human disease. In Maggi CA, editor: *Nervous control of the urogenital system*, London, 1993, Harwood Academic, pp 227-90.
23. de Groat WC, Araki I, Vizzard MA, Yoshiyama M, et al: Developmental and injury induced plasticity in the micturition reflex pathway, *Behav Brain Res* 92:127-40, 1998.
24. Araki I, de Groat WC: Developmental synaptic depression underlying reorganization of visceral reflex pathways in the spinal cord, *J Neurosci* 17:8402-07, 1997.
25. Sugaya K, Roppolo JR, Yoshimura N, Card JP, de Groat WC: The central neural pathways involved in the neonatal rat as revealed by the injection of pseudorabies virus into the bladder, *Neurosci Lett* 223:197-200, 1997.
26. Sugaya K, de Groat WC: Micturition reflexes in the in-vitro neonatal rat brainstem-spinal cord-urinary bladder preparation, *Am J Physiol* 266:R658-67, 1994.
27. Yeung CK: Pathophysiology of bladder dysfunction. In Gearheart JP, Rink RC, Mouriquand PDE, editors: *Pediatric urology*, Philadelphia, 2001, Saunders, pp 453-69.
28. Goellner MH, Ziegler EE, Fomon SJ: Urination during the first three years of life. *Nephron* 28:174-78, 1981.
29. Yeung CK: The normal infant bladder, *Scand J Urol Nephrol Suppl* 173:19-23, 1995.
30. Holmdahl G, Hanson E, Hanson M, Hellstrom AL, et al: Four-hour voiding observation in health infants, *J Urol* 156:1809-12, 1996.

31. Koff SA: Non-neuropathic vesicourethral dysfunction in children. In O'Donnell B, Koff SA, editors: *Pediatric urology*, Oxford, 1997, Butterworth-Heinemann, pp 217-228.
32. Yeates WK: Bladder function in normal micturition. In Kolvin I, MacKeith RC, Meadow SR, editors: *Bladder control and enuresis*, London, 1973, W Heinemann Medical Books Ltd, pp 28-36.
33. Koff SA: Estimating bladder capacity in children, *Urology* 21:248, 1983.
34. Hjalmas K: Urodynamics in normal infants and children, *Scand J Urol Nephrol Suppl* 114:30-37, 1988.
35. Hjalmas K: Micturition in infants and children with normal lower urinary tract: a urodynamic study, *Scand J Urol Nephrol* 37:9-17, 1976.
36. Bachelard M, Sillen U, Hansson S, Hermansson G, et al: Urodynamic pattern in asymptomatic infants: siblings of children with vesicoureteric reflux, *J Urol* 162:1733-37, 1999.
37. Sillen U, Solsnes E, Hellstrom AL, Sandberg K: The voiding pattern of healthy preterm neonates, *J Urol* 163:278-81, 2000.
38. Yeung CK, Godley ML, Duffy PG, Ransley PG: Natural filling cystometry in infants and children, *Br J Urol* 75:531-37, 1995.
39. Norgaard JP, van Gool JD, Hjalmas K, Djurhuus JC, Hellstrom AL: Standardization and definitions in lower urinary tract dysfunction in children, *Br J Urol* 81:1-16, 1998.
40. van Gool JD, de Jonge GA: Urge syndrome and urge incontinence, *Arch Dis Child* 64:1629-34, 1989.
41. Vincent SA: Postural control of urinary incontinence—the Curtsey sign, *Lancet* 2:631-32, 1966.
42. O'Reagan S, Yazback S, Hamberger B, Schick E: Constipation—a commonly unrecognised cause of enuresis, *Am J Dis Child* 140:260-61, 1986.
43. Hinman F, Baumann FW: Vesical and ureteral damage from voiding dysfunction in boys without neurologic or obstructive disease, *J Urol* 109:727-32, 1973.
44. Hinman F: Non-neurogenic neurogenic bladder (the Hinman syndrome)—15 years later, *J Urol* 136:769-77, 1986.
45. Allen TD: The non-neurogenic neurogenic bladder, *J Urol* 117:232-38, 1977.
46. Dorfman LE, Bailey J, Smith JP: Subclinical neurogenic bladder in children, *J Urol* 101:48-54, 1969.
47. Williams DI, Hirst G, Doyle D: The occult neuropathic bladder, *J Pediatr Surg* 9:35-41, 1975.
48. Jayanthi VR, Khoury AE, McLorie GA, Agarwal SK: The non-neurogenic neurogenic bladder of early infancy, *J Urol* 158:1281-85, 1997.
49. Hinman F: Non-neurogenic bladder (Hinman syndrome). In O'Donnell B, Koff SA, editors: *Pediatric urology*, Oxford, UK, 1997, Butterworth-Heinemann, pp 245-48.
50. Ochoa B, Gorlin RJ: Urofacial (Ochoa) syndrome, *Am J Med Genet* 27:661-67, 1987.
51. Ochoa B: The urofacial (Ochoa) syndrome revisited, *J Urol* 148:580-83, 1992.
52. Kjalmas K, Arnold T, Bower W, et al: Nocturnal enuresis: an international evidence based management strategy, *J Urol* 171:2545-61, 2004.
53. Neveus T, Hansell P, Stenberg A: Vasopressin and hypercalciuria in enuresis: a reappraisal, *BJU Int* 90:725-29, 2002.
54. Yeung CK, Sreedhar B, Leung VT, Metriweli C: Ultrasound bladder measurements in patients with primary nocturnal enuresis: a urodynamic and treatment outcome correlation, *J Urol* 171:2589-94, 2004.
55. Venhola M, Reunanen M, Taskinen S, Lahdes-Vasama T, Uhari M: Interobserver and intra-observer agreement in interpreting urodynamic measurements in children, *J Urol* 169:2344-46, 2003.
56. Nijman JM: The interpretation of urodynamic investigations in children. Second course on pediatric urodynamics International Children's Continence Society Course, Utrecht, 1997, pp 45-53.
57. Yeung CK: Continuous real-time ambulatory urodynamic monitoring in infants and young children using infrared telemetry, *Br J Urol* 81:76-80, 1998.
58. Bower YF, Yip SK, Yeung CK: Dysfunctional elimination symptoms in childhood and adulthood, *J Urol* 174:1623-27, 2006.
59. Karaman MI, Kaya C, Caskurlu T, Guney S, Ergenekon E: Urodynamic findings in children with cerebral palsy, *Int J Urol* 12:717-20, 2005.
60. Sakakibara R, Uchiyama T, Arai K, Yamanishi T, Hattori T: Lower urinary tract dysfunction in Machado-Joseph disease: a study of 11 clinical-urodynamic observations, *J Neurol Sci* 218:67-72, 2004.
61. Silveri M, de Gennaro M, Gatti C, Bizzarri C, et al: Voiding dysfunction in x-linked adrenoleukodystrophy: symptom score and urodynamic findings, *J Urol* 171:2651-53, 2004.
62. Kaefer M, Pabby A, Kelly M: Improved bladder function after prophylactic treatment of the high risk neurogenic bladder in newborns with myelomeningocele, *J Urol* 162:1068-71, 1999.
63. Wu HY, Baskin LS, Kogan BA: Neurogenic bladder dysfunction due to myelomeningocele: neonatal versus childhood treatment, *J Urol* 157:2295-97, 1997.
64. Tanaka H, Kakizaki H, Kobayashi S, Shibata T, et al: The relevance of urethral resistance in children with myelodysplasia: its impact on upper urinary tract deterioration and the outcome of conservative management, *J Urol* 161:929-32, 1999.
65. Bauer SB, Hallett M, Khoshbin S, et al: Predictive value of urodynamic evaluation in newborns with myelodysplasia, *JAMA* 252:650-52, 1984.
66. Sidi AA, Dykstra DD, Gonzalez R: The value of urodynamic testing in the management of neonates with myelodysplasia: a prospective study, *J Urol* 135:90-93, 1986.
67. Bauer SB: Early evaluation and management of children with spina bifida. In King LR, editor: *Urological surgery in neonates and young infants*, Philadelphia, 1988, WB Saunders, pp 252-64.
68. Snodgrass WT, Adams R: Initial urologic management of myelomeningocele, *Urol Clin North Am* 31:427-34, 2004.
69. McGuire EJ, Woodside JR, Borden TA, Weiss RM: Prognostic value of urodynamic testing in myelodysplastic patients, *J Urol* 126:205-09, 1981.
70. Lapides J, Diokno AC, Silber SJ, Lowe BS: Clean intermittent self-catheterization in the treatment of urinary tract disease, *J Urol* 107:458-61, 1972.
71. Campbell JB, Moore KN, Voaklander DC, Mix LW: Complications associated with clean intermittent catheterization in children with spina bifida, *J Urol* 171:2420-22, 2004.
72. Lindehall B, Abrahamsson K, Hjalmas K, Jodal U, et al: Complications of clean intermittent catheterization in boys and young males with neurogenic bladder dysfunction, *J Urol* 172:1686-88, 2004.
73. Schulman SL: Voiding dysfunction in children, *Urol Clin North Am* 31:481-90, 2004.
74. Youdim K, Kogan BA: Preliminary study of the safety and efficacy of extended-release oxybutynin in children, *Urology* 59:428-32, 2002.
75. Ellsworth PI, Borgstein NG, Nijman RJ, Reddy PP: Use of tolterodine in children with neurogenic detrusor overactivity: relationship between dose and urodynamic response, *J Urol* 174:1647-51, 2005.
76. Castro-Gago M, Novo I, Cimadevila A, Pena J, et al: Management of neurogenic bladder dysfunction secondary to myelomeningocele, *Eur J Pediatr* 150:62-65, 1990.
77. Ferrara P, D'Aleo CM, Tarquini E, Salvatore S, Salvaggio E: Side-effects of oral or intravesical oxybutynin chloride in children with spina bifida, *BJU Int* 87:674-78, 2001.
78. Seki N, Ikawa S, Takano N, Naito S: Intravesical instillation of resiniferatoxin for neurogenic bladder dysfunction in a patient with myelodysplasia, *J Urol* 166:2368-69, 2001.
79. Abrams P, Amarenco G, Bakke A, et al: Tamsulosin: efficacy and safety in patients with neurogenic lower urinary tract dysfunction due to suprasacral spinal cord injury, *J Urol* 170:1242-51, 2003.
80. Schulte-Baukloh H, Michael T, Miller K, Knispel HH: Alfuzosin in the treatment of high leak-point pressure in children with neurogenic bladder, *BJU Int* 90:716-20, 2002.
81. Bogaert G, Beckers G, Lombaerts R: The use and rationale of selective alpha blockade in children with non-neurogenic neurogenic bladder dysfunction, *Int Braz J Urol* 30:128-34, 2004.
82. Schurch B, Corcos J: Botulinum toxin injections for paediatric incontinence, *Curr Opin Urol* 15:264-67, 2005.

83. Kuo HC: Effect of botulinum a toxin in the treatment of voiding dysfunction due to detrusor underactivity, *Urology* 61:550-54, 2003.
84. Smith CP, Nishiguchi J, O'Leary M, Yoshimura N, Chancellor MB: Single-institution experience in 110 patients with botulinum toxin A injection into bladder or urethra, *Urology* 65:37-41, 2005.
85. Bauer SB: The management of the myelodysplastic child: a paradigm shift, *BJU Int* 92:23-28, 2003.
86. Hafez AT, McLorie G, Gilday D, et al: Long-term evaluation of metabolic profile and bone mineral density after ileocystoplasty in children, *J Urol* 170:1639-42, 2003.
87. Vajda P, Pinter AB, Harangi F, Farkas A, et al: Metabolic findings after colocystoplasty in children, *Urology* 62:542-46, 2003.
88. DeFoor W, Minevich E, Reeves D, Tackett L, et al: Gastrocystoplasty: long-term followup, *J Urol* 170:1647-50, 2003.
89. Liard A, Seguier-Lipszyc E, Mathiot A, Mitrofanoff P: The Mitrofanoff procedure: 20 years later, *J Urol* 165:2394-98, 2001.
90. Wein AJ: Pathophysiology and categorization of voiding dysfunction. In Walsh PC, Retik AB, Vaughan ED, Wein AJ, editors: *Campbell's urology*, Philadelphia, 1998, WB Saunders, pp 917-26.
91. Lapides J: Neuromuscular, vesical and urethral dysfunction. In Campbell MF, Harrison H, editors: *Urology*, Philadelphia, 1970, WB Saunders, pp 1343-79.
92. Bellinger MF: Myelomeningocele and neuropathic bladder. In Gillenwater JY, Grayhack JT, Howards SS, Ducckett JW, editors: *Adult and pediatric surgery*, St. Louis, 1996, Mosby-Year Book, pp 2489-528.
93. Dewan PA, Goh DG: Variable expression of the congenital obstructive posterior urethral membrane, *Urology* 45:507-09, 1995.
94. Dhillon HK, Yeung CK, Ransley PG, Duffy PG: Cowper's gland cysts—a cause of transient intra-uterine bladder outflow obstruction?, *Fetal Diagn Ther* 8:51-55, 1993.
95. Bachelard M, Sillen U, Hansson S, Hermansson G, et al: Urodynamic pattern in infants with urinary tract infection, *J Urol* 160:522-26, 1998.
96. Mazzola BL, von Vigier RO, Marchand S, Tonz M, Bianchetti MG: Behavioral and functional abnormalities linked with recurrent urinary tract infections in girls, *J Nephrol* 16:133-38, 2003.
97. Wan J, Kaplinsky R, Greenfield S: Toilet habits of children evaluated for urinary tract infection, *J Urol* 154:797-99, 1995.
98. Hellerstein S, Nickell E: Prophylactic antibiotics in children at risk for urinary tract infection, *Pediatr Nephrol* 17:506-10, 2002.
99. Bakker E, Van Gool J, van Sprundel M, van der Auwera JC, Wyndaele JJ: Risk factors for recurrent urinary tract infection in 4332 Belgian schoolchildren aged between 10 and 14 years, *Eur J Pediatr* 163:234-38, 2004.
100. Homayoon K, Chen JJ, Cummings JM, Steinhardt GF: Voiding dysfunction: outcome in infants with congenital vesicoureteral reflux, *Urology* 66:1091-94, 2005.
101. Podesta ML, Castera R, Ruarte AC: Videourodynamic findings in young infants with severe primary reflux, *J Urol* 171:829-33, 2004.
102. Godley ML, Desai D, Yeung CK, Dhillon HK, et al: The relationship between early renal status, and the resolution of vesico-ureteric reflux and bladder function at 16 months, *BJU Int* 87:457-62, 2001.
103. Yeung CK, Sreedhar B, Sihoe JDY, Sit FKY: Renal and bladder functional status at diagnosis as predictive factors for the outcome of primary vesicoureteral reflux in children, *J Urol* 176:1152-57, 2006.
104. Koff SA, Wagner TT, Jayanthi VR: The relationship among dysfunctional elimination syndromes, primary vesicoureteral reflux and urinary tract infections in children, *J Urol* 160:1019-22, 1998.
105. Dacher JN, Savoye-Collet C: Urinary tract infection and functional bladder sphincter disorders in children, *Eur Radiol* 14:L101-06, 2004.
106. Pfister C, Dacher JN, Gaucher S, Liard-Zmuda A, et al: The usefulness of a minimal urodynamic evaluation and pelvic floor biofeedback in children with chronic voiding dysfunction, *BJU Int* 84:1054-57, 1999.
107. Clayden GS, Keshtgar AS, Carcani-Rathwell I, Abhyankar A: The management of chronic constipation and related faecal incontinence in childhood, *Arch Dis Child Educ Pract Ed* 90:ep58-67, 2005.
108. Ayan S, Kaya K, Topsakal K, Kilicarslan H, et al: Efficacy of tolterodine as a first-line treatment for non-neurogenic voiding dysfunction in children, *BJU Int* 96:411-14, 2005.
109. Chapple CR, Abrams P: Comparison of darifenacin and oxybutynin in patients with overactive bladder: assessment of ambulatory urodynamics and impact on salivary flow, *Eur Urol* 48:102-09, 2005.
110. Donohoe JM, Combs AJ, Glassberg KI: Primary bladder neck dysfunction in children and adolescents II: results of treatment with alpha-adrenergic antagonists, *J Urol* 173:212-16, 2005.
111. Cain MP, Wu SD, Austin PF, Herndon CD, Rink RC: Alpha blocker therapy for children with dysfunctional voiding and urinary retention, *J Urol* 170:1514-15, 2003.
112. Kramer SA, Rathbun SR, Elkins D, Karnes RJ, Husmann DA: Double-blind placebo controlled study of alpha-adrenergic receptor antagonists (doxazosin) for treatment of voiding dysfunction in the pediatric population, *J Urol* 173:2121-24, 2005.
113. Austin PF, Homsy YL, Masel JL, Cain MP, et al: Alpha-adrenergic blockade in children with neuropathic and nonneuropathic voiding dysfunction, *J Urol* 162:1064-67, 1999.
114. Yucel S, Akkaya E, Guntekin E, et al: Can alpha-blocker therapy be an alternative to biofeedback for dysfunctional voiding and urinary retention? A prospective study, *J Urol* 174:1612-15, 2005.
115. Yang SS, Wang CC, Chen YT: Effectiveness of alpha1-adrenergic blockers in boys with low urinary flow rate and urinary incontinence, *J Formos Med Assoc* 102:551-55, 2003.
116. Yagci S, Kibar Y, Akay O, et al: The effect of biofeedback treatment on voiding and urodynamic parameters in children with voiding dysfunction, *J Urol* 174:1994-97, 2005.
117. Nelson JD, Cooper CS, Boyt MA, Hawtrey CE, Austin JC: Improved uroflow parameters and post-void residual following biofeedback therapy in pediatric patients with dysfunctional voiding does not correspond to outcome, *J Urol* 172:1653-56, 2004.
118. Bani-Hani AH, Vandersteen DR, Reinberg YE: Neuromodulation in pediatrics, *Urol Clin North Am* 32:101-07, 2005.
119. Pohl HG, Bauer SB, Borer JG, et al: The outcome of voiding dysfunction managed with clean intermittent catheterization in neurologically and anatomically normal children, *BJU Int* 89:923-27, 2002.
120. Yeung CK, Sreedhar B, Sihoe JDY, Sit FKY, Lau J: Differences in characteristics of nocturnal enuresis between children and adolescence: a critical appraisal from a large epidemiological study, *BJU Int* 97:1069-73, 2006.
121. Forsythe WI, Redmond A: Enuresis and spontaneous cure rate—study of 1129 enuretics, *Arch Dis Child* 49:259-63, 1974.
122. Feehan H, McGee R, Stanton W, Silva PA: A 6 year follow-up of childhood enuresis: prevalence in adolescence and consequences for mental health, *J Paediatr Child Health* 26:75-79, 1990.
123. Yeung CK, Sihoe JDY, Sit FKY, Diao M, Yew SY: Urodynamic findings in adults with primary nocturnal enuresis, *J Urol* 171:2595-98, 2004.
124. Hirasing RA, Van LF, Bolk BL, Janknegt RA: Enuresis nocturna in adults, *Scand J Urol Nephrol* 31:533-36, 1997.
125. Rittig S, Knudsen UB, Norgaard JP, Pedersen EB, Djurhuus JC: Abnormal diurnal rhythm of plasma vasopressin and urinary output in patients with enuresis, *Am J Physiol* 256:F664-71, 1989.
126. Norgaard JP, Pedersen EB, Djurhuus JC: Diurnal anti-diuretic hormone levels in enuretics, *J Urol* 134:1029-31, 1985.
127. Moffatt MEK, Harlos S, Kirshen AJ, Burd L: Desmopressin acetate and nocturnal enuresis: how much do we know?, *Pediatrics* 92:420-25, 1993.
128. Rittig S, Knudsen UB, Sorensen S, Djurhuus JC, Norgaard JP: Long-term double blind crossover study of desmopressin intranasal spray in the management of nocturnal enuresis. In Meadow SR, editor: *Desmopressin in nocturnal enuresis*, London, 1989, Horus Medical Publications, pp 43-55.
129. Eller DA, Austin PF, Tanguay S, Homsy YL: Daytime functional bladder capacity as a predictor of response to desmopressin in monosymptomatic nocturnal enuresis, *Eur Urol* 33 Suppl 3:25-29, 1998.

130. Rushton HG, Belman AB, Zaontz MR, Skoog SJ, Sihelnik S: The influence of small functional bladder capacity and other predictors on the response to desmopressin in the management of monosymptomatic nocturnal enuresis, *J Urol* 156:651-55, 1996.
131. Starfield B: Functional bladder capacity in enuretic and nonenuretic children, *J Pediatr* 70:777-81, 1967.
132. Jarvelin MR, Huttunen NP, Seppanen J, Seppanen U, Moilanen I: Screening of urinary tract abnormalities among day and night-wetting children, *Scand J Urol Nephrol* 24:181-89, 1990.
133. Norgaard JP: Urodynamics in enuresis I: reservoir function, *Neurourol Urodyn* 8:199-211, 1989.
134. Yeung CK, Chiu HN, Sit FKY: Bladder dysfunction in children with refractory monosymptomatic primary nocturnal enuresis, *J Urol* 162:1049-55, 1999.
135. Watanabe H, Kawauchi A, Kitamori T, Azuma Y: Treatment system for nocturnal enuresis according to an original classification system, *Eur Urol* 25:43-50, 1994.
136. Rittig S, Schaumburg H, Schmidt F, et al: Long-term home studies of water balance in patients with nocturnal enuresis, *Scand J Urol Nephrol Suppl* 31:25-27, 1997.
137. Ornitz EM, Russell AT, Hanna GL, et al: Prepulse inhibition of startle and the neurobiology of primary nocturnal enuresis, *Biol Psychiatry* 45:1455-66, 1999.
138. Ornitz EM, Russell AT, Gabikian P, Gehricke JG, Guthrie D: Prepulse inhibition of startle, intelligence and familial primary nocturnal enuresis, *Acta Paediatr* 89:475-81, 2000.
139. Diao M, Yeung CK, Sihoe JDY, et al: Brainstem and bladder dysfunctions in nocturnal enuresis. Proceedings of the 2nd Joint Meeting of European Society for Paediatric Urology (ESPU) and American Academy of Pediatrics. Uppsala, Sweden, 2005.
140. Redsell SA, Collier J: Bedwetting, behaviour and self-esteem: a review of the literature, *Child Care Health Dev* 27:149-62, 2001.
141. Longstaffe S, Moffatt MEK, Whalen JC: Behavioral and self-concept changes after six months of enuresis treatment: a randomized, controlled trial, *Pediatrics* 105:935-40, 2000.
142. Glazener CMA, Evans JHC: Simple behavioural and physical interventions for nocturnal enuresis in children, *Cochrane Database Syst Rev* CD003637:DOI:10.1002/14651858.CD003637.pub2, 2004.
143. Devlin JB, O'Cathain C: Predicting treatment outcome in nocturnal enuresis, *Arch Dis Child* 65:1158-61, 1990.
144. Glazener CMA, Evans JHC, Peto RE: Alarm interventions for nocturnal enuresis in children, *Cochrane Database Syst Rev* CD002911:DOI:10.1002/14651858.CD002911.pub2, 2005.
145. Bosson S, Lyth N: Nocturnal enuresis, *Clin Evid* 9:407-14, 2003.
146. Mellon MW, McGrath ML: Empirically supported treatments in pediatric psychology: nocturnal enuresis, *J Pediatr Psychol* 25:193-214, 2000.
147. Moffatt MEK: Nocturnal enuresis: a review of the efficacy of treatments and practical advice for clinicians, *J Dev Behav Pediatr* 18:49-56, 1997.
148. Houts AC, Berman JS, Abramson H: Effectiveness of psychological and pharmacological treatments for nocturnal enuresis, *J Consult Clin Psychol* 62:737-45, 1994.
149. Dische S, Yule W, Corbett J, Hand D: Childhood nocturnal enuresis: factors associated with outcome of treatment with an enuresis alarm, *Dev Med Child Neurol* 25:67-80, 1983.
150. Bonde HV, Andersen JP, Rosenkilde P: Nocturnal enuresis: change of nocturnal voiding pattern during alarm treatment, *Scand J Urol Nephrol* 28:349-52, 1994.
151. Hansen AF, Jorgensen TM: Alarm treatment: influence on functional bladder capacity, *Scand J Urol Nephrol Suppl* 31:59-60, 1997.
152. Morgan RT: Relapse and therapeutic response in the conditioning treatment of enuresis: a review of recent findings on intermittent reinforcement, overlearning and stimulus intensity, *Behav Res Ther* 16:273-79, 1978.
153. Azrin NH, Sneed TJ, Foxx RM: Dry-bed training: rapid elimination of childhood enuresis, *Behav Res Ther* 12:147-56, 1974.
154. Butler RJ, Brewin CR, Forsythe WI: A comparison of two approaches to the treatment of nocturnal enuresis and the prediction of effectiveness using pre-treatment variables, *J Child Psychol Psychiatry* 29:501-09, 1988.
155. Glazener CMA, Evans JHC, Peto RE: Complex behavioural and educational interventions for nocturnal enuresis in children, *Cochrane Database Syst Rev* CD004668:DOI:10.1002/14651858.CD004668, 2004.
156. Sukhai RN, Mol J, Harris AS: Combined therapy of enuresis alarm and desmopressin in the treatment of nocturnal enuresis, *Eur J Pediatr* 148:465-67, 1989.
157. Bradbury M: Combination therapy for nocturnal enuresis with desmopressin and an alarm device, *Scand J Urol Nephrol Suppl* 31:61-63, 1997.
158. Leebeek-Groenewegen A, Blom J, Sukhai R, Van DH: Efficacy of desmopressin combined with alarm therapy for monosymptomatic nocturnal enuresis, *J Urol* 166:2456-58, 2001.
159. Ng CFN, Wong SN, The Hong Kong Childhood Enuresis Study Group: Comparing alarms, desmopressin, and combined treatment in Chinese enuretic children, *Pediatr Nephrol* 20:163-69, 2005.
160. Glazener CMA, Evans JHC: Desmopressin for nocturnal enuresis in children, *Cochrane Database Syst Rev* CD002112: DOI:10.1002/14651858.CD002112, 2002.
161. Tullus K, Bergstrom R, Fosdal I, Winnergard I, Hjalmas K: Efficacy and safety during long-term treatment of primary monosymptomatic nocturnal enuresis with desmopressin. Swedish Enuresis Trial Group, *Acta Paediatr* 88:1274-78, 1999.
162. Bernstein SA, Williford SL: Intranasal desmopressin-associated hyponatremia: a case report and literature review, *J Fam Pract* 44:203-08, 1997.
163. Caione P, Arena F, Biraghi H, et al: Nocturnal enuresis and daytime wetting: a multicentric trial with oxybutynin and desmopressin, *Eur Urol* 31:459-63, 1997.
164. Neveus T: Oxybutynin, desmopressin and enuresis, *J Urol* 166:2459-62, 2001.
165. Glazener CMA, Evans JHC, Peto R: Tricyclic and related drugs for nocturnal enuresis in children, *Cochrane Database Syst Rev* CD002117:DOI:10.1002/14651858.CD002117, 2003.

CHAPTER 39

Acute Renal Failure: Prevention, Causes, and Investigation

Veronique Phan, Patrick D. Brophy, and Geoffrey M. Fleming

INTRODUCTION

Pediatric acute renal failure (ARF) is a dynamic entity that has many causes. The elucidation of the pathophysiology underlying ARF is under intense investigation. Recent developments in the classification schemes and cohesiveness of definitions will undoubtedly bring forth clarity regarding the understanding of the causes of, the prevention of, and, ultimately, the interventions for ARF. Indeed, new biomarkers are on the horizon that will better allow predictive interventions for childhood ARF. This chapter focuses in generalities on the causes of ARF. For a more in-depth review of these causes, readers are referred to individual chapters within this text.

THE DEFINITION OF ACUTE RENAL FAILURE

ARF is classically defined as an abrupt (hours to weeks) and prolonged loss of renal function that is reversible in the majority of cases.[1] More than 30 different definitions of ARF exist in the literature.[2] Although some define ARF as an increase in serum creatinine that ranges from mild to significant,[3] others define ARF as an increase in serum urea or a decrease in urine output.[4] Finally, some define ARF as a need for dialysis.[5] Most of these definitions have not been validated in prospective trials, and none has been validated in children. Indeed, the current understanding of the pathophysiology underlying ARF may favor the use of the term *acute kidney injury* rather than *ARF*.

The lack of consensus on the definition of ARF has led to a variety of quoted incidence rates, risk factors, and morbidity and mortality rates. Recently, a group of pediatric and adult nephrologists and intensivists founded the Acute Dialysis Quality Initiative and proposed a consensus definition called the *RIFLE classification*.[6] This definition is based on serum creatinine and urine output, and it was derived to reflect the dynamic process of ARF, which can progress from mild to severe forms. The RIFLE classification aims to describe different degrees of severity of renal dysfunction; five levels are defined, from a mild form (RIFLE-Risk) to a more severe form of renal disease (RIFLE-Loss)[6] (Table 39-1). Another classification has been proposed by AKIN (Acute Kidney Injury Network) and may be viewed at http://ccforum.com/content/11/2/R31. The identification of ARF early during the course of the disease may prove useful for preventing the progression of renal failure.

In recent years, retrospective studies in the adult population using the RIFLE classification have been published and reported a good predictive correlation between the different degrees of ARF and mortality.[7,8] To date, however, there is still no prospective trial that validates this definition in either an adult or a pediatric population. However, in the near future, a pediatric modified RIFLE criteria will be evaluated and validated.

THE EPIDEMIOLOGY OF ACUTE RENAL FAILURE IN CHILDREN

The incidence of ARF varies according to the population studied and the definition of ARF employed. A retrospective study from Italy reported an incidence rate of ARF of 2.7% (defined as the need for dialysis) among children undergoing cardiopulmonary bypass surgery.[9] Another from the United Kingdom reported an incidence of ARF (defined as the need for dialysis) of 3.2 per 100,000 children, infants, and young children.[10] In the prospective study validating the Pediatric Logistic Organ Dysfunction score in pediatric intensive care units (PICU), the incidence of ARF (defined as a serum creatinine level above 55 μmol/L to 140 μmol/L, depending on the age of the child) was 129 per 1000 admissions.[11] A prospective trial from Spain reported an incidence rate of ARF (defined as a serum creatinine level superior to the 95th percentile) of 2.4% in the PICU. Another PICU prospective trial performed in Canada reported an incidence rate of ARF of 44.7 per 1000 admissions.[12] In the face of the lack of common defining terms of pediatric ARF, clear incidence and prevalence data are difficult to establish on the basis of the literature.

PATHOPHYSIOLOGY OF ACUTE RENAL FAILURE

Background

Two excellent reviews were published in recent years about the pathophysiology of ischemic ARF; readers are referred to

TABLE 39-1 RIFLE Criteria

Risk: Serum creatinine ×1.5 normal and/or urine output <0.5 ml/kg/hour ×6 consecutive hours
Injury: Serum creatinine ×2.0 and/or urine output <0.5 ml/kg/hour ×12 consecutive hours
Renal failure: Serum creatinine ×3.0 and/or urine output <0.3 ml/kg/hour ×24 consecutive hours and/or anuria ×12 consecutive hours
Renal loss: Complete loss of renal function (need for dialysis) ×4 consecutive weeks
End-stage renal disease: Need for dialysis ×3 consecutive months

Renal failure is a dynamic process, and a patient can progress from a mild form (e.g., injury) to a more severe form of renal disease (e.g., loss).
From Bellomo R, et al: *Crit Care* 8(4):R204-12, 2004.

these articles for a more in-depth review.[1,13] Some of these important pathophysiologic features will now be discussed.

Renal Blood Flow Autoregulation

Renal blood flow is under autoregulatory processes, which is true in most organs. Autoregulatory mechanisms act to preserve renal blood flow during periods of hypotension or hypoperfusion. More specifically, the preservation of glomerular capillary perfusion pressure is the goal of the autoregulatory process. To achieve this, afferent and efferent glomerular arterioles are maintained at differential vascular resistances to produce a pressure gradient at the level of the glomerular capillary bed. In states of hypoperfusion, the afferent arteriole dilates, and the efferent arteriole vasoconstricts to maintain the transglomerular pressure gradient, thereby maintaining glomerular filtration.[1,13]

Many putative mediators have been proposed as regulators of renal blood flow. The renin-angiotensin system is a well-documented and established mediator of vascular tone, both locally in the kidney and systemically. As glomerular filtration decreases, the macula densa senses a reduction in solute and water delivery to the distal tubule, which stimulates the release of renin, as does increased catecholamine activity, which usually accompanies hypotension.[1,13] Renin acts to increase the release of angiotensinogen from the liver, and it cleaves this peptide into angiotensin I. Angiotensin I is converted by the angiotensin-converting enzyme in the lungs to angiotensin II, a potent vasoconstrictor both systemically and locally at the level of the afferent and efferent glomerular arterioles. Additional vasoconstrictors implicated in the autoregulatory process include endothelin and thromboxane A_2 (both of which are derived from vascular endothelium) and adenosine generated by injured endothelium and tubular epithelium.[1,13] Endothelin is released from vascular endothelium and causes vasoconstriction in response to hypoxia via the ET_A receptor. Adenosine, which produces a paradoxic (as compared with other vascular beds) vasoconstriction in the glomerular arterioles, is produced during tissue injury. Its production occurs with the degradation of adenosine triphosphate (ATP) to adenosine monophosphate (AMP) via the enzyme adenosine kinase. Thromboxane A_2 is produced from the metabolism of prostanoids, specifically by the conversion of prostaglandin H_2 by thromboxane synthase. In addition to its direct effect on the vasculature, which is mediated by G-protein–coupled alpha-receptors, catecholaminergic activity will also affect vasoconstriction through indirect mechanisms by altering the production of both vasodilators and vasoconstrictors.[1,13]

Vasoconstriction of both afferent and efferent arterioles does not produce the gradient that is necessary for glomerular filtration.[1,13] Isolated afferent vasodilatation is necessary to produce this gradient. First, prostaglandins appear to play a substantial role in the selective vasodilatation that is necessary to produce the transglomerular capillary gradient responsible for filtration. Prostaglandin synthesis and release are stimulated by the renin-angiotensin system, and these processes are also under local vascular endothelial control. The inhibition of prostaglandin synthesis as is seen with aspirin and nonsteroidal anti-inflammatory drug (NSAID) use is implicated in acute tubular necrosis and ARF.[1,13] In pediatrics, this is most evident in the neonatal intensive care unit in the management of patent ductus arteriosis with indomethacin.[14] Additional mediators of vasodilatation include endothelium-derived relaxation factor, which is now known as nitric oxide. Nitric oxide is produced locally by vascular endothelium by both inducible nitric oxide synthase and constitutive nitric oxide synthase. Diffuse endothelial damage, as is seen in states of inflammation such as sepsis, alters organ autoregulatory function through diminished nitric oxide production.[1,13] Additionally, the macula densa has a direct reflex vasodilatation effect on the afferent arteriole; this is called the *myogenic reflex*. The myogenic reflex causes relaxation in response to the same stimuli as renin release. Finally, atrial natriuretic peptide is released from myocytes in response to atrial stretch in states of volume overload. Atrial natriuretic peptide acts to dilate the afferent arterioles and increase glomerular filtration.[1,13]

The Classic Theory of Ischemic Renal Injury

This theory focuses on the interaction between two important elements of the kidney: the vascular component and the tubules. A reduction in glomerular filtration rate (GFR) is the result of a persistent vasoconstriction that leads to congestion in the outer medulla and to the increased delivery of solute to the macula densa, which results in the activation of the tubuloglomerular feedback mechanism. This vasoconstriction is the result of mediators such as endothelin, adenosine, and angiotensin II, as previously mentioned.[1,13] This vasoconstriction is augmented by a decrease in vasodilatation via a decrease in nitric oxide as a result of a decrease in constitutive nitric oxide synthase activity. Both mechanisms decrease regional perfusion to the outer medulla, causing tubular injury, which in turn results in tubular cellular swelling, increased cell adhesions, and leukocyte activation, leading to further decreases in blood flow.

Response to Hypoxia and Ischemia

Vascular Response and Cell Energetics: During normal function, the kidneys receive approximately 20% to 30% of cardiac output and consume 7% of delivered oxygen. In times of physiologic stress, however, oxygen consumption may increase dramatically with little means of increasing total renal blood flow as compared with myocardial perfusion, which may increase as much as 10-fold to meet metabolic demands.[1,13] These factors place the metabolically active nephron units at risk for oxygen debt caused by global hypoperfusion and/or hypoxemia. Cortical nephrons are at the greatest risk, partially because their blood supply is the most distal from the renal artery, and they are the most metabolically active nephrons as compared with medullary ones. However, renal blood flow and glomerular perfusion pressure are only one aspect of ARF.[1,13] During these periods, as a result of either cardiovascular shock or the vasoconstrictive autoregulatory process, the metabolically active tubular epithelium is placed under hypoxic/ischemic stress. During these periods, ATP stores are consumed rapidly, and energy availability becomes dependent on the local mitochondrial oxidative phosphorylation-mediated regeneration of ATP from adenosine diphosphate. Additionally, a second phase of ATP recovery occurs via neosynthesis and regeneration from purine precursors and AMP. Hence, recovery from an ischemic event is dependent on the length of the insult and the metabolic status of the patient before the insult. An unstressed patient with normal cardiac output will recover quickly from aortic or renal cross clamping with a rapid local regeneration of ATP as well as the neosynthesis of ATP from purine analogs delivered to the kidney.[1,13] However, a patient in low cardiac output with a high metabolic demand (e.g., a patient with sepsis) will not recover as rapidly from an acute ischemic event, because the ability to regenerate ATP from local precursors is diminished. During periods of extensive deprivation, AMP is shunted off to form adenosine and inosine, from which the regeneration of ATP requires extensive metabolic remodeling.[1,13] Hence, energetic recovery is hampered, and the injury period is extended beyond the period of acute ischemia.

Free Radical Injury

During periods of recovery from oxidative stress, toxic byproducts are created, such as oxygen free radicals. Highly reactive species such as hydroxyl radical and superoxide anion cause direct injury to proteins by oxidizing amino acid residues and changing the structure or function of important enzymes. Additionally, the lipoprotein bilayer and the ultrastructure of the cell are affected, thereby causing cell rupture and an increase in permeability that reduce the cell's ability to isolate the cytosol from the surrounding milieu. Thirdly, direct DNA damage can occur, which limits the ability of a cell to perform important reparative functions.[1,13] Hence, through a variety of mechanisms, further cell death is incurred during the reperfusion phase after an acute ischemic event.

Tubular Changes

Polarity: Renal tubular epithelium, as previously mentioned, is highly metabolically active. This energetic activity is predominantly used to fuel the active transport of solutes against a concentration gradient. The straight proximal segment of renal tubule (S3 segment) is highly susceptible to injury, because it contains many sodium-potassium ATPase transport channels. These channels are found predominantly on the basolateral surface of the cell, and they are anchored in place by cytoskeletal elements. Injury to the cell either through primary ischemia/hypoxia or as a result of reactive oxygen species causes the sodium-potassium ATPase to mislocate through the fluid lipoprotein bilayer and reside on the apical surface.[1,13] Additionally, energy needs for this ATPase are not met, and their function is reduced. Furthermore, intracellular calcium regulation is vital to normal function, with calcium sequestered predominantly in the extracellular milieu. This calcium gradient is maintained as well via the metabolically active transport channels, including a calcium ATPase. Hence, protein migration from the basolateral to the apical surface and the reduced activity of the ion channels disrupt the polarity of the electrochemical gradient established by the tubular epithelium, which is vital to normal function.[1,13] This loss in polarity may explain the increased solute delivery to the distal nephron.[15] Changes in cytoskeleton structure are also seen in arteries, arterioles, and the vasa recta. These changes may play a role in the loss of autoregulation of renal blood flow and vascular activity.[16]

Renal Tubule Obstruction and Backflow: Insults to the renal tubular epithelium result in cell death and diminished or absent regeneration. The cellular debris sloughs off and enters the tubular lumen. In some cases, this debris is felt to obstruct the tubular lumen (especially in the inferior segment of the loop of Henle) and to raise tubule intraluminal pressure, thereby further reducing the gradient from the glomerular capillary to Bowman's space, which is necessary for effective filtration. This obstruction may also cause the backflow of ultrafiltrate, which is no longer contained as a result of the loss of the integrity of the tubular epithelium; this fluid extrudes into the surrounding interstitium.[1,13] Extruded fluid may alter the interstitial milieu substantially, affecting corticomedullary osmolarity gradients and local electrochemical gradients as well as causing direct cell injury and further propagating renal dysfunction.

Inflammation: The tubular cells, apart from the changes in cytoskeleton, produce proinflammatory cytokines such as tumor necrosis factor α, interleukins 6 and 8, transforming growth factor β, and chemokines.[1,13] These proinflammatory molecules may contribute to the vasoconstriction and interstitial inflammation.

Summary of the Classic Theory

In summary, there are four phases to the progression of parenchymal injury during ischemic acute renal failure.[17] The first phase—initiation—follows the decrease in perfusion and ATP depletion. The second phase—extension—is marked by ischemia reperfusion injuries that may cause further damage. During this phase, inflammation is observed and effects the prolongation of ischemia and the aggravation of injury. The proximal tubules regenerate, but cells from the S3 segment of the same proximal tubule and from the medullary thick ascending limb undergo necrosis and apoptosis. The effect of therapy, if it is applied during the extension phase in experimental models, supports the notion that the severity of injury during this phase is proportional to the prognosis of the injury.[18] During the third phase—maintenance—necrosis and apoptosis persist via inflammation and cell injury. Finally, during the last phase—recovery—several mechanisms occur concomitantly, such as repair, regeneration, and the proliferation of injured cells.

ACUTE RENAL FAILURE: CLASSIFICATION, DEMOGRAPHICS, AND RISK

There are multiple causes of ARF, and they depend on many factors, such as geographic area, hospitals (referral versus local), endemic diseases, and accessibility to health care services.

The Traditional Classification of Acute Renal Failure: Prerenal, Renal, and Postrenal

Classically, ARF is divided into prerenal, renal, and postrenal categories and further subdivided into oliguric and nonoliguric renal failure. To better understand these categorizations, it is useful to review the mechanisms by which the functioning units—nephrons—are injured. These classification categories often include overlapping processes. For example, a low cardiac output state would be primarily categorized as prerenal ARF. However, after circulating blood volume and cardiac output are restored, ARF may persist as a result of residual injury to nephrons; this would then be classified as renal ARF. Most definitions of ARF include a change in creatinine clearance and a measurement of urine production that is usually normalized to body weight. Although such definitions are applicable clinically, they monitor the end-product function of the kidney, and they do not help identify the underlying pathophysiologic mechanism of injury.

Other Classifications of Acute Renal Failure

ARF can also be subcategorized as primary or secondary. ARF is primary when the kidney disease is caused, for example, by a glomerulonephritis or hemolytic uremic syndrome (HUS). ARF is secondary when it is caused by a systemic disease such as sepsis or shock. Traditionally, primary ARF is caused by acute glomerulonephritis and HUS[19,20] were the most common causes of ARF in children. In recent years, with advances in the treatment of other childhood pathologies, secondary ARF caused by sepsis, nephrotoxic drugs, or renal ischemia in children undergoing bone marrow transplant, solid organ transplantation, or cardiac surgery represent the majority of cases of ARF.[21,22] This is particularly true in developed countries.

Demographics

The development of ARF is also influenced by the type of hospital. Referring, tertiary care pediatric hospitals are more likely to see ARF in children undergoing procedures such as organ transplantation, bone marrow transplantation, cardiac surgery, and the treatment of oncology pathologies[21,22] as compared with regional hospitals not offering these treatments.

Geographic location and cultural traditions are also likely to influence the causes of ARF[19,22,23] (Table 39-2). In developing countries, infectious diseases are the main causes of ARF. Two studies from Nigeria observed that 71% of cases of ARF were secondary.[23,24] Malaria was the most common cause of ARF. Other common causes were gastroenteritis and human immunodeficiency virus nephropathy.[24] In India, HUS and glomerulonephritis still represent most cases of ARF.[19] Some longstanding local customs,[25] such as the use of herbal medicines in developing countries, are associated with ARF. In recent years as a result of the migration of many people, herbal-medicine–induced ARF is seen with increasing frequency in developed countries.[26,27]

Risk Factors

Risk factors for ARF are multiple, and they are likely to be different according to the patient population being studied. What transpires from the literature is that, in most circumstances, more than one risk factor is usually present before the development of ARF.[28,29]

TABLE 39-2 **Causes of Pediatric Acute Renal Failure: Demographic Comparison**

Study	Oluwu et al[23]	Arora et al[19]	Hui-Stickle et al[22]
Location	Kenya	India	United States
Number of patients	123	80	248
Causes			
Hemolytic uremic syndrome	2 (1.6%)	25 (31%)	3 (1.2%)
Acute glomerulonephritis	10 (8.1%)	18 (22.5%)	9 (3.6%)
Acute tubular necrosis	—	19 (23.8%)	—
Urology	7 (5.7%)	7 (8.7%)	20 (8.0%)
Renal ischemia or nephrotoxic drugs in the context of the following:			
After cardiac surgery	—	11 (13.4%)	43 (17.3%)
Hematology/oncology	17 (13.4%; renal Burkitt's lymphoma)	—	33 (13.3%)
Hepatic/intestinal transplantation	—	—	11 (4.4%)
Genetic diseases	—	—	19 (7.7%)
Infections (malaria)	37 (30%)	—	—
Sepsis	25 (20.3%)	—	27 (11%)

Risk factors of ARF in the adult population are septic shock (40% to 50%),[30,31,28] other types of shock (cardiogenic, hypovolemic),[30] and nephrotoxic drugs.[30] A large international multicenter prospective observational study of 29,269 critically ill adults confirmed these observations. In this cohort, risk factors for ARF included septic shock (47.5%), cardiogenic shock (27%), hypovolemia (26%), and nephrotoxic drugs such as aminoglycosides, antifungal agents, calcineurin inhibitors, and angiotensin-converting enzyme inhibitors in cases of associated hypovolemia (19%).[4]

Few data about the risk factors of ARF in children are available. One prospective trial in critically ill children in Spain observed that sepsis was present in 40% of cases and that hypovolemia was present in 1.6%.[32] In one Canadian prospective study, risk factors included cardiovascular dysfunction such as hypotension and hematologic dysfunction.[12] Another study looking at postcardiac bypass surgery demonstrated that low cardiac output was the main risk factor for ARF in this particular population.[33]

CAUSES OF ACUTE RENAL FAILURE

The classic divisions of ARF are useful for establishing a differential diagnosis. Table 39-3 provides a schematic for the three classifications.[34,35]

Prerenal Acute Renal Failure

Prerenal ARF predominantly includes states of reduced renal blood flow. The cause of reduced renal blood flow may be a reduction in circulating volume as is seen in hypovolemic shock (i.e., profound diarrhea in the neonate). Alternatively, it may involve low cardiac output or cardiogenic shock as is seen in postsurgical cardiac patients or those with primary myocarditis/cardiomyopathy. Finally, prerenal ARF may be the result of a combination of these factors as is seen in distributive or septic shock.[36,37] After it has been established and is prolonged, prerenal ARF may be manifested as intrinsic renal ARF in the form of acute tubular necrosis or the even worse nonreversible cortical necrosis. If suspected, acute and timely fluid management and the restoration of effective circulating volume (pressor or cardiac support) are imperative to ensure that intrinsic disease is not established.

Renal (Intrinsic Renal Disease) Acute Renal Failure

Glomerular, Tubular, and Interstitial Diseases

Glomerulonephritis: The term *glomerulonephritis* refers to a broad array of disease processes that affect the glomerular filtration unit and thereby reduce renal function. These diseases include inflammatory processes that result in the swelling of glomerular epithelial cells and a reduction in the intracellular gaps necessary for the filtration of plasma. Additionally, immune deposits along the basement membrane form barriers to filtration. Glomerulonephritis may be classified by the type and site of immune deposits and whether it is associated with drugs, infections, or autoimmune diseases.[38] Antibodies may form complexes with circulating extrarenal antigens that deposit on the basement membrane, or antibody-antigen complexes may form at the level of the basement membrane. Finally, antibodies may react with renal

TABLE 39-3 Causes of Acute Renal Failure

Prerenal
Intravascular volume depletion Bleeding, trauma Gastrointestinal losses: diarrhea, vomiting Renal losses: diabetes insipidus Skin/mucous membrane losses: burns, fever (prolonged) Third space losses: pancreatitis, hypoalbuminemia, crush injuries, systemic inflammatory response syndrome (SIRS)
Decreased cardiac output Congestive heart failure Cardiomyopathy
Sepsis
Drugs (overdose), anesthetics
Anaphylaxis
Renal vasoconstriction Liver disease, sepsis, hypercalcemia
Drugs
Angiotensin-converting enzyme inhibitors
Nonsteroidal anti-inflammatory drugs
Renal (intrinsic)
Acute tubular necrosis
Hemolytic-uremic syndrome
Glomerulonephritis/rapidly progressive glomerulonephritis Postinfectious glomerulonephritis Systemic lupus erythematosus Membranoproliferative glomerulonephritis Immunoglobulin A nephropathy Henoch-Schönlein purpura
Pulmonary-renal syndromes Wegener's granulomatosis Goodpasture's syndrome
Acute interstitial nephritis
Nephrotoxins Drugs: aminoglycosides, cyclosporine A, amphotericin B, cisplatinum Toxins: ethylene glycol, heavy metals, herbal remedies Pigments: hemolysis, rhabdomyolysis
Postrenal (obstructive)
Ureter
Nephrolithiasis, sloughed renal papillae Postoperative ureteric surgery Hemorrhage, tumor
Bladder Calculi, blood clots, bladder catheter obstruction Neurogenic bladder Tumor
Urethral Valves, phimosis, strictures

From Brady HR, Clarkson MR, Lieberthal W, in Brenner BM, editor: *Brenner & Rector's the kidney*, ed 7, Philadelphia, 2004, Saunders, pp 1215-70; and Andreoli SP, in Avner ED, Harmon WE, Niaudet P, editors: *Pediatric nephrology*, ed 5, Baltimore, 2004, Lippincott Williams & Wilkins, pp 1233-4.

antigens as is seen in autoimmune disease. The exact mechanisms of injury will be reviewed in greater detail in Chapters 11, 20, and 21. Briefly, antibody-antigen–mediated injury occurs as a result of the activation of complement attack complexes and direct cell injury. Additionally, the infiltration of neutrophils and macrophages promotes cytokine amplification and the exocytosis of proteolytic enzymes and reactive oxygen species. The local release of growth factors promotes inappropriate epithelial cell proliferation, which worsens disease rather than regenerating damaged tissues. Finally, fibrin deposition occurs as an end product of injury and of the activation of elements of the coagulation cascade; these deposits further inhibit filtration.[39]

Hemolytic Uremic Syndrome: As mentioned previously, HUS was the most common cause of ARF in children. In recent years, its incidence has decreased in developed countries. It can be associated with diarrhea (HUS-D+) or without (HUS D–). In this chapter, the HUS-D+ form will be primarily discussed, because it is the more common of the two. The diagnosis of HUS can be entertained if a patient presents with a microangiopathic hemolytic anemia, thrombocytopenia, and ARF. It is more frequent during the summer months and in rural areas.[40]

Clinical Presentation: Ninety percent of HUS-D+ is seen in patients with enterohemorrhagic infection resulting from *Escherichia coli* infection.[41] The most common serotype in North America is *E. coli* O157:H7.[42] In other regions of the world, other serotypes are more common. The infection begins after the ingestion of enterohemorrhagic *E. coli*. The main source of contamination is meat from infected animals (e.g., cattle, sheep) or contaminated water, food, or beverages. HUS develops in 5% to 10% of children who are infected with *E. coli* O157:H7, and they are usually less than 10 years old.[43] Risk factors for HUS are a high white cell count, the use of antibiotic or antimotility agents, and an age of less than 10 years.[40] The majority of childhood cases present with bloody colitis. Five to 10 days after the colitis, microangiopathic hemolytic anemia and thrombocytopenia can be observed. Close to 50% of patients will require dialysis during the acute phase, but few will remain on chronic dialysis. However, these patients require follow-up, because long-term complications are often encountered. A meta-analysis of patients with HUS demonstrated that mortality or end-stage renal disease was seen in 12%, whereas 25% developed hypertension, proteinuria, chronic renal disease, or some combination of the three.[44]

Pathophysiology: Shiga toxins produced by enterohemorrhagic *E. coli* are key in the pathophysiology of the disease, and they belong to the family of AB toxins.[45] Shiga toxins and lipopolysaccharides cross the inflamed colon and circulate via the vascular system. The toxins bind to glycoprotein receptor (Gb3), which is found in the kidney and intestine. In the kidney, Gb3 receptors are found in the endothelial cells of the glomeruli, and the resulting internalization of the toxins leads to cell death.

Most authors would argue that damage to the endothelium is pivotal to the development of HUS. The pathophysiology of this insult is still partly unknown. Shiga toxin subtypes (STX2 or STXC) and their levels are responsible for endothelial injuries. Cytolethal distending toxin produced by those enterobacteria can contribute to the endothelial injury by interference with the cell cycle, thereby resulting in the inhibition of cell proliferation and ultimately cell death.[46] This cascade of events triggers the secondary activation of platelets and results in microangiopathic hemolytic anemia. Other mediators of the coagulation cascade seen in HUS have been implicated, such as a reduction in thrombomodulin (coagulation inhibitor) induced by STX2,[47] tumor necrosis factor α, and lipopolysaccharides.

Prevention and Early Detection: Prevention is key, because no efficacious treatments exist. Safe meat processing methods, food handling (avoiding contact between uncooked meats and vegetables, washing hands after handling meat), cooking standards, and the irradiation of raw meat products are essential in the fight against HUS.

Because there is a window of opportunity for treatment between ingestion and the appearance of symptoms, many researchers have focused on the early detection of infection, at the start of symptoms (i.e., the colitis stage). New methods of detection of Shiga toxins in the stools or blood have been designed, including serum flow cytometry[48] and immunoassays.[49]

Treatment of Hemolytic Uremic Syndrome: The treatment of HUS is discussed in detail in Chapter 25. Passive immunity via monoclonal antibodies directed against Shiga toxins may be a novel way of approaching the treatment of children with HUS.[50] Studies in children have not yet been published.

Interstitial Nephritis: Acute tubulointerstitial nephritis (AIN) refers to the sudden onset and rapid decline in renal function that results from acute inflammatory processes in the kidney. The pathologic presentation is characterized by the inflammation of the renal interstitium, interstitial edema, and damage to tubular epithelial cells. The prevalence of AIN in the pediatric population is unclear. A single pediatric center analysis over a 3-year period found that AIN (confirmed by percutaneous renal biopsy) was present in 7% of samples.[51] The prevalence in adults is varied on the basis of presentation, with 1% presenting with proteinuria and/or hematuria and 15% presenting with ARF.[52]

Presentation and Diagnosis: Patients with AIN commonly present with nonspecific symptoms, including fever, abdominal pain, nausea, vomiting, anorexia, weight loss, polydipsia, polyuria, hypertension, headaches, and skin rash.[51,53-57] Hematologic, biochemical, and urinary findings include anemia, leukocytosis, eosinophilia, elevated erythrocyte sedimentation rate, ARF (elevated serum creatinine with a decreased calculated or measured glomerular filtration rate),[53-55] an elevated fractional excretion of sodium, hematuria, and pyuria.[51,53-57] Proteinuria, although often prominent, is usually in the non-nephrotic range of less than 2 g per 24 hours (>4 mg/m^2/hr but <40 mg/m^2/hr) or a urine protein-to-creatinine ratio of greater than 0.20 mg/mg but less than 2.0 mg/mg (>20 mg/mmol but <200 mg/mmol).[53-56] Most commonly, renal ultrasonography is used to image the kidneys in cases of ARF in which AIN may be in the differential diagnosis. In AIN, the kidneys often appear to be universally enlarged as compared with the similar renal measurements in normal, age-matched pediatric patients.[58,59] In addition to the nephromegaly, the kidneys may appear to be diffusely echogenic, particularly in the renal cortices.[58,59] Percutaneous kidney biopsy remains the "gold standard" for diagnosis. Previous studies have demonstrated the value of biopsy in pediatric patients diagnosed with AIN in terms of the accuracy of diagnosis and hence appropriate treatment.[60]

Management: Treatment of ARF that results from AIN is initially supportive in nature.[51,53-57,61] The discontinuation of medications that may be responsible for AIN should be considered. If a medication is necessary for the treatment of an underlying disorder and an appropriate substitute agent is available, then substitution of the suspected medication is justified. If an infectious cause is suspected, then prompt medical treatment with appropriate antibiotics, antifungals, or antiviral medications should be initiated. For those patients presenting with ARF and indications for dialytic therapies, renal replacement therapy should be provided until the patient's renal function recovers.[51,53-57,61] Both T- and B-cell mechanisms are involved in the development of AIN in humans.[52,61,62] For AIN that is unresponsive to drug discontinuation or to the treatment of a suspected infection, corticosteroids should be used. Previous adult studies have demonstrated a faster return to baseline creatinine when corticosteroids are employed.[51,53-57,61]

Acute Tubular Necrosis and Cortical Necrosis: Acute tubular necrosis (ATN) and cortical necrosis may result from direct tubular epithelial injury, as with drug-induced nephrotoxicity, or indirectly from ischemic injury induced by vasoconstrictor autoregulatory mechanisms.[63] The mechanisms underlying ATN are described in the first part of this chapter.

Sepsis and Shock: Sepsis and severe septic shock promote renal failure through a variety of mechanisms. First, hypotension and low cardiac output states foster a reduction in renal blood flow that often falls below the autoregulatory capacity of the kidney. Central venous pressure often rises as a result of myocardial dysfunction and the volume resuscitation necessary to maintain cardiac output. This increased central venous pressure in conjunction with systemic hypotension reduces organ perfusion pressure. The vascular endothelium is diffusely injured, and important functions are lost, such as physical barriers to capillary leak, the loss of nitric-oxide–mediated organ autoregulatory mechanisms, and the loss of the pro- and anticoagulant balance of the coagulation system.[64] Disseminated intravascular coagulation causes a diffuse microangiopathic thrombosis that affects the kidneys in a way that is similar to HUS. In addition, elevated cytokine levels promote further endothelial damage and vasoconstriction and increase metabolic rates. Catecholamine levels are also increased by both endogenous mechanisms and infusions of inotropes and vasopressors, which again affect metabolic rate and vascular autoregulation in addition to increasing renin-angiotensin activity. The influx of polymorphonuclear neutrophils may also exacerbate free radical injury through the generation of superoxide anion and of weaker reactive oxygen species such as hydrogen peroxide and hypochlorous acid.[64] Finally, antimicrobials administered during sepsis may have nephrotoxic effects through the mechanisms discussed later in this chapter. Hence, sepsis-induced ARF is multifactorial,[65] and it is difficult to adequately categorize using the pre-/intra-/postrenal nomenclature.

Pathophysiology of Acute Tubular Necrosis Associated With Sepsis: Inflammation as a result of sepsis is also linked to the development of acute renal injury and ARF.[66] In response to sepsis, individual susceptibility seems to play an important role. In critically ill patients, the hyperinflammation response observed in sepsis can be decreased and even abolished, thereby resulting in a downregulation of the immune system. In sepsis, nitric oxide synthesis is increased via cytokine induction, which causes a vasodilatation.[67] In response to this vasodilatation, the sympathetic nervous system and the angiotensin-aldosterone system are stimulated and vasopressin is released. This response induces vasoconstriction, thereby leading to ARF. At the level of the kidney, during the initial stage of ARF, vasoconstriction as a result of endothelin secreted by tumor necrosis factor α[68] precedes tubular damage, because sodium and water reabsorption are preserved. Other mechanisms related to sepsis and endotoxins play a role in the development of ARF. Endothelial damage may be associated with microthrombi and may increase the release of von Willebrand factor.[69] The subsequent vasodilatory response to counteract this vasoconstriction is blunted by decreased nitric oxide synthase activity in the damaged endothelium.[70]

Drug-Induced Acute Renal Failure: Drug-induced ARF is an important mechanism of renal failure, because it may be preventable with vigilance. Drug-induced ARF accounted for 16% of pediatric renal failure cases in a recent epidemiology study,[22] and drug-induced ARF becomes more prevalent in sicker populations.[71] The risks of ARF are compounded by inadequate circulating volume, low cardiac output states, and multiple nephrotoxic drugs administered to critically ill patients; hence, drug-induced ARF increases in prevalence in the intensive care unit. ARF induced by drugs occurs by two predominant mechanisms. First, direct toxicity to renal tubular epithelium is seen with aminoglycosides and amphotericin. Second, interference with autoregulatory mechanisms often leads to unrestricted vasoconstriction and reduced renal blood flow and ischemic injury, as is seen with NSAID toxicity. The prevention of drug-induced ARF is more effective than therapies for individual toxicities, and the recognition of high-risk patients is necessary to reduce the incidence. A few individual drug categories are discussed later in this chapter as a result of their frequency of use or toxicity, but this list is not meant to be exhaustive, and other references may offer further clinical information.[72]

Nonsteroidal Anti-Inflammatory Drugs: NSAIDs are commonly used in pediatrics for fever control and musculoskeletal pain. Although ARF does not occur with great frequency, it has been associated with NSAID use in children, and it is clinically recognized as acute tubular necrosis and interstitial nephritis. Most renal injury from NSAID use is caused by alterations in renal blood flow. However, some patients develop interstitial nephritis and nephritic syndrome,[71] with a reversal of the disease seen after withdrawal of the NSAID. As discussed previously, renal blood flow is maintained by a balance between vasoconstrictor and vasodilator mediators in the kidney. The predominant vasodilators are the prostanoid regulators, such as prostaglandins I_2 and E_2. Each appears to be produced locally to vasodilate the afferent arteriole and counterbalance the vasoconstrictor properties of other prostanoids, such as thromboxane A_2. Renal production of the various prostanoids requires the cyclooxygenase enzyme (COX), of which two isoforms have been extensively studied.

COX-1 is felt to be constitutive and resides in all regions of the kidney, including the vascular endothelium and the tubular epithelium from Bowman's space to the distal collecting ducts.[73] COX-2 activity appears to be inducible during periods of stress, and it resides in the renal medullary tubular epithelium and the macula densa. The nonselective NSAID inhibition of both COX-1 and COX-2 isoforms results in reduced GFR and reduced natriuresis, which may lead to significant reductions in renal function and edema, respectively. The predominant mechanism appears to be ischemic and to be mediated by reduced vasodilatory prostaglandin formation. Renal injury appears to be more prevalent in states of high renin-angiotensin activity, such as volume depletion and congestive heart failure, where vasoconstrictor effects are unable to be balanced by prostaglandin I_2 and E_2 production.[74] COX-2 activity has been implicated in a complex interaction with the renin-angiotensin system, where it is both the stimulus of renin production and a product of renin release. Additionally, COX-2 activity is under negative feedback control by renin. Hence, although the COX-2 inhibitors were hoped to be renal sparing, further study has shown renal failure is possible with these drugs and that it may also be more prevalent in states of high renin-angiotensin activity.[73] Finally, NSAID use during pregnancy has also been implicated in in utero renal injury and failure. The proposed mechanisms of injury are felt to be similar to postnatal exposure (i.e., vasoconstriction-mediated reduced renal blood flow). Additionally, the role of prostaglandins during organogenesis is not yet completely defined, but it may play a role in in utero NSAID renal injury.[74,75]

Acetaminophen: Acetaminophen toxicity is the leading cause of acquired liver failure in children, and its nephrotoxic effects are often overshadowed by hepatotoxicity. Nephrotoxicity occurs in 2% to 10% of toxic acetaminophen ingestions.[76] Although it may be viewed as benign as a result of its over-the-counter accessibility, toxic doses are easily achieved, especially with "maximum strength" preparations, and cumulative toxicity may occur with repeat dosing. Although the associated liver toxicity is well described and understood, acetaminophen-induced renal injury is not as well understood, and two mechanisms are proposed. Normally, acetaminophen is sulfated (34%) or glucuronidated (63%) and excreted in urine. In cases of toxic ingestion, the pathway is depleted of an essential component (glucuronide), and acetaminophen is shunted into the cytochrome P450 system. Less than 5% of acetaminophen is normally metabolized to mercapturic acid by the P450 system, which requires glutathione as a cofactor. With large amounts of acetaminophen shunted into the P450 system, glutathione is quickly depleted, and the toxic metabolite *N*-acetyl-*p*-benzoquinoneimine (NAPQI) is produced.[76] NAPQI is known to cause direct cytotoxic effects, and it is postulated to be the cause of tubular epithelial necrosis.[77] Recent data from an in vitro model demonstrate a third COX isoform, COX-3.[78] This COX-3 isoform is produced by alternative COX-1 mRNA splicing. The COX-3 enzyme studied had weak but measurable inhibition by acetaminophen, although the evidence is not conclusive for a separate COX site of inhibition.[79] One could postulate that COX-3 inhibition by acetaminophen may affect prostanoid activity in the kidney, thereby rendering it more susceptible to vasoconstriction injury and compounding the direct cytotoxic effects of NAPQI. There is no specific therapy for acetaminophen-induced renal injury beyond *N*-acetylcysteine administration, which is the mainstay for hepatotoxicity.

Antibiotics and Antifungal Agents: Aminoglycosides are frequently used in clinical practice, and they are associated with renal toxicity in 5% to 20% of therapeutic courses in adult[80] and pediatric patients.[14,71] Aminoglycosides are excreted into the tubular lumen, where they quickly bind to the membrane surface of tubular epithelial cells. Binding to the membrane surface induces a series of changes. First, it alters the brush border architecture and leads to an enzymuria. Second, the drug undergoes endocytosis and concentrates within renal tubular epithelial cells in lysosomes. Within these lysosomes, phospholipids undergo hydrolysis, and electron-dense myeloid bodies become evident. The rupture of lysosomes further increases intracellular damage, now exposing mitochondrial membranes to phospholipid hydrolysis. Diffuse intracellular architectural injury leads to cellular swelling, a loss of electrochemical gradients, and subsequent tubular epithelial cell necrosis.[71,80] The dose and duration of therapy are important contributors to aminoglycoside nephrotoxicity; thus, care in dosing calculations and the evaluation of drug levels (where available) are important considerations for the prevention of ARF.

Amphotericin B induces renal failure through two mechanisms: reduced GFR and direct cytotoxicity. Direct cytotoxicity to the renal tubular epithelium results in a tubular acidosis, a reduction of sodium and potassium reabsorption, and an activation of tubuloglomerular feedback.[71,80] The activation of the tubuloglomerular feedback reflex by the reduced delivery of sodium chloride to the macula densa reduces glomerular filtration by uncoupling afferent and efferent arteriolar tone. Additionally, amphotericin B causes direct vasoconstriction through alterations in calcium flux into smooth muscle cells.[80] Hence, measures to reduce amphotericin B nephrotoxicity include sodium chloride loading at infusion and calcium channel blockade in conjunction with limiting the dose and duration of therapy as clinically indicated. Newer liposomal preparations are less nephrotoxic, but they have the disadvantage of inadequate urinary fungal coverage.

Antiviral agents are used in a variety of clinical scenarios, and they may have renal toxicity associated with their use. Cidofovir and foscarnet both cause direct tubular injury and cytotoxicity through two different mechanisms. Cidofovir is a nucleotide analog that is taken up through basolateral anion transporters and that interferes with membrane phospholipids. Foscarnet interferes with cellular energetics by inhibiting sodium-phosphorus cotransport. Acyclovir interferes with renal function through precipitation in distal tubules, which results in tubular obstruction with ultrafiltrate backleak and nephron dysfunction.[71] The adequate replacement of circulating volume is the primary preventative therapy, although alkalinization of the urine may also be beneficial with acyclovir.[80]

Angiotensin-Converting Enzyme Inhibitors and Angiotensin Receptor Blockers: Angiotensin-converting enzyme inhibitors (ACEIs) and angiotensin receptor blockers (ARBs) induce renal dysfunction through alterations in renal blood flow.[71] These drugs limit a portion of the vasoconstrictor arm of the autoregulatory mechanism of the kidney. During periods of reduced renal blood flow, the patient on ACEIs or ARBs is unable to produce the vasoconstriction necessary to promote and maintain adequate renal blood flow and, hence, glomerular filtration pressure. This effect may be compounded by the concomitant use of inhibitors of selective vasodilation, such as NSAIDs.[71] The predominant therapy for ACEI- or ARB-induced renal dysfunction is the discontinuation of the drug, adequate volume repletion, and/or inotropic support.

Calcineurin Inhibitors: Cyclosporine and tacrolimus have gained popularity in all types of transplantation, from stem cell to solid organ transplantation. Drug concentrations are carefully monitored to prevent over- or underdosing. As is often the case, multiple drugs interact with calcineurin inhibitors, and levels can rise precipitously. As patients become toxic from these drugs, a profound vasoconstriction ensues, resulting in a subsequent reduction in GFR. The mechanism of vasoconstriction is felt to include loss of vasodilating nitric oxide and prostaglandin E activity as well as increased vasoconstriction from thromboxane A_2 and endothelin activity. A clinical clue to calcineurin toxicity may be systemic hypertension; however, trough level measurement is necessary for diagnosis. Therapy for calcineurin inhibitor toxicity has included calcium-channel blockers,[81] which are felt to reverse the endothelin-mediated calcium influx into vascular smooth muscle. Additionally, methylxanthine infusions such as theophylline and aminophylline have been studied and are felt to improve GFR by adenosine antagonism, which may mediate some portion of the vasoconstriction.[82-84]

Antineoplastic Agents: Antineoplastic agents target cells undergoing division; hence, any regenerative cellular group is at risk for toxicity.[85] Renal tubular injury is the predominant mechanism of injury of most antineoplastic agents, although this is accompanied by vasoconstriction for some agents, such as cisplatin and methotrexate.[71] Additionally, tubular obstruction may occur with crystalline formation and epithelial sloughing. Many chemotherapeutic regimens include a prehydration period and urine alkalinization protocol to minimize renal toxicity.[71] Renal toxicity appears to be cumulative for many of these agents.

Pigment Nephropathies: *Pigment nephropathies,* which is the name given to ARF induced by myoglobinuria and hemoglobinuria, have multiple proposed mechanisms of injury.[86] Myoglobin, which is released from muscle during crush or overuse injuries (e.g., status epilepticus), is proposed to cause injury through direct cytotoxicity, tubular cast formation with tubular obstruction, and vasoconstriction. Iron in the ferric state is felt to produce free radical cell injury.[86-88] The degree of injury is correlated with the rise in free myoglobin, and it is postulated to be accentuated by other intracellular products released in a way that is similar to tumor lysis syndrome. Hemoglobinuria occurs after hemolysis, and it is rarely a cause of significant renal injury in the healthy kidney. However, it will cause significant disease in conjunction with additional nephrotoxic mechanisms.[88]

Nondialytic therapy for pigment nephropathy relies predominantly on prevention. Approaches to the prevention of ARF include the adequate repletion of intravascular volume and the treatment of low cardiac output states to prevent injury from low blood flow. A vigorous diuresis is encouraged with both loop and osmotic diuretics. Mannitol may provide benefits beyond osmotic diuresis, because it is postulated to be a free-radical scavenger. Finally, maintaining a slightly alkaline urine pH may help with the excretion and prevention of crystallization of both uric acid and phosphorus, which may accompany these cell lysis states.[87,89]

Contrast Nephropathy: Contrast nephropathy is the cause of ARF that requires hospitalization in 12% of adult patients after they have undergone imaging that requires a contrast agent,[90] and it is associated with an increase risk of mortality during the year after the episode of ARF.[91] The incidence in children is unknown. Patients with chronic renal disease or diabetes are more at risk.[91] The volume of administration and the use of high osmolar contrast agents are associated with a higher risk of contrast nephropathy as compared with the lower osmolar agents.[92,93] The ionicity of the contrast agent is still a matter of debate, but nonionic agents are thought to be safer in patients with chronic renal disease.[94]

Pathophysiology: The pathophysiology of contrast nephropathy is still largely unknown. One theory implicates a severe vasoconstriction after the administration of the agent. Endothelin,[95] a decrease in nitric oxide, and adenosine[96] are thought to be responsible for the vasoconstriction that results in medullary ischemia and acute tubular necrosis. Another theory directly implicates the cytotoxicity of the agent on the tubular cell via oxygen free radicals.[97]

Clinical Manifestation: A rise in serum creatinine occurs 1 to 2 days after the procedure, and it is usually not accompanied by a decrease in urine output.[98] Dialysis is required in a minority of patients.

Prevention: No treatment exists other than support if ARF occurs. However, during recent years, attention has focused on the prevention of contrast nephropathy.[71,99] A recent meta-analysis of prevention strategies recommends intravenous hydration, bicarbonate, and the use of low or iso-osmolar contrast agents in the smallest volume possible in patients who are at risk of contrast nephropathy. *N*-acetylcysteine and ascorbic acid have also been suggested for use in the higher-risk populations.[94] These treatments have not been validated in children.

Tumor Lysis Syndrome: Tumor lysis syndrome (TLS) is seen in patients undergoing the first cycle of chemotherapy when rapid tumor destruction occurs. It is more frequent in patients with certain neoplasias, such as lymphoma and acute myelogenous leukemia. The patient usually presents with an increased serum uric acid level, hyperkalemia, hyperphosphatemia, and resulting hypocalcemia. The increased tumor necrosis can lead to ARF.[71,99]

Pathophysiology of Acute Renal Failure: Multiple mechanisms can explain the ARF seen with TLS. The hyperuricemia leads to hyperuricosuria, and the precipitation of uric acid in the tubules leads to occlusion and decreased filtration.[100] This precipitation is enhanced in acidic urine and in hypovolemic states. Hyperphosphatemia may also contribute to ARF as a result of the precipitation of phosphate and calcium crystals in the tubules.[101]

Clinical Presentation: The incidence of TLS in patients with high-risk neoplasia is around 10%.[102] Patients usually present with a metabolic disorder that is linked to the rapid cell turnover, such as hyperuricemia, hyperkalemia, hyperphosphatemia, and resulting hypocalcemia. The difficulty lies in early diagnosis. A recent study looked at independent risk factors of TLS.[102] After univariate analysis, elevated prechemotherapy serum uric acid, creatinine, lactate dehydrogenase, white blood cell count, gender, and a history of chronic myelomonocytic leukemia were significant predictors of TLS development. In multivariate analysis, lactate dehydrogenase, uric acid, and gender remained significant predictors of TLS. Agents used in chemotherapy, such as cisplatin, etoposide, fludarabine, and methotrexate, also compound the ARF risk,[103,104] as do alternative therapies such as rituximab[105] and irradiation.[106]

Treatment: Prevention is also key in this situation. The early recognition of patients at risk for TLS is critical. The avoidance of nephrotoxic drugs and volume depletion is important.[107] Controlling uric acids level is also important: drugs such as allopurinol and, more recently, recombinant urate oxidase (rasburicase) are efficacious.[108,109] Hemolytic anemia has been reported in patients with glucose-6-phosphate dehydrogenase deficiency using Rasburicase.[110] Alkalinization should be used with caution; it will reduce uric acid precipitation in the tubule, but it may increase the precipitation of calcium phosphate crystals. Targeting the urinary pH to around 7 is usually sufficient, and alkalinization should be stopped after a normal serum uric acid level is reached.[100] If ARF occurs and dialysis is required, intermittent hemodialysis is most efficacious. However, because rebound often occurs, continuous venovenous hemofiltration (CVVH) is recommended.[100] Some even use CVVH as prophylaxis before ARF,[111] but drug adjustment is needed, and this approach is still not universally accepted.

Tumor Invasion: Wilms' tumor is the most common pediatric kidney tumor, but the tumor itself causes relatively little disruption of renal function. Many patients with Wilms' tumor have hypertension and hematuria at presentation as a result of the compression of the renal vasculature.[85] However, there is a significant association with genitourinary anomalies (e.g., renal hypoplasia) and horseshoe kidney, which have higher rates of renal dysfunction at baseline. Other primary renal tumors are uncommon, but they may occur in children and cause renal failure through the disruption of normal function and architecture. Additionally, metastatic tumor invasion will disrupt renal architecture and function and cause renal failure.[85]

Trauma: Renal trauma is estimated to occur in 10% to 20% of pediatric blunt traumas and much more rarely for penetrating injuries. However, renal trauma does not usually cause significant clinical renal failure, except in situations of single kidneys. Renal trauma is graded according to the organ injury scoring system adopted by the American Association for the Surgery of Trauma, and it is based on both clinical and computed tomography (CT) findings. Grade I trauma is contusion with microscopic or mild gross hematuria, and it is part of a spectrum up to grade V, which includes complete shattering of the organ or avulsion of the renal hilum and devascularization. Most renal trauma is managed nonoperatively, and the frequent reassessment of the injury is required. Indications for CT scan include more than 5 red blood cells per high powered field in penetrating trauma or more than 50 red blood cells per high-powered field in blunt trauma. Gross hematuria or hemodynamic instability at any time is an indication for CT scanning. Trauma surgeons may use angiographic-guided embolization in some circumstances or open operative management for the most severe grades of renal injury. Patients usually undergo a 12- to 24-hour observation period, because clinically significant bleeding is most often detectable during this time period. An excellent review of renal trauma and its staging and management is available in the literature.[112,113]

Vascular Involvement in Intrinsic Renal Disease

Vasculitis: Renal disease associated with vasculitis is varied, and it is dependent on the size of the vessel involved in the inflammatory process.[114] Large vessel involvement leads to renal artery stenosis, as seen in Takayasu arteritis and temporal arteritis. As the vessels involved become smaller, the frequency of glomerulonephritis increases.[115] For the majority of these presentations, clinical and laboratory indices will direct the clinician toward intrinsic renal disease as a cause for ARF. In many cases, acute, directed, and specific management may allow for the rescue of the patient from ARF and for the further prevention of renal disease.

Thrombosis: Renal artery thrombosis and renal vein thrombosis disrupt renal function by their effects on renal blood flow. Thrombosis may cause clinically evident disease if it involves both of the kidneys or a solitary functioning organ.[116,117] Renal artery thrombosis reduces renal blood flow and diminishes the glomerular capillary perfusion gradient. It is most often seen in association with an indwelling aortic catheter, such as umbilical artery catheter used predominantly in the neonatal intensive care unit. Patients may present with hypertension, and urinary sediment may contain gross blood or microscopic evidence of hematuria. Renal ultrasound without doppler may be normal; however, functional scans such as dimercaptosuccinic acid scans will show little or no renal blood flow. Conversely, renal vein thrombosis will demonstrate an enlarged edematous kidney on ultrasound; this will affect renal blood flow by increasing venous pressures and thereby reducing the transglomerular pressure gradient. Renal venous hypertension additionally affects the kidney by increasing interstitial fluid content, which may result in the gross disruption of renal architecture. Renal vein thrombosis is typically associated with low blood flow states and hyperviscosity, such as severe dehydration and polycythemia[118]; however, it may also be associated with indwelling catheters and the extension of deep venous thrombosis, or it may occur in utero. Both renal artery and renal vein thrombosis are possible complications of transplantation. The treatment of renal arterial or vein thrombosis may be attempted using clot-breaking agents such as tissue plasminogen activator.[119,120] This approach is not without significant potential bleeding complications, and it should only be attempted in the setting of bilateral renal occlusion.

Postrenal Acute Renal Failure

Obstruction to the flow of tubular ultrafiltrate can cause significant renal dysfunction. Glomerular filtration is a product of the balance between hydrostatic and oncotic pressure gradients at Bowman's space. Intratubular pressure is normally very low, and it is nearly negligible as compared with the driving pressure across the glomerular capillary bed. However, with obstruction to tubular ultrafiltrate flow, the pressure in Bowman's space rises and becomes a significant effector of glomerular filtration. In other words, glomerular filtration is reduced as afferent and efferent vascular autoregulatory mechanisms are maximized, and elevated pressure within Bowman's space reduces the overall difference in pressure that drives ultrafiltration. Obstruction to ultrafiltrate flow may occur at the tubular level (as is seen with ATN or crystal precipitation), or it may occur postrenally in the ureter or the bladder. Unilateral obstruction induces changes in renal function, but it may not be clinically evident with a compensatory change in the unaffected kidney.[121] However, in cases of bilateral obstruction or obstruction occurring in a solitary kidney, clinically significant changes in renal function will occur, thereby leading to ARF. Additionally, the duration of obstruction will affect renal function and recovery. For example, longstanding intrauterine bilateral obstruction is quite different from acute obstruction as a result of nephrolithiasis.[122] The site of obstruction, as indicated previously, may occur from the tubule to the urethra. It may be congenital or acquired, but it is most frequently unilateral. The ureter may be obstructed at multiple sites, although congenital obstruction usually occurs at the ureteropelvic junction. Ureteral obstruction may occur as a result of urinary stones, intraabdominal or retroperitoneal masses, traumatic disruption, or surgical trauma (e.g., inadvertent ligation), or it may be syndromic as is seen with prune belly syndrome.[122,123] Obstruction as a result of bladder dysfunction is more likely to cause bilateral disease, and it may result from bladder atony caused by drugs or neurogenic bladder. Obstruction of the urethral orifice may be the result of debris such as clot or urinary stones or of a congenital malformation as in the case of posterior urethral valves.

A postobstructive diuresis occurs after the relief of the obstruction, and this deserves special mention. In this scenario, the GFR is rapidly returned to normal, but there is a significant delay in the return of tubular functions. Hence, ultrafiltrate contains large quantities of sodium, chloride, and bicarbonate; there is a reduced excretion of potassium and hydrogen ions, and there is a low tonicity as a result of reduced medullary osmotic gradients required for water reabsorption. Clinically, the urine sodium is often in excess of 75 milliequivalents per liter, and the volume of urine produced requires urinary replacement to prevent intravascular depletion. The measurement of urine electrolytes will guide replacement fluid composition. Close monitoring of serum electrolytes will additionally guide urine replacement, and supplementation with calcium and bicarbonate may be required. The diuresis occurs over 24 to 36 hours, during which time creatinine clearance will improve rapidly and urinary replacement needs will taper off.

INVESTIGATIONS

Multiple investigations are used to differentiate the type of ARF. History is important. Simple tests using either urine or serum or a combination of both will help with refining the diagnosis. Many entities leading to ARF demonstrate specific patterns of biochemical and urinary findings that are useful when developing a differential diagnosis. Ultimately, renal biopsy may be the gold standard required to identify a specific pathologic process and hence to define therapeutic regimens.

Urine and Blood Tests

ARF is characterized by increases in blood urea nitrogen and serum creatinine levels. The evaluation of the pediatric patient takes on a different dimension as compared with adult patients with ARF. The normal creatinine values in pediatric patients are varied and depend on age and body mass.[124] Indeed, ARF in pediatric patients may go undiagnosed if the attending physician does not take into account the size and age of the patient, because many laboratories do not specify age-appropriate creatinine ranges. Creatinine clearance in children and adolescents may be approximated by using the Schwartz equation.[125] Clues may be provided regarding the underlying cause of ARF on the basis of the pattern of change in serum creatinine. Rapid rises in serum creatinine may accompany hemodynamic instability as is found in prerenal ARF, whereas a rapid rise in creatinine found in the patient with systemic symptoms (i.e., a facial rash) may implicate rapidly progressive glomerulonephritis.[126] Renal ischemic changes may not be recognized until 1 to 2 days later, when serum creatinine levels begin to rise,[98] as may be the case in contrast-induced nephropathy or postoperative cardiac surgery. Whereas creatinine levels peak at 5 days and return to normal by 7 days in patients with contrast nephropathy, they may peak at 10 days and return to normal in 14 days in patients with ischemic ARF.

Value of the Serum Urea/Creatinine Ratio

Urea is passively reabsorbed in the proximal tubule as a result of the increased sodium and water reabsorption seen in hypovolemia. Thus, a high serum urea/creatinine ratio is suggestive of prerenal ARF. Serum urea and creatinine are reported in mg/dL; a ratio exceeding 20 : 1 suggests prerenal causes, and a ratio of 10 : 1 to 15 : 1 suggests ATN. When serum creatinine is reported in μmol/L, and urea is reported in mmol/L; a urea/creatinine ratio of more than 0.10 and a urea value of more than 10 mmol/L (60 mg/dL) are suggestive of prerenal ARF.[127,128]

The value of this ratio is limited especially in situations of high catabolism, corticosteroid administration, and gastrointestinal bleeding. Under these circumstances, urea will be elevated; therefore, the ratio will be elevated in the absence of hypovolemia. A high ratio can also be seen if muscle mass is decreased. A normal ratio cannot exclude prerenal causes, especially in the presence of liver disease or decreased protein intake.

Fractional Excretion of Sodium

Often by history, prerenal ARF can be differentiated from other causes. It is important to make this distinction not only for diagnostic purposes but also because this will affect management. Urine sodium can be used to estimate the patient's volume status. In situations of hypovolemia, urine sodium is usually less than 20 Meq/L.[129] However, low urine sodium may be found in normovolemia associated with acute glomerulonephritis.[130] The contrary can also be seen, when high urine sodium is noted in the face of hypovolemia in cases of diuretic use, Bartter's syndrome, adrenal insufficiency, tubulointerstitial nephritis, and chronic renal disease, among others.[131-133] Water reabsorption can also influence urine sodium. For example, in polyuric patients with diabetes insipidus, a daily normal excretion of sodium can be associated with low urine sodium as a result of dilution and thus labeled as hypovolemia. To avoid this situation, the renal handling of water can be assessed with the use of the fractional excretion of sodium (FE_{Na}).

FE_{Na} is easily calculated from a random urine sample. It is often used in cases of ARF. In cases of hypovolemia, most sodium should be reabsorbed in the proximal tubule, and, thus, the FE_{Na} should be less than 1%. If the tubules are damaged, as is seen in ATN, the FE_{Na} is often in the range of 2% to 3%.[129,134] The FE_{Na} can be calculated as follows[130]:

$$Fe_{Na}\,(\%) = \frac{\text{Quantity of Na}^+\text{ excreted}}{\text{Quantity of Na}^+\text{ filtered}} \times 100$$

$$FE_{Na}\,(\%) = \frac{U_{Na} \times V}{P_{Na} \times \left(Ucr \times \dfrac{V}{Pcr}\right)} \times 100$$

$$= \frac{U_{Na} \times Pcr}{P_{Na} \times U_{cr}} \times 100$$

In this equation, the amount of sodium excreted is equal to the product of the urine concentration of sodium (U_{Na}) and the urine volume (V); the amount of sodium filtered is equal to the product of the plasma concentration of sodium (P_{Na}) and the glomerular filtration rate ($Ucr \times V/Pcr$).

FE_{Na} can be less than 1% in conditions other than hypovolemia, such as congestive heart failure, nephrotic syndrome, or hepatic cirrhosis.[129] It can also be less than 1% in contrast nephropathy or heme pigmentation nephropathy.[129]

Urine sodium and FE_{Na} are unreliable if the patient is taking diuretics. If measured, urine should be collected on the basis of the half-life of the diuretics being administered. For example, in the case of furosemide, the urine sample should be taken a minimum of 6 hours after the drug has been taken. Caution should also be exercised in the neonatal population when using this ratio. FE_{Na} is appropriately elevated in newborns making the transition from intra- to extrauterine life. This ratio is even less reliable in those infants who are born preterm.

Fractional Excretion of Urea

Because of the limited value of the FE_{Na} in circumstances in which diuretics have been administered, the concept of measuring the fractional excretion of urea (FE_{UN}) has been proposed. In states of clinical dehydration, the urinary excretion of urea should also decrease.[135] The FE_{UN} should be less than 35% in hypovolemic states of prerenal ARF, whereas, in the case of ATN, it should be greater than 50%. A hospital-based prospective study conducted a comparative analysis of FE_{Na} and FE_{UN} with regard to their respective abilities to differentiate between prerenal ARF and ATN in the presence of diuretics.[136] In this study, FE_{UN} (<35%) had a better sensitivity and specificity (85% and 92%, respectively) for differentiating ARF resulting from prerenal causes as compared with ATN, particularly when diuretics were employed. More importantly, a high positive predictive value of 98% was noted for FE_{UN}. Studies evaluating FE_{UN} in children with ARF are limited.

Other Laboratory Values

Other laboratory patterns may also provide insight into the underlying cause of ARF. Complete blood cell counts, peripheral blood smears, and biochemical testing (electrolytes and hepatic panels, C-reactive protein, creatine kinase) as well as serologic panels may be indicative of particular causes. Specialized testing may be indicated in the face of suspected intoxication or overdose.

Routine complete blood cell counts are imperative for the evaluation of ARF, because anemia is almost always noted.[137-139] Examination of the peripheral blood smear may provide clues about the underlying cause. The presence of spherocytes may be indicative of lupus nephritis, whereas schistocytes may implicate HUS, drug-induced hemolysis, or sepsis-associated disseminated intravascular coagulopathy.[140] With severe anemia in the absence of hemorrhage, hemolysis should be suspected and other blood count parameters evaluated, including platelets, which may be suggestive of thrombotic microangiopathy. Decreased complement levels (particularly C3 and C4) and high titers of antiglomerular basement membrane antibodies, antineutrophil cytoplasmic antibodies, antinuclear antibodies, and circulating immune complexes are useful for the diagnosis of suspected glomerulonephritis or vasculitis.[126,141,143] Indeed, a low C3 level is found in postinfectious glomerulonephritis and will normalize within 6 to 8 weeks, whereas a low C3 will persist in a case of membranoproliferative glomerulonephritis.[144,145] Thus, following the disease pattern temporally can be important for making the correct diagnosis and hence implementing appropriate therapy.[126] A review of the differential white blood cell panel can also provide clues regarding potential underlying abnormalities. For example, systemic eosinophilia may suggest allergic interstitial nephritis.

Biochemical abnormalities may be appreciated in a variety of different patterns of ARF. For example, rhabdomyolysis (crush injury) may be manifested with ARF along with hyperphosphatemia, hypocalcemia, increased concentrations of serum uric acid and creatine kinase, and hyperkalemia.[87] TLS may present with similar electrolyte abnormalities; however, the creatine kinase is not usually elevated in this situation.[100,101]

Acutely, hyperkalemia is one of the most important electrolyte disturbances to note, because serum potassium concentration is frequently elevated in patients with ARF. This potentially life-threatening complication can result from hypofiltration and abnormal tubular function, decreased tubular secretion, and, in some cases, excessive cellular release (e.g., crush injury/rhabdomyolysis).[87] This is one of the primary indications for the implementation of renal replacement therapy. Hypokalemia can also be seen in the presence of significant volume depletion resulting from vomiting, diarrhea, and diuretics.[99] Entities that result in hypercalcemia (i.e., primary hyperparathyroidism) can also induce ARF.[142]

Measurement of the anion and osmolar gaps is important for the evaluation of ARF, especially when ingestion is suspected. The widening of both of these gaps may point toward ethylene or diethylene glycol poisoning and indicate the further evaluation of the patient's urine for crystal formation.[146]

In general, careful scrutiny of the electrolyte and biochemical levels as well as the complete blood cell count is absolutely required for the diagnosis and management of pediatric ARF.

Urinalysis and Urine Sediment

Qualitative urinalysis is a standard of care when assessing any child with suspected renal disease.[147] Diagnostic clues provided by this analysis can guide further investigations and, ultimately, therapy. Perhaps one of the most important components of the urinalysis is the examination for protein. The presence of urinary protein excretion and its subsequent quantification with urine protein/creatinine ratio or 24-hour assessment is integral to the workup of ARF. Children typically excrete less than 4 $mg/m^2/hour$ of protein (urine protein/creatinine ratio: <0.20 mg/mg or <20 mg/mmol).[126] Increased excretion may be reflected in the face of ischemic or nephrotoxic ARF, thus demonstrating the excretion of debris from tubular damage and a failure to absorb normally filtered protein at the level of the proximal tubule. Indeed, tubular and glomerular protein loss may be differentiated by the use of urinary protein electrophoresis. Increasing amounts of protein in the urine may be reflective of injury to the glomerular barrier, thereby suggesting a glomerulonephritis[126] or AIN as a root cause of the ARF. The correlation of urinary protein loss, other associated urinary findings (e.g., hematuria), biochemical indices (e.g., hypoalbuminemia) and clinical presentation are paramount for establishing the underlying cause of ARF.

The urinary sediment is also an essential part of the workup of pediatric ARF, because it may provide clues regarding the underlying pathophysiology involved. Indeed, every nephrologist should be able to prepare and review spun urines to identify histologic clues for diagnosis.[148] Abnormalities in urinary sediment are strong indicators of intrinsic ARF. The classical finding of red blood cell casts in the face of rising serum creatinine would be strongly indicative of an acute glomerulonephritis[126,147] and would mandate early biopsy for the consideration of treatment with corticosteroids and cytotoxic agents. A relatively bland acellular urine with or without clear hyaline casts (typically composed of Tamm-Horsfall protein secreted by epithelial cells from the loop of Henle) in the face of a history of low effective circulating blood volume would reaffirm the potential diagnosis of prerenal ARF.[147,149] Benign sediment may be seen in pediatric patients with postrenal ARF; however, hematuria and pyuria can occur, because many patients will have intraluminal obstruction as a result of stones or blood clots. In general, urine sediment and supernatant should be analyzed for the presence of crystals, cells, cellular debris, casts, protein, and blood by-products.

Pediatric patients presenting with tea-colored urine may have an underlying glomerulonephritis with dysmorphic red blood cells and red blood cell casts,[126] but a pigment nephropathy (hemoglobinuria/myoglobinuria) cannot be excluded without further analysis of the urine and plasma.[150] Indeed, even patients with combined liver and kidney disease may present with darkened, ruddy-looking urine as a result of bilious components. Reddish-brown granular and tubular epithelial casts may be found in the urine of patients with nephrotoxic or ischemic ATN.[147,149] The root cause of ARF for all of these presentations of darkened urine may be misleading without a closer analysis of the urine.

Another important finding of the urinalysis may be eosinophiluria. Although the majority of causes of eosinophiluria are the result of the infection of the upper or lower urinary tract, it may be seen in up to 25% of cases of AIN.[151,152] Eosinophiluria and white blood cells casts are strongly suspicious for the presence of interstitial nephritis. Urate or calcium oxalate crystals may be indicative of tumor lysis syndrome or ethylene glycol poisoning, respectively. Broad granular/waxy casts (likely representing dilated tubules) are a more consistent finding in chronic renal failure,[147] but they nonetheless may be very useful in diagnostic efforts for the evaluation of ARF.

Tables 39-4 and 39-5[34] provide guides to commonly associated microscopic urinary sediment and urinalysis findings associated with prerenal, renal, and postrenal ARF.

Novel Markers of Acute Renal Failure

Serum creatinine is an easily measured marker of ARF. However, it is generally appreciated that serum creatinine is a relatively inaccurate marker of ARF, because a rise in creatinine signifies that damage has already occurred. With improved molecular biology techniques, understanding the molecular underpinnings of ARF has been greatly enhanced during the last few years. This increased knowledge has led to the discovery of early markers of ARF. The principal use of these markers is to detect early signs of injury that could lead the clinician to alter management to prevent further damage to the kidneys. Early markers may also serve to predict the severity of injury and to help with monitoring the effect of an intervention.

An excellent review of biomarkers in ARF has recently been published.[153] Biomarkers should ideally be noninvasive, reproducible, accurate, and reliable, and they should have a high predictive ability (i.e., they should be specific and sensitive). They should also be easy to perform, and the results should be rapidly available. To date, few markers have been used in prospective clinical studies; the most promising ones will be discussed.

Cystatin C

Cystatin C is a cysteine protease inhibitor protein that, unlike serum creatinine, is freely filtered, completely reabsorbed, and catabolized by the tubular epithelial cells; it is not secreted. It is stable and not influenced by body mass, gender, or age. More interestingly, its measurement is simple, automated, and easily available.[154] One prospective study in an adult population at risk for ARF showed that an increase of 50% in serum cystatin C level predicted ARF 1 to 2 days before a rise in serum creatinine.[155] Another study demonstrated that cystatin C had a better correlation with GFR than serum creatinine in critically ill adults.[156] Cystatin C levels were also able to predict the need for renal replacement therapy, but they could not differentiate among various causes

TABLE 39-4 **Characteristics of Urinary Sediment in Acute Renal Failure**

Acute Renal Failure Diagnosis	Normal to Few Red and White Blood Cells	Granular Casts	Red Blood Cell Casts	White Blood Cell Casts	Eosinophiluria >5%	Crystalluria
Prerenal azotemia	Yes					
Hemolytic uremic syndrome/ thrombotic thrombocytopenic purpura	Yes					
Arterial thrombus	Yes					
Postrenal azotemia	Yes					
Acute tubular necrosis		Yes				
Glomerulonephritis		Yes	Yes	Yes		
Vasculitis		Yes	Yes			
Acute interstitial nephritis		Yes	Yes (rare)	Yes	Yes	
Pyelonephritis (severe)				Yes		
Leukemic/lymphomatous infiltrate				Yes		
Urate nephropathy						Yes
Calcium oxalate						Yes
Medications (acyclovir/sulfonamides)						Yes
Radiocontrast agents						Yes

From Brady HR, Clarkson MR, Lieberthal W, in Brenner BM, editor: *Brenner & Rector's the kidney,* ed 7, Philadelphia, 2004, Saunders, pp 1215-70.

TABLE 39-5 **Characteristics of Urinalysis in Acute Renal Failure**

Acute Renal Failure Diagnosis	Urinalysis
Prerenal causes	Normal
Renal (intrinsic) causes	
Acute tubular necrosis	Granular casts and epithelial cells
Glomerulonephritis	Red blood cells, red blood cell casts, and marked proteinuria
Interstitial nephritis	Red and white blood cells with or without eosinophils and granular casts
Vascular disorders	Normal or red blood cells and proteinuria
Postrenal causes	Normal or red blood cells, red blood cell casts, and pyuria

From Brady HR, Clarkson MR, Lieberthal W, in Brenner BM, editor: *Brenner & Rector's the kidney,* ed 7, Philadelphia, 2004, Saunders, pp 1215-70.

of ARF. Cystatin C measurement has also been useful in kidney transplantation.[157] In children, cystatin C has been demonstrated to correlate with ARF in children suffering from malaria.[158] So far, no prospective study of the value of cystatin C for predicting ARF in children has been published.

Kidney Injury Molecule

Kidney injury molecule 1 (KIM-1) is a transmembrane receptor that undergoes cleavage and that is found in the urine after ischemic injury.[159] In a small study, KIM-1 measurement was able to differentiate ischemic renal injury from prerenal causes and chronic kidney disease.[159] To date, no large study has validated the predictive value of KIM-1 in ARF in adults. KIM-1 is also undergoing analysis and evaluation for its usefulness as a predictive tool for ARF in children.

Neutrophil Gelatinase-Associated Lipocalin

Neutrophil gelatinase-associated lipocalin (NGAL) is protein bound to gelatinase, and it was first described in neutrophils.[160] Circulating NGAL is normally reabsorbed at the level of the proximal tubule, and, after ischemia, NGAL is secreted in the thick ascending limb and found in the urine. A study in 71 children undergoing cardiopulmonary bypass surgery measured urinary NGAL 2 hours after surgery.[161] Twenty children had an increase in urinary NGAL, and this increase preceded a rise in serum creatinine by 2 to 4 days. The specificity and sensitivity were excellent (98% and 100%, respectively).

NGAL has been recently proven to be a useful predictor of ARF in patients with HUS.[162] NGAL may be increased in patients with infections. Thus, its value for diagnosing early ARF in complicated, septic patients may be limited. Urinary NGAL measurement has recently become commercially available.

Interleukin 18

Interleukin-18 is a cytokine found in the urine after ischemia. It is cleaved to its mature (active) form by a proinflammatory cysteine protease, caspase I.[163] Many studies have observed an increase in urinary interleukin 18 that predicts an increase in serum creatinine in diverse patient populations.[164-166] It has also been used to differentiate among the diverse causes of ARF.[164] When combined with NGAL, it predicted the duration of ARF in children after cardiac surgery.[161] A determination of the level of this substance is easy to perform, and a commercial assay is available.

Other Markers

Markers, such as sodium/hydrogen exchanger isoform 3, *N*-acetyl-β-glucosaminidase, and matrix metalloproteinase 9 may be useful for the early detection of ARF, but presently the assays are not easily performed nor is there enough preliminary data to support their use.[159,167]

Use of These Markers

The value of these markers for predicting ARF is under intense study. Although urinary interleukin 18 and NGAL are good predictors of ARF, in situations of complex pediatric patients (i.e., PICU patients), their value may be diminished. Serum cystatin C measurement is promising, but large prospective studies in patient populations with complex diseases need to be performed before its use can be fully established. Before these markers make a significant impact on clinical management in pediatric patients developing ARF, there is a need for simple, accurate, inexpensive, and rapid methods of measuring them. Additionally, prospective studies in diverse pediatric patient groups developing ARF are required.

Imaging

A variety of imaging studies are available in the arsenal that is used to identify and manage pediatric ARF. Urinary tract imaging by either ultrasonography (US), CT, magnetic resonance imaging, or, occasionally, plain film of the abdomen is recommended for most patients with ARF. The choice of which study best suits the patient is guided by the clinical and laboratory examination. Not all patients will need all studies. These studies may help distinguish between acute and chronic kidney disease. Each of these modalities has particular advantages and disadvantages in terms of diagnostic abilities and potential side effects to the pediatric patient population.[168,169] The interpreter of such studies (a radiologist in most cases) will also add variability with regard to the use and diagnostic criteria of each of these modalities. It is important to discuss each case with the interpreting physician, especially when the circumstance of the ARF is unclear. The provision of an adequate history is paramount in such circumstances.

Another important variable that must be considered, especially in smaller pediatric patients, is the potential requirement for sedation. Many imaging studies require the patient to lie very still, and this adds a degree of complexity that is not necessarily noted in the adult population.

Ultrasonography

US remains the imaging modality of choice for pediatric patients with newly diagnosed or worsening renal failure. The resolution of anatomic detail is generally excellent. US avoids exposure to contrast agents or radiation, thus making it a preferred alternative to helical CT scanning for the assessment of renal colic in children. However, the assessment of renal function is very limited. In ARF, its primary role is to initially identify postrenal causes (because obstruction may potentially be ruled out by the absence of hydronephrosis) and to provide an estimation of bladder size and thickness.[170-172] US abnormalities may not be appreciated in cases of prerenal ARF, but intrinsic renal ARF can be appreciated by a variety of anatomic changes. The measurement of the renal size may give an indication of the chronicity of renal failure. Enlarged kidneys (standardized to the patient's age and size) are suggestive of ARF caused by medical renal diseases such as AIN, renal vein thrombosis, or infectious processes. Chronic kidney disease is suggested by the presence of kidneys that are small for the patient's age. US is excellent for the assessment of changes in the echo texture of the kidneys, because an increase in echogenicity may indicate acute or chronic kidney disease.[173] One caveat to note is that, in the neonatal population, echogenicity may be present as a result of the age of the patient. An experienced radiologist is invaluable in such circumstances.[174]

US with Doppler capabilities may also take on a more significant role in the evaluation of renal vascular disorders. The use of resistive indices in the assessment of children has not been standardized, and it is not reliable at present.[175] However, because blood flow to the kidneys is reduced in most cases of ARF, Doppler flow scanning may allow for the detection of abnormal or low renal blood flow states that can be indicative of renal artery stenosis or complete thrombosis and therefore the absence of renal circulation.[176,177]

US has numerous advantages over other modalities. It can be performed at the bedside; minimal or no sedation is usually required for smaller children; it is noninvasive; it does not expose patients to radiation or contrast agents (which can be nephrotoxic and contraindicated in ARF)[178,179]; and it provides detailed renal anatomic information. Limitations include the lack of functional information in terms of ARF assessment, although, if Doppler capabilities are present and both ureter jets are observed, global renal function may be assumed to be present.[180] Finally, it is more operator dependent than other modalities.

Nuclear Medicine

The use of radionuclide imaging using I^{131}-labeled iodohippurate or ^{99m}Tc-labeled diethylene-triamine pentaacetic acid (^{99m}Tc-DIPA) can be employed to assess tubular function and blood flow in ARF.[181] However, the utility of these tests may be similar to that of Doppler flow scanning. Significant delays in nuclide excretion by tubules can occur in both prerenal and intrinsic renal ARF, thereby limiting its usefulness in this setting unless blood flow is completely absent.[182] Recently, it has proven to be useful for diagnosing exercise-induced ARF.[183] In general, these tests have demonstrated inconsistent or poor results in studies, so they are mainly used during the postrenal transplant period.[182,184]

Computed Tomography Scanning

CT scanning offers advantages when US is limited by technical issues. It is also valuable for trauma assessment when the kidneys are involved.[112,113] Noncontrast CT scans are valuable for demonstrating the renal pelvis and proximal ureter using sequential transverse sections to identify sites of ureteral obstruction. They can also help identify primary causes of obstruction, such as stones, tumors, or congenital abnormalities. Residual renal function may be identified using contrast-enhanced CT scans. In this setting, the pattern of a delayed and prolonged nephrogram may be demonstrated.[185] Although this is technically useful, the potential of contrast nephropathy worsening renal dysfunction and the potential requirement of anesthesia in children for adequate studies does add limitations to its usefulness. Finally, repetitive scans can lead to a high cumulative radiation exposure that may put children at risk for radiation toxicity over the long term.

Magnetic Resonance Imaging

In recent years, magnetic resonance urography (MRU) has provided significant advances in the assessment of pediatric renal disease and ARF.[185,186] MRU can identify collecting system morphology regardless of excretory function. Also, with its high sensitivity and specificity, it has been used to effectively identify causes of postrenal ARF in terms of obstruction.[187] Both static and dynamic (gadolinium-enhanced) techniques are used for MRU evaluation.[188] The addition of furosemide may be important to improve image quality by enhancing the distribution and excretion of contrast media in the collecting system.[188,189] In the presence of small kidneys and oliguria, a clinically useful urographic effect may be not appreciated with the use of MRU.[190,191]

Other Techniques

A renal angiogram is helpful for pediatric patients with ARF caused by vascular disorders, including renal artery stenosis with ARF, renal artery thrombus, and acute aortorenal occlusion. These procedures have been evaluated and established in children with renal vascular disease, and they have proven to be highly reliable.[192]

Magnetic resonance angiography of the kidneys is extremely useful for detecting renal artery stenosis, and its role has been extended to the evaluation of acute renovascular crises.[192] Magnetic resonance angiography is a time-efficient and safe test as compared with conventional arteriography, and it does not require the administration of nephrotoxic contrast material. However, contrast angiography remains the gold standard for the definitive diagnosis of renal vasculopathies in children.[193,194] There is a general consensus that intravenous pyelography is best avoided in patients with ARF because it is ineffective and may add contrast nephropathy to already compromised renal function.

Renal Biopsy

Renal biopsy is considered the gold standard for diagnosing the underlying cause of ARF. This is especially true in pediatric patients in whom both prerenal and postrenal causes of ARF have been excluded. Practically speaking, the benefits and risk factors of renal biopsy need to be carefully considered.[195]

Risk factors include infection, bleeding/transfusion, loss of the kidney, inadequate sampling, and any anesthetic risks, depending on whether conscious or general sedation is used. This is especially true in critical care situations in which patients are already at increased risk for bleeding complications. Renal biopsy should be considered in situations in which the underlying pattern of disease in terms of history and biochemical and imaging studies is unclear; the biopsy will shed light on the potential therapeutic options that are available. This is especially critical in the case of pediatric patients with a clinical presentation of rapidly progressive glomerulonephritis. Early diagnosis and appropriate intervention in this renal medical emergency may prevent the progression from ARF to chronic kidney disease. Another important group to consider is pediatric renal transplant patients with ARF. The early biopsy diagnosis of acute cellular rejection may direct therapeutic intervention and thus prevent a further decline in renal function.[196-203]

PROGNOSTIC FACTORS OF ACUTE RENAL FAILURE

Classic Prognostic Factors

Anuria, the need for dialysis, the use of inotropic medications, and an age of less than 1 year have all been described as prognostic factors predicting worse outcomes among children developing ARF.[19,22] Hospital-acquired ARF was shown to have a worse outcome than ARF presenting at admission to the hospital among adult patients.[204-206] In critically ill adult patients, the delayed occurrence of ARF (after admission to the intensive care unit) is also a negative prognostic factor.[207] In children, no large study has demonstrated that delayed or hospital-acquired ARF has a worse prognosis than ARF that is present before either hospitalization or admission to the PICU.[12]

New Prognostic Factors

The severity of fluid overload in patients at the initiation of CVVH has received a lot of attention during the last few years. One of the first studies to address the importance of fluid overload with regard to the outcomes of pediatric patients suffering from ARF was performed retrospectively in a cohort of 21 pediatric patients with ARF that was treated by CVVH. In that study, increased fluid overload was associated with increased mortality.[208] A larger retrospective study involving 113 children who were treated with CVVH observed the same association of the severity of fluid overload with mortality, particularly among patients developing multiple organ failure.[209] Goldstein and colleagues[210] followed these studies with a prospective observational multicenter study of 157 children treated with CVVH and observed again that the severity of fluid overload was associated with a worse outcome, even after adjusting for severity of disease.[210] These authors suggest that CVVH be initiated earlier and that inotropic agents should be used more rapidly instead of fluid after the initial resuscitation.

To date, no prospective trial in children controlling for fluid overload has been performed to assess whether fluid overload is indeed a risk factor for mortality in children with ARF or just a risk marker of disease severity. A recent trial comparing a strict fluid management practice with a more liberal one in adult patients with acute lung injury noted a higher serum urea and creatinine in the strict fluid management arm but no difference in the number of patients who required dialysis.[211] However, patients requiring dialysis were excluded from the study.

CLINICAL IMPACT OF ACUTE RENAL FAILURE

The clinical impact of ARF varies according to the population being studied. The few data available in children suggest that morbidity and mortality attributable to ARF may be important. A few retrospective studies reported a mortality rate of up to 78% when renal replacement therapy was needed.[22,212,213] In prospective trials, mortality associated with ARF but not attributed to ARF ranged from 13% to 36%.[11,12,32]

Long-term data regarding renal function after ARF are limited. Recently, the long-term outcome of 21 cases of meningococcal sepsis-associated ARF requiring renal replacement therapy (hemofiltration and hemodialysis of peritoneal dialysis) was reported.[214] In this series, all patients were dialyzed for ARF and not solely to clear inflammatory mediators. Among the 15 survivors, 12 were available for further study. Four of these 12 children had evidence of abnormal renal function 2 to 7 years after ARF, and one required renal transplantation. Another study was able to retrace 29 of 139 children after ARF who survived 12 months after the initial hospitalization. Sixteen children progressed to end-stage renal disease over the course of 3 to 5 years. Those who had primary renal disease or urologic malformation demonstrated the worst renal outcomes. More importantly, 59% had signs of chronic renal injury (microalbuminuria and hypertension); however, only 35% were followed by a nephrologist.[215]

CONCLUSION

ARF is frequently seen in the pediatric population. It is associated with increased mortality and long-term morbidity rates. The epidemiology has changed over the last decade. Secondary ARF as a result of bone marrow transplantation, solid organ transplantation, and sepsis is more frequent in developed countries than is ARF resulting from classic causes such as HUS. Both classic and newer risk factors (e.g., fluid overload) have been described, and they vary according to the population being studied. Novel markers of renal injury and a consensus definition of ARF may help to detect ARF early during its development and thus allow interventions to either prevent or treat the disease early during its course.

REFERENCES

1. Lameire N, Van Biesen W, Vanholder R: Acute renal failure, *Lancet* 365(9457):417-30, 2005.
2. Bellomo R, Kellum J, Ronco C: Acute renal failure: time for consensus, *Intensive Care Med* 27(11):1685-8, 2001.
3. Singri N, Ahya SN, Levin ML: Acute renal failure, *JAMA* 289(6):747-51, 2003.
4. Uchino S, et al: Acute renal failure in critically ill patients: a multinational, multicenter study, *JAMA* 294(7):813-8, 2005.
5. Flynn JT, et al: Peritoneal dialysis for management of pediatric acute renal failure, *Perit Dial Int* 21(4):390-4, 2001.
6. Bellomo R, et al: Acute renal failure—definition, outcome measures, animal models, fluid therapy and information technology needs: the Second International Consensus Conference of the Acute Dialysis Quality Initiative (ADQI) Group, *Crit Care* 8(4):R204-12, 2004.
7. Bell M, et al: Optimal follow-up time after continuous renal replacement therapy in actual renal failure patients stratified with the RIFLE criteria, *Nephrol Dial Transplant* 20(2):354-60, 2005.
8. Abosaif NY, et al: The outcome of acute renal failure in the intensive care unit according to RIFLE: model application, sensitivity, and predictability, *Am J Kidney Dis* 46(6):1038-48, 2005.
9. Picca S, et al: Risks of acute renal failure after cardiopulmonary bypass surgery in children: a retrospective 10-year case-control study, *Nephrol Dial Transplant* 10(5):630-6, 1995.
10. Moghal NE, Brocklebank JT, Meadow SR: A review of acute renal failure in children: incidence, etiology and outcome, *Clin Nephrol* 49(2):91-5, 1998.
11. Leteurtre S, et al: Validation of the paediatric logistic organ dysfunction (PELOD) score: prospective, observational, multicentre study, *Lancet* 362(9379):192-7, 2003.
12. Bailey D, Gavin F, Phan V, Litalien C, Mérouani A, Lacroix J: Facteurs de risque de l'insuffisance rénale aiguë chez l'enfant sévèrement malade: étude prospective épidémiologique. 33ème Congrès annuel de la Société de Réanimation de Langue Française, Paris, *Réanimation* 14:S199, 2005.
13. Bonventre JV, Weinberg JM: Recent advances in the pathophysiology of ischemic acute renal failure, *J Am Soc Nephrol* 14(8):2199-210, 2003.
14. Andreoli SP: Acute renal failure in the newborn, *Semin Perinatol* 28(2):112-23, 2004.
15. Kwon O, et al: Backleak, tight junctions, and cell-cell adhesion in postischemic injury to the renal allograft, *J Clin Invest* 101(10):2054-64, 1998.
16. Kwon O, Phillips CL, Molitoris BA: Ischemia induces alterations in actin filaments in renal vascular smooth muscle cells, *Am J Physiol Renal Physiol* 282(6):F1012-9, 2002.
17. Sutton TA, Fisher CJ, Molitoris BA: Microvascular endothelial injury and dysfunction during ischemic acute renal failure, *Kidney Int* 62(5):1539-49, 2002.
18. Rosen S, Heyman SN: Difficulties in understanding human "acute tubular necrosis": limited data and flawed animal models, *Kidney Int* 60(4):1220-4, 2001.
19. Arora P, et al: Prognosis of acute renal failure in children: a multivariate analysis, *Pediatr Nephrol* 11(2):153-5, 1997.
20. Flynn JT: Causes, management approaches, and outcome of acute renal failure in children, *Curr Opin Pediatr* 10(2):184-9, 1998.
21. Bunchman TE, et al: Pediatric acute renal failure: outcome by modality and disease, *Pediatr Nephrol* 16(12):1067-71, 2001.
22. Hui-Stickle S, Brewer ED, Goldstein SL: Pediatric ARF epidemiology at a tertiary care center from 1999 to 2001, *Am J Kidney Dis* 45(1):96-101, 2005.
23. Olowu WA, Adelusola KA: Pediatric acute renal failure in southwestern Nigeria, *Kidney Int* 66(4):1541-8, 2004.
24. Anochie IC, Eke FU: Acute renal failure in Nigerian children: Port Harcourt experience, *Pediatr Nephrol* 20(11):1610-4, 2005.
25. Mabina MH, Moodley J, Pitsoe SB: The use of traditional herbal medication during pregnancy, *Trop Doct* 27(2):84-6, 1997.
26. Kadiri S, et al: The causes and course of acute tubular necrosis in Nigerians, *Afr J Med Med Sci* 21(1):91-6, 1992.
27. Jha V, Chugh KS: Nephropathy associated with animal, plant, and chemical toxins in the tropics, *Semin Nephrol* 23(1):49-65, 2003.
28. Liano F, et al: The spectrum of acute renal failure in the intensive care unit compared with that seen in other settings. The Madrid Acute Renal Failure Study Group, *Kidney Int Suppl* 66:S16-24, 1998.
29. Uchino S, et al: Diuretics and mortality in acute renal failure, *Crit Care Med* 32(8):1669-77, 2004.
30. Brivet FG, et al: Acute renal failure in intensive care units—causes, outcome, and prognostic factors of hospital mortality; a prospective, multicenter study. French Study Group on Acute Renal Failure, *Crit Care Med* 24(2):192-8, 1996.
31. Cosentino F, Chaff C, Piedmonte M: Risk factors influencing survival in ICU acute renal failure, *Nephrol Dial Transplant* 9(Suppl 4):179-82, 1994.
32. Medina Villanueva A, et al: [Acute renal failure in critically-ill children. A preliminary study], *An Pediatr (Barc)* 61(6):509-14, 2004.
33. Skippen PW, Krahn GE: Acute renal failure in children undergoing cardiopulmonary bypass, *Crit Care Resusc* 7(4):286-91, 2005.
34. Brady HR, Clarkson MR, Lieberthal W: Acute renal failure. In Brenner BM, editor: *Brenner & Rector's the kidney*, ed 7, Philadelphia, 2004, Saunders, pp 1215-70.

35. Andreoli SP: Clinical evaluation and management. In Avner ED, Harmon WE, Niaudet P, editors: *Pediatric nephrology,* ed 5, Baltimore, 2004, Lippincott Williams & Wilkins, pp 1233-4.
36. Blantz RC: Pathophysiology of pre-renal azotemia, *Kidney Int* 53:512-23, 1998.
37. Badr KF, Ichikawa I: Prerenal failure: a deleterious shift from renal compensation to decompensation, *N Engl J Med* 319:623-9, 1988.
38. Lau KK, Wyatt RJ: Glomerulonephritis. *Adolesc Med Clin* 16(1):67-85, 2005.
39. Davis ID, Avner ED: Introduction to glomerular diseases. In Behrman RE, Kliegman RM, Jenson HB, editors: *Nelson textbook of pediatrics,* ed 17, Philadelphia, 2004, Saunders, pp 1734-5.
40. Tarr PI, Gordon CA, Chandler WL: Shiga-toxin-producing *Escherichia coli* and haemolytic uraemic syndrome, *Lancet* 365(9464): 1073-86, 2005.
41. Siegler R, Oakes R: Hemolytic uremic syndrome; pathogenesis, treatment, and outcome, *Curr Opin Pediatr* 17(2):200-4, 2005.
42. Khan A, et al: Shiga toxin producing *Escherichia coli* infection: current progress & future challenges. *Indian J Med Res* 118:1-24, 2003.
43. Bender JB, et al: Surveillance by molecular subtype for *Escherichia coli* O157:H7 infections in Minnesota by molecular subtyping, *N Engl J Med* 337(6):388-94, 1997.
44. Garg AX, et al: Long-term renal prognosis of diarrhea-associated hemolytic uremic syndrome: a systematic review, meta-analysis, and meta-regression, *JAMA* 290(10):1360-70, 2003.
45. Paton AW, et al: A new family of potent AB(5) cytotoxins produced by Shiga toxigenic *Escherichia coli, J Exp Med* 200(1):35-46, 2004.
46. Karch H, et al: New aspects in the pathogenesis of enteropathic hemolytic uremic syndrome, *Semin Thromb Hemost* 32(2):105-12, 2006.
47. Fernandez GC, et al: Decrease of thrombomodulin contributes to the procoagulant state of endothelium in hemolytic uremic syndrome, *Pediatr Nephrol* 18(10):1066-8, 2003.
48. Tazzari PL, et al: Flow cytometry detection of Shiga toxins in the blood from children with hemolytic uremic syndrome, *Cytometry B Clin Cytom* 61(1):40-4, 2004.
49. Lin FY, Sherman PM, Li D: Development of a novel hand-held immunoassay for the detection of enterohemorrhagic *Escherichia coli* O157:H7, *Biomed Microdevices* 6(2):125-30, 2004.
50. Sheoran AS, et al: Human antibody against shiga toxin 2 administered to piglets after the onset of diarrhea due to *Escherichia coli* O157:H7 prevents fatal systemic complications, *Infect Immun* 73(8):4607-13, 2005.
51. Greising J, Trachtman H, Gauthier B, Valderrama E: Acute interstitial nephritis in adolescents and young adults, *Child Nephrol Urol* 10:189-95, 1990.
52. Cavallo T: Tubulointerstitial nephritis. In Jennette JC, Olson LL, Schwartz MM, Silva FG, editors: *Heptinstall's pathology of the kidney,* ed 5, Philadelphia, 1998, Lippincott-Raven Publishers, pp 667-723.
53. Ellis D, Fried WA, Yunis EJ, Blau EB: Acute interstitial nephritis in children: a report of 13 cases and review of the literature, *Pediatrics* 67(6):862-70, 1981.
54. Kobayashi Y, Honda M, Yoshikawa N, Ito H: Acute tubulointerstitial nephritis in 21 Japanese children, *Clin Nephrol* 54(3):191-7, 2000.
55. Kobayashi Y, Honda M, Yoshikawa N, Ito H: Immunohistological study in sixteen children with acute tubulointerstitial nephritis, *Clin Nephrol* 50(1):14-20, 1998.
56. Burghard R, Brandis M, Hoyer PF, Ehrich JHH, et al: Acute interstitial nephritis in childhood, *Eur J Pediatr* 142:103-10, 1984.
57. Hawkins EP, Berry PL, Silva FG: Acute tubulointerstitial nephritis in children: clinical, morphologic, and lectin studies. A report of the Southwestern Pediatric Nephrology Study Group, *Am J Kidney Dis* 14(6):466-71, 1989.
58. Winkler P, Altrogge H: Sonographic signs of nephritis in children: a comparison of renal echography with clinical evaluation, laboratory data and biopsy, *Pediatr Radiol* 15:231-7, 1985.
59. Hiraoka M, Hori C, Tsuchida S, Tsukahara H, Sudo M: Ultrasonographic findings of acute tubulointerstitial nephritis, *Am J Nephrol* 16(2):154-8, 1996.
60. Ellis D, Fried WA, Yunis EJ, Blau EB: Acute interstitial nephritis in children: a report of 13 cases and review of the literature, *Pediatrics* 67(6):862-70, 1981.
61. Dell KM, Kaplan BS, Meyers CM: Tubulointerstitial nephritis. In Barrett TM, Avner ED, Harmon WE, editors: *Pediatric nephrology,* ed 4, Baltimore, 1999, Lippincott Williams & Wilkins, pp 823-34.
62. Jones CL, Eddy AA: Tubulointerstitial nephritis, *Pediatr Nephrol* 6(6):572-86, 1992.
63. Vogt BA, Avner ED: Renal failure. In Behrman RE, Kliegman RM, Jenson HB, editors: *Nelson textbook of pediatrics,* ed 17, Philadelphia, 2004, Saunders, pp 1768.
64. Klenzak J, Himmelfarb J: Sepsis and the kidney, *Crit Care Clin* 21(2):211-22, 2005.
65. De Vriese AS: Prevention and treatment of acute renal failure in sepsis, *J Am Soc Nephrol* 14(3):792-805, 2003.
66. Schrier RW, Wang W: Acute renal failure and sepsis, *N Engl J Med* 351(2):159-69, 2004.
67. Landry DW, Oliver JA: The pathogenesis of vasodilatory shock, *N Engl J Med* 345(8):588-95, 2001.
68. Kon V, Badr KF: Biological actions and pathophysiologic significance of endothelin in the kidney, *Kidney Int* 40(1):1-12, 1991.
69. Reinhart K, et al: Markers of endothelial damage in organ dysfunction and sepsis, *Crit Care Med* 30(5 Suppl):S302-12, 2002.
70. Wang W, et al: Endothelial nitric oxide synthase-deficient mice exhibit increased susceptibility to endotoxin-induced acute renal failure, *Am J Physiol Renal Physiol* 287(5):F1044-8, 2004.
71. Taber SS: Drug-associated renal dysfunction, *Crit Care Clin* 22(2):357-74, 2006.
72. Tune BM, Reznik VM, Mendoza SA: Renal complications of drug therapy. In Holliday MA, Barratt TM, Avner ED, editors: *Pediatric nephrology,* ed 3, Baltimore, 1994, Williams and Wilkins, pp 1212-26.
73. Cheng HF, Harris RC: Renal effects of non-steroidal anti-inflammatory drugs and selective cyclooxygenase-2 inhibitors, *Curr Pharm Des* 11(14):1795-804, 2005.
74. Cuzzolin L, Dal Cere M, Fanos V: NSAID-induced nephrotoxicity from the fetus to the child, *Drug Saf* 24(1):9-18, 2001.
75. Benini D, et al: In utero exposure to nonsteroidal anti-inflammatory drugs: neonatal renal failure, *Pediatr Nephrol* 19(2):232-4, 2004.
76. Blakely P, McDonald BR: Acute renal failure due to acetaminophen ingestion: a case report and review of the literature, *J Am Soc Nephrol* 6(1):48-53, 1995.
77. Mour G, et al: Acute renal dysfunction in acetaminophen poisoning, *Ren Fail* 27(4):381-3, 2005.
78. Chandrasekharan NV, et al: COX-3, a cyclooxygenase-1 variant inhibited by acetaminophen and other analgesic/antipyretic drugs: cloning, structure, and expression, *Proc Natl Acad Sci U S A* 99(21):13926-31, 2002.
79. Schwab JM, Schluesener HJ, Laufer S: COX-3: just another COX or the solitary elusive target of paracetamol?, *Lancet* 361(9362):981-2, 2003.
80. Joannidis M: Drug-induced renal failure in the ICU, *Int J Artif Organs* 27(12):1034-42, 2004.
81. Silverstein DM, Palmer J, Baluarte HJ, Brass C, et al: Use of calcium-channel blockers in pediatric renal transplant recipients, *Pediatr Transplant* 3(4):288-92, 1999.
82. McLaughlin GE, Land MP, Rossique-Gonzalez M: Effect of aminophylline on urine flow in children with tacrolimus-induced renal insufficiency, *Transplant Proc* 32(4):817-20, 2000.
83. Thomas NJ, Carcillo JA: Theophylline for acute renal vasoconstriction associated with tacrolimus: a new indication for an old therapeutic agent?, *Pediatr Crit Care Med* 4(3):392-3, 2003.
84. McLaughlin GE, Abitbol CL: Reversal of oliguric tacrolimus nephrotoxicity in children, *Nephrol Dial Transplant* 20(7):1471-5, 2005.
85. Keaney CM, Springate JE: Cancer and the kidney, *Adolesc Med Clin* 16(1):121-48, 2005.
86. Poels PJ, Gabreels FJ: Rhabdomyolysis: a review of the literature, *Clin Neurol Neurosurg* 95(3):175-92, 1993.

87. Malinoski DJ, Slater MS, Mullins RJ: Crush injury and rhabdomyolysis, *Crit Care Clin* 20(1):171-92, 2004.
88. Patel DR, Torres AD, Greydanus DE: Kidneys and sports, *Adolesc Med Clin* 16(1):111-9, 2005.
89. Kapadia FN, Bhojani K, Shah B: Special issues in the patient with renal failure, *Crit Care Clin* 19(2):233-51, 2003.
90. Nash K, Hafeez A, Hou S: Hospital-acquired renal insufficiency, *Am J Kidney Dis* 39(5):930-6, 2002.
91. Rihal CS, et al: Incidence and prognostic importance of acute renal failure after percutaneous coronary intervention, *Circulation* 105(19):2259-64, 2002.
92. Barrett BJ, Carlisle EJ: Metaanalysis of the relative nephrotoxicity of high- and low-osmolality iodinated contrast media, *Radiology* 188(1):171-8, 1993.
93. Solomon R: The role of osmolality in the incidence of contrast-induced nephropathy: a systematic review of angiographic contrast media in high risk patients, *Kidney Int* 68(5):2256-63, 2005.
94. Pannu N, Wiebe N, Tonelli M: Prophylaxis strategies for contrast-induced nephropathy, *JAMA* 295(23):2765-79, 2006.
95. Cantley LG, et al: Role of endothelin and prostaglandins in radiocontrast-induced renal artery constriction, *Kidney Int* 44(6):1217-23, 1993.
96. Pflueger A, et al: Role of adenosine in contrast media-induced acute renal failure in diabetes mellitus, *Mayo Clin Proc* 75(12):1275-83, 2000.
97. Persson PG: [The Cancer Foundation: donations greater than ever], *Lakartidningen* 103(6):391, 2006.
98. Rudnick MR, et al: Nephrotoxic risks of renal angiography: contrast media-associated nephrotoxicity and atheroembolism—a critical review, *Am J Kidney Dis* 24(4):713-27, 1994.
99. Peixoto AJ: Critical issues in nephrology, *Clin Chest Med* 24(4):561-81, 2003.
100. Davidson MB, et al: Pathophysiology, clinical consequences, and treatment of tumor lysis syndrome, *Am J Med* 116(8):546-54, 2004.
101. Spinazze S, Schrijvers D: Metabolic emergencies, *Crit Rev Oncol Hematol* 58(1):79-89, 2006.
102. Mato AR, et al: A predictive model for the detection of tumor lysis syndrome during AML induction therapy, *Leuk Lymphoma* 47(5):877-83, 2006.
103. McCroskey RD, et al: Acute tumor lysis syndrome and treatment response in patients treated for refractory chronic lymphocytic leukemia with short-course, high-dose cytosine arabinoside, cisplatin, and etoposide, *Cancer* 66(2):246-50, 1990.
104. Seymour JF, et al: Cisplatin, fludarabine, and cytarabine: a novel, pharmacologically designed salvage therapy for patients with refractory, histologically aggressive or mantle cell non-Hodgkin's lymphoma, *Cancer* 94(3):585-93, 2002.
105. Dillman RO: Infusion reactions associated with the therapeutic use of monoclonal antibodies in the treatment of malignancy, *Cancer Metastasis Rev* 18(4):465-71, 1999.
106. Fleming DR, Henslee-Downey PJ, Coffey CW: Radiation induced acute tumor lysis syndrome in the bone marrow transplant setting, *Bone Marrow Transplant* 8(3):235-6, 1991.
107. Sallan S: Management of acute tumor lysis syndrome, *Semin Oncol* 28(2 Suppl 5):9-12, 2001.
108. Wang LY, et al: Recombinant urate oxidase (rasburicase) for the prevention and treatment of tumor lysis syndrome in patients with hematologic malignancies, *Acta Haematol* 115(1-2):35-8, 2006.
109. Goldman SC, et al: A randomized comparison between rasburicase and allopurinol in children with lymphoma or leukemia at high risk for tumor lysis, *Blood* 97(10):2998-3003, 2001.
110. Brant JM: Rasburicase: an innovative new treatment for hyperuricemia associated with tumor lysis syndrome, *Clin J Oncol Nurs* 6(1):12-6, 2002.
111. Saccente SL, Kohaut EC, Berkow RL: Prevention of tumor lysis syndrome using continuous veno-venous hemofiltration, *Pediatr Nephrol* 9(5):569-73, 1995.
112. Buckley JC, McAninch JW: The diagnosis, management, and outcomes of pediatric renal injuries, *Urol Clin North Am* 33:33-40, 2006.
113. Alsikafi NF, Rosenstein DI: Staging, evaluation, and nonoperative management of renal injuries, *Urol Clin North Am* 33:13-19, 2006.
114. Samarkos M, Loizou S, Vaiopoulos G, Davies KA: The clinical spectrum of primary renal vasculitis, *Semin Arthritis Rheum* 35:95-111, 2005.
115. Dedeoglu F, Sundel RP: Vasculitis in children, *Pediatr Clin North Am* 52(2):547-75, 2005.
116. Keating MA, Althausen AF: The clinical spectrum of renal vein thrombosis, *J Urol* 133:938-45, 1985.
117. Amigo M: Kidney disease in antiphospholipid syndrome, *Rheum Dis Clin North Am* 32(3):509-22, 2006.
118. Glassock RJ, Duffee J, Kodroff MB, Chan JC: Dehydration, renal vein thrombosis and hyperkalemic renal tubular acidosis in a newborn, *Am J Nephrol* 3:329-37, 1983.
119. Song JY, Valentino L: A pregnant patient with renal vein thrombosis successfully treated with low-dose thrombolytic therapy: a case report, *Am J Obstet Gynecol* 192(6):2073-5, 2005.
120. Chevalier RL: What treatment do you advise for bilateral or unilateral renal thrombosis in the newborn, with or without thrombosis of the inferior vena cava?, *Pediatr Nephrol* 5(6):679, 1991.
121. Palevsky PM: Acute renal failure, *J Am Soc Nephrol* 2(2):41-76, 2003.
122. Strand WR: Initial management of complex pediatric disorders: prunebelly syndrome, posterior urethral valves, *Urol Clin North Am* 31(3):399-415, 2004.
123. Bellomo R: Defining, quantifying, and classifying acute renal failure, *Crit Care Clin* 21(2):223-37, 2005.
124. Wong AF, Bolinger AM, Gambertoglio JG: Pharmacokinetics and drug dosing in children with decreased renal function. In Holliday MA, Barratt TM, Avner ED, editors: *Pediatric nephrology*, ed 3, Baltimore, 1994, Williams and Wilkins, pp 1306.
125. Schwartz GM, Brion LP, Spitzer A: The use of plasma creatinine concentration for estimating glomerular filtration rate in infants, children, and adolescents, *Pediatr Clin North Am* 34:571-90, 1987.
126. Lau KK, Wyatt RJ: Glomerulonephritis, *Adolesc Med Clin* 16(1):67-85, 2005.
127. Morgan DB, Carver ME, Payne RB: Plasma creatinine and urea: creatinine ratio in patients with raised plasma urea, *Br Med J* 2(6092):929-32, 1977.
128. Acute renal failure: urea:creatinine ratio was not very helpful in diagnosing prerenal failure. Evidence-Based On-Call database. Available at: www.eboncall.org/CATs/1844.htm. Accessed August 30, 2007.
129. Rose BD: Meaning and application of urine chemistries. In Rose BD, editor, *Clinical physiology of acid-base and electrolyte disorders*, ed 5, New York, 2001, McGraw-Hill, p 405-14.
130. Miller TR, et al: Urinary diagnostic indices in acute renal failure: a prospective study, *Ann Intern Med* 89(1):47-50, 1978.
131. Jeck N, et al: The diuretic- and Bartter-like salt-losing tubulopathies, *Nephrol Dial Transplant* 15(Suppl 6):19-20, 2000.
132. Rodriguez-Soriano J, et al: Hyperkalemic distal renal tubular acidosis in salt-losing congenital adrenal hyperplasia, *Acta Paediatr Scand* 75(3):425-32, 1986.
133. Danovitch GM, Jacobson E, Licht A: Absence of renal sodium adaptation in chronic renal failure, *Am J Nephrol* 1(3-4):173-6, 1981.
134. Zarich S, Fang LS, Diamond JR: Fractional excretion of sodium. Exceptions to its diagnostic value, *Arch Intern Med* 145(1):108-12, 1985.
135. Goldstein MH, Lenz PR, Levitt MF: Effect of urine flow rate on urea reabsorption in man: urea as a "tubular marker," *J Appl Physiol* 26(5):594-9, 1969.
136. Carvounis CP, Nisar S, Guro-Razuman S: Significance of the fractional excretion of urea in the differential diagnosis of acute renal failure, *Kidney Int* 62(6):2223-9, 2002.
137. du Cheyron D, Parienti JJ, Fekih-Hassen M, Daubin C, Charbonneau P: Impact of anemia on outcome in critically ill patients with severe acute renal failure, *Intensive Care Med* 31(11):1529-36, 2005.
138. Park J, Gage BF, Vijayan A: Use of EPO in critically ill patients with acute renal failure requiring renal replacement therapy, *Am J Kidney Dis* 46(5):791-8, 2005.

139. Anochie IC, Eke FU: Acute renal failure in Nigerian children: Port Harcourt experience, *Pediatr Nephrol* 20(11):1610-4, 2005.
140. Blake JS, Butani L: Rapidly progressive lupus glomerulonephritis and concomitant microangiopathy in an adolescent, *Lupus* 11(8):533-5, 2002.
141. Little MA, Pusey CD: Rapidly progressive glomerulonephritis: current and evolving treatment strategies, *J Nephrol* 17(Suppl 8): S10-9, 2004.
142. Moysés-Neto M, Guimarães FM, Ayoub FH, Vieira-Neto OM, et al: Acute renal failure and hypercalcemia, *Ren Fail* 28(2):153-9, 2006.
143. Couser WG: Rapidly progressive glomerulonephritis: classification, pathogenetic mechanisms, and therapy, *Am J Kidney Dis* 11(6):449-64, 1988.
144. Smith KD, Alpers CE: Pathogenic mechanisms in membranoproliferative glomerulonephritis, *Curr Opin Nephrol Hypertens* 14(4):396-403, 2005.
145. Sotsiou F, Dimitriadis G, Liapis H: Diagnostic dilemmas in atypical postinfectious glomerulonephritis, *Semin Diagn Pathol* 19(3):146-59, 2002.
146. Brophy PD, Tenenbein M, Gardner J, Bunchman TE, Smoyer WE: Childhood diethylene glycol poisoning treated with alcohol dehydrogenase inhibitor fomepizole and hemodialysis, *Am J Kidney Dis* 35(5):958-62, 2000.
147. Patel HP: The abnormal urinalysis, *Pediatr Clin North Am* 53(3):325-37, 2006.
148. Tsai JJ, Yeun JY, Kumar VA, Don BR: Comparison and interpretation of urinalysis performed by a nephrologist versus a hospital-based clinical laboratory, *Am J Kidney Dis* 46(5):820-9, 2005.
149. Simerville JA, Maxted WC, Pahira JJ: Urinalysis: a comprehensive review, *Am Fam Physician* 71(6):1153-62, 2005.
150. Gerber GS, Brendler CB: Evaluation of the urologic patient: history, physical examination, and urinalysis. In Walsh PC, editor: *Campbell's urology*, ed 8, Philadelphia, 2002, Elsevier, pp 100-104.
151. Corwin HL, Korbet SM, Schwartz MM: Clinical correlates of eosinophiluria, *Arch Intern Med* 145(6):1097-9, 1985.
152. Corwin HL, Bray RA, Haber MH: The detection and interpretation of urinary eosinophils, *Arch Pathol Lab Med* 113(11):1256-8, 1989.
153. Zhou H, et al: Acute kidney injury biomarkers—need, present status, and future promise, *J Am Soc Nephrol* 5(2):63-71, 2006.
154. Herget-Rosenthal S, et al: Prognostic value of tubular proteinuria and enzymuria in nonoliguric acute tubular necrosis, *Clin Chem* 50(3):552-8, 2004.
155. Herget-Rosenthal S, et al: Early detection of acute renal failure by serum cystatin C, *Kidney Int* 66(3):1115-22, 2004.
156. Villa P, et al: Serum cystatin C concentration as a marker of acute renal dysfunction in critically ill patients, *Crit Care* 9(2):R139-43, 2005.
157. White C, et al: Estimating glomerular filtration rate in kidney transplantation: a comparison between serum creatinine and cystatin C-based methods, *J Am Soc Nephrol* 16(12):3763-70, 2005.
158. Burchard GD, et al: Renal dysfunction in children with uncomplicated, Plasmodium falciparum malaria in Tamale, Ghana, *Ann Trop Med Parasitol* 97(4):345-50, 2003.
159. Han WK, et al: Kidney injury molecule-1 (KIM-1): a novel biomarker for human renal proximal tubule injury, *Kidney Int* 62(1):237-44, 2002.
160. Kjeldsen L, Cowland JB, Borregaard N: Human neutrophil gelatinase-associated lipocalin and homologous proteins in rat and mouse, *Biochim Biophys Acta* 1482(1-2):272-83, 2000.
161. Mishra J, et al: Neutrophil gelatinase-associated lipocalin (NGAL) as a biomarker for acute renal injury after cardiac surgery, *Lancet* 365(9466):1231-8, 2005.
162. Trachtman H, et al: Urinary neutrophil gelatinase-associated lipocalcin in D+HUS: a novel marker of renal injury, *Pediatr Nephrol* 21(7):989-94, 2006.
163. Melnikov VY, et al: Impaired IL-18 processing protects caspase-1-deficient mice from ischemic acute renal failure, *J Clin Invest* 107(9):1145-52, 2001.
164. Parikh CR, et al: Urinary interleukin-18 is a marker of human acute tubular necrosis, *Am J Kidney Dis* 43(3):405-14, 2004.
165. Parikh CR, et al: Urine IL-18 is an early diagnostic marker for acute kidney injury and predicts mortality in the intensive care unit, *J Am Soc Nephrol* 16(10):3046-52, 2005.
166. Parikh CR, et al: Urinary IL-18 is an early predictive biomarker of acute kidney injury after cardiac surgery, *Kidney Int* 70(1):199-203, 2006.
167. du Cheyron D, et al: Urinary measurement of Na+/H+ exchanger isoform 3 (NHE3) protein as new marker of tubule injury in critically ill patients with ARF, *Am J Kidney Dis* 42(3):497-506, 2003.
168. Palmer LS: Pediatric urologic imaging, *Urol Clin North Am* 33(3):409-23, 2006.
169. Sty JR, Pan CG: Genitourinary imaging techniques, *Pediatr Clin North Am* 53(3):339-61, 2006.
170. Kiely EA, Hartnell GG, Gibson RN, et al: Measurement of bladder volume by real-time ultrasound, *Br J Urol* 60:33-5, 1987.
171. Ireton RC, Krieger JN, Cardenas DD, et al: Bladder volume determination using a dedicated, portable ultrasound scanner, *J Urol* 143:909-11, 1990.
172. Mainprize TC, Drutz HP: Accuracy of total bladder volume and residual urine measurements: comparison between real-time ultrasound and catheterization, *Am J Obstet Gynecol* 160:1013-6, 1989.
173. Coleman BG: Ultrasonography of the upper genitourinary tract, *Urol Clin North Am* 12:633-44, 1985.
174. Mercado-Deane MG, Beeson JE, John SD: US of renal insufficiency in neonates, *Radiographics* 22(6):1429-38, 2002.
175. Vade A, Dudiak C, McCarthy P, Hatch DA, Subbaiah P: Resistive indices in the evaluation of infants with obstructive and nonobstructive pyelocaliectasis, *J Ultrasound Med* 18(5):357-61, 1999.
176. Krumme B, Blum U, Schwertfeger E, et al: Diagnosis of renovascular disease by intra- and extrarenal Doppler scanning, *Kidney Int* 50:1288-92, 1996.
177. Platt JF, Rubin JM, Ellis JH: Lupus nephritis: predictive value of conventional and Doppler US and comparison with serologic and biopsy parameters, *Radiology* 203:82-6, 1997.
178. Waybill MM, Waybill PN: Contrast media-induced nephrotoxicity: identification of patients at risk and algorithms for prevention, *J Vasc Interv Radiol* 12:3-9, 2001.
179. Gerlach AT, Pickworth KK: Contrast medium-induced nephrotoxicity: pathophysiology and prevention, *Pharmacotherapy* 20:540-8, 2000.
180. Burge HJ, Middleton WD, McClennan BL, et al: Ureteral jets in healthy subjects and in patients with unilateral ureteral calculi: comparison with color Doppler US, *Radiology* 180:437-42, 1991.
181. Goldfarb CR, Srivastava NC, Grotas AB, Ongseng F, Nagler HM: Radionuclide imaging in urology, *Urol Clin North Am* 33(3):319-28, 2006.
182. Sherman RA, Byun KJ: Nuclear medicine in acute and chronic renal failure, *Semin Nucl Med* 12:265-79, 1982.
183. Nishida H, Kaida H, Ishibashi M, Baba K, et al: Evaluation of exercise-induced acute renal failure in renal hypouricemia using Tc-99m DTPA renography, *Ann Nucl Med* 19(4):325-9, 2005.
184. Coulthard MG, Keir MJ: Reflux nephropathy in kidney transplants, demonstrated by dimercaptosuccinic acid scanning, *Transplantation* 82(2):205-10, 2006.
185. Kawashima A, Glockner JF, King BF Jr: CT urography and MR urography, *Radiol Clin North Am* 41(5):945-61, 2003.
186. Huang AJ, Lee VS, Rusinek H: MR imaging of renal function, *Radiol Clin North Am* 41(5):1001-17, 2003.
187. Nolte-Ernsting CCA, Adam GB, Gunther RW: MR urography: examination techniques and clinical applications, *Eur Radiol* 11:355-72, 2001.
188. Borthne AS, Pierre-Jerome C, Gjesdal KI, Storaas T, et al: Pediatric excretory MR urography: comparative study of enhanced and non-enhanced techniques, *Eur Radiol* 13(6):1423-7, 2003.
189. Jung P, Brauers A, Nolte-Ersting CA, Jakse G, Gunther RW: Magnetic resonance urography enhanced by gadolinium and diuretics: a comparison with conventional urography in diagnosing the cause of ureteric obstruction, *BJU Int* 86:960-5, 2000.
190. Wefer AE, Wefer J, Fricks B, Truss MC, Galanski M: Advances in uroradiological imaging, *BJU Int* 89:477-87, 2002.

191. Dagher PC, Herget-Rosenthal S, Ruehm SG, Jo SK, et al: Newly developed techniques to study and diagnose acute renal failure, *J Am Soc Nephrol* 14(8):2188-98, 2003.
192. Stanley JC, Criado E, Upchurch GR Jr, Brophy PD, et al: Pediatric renovascular hypertension: 132 primary and 30 secondary operations in 97 children, *J Vasc Surg* 44(6):1219-28, 2006.
193. Marcos HB, Choyke PL: Magnetic resonance angiography of the kidney. *Semin Nephrol* 20:450-5, 2000.
194. Weise WJ, Jaffrey JB: CT angiography and magnetic resonance imaging are the best less-invasive tests for renal artery stenosis, *ACP J Club* 136:69, 2002.
195. Al Makdama A, Al-Akash S: Safety of percutaneous renal biopsy as an outpatient procedure in pediatric patients, *Ann Saudi Med* 26(4):303-5, 2006.
196. Vande Walle J, Mauel R, Raes A, Vandekerckhove K, Donckerwolcke R: ARF in children with minimal change nephrotic syndrome may be related to functional changes of the glomerular basal membrane, *Am J Kidney Dis* 43(3):399-404, 2004.
197. Subtirelu MM, Flynn JT, Schechner RS, Pullman JM, et al: Acute renal failure in a pediatric kidney allograft recipient treated with intravenous immunoglobulin for parvovirus B19 induced pure red cell aplasia, *Pediatr Transplant* 9(6):801-4, 2005.
198. Demirkaya E, Atay AA, Musabak U, Sengul A, Gok F: Ceftriaxone-related hemolysis and acute renal failure, *Pediatr Nephrol* 21(5):733-6, 2006.
199. Korbet SM: Percutaneous renal biopsy, *Semin Nephrol* 22(3):254-67, 2002.
200. Conley SB: Renal biopsy in the 1990s, *Pediatr Nephrol* 10(4):412-13, 1996.
201. Solez K, Racusen LC: Role of the renal biopsy in acute renal failure, *Contrib Nephrol* 132:68-75, 2001.
202. Preston RA, Stemmer CL, Materson BJ, et al: Renal biopsy in patients 65 years of age or older: an analysis of the results of 334 biopsies, *J Am Geriatr Soc* 38(6):669-74, 1990.
203. Jennette JC, Falk RJ: Diagnosis and management of glomerular diseases, *Med Clin North Am* 81(3):653-77, 1997.
204. Dharan KS, et al: Prediction of mortality in acute renal failure in the tropics, *Ren Fail* 27(3):289-96, 2005.
205. Sesso R, et al: Prognosis of ARF in hospitalized elderly patients, *Am J Kidney Dis* 44(3):410-9, 2004.
206. Nolan CR, Anderson RJ: Hospital-acquired acute renal failure, *J Am Soc Nephrol* 9(4):710-8, 1998.
207. Guerin C, et al: Initial versus delayed acute renal failure in the intensive care unit. A multicenter prospective epidemiological study. Rhone-Alpes Area Study Group on Acute Renal Failure, *Am J Respir Crit Care Med* 161(3 Pt 1):872-9, 2000.
208. Goldstein SL, et al: Outcome in children receiving continuous venovenous hemofiltration, *Pediatrics* 107(6):1309-12, 2001.
209. Foland JA, et al: Fluid overload before continuous hemofiltration and survival in critically ill children: a retrospective analysis, *Crit Care Med* 32(8):1771-6, 2004.
210. Goldstein SL, et al: Pediatric patients with multi-organ dysfunction syndrome receiving continuous renal replacement therapy, *Kidney Int* 67(2):653-8, 2005.
211. National Heart, Lung, and Blood Institute Acute Respiratory Distress Syndrome (ARDS) Clinical Trials Network; Wiedemann HP, Wheeler AP, Bernard GR, Thompson BT, et al: Comparison of two fluid-management strategies in acute lung injury, *N Engl J Med* 354(24):2564-75, 2006.
212. Smoyer WE, McAdams C, Kaplan BS, Sherbotie JR: Determinants of survival in pediatric continuous hemofiltration, *J Am Soc Nephrol* 6(5):1401-9, 1995.
213. Wong W, McCall E, Anderson B, Segedin E, Morris M: Acute renal failure in the paediatric intensive care unit, *N Z Med J* 109(1035):459-61, 1996.
214. Slack R, Hawkins KC, Gilhooley L, Addison GM, et al: Long-term outcome of meningococcal sepsis-associated acute renal failure, *Pediatr Crit Care Med* 6(4):477-9, 2005.
215. Askenazi DJ, Feig DI, Graham NM, Hui-Stickle S, Goldstein SL: 3-5 year longitudinal follow-up of pediatric patients after acute renal failure, *Kidney Int* 69(1):184-9, 2006.

CHAPTER

40 Management of Acute Renal Failure

Stuart L. Goldstein

INTRODUCTION

Acute renal failure (ARF) management in children requires special considerations not commonly encountered in the care of adult patients. Pediatric patients with ARF may range in weight from a 1.5-kg neonate to a 200-kg young adult. In addition, disease states that may require acute renal replacement therapy in the absence of significant renal dysfunction, such as inborn errors of metabolism or postoperative care of an infant with congenital cardiac defects, are more prevalent in the pediatric setting. Optimal care for the pediatric patient requiring renal replacement therapy requires an understanding of the causes and patterns of pediatric ARF and multiorgan dysfunction syndrome and recognition of the local expertise with respect to the personnel and equipment resources. The aim of this chapter is to review pediatric ARF management with an emphasis on emerging practice patterns with respect to modality and the timing of treatment.

FLUID AND ELECTROLYTE CONSIDERATIONS

Careful attention to fluid and electrolyte management in pediatric ARF is critical to prevent or mitigate associated comorbidities, and is dependent on an accurate assessment of the underlying cause of ARF. For example, patients with pre-renal azotemia most often have reversible ARF, which is responsive to fluid resuscitation, whereas patients with acute tubular necrosis should be treated with volume, sodium, and potassium restriction, to prevent development of worsening fluid overload and hyperkalemia. Finally, patients with ARF secondary to nephrotoxic medications or interstitial nephritis often demonstrate polyuria.

The standard practice of providing "maintenance fluids" based on patient size or caloric requirement (e.g., the Holliday-Seger method[1] or 1600 ml/m^2 of body surface area) was derived from patients with normal renal function and the amount of urine volume needed to excrete a normal daily solute load. Such maintenance fluid algorithms are not appropriate and can be dangerous for children with ARF. The fluid prescription for children with ARF should be directed by the individual clinical situation. A safe starting point in most cases is insensible losses plus replacement of ongoing losses. A daily volume of 400 ml/m^2 of body surface area to replace insensible fluid losses should be prescribed for patients with a normal basal metabolic rate, whereas higher volumes may be required for febrile patients. Lower insensible loss volume replacement may be appropriate for patients receiving invasive mechanical ventilation who have decreased respiratory insensible fluid loss. Patients with oligoanuric renal failure should not receive potassium or phosphorus unless they exhibit hypokalemia or hypophosphatemia. Sodium administration should be restricted to 2 to 3 meq/kg body weight per day to prevent fluid retention and hypertension in children with oligoanuric ARF. Accurate and strict accounting of urine and extrarenal fluid losses is essential for optimal management of ARF. Depending on the clinical situation, replacement of all or only part of a patient's ongoing losses may be warranted. For example, patients with fluid overload might be managed appropriately with a fluid rate that contains insensible losses plus half of ongoing losses in order to provide sufficient glucose and electrolytes, and to allow the patient to attain negative fluid balance. Patient weight and serum electrolyte concentrations should be measured at least daily in order to modify the fluid and electrolyte prescription appropriately.

Optimal fluid repletion strategies for patients also with intravascular volume contraction require a rational approach. Clinical signs and symptoms including tachycardia, degree of skin turgor, mucus membrane hydration, and mental status can be used to estimate patient fluid deficits. Aggressive rehydration is warranted for patients with significant circulatory compromise in order to restore organ perfusion. For patients with less severe dehydration, the fluid deficit can be replaced over 24 to 48 hours while continuing to replace insensible and ongoing fluid losses.

Significant clinical research has been conducted recently to assess various fluid repletion strategies based on physiologic directed endpoint in patients in shock. Recent data from adult patients with septic shock demonstrate that goal-directed fluid therapy using physiologic endpoints could significantly improve patient survival.[2,3] Adult patients who received early goal-directed fluid therapy in the emergency center received more fluid in the emergency center, but received less fluid overall during hospitalization and had better survival in the ICU compared to patients who received standard therapy. Fluid resuscitation in critically ill children is essential for patients with acute hypovolemia and septic shock.[4] The subacute effects of fluid overload, however, are more uncertain. Several studies have suggested an association between excessive fluid retention and negative patient outcome. Adult surgical ICU patients who develop fluid retention have increased morbidity, increased requirements for blood products, prolonged dependency on pressors, and a twofold increase in death.[5] Fluid overload has also been associated with decreased survival in adult patients with adult respiratory distress syndrome.[6,7]

PHARMACOLOGIC THERAPY

Acute renal failure management should begin prior to consultation of a nephrologist and provision of renal replacement therapy. Maintenance of adequate urine volumes and prevention/treatment of metabolic derangements comprise the goals of pharmacologic therapy in children with ARF. Preservation or restoration of renal perfusion with appropriate inotropic agents is essential and the first pharmacologic measure to maintain urine output in critically ill patients unresponsive to volume repletion.[8]

Vasopressors

The effects of dopamine are varied and complex, leading to controversy with respect to its utility in the setting of ARF. At low or so-called "renal doses" of 0.5 to 2 mcg/kg/min, dopamine increases renal plasma flow and sodium excretion. At 2 to 5 mcg/kg/min, dopamine binds β-adrenergic receptors and at doses above 5 mcg/kg/min, dopamine's α-adrenergic receptor binding becomes activated. These complex actions render it difficult to ascertain whether any observed renal benefit from dopamine occurs as a result of its dopaminergic or inotropic effect. However, well-designed prospective randomized studies of adult patients at risk for acute tubular necrosis have called into question the utility of "renal-dose" dopamine in reversing oliguria,[9,10] and many centers have abandoned its use in the setting of ATN.[11,12]

Dobutamine does not exhibit a direct effect on the kidney, but rather acts primarily on the β-1 adrenergic receptors. The benefit of dobutamine for patients with ARF resides in its ability to increase cardiac output, leading to an increase in renal blood flow.

Norepinephrine also exerts complex systemic and renal actions,[13] which have the contradictory effects of decreasing renal blood flow in healthy individuals but improving systemic pressure and leading to renal vasodilatation. Norepinephrine appears to be the most beneficial vasopressor in euvolemic patients with hypotension, such as those with septic shock, leading to improved glomerular filtration rate.

Vasopressin increases systemic vascular resistance by direct action on the vascular smooth muscle cells. Vasopressin has been shown to be especially effective in maintaining renal perfusion in patients with septic shock who were unresponsive to catecholamines.[14]

Prospective randomized studies of adult patients at risk for acute tubular necrosis have called into question the utility of intravenous furosemide in reversing oliguria.[15,16] However, the practice of providing furosemide, either as an intermittent bolus or as a continuous infusion (0.1 to 0.3 mg/kg/hr) in combination with a thiazide diuretic, has potential to maintain urine output in patients at risk of developing anuria.

Another recent study supports the use of fenoldopam, a dopamine α-1 agonist, to prevent ARF in certain critically ill adult populations.[17,18] No published pediatric study exists on the effect of fenoldopam in pediatric ARF.

Many other agents, which are still considered to be experimental, have shown inconsistent results regarding prevention or amelioration of a course of ARF. N-acetylcysteine has been studied most extensively in the setting of contrast-induced nephropathy prevention. Results from an early successful trial,[19] in which only 2% of patients who received N-acetylcysteine versus 21% who received placebo demonstrated increased serum creatinine have not been reproduced.[20,21] Less well-studied agents, including insulin-like growth factor I[22] and thyroxine[23] have not been effective in improving an ARF course.

RENAL REPLACEMENT THERAPY

Provision of renal replacement therapy as intermittent hemodialysis (HD), peritoneal dialysis, or continuous renal replacement therapy (CRRT) is now a mainstay of treatment for the child with ARF. Technological advances aimed at providing accurate ultrafiltration with volumetric control incorporated into hemodialysis and CRRT equipment and disposable lines, circuits, and dialyzers sized for the entire pediatric weight spectrum have made renal replacement therapy safer in the pediatric setting.[24] Transition from the use of adaptive CRRT equipment to production of hemofiltration machines with volumetric control allowing for accurate ultrafiltration (UF) flows has likewise led to a change in prevalence patterns of pediatric renal replacement therapy modality. Accurate UF and blood flow rates are crucial for pediatric renal replacement therapy since the extracorporeal circuit volume can comprise more than 15% of a small pediatric patient's total blood volume and small UF inaccuracies may represent a large percentage of a small pediatric patient's total body water. Polls of U.S. pediatric nephrologists demonstrate increased CRRT use over peritoneal dialysis as the preferred modality for treating pediatric ARF. In 1995, 45% of pediatric centers ranked peritoneal dialysis (PD) and 18% ranked CRRT as the most common modality used for initial ARF treatment. In 1999, 31% of centers chose PD versus 36% of centers that reported CRRT as their primary initial modality for ARF treatment.[25]

In the last decade, survival rates stratified by renal replacement therapy modality have been stable; survival rates for patients receiving hemodialysis (73% to 89%) are higher than those receiving PD (49% to 64%) or CRRT (34% to 42%).[26,27] Worse survival in patients who receive PD or CRRT likely results from greater hemodynamic instability, which may preclude prescription of acute HD as such patients may not be able to tolerate associated rapid UF rates. However, a prospective pediatric study that controls for patients' illness severity comparing survival across modalities does not exist.

Acute drug intoxications and hyperammonemia secondary to inborn errors of metabolism are often best treated with hemodialysis since rapid drug removal is important to prevent morbidity, and hemodialysis is the most efficient RRT modality.[28,29] However, recent studies demonstrate that

CRRT with either the CVVHD or CVVH modality is the preferred treatment for hyperammonemia.[30-32]

Technical and Logistic Aspects of Renal Replacement Therapy Modalities

Choice of Therapy

In general, factors that determine the most optimal modality for a clinical situation include patient size, hemodynamic stability, and institutional expertise. PD and CRRT are better suited for patients with hemodynamic instability, since daily total ultrafiltration goals can be achieved over a 24-hour period instead of a 3- to 4-hour intermittent hemodialysis treatment. Table 40-1 outlines various advantages and disadvantages of various acute renal replacement therapy modalities.

Vascular Access

Provision of intermittent HD and CRRT requires vascular access. In the acute setting, the most common sites for catheter placement are the internal jugular, subclavian, and femoral veins. Avoidance of the subclavian vein is preferable in order to prevent subclavian vein stenosis in patients who may not recover renal function who would need permanent vascular access in the ipsilateral upper extremity. A study of adult patients reported increased recirculation and worse performance in catheters placed in the femoral vein versus subclavian or jugular veins,[33] but these data have not been reproduced in children. Catheter size should also be matched to patient size. In pediatric patients, catheter size must be matched to the size of the patient in order to provide for optimal blood flow while causing the least amount of vascular trauma. Table 40-2 lists catheter configurations and patient size combinations. The access prescription should allow for blood pump flow rates of 3 to 5 ml/kg/minute. A general guideline for maximal flow rate by catheter size follows: 5 French (20 to 30 ml/min), 7 French (40 to 60 ml/min), 8 French (80 to 100 ml/min), 9 French (120 to 130 ml/min), 10 French (150 to 200 ml/min), and 11 French (300 to 400 ml/min). In neonates, two separate single-lumen 5 French catheters are often required to provide acute renal replacement therapy. The umbilical vessels should be used as a last resort for acute RRT in neonates, since consistent adequate flow cannot be ensured.

TABLE 40-1 Advantages and Disadvantages of Various Acute Renal Replacement Therapy Modalities

Modality	Advantages	Disadvantages
Intermittent HD	Short treatment times Accurate UF	Vascular access necessary Hemodynamic instability Heparin anticoagulation
Peritoneal Dialysis	No need for vascular access Minimal equipment needs Minimal training needs Feasible in small infants Continuous treatment	Less efficient than HD/CRRT Variable UF dependent on BP
CRRT	Accurate UF that can be altered to account for changes in intake/patient BP Smaller circuit volumes Citrate anticoagulation	Vascular access necessary

BP, Blood pressure; *HD*, hemodialysis; *UF*, ultrafiltration; *CRRT*, continuous renal replacement therapy.

Peritoneal Dialysis

Acute PD requires much less technical expertise, expense, and equipment compared to intermittent hemodialysis and CRRT. PD catheters can be placed quickly and easily. Initial dwell volumes should be limited to 10 cc/kg of patient body weight in order to minimize intraabdominal pressure and potential for fluid leakage along the catheter tunnel. Although PD may deliver less-efficient solute removal than hemodialysis or CRRT, its relative simplicity and minimal associated side effects allow for renal replacement therapy provision in settings lacking pediatric dialysis–specific support and personnel. Tenckhoff catheters with one or two cuffs are the preferred catheter configuration for acute PD, even though the cuff may be left outside the patient's body in patients receiving acute PD after cardiac bypass surgery. Trocar catheters are obsolete secondary to inconsistent function.

CRRT

Continuous renal replacement therapy is defined as any extracorporeal blood purification therapy intended to substitute for impaired renal function over an extended period of time and prescribed for 24 hours per day. In general, CRRT may be divided into several basic modalities and definitions that are detailed below. The molecular transport mechanism employed with each modality is described first.

TABLE 40-2 Acute Catheter Configuration and Patient Size Combination

Patient Size	Catheter Size and Source	Site of Insertion
Neonate	Single-lumen 5 French (COOK) Dual-lumen 7.0 French (COOK/MEDCOMP)	Femoral artery or vein Femoral vein
3-6 kg	Dual-lumen 7.0 French (COOK/MEDCOMP) Triple-lumen 7.0 French (MEDCOMP)	Internal/external—Jugular, subclavian, or femoral vein Internal/external—Jugular, subclavian, or femoral vein
6-15 kg	Dual-lumen 8.0 French (KENDALL, ARROW)	Internal/external—Jugular, subclavian, or femoral vein
>15 kg	Dual-lumen 9.0 French (MEDCOMP)	Internal/external—Jugular, subclavian, or femoral vein
>30 kg	Dual-lumen 10.0 French (ARROW, KENDALL)	Internal/external—Jugular, subclavian, or femoral vein

Continuous Venovenous Hemofiltration

In continuous venovenous hemofiltration (CVVH), the ultrafiltration produced is replaced completely or in part by sterile filter replacement fluid. This technique provides a substantial amount of convection-based clearance, which allows for increased clearance of larger molecules, compared to purely diffusive techniques, and may therefore offer advantages in clearing pro- and anti-inflammatory cytokines. Small molecule clearances are similar between convective and diffusive modalities. The only potential drawback to CVVH is the need for increased blood pump flow rates to decrease the impact of increased ultrafiltration on intrafilter hemoconcentration.

Continuous Venovenous Hemodialysis

In continuous venovenous hemodialysis, the extracorporeal circuit is characterized by slow countercurrent dialysate flow into the ultrafiltrate-dialysate compartment of the membrane. Fluid replacement is not routinely administered. Solute clearance is diffusive. The pump from the filter controls not only the dialysate flow rate but also the UF volume.

Continuous Venovenous Hemodiafiltration

Continuous venovenous hemodiafiltration is a technique of CRRT whereby the CVVH circuit is modified by the addition of slow countercurrent dialysate flow to the ultrafiltrate-dialysate compartment of the membrane. Fluid replacement is routinely administered as clinically indicated to maintain desired fluid balance, as UF rate is greater than expected patient weight loss. Solute removal is both diffusive and convective.

Various CRRT aspects, including CRRT dose, dialysis/hemofiltration fluid composition, and anticoagulation methods have been studied in recent years. Until recently, most CRRT hemofiltration fluid or dialysis fluid used lactate as a buffer. A crossover study in adult patients receiving CRRT revealed that lactate-based solutions could lead to a rising serum lactate level in patients,[34] a phenomenon that could lead to unnecessary investigation for tissue ischemia. Bicarbonate-buffered solutions can be made by hospital pharmacies, but are also now available from industry sources.[35] A recent pediatric study has highlighted the potential patient safety implications with pharmacy-prepared solutions that can arise from compounding errors.[36] Thus, a solution composition validation program should exist in centers that opt to use pharmacy-made solutions for CRRT.

Small molecule clearance is similar for all CRRT modalities and is primarily limited by the rate of dialysis fluid or replacement fluid. Post-filter replacement fluid may achieve higher clearance than pre-dilution replacement fluid in CRRT, since the blood is diluted in the latter modality. Intermittent hemodialysis provides the most efficient small solute removal per unit time and is limited by the blood pump flow rate and dialyzer characteristics. However, both CRRT and PD may deliver greater daily small solute clearance if they are provided continuously over a 24 hour period.

A typical starting standard CRRT prescription would be a blood pump blood flow rate of 3-5 ml/kg/min and a small molecule clearance rate of 2000 ml/hr/1.73 m^2.

Several CRRT machines suitable for pediatric use are listed in Table 40-3. Membranes used in hemofiltration are designed with high hydraulic permeability to promote maximum ultrafiltration. They are manufactured from polymeric thermoplastics such as polysulfone, polyamide, polyacrylonitrile, and polymethylmethacrylate. The hemofiltration membrane is a composite structure consisting of an inner thin layer adjacent to the blood path surrounded by a supporting superstructure that provides mechanical integrity without restricting the passage of water or any solutes small enough to pass through the pores of the inner layer. Hemodialysis membranes contain long, tortuous interconnecting channels that result in higher resistance to fluid flow. The hemofiltration membrane consists of straight channels of increasing diameter that offer lower resistance to fluid flow. These membranes permit clearance of non–protein-bound molecules that have a molecular weight of less than 50,000 daltons.

All HF machines currently available in the market can provide circuit volumes that offer the adaptability to sustain therapy for smaller and larger size individuals. The Baxter, Braun, and the Fresenius machines allow for individual choice of hemofilter membrane while the PRISMA®/PRISMAFLEX® uses a single membrane (AN-69) incorporated into a cassette containing blood tubing and pressure pods. Table 40-4 lists the properties of various hemofilters and the choice of which is based on the local standard of care as opposed to clinical outcome.

TABLE 40-3 **Continuous Renal Replacement Therapy Machines**

				VOLUME TUBING SET	
Company	Machine	Blood Flow	Dialysate/Filtrate Flow	Neonatal	Pediatric
Edwards Lifesciences	Aquarius	10 to 450 ml/min	0 or 100 to 12,000 ml/hr	—	64 ml
Gambro	Prisma	10 to 180 ml/min	0 or 100 to 4500 ml/hr (CVVH)	50 ml*	90 ml*
	Prismaflex	10 to 450 ml/min	0 or100 to 2500 ml/hr (CVVHD) 0 to 8000 ml/hr (CVVH/CVVHD) 0 to 10,000 ml/hr (CVVHDF)	Not yet available	Not yet available
Baxter	Accura BM 25	30 to 450 ml/min 5 to 150 ml/min	0 or 100 to 10,000 ml/hr 0 or 50 to 9000 ml/hr	 47 ml	 79 ml

* Including hemofilter.

TABLE 40-4 **Continuous Renal Replacement Therapy Hemofilters**

Hemofilter	Properties/Surface Area	Priming Volume
Amicon	Polysulfone/0.07 m^2	15 ml
Minifilter Plus		
Renaflo II	Polysulfone	
HF 400	0.3 m^2	28 ml
HF 700	0.7 m^2	53 ml
HF 1200	1.25 m^2	83 ml
Gambro		
Multiflow 100	AN-69/0.8 m^2	107 ml
Multiflow 60	AN-69/0.6 m^2	84 ml
Multiflow 10	AN-69/0.3 m^2	50 ml
HF1000	Polysulfone/1.16 m^2	128 ml
Asahi PAN	Poly acrylonitrile	
0.3	0.3 m^2	33 ml
0.6	0.6 m^2	63 ml
1.0	1.0 m^2	78 ml

Anticoagulation

Anticoagulation of the CRRT circuit is essential to provide the therapy. Heparin and citrate are the two most common forms of anticoagulation. A standard CRRT heparin anticoagulation protocol is to start with a bolus of 25 units per/kg and then provide a continuous infusion of 10 units/kg/hour. Follow activated clotting times every 2 to 4 hours to keep ACT between 180 and 240 seconds. If the ACT is < 180 seconds increase the heparin infusion by 1 unit/kg/hour, if the ACT > 240 seconds, decrease the heparin infusion rate by 1 unit/kg/hour. The side effects of heparin include systemic anticoagulation and the rare occurrence of induction of heparin-induced thrombocytopenia.

Citrate anticoagulation occurs by decreasing the ionized calcium in the blood. CRRT circuits can undergo regional anticoagulation, where citrate is infused into the access line of the CRRT circuit and calcium is infused into a separate systemic central venous line or at the return line to maintain physiologic ionized calcium in the patient. A well-studied pediatric CRRT citrate anticoagulation protocol uses Baxter Anticoagulant Citrate Dextrose-A (ACD-A) solution infused (in ml/hr) at 1.5 times the blood pump rate (in ml/min). For example, if the blood pump rate is 100 ml/min, then the ACD-A rate should start at 150 ml/hour. To prevent patient systemic hypocalcemia, a solution of calcium chloride (8 grams in one liter NS) is infused back to the patient at 0.4 times the ACD-A rate. So, in the example, the $CaCl_2$ rate would be 60 ml/hour. Both patient and CRRT circuit ionized calcium levels should be measured every 4-6 hours to keep the levels at greater than 1 mmol/L and at 0.2-0.4 mmol/L, respectively. Serum total calcium should also be checked daily to assess for citrate lock. The potential complications of regional citrate anticoagulation include metabolic alkalosis (especially if used in combination with bicarbonate buffered CRRT replacement/dialysis solutions) and citrate lock. Citrate lock is a phenomenon where the delivery of citrate exceeds the patient's hepatic clearance. As a result, citrate concentrations increase in the blood and act as a buffer to bind calcium. Citrate lock is identified by decreasing serum ionized calcium in the presence of rising total calcium. The treatment for citrate lock is to discontinue citrate for 4 hours and then restart at a lower citrate delivery rate. Recent pediatric studies have reported practical and safe citrate anticoagulation protocols.[35,37,38]

Infants

Infants and neonates with ARF present unique problems for renal replacement therapy provision. As noted earlier, delivery of hemodialysis or CRRT to these small patients entails a significant portion of their blood volume to be pumped through the extracorporeal circuit. Therefore, extracorporeal circuit volumes that comprise more than 10% to 15% of patient blood volume (60 to 70 ml/kg dry body weight) should be primed with whole blood to prevent hypotension and anemia. Patient blood volume is 70 ml/kg of body weight for infants less than one year of age and 60 ml/kg for older children. Table 40-4 lists some smaller filters available for neonates, but many of these still comprise a significant proportion of neonate blood volume and still require blood priming.[39] Since the prime volume is not discarded, it is important to not re-infuse the blood into the patient at the end of the treatment in order to prevent volume overload and hypertension. Patients who receive CRRT with an AN-69 are at risk for the bradykinin release syndrome (BRS) when circuits require blood priming. The BRS leads to hypotension and can be mitigated by normalizing the blood pH and giving a calcium bolus to the patient to counter the citrate in the blood unit.[40]

Congenital Heart Disease

Infants with ARF after corrective congenital heart surgery comprise a well-studied cohort. These patients represent a nearly unique group in that the timing of the event leading to ARF, namely cardiopulmonary bypass (CPB), is precisely known. In this sense, children undergoing cardiopulmonary bypass are akin to adults receiving nephrotoxic radiologic contrast or emergent surgery for aortic aneurysms; they all provide an opportunity to follow the time course of ARF from beginning to end in patients without significant underlying renal disease.

The incidence of infant ARF after CPB ranges from 2.7% to 5.3% with survival rates ranging from 21% to 70%.[41-43] Risk factors for mortality include increasing underlying complexity of the congenital heart disease and poor cardiac function. A recent trend toward providing PD therapy earlier in the post-CPB course has been reported, with one study of 20 patients demonstrating 80% patient survival.[44] While improved survival with early PD initiation may result from prevention of fluid overload, some posit improved survival with early PD initiation results from increased clearance of CPB-induced pro-inflammatory cytokines, although further study is required to support this hypothesis.[45]

Multiorgan Dysfunction Syndrome

The critically ill patient population with multiorgan dysfunction syndrome has been a focus of significant outcome study in recent years. The concept that worsening fluid overload is associated with worse outcome in critically ill pediatric patients with multiorgan dysfunction syndrome who require renal replacement therapy has been the focus of recent pediatric studies. Both single-center data[27,46-48] and a multicenter effort, the Prospective Pediatric Continuous Renal Replacement Therapy Registry Group[49] demonstrate that worsening fluid overload is an independent risk factor for mortality, irrespective of severity of illness, in patients who receive CRRT.[50] These data, coupled with the predilection for early multiorgan system failure and death in critically ill children with ARF,[51,52] may argue for early and aggressive initiation of renal replacement therapy in association with a goal-directed fluid repletion strategy in patients with multiorgan dysfunction syndrome.

Stem Cell Transplantation

Stem cell transplant recipients are at risk for ARF from a number of causes including nephrotoxic medications, radiation-induced nephropathy, and a hepatorenal-like syndrome associated with vaso-occlusive disease. Early recognition of ARF and prevention of fluid overload in patients with a recent stem cell transplant is critical since the need for mechanical ventilation in these patients is associated with increased mortality. Recent pediatric studies have demonstrated that aggressive fluid control with early initiation of diuretics and CRRT can lead to improved survival in children with stem cell transplantation and ARF.[53,54]

REFERENCES

1. Holliday MA, Segar WE: The maintenance need for water in parenteral fluid therapy, *Pediatrics* 19:823-32, 1957.
2. Rivers E, Nguyen B, Havstad S, et al: Early goal-directed therapy in the treatment of severe sepsis and septic shock, *N Engl J Med* 345:1368-77, 2001.
3. Trzeciak S, Dellinger RP, Abate NL, et al: Translating research to clinical practice: a 1-year experience with implementing early goal-directed therapy for septic shock in the emergency department, *Chest* 129:225-32, 2006.
4. Carcillo JA, Fields AI: Clinical practice parameters for hemodynamic support of pediatric and neonatal patients in septic shock, *Crit Care Med* 30:1365-78, 2002.
5. Simmons RS, Berdine GG, Seidenfeld JJ, et al: Fluid balance and the adult respiratory distress syndrome, *Am Rev Respir Dis* 135:924-29, 1987.
6. Humphrey H, Hall J, Sznajder I, et al: Improved survival in ARDS patients associated with a reduction in pulmonary capillary wedge pressure, *Chest* 97:1176-80, 1990.
7. Schuller D, Mitchell JP, Calandrino FS, et al: Fluid balance during pulmonary edema. Is fluid gain a marker or a cause of poor outcome? *Chest* 100:1068-75, 1991.
8. Lameire NH, De Vriese AS, Vanholder R: Prevention and nondialytic treatment of acute renal failure, *Curr Opin Crit Care* 9:481-90, 2003.
9. Lassnigg A, Donner E, Grubhofer G, et al: Lack of renoprotective effects of dopamine and furosemide during cardiac surgery, *J Am Soc Nephrol* 11:97-104, 2000.
10. Baldwin L, Henderson A, Hickman P: Effect of postoperative low-dose dopamine on renal function after elective major vascular surgery, *Ann Intern Med* 120:744-47, 1994.
11. Schenarts PJ, Sagraves SG, Bard MR, et al: Low-dose dopamine: a physiologically based review, *Curr Surg* 63:219-25, 2006.
12. Lauschke A, Teichgraber UK, Frei U, et al: "Low-dose" dopamine worsens renal perfusion in patients with acute renal failure, *Kidney Int* 69:1669-74, 2006.
13. Schetz M: Vasopressors and the kidney, *Blood Purif* 20:243-51, 2002.
14. Tsuneyoshi I, Yamada H, Kakihana Y, et al: Hemodynamic and metabolic effects of low-dose vasopressin infusions in vasodilatory septic shock, *Crit Care Med* 29:487-93, 2001.
15. Shilliday IR, Quinn KJ, Allison ME: Loop diuretics in the management of acute renal failure: a prospective, double-blind, placebo-controlled, randomized study, *Nephrol Dial Transplant* 12:2592-96, 1997.
16. Klinge J: Intermittent administration of furosemide or continuous infusion in critically ill infants and children: does it make a difference? *Intensive Care Med* 27:623-24, 2001.
17. Samuels J, Finkel K, Gubert M, et al: Effect of fenoldopam mesylate in critically ill patients at risk for acute renal failure is dose dependent, *Ren Fail* 27:101-105, 2005.
18. Tumlin JA, Finkel KW, Murray PT, et al: Fenoldopam mesylate in early acute tubular necrosis: a randomized, double-blind, placebo-controlled clinical trial, *Am J Kidney Dis* 46:26-34, 2005.
19. Safirstein R, Andrade L, Vieira JM: Acetylcysteine and nephrotoxic effects of radiographic contrast agents—a new use for an old drug, *N Engl J Med* 343:210-12, 2000.
20. Boccalandro F, Amhad M, Smalling RW, et al: Oral acetylcysteine does not protect renal function from moderate to high doses of intravenous radiographic contrast, *Catheter Cardiovasc Interv* 58:336-41, 2003.
21. Briguori C, Manganelli F, Scarpato P, et al: Acetylcysteine and contrast agent-associated nephrotoxicity, *J Am Coll Cardiol* 40:298-303, 2002.
22. Hladunewich MA, Corrigan G, Derby GC, et al: A randomized, placebo-controlled trial of IGF-1 for delayed graft function: a human model to study postischemic ARF, *Kidney Int* 64:593-602, 2003.
23. Acker CG, Singh AR, Flick RP, et al: A trial of thyroxine in acute renal failure, *Kidney Int* 57:293-98, 2000.
24. Bunchman TE, Maxvold NJ, Kershaw DB, et al: Continuous venovenous hemodiafiltration in infants and children, *Am J Kidney Dis* 25:17-21, 1995.
25. Warady BA, Bunchman T: Dialysis therapy for children with acute renal failure: survey results, *Pediatr Nephrol* 15:11-13, 2000.
26. Bunchman TE, McBryde KD, Mottes TE, et al: Pediatric acute renal failure: outcome by modality and disease, *Pediatr Nephrol* 16:1067-71, 2001.
27. Goldstein SL, Currier H, Graf C, et al: Outcome in children receiving continuous venovenous hemofiltration, *Pediatrics* 107:1309-12, 2001.
28. Brusilow SW, Danney M, Waber LJ, et al: Treatment of episodic hyperammonemia in children with inborn errors of urea synthesis, *N Engl J Med* 310:1630-34, 1984.
29. McBryde KD, Kudelka TL, Kershaw DB, et al: Clearance of amino acids by hemodialysis in argininosuccinate synthetase deficiency, *J Pediatr* 144:536-40, 2004.
30. Askenazi DJ, Goldstein SL, Chang IF, et al: Management of a severe carbamazepine overdose using albumin-enhanced continuous venovenous hemodialysis, *Pediatrics* 113:406-409, 2004.
31. Picca S, Dionisi-Vici C, Abeni D, et al: Extracorporeal dialysis in neonatal hyperammonemia: modalities and prognostic indicators, *Pediatr Nephrol* 16:862-67, 2001.
32. Schaefer F, Straube E, Oh J, et al: Dialysis in neonates with inborn errors of metabolism, *Nephrol Dial Transplant* 14:910-18, 1999.
33. Little MA, Conlon PJ, Walshe JJ: Access recirculation in temporary hemodialysis catheters as measured by the saline dilution technique, *Am J Kidney Dis* 36:1135-39, 2000.
34. Zimmerman D, Cotman P, Ting R, et al: Continuous veno-venous haemodialysis with a novel bicarbonate dialysis solution: prospective cross-over comparison with a lactate buffered solution, *Nephrol Dial Transplant* 14:2387-91, 1999.
35. Bunchman TE, Maxvold NJ, Barnett J, et al: Pediatric hemofiltration: Normocarb dialysate solution with citrate anticoagulation, *Pediatr Nephrol* 17:150-54, 2002.
36. Barletta JF, Barletta GM, Brophy PD, et al: Medication errors and patient complications with continuous renal replacement therapy, *Pediatr Nephrol* 21:842-45, 2006.
37. Brophy PD, Somers MJ, Baum MA, et al: Multi-centre evaluation of anticoagulation in patients receiving continuous renal replacement therapy (CRRT), *Nephrol Dial Transplant* 20:1416-21, 2005.

38. Bunchman TE, Maxvold NJ, Brophy PD: Pediatric convective hemofiltration: Normocarb replacement fluid and citrate anticoagulation, *Am J Kidney Dis* 42:1248-52, 2003.
39. Goldstein SL, Hackbarth R, Bunchman TE, et al: Evaluation of the PRISMA M10 circuit in critically ill infants with acute kidney injury: a report from the Prospective Pediatric CRRT Registry Group, *Int J Artif Organs* 29:1105-108, 2006.
40. Brophy PD, Mottes TA, Kudelka TL, et al: AN-69 membrane reactions are pH-dependent and preventable, *Am J Kidney Dis* 38:173-78, 2001.
41. Book K, Ohqvist G, Bjork VO, et al: Peritoneal dialysis in infants and children after open heart surgery, *Scand J Thorac Cardiovasc Surg* 16:229-33, 1982.
42. Rigden SP, Barratt TM, Dillon MJ, et al: Acute renal failure complicating cardiopulmonary bypass surgery, *Arch Dis Child* 57:425-30, 1982.
43. Picca S, Principato F, Mazzera E, et al: Risks of acute renal failure after cardiopulmonary bypass surgery in children: a retrospective 10-year case-control study, *Nephrol Dial Transplant* 10:630-36, 1995.
44. Sorof JM, Stromberg D, Brewer ED, et al: Early initiation of peritoneal dialysis after surgical repair of congenital heart disease, *Pediatr Nephrol* 13:641-45, 1999.
45. Bokesch PM, Kapural MB, Mossad EB, et al: Do peritoneal catheters remove pro-inflammatory cytokines after cardiopulmonary bypass in neonates? *Ann Thorac Surg* 70:639-43, 2000.
46. Goldstein SL, Somers MJ, Baum MA, et al: Pediatric patients with multi-organ dysfunction syndrome receiving continuous renal replacement therapy, *Kidney Int* 67:653-58, 2005.
47. Gillespie RS, Seidel K, Symons JM: Effect of fluid overload and dose of replacement fluid on survival in hemofiltration, *Pediatr Nephrol* 19:1394-99, 2004.
48. Foland JA, Fortenberry JD, Warshaw BL, et al: Fluid overload before continuous hemofiltration and survival in critically ill children: a retrospective analysis, *Crit Care Med* 32:1771-76, 2004.
49. Goldstein SL, Somers MJ, Brophy PD, et al: The Prospective Pediatric Continuous Renal Replacement Therapy (ppCRRT) Registry: design, development and data assessed, *Int J Artif Organs* 27:9-14, 2004.
50. Kim JJ, Denfield SW, McKenzie ED, et al: Mechanical circulatory support as a bridge to combined dual organ transplantation in children, *J Heart Lung* 25:1480-82, 2006.
51. Proulx F, Fayon M, Farrell CA, et al: Epidemiology of sepsis and multiple organ dysfunction syndrome in children, *Chest* 109:1033-37, 1996.
52. Proulx F, Gauthier M, Nadeau D, et al: Timing and predictors of death in pediatric patients with multiple organ system failure, *Crit Care Med* 22:1025-31, 1994.
53. Michael M, Kuehnle I, Goldstein SL: Fluid overload and acute renal failure in pediatric stem cell transplant patients, *Pediatr Nephrol* 19:91-95, 2004.
54. DiCarlo JV, Alexander SR, Agarwal R, et al: Continuous venovenous hemofiltration may improve survival from acute respiratory distress syndrome after bone marrow transplantation or chemotherapy, *J Pediatr Hematol Oncol* 25:801-805, 2003.

CHAPTER 41

Epidemiology and Consequences of Childhood Hypertension

Empar Lurbe, Juan J. Alcon, and Josep Redon

INTRODUCTION

During the last few years there has been a renewed interest in measuring blood pressure (BP) in children and adolescents after the recognition that besides the presence of secondary hypertension, in most cases caused by renal diseases, essential hypertension is common in adolescents. Furthermore, the long-term health risk for hypertensive children and adolescents can be substantial. This chapter will review the epidemiology and consequences of hypertension in the pediatric age group.

Hypertension in children has specific characteristics that need to be highlighted.[1] To begin with, hypertension in children, as defined by casual BP values, is not well correlated to any particular form of hypertensive target-organ damage. No single cut-off point defines hypertension in a pediatric patient, making identification of childhood hypertension difficult. Physicians have traditionally used population-based percentiles to define pediatric hypertension. Next, pediatric hypertension is associated with a broad spectrum of underlying diseases that change from childhood through adolescence. Definable causes of hypertension are the rule in the early years of life, whereas essential hypertension is more common in adolescence. Consequently, techniques for the evaluation and diagnosis of hypertension differ, at least in part, by age group.

DEFINITION OF HYPERTENSION

Two facts regarding levels and distribution of casual BP in childhood and adolescence are well accepted: blood pressure increases steadily during growth and maturation, and adolescence is a fast growth period during which body mass and BP change rapidly.[2] For these reasons, reference BP values specific to gender, age, and/or height have been introduced for children and adolescents (Table 41-1).

In 1977, the first age-related norms for BP in children were developed by the Task Force for Blood Pressure in Children, a group sponsored by the National Heart, Lung and Blood Institute and by the National Institutes of Health.[3] In 1987, a revision of the standards evaluated data from more than 70,000 Caucasian, African-American, and Hispanic children.[4] Age-specific percentile curves of BP measurements for boys and girls ranging in age from birth to 18 years were created. In addition, these revised standards defined the proper techniques for measuring BP in infants, children, and adolescents. All measurements used in constructing the Task Force's tables were made with a standard mercury sphygmomanometer placed on the child's right arm, using a cuff size that covered 80% to 100% of arm circumference. In 1996, the Task Force became aware of the importance of considering age and height together when defining reference values.[5] This approach avoids misclassifying children at the extremes of normal growth since tall children will not be misclassified as hypertensive, and very short children with high normal BP or even hypertension will not be missed. In children of the same age, the upper limit of systolic BP normality for the third percentile of height is 8 to 9 mm Hg lower than the values for the 90th percentile. At the same time, the Task Force redefined diastolic BP as the fifth rather than the fourth Korotkoff sound for children in all age groups. No changes to the standards for systolic BP and diastolic BP for infants younger than 1 year were reported in the 1996 update.

Recently, the fourth report of the Task Force[6] defined as normal systolic and diastolic BP lower than the 90th percentile for age, gender, and height. Hypertension is defined as average SBP and/or DBP that is greater than or equal to the

TABLE 41-1 Classification of Hypertension in Children and Adolescents

	SBP or DBP Percentile
Normal	<90th
High-normal (prehypertension)	≥90th to <95th ≥120/80 even if below 90th percentile in adolescents
Stage 1 hypertension	95th percentile to 99th percentile plus 5 mm Hg
Stage 2 hypertension	>99th percentile plus 5 mm Hg

Source: National High Blood Pressure Education Program Working Group on High Blood Pressure in Children and Adolescents: the fourth report on the diagnosis, evaluation and treatment of high blood pressure in children and adolescents. *Pediatrics* 114:555-76, 2004.

95th percentile for age, gender, and height on three or more occasions. Average SBP and/or DBP levels that are 90th percentile or greater but less than the 95th percentile had been designated as prehypertension. As with adults, it is now recommended that children and adolescents with BP levels of 120/80 mm Hg or greater, even if below the 90th percentile, should be considered prehypertensive as well.

An additional point of interest included in the most recent Task Force report was the introduction of comments concerning oscillometric devices for measuring BP. The BP tables are based on auscultatory measurements; therefore, the preferred method of measurement is auscultation. Oscillometric devices are convenient and minimize observer error, but they do not provide measurements that are identical to auscultation. Therefore, to confirm hypertension, BP in children should be measured with a standard clinical sphygmomanometer using a stethoscope placed over the brachial artery pulse.

PREVALENCE

The prevalence of hypertension in children is reported to be 1%.[4] In recent years, the prevalence in school-aged children appeared to be increasing, perhaps resulting from greater prevalence of obesity. The majority of these children have mild hypertension, most often primary. A small group of children have much higher blood pressures, usually due to a secondary cause.

Hypertension in children and adolescents depends on the demographic characteristics of the subjects analyzed, age, gender, and body weight, as well as ethnicity. Prevalence increases in parallel with age; the highest prevalence is in older children and boys have a larger prevalence than do girls in all the screening studies. Body weight has the greatest impact on the rate of hypertension. The role of ethnicity in prevalences is controversial: compared to Caucasians, a higher BP in Hispanics and African Americans, and a lower BP in Asians has been observed.[7] In a study carried out in a school-based screening, however, ethnic differences in the prevalence of hypertension were not significant after controlling for overweight/obesity. Prevalence increased progressively as the body mass index (BMI) percentile increased from 2% in a BMI percentile below the 5th to 11% in those children in a percentile above the 95th.[8]

In addition to characteristics of subjects, the number of BP measurements is crucial in the prevalence of hypertension. Two studies, by the Task Force in 1987[4] and by Sinaiko et al.[9] in 1989, found the prevalence of hypertension in the general population to be only 1%. In a study published in 2001,[10] using the Task Force standards of 1996,[5] the combined prevalence of systolic and diastolic hypertension in junior high school–aged children did not substantially change from the previously reported level. Statistically, 5% of children had a BP measurement above the 95th percentile recorded during a single office visit. Blood pressure, however, tended to normalize on subsequent measurements due to the accommodation of the child to the measurement procedure and to the statistical phenomenon of regression toward the mean.[11] Consequently, the prevalence of hypertension decreased to 1% after only one repeated examination. The diagnostic algorithm of hypertension is found in Figure 41-1.

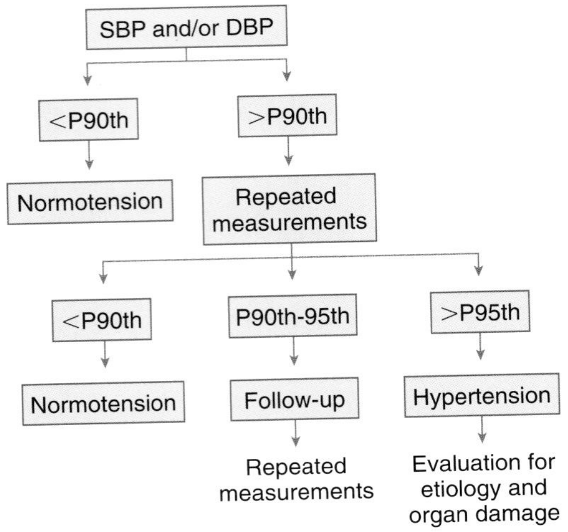

Figure 41-1 Diagnostic algorithm of hypertension in children and adolescents. P90th/95th, 90th/95th percentile.

SIGNIFICANCE OF AMBULATORY BLOOD PRESSURE

In young people, BP variability and observer bias limit the reliability of office measurements that have the potential for inaccuracies.[12] Automated techniques of BP measurement may overcome these limitations; therefore, ambulatory BP monitoring became an established instrument for the diagnosis of hypertension in children and adolescents.[13]

Simultaneous measurements of office and ambulatory BP delineate four conditions. In normotensive and hypertensive children, both the conventional and the daytime ambulatory BP are consistently normal or elevated, respectively. White-coat hypertension, also known as isolated clinic hypertension, is the transient elevation of a patient's BP in response to the observer measuring BP[14,15]; daytime ambulatory BP is normal in the presence of office hypertension. In adults, 37% of patients with white-coat hypertension evolved to persistent hypertension over a follow-up period of 0.5 to 6.5 years.[16] The opposite phenomenon, masked hypertension or isolated ambulatory hypertension, consists of an elevated daytime or awake ambulatory BP, but a normal office BP measurement.[17,18] In adults, masked hypertension is associated with increased left ventricular mass[19] and a negative cardiovascular prognosis.[20]

In the largest pediatric study to date, Sorof and Portman[21] reported in children referred for evaluation of hypertension that the frequency of white-coat hypertension was 35% (40/115) for all referred patients and 22% (11/51) for patients with confirmed clinical hypertension. Although these results suggest that the phenomenon of white-coat hypertension does occur commonly in children, it should be emphasized that white-coat hypertension may not be an entirely benign condition, and in fact may represent a prehypertensive state. There are currently no data on the long-term follow-up of children found to have white-coat hypertension on initial assessment.

In a recent study of 592 healthy Spanish children and adolescents,[22] 535 subjects were normotensive using both office as well as daytime ambulatory BP measurement (90.4%), and 45 had masked hypertension (7.6%). Compared to normotensive controls, participants with masked hypertension had a higher ambulatory pulse rate, were more obese, and were 2.5 times more likely to have a parental history of hypertension. Among 34 patients with masked hypertension (median follow-up 37 months), 18 became normotensive, 13 had persistent masked hypertension, and 3 developed sustained hypertension. Patients with persistent masked hypertension or who progressed from masked to sustained hypertension had a higher left ventricular mass index, and a higher percentage had a left ventricular mass index above the 95th percentile than normotensive controls.

Individuals with masked hypertension had a higher ambulatory pulse rate than did normotensive subjects, were more obese, and were more than twice as likely to have a parental history of hypertension. These three characteristics, alone or in combination, predict the development of hypertension and increase cardiovascular risk later in life. Tachycardia and high BMI are usually accompanied by the stimulation of the sympathetic nervous system, which together with elevated daytime BP and obesity might underlie the development of left ventricular hypertrophy in youths with masked hypertension even before these proceed to sustained hypertension.[23,24] Approximately 50% of this population with persistent masked hypertension had a positive parental history of hypertension. This is in agreement with previous epidemiological studies demonstrating that children with a positive familial history of hypertension had a higher BP than those without such a history.[25] This association was even more pronounced when parents became hypertensive early in life.[26] In children and adolescents, masked hypertension is a precursor of sustained hypertension and left ventricular hypertrophy. This condition warrants follow-up and, once it becomes persistent, is an indication for BP-lowering treatment.

Apart from the ability of ambulatory BP monitoring to obtain more accurate and reproducible BP values,[27] another advantage of this method is the assessment of BP during sleep and, therefore, the estimation of circadian variability.[28] There is a physiological nocturnal fall of BP during sleep in response to the reduction of the sympathetic tone. Patients with renal disease and/or volume expansion are consistently found to have abnormalities in circadian BP variability with a high prevalence of the so-called nondipping pattern, that is, a blunted nocturnal fall. Although this may be related to the severity of hypertension, as in subjects with renovascular hypertension, in the majority of the other underlying causes the degree of hypertension does not predict the amount of circadian variation.[29,30]

ETIOLOGY

Sustained hypertension in children and adolescents is usually classified as secondary, with a specific potentially correctable cause, or as essential, that is, without an identifiable cause.[4] The most common causes of hypertension change during childhood. Essential hypertension is rarely seen in infants and young children, but its prevalence increases significantly in adolescence.[31] A good general rule to follow is that the likelihood of identifying a secondary cause of hypertension is inversely related to the age of the child and directly related to the degree of BP elevation. Consequently, the evaluation of children with hypertension, especially young children and those with severe hypertension, should be comprehensive and aimed at identifying known causes of the disease.

TABLE 41-2 Most Common Causes of Hypertension by Age Group

<1 Month	>6-10 Years
Renal arterial thrombosis	Renal parenchymal disease
Coarctation of the aorta	Renovascular disease
Congenital renal disease	Essential hypertension
Bronchopulmonary dysplasia	
>1 Month to <6 Years	>10-18 Years
Renal parenchymal disease	Essential hypertension
Coarctation of the aorta	Renal parenchymal disease
Renovascular disease	Renovascular disease

Definable causes of hypertension are associated with a broad spectrum of diseases. The distribution of causes clearly varies with age (Table 41-2). Renal parenchymal disorders predominate, accounting for a majority of secondary causes.[32] Renal parenchymal disorders with renovascular disease, and coarctation of the aorta account for 70% to 90% of all cases.[33,34] These figures vary depending on age structure, type of referral center, and referral bias. Additionally, hypertension is often related to prescribed drugs with hypertensiogenic potential. Infrequent causes of sustained hypertension, such as tumors and central nervous system and endocrine system disorders, must be considered only when the more common causes of secondary hypertension have been eliminated. An emerging cause of secondary hypertension is a single gene mutation that produces profound elevation of BP.[35]

Hypertension in term or preterm neonates may be seen in up to 2% of all infants in modern neonatal intensive care units. Although the definition of hypertension in this age group has not been completely standardized, useful data have been published[36] and may be used to facilitate the identification of such infants. As in older children, the causes of hypertension in neonates are numerous, with the two largest categories being renovascular and parenchymal diseases. More specifically, umbilical artery catheter–associated thromboembolism affecting either the aorta and/or the renal arteries probably accounts for the majority of cases of hypertension seen in the typical neonatal intensive care unit.[37] A careful history and physical examination will usually identify the cause in most cases, without the need for extensive laboratory or radiological testing.

In very young children (<6 years), hypertension is most often the result of such renal parenchymal disease as glomerulonephritis, renal scarring, polycystic kidney diseases, and renal dysplasia. Renal artery stenosis and cardiovascular disorders like coarctation of the aorta, less frequent causes of hypertension in this age group, are usually detected within the first decade of life. Late in the first decade and throughout the second, essential hypertension is the most common cause of sustained hypertension, particularly in those children with mild asymptomatic disease.[38,39]

When confronted with an infant, child, or adolescent with hypertension, the first question to be asked concerns the chronicity of the problem. Clearly, the most helpful information to have when one is attempting to establish the hypertension chronicity is past BP readings. Unfortunately, these are usually unavailable since routine BP measurements in children over 3 years of age are not yet uniformly obtained. In the absence of previous readings, one needs to look for the evidence of target-organ damage.

Faced with a child with chronic hypertension of unknown etiology, a diagnostic evaluation is based to some degree on the level of BP, age, clinical findings, and family history. Careful selection of the necessary tests often shortens the diagnostic process (see Chapter 42).

HYPERTENSION IN KIDNEY DISEASES

The use of office BP has demonstrated that children with renal disease frequently have levels in the hypertensive range.[40,41] Hypertension is more prevalent in patients with polycystic kidney disease or with glomerulonephritis than in those with structural renal disease. An increase in BP as a consequence of kidney disease contributes to the progression of renal damage. A rapid progression of renal damage may result in end-stage renal insufficiency during childhood.

Both renal insufficiency and cardiovascular damage contribute to the high mortality rate in patients with hypertensive renal disease. With the decline in the number of functional nephrons, a further increase in BP occurs, creating a vicious cycle that progresses to end-stage renal disease. Furthermore, progressive vascular disease compromises renal blood supply and contributes still further to the vicious cycle by increasing renal damage.

Since hypertension is prevalent in renal disease and the benefits of strict BP control are great, an accurate measurement of BP and the assessment of the response to antihypertensive treatment are important. The regular use of ambulatory BP monitoring in patients with renal disease not only permits a better assessment of BP control, but also frequently uncovers circadian variability abnormalities. A blunted nocturnal BP fall, the nondipper pattern, is characteristic for renal failure, regardless of etiology. The role of the pattern as either a marker or a pathogenic factor for kidney damage has been stressed in many studies.[42]

Patients with a decrease in glomerular filtration rate (GFR) are likely to show less of a nocturnal dip in BP, and frequently show an increase in nocturnal versus daytime BP levels when compared with the BP profiles from normotensives or hypertensives with a normal GFR.[43-45] The prevalence of nondipping rises with worsening renal function, reaching statistical significance once plasma creatinine exceeds 400 micromol/l.[45] When end-stage renal disease is reached, more than 70% of patients exhibit the nondipper pattern. This figure remains constant during renal replacement therapy.

After renal transplantation, an insufficient nocturnal BP decline is found almost universally in adults as well as in children.[46-51] Some of these patients may experience reverse dipping, with nighttime BP exceeding daytime BP. In a study by Sorof et al.,[49] 72% showed an attenuated decline in nocturnal systolic BP, with 24% having greater nighttime than daytime BP.

Even in the absence of renal insufficiency, the prevalence of the nondipper pattern is high in certain diseases such as autosomic dominant polycystic kidney disease,[52] reflux nephropathy,[53,54] and type 1 diabetes.[55] The greatest amount of information has been obtained for type 1 diabetes.

The spectrum of abnormalities of circadian BP variability through all nephropathy stages of type 1 diabetes shows a persistently blunted nocturnal BP fall in about 58% of the microalbuminuric and 80% of the proteinuric subjects. The reduced BP nocturnal fall is independent of the disease duration.[56] In type 1 diabetes, the presence of persistent microalbuminuria represents an early BP dysregulation during sleep even in the absence of hypertension. When overt nephropathy is established, hypertension is present and abnormalities in the circadian BP profile are more conspicuous. A pathogenic role of nocturnal systolic BP has been related to the development of microalbuminuria in normotensive type 1 diabetics.[57] An increase in BP during sleep precedes the development of microalbuminuria, whereas in those whose BP decreased normally during sleep the progression to microalbuminuria was less frequent.

The mechanisms underlying the abnormal circadian variation are not well understood. A role of sympathetic overdrive has been rendered unlikely by a study comparing plasma norepinephrine values in dipper and nondipper end-stage renal disease subjects.[58] Some authors affirm that the nondipper pattern in subjects with end-stage renal disease may be related to autonomic neuropathy or glucocorticoid treatment rather than to end-stage renal disease itself.[59]

Whether abnormal circadian variability contributes to further kidney damage is a matter of debate. Some evidence supports the potential role of systemic BP transmission as a mechanism of inducing renal damage, whereas other evidence supports the nondipping pattern as a consequence of the renal damage itself. Neither the cause nor the consequence interpretation of these data is mutually exclusive. In some cases, higher BP values during nighttime may contribute to the progression toward renal insufficiency, while in other cases the values are but a consequence of altered renal function itself. In the latter, higher BP may also participate in accelerating the loss of renal function, contributing in turn to more severe hypertension.

Published information regarding the prognostic value of abnormalities in circadian BP variability in the development of renal damage is still scarce in adults and absent in children. Existing data have been obtained from studies in small cohorts. Timio et al.[60] observed the impact of the nondipping pattern on renal function in a longitudinal study.[60] They observed that the slope of 1/Scr was steeper and urinary albumin excretion more pronounced in nondipper subjects, indicating a role of nocturnal BP as a prognostic marker and suggesting an impact of the nocturnal BP burden on progressive renal dysfunction. Hence, the assessment of nocturnal BP may become an important component in the attempt to optimize the nephroprotective effect of antihypertensive therapy. Furthermore, the presence of nocturnal hypertension can contribute not only accelerated progression of renal failure, but also to the development of more severe hypertensive cardiovascular disease.

However, the optimal nocturnal BP goal has not yet been defined in prospective studies. Moreover, while casual and 24-hour ambulatory BP values consistently above the 95th percentile for age, gender, and height are considered an indication to initiate antihypertensive treatment in children and adolescents,[5] the isolated presence of a nondipping pattern with absolute BP values below the 95th percentile has not been deemed sufficient cause to start treatment. Future studies are required to address this specific point.

CONSEQUENCES

Although it is generally agreed that early essential hypertension poses little immediate risk to most children, it carries the potential for future end-organ damage. In children, the accurate identification of hypertension at the earliest possible age would, therefore, give health care providers the opportunity to initiate preventive measures, thereby reducing the chance of developing end-organ damage and its concomitant morbidity and mortality. Consequently, repeated BP measurements over time should become a routine part of pediatric well-child care.

Because overt morbid cardiovascular events are rare in the majority of hypertensive children, attention has focused on other markers of hypertension injury, such as early renal damage, increased left ventricular mass index, and functional or organic vascular abnormalities. Cardiovascular damage develops in parallel to renal damage, although the cardiovascular sequelae of childhood onset hypertension, such as left ventricular hypertrophy and dysfunction and atherosclerosis, may not become clinically relevant before adulthood.

Heart

The abnormal increase of left ventricular mass and/or geometry has been recognized as one of the most important markers of risk for hypertension-induced cardiovascular morbidity and mortality in adults. In children and adolescents, the relationship between hypertension and left ventricular mass is more difficult to recognize because children and adolescents grow rapidly and their BP physiologically increases with age.

Cross-sectional studies have shown that the major determinants of left ventricular growth are body size and sex, with a smaller contribution made by BP.[61,62] The important contribution of the somatic growth and the recognition that lean body mass contributes somewhat more to cardiac growth than fat mass were nicely demonstrated in the Bogalusa Heart Study.[63] In a longitudinal study, left ventricular mass tracked from early to late adolescence to about the same degree as other important risk factors, such as BP and cholesterol.[64] Recently, the potential role of obesity in the increment of left ventricular mass has been highlighted. Obesity and left ventricular mass are related in childhood, and this association tracks and becomes stronger in young adulthood. Moreover, the increase in left ventricular mass from childhood to young adult age is related to the degree of increase in body mass index.[65]

Studies of normal and hypertensive children have found that systolic BP and left ventricular mass index are positively associated across a wide range of BP values, with no clear threshold to predict pathologically increased left ventricular mass index. Sensitivity and response to hemodynamic load seem to vary with age, sex, and ethnicity, which explains some of the differences among published results.

Although epidemiological studies do not help to establish the difference between appropriate and excessive increases in left ventricular mass, operational thresholds have been established. Both the allometric definition of excessive mass ($>38.5\ g/m^{2.7}$) as well as the percentile distribution of mass and geometry have been recommended. Using these operational thresholds, a few studies have analyzed the prevalence of left ventricular hypertrophy in healthy as well as hypertensive children and adolescents. In hypertensive children, the prevalence of left ventricular hypertrophy ranges from 24% to 40% in different pediatric studies.[66-70]

The relationship between left ventricular mass index and systolic BP is more evident when BP is measured using 24-hour ambulatory BP monitoring. Consequently, the hemodynamic load seems to play a more important role in the growth of left ventricular mass than previously recognized by using office BP. Accordingly, left ventricular mass tends to be greater in those groups with a higher ambulatory BP. In one cross-sectional study, both subjects with sustained hypertension as well as masked hypertensives had significantly higher left ventricular mass index than confirmed normotensive subjects.[69] Moreover, in a group with adolescents who had sustained masked hypertension, the left ventricular mass index was significantly higher than that observed in normotensive adolescents.[22]

Cardiac end-organ damage from hypertension exists in children, and left ventricular mass assessment seems to be important in the management of childhood hypertension, since it is the most prominent evidence of target-organ damage in childhood hypertension. The Task Force for BP in children has recommended performing echocardiography in all hypertensive children and in prehypertensive children with diabetes or kidney disease.[6]

The presence of left ventricular hypertrophy is an indicator to initiate or intensify antihypertensive therapy. Studies assessing the effect of medical therapy of pediatric hypertension on left ventricular mass need to be performed in the future to further reinforce the necessity of monitoring left ventricular mass.

Kidney

Evidence of the importance of BP values in the progression of renal disease has come from several clinical studies in children with or without established renal insufficiency. In a randomized multicenter study[41] in children with chronic renal failure, a significant difference in the loss of the GFR was related to systolic BP. In those with systolic BP above 120 mm Hg, a steeper decline of GFR was observed. In this study, the decrease in creatinine clearance strongly correlated with absolute BP rather than with height-corrected BP. The correlation between the decrease in creatinine clearance and BP was found even when BP was generally well controlled according to conventional criteria used to define BP control.

These data suggest that BP in the low normal range should probably be the target BP for patients with renal disease[71,72] (see Chapter 45).

Besides the GFR reduction, an increase in urinary albumin excretion is a marker of hypertension-induced renal damage. Proteinuria is a marker of glomerular damage in primary and secondary glomerulopathies that can increase as a consequence of elevated BP values, so it should be targeted by lowering BP. More than 20 years ago, the Framingham Study demonstrated that an increase in urinary proteins was associated with a high risk of cardiovascular events, including coronary heart disease as well as stroke.[73] Even small amounts of urinary albumin excretion (UAE) (microalbuminuria) are correlated with the progression of nephropathy and to a higher cardiovascular risk. Initially, information came from cross-sectional studies that demonstrated a clustering of cardiovascular risk factors and organ damage associated with a subtle increase in UAE. In follow-up studies, a given value of UAE measured at the beginning was associated with total and with cardiovascular mortality or morbidity over time. Furthermore, the level of albuminuria during antihypertensive treatment was closely related to cardiovascular risk during treatment, implying that changes in albuminuria translate to changes in risk.[74] Hence, the assessment of increases in UAE is a powerful method to identify those adults at risk for multiple cardiovascular risk factor intervention. Changes in UAE seem to run in parallel to cardiovascular risk, and prompt intervention to avoid the progressive increment of UAE may result in better protection against hypertension-induced morbidity and mortality.[75] The role of microalbuminuria assessment in pediatrics, however, is limited to diabetic children and adolescents. Its significance in pediatric essential hypertension has yet to be established, and routine urinary albumin assessment is, therefore, not yet recommended.[6]

Vessels

Hypertension-induced abnormalities in arterial structure and function are important because they underlie many adverse effects. Assessment of vascular damage, however, received little attention prior to the advent of the advanced ultrasound technology which permits noninvasive study of vascular walls and lumen. Intima-media thickness measurement at the carotid artery is the most common of the methods to assess structural abnormalities. Since age and sex influence the values of intima-media thickness, measured values should be related to percentiles or expressed as standard deviation scores.[76]

In the few pediatric studies available, hypertensive children and adolescents tended to exhibit an increased intima-media thickness compared to normotensive controls,[67,77,78] although one study did not observe differences among normotensives, white-coat, masked, or sustained hypertensives.[69] Moreover, a relationship between intima-media thickness and endothelial function has been established in the Cardiovascular Risk in Young Finns Study.[79] The impact of other cardiovascular risk factors besides hypertension, such as cholesterol levels or smoking, needs to be considered in the interpretation of intima-media thickness levels, since these have been associated with intima-media thickness as well.[80] Moreover, measurement is not trivial and subject to some observer bias. Hence, despite the increasing evidence for its predictive value in cardiovascular disease, carotid intima-media thickness assessments have not yet been recommended universally for routine clinical use.[6]

CONCLUSIONS

The goal of BP measurement in children and adolescents is to provide strategies for promoting cardiovascular health, and should be integrated into a comprehensive pediatric health care program. Understanding the persistence of BP elevation over time and its progression into clinical hypertension would aid in the early identification and prevention of hypertension. An early diagnosis and proper evaluation are essential to reducing not only the late but also the early consequences of hypertension.

REFERENCES

1. Lurbe E, Rodicio JL: Hypertension in children and adolescents, *J Hypertens* 22:1423-25, 2004.
2. Lauer RM, Anderson AR, Beaglehole R, Burns TL: Factors related to tracking of blood pressure in children, *Hypertension* 6:307-14, 1984.
3. National Heart, Lung and Blood Institute: Report of the task force on blood pressure control in children, *Pediatrics* 59:797-820, 1977.
4. National Heart, Lung and Blood Institute: Report of the second task force on blood pressure control in children—1987, *Pediatrics* 79:1-25, 1987.
5. Update on the 1987 Task Force Report on High Blood Pressure in Children and Adolescents: a Working Group Report from the National High Blood Pressure Education Program, *Pediatrics* 98:649-58, 1996.
6. National High Blood Pressure Education Program Working Group on High Blood Pressure in Children and Adolescents: the fourth report on the diagnosis, evaluation and treatment of high blood pressure in children and adolescents, *Pediatrics* 114:555-76, 2004.
7. Harshfield GA, Wilson ME: Ethnic differences in childhood blood pressure. In Portman RJ, Sorof JM, Ingelfinger JR, editors: *Pediatric hypertension*, Totowa, NJ, 2004, Humana Press, pp. 293-305.
8. Sorof JM, Lai D, Turner J, Poffenbarger T, Portman R: Overweight, ethnicity and the prevalence of hypertension in school-aged children, *Pediatrics* 113:475-82, 2004.
9. Sinaiko AR, Gomez-Marin O, Prineas RJ: Prevalence of "significant" hypertension in junior high school-aged children: the children and adolescent Blood Pressure Program, *J Pediatr* 114:664-69, 1989.
10. Adrogue H, Sinaiko A: Prevalence of hypertension in junior high school–aged children: Effect of new recommendations in the 1996 update task force report, *Am J Hypertens* 14:412-14, 2001.
11. Gardner LS, Heady JA: Some effects of within-person variability in epidemiological studies, *J Chronic Dis* 26:781-95, 1973.
12. O'Brien E, Asmar R, Beilin L, Imai Y, et al: European Society of Hypertension recommendations for conventional, ambulatory and home blood pressure measurement, *J Hypertens* 21:821-48, 2003.
13. Lurbe E, Sorof JM, Daniels SR: Clinical and research aspects of ambulatory blood pressure monitoring in children, *J Pediatr* 144:7-16, 2004.
14. Cavallini MC, Roman MJ, Pickering TG, Schwartz JE, et al: Is white coat hypertension associated with arterial disease or left ventricular hypertrophy? *Hypertension* 26:413-19, 1995.
15. Sorof JM, Poffenbarger T, Franco K, Portman R: Evaluation of white-coat hypertension in children: importance of the definitions of

normal ambulatory blood pressure and the severity of casual hypertension, *Am J Hypertens* 14:855-60, 2001.
16. Verdecchia P, Schillaci G, Borgioni C, Ciucci A, et al: Identification of subjects with white-coat hypertension and persistently normal ambulatory blood pressure, *Blood Press Monit* 1:217-22, 1996.
17. Pickering TG, Davidson K, Gering W, Schwartz JE: Masked hypertension, *Hypertension* 40:795-96, 2002.
18. Mancia G: Reversed white-coat hypertension: definition, mechanisms and prognostic implications, *J Hypertens* 20:579-81, 2002.
19. Sega R, Trocino G, Lanzarotti A, Carugo S, et al: Alterations of cardiac structure in patients with isolated office, ambulatory, or home hypertension: data from the general population (Pressione Arteriose Monitorate E Loro Associazioni [PAMELA] Study), *Circulation* 104:1385-92, 2001.
20. Björklund K, Lind L, Zethelius B, Andrén B, Lithell H: Isolated ambulatory hypertension predicts cardiovascular morbidity in elderly men, *Circulation* 107:1297-302, 2003.
21. Sorof JM, Portman RJ: White coat hypertension in children with elevated casual blood pressure, *J Pediatr* 137:493-97, 2000.
22. Lurbe E, Torro I, Alvarez V, Nawrot T, et al: Prevalence, persistence, and clinical significance of masked hypertension in youth, *Hypertension* 45:493-98, 2005.
23. Palatini P, Julius S: Heart rate and the cardiovascular risk, *J Hypertens* 15:1-37, 1997.
24. Julius S, Valentini M, Palatini P: Overweight and hypertension: a 2 way street? *Hypertension* 35:807-13, 2000.
25. Lauer RM, Clarke WR: Childhood risk factors for high adult blood pressure: the Muscatine Study, *Pediatrics* 84:633-41, 1989.
26. Hunt SC, Williams RR, Barlow GK: A comparison of positive family history definitions for defining risk of future disease, *J Chronic Dis* 39:809-21, 1986.
27. Lurbe E, Redon J, Liao Y, Tacons J, et al: Ambulatory blood pressure monitoring in normotensive children, *J Hypertens* 12:1417-23, 1994.
28. Lurbe E, Thijs L, Redón J, Alvarez V, et al: Diurnal blood pressure curve in children and adolescents, *J Hypertens* 14:41-46, 1996.
29. Middeke M, Schrader J: Nocturnal blood pressure in normotensive subjects and those with white-coat, primary and secondary hypertension, *BMJ* 308:630-32, 1994.
30. Imai Y, Abe K, Munakata M, Sakuma H, et al: Does ambulatory blood pressure monitoring improve the diagnosis of secondary hypertension? *J Hypertens* 8 (Suppl):S71-75, 1990.
31. Vogt BA: Hypertension in children and adolescents: definition, pathophysiology, risk factors and long-term sequelae, *Curr Therap Res* 62:283-97, 2001.
32. Goonasekera CDA, Dillon MJ: Measurement and interpretation of blood pressure, *Arch Dis Child* 82:261-65, 2000.
33. Arar MY, Hogg RJ, Arant BS, Seikaly MG: Etiology of sustained hypertension in children in the Southwestern United States, *Pediatr Nephrol* 8:186-89, 1994.
34. Lieberman E: Hypertension in childhood and adolescence. In Kaplan N, editor: *Clinical hypertension*, ed 5, Baltimore, 1990, Williams and Wilkins, pp. 407-33.
35. Yiu V, Dluhy RP, Lifton RP, Guay-Woodford LM: Low-peripheral plasma renin activity as a critical marker in pediatric hypertension, *Pediatr Nephrol* 11:343-46, 1997.
36. Zubrow AB, Hulman S, Kushner H, Falkner B: Determinants of blood pressure in infants admitted to neonatal intensive care units: a prospective multicenter study, *J Perinatol* 15:470-79, 1995.
37. Flynn J: Neonatal hypertension: diagnosis and management, *Pediatr Nephrol* 14:332-41, 2000.
38. Kay JD, Sinaiko AR, Daniels SR: Pediatric hypertension, *Am Heart J* 142:422-32, 2001.
39. Luma GB, Spiotta RT: Hypertension in children and adolescents, *Am Fam Physician* 73:1558-68, 2006.
40. Fivush BA, Jabs K, Neu AM, Sullivan EK, et al: Chronic renal insufficency in children and adolescents: the 1996 annual report of NAPRTCS, *Pediatr Nephrol* 12:328-37, 1998.
41. Wingen A, Fabian-Bach C, Schaefer F, Mehls O: European study group for nutritional treatment of chronic renal failure in childhood. Randomized multicenter study of a low protein diet on the progression of chronic renal failure in children, *Lancet* 349:1117-23, 1997.
42. Lurbe E, Redón J: Assessing ambulatory blood pressure in renal diseases: facts and concerns, *Nephrol Dial Transplant* 14:2564-68, 1999.
43. Portaluppi F, Montanari L, Massari M, Di Chiara V, Capanna M: Loss of nocturnal decline of blood pressure in hypertension due to chronic renal failure, *Am J Hypertens* 4:20-26, 1991.
44. Luik AJ, Struijk DG, Gladziwa U: Diurnal blood pressure variations in haemodyalisis and CAPD patients, *Nephrol Dial Transplant* 9:1616-21, 1994.
45. Farmer CK, Goldsmith DJ, Cox J, Dallyn P, et al: An investigation of the effect of advancing uraemia, renal replacement therapy and renal transplantation on blood pressure diurnal variability, *Nephrol Dial Transplant* 12:2301-307, 1997.
46. Faria Mdo S, Nunes JP, Ferraz JM, Fernandes J, et al: 24-hour blood pressure profile early after renal transplantation, *Rev Port Cardiol* 14:227-31, 1995.
47. Lingens N, Dobos E, Lemmer B, Scharer K: Nocturnal blood pressure elevation in transplanted pediatric patients, *Kidney Int Suppl* 55:S175-76, 1996.
48. Mistnefes M, Portman R: Ambulatory blood pressure monitoring in pediatric renal transplantation, *Pediatr Transplant* 7:86-92, 2003.
49. Sorof J, Poffenbarger T, Portman R: Abnormal 24-hour blood pressure patterns in children after renal transplantation, *Am J Kidney Dis* 35:681-86, 2000.
50. Calzolari A, Giordano U, Matteucci M, Pastore E, et al: Hypertension in young patients alter renal transplantation: ambulatory blood pressure monitoring versus casual blood pressure, *Am J Hypertens* 11:497-501, 1998.
51. Morgan H, Khan I, Hashmi A, Hebert D, et al: Ambulatory blood pressure monitoring after renal transplantation in children, *Pediatr Nephrol* 16:843-47, 2001.
52. Li Kam, Wa TC, Macnicol AM, Watson ML: Ambulatory blood pressure in hypertensive patients with autosomal dominant polycystic kidney disease, *Nephrol Dial Transplant* 12:2075-80, 1997.
53. Lama G, Tedesco MA, Graziano L, Calabrese E, et al: Reflux nephropathy and hypertension: correlation with the progression of renal damage, *Pediatr Nephrol* 18:241-45, 2003.
54. Patzer L, Seeman T, Luck C, Wühl E, et al: Day and night time blood pressure elevation in children with higher grades of renal scarring, *J Pediatr* 142:117-22, 2003.
55. Lurbe A, Redon J, Pascual JM, Tacons J, et al: Altered blood pressure during sleep in normotensive subjects with type I diabetes, *Hypertension* 21:227-35, 1993.
56. Lurbe E, Redon J, Pascual JM, Tacons J, Alvarez V: The spectrum of circadian blood pressure changes in type 1 diabetic patients, *J Hypertens* 19:1421-28, 2001.
57. Lurbe E, Redon J, Kesani A, Pascual JM, et al: Increase in nocturnal blood pressure and progression to microalbuminuria in type 1 diabetes, *N Engl J Med* 347:797-805, 2002.
58. van de Borne P, Tielemans C, Collart F, et al: Twenty-four-hour blood pressure and heart rate patterns in chronic hemodialysis patients, *Am J Kidney Dis* 22:419-25, 1993.
59. Redon J, Lurbe E: Ambulatory blood pressure and the kidney: implications for renal dysfunction. In Epstein M, editor: *Calcium antagonists in clinical medicine*, Philadelphia, 2002, Hanley & Belfus, pp. 665-79.
60. Timio M, Venanzi S, Lolli S, Lippi G, et al: "Non dipper" hypertensive patients and progressive renal insufficiency: a 3 year longitudinal study, *Clin Nephrol* 43:382-87, 1995.
61. Malcolm DD, Burns TL, Mahoney LT, Lauer RM: Factors affecting left ventricular mass in childhood: the Muscatine Study, *Pediatrics* 92:703-709, 1993.
62. de Simone G, Devereux RB, Daniels SR, Koren MJ, et al: Effect of growth on variability of left ventricular mass: assessment of allometric signals in adults and children and their capacity to predict cardiovascular risk, *J Am Coll Cardiol* 25:1056-62, 1995.
63. Urbina EM, Gidding SS, Bao W, Pickoff AS, et al: Effect of body size, ponderosity, and blood pressure on left ventricular growth in children and young adults in the Bogalusa Heart Study, *Circulation* 91:2400-406, 1995.
64. Schieken RM, Schwartz PF, Goble MM: Tracking of left ventricular mass in children: race and sex comparisons: the MCV Twin Study. Medical College of Virginia, *Circulation* 97:1901-906, 1998.

65. Sivanandam S, Sinaiko AR, Jacobs DR Jr, Steffen L, et al: Relation of increase in adiposity to increase in left ventricular mass from childhood to young adulthood, *Am J Cardiol* 98:411-15, 2006.
66. Flynn JT, Alderman MH: Characteristics of children with primary hypertension seen at a referral center, *Pediatr Nephrol* 20:961-66, 2005.
67. Litwin M, Niemirska A, Sladowska J, Antoniewicz J, et al: Left ventricular hypertrophy and arterial wall thickening in children with essential hypertension, *Pediatr Nephrol* 21:811-19, 2006.
68. Daniels SR, Loggie JM, Khoury P, Kimball TR: Left ventricular geometry and severe left ventricular hypertrophy in children and adolescents with essential hypertension, *Circulation* 97:1907-11, 1998.
69. Stabouli S, Kotsis V, Toumanidis S, Papamichael C, et al: White-coat and masked hypertension in children: association with target-organ damage, *Pediatr Nephrol* 20:1151-55, 2005.
70. Sorof JM, Cardwell G, Franco K, Portman RJ: Ambulatory blood pressure and left ventricular mass index in hypertensive children, *Hypertension* 39:903-908, 2002.
71. Toto RD: Treatment of hypertension in chronic kidney disease, *Semin Nephrol* 25:435-39, 2005.
72. Sarnak MJ, Greene T, Wang X, Beck G, et al: The effect of a lower target blood pressure on the progression of kidney disease: long-term follow-up of the modification of diet in renal disease study, *Ann Intern Med* 142:342-51, 2005.
73. Kannel WB, Stampfer MJ, Castelli WP, Verter J: The prognostic significance of proteinuria: the Framingham study, *Am Heart J* 108:1347-52, 1984.
74. Redon J, Ruilope LM: Microalbuminuria as an intermediate endpoint in essential hypertension: evidence is coming, *J Hypertens* 22:1679-81, 2004.
75. Redon J: Urinary albumin excretion: lowering the threshold of risk in hypertension, *Hypertension* 46:19-20, 2005.
76. Jourdan C, Wühl E, Litwin M, Fahr K, et al: Normative values for intima-media thickness and distensibility of large arteries in healthy adolescents, *J Hypertens* 23:1707-15, 2005.
77. Sass C, Herbeth B, Chapet O, Siest G, et al: Intima-media thickness and diameter of carotid and femoral arteries in children, adolescents and adults from the Stanislas cohort: effect of age, sex, anthropometry and blood pressure, *J Hypertens* 16:1593-602, 1998.
78. Sorof JM, Alexandrov AV, Cardwell G, Portman RJ: Carotid artery intimal-medial thickness and left ventricular hypertrophy in children with elevated blood pressure, *Pediatrics* 111:61-66, 2003.
79. Juonala M, Viikari JSA, Laitinen T, Marniemi J, et al: Interrelations between brachial endothelial function and carotid intima-media thickness in young adults. The Cardiovascular Risk in Young Finns Study, *Circulation* 110:2918-23, 2004.
80. Davis PH, Dawson JD, Riley WA, Lauer RM: Carotid intimal-medial thickness is related to cardiovascular risk factors measured from childhood through middle age: the Muscatine Study, *Circulation* 104:2815-19, 2001.

CHAPTER

42 Investigation of Hypertension in Childhood

Charlotte Hadtstein and Elke Wühl

INTRODUCTION

The rational investigation of hypertension is of special importance in childhood. Hypertensive children are more likely to suffer from a specific underlying disease than adults, are at greater risk of long-term target-organ damage, and should not be subjected to unnecessary diagnostic procedures. However, the investigation of pediatric hypertension poses numerous practical and scientific problems in three main areas: measuring blood pressure (BP), defining hypertension, and deciding about the extent of further investigations in the hypertensive patient. The changing cardiovascular physiology, pathology, and body dimensions in childhood add complexity in each of these areas. This chapter deals first with the various techniques for measuring BP with respective advantages and pitfalls. Subsequently, the current definitions of hypertension are discussed, including the pediatric population distribution–based approach to normal BP ranges. For each method, the availability and usefulness of normal values are presented. Finally, we give a guide to the initial and follow-up investigation of the hypertensive child, with a discussion of established and novel diagnostic tests as well as markers of target-organ damage.

Key international statements on the standards of the investigation of hypertension in adults which are referred to here include the seventh report of the Joint National Committee (JNC) on Prevention, Detection, Evaluation, and Treatment of High Blood Pressure,[1] the 1999 World Health Organization/International Society of Hypertension guidelines for managing hypertension,[2] and the guidelines of the British Hypertension Society. While these guidelines focus mainly on management and treatment of hypertension[3] without specific reference to children, the fourth report by the JNC[4] provides the only specifically pediatric guideline. However, some recommendations in the fourth report pertain to the large proportion of essential hypertensives in North America, which limits their applicability in certain other pediatric populations.

TECHNICAL ASPECTS OF BLOOD PRESSURE MEASUREMENT IN CHILDREN

General Considerations

The great intra- and inter-individual variability as well as inter-observer variability of BP measurements have led to the consensus that both measuring devices and techniques should be standardized. All types of BP measurements should be performed after adequate preparation of the patient including resting for 5 minutes, sitting in an upright supported position, and an arm support to ensure the cubital fossa is at heart level. At least three measurements should be taken at each visit. While adult and pediatric recommendations are in agreement about this standardization,[1,4] it can make measurements in toddlers a significant effort. Young infants can only be examined in the supine position. The right arm is preferred to avoid false low readings in children with coarctation of the aorta.

Concerning cuff size, the inflatable bladder should cover 80% to 100% of the arm circumference and its width should be at least 38% of arm circumference.[4] However, a width-to-length ratio of at least 1 : 2 is not yet compulsory and therefore not universally found. If in doubt about which size to use, a cuff that is too large appears to cause less underestimation of BP compared to the overestimation caused by an undersized cuff.[5]

Adolescents should avoid caffeine and tobacco for 30 minutes beforehand, and acute BP effects of drugs such as theophylline or epinephrine should be recognized in all age groups.

Casual (Clinic) Blood Pressure Measurement

Blood pressure measurements that are taken intermittently in the clinical setting are usually referred to as “casual” or “clinic” measurements. The most established method is the *auscultatory measurement*, classically performed with the mercury sphygmomanometer, but largely replaced in recent years by aneroid manometry due to safety concerns about the use of mercury. Satisfactory accuracy of aneroid manometry depends heavily on regular servicing of the devices, which is often not achieved in clinical practice.[6-9] For auscultatory measurements the fifth Korotkoff sound has been established as diastolic BP in all children of all ages since the 1980s.[10]

A problem inherent to auscultatory measurements is significant observer bias. Even experienced, well-trained observers tend to round figures and approximate the measured towards expected and target values. The phenomenon of terminal digit preference is common even in specialized hypertension centers and in clinical trial settings.[11-13] For the purposes of clinical trials, observer bias can be overcome by use of "random zero" devices, which blind the examiner with respect to the absolute BP value until the end of the measurement, but are generally too complicated for everyday use.[14]

In recent years, automated *oscillometric BP* devices have gained popularity in clinic and home settings alike. Oscillometric measurements reduce observer bias due to greater automation, and are more convenient to use, particularly in smaller children. Freeing the attention of the examiner from the manometer display towards distraction of the child can be a key component of successful BP measurements in toddlers. In this context, the ability to adjust inflating pressures is an important feature of newer devices to avoid lengthy unpleasant arm compression in infants. However, values obtained by oscillometry may vary significantly from the auscultatory technique, as rather than recording Korotkoff sounds, the pressure at which the greatest oscillation occurs is taken to be the mean arterial pressure (MAP). Systolic and diastolic values are calculated via algorithms, which are company-owned trade secrets, and therefore cannot be verified or standardized independently. The correlation of oscillometric to auscultatory and intra-arterial measurements therefore needs to be evaluated on a model-by-model basis using the rigorous standards of the British Hypertension Society (BHS) and Association for the Advancement of Medical Instrumentation (AAMI)[15,16] or the newer guidelines of the European Society of Hypertension (ESH).[17] For instance, the Dinamap 8100 has been found to measure on average approximately 10 mm Hg higher than auscultation.[14] Another important drawback of oscillometric measurements in children is the fact that to date reference values have been obtained from much smaller population samples than for auscultatory measurements.[4,18,19]

Hence, the choice between auscultatory and oscillometric measurements demands weighing the advantages of accuracy and experience against ease and practicability. The JNC's fourth report recommends auscultation as the preferred method for diagnosing hypertension in children, mainly on the grounds that reference values are based on this method. It is proposed that oscillometric measurements above the 90th percentile should be repeated by auscultation.[4]

However, in addition to device-related limits to accuracy, single casual BP measurements have poor reproducibility.[20,21] This is due both to the natural variation of BP over time, as well as the "white-coat effect," the response to the medical setting. White-coat hypertension occurs in up to 45% of children.[22-25] Taking at least three readings at every session is therefore strongly recommended.[1,2,4] In addition, BP should be measured on several separate occasions if clinic BPs alone are used for diagnosis and treatment of hypertension. Vollmer et al.[26] found that three to five clinic visits were necessary to achieve a similar reproducibility of clinic measurements compared to ambulatory BP measurement in detecting changes of BP.

Home Blood Pressure Measurement

Home BP monitoring is becoming an increasingly popular way of obtaining multiple BP readings away from the white-coat clinic setting. Additionally, it is a valuable way of involving patients in the management of this "invisible" disease, and probably improves adherence to long-term medication.[27] From the THOP (Treatment of Hypertension Based on Home or Office Blood Pressure) trial there is evidence that integrating home measurements into clinical decision making reduces unnecessary medications and can produce some cost savings.[28]

The above considerations about technical accuracy of auscultatory versus oscillometric BP measurements equally apply at home, but the different setting also raises new issues. For example, adequate training of relatives in the auscultatory method is time consuming and may not always be possible. Also, there is evidence of significant misreporting by patients, which may in part be overcome by the use of oscillometric devices with internal memory.[29] At the very least, a written patient record should be kept. In the foreseeable future, BP telemonitoring may open a new dimension of effective and objective home BP monitoring.

Most importantly, even though home measurements are more reproducible than clinic readings, they are significantly lower,[21,30] and therefore require independent reference values. Normative home BP data have recently been published for 778 Greek children.[30a]

Ambulatory Blood Pressure Monitoring

Ambulatory BP monitoring (ABPM) involves repetitive noninvasive BP measurements using portable devices in outpatients over an entire day. Auscultatory and oscillometric devices are available, but technical aspects strongly favor oscillometry. As auscultatory devices are based on microphone recordings, displacement of the microphone during physical activity leads to a high proportion of unsuccessful readings in children.[31] Normative data for ABPM are extremely important in view of the specific technology and circumstances of the measurements. Unlike adults, children have significantly higher mean daytime BP values than clinic readings due to their greater physical activity.[32,33] A patient diary should be kept in order take account of times of physical activity, sleep, and drug intake. Clinical experience suggests good tolerance of ABPM in the large majority of children as young as 3 to 5 years old.[21,34] Some patients find it hard to tolerate repetitive measurements at night, which may cause falsely high readings due to disturbed sleep. With ABPM the white-coat effect is markedly reduced, although not completely eliminated since the device is usually put in place in the clinic setting.[35]

Improved prediction of end-organ damage by mean BP from ABPM compared to clinic readings has been demonstrated in hypertensive adults,[36,37] and to some extent in the general adult population.[38] In children, left ventricular hypertrophy also shows a superior correlation to ABPM over clinic BP,[39] most likely due to the much better approximation of true BP load achieved by multiple readings as compared to single casual measurements. As the superiority of ABPM becomes smaller when compared to repetitive clinic readings, some have argued against its overuse on these grounds.[40] However, multiple clinic measurements are difficult to obtain in practice, particularly in children, so the benefit of obtaining multiple readings by ABPM in a single session remains. The superior sensitivity of ABPM is also demonstrated by the fact that ethnic differences in children's BPs have only been detected by ABPM, but not by casual measurements.[41-43]

When good readings can be obtained during the night, ABPM permits assessment of the circadian BP profile. Several studies in both normotensive and hypertensive adults have demonstrated that loss of the nocturnal decrease of BP ("dipping" phenomenon) to be an important predictor of mortality[44,45] and end-organ damage,[46,47] independently of absolute BP levels.

Over the past 15 years, ABPM has become increasingly recognized as a valuable tool in the investigation of pediatric hypertension. This relates to clinical aspects such as the minimized white-coat effect and the superior prediction of clinical outcomes as well as to the novel research possibilities introduced by the ability to study the diurnal variability of BP. Financial constraints have slowed the spreading of ABPM in many parts of the world. Most U.S. insurance companies, for example, currently do not cover ABPM costs (about US$400 per scan).

NORMAL BLOOD PRESSURE RANGES AND DEFINITION OF HYPERTENSION IN CHILDREN

General Considerations

Due to the continuous distribution of BP, there has been considerable debate about what constitutes a normal BP in adults. Systolic BP of 135 mm Hg was considered "normal" in the JNC III guidelines in 1984 and "high normal" in JNC VI 1997, but was labeled "prehypertensive" in JNC VII in 2003.[1,48,49] Even below the arbitrary cut-off levels that define hypertension, cardiovascular risk is proportional to BP. However, the benefits of lowering BP become progressively smaller with lower starting BP. Recent guidelines have set lower BP targets for populations at increased cardiovascular risk such as patients with diabetes and/or chronic kidney disease (CKD).

In children, the matter is further complicated by the marked dependence of BP on height, age, and gender, and the lack of cardiovascular mortality outcome data. From the earliest consensus statements, the definition of hypertension has therefore been based on population distributions. A systolic and/or diastolic BP above the 95th percentile on several occasions is the accepted cut-off for hypertension. However, while early reports regarded children on the 95th percentile as merely high-normal and not hypertensive,[50] the latest guidelines label BPs between the 90th and 95th percentile and any value above 120/80 mm Hg as "prehypertensive," reflecting the trends in adult medicine[4] (Table 42-1). Prehypertension is considered a treatment indication for children and adolescents at high risk, such as those with CKD, diabetes mellitus, heart failure, or left ventricular hypertrophy.

TABLE 42-1 Definition of Hypertension in Children

Prehypertension	SBP or DBP 90th-95th percentile or >120/80 mm Hg
Hypertension	SBP or DBP >95th percentile
Stage 1	SBP or DBP 95th-99th percentile + 5 mm Hg
Stage 2	SBP or DBP >99th percentile + 5 mm Hg

DBP, Diastolic blood pressure; *SBP*, systolic blood pressure.
Source: National High Blood Pressure Education Program Working Group on High Blood Pressure in Children and Adolescents: The fourth report on the diagnosis, evaluation, and treatment of high blood pressure in children and adolescents, *Pediatrics* 114:555-76, 2004.

Inherent to the population-based approach are questions about the validity of normative data in different ethnic contexts. This does not appear to be a major problem for casual measurements as shown among schoolchildren and young adults in the three major ethnic groups in the southern United States[42,43]; however, it is relevant to ABPM.[41] The growing epidemic of childhood obesity poses even more profound problems for the establishment of new population-based data, as BP in the general population is increasing over time.[51] Calls for end-organ damage- or mortality-based definitions are therefore unanimous,[52] yet in practice almost impossible to obtain in the pediatric age range.

Casual Blood Pressure

Extensive pediatric normative data on auscultatory clinic measurements have been provided for the United States,[4] based on more than 70,000 children of the National Health and Nutrition Examination Survey (NHANES) and additional studies. Blood pressure percentiles have been calculated for each sex, age group, and seven height percentile categories (see Appendix). Height percentiles are based on the growth charts of the Center for Disease Control and Prevention (www.cdc.gov/growthcharts). Reference values for European children were published in 1991, obtained from more than 28,000 subjects.[53] The largest sample to date of normative data for oscillometric measurements is based on 7208 schoolchildren measured with the Dinamap Model 8100.[18]

For infants under 1 year there is a distinct lack of data. Auscultatory normal ranges have been provided by the Task Force on Blood Pressure Control in Children[54]; however, the fourth Korotkoff sound was used in this study, which was performed between 1976 and 1984. Oscillometric normal ranges have been reported for the 0- to 5-year age group by Park and colleagues.[19,55]

Home Blood Pressure

Even when the same devices are used, home BP readings are consistently lower than clinic measurements, both in adults[56] and in children.[21,30] In adults, home BP over 135/85 mm Hg is therefore considered hypertensive, while in the clinic it would still be regarded as "prehypertensive." In children, no normal data have been collected for home BP measurements, and there are no accepted cut-offs. The dilemma of using clinic reference values became evident in the THOP trial where management based on home BP using clinic cut-offs led to higher overall BP in the home monitoring group.[28] Using the 95th percentile for daytime ambulatory BP is even more problematic since these are even higher than clinic readings due to inclusion of measurements under nonresting conditions.

Ambulatory Blood Pressure Monitoring

The most comprehensive normative data for ABPM is based on data by Soergel et al.[32] from 1141 European children using oscillometric devices. A sample of similar size was collected in England for the less commonly used auscultatory ABPM method.[31] Again, device-specific normative values should ideally be collected for oscillometric monitors; for instance, the Dinamap and Spacelabs monitors do not vary from sphygmomanometric measurements in the same direction.[34]

The large number of readings taken by ABPM allows defining hypertension in various statistical ways. In general, 24-hour mean values are very robust and reproducible.[20,21] However, it is useful to assess both daytime and nighttime mean BP. To that end, either fixed definitions (e.g., 8 A.M. to 8 P.M. for daytime and 12 midnight to 6 A.M. for nighttime), or the actual patient record can be used; however, the latter may not always be available or reliable. If the patient reports poor sleep due to disturbance by the measurement, nighttime BP should be interpreted with care. When using oscillometric ABPM devices, we recommend using MAP, rather than systolic or diastolic BP, as the latter are calculated rather than measured. The use of MAP simplifies the interpretation of the large number of values generated by ABPM. The percentiles of 24-hour, daytime, and nighttime MAP are given in Table 42-2.

Due to the closer correlation of BP with height than with age, height should be used as a reference parameter.[32] For longitudinal observations or comparisons of nonmatched groups, we strongly recommend the use of standard deviation scores (SDS or Z-scores). For this purpose normalized reference values based on the European population have been provided by Wühl et al.[33]

ABPM also allows the calculation of BP "load," that is, the percentage of systolic and diastolic BP measurements above the 95th percentile. In adults, BP load is correlated to target-organ damage,[57,58] although cut-offs for normal load vary between 25% and 50%. For children, a BP load of more than 30% has been suggested as hypertensive.[59] However, the number of pediatric studies evaluating BP load as a diagnostic tool is limited. In a recent analysis of 728 pediatric ABPM profiles for correlation between hypertension defined by mean BP above the 95% or BP load greater than 30%, agreement was only moderate to good. Maximum agreement was achieved when 50% BP load was used as a cut-off level.[60] Using the 30% limit will label many children with normotensive mean 24-hour BP values as hypertensive. Therefore, BP load as the sole definition for hypertension or alternate use of both definitions for hypertension should be avoided.

Comparing Methods: When to Use Which?

The technical and clinical arguments for and against different techniques of BP assessment are summarized in Table 42-3. The availability of methodologies with variable reproducibility and concordance can result in diagnostic and therapeutic dilemmas when results are not in agreement.

A high clinic BP but normal ABPM is readily explained as *white-coat hypertension*. In adults, there is some evidence suggesting that white-coat hypertensives are at increased risk of left ventricular hypertrophy, intima media thickening, stroke, and later development of full-blown hypertension; however, many adult studies also show no increased risk, and there is no conclusive evidence in children (for an overview, see Angeli et al.[61] and Stergiou et al.[62]). In addition to the exaggerated sympathetic response in the clinic setting, several other factors can contribute white-coat hypertension, such as day-to-day variation of BP, reading and device inaccuracies, and insufficient standardization of measurement. The reverse finding of *masked hypertension*, that is, hypertension by ABPM but not clinic measurement, has been recognized more recently. It is more consistently associated with end-organ damage than white-coat hypertension, underlining the greater predictive power of ABPM compared to clinic BPs.[22,63] However, the moderate reproducibility of masked hypertension again points to the fact that measurement errors and biological BP variability play a role in borderline BP phenomena.

Disagreement between measurement methods is much more common than one might think. White-coat hypertension has been observed in up to 45% of children.[22-25] The magnitude of the white-coat effect rises with the absolute BP,[30] and is therefore an even greater source of error in hypertensive than in normotensive children. In 118 children with chronic renal failure and high-normal or elevated BP on antihypertensive treatment, we found that 27 were hypertensive by ABPM. Of these, only 29 (70%) were detected by simultaneous clinic measurements and 14 (52%) by home measurements. White-coat hypertension was found in 30%, and "home hypertension" in 17.5%. Thus, clinic measurements have a higher sensitivity, but lower specificity than home measurements for detecting hypertension, as defined by ABPM. The greater sensitivity of clinic BP makes it a useful screening tool, while ambulatory and home measurements show greater specificity, and are therefore especially suited to confirming a suspected diagnosis of hypertension.[30]

We therefore think that the choice of BP monitoring method should take into account the pre-test risk of hypertension, where "risk" means both the likelihood of hypertension being present, as well as the potential health risk of missing hypertension due to pre-existing disease. A practical guide in the form of a flow diagram is given in Figure 42-1. Children at low risk include those at routine medical examinations or with presenting complaints unlikely to be associated with hypertension. Children with obesity, CKD stages 1 to 3, well-controlled diabetes, autonomic dysfunction, or long-term steroid treatment should be considered at intermediate risk. High-risk patients include both those with a high likelihood of hypertension as well as those with end-stage renal failure, renal allograft recipients, or end-organ damage such as left ventricular hypertrophy, hypertensive retinopathy, or diabetics with microalbuminuria.

Other authors have suggested performing ABPM in every patient with three repeated casual measurements above the 95th percentile, and to continue home BP measurements in

TABLE 42-2 75th, 90th, and 95th Percentiles of 24-Hour Systolic, Diastolic, and Mean Arterial Blood Pressure in Ambulatory Blood Pressure Monitoring by Gender

	24-HOUR SYSTOLIC BP			24-HOUR DIASTOLIC BP			24-HOUR MEAN ARTERIAL PRESSURE		
Height	75th	90th	95th	75th	90th	95th	75th	90th	95th
Boys									
120	109	114	117	70	74	77	82	86	89
125	110	115	118	70	74	77	82	87	90
130	111	116	119	70	74	77	83	87	90
135	112	117	120	70	74	77	84	88	90
140	113	118	121	71	75	77	84	88	91
145	115	119	123	71	75	77	85	89	91
150	116	121	124	71	75	77	85	89	91
155	118	123	126	71	75	77	86	90	92
160	119	124	127	71	75	77	87	90	93
165	121	126	129	71	75	77	87	91	93
170	123	128	131	71	75	78	88	92	94
175	125	130	133	72	75	78	89	93	95
180	127	131	134	72	76	78	90	94	96
185	128	133	135	72	76	78	91	94	96
Girls									
120	108	112	114	69	71	72	81	84	85
125	109	113	116	69	71	73	81	84	86
130	110	114	117	69	72	73	82	85	87
135	111	115	118	70	72	74	82	86	87
140	112	116	119	70	73	75	83	86	88
145	113	117	120	70	73	75	83	87	89
150	115	119	121	70	74	76	84	87	89
155	116	120	122	71	74	76	85	88	90
160	117	121	123	71	74	76	85	88	90
165	118	122	124	71	74	76	86	89	91
170	119	123	125	71	74	76	87	90	91
175	120	124	126	72	74	76	87	90	92

those found only to have white-coat hypertension, while repeating ABPM at regular intervals in confirmed hypertensives.[64] The current American guidelines even restrict the use of ABPM to specialist centers. However, the high incidence of masked hypertension and the well-documented risk of hypertension on disease progression[65] are strong arguments for a more widespread use of ABPM in intermediate- and high-risk populations.

Blood Pressure Variability

Concerning data on BP variability from ABPMs, there is little standardization in the parameters used among different studies. Moreover, variability parameters strongly depend on the quality of recording, as given by the number and frequency of successful measurements as well as appropriate definitions of day and night periods. Hence, variability measures tend to be less reproducible than mean BPs.[66]

The most robust of these measurements is the nocturnal BP fall (dipping), usually expressed as a percentage of the individual's mean daytime BP. Loss of nighttime dipping is an important feature of secondary hypertension,[67,68] especially as it has been associated with worse cardiovascular outcome, progression of renal failure, and changes in the autonomic nervous system.[44-47,69] In the mid-European study, population nighttime dipping was 13% ± 6% for systolic and 23% ± 9% for diastolic BP, based on a standard night definition of midnight to 6 A.M.[32] Lurbe et al.[70] found very similar values (12% systolic and 22% diastolic dipping) in 241 children based on individual sleep time. Moreover, there may be ethnic differences in diurnal BP variability. For instance, higher nighttime

TABLE 42-3 **Overview of Blood Pressure Measurement Techniques**				
	TECHNICAL ASPECTS		CLINICAL ASPECTS	
	Advantages	**Drawbacks**	**Advantages**	**Drawbacks**
Clinic BP			Reliable normative data available	White coat effect, limited number of readings
Auscultatory	Direct measurement of Korotkoff sounds		Noninvasive, quick to perform	Observer bias, terminal digit preference
Mercury	Most "evidence based"	Safety hazard		
Aneroid	Mercury-free	More frequent calibration	Easily portable	
Oscillometric	Easy to use	Indirect measurement, unknown algorithms, validation monitor by monitor	Automation reduces observer bias, able to direct attention toward distraction of toddlers	Only limited reference values
Home BP		Cost of device, no control over calibration, servicing, and measuring technique	Multiple measurements, involving patients in disease management, no white coat effect	Training required, lack of reference data, false reporting, may cause anxiety
ABPM		Considerable cost, patient not in standardized position	Multiple measurements in shorter time frame give greater reproducibility and predictive power, detection of white coat hypertension and hypotensive episodes, nighttime evaluation	Uncomfortable, patient cooperation required, regular maintenance
Auscultatory	Direct measurement of Korotkoff sounds gives more accurate readings	High percentage of errors due to displacement and microphone errors		
Oscillometric	More robust against displacement		Reliable normative data available	

BP, Blood pressure; *ABPM*, ambulatory blood pressure measurement.

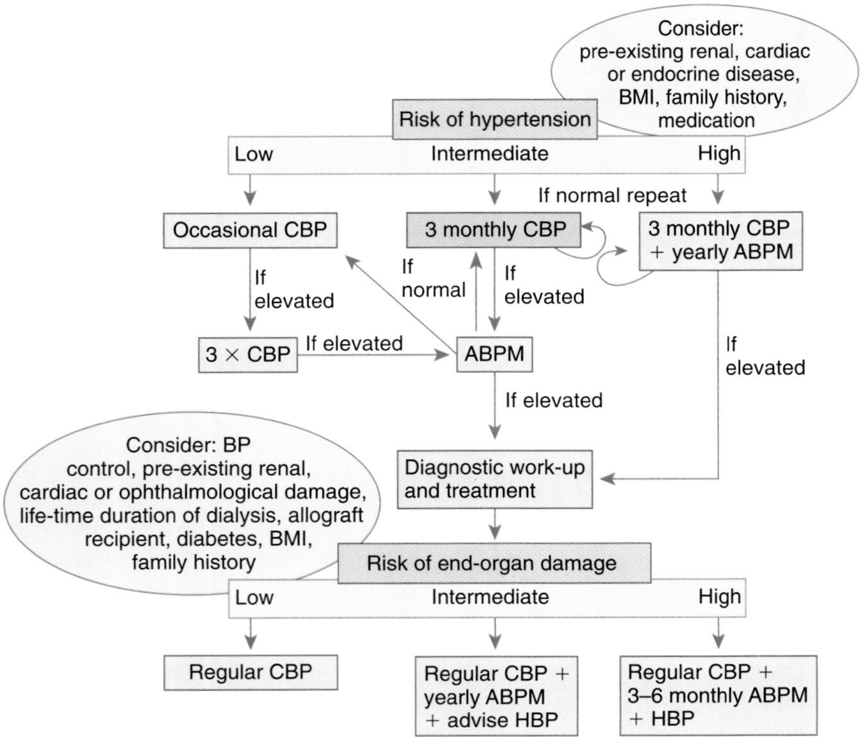

Figure 42-1 Flow diagram for suggesting method and frequency of blood pressure measuring during screening, follow-up, and treatment. *ABPM*, 24-hour ambulatory blood pressure monitoring; *BP*, blood pressure; *CBP*, clinic blood pressure; *HBP*, home blood pressure measurement.

TABLE 42-4 **Important Points in Medical History**

Symptoms of hypertension	Headache, epistaxis, flush, visual disturbance, vertigo, decline of school performance
Clues toward underlying cause Renal disease	Edema, polyuria, nocturia, hematuria, fatigue, muscle weakness, weight loss, failure to thrive History of oligohydramnios or recurrent urinary tract infections, family history of renal failure
Renovascular disease	Neonatal history of umbilical arterial catheter, neonatal asphyxia, or episodes of severe hypotension
Tumor	Weight loss, flushing, sweating
Systemic disease	Skin abnormalities (systemic lupus erythematosus, neurofibromatosis, scleroderma), family history, such as hyperthyroidism
Clues toward iatrogenic hypertension	Previous medical history Medication: anti-inflammatory agents, decongestants, stimulants (e.g., for attention deficit disorder), tricyclic antidepressants, immunosuppressives, hormonal contraceptives
Clues toward essential hypertension	Weight gain and diet, physical activity Smoking/alcohol Family history of cardiovascular disease or diabetes Sleep disturbance (sleep apnea)
Important questions at follow-up visits	Medication side effects, such as fatigue (β blockers), cough (angiotensin-converting enzyme [ACE] inhibitors), enuresis (diuretics) Compliance with therapeutic lifestyle changes. Compliance with medication

BP has been demonstrated in African Americans; however, no normal ranges are available for this population.[41]

However, as not all children show a nighttime dip, modeling of a smoothed 24-hour curve is a way of analyzing more complex patterns without external definitions of daytime and nighttime. Normal values for one such method, Fourier analysis, have been presented for the European study cohort. In this approach circadian (24 hours) and ultradian (12 hours, 8 hours, and 6 hours) cosine oscillations are combined to model BP changes over the day.[30] In the majority of normal individuals rapid, ultradian oscillations could be detected superimposed on the circadian rhythm; such fluctuations may provide novel information on the function of the autonomous nervous system. Notably, alterations of ultradian BP oscillations have been correlated with the degree of renal damage in children with CKD.[71] Other methods to quantify variability in ambulatory BP such as standard deviation of measurements and fast Fourier transformation– and cumulative sum–derived circadian alteration magnitudes have also been examined, although without adequate power to produce population-based normal values. In adults, there are data to suggest a predictive value of daytime ABPM variability on the progression of intima media thickening in patients and cardiovascular mortality in the general population.[72,73]

FURTHER EVALUATION OF HYPERTENSIVE PATIENT: DETECTING UNDERLYING DISEASE AND RISK FACTORS FOR ESSENTIAL HYPERTENSION

Once hypertension is confirmed, the initial evaluation of the hypertensive child is directed towards detection of an underlying disease and the search for risk factors of essential hypertension. Due to the high incidence of secondary hypertension in childhood, a more rigorous investigation than in adults is justified; however, it should be initiated in a stepwise fashion in order to avoid unnecessary burdens. In addition, monitoring for target-organ damage should be initiated as soon as hypertension becomes apparent, and continued at regular intervals dependent on the extent of damage and the degree of hypertension. Only in symptomatic patients and those with severe hypertension should the diagnostic evaluation be postponed until treatment has been initiated. Full investigation of the hypertensive child requires the multidisciplinary work of pediatric nephrologists, radiologists, endocrinologists, cardiologists, and ophthalmologists.

History and Examination

History and physical examination are two important diagnostic steps that should always precede costly and invasive examinations. The most important items to consider are summarized in Tables 42-4 and 42-5.

Primary Laboratory and Imaging Investigations

Despite the extensive list of possible clues in history and examination, these are rarely conclusive and laboratory tests should always be performed. An overview is given in Figure 42-2. The initial laboratory work-up of all children with persistent BP above the 95th percentile is not overly extensive, and may only be omitted if the patient has a very high likelihood of essential hypertension (e.g., a grossly obese teenager with mild hypertension and a strong family history of obesity and early-onset hypertension). In these patients, fasting lipids and fasting glucose should be determined as cardiovascular risk factors and glycosylated hemoglobin ($HbA1_c$) a useful screening test for latent diabetes mellitus type 2. Even with a family history of obesity, endocrinological causes of overweight should be explored if clinical features of Cushing syndrome are present.

TABLE 42-5 Possible Physical Signs in Hypertensive Patient

	Finding	Possible Etiology
General observation		
Body habitus	Obesity Truncal obesity Thinness Short stature Webbed neck Widely spaced nipples	Metabolic syndrome, primary HTN Cushing syndrome Hyperthyroidism, pheochromocytoma Chronic renal disease—Turner, Williams, or Gordon syndrome Turner or Gordon syndrome Turner syndrome
Face	Rounded facies/moon face Elfin facies VIIth cranial nerve palsy	Cushing syndrome Williams syndrome Hypertensive encephalopathy
Skin	Edema, pale mucous membranes Pallor, flushing, diaphoresis Acne, hirsutism, striae Acanthosis nigricans Café-au-lait spots, neurofibromas Butterfly rash Adenoma sebaceum, ash leaf spots Vasculitis	Renal failure Pheochromocytoma Cushing syndrome Type 2 diabetes mellitus Neurofibromatosis SLE Tuberous sclerosis SLE, Henoch-Schönlein nephritis, collagen vascular diseases
Head and neck	Goiter	Hyperthyroidism
Eyes	Hypertensive retinal changes Exophthalmus External ocular nerve palsies	Severe or longstanding HTN Hyperthyroidism Severe HTN, hyperthyroidism
Throat	Adenotonsillar hypertrophy	Sleep apnea
Cardiovascular system	Tachycardia Apical heave, enlarged heart Cardiac friction rub Loss of foot pulses, leg BP more than 10 mm Hg below arm BP, heart murmur Edema, heart murmur Abdominal bruit	Hyperthyroidism, pheochromocytoma, neuroblastoma, primary HTN Left ventricular hypertrophy Pericarditis due to SLE, uremia, or collagen vascular disease Coarctation of aorta Heart failure Renal artery stenosis
Abdomen and urogenital system	Abdominal mass, palpable kidneys Hepatomegaly Flank tenderness Ambiguous genitalia, virilization	Wilms tumor, neuroblastoma, pheochromocytoma, polycystic kidney disease, severe hydronephrosis, multicystic-dysplastic kidney Autosomal recessive polycystic kidney disease, heart failure Acute glomerulonephritis or obstruction, pyelonephritis Congenital adrenal hyperplasia
Musculoskeletal system	Joint swelling Rickets Brachydactyly Muscle weakness	SLE, collagen vascular disease Chronic renal failure Hypertension brachydactyly syndrome, Gordon syndrome Hyperaldosteronism, Liddle syndrome

BP, Blood pressure; *HTN*, hypertension; *SLE*, systemic lupus erythematosus.
Sources: Adapted from references 64 and 105, and from the OMIM database.

All other children should have their serum creatinine, blood urea nitrogen, electrolytes, and blood gases measured in order to rule out significant kidney disease. Low potassium and metabolic alkalosis may point towards monogenetic forms of hypertension (e.g., Liddle syndrome, glucocorticoid remediable aldosteronism, and apparent mineralocorticoid excess). Hypokalemia is sometimes also encountered in renovascular hypertension due to secondary hyperaldosteronism. High serum potassium and metabolic acidosis are usually due to renal failure, but are also found in Gordon syndrome.

The urine should be tested for leukocytes, hematuria, and the presence of deformed erythrocytes and casts as part of the screening for renal disease. Proteinuria is best determined on a 24-hour collection, but the protein/creatinine ratio in spot urine is an adequate alternative for screening, especially in small children.

At presentation, every child with hypertension should have a renal ultrasound. Sonography provides a noninvasive way of identifying a number of features to direct further investigation, such as enlarged bilateral kidneys (glomerulonephritis, pyelonephritis), renal cysts (polycystic kidney disease, multicystic dysplastic kidney disease), dysplasia, obstruction, nephrocalcinosis (tubular defects), unilateral small kidney (renovascular disease, vesico-ureteric reflux, renal scarring), and renal masses (Wilms tumor, neuroblastoma). In obese children, ultrasound may reveal associated abnormalities such as fatty changes of the liver.

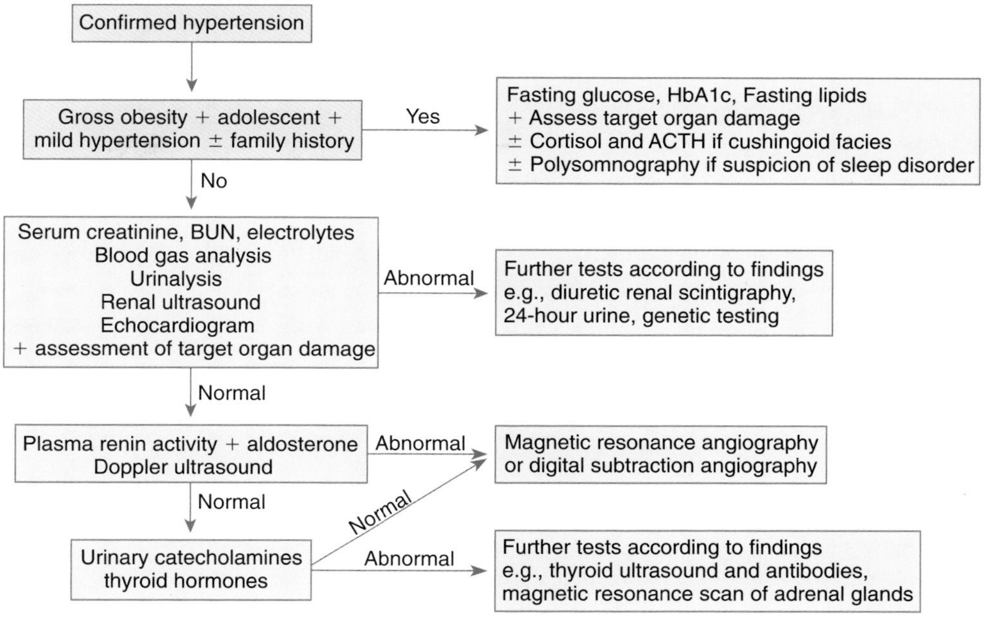

Figure 42-2 Diagnostic workup of confirmed hypertension in children. For Assessment of target organ damage, see Figure 42-3. *ACTH*, Adrenocorticotropic hormone; *BUN*, blood urea nitrogen; *HbA1c*, glycosylated hemoglobin.

Further Laboratory and Imaging Studies

After the primary laboratory and imaging studies, further tests may be indicated if the cause of hypertension is still unclear. If fasting glucose or $HbA1_c$ is high normal or elevated, a glucose tolerance test is usually indicated for clarification. If hyperlipidemia is present, high- and low-density lipoprotein fractions help to determine the need for statin therapy.

A low plasma renin activity (PRA) is an important clue towards monogenetic forms of hypertension (see also Chapter 43). A high PRA is a specific but not very sensitive test for renovascular disease, as about 15% of children with renal artery stenosis have normal renin.[74,75] Samples for PRA must be taken in the supine position after a period of rest and interpreted with appropriate pediatric reference ranges.[74,76]

If the history or clinical picture is suggestive of endocrine disease, appropriate tests such as thyroid hormones, serum aldosterone, and plasma and urine steroid levels should be used. Similarly, a clinical suspicion of pheochromocytoma should prompt plasma or urine catecholamine testing. Traditionally, 24-hour urine vanillylmandelic acid has been used widely due to its high specificity (specificity 95%, but only 64% sensitivity), and this is still a valuable test for children with a low risk of pheochromocytoma. For patients at high risk—such as children with multiple endocrine neoplasia (MEN) syndromes, von Hippel-Landau syndrome, neurofibromatosis, or paraganglionic syndromes—plasma-free metanephrines have superseded plasma catecholamines due to their very high sensitivity (sensitivity 99% and 69%, respectively).[77,78] Usually, however, such tests are only necessary if the primary investigations have not unveiled a cause of hypertension (see Figure 42-2). Overuse of very sensitive but not very specific tests, such as plasma metanephrines, leads to a high rate of false-positive results.[79]

Additional renal imaging is necessary to exclude renovascular disease. This should be suspected especially in small children, patients with marked hypertension, and elevated plasma renin activity, and those with a history of neonatal umbilical artery catheterization, neonatal asphyxia, severe hypotensive episodes, or in neurofibromatosis type 1. There is no standard order of investigations, as a range of imaging techniques exists, and local availability and expertise play a considerable role. For adults, a two-step approach has been suggested, starting with Doppler ultrasound, conventional renography (usually with DMSA), or ACE inhibitor renography, and proceeding to spiral CT for patients with normal renal function or magnetic resonance angiography (MRA) for patients with impaired renal function.[80]

In children, we advise the use of Doppler ultrasound as the first-line examination. Even though in many larger children interpretation of native kidneys may be difficult, often helpful information can be gained in smaller children and in transplant recipients. Due to the lower exposure to radiation, MRA should be preferred over CT as the second-line examination. Only in special cases should renal vein renin measurements and intra-arterial digital subtraction angiography be performed, even though the latter is considered the "gold standard," because both techniques are invasive and require a large degree of skill and expertise.[81]

Other forms of renal imaging may be necessary if a suggestive history is present, such as micturating cysto-urethrography if there is a history of febrile urinary tract infections, or if renal ultrasound is suggestive of structural abnormalities. For instance, an abdominal magnetic resonance scan might be undertaken to exclude a tumor or a diuretic radionucleotide scan to determine the extent of ureteric obstruction.

Assessment of End-Organ Damage in Pediatric Hypertension

As soon as hypertension is confirmed and diagnostic procedures initiated, the assessment of end-organ damage should also be started and continued at regular intervals depending

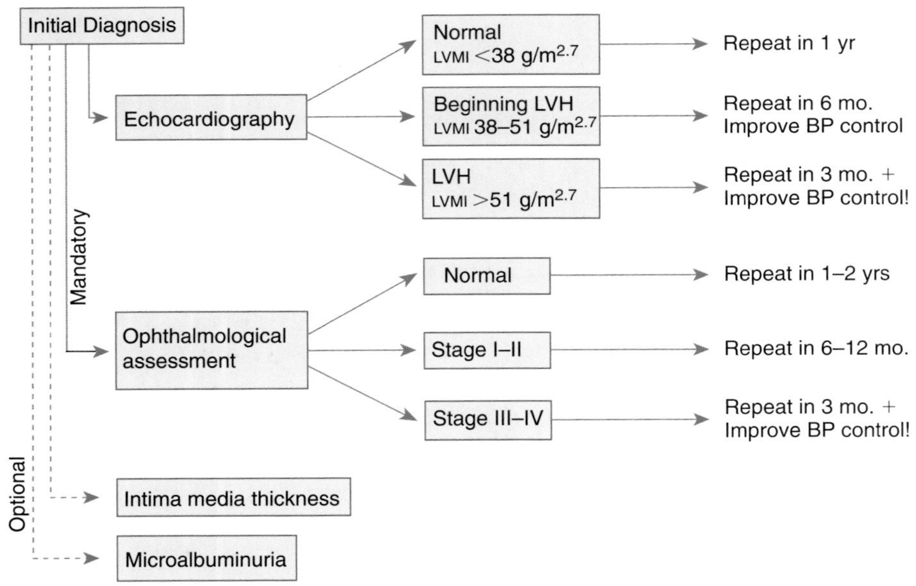

Figure 42-3 Assessment of target organ damage at diagnosis and follow-up. Hypertensive retinopathy is graded on the Keith-Wagener-Barker classification. *BP*, Blood pressure; *LVH*, left ventricular hypertrophy; *LVMI*, left ventricular mass index.

on initial findings and the degree of hypertension. The presence, absence, or new development of end-organ damage is an important guide in the choice and intensity of antihypertensive therapy. Current guidelines recommend echocardiography and retinal examination as necessary examinations in assessing end-organ damage.[4] More recently, carotid artery intima media thickness and microalbuminuria have been propagated as additional markers of vascular damage. Due to their noninvasiveness and sensitivity, we feel they should be included in the staging and monitoring of the cardiovascular status in hypertensive children. A flow diagram of target-organ damage assessment is given in Figure 42-3.

Cardiac Evaluation

Left ventricular hypertrophy is second only to age in being the most powerful predictor of cardiovascular events in adults, predisposing to coronary heart disease, sudden death, congestive heart failure, and stroke. The best noninvasive assessment of cardiac mass is the estimation of left ventricular mass (LVM) by echocardiographic standardized measurements with the Devereux formula, indexed to height (in meters) to the power of 2.7.[82-84] By convention, an LVM index greater than 51 $g/m^{2.7}$ is defined as left ventricular hypertrophy (LVH) in adults, as this has been associated with a four-fold increase in cardiovascular risk.[85]

Left ventricular hypertrophy is found in a large number of children with secondary hypertension, as well as with mild, untreated essential hypertension.[39,86] Therefore, all children with hypertension should have at least one echocardiogram,[4] rather than just an ECG, which has unsatisfactory sensitivity and specificity for detecting LVH.[87]

Controversy exists about the cut-off levels of LVM to define LVH in children. The JNC fourth report[4] suggests using the adult cut-off (i.e., 51 $g/m^{2.7}$), but this is very conservative since the 95th percentile of LVM in children is approximately 38 $g/m^{2.7}$. The adult 97th percentile of 51 $g/m^{2.7}$ is far above the 99th pediatric percentile.[86] Hence, although studies linking LVM to cardiovascular outcomes do not exist in children, it appears reasonable to define, analogously to BP limits, any LVM above the 95th percentile as significant LVH, and thus to be considered for intensified antihypertensive treatment. An LVM index of 38 to 51 would indicate mild to moderate, and an index above 51 severe LVH.

Ophthalmological Evaluation

Hypertensive retinal changes are not only a marker of hypertensive vessel damage but can seriously endanger a patient's eyesight. Proper fundoscopic examination is required to detect hypertensive retinopathy, which is graded into four stages.[88] Although this classification has been criticized as too insensitive for mild changes,[89] it is robust and predictive of cardiovascular mortality in adults.[90] Three pediatric studies found a high prevalence of retinal changes (between 30 and 50%) in hypertensive infants, children, and adolescents.[89,91,92] Grade I and II changes are caused by persistent mild hypertension, while grade III and IV changes usually occur during hypertensive crises and may cause permanent loss of vision.[89] There is no specific treatment, but grade I and II changes particularly appear to reverse more easily in children than adults upon lowering of BP. However, younger individuals are at greater risk of hypertensive choroidopathy, which may contribute to visual loss. Hypertension is also associated with retinal vein hemorrhage and raised intraocular pressure, altogether warranting professional ophthalmologic examination of newly diagnosed hypertensive children.

Vascular Evaluation

In addition to left ventricular mass indexing, a range of peripheral vessel examinations are abnormal in hypertensive subjects such as intima media thickness (IMT) of the carotid arteries or the aorta, flow-mediated dilatation of forearm vessels, stiffness indexes derived from pulse wave analysis, and coronary artery calcification. Intima media thickening is a result of high BP leading to fibromuscular thickening in response to higher tension on vessel walls. It is of long-term significance, as higher childhood BP is associated with higher IMT even 20 years later into adulthood,[93] where IMT is an independent predictor of myocardial infarction and stroke.[94] The noninvasive nature of the technique makes it an attractive option for a clinically useful sign of target-organ damage and predictor of outcome.

In children, IMT is increased in essential and secondary hypertension, as well as in normotensive children with classical cardiovascular risk factors such as increased BMI.[95-97] Interestingly, in a recent study of age and BMI matched children, ambulatory BP remained a strong correlate of IMT despite BMI matching, indicating that even though intima media thickening is found simultaneously with nonhypertensive risk factors, BP per se does play an important role.[98] In children with chronic renal failure, intima media thickening may be partly reversible after renal transplantation.[96]

Microalbuminuria

As hypertension is a leading cause of renal failure in adults, early markers of subtle renal damage have been investigated in order to detect early kidney involvement. The main marker used in this field is microalbuminuria, as it has been identified as an important risk predictor in diabetics.[99,100] Opinions about the use of specialized assays for microalbuminuria in children vary. While the current U.S. guidelines do not recommend them as standard,[4] others consider them part of basic investigations[101] due to the predictive power of cardiovascular events in adults.[102] As newer results also show a correlation of reduction of microalbuminuria and improved cardiovascular mortality in nondiabetic adults, it appears justified to regard reduction of microalbuminuria as an independent treatment goal.[103] This relates both to adults and to children with hypertension of other than renal origin. In children with CKD, proteinuria is usually an intrinsic feature of the underlying kidney disorder.

Follow-Up

In patients with left ventricular hypertrophy or inadequately controlled BP, cardiac assessment should be repeated at least every 6 months. In addition, ophthalmological examinations should be regularly performed in patients with hypertensive retinopathy, especially in stages III and IV, but also in stages I and II (at least yearly in the latter). However, even patients with well-controlled hypertension and no end-organ damage at presentation should receive regular cardiological and ophthalmological follow-up, albeit at larger intervals, such as every 12 to 24 months. A diagram of follow-up schedules for assessment of target-organ damage depending on primary results is given in Figure 42-3.

In our experience, yearly ABPMs are helpful in optimizing 24-hour BP control in patients under antihypertensive medication, and to diagnose early changes in BP rhythmicity in patients with secondary hypertension. The finding of persistent nighttime hypertension should prompt the physician to change the timing and/or dosing of antihypertensive drugs.

Target Blood Pressure

Successful treatment of hypertension involves not only the reduction of BP, but also modifying other cardiovascular risk factors such as obesity and (even ambient) smoking. However, the definition of treatment goals is important for guiding therapy. After considerable international divergence about target BP in earlier consensus statements, adult guidelines now uniformly recommend BP lowering below 140/85 mm Hg in "uncomplicated" patients, and below 130/80 mm Hg in patients with diabetes, renal impairment, or established cardiovascular disease. This is based on limited evidence from specifically designed trials such as the Hypertension Optimal Treatment study,[104] and due to a large body of indirect evidence of an association of lower BP with lower cardiovascular risk.

In children, the North American guidelines stipulate lowering BP below the 90th percentile. We also agree with this recommendation, but would base it on 24-hour mean ABPM values rather than clinic measurements, as these give a much better indication of all-day control of hypertension.

The optimal BP target in children with CKD is as yet unknown. The ongoing ESCAPE trial, which evaluates the effect of different BP targets in children with CKD, will soon provide valuable information on this issue. For the time being, we propose to adopt the adult approach of aiming for more stringent BP control in children with CKD, targeting 24-hour MAP to below the 75th percentile. The 75th percentiles for systolic, diastolic, and mean arterial BP are given in Table 42-2.

CONCLUSION

The investigation of hypertension in children requires special consideration, as BP measurements vary according to methods and settings. Attention to detail with regard to use of well-calibrated and validated devices is therefore needed, in addition to use of the correct reference ranges where available. While the debate over auscultatory versus oscillometric devices is still ongoing, the establishment of a new gold standard for casual BP measurement devices, their validation in clinical practice, and new reference data are urgently needed. In the meantime, ABPM overcomes some of the problems of inaccurate measurements through a greater number of readings. Additional benefits of ABPM include the attenuation of white-coat effects, the identification of masked hypertension, and information about circadian and ultradian BP variability. Masked hypertension appears not to be as innocent as white-coat hypertension, and altered BP variability is an additional risk factor for adverse outcomes. Self-monitoring of BP at home is an alternative and cheaper way of gaining a greater number of readings as well as enhancing patient care by involving the patients and their families.

With the variety of techniques used in clinical practice, it is important to remember that correct reference ranges are essential to diagnosing hypertension. While outcome-based data are unavailable for children, the 95th percentile is a flexible age-, gender-, and height-specific cut-off for the definition of hypertension. Problems of this population-based approach are likely to increase in the future, with the obesity epidemic skewing "normal" weight and BP distributions.

Once hypertension is confirmed, a sequential diagnostic approach can uncover an underlying cause in a high percentage of children. A multidisciplinary, specialized team is needed to provide adequate diagnostic facilities for the wide spectrum of pediatric diseases that cause hypertension. The risk factors for essential hypertension and other cardiovascular risk factors should be assessed in all children, as primary and secondary hypertension may overlap, and successful treatment is aimed not only at lowering the BP below the 90th percentile, but also at reducing known cardiovascular risk factors.

Finally, regular assessments of end-organ status should be an integral part of the management of hypertensive children. Sensitive, noninvasive diagnostic tools are available and should be utilized to tailor antihypertensive treatment, not only by absolute BP values, but also by these intermediate cardiovascular endpoints.

APPENDIX: PERCENTILES FOR CASUAL BLOOD PRESSURE USING AUSCULTATORY MEASUREMENTS*

Blood Pressure for Boys by Age and Height Percentile

		SYSTOLIC (mm Hg)							DIASTOLIC BP (mm Hg)						
		PERCENTILE OF HEIGHT							PERCENTILE OF HEIGHT						
Age (year)	BP Percentile	5th	10th	25th	50th	75th	90th	95th	5th	10th	25th	50th	75th	90th	95th
1	50th	80	81	83	85	87	88	89	34	35	36	37	38	39	39
	90th	94	95	97	99	100	102	103	49	50	51	52	53	53	54
	95th	98	99	101	103	104	106	106	54	54	55	56	57	58	58
	99th	105	106	108	110	112	113	114	61	62	63	64	65	66	66
2	50th	84	85	87	88	90	92	92	39	40	41	42	43	44	44
	90th	97	99	100	102	104	105	106	54	55	56	57	58	58	59
	95th	101	102	104	106	108	109	110	59	59	60	61	62	63	63
	99th	109	110	111	113	115	117	117	66	67	68	69	70	71	71
3	50th	86	87	89	91	93	94	95	44	44	45	46	47	48	48
	90th	100	101	103	105	107	108	109	59	59	60	61	62	63	63
	95th	104	105	107	109	110	112	113	63	63	64	65	66	67	67
	99th	111	112	114	116	118	119	120	71	71	72	73	74	75	75
4	50th	88	89	91	93	95	96	97	47	48	49	50	51	51	52
	90th	102	103	105	107	109	110	111	62	63	64	65	66	66	67
	95th	106	107	109	111	112	114	115	66	67	68	69	70	71	71
	99th	113	114	116	118	120	121	122	74	75	76	77	78	78	79
5	50th	90	91	93	95	96	98	98	50	51	52	53	54	55	55
	90th	104	105	106	108	110	111	112	65	66	67	68	69	69	70
	95th	108	109	110	112	114	115	116	69	70	71	72	73	74	74
	99th	115	116	118	120	121	123	123	77	78	79	80	81	81	82
6	50th	91	92	94	96	98	99	100	53	53	54	55	56	57	57
	90th	105	106	108	110	111	113	113	68	68	69	70	71	72	72
	95th	109	110	112	114	115	117	117	72	72	73	74	75	76	76
	99th	116	117	119	121	123	124	125	80	80	81	82	83	84	84
7	50th	92	94	95	97	99	100	101	55	55	56	57	58	59	59
	90th	106	107	109	111	113	114	115	70	70	71	72	73	74	74
	95th	110	111	113	115	117	118	119	74	74	75	76	77	78	78
	99th	117	118	120	122	124	125	126	82	82	83	84	85	86	86
8	50th	94	95	91	99	100	102	102	56	57	58	59	60	60	61
	90th	107	109	110	112	114	115	116	71	72	72	73	74	75	76
	95th	111	112	114	116	118	119	120	75	76	77	78	79	79	80
	99th	119	120	122	123	125	127	127	83	84	85	86	87	87	88
9	50th	95	96	98	100	102	103	104	57	58	59	60	61	61	62
	90th	109	110	112	114	115	117	118	72	73	74	75	76	76	77
	95th	113	114	116	118	119	121	121	76	77	78	79	80	81	81
	99th	120	121	123	125	127	128	129	84	85	86	87	88	88	89
10	50th	97	98	100	102	103	105	106	58	59	60	61	61	62	63
	90th	111	112	114	115	117	119	119	73	73	74	75	76	77	78
	95th	115	116	117	119	121	122	123	77	78	79	80	81	81	82
	99th	122	123	125	127	128	130	130	85	86	86	88	88	89	90
11	50th	99	100	102	104	105	107	107	59	59	60	61	62	63	63
	90th	113	114	115	117	119	120	121	74	74	75	76	77	78	78
	95th	117	118	119	121	123	124	125	78	78	79	80	81	82	82
	99th	124	125	127	129	130	132	132	86	86	87	88	89	90	90
12	50th	101	102	104	106	108	109	110	59	60	61	62	63	63	64
	90th	115	116	118	120	121	123	123	74	75	75	76	77	78	79
	95th	119	120	122	123	125	127	127	78	79	80	81	82	82	83
	99th	126	127	129	131	133	134	135	86	87	88	89	90	90	91

Continued

*National High Blood Pressure Education Program Working Group on High Blood Pressure in Children and Adolescents. The fourth report on the diagnosis, evaluation, and treatment of high blood pressure in children and adolescents, *Pediatrics* 114:555-76, 2004. Used with permission.

Blood Pressure for Boys by Age and Height Percentile—cont'd

		SYSTOLIC (mm Hg)							DIASTOLIC BP (mm Hg)						
		PERCENTILE OF HEIGHT							PERCENTILE OF HEIGHT						
Age (year)	**BP Percentile**	**5th**	**10th**	**25th**	**50th**	**75th**	**90th**	**95th**	**5th**	**10th**	**25th**	**50th**	**75th**	**90th**	**95th**
13	50th	104	105	106	108	110	111	112	60	60	61	62	63	64	64
	90th	117	118	120	122	124	125	126	75	75	76	77	78	79	79
	95th	121	122	124	126	128	129	130	79	79	80	81	82	83	83
	99th	128	130	131	133	135	136	137	87	87	88	89	90	91	91
14	50th	106	107	109	111	113	114	115	60	61	62	63	64	65	65
	90th	120	121	123	125	126	128	128	75	76	77	78	79	79	80
	95th	124	125	127	128	130	132	132	80	80	81	82	83	84	84
	99th	131	132	134	136	138	139	140	87	88	89	90	91	92	92
15	50th	109	110	112	113	115	117	117	61	62	63	64	65	66	66
	90th	122	124	125	127	129	130	131	76	77	78	79	80	80	81
	95th	126	127	129	131	133	134	135	81	81	82	83	84	85	85
	99th	134	135	136	138	140	142	142	88	89	90	91	92	93	93
16	50th	111	112	114	116	118	119	120	63	63	64	65	66	67	67
	90th	125	126	128	130	131	133	134	78	78	79	80	81	82	82
	95th	129	130	132	134	135	137	137	82	83	83	84	85	86	87
	99th	136	137	139	141	143	144	145	90	90	91	92	93	94	94
17	50th	114	115	113	118	120	121	122	65	66	66	67	68	69	70
	90th	127	128	130	132	134	135	136	80	80	81	82	83	84	84
	95th	131	132	134	136	138	139	140	84	85	86	87	87	88	89
	99th	139	140	141	143	145	146	147	92	93	93	94	95	96	97

Blood Pressure for Girls by Age and Height Percentile

Age (year)	BP Percentile	SYSTOLIC (mm Hg) PERCENTILE OF HEIGHT 5th	10th	25th	50th	75th	90th	95th	DIASTOLIC BP (mm Hg) PERCENTILE OF HEIGHT 5th	10th	25th	50th	75th	90th	95th
1	50th	83	84	85	86	88	89	90	38	39	39	40	41	41	42
	90th	97	97	98	100	101	102	103	52	53	53	54	55	55	56
	95th	100	101	102	104	105	106	107	56	57	57	58	59	59	60
	99th	108	108	109	111	112	113	114	64	64	65	65	66	67	67
2	50th	85	85	87	88	89	91	91	43	44	44	45	46	46	47
	90th	98	99	100	101	103	104	105	57	58	58	59	60	61	61
	95th	102	103	104	105	107	108	109	61	62	62	63	64	65	65
	99th	109	110	111	112	114	115	116	69	69	70	70	71	72	72
3	50th	86	87	88	89	91	92	93	47	48	48	49	50	50	51
	90th	100	100	102	103	104	106	106	61	62	62	63	64	64	65
	95th	104	104	105	107	108	109	110	65	66	66	67	68	68	69
	99th	111	111	113	114	115	116	117	73	73	74	74	75	76	76
4	50th	88	88	90	91	92	94	94	50	50	51	52	52	53	54
	90th	101	102	103	104	106	107	108	64	64	65	66	67	67	68
	95th	105	106	107	108	110	111	112	68	68	69	70	71	71	72
	99th	112	113	114	115	117	118	119	76	76	76	77	78	79	79
5	50th	89	90	91	93	94	95	96	52	53	53	54	55	55	56
	90th	103	103	105	106	107	109	109	56	67	67	68	69	69	70
	95th	107	107	108	110	111	112	113	70	71	71	72	73	73	74
	99th	114	114	116	117	118	120	120	78	78	79	79	80	81	81
6	50th	91	92	93	94	96	97	98	54	54	55	56	56	57	58
	90th	104	105	106	108	109	110	111	68	68	69	70	70	71	72
	95th	108	109	110	111	113	114	115	72	72	73	74	74	75	76
	99th	115	116	117	119	120	121	122	80	80	80	81	82	83	83
7	50th	93	93	95	96	97	99	99	55	56	56	57	58	58	59
	90th	106	107	108	109	111	112	113	69	70	70	71	72	72	73
	95th	110	111	112	113	115	116	116	73	74	74	75	76	76	77
	99th	117	118	119	120	122	123	124	81	81	82	82	83	84	84
8	50th	95	95	96	98	99	100	101	57	57	57	58	59	60	60
	90th	108	109	110	111	113	114	114	71	71	71	72	73	74	74
	95th	112	112	114	115	116	118	118	75	75	75	76	77	78	78
	99th	119	120	121	122	123	125	125	82	82	83	83	84	85	86
9	50th	96	97	98	100	101	102	103	58	58	58	59	60	61	61
	90th	110	110	112	113	114	116	116	72	72	72	73	74	75	75
	95th	114	114	115	117	118	119	120	76	76	76	77	78	79	79
	99th	121	121	123	124	125	127	127	83	83	84	84	85	86	87
10	50th	98	99	100	102	103	104	105	59	59	59	60	61	62	62
	90th	112	112	114	115	116	118	118	73	73	73	74	75	76	76
	95th	116	116	117	119	120	121	122	77	77	77	78	79	80	80
	99th	123	123	125	126	127	129	129	84	84	85	86	86	87	88
11	50th	100	101	102	103	105	106	107	60	60	60	61	62	63	63
	90th	114	114	116	117	118	119	120	74	74	74	75	76	77	77
	95th	118	118	119	121	122	123	124	78	78	78	79	80	81	81
	99th	125	125	126	128	129	130	131	85	85	86	87	87	88	89
12	50th	102	103	104	105	107	108	109	61	61	61	62	63	64	64
	90th	116	116	117	119	120	121	122	75	75	75	76	77	78	78
	95th	119	120	121	123	124	125	126	79	79	79	80	81	82	82
	99th	127	127	128	130	131	132	133	86	86	87	88	88	89	90
13	50th	104	105	106	107	109	110	110	62	62	62	63	64	65	65
	90th	117	118	119	121	122	123	124	76	76	76	77	78	79	79
	95th	121	122	123	124	126	127	128	80	80	80	81	82	83	83
	99th	128	129	130	132	133	134	135	87	87	88	89	89	90	91
14	50th	106	106	107	109	110	111	112	63	63	63	64	65	66	66
	90th	119	120	121	122	124	125	125	77	77	77	78	79	80	80
	95th	123	123	125	136	127	129	129	81	81	81	82	83	84	84
	99th	130	131	132	133	135	136	136	88	88	89	90	90	91	92

Continued

Blood Pressure for Girls by Age and Height Percentile—cont'd

		SYSTOLIC (mm Hg)							DIASTOLIC BP (mm Hg)						
		PERCENTILE OF HEIGHT							PERCENTILE OF HEIGHT						
Age (year)	BP Percentile	5th	10th	25th	50th	75th	90th	95th	5th	10th	25th	50th	75th	90th	95th
15	50th	107	108	109	110	111	113	113	64	64	64	65	66	67	67
	90th	120	121	122	123	125	126	127	78	78	78	79	80	81	81
	95th	124	125	126	127	129	130	131	82	82	82	83	84	85	85
	99th	131	132	133	134	136	137	138	89	89	90	91	91	92	93
16	50th	108	108	110	111	112	114	114	64	64	65	66	66	67	68
	90th	121	122	123	124	126	127	128	78	78	79	80	81	81	82
	95th	125	126	127	128	130	131	132	82	82	83	84	85	85	86
	99th	132	133	134	135	137	138	139	90	90	90	91	92	93	93
17	50th	108	109	110	111	113	114	115	64	65	65	66	67	67	68
	90th	122	122	123	125	126	127	128	78	79	79	80	81	81	82
	95th	125	126	127	139	130	131	132	82	83	83	84	85	85	86
	99th	133	133	134	136	137	138	139	90	90	91	91	92	93	93

REFERENCES

1. Chobanian AV, Barkis GL, Black DL, Cushman WC, et al: The Seventh Report of the Joint National Committee on Prevention, Detection, Evaluation, and Treatment of High Blood Pressure: the JNC 7 Report, *JAMA* 289(19):2560-71, 2003.
2. 1999 World Health Organization–International Society of Hypertension Guidelines for the Management of Hypertension, *J Hypertens* 17:151-83, 1999.
3. Williams B, Poulter NR, Brown MJ, Davis M, et al: The BHS Guidelines Working Party guidelines for management of hypertension: report of the fourth working party of the British Hypertension Society, *J Hum Hypertens* 18:139-85, 2004.
4. National High Blood Pressure Education Program Working Group on High Blood Pressure in Children and Adolescents: The fourth report on the diagnosis, evaluation, and treatment of high blood pressure in children and adolescents, *Pediatrics* 114:555-76, 2004.
5. Cuspidi C, Meani S, Fusi V, Valerio C, et al: Isolated ambulatory hypertension and changes in target organ damage in treated hypertensive patients, *J Hum Hypertens* 19:471-77, 2005.
6. Canzanello VJ, Jensen PL, Schwartz GL: Are aneroid sphygmomanometers accurate in hospital and clinic settings? *Arch Intern Med* 161:729-31, 2001.
7. Bailey RH, Knaus VL, Bauer JH: Aneroid sphygmomanometers. An assessment of accuracy at a university hospital and clinics, *Arch Intern Med* 151:1409-12, 1991.
8. Yarows SA, Qian K: Accuracy of aneroid sphygmomanometers in clinical usage: University of Michigan experience, *Blood Press Monit* 6:101-106, 2001.
9. Hussain A, Cox JG: An audit of the use of sphygmomanometers, *Br J Clin Pract* 50:124, 1996.
10. National High Blood Pressure Education Program Working Group on Hypertension Control in Children and Adolescents: Update on the 1987 task force report on high blood pressure in children and adolescents: a working group report from the national high blood pressure educational program, *Pediatrics* 98 (4):649-58, 1996.
11. Graves JW, Bailey KR, Grossardt BR, Gullerud RE, et al: The impact of observer and patient factors on the occurrence of digit preference for zero in blood pressure measurement in a hypertension specialty clinic: evidence for the need of continued observation, *Am J Hypertens* 19:567-72, 2006.
12. Nietert PJ, Wessell AM, Feifer C, Ornstein SM: Effect of terminal digit preference on blood pressure measurement and treatment in primary care, *Am J Hypertens* 19:147-52, 2006.
13. Wingfield D, Cooke J, Thijs L, Staessen JA, et al: Terminal digit preference and single-number preference in the Syst-Eur trial: influence of quality control, *Blood Press Monit* 7:169-77, 2002.
14. Wright BM, Dore CF: A random-zero sphygmomanometer, *Lancet* 1:337-38, 1970.
15. O'Brien E, Petrie J, Littler W, de Swiet M, et al: The British Hypertension Society protocol for the evaluation of automated and semi-automated blood pressure measuring devices with special reference to ambulatory systems, *J Hypertens* 8:607-19, 1990.
16. American National Standard Institution (ANSI)/Association for the Advancement of Medical Instrumentation (AAMI): *SP10:20022—manual, electronic or automated sphygmomanometers*, 2003.
17. O'Brien E, Pickering T, Asmar R, Myers M, et al: Working Group on Blood Pressure Monitoring of the European Society of Hypertension International Protocol for validation of blood pressure measuring devices in adults, *Blood Press Monit* 7:3-17, 2002.
18. Park MK, Menard SM, Schoolfield J: Oscillometric blood pressure standards for children, *Pediatr Cardiol* 26:601-607, 2005.
19. Park MK, Menard SM: Normative oscillometric blood pressure values in the first 5 years in an office setting, *Am J Dis Child* 143 (7):860-64, 1989.
20. Stergiou GS, Efstathiou SP, Argyraki CK, Gantzarou AP, et al: Clinic, home and ambulatory pulse pressure: comparison and reproducibility, *J Hypertens* 20:1987-93, 2002.
21. Stergiou GS, Alamara CV, Salgami EV, Vaindirlis IN, et al: Reproducibility of home and ambulatory blood pressure in children and adolescents, *Blood Press Monit* 10:143-47, 2005.
22. Toumanidis S, Stabouli S, Kotsis V, Toumanidis S, et al: White-coat and masked hypertension in children: association with target organ damage, *Pediatr Nephrol* 20:1151-55, 2005.
23. Hornsby JL, Morgan PF, Taylor AT, Treibner FA: White coat hypertension in children, *J Fam Pract* 3:617-23, 1991.
24. Sorof JM, Portman RJ: White coat hypertension in children with elevated casual blood pressure, *J Pediatr* 137:493-97, 2000.
25. Matsuoka S, Kawamura K, Honda M, Awazu M: White coat effect and white coat hypertension in pediatric patients, *Pediatr Nephrol* 17:950-53, 2002.
26. Vollmer WM, Appel LJ, Svetkey LP, Moore TJ, et al: Comparing office-based and ambulatory blood pressure monitoring in clinical trials, *J Hum Hypertens* 19:77-82, 2005.
27. Ogedegbe G, Schoenthaler A: A systematic review of the effects of home blood pressure monitoring on medication adherence, *J Clin Hypertens (Greenwich)* 8:174-80, 2006.
28. Staessen JA, Den Hond E, Celis H, Fagard R, et al: Antihypertensive treatment based on blood pressure measurement at home or in the physician's office: a randomized controlled trial, *JAMA* 291:955-64, 2004.
29. Nordman A, Frach B, Walker T, Martina B: Comparison of self-reported home blood pressure measurements with automatically stored values and ambulatory blood pressure, *Blood Press* 9 (4):200-205, 2000.
30. Wühl E, Hadtstein C, Mehls O, Schaefer F, ESCAPE Trial Group: Home, clinic, and ambulatory blood pressure monitoring in children with chronic renal failure, *Pediatr Res* 55:492-97, 2004.

30a. Stergiou GS, Yiannes NG, Rarra VC, Panagiotakos DB: Home blood pressure normalcy in children and adolescents: The Arsakeion School Study, *J Hypertens* 25:1375-79, 2007.

31. O'Sullivan JJ, Derrick G, Griggs P, Foxall R, et al: Ambulatory blood pressure in schoolchildren, *Arch Dis Child* 80:529-32, 1999.
32. Soergel M, Kirschstein M, Busch C, Danne T, et al: Oscillometric twenty-four-hour ambulatory blood pressure values in healthy children and adolescents: a multicenter trial including 1141 subjects, *J Pediatr* 130:178-84, 1997.
33. Wühl E, Witte K, Soergel M, Mehls O, Schaefer F: Distribution of 24-h ambulatory blood pressure in children: normalized reference values and role of body dimensions. German Working Group on Pediatric Hypertension, *J Hypertens* 20(10):1995-2007, 2002.
34. Bald M, Kubel S, Rascher W: Validity and reliability of 24h blood pressure monitoring in children and adolescents using a portable, oscillometric device, *J Hum Hypertens* 8:363-66, 1994.
35. Owens P, Atkins N, O'Brien E: Diagnosis of white coat hypertension by ambulatory blood pressure monitoring, *Hypertension* 34:267-72, 1999.
36. Staessen JA, Thijs L, Fagard B, O'Brien ET, et al: Predicting cardiovascular risk using conventional ambulatory blood pressure in older patients with systolic hypertension, *JAMA* 282:539-46, 1999.
37. Clement DL, de Buyzere ML, de Bacquer DA, de Leeuw PW, et al: Prognostic value of ambulatory blood-pressure recordings in patients with treated hypertension, *N Engl J Med* 348(24):2407-15, 2004.
38. Sega R, Facchetti R, Bombelli M, Cesana G, et al: Prognostic value of ambulatory and home blood pressures compared with office blood pressure in the general population: follow-up results from the Pressioni Artereiose Monitorate e Loro Asssociazioni (PAMELA) study, *Circulation* 111:1777-83, 2005.
39. Sorof JM, Cardwell G, Franco K, Portman RJ: Ambulatory blood pressure and left ventricular mass index in hypertensive children, *Hypertension* 39:903-908, 2002.
40. Palatini P: Too much of a good thing? A critique of overemphasis on the use of ambulatory blood pressure monitoring in clinical practice, *J Hypertens* 20:1917-23, 2002.
41. Profant J, Dimsdale JE: Race and diurnal blood pressure patterns. A review and meta-analysis, *Hypertension* 33:1099-104, 1999.
42. Park MK, Menard SM, Yuan C: Comparison of blood pressure in children from three ethnic groups, *Am J Cardiol* 87:1305-308, 2001.

43. Baron AE, Freyer B, Fixler DE: Longitudinal blood pressure in blacks, whites, and Mexican Americans during adolescence and early adulthood, *Am J Epidemiol* 123:809-17, 1986.
44. Liu M, Takahashi H, Morita Y, Maruyama S, et al: Non-dipping is a potent predictor of cardiovascular mortality and is associated with autonomic dysfunction in haemodialysis patients, *Nephrol Dial Transplant* 18:563-69, 2003.
45. Ohkubo T, Hozawa A, Yamaguchi J, Kikuya M, et al: Prognostic significance of the nocturnal decline in blood pressure in individuals with and without high 24-h blood pressure: the Ohasama study, *J Hypertens* 20 (11):2183-89, 2002.
46. Farmer CKT, Goldsmith DJA, Cox J, Dallyn P, et al: An investigation of the effects of advancing uraemia, renal replacement therapy and renal transplantation on blood pressure variability, *Nephrol Dial Transplant* 12:2301-307, 1997.
47. Timio M, Venanzi S: "Non-dipper" hypertensive patients and progressive renal insufficiency: a 3-year longitudinal study, *Clin Nephrol* 43(6):382-87, 1995.
48. Dustan HP, Gifford RW, Frohlich ED, Joint National Committee on Prevention Detection Evaluation and Treatment of High Blood Pressure: The 1984 report of the Joint National Committee on Detection, Evaluation and Treatment of High Blood Pressure, *Arch Intern Med* 144:1045-57, 1984.
49. Sheps SG, Black H, Cohen JD, Joint National Committee on Prevention Detection Evaluation and Treatment of High Blood Pressure: The sixth report of the Joint National Committee on Prevention, Detection, Evaluation, and Treatment of High Blood Pressure, *Arch Intern Med* 157:2413-46, 1997.
50. Task Force on Blood Pressure Control in Children: report of the Task Force on Blood Pressure Control in Children, *Pediatrics* 59 (5):795-820, 1977.
51. Muntner P, He J, Cutler JA, Wildman RP, Whelton PK: Trends in blood pressure among children and adolescents, *JAMA* 291:2107-13, 2004.
52. Staessen JA, Asmar R, de Buyzere ML, Imai Y, et al: Task Force II: blood pressure measurement and cardiovascular outcome, *Blood Press Monit* 6:355-70, 2001.
53. de Man SA, André JL, Bachmann HJ, Grobbee DE, et al: Blood pressure in childhood: pooled findings of six European studies, *J Hypertens* 9:109-14, 1991.
54. Task Force on Blood Pressure Control in Children: Report of the second task force on blood pressure control in children—1987, *Pediatrics* 97(1):1-25, 1987.
55. Park MK, Lee DH: Normative arm and calf blood pressure values in the newborn, *Pediatrics* 83:240-43, 1989.
56. Mancia G, Sega R, Bravi C, De Vito G, et al: Ambulatory blood pressure normality: results from the PAMELA study, *J Hypertens* 13:1377-90, 1995.
57. White WB, Dey HM, Schulman P: Average daily blood pressure load as determinant of cardiac function in patients with mild to moderate hypertension, *Am Heart J* 118:782-95, 1989.
58. White WB, Schulman P, McCabe EJ, Dey HM: Average daily blood pressure, not office blood pressure, determines cardiac function in patients with hypertension, *JAMA* 261:873-77, 1989.
59. Nehal US, Ingelfinger JR: Pediatric hypertension: recent literature, *Curr Opin Pediatr* 14:189-96, 2002.
60. Koshy S, Macarthur C, Luthra S, Gajaria M, Geary D: Ambulatory blood pressure monitoring: mean blood pressure and blood pressure load, *Pediatr Nephrol* 20:1484-86, 2005.
61. Angeli F, Verdeccia P, Gattobigio R, Saradone M, Reboldi G: White coat hypertension in adults, *Blood Press Monit* 10:301-305, 2005.
62. Stergiou GS, Yiannes NJ, Rarra VC, Alamara CV: White-coat hypertension and masked hypertension in children, *Blood Press Monit* 10:297-300, 2005.
63. Lurbe E, Torro I, Alvarez V, Nawrot T, et al: Prevalence, persistence and clinical significance of masked hypertension in youth, *Hypertension* 45:493-98, 2005.
64. Swinford RD, Portman RJ: Diagnostic evaluation of pediatric hypertension. In Portman RJ, Sorof JM, Ingelfinger JR, editors: *Pediatric hypertension*, Totowa, NJ, 2004, Humana Press, pp. 405-20.
65. Wingen AM, Fabian Bach C, Schaefer F, Mehls O, European Study Group for Nutritional Treatment of Chronic Renal Failure in Childhood: Randomised multicentre study of a low-protein diet on the progression of chronic renal failure in children, *Lancet* 349 (9059):1117-23, 1997.
66. Lurbe E, Thijs L, Redon J, Alvarez V, et al: Diurnal blood pressure curve in children and adolescents, *J Hypertens* 14:41-46, 1995.
67. Portaluppi F, Montanari L, Ferlini M, Gilli P: Altered circadian rhythms of blood pressure and heart rate in non-hemodialysis chronic renal failure, *Chronobiol Int* 7(4):321-27, 1990.
68. Carvalho MJ, van den Meiracker AH, Boomsma F, Lima M, et al: Diurnal blood pressure variation in progressive autonomic failure, *Hypertension* 35 (4):892-97, 2000.
69. Narkiewicz K, Winnicki M, Schroeder K, Phillips BG, et al: Relationship between muscle sympathetic nerve activity and diurnal blood pressure profile, *Hypertension* 39 (1):168-72, 2002.
70. Lurbe E, Redon J, Liao Y, Tacons J, et al: Ambulatory blood pressure monitoring in normotensive children, *J Hypertens* 12:1417-23, 1994.
71. Wühl E, Hadtstein C, Mehls O, Schaefer F, ESCAPE Trial Group: Ultradian but not circadian blood pressure rhythms correlate with renal dysfunction in children with chronic renal failure, *J Am Soc Nephrol* 16:746-54, 2005.
72. Sander D, Kukla C, Klingelhofer J, Winbeck K, Conrad B: Relationship between circadian blood pressure patterns and progression of early carotid atherosclerosis: a 3-year follow-up study, *Circulation* 102:1536-41, 2000.
73. Kikuya M, Hozawa A, Ohokubo T, Tsuji I, et al: Prognostic significance of blood pressure and heart rate variabilities. The Ohasama Study, *Hypertension* 36:901-906, 2000.
74. Dillon MJ, Ryness JM: Plasma renin activity and aldosterone concentration in children, *BMJ* 5992:316-19, 1975.
75. Guzzetta PC, Potter BM, Ruley EJ, Majd M, Bock GH: Renovascular hypertension in children: current concepts in evaluation and treatment, *J Pediatr Surg* 24:1236-49, 1989.
76. Harshfield GA, Alpert BS, Pulliam DA: Renin-angiotensin-aldosterone system in healthy subjects aged ten to eighteen years, *J Pediatr* 122:563-67, 1993.
77. Lenders JWM, Pacak K, Walther MM, Linehan WM, et al: Biochemical diagnosis of pheochromocytoma. Which test is best? *JAMA* 287:1427-34, 2002.
78. Weise M, Merke DP, Pacak K, Walther MM, Eisenhofer G: Utility of plasma free metanephrines for detecting childhood pheochromocytoma, *J Clin Endocrinol Metab* 87:1955-60, 2002.
79. Sakawa AM, Jaeschke R, Singh RJ, Young WF Jr: A comparison of biochemical tests for pheochromocytoma: measurement of fractionated plasma metanephrines compared with the combination of 24-hour urinary metanephrines and catecholamines, *J Clin Endocrinol Metab* 88:553-58, 2003.
80. Pedersen EB: New tools in diagnosing renal artery stenosis, *Kidney Int* 57:2657-77, 2000.
81. Dillon MJ: The diagnosis of renovascular hypertension, *Pediatr Nephrol* 11:366-72, 1997.
82. Sahn DJ, DeMaria A, Kisslo J, Weyman A: Recommendations regarding quantitation in M-mode echocardiography: results of a survey of echocardiographic measurements, *Circulation* 58:1072-83, 1978.
83. Devereux RB, Alonso DR, Lutas EM, Gottlieb GJ, et al: Echocardiographic assessment of left ventricular hypertrophy: comparison to necropsy findings, *Am J Cardiol* 57:450-58, 1986.
84. de Simone G, Daniels SR, Devereux RB, Meyer RA, et al: Left ventricular mass and body size in normotensive children and adults: assessment of allometric relations and impact of overweight, *J Am Coll Cardiol* 20:1251-60, 1992.
85. de Simone G, Devereux RB, Daniels SR, Koren MJ, et al: Effect of growth on variability of left ventricular mass: assessment of allometric signals in adults and children and their capacity to predict cardiovascular risk, *J Am Coll Cardiol* 25:1056-62, 1995.
86. Matteucci MC, Wühl E, Picca S, Mastrostefano A, et al: Left ventricular geometry in children with mild to moderate chronic renal insufficiency, *J Am Soc Nephrol* 17:218-26, 2006.
87. Okin PM, Wright JT, Nieminen MS, Jern S, et al: Ethnic differences in electrocardiographic criteria for left ventricular hypertrophy: the LIFE study. Lorstartan Intervention for Endpoint, *Am J Hypertens* 15:663-71, 2002.

88. Keith NM, Wagener HP, Barkere NW: Some different types of essential hypertension: their course and prognosis, *Am J Med Sci* 197:332-43, 1939 (also 197:332-43, 1974).
89. Raczynska K, Potaz P, Aleszewicz-Baranowska J: [Epidemiology of hypertensive retinopathy in young patients after coarctation of the aorta repair], *Klin Oczna* 106:456-59, 2004.
90. Svardsudd K, Wedel H, Aurell E, Tibblin G: Hypertensive eye ground changes. Prevalence, relation to blood pressure and prognostic importance. The study of men born in 1913, *Acta Med Scand* 204:159-67, 1978.
91. Daniels SR, Lipman MJ, Burke MJ, Loggie JM. Determinants of retinal vascular abnormalities in children and adolescents with essential hypertension, *J Hum Hypertens* 7:223-28, 1993.
92. Skalina ME, Annable WL, Kliegman RM, Fanaroff AA: Hypertensive retinopathy in the newborn infant, *J Pediatr* 103:781-86, 1983.
93. Raitakari OT, Juonala M, Kähönen M, Taittonen L, et al: Cardiovascular risk factors in childhood and carotid artery intima-media thickness in adulthood. The Cardiovascular Risk in Young Finns Study, *JAMA* 290:2277-83, 2003.
94. O'Leary DH, Polak JF, Kronmal RA, Manolio TA, et al: Carotid-artery intima and media thickness as a risk factor for myocardial infarction and stroke in older adults, *N Engl J Med* 340:14-22, 1999.
95. Davis PH, Dawson JD, Mahoney LT, Lauer RM: Increased carotid intima-medial thickness and coronary calcification are related in young and middle-aged adults: the Muscatine Study, *Circulation* 100:838-42, 1999.
96. Litwin M, Wühl E, Jourdan C, Trelewicz J, et al: Altered morphologic properties of large arteries in children with chronic renal failure and after renal transplantation, *J Am Soc Nephrol* 16:1494-500, 2005.
97. Litwin M, Trelewicz J, Wawer Z, Antoniewicz J, et al: Intima-media thickness and arterial elasticity in hypertensive children: controlled study, *Pediatr Nephrol* 19:767-74, 2004.
98. Lande MB, Carson NL, Roy J, Meagher CC: Effects of childhood primary hypertension on carotid intima media thickness. A matched controlled study, *Hypertension* 48:40-44, 2006.
99. Mogensen CE, Christensen CK: Predicting diabetic nephropathy in insulin-dependent patients, *N Engl J Med* 311:89-93, 1984.
100. Parving HH, Oxenboll B, Svendsen PA, Christansen JS, Andersen AR: Early detection of patients at risk of developing diabetic nephropathy. A longitudinal study of urinary albumin excretion, *Acta Endocrinol (Copenh)* 100:550-55, 1982.
101. Varda NM, Gregoric A: A diagnostic approach for the child with hypertension, *Pediatr Nephrol* 20:499-506, 2005.
102. Bigazzi R, Bianchi S, Baldari D, Campese VM: Microalbuminuria predicts cardiovascular events and renal insufficiency in patients with essential hypertension, *J Hypertens* 16:1325-33, 1998.
103. Schrader J, Luders S, Kulschewski A, Hammersen F, et al: Microalbuminuria and tubular proteinuria as risk predictors of cardiovascular morbidity and mortality in essential hypertension: final results of a prospective long-term study (MARPLE Study), *J Hypertens* 24:447-49, 2006.
104. Hansson L, Zanchetti A, Carruthers SG, Dahlof B, et al: Effects of intensive blood-pressure lowering and low-dose aspirin in patients with hypertension: principal results of the Hypertension Optimal Treatment (HOT) randomised trial. HOT Study Group, *Lancet* 351(9118):1755-56, 1998.
105. Flynn JT: Evaluation and management of hypertension in childhood, *Prog Pediatr Cardiol* 12:177-88, 2001.

CHAPTER

43 Etiology of Childhood Hypertension

Julie R. Ingelfinger

INTRODUCTION

Identifying a definable cause for elevated blood pressure in hypertensive children and adolescents is an important clinical goal,[1-3] because a specific diagnosis suggests potential for cure, at least in some cases (see Chapter 42). Yet, as blood pressure is increasingly measured and followed by those providing health care to children, the presumed diagnosis of primary hypertension has become more common. Primary or essential hypertension appears to be multifactorial, and one may predict that many people with a diagnosis of what is now called primary hypertension will turn out to have underlying conditions that will be defined in the future. However, it is also clear that multiple genes and many environmental factors contribute to primary hypertension. Among the latter are those nongenetic factors that stem from the in utero milieu or arise during development and that may affect blood pressure over time, a concept under wide discussion as the developmental origins of health and disease, or DOHaD.

We are in the midst of an epidemic of obesity and metabolic syndrome, and that epidemic has profound implications for how we view hypertension.[1,4,5] Hypertension tracks with obesity and is part of the metabolic syndrome. Classifications of blood pressure and hypertension should consider the issues surrounding how best to prevent, forestall, and treat metabolic syndrome.

There are multiple ways in which hypertension can be classified, and how we think about the evaluation of hypertension depends substantially on the method of classification. This chapter will consider several ways in which to categorize blood pressure elevation, and will also briefly discuss several types of hypertension.

CLASSIFICATION BY MAGNITUDE OF BLOOD PRESSURE ELEVATION

Hypertension is often considered in concert with the degree of blood pressure (BP) elevation. Indeed, the 2004 National Heart, Lung, and Blood Institute Task Force update[1] took the actual level of blood pressure for age and height into consideration in their classification of hypertension. The Task Force defined hypertension according to BP levels for age and height, as discussed in Chapter 41 (and listed in Table 41-1). These definitions included a new category, prehypertension,[6] defined as BP between the 90th and 95th percentiles, or over 120/80 mm Hg for any age. The reasoning behind this change in definition is that BP tends to track along a given centile over time, so that many children with BPs in higher ranges are destined to become frankly hypertensive at a later time. The other categories are listed as follows: stage 1, BP between the 95th and 99th centiles plus 5 mm Hg, at which point evaluation and nonpharmacological therapy are recommended; stage II, BP over the 99th centile; and stage III, even higher BP. This is a useful classification, as the higher the BP, the more aggressive the evaluation of hypertension should be. However, such a classification does little to uncover the genesis of the hypertension and, as such, fails to help the clinician uncover a definable cause.

While the degree of BP elevation fails to define etiology, it should be used to inform and guide the evaluation of hypertension (see Chapter 42). Stated simply, the higher the BP and the younger the child, the more actively the clinician should recommend and carry out an extensive evaluation to uncover a definable cause of hypertension. It is also clear that mild increases in BP for age and size are less likely to be associated with a definable cause of hypertension when compared to very high BPs.

Classifying BP by degree of elevation may help to direct therapy. Therapy is discussed in Chapter 44.

DEFINING HYPERTENSION BY ORGANS OR SYSTEMS

A long-established method for classifying hypertension is an organ- or system-based approach that considers hypertension according to the organ or tissue involved. Many of the diagnoses categorized in this fashion have defining characteristic history, signs, and symptoms. The main categories usually chosen include central, cardiac, pulmonary, renal, endocrine, iatrogenic, and other types of hypertension, as listed in Table 43-1.[7,8] One of the first classifications by system was provided by Londe,[9] who reported that about 80% of definable hypertension in childhood was renal parenchymal in origin, with another 10% caused by renovascular lesions, a categorization that has been confirmed by others[7] and sustained for several decades.

The most common causes of hypertension among children of various age groups are listed in Table 41-2.[10] Several of the most common categories will now be discussed from the viewpoint of distinguishing characteristics that may inform the clinical approach to diagnosis and management.

TABLE 43-1 Classification of Childhood Hypertension

Primary Hypertension
Undefined, primary or essential hypertension
Associated with metabolic syndrome
Associated with obesity without full metabolic syndrome
Definable Hypertension
Renal Renal parenchymal Glomerulonephritides Polycystic kidney disease (PKD) Pyelonephritis Obstructive uropathy Transporter mutations Gordon syndrome Liddle syndrome
Vascular Renovascular Main renal arteries Branch arteries Coarctation of aorta Thoracic Abdominal Midaortic syndrome Vasculopathies
Endocrine Adrenal Adrenal adenoma Glucocorticoid responsive aldosteronism (GRA) Apparent mineralocorticoid excess (AME) Congenital adrenal hyperplasia (CAH) Thyroid Hyperthyroidism Hypothyroidism Parathyroid Associated with hyperparathyroidism Pituitary Cushing syndrome Pituitary tumors
Central Sympathetic nervous system abnormalities Conditions associated with increased intracranial pressure Vasomotor center abnormalities
Iatrogenous Medications Substances (some of which are drugs) Injury related

Adapted from Dillon MJ: Secondary forms of hypertension disease. In Portman RJ, Sorof JM, Ingelfinger JR, editors: *Pediatric hypertension*, Totowa, NJ, 2005, Humana Press, pp. 159-79; Ingelfinger JR: Hypertension in children: endocrine considerations. In Lifshitz F, editor: *Pediatric endocrinology*, ed 5, New York, 2007, Informa Health Care, pp. 261-78; Londe S: Causes of hypertension in the young, *Pediatr Clin North Am* 25:55-58, 1978; and Update on the 1987 Task Force Report on High Blood Pressure in Children and Adolescents: a Working Group Report from the National High Blood Pressure Education Program, *Pediatrics* 98:649-58, 1996.

Acute or Transient Hypertension

Acute or sudden-onset hypertension occurs during the course of various forms of acute nephritis, such as postinfectious nephritis and other nephropathies.[7,11-13] Such hypertension often resolves once the acute illness has resolved (although the hypertension warrants therapy). Table 43-2 lists some causes of acute or transient hypertension. Acute hypertension occurs with acute pyelonephritis, with many forms of acute kidney dysfunction, following renal transplant, and with vascular events. Acute obstruction of the urinary tract may also be associated with acute hypertension. Additionally, both salt and water overload, as well as severe salt and water depletion, may be associated with acute hypertension. Increased intracranial pressure, as well as seizures and Guillain-Barré syndrome also may be accompanied by hypertension. One should never forget that iatrogenic causes of BP elevation may occur either because of medical intervention or patient-related use of medications, certain substances, or certain foods.

Renal Parenchymal Hypertension

Most children with renal parenchymal hypertension present with signs of renal disease rather than hypertension.[14] However, some children with renal parenchymal disease first present with severely elevated BP.[11-13] The most common forms of renal parenchymal disease associated with hypertension are pyelonephritic scarring and various acute or chronic glomerulonephritides.[7,15] Other renal diseases associated with hypertension include obstructive uropathy, polycystic kidney disease, and hemolytic uremic syndrome. Reflux nephropathy, particularly if there is renal scarring, has also been associated with hypertension.[16-18] Children with reflux nephropathy may develop hypertension over time. It has been observed in both referral and unselected patient cohorts that the number of children with reflux nephropathy who develop elevated BP increases with age, and is positively associated with renal damage early in life.

While single kidney has been associated with hypertension, this is most often when concomitant problems are present in the single kidney itself, such as renal dysplasia, reflux nephropathy, or other acquired nephropathies.[19,20]

Hypertension, frequently difficult to treat, is often encountered in patients with both autosomal dominant and autosomal recessive polycystic kidney disease.[21,22] Indeed, hypertension in children with polycystic kidneys can be quite difficult to control.

Persistent hypertension is a hallmark of chronic glomerulonephritides.[7] Hypertension is most common in focal-segmental glomerulosclerosis, membranoproliferative glomerulonephritis, crescentic glomerulonephritis, and glomerulonephritis in conjunction with systemic diseases (e.g., lupus glomerulonephritis).

In hypertension associated with chronic renal disease, there may be increased cardiac output and an increased intravascular volume in association with decreased glomerular filtration rate and sodium excretion, along with increased extracellular fluid, increased renal nerve activity, and increased adrenergic activity impacting the heart.[14,23-26] In addition, chronic renal disease is associated with increased peripheral vascular resistance, along with increased adrenergic stimuli, and an increase in angiotensin II, endothelin, endothelium-derived contracting factors, and thromboxane, and a decrease in prostacyclin, nitric oxide, and endothelial-derived hyperpolarizing factors.[14,23-26]

Hypertension is common after renal transplantation, both in the immediate posttransplant period and later.[27-31] While

TABLE 43-2 Hypertension: Acute and/or Transient
Renal and Renovascular
Vascular: thrombotic (renal artery or renal vein), embolic (clot, infectious), vasculitic severe hypertensive damage, microthrombi), trauma-related, iatrogenic (related to surgery, radiographic procedures), compression of vessels, AV fistulae
Parenchymal: acute nephritides (postinfectious GN, HSP, exacerbation of chronic disease, HUS, acute interstitial GN, FSGS (on occasion), RPGN
Acute renal failure: ATN, rapidly progressive glomerulonephritides, RVT, drug induced, any renal parenchymal cause if ARF ensues
Post-transplant: vascular compromise, acute rejection, medication-related, and so on
Acute obstruction
Acute pyelonephritis
Vascular
Renovascular as noted above
Acute aortic compression or compromise due to trauma or surgery
Salt and Water Overload
Iatrogenoic (plasma, saline, too much fluid)
Associated with ARF or with administration of salt-retaining hormones
Severe Intravascular Depletion
Salt and water depletion, severe
Nephrotic relapse with marked intravascular depletion
Neurological
Increased intracranial pressure Seizures Guillain-Barré syndrome Spinal cord injury Dysautonomia Poliomyelitis Other infections
Iatrogenic
Oral contraceptive drugs Nonsteroidal anti-inflammatory drugs Sympathomimetic drugs Cocaine Erythropoietin Ethanol
Food related: caffeine, tyramines, licorice—all said to be associated with increased blood pressure

ATN, Acute tubular necrosis; *AARF*, acute renal failure (also known as *AKI*, acute kidney injury); *FSGS*, focal segmental glomerulonephritis; *GN*, glomerulonephritis; *HUS*, hemolytic uremic syndrome; *HST*, Henoch-Shönlein purpura; *PVT*, renal vein thrombosis.
Adapted from Dillon MJ: Secondary forms of hypertension disease. In Portman RJ, Sorof JM, Ingelfinger JR, editors: *Pediatric hypertension*, Totowa, NJ, 2005, Humana Press, pp. 159-79.

posttransplant hypertension is more common in children who had hypertension prior to transplantation, it may accompany acute rejection and may be related to iatrogenic causes secondary to medications and to salt and water overload. In particular, the very agents used to prevent rejection, particularly calcineurin inhibitors and glucocorticoids, are associated with hypertension. Posttransplant hypertension is also common with recurrent disease and during chronic allograft rejection or allograft nephropathy. The role of the native kidneys in posttransplant hypertension has been controversial, although hypoperfusion with release of vasoconstrictors has long been considered a major factor.[31]

Calcineurin inhibitor–related hypertension is thought to be multifactorial, with activation of the renin-angiotensin system,[31,32] inhibition of nitric oxide,[31,33] and increased sympathetic nervous system activity among the factors.[31,34] Glucocorticoids have long been appreciated as causing hypertension in solid-organ recipients.[31]

Renovascular Hypertension

Compromised blood flow to one, both, or a portion of the kidneys leads to renovascular hypertension.[7,35-37] Renovascular disease is an important cause of hypertension in children and is potentially correctable. Given advances in relatively noninvasive evaluation and in therapy, and less-invasive procedures such as transluminal angioplasty and stenting, as well as in renovascular surgery, it is important to consider this diagnosis. It is unusual to have mild hypertension in renovascular disease,[38] a fact that should be considered in evaluation. Another issue is that several of the diagnoses associated with renovascular disease, such as neurofibromatosis type 1 (NF1), may be progressive.[39,40] Thus, one artery may be involved early in the course of the disease, and other arteries subsequently.

Evaluation for renovascular disease should be considered in infants or children with other known predisposing factors, including neurofibromatosis.[36,39-41] A number of newer diagnostic techniques, such as magnetic resonance angiography and 3-D CT, are widely used in adults; but experience in their use in pediatric patients remains limited in many centers. Consequently, the recommended approaches (see Chapter 42) still note the use of formal intraarterial angiography, digital-subtraction angiography, and scintigraphy (with or without ACE inhibition) as acceptable, if not the "gold standard."[1,36,42] However, the use of less-invasive technologies such as 3-D CT and magnetic resonance angiography are desirable whenever the expertise for both carrying out the study and interpreting it are present. Opinions concerning the utility of renal vein renin studies still vary, and use is center dependent. Because technologies are evolving rapidly, children should be referred for imaging studies to those with expertise in imaging children with hypertension.

Among children, fibromuscular dysplasia is the most common form of renovascular disease. Neurofibromatosis is associated with intimal hyperplasia.[38] A variety of other entities have been associated with renovascular disease in children—Takayasu disease,[43] Moyamoya syndrome,[44] and systemic vasculitides including Kawasaki disease.[45] Renal artery trauma may lead to renovascular hypertension, whether from embolism in the neonatal period, from surgical injury, or from random accidents.[7] In general, children may have involvement of small, segmental vessels to a greater extent than is seen in adults.[7]

The presentation of renal artery disease varies from asymptomatic to hypertensive crisis. Some of the reported symptoms include headache, failure to thrive, and lack of urinary concentration manifested as polyuria or enuresis. While flank or abdominal bruits may be heard, these are not always present.[7,36]

Evaluation should determine the functional significance of the lesion(s) and whether they are approachable or correctable. Management focuses on correction followed by medical control, if full correction is not feasible. Details concerning evaluation are discussed in Chapter 42, and treatment is discussed in Chapter 44.

Coarctation of the Aorta

Narrowing of a segment of the aorta is called *coarctation* and most commonly occurs in the juxtaductal area of the thoracic aorta, just distal to the origin of the left subclavian artery.[46,47] Coarctation accounts for nearly one-third of the cases of hypertension in infancy and about 10% of those in referral centers, but accounts for fewer in other series.[9] While thoracic coarctation is by far most common, coarctation may occur in the abdominal aorta.

In about half the cases of coarctation, the narrowing is severe enough to cause symptoms in the neonatal period.[46,47] Otherwise, coarctation may not be recognized for years. Certain syndromes are associated with coarctation of the aorta, such as Turner syndrome,[48] Williams Beuren syndrome,[49] and PHACE syndrome,[50] which includes posterior fossa malformations (P), hemangiomas (H), arterial anomalies (A), coarctation of the aorta and cardiac defects (C), and eye abnormalities (E). Mid-aortic syndrome, with massive narrowing of the abdominal aorta, often in concert with narrowing of the renal arteries, as well as the inferior mesenteric artery, superior mesenteric artery, and celiac vessels, generally requires major surgical repair.[51]

The genesis of hypertension in coarctation of the aorta is multifactorial.[46,47] Certainly, a major narrowing in the aorta leads to lower BP in the areas below the narrowing. There is, however, much evidence that decreased flow to the kidneys, compensation for that phenomenon, and neural factors are involved. Postcoarctectomy hypertension may also be present and has been the subject of substantial research. Even though coarctation repair is often via noninvasive means, post-repair BP still requires monitoring. Many children still require antihypertensive therapy following repair of coarctation.

Renal Tumors and Hypertension

A variety of tumors, particularly renal and neural tumors, may be associated with hypertension, either owing to direct impingement on renal vessels or because of release of hormones.[7] More than half of Wilms tumor cases are associated with hypertension.[52,53] Reninomas and hemangiopericytomas are small tumors that cause increased release of renin (and may be hard to identify); these may lead to difficult-to-manage hypertension.[54] Occasionally, hamartomas of the kidney are associated with hypertension. Additionally, neuroblastomas and other neural tumors are associated with hypertension.

Endocrine Causes of Hypertension

Most hypertension in children is *not* endocrine in nature, but considering the possibility of adrenal, thyroid, pituitary, and other endocrine etiologies for elevated BP will lead to the identification of some cases of secondary hypertension.[8,55] These are listed in Table 43-1. Pheochromocytomas and paragangliomas are rare but important causes of secondary hypertension.[56]

Whether metabolic syndrome should be classified within primary hypertension or as endocrine hypertension is unclear.[57-59] What is evident, however, is that this syndrome, also called syndrome X, is characterized by insulin resistance. As it has high association with obesity, dyslipidemia, type 2 diabetes, and hyperandrogenism, we mention it here.

Iatrogenic Causes of Hypertension

A wide variety of substances and events may increase BP, often acutely, but sometimes chronically.[60-65] Thus, it is crucial to explore the potential for both general categories as causing either *de novo* or worsening hypertension. A huge number of medications may be associated with increases in BP. These include oral contraceptive agents, sympathomimetic drugs, NSAIDs, calcineurin inhibitors, and glucocorticoids. Erythropoietin is also associated with hypertension. Street drugs are associated with hypertension, particularly cocaine. Some causes are listed in Table 43-2. A more exhaustive list may be found in a review by Messerli and Frohlich;[66] it is essential to review medications and to obtain toxic screens when concerned.

CLASSIFICATION BY PHYSIOLOGY AND MAJOR CONTRIBUTORY PATHWAYS

Yet another way to classify hypertension is by defining its physiology. However, while the physiology for certain conditions that cause elevated BP is well understood (e.g., renovascular hypertension), it is not well defined for others (e.g., primary hypertension). Among the well-known pathways that contribute to elevated BP are the renin-angiotensin system, volume pathways, neural pathways, and of multiple other hormones.[67-70] Markers for many of these contributing factors cannot readily be measured clinically at present. However, there are a few markers that are worth considering, as determining their levels of expression may inform both further diagnostic evaluation and subsequent therapy.

It is helpful to classify BP elevation in children by renin level,[67] profiling the renin level against sodium excretion and considering family history. A high renin level for age is suggestive of renovascular disease or parenchymal disease. However, while elevated levels, on average, are higher in patients with renal artery stenosis, the substantial overlap in high plasma renin activity (PRA) levels between patients with renal artery stenosis and essential hypertension limits its usefulness as a screening tool. Many children with renovascular hypertension will have a totally normal screening examination, though PRA may be elevated and plasma potassium decreased; approximately 15% of children with arteriographically evident renal artery stenosis have normal PRA values.[38] In contrast, an extremely low plasma renin level may suggest one of the several forms of monogenic hypertension. These low-renin forms of hypertension[67] have very different etiologies and include glucocorticoid responsive aldosteronism, apparent mineralocorticoid excess, Liddle syndrome, Gordon syndrome, 11-β-hydroxylase deficiency, and 17-α-hydroxylase deficiency (see subsequent discussion). Assays for direct measurement of renin, a different assay from PRA, are now commonly available, although extensive normative data in children and adolescents are not yet available.

Should BP be profiled with other markers in children? None are quite so directive presently as renin. However, it has been suggested that the use of risk factors as markers may be helpful. For example, uric acid[70] appears to be a risk factor that may be linked to primary hypertension. Both an animal model (in the rat) and epidemiologic data suggest that increased uric acid is linked to hypertension. The rat model creates mild increases in plasma uric acid by feeding animals oxonic acid, which inhibits uric acid oxidase. The treated animals develop hypertension and arteriolosclerosis, which is reversed by administering allopurinol (reviewed in Feig and Johnson[70] and Feig et al.[71]). Kahn et al.[72] were the first to suggest an association between uric acid and hypertension, but there is now a growing number of studies in adults supporting this viewpoint (reviewed in Feig and Johnson[70] and Feig et al.[71]). The association of increased uric acid and hypertension is even more prominent in teenagers, as noted in the Moscow Children's Hypertension Study,[73] the Hungarian Children's Health Study,[74] and a smaller U.S. study by Gruskin.[75] In a more recent study, Feig and Johnson[76] reported that in a racially diverse cohort of children, uric acid was significantly elevated in primary hypertension, and slightly but significantly increased in secondary hypertension, but lower in normal children and those with white-coat hypertension.

While cardiac output, peripheral vascular resistance, and neural and vasoactive systems are known to be involved in determining BP, most are not seen as being specific markers for a cause of hypertension.

CLASSIFICATION BY GENETIC CONTRIBUTIONS TO HYPERTENSION

Clinically, the forms of hypertension that are genetic include a group of relatively rare conditions in which one gene is involved. Most of these conditions were well described before the genetic abnormalities were delineated. These are listed in Table 43-3. Interestingly, most of these conditions either involve the adrenal gland or its response to an aberrant gene. Table 43-4 suggests when to consider genetic hypertension.

Monogenic Forms of Hypertension

Mutations in various specific genes may cause hypertension. In these conditions, the abnormal gene function or product results in specific physiology that results in hypertension, frequently *severe*, early in life.[67,77]

Since several of these conditions are associated with low PRA, as noted above, a low PRA or level, particularly when profiled against urinary sodium excretion, should be investigated further. Table 43-3 lists several forms of monogenic hypertension. If a child has a family history that includes multiple relatives with hard-to-control, early-onset hypertension, monogenic forms of hypertension should be considered. These are now discussed briefly.

Apparent Mineralocorticoid Excess

Hypertension, often severe, in association with low renin, metabolic alkalosis, and hypokalemia, is characteristic of apparent mineralocorticoid excess (AME, OMIM #218030), first defined as a syndrome by New and colleagues.[77-90] AME often presents early in childhood, and its diagnosis is elusive. Indeed, end-organ damage may be present by the time of diagnosis.

In AME, a mutation in 11-β-hydroxysteroid dehydrogenase 2 (*11-β-HSD2*)[81] results in very low levels of this enzyme, which catalyzes the conversion of cortisol to cortisone. Cortisol, as well as aldosterone, can bind to the mineralocorticoid receptor. The increased cortisol is capable of activating the mineralocorticoid receptor, and, consequently, leads to a picture of aldosterone excess. Renin levels are strikingly low.

In addition to marked hypertension, children with classic AME may have failure to thrive and polyuria. The restriction of dietary sodium may be helpful, as volume expansion is part of the physiology.

Glucocorticoid-Responsive Aldosteronism

Over 50 years ago it was noted that some patients with low renin hypertension and high aldosterone or aldosterone metabolites responded to dexamethasone with a decrease in BP levels. Thus, glucocorticoid-responsive aldosteronism (GRA) was differentiated from other forms of hypertension.[82,83] This form of hypertension, (OMIM#103900) occurs because the presence of a chimeric gene (fusion of the 11-β-hydroxylase and aldosterone synthase genes via unequal crossing-over event)[84,85] leads to aldosterone synthesis stimulated via corticotropin rather via angiotensin II or potassium. In GRA, both aldosterone synthesis and secretion are usually high,[86,87] leading to salt and water retention and volume expansion.

This diagnosis should be considered if a child with hypertension has a family history of severe and "resistant" hypertension, particularly when relatives have had early stroke or myocardial infarction. The clinical course in 20 children with known GRA (confirmed either because they had affected relatives with the mutation or in the course of hypertension evaluation) observed that 80% were hypertensive, some even in the first month of life.[88]

Aldosterone levels in both urine and plasma (or serum) may be elevated, but not invariably. Cortisol is converted to 18-hydroxy and 18-oxo metabolites in this condition. These compounds can be measured in urine,[89] which will contain very high levels of 18-oxotetrahydrocortisol (TH18oxoF) and 18-hydroxycortisol, and the TH18oxoF/urinary tetrahydroaldosterone (THAD) ratio is elevated.

Liddle Syndrome

In 1963, Liddle described an autosomal form of severe BP elevation (OMIM #177200) in a family with hypokalemia, low renin, and low aldosterone levels.[90] Hypokalemia was not uniformly present, and inhibiting the aldosterone receptor was ineffective. In contrast, low-salt diet and use of distal nephron sodium transporters were effective in controlling the hypertension. Red blood cell transport studies subsequently suggested aberrant membrane sodium transport.[91] The data taken together suggested that the condition was likely related to an abnormality in the renal handling of salt and water transport. Further, the hypertension and

TABLE 43-3 Low-Renin Hypertension, Including Monogenic Disorders

	Hormonal Findings	Source	Genetics	Comment
Steroidogenic Enzyme Defects				
Steroid 11β-hydroxylase deficiency	↓ PRA and aldosterone; high serum androgens/urine 17 ketosteroids; elevated DOC and 11-deoxycortisol	Adrenal: zona fasciculata	CYP11B1 mutation (encodes cytochrome P_{450}11β/18 of ZF); impairs synthesis of cortisol and ZF 17-deoxysteroids	Hypertensive virilizing CAH; most patients identified by the time they are hypertensive. Increased BP may also occur from medication side effects
Steroid 11α-hydroxylase/17,20-lyase deficiency	↓ PRA and aldosterone; low serum/urinary 17-hydroxysteroids; decreased cortisol, ↑ corticosterone (B), and DOC in plasma; serum androgens and estrogens very low; serum gonadotropins very high	Adrenal: zona fasciculata Gonadal: interstitial cells (Leydig in testis, theca in ovary)	CYP17 mutation (encodes cytochrome P_{450}C17) impairs cortisol and sex steroid production	CAH with male pseudohermaphroditism; female external genital phenotype in males; primary amenorrhea in females
Hyperaldosteronism				
Primary aldosteronism	↓ PRA; ↑ plasma aldosterone, 18-OH- and 18-oxoF; normal 18-OH/aldosterone ratio	Adrenal adenoma: clear cell tumor with suppression of ipsilateral ZG	Unknown; very rare in children; female:male ratio is 2.5-3/1	Conn syndrome with aldosterone-producing adenoma; muscle weakness and low K^+ in sodium-replete state
Adrenocortical hyperplasia	As above; source of hormone established by radiology or scans	Adrenal: focal or diffuse adrenal cortical hyperplasia	Unknown	As above
Idiopathic primary aldosteronism	High plasma aldosterone; elevated 18-OHF/aldosterone ratio	Adrenal: hyperactivity of ZG of adrenal cortex	Unknown	As above
Glucocorticoid-remediable aldosteronism (GRA)	Plasma and urinary aldo responsive to ACTH; dexamethasone suppressible within 48 hours; ↑ urine and plasma 18-OHS,18-OHF, and 18-oxoF	Adrenal: abnormal presence of enzymatic activity in adrenal ZF, allowing completion of aldo synthesis from 17-deoxy steroids	Chimeric gene that is expressed at high level in ZF (regulated like CYP11B1) and has 18-oxidase activity (CYP11B2 functionality)	Hypokalemia in sodium-replete state
Apparent mineralocorticoid excess (AME)	↑ plasma ACTH and secretory rates of all corticosteroids; nl serum F (delayed plasma clearance)	↑ plasma F bioactive in periphery (F → E) of bi-directional 11β-OHSD or slow clearance by α/β reduction to allo dihydro-F	Type 2 11β-OHSD mutations	Cardiac conduction changes; LVH, vessel remodeling; some calcium abnormalities; nephrocalcinosis; rickets
Nonsteroidal Defects				
Liddle's syndrome	Low plasma renin, low or normal K^+; negligible urinary aldosterone	Not a disorder of steroidogenesis, but of transport	Autosomal dominant Abnormality in epithelial sodium transporter, ENaC	Responds to triamterene
Pseudohypoaldosteronism II—Gordon syndrome	Low plasma renin, normal or elevated K^+	Not a disorder of steroidogenesis, but of transport	Autosomal dominant Abnormality in WNK1 or WNK4	Responds to thiazides

18 OHS, 18 hydro compound S; *18-OXOF,* 18-oxotetrahydrocortisol; *ACTH,* adrenocorticotropic hormone; *BP,* blood pressure; *CAH,* congenital adrenal hyperplasia; *compound E,* cortisone; *compound F,* cortisol; *compound S,* 11-deoxycortisol; *CYP 11B1,* 11β-hydroxylase; *CYP 11B2,* aldosterone synthase; *CYP 17,* 17 hydroxylase/17,20 lyase; *DOC,* deoxycorticosterone; *LVH,* left ventricular hypertrophy; *nl,* normal; *ZF,* zona fasciculata; *ZG,* zona glomerulosa.
Adapted from Ingelfinger JR: Hypertension in children: endocrine considerations. In Lifshitz F, editor: *Pediatric endocrinology,* ed 5, New York, 2007, Informa Health Care, pp. 261-78.

TABLE 43-4 When to Suspect a Hypertensive Genetic Disorder

At-risk members of kindreds with a known monogenic hypertensive disorder (e.g., multiple endocrine neoplasia, syndromes)
Hypokalemia in hypertensive children and their first-degree relatives
Hypertension in very young children, particularly if plasma renin is suppressed
Physical findings suggestive of syndromes or hypertensive disorders (e.g., retinal angiomas, neck mass, or hyperparathyroidism in patient with a pheochromocytoma)

Adapted from Dluhy RG: Screening for genetic causes of hypertension, *Curr Hypertens Rep* 4:439-444, 2002; and Ingelfinger JR: Hypertension in children: endocrine considerations. In Lifshitz F, editor: *Pediatric endocrinology*, ed 5, New York, 2007, Informa Health Care, pp. 261-78.

hypokalemia resolved in one patient who underwent a kidney transplant.[92]

It is now widely known that the epithelial sodium channel, ENaC, composed of α, β, and γ subunits, is important for mineralocorticoid-dependent sodium transport in the kidney. Activating mutations of the epithelial sodium channel within the β and γ subunits (which lie in close proximity on chromosome 16) have now been shown to be the cause of Liddle syndrome.[93,94]

Pseudohypoaldosteronism Type II (Gordon Syndrome)

Pseudohypoaldosteronism type II (also called *Gordon syndrome* or *familial hyperkalemia*) is an autosomal-dominant form of hypertension associated with hyperkalemia (OMIM #145260) with a normal glomerular filtration rate, and occasionally with increased renal salt reabsorption and acidemia.[95,96] Mutations in the *WNK1* and *WNK4* kinase genes, located on human chromosomes 12 and 17, respectively,[97,98] are the cause of this rare form of hypertension. People with *WNK1* mutations have mutations in introns, while WNK4 cases are due to missense mutations.[97-98] (Note that the name WNK derives from a description—the absence of a key lysine in kinase subdomain II [with no K kinases]).

WNK4 appears to act as a multifunctional regulator of diverse ion transporters in the kidney, which explains the clinical picture of electrolyte abnormalities and hypertension. Many affected patients have hyperchloremia, metabolic acidosis, and markedly decreased plasma renin activity. *WNK4* mutations appear to act as a loss-of-function mutation for the Na^+-Cl^- cotransporter but a gain-of-function mutation when it comes to the apical secretory K^+ channel ROMK and the claudins.

Hypertension and electrolyte abnormalities usually improve when triamterene or thiazide diuretics are employed, while aldosterone receptor antagonists are ineffective.

WNK1 mutations are also a cause of PHA II. A kindred in which affected patients had large intronic deletions that increased WNK1 expression was observed.

Since WNKs regulate the handling of potassium and hydrogen, patients with *WNK* mutations have increased sodium resorption and volume expansion. Recent research indicates that WNK1 may be an important regulator in BP within the general population.[99,100]

Other Types of Monogenic Hypertension

Hypertension and brachydactyly[101,102] (Bilginturan syndrome, OMIM #112410), is characterized by short stature, short metacarpals, and elevated BP. No responsible gene or mutation has been discovered, although linkage studies suggest that a responsible gene may be on chromosome 12p. There is no specific treatment.

Polygenic Hypertension

Essential or primary hypertension appears to be the end result of the interaction of multiple genes and environmental events. Estimates suggest that more than a billion people worldwide have hypertension, mostly "primary." Primary hypertension was recognized as having a strong genetic component in the premolecular era—it is likely that genetic factors account for 60% to 70% of familial hypertension.[92-94] It was originally estimated that 5 to 10 genes might be involved in setting BP level, but it now seems possible that even more contribute.[103-105]

Familial aggregation of BP (and hypertension) has been recognized for decades. The search for genes controlling BP has increased. Despite the concept that genes are integrally involved in the development of essential hypertension, identifying genes and mechanisms remains elusive. That being said, a number of genes have been associated consistently with primary hypertension, as listed in Table 43-5.[106] Presently, studies to identify potential risk alleles and candidate genes in hypertensive children have limited clinical utility but do have future promise.

DEVELOPMENTAL ORIGINS OF HEALTH AND DISEASE: PERINATAL PROGRAMMING AND HYPERTENSION

That both the intrauterine milieu and the postnatal experience can have a profound influence on future health is well recognized, although the extent to which this occurs is hotly debated.[107-113] The concept that as the vasculature and the kidney are forming, events that impact vasculogenesis and nephrogenesis may lead to alterations that "program" the offspring to increased cardiovascular risk was introduced by Barker and colleagues[107] who observed an inverse association between cardiovascular disease in midlife and birth weight and placental weight. Much evidence has been amassed suggesting that perinatal malnutrition or other adverse in utero events can lead to increased risk for cardiovascular disease.

The link may lie in nephron number. Among the first to note a potential link between nephron number and later hypertension, as well as renal disease, were Brenner et al.[114] Subsequently, Keller et al.[113] looked at nephron numbers at autopsy in a small study, and found fewer nephrons but larger glomeruli in hypertensive persons as compared to normotensive people. Several studies have since reported an association among low birth weight, nephron number, and future cardiovascular disease.[112,115-118]

Laboratory work has been useful in suggesting how developmental events may result in later hypertension. A variety

TABLE 43-5 **Genes Associated with Hypertension**

OMIM Number	Gene	Function	Gene Map Locus
106180	ACE, angiotensin-converting enzyme; kininase 2	Converts Ang I to Ang II and involved in bradykinin breakdown	17q23
601699.0001	PTGIS Prostaglandin I2 synthase or prostacyclin synthase	Vasodilator and inhibitor of platelet aggregation	20q13.11-q13.13
106150	Angiotensinogen; AGT	Substrate of renin angiotensin system; source of angiotensins	1q42-q43
106165	AGTR1, angiotensin receptor 1	Vascular receptor for angiotensin II	3q21-q25
139130	GNB3, the beta unit of guanine nucleotide binding protein	Abnormalities in gene may be responsible for G-protein hyperresponsiveness in hypertension	12p13
191191	TNFR2, tumor necrosis factor receptor 2	May be linked with hypertension	1p36.3-p36.2
600423	Endothelin-converting enzyme 1; ECE1	Involved in processing of endothelin	1p36.1
102680	Adducin-1; ADD-1	Cytoskeletal protein	4p16.3
605325.0001	CYP3A5	CYP3A5*1/*3 polymorphism is associated with hypertension	7q22.1
http://www.ncbi.nlm.nih.gov/entrez/dispomim.cgi?id=605325&a=605325_AllelicVariant0001 163729.0001	Cytochrome P450, subfamily IIIA, polypeptide 5		
	NOS3 Nitric oxide synthase 3	Mutation associated with therapy-resistant hypertension	7q36
171190	Phenylethanolamine *N*-methyltransferase, PNMT, PENT	May be involved in essential hypertension	17q21-q22

Note: Additionally, listed in OMIM, susceptibility loci for essential hypertension have been mapped to chromosomes 17 (HYT1; 603918), 15q (HYT2; 604329), 2p25-p24 (HYT3; 607329), 12p (HYT4; 608742), 20q (HYT5; 610261), and 5p (HYT6; 610262).
Source: Ingelfinger JR: The molecular basis of pediatric hypertension, *Pediatr Clin North Amer* 53(5):1011-28, 2006.

of studies using maternal exposure to medications (e.g., glucocorticoids) during pregnancy or maternal malnutrition suggest that events during gestation can result in later hypertension, nephron deficit, and renal disease (summarized in Vehaskari and Woods[109] and Hoy et al.[117]). Renal development is an exceedingly complex process that can be interrupted easily by toxic insults. Severe toxic exposure may be lethal to the fetus, but the effects of malnutrition or more subtle exposures are far less obvious. In early inquiries about how programming occurs, some studies have examined candidate genes and systems known to be important in renal development. Thus, various research groups have explored changes in the placenta or fetal kidney.

Maternal protein restriction can alter placental steroid metabolism, for example, decreasing the amount of 11β-hydroxysteroid dehydrogenase, which normally inactivates cortisol or corticosterone; as a result, the fetus is exposed to more maternal cortisone.[119] A higher amount of cortisol will be able to act on nuclear receptors, which might affect nephrogenesis. Experimentally, in the rat, Ortiz et al.[120] found that, depending on the time of injection, dexamethasone could affect glomerular number and later BP.

Another approach is based on the concept that since enhanced sodium retention can lead to hypertension, one should look for alterations in sodium transporters in animals exposed to the effects of low-protein maternal diet. Manning et al.[121] took this approach and found that animals exposed to a low-protein diet had increased expression of two sodium transporters, renal bumetanide–sensitive Na^+-K^+-$2Cl^-$ cotransporter (BSC1), and the thiazide-sensitive sodium chloride cotransporter (TSC). This was seen early, at 4 weeks of age, before the onset of hypertension.

A number of studies have examined the intrarenal renin-angiotensin system (RAS) in the offspring of protein-restricted mothers.[122-124] The kidneys of offspring of low-protein mothers appear to have lower levels of renin mRNA, protein, renin immunostaining, and angiotensin II. Since intrarenal angiotensin II is necessary for normal nephrogenesis, it appears that the alteration in this pathway may be a mechanism by which programming occurs. Further, this finding is consistent with the changes seen to a more pronounced degree when a fetus is exposed to medications that interrupt the RAS, interfere with the production of angiotensin II, or block its receptors.[125] Other factors that may be important include changes in growth factors[126] and increased apoptosis.[127] Another hypothesis is that the balance between nitric oxide (NO) and reactive oxygen species (ROS) is altered when there is perinatal maternal malnutrition,[128] which would affect the fetus. To date, effects of perinatal manipulation of NO and ROS on adult BP have not been delineated. As more is understood about the genes and systems involved in the development of the mammalian kidney, better understanding of perinatal programming is likely to emerge. An additional issue is the rate of postnatal growth. There is evidence that adults who go on to have cardiovascular events had low birth weights and grew slowly early on but subsequently showed rapid growth and weight gain, leading to insulin resistance. Thus, the rate or tempo of growth may be important.[129]

From the viewpoint, however, of classifying hypertension, it is not possible to categorize a child as having hypertension owing to perinatal programming. However, it may be reasonable to state that perinatal programming contributes to what we call primary hypertension.

SUMMARY

Since the conditions that cause hypertension in children are multiple, and the symptoms are often nonspecific, it makes sense to consider a wide differential diagnosis and to seek causes of definable hypertension, and particularly the younger the child and the higher the BP. History, family history, and physical examination must be performed carefully in order to focus the evaluation. Careful attention to these several components of clinical medicine may guide assessment of the hypertensive child.

REFERENCES

1. National High Blood Pressure Education Program Working Group on High Blood Pressure in Children and Adolescents: Fourth report on the diagnosis, evaluation and treatment of high blood pressure in children and adolescents, *Pediatrics* 114:555-76, 2004.
2. Rowan S, Adrogues H, Mathur A, Kamat D: Pediatric hypertension: a review for the primary care provider, *Clin Pediatr (Phila)* 44(4):289-96, 2005.
3. Varda NM, Gregoric A: A diagnostic approach for the child with hypertension, *Pediatr Nephrol* 20(4):499-506, 2005.
4. Sorof JM, Lai D, Turner J, Poffenbarger T, Portman RJ: Overweight, ethnicity, and the prevalence of hypertension in school-aged children, *Pediatrics* 113(3 Pt 1):475-82, 2004.
5. Daniels SR, Arnett DK, Eckel RH, Gidding SS, et al: Overweight in children and adolescents: pathophysiology, consequences, prevention, and treatment, *Circulation* 111(15):1999-2012, 2005.
6. Chobanian AV, Bakris GL, Black HR, Cushman WC, et al: The Seventh Report of the Joint National Committee on Prevention, Detection, Evaluation, and Treatment of High Blood Pressure, *JAMA* 289(19):2560-72, 2003. Epub May 14, 2003.
7. Dillon MJ: Secondary forms of hypertension disease. Portman RJ, Sorof JM, Ingelfinger JR, editors: *Pediatric hypertension*, Totowa, NJ, 2005, Humana Press, pp. 159-79.
8. Ingelfinger JR: Hypertension in children: endocrine considerations. In Lifshitz F, editor: *Pediatric endocrinology*, ed 5, New York, 2007, Informa Health Care, pp. 261-78.
9. Londe S: Causes of hypertension in the young, *Pediatr Clin North Am* 25:55-58, 1978.
10. Update on the 1987 Task Force Report on High Blood Pressure in Children and Adolescents: a Working Group Report from the National High Blood Pressure Education Program, *Pediatrics* 98:649-58, 1996.
11. Adelman RD, Coppo R, Dillon MJ: The emergency management of severe hypertension, *Pediatr Nephrol* 14(5):422-27, 2000.
12. Mentser M, Bunchman T: Nephrology in the pediatric intensive care unit, *Semin Nephrol* 18(3):330-40, 1998.
13. Fivush B, Neu A, Furth S: Acute hypertensive crisis in children: emergencies and urgencies, *Curr Opin Pediatr* 9:233-36, 1996.
14. Schaefer F, Mehls O: Hypertension in chronic kidney disease. In Portman RJ, Sorof JM, Ingelfinger JR, editors: *Pediatric hypertension*, Totowa, NJ, 2005, Humana Press, pp. 371-87.
15. Gill JR Jr, Bartter FC: Overproduction of sodium-retaining steroids by the zona glomerulosa is adrenocorticotropin-dependent and mediates hypertension in dexamethasone-suppressible aldosteronism, *J Clin Endocrinol Metab* 53:331-37, 1981.
16. Wallace DMH, Rothwell DL, Williams DI: Long term follow up of surgically treated vesico ureteric reflux, *Br J Urol* 50:479-84, 1978.
17. Zhang Y, Bailey RR: A long-term followup of adults with reflux nephropathy, *N Z Med J* 108:142-44, 1995.
18. Goonasekera CDA, Shah V, Wade AM, Barratt TM, Dillon MJ: 15-year follow-up of renin and blood pressure in reflux nephropathy, *Lancet* 347:640-43, 1996.
19. Mei-Zahav M, Korzets Z, Cohen I, Kessler O, et al: Ambulatory blood pressure monitoring in children with a solitary kidney—a comparison between unilateral renal agenesis and uninephrectomy, *Blood Press Monit* 6:263-67, 2001.
20. Seeman T, Patzer L, John U, Dusek J, et al: Blood pressure, renal function, and proteinuria in children with unilateral renal agenesis, *Kidney Blood Press Res* 29(4):210-15, 2006. Epub September 8, 2006.
21. Rahill WJ, Rubin MI: Hypertension in infantile polycystic renal disease, *Clin Pediatr* 11:232-35, 1971.
22. Nash DA: Hypertension in polycstic kidney disease without renal failure, *Arch Intern Med* 137:1571-75, 1977.
23. D Amico M, Locatelli F: Hypertension in dialysis: pathophysiology and treatment, *J Nephrol* 25:438-45, 2002.
24. Mitsnefes MM, Daniels SR, Schwartz SM, Khoury P, Strife CF: Changes in left ventricular mass in children and adolescents during chronic dialysis, *Pediatr Nephrol* 16:318-25, 2001.
25. Horl MP, Horl WH: Hemodialsis associated hypertension: pathophysiology and therapy, *Am J Kidney Dis* 39:227-44, 2002.
26. Vandevoorde RG, Barletta GM, Chand DH, Dresner IG, et al: Blood pressure control in pediatric hemodialysis: the Midwest Pediatric Nephrology Consortium Study, *Pediatr Nephrol* 22:547-53, 2006. Epub November 7, 2006.
27. Sorof JM, Poffenbarger T, Portman R: Abnormal 24-hour blood pressure pattern in children after renal transplantation, *Am J Kidney Dis* 35:681-86, 2000.
28. Mitsnefes MM, Schwartz SM, Daniels SR, Kimball TR, et al: Changes in left ventricular mass index in children and adolescents after renal transplantation. *Pediatr Transplant* 5:279-84, 2001.
29. Calo LA, Dall'Amico R, Pagnin E, Bertipaglia L, et al: Oxidative stress and post-transplant hypertension in pediatric kidney-transplanted patients, *J Pediatr* 149(1):53-57, 2006.
30. McGlothan KR, Wyatt RJ, Ault BH, Hastings MC, et al: Predominance of nocturnal hypertension in pediatric renal allograft recipients, *Pediatr Transplant* 10(5):558-64, 2006.
31. Morales JM: Influence of the new immunosuppressive combinations on arterial hypertension after renal transplantation, *Kidney Int* 62(Suppl)82:81-87, 2002.
32. Lassila M: Interaction of cyclosporine A and the renin-angiotensin system; new perspectives, *Curr Drug Metab* 3(1):61-71, 2002.
33. Lanse DM, Conger JM: Effects of endothelin receptor antagonist on cyclosporine-induced vasoconstriction in isolated rat renal arterioles, *J Clin Invest* 91:2144-49, 1993.
34. Scherrer U, Vissing SF, Morgan BJ, et al: Cyclosporine-induced sympathetic activation and hypertension after heart transplantation, *N Engl J Med* 323(11):693-99, 1990.
35. Deal JE, Snell ME, Barratt TM, Dillon MJ: Renovascular disease in childhood, *J Pediatr* 121:378-84, 1992.
36. Dillon MJ: The diagnosis of renovascular disease, *Pediatr Nephrol* 11:366-72, 1997.
37. Ingelfinger JR: Renovascular disease in children, *Kidney Int* 43(2):493-505, 1993.

38. Hiner LB, Falkner B: Renovascular hyper-tension in children, *Pediatr Clin North Am* 40:123-40, 1993.
39. Mena E, Bookstein JJ, Holt JF, Fry WJ: Neurofibromatosis and renovascular hypertension in children, *Am J Roentgenol Radium Ther Nucl Med* 118(1):39-45, 1973.
40. Kohane DS, Ingelfinger JR, Nimkin K, Wu CL: Case records of the Massachusetts General Hospital. Case 16-2005. A nine-year-old girl with headaches and hypertension, *N Engl J Med* 352(21):2223-31, 2005.
41. Wells TG, Belsha CW: Pediatric renovascular hypertension, *Curr Opin Pediatr* 8:128-34, 1996.
42. Vo NJ, Hammelman BD, Racadio JM, Strife CF, et al: Anatomic distribution of renal artery stenosis in children: implications for imaging, *Pediatr Radiol* 36(10):1032-36, 2006. Epub July 4, 2006.
43. Fieldston E, Albert D, Finkel T: Hypertension and elevated ESR as diagnostic features of Takayasu arteritis in children, *J Clin Rheumatol* 9(3):156-63, 2003.
44. Choi Y, Kang BC, Kim KJ, Cheong HI, et al: Renovascular hypertension in children with moyamoya disease, *J Pediatr* 131(2):258-63, 1997.
45. Foster BJ, Bernard C, Drummond KN: Kawasaki disease complicated by renal artery stenosis, *Arch Dis Child* 83(3):253-55, 2000.
46. Ing FF, Starc TJ, Griffiths SP, Gersony WM: Early diagnosis of coarctation of the aorta in children: a continuing dilemma, *Pediatrics* 98:378-82, 1996.
47. Rothman A: Coarctation of the aorta: an update, *Curr Probl Pediatr* 28:33-60, 1998.
48. Nathwani NC, Unwin R, Brook CG, Hindmarsh PC: Blood pressure and Turner syndrome, *Clin Endocrinol (Oxf)* 52(3):363-70, 2000.
49. Pober BR, Lacro RV, Rice C, Mandell V, Teele RL: Renal findings in 40 individuals with Williams syndrome, *Am J Med Genet* 46:271-74, 1993.
50. Wendelin G, Kitzmuller E, Salzer-Muhar U: PHACES: a neurocutaneous syndrome with anomalies of the aorta and supraaortic vessels, *Cardiol Young* 14(2):206-209, 2004.
51. Lewis VD 3rd, Meranze SG, McLean GK, O'Neill JA Jr, et al: The midaortic syndrome: diagnosis and treatment. The midaortic syndrome: diagnosis and treatment, *Radiology* 167(1):111-13, 1988.
52. Maas MH, Cransberg K, van Grotel M, Pieters R, et al: Renin-induced hypertension in Wilms tumor patients, *Pediatr Blood Cancer* 48:500-03, 2007.
53. Haddy TB, Mosher RB, Reaman GH: Hypertension and prehypertension in long-term survivors of childhood and adolescent cancer, *Pediatr Blood Cancer* 49:79-83, 2007.
54. Shao L, Manalang M, Cooley L: Juxtaglomerular cell tumor in an 8-year-old girl, *Pediatr Blood Cancer* 2006, Epub ahead of print.
55. Rodd CJ, Sockalosky JJ: Endocrine causes of hypertension in children, *Pediatr Clin North Am* 40(1):149-64, 1993.
56. Pham TH, Moir C, Thompson GB, Zarroug AE, Hamner, et al: Pheochromocytoma and paraganglioma in children: a review of medical and surgical management at a tertiary care center, *Pediatrics* 118(3):1109-17, 2006.
57. Rocchini AP: Obesity hypertension, *Am J Hypertens* 15(2 Pt 2):50S-52S, 2002.
58. Ten S, Maclaren N: Insulin resistance syndrome in children, *J Clin Endocrinol Metab* 89(6):2526-39, 2004.
59. Burke V. Obesity in childhood and cardiovascular risk, *Clin Exp Pharmacol Physiol* 33(9):831-37, 2006.
60. Gillman MW, Cook NR, Evans DA, Rosner B, Hennekens CH: Relationship of alcohol intake with blood pressure in young adults, *Hypertension* 25(5):1106-10, 1995.
61. Stewart PM, Wallace AM, Valentino R, Burt D, et al: Mineralocorticoid activity of liquorice: 11-beta-hydroxysteroid dehydrogenase deficiency comes of age, *Lancet* 2(8563):821-24, 1987.
62. Blachley JD, Knochel JP: Tobacco chewer's hypokalemia: licorice revisited, *N Engl J Med* 302(14):784-85, 1980.
63. Jee SH, He J, Whelton PK, Suh I, Klag MJ: The effect of chronic coffee drinking on blood pressure: a meta-analysis of controlled clinical trials, *Hypertension* 33(2):647-52, 1999.
64. Nurminen ML, Niittynen L, Korpela R, Vapaatalo H: Coffee, caffeine and blood pressure: a critical review, *Eur J Clin Nutr* 53(11):831-39, 1999.
65. Rezvani M, Hartfield D: Cocaine toxicity after laryngoscopy in an infant, *Can J Clin Pharmacol* 13(2):e232-35, 2006.
66. Messerli FH, Frohlich ED: High blood pressure. A side effect of drugs, poisons and food, *Arch Intern Med* 139:682-87, 1979.
67. Yiu VW, Dluhy RG, Lifton RP, Guay-Woodford LM: Low peripheral plasma renin activity as a critical marker in pediatric hypertension, *Pediatr Nephrol* 11:343-46, 1997.
68. Segar JL, Robillard JE: Neurohumoral regulation of blood pressure. In Portman RJ, Sorof JM, Ingelfinger JR, editors: *Pediatric hypertension*, Totowa, NJ, 2004, Humana Press, pp. 3-21.
69. Jones JE, Natarajan AR, Jose PA: Cardiovascular and autonomic influences on blood pressure. In Portman RJ, Sorof JM, and Ingelfinger JR, editors: *Pediatric hypertension*, Totowa, NJ, 2004, Humana Press, pp. 23-43.
70. Feig DE, Johnson RJ: The role of uric acid in pediatric hypertension, *J Ren Nutr* 17(1):79-83, 2007.
71. Feig DI, Mazzali M, Kang D-H, et al: Serum uric acid: a risk factor and a target for treatment? *J Am Soc Nephrol* 17:69-73, 2006.
72. Kahn HA, Medalie JH, Neufeld HN, Riss E, Goldbourt U: The incidence of hypertension and associated factors: the Israel ischemic heart study, *Am Heart J* 84:171-82, 1972.
73. Rovda Iu I, Kazakova LM, Plaksina EA: [Parameters of uric acid metabolism in healthy children and in patients with arterial hypertension], *Pediatriia* 8:19-22, 1990.
74. Torok E, Gyarfas I, Csukas M: Factors associated with stable high blood pressure in adolescents, *J Hypertens* 3:S38990, 1985.
75. Gruskin AB: The adolescent with essential hypertension, *Am J Kidney Dis* 6:86-90, 1985.
76. Feig DI, Johnson RJ: Hyperuricemia in childhood primary hypertension, *Hypertension* 42:247-52, 2003.
77. New MI, Geller DS, Fallo F, Wilson RC: Monogenic low renin hypertension, *Trends Endocrinol Metab* 16(3):92-97, 2005.
78. Cerame BI, New MI: Hormonal hypertension in children: 11b-hydroxylase deficiency and apparent mineralocorticoid excess, *J Pediatr Endocrinol* 13:1537-47, 2000.
79. New MI, Levine LS, Biglieri EG, Pareira J, Ulick S: Evidence for an unidentified ACTH-induced steroid hormone causing hypertension, *J Clin Endocrinol Metab* 44:924-33, 1977.
80. New MI, Oberfield SE, Carey RM, Greig F, et al: A genetic defect in cortisol metabolism as the basis for the syndrome of apparent mineralocorticoid excess. In Mantero F, Biglieri EG, Edwards CRW, editors: *Endocrinology of hypertension*, Serono Symposia No. 50, New York, 1982, Academic Press, 85-101.
81. Mune T, Rogerson FM, Nikkila H, Agarwal AK, White PC: Human hypertension caused by mutations in the kidney isozyme of 11 beta-hydroxysteroid dehydrogenase, *Nat Genet* 10:394-99, 1995.
82. Sutherland DJ, Ruse JL, Laidlaw JC: Hypertension, increased aldosterone secretion and low plasma renin activity relieved by dexamethasone, *CMAJ* 95:1109-19, 1966.
83. New MI, Peterson RE: A new form of congenital adrenal hyperplasia, *J Clin Endocrinol Metab* 27:300-305, 1967.
84. Lifton RP, Dluhy RG, Powers M, et al: Chimeric 11?-hydroxylase/aldosterone synthase gene causes GRA and human hypertension, *Nature* 355:262-65, 1992.
85. Lifton RP, Dluhy RG, Powers M, et al: Hereditary hypertension caused by chimeric gene duplications and ectopic expression of aldosterone synthetase, *Nat Genet* 2:66-74, 1992.
86. Oberfield SE, Levine LS, Stoner E, et al: Adrenal glomerulosa function in patients with dexamethasone-suppressible normokalemic hyperaldosteronism, *J Clin Endocrinol Metab* 53:158-64, 1981.
87. Gomez-Sanches CE, Gill JR Jr, Ganguly A, Gordon RD: Glucocorticoid-suppressible aldosteronism: a disorder of the adrenal transitional zone, *J Clin Endocrinol Metab* 67:444-48, 1988.
88. Dluhy RG, Anderson B, Harlin B, Ingelfinger J, Lifton R: Glucocorticoid-remediable aldosteronism is associated with severe hypertension in early childhood, *J Pediatr* 138(5):715-20, 2001.
89. Ulick S, Chan CK, Gill JR Jr, Gutkin M, et al: Defective fasciculate zone function as the mechanisms of glucocorticoid-remediable aldosteronism, *J Clin Endocrinol Metab* 71:1151-57, 1990.

90. Liddle GW, Bledsoe T, Coppage WS: A familial renal disorder simulating primary aldosteronism ut with negligible aldosterone secretion, *Trans Assoc Phys* 76:199-213, 1963.
91. Wang C, Chan TK, Yeung RT, Coghlan JP, et al: The effect of triamterene and sodium intake on renin, aldosterone, and erythrocyte sodium transport in Liddle's syndrome, *J Clin Endocrinol Metab* 52:1027-32, 1981.
92. Botero-Velez M, Curtis JJ, Warnock DG: Brief report: Liddle's syndrome revisited—a disorder of sodium reabsorption in the distal tubule, *N Engl J Med* 330:178-81, 1994.
93. Shimkets RA, Warnock DG, Bositis CM, et al: Liddle's syndrome: heritable human hypertension caused y mutations in the b subunit of the epithelial sodium channel, *Cell* 79:407-14, 1994.
94. Hansson JH, Nelson-Williams C, Suzuki H, et al: Hypertension caused by a truncated epithelial sodium channel gamma subunit: genetic heterogeneity of Liddle syndrome, *Nat Genet* 11:76-82, 1995.
95. Gordon RD: The syndrome of hypertension and hyperkalemia with normal glomerular filtration rate: Gordon's syndrome, *Aust N Z J Med* 16(2):183-84, 1986.
96. Take C, Ikeda K, Kurasawa T, Kurokawa K: Increased chloride reabsorption as an inherited renal tubular defect in familial type II pseudohypoaldosteronism, *N Engl J Med* 324:472-76, 1991.
97. Mansfield TA, Simon DB, Farfel Z, et al: Multilocus linkage of familial hyperkalaemia and hypertension, pseudohypoaldosteronism type II, to chromosomes 1q31-42 and 17p11-q21, *Nat Genet* 16:202-205, 1997.
98. Wilson FH, Disse-Nicodeme S, Choate KA, et al: Human hypertension caused by mutations in WNK kinases, *Science* 293:1107-12, 2001.
99. Tobin MD, Raleigh SM, Newhouse S, Braund P, et al: Association of WNK1 gene polymorphisms and haplotypes with ambulatory blood pressure in the general population, *Circulation* 112:3423-29, 2005.
100. Hadchouel J, Delaloy C, Faure S, Achard JM, Jeunemaitre X: Familial hyperkalemic hypertension, *J Am Soc Nephrol* 17(1):208-17, 2006.
101. Bilginturan N, Zileli S, Karacadag S, Pirnar T: Hereditary brachydactyly associated with hypertension, *J Med Genet* 10(3):253-59, 1973.
102. Schuster H, Wienker TF, Toka, et al: Autosomal dominant hypertension and brachydactyly in a Turkish kindred resembles essential hypertension, *Hypertension* 28:1085-92, 1996.
103. Garcia EA, Newhouse JM, Caulfield MJ, Munroe PB: Genes and hypertension, *Curr Pharm Des* 9:1679-89, 2003.
104. Mein CA, Caulfield MJ, Dobson RJ, Munroe PB: Genetics of essential hypertension, *Hum Mol Genet* 13:R169-75, 2004.
105. Staessen JA, Wang J, Bianchi G, Birkenhager WH: Essential hypertension, *Lancet* 361:1629-41, 2003.
106. Ingelfinger JR, The molecular basis of pediatric hypertension, *Pediatr Clin North Am* 53(5):1011-28, 2006.
107. Barker DJ, Eriksson JG, Forsen T, Osmond C: Fetal origins of adult disease: strength of effects and biological basis, *Int J Epidemiol* 31:1235-39, 2002.
108. Brenner BM: Nephron adaptation to renal injury or ablation, *Am J Physiol* 249:F324-27, 1985.
109. Vehaskari VM, Woods LL: Prenatal programming of hypertension: lessons from experimental models, *J Am Soc Nephrol* 16(9):2545-56, 2005.
110. Baum M, Ortiz L, Quan A: Fetal origins of cardiovascular disease, *Curr Opin Pediatr* 12:166-70, 2003.
111. Silver LE, Decamps PJ, Kost LM, Platt LD, Castro LC: Intrauterine growth restriction is accompanied by decreased renal volume in the human fetus, *Am J Obstet Gynecol* 188:1320-25, 2003.
112. Manalich R, Reyes L, Herera M, Melendi C, Fundora I: Relationship between weight at birth and the number and size of renal glomeruli in humans: a histomorphometric study, *Kidney Int* 58:770-73, 2000.
113. Keller G, Zimmer G, Mall G, Ritz E, Amann K: Nephron number in patients with primary hypertension, *N Engl J Med* 348:101-108, 2003.
114. Brenner BM, Garcia DL, Anderson S. Glomeruli and blood pressure. Less of one, more the other? *Am J Hypertens* 1:335-47, 1988.
115. Cass A, Cunningham J, Snelling P, Wang Z, Hoy W: End-stage renal disease in indigenous Australians: a disease of disadvantage, *Ethn Dis* 12(3):373-78, 2002.
116. Hoy WE, Hughson MD, Singh GR, Douglas-Denton R, Bertram JF: Reduced nephron number and glomerulomegaly in Australian Aborigines: a group at high risk for renal disease and hypertension, *Kidney Int* 70(1):104-10, 2006.
117. Hoy WE, Hughson MD, Bertram JF, Douglas-Denton R, Amann K: Nephron number, hypertension, renal disease, and renal failure, *J Am Soc Nephrol* 16 (9):2557-64, 2005.
118. Vehaskari VM: Developmental origins of adult hypertension: new insights into the role of the kidney, *Pediatr Nephrol* 22(4):490-95, 2007. Epub November 18, 2006.
119. Seckl JR, Benediktsson R, Lindsay RS, Brown RW: Placental 11 beta-hydroxysteroid dehydrogenase and the programming of hypertension, *J Steroid Biochem Mol Biol* 55:447-55, 1995.
120. Ortiz LA, Quan A, Weinberg A, Baum M: Effect of prenatal dexamethasone on rat renal development, *Kidney Int* 59(5):1663-69, 2001.
121. Manning J, Beutler K, Knepper MA, Vehaskari VM: Upregulation of renal BSC1 and TSC in prenatally programmed hypertension, *Am J Physiol Am J Physiol* 283(1):F202-206, 2002.
122. Woods LL, Ingelfinger JR, Nyengaard JR, Rasch R: Maternal protein restriction suppresses the newborn renin-angiotensin system and programs adult hypertension in the rat, *Pediatr Res* 49:460-67, 2001.
123. Sahajpal V, Ashton N: Renal function and angiotensin AT1 receptor expression in young rats following intrauterine exposure to a maternal low-protein diet, *Clin Sci* 104 (6):607-14, 2003.
124. Vehaskari VM, Aviles DH, Manning J: Prenatal programming of adult hypertension in the rat, *Kidney Int* 59:238-45, 2001.
125. Sedman AB, Kershaw DB, Bunchman TE: Recognition and management of angiotensin converting enzyme inhibitor fetopathy, *Pediatr Nephrol* 9(3):382-85, 1995.
126. Rees WD, Hay SM, Buchan V, Antipatis C, Palmer RM: The effects of maternal protein restriction on the growth of the rat fetus and its amino acid supply, *Br J Nutr* 81:243-50, 1999.
127. Welham SJ, Wade A, Woolf AS: Protein restriction in pregnancy is associated with increased apoptosis of mesenchymal cells at the start of rat metanephrogenesis, *Kidney Int* 61(4):1231-42, 2002.
128. Racasan S, Braam B, Koomans HA, Joles JA: Programming blood pressure in adult SHR by shifting perinatal balance of NO and reactive oxygen species toward NO: the inverted Barker phenomenon, *Am J PhysiolAm J Physiol Renal Physiol* 288(4):F626-36, 2005.
129. Barker DJP, Osmond C, Forsén TJ, Kajantie E, Eriksson JG: Trajectories of growth among children who have coronary events as adults, *N Engl J Med* 353:1802-809, 2005.

CHAPTER 44

Treatment of Childhood Hypertension

Donald L. Batisky, Renee F. Robinson, and John D. Mahan

INTRODUCTION

In this chapter, we present a clinical approach to the treatment of the infant, child, and adolescent with hypertension (HTN). After the clinical approaches are presented, we will discuss the various therapeutic options that are available. Broadly, these options include nonpharmacologic approaches as well as pharmacologic interventions. Currently, the nonpharmacologic options are considered therapeutic lifestyle changes (TLC), in the terminology of the Fourth Report on the Diagnosis, Evaluation and Treatment of High Blood Pressure in Children and Adolescents.[1] TLC are particularly appropriate for children with prehypertension or mild HTN, especially if the etiology is primary or essential.

Within the pediatric age groups, patients span the spectrum from premature and newborn through young adult. Along this spectrum, the role of the specific etiology of HTN is paramount although there are quite different etiologies of HTN in the various age groups that must be considered, particularly when making decisions about initial therapy. Other modifiers for treatment decision making include whether the patient is symptomatic and whether the specific cause of the HTN is defined quickly enough to be considered in the initial treatment decision.

The Infant

Table 44-1 lists a differential diagnosis for elevated blood pressure (BP) in infancy.[2] The infant with elevated BP is likely to have either a secondary cause or an iatrogenic cause for elevated BP. The symptomatic infant with HTN may manifest with a variety of either nonspecific symptoms such as feeding intolerance, irritability, and excessive crying or fussiness, or specific symptoms such as those related to intravascular volume overload due to renal failure. Elevated BP in the newborn period, especially in the neonatal intensive care unit, tends to fall into one of two categories. The first group includes the ill-appearing newborn who may be premature or term with complications such as asphyxia, meconium aspiration, recent sepsis, or multisystem organ injury. These infants need to be assessed within the context of their overall condition. The premature infant needs to be assessed relative to gestational age as well. Caution must be exercised when deciding on therapeutic interventions in premature infants, because renal perfusion and function may be tenuous in these infants and there may be effects on ongoing renal development with certain classes of medications, namely with inhibition of the renin-angiotensin system (RAS).[3] The presence and placement of umbilical artery catheter (UAC) in the newborn infant places the child at risk for HTN from renal infarction.[4] Occasionally, a newborn presents with no obvious complicating features and a secondary cause, such as coarctation of the aorta, or a renal artery or parenchymal disorder.

The other group of infants with HTN encountered in the NICU or post-NICU setting are those who are out of the acute phase of prematurity or acute illness and are noted to have elevated BP when they are a little older. These infants may have had a UAC or renal injury in the past, may have chronic lung disease, and/or may be on therapy for lung disease with β-agonists or corticosteroids. These infants warrant careful evaluation for other possible causes of elevated BP, such as a coexistent underlying renal disorder. HTN in these patients may be noted incidentally or it may be associated with nonspecific symptoms.

Treatment strategies most appropriate for infants with HTN involve (1) quickly uncovering the etiology of the HTN, (2) addressing the likely cause if surgical or medication adjustments are possible, and (3) controlling elevated BP with direct vasodilators or angiotensin-converting enzyme inhibitors (ACEIs).

The Young Child

Table 44-2 lists common causes of HTN in age groups beyond infancy.[5,6] The child aged under 6 years is much more likely to have a secondary cause for HTN, and conditions that often present symptomatically include glomerulonephritis, other renal diseases such as nephrotic syndrome, and endocrinologic causes such as thyroid disease or catecholamine excess syndromes. Conditions that may be asymptomatic include anomalies of the urinary tract or the cardiovascular system, such as coarctation of the aorta. As the epidemic of obesity continues to expand, overweight and obese children even in this age group are at risk for HTN, which often is asymptomatic. When evaluating an obese child, it is important to assess for comorbid conditions, and HTN may be seen in as many as 30% of overweight and obese children.[7] As noted in the Fourth Report, other comorbid issues that may have an impact on therapy in obesity-associated HTN include lipid abnormalities, glucose intolerance, and sleep disturbances.[1]

Treatment strategies most appropriate for young children with HTN involve (1) a thorough evaluation to determine

TABLE 44-1 Etiologies of High Blood Pressure in Infants

Renovascular	Thromboembolism Renal artery stenosis Renal venous compression Renal arterial compression
Renal parenchymal disease	Congenital Polycystic kidney disease Multicystic/dysplastic kidney Ureteral-pelvic junction obstruction Acquired Acute tubular necrosis Hemolytic-uremic syndrome
Cardiac	Coarctation of aorta
Pulmonary	Bronchopulmonary dysplasia
Endocrinologic	Congenital adrenal hyperplasia Pseudohypoaldosteronism type II
Medication/intoxication	Maternal Opioids (cocaine, heroin) Infant Dexamethasone Theophylline Caffeine Pancuronium Phenylephrine
Neoplastic	Wilms tumor Mesoblastic nephroma Neuroblastoma
Neurologic	Pain Intracranial hypertension Seizures

TABLE 44-2 Most Likely Causes of Hypertension Based on Age

Young child	1-6 years	Renal parenchymal disease Renovascular disease Iatrogenic Endocrinologic causes Coarctation of aorta Essential
School-age child	6-12 years	Renal parenchymal disease Essential Iatrogenic Renovascular disease Endocrinologic causes Coarctation of aorta
Adolescent	12-18 years	Essential Iatrogenic Renal parenchymal disease Renovascular disease Endocrinologic causes Coarctation of aorta

the etiology of the HTN, (2) addressing the likely cause if surgical or medication adjustments are possible, and (3) controlling elevated BP with vasodilators, from the calcium channel blocker (CCB) or ACEI categories, when necessary.

The School-Aged Child

Children in this age group (6 to 12 years) may also present with secondary HTN that points to renal, cardiovascular, or endocrinologic etiologies or may ultimately prove to have primary or essential HTN. The child's signs and symptoms may assist in directing the diagnostic workup as well as influencing therapeutic decisions. Symptomatic or severe asymptomatic HTN is most likely, but not exclusively, secondary in origin, and the treatment strategies are directed to the underlying cause of the HTN. Asymptomatic causes include anomalies of the renal and cardiovascular systems. More obese school children are being assessed and identified. As the prevalence of overweight and obese children rises, HTN as part of the metabolic syndrome has been increasingly noted as well. Medications that may lead to HTN are important etiologies in this age group as well.

As children become involved in school, some will also be diagnosed with learning and behavioral problems. For many of the medications used for treatment of behavioral problems, the risk of cardiovascular complications and HTN must be considered and discussed with families.[8] In clinical practice, one of two scenarios may be seen. In the first instance, a hypertensive child is diagnosed with attention deficit disorder (ADD) or attention deficit hyperactivity disorder (ADHD), and considered to be a candidate for treatment with medications with some cardiovascular and HTN risk. The other scenario is that of a child diagnosed with ADD or ADHD who subsequently develops elevated BP while on treatment. In both scenarios, close monitoring of BP is prudent; however, the indications for intervention are not well defined. Depending on the agent used for control of behavior, there may be an alternative medication choice. For many affected children, it is likely that the addition of an antihypertensive medication or stepping up such therapy rather than eliminating the ADD/ADHD medication will be most appropriate. The absolute best choice of antihypertensive medication in this situation is unclear but many therapies appear to be effective.

Treatment strategies most appropriate for school-age children with HTN involve (1) a thorough evaluation to determine the etiology of the HTN and understanding the more common appearance of essential and obesity-associated HTN in this age group today, (2) addressing the rare patients where surgical or medication adjustments may be useful, (3) introducing TLC in patients when appropriate, and (4) controlling elevated BP with vasodilators from the CCB and ACEI groups, with additional medications as necessary.

The Adolescent

The most common reason for an adolescent (age 12 to 18 years) to have HTN is primary or essential HTN.[9] Many times essential HTN is asymptomatic, and often it is linked to obesity, sedentary lifestyle, diet, and a positive family history of HTN. A recent report has shown that HTN is not always "silent" in this age group.[10] Elevated BP in the asymptomatic adolescent may be detected during physical examinations as part of routine health maintenance evaluations, from a preparticipation sports physical or during evaluation for other problems. When persistent and asymptomatic, HTN is especially challenging to treat in this age group. TLC may be most appropriate for the adolescent with mild and most likely essential HTN, but not easy to accomplish. While adolescents may be more independent and not reliant on parents for administration of medication, they often also have a sense of invincibility and resist the advice of parents, caregivers, and authority figures.

Symptoms of HTN are uncommon in the adolescent with HTN, but may include various types of pain and discomfort (abdominal pain, chest pain, headaches, nausea/vomiting, and palpitations), sleep disturbances, and respiratory and neurosensory complaints.[7] Symptoms that are suggestive of a secondary cause of HTN include symptoms of renal, cardiovascular, and endocrinologic involvement. Another important etiology to consider is illicit drug and substance use and abuse.

Table 44-3 lists a variety of agents that are associated with high BP or aggravation of BP. It includes illicit drugs, some herbal supplements, and a variety of over-the-counter and prescribed medications.[11]

Treatment strategies most appropriate for adolescents with HTN involve (1) a thorough evaluation to define whether HTN is primary (most likely if mild or associated with obesity) or secondary, (2) addressing the rare patients for whom surgical or medication adjustments may be useful, (3) educating families and patients and stressing the value of TLC when appropriate, and (4) controlling elevated BP with long half-life agents, typically vasodilators from the CCB, ACEI, and angiotensin receptor blocker (ARB) groups, with additional medications as necessary.

TABLE 44-3 **Various Substances Associated with High Blood Pressure**

Illicit drugs	Ephedra (ma-huang) Herbal ecstasy Anabolic steroids Cocaine Amphetamines Phencyclidine (PCP, "angel dust")
Herbal supplements	*Citrus aurantium* (bitter orange) Gingko Ginseng Licorice St. John's wort
Decongestants	Oxymetazoline Phenylephrine Phenylpropanolamine Pseudoephedrine
Pain relievers	Acetaminophen (regular use) Nonsteroidal anti-inflammatory drugs (NSAIDs) • Naproxen (Naprosyn) • Naproxen sodium (Aleve) • Meloxicam (Mobic) • Ibuprofen (Advil, Motrin)
Prescription medications	Antidepressants • Desipramine (Norpramin) • Phenelzine (Nardil) • Bupropion (Wellbutrin, Wellbutrin SR, Zyban) • Venlafaxine (Effexor, Effexor XR) COX-2 inhibitors • Celecoxib (Celebrex) Immunosuppressants • Corticosteroids (Medrol, prednisone) • Cyclosporine (Neoral, Sandimmune) • Tacrolimus (Prograf, Protropic)
Oral contraceptives	Alesse Ortho-Novum Ortho Tri-Cyclen Triphasil Yasmin
Other	Sibutramine (Meridia) Epoetin alfa (Epogen, Procrit) Methylphenidate (Ritalin) Yohimbine (Yocon)

Source: Mayo Clinic Staff: High blood pressure, available at www.mayoclinic.com/health/blood-pressure/HI00053.

TREATMENTS

Treatment Priorities

The paramount treatment consideration is the underlying etiology or mechanism of HTN (Table 44-4). While there is not an agreed-upon, single best agent for treatment of HTN, one must take into account specific age and patient issues that may be important. There may be compelling underlying disorder–specific reasons to choose one class of medication over another. For instance, a patient with diabetes mellitus may be well suited for treatment with an ACEI or ARB. A patient with migraine headaches may do well with a β-blocker or CCB. On the other hand, one should not use a β-blocker in a patient with asthma or diabetes mellitus, and ACEIs and ARBs need to be used cautiously with teenage girls who may become pregnant. The effects of ACE inhibition on a developing fetus have been underscored by a recent article showing that there may be harmful effects on fetuses exposed even during the first trimester of pregnancy.[12]

In school-age children and adolescents, convenience via once-a-day dosing can be a very important next consideration. Minimizing the risk of side effects, particularly in older children and those who are completely asymptomatic, may also be of great value. Careful explanation of potential side effects, the value of close attention to side effects, and the number of alternative medications must also be stressed to families and adolescents. The family and, in particular, the adolescent patient, should understand the role and importance of the therapies, asking questions, reporting potential concerns and side effects, and the need for continued monitoring of BP to assess the response to treatment. The family should understand the treatment goals. Lastly, the family and patient should understand the collaborative effort among the patient, family, and caregivers needed to successfully treat HTN in children and adolescents.

Children and adolescents with loss of renal function need careful attention as well. The broad term "chronic kidney disease" (CKD) includes children and adolescents with a wide range of impaired renal function. If there is renal injury, high BP may result. With impaired glomerular filtration rate (GFR) and elevated BP, controlling BP may be helpful in preserving GFR. Depending on the reason for the impaired GFR, certain types of medications may be specifically indicated. On the other hand, once there is progressive loss of

TABLE 44-4 **Considerations in Hypertension Treatment in Children and Adolescents**

Most important consideration	Underlying mechanism of HTN (likelihood influenced by age)
Secondary considerations (in or order of decreasing importance)	Likelihood of success with therapy Convenience of once or twice a day dosing Ease of administration Risk of side effects Cost

GFR, those same medications may pose risks for the patient. The child or adolescent with end-stage renal disease (ESRD) needs to be carefully assessed as well. For patients on dialysis, high BP can often be controlled by attending to the volume status of the patient. Patients may be treated either with peritoneal dialysis or hemodialysis, and there are challenges in volume regulation with both modalities. Sometimes there is a need for adjunctive pharmacologic intervention with these patients as well. Children and adolescents who receive renal transplants are also at risk for HTN. While these are important and complex areas, complete attention to these situations is beyond the scope of this discussion. There are good sources with extensive discussions devoted to the subject of HTN in the pediatric patient with chronic kidney disease and ESRD.[13,14]

Treatment Considerations Based on the Fourth Report

In the recent Fourth Report, BP is stratified into normal BP, prehypertension, or HTN, and HTN is further stratified into stage 1 and stage 2 HTN. This is consistent with the Seventh Report of the Joint National Committee on Prevention, Detection, Evaluation, and Treatment of High Blood Pressure (JNC 7) report.[15] In this system, patients with normal BP are educated on healthy lifestyles. The specific intervention for the patient with prehypertension is TLC. Patients with stage 1 HTN usually begin with TLC, but they may eventually reach a point when pharmacologic treatment is prescribed, especially if there are compelling indications. Weight reduction is considered to be a priority in patients who are overweight or obese, as it can lead to a reduction in BP, and it has no side effects, yet it is often quite challenging to obtain cooperation from not only the patient, but also the patient's family. The patient with stage 2 HTN is likely to be prescribed medication sooner, yet TLC remains important adjunctive therapy, and when obesity is a component, it must be addressed.[1]

Summary of Age and Other Factors Involved in Treatment Strategies

When the decision is made to treat a pediatric patient with HTN, a number of factors need to be considered, and the relative ranking of treatment considerations is probably consistent across the age groups (see Table 44-4). One of the first is the age of the patient. The age of the patient helps to frame consideration of the most likely etiologies, determine the type of evaluation, and influence initial treatment options. The treatment priority is the underlying cause of the HTN and the likelihood of success with the particular intervention. Nonpharmacologic treatments, or TLC, should always be at least a part of the patient's management, and sometimes TLC is enough to control the BP, especially in the prehypertensive, or mild stage 1 patient. Essential HTN may be completely corrected or significantly improved by TLC. When the issue of medication to control BP is considered, the importance of the likelihood of success, convenience of once a day or twice a day dosing, ease of administration, low risk of side effects, and cost should be considered. There are a few indications for surgical management of HTN, especially when there is narrowing of blood vessels, that is, coarctation of the aorta or renovascular HTN (renal artery stenosis).

Other compelling reasons include presence of target organ damage (i.e., left ventricular hypertrophy) and comorbid conditions such as CKD and diabetes mellitus. Patients who have a strong family history of HTN should also be considered for therapy.

A review of nonpharmacologic options is followed by a review of the pharmacologic options and evidence in children and adolescents.

Nonpharmacologic Treatment of Hypertension

When essential HTN or prehypertension is detected in a child, nonpharmacologic approaches to lowering BP are often preferable to medications for both the family/patient and the physician.[1,16] Long-term use of medications may be associated with significant side effects and generate associated morbidity and/or mortality. The attractiveness of nonpharmacologic measures to lower BP include the opportunity to respond to underlying pathophysiology, the engagement of the family/patient's effort, and a number of associated long-term health benefits for the child.[17]

Several nonpharmacologic measures have been demonstrated to be successful in lowering BP in adults and children. These include weight loss, exercise, stress reduction, and alterations in diet, including sodium, potassium, and chloride.

Weight Loss

The association between obesity and HTN has been recognized for some time[18] and has been confirmed in a number of well-controlled studies. Independent of age, gender, and race/ethnicity, higher weight is associated with higher BP values in children.[19] Freedman et al.[20] noted that children with obesity were 4.5 times more likely to have elevated systolic BP (SBP) and 2.4 times more likely to have elevated diastolic BP (DBP). Sorof et al.[21] noted three times more HTN in obese compared to nonobese adolescents in a school screening study. In addition to the link to HTN, obesity in children has been strongly correlated with type 2 diabetes, dyslipidemias, obstructive sleep apnea, left ventricular hypertrophy, orthopedic problems, and psychological disorders, and these comorbidities often complicate the lives of children with HTN.[22,23] Vascular changes related to obesity and HTN can be detected early in childhood.[24]

The type of obesity, or body fat distribution, can have a significant effect on BP. Body mass index (BMI) (weight in kilograms/height in meters^2) is a clinically useful method to assess the relation of body mass to height and can serve to help define if increased weight is due to increased adipose tissue. The normal range of BMI varies by age and gender and must be considered in studies of obesity and BP in children. Figure 44-1 displays the BMI-for-age percentiles for both males and females. These charts may be obtained at the referenced website.[25] Several population-based studies in adults have demonstrated that upper body obesity is more tightly linked to HTN than either total body weight or BMI, and that the risk of developing HTN is higher in individuals with upper body obesity. Shear et al.[26] confirmed that BP correlated more closely with upper body fat than total body weight in an investigation of children and young adults over 20 years ago, but there has been no recent information on this topic.

The mechanisms that underlie the link between obesity and HTN in children and adolescents are multifactorial:

1. Insulin resistance leads to salt and water retention and is well correlated to HTN.[27]
2. Activation of the sympathetic nervous system can lead to euglycemic hyperinsulinism, increased heart rate, BP, and plasma catecholamines.[28]
3. Activation of the renin-angiotensin system (RAS) induces altered adrenal sensitivity to angiotensin II and

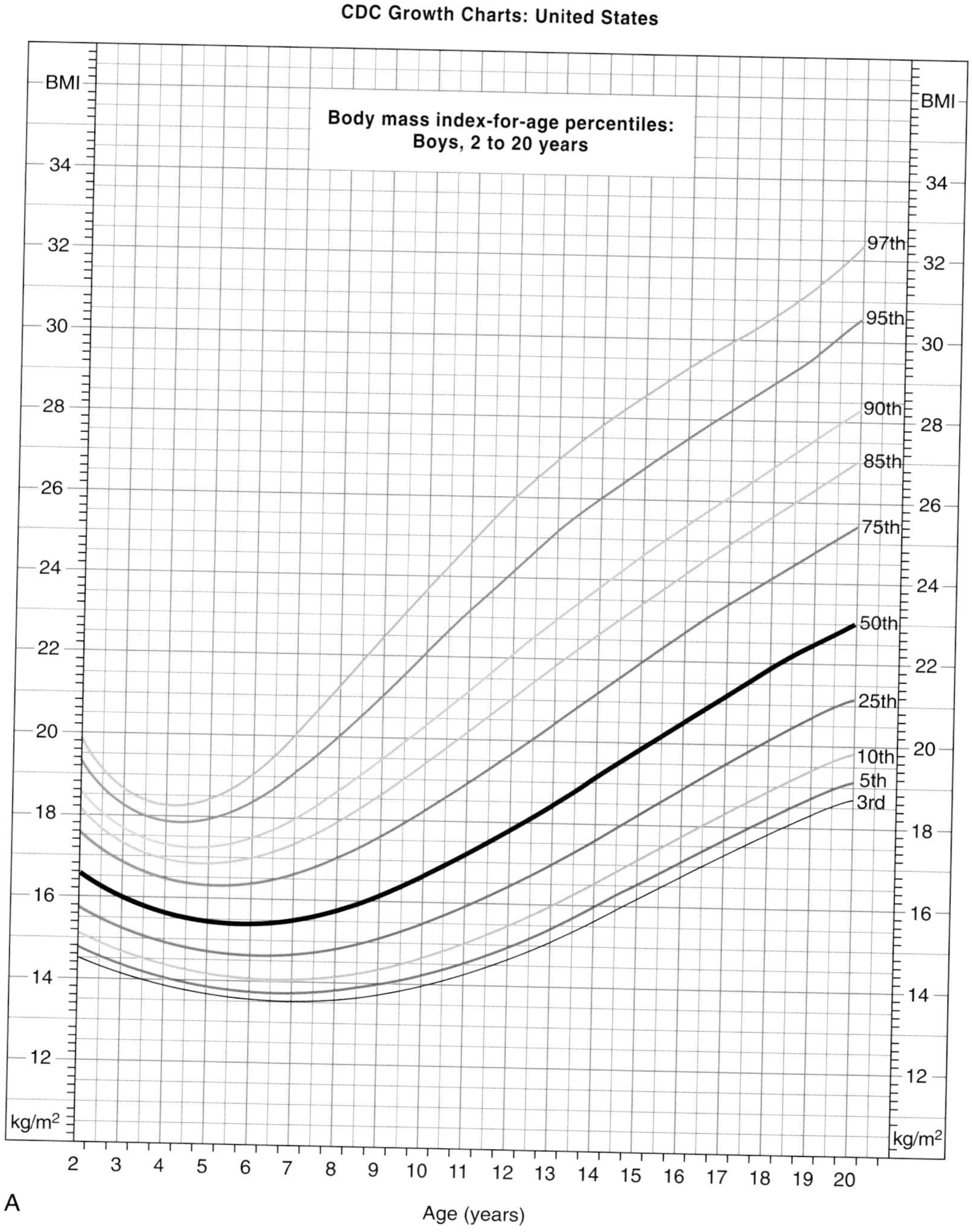

Figure 44-1 Body mass index percentiles for age. **(A)** Boys. **(B)** Girls.

CDC Growth Charts: United States

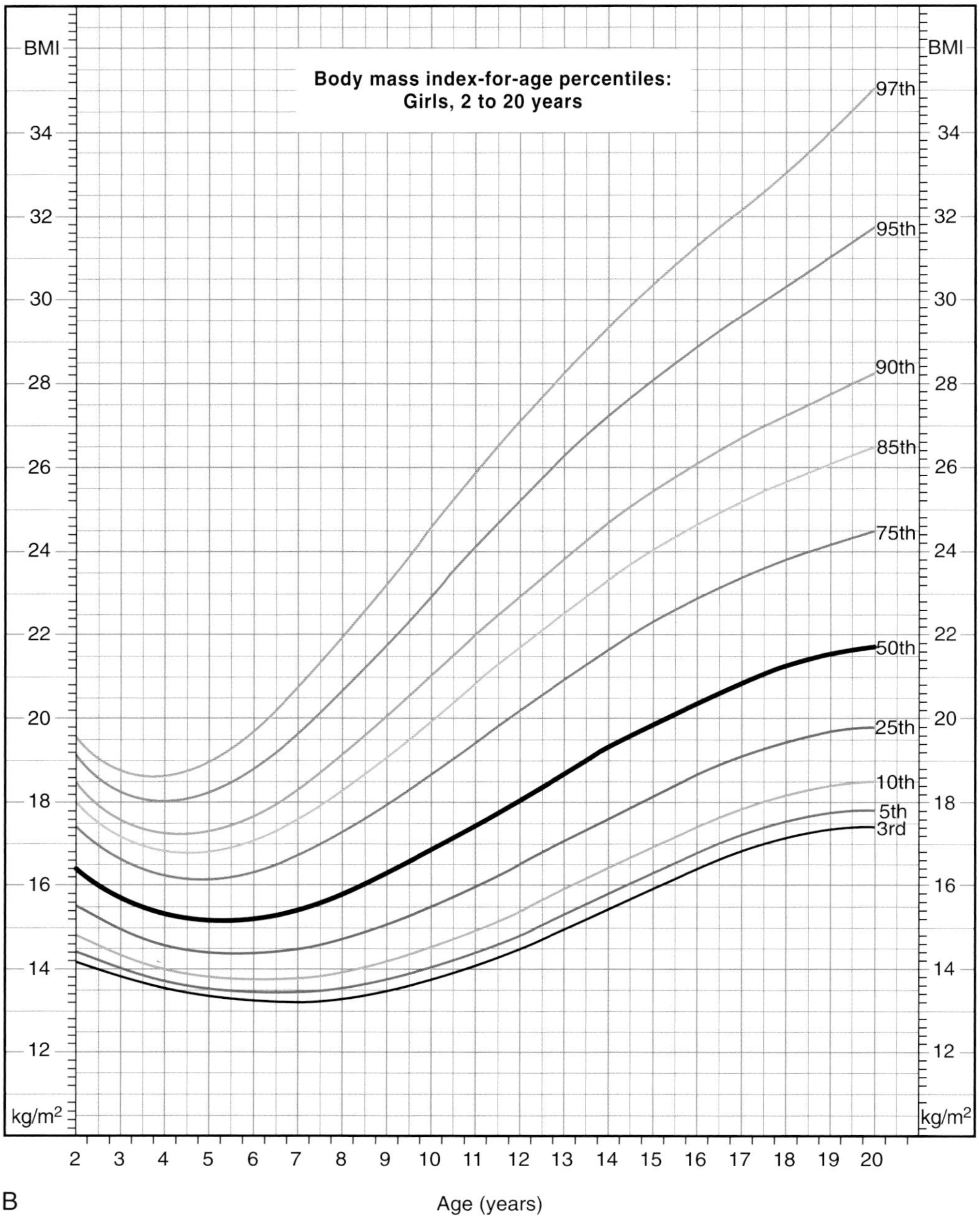

B

Figure 44-1, cont'd

increased levels of aldosterone related to BP levels in obese adolescents.[29]

4. Noninsulin-related alterations in sodium handling may also occur secondary to fat encapsulation of the kidney and resultant increased interstitial fluid pressure, decreased tubular flow rates and enhanced tubular sodium absorption.[30]
5. Leptin, secreted by adipocytes, is elevated in most obese individuals and may lead to increased sympathetic outflow.[31]
6. Altered vascular reactivity in obese children may also affect BP by enhanced vascular resistance response to exercise, persistent decreased vascular compliance or fixed vascular changes.[32]
7. Abnormal hypothalamic-pituitary-adrenal (HPA) axis function and cortisol release has been demonstrated in adults with HTN but has not been investigated yet in children.[33]

The issue of hyperuricemia and its relationship to HTN in the pediatric population is interesting. There have been large studies such as the Moscow Children's Hypertension Study and National Health and Nutrition Examination Survey III that have reported an association between serum uric acid and HTN. In Feig and Johnson's[34] study of 125 children with newly diagnosed and previously untreated HTN, hyperuricemia was correlated with primary HTN, yet BMI—although higher in patients with primary HTN—seemed to contribute little to the observed effect of serum uric acid on BP.

Weight loss is associated with improved BP in children and adolescents with HTN. In adult studies it is clear that obese subjects with HTN experience reduced BP related to weight loss, independent of the effects of alterations of sodium intake and excretion. For individuals at risk of HTN, weight loss is associated with a decreased incidence of subsequent HTN compared to control subjects who do not lose weight.[35]

Obesity, in particular upper body obesity, is clearly an independent risk factor for HTN in children and adolescents. Weight loss in obese individuals with HTN is associated with improved BP values, and for many individuals, only modest decrements in body weight (e.g., only 10% loss of body weight), even if not back to ideal body weight, may completely normalize BP. The strongest evidence points to the effects of insulin resistance, enhanced sodium retention, and altered sympathetic vascular tone as the predominant mechanisms to explain the obesity-HTN connection in children and adolescents.

Efforts directed at weight loss, even if only partially successful, appear to be capable of reversing hyperinsulinemia, sodium retention, and a variety of other pathogenetic factors, and should be incorporated into the management of any child with HTN who is obese or at risk for obesity due to elevated weight for height or familial and genetic predisposition.

Exercise

The benefit of exercise in lowering BP in children and adolescents has been recognized for some time,[36] and emerging evidence suggests that regular exercise in childhood may improve BP later in adult life.[37] There is now good information about specific aspects of exercise programs that can provide beneficial effects in children with essential HTN and, although initially a concern, there is no evidence that significant exercise is associated with any deleterious effects on BP or cardiovascular status (CV) in children with mild HTN.

Significant aerobic exercise over time is associated with improved BP in children with essential HTN. In 1982, Frank et al.[38] described the effects of a combination diet and exercise program in 48 Caucasian and African-American children with HTN, ages 8 to 18, in the Bogalusa Heart Study. The subjects were also provided dietary counseling and antihypertensive medications and had significant (~9 mm Hg) decreases in both SBP and DBP.

Both endurance and weight-training types of exercise programs have beneficial effects on SBP and DBP in children and adolescents with essential HTN. Hagberg and colleagues[39] carefully assessed the impact of aerobic and weight-training programs in a group of Caucasian and African-American adolescents with essential HTN. They noted significant effects (8- to 12-mm Hg drop in SBP and 6- to 7-mm Hg drop in DBP) after 5 to 6 months of aerobic training (30 to 50 minutes of supervised vigorous aerobic activity three times per week). The addition of a substantial regular weight-training program of 5 months' duration in a subset of subjects was associated with further reductions of SBP (4 mm Hg) but not DBP. Interestingly, after 9 to 12 months of detraining, the subjects returned to their baseline BP.

As little as 3 months of aerobic training is associated with improved BP independent of changes in weight in children with essential HTN. As demonstrated convincingly by Danforth et al.,[40] 30 minutes of aerobic exercise three times per week for 3 months decreased both SBP and DBP by 9 mm Hg each in a group of 12 African-American children with mild HTN.

The benefits of exercise programs may be more apparent in boys with HTN than girls with HTN and, not surprisingly, the quality and rigor of the activity are important in achieving a beneficial effect. Hansen and colleagues[41] studied 69 boys and girls, ages 9 to 11, with mild HTN. They all participated in three additional 50-minute sessions of physical education in school each week for 8 months. Although there were no significant changes after 3 months, by 8 months the boys experienced an average 6-mm Hg decrease in SBP, but no change in DBP, while there was no change in BP in the girls. The extent of participation among subjects was difficult to control, as it is in real life, and may account for the different results between the genders.

In children and adolescents, regular aerobic exercise is associated with reductions of both SBP and DBP, and resistance training may, when added to aerobic exercise, provide additional beneficial effects on BP. Moreover, there is no evidence from carefully controlled studies that there are deleterious effects of aerobic or resistance training in children with essential HTN. Accordingly, children with no evidence of HTN-induced end-organ damage should not be excluded from aerobic or resistance training and, in fact, exercise programs should be incorporated into treatment programs in children with essential HTN. Unfortunately, there are no good data that address the safety and efficacy of exercise programs on BP in children with secondary HTN or severe essential HTN. Evidence from studies in adults with secondary HTN demonstrates improved BP with carefully controlled exercise programs, and there is no reason to think that the same types of benefits would not occur in children.

Stress Reduction

There has been long-standing interest in the effects of stress in elevating BP, and in the potential benefits of stress reduction for the treatment of individuals at risk for HTN, as well as for those with established essential HTN. Given the evidence that children with BP values in the upper ranges of normal trend over time to significant HTN in adulthood, and that children with mild HTN may demonstrate improved BP with a variety of nonpharmacologic lifestyle interventions, stress-reduction techniques are particularly attractive options for this population. Moreover, stress reduction offers the promise of an intervention that is directed to underlying pathophysiology in children at risk for adult HTN, since a number of studies have demonstrated that BP responses to stress in children and adolescents can predict subsequent elevations in resting BP over time.[42]

Biofeedback and relaxation training have been proven to be effective for a variety of medical conditions in children, including fecal soiling, urinary incontinence, headache, asthma, and chronic pain, and there are now several studies documenting the effectiveness of such strategies in children with mild HTN. Regular use of relaxation techniques has been associated with significant improvements in BP in children with mild HTN, via musical relaxation therapy,[43] prayer and church attendance,[44] and meditation.[45] The benefits of such approaches were typically modest, but well received by the subjects and the effects in the well-detailed study of Sidorenko[43] noted the most significant benefits in subjects with the highest baseline BP values.

Dietary Alterations (Sodium, Potassium)

Modifications of sodium and/or potassium intake have proven to be effective in lowering BP in adults and children[46] with HTN. There is now a consensus that efforts designed to reduce sodium intake and improve potassium intake should be part of any prevention approach to individuals at risk for HTN.[47] The interplay of environmental factors, including dietary intake, and genetic inheritance affect BP in children. In particular, the impact of sodium handling and genetic phenotypes in young children affect parameters, such as BP, that are important CV risk factors.[48] In addition, positive changes in sodium and potassium intake can reduce BP over time.[47]

The weight of many observational studies in children and adolescents, reviewed by Simons-Morton and Obarzanck,[49] demonstrates a striking positive association between sodium intake, urine sodium excretion, and BP. In individuals who are at greatest risk for CV complications (e.g., hypertensive children, African Americans, those with a positive family history of HTN), there is an increased incidence of salt sensitivity and exaggerated BP elevations with salt loading.[50] The impact of potassium intake on BP in children is not as clear-cut,[49] but there is evidence that the most beneficial effect with high potassium intake is seen in children with salt-sensitive HTN.[51]

Although larger population studies of children and adolescents where electrolyte intake was altered have demonstrated modest improvements in SBP and DBP at best, certain subgroups may experience more profound benefits. Obese adolescents with HTN appear to benefit more from sodium restriction and African-American children experience more impressive declines in BP values with sodium restriction than do Caucasian children.[52]

Altering sodium and potassium intake may be very effective in minimizing the risk of development of HTN in susceptible children and adolescents. A significant limitation of this approach is the difficulties in compliance with such simple dietary recommendations. More work on methods to understand the factors that affect adherence to medical recommendations in children and adolescents, and better approaches to induce at-risk and affected children to comply with such simple recommendations, are needed to realize the value of these simple measures.

Therapeutic Lifestyle Changes Approach—Summary

TLCs are health-promoting behaviors such as diet, exercise, and weight reduction, which may improve BP in children with mild to moderate HTN and minimize the chances of developing HTN in children with intermittent HTN associated with stress or those at risk for developing HTN later in childhood or adulthood. The recent Fourth Report from the National High Blood Pressure Education Program Working Group on High Blood Pressure in Children and Adolescents guidelines[1] recognize the benefits of these nonpharmacologic approaches, and endorse these options for children with mild HTN as well as children with prehypertension.

Weight loss, although never easy, offers significant benefits. Even with only modest changes in body weight, children may reap significant improvements in BP. This approach should be a mainstay of treatment for all children at risk for HTN as well as children with HTN. Regular aerobic exercise also offers significant benefits independent of the effects on weight, and should be prescribed as a thoughtful, regular, measurable part of the approach to treatment of children at risk for developing HTN, those with mild HTN, and those with significant HTN who have experienced improved BP on medications.

Stress reduction has long been neglected as a prescribed therapeutic option for children at risk of HTN as well as for those with established HTN. Given the lack of toxicity and real benefits, individualized approaches and formal training programs should be considered in formulation of treatment programs for these children. The impact of diet and dietary intake of electrolytes is an area of intense interest and these manipulations appear to be particularly useful in the management of children at risk for developing HTN as well as those with mild essential HTN. These principles, as part of a "heart-healthy" diet program, should also be incorporated into any dietary counseling, and should be monitored in these populations with regular determinations of urinary electrolytes and feedback designed to change behavior and BP over time.

Pharmacologic Treatment of Hypertension in Children and Adolescents

HTN results from multiple mechanisms, including arterial vascular vasoconstriction, increased sympathetic nervous system activity, direct cardiovascular inotropic effect, and aldosterone-enhanced salt and water retention. The pharmacologic interventions discussed next are directed at these mechanisms to lower BP.

Pharmacologic treatment of HTN in children and adolescents has been hampered by the lack of available safety and efficacy data and age-appropriate drug formulations.[1,53,54] The Fourth Report recommends a stepped-care drug therapy approach to reduce BP in children and adolescents unresponsive to nonpharmacologic therapy, in those not at goal despite current pharmacologic therapy, in children and adolescents with severe HTN despite current pharmacologic therapy, and/or in those with evidence of end-organ damage (e.g., left ventricular hypertrophy). Ten classes of medications are used to treat HTN: ACEIs, ARBs, CCBs, β-adrenergic blockers, α-adrenergic blockers, α-adrenergic agonists, vasodilators, peripheral adrenergic agents, diuretics, and combination products. Medication therapy is primarily based on underlying disease state and concomitant medical condition(s) (Table 44-5). In the absence of a secondary disease or other con-

TABLE 44-5 Indications/Contraindications for Pharmacologic Selection

Class	Indications	Contraindications
Angiotensin-converting enzyme inhibitors	Concurrent diabetes mellitus	Renal artery stenosis Bilateral renal artery stenosis Pregnancy
Angiotensin II receptor antagonists		Renal artery stenosis Bilateral renal artery stenosis Pregnancy or GFR < 30 ml ml/min/1.73 m² (losartan)
β-adrenergic antagonists		Asthma Heart failure Concurrent diabetes mellitus
Calcium channel blockers		
Centrally acting α-adrenergic antagonists	Use in children with attention deficit and hyperactivity disorder (clonidine)	
Loop diuretics		Renal insufficiency (GFR < 30)
Peripheral α-adrenergic antagonists	Children with insulin-resistant syndrome	
Potassium-sparing diuretics	Hypertension secondary to mineralocorticoid excess	
Thiazide diuretics Vasodilators		Renal insufficiency (GFR < 30)

GFR, glomerular filtration rate.

traindications (e.g., in uncomplicated primary or essential HTN), ACEIs, long-acting dihydropyridine CCBs, β-adrenergic blockers, and diuretics are considered first-line therapy. Due to the relatively low side-effect profile, long duration of action (e.g., once-daily dosing), and ease of use (e.g., liquid preparations for pediatric patients), ACEIs and long-acting dihydropyridine CCBs are used more often. Concomitant disease (e.g., asthma), and drug side-effect profiles (e.g., drowsiness) may limit β-adrenergic blocker and diuretic utilization in children or adolescents. α-adrenergic blockers, α-adrenergic agonists, angiotensin receptor blockers, vasodilators, and peripheral adrenergic agents are usually reserved for refractory HTN uncontrolled by ACEIs, CCBs, β-adrenergic blockers, and/or diuretics.

Table 44-6 lists side-effects profiles for various classes of medication. Table 44-7 lists published guidelines for treatment of pediatric HTN, and Table 44-8 lists intravenous drugs used in management of hypertensive emergency.

Angiotensin-Converting Enzyme Inhibitors

Angiotensin-converting enzymes (ACEs) catalyze the conversion of angiotensin I to angiotensin II and the degradation of the vasodilatory peptide bradykinin.[55] ACEIs reversibly inhibit the enzyme ACE, resulting in vasodilatation and decreased sympathetic nervous system activity. Inhibition of the breakdown of bradykinin results in the accumulation of substance P, and is thought to contribute to the cardiac and renal protective effects of ACEIs. ACE inhibition has a dose-dependent effect on BP, and a beneficial effect on both pediatric BP and cardiovascular function.[56,57] ACEIs are commonly prescribed for their renal protective effects (reduced protein excretion) in children and adolescents with concurrent diabetes and/or renal disease (contraindicated in bilateral renal artery stenosis[31]; see also Chapter 45). ACEIs preserve renal function in both normotensive and hypertensive diabetic adolescents and in adults with or without diabetic nephropathy.[58,59] ACEIs are considered the drug of choice in patients with congestive heart failure, left ventricular dysfunction, diabetes, or mild to moderate renal insufficiency (for renal protection), and ACEIs are a good choice in patients with concurrent hyperlipidemia.[60] They are generally well tolerated, and the pharmacokinetic parameters in children and adolescents appear to be similar to those in adults.[61] Clearance is positively correlated with renal function; however, in patients with renal dysfunction, hepatic metabolism is increased.[62] Potency and duration of action of ACEIs are greater in neonates and infants.[63] Reduced doses and more consistent monitoring are necessary in infants and neonates to avoid side effects (e.g., hypotension, anuria, oliguria, neurologic complications, and renal failure) (Table 44-6).[63,64] However, as the vascular status of the kidney improves with growth and development, the dose often requires adjustment to maintain the same effect.

ACEIs are generally well tolerated, and acute drug effects (ADEs) are generally rare.[65] While these agents have been linked with chronic cough, in the pediatric trial of enalapril, fewer than 3% of subjects reported this adverse effect.[65] Hyperkalemia, thrombocytopenia, neutropenia, decreased GFR, hypotension secondary to volume depletion, transient anuria, angioedema (0.1% to 0.2% of patients), loss of taste, transient vomiting, blood dyscrasias, transient proteinuria, and renal insufficiency have been described in adult and pediatric patients.[65,66] ACEI use during all trimesters of pregnancy should be avoided due to risk of fetopathy (e.g., fetal hypotension, oligohydramnios, cardiac and renal defects).[12] Pulmonary hypoplasia, renal tubular dysplasia, hypotension, and anuria have also been documented with maternal use in the second and third trimesters, but had not previously been associated with use at conception or during the first trimes-

TABLE 44-6 Side Effects Associated with Pharmacologic Management

Class	Side Effects Reported	Potentially Severe Side Effects
Angiotensin-converting enzyme inhibitors	Cough, headache, hypotension, hyperkalemia, angioedema, rash, anemia, nasopharyngitis (fosinopril)	Renal failure (↑ incidence in neonates or children with preexisting renal dysfunction) Fetopathy/neonatal toxicity Neutropenia Fatal liver damage (quinapril)
Angiotensin II receptor antagonists	Hypotension, hyperkalemia, angioedema, rash, anemia	Renal failure (↑ incidence in neonates or children with preexisting renal dysfunction) Fetopathy/neonatal toxicity Neutropenia
β-adrenergic antagonists	Fatigue, sedation, bradycardia, hypercholesterolemia, mask hypoglycemia	Bronchial constriction Heart failure
Calcium channel blockers	Flushing, headache, fatigue, edema, palpitations, tachycardia	Cardiovascular events—myocardial infarction, congestive heart failure (adult data from Joint National Report, Sixth Report)
Centrally acting α-adrenergic antagonists	Sedation, dry mouth, headache	Rebound hypertension
Loop diuretics	Fatigue, nausea, muscle cramps, dehydration	Hypokalemia, hyponatremia, hyperlipidemia, metabolic alkalosis, and hearing loss
Peripheral α-adrenergic antagonists	Anticholinergic effects, drowsiness/dizziness, fluid retention, headache, stress incontinence	Orthostatic hypotension (first dose)
Potassium-sparing diuretics	Fatigue, nausea, muscle cramps, dehydration	Hyperkalemia, hyponatremia, hyperlipidemia
Thiazide diuretics	Fatigue, nausea, muscle cramps, dehydration	Hypokalemia, hyponatremia, hyperlipidemia, and metabolic alkalosis
Vasodilators	Edema, hypertrichosis (minoxidil)	Lupus-like syndrome (hydralazine)

Sources: Jung FF, Ingelfinger JR: Hypertension in childhood and adolescence, *Pediatr Rev* 14 (5):169-79, 1993; Stokes GS: Age-related effects of antihypertensive therapy with alpha-blockers, *J Cardiovasc Pharmacol* 12(Suppl 8):S109-15, 1988; and Blowey DL: Safety of the newer antihypertensive agents in children, *Expert Opin Drug Saf* 1 (1):39-43, 2002.

ter.[61] A recent report shows that infants exposed during the first trimester are at higher risk for malformations of the cardiovascular and central nervous systems.[12] Therefore, caution should be exercised with use of ACEIs in adolescent girls who have achieved menarche.

Of the available ACEIs, captopril is most extensively tested and used in neonates, children, and adolescents.[62,67] Captopril reduced both SBP and DBP in children and adolescents with mild, moderate, and severe HTN.[57] In infants with renin-induced HTN, it was effective in both short- and long-term treatment of HTN (2 years).[67] However, its utility is limited by its relatively short duration of action; therefore, multiple daily doses are usually required to sustain BP decreases.

Enalapril, lisinopril, ramipril, quinapril, moexipril, and fosinopril have been tested and used in the pediatric population. These agents lack the sulfhydryl group found on captopril, resulting in a longer elimination half-life and once daily dosing.[68] Enalapril is more effective and is associated with fewer ADEs than captopril.[65] It is effective both as monotherapy and when used in conjunction with other antihypertensive agents (e.g., diuretics) to manage pediatric HTN.[68] It effectively reduces BP, edema, hypoalbuminemia, and hypercholesterolemia in children with nephrotic range proteinuria.[69] BP reduction does not appear affected by pubertal status, age, gender, and race/ethnicity.[65] However, as with other ACEIs, variability in neonatal and infant metabolism may result in toxicity and subsequent hypotensive crisis if unmonitored.[64,70]

Safety and efficacy of lisinopril have been studied children and adolescents 6 to 16 years of age.[71] A strong dose–response relationship was noted between low and high doses and change in torrs (mm Hg).[71] Plasma concentrations and reported adverse events appear to be similar to those found in adults. Safety and efficacy of ramipril have been studied in children and adolescents from 1 to 20 years of age.[72] BP was reduced (casual BP and ambulatory blood pressure monitoring [ABPM]), GFR preserved, and no ADEs were reported in hypertensive children treated with ramipril. However, no consistent relationship among changes in albumin, BP, primary renal disease, and sodium excretion was noted in this population. A placebo-controlled study is currently underway to define the dose–response of ramipril and to prove its efficacy. There are pharmacokinetic and stability studies of quinapril in children as young as 6 years of age[73,74] but no published safety and efficacy data in children with HTN. Safety and efficacy of fosinopril have been studied in children and adolescents 6 to 16 years of age.[75] All three doses were effective in reducing BP, and no dose response was noted.[75] Fosinopril was generally well tolerated during the trial and open-label period.[75] Headache was the most common adverse event reported in 20% of patients. Serum creatinine values were elevated in approximately 9% of patients; however, elevations were transient and did not exceed the upper limit of normal.[75]

TABLE 44-7 **Published Dosing Recommendations for Treating Pediatric Hypertension**

Drug	Initial Dose (mg/kg/day)	Maximum Dose	Dosing Frequency
Angiotensin-Converting Enzyme Inhibitors			
Captopril			
Infants	0.02-0.5	6	Q 8-12 hr
Children	0.15-1.5	6	Q 6-8 hr
Enalapril (liquid bioavailability equal to tablets)			
Infants	0.04-0.08	5 mg/daily	Q 12-24 hr
Children	0.08-0.58	40 mg/daily	Q 12-24 hr
Lisinopril	0.7 mg/kg	5 mg	Q 24 hr
Quinapril (data based on pharmacokinetic data in children <6 years of age and unpublished reports)	0.2 mg/kg/dose	20 mg/day	Q 24 hr
Fosinopril	0.1 mg/kg/dose	0.3 mg/kg/day up to 80 mg/day	Q 24 hr
Angiotensin Receptor Blockers			
Irbesartan (tested in children 6-16 years of age)	75 mg	300 mg	Q 24 hr
Losartan (tested in children ≥6 years of age)	0.7	100 mg/day	Q 24 hr
Calcium Channel Blockers			
Felodipine ER	0.1	0.6 (up to 20 mg/day)	Q 24 hr
Isradipine	0.2	0.8 (up to 20 mg/day)	Q 6-8 hr
Nifedipine XL	0.25	3 (up to 180 mg/day)	Q 12-24 hr
Verapamil	3	8 (up to 480 mg/day)	Q 12 hr
Amlodipine	0.1-0.2	0.6 (up to 20 mg/day)	Q 24 hr
Diuretics			
Hydrochlorothiazide	1-2	37.5 mg/day >2 yr 100 mg/day ≤2 yr	Q 12 hr
Metalozone	0.1	3	Q 24 hr
Furosemide	2	6 mg/kg/day	Q 6-12 hr
Bumetanide	0.02-0.05	0.3	Q 6-12 hr
Spironolactone	1-1.5	3.3 mg/kg/day	Q 6-12 hr
Triamterene	2	3	Q 12-24 hr
Vasodilators			
Hydralazine	0.75	200 mg/day	Q 6 hr
Minoxidil	0.1-0.2	50 mg/day	Q 12 hr
Adrenergic-Blocking Agents			
Labetolol	1-3	1 to 3	Q 6-8 hr
Prazosin	0.05-0.1	0.5	Q 6-8 hr
Propranolol	1	16 mg/kg/day	Q 12 hr
Atenolol	1	6	Q 24 hr
Metoprolol (Adolescents)	100	200	Q 24 hr
Bisoprolol fumarate/hydrochlorothiazide (fixed dose combination)	2.5/6.25 mg	10/6.25 mg	Q 24 hr
Adrenergic Stimulants			
Clonidine			
Methyldopa	10	3 g/day	Q 6-12 hr

Sources: Kelsey RM, Barnard M, Alpert BS: Race, SES and cardiovascular reactivity to cold stress as longitudinal predictors of blood pressure in adolescents, *Am J Hypertens* 14:250A, 2001; Wells T, Rippley R, Hogg R, Sakarcan A, et al: The pharmacokinetics of enalapril in children and infants with hypertension, *J Clin Pharmacol* 41 (10):1064-74, 2001; Wells T, Frame V, Soffer B, Shaw W, et al: A double-blind, placebo-controlled, dose–response study of the effectiveness and safety of enalapril for children with hypertension, *J Clin Pharmacol* 42 (8):870-80, 2002; Herrera P, Soffer B, Zhang Z, Miller K, et al: Effects of the ACE inhibitor, lisinopril in children age 6-16 years, *Am J Hypertens* 15 (4):32A, 2002; Flynn JT, Pasko DA: Calcium channel blockers: pharmacology and place in therapy of pediatric hypertension, *Pediatr Nephrol* 15 (3-4):302-16, 2000; Khattak S, Rogan JW, Saunders EF, Theis JG, et al: Efficacy of amlodipine in pediatric bone marrow transplant patients, *Clin Pediatr (Phila)* 37 (1):31-35, 1998; and Sorof JM, Cargo P, Graepel J, Humphrey D, et al: Beta-blocker/thiazide combination for treatment of hypertensive children: a randomized double-blind, placebo-controlled trial, *Pediatr Nephrol* 17 (5):345-50, 2002; Falkner B, Lowenthal DT, Affrime MB: The pharmacodynamic effectiveness of metoprolol in adolescent hypertension, *Pediatr Pharmacol (N Y)* 2 (1):49-55, 1982; Soffer B, Zhang Z, Miller K, Vogt BA, Shahinfar S: A double-blind, placebo-controlled, dose–response study of the effectiveness and safety of lisinopril for children with hypertension, *Am J Hypertens* 16 (10):795-800, 2003; Rippley RK, Connor J, Boyle J, Bradstreet TE, et al: Pharmacokinetic assessment of an oral enalapril suspension for use in children, *Biopharm Drug Dispos* 21 (9):339-44, 2000.

TABLE 44-8 **Intravenous Drugs Recommended for Treatment of Hypertensive Emergency**

Drug	Dose	Onset of Action	Duration of Action
Angiotensin-Converting Enzyme Inhibitors			
Enalaprilat (IV) Children	0.005-0.01 mg/kg Q 8-24 hr	Within 15 minutes	12-24 hr
Calcium Channel Blockers			
Nicardipine (IV)	0.5-3 mcg/kg/min	Within 15 minutes	15-30 min
Vasodilators			
Hydralazine (IV) Sodium nitroprusside (IV)	0.1-0.5 mg/kg 0.5-8 mcg/kg/min	10-30 min Within seconds	4-12 hr Minute
Adrenergic-Blocking Agents			
Labetolol (IV) Esmolol (IV)	0.5-3 mg/kg/hr 2-6 mcg/kg/min	5-10 min Within seconds	2-3 hr 10-20 min
Adrenergic Stimulant			
Clonidine (IV)	2-6 mcg/kg	10 min	15-30 min
Dopamine I Receptor Agonists			
Fenoldopam (IV)	0.5-2 mcg/kg/min	15 min	15-30 min

Sources: Piovan D, Padrini R, Svalato Moreolo G, Magnolfi G, et al: Verapamil and norverapamil plasma levels in infants and children during chronic oral treatment, *Ther Drug Monit* 17 (1):60-67, 1995; Shaddy RE, Curtin EL, Sower B, Tani LY, et al: The Pediatric Randomized Carvedilol Trial in Children with Heart Failure: rationale and design, *Am Heart J* 144 (3):383-89, 2002; Talseth T: Clinical pharmacokinetics of hydralazine, *Clin Pharmacokinet* 2 (5):317-29, 1977; Blowey DL: Safety of the newer antihypertensive agents in children, *Expert Opin Drug Saf* 1 (1):39-43, 2002; and Adelman RD, Coppo R, Dillon MJ: The emergency management of severe hypertension, *Pediatr Nephrol* 14 (5):422-27, 2000.

Angiotensin Receptor Blockers

Angiotensin receptor blockers have not been extensively used in the pediatric population.[76] ARBs interfere with the binding of ANG II to type 1 ANG II receptors. Blockade of the ANG II receptor is believed to achieve more specific and complete[77] lowering of BP without production of substance P and its associated ADEs (e.g., cough). Monitoring parameters, contraindications (e.g., during pregnancy, and in patients with renal artery stenosis), and adverse events associated with ARB use (e.g., angioedema) are the same as expected with ACEI therapy except cough (Tables 44-4 and 44-5).[78] More studies are necessary to determine if ARBs will have similar renal protective effects as ACEIs and decrease cardiovascular morbidity and mortality as well as ACEIs.

Losartan monotherapy and concomitant hydrochlorothiazide therapy were both found to be more effective than amlodipine in lowering CV risk and preserving renal function in adults with impaired renal function (i.e., reducing albuminuria) treated for 12 weeks.[79] Losartan therapy was associated with prolonged and sustained BP reduction in children aged under 18 years.[80] It was well tolerated in most children and adverse events were generally mild and responded to dose reduction. Significant adverse events (increased serum creatinine, blurred vision, and syncope) were reported in 11% of patients; however, concurrent administration of immunosuppressants may have been the cause.[81]

Irbesartan safety and efficacy have been studied in children and adolescents 6 to 16 years of age.[76] BP values decreased with monotherapy and plasma concentrations were similar among both children and adolescents. However, patients with significant renal disease (creatinine clearance less than 25 ml/min/1.73 m^2) were not included in the trial and a majority of patients were African American (10/11 in participating children and 9/12 in the adolescent group).[76] Lastly, safety and efficacy data for valsartan are limited to adult studies; studies in children have been conducted but not published yet.[77]

Calcium Channel Blockers

Ionized calcium in the body serves as a link between electrical and chemical stimulation, and is vital in both striated and smooth muscle contraction. CCBs reduce BP by inhibiting the influx of calcium ions into the smooth muscle cellular membrane in a dose-dependent fashion.[68,82] Inhibition or blocking of calcium ions in smooth muscle results in peripheral arteriole dilation and decreased peripheral resistance.[68,82] Blockade of calcium may also cause a transient increase in heart rate, cardiac output, renal plasma blood flow, and GFR (Table 44-6).[82]

CCBs are classified according to underlying molecular structure and clinical application into two classes: nondihydropyridines (tertiary amines) and dihydropyridines. Nondihydropyridines are primarily used in the treatment of atrioventricular nodal conduction and repetitive membrane polarization arrythmias.[83] Dihydropyridines are more effective vasodilators and used primarily in the treatment of peripheral vascular diseases and HTN. Cardiac response to vascular changes is variable, while peripheral vascular resistance remains low throughout therapy.[84] Most dihydropyridines (felodipine, nicardipine, nisoldipine, and nifedipine) cause reflex tachycardia, which returns to normal within a few weeks, whereas nondihydropyridines (verapamil, diltiazem) and some dihydropyridine drugs (isradipine and amlodipine) cause little or no change in heart rate. Both the nondihydropyridines and dihydropyridines are metabolized to inactive metabolites; therefore, dosage modification is not required in patients with impaired renal function.[68,82,84] CCBs are also considered a good first choice for patients with hyperlipidemia and do not appear to affect serum lipids. Dihydropyridine CCBs do not lower pressure and may even increase proteinuria. They are therefore not considered agents of first choice in chronic kidney diseases (see Chapter 45).[82] CCBs are very effective in patients with low renin (i.e., volume expanded, volume dependent), and where HTN is mediated via afferent arteriolar vasoconstriction (e.g., cyclosporine-induced HTN).[85] Increased sodium and water excretion is seen with initiation of drug therapy and is often maintained. Adverse events associated with dihydropyridine therapy include fatigue, headache, facial flushing, dizziness, edema, abdominal pain, chest pain, nausea, vomiting, and peripheral edema.[86] The number of reported ADEs associated with dihydropyridine therapy (e.g., headache, flushing, dizziness, gingival hyperplasia, and leg cramps) is significantly higher in transplant recipients than in those with essential HTN.[87]

Nifedipine, amlodipine, felodipine, and isradipine are the most commonly prescribed CCBs for the treatment of chronic pediatric HTN (Table 44-7).[83-87] Nifedipine comes in two formulations: an immediate release preparation (IR) and an extended-release preparation (ER). The IR preparation is rapidly absorbed and commonly used in the treatment of hypertensive emergencies, and the ER preparation is used in chronic HTN.[88] Nifedipine is associated with more ADEs in the pediatric population than newer agents such as amlodipine.[86,88]

The most commonly prescribed CCB for the treatment of chronic pediatric HTN is amlodipine.[86,88] It is the only CCB with a tested oral formulation compounding recipe.[89] Amlodipine safely and effectively lowers BP (casual and ambulatory BP values decrease) in children and adolescents.[86] Antihypertensive effects are similar in those with normal and impaired renal function. No significant differences in mean SBP, mean DBP, daily ABPM values, or medication adherence was noted in renal transplant recipients receiving amlodipine, nifedipine, or felodipine.[90] Serum amlodipine concentrations do not significantly increase or require adjustment in patients with renal insufficiency or between dialysis sessions. Amlodipine was effective in reducing SBP and DBP in pediatric bone marrow transplant patients without impacting immunosuppressant therapy (e.g., cyclosporine).[91] ADEs reported with amlodipine therapy (e.g., edema, flushing, and headache) were infrequent and mild; however, many children and adolescents reporting side effects discontinued therapy.[86,90] Transient increases in heart rate did not appear to impact medication adherence.[86,90]

The safety and efficacy of felodipine have been studied in children and adolescents with primary and secondary HTN.[80,88] This highly protein-bound (99%) CCB effectively reduces SBP with fewer adverse effects than extended-release nifedipine.[88] Overall compliance, measured by the medication event monitoring system (MEMS, Aprex), was greater with felodipine therapy than extended-release nifedipine therapy (95.6% vs. 78.9%).[92] Felodipine's powder-filled capsules may contribute to the improved adherence noted. Felodipine capsules can be opened for dose titration and administration in young children. Safety and efficacy of the CCB isradipine has been studied in infants, children, and adolescents.[88,93] Mean change in SBP and DBP were statistically significant and ranged from 12.8% to 24.7%, respectively.[88,93] More than half of children with secondary HTN who received isradipine were controlled on monotherapy.[93] Transplant recipients required lower doses (0.31 ± 0.18 mg/kg/day) than patients with essential HTN (0.46 ± 0.28 mg/kg/day).[88] Concurrent administration of isradipine did not appear to affect cyclosporine levels and may therefore be preferred to felodipine in transplant HTN.[88]

Adrenergic Agents

β-adrenergic antagonists decrease BP through several mechanisms. β-adrenergic antagonists inhibit cardiac β-receptors resulting in negative inotropic and chronotropic effects that decrease cardiac output, reduce sympathetically mediated pressor reflexes to gradually reset baroreceptor levels, inhibit renin secretion, and redistribute intravascular volume to decrease plasma volume, subsequently reducing peripheral vascular resistance.[94] β-adrenergic antagonists are classified as cardioselective β-adrenergic antagonists (e.g., acebutolol, atenolol, bisoprolol, metoprolol, and betaxolol) and nonselective β-adrenergic antagonists (e.g., carvedilol, labetolol, nadolol, propranolol, and timolol). Cardioselective agents have a greater affinity for β_1-adrenergic receptors located in the heart, whereas nonselective agents work on β_1-adrenergic receptors and β_2-adrenergic receptors located in bronchial musculature. However, at high doses cardioselectivity is lost. The significant differences in pharmacologic properties of agents within this group (cardioselectivity, lipid solubility, intrinsic sympathomimetic activity, membrane stabilization, and potency) impact drug selection. In addition, effects do not correlate with β-adrenergic antagonist plasma concentration and exceed expected duration of drug action based on plasma half-life.

β-adrenergic antagonists are not considered first-line agents for many populations due to their extensive ADE profile.[94] β-adrenergic antagonists should not be considered first-line therapy in athletes (because of decreased cardiac output and athletic reserve); patients with concurrent asthma, chronic lung disease, or congestive heart failure (because of potential bronchospasm and pulmonary insufficiency); and diabetic patients (because of masking of the signs and symptoms of hypoglycemia such as tachycardia, palpitations, and hunger).[1,94] β-adrenergic antagonists are also believed to be less effective in African Americans; however, this has not been substantiated in pediatric patients.[1] Other ADEs include postural hypotension, bradycardia, fatigue, depression, impotence, hyperkalemia, increased serum triglycerides, hallucinations, cold extremities, and decreased HDL cholesterol.[1,94] In addition, sudden withdrawal of β-adrenergic antagonists can lead to exacerbation of myocardial infarction, and aggravate allergic reactions resulting in bronchospasm. Combination products have been used in adolescents with HTN; however, difficulty titrating dose and achieving target BP, and increased side effects limit consideration as a first-line therapy.[94,95]

Few β-adrenergic antagonists have been studied in children: propranolol, atenolol, metoprolol, labetalol, and carvedilol. Propranolol is the most extensively used β-adrenergic antagonists in neonates, children, and adolescents.[96] It is effective (decreases SBP, DBP, heart rate, and cardiac contractility), and is associated with side effects that may influence adherence (i.e., decreased mental concentration, impaired athletic performance, and anorexia).[96] Patients with HTN secondary to renal dysfunction/disease require larger doses than children with essential HTN.[96] As with ACEI therapy, pretreatment plasma renin does not correlate with BP changes. Safety and efficacy of atenolol have been established in adolescents and adults with HTN.[97] Metoprolol safety and efficacy have been studied in adolescents with primary and secondary HTN.[98] Significant decreases in SBP, DBP, heart rate, and cardiovascular response to mental stress were found.[98] Although a pharmacokinetic study has been conducted in six children aged 5 to 13 years, published safety and efficacy data for betaxolol are limited to adult studies.[99]

In addition to their β-receptor activity, labetolol[100] and carvedilol[101] possess peripheral α-blocking activity. Safety and efficacy of labetolol have been established in children and adolescents with chronic HTN.[101] It has been shown to be effective in patients unresponsive to other β-adrenergic antagonists, and does not appear to have the negative effects on lipids and exercise tolerance seen with other β-adrenergic antagonists.[72,82] Although approved for acute and chronic HTN in adults, carvedilol is primarily used in the treatment of congestive heart failure in children.

Diuretics

Diuretics primarily play a role in multiple-drug regimens where salt and water retention are concerns. They lower BP by reducing plasma volume and peripheral vascular resistance via inhibition of sodium and water reabsorption and increased excretion in the nephron.[102] With chronic dosing, sodium balance is maintained and extracellular plasma volume returns to normal; however, change in BP is maintained through the decline in peripheral vascular resistance.[102] Diuretics are no longer considered first-line therapy due to their side effect profile (fatigue, nausea, muscle cramps, and other side effects related to hypokalemia, hyponatremia, hyperlipidemia, and metabolic alkalosis).[102] Impaired renal autoregulation has also been noted.

Diuretics can be classified into three categories: thiazide diuretics, loop diuretics, and potassium-sparing diuretics. Selection of an agent is based on baseline GFR (if <30%, thiazides are ineffective), electrolytes (baseline hyper- or hypokalemia) and concurrent medication selection (concomitant potassium-sparing therapy).[102] Adolescents in general do not usually respond well to diuretic monotherapy. They have an over-responsive sympathetic nervous system, and salt and water retention is not the usual underlying cause. African American children and adolescents, however, may have salt-sensitive HTN and benefit from diuretic therapy.[1] All diuretics should also be avoided in salt-losing states such as adrenal disorders, salt-losing nephropathy, and athletes practicing in warm climates.

Thiazide diuretics are secreted into the tubular lumen and exert their diuretic effect by inhibiting Na^+-Cl^- co-transport in the early distal convoluted tubule.[102] The drug must be present within the lumen to exert diuretic effect. They are the diuretic of choice when GFR is greater than 50% and are considered ineffective when clearance is less than 30 ml ml/min (Table 44-5). Thiazide diuretics are primarily used in conjunction with CCBs, ACEIs, and/or β-adrenergic blockers in the treatment of primary and secondary HTN unresponsive to monotherapy, and as monotherapy in children and adolescents with mild HTN.[92] Use of thiazide diuretics in adolescents and children has come into question due to their potential long-term effects on lipids and bone growth.[1,91,103]

Loop diuretics are more potent than thiazide diuretics but, as with thiazide diuretics, effectiveness decreases as renal function decreases.[82,103] Loop diuretics are used primarily in patients with underlying renal disease, fluid retention, and renal insufficiency (creatinine clearance 30 to 50 ml ml/min).[102,103] Rate of clearance is even lower in premature infants. Dosage intervals need to be adjusted and monitoring increased as there is potential ototoxicity.[102,103] Spironolactone is the only potassium-sparing diuretic commonly given to children.[4] It is primarily used in the treatment of HTN secondary to mineralocorticoid excess and as concomitant therapy in children taking medications that increase aldosterone secretion such as CCBs and vasodilators. Spironolactone does not appear to be as effective as thiazide or loop diuretics when HTN is not related to mineralocorticoid excess.

Other Medications

Other agents that are not often used as first-line treatment of chronic pediatric HTN include α-adrenergic receptor antagonists, α-adrenergic agonist vasodilators, peripheral adrenergic neuron antagonists, and combination products. α-adrenergic receptor antagonists (e.g., prazosin, doxazosin, and terazosin) decrease total peripheral resistance and venous return through arteriolar relaxation secondary to increased cyclic AMP and GMP.[104] These agents are usually reserved for severe or drug-resistant HTN and are not traditionally used in children or adolescents due to their side effect profile.[105,106] Side effects associated with α-adrenergic receptor antagonist therapy include anticholinergic effects, dizziness, vertigo, headache, palpitations, fluid retention, drowsiness, weakness, stress incontinence, and priapism.[104,105] Syncope with first dose is most common with prazosin therapy and in patients receiving diuretic or β-adrenergic receptor antagonist. They cause less tachycardia than direct vasodilators, but more frequent postural hypotension. In addition, blood lipid levels are not influenced by α-adrenergic receptor antagonist therapy, which makes these agents a good choice in patients with hyperlipidemia.

Centrally acting α_2-adrenergic agonists (e.g., clonidine and guanabenz) stimulate α_2-adrenergic receptors in the central nervous system reducing electrical activity along the sympathetic tract, decreasing peripheral vascular resistance and heart rate (secondary to increased vagal tone).[107] However, they do not inhibit sympathetic reflex responses as completely as peripheral sympatholytic drugs. The α_2-adrenergic agonists are primarily used as concomitant therapy in adolescents with resistant HTN and in children and adolescents receiving a stimulant for attention deficit and hyperactivity disorder (i.e., clonidine).[107,108] These agents are often avoided due to their extensive side effect profile: drowsiness, rebound HTN, dry mouth, bradycardia, heart block, and dermatitis with patch administration.[107,108] Gradual withdrawal is necessary; abrupt withdrawal may result in rebound HTN, headache, and tremor. Peripheral adrenergic neuron antagonists (e.g., guanethidine) act by depleting catecholamine and 5-hydroxytryptophan in the central nervous system, decreasing peripheral resistance and cardiac output. Although successful at reducing BP, these agents have a cumulative effect, and elevated doses are associated with orthostatic hypotension, exercise hypotension, diarrhea, bradycardia, sodium and water retention, depression, and tardive dyskinesias at high doses.

Vasodilators, such as hydralazine and minoxidil, act directly on vascular smooth muscle of the precapillary arterioles to reduce vascular wall tension and peripheral vascular resistance.[109] Although successful at reducing BP in children and adolescents these agents are best reserved for severe and drug-resistant HTN.[110] Utility of these agents is limited by side effect profile: reflex tachycardia, severe fluid retention (minoxidil), headache, flushing, dizziness, lupus erythematosus-like syndrome (hydralazine), palpitations, increased cardiac output, hirsutism (minoxidil), and salt and water retention.[109,110] Concurrent administration with a β-blocker or a loop diuretic may minimize tachycardia, whereas concomitant loop diuretic therapy may diminish sodium and water retention.

Lastly, combination products have traditionally not been tested in pediatrics. This is most likely because of the need for dose titration in children and adolescents. However, fixed combinations appear to be well tolerated in the adult population, and will likely be studied in children and adolescents in the future.[111,112]

CONCLUSION

The pediatric patient with HTN requires careful attention for optimal treatment. Treatment is usually a combination of nonpharmacologic and pharmacologic strategies, but many details go into the decision-making process. Of most importance is the underlying etiology; this will primarily influence the treatment choice, although other factors, such as response to therapy, convenience of once- or twice-daily dosing, ease of administration, risk of side effects, and cost will influence therapy choice as well. TLC should not be neglected and may be sufficient, if taken seriously by the patient and his/her family, to successfully treat mild HTN or prevent the child with pre-HTN from progressing to stage 1 HTN. The best methods to encourage and effect change in body weight, exercise level, stress, and electrolyte intake in children and adolescents require much more attention and validation. The availability of medications suitable and well studied in children and adolescents was a problem in the past. As more medications are approved for use after successful clinical trials, there should be more opportunities to establish optimal evidence-based choices for treatment among the various pharmacologic options. The Fourth Report provides guidance on the treatment of HTN in children and adolescents; well-tested and evidence-based optimal strategies will require much more work.

REFERENCES

1. National High Blood Pressure Education Program Working Group on High Blood Pressure in Children and Adolescents: The Fourth Report on the Diagnosis, Evaluation, and Treatment of High Blood Pressure in Children and Adolescents—2004, *Pediatrics* 114(2):555-76, 2004.
2. Ettinger LM, Flynn JT: Hypertension in the neonate, *NeoReviews* 3(8):e151-56, 2002.
3. Ingelfinger JR: Perinatal programming and blood pressure. In Portman RJ, Sorof JM, Ingelfinger JR, editors: *Pediatric hypertension*, Totowa, NJ, 2004, Humana Press, pp. 241-50.
4. Flynn JT, Neonatal hypertension: diagnosis and management, *Pediatr Nephrol* 14:332-41, 2000.
5. Flynn JT: Evaluation and management of hypertension in childhood, *Prog Pediatr Cardiol* 12:177-88, 2001.
6. Bartosh SM, Aronson AJ: Childhood hypertension. An update on etiology, diagnosis, and treatment, *Pediatr Clin North Am* 46:235-52, 1999.
7. Sorof JM, Lai D, Turner J, Poffenbarger T, Portman RJ: Overweight, ethnicity, and the prevalence of hypertension in school-aged children, *Pediatrics* 113(3 pt 1):475-82, 2004.
8. Nissen SE: ADHD drugs and cardiovascular risk, *N Engl J Med* 354(14):1445-48, 2006.
9. Flynn JT: Hypertension in adolescents, *Adolesc Med Clin* 16:11-29, 2005.
10. Croix B, Feig DI: Childhood hypertension is not a silent disease, *Pediatr Nephrol* 21(4):527-32, 2006.
11. Mayo Clinic Staff: High blood pressure, available at www.mayoclinic.com/health/blood-pressure/HI00053.
12. Cooper WO, Hernandez-Diaz S, Arbogast PG, Dudley JA, et al: Major congenital malformations after first-trimester exposure to ACE inhibitors, *N Engl J Med* 354(23):2443-51, 2006.
13. Schafer F, Mehls O: Hypertension in chronic kidney disease. In Portman RJ, Sorof JM, Ingelfinger JR, editors: *Pediatric hypertension*, Totowa, NJ, 2004, Humana Press, pp. 371-87.
14. Scharer K: Hypertension in end-stage renal disease. In Portman RJ, Sorof JM, Ingelfinger JR, editors: *Pediatric hypertension*, Totowa, NJ, 2004, Humana Press, pp. 389-402.
15. Chobanian AV, Bakris GL, Black HR, Cushman WC, et al: *JAMA* 289(19):2560-72, 2003.
16. Portman RJ, McNiece KL, Swinford RD, Braun MC, Samuels JA: Pediatric hypertension: diagnosis, evaluation, management, and treatment for the primary care physician, *Curr Probl Pediatr Adolesc Heath Care* 7:262-94, 2005.
17. Williams CL, Hayman LL, Daniels SR, Robinson TN, et al: Cardiovascular health in childhood. A statement for health professionals from the Committee on Atherosclerosis, Hypertension and Obesity in the Young (AHOY) of the Council on Cardiovascular Disease in the Young, American Heart Association, *Circulation* 106:143-60, 2002.
18. Rosner B, Prineus R, Daniels SR, Loggie J: Blood pressure differences between blacks and whites in relation to body size among US children and adolescents, *Am J Epidemiol* 151:1007-19, 2000.
19. Paradis G, Lambert M, O'Loughlin J, Lavallee C, et al: Blood pressure and adiposity in children and adolescents, *Circulation* 110:1832-38, 2004.
20. Freedman DS, Dietz WH, Srinivasan SR, Berenson GS: The relation of overweight to cardiovascular risk factors among children and adolescents: the Bogalusa Heart Study, *Pediatrics* 103:1175-82, 1999.
21. Sorof JM, Poffenbarger T, Franco K, Bernard L, Portman RJ: Isolated systolic hypertension, obesity, and hyperkinetic hemodynamic states in children. *J Pediatr* 140:660-66, 2002.
22. Daniels SR, Arnett DK, Eckel RH, Gidding SS, et al: Overweight in children and adolescents: pathophysiology, consequences, prevention and treatment, *Circulation* 111:1999-2012, 2005.
23. Schiel R, Beltschikow W, Kramer G, Stein G: Overweight, obesity and elevated blood pressure in children and adolescents, *Eur J Med Res* 11:97-101, 2006.

24. Reinehr T, Kiess W, de Sousa G, Stoffel-Wagner B, Wunsch R: Intima media thickness in childhood obesity: relation to inflammatory marker, glucose metabolism and blood pressure, *Metabolism* 55:113-18, 2006.
25. National Center for Health Statistics: National Health and Nutrition Examination Survey, CDC growth charts, United States, available at www.cdc.gov/nchs/about/major/nhanes/growthcharts/charts.htm.
26. Shear CL, Freedman DS, Burke GL, Harsha DW, Berenson GS: Body fat patterning and blood pressure in children and young adults: the Bogalusa Heart Study, *Hypertension* 9:236-44, 1987.
27. Rocchini AP, Katch V, Kveselis D: Insulin and renal sodium handling in obese adolescents, *Hypertension* 14:367-74, 1989.
28. Rocchini AP, Katch V, Anderson J: Blood pressure and obese adolescents: effect of weight loss, *Pediatrics* 82:116-23, 1988.
29. Rocchini AP, Moorehead C, DeRemer S, Goodfriend TL, Ball DL: Hyperinsulinemia and the aldoserone and pressor responses to angiotensin II, *Hypertension* 15:861-66, 1990.
30. Hall JE, Brands MW, Henegar JR, Shek EW: Abnormal kidney function as a cause and consequence of obesity hypertension, *Clin Exp Pharmacol Physiol* 25:58-64, 1998.
31. Collins S, Kuhn CM, Petro AE, Swick AG, et al: Role of leptin in fat regulation, *Nature* 380:667-74, 1996.
32. Meyer AA, Kundt G, Steiner M, Schuff-Werner P, Kienast W: Impaired flow-mediated vasodilation, carotid artery intima-media thickening, and elevated endothelial plasma markers in obese children: the impact of cardiovascular risk factors, *Pediatrics* 117:1560-67, 2006.
33. Bjorntop P, Rosmond R: Neuroendocrine abnormalities in visceral obesity, *Int J Obes Relat Metab Disord* 24(Suppl 2):S80-85, 2000.
34. Feig DI, Johnson RJ: Hyperuricemia in childhood primary hypertension, *Hypertension* 42:247-52, 2003.
35. Hypertension Prevention Treatment Group: The Hypertension Trial: three-year effects of dietary changes on blood pressure, *Arch Intern Med* 150:153-62, 1990.
36. Alpert BS, Wilmore JH: Physical activity and blood pressure in adolescents, *Pediatr Exerc Sci* 6:361-80, 1994.
37. Hernelahti M, Levalahti E, Simonen RL, Kaprio J, et al: Relative roles of heredity and physical activity in adolescence and adulthood on blood pressure, *J Appl Physiol* 97:1046-52, 2004.
38. Frank GC, Farris RP, Ditmarsen P, Voors AW, Berenson GS: An approach to primary preventive treatment for children with high blood pressure in a total community, *J Am Coll Nutr* 1:357-74, 1982.
39. Hagberg JM, Eshani AA, Goldberg D, Hernadez A, et al: Effect of weight training on blood pressure and hemodynamics in hypertensive adolescents, *J Pediatr* 104:147-51, 1984.
40. Danforth JS, Allen KD, Fitterling JM: Exercise as a treatment of hypertension in low-socioeconomic-status black children, *J Consult Clin Psychol* 58:237-39, 1990.
41. Hansen HS, Froberg K, Hyldebrandt N, Nielsen JR: A controlled study of eight months of physical training and reduction of blood pressure in children: the Odense schoolchild study, *BMJ* 303:682-85, 1991.
42. Kelsey RM, Barnard M, Alpert BS: Race, SES and cardiovascular reactivity to cold stress as longitudinal predictors of blood pressure in adolescents, *Am J Hypertens* 14:250A, 2001.
43. Sidorenko VN: Effects of the medical resonance therapy music on hemodynamic parameter in children with autonomic nervous system disturbances, *Integrative Physiol Behav Sci* 35:208-11, 2000.
44. Walsh A: Religion and hypertension: testing alternative explanations among immigrants, *Behav Med* 24:122-30, 1998.
45. Barnes VA, Davis HC, Murzynowski JB, Treiber FA: Impact of meditation on resting and ambulatory blood pressure and heart rate in youth, *Psychom Med* 66:909-14, 2004.
46. Sinaiko AR, Gomez-Marin O, Prineas R: Effect of low sodium diet or potassium supplementation on adolescent blood pressure, *Hypertension* 21:989-94, 1993.
47. Whelton PK, He J, Appel LJ: Primary prevention program of hypertension, clinical and public health advisory from the National High Blood Pressure Education Program, *JAMA* 288:1882-88, 2002.
48. Guerra A, Monteiro C, Breitenfeld L: Genetic and environmental factors regulating blood pressure in childhood: prospective study from 0 to 3 years, *J Hum Hypertens* 11:233-38, 1997.
49. Simons-Morton DG, Obarzanck E: Diet and blood pressure in children and adolescents, *Pediatr Nephrol* 11:244-49, 1997.
50. Falkner B, Kushner H, Khalsa DK: Sodium sensitivity, growth and family history of hypertension in young blacks, *J Hypertens* 4 (Suppl):S381-83, 1986.
51. Wilson DK, Bayer L, Krishnamoorthy JS, Ampey-Thornhill G, et al: The prevalence of salt-sensitivity in an African American adolescent population, *Ethn Dis* 9:950-58, 1999.
52. Wilson DK, Becker JA, Alpert BS: Prevalence of sodium sensitivity in black versus white adolescents, *Circulation* 1 (Suppl):13-16, 1992.
53. Nahata MC: Lack of pediatric drug formulations, *Pediatrics* 104(3 Pt 2):607-609, 1999.
54. Flynn JT: Pediatric use of antihypertensive medications: much more to learn, *Curr Ther Res Clin Exp* 62(4):314-28, 2001.
55. Chinard FP: Estimation of extravascular lung water by indicator-dilution techniques, *Circ Res* 37(2):137-45, 1975.
56. Bouissou F, Meguira B, Rostin M, Fontaine C, et al: Long term therapy by captopril in children with renal hypertension, *Clin Exp Hypertens A* 8(4-5):841-45, 1986.
57. Sinaiko AR, Kashtan CE, Mirkin BL: Antihypertensive drug therapy with captopril in children and adolescents, *Clin Exp Hypertens A* 8(4-5):829-39, 1986.
58. Doyle AE: Role of angiotensin-converting enzyme inhibitors in preventing or reducing end-organ damage in hypertension, *J Cardiovasc Pharmacol* 19(Suppl 5):S21-27, 1992.
59. Laffel LM, McGill JB, Gans DJ: The beneficial effect of angiotensin-converting enzyme inhibition with captopril on diabetic nephropathy in normotensive IDDM patients with microalbuminuria. North American Microalbuminuria Study Group, *Am J Med* 99(5):497-504, 1995.
60. National High Blood Pressure Education Program Working Group report on hypertension in diabetes, *Hypertension* 23 (2):145-58; discussion 159-60, 1994.
61. Wells T, Rippley R, Hogg R, Sakarcan A, et al: The pharmacokinetics of enalapril in children and infants with hypertension, *J Clin Pharmacol* 41(10):1064-74, 2001.
62. Sinaiko AR, Mirkin BL, Hendrick DA, Green TP, O'Dea RF: Antihypertensive effect and elimination kinetics of captopril in hypertensive children with renal disease, *J Pediatr* 103(5):799-805, 1983.
63. O'Dea RF, Mirkin BL, Alward CT, Sinaiko AR: Treatment of neonatal hypertension with captopril, *J Pediatr* 113(2):403-406, 1983.
64. Schilder JL, Van den Anker JN: Use of enalapril in neonatal hypertension, *Acta Paediatr* 84(12):1426-28, 1995.
65. Wells T, Frame V, Soffer B, Shaw W, et al: A double-blind, placebo-controlled, dose-response study of the effectiveness and safety of enalapril for children with hypertension, *J Clin Pharmacol* 42(8):870-80, 2002.
66. Pryde PG, Sedman AB, Nugent CE, Barr M Jr: Angiotensin-converting enzyme inhibitor fetopathy, *J Am Soc Nephrol* 3(9):1575-82, 1993.
67. Bifano E, Post EM, Springer J, Williams ML, Streeten DH: Treatment of neonatal hypertension with captopril, *J Pediatr* 100(1):143-46, 1982.
68. Sinaiko AR: Clinical pharmacology of converting enzyme inhibitors, calcium channel blockers and diuretics, *J Hum Hypertens* 8(5):389-94, 1994.
69. Prasher PK, Varma PP, Baliga KV: Efficacy of enalapril in the treatment of steroid resistant idiopathic nephrotic syndrome, *J Assoc Physicians India* 47(2):180-82, 1999.
70. Cook J, Daneman D, Spino M, Sochett E, et al: Angiotensin converting enzyme inhibitor therapy to decrease microalbuminuria in normotensive children with insulin-dependent diabetes mellitus, *J Pediatr* 117(1 Pt 1):39-45, 1990.
71. Herrera P, Soffer B, Zhang Z, Miller K, et al: Effects of the ACE inhibitor, lisinopril in children age 6-16 years, *Am J Hypertens* 15(4):32A, 2002.

72. Seeman T, Dusek J, Vondrak K, Flogelova H, et al: Ramipril in the treatment of hypertension and proteinuria in children with chronic kidney diseases, *Am J Hypertens* 17(5):415-20, 2004.
73. Blumer JL, Daniels SR, Dreyer WJ, Batisky D, et al: Pharmacokinetics of quinapril in children: assessment during substitution for chronic angiotensin-converting enzyme inhibitor treatment, *J Clin Pharmacol* 43(2):128-32, 2003.
74. Freed AL, Silbering SB, Kolodsick KJ, Rossi DT, et al: The development and stability assessment of extemporaneous pediatric formulations of Accupril, *Int J Pharm* 304(1-2):135-44, 2005.
75. Li JS, Berezny K, Kilaru R, Hazan L, et al: Is the extrapolated adult dose of fosinopril safe and effective in treating hypertensive children? *Hypertension* 44(3):289-93, 2004.
76. Sakarcan A, Tenney F, Wilson JT, Stewart JJ, et al: The pharmacokinetics of irbesartan in hypertensive children and adolescents, *J Clin Pharmacol* 41(7):742-49, 2001.
77. McConnaughey MM, McConnaughey JS, Ingenito AJ: Practical considerations of the pharmacology of angiotensin receptor blockers, *J Clin Pharmacol* 39(6):547-59, 1999.
78. Furberg CD, Herrington DM, Psaty BM: Are drugs within a class interchangeable? *Lancet* 354(9185):1202-204, 1999.
79. Fernandez-Andrade C, Russo D, Iversen B, Zucchelli P, et al: Comparison of losartan and amlodipine in renally impaired hypertensive patients, *Kidney Int Suppl* 68:S120-24, 1998.
80. Trachtman H, Frank R, Mahan JD, Portman R, et al: Clinical trial of extended-release felodipine in pediatric essential hypertension, *Pediatr Nephrol* 18(6):548-53, 2003.
81. Ellis D, Moritz ML, Vats A, Janosky JE: Antihypertensive and renoprotective efficacy and safety of losartan. A long-term study in children with renal disorders, *Am J Hypertens* 17(10):928-35, 2004.
82. Jung FF, Ingelfinger JR: Hypertension in childhood and adolescence, *Pediatr Rev* 14(5):169-79, 1993.
83. Piovan D, Padrini R, Svalato Moreolo G, Magnolfi G, et al: Verapamil and norverapamil plasma levels in infants and children during chronic oral treatment, *Ther Drug Monit* 17(1):60-67, 1995.
84. Wells TG, Sinaiko AR: Antihypertensive effect and pharmacokinetics of nitrendipine in children, *J Pediatr* 118:638-43, 1991.
85. Luke RG: Pathophysiology and treatment of posttransplant hypertension, *J Am Soc Nephrol* 2(2 Suppl 1):S37-44, 1991.
86. Tallian KB, Nahata MC, Turman MA, Mahan JD, et al: Efficacy of amlodipine in pediatric patients with hypertension, *Pediatr Nephrol* 13(4):304-10, 1999.
87. Silverstein DM, Palmer J, Baluarte HJ, Brass C, et al: Use of calcium-channel blockers in pediatric renal transplant recipients, *Pediatr Transplant* 3(4):288-92, 1999.
88. Flynn JT, Pasko DA: Calcium channel blockers: pharmacology and place in therapy of pediatric hypertension, *Pediatr Nephrol* 15(3-4):302-16, 2000.
89. Nahata MC, Morosco RS, Hipple TF: Stability of amlodipine besylate in two liquid dosage forms, *J Am Pharm Assoc (Wash)* 39(3):375-77, 1999.
90. Rogan JW, Lyszkiewicz DA, Blowey D, Khattak S, et al: A randomized prospective crossover trial of amlodipine in pediatric hypertension, *Pediatr Nephrol* 14(12):1083-87, 2000.
91. Khattak S, Rogan JW, Saunders EF, Theis JG, et al: Efficacy of amlodipine in pediatric bone marrow transplant patients, *Clin Pediatr (Phila)* 37(1):31-35, 1998.
92. Moncica I, Oh PI, ul Qamar I, Scolnik D, et al: A crossover comparison of extended release felodipine with prolonged action nifedipine in hypertension, *Arch Dis Child* 73(2):154-56, 1995.
93. Flynn JT, Warnick SJ: Isradipine treatment of hypertension in children: a single-center experience, *Pediatr Nephrol* 17(9):748-53, 2002.
94. Kornbluth A, Frishman WH, Ackerman M: Beta-adrenergic blockade in children, *Cardiol Clin* 5(4):629-49, 1987.
95. Sorof JM, Cargo P, Graepel J, Humphrey D, et al: Beta-blocker/thiazide combination for treatment of hypertensive children: a randomized double-blind, placebo-controlled trial, *Pediatr Nephrol* 17(5):345-50, 2002.
96. Griswold WR, McNeal R, Mendoza SA, Sellers BB, Higgins S: Propranolol as an antihypertensive agent in children, *Arch Dis Child* 53(7):594-96, 1978.
97. Frishman WH, Brobyn R, Brown RD, Johnson BF, et al: A randomized placebo-controlled comparison of amlodipine and atenolol in mild to moderate systemic hypertension, *J Cardiovasc Pharmacol* 12(Suppl 7):S103-106, 1988.
98. Falkner B, Lowenthal DT, Affrime MB: The pharmacodynamic effectiveness of metoprolol in adolescent hypertension, *Pediatr Pharmacol (NY)* 2(1):49-55, 1982.
99. Palminteri R, Assael BM, Bianchetti G, Gomeni R, et al: Betaxolol kinetics in hypertensive children with normal and abnormal renal function, *Clin Pharmacol Ther* 35(2):141-47, 1984.
100. Bunchman TE, Lynch RE, Wood EG: Intravenously administered labetalol for treatment of hypertension in children, *J Pediatr* 120(1):140-44, 1992.
101. Shaddy RE, Curtin EL, Sower B, Tani LY, et al: The Pediatric Randomized Carvedilol Trial in Children with Heart Failure: rationale and design, *Am Heart J* 144(3):383-89, 2002.
102. Ellison DH: Intensive diuretic therapy: high doses, combinations and constant infusions. In DW Seldin, G Giebisch, editors: *Diuretic agents: clinical physiology and pharmacology*, San Diego, 1997, Academic Press, 1997, pp. 281-300.
103. Sadowski RH, Falkner B: Hypertension in pediatric patients, *Am J Kidney Dis* 27(3):305-15, 1996.
104. Stokes GS: Age-related effects of antihypertensive therapy with alpha-blockers, *J Cardiovasc Pharmacol* 12(Suppl 8):S109-15, 1988.
105. Sorof JM: Systolic hypertension in children: benign or beware? *Pediatr Nephrol* 16(6):517-25, 2001.
106. Hiner LB, Falkner B: Renovascular hypertension in children, *Pediatr Clin North Am* 40(1):123-40, 1993.
107. Falkner B, Onesti G, Lowenthal DT, Affrime MB: Effectiveness of centrally acting drugs and diuretics in adolescent hypertension, *Clin Pharmacol Ther* 32(5):577-83, 1982.
108. Falkner B, Lowenthal DT, Onesti G: Dynamic exercise response in hypertensive adolescent on clonidine therapy: clonidine therapy in adolescent hypertension, *Pediatr Pharmacol (NY)* 1(2):121-28, 1980.
109. Talseth T: Clinical pharmacokinetics of hydrallazine, *Clin Pharmacokinet* 2(5):317-29, 1977.
110. Sinaiko AR, Mirkin BL: Management of severe childhood hypertension with minoxidil: a controlled clinical study, *J Pediatr* 91(1):138-42, 1977.
111. Cifkova R, Nakov R, Novozamska E, Hejl Z, et al: Evaluation of the effects of fixed combinations of sustained-release verapamil/trandolapril versus captopril/hydrochlorothiazide on metabolic and electrolyte parameters in patients with essential hypertension, *J Hum Hypertens* 14(6):347-54, 2000.
112. von Vigier RO, Mozzettini S, Truttmann AC, Meregalli P, et al: Cough is common in children prescribed converting enzyme inhibitors, *Nephron* 84(1):98, 2000.
113. Blowey DL: Safety of the newer antihypertensive agents in children, *Expert Opin Drug Saf* 1(1):39-43, 2002.
114. Soffer B, Zhang Z, Miller K, Vogt BA, Shahinfar S: A double-blind, placebo-controlled, dose-response study of the effectiveness and safety of lisinopril for children with hypertension, *Am J Hypertens* 16(10):795-800, 2003.
115. Rippley RK, Connor J, Boyle J, Bradstreet TE, et al: Pharmacokinetic assessment of an oral enalapril suspension for use in children, *Biopharm Drug Dispos* 21(9):339-44, 2000.
116. Adelman RD, Coppo R, Dillon MJ: The emergency management of severe hypertension, *Pediatr Nephrol* 14(5):422-27, 2000.

CHAPTER 45

Progression of Chronic Kidney Disease and Renoprotective Therapy in Children

Elke Wühl and Franz Schaefer

INTRODUCTION

The progression of renal malfunction towards end stage renal failure is common among patients with chronic kidney disease (CKD), and, after significant impairment of renal function has occurred, it tends to progress, irrespective of the underlying kidney disorder.

It was first shown in the 1930s that the removal of three quarters of the renal mass in rats leads to a slowly progressive deterioration of the function of the remaining nephrons with progressive glomerulosclerosis.[1] The glomerular lesions of the remnant kidney were associated with abnormal glomerular permeability and proteinuria. At that time, proteinuria was considered a mere marker of the extent of glomerular damage, despite the findings of Volhard and Fahr in 1914[2] and von Mollendorf and Stohr[3] in 1924 demonstrating that renal damage was globally related to pathologic amounts of protein excreted in the urine. In 1954, Oliver and colleagues[4] recognized protein droplets in the cytoplasm of tubular cells. It was proposed that proteinuria could lead to structural and functional nephron damage. During the late 1960s, Hostetter and coworkers[5] described the pathophysiology of renal adaptation to nephron loss in the rat remnant kidney model; they found that, after the removal of nephron mass, arteriolar resistance lowers and plasma flow increases in remnant glomeruli. The tone of afferent arterioles was found to drop by a greater degree than those of the efferent arterioles, thereby increasing glomerular capillary pressure and leading to increased filtration rate per nephron. These authors also demonstrated that therapies attenuating these changes reduce glomerular filtration rate (GFR) decline and structural alterations.

Today, there is clear evidence from clinical studies that both hypertension and proteinuria are key players in the pathophysiology of CKD progression in humans.[6-8] The renin-angiotensin system is intrinsically involved in the process, and other potential contributors include the genetic background, renal anemia, altered mineral homeostasis, dyslipidemia, inflammation, and oxidative stress as well as general cardiovascular risk factors such as diabetes, smoking, and obesity.

The phenomenon of renal failure progression after kidney injury is a current focus of renal research in adults as well as in children. This chapter summarizes the current state of knowledge regarding the pathophysiology of renal disease progression and discusses the evidence base of renoprotective strategies for pediatric CKD.

NATURAL COURSE OF PROGRESSION OF CHRONIC RENAL FAILURE IN CHILDREN WITH CHRONIC KIDNEY DISEASE

Limited information about the natural course of CKD progression in children is available to date. The prospective, population-based ItalKid registry was started in 1990, and, during the first 10 years, 1197 patients with CKD of various origin were registered, including 23% who had severe kidney disease with renal insufficiency.[9] The incidence of renal

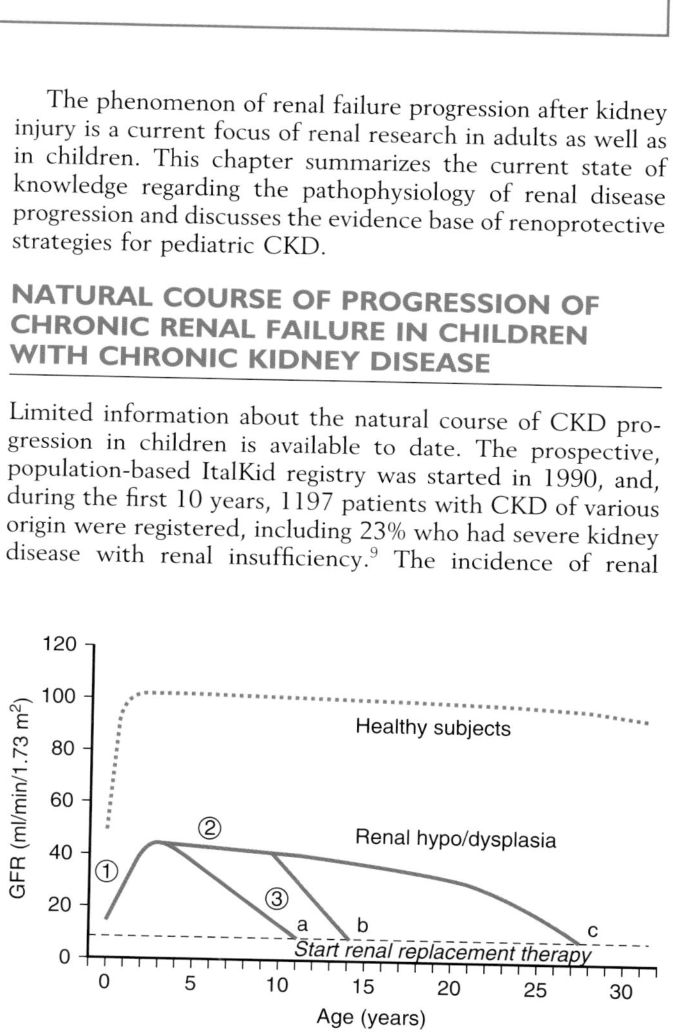

Figure 45-1 Natural time course of renal disease progression in children with renal hypodysplasia. ①, Period of improving renal function during infancy. ②, Period of stable renal function. ③, Period of renal function deteriorating toward end-stage renal disease. The third phase is characterized either by rapid decline soon after infancy *(a)*, decline at an early pubertal age *(b)*, or a steady, slow decline of renal function *(c)*. Reproduced from Gonzalez Celedon C, Bitsori M, Tullus K: Progression of chronic renal failure in children with dysplastic kidneys, *Pediatr Nephrol* 22(7):1014-20, 2007.

replacement therapy was 7.3 per year per 100 patients, and the risk of developing end-stage renal disease (ESRD) by age 20 was 68%. The decline of renal function was not linear; rather, it was characterized by a sharp decline during puberty and at an early postpubertal age. The probability of kidney survival decreased with lower GFR at baseline. This finding supports the general clinical impression that, in many children with renal hypodysplasia, renal function deteriorates more rapidly around the time of puberty.

A recent retrospective analysis of 176 patients with renal hypodysplasia suggests that the natural time course of chronic renal failure progressing to ESRD in children can be divided into three time periods: (1) an initial period that usually lasts for the first 3 years of life and that is characterized by renal function that actually improves (+6.3 ml per year, on average); (2) a subsequent period of stable renal function that is attained by 50% of patients for a mean of 8 years; and (3) a phase during which renal function gradually deteriorates and becomes ESRD[10] (Figure 45-1). The latter period started just after infancy in 48% of patients and around puberty in 23% of patients. In 30% of patients, renal function remained stable even beyond puberty. Figure 45-1 shows the patterns of renal function in patients with renal hypodysplasia. Correlates of deteriorating renal function were proteinuria, hypertension, previous febrile urinary tract infections, and lower GFR at onset.[10]

A retrospective analysis of the prestudy GFR data of patients participating in the European Study on Nutritional Treatment of Chronic Renal Failure in Childhood[11] suggests that the initial period of improving renal function may last even longer, for a mean of 5 years (personal communication, O. Mehls, 2007).

MECHANISMS OF RENAL DISEASE PROGRESSION

According to the Brenner hypothesis, any critical loss of functioning renal mass, irrespective of the nature of the initial injury, leads to glomerular hyperfiltration with an increased single-nephron GFR (Figure 45-2). The remaining nephrons lose their ability to autoregulate glomerular pressure, which results in the transmission of systemic hypertension to the glomerulus. Elevated intraglomerular pressure induces glomerular and tubular hypertrophy. Increased intraglomerular pressure induces proteinuria, which is the pathophysiologic link between glomerular, interstitial,[12] and tubular damage.[13] The degree of proteinuria in glomerular disease correlates with the rate of renal failure progression.[14]

Recent research has attributed a central role to the podocytes, which are terminally differentiated and unable to respond to injury by proliferation and repair.[15] The key role of this glomerular cell type in the pathophysiology of CKD progression has been explored as a result of a growing number of specific genetic disorders that affect the development, terminal differentiation, and postnatal function of the podocytes and that result in congenital or infantile nephrotic syndrome, which inevitably leads to glomerulosclerosis and progressive renal failure. The loss of lesioned podocytes may lead to focal and segmental adhesions of the denuded basement membrane to Bowman's capsule, with a concomitant spreading of the ultrafiltrate into the tubulointerstitial compartment, where it causes inflammatory injury (i.e., "misdirected filtration").

The formation and maintenance of the glomerular filtration barrier require a complex interaction between podocytes and glomerular capillary endothelial cells. Vascular endothelial growth factor overexpression by podocytes has been noted in proteinuric states, and antibodies that block this factor prevent glomerular hyperfiltration, hypertrophy, and proteinuria. Endothelial cell injury resulting from disease-specific or nonspecific uremia-associated vasculotoxic and inflammatory insults is frequently involved in progressive glomerular damage.[16] Vascular endothelial cells release endothelin, platelet-derived growth factor, and fibroblast growth factor in response to fluid shear stress.[17] Moreover, injured endothelial cells express increased angiotensinogen and transforming growth factor-β (TGF-β),[18] which are factors that cause inflammation and fibrosis. In chronic glomerular injury, endothelial cells lose part of their anticoagulant properties and intensify their procoagulant activity by the increased expression of plasminogen activator inhibitor 1. By the release of adhesion molecules such as intercellular adhesion molecule 1, endothelial cells facilitate macrophage infiltration and the attraction and proliferation of inflammatory cells. In addition,

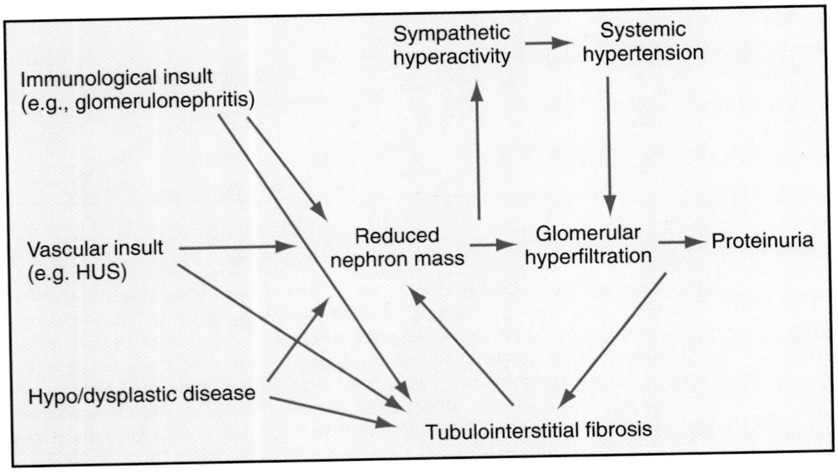

Figure 45-2 Mechanisms of progressive renal disease in pediatric nephropathies.

damage to endothelial cells may denude the glomerular basement membrane, which results in the induction of local platelet aggregation and the activation of coagulation with fibrin deposition and microthrombi formation.

The reabsorption of filtered proteins by the tubuloepithelial cells can induce direct injury to intracellular lysosomal pathways, oxidative stress, and the increased local expression of growth factors[19,20] such as insulin-like growth factor 1, TGF-β, and hepatocyte growth factor. Moreover, stressed epithelial cells release an array of chemotactic factors, including monocyte chemoattractant protein 1, regulated upon activation, normal T-cell expressed and secreted (RANTES), connective tissue growth factor, fibronectin, and endothelin-1, which promote tubulointerstitial inflammation and fibrosis through the recruitment and activation of macrophages.[21-27] Macrophages infiltrating the renal parenchyma in turn perpetuate the production of further cytokines and growth factors. The proteins of the complement system represent another component of proteinuria that may cause tubular damage, and, after tubular cells are injured, they may activate the alternative complement pathway.

Both in the glomerulus and in the tubular apparatus, chronic inflammatory processes promote cell transdifferentiation toward a fibroblast phenotype, driven by a high tone of TGF-β (i.e., epithelial mesenchymal transformation). Myofibroblastic transformation is characterized by the release of proteinases, cytokines, and oxidants.[28,29] Moreover, myofibroblasts and local fibroblasts begin to deposit fibronectin and laminin, which make up the molecular framework for interstitial collagen deposition,[30] and they secrete extracellular matrix components, including type IV collagen and collagens I, III, and V (i.e., "scar" collagens), which result in scar formation.[31] In addition, the activity of matrix-degrading enzymes is inhibited by the overproduction of inhibitory peptides (i.e., plasminogen activator inhibitor 1, tissue inhibitors of metalloproteinases).[32,33] As a result of increased synthesis and reduced degradation, excessive tubulointerstitial collagen accumulation occurs. The fibrous masses in the tubulointerstitium are believed to compromise oxygen supply to the tubular cells, thereby further contributing to tubular atrophy and nephron loss.

Glomerular sclerosis, tubulointerstitial fibrosis, and tubular atrophy result in a further loss of functioning renal mass, thereby closing a vicious circle by further increasing the intraglomerular pressure and the hypertrophy of the remaining glomeruli (Figure 45-3).

Angiotensin II (Ang II), the primary effector of the renin-angiotensin system, is mechanistically involved in most of the mechanisms described previously. Ang II is produced both systemically and locally in the kidney, and it exerts multiple endocrine, intercrine, autocrine, and paracrine effects. Intrarenal Ang II concentrations are a thousand-fold higher than those found in the circulation. The major source of intrarenal Ang II is autocrine/paracrine synthesis by tubular, juxtaglomerular, and glomerular cells.[34-36] Renin release from the juxtaglomerular apparatus drives systemic Ang II generation, and it is involved in blood pressure upregulation; however, it probably has little to do with intrarenal Ang II action. Most of the intrarenal effects of Ang II are mediated via the Ang II type 1 receptor.[37] Ang II is a potent vasoconstrictor that augments intraglomerular pressure by preferentially increasing the efferent arteriolar tone. Ang II also increases intracellular calcium in podocytes,[38,39] thereby inducing cytoskeletal changes and altered podocyte function with the induction of protein ultrafiltration, even in the absence of structural glomerular damage.[40,41] Moreover, Ang II increases the proliferation of smooth muscle cells and increases the glomerular and tubular expression of various growth factors, cytokines, and chemokines, most importantly of the TGF-β/connective tissue growth factor system but also of tumor necrosis factor-

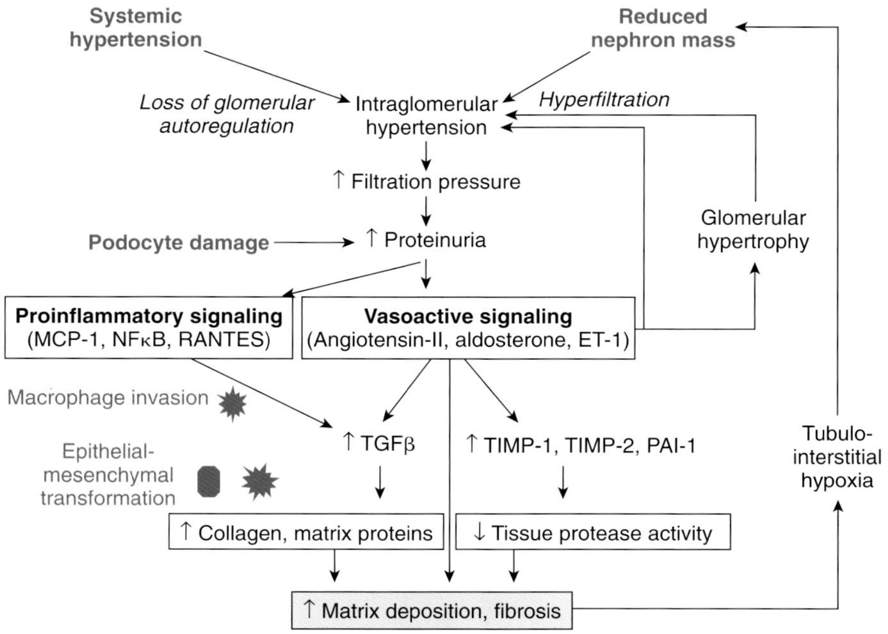

Figure 45-3 Pathophysiologic consequences of hypertension and proteinuria in chronic kidney disease.

α, platelet-derived growth factor, basic fibroblast growth factor, and vascular cell adhesion molecule 1. Ang II also stimulates oxidative stress, which perpetuates the upregulation of cytokines, adhesion molecules, and chemoattractants.[42,43] Finally, intrarenal Ang II stimulates neuronal afferences, which are believed to activate the central nervous structures that regulate the sympathetic tone. Hence, Ang II is pathophysiologically involved in the state of sympathetic hyperactivation that is characteristic of CKD and that constitutes another important mechanism of renal disease progression and cardiovascular morbidity.[44,45]

In patients with reduced nephron mass and anemia, the hypoxia of tubular cells is favored by an increased oxygen consumption by the tubular cells of the remaining nephrons, a decreased number of interstitial capillaries,[46] and the accumulation of extracellular matrix between interstitial capillaries and tubular cells, which hampers oxygen diffusion. In turn, hypoxia stimulates the production of profibrotic molecules such as TGF-β or endothelin-1 by tubular cells, further increases the synthesis of extracellular matrix by fibroblastic cells, and ultimately leads to tubuloepithelial cell loss with the formation of atubular glomeruli.[47,48]

In addition, hypoxia enhances the local production of reactive oxygen species. Oxidative stress also induces the release of proinflammatory and profibrotic molecules, thereby enhancing the production of extracellular matrix by fibroblasts and favoring cell death.

FACTORS THAT MODIFY THE RISK OF RENAL DISEASE PROGRESSION

Age at Attainment of Renal Mass Deficit

The age at which a significant loss of renal mass occurs may influence the degree of glomerular hypertrophy and the long-term renal prognosis. Patients who are born with unilateral renal agenesis are at greater risk for proteinuria, hypertension, and renal insufficiency than subjects who undergo unilateral nephrectomy by trauma or kidney donation during later life, which suggests that the number of functional nephrons in congenital solitary kidneys may be decreased, possibly by hypogenesis.[49] Compensatory renal growth after unilateral nephrectomy for Wilms' tumor was most marked in patients who underwent surgery at a very young age. Marked kidney growth was associated with microalbuminuria in more than 30% of these patients.[50] The possibility that nephrons in infantile solitary kidneys are subject to greater hypertrophic stress is supported by quantitative morphometric studies showing glomerular volumes that are five to six times greater than normal.[51]

Gender

Among adult patients with CKD, men tend to exhibit more rapid renal failure progression and poorer renal survival rates than women. Although the gender effect is not very marked and has varied among individual studies, an overall female renal survival advantage has been suggested by meta-analysis for autosomal dominant polycystic kidney disease, immunoglobulin A nephropathy, and membranous nephropathy.[52] The advantage seems to be lost in postmenopausal women, which suggests a renoprotective effect of female sex steroids; however, some impact of secondary factors such as lipid levels or the prevalence of smoking cannot be ruled out. Although a sexual dimorphism in the course of renal function has not been observed to date in children, the apparent acceleration of GFR loss around puberty deserves further study with respect to possible gender differences.

Underlying Renal Disease and Genetic Pathology

Although the pathophysiologic principles of renal disease progression described previously generally apply to all cases of CKD, the time course of renal failure for individual disease entities is highly variable. It is evident that patients with aggressive, incompletely controlled immunologic nephropathies will have a more rapid progression of renal failure than subjects with renal hypoplasia. However, even within groups of patients suffering from pathogenetically homogeneous hereditary kidney diseases, the rate of renal failure progression can vary markedly among individuals. In a growing number of these entities, the progression phenotype can be linked to the underlying genetic defect. In disease entities caused by defects in more than one gene, progression patterns may differ according to the gene involved. For example, in adults with autosomal dominant polycystic kidney disease, individuals with mutations in the PKD1 gene typically have a more severe disease course with an earlier need for renal replacement therapy than those with mutations in the PKD2 gene. A gene-phenotype correlation is also obvious in children with the nephronophthisis complex. In children with mutations in the NPHP1 gene, ESRD is attained at a mean age of 13 years as compared with 8 months in those with NPHP2 mutations and 19 years in those with NPHP3 mutations[53] (see Chapter 8). Even within the same gene, the localization and type of the causative mutations are key determinants of the renal prognosis. The highly variable times of disease onset and progression to ESRD in steroid-resistant nephrotic syndrome caused by different mutations in the NPHS2 gene (see Chapter 13) and in Alport syndrome related to COL4A5 gene mutations (see Chapter 14) are classic examples of genotype-phenotype correlations in recessive and dominant forms of hereditary kidney disorders.

Polymorphic Genetic Variation

In addition to the crucial causative role of genetic defects in many if not most pediatric kidney diseases, it is currently held that common polymorphic variants in various genes determine an individual's susceptibility to renal injury and renal disease progression and his or her response to renoprotective treatment. One of the first common variants studied in the context of renal disease progression is the insertion/deletion polymorphism of the angiotensin-converting enzyme (ACE) gene. The DD genotype has been shown to predispose an individual to progressive renal failure in the immunoglobulin A nephropathy.[54,55] Some (but not all) studies found an elevated risk for parenchymal damage that appears to be increased with the DD genotype in children with congenital urologic abnormalities, particularly vesicoureteral reflux.[56-58] A prospective study in children with CKD caused by renal hypodysplasia associated the DD genotype with poor renal survival.[56] There is still inconclusive data regarding any effects of polymorphisms in the ACE, angiotensinogen, or Ang II type 1 receptor genes on proteinuria and renal failure progression in children with nephrotic syndrome and focal-segmental sclerosis.[59-61]

In adults with nondiabetic proteinuric nephropathies, the ACE polymorphism has been claimed to predict the renoprotective efficacy of ACE inhibition. Proteinuria, the rate of GFR decline, and the progression to ESRD were lowered by ACE inhibitors in patients with the DD genotype but not in those with the II or ID genotype.[62,63]

Several polymorphisms have been involved in the pathogenesis of hypertension (see Chapter 43); these may indirectly affect the evolution of renal function in chronic kidney disorders. Also, common variants exist in various genes encoding the cytokines, growth factors, and regulatory peptides involved in CKD progression, but none of these have been consistently associated with disease progression to date.

The kidney has a natural capacity to remodel into its original architecture after injury as evidenced by the partial reversal of glomerulosclerosis observed after the removal of the pathogenic mechanism (e.g., by successful pancreas transplantation in type I diabetes[64]) or by the efficient high-dose blockade of the renin-angiotensin system (RAS) in uremic[65] or hypertensive rodents.[66] In renal transplantation, the upregulation of heme oxygenase-1, a molecule that displays cytoprotective activity, is a beneficial response to acute renal injury.[67] A polymorphism in the promoter region of the donor's HO-1 gene has been associated with graft survival.[68,69] The further molecular exploration of such reconstitutive mechanisms may uncover significant genetic variability affecting the course of renal disease.

Hypertension

Hypertension is an independent risk factor for renal failure progression in adults.[6-8] Although the degree of hypertension is a marker of the underlying renal disease severity, interventional studies (described later) have provided evidence that high blood pressure actively contributes to renal failure progression in human CKD. In pediatric nephropathies, renal hypertension is common, but it is typically less severe than that seen with adult kidney disorders. Hypertension prevalence estimates in children with CKD range from 20% to 80%, depending on the degree of renal dysfunction.[70,71] However, even children with stage 2 CKD or renal hypodysplasia (conditions that are usually not strongly associated with hypertension) may present with elevated blood pressure.[72] A systolic blood pressure of more than 120 mm Hg has been associated with a faster GFR decline in a large prospective study of children with CKD[11] (Figure 45-4).

Investigations into the physiologic diurnal variation of blood pressure by ambulatory blood pressure monitoring have revealed that the integrity of the nocturnal fall of blood pressure (i.e., the "dipping" pattern) plays a significant role in renal failure progression in addition to and independent of the absolute blood pressure level. Nondipping, which is a well-known independent cardiovascular risk factor and a common characteristic of renoparenchymal hypertension, is associated with a more rapid progression of renal failure in adult patients with CKD.[73,74] Nondipping is believed to reflect a state of sympathetic hyperactivation in CKD. Although the association appears to be firm, it is as yet unclear whether the pharmacologic restoration of the dipping pattern will be of any long-term clinical benefit for cardio-

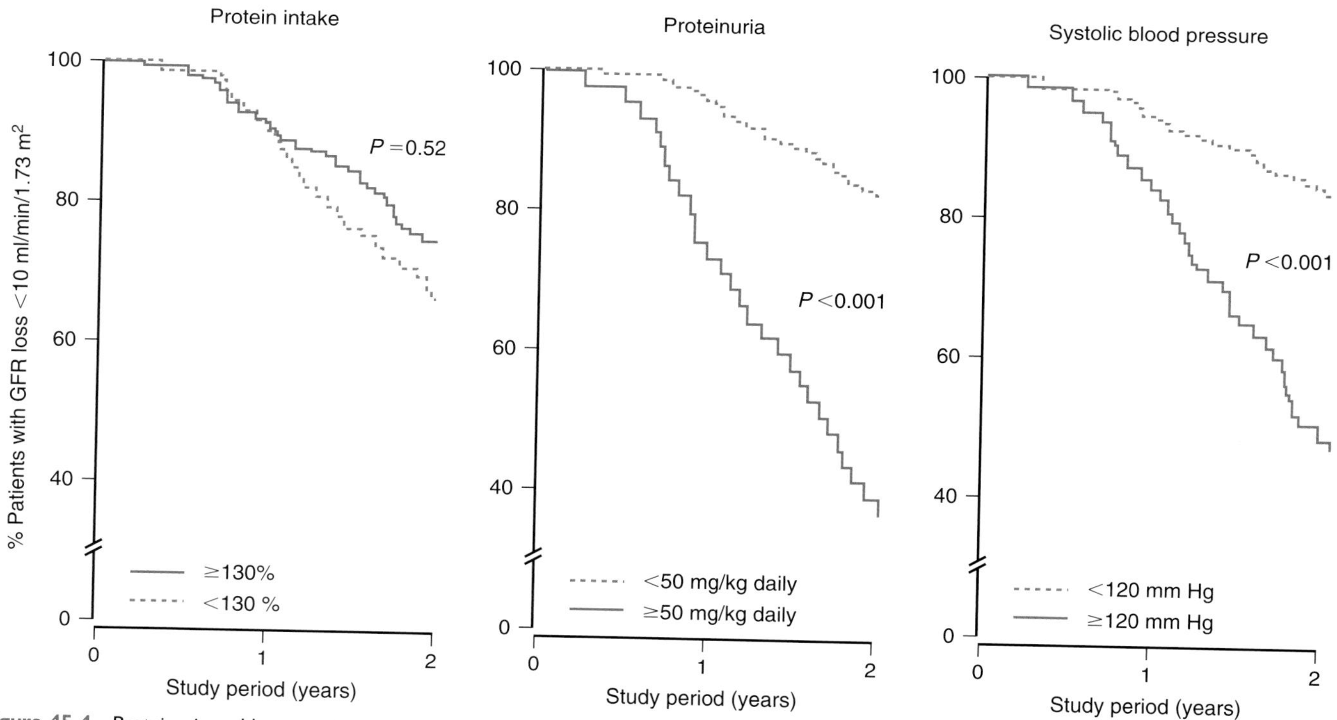

Figure 45-4 Proteinuria and hypertension predict the risk for renal disease progression in children with chronic kidney disease. Reproduced from Wingen AM, Fabian-Bach C, Schaefer F, Mehls O: Randomised multicentre study of a low-protein diet on the progression of chronic renal failure in children. European Study Group of Nutritional Treatment of Chronic Renal Failure in Childhood, *Lancet* 349:1117-23, 1997.

vascular health in general and renal function preservation in patients with CKD.

Proteinuria

Population-based studies in healthy individuals have demonstrated that proteinuria is an independent risk factor for ESRD and overall mortality.[75-77] In adults with diabetic and nondiabetic kidney disorders, proteinuria is clearly predictive of the renal prognosis.[14,78,79] In the Ramipril Efficacy in Nephropathy trial,[80] urinary protein excretion was the only baseline variable that correlated with GFR decline and progression to ESRD. The spectrum of underlying renal disorders in children markedly differs from that of adults. Congenital renal hypodysplasia with or without urinary tract abnormalities is the leading underlying pediatric renal disorder, affecting more than 60% of children with CKD. The European Study Group for Nutritional Treatment of Chronic Renal Failure in Childhood first demonstrated in 200 children with stage 3 or 4 CKD that proteinuria and hypertension are also major determinants of GFR decline in pediatric nephropathies[11] (see Figure 45-4). The ItalKid Project confirmed that proteinuria also predicts renal disease progression in children with renal hypodysplasia.[81] In the ongoing ESCAPE trial, residual proteinuria during ACE inhibition appears to be quantitatively associated with renal failure progression.[82] In a group of Polish children with chronic renal failure of nonglomerular origin without significant proteinuria, the protein excretion level did not play a major role in the progression of the condition. The main risk factors for chronic renal failure progression in that group were rapid somatic growth, age, and blood pressure.[83]

Dyslipidemia and Insulin Resistance

Epidemiologic studies may give some evidence that dyslipidemia is an independent risk factor not only for cardiovascular disease but also for progressive chronic renal failure.[84] The dyslipidemic pattern differs between the major renal disease entities,[85] and the degree of dyslipidemia parallels the degree of renal function impairment. Underlying mechanisms of uremic dyslipidemia include insulin resistance,[86] hyperparathyroidism,[87] malnutrition, acidosis,[88] and the impaired catabolism of triglyceride-rich lipoproteins by the decreased activity of lipoprotein lipase and hepatic triglyceride lipase,[89,90] but lipoprotein synthesis appears to be unaltered. In line with findings in adults, in children with CKD, serum triglycerides are elevated, and the total cholesterol level is close to normal.

In animal models, hypercholesterolemia clearly accelerates the rate of progression of kidney disease.[91] A high-fat diet causes macrophage infiltration and foam cell formation in rats, which leads to glomerulosclerosis.[92] Dyslipidemia may damage glomerular capillary endothelial and mesangial cells as well as podocytes. Mesangial cells express receptors for low-density lipoproteins and oxidized low-density lipoproteins, which, upon activation, induce mesangial cell proliferation, increase mesangial matrix deposition, and enhance the production of chemokines, cytokines, and growth factors. Circulating lipids bind to extracellular matrix molecules,[91] undergo oxidation, and increase the formation of reactive oxygen species.[93] Macrophages phagocytose oxidized lipids and undergo the transition to become foam cells. Macrophage-derived foam cells release cytokines that recruit more macrophages to the lesion and influence lipid deposition, endothelial cell function, and vascular smooth muscle cell proliferation.

In unilaterally nephrectomized rats, a link between dyslipidemia and oxidative stress in the pathogenesis of renal damage was shown in which hyperlipidemia increased glomerular and tubulointerstitial infiltration and aggravated glomerulosclerosis.[94]

It has also been observed that the insulin resistance syndrome may underlie or mediate the association between lipids and the loss of renal function. In humans, a strong relationship between the metabolic syndrome and the risk for chronic renal disease and microalbuminuria was found in a large nondiabetic general population.[95] A relationship between serum cholesterol levels and GFR decline was also shown in adult patients with type 1 diabetes and overt nephropathy[96]; patients with a total cholesterol level of more than 7 mmol/L showed an at least three times faster decline in GFR than subjects with lower cholesterol levels. In nondiabetic patients, a strong correlation between triglyceride-rich apolipoprotein-B-containing lipoproteins and the rate of renal disease progression was observed,[97] and patients with low high-density lipoprotein cholesterol levels and hypertriglyceridemia had an increased risk of progressive kidney disease.[84]

However, the evidence for dyslipidemia as an independent risk factor for renal disease development or progression is not as strong in clinical studies as it is in experimental settings. It is unclear whether dyslipidemia increases the renal risk in those patients without other risk factors for kidney disease, because most studies have been performed in patients with preexisting renal disease or associated renal risk factors, such as hypertension or diabetes.

TREATMENT STRATEGIES IN RENAL DISEASE PROGRESSION

On the basis of the current understanding of the mechanisms of renal disease progression, several principal renoprotective strategies have emerged in recent years. These are based mainly on clinical evidence established in adult patients, but growing evidence supports their efficacy also for the treatment of children. The efficient control of blood pressure and the minimization of proteinuria appear to be the two most important measures for the preservation of residual kidney function. Other issues, such as the prevention and treatment of renal anemia, uremic dyslipidemia, and disorders of mineral metabolism, have an experimental basis, although their clinical importance is currently less clear.

Blood Pressure Control

Numerous studies in adults have provided proof of the concept that consequent antihypertensive therapy slows down the rate of renal failure progression.[98] There seems to be a close linear relationship between the blood pressure level achieved by antihypertensive treatment and the rate of renal failure progression in patients with CKD (Figure 45-5). This relationship appears to persist well into the normal range of blood pressure.[99,100]

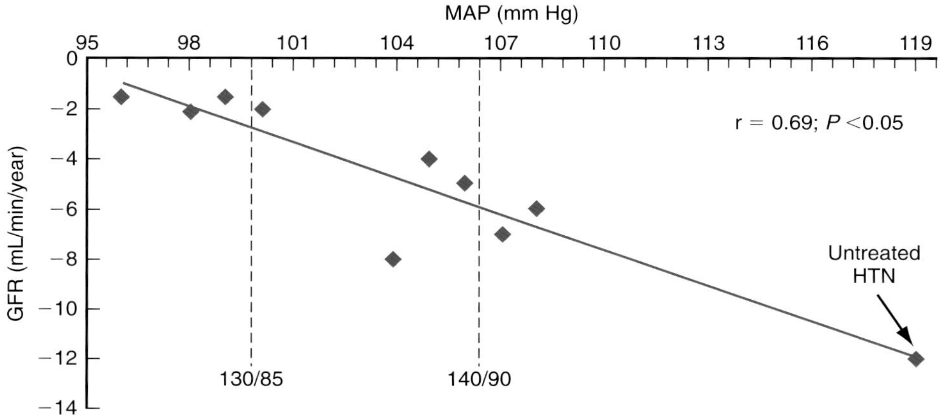

Figure 45-5 Relationship between achieved blood pressure control and declines in glomerular filtration rate in clinical trials of diabetic and nondiabetic renal disease. Each dot represents one trial. Reproduced from Bakris GL, Williams M, Dworkin L, Elliot WJ, et al: Preserving renal function in adults with hypertension and diabetes: a consensus approach. National Kidney Foundation Hypertension and Diabetes Executive Committees Working Group, *Am J Kidney Dis* 36:646-61, 2000.

The firm evidence of a favorable effect of intensified blood pressure control in patients with CKD has resulted in generally lower target blood pressure recommendations for this patient population. In the most recent guidelines from the Joint National Committee in the United States[101] and the Guidelines of the European Hypertension Society,[102] 120/80 mm Hg has been defined as the upper limit of the optimal blood pressure range, and any blood pressure greater than 130/80 mm Hg in CKD patients should be actively lowered by therapeutic intervention. These blood pressure targets are equivalent to the 50th to the 75th distribution percentile in the general young adult population. It is as yet unknown whether these blood pressure targets hold true for the pediatric population and whether glomerular damage in children correlates with absolute or age-specific relative blood pressure. Assuming that equivalent blood pressure percentiles should be targeted in children as they are in adults, the adult recommendations would, for example, correspond with an acceptable upper blood pressure level of 106/66 mm Hg (75th percentile) in an 8-year-old child with CKD. The ESCAPE trial will provide pediatric evidence of whether intensified blood pressure control (targeting to below the 50th percentile of 24-hour mean arterial pressure) will confer a renoprotective advantage over a more conventional target range (i.e., the 50th to the 95th percentile).[103] The results of this 5-year randomized trial will be available in late 2007.

Proteinuria Control

In line with the experimental evidence given previously, multiple clinical studies have confirmed that proteinuria is not only a marker but also an important mechanism of kidney disease progression. Its reduction is associated with a slowing of GFR loss in the long term.[14,104-106] In the Modification of Diet in Renal Disease (MDRD) trial, for each 1 g/d reduction in proteinuria observed after 4 months of treatment with antiproteinuric therapies (i.e., blood pressure and dietary interventions), subsequent GFR decline was slowed by about 1 ml/min per year.[14] In the Ramipril Efficacy in Nephropathy study, a reduction of proteinuria after 3 months of ACE inhibitor therapy by 1 g/d resulted in a slowing down of GFR decline by 2 ml/min per year.[107] The goal of antiproteinuric treatment is to reduce proteinuria as much as possible, ideally to less than 300 mg/m²/day. This degree of proteinuria reduction appears to be associated with the maximal renoprotective effect.[108,109]

Several antiproteinuric therapies have proven to be effective. First, blood pressure control lowered proteinuria in three large trials: the MDRD study,[14] the Appropriate Blood Pressure Control in Diabetes study,[110] and the African American Study of Kidney Disease and Hypertension study.[105] A low blood pressure goal (i.e., <125/75 mm Hg in adults) either reduced proteinuria absolutely by 50%[14] or prevented the two- to threefold increases in proteinuria that have been observed in patients with the more conventional blood pressure goal of 140/90 mm Hg.[110] A low blood pressure goal appears to be very well tolerated by the vast majority of patients. In terms of cardiovascular outcomes, the "J curve" phenomenon (i.e., a slight increase in cardiovascular events among patients achieving a very low blood pressure level) seems to be confined to older patients with advanced atherosclerosis.

Pharmacologic Options

Although the different classes of antihypertensive agents are comparable with respect to their blood pressure lowering efficacy, they differ markedly regarding their effects on proteinuria and CKD progression.[105,108,111,112]

By virtue of their pharmacologic properties, ACE inhibitors and, more recently, Ang II type I receptor blockers (ARB) have become the pharmacotherapeutics of choice for both adults and children with CKD. RAS antagonists have an excellent safety profile that is almost indistinguishable from that of placebo. In adults with essential hypertension, treatment with RAS antagonists has been associated with the best quality of life among all antihypertensive agents. In the ESCAPE trial cohort, which comprised 184 children with CKD completing 5 years of ramipril treatment out of 385 patients started, the drug was permanently discontinued as a result of symptomatic hypotension in 3 patients, hyperkalemia in 5 patients, and persistent cough in 2 patients[103] (also unpublished results).

RAS antagonists suppress the local Ang II tone (ACE inhibitors) or action (ARBs). This results in a reduction of intraglomerular pressure and proteinuria; a diminished local release of TGF-β and other growth factors, cytokines, and chemokines, with consequently attenuated glomerular hypertrophy and sclerosis; tubulointerstitial inflammation and fibrosis[72]; and a normalized central nervous sympathetic tone as a result of reduced renal afferent nerve stimulation.

Several randomized trials in adults with diabetic or nondiabetic kidney disease have demonstrated a more effective reduction of proteinuria (usually by 30% to 40%) with ACE inhibitor therapy as compared with treatment with placebo or other antihypertensive agents.[108] In the long term, this is associated with a significantly reduced rate of renal failure progression.[104,108,113-121]

Very similar results were obtained in randomized comparisons of ARBs with placebo or conventional antihypertensive agents in patients with diabetic nephropathy.[112,122,123] It has been reasoned that ACE inhibitors may have a specific renoprotective advantage by inducing the accumulation of vasodilatory and antifibrotic bradykinins, but the course of GFR was similar in two clinical trials comparing ACE inhibitors and ARB therapy.[124,125] The size of the advantage of RAS antagonists over other antihypertensive agents is still being debated.[126] The risk of doubling serum creatinine or attaining ESRD is typically reduced by 30% to 40%, but the superiority of RAS antagonists is related to the prevailing degree of proteinuria (Figure 45-6). In adults, ACE inhibitors are believed to provide better renoprotection than other antihypertensive agents in patients with proteinuria exceeding 500 mg/day.

Also, there is some evidence that previous studies may not have used sufficiently high ACE inhibitor doses to achieve effective RAS suppression at the kidney tissue level and to obtain a maximal renoprotective effect. Moreover, at least a subset of patients appears to develop partial secondary resistance to ACE inhibition (i.e., "aldosterone escape" by the compensatory upregulation of ACE-independent Ang II production).[127-129] It is currently an open issue whether such patients would benefit from the primary use of ARBs alone or in combination with ACE inhibitors.

Although the maximal antiproteinuric and renoprotective effects of ACE inhibitors and ARBs seem to occur at doses that are supramaximal with respect to maximal antihypertensive action, regulatory authority approval is usually available only for the indication of hypertension in the respective dose range. Therefore, it is generally recommended to administer these drugs after confirming tolerability with a short run-in period at the highest approved doses.[105,130]

The antiproteinuric response within the first 2 to 3 months of administration appears to be predictive of the long-term renoprotective effect,[107] and it can be used to tailor the appropriate drug dose. The specific glomerulodynamic effects of RAS antagonists induce an immediate drop of the GFR (usually by approximately 10% to 15%) when these drugs are first administered. In patients with CKD, this may cause a significant increase in serum creatinine. It is important to know that a marked initial GFR decline is actually a positive predictor of the long-term renoprotective effect.[131] Rapid acute renal failure soon after the administration of an RAS antagonist is a very rare event, and it is usually related to concomitant volume depletion or previously unidentified bilateral renal artery stenoses.

Limited information is available regarding the efficacy of RAS antagonism for renoprotection in children with CKD. Small uncontrolled studies showed stable renal function in children after hemolytic uremic syndrome during long-term ACE inhibition,[132] with a stable GFR seen during 2.5 years of losartan treatment in children with proteinuric CKD[133] and attenuated histopathologic progression seen in children with immunoglobulin A nephropathy receiving combined RAS blockade.[134] So far, the ESCAPE trial has demonstrated efficient blood pressure and proteinuria reduction with the use of ramipril in 400 children with CKD.[103] However, an interim analysis of the 3-year results revealed a gradual rebound of proteinuria after the second treatment year. This effect was dissociated from persistently good blood pressure control, and it may limit the long-term renoprotective efficacy of ACE inhibitor monotherapy in pediatric chronic kidney disorders.[82]

Calcium channel blockers (CCBs) are safe and able to achieve blood pressure goals in patients with CKD. However, CCBs of the dihydropyridine type (i.e., amlodipine, nifedipine) fail to reduce the progression of chronic renal failure and may even increase proteinuria. Therefore, dihydropyri-

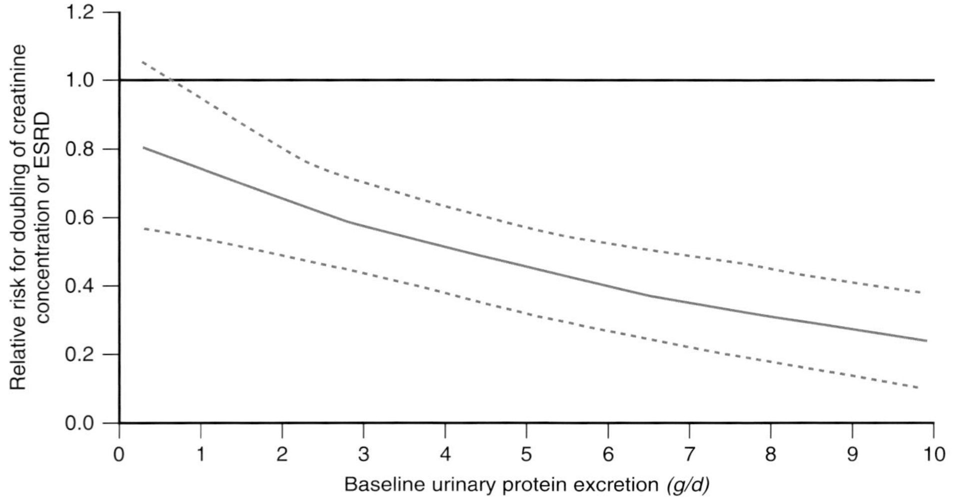

Figure 45-6 Reduction of the risk of the development of progressive renal failure in adult patients with nondiabetic nephropathies receiving angiotensin-converting enzyme inhibitor treatment as compared with controls, stratified according to baseline proteinuria. *Solid line* represents mean; *dotted lines* represent 95% confidence intervals of relative risk.[108,109]

dine CCBs may be acceptable as first-line antihypertensive monotherapy only in nonproteinuric patients.[106] They may be used in combination with RAS antagonists to improve blood pressure control in severely hypotensive patients.[130] By contrast, nondihydropyridine CCBs (i.e., diltiazem, verapamil) have some antiproteinuric effect and might therefore provide additional renoprotection.

CKD is often associated with a state of the overactivation of the sympathetic nervous system, and antiadrenergic drugs play an important role in the management of this condition. Drugs that are beta-blockers are effective for lowering blood pressure in patients with CKD; metoprolol and atenolol were the first antihypertensive agents with which beneficial effects on the decline of renal function in patients with CKD were seen.[114] In the African American Study of Kidney Disease and Hypertension trial, the beta-blocker metoprolol had an antiproteinuric effect that was almost comparable to that of ramipril and in marked contrast with amlodipine.[105] The antiproteinuric action may be the result of sympathicoplegic effects. Newer beta-blockers such as carvedilol have even improved antiproteinuric effects as compared with atenolol.[135,136]

Combination Therapies

Because hypertension is a multifactorial disorder, monotherapy is often not effective for lowering blood pressure to the target range. Treatment with a single antihypertensive agent usually controls blood pressure in less than half of patients. According to the Joint National Committee guidelines, subjects with blood pressure of more than 20/10 mm Hg above the normal range (i.e., >160/100 mm Hg in adults) should be started on combination drug therapy.[101] In patients with CKD, RAS antagonists are most commonly combined with a diuretic or a CCB, whereas their combination with a beta-blocker usually does not exert an additive effect on blood pressure control. Fixed-dose combination preparations are becoming increasingly popular in antihypertensive therapy, and they may help to maximize treatment adherence and efficacy.

Combined RAS blockade using ACE inhibitors and ARBs concomitantly has only a minor effect on blood pressure (3 to 4 mm Hg as compared with monotherapy) but increases the antiproteinuric effect of ACE inhibitor or ARB monotherapy by 30% to 40%.[124,137-139] A single prospective randomized trial performed in adults with nondiabetic nephropathies suggested that combination therapy may also provide better long-term renoprotection.[124] However, in most ACE inhibitor/ARB combination studies, it remained unclear whether maximally efficient single-drug doses were used, which is a formal prerequisite to demonstrating the true synergism of the two drug classes. The few published studies that assessed the effects of single-drug dose escalation followed by the combined administration of an ACE inhibitor and an ARB at maximally effective single doses found synergistic antiproteinuric effects of combined treatment.[140] Alternatively, a recent study demonstrated additional proteinuria reduction by escalating candesartan exposure to an ultra-high dose.[141] Notably, raising the dose from 16 to 32 mg daily had no effect on proteinuria, whereas a further increase from 32 to 64 mg was highly effective, thereby suggesting that the dose-response relationship may be nonlinear. Hence, the issue of whether ACE inhibitor/ARB combination therapies have a synergistic renoprotective potential remains an exciting field of clinical research.

Antihypertensive Chronotherapy

In view of the fact that nocturnal blood pressure nondipping is an independent risk factor for CKD progression, effects of the timing of the application of antihypertensive drugs may be an issue of interest. Even using agents with a long half-life and a once-daily recommended dose with evening administration lowers nighttime blood pressure more effectively, thereby increasing the day-to-night ratio and partially restoring the physiologic nocturnal dipping pattern. However, these effects seem to differ for individual antihypertensive drug classes. Whereas the bedtime administration of CCBs and ACE inhibitors tends to restore the dipping pattern, the evening dosing of beta-blockers has no effect on the circadian blood pressure rhythm.[142] In a substudy of the HOPE trial, adult patients were evaluated by ambulatory blood pressure monitoring after the evening administration of the ACE inhibitor ramipril. A more marked blood pressure reduction during the nighttime was observed, and this is compatible with the notion that the beneficial effects of ramipril on cardiovascular morbidity and mortality in the HOPE study were related to the 8% increase in the day-to-night ratio of blood pressure obtained with evening dosing.[143] Although antihypertensive chronotherapy has not been demonstrated to affect CKD progression as of yet, it is of note that the antiproteinuric efficacy of the ARB valsartan was found to correlate with an increase in the blood pressure day-to-night ratio that was induced by evening dosing.[144]

Other Supportive Treatment Strategies

In rats undergoing acute ischemic renal injury, pretreatment with recombinant human erythropoietin (EPO) reduced renal dysfunction and morphologic damage. These protective effects appear to be mainly mediated by a reduction of apoptotic cell death.[145] In addition, recent studies of patients with CKD provided some evidence that the correction of renal anemia with the use of EPO results in better renal survival.[146] This renoprotective effect of EPO might be related to an attenuation of interstitial fibrosis and tubuloepithelial cell loss by improved oxygen supply and reduced oxidative stress via the correction of anemia. In addition, EPO may exert direct protective effects on tubular cells and help to maintain the integrity of the interstitial capillary network. Other possible components of the repair and regeneration of injured renal tissue are stem cells and progenitor cells. The infiltration of resident stem cells may contribute to the replacement of lost or damaged tissue. Although the regulation of circulating progenitor cells and their quantitative role in acute and chronic tissue repair is far from being completely understood, EPO in animal models induced mobilization and the differentiation of endothelial progenitor cells and ameliorated tissue injury.[147] Endothelial progenitor cells can also be increased by the pharmacologic administration of statins[148] or ARBs.[149]

The treatment of uremic dyslipidemia is another component of renoprotective therapy. General measures to prevent dyslipidemia in CKD patients include the prevention or treatment of malnutrition and the correction of metabolic acidosis, hyperparathyroidism, and anemia, all of which may contribute to dyslipidemia.[87,150,151] In addition, referring to evidence from the general population, therapeutic lifestyle modification (i.e., diet, exercise, weight reduction) is recommended for adults and children with CKD-related dyslipidemia.[152] However, the lipid-lowering effect of lifestyle modifications in patients with CKD is usually not impressive. Dietary supplementation with fish oil effectively improved lipid profiles in a small cohort of children receiving renal replacement therapy.[153] Lipid-lowering medical treatment is commonly prescribed for adults with CKD on the basis of the evident benefit of this approach for the primary and secondary prevention of cardiovascular disease in the general adult population. Statin therapy is effective for reducing cardiovascular morbidity and mortality in adults with moderate to severe CKD although not for patients with ESRD.[154,155]

With respect to renoprotection, experimental evidence suggests that statins may retard renal disease progression not only by their lipid-lowering effects but also by their lipid-independent pleiotropic effects. Statins inhibit signalling molecules at several points in inflammatory pathways. Anti-inflammatory effects and improved endothelial function are thought to be partially responsible both for cardiovascular disease risk reduction and improved renal function.[156] Furthermore, there is also evidence for the synergistic effects of statins and RAS inhibitors on the prevention of renal disease progression.[157] However, a recent meta-analysis of published clinical trials concluded that the intrinsic antiproteinuric and renoprotective effects of statins are quantitatively small although still significant.[158] No studies to date have evaluated the usefulness of statins for children with progressive nephropathies.

Experimental studies have suggested a parathyroid-hormone-independent beneficial effect of phosphate restriction on renal failure progression. A high calcium phosphorus product may be detrimental to renal survival by aggravating intrarenal vasculopathy and by causing tubulointerstitial calcifications, which may stimulate tubulointerstitial inflammation and fibrosis. In view of these pathophysiologic associations, it is currently under investigation whether calcium-free phosphate binders may have some renoprotective potential for patients with CKD. Sevelamer may prove beneficial beyond phosphate lowering as a result of its pleiotropic effects, which include lipid-lowering and anti-inflammatory properties. Treatment with nonhypercalcemic doses of active vitamin D attenuates renal failure progression in animal models of chronic kidney disease.[159] This effect may be brought about by the immune modulatory and antifibrotic properties of vitamin D. Although these exciting experimental findings provide even more arguments for close monitoring and early intervention to maintain mineral, vitamin D, and parathyroid hormone homeostasis in patients with CKD, it should be kept in mind that neither a causative association of mineral metabolism disorders with renal failure progression nor a beneficial effect of respective interventions has been affirmed in the human setting to date.

CONCLUSIONS

The progression of childhood CKD to end-stage renal failure is common, and, after a significant impairment of renal function has occurred, it progresses irrespective of underlying renal disease. The onset of CKD and the progression rate in defined disease entities may be influenced by genetic factors. Hypertension and proteinuria are the most important independent risk factors for renal disease progression. Therefore, therapeutic strategies to prevent progression should comprise blood pressure control, probably aiming for a target blood pressure below the 75th percentile. RAS antagonists preserve kidney function not only by lowering blood pressure but also by their antiproteinuric and anti-inflammatory properties. Intensified blood pressure control may exert additional renoprotective effects. Other factors that contribute in a multifactorial manner to renal disease progression include anemia, dyslipidemia, and disorders of mineral metabolism. Measures to preserve renal function should therefore also comprise the maintenance of hemoglobin, serum lipid, and calcium-phosphorus ion product levels in the normal range.

REFERENCES

1. Chanutin A, Ferris EB: Experimental renal insufficiency produced by partial nephrectomy. 1. Control diet, *Arch Intern Med* 49:767-87, 1932.
2. Volhard F, Fahr TH: *Die Bright'sche Nierenkrankheit*, Berlin, 1914, Julius Springer Verlag.
3. von Mollendorf W, Stohr P: *Lehrbuch der Histologie*, Jena, Germany, 1924, Fischer-Verlag.
4. Oliver J, Macdowell M, Lee YC: Cellular mechanisms of protein metabolism in the nephron. I. The structural aspects of proteinuria, tubular absorption, droplet formation, and the disposal of proteins, *J Exp Med* 99:589-604, 1954.
5. Hostetter TH, Olson JL, Rennke HG, Venkatachalam MA, Brenner BM: Hyperfiltration in remnant nephrons: a potentially adverse response to renal ablation, *Am J Physiol* 241:F85-93, 1981.
6. Klag MJ, Whelton PK, Randall BL, Neaton JD, et al: Blood pressure and end-stage renal disease in men, *Hypertension* 13:180-93, 1996.
7. Iseki K, Ikemiya Y, Iseki C, Takishita S: Proteinuria and the risk of developing end-stage renal disease, *Kidney Int* 63:1468-74, 2003.
8. Locatelli F, Marcelli D, Comelli M, Alberti D, et al: Proteinuria and blood pressure as causal components of progression to end-stage renal failure. Northern Italian Cooperative Study Group, *Nephrol Dial Transplant* 11:461-7, 1996.
9. Ardissino G, Dacco V, Testa S, Bonaudo R, et al: Epidemiology of chronic renal failure in children: data from the ItalKid Project, *Pediatrics* 111:382-7, 2003.
10. Gonzalez Celedon C, Bitsori M, Tullus K: Progression of chronic renal failure in children with dysplastic kidneys, *Pediatr Nephrol* 22(7):1014-20, 2007.
11. Wingen AM, Fabian-Bach C, Schaefer F, Mehls O: Randomised multicentre study of a low-protein diet on the progression of chronic renal failure in children. European Study Group of Nutritional Treatment of Chronic Renal Failure in Childhood, *Lancet* 349:1117-23, 1997.
12. Remuzzi G, Bertani T: Pathophysiology of progressive nephropathies, *N Engl J Med* 339:1448-56, 1998.
13. Olbricht CJ, Cannon LK, Garg LC, Tisher CC: Activities of cathepsins B and L in isolated nephron segments from proteinuric and nonproteinuric rats, *Am J Physiol* 250:F1055-62, 1986.

14. Peterson JC, Adler S, Burkart JM, Greene T, et al: Blood pressure control, proteinuria, and the progression of renal disease: the modification of diet in renal disease study, *Ann Intern Med* 123:754-62, 1995.
15. Kriz W: Progressive renal failure—inability of podocytes to replicate and the consequences for development of glomerulosclerosis, *Nephrol Dial Transplant* 11:1738-42, 1996.
16. Takano T, Brady HR: The endothelium in glomerular inflammation, *Curr Opin Nephrol Hypertens* 4:277-86, 1995.
17. Malek AM, Greene AL, Izumo S: Regulation of endothelin 1 gene by fluid shear stress is transcriptionally mediated and independent of protein kinase C and cAMP, *Proc Natl Acad Sci U S A* 90:5999-6003, 1993.
18. Lee LK, Meyer TW, Pollock AS, Lovett DH: Endothelial cell injury initiates glomerular sclerosis in the rat remnant kidney, *J Clin Invest* 96:953-64, 1995.
19. Hirschberg R, Wang S: Proteinuria and growth factors in the development of tubulointerstitial injury and scarring in kidney disease, *Curr Opin Nephrol Hypertens* 14:43-52, 2005.
20. Wang SN, Lapage J, Hirschberg R: Glomerular ultrafiltration and apical tubular action of IGF-1, TGF-beta, and HGF in nephrotic syndrome, *Kidney Int* 56:1247-51, 1999.
21. Wang SN, Hirschberg R: Growth factor ultrafiltration in experimental diabetic nephropathy contributes to interstitial fibrosis, *Am J Physiol Renal Physiol* 278:F554-60, 2000.
22. Wang SN, Lapage J, Hirschberg R: Loss of tubular bone morphogenetic protein-7 in diabetic nephropathy, *J Am Soc Nephrol* 12:2392-9, 2001.
23. Donadelli R, Abbate M, Zanchi C, Corna D, et al: Protein traffic activates NF-kB gene signaling and promotes MCP-1-dependent interstitial inflammation, *Am J Kidney Dis* 36:1226-41, 2000.
24. Morigi M, Macconi D, Zoja C, Donadelli R, et al: Protein overload-induced NF-kappaB activation in proximal tubular cells requires H(2)O(2) through a PKC-dependent pathway, *J Am Soc Nephrol* 13:1179-89, 2002.
25. Zoja C, Donadelli R, Colleoni S, Figliuzzi M, et al: Protein overload stimulates RANTES production by proximal tubular cells depending on NF-kappaB activation, *Kidney Int* 53:1608-15, 1998.
26. Zoja C, Morigi M, Figliuzzi M, Bruzzi I, et al: Proximal tubular cell synthesis and secretion of endothelin-1 on challenge with albumin and other proteins, *Am J Kidney Dis* 26:934-41, 1995.
27. Kees-Folts D, Sadow JL, Schreiner GF: Catabolism of albumin is associated with the release of an inflammatory lipid, *Kidney Int* 45:1697-709, 1994.
28. Floege J, Burns MW, Alpers CE, Yoshimura A, et al: Glomerular cell proliferation and PDGF expression precede glomerulosclerosis in the remnant kidney model, *Kidney Int* 41:297-309, 1992.
29. Couser WG: Pathogenesis of glomerular damage in glomerulonephritis, *Nephrol Dial Transplant* 13:10-5, 1998.
30. Strutz F, Neilson EG: New insights into mechanisms of fibrosis in immune renal injury, *Springer Semin Immunopathol* 24:459-79, 2003.
31. Kelly CJ, Neilson EG: Tubulointerstitial diseases. In Brenner BM, editor: *The kidney*, Philadelphia, 2004, Saunders, pp 1483-512.
32. Eddy AA, Fogo A: Plasminogen activator inhibitor-1 in chronic kidney disease: evidence and mechanisms of action, *J Am Soc Nephrol* 17:2999-3012, 2006.
33. Catania JM, Chen G, Parrish AR: Role of matrix metalloproteinases in renal pathophysiologies, *Am J Physiol Renal Physiol* 292:F905-11, 2007.
34. Schalekamp MA, Danser AH: Angiotensin II production and distribution in the kidney: I. A kinetic model, *Kidney Int* 69:1543-52, 2006.
35. Schalekamp MA, Danser AH: Angiotensin II production and distribution in the kidney—II. Model based analysis of experimental data. *Kidney Int* 69:1553-57, 2006.
36. Navar LG, Nishiyama A: Why are angiotensin concentrations so high in the kidney?, *Curr Opin Nephrol Hypertens* 13:107-15, 2004.
37. Schmitz D, Berk BC: Angiotensin II signal transduction stimulation of multiple mitogen activated protein kinase pathways, *Trends Endocrinol Metab* 8:261-6, 1997.
38. Henger A, Huber T, Fischer KG, Nitschke R, et al: Angiotensin II increases the cytosolic calcium activity in rat podocytes in culture, *Kidney Int* 52:687-93, 1997.
39. Nitschke R, Henger A, Ricken S, Gloy J, et al: Angiotensin II increases the intracellular calcium activity in podocytes of the intact glomerulus, *Kidney Int* 57:41-9, 2000.
40. Bohrer MP, Deen WM, Robertson CR, Brenner BM: Mechanism of the angiotensin II-induced proteinuria in the rat, *Am J Physiol* 233: F13-21, 1977.
41. Yoshioka T, Mitarai R, Kon V, Deen WM, et al: Role of angiotensin II in overt functional proteinuria, *Kidney Int* 52:687-93, 1997.
42. Taal MW, Omer SA, Nadim MK, Mackenzie HS: Cellular and molecular mediators in common pathway mechanisms of chronic renal disease progression, *Curr Opin Nephrol Hypertens* 9:323-31, 2000.
43. Taal MW, Chertow GM, Rennke HG, Gurnani A, et al: Mechanisms underlying renoprotection during renin-angiotensin system blockade, *Am J Physiol Renal Physiol* 280:F343-55, 2001.
44. Converse RL, Jacobsen TN, Toto RD, Jost CMT, et al: Sympathetic overactivity in patients with chronic renal failure, *N Engl J Med* 327:1912-8, 1992.
45. Hausberg M, Kosch M, Harmelink P, Barenbrock M, et al: Sympathetic nerve activity in end-stage renal disease, *Circulation* 165:1974-79, 2002.
46. Kang DH, Kanellis J, Hugo C, Truong L, et al: Role of the microvascular endothelium in progressive renal disease, *J Am Soc Nephrol* 13:806-16, 2002.
47. Orphanides C, Fine LG, Norman JT: Hypoxia stimulates proximal tubular cell matrix production via a TGF-β1-independent mechanism, *Kidney Int* 52:637-47, 1997.
48. Fine LG, Orphanides C, Norman JT: Progressive renal disease: the chronic hypoxia hypothesis, *Kidney Int Suppl* 65:S74-8, 1998.
49. Argueso L, Ritchey ML, Boyle ET Jr, Milliner DS, et al: Prognosis of patients with unilateral renal agenesis, *Pediatr Nephrol* 6:412-6, 1992.
50. Di Tullio MT, Casale F, Indolfe P, Polito C, et al: Compensatory hypertrophy and progressive renal damage in children nephrectomized for Wilms' tumor, *Med Pediatr Oncol* 26:325-8, 1996.
51. Bhathena DB, Julian BA, McMorrow RG, Baehler RW: Focal sclerosis of hypertrophic glomeruli in solitary functioning kidneys of humans, *Am J Kidney Dis* 5:226-32, 1985.
52. Neugarten J, Acharya A, Silbiger SR: Effect of gender on the progression of nondiabetic renal disease: a meta-analysis, *J Am Soc Nephrol* 11:319-29, 2000.
53. Hildebrandt F, Otto E, Omran H: Nephronophthise und verwandte Krankheiten, *Med Genet* 12:225-31, 2000.
54. Bantis C, Ivens K, Kreusser W, Koch M, et al: Influence of genetic polymorphisms of the renin-angiotensin system on IgA nephropathy, *Am J Nephrol* 24:258-67, 2004.
55. Maruyama K, Yoshida M, Nishio H, Shirakawa T, et al: Polymorphisms of renin-angiotensin system genes in childhood IgA nephropathy, *Pediatr Nephrol* 16:350-5, 2001.
56. Hohenfellner K, Hunley TE, Brezinska R, Brodhag P, et al: ACE I/D gene polymorphism predicts renal damage in congenital uropathies, *Pediatr Nephrol* 13:514-8, 1999.
57. Erdogan H, Mir S, Serdaroglu E, Berdeli A, Aksu N: Is ACE gene polymorphism a risk factor for renal scarring with low grade reflux?, *Pediatr Nephrol* 19:734-7, 2004.
58. Dudley J, Johnston A, Gardner A, McGraw M: The deletion polymorphism of the ACE gene is not an independent risk factor for renal scarring in children with vesico-ureteric reflux, *Nephrol Dial Transplant* 17:652-4, 2002.
59. Serdaroglu E, Mir S, Berdeli A, Aksu N, Bak M: ACE gene insertion deletion polymorphism in childhood idiopathic nephrotic syndrome, *Pediatr Nephrol* 20:1738-43, 2005.
60. Tabel Y, Berdeli A, Mir S, Serdaroglu E, Yilmaz E: Effects of genetic polymorphisms of the renin-angiotensin system in children with nephrotic syndrome, *J Renin Angiotensin Aldosterone Syst* 6:138-144, 2005.
61. Oktem F, Srin A, Bilge I, Emre S, et al: ACE I/D gene polymorphism in primary FSGS and steroid-sensitive nephrotic syndrome, *Pediatr Nephrol* 19:384-9, 2004.

62. Perna A, Ruggenenti P, Testa A, Spoto B, et al: ACE genotype and ACE inhibitors induced renoprotection in chronic proteinuric nephropathies1, *Kidney Int* 57:274-81, 2000.
63. Ruggenenti P, Perna A, Zoccali C, Gherardi G, et al: Chronic proteinuric nephropathies. II. Outcomes and response to treatment in a prospective cohort of 352 patients: differences between women and men in relation to the ACE gene polymorphism. Gruppo Italiano di Studi Epidemologici in Nefrologia (Gisen), *J Am Soc Nephrol* 11:88-96, 2000.
64. Fioretto P, Steffes MW, Sutherland DE, Goetz FC, Mauer M: Reversal of lesions of diabetic nephropathy after pancreas transplantation, *N Engl J Med* 339:115-7, 1998.
65. Adamczak M, Gross ML, Krtil J, Koch A, et al: Reversal of glomerulosclerosis after high-dose enalapril treatment in subtotally nephrectomized rats, *J Am Soc Nephrol* 14:2833-42, 2003.
66. Boffa JJ, Lu Y, Placier S, Stefanski A, et al: Regression of renal vascular and glomerular fibrosis: role of angiotensin II receptor antagonism and matrix metalloproteinases, *J Am Soc Nephrol* 14:1132-44, 2003.
67. Sikorski EM, Hock T, Hill-Kapturczak N, Agarwal A: The story so far: molecular regulation of the heme oxygenase-1 gene in renal injury, *Am J Physiol Renal Physiol* 286:F425-41, 2004.
68. Exner M, Bohmig GA, Schillinger M, Regele H, et al: Donor heme oxygenase-1 genotype is associated with renal allograft function, *Transplantation* 77:538-42, 2004.
69. Baan C, Peeters A, Lemos F, Uitterlinden A, et al: Fundamental role for HO-1 in the self-protection of renal allografts, *Am J Transplant* 4:811-8, 2004.
70. Seeman T, Simkova E, Kreisinger J, Vondrak K, et al: Control of hypertension in children after renal transplantation, *Pediatr Transplant* 10:316-22, 2006.
71. Lingens N, Dobos E, Witte K, Busch C, et al: Twenty-four-hour ambulatory blood pressure profiles in pediatric patients after renal transplantation, *Pediatr Nephrol* 11:23-6, 1997.
72. Schaefer F, Mehls O: Hypertension in chronic kidney disease. In Portman RJ, Sorof JM, Ingelfinger JR, editors: *Pediatric hypertension*, Totowa, NJ, 2004, Humana Press, pp 371-87.
73. Jacob P, Hartung R, Bohlender J, Stein G: Utility of 24-h ambulatory blood pressure measurement in a routine clinical setting of patients with chronic renal disease, *J Hum Hypertens* 18:745-51, 2004.
74. Timio M, Venanzi S, Lolli S, Lippi G, et al: "Non-dipper" hypertensive patients and progressive renal insufficiency: a 3-year longitudinal study, *Clin Nephrol* 43:382-7, 1995.
75. Tarver-Carr M, Brancati F, Eberhardt M, Powe N: Proteinuria and the risk of chronic kidney disease (CKD) in the United States, *J Am Soc Nephrol* 11:168A, 2000.
76. Hoy WE, Wang Z, vanBuynder P, Baker PR, Mathews JD: The natural history of renal disease in Australian Aborigines. Part I. Changes in albuminuria and glomerular filtration rate over time. *Kidney Int* 60:243-8, 2001.
77. Iseki K, Kinjo K, Iseki C, Takishita S: Relationship between predicted creatinine clearance and proteinuria and the risk of developing ESRD in Okinawa, Japan, *Am J Kidney Dis* 44:806-14, 2004.
78. Risdon RA, Sloper JC, de Wardener HE: Relationship between renal function and histological changes found in renal biopsy specimens from patients with persistent glomerular nephritis, *Lancet* 2:363-6, 1968.
79. Remuzzi G, Ruggenenti P, Perico N: Chronic renal disease: renoprotective benefits of renin-angiotensin system inhibition, *Ann Intern Med* 136:604-15, 2002.
80. Ruggenenti P, Perna A, Mosconi L, Matalone M, et al: Proteinuria predicts end-stage renal failure in non-diabetic chronic nephropathies. The "Gruppo Italiano di Studi Epidemiologici in Nefrologia" (GISEN), *Kidney Int Suppl* 63:S54-7, 1997.
81. Ardissino G, Testa S, Dacco V, Vigano S, et al: Proteinuria as a predictor of disease progression in children with hypodysplastic nephropathy, *Pediatr Nephrol* 19:172-7, 2004.
82. Wühl E, Mehls O, Schaefer F; ESCAPE Trial Group: Long-term dissociation of antiproteinuric and antihypertensive efficacy of ACE inhibition in children with chronic renal failure. COD.OC 16 [Abstract], *Pediatr Nephrol* 21:1505, 2006.
83. Litwin M: Risk factors for renal failure in children with non-glomerular nephropathies, *Pediatr Nephrol* 19:178-86, 2004.
84. Muntner P, Coresh J, Clinton Smith J, Eckfeldt J, Klag MJ: Plasma lipids and risk of developing renal dysfunction: the Atherosclerosis Risk in Communities Study, *Kidney Int* 58:293-301, 2000.
85. Saland MJ, Ginsberg H, Fisher EA: Dyslipidemia in pediatric renal disease: epidemiology, pathophysiology, and management, *Curr Opin Pediatr* 14:197-204, 2002.
86. Cheng SC, Chu TS, Huang KY, Chen YM, et al: Association of hypertriglyceridemia and insulin resistance in uremic patients undergoing CAPD, *Perit Dial Int* 21:282-9, 2001.
87. Mak RH: 1,25-Dihydroxyvitamin D3 corrects insulin and lipid abnormalities in uremia, *Kidney Int* 53:1353-57, 1998.
88. Mak RH: Effect of metabolic acidosis on hyperlipidemia in uremia, *Pediatr Nephrol* 13:891-3, 1999.
89. Chan PC, Persaud J, Varghese Z, Kingstone D, et al: Apolipoprotein B turnover in dialysis patients: its relationship to pathogenesis of hyperlipidemia, *Clin Nephrol* 31:88-95, 1989.
90. Horkko S, Huttunen K, Kesaniemi YA: Decreased clearance of low-density lipoproteins in uremic patients under dialysis treatment, *Kidney Int* 47:1732-40, 1995.
91. Abrass CK: Cellular lipid metabolism and the role of lipids in progressive renal disease, *Am J Nephrol* 24:46-53, 2004.
92. Hattori M, Nikotic-Paterson DJ, Miyazaki K, Isbel NM, et al: Mechanisms of glomerular macrophage infiltration in lipid-induced renal injury, *Kidney Int Suppl* 71:S47-50, 1999.
93. Chait A, Heinecke JW: Lipoprotein modification: cellular mechanisms, *Curr Opin Lipidol* 5:363-70, 1994.
94. Scheuer H, Gwinner W, Hohbach J, Grone EF, et al: Oxidant stress in hyperlipidemia-induced renal damage, *Am J Physiol Renal Physiol* 278:F63-74, 2000.
95. Chen J, Muntner P, Hamm LL, Jones DW, et al: The metabolic syndrome and chronic kidney disease in US adults, *Ann Intern Med* 140:167-74, 2004.
96. Mulec H, Johnson SA, Bjorck S: Relation between serum cholesterol and diabetic nephropathy, *Lancet* 335:1537-8, 1990.
97. Sammuelson O, Attman P, Knicht-Gibson C, Larsonn R, et al: Complex apolipoprotein B-containing lipoprotein particles are associated with a higher rate of progression of human chronic renal insufficiency, *Am J Soc Nephrol* 9:1482-8, 1998.
98. Bakris GL, Williams M, Dworkin L, Elliot WJ, et al: Preserving renal function in adults with hypertension and diabetes: a consensus approach. National Kidney Foundation Hypertension and Diabetes Executive Committees Working Group, *Am J Kidney Dis* 36:646-61, 2000.
99. Peterson JC, Adler S, Burkart JM, Greene T, et al: Blood pressure control, proteinuria, and the progression of renal disease. The Modification of Diet in Renal Disease Study, *Ann Intern Med* 123:754-62, 1995.
100. Sarnak MJ, Greene T, Wang X, Beck G, et al: The effect of a lower target blood pressure on the progression of kidney disease: long-term follow-up of the modification of diet in renal disease study, *Ann Intern Med* 142:342-51, 2005.
101. Chobanian AV, Barkis GL, Black DL, Cushman WC, et al: The Seventh Report of the Joint National Committee on Prevention, Detection, Evaluation, and Treatment of High Blood Pressure: The JNC 7 Report, *JAMA* 289:2560-71, 2003.
102. European Society of Hypertension—European Society of Cardiology Guidelines Committee: 2003 European Society of Hypertension—European Society of Cardiology guidelines for the management of arterial hypertension, *J Hypertens* 21:1011-53, 2003.
103. Wühl E, Mehls O, Schaefer F; ESCAPE Trial Group: Antihypertensive and antiproteinuric efficacy of ramipril in children with chronic renal failure, *Kidney Int* 66:768-76, 2004.
104. The GISEN Group (Gruppo Italiano di Studi Epidemiologici in Nefrologia): Randomised placebo-controlled trial of effect of ramipril on decline in glomerular filtration rate and risk of terminal renal failure in proteinuric, non-diabetic nephropathy, *Lancet* 349:1857-63, 1997.
105. Wright JT Jr, Bakris G, Greene T, Agodoa LY, et al: African American Study of Kidney Disease and Hypertension: effect of blood pressure lowering and antihypertensive drug class on progression of

hypertensive kidney disease: results from the AASK trial, *JAMA* 288:2421-31, 2003.
106. Remuzzi G, Ruggenenti P, Benigni A: Understanding the nature of renal disease progression, *Kidney Int* 51:2-15, 1997.
107. Ruggenenti P, Perna A, Remuzzi G: Retarding progression of chronic renal disease: the neglected issue of residual proteinuria, *Kidney Int* 63:2254-61, 2003.
108. Jafar TH, Schmid CH, Landa M, Giatras J, et al, for the ACE Inhibition in Progressive Renal Disease Study Group: Angiotensin-converting enzyme inhibitors and progression of nondiabetic renal disease. A meta-analysis of patient-level data, *Ann Intern Med* 135:73-87, 2001.
109. Ruggenenti P, Schieppati A, Remuzzi G: Progression, remission, regression of chronic renal diseases, *Lancet* 357:1601-8, 2001.
110. Schrier RW, Estacio RO, Esler A, Mehler P: Effects of aggressive blood pressure control in normotensive type 2 diabetic patients on albuminuria, retinopathy and strokes, *Kidney Int* 61:1086-97, 2002.
111. Brenner BM, Cooper ME, DeZeeuw D, Keane WF, et al; RENAAL Study Investigators: Effects of losartan on renal and cardiovascular outcomes in patients with type 2 diabetes and nephropathy, *N Engl J Med* 345:861-9, 2001.
112. Lewis EJ, Hunsicker LG, Raymond PB, Rohde RD, for the Collaborative Study Group: The effect of angiotensin-converting-enzyme inhibition on diabetic nephropathy, *N Engl J Med* 329:1456-62, 1993.
113. Maschio G, Alberti D, Janin G, Locatelli F, et al: Effect of angiotensin-converting-enzyme inhibitor benazepril on the progression of chronic renal insufficiency, *N Engl J Med* 334:939-45, 1996.
114. Parving HH, Andersen AR, Smidt UM, Svendsen PA: Early aggressive antihypertensive treatment reduces rate of decline in kidney function in diabetic nephropathy, *Lancet* 1:1175-9, 1983.
115. Zucchelli P, Zuccalà A, Borghi M, Fusaroli M, et al: Long-term comparison between captopril and nifedipine in the progression of renal insufficiency, *Kidney Int* 42:452-8, 1992.
116. Kamper AL, Strandgaard S, Leyssac P: Effect of enalapril on the progression of chronic renal failure: a randomized controlled trial, *Am J Hypertens* 5:423-30, 1992.
117. van Essen GG, Apperloo AJ, Rensma PL, Stegeman CA, et al: Are angiotensin converting enzyme inhibitors superior to beta blockers in retarding progressive renal function decline?, *Kidney Int Suppl* 63:S58-62, 1997.
118. Hannedouche T, Landais P, Goldfarb B, el Esper N, et al: Randomised controlled trial of enalapril and beta blockers in non-diabetic chronic renal failure, *BMJ* 309:833-7, 1994.
119. Bannister KM, Weaver A, Clarkson AR, Woodroffe AJ: Effect of angiotensin converting enzyme and calcium channel inhibition on progression of IgA nephropathy, *Contrib Nephrol* 111:184-92, 1995.
120. Ihle BU, Whitworth JA, Shahinfar S, Cnaan A, et al: Angiotensin-converting-enzyme inhibition in non-diabetic progressive renal insufficiency: a controlled double-blind trial, *Am J Kidney Dis* 27:489-95, 1996.
121. Ruggenenti P, Perna A, Gherardi G, Garini G, et al: Renoprotective properties of ACE-inhibition in non-diabetic nephropathies with non-nephrotic proteinuria, *Lancet* 354:359-64, 1999.
122. Viberti G, Mogensen CE, Groop LC, Pauls JF: Effect of captopril on progression to clinical proteinuria in patients with insulin-dependent diabetes mellitus and microalbuminuria. European Microalbuminuria Captopril Study Group, *JAMA* 271:275-9, 1994.
123. Parving HH, Hommel E, Smidt UM: Protection of kidney function and decrease in albuminuria by captopril in insulin-dependent diabetics with nephropathy, *BMJ* 297:1086-91, 1988.
124. Nakao N, Yoshimura A, Morita H, Takada M, et al: Combination treatment of angiotensin-II receptor blocker and angiotensin-converting-enzyme inhibitor in non-diabetic renal disease (COOPERATE): a randomised controlled trial, *Lancet* 361:117-24, 2003.
125. Barnett AH, Bain SC, Bouter P, Karlberg B, et al; Diabetics Exposed to Telmisartan and Enalapril Study Group: Angiotensin-receptor blockade versus converting-enzyme inhibition in type 2 diabetes and nephropathy, *N Engl J Med* 351:1952-61, 2004.
126. Casas JP, Weiliang C, Loukogeorgakis S, Vallance P, et al: Effect of inhibitors of the renin-angiotensin system and other antihypertensive drugs on renal outcomes: systematic review and meta-analysis, *Lancet* 366:2026-33, 2005.
127. Mooser V, Nussberger J, Juillerat L, Burnier M, et al: Reactive hyperreninemia is a major determinant of plasma angiotensin II during ACE inhibition, *J Cardiovasc Pharmacol* 15:276-82, 1990.
128. van den Meiracker AH, Man in 't Veld AJ, Admiraal PJ, Ritsema van Eck HJ, et al: Partial escape of angiotensin converting enzyme (ACE) inhibition during prolonged ACE inhibitor treatment: does it exist and does it affect the antihypertensive response?, *J Hypertens* 10:803-12, 1992.
129. Shiigai T, Shichiri M: Late escape from the antiproteinuric effect of ACE inhibitors in nondiabetic renal disease, *Am J Kidney Dis* 37:477-83, 2001.
130. Wilmer WA, Rovin BH, Hebert CJ, Rao SV, et al: Management of glomerular proteinuria: a commentary, *J Am Soc Nephrol* 14:3217-32, 2003.
131. Bakris GL, Weir MR: Angiotensin-converting enzyme inhibitor-associated elevations in serum creatinine: is this a cause for concern?, *Arch Intern Med* 160:685-93, 2000.
132. Van Dyck M, Proesmans W: Renoprotection by ACE inhibitors after severe hemolytic uremic syndrome, *Pediatr Nephrol* 19:688-90, 2004.
133. Ellis D, Vats A, Moritz ML, Reitz S, et al: Long-term antiproteinuric and renoprotective efficacy and safety of losartan in children with proteinuria, *J Pediatr* 143:89-97, 2003.
134. Tanaka H, Suzuki K, Nakahata T, Tsugawa K, et al: Combined therapy of enalapril and losartan attenuates histologic progression in immunoglobulin A nephropathy, *Pediatr Int* 46:576-9, 2004.
135. Marchi F, Ciriello G: Efficacy of carvedilol in mild to moderate essential hypertension and effects on microalbuminuria: a multicenter, randomized, open-label, controlled study versus atenolol, *Adv Ther* 12:212-21, 1995.
136. Fassbinder W, Quarder O, Waltz A: Treatment with carvedilol is associated with a significant reduction in microalbuminuria: a multicenter randomized study, *Int J Clin Pract* 53:519-22, 1999.
137. Doulton TW, He FJ, MacGregor FA: Systemic review of combined angiotensin-converting enzyme inhibition and angiotensin receptor blockade in hypertension, *Hypertension* 45:880-6, 2005.
138. Campbell R, Sangalli F, Perticucci E, Aros C, et al: Effects of combined ACE inhibitor and angiotensin II antagonist treatment in human chronic nephropathies, *Kidney Int* 63:1094-103, 2003.
139. MacKinnon M, Shurraw S, Akbari A, Knoll GA, et al: Combination therapy with an angiotensin receptor blocker and an ACE inhibitor in proteinuric renal disease: a systematic review of the efficacy and safety data, *Am J Kidney Dis* 48:8-20, 2006.
140. Laverman GD, Navis G, Henning RH, de Jong PE, de Zeeuw D: Dual renin-angiotensin system blockade at optimal doses for proteinuria, *Kidney Int* 62:1020-5, 2002.
141. Schmieder RE, Klingbeil AU, Fleischmann EH, Veelken R, Delles C: Additional antiproteinuric effect of ultrahigh dose candesartan: a double-blind, randomized, prospective study, *J Am Soc Nephrol* 16:3038-45, 2005.
142. Hermida RC, Diana EA, Calvo C: Administration-time-dependent effects of antihypertensive treatment on the circadian pattern of blood pressure, *Curr Opin Nephrol Hypertens* 14:453-9, 2005.
143. Svensson P, de Faire U, Sleight P, Yusuf S, Ostergren J: Comparative effects of ramipril on ambulatory and office blood pressures: a HOPE substudy, *Hypertension* 38:e28-32, 2001.
144. Hermida RC, Calvo C, Ayala DE, Lopez JE: Decrease in urinary albumin excretion associated with the normalization of nocturnal blood pressure in hypertensive subjects, *Hypertension* 46:960-8, 2005.
145. Sharples EJ, Patel N, Brown P, Stewart K, et al: Erythropoietin protects the kidney against the injury and dysfunction caused by ischemia-reperfusion, *J Am Soc Nephrol* 15:2115-24, 2004.
146. Gouva C, Nikolopoulos P, Ioannidis JP, Siamopoulos KC: Treating anemia early in renal failure patients slows the decline of renal function: a randomized controlled trial, *Kidney Int* 66:753-60, 2004.
147. Haller H, de Groot K, Bahlmann F, Elger M, Fliser D: Stem cells and progenitor cells in renal disease, *Kidney Int* 68:1932-6, 2005.

148. Dimmeler S, Aicher A, Vasa M, Mildner-Rihm C, et al: HMG-CoA reductase inhibitors (statins) increase endothelial progenitor cells via the PI 3-kinase/Akt pathway, *J Clin Invest* 108:391-397, 2001.
149. Bahlmann FH, de Groot K, Mueller O, Hertel B, et al: Stimulation of endothelial progenitor cells: a new putative therapeutic effect of angiotensin II receptor antagonists, *Hypertension* 45:526-9, 2005.
150. Mak RH: Metabolic effects of erythropoietin in patients on peritoneal dialysis, *Pediatr Nephrol* 12:660-5, 1998.
151. Mak RH: Effect of metabolic acidosis on insulin action and secretion in uremia, *Kidney Int* 54:603-7, 1998.
152. K/DOQI clinical practice guidelines for bone metabolism and disease in chronic kidney disease, *Am J Kidney Dis* 42(Suppl 3): S1-201, 2003.
153. Goren A, Stankiewicz H, Goldstein R, Drukker A: Fish oil treatment of hyperlipidemia in children and adolescents receiving renal replacement therapy, *Pediatrics* 88:265-8, 1991.
154. Holdaas H, Wanner C, Abletshauser C, Gimpelewicz C, Isaacsohn J: The effect of fluvastatin on cardiac outcomes in patients with moderate to severe renal insufficiency: a pooled analysis of double-blind, randomized trials, *Int J Cardiol* 117:64-74, 2007.
155. Wanner C, Krane V, März W, Olschewski M, et al; German Study Group for Growth Hormone Treatment in Chronic Renal Failure: Atorvastatin in patients with type 2 diabetes mellitus undergoing hemodialysis, *N Engl J Med* 353:238-48, 2005.
156. Epstein M, Campese VM: Pleiotropic effects of 3-hydroxy-3-methylglutaryl coenzyme a reductase inhibitors on renal function, *Am J Kidney Dis* 45:2-14, 2005.
157. Zoja C, Corna D, Rottoli D, Cattaneo D, et al: Effect of combining ACE inhibitor and statin in severe experimental nephropathy, *Kidney Int* 61:1635-45, 2002.
158. Sandhu S, Wiebe N, Fried LF, Tonelli M: Statins for improving renal outcomes: a meta-analysis, *J Am Soc Nephrol* 17:2006-16, 2006.
159. Tian J, Liu Y, Williams LA, de Zeeuw D: Potential role of active Vitamin D in retarding the progression of chronic kidney disease, *Nephrol Dial Transplant* 22:321-28, 2007.

CHAPTER

46 Growth and Puberty in Chronic Kidney Disease

Dieter Haffner and Richard Nissel

INTRODUCTION

Growth failure remains a challenging problem of the management of children with chronic kidney disease (CKD). Despite tremendous progress with regard to both conservative treatment and renal replacement therapy, 30% to 60% of children with end-stage renal disease (ESRD) still grow up to become stunted adults.[1-9] Growth failure markedly hampers the psychosocial integration of pediatric patients with CKD. Moreover, the degree of growth retardation is associated with the excessive mortality of children with CKD.[10,11]

There is no single cause of growth failure in children with CKD (Table 46-1). Children may have various acquired or congenital renal abnormalities that manifest during early or late childhood and that differ widely with regard to their severity and rate of progression, with various concomitant complications such as metabolic acidosis, electrolyte disturbances, and malnutrition. Furthermore, children with CKD may undergo various medical interventions and different modes of renal replacement therapy of variable timing and duration during their growth period. Hence, growth in children with CKD is not only influenced by renal dysfunction but also by specific disease-related comorbidities and treatment modalities. This review summarizes the current knowledge of the phenotype, pathophysiology and therapeutic options for growth failure in children with CKD.

CLINICAL PRESENTATION

The physiologic growth pattern can be divided into the periods of infancy, mid childhood, and puberty. Whereas during infancy growth mainly depends on nutritional intake, growth during mid childhood is driven by the somatotropic hormone axis. During puberty, growth is additionally influenced by the gonadotropic hormone axis, which stimulates growth via the increased proliferation of growth plate chondrocytes and the modulation of growth hormone (GH) secretion from the pituitary gland[12] (Figure 46-1).

Children with congenital CKD are prone to marked growth retardation during the first 2 years of life, which is followed by a rather percentile-parallel growth during mid childhood. During the last 2 to 3 prepubertal years, height velocity again decreases disproportionately, thereby resulting in further growth impairment. The onset of the pubertal growth spurt is delayed and its magnitude impaired, thus resulting in a further loss of growth potential and a reduced final height (see Figure 46-1).

Infancy

Approximately one third of total postnatal growth occurs during the first 2 years of life. Therefore, any circumstances that lead to decreased growth rates during this period result in severe growth retardation and a potentially irreversible loss of growth potential.[13-15] The decrease in mean standardized height can amount up to 0.6 standard deviation (SD) per month in infants with ESRD.[16] During recent years, the increasing acceptance of renal replacement therapy, even in multimorbid infants, has increased the challenge of achieving normal growth in this age group.

A mechanistic insight into the growth patterns of patients with CKD has been provided by the application of the infancy/childhood/puberty model of statural growth.[17] Growth failure during early life leads to a reduced standardized height by −3 SD scores at 3 years of age. Approximately one-third of this impairment apparently occurs during fetal life, and one-third occurs during the first postnatal months. Between 9 and 18 months of age, height decreases by a further 1 SD as a consequence of either a delayed onset of the subsequent childhood growth phase or a regression to the infancy phase pattern. By contrast, growth during the second and third quarters of the first postnatal year and from 18 months to 5 years of age was generally percentile parallel and thus less likely to be affected by CKD and its sequelae. It has been suggested that the growth failure during fetal life and the first postnatal months reflects metabolic and nutritional influences and that the impaired growth around the first birthday may be related to a partial insensitivity to GH.

Malnutrition in children with CKD is caused by inadequate nutritional intake and frequently by recurrent vomiting. In addition, catabolic episodes as a result of infection, loss of water and electrolytes, and renal osteodystrophy are major contributing factors to growth impairment during this period. If these disturbances are adequately controlled, severe stunting can be avoided in the majority of patients.[18-20] However, most infants with severe CKD need supplementary

TABLE 46-1 Causes of Growth Failure in Children with Chronic Kidney Disease

Genetic factors • Parent height • Gender • Syndromal disorders (with kidney involvement as a part)
Age at onset of chronic kidney disease
Residual renal function
Treatment modalities for chronic kidney disease
Energy malnutrition
Water and electrolyte disturbances
Metabolic acidosis
Renal anemia
Hormonal disturbances affecting the following: • The somatotropic hormone axis • The gonadotropic hormone axis • Parathyroid hormone and vitamin D metabolism/action (renal osteodystrophy) • Other hormones

feeding to obtain adequate nutrient, water, and electrolyte intake.[19]

Mid Childhood

Patients with congenital CKD usually show percentile parallel growth during the mid-childhood years. Growth is closely correlated with the degree of renal dysfunction during this period. Although there is no critical threshold for the glomerular filtration rate (GFR), growth patterns are typically stable if the GFR remains above 25 ml/min/1.73 m^2, and they tend to diverge from the percentiles if the GFR falls below this level.[21,22] A mean cumulative loss of 6 cm from the predicted final height was observed in children with a mean GFR below 25 ml/min/1.73 m^2 between early childhood and the age of 10 years.[21] Sequelae of CKD such as anemia, metabolic acidosis, and malnutrition seem to be less important during mid childhood.

It must be questioned whether the percentile-parallel growth pattern below the third percentile in stunted children with CKD during the mid-childhood period reflects normal growth. Children who receive kidney allografts and steroid-free immunosuppression exhibit significant catchup growth that is compatible with the notion of the continued suppression of an intrinsic catch-up growth potential in the uremic state.[23,24]

Conflicting information has been provided with respect to segmental growth in patients with CKD. de Graaff and colleagues[25] investigated body proportions in 37 children with CKD. To assess body proportions, the various body segments were related to height and expressed as shape values.[25] All children had normal shape values, which indicated normal body proportions. By contrast, a prospective detailed and standardized evaluation of body morphology in 190 boys with CKD noted age-related disproportionate growth patterns in children with a long-term history of CKD and renal replacement therapy.[26] Growth impairment and disproportionality were most obvious during early childhood. Sitting height was mostly preserved, whereas the growth of the legs and arms was most severely affected. The discrepant findings in the two studies may be related to methodologic differences and stresses the need for further study of this issue.

Pubertal Development and Pubertal Growth

Pubertal Development

The onset of the clinical signs of puberty as well as the start of the pubertal growth spurt in children with CKD stage V appears to be delayed by approximately 2 years.[27] Unfortunately, the determination of bone age is only a crude marker to estimate the onset of puberty in these children. Indeed, the distribution of bone age at pubertal onset varies at least as much as the distribution of chronologic age in these patients. At least 50% of adolescents with ESRD show delayed onset of puberty and achieve the pubertal milestones later in life than their healthy peers.[28] Pubertal onset is also delayed in adolescents after renal transplantation (RTx). In the Cooperative Study for Pubertal Development in Chronic Renal Failure, the onset of puberty was globally delayed by 2 to 2.5 years.[29] The start of genital growth (Tanner stage G2) was delayed by 1.8 years in boys on dialysis and by 2.5 years in boys who had undergone transplant procedures. Full genital maturation was achieved with a delay of 2.2 and 3.2 years in these groups, respectively. Hence, the progression through the pubertal stages appears to be normal or only slightly slowed. Menarche occurs in almost half of the girls treated by dialysis or transplantation beyond the upper limit of the normal age range (i.e., 15 years).[2] Despite the presentation of pubertal stage IV or V, a substantial proportion of dialysis patients present with permanently impaired reproductive function. Autopsy studies in uremic boys revealed germ cell depletion in the testicular tubules.[30] In contrast with adult dialysis patients, semen quality is severely affected, and spermatogenesis does not improve after RTx in patients exposed to uremia before or during adolescence, which is the crucial period for spermatogenesis.[31,32] In adult women on hemodialysis, pathologic changes of the endometrium are frequently seen.[33] In addition, several studies revealed reduced sperm cell count, erectile dysfunction, decreased libido, and decreased fertility in uremic patients on dialysis or after RTx.[34] Consequently, the frequency of conception is decreased among adolescents and women with ESRD. In children of female patients with CKD who manage to become pregnant, intrauterine growth retardation and reduced birth weight are frequent.[35]

Pubertal Growth

Total height gain during the pubertal growth spurt is subnormal in patients with CKD.[1,3,6,14,29,36,37] In 29 patients with CKD who attained ESRD before the age of 15 years, the pubertal growth spurt started with a mean delay of 2.5 years.[29] The degree of delay was related to the duration of uremia. Although an acceleration of height velocity comparable with that seen in healthy adolescents was observed, the mean height velocity at the start of the pubertal growth spurt was reduced, and its duration was shortened by approximately 1.5 years. Consequently, total pubertal height in children with ESRD is reduced by 50% as compared with healthy,

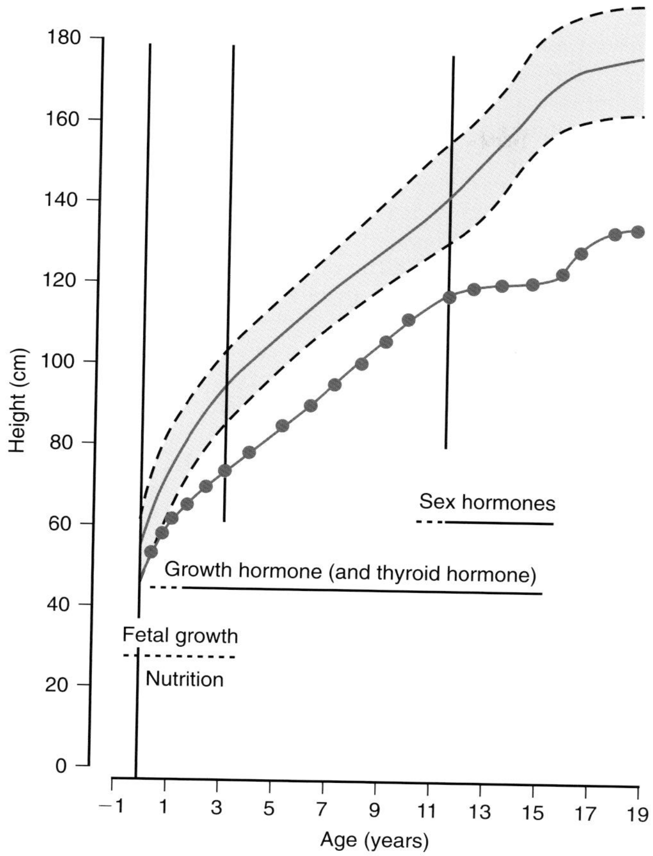

Figure 46-1 Typical growth pattern in congenital chronic renal failure. Relative loss during the nutrient-dependent infantile and gonadal hormone-dependent puberty phases and percentile-parallel growth during the mainly growth-hormone-dependent growth period during mid childhood are shown. The shaded area represents the normal range (3rd to 97th percentiles). (Reproduced from Mehls O, Schaefer F: Endocrine, metabolic and growth disorders—patterns of growth and maturation in chronic renal failure—impact of developmental stage. In Holliday MA, Barratt TM, Avner ED, editors: *Pediatric nephrology*, Baltimore, 1994, Williams & Wilkins, pp 1260-63.)

late-maturing controls. Therefore, a further loss of standardized height of about 1 SD can usually be expected in patients with ESRD during puberty.

Final Height and Height Prediction

Reduced adult heights have been reported in about 30% to 50% of patients with CKD, although a trend for improved final heights was observed during the past decade.[1-7,38-43] Mean final height in patients with CKD stage III to V ranged between −0.6 and −3.5 SD. In general, patients receiving RTx or additional treatment with recombinant human GH (rhGH) showed improved mean levels of final height as compared with patients receiving long-term dialysis or without concomitant rhGH therapy.[8] The age at onset of ESRD (positive effect), the duration of chronic renal failure (negative effect), male gender (negative effect), and the presence of congenital nephropathies (negative effect) are the most relevant predictors of final height. Among the different renal disease entities, patients with nephropathic cystinosis or primary hyperoxaluria show the most markedly compromised final heights.[44,45]

The applicability of adult height prediction methods is a question of special interest in children with CKD. In several studies, a mean overprediction of eventual final height of 3 to 10 cm has been reported.[4,6,8] The overprediction of final height in children with CKD is thought to be the result of unpredictable changes in treatment modalities and of renal osteodystrophy compromising the assessment of skeletal maturation. No significant relationship between the degree of bone age delay at the time of transplantation or the start of the pubertal growth spurt with eventual catch-up growth was observed.[6] This is probably caused by the apparent dissociation between bone maturation and pubertal growth in patients who have undergone transplantation, which is thought to be related to endocrine alterations and to the growth-suppressing effects of glucocorticoid treatment.[4,29,46]

CAUSES OF GROWTH FAILURE IN CHRONIC KIDNEY DISEASE

Underlying Renal Disease

Hypoplastic and Dysplastic Nephropathies

Congenital renal dysplasia or hypoplasia with or without urinary tract obstruction is the most common cause of ESRD during infancy and childhood. Renal dysplasia is often associated with electrolyte and water losses, and both factors may contribute to growth failure in these patients. Although the progression of chronic renal failure differs widely, children with renal dysplasia or hypoplasia usually show a constant decline in renal function over time. For the care of these patients, it is important to compensate water and electrolyte losses. In addition, the appropriate treatment of concomitant urinary tract infections and hypertension is indicated. Pharmacologic renoprotective therapy with renin-angiotensin system antagonists may slow the progression of renal failure and thereby have a positive long-term effect on growth in these children.[47]

Glomerulopathies

In children with glomerulopathies, growth rates may even decline in cases of rather mild renal insufficiency.[48] The nephrotic state per se and glucocorticoid treatment are known risk factors for further growth delay in these patients. Prolonged high corticosteroid doses leads to severe growth failure. Although partial catch-up growth can be seen after the cessation of glucocorticoid treatment, this is usually restricted to young (prepubertal) patients.[49-52] The congenital nephrotic syndrome is usually associated with severe stunting during the first months of life. This may even be the case in patients with preserved renal function (e.g., congenital nephrotic syndrome of the Finnish type), and it seems to result from persistent edema, recurrent infections, losses of peptide and protein-bound hormones, and protein-calorie malnutrition.[53] In Finnish-type nephrotic syndrome, adequate nutritional support is vital, and bilateral nephrectomy and the initiation of peritoneal dialysis may be necessary to stabilize growth. In other types of congenital nephrotic syndrome, unilateral nephrectomy and treatment with prostaglandin synthesis inhibitors and renin-angiotensin system antagonists can reduce proteinuria and thereby stabilize growth and the overall clinical condition.[54,55]

Tubular and Interstitial Nephropathies

Tubular dysfunction characterized by losses of electrolytes, bicarbonate, and water can lead to severe growth failure, even in the presence of normal glomerular function. The growth-suppressive effects of isolated tubular defects are illustrated by the severe growth failure that is typically seen in patients with renal tubular acidosis, Bartter syndrome, nephrogenic diabetes insipidus, and idiopathic hypercalciuria.[56-61] Early and consequent supplementation of electrolyte, water, and bicarbonate losses prevents growth failure or results in catch-up growth in these patients. The most severe growth failure usually occurs in patients with complex tubular disorders such as idiopathic Fanconi syndrome.[62] In these patients, only partial catch-up growth can usually be achieved, even with vigorous water and electrolyte supplementation.

Systemic metabolic disorders that result in complex tubular dysfunction, the progressive loss of renal function, and the involvement of other vital organs (e.g., liver, bone, brain) usually lead to severe growth failure.[63,64]

In children with nephropathic cystinosis, growth failure occurs as early as infancy, when glomerular function is typically not yet compromised. Progressive growth failure is further sustained by the generalized deposition of cystine crystals altering the function of the growth plate, the bone marrow, the hypothalamus, and the pituitary and thyroid glands. The early initiation of treatment with cystine-depleting agents (cysteamine) results in an improvement of growth rates and at least a delay of the development of chronic renal failure.[65]

In patients with primary hyperoxaluria, supplementary treatment with citrate and pyridoxine can delay the progression of renal failure and possibly improve longitudinal growth.[64] In patients with systemic oxalosis, combined liver and kidney transplantation is a curative option; however, real catch-up growth after combined transplantation is rarely observed, even in prepubertal patients with oxalosis patients.[45]

In patients with chronic or recurrent interstitial nephropathies, the development of growth failure is rare and usually only of mild degree. Recurrent urinary tract infection as a result of bilateral vesicoureteric reflux may lead to moderate growth retardation. Antireflux surgery and antibiotic prophylaxis have been reported to induce catch-up growth in these patients.[66,67]

Protein-Calorie Malnutrition

Nutritional imbalances—particularly protein-energy malnutrition—are frequently seen in children with CKD. Infants and young children are especially vulnerable to malnutrition as a result of low nutritional stores and high energy demands, which are in turn necessary to allow high growth rates in this age group. Malnutrition is a crucial clinical issue, because it is significantly associated with increased mortality in children with CKD.[10,11] Recently, the term *malnutrition-inflammation complex syndrome (MICS)* has been coined to describe the association between chronic inflammation and malnutrition in children and adults receiving dialysis treatment.[68] Possible causes of MICS include comorbid illnesses, oxidative and carbonyl stress, nutrient loss through dialysis, anorexia, low nutrient intake, uremic toxins, cytokine induction by exposure to bioincompatible dialysis materials, decreased clearance of inflammatory cytokines, volume overload, and other dialysis-related factors. MICS is considered to be the main cause of erythropoietin hyporesponsiveness, of the high rate of cardiovascular atherosclerotic disease, of a decreased quality of life, and of increased mortality and hospitalization rates among dialysis patients. However, there is no consensus about how to determine the degree of severity of MICS or how to manage it. Anorexia manifests early during the course of renal failure, and it usually progresses with declining renal function.[22] In addition, protein synthesis is decreased in patients with uremia, and catabolism is increased. At any given protein intake, the conversion of dietary protein to body protein is diminished in uremic as compared with pair-fed control animals.[69] In patients with CKD, spontaneous energy intake is correlated with growth rates if it is less than 80% of the recommended dietary allowance.[70,71] However, a further augmentation of energy above this level results in increasing obesity rather than the additional stimulation of longitudinal growth.[70-73]

Metabolic Acidosis

With the progression of renal failure, defects develop in the homeostatic function of the kidney that is responsible for the maintenance of external acid–base balance. Metabolic acidosis usually occurs when the GFR is below 50% of normal. However, this is markedly influenced by nutritional intake (protein and acid load), catabolism, and alterations in electrolyte balance. Metabolic acidosis is associated with several metabolic and endocrine consequences that are thought to contribute to uremic growth failure. The presence of metabolic acidosis is significantly associated with decreased longitudinal growth and increased protein breakdown in children with CKD[74-77] (Figure 46-2). In experimental uremia, meta-

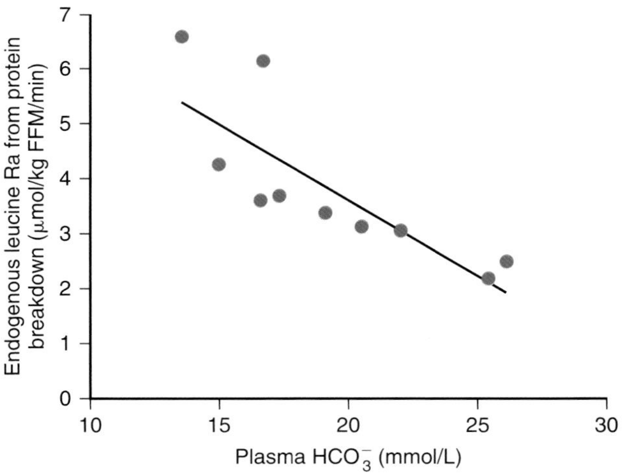

Figure 46-2 Relationship between plasma bicarbonate and the endogenous leucine rate of appearance (i.e., whole-body protein breakdown) in a population comprised of children with chronic renal failure ($r^2 = 0.65$; $p < 0.01$). (Reproduced from Boirie Y, Broyer M, Gagnadoux MF, Niaudet P, Bresson JL: Alterations of protein metabolism by metabolic acidosis in children with chronic renal failure, *Kidney Int* 58:236-41, 2000.)

bolic acidosis results in increased glucocorticoid production, increased protein degradation, and profound effects on the somatotropic hormone axis. The latter is characterized by the downregulation of spontaneous GH secretion of the pituitary gland, decreased expression of the GH-receptor and the insulin-like growth factor I (IGF-I) receptor in various target organs, and decreased IGF-I serum concentrations.[78-80] Hence, metabolic acidosis induces a state of GH insensitivity that further contributes to impaired longitudinal growth in patients with CKD.

Disturbances of Water and Electrolyte Metabolism

Children with congenital renal abnormalities often show losses of water and electrolytes. Although the relationship between salt loss and growth failure has not been formally proven in children with CKD, children with isolated tubular disorders that result in urinary salt losses show severe growth retardation, which can be at least partly resolved by adequate sodium chloride supplementation. The same applies to patients with a reduced chloride diet or with familial chloride diarrhea.[81] In rats, sodium depletion leads to diminished protein synthesis and the impairment of longitudinal growth.[82,83] Polyuria may also aggravate growth retardation. Again, the finding of growth impairment in patients with diabetes insipidus supports the concept that polyuria may also contribute to growth failure in patients with CKD.

Renal Osteodystrophy

It is widely accepted that skeletal deformities caused by renal osteodystrophy contribute to uremic growth failure.[84] Pronounced secondary hyperparathyroidism can interfere with longitudinal growth by the destruction of the growth plate architecture, epiphyseal displacement, and metaphyseal fractures. Severe destruction of the metaphyseal bone architecture may result in complete growth arrest. Treatment with 1,25-dihydroxyvitamin D_3 improves growth in uremic rats.[85] However, no consistent improvement of longitudinal growth could be demonstrated in children with CKD receiving 1,25-dihydroxyvitamin D_3.[86-88]

It is not clear to what extent the degree of secondary hyperparathyroidism contributes to uremic growth failure. Parathyroid hormone (PTH) is an anabolic hormone that stimulates the proliferation and differentiation of growth plate chondrocytes. This is at least partly mediated by the PTH-related stimulation of local IGF-I synthesis.[46] Furthermore, PTH stimulates the expression of the vitamin D receptor in growth plate chondrocytes. However, PTH resistance occurs in uremic bones and growth plates.[89] Low bone turnover in children with CKD and in uremic animals that is associated with low PTH levels results in diminished longitudinal growth.[90] Interestingly, longitudinal growth in prepubertal patients with CKD receiving conservative treatment as well as in patients on dialysis was found to correlate with the degree of secondary hyperparathyroidism.[90,91] Alternatively, the excessive secretion of PTH can lead to the destruction of the growth plate architecture and complete growth arrest in patients with CKD. Therefore, both low bone turnover (i.e., low PTH levels) and high bone turnover (i.e., secondary hyperparathyroidism) may contribute to growth impairment in patients with CKD. A putative positive effect of increased PTH levels on longitudinal growth must be counterbalanced with the clinical consequences of longstanding hyperparathyroidism (i.e., recurrent episodes of hypercalcemia and the increased risk for ectopic calcifications).[92]

Anemia

Longstanding anemia in patients with CKD has profound systemic consequences, including anorexia and catabolism caused by altered energy turnover and multiple system dysfunctions. The retardation of growth and development is a hallmark of untreated chronic anemias of nonrenal origin (e.g., thalassemia major). Theoretically, anemia may interfere with growth via various mechanisms, such as poor appetite, intercurrent infections, cardiac complications, and severely reduced oxygen supply to cartilage. The advent of recombinant human erythropoietin during the late 1980s permitted researchers to study the effects of anemia correction on longitudinal growth in patients with CKD. The partial correction of anemia in children with CKD leads to improved exercise capacity and a decreased heart rate and resting oxygen consumption level.[93,94] Although short-term stimulatory effects of erythropoietin treatment on longitudinal growth have been reported anecdotally, no persistent catch-up growth could be demonstrated in several multicenter clinical trials.[94-97]

Endocrine Changes

Uremia interferes with the metabolism and with the regulation of various peptide hormones. This leads to inappropriate concentrations of circulating hormones and/or altered hormone action on target tissues. Distinct alterations of the somatotropic and gonadotropic hormone axes have been identified that are believed to contribute importantly to uremic growth failure.

Gonadotropic Hormone Axis

Gonadal Hormones Adolescents and adults with ESRD usually show low or low-normal total and free testosterone (T) and dihydrotestosterone (DHT) plasma concentrations.[98-102] Decreased T and DHT levels are thought to be caused by decreased synthesis, increased metabolic clearance rate, or both.[103,104] The impaired conversion of T to DHT as a result of reduced 5α-reductase activity has been reported.[105] Because the conversion of T to DHT is essential for the development of secondary sexual characteristics in boys, this finding may at least partly explain the delayed pubertal development that is seen in boys with advanced renal failure.

Concentrations of sex hormone binding protein are higher and concentrations of unbound T are lower than those seen in healthy children,[101] possibly as a result of the decreased clearance of the sex hormone binding protein in uremia.[99] In addition, the plasma concentrations of inhibin (a gonadotropin feedback inhibitor produced by Sertoli cells) are increased in pubertal boys with CKD.[106]

Plasma estradiol levels tend to be decreased in proportion with GFR reduction in women with preterminal chronic renal failure.[107] Similarly, adolescent girls show low-normal or decreased estradiol levels for their pubertal ages.[108,109]

Gonadotropins Increased luteinizing hormone (LH) and follicle-stimulating hormone plasma concentrations have been found in adults and adolescents with CKD.[99,100,107,108,110] The combination of increased gonadotropins and decreased or low-normal gonadal hormone levels suggests a state of compensated hypergonadotropic hypogonadism in uremia.[99] However, the degree of hypergonadotropism in CKD is usually inadequate relative to the degree of hypogonadism, which is compatible with an additional defect of pituitary gonadotropin release. The analysis of spontaneous pulsatile LH secretion has provided new insights into the pathophysiology of the gonadotropic hormone axis in uremia.[111] In both patients with CKD and the uremic rat model, the elevation of mean plasma LH levels is entirely the result of decreased renal metabolic clearance.[112,113] The plasma half-life of LH is inversely correlated with residual renal function. By contrast, the actual LH secretion was found to have decreased by approximately 70% both in patients with CKD and in the rat model.[112,114] After RTx, LH pulsatility normalizes.[112] Because the onset of puberty is heralded by the appearance of nocturnal LH secretion episodes, the observed defective pulsatile LH release in cases of uremia suggests that the delayed pubertal onset in patients with CKD is caused by a primary hypothalamic defect. Indeed, experimental evidence suggests the reduced release of hypothalamic gonadotropin-releasing hormone (GnRH) into the hypophyseal portal circulation.[113,115] The altered function of the GnRH pulse generator may be related to the increased tone of the inhibitory neurotransmitter gamma-aminobutyric acid in the hypothalamic medial preoptic area.[116] Uremic serum inhibits gonadotropin release in vitro, thus pointing to a circulating inhibitor of GnRH neuron activity.[117]

In addition to the quantitative alterations of gonadotropin release, the biologic quality of circulating gonadotropins is also affected in uremia. In pubertal and adult patients with CKD, the ratio of bioactive to immunoreactive plasma LH is diminished, thereby suggesting a shift toward bioinactive isoforms as a result of the impaired glycosylation of the imbalanced accumulation of less-active isoforms.[110,112,115,118]

In summary, the insufficient activation of the hypothalamic GnRH pulse generator, which is likely mediated via circulating inhibitors, appears to be the key abnormality underlying delayed puberty and altered sexual functions in patients with CKD. The neuroendocrine pathology resembles the regression of the gonadotropic hormone axis to the prepubertal state in patients with anorexia nervosa.

Somatotropic Hormone Axis

Growth Hormone Secretion and Metabolism Fasting GH concentrations are normal or even increased in pediatric and adult patients with CKD, depending on the degree of renal failure.[119] GH is a 22-kilodalton protein that is almost freely filtered by the glomerulus (sieving coefficient, ~0.82) and thereby ultimately cleared from the circulation.[120] Indeed, the steady-state infusion of GH in humans has shown that the metabolic clearance rate of GH is linearly correlated with the GFR and reduced by approximately 50% in patients with ESRD.[121,122]

The deconvolution analysis of endogenous GH secretion has revealed that the increase in GH plasma levels is not caused by increased GH release but rather by an increased plasma half-life of the hormone. However, GH secretion rates in children and adolescents with CKD vary widely. Whereas a high-normal endogenous GH secretion rate was observed in prepubertal patients with ESRD, GH secretion was clearly decreased in pubertal patients with CKD, thereby suggesting the deficient stimulation of GH release by gonadal steroids during puberty.[123-125] The variability of GH secretion in patients with CKD may also be the result of differences in nutritional intake and the degree of metabolic acidosis. Both factors significantly influence GH secretion in both rodents and humans.[78]

Growth Hormone Receptor and Growth Hormone Signaling GH-induced hepatic IGF-I synthesis is significantly reduced in uremic animals.[126,127] In principle, diminished GH-induced IGF-I synthesis may be the result of decreased GH receptor expression and/or a postreceptor signaling defect.

In humans, levels of circulating GH binding protein (GHBP) are thought to reflect the GH receptor expression, because GHBP is produced by the partial proteolytic cleavage of the extracellular receptor domain. GHBP plasma levels are decreased in children and adults with CKD in relation to residual renal function.[128,129] Reduced hepatic GH receptor mRNA and growth plate receptor protein levels have been reported in some but not all studies in uremic animals.[126,127,130-133] Although several studies found reduced GH receptor gene expression, unaltered, hepatic GH receptor protein expression and binding activity were found despite subnormal mRNA expression when controlling for uremia-associated anorexia by pair feeding.[126] By contrast, reduced GH receptor protein abundance was found in the growth plate cartilage of uremic animals as compared with pair-fed, sham-operated animals.[133] These discrepancies may be related to differences in the degree of renal insufficiency or nutritional state or in the presence of metabolic acidosis in the rat model of CKD.

Another mechanism of GH resistance in uremia is the presence of a postreceptor GH signaling defect. GH activates several signaling pathways via the Janus kinase (JK)/signal transducer and activator of transcription (STAT) pathway[134] (Figure 46-3). The binding of GH to its receptor activates JAK2, a receptor-associated tyrosine kinase that phosphorylates the GH receptor and several proteins of the STAT family. Phosphorylated STATs form dimers that enter the nucleus, where they activate or repress their target genes, such as IGF-I and some suppressors of cytokine signaling (SOCS). The latter are GH-induced negative feedback regulators that dephosphorylate the activated signaling proteins. In chronically uremic rats, the GH-induced phosphorylation of JAK2 and the downstream molecules STAT5, STAT3, and STAT1 are diminished, and the nuclear accumulation of phosphorylated STATs is reduced.[126] This defect is possibly caused by the exaggerated expression of suppressors of GH signaling (i.e., SOCS2 and SOCS3). Because these regulatory proteins are coinduced by inflammatory cytokines, it has been suggested that GH resistance in uremia is at least partly related to a microinflammatory state.

Insulin-Like Growth Factor Plasma Binding and Tissue Action There is strong evidence that insensitivity to IGF-I

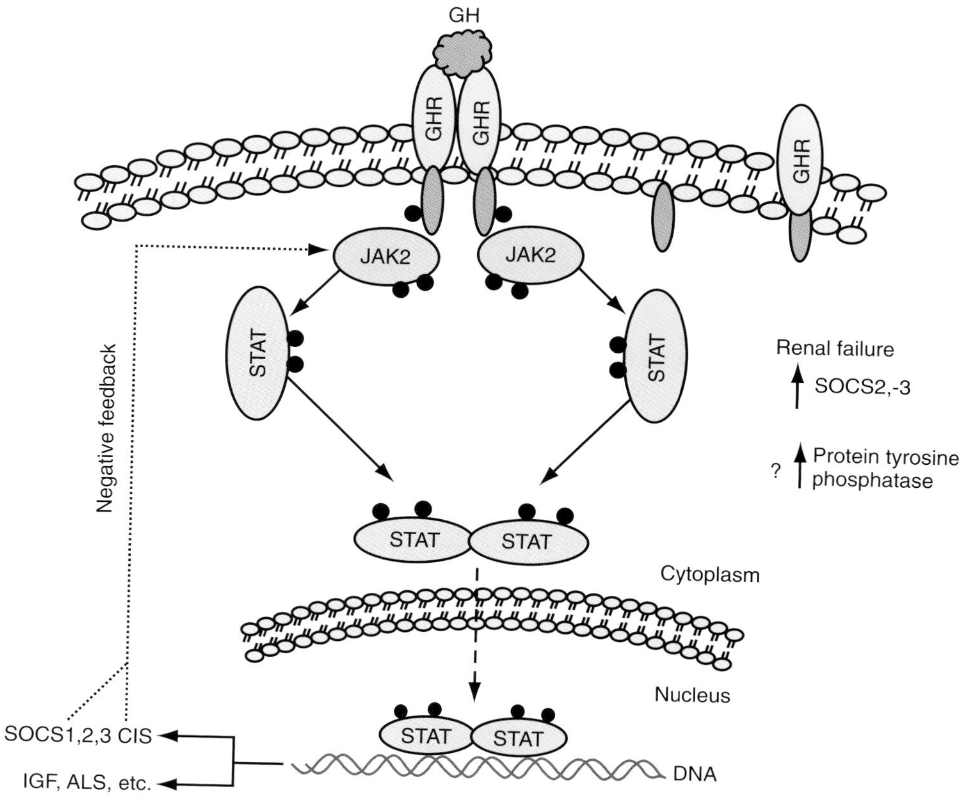

Figure 46-3 Growth hormone (GH)-mediated JAK2/STAT signal transduction. GH activates several signaling pathways via Janus kinase2 (JAK2), including the JAK/STAT (signal transducer and activator of transcription) pathway. The binding of GH to its receptor (GHR) activates JAK2, which then self-phosphorylates, and this is followed by phosphorylation of the GHR and subsequently STATs 1a, 3, 5a, and 5b, which are members of a larger family of cytoplasmic transcription factors. These phosphorylated STATs form dimers that enter the nucleus, where they bind to specific DNA sequences and activate their target genes, including insulin-like growth factor-1 (IGF-1) and some suppressors of cytokine signaling (SOCS). The deletion of STAT5 expression leads to retarded body growth, and STAT5b is required for GH-mediated IGF-1 gene expression. In renal failure, the phosphorylation of JAK2 and the downstream signaling molecules STAT5, STAT3, and STAT1 are impaired, as are the nuclear levels of phosphorylated STAT proteins. This important cause of uremic GH resistance may result in part from the upregulation of suppressors of cytokine signaling (SOCS) 2 and 3 expression with suppressed GH signaling and also from increased protein tyrosine phosphatase activity, with enhanced dephosphorylation and the deactivation of the signaling proteins. (Reproduced with permission of Rabkin R, Sun DF, Chen Y, Tan J, Schaefer F: Growth hormone resistance in uremia, a role for impaired JAK/STAT signaling, *Pediatr Nephrol* 20:313-18, 2005.)

is an important cause of GH resistance in uremia.[135-139] According to the dual effector theory, the stimulatory effects of GH on longitudinal growth are mediated by the stimulation of both the systemic (endocrine mechanism) and the local (paracrine mechanism) synthesis of somatomedins (i.e., IGF-I and IGF-II) in target organs (e.g., liver, muscle, epiphyseal chondrocytes).[140] Serum concentrations of IGF-I and IGF-II in children with CKD are usually within the normal range, whereas in patients with ESRD plasma IGF-I is slightly reduced and IGF-II is mildly increased.[141] Although total immunoreactive IGF in uremic serum is unaltered, the levels of free (biologically active) IGF-I are reduced, and somatomedin bioactivity is diminished in relation to the degree of renal failure.[142,143] The discrepancy of normal immunoreactivity but reduced bioactivity of IGF-I points to circulating IGF inhibitors.[143] Although a low-molecular-weight inhibitor protein (~1 kDa) in uremic serum has been reported, the prevailing inhibitory effect of uremic serum is the result of an excess of high-affinity IGF binding proteins (IGFBPs). Six IGFBPs (1 through 6) have been reported, representing more than 96% of total IGF binding within the circulation. IGFBPs are eliminated by the kidney. In uremic children, plasma concentrations of IGFBP-1, -2, -4, and -6 are elevated and inversely correlated with residual renal function[141,144-149] (Figure 46-4). Whereas the concentration of immunoreactive IGFBP-5 is not altered in uremic serum, the majority of IGFBP-5 is fragmented.[149] Likewise, ligand blotting revealed that the elevation of immunoreactive IGFBP-3 is the result of the accumulation of low-molecular-weight fragments (14 to 19 kDa), whereas intact IGFBP-3 (38 to 41 kDa) is even markedly diminished.[150,151] IGFBP-1, -2, and -6 inhibit IGF bioactivity in vitro.[152] Taken together, the molar excess of IGFBPs as compared with IGFs is approximately 25% in healthy children, 150% in children with CKD, and 200% in children with ESRD.[153] Reduced IGF bioactivity can be returned to normal by removing unsaturated IGFBP.[143] In subtotally nephrectomized rats, elevated IGFBP-1 and -2 levels are the result of a combination of reduced renal metabolic clearance and increased hepatic synthesis.[154] Notably, the degree of growth retardation in children with CKD was

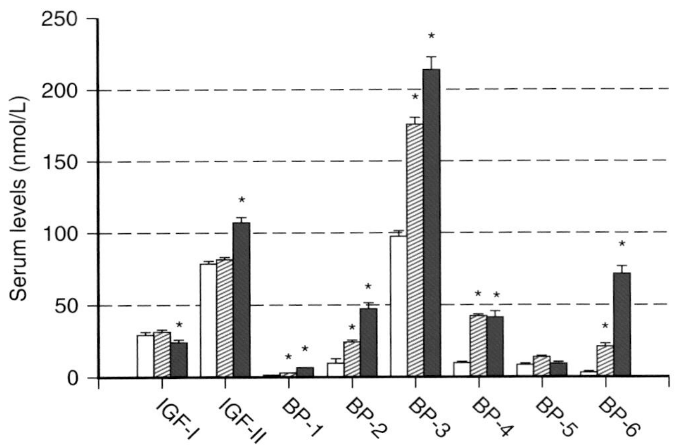

Figure 46-4 Comparison of the molar serum concentrations of insulin-like growth factors (IGFs) and IGF binding proteins (IGFBPs) in children with preterminal chronic renal failure *(hatched bars)* and children with end stage renal disease *(filled bars)*. The respective mean molar concentration in normal age-matched children is given in open bars for comparison. Data are given as the mean plus the standard error of the mean. *Significant ($p < 0.05$ by analysis of variance) versus control. (Reproduced from Ulinski T, Mohan S, Kiepe D, et al: Serum insulin-like growth factor binding protein (IGFBP)-4 and IGFBP-5 in children with chronic renal failure: relationship to growth and glomerular filtration rate. The European Study Group for Nutritional Treatment of Chronic Renal Failure in Childhood. German Study Group for Growth Hormone Treatment in Chronic Renal Failure, *Pediatr Nephrol* 14:589-97, 2000.)

inversely correlated with IGFBP-1, -2, and -4 serum concentrations.[135,141,149] In summary, these data are in favor of the concepts that serum IGFBPs increase with declining renal function in patients with CKD and that the greater excess of IGFBPs in patients with ESRD as compared with patients with pre-end-stage CKD contributes to the higher degree of growth failure and reduced response to rhGH therapy in these children.

In addition to the uremia-related disturbances of IGF plasma binding proteins, a postreceptor defect of IGF-I signaling may also contribute to IGF-I resistance. In chronically uremic rats, exogenous IGF-I did not translate into the increased synthesis of muscle protein, whereas the number of IGF-I receptors was significantly increased, and the IGF-I-induced receptor autophosphorylation and tyrosine kinase activity were reduced.[136] However, no abnormality in IGF-I-receptor expression, receptor autophosphorylation, or tyrosine kinase activity was identified, thereby suggesting a more distal defect of IGF-I signaling in uremia.[155]

In summary, the markedly deficient IGF-I synthesis and the modest elevation of GH levels as a result of decreased metabolic clearance in the presence of increased IGF plasma-binding capacity strongly supports the concept of a multilevel homeostatic failure of the GH/IGF-I system in uremia.

Corticosteroid Treatment

Long-term glucocorticoid treatment in patients after RTx leads to diminished longitudinal growth by the impairment of the somatotropic hormone axis on various levels. High-dose glucocorticoid treatment suppresses the pulsatile GH release of the pituitary gland, mainly by a reduction of the amplitude.[102,156] The physiologic increase in GH secretion during puberty is reduced in allograft recipients receiving glucocorticoid treatment, and the association between sex steroid plasma concentrations and GH release observed in healthy adolescents is blunted in these patients.[102] Studies in humans and animals have revealed that these changes are mainly the result of increased hypothalamic somatostatin release.[157] In addition to the reduced GH release, corticosteroids repress the GH receptor mRNA and protein in animals and most likely also in humans.[158,159] Consequently, hepatic IGF-I mRNA levels are reduced in animals receiving glucocorticoids. However, plasma concentrations of IGF-I in patients treated with glucocorticoids are normal or only slightly reduced. In individual children receiving corticosteroid treatment, impaired longitudinal growth occurs despite normal GH secretion and plasma IGF-I levels, which suggests an insensitivity to GH and IGF-I on the level of the growth plate. Indeed, a direct growth-inhibiting effect of dexamethasone on the growth plate was shown by local injection in rabbits.[160] In cultured growth plate chondrocytes, glucocorticoids decrease DNA synthesis and cell proliferation in a dose-dependent fashion that is associated with the reduced expression of the GH receptor and diminished paracrine IGF-I synthesis.[161-163] In addition, pharmacologic doses of glucocorticoids also impair the proliferative response to the calciotropic hormones calcitriol and PTH.[46] This is at least partly related to a diminished release of paracrine IGF-I secretion by these hormones. IGF-I modulates its own activity in cultured rat growth plate chondrocytes by the synthesis of both inhibitory (IGFBP-3) and stimulatory (IGFBP-5) binding proteins.[164,165] This modulation is modified by glucocorticoid treatment.[163] Therefore, glucocorticoid treatment not only interferes with the somatotropic hormone axis with respect to GH secretion and GH/IGF-I receptor signaling but also by the modulation of paracrine IGF-I synthesis and binding by IGF-binding proteins.

TREATMENT OF GROWTH FAILURE IN CHRONIC KIDNEY DISEASE

General Measures

In infants and young children with CKD, the most important measure for avoiding uremic growth failure is the provision of adequate caloric intake. This often necessitates supplementary feeding via nasogastric tube or gastrostomy. During later childhood, adequate nutrition is a permissive factor for growth, but catch-up growth can only rarely be provided by dietary manipulations alone.[166] In general, the caloric intake target should be to provide 80% to 100% of the recommended daily allowance (RDA) of healthy children.[70,71,167] To account for the sometimes extreme degree of stunting, the caloric intake should be related to the patient's "height age" rather than to his or her chronologic age. Increasing caloric intake in patients with CKD above 100% of the RDA does not induce catchup growth but rather results in obesity and may thereby negatively contribute to long-term cardiovascular morbidity in these patients.[70-73] Protein intake should be 100% of the RDA. In patients on peritoneal dialysis, a slightly higher intake (+0.2 g/kg/day) is recommended to compensate for dialytic protein losses. Higher protein intake should be avoided because, despite many attempts, anabolizing or growth-promoting effects of high-protein diets have neither been demonstrated in animal models nor in children with CKD; on the contrary, high-protein diets may be detrimental by aggravating metabolic acidosis and augmenting the dietary phosphorus load.

Metabolic acidosis should be vigorously treated by alkaline supplementation. In addition, the supplementation of water and electrolytes is essential for patients presenting with polyuria and/or salt-losing nephropathies.[167-169] The supplementation of sodium chloride is also important for young children on peritoneal dialysis, because significant amounts of sodium chloride (i.e., 2 to 5 mmol/kg body weight) may be eliminated via ultrafiltration.

Dialysis

Although dialysis treatment partly corrects the uremic state, longitudinal growth is usually not improved by the institution of dialysis.[170-172] In general, a gradual loss of standardized height must be expected in children and adolescents treated with long-term peritoneal or hemodialysis.[173,174] Losses of up to 1 SD per year have been reported in dialyzed infants.[16] High-flux hemodialysis and hemofiltration techniques do not result in better growth rates. Residual renal function seems to be a better predictor of longitudinal growth than dialytic clearance.[175,176] The same holds true for continuous peritoneal dialysis (i.e., continuous cycling peritoneal dialysis or automated peritoneal dialysis).[175,176] Notably, a high peritoneal transporter status is associated with subnormal longitudinal growth in children on chronic peritoneal dialysis.[175] A high transporter status, which is associated with increased morbidity and mortality in adults, is thought to be an indicator of microinflammation, a condition that may suppress growth by causing GH resistance (described previously).[177] Recently, evidence was obtained that intensified dialysis as applied by prolonged thrice weekly or short daily hemodialysis sessions may induce catch-up growth.[178,179] However, this concept has to be confirmed in prospective clinical trials.

Transplantation

Because many of the metabolic and endocrine disorders contributing to uremic growth failure are resolved by RTx, catch-up growth should be expected in children who are growth retarded at the time of RTx. However, growth rates in children after RTx vary widely, from progressive stunting to impressive catch-up growth that results in normal adult height.[6,37,39,41-43,180-187] The main factors that influence growth after RTx are age, impairment of renal function, and glucocorticoid dosage; all these factors are inversely associated with longitudinal growth after RTx. Even low-dose glucocorticoid treatment (<4 mg/m^2/day) results in growth suppression in children after RTx. However, a relationship between glucocorticoid dosage and posttransplant growth was not unanimously observed,[6,29] probably as a result of small dose ranges and large pharmacokinetic and pharmacodynamic variability.[188] Seikku and colleagues[189] recently compared the time-averaged concentration profile of methylprednisolone with the bioactivity of circulating glucocorticoids in 16 pediatric allograft patients. Posttransplant growth was inversely associated with both the time-averaged methylprednisolone concentration profile and the serum glucocorticoid bioactivity. Hence, the time course of actual exposure to bioactive glucocorticoids appears to be the relevant determinant of growth after RTx.

The introduction of cyclosporin A for posttransplant maintenance immunosuppression two decades ago permitted a substantial reductions of glucocorticoid dose requirements.[41] The introduction of triple immunosuppressive therapy that included cyclosporin A, azathioprine, and prednisolone was associated with a tendency toward improved adult height outcomes in some (albeit not all) studies as compared with the precyclosporin era, when progressive posttransplant stunting was common.[6,41-43] However, standardized height does not globally improve in patients receiving triple immunosuppression therapy. A recent comprehensive analysis of prepubertal and pubertal growth after RTx in 37 children receiving cyclosporin A, azathioprine, and prednisolone observed a significant increase of height velocity in prepubertal children from 4.9 to 8.0 cm/year, resulting in a standardized height improvement by 0.6 SD within 2 years after RTx[6] (Figure 46-5). In children who underwent RTx before and after the onset of puberty, pubertal peak height velocity was even greater than it was in healthy children[6] (Figures 46-5 and 46-6). However, because the pubertal growth spurt was markedly delayed (by 1.5 years) and abbreviated (by 1.6 years), total pubertal height gain was reduced by approximately 20%. The main factors influencing cumulative pubertal height gain were age at the start of the pubertal growth spurt (negative), the age at RTx (negative), and GFR (positive). These three factors explained about 60% of the overall variability of pubertal height gain. Interestingly, the strong negative association between the age at RTx and the pubertal height gain was also seen in patients who underwent RTx well before puberty. Indeed, age at RTx explained 50% of the total variability of pubertal height gain. This novel finding suggests that, in children with ESRD, early RTx is not only mandatory for optimal prepubertal growth but also for appropriate pubertal growth.

Several controlled and uncontrolled studies have shown that growth can be improved when the same total dose of corticosteroids is given on alternate days rather than in a daily fashion.[190-193] Whereas a mean change in standardized height of 0.25 to 0.5 SD per year has been demonstrated in patients on alternate-day steroids, no change was observed on daily treatment in two multicenter trials.[192,193]

The most impressive catch-up growth has been demonstrated after complete steroid withdrawal, with improvements of 0.6 to 0.8 SD during the first year after RTx.[23,184] Although complete steroid withdrawal was associated with unacceptably high rejection rates in children with azathioprine and cyclosporin A medication,[194,195] withdrawal appears to be much safer with the currently preferred immunosuppressants. Complete steroid withdrawal in more than 90% of RTx patients receiving high-dose tacrolimus monotherapy resulted in marked catch-up growth and the normalization of height in the majority of prepubertal patients.[184] In a retrospective case-control study, glucocorticoids were weaned off in 12 selected patients who were continued on cyclosporin A and mycophenolate mofetil without acute allograft rejections and with stable graft function for at least 1 year after RTx.[196] After steroid withdrawal, prepubertal patients

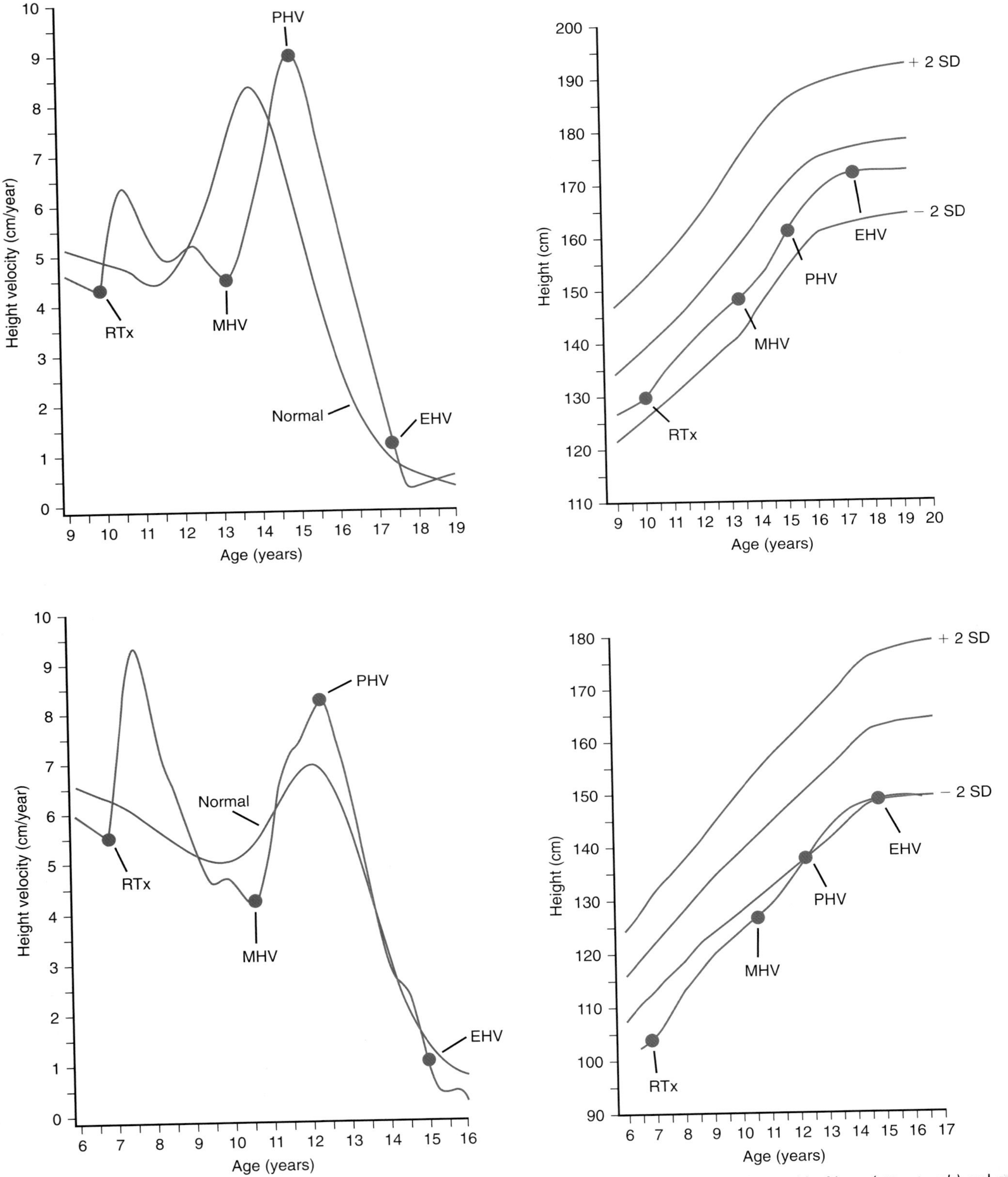

Figure 46-5 Synchronized mean height velocity curves *(left panels)* and synchronized mean growth curves *(right panels)* of boys *(upper panels)* and g *(lower panels)* who received renal transplants before the onset of puberty as compared with normal children. *RTx,* Renal transplantation; *MHV,* minimal presp height velocity; *PHV,* peak height velocity; *EHV,* end point height velocity. (Reproduced from Nissel R, Brazda I, Feneberg R, et al: Effect of renal transplan tion in childhood on longitudinal growth and adult height, *Kidney Int* 66:792-800, 2004.)

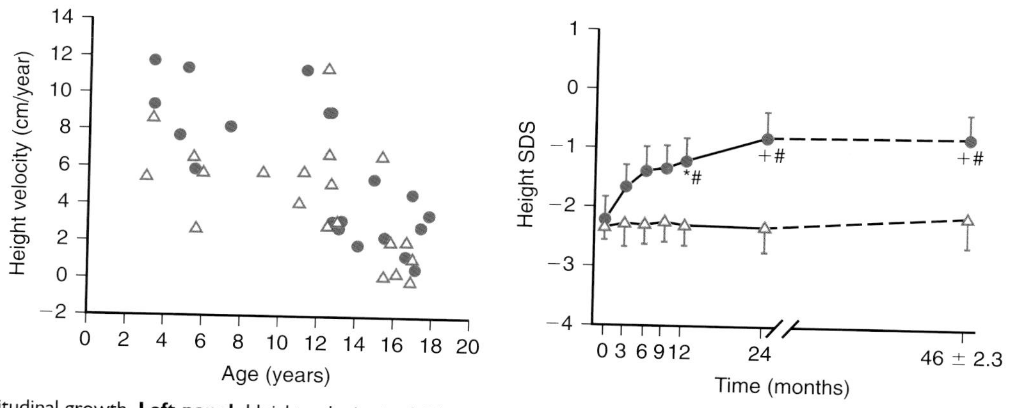

Figure 46-6 Longitudinal growth. **Left panel,** Height velocity in children during the first year after steroid withdrawal (*closed symbols; n* = 20) as compared with those remaining on steroids (case controls; *open triangles; n* = 20). **Right panel,** Mean (± standard error of the mean) height standard deviation score (SDS) at baseline, in 3-month intervals for 1 year after study entry, at 2 years, and at 46 ± 2.3 months after study entry in prepubertal patients no longer taking steroids (*closed symbols; n* = 6) and controls (*open triangles; n* = 6). Although height SDS remained unchanged in patients taking steroids, there was a significant increase of height SDS in patients off steroids. $^{*}p < 0.05$ versus baseline; $^{\#}p < 0.05$ versus controls; $^{+}p < 0.01$ versus baseline. (Reproduced from Höcken B, John U, Plank C, et al: Successful withdrawal of steroids in pediatric renal transplant recipients receiving cyclosporine A and mycophenolate mofetil treatment: results after four years, *Transplantation* 78:228-34, 2004.)

exhibited significant catchup growth with a mean increase in standardized height of 1.5 SD, whereas standardized height did not improve in patients who continued steroid medication[196] (Figure 46-6). Another historic case-control study compared posttransplant growth in 107 patients receiving either interleukin-2 receptor antibodies and tacrolimus in combination with either steroids or with mycophenolate mofetil.[197] In this study, steroid withdrawal was associated with improved growth in patients who were less than 5 years old (+1.5 SD versus –0.4 SD) and in patients between the ages of 5 and 15 years (+0.7 SD versus +0.2 SD). It still remains questionable whether steroid withdrawal may lead to complete catch-up growth; in clinical practice, this is not seen consistently. Interestingly, incomplete catch-up growth is observed after the transient local application of glucocorticoids to the tibial growth plate in rabbits, thus suggesting the induction of a permanent growth deficit.[160]

Pape and colleagues[198] investigated retrospectively whether growth during the 5 years after RTx differs between patients receiving living-related donor grafts and those receiving cadaveric donor grafts. Although standardized height was comparable at the time of RTx in both groups, it was significantly higher among living-related donor recipients 5 years later. Living-related donor graft recipients appeared to exhibit better catch-up growth even independent of GFR as compared with cadaveric donor allograft recipients. These findings argue for preferential living-related donor grafts for children with respect to posttransplant growth.

In conclusion, posttransplant catch-up growth is usually restricted to young children, and it occurs far from regularly. Efforts to avoid a height deficit before RTx are required to improve final height in children after RTx; these strategies include rhGH treatment, early (preemptive) RTx, and the use of efficacious immunosuppressive strategies for optimized graft function and early withdrawal from or even the complete avoidance of steroids.

Hormonal Treatment

Calcitriol

Calcitriol deficiency is a major cause of secondary hyperparathyroidism and renal osteodystrophy. Although calcitriol supplementation reverses the biochemical, radiographic, and histological signs of high turnover bone disease, the improvement of longitudinal height was not consistently observed in clinical trials. Alternatively, there is limited experimental and clinical evidence that a low turnover bone state, which is the typical complication of calcitriol therapy, may compromise longitudinal growth. Therefore, plasma PTH levels should be kept at two to three times the upper-normal range in patients with CKD stages IV and V and within the upper limit of the normal range in patients with CKD stages I through III.[84] Although these recommendations have not been formally proven in prospective clinical trials, these target levels are thought to allow for the sufficient control of secondary hyperparathyroidism (and thus avoid adynamic bone disease) and therefore optimal growth in children with CKD.[84,92,199]

Growth Hormone

Chronic uremia is accompanied by a state of combined resistance to endogenous GH and IGF-I (described previously). In pivotal studies in uremic rats, Mehls and colleagues[200,201] demonstrated that GH insensitivity can be overcome by the administration of GH at pharmacologic doses. In addition, animal studies demonstrated that the glucocorticoid-induced GH resistance can be overcome by rhGH treatment.[202] These studies have provided the rationale for treating growth-retarded children with CKD with rhGH. The administration of rhGH markedly increases systemic (mainly hepatic) and local (in growth cartilage) IGF-I production, whereas IGFBPs are only modestly stimulated, thus resulting in the normalization of the diminished bioactivity of IGF-I and the stimulation of longitudinal growth[203,204] (Figure 46-7). The efficacy and safety of long-term treatment with rhGH in children

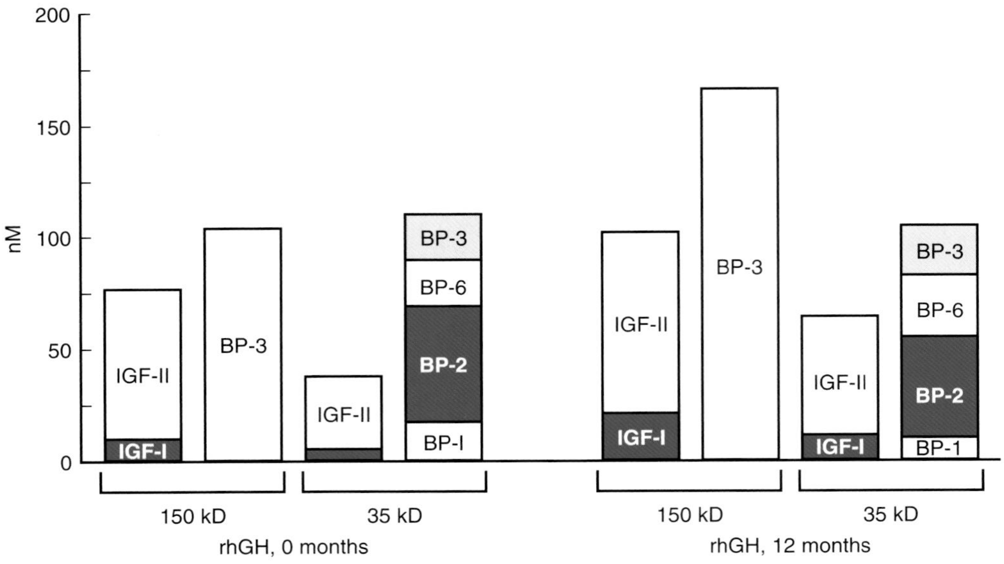

Figure 46-7 Balance between insulin-like growth factor binding proteins (IGFBPs) and insulin-like growth factors (IGFs) in the serum of children with chronic renal failure (CRF) before and after treatment with recombinant human growth hormone (rhGH). Levels (nanomoles per L) of IGF-I, IGF-II, IGFBP-1, IGFBP-2, IGFBP-3, and IGFBP-6 in the 150- and 35-kDa fractions of serum are presented. Protein levels were measured in the whole serum of 30 children with CRF before (0 months) and during (12 months) treatment with rhGH. Mean IGFBP-1, IGFBP-2, and IGFBP-6 levels were assigned entirely to the 35-kDa serum fractions. The percentages of IGFBP-3 and IGFs at 150 kDa (fractions 23 through 27) and at 35 kDa (fractions 28 through 30) in sera from children with CRF before and after 12 months of rhGH treatment were calculated; these percentages were then applied to the mean whole serum levels to calculate the amounts of each protein at 150 and 35 kDa. Both intact IGFBP-3 and IGFBP-329 were abundant in the 150-kDa fractions; IGFBP-329 was much more abundant than intact IGFBP-3 in the 35-kDa fractions. (Reproduced from Powell DR, Durham SK, Liu F, et al: The insulin-like growth factor axis and growth in children with chronic renal failure: a report of the Southwest Pediatric Nephrology Study Group, *J Clin Endocrinol Metab* 83:1654-61, 1998.)

with CKD before and after RTx have been established extensively.

Prepubertal Children with Preterminal Renal Failure and on Dialysis

Several uncontrolled and controlled studies in growth-retarded prepubertal children with CKD before dialysis have demonstrated that rhGH increases height velocity during the first treatment year approximately twofold as compared with baseline or with placebo-treated children.[205-212] During the subsequent treatment years, standardized height continues to increase, whereas height velocity gradually declines. After 5 to 6 years of rhGH treatment, mean standardized height was increased from −2.6 to −0.7 SD in North American patients, from −3.4 to −1.9 in German patients, and from −3.0 to −0.5 in Dutch patients.[210-212]

Because no acceleration in bone maturation was observed in these studies, predicted adult height steadily increased during rhGH treatment. In the German study, the mean increase in predicted adult height amounted to 10.3 cm after 5 years of rhGH treatment.[210] Several studies demonstrated that the growth response to rhGH treatment is significantly less in dialysed children as compared with children with pre-end-stage CKD,[210,213,214] even when patients were adequately matched with respect to possible confounders such as age, gender, and baseline height retardation.[213] In the German study, the mean change in standardized height during the first two treatment years was +0.8 SD and +1.3 SD in patients on dialysis and conservative treatment, respectively[210] (Figure 46-8). No difference in response was observed between children on peritoneal dialysis or hemodialysis.[215] The differences in growth response between dialyzed children and patients with pre-end-stage CKD may be explained by a higher degree of GH insensitivity as indicated by the lower expression of GH receptors and higher levels of IGFBPs.[129] Approximately 50% of the overall variability of growth response could be explained by age, residual GFR, pretreatment growth rate, and genetic target height.[210] Interestingly, the absolute increase in height velocity (i.e., cm per year) is independent of age, whereas the change in height SD declines with increasing age as a result of the widening distribution range of height across childhood.[210]

The growth response in children with nephropathic cystinosis is comparable to that of children with other underlying diseases.[44,216] There is limited data regarding the efficacy of rhGH therapy in infants with CKD. A placebo-controlled study of patients with CKD who were younger than 2.5 years old showed a mean increase in standardized height of 2 SD in the rhGH group as compared with −0.2 SD in controls.[217] This observation confirms the results of a previous uncontrolled study and supports of the concept of early rhGH initiation in infants and young children if adequate energy intake fails to allow for normal growth.[218]

Prepubertal Children after Renal Transplantation

Several uncontrolled and controlled randomized studies have demonstrated a positive effect of rhGH treatment on height velocity in prepubertal children after RTx who are receiving concomitant glucocorticoid treatment[205-207,219-233] (Table 46-2). The magnitude of the growth response is intermediate between that of patients with pre-end-stage CKD and those on dialysis, with a cumulative height increment of 1.0 to 1.5 SD during the first 3 treatment years.[227]

Pubertal Growth and Final Height

The analysis of pubertal growth in patients with CKD is complicated by the fact that the pubertal growth spurt is usually delayed by approximately 2 years and shortened by approximately 1.5 years as compared with healthy children.[29] In addition, children with CKD are often prone to changes in treatment modalities (i.e., start of dialysis and RTx). GH is usually discontinued at the time of RTx, but it is sometimes reinstituted in cases of insufficient posttransplant growth. Hence, any analysis of pubertal growth in children with CKD would ideally require an appropriate untreated control group. Alternatively, it is considered ethically unjustified to permanently withhold GH, which is the only growth-promoting treatment with well-established short-term efficacy for children with chronic renal failure, from severely growth-retarded children.

During the physiologic deceleration of growth velocity before the onset of the pubertal growth spurt, the growth response during long-term rhGH treatment may appear disappointing, frequently causing physicians to stop treatment. However, a marked pubertal growth spurt can be expected if rhGH treatment is continued in these patients[212] (Figure 46-9). RhGH treatment also stimulates longitudinal growth in pubertal renal allograft recipients. In a Dutch study, the average height increment from the start of rhGH treatment to the final height was doubled as compared with a matched control group (19 versus 9.4 cm).[234] In a German multicenter study, 38 prepubertal patients treated with rhGH were followed until final adult height was achieved as comparison with 50 matched untreated children.[8] During the prepubertal growth period, height velocity was markedly stimulated by rhGH[8] (Figure 46-10). After this prepubertal peak, height velocity gradually decreased toward the start of the pubertal growth spurt. The cumulative prepubertal height gain in the rhGH-treated children was twice that of the untreated controls, and the onset of the pubertal growth spurt was not advanced (Figures 46-10 and 46-11, *A*). After the onset of the pubertal spurt, bone maturation accelerated in rhGH-treated boys, resulting in a slight shortening of the growth spurt by approximately 6 months. Because the amplitude of the pubertal growth spurt was slightly higher in the rhGH-treated children (see Figure 46-10), the total pubertal height gain remained unaffected (see Figure 46-11, *B*). Regardless of rhGH treatment, the pubertal height gain was only 65% of that observed in healthy children. The apparent inefficacy of rhGH administration during puberty in this analysis may in part be explained by the fact that rhGH treatment was stopped during puberty (mainly because of RTx) in 50%

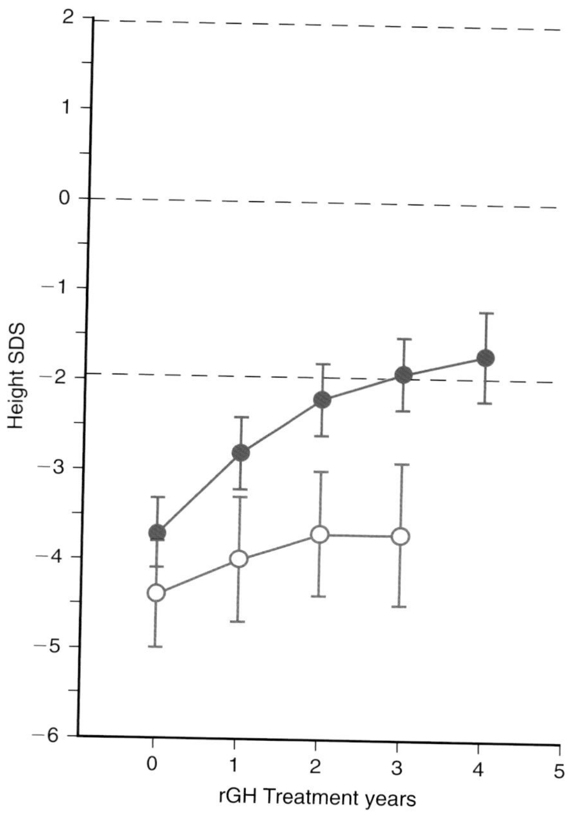

Figure 46-8 Superior efficacy of recombinant human growth hormone treatment in children with pre-end stage chronic renal failure (*closed circles; n* = 19) as compared with children on dialysis (*open circles; n* = 6). *SDS*, Standard deviation score. (Reproduced from Haffner D, Wühl E, Schaefer F, Nissel R, et al: Factors predictive of the short- and long-term efficacy of growth hormone treatment in prepubertal children with chronic renal failure. The German Study Group for Growth Hormone Treatment in Chronic Renal Failure, *J Am Soc Nephrol* 9:1899-907, 1998.)

TABLE 46-2 **Controlled Studies of Treatment with Recombinant Human Growth Hormone in Prepubertal Children After Renal Transplantation**

		Growth Velocity (cm/year)		
	Number of Patients	Recombinant Human Growth Hormone	Controls	*p* Value
Hokken-Koelega et al.[228]	6	5.3	1.5	<.0001
Maxwell et al.[232]	15	8.1	3.7	<.005
Guest et al.[231]	90	7.7	4.6	<.0001
Fine et al.[233]	67	9.0	4.2	<.0001

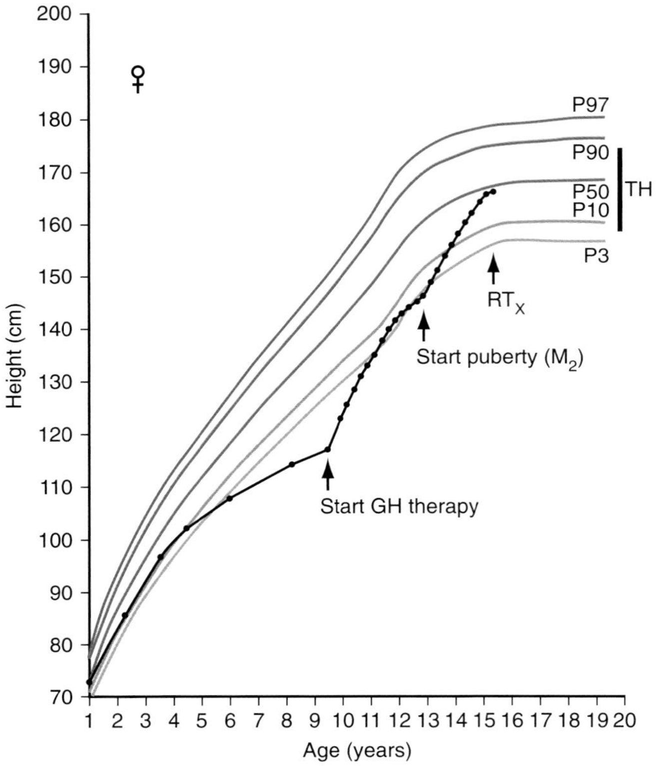

Figure 46-9 Individual growth chart of a girl treated with growth hormone therapy for many years showing a prepubertal dip in height velocity during the period before the start of puberty. *RTx*, Renal transplantation; *TH*, target height. (Reproduced from Hokken-Koelega AC, Mulder P, De JR, Lilien M, et al: Long-term effects of growth hormone treatment on growth and puberty in patients with chronic renal insufficiency, *Pediatr Nephrol* 14:701-06, 2000.)

of patients. Indeed, the total pubertal height gain was positively correlated with the duration of rhGH treatment during this growth period. The rhGH-treated children showed sustained catch-up growth (mean total gain, 1.6 SD), whereas the control children developed progressive growth failure (mean total loss, 0.6 SD; Figure 46-12). Despite their lower height at the start, the mean adult height of rhGH-treated boys (165.2 cm) and girls (156.2 cm) was significantly higher than that of control boys (162.1 cm) and girls (151.9 cm). Two thirds of the rhGH-treated children reached an adult height above the 3rd percentile. The figures obtained in the German study are in line with several recent reports[212,230,234-240] (Table 46-3). The cumulative height gain during rhGH treatment was positively affected by the duration of rhGH therapy and the initial target height deficit, and it was negatively affected by the duration of dialysis.[8] The relative height gain attained during rhGH treatment appears to be maintained until the final height is achieved in patients undergoing RTx.

General Treatment Strategies

The growth response to rhGH treatment is positively associated with residual renal function, target height, initial target height deficit, and duration of rhGH treatment and inversely associated with the age at the start of treatment.[210] Daily dosing is more effective than three administrations per week.[241] A dose of 4 IU/m²/day is more efficient than 2 IU/m²/day, whereas 8 IU/m²/day has no further effect.[234,242] Therefore, a fixed daily dose of 4 IU/m²/day (i.e., 12 mg/m²/day) should be used. Whereas the discontinuation of rhGH results in catch-down growth in approximately 75% of patients with CKD, this phenomenon is rarely observed when rhGH treatment is discontinued after RTx.[237,243] The clear

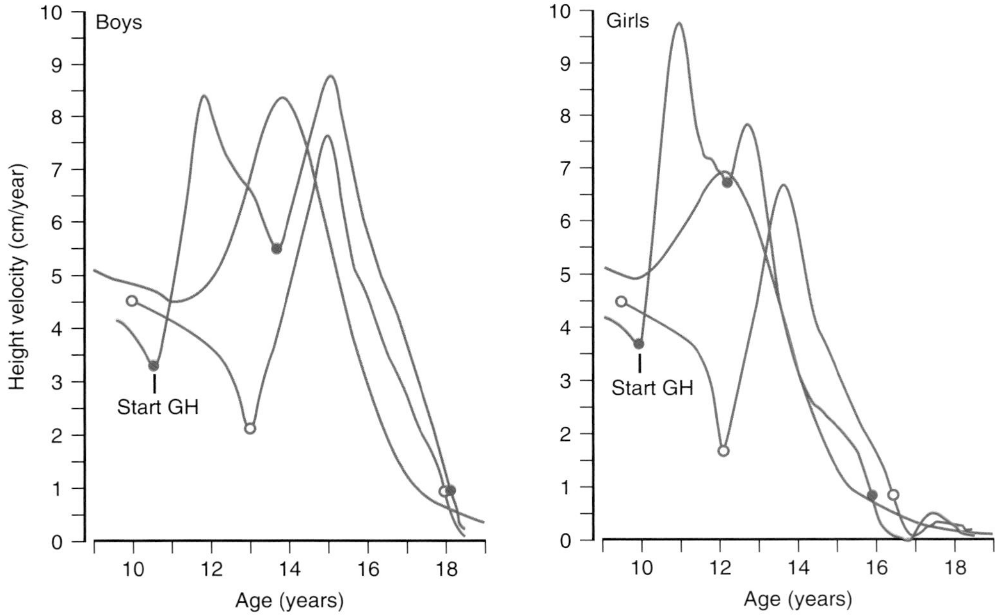

Figure 46-10 Synchronized mean height velocity curves of 32 boys *(left panel)* and 6 girls *(right panel)* with chronic renal failure during treatment with recombinant human growth hormone (rhGH; *closed circles*) as compared with 50 children with chronic renal failure not treated with rhGH *(open circles)* and 232 normal children *(thin lines)*. The dots indicate the time of the first observation, which corresponds with the start of rhGH treatment in the growth-hormone-treated children, minimal prespurt height velocity, and the time of the end of the pubertal growth spurt. (Reproduced from Haffner D, Schaefer F, Nissel R, Wühl E, et al: Effect of growth hormone treatment on the adult height of children with chronic renal failure. German Study Group for Growth Hormone Treatment in Chronic Renal Failure, *N Engl J Med* 343:923-30, 2000.)

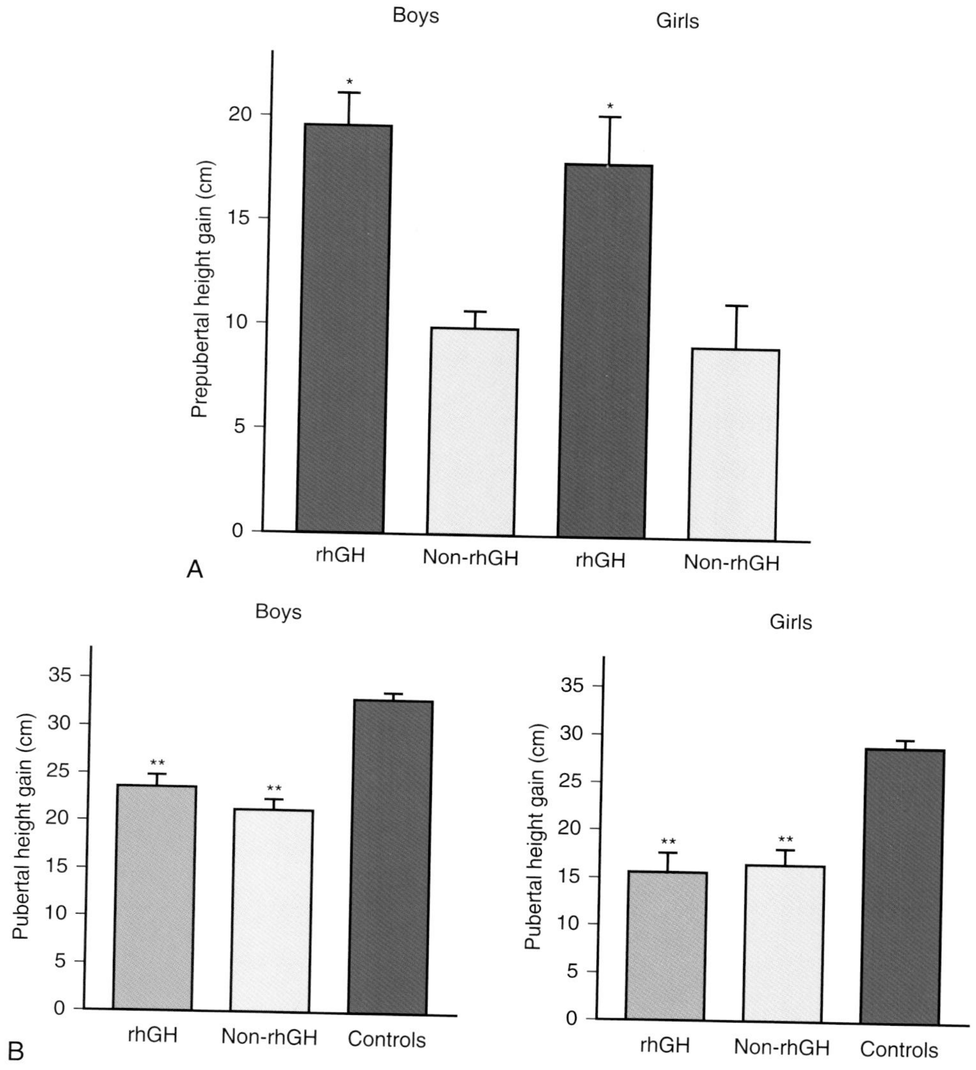

Figure 46-11 **A,** Prepubertal and **B,** pubertal height gain in children evaluated from around 10 years of age to final height with or without treatment with recombinant human growth hormone (rhGH) as compared with controls. Prepubertal height gain was measured from first observation until the start of the pubertal growth spurt. *$p < 0.0001$ with rhGH treatment versus no rhGH treatment; **$p < 0.0001$ patients with chronic renal failure versus controls. (Reproduced from Haffner D, Schaefer F, Nissel R, Wühl E, et al: Effect of growth hormone treatment on the adult height of children with chronic renal failure. German Study Group for Growth Hormone Treatment in Chronic Renal Failure, *N Engl J Med* 343:923-30, 2000.)

relationship between residual renal function and rhGH efficacy supports the concept of starting rhGH early during the course of chronic renal failure. Because the absolute height gain during rhGH treatment (in cm per year) is independent of age but the reference range increases with age, rhGH treatment should be started as early as growth retardation becomes evident (i.e., height below the 3rd percentile)[210] (Figure 46-13). Whether a low growth rate (i.e., height velocity below the 5th percentile) should also be an indication to start rhGH therapy even before height drops below the 3rd percentile is an open issue. Such early preventive therapy is probably more cost effective than starting at a more advanced age, when growth retardation has become evident and higher absolute rhGH doses must be applied. Because rhGH treatment is also effective for young children and infants with CKD, this treatment modality should not be withheld in this age group if malnutrition, metabolic acidosis, renal osteodystrophy, and electrolyte losses have been treated sufficiently.

The primary treatment target should be to return height into the patient's individual genetic percentile channel. Treatment may be suspended after this target is reached, but growth should be monitored closely, as outlined previously. For patients receiving rhGH while also receiving conservative treatment, rhGH should be continued after the initiation of dialysis; after RTx, rhGH should be stopped to monitor spontaneous growth during the next 12 months. If growth appears to be subnormal, the weaning of glucocorticoids should be the first therapeutic consideration, and the reinstitution of rhGH should be restricted to those patients with lacking or insufficient catch-up growth after steroid withdrawal or with a permanent need for maintenance glucocorticoid medication. For patients with imminent puberty or those with early skeletal maturation, determining whether pharmacologic intervention with GnRH analogues or aromatase inhibitors is indicated to extend the prepubertal growth phase will require assessment in prospective clinical trials.

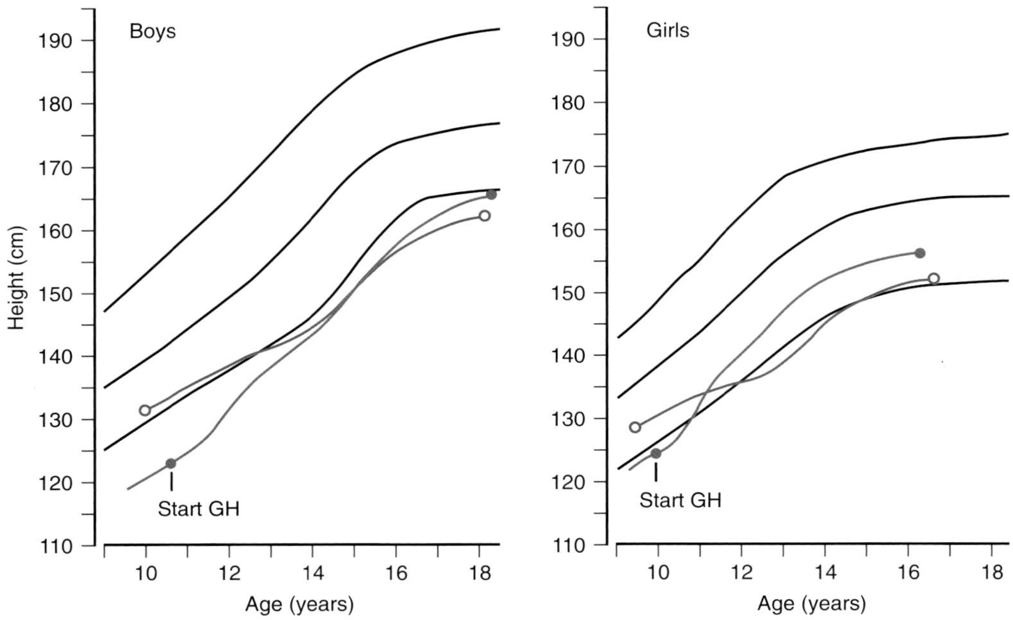

Figure 46-12 Synchronized mean height curves of 32 boys *(left panel)* and 6 girls *(right panel)* with chronic renal failure during treatment with recombinant human growth hormone (rhGH; *closed circles*) as compared with 50 children with chronic renal failure who were not treated with rhGH *(open circles)*. Normal values are indicated by the 3rd, 50th, and 97th percentiles. The dots indicate the time of the first observation, which corresponds with the start of rhGH treatment in the growth-hormone-treated children, and the time of the end of the pubertal growth spurt. (Reproduced from Haffner D, Schaefer F, Nissel R, Wühl E, et al: Effect of growth hormone treatment on the adult height of children with chronic renal failure. German Study Group for Growth Hormone Treatment in Chronic Renal Failure, *N Engl J Med* 343:923-30, 2000.)

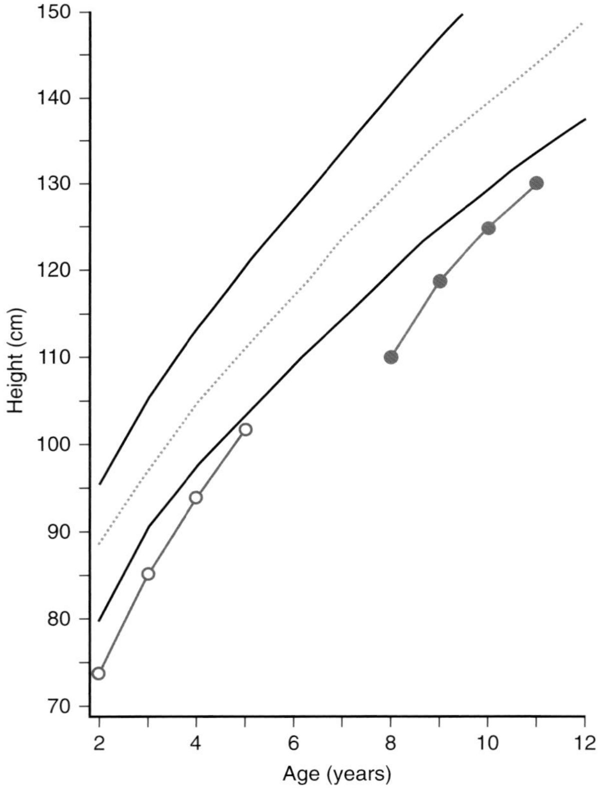

Figure 46-13 Age-dependent efficacy of recombinant human growth hormone (rhGH) treatment exemplified by individual growth curves predicted for two patients (aged 2 years and 8 years) started on rhGH at a basal height of –3.5 standard deviations and a height velocity of –2.0 standard deviations. The dotted line indicates the 50th percentile of a normal population, and the solid lines bounding the dotted line denote the 3rd and 97th percentiles. Growth is accelerated over baseline height velocity in both patients by 4.5 cm during the first year, 1.9 cm during the second year, and 1.0 cm during the third year (empiric means of all patients on conservative treatment were tracked for 3 years). The young child reaches the third percentile within the 3rd year, whereas the older child does not. (Reproduced from Haffner D, Wuhl E, Schaefer F, Nissel R, et al: Factors predictive of the short- and long-term efficacy of growth hormone treatment in prepubertal children with chronic renal failure. The German Study Group for Growth Hormone Treatment in Chronic Renal Failure, *J Am Soc Nephrol* 9:1899-907, 1998.)

TABLE 46-3 **Synopsis of Studies Reporting Adult Height Data after Treatment with Recombinant Human Growth Hormone for Growth Failure in Patients with Chronic Kidney Disease**

Study	Number of Patients	Chronic Renal Failure Treatment Modalities	Age at Start of rhGH Treatment (years)	Pubertal Status at Start of rhGH Treatment	Duration of Follow-up (years)	Duration of rhGH Treatment (years)	Initial Height SDS	Final Height SDS	Change in Height SDS
Dutch[212]	4	Conservative treatment/dialysis	<11.0	Prepubertal	>5.0	>5.0	NI	−0.2*	**NI**
Dutch[238]	65	Conservative treatment/dialysis	NI	Prepubertal	NI	5.8	−2.8.	−1.4	**+1.4**
KIGS[235]	12	Conservative treatment/dialysis	11.9	Prepubertal	NI	5.0	NI	NI	**+1.0**
KIGS[240]	75	Conservative treatment/dialysis	10.7	Prepubertal	NI	6.1	−3.5.	−2.6.	**+0.9**
UK[237]	2	Conservative treatment	9.9*	Prepubertal	10.0*	0.4*	−2.2*	−1.1*	**+1.1***
	5	Transplant	11.9	Prepubertal	>6.0	2.9	−3.3	−3.0	**+0.3**
	6	Transplant	15.6	Pubertal	>5.0	1.4	−3.4	−2.5	**+0.9**
NAPRTCS[236]	9	Conservative treatment	NI	NI	3.2	<3.2	−3.0	−2.2	**+0.7**
	22	Dialysis	NI	NI	4.1	<4.1	−3.6	−3.2	**+0.4**
	72	Transplant	NI	NI	3.7	<3.7	−3.0	−2.5	**+0.5**
German[8]	38	47% conservative treatment; 24% dialysis; 29% transplant†	10.4	Prepubertal	7.6	5.3	−3.1	−1.6	**+1.4**
Belgian[230]	17	Transplant	NI	NI	NI	3.4	−3.0	−1.8	**+1.2**
Dutch[234]	18	Transplant	15.5	Pubertal	NI	NI	NI	NI	**Total height gain 19 cm**
NAPRTCS[239]	71	Transplant	NI	NI	NI	NI	−2.7	−1.8	**+0.9**

rhGH, Recombinant human growth hormone; *SDS*, standard deviation score; *NI*, no information given.
* Median
† Percentage distribution of patient years spent in each treatment category.

Potential Adverse Events of Recombinant Human Growth Hormone Therapy

The safety of long-term rhGH treatment in patients with CKD has been evaluated in several clinical studies and registries. In a recent comparison of adverse event rates in a large cohort of patients with CKD who were receiving conservative treatment, who were on dialysis, and who had undergone RTx with and without concomitant rhGH treatment, rhGH use was not significantly associated with a higher incidence of malignancy, slipped capital femoral epiphysis, avascular necrosis, glucose intolerance, pancreatitis, progressive deterioration of renal function, acute allograft rejection, or fluid retention.[244] Of the targeted adverse events, the only significant relation with rhGH treatment was the occurrence of intracranial hypertension (ICH) in patients with CKD; however, in all three instances, ICH occurred after the discontinuation of rhGH. In another survey, ICH was noted in 15 out of 1670 patients with CKD receiving rhGH treatment (0.9%).[245] Although the clinical symptoms weaned off after the cessation of rhGH treatment, two patients had persistent blindness. In four patients, symptoms of ICH recurred after the reinstitution of rhGH treatment. The apparent slightly increased risk of ICH in patients with CKD provides a rationale for recommending a baseline fundoscopy and for starting treatment with 50% of the maintenance rhGH dose for the first few weeks of treatment. The state of hydration should be carefully monitored in patients with CKD who are receiving rhGH, because overhydration seems to be a predisposing factor for ICH. In the presence of symptoms like headache or vomiting, an immediate workup for ICH, including fundoscopy, should be performed.

Insulin secretion increases during the first rhGH treatment year, and hyperinsulinemia persists during long-term treatment. This increase is most pronounced in patients after RTx who are receiving concomitant glucocorticoid therapy. However, normal oral glucose tolerance has been found to be preserved during up to 5 years of rhGH administration in patients with CKD who are receiving conservative treatment and dialysis and who have undergone RTx.[246] Theoretically, hyperinsulinemia may contribute to the development of atherosclerosis or induce diabetes mellitus by the exhaustion of β cells. However, no increased incidence of diabetes mellitus has been observed to date in patients with CKD who are receiving rhGH.[244]

An aggravation of secondary hyperparathyroidism has rarely been reported in patients with CKD receiving rhGH treatment.[247,248] The mechanism of PTH stimulation levels during rhGH treatment remains unclear. GH may have a direct stimulatory effect on the parathyroid gland. Alternatively, rhGH may induce discrete changes in ionized calcium as a result of the increased deposition of calcium in the skeleton and thereby stimulate PTH secretion. Finally, increased longitudinal bone growth by rhGH treatment may unmask preexisting renal osteodystrophy. Therefore, the careful evaluation of bone metabolism and the adequate treatment of hyperparathyroidism should be performed before the initiation of rhGH therapy in patients with CKD.

Concern has been raised that, in the long term, rhGH-induced hyperfiltration may lead to the accelerated progression of renal failure in patients with CKD. However, no evidence for accelerated GFR loss in rhGH-treated patients has been detected in several studies of patients with CKD before and after RTx.[208,231,233,242,249]

Furthermore, rhGH therapy has not been associated with a significant increase in acute rejection episodes in RTx patients as compared with rejection rates before rhGH treatment or in untreated controls.[228,231] Although some authors have suggested that patients with a history of more than one acute rejection episode are at an increased risk of acute rejection after the initiation of rhGH therapy, no definitive evidence of a causal relationship has been found.[231,233]

REFERENCES

1. Chantler C, Broyer M, Donckerwolcke RA, et al: Growth and rehabilitation of long-term survivors of treatment for end-stage renal failure in childhood, *Proc Eur Dial Transplant Assoc* 18:329-42, 1981.
2. Rizzoni G, Broyer M, Brunner FP, et al: Combined report on regular hemodialysis and transplantation in Europe, 1985, *Proc Eur Dial Transplant Assoc* 23:55-83, 1986.
3. van Diemen-Steenvoorde R, Donckerwolcke RA, Brackel H, Wolff ED, de Jong MC: Growth and sexual maturation in children after kidney transplantation, *J Pediatr* 110:351-56, 1987.
4. Schaefer F, Gilli G, Schärer K: Pubertal growth and final height in chronic renal failure. In Schärer K, editor: *Growth and endocrine changes in children and adolescents with chronic renal failure*, Basel, 1989, Karger, pp 59-69.
5. Fine RN, Ho M, Tejani A: The contribution of renal transplantation to final adult height: a report of the North American Pediatric Renal Transplant Cooperative Study (NAPRTCS), *Pediatr Nephrol* 16:951-56, 2001.
6. Nissel R, Brazda I, Feneberg R, et al: Effect of renal transplantation in childhood on longitudinal growth and adult height, *Kidney Int* 66:792-800, 2004.
7. Andre JL, Bourquard R, Guillemin F, Krier MJ, Briancon S: Final height in children with chronic renal failure who have not received growth hormone, *Pediatr Nephrol* 18:685-91, 2003.
8. Haffner D, Schaefer F, Nissel R, Wuhl E, et al: Effect of growth hormone treatment on the adult height of children with chronic renal failure. German Study Group for Growth Hormone Treatment in Chronic Renal Failure, *N Engl J Med* 343:923-30, 2000.
9. Seikaly MG, Salhab N, Gipson D, Yiu V, Stablein D: Stature in children with chronic kidney disease: analysis of NAPRTCS database, *Pediatr Nephrol* 21:793-99, 2006.
10. Furth SL, Hwang W, Yang C, Neu AM, et al: Growth failure, risk of hospitalization and death for children with end-stage renal disease, *Pediatr Nephrol* 17:450-55, 2002.
11. Wong CS, Gipson DS, Gillen DL, et al: Anthropometric measures and risk of death in children with end-stage renal disease, *Am J Kidney Dis* 36:811-19, 2000.
12. Mehls O, Schaefer F: Endocrine, metabolic and growth disorders—patterns of growth and maturation in chronic renal failure—impact of developmental stage. In Holliday MA, Barratt TM, Avner ED, editors: *Pediatric nephrology*, Baltimore, 1994, Williams & Wilkins, pp 1260-63.
13. Jones RW, Rigden SP, Barratt TM, Chantler C: The effects of chronic renal failure in infancy on growth, nutritional status and body composition, *Pediatr Res* 16:784-91, 1982.
14. Kleinknecht C, Broyer M, Huot D, Marti-Henneberg C, Dartois AM: Growth and development of nondialyzed children with chronic renal failure, *Kidney Int Suppl* 15:S40-47, 1983.

15. Warady BA, Kriley M, Lovell H, Farrell SE, Hellerstein S: Growth and development of infants with end-stage renal disease receiving long-term peritoneal dialysis, *J Pediatr* 112:714-19, 1988.
16. Schaefer F, Mehls O: Endocrine, metabolic and growth disorders. In Holliday MA, Barratt TM, Avner ED, editors: *Paediatric nephrology*, Baltimore, 1994, Williams & Wilkins, pp 1241-86.
17. Karlberg J, Schaefer F, Hennicke M, Wingen AM, et al: Early age-dependent growth impairment in chronic renal failure. European Study Group for Nutritional Treatment of Chronic Renal Failure in Childhood, *Pediatr Nephrol* 10:283-87, 1996.
18. Abitbol CL, Zilleruelo G, Montane B, Strauss J: Growth of uremic infants on forced feeding regimens, *Pediatr Nephrol* 7:173-77, 1993.
19. Kari JA, Gonzalez C, Ledermann SE, Shaw V, Rees L: Outcome and growth of infants with severe chronic renal failure, *Kidney Int* 57:1681-87, 2000.
20. Ledermann SE, Spitz L, Moloney J, Rees L, Trompeter RS: Gastrostomy feeding in infants and children on peritoneal dialysis, *Pediatr Nephrol* 17:246-50, 2002.
21. Schaefer F, Wingen AM, Hennicke M, Rigden S, Mehls O: Growth charts for prepubertal children with chronic renal failure due to congenital renal disorders. European Study Group for Nutritional Treatment of Chronic Renal Failure in Childhood, *Pediatr Nephrol* 10:288-93, 1996.
22. Norman LJ, Coleman JE, Macdonald IA, Tomsett AM, Watson AR: Nutrition and growth in relation to severity of renal disease in children, *Pediatr Nephrol* 15:259-65, 2000.
23. Klare B, Strom TM, Hahn H, et al: Remarkable long-term prognosis and excellent growth in kidney-transplant children under cyclosporine monotherapy, *Transplant Proc* 23:1013-17, 1991.
24. Ellis D: Growth and renal function after steroid-free tacrolimus-based immunosuppression in children with renal transplants, *Pediatr Nephrol* 14:689-94, 2000.
25. de Graaff LC, Mulder PG, Hokken-Koelega AC: Body proportions before and during growth hormone therapy in children with chronic renal failure, *Pediatr Nephrol* 18:679-84, 2003.
26. Zivicnjak M, Franke D, Filler G, et al: Growth impairment shows an age-dependent pattern in boys with chronic kidney disease, *Pediatr Nephrol* 22:420-29, 2007.
27. Schärer K: Growth and development of children with chronic renal failure. Study Group on Pubertal Development in Chronic Renal Failure, *Acta Paediatr Scand Suppl* 366:90-92, 1990.
28. Schärer K, Chantler C, Brunner FP, et al: Combined report on regular dialysis and transplantation of children in Europe, 1974, *Proc Eur Dial Transplant Assoc* 12:65-108, 1976.
29. Schaefer F, Seidel C, Binding A, et al: Pubertal growth in chronic renal failure, *Pediatr Res* 28:5-10, 1990.
30. Burke BA, Lindgren B, Wick M, Holley K, Manivel C: Testicular germ cell loss in children with renal failure, *Pediatr Pathol* 9:433-44, 1989.
31. Schaefer F, Walther U, Ruder H: Reduced spermaturia in adolescent and young adult patients after renal transplantation, *Nephrol Dial Transplant* 6:840, 1991.
32. Inci K, Duzova A, Aki FT, et al: Semen variables and hormone profiles after kidney transplantation during adolescence, *Transplant Proc* 38:541-42, 2006.
33. Matuszkiewicz-Rowinska J, Skorzewska K, Radowicki S, et al: Endometrial morphology and pituitary-gonadal axis dysfunction in women of reproductive age undergoing chronic haemodialysis—a multicentre study, *Nephrol Dial Transplant* 19:2074-77, 2004.
34. Palmer BF: Sexual dysfunction in uremia, *J Am Soc Nephrol* 10:1381-88, 1999.
35. Hou S: Pregnancy in chronic renal insufficiency and end-stage renal disease, *Am J Kidney Dis* 33:235-52, 1999.
36. Rees L, Greene SA, Adlard P, et al: Growth and endocrine function after renal transplantation, *Arch Dis Child* 63:1326-32, 1988.
37. Broyer M, Guest G: Growth after kidney transplantation—a single center experience. In Schärer K, editor: *Growth and endocrine changes in children and adolescents with chronic renal failure*, Basel, 1989, Karger, pp 36-45.
38. Gilli G, Mehls O, Schärer K: Final height of children with chronic renal failure, *Proc Eur Dial Transplant Assoc* 21:830-36, 1984.
39. Fennell RS III, Love JT, Carter RL, et al: Statistical analysis of statural growth following kidney transplantation, *Eur J Pediatr* 145:377-79, 1986.
40. Hokken-Koelega AC, van Zaal MA, van BW, et al: Final height and its predictive factors after renal transplantation in childhood, *Pediatr Res* 36:323-28, 1994.
41. Offner G, Latta K, Hoyer PF, et al: Kidney transplanted children come of age, *Kidney Int* 55:1509-17, 1999.
42. Ninik A, McTaggart SJ, Gulati S, Powell HR, et al: Factors influencing growth and final height after renal transplantation, *Pediatr Transplant* 6:219-23, 2002.
43. Englund MS, Tyden G, Wikstad I, Berg UB: Growth impairment at renal transplantation—a determinant of growth and final height, *Pediatr Transplant* 7:192-99, 2003.
44. Wühl E, Haffner D, Offner G, Broyer M, et al: Long-term treatment with growth hormone in short children with nephropathic cystinosis, *J Pediatr* 138:880-87, 2001.
45. Nissel R, Latta K, Gagnadoux MF, et al: Body growth after combined liver-kidney transplantation in children with primary hyperoxaluria type 1, *Transplantation* 82:48-54, 2006.
46. Klaus G, Jux C, Fernandez P, Rodriguez J, et al: Suppression of growth plate chondrocyte proliferation by corticosteroids, *Pediatr Nephrol* 14:612-15, 2000.
47. Wühl E, Mehls O, Schaefer F: Antihypertensive and antiproteinuric efficacy of ramipril in children with chronic renal failure, *Kidney Int* 66:768-76, 2004.
48. Hodson EM, Shaw PF, Evans RA, et al: Growth retardation and renal osteodystrophy in children with chronic renal failure, *J Pediatr* 103:735-40, 1983.
49. Schärer K, Essigmann HC, Schaefer F: Body growth of children with steroid-resistant nephrotic syndrome, *Pediatr Nephrol* 13:828-34, 1999.
50. Lam CN, Arneil GC: Long-term dwarfing effects of corticosteroid treatment for childhood nephrosis, *Arch Dis Child* 43:589-94, 1968.
51. Foote KD, Brocklebank JT, Meadow SR: Height attainment in children with steroid-responsive nephrotic syndrome, *Lancet* 2:917-19, 1985.
52. Rees L, Greene SA, Adlard P, et al: Growth and endocrine function in steroid sensitive nephrotic syndrome, *Arch Dis Child* 63:484-90, 1988.
53. Holtta TM, Ronnholm KA, Jalanko H, la-Houhala M, et al: Peritoneal dialysis in children under 5 years of age, *Perit Dial Int* 17:573-80, 1997.
54. Licht C, Eifinger F, Gharib M, Offner G, et al: A stepwise approach to the treatment of early onset nephrotic syndrome, *Pediatr Nephrol* 14:1077-82, 2000.
55. Kovacevic L, Reid CJ, Rigden SP: Management of congenital nephrotic syndrome, *Pediatr Nephrol* 18:426-30, 2003.
56. Nash MA, Torrado AD, Greifer I, Spitzer A, Edelmann CM Jr: Renal tubular acidosis in infants and children. Clinical course, response to treatment, and prognosis, *J Pediatr* 80:738-48, 1972.
57. Tsuru N, Chan JC: Growth failure in children with metabolic alkalosis and with metabolic acidosis, *Nephron* 45:182-85, 1987.
58. Morris RC, Sebastian AC: Renal tubular acidosis and Fanconi syndrome. In Stanbury JB, Wyngaarden JB, Frederickson DS, editors: *The metabolic basis of inherited disease*, New York, 1983, McGraw-Hill, pp 1808.
59. Niaudet P, Dechaux M, Trivin C, Loirat C, Broyer M: Nephrogenic diabetes insipidus: clinical and pathophysiological aspects, *Adv Nephrol Necker Hosp* 13:247-60, 1984.
60. Simopoulos AP: Growth characteristics in patients with Bartter's syndrome, *Nephron* 23:130-35, 1979.
61. Haffner D, Weinfurth A, Manz F, et al: Long-term outcome of paediatric patients with hereditary tubular disorders, *Nephron* 83:250-60, 1999.
62. Haffner D, Weinfurth A, Seidel C, et al: Body growth in primary de Toni-Debre-Fanconi syndrome, *Pediatr Nephrol* 11:40-45, 1997.
63. Winkler L, Offner G, Krull F, Brodehl J: Growth and pubertal development in nephropathic cystinosis, *Eur J Pediatr* 152:244-49, 1993.

64. Leumann E, Hoppe B: The primary hyperoxalurias, *J Am Soc Nephrol* 12:1986-93, 2001.
65. Kimonis VE, Troendle J, Rose SR, Yang ML, et al: Effects of early cysteamine therapy on thyroid function and growth in nephropathic cystinosis, *J Clin Endocrinol Metab* 80:3257-61, 1995.
66. Smellie JM, Preece MA, Paton AM: Normal somatic growth in children receiving low-dose prophylactic co-trimoxazole, *Eur J Pediatr* 140:301-04, 1983.
67. Merrell RW, Mowad JJ: Increased physical growth after successful antireflux operation, *J Urol* 122:523-27, 1979.
68. Bamgbola FO, Kaskel FJ: Uremic malnutrition-inflammation syndrome in chronic renal disease: a pathobiologic entity, *J Ren Nutr* 13:250-58, 2003.
69. Mehls O, Ritz E, Gilli G, et al: Nitrogen metabolism and growth in experimental uremia, *Int J Pediatr Nephrol* 1:34-41, 1980.
70. Arnold WC, Danford D, Holliday MA: Effects of caloric supplementation on growth in children with uremia, *Kidney Int* 24:205-09, 1983.
71. Betts PR, Magrath G, White RH: Role of dietary energy supplementation in growth of children with chronic renal insufficiency, *Br Med J* 1:416-18, 1977.
72. Coleman JE, Watson AR: Gastrostomy buttons for nutritional support in children with cystinosis, *Pediatr Nephrol* 14:833-36, 2000.
73. Ledermann SE, Shaw V, Trompeter RS: Long-term enteral nutrition in infants and young children with chronic renal failure, *Pediatr Nephrol* 13:870-75, 1999.
74. May RC, Kelly RA, Mitch WE: Metabolic acidosis stimulates protein degradation in rat muscle by a glucocorticoid-dependent mechanism, *J Clin Invest* 77:614-21, 1986.
75. May RC, Hara Y, Kelly RA, Block KP, et al: Branched-chain amino acid metabolism in rat muscle: abnormal regulation in acidosis, *Am J Physiol* 252:E712-18, 1987.
76. Bailey JL, Wang X, England BK, Price SR, et al: The acidosis of chronic renal failure activates muscle proteolysis in rats by augmenting transcription of genes encoding proteins of the ATP-dependent ubiquitin-proteasome pathway, *J Clin Invest* 97:1447-53, 1996.
77. Boirie Y, Broyer M, Gagnadoux MF, Niaudet P, Bresson JL: Alterations of protein metabolism by metabolic acidosis in children with chronic renal failure, *Kidney Int* 58:236-41, 2000.
78. Challa A, Krieg RJ Jr, Thabet MA, Veldhuis JD, Chan JC: Metabolic acidosis inhibits growth hormone secretion in rats: mechanism of growth retardation, *Am J Physiol* 265:E547-E53, 1993.
79. Challa A, Chan W, Krieg RJ Jr, et al: Effect of metabolic acidosis on the expression of insulin-like growth factor and growth hormone receptor, *Kidney Int* 44:1224-27, 1993.
80. Brungger M, Hulter HN, Krapf R: Effect of chronic metabolic acidosis on the growth hormone/IGF-1 endocrine axis: new cause of growth hormone insensitivity in humans, *Kidney Int* 51:216-21, 1997.
81. Grossman H, Duggan E, McCamman S, Welchert E, Hellerstein S: The dietary chloride deficiency syndrome, *Pediatrics* 66:366-74, 1980.
82. Wassner SJ: Altered growth and protein turnover in rats fed sodium-deficient diets, *Pediatr Res* 26:608-13, 1989.
83. Wassner SJ: The effect of sodium repletion on growth and protein turnover in sodium-depleted rats, *Pediatr Nephrol* 5:501-04, 1991.
84. Klaus G, Watson A, Edefonti A, et al: Prevention and treatment of renal osteodystrophy in children on chronic renal failure: European guidelines, *Pediatr Nephrol* 21:151-59, 2006.
85. Mehls O, Ritz E, Gilli G, Wangdak T, Krempien B: Effect of vitamin D on growth in experimental uremia, *Am J Clin Nutr* 31:1927-31, 1978.
86. Mehls O, Ritz E, Gilli G, Heinrich U: Role of hormonal disturbances in uremic growth failure, *Contrib Nephrol* 50:119-29, 1986.
87. Chesney RW, Moorthy AV, Eisman JA, Jax DK, et al: Increased growth after long-term oral 1alpha,25-vitamin D3 in childhood renal osteodystrophy, *N Engl J Med* 298:238-42, 1978.
88. Chesney RW, Hamstra A, Jax DK, Mazess RB, DeLuca HF: Influence of long-term oral 1,25-dihydroxyvitamin D in childhood renal osteodystrophy, *Contrib Nephrol* 18:55-71, 1980.
89. Kreusser W, Weinkauff R, Mehls O, Ritz E: Effect of parathyroid hormone, calcitonin and growth hormone on cAMP content of growth cartilage in experimental uraemia, *Eur J Clin Invest* 12:337-43, 1982.
90. Kuizon BD, Goodman WG, Juppner H, et al: Diminished linear growth during intermittent calcitriol therapy in children undergoing CCPD, *Kidney Int* 53:205-11, 1998.
91. Schmitt CP, Ardissino G, Testa S, Claris-Appiani A, Mehls O: Growth in children with chronic renal failure on intermittent versus daily calcitriol, *Pediatr Nephrol* 18:440-44, 2003.
92. Waller SC, Ridout D, Cantor T, Rees L: Parathyroid hormone and growth in children with chronic renal failure, *Kidney Int* 67:2338-45, 2005.
93. Martin GR, Ongkingo JR, Turner ME, Skurow ES, Ruley EJ: Recombinant erythropoietin (Epogen) improves cardiac exercise performance in children with end-stage renal disease, *Pediatr Nephrol* 7:276-80, 1993.
94. Morris KP, Sharp J, Watson S, Coulthard MG: Non-cardiac benefits of human recombinant erythropoietin in end stage renal failure and anaemia, *Arch Dis Child* 69:580-86, 1993.
95. Rees L, Rigden SP, Chantler C: The influence of steroid therapy and recombinant human erythropoietin on the growth of children with renal disease, *Pediatr Nephrol* 5:556-58, 1991.
96. Jabs K: The effects of recombinant human erythropoietin on growth and nutritional status, *Pediatr Nephrol* 10:324-27, 1996.
97. Schaefer F, André JL, Krug C: Growth and skeletal maturation in dialysed children treated with recombinant human erythropoietin (rhEPO)—a multicenter study. *Pediatr Nephrol* 5, C61, 1991.
98. Schärer K, Broyer M, Vecsei P, Roger M, et al: Damage to testicular function in chronic renal failure of children, *Proc Eur Dial Transplant Assoc* 17:725-29, 1980.
99. Oertel PJ, Lichtwald K, Hafner S, Rauh W, et al: Hypothalamo-pituitary-gonadal axis in children with chronic renal failure, *Kidney Int Suppl* 15:S34-39, 1983.
100. Handelsman DJ: Hypothalamic-pituitary gonadal dysfunction in renal failure, dialysis and renal transplantation, *Endocr Rev* 6:151-82, 1985.
101. Belgorosky A, Ferraris JR, Ramirez JA, Jasper H, Rivarola MA: Serum sex hormone-binding globulin and serum nonsex hormone-binding globulin-bound testosterone fractions in prepubertal boys with chronic renal failure, *J Clin Endocrinol Metab* 73:107-10, 1991.
102. Schaefer F, Hamill G, Stanhope R, Preece MA, Scharer K: Pulsatile growth hormone secretion in peripubertal patients with chronic renal failure. Cooperative Study Group on Pubertal Development in Chronic Renal Failure, *J Pediatr* 119:568-77, 1991.
103. Corvol P, Bertagna X, Bedrossian J: Increased steroid metabolic clearance rate in anephric patients, *Acta Endocrinol (Copenh)* 75:756-62, 1974.
104. Stewart-Bentley M, Gans D, Horton R: Regulation of gonadal function in uremia, *Metabolism* 23:1065-72, 1974.
105. Van KE, Thijssen JH, Schwarz F: Sex hormones in male patients with chronic renal failure. I. The production of testosterone and of androstenedione, *Clin Endocrinol (Oxf)* 8:7-14, 1978.
106. Mitchell R, Schaefer F, Morris ID, Scharer K, et al: Elevated serum immunoreactive inhibin levels in peripubertal boys with chronic renal failure. Cooperative Study Group on Pubertal Development in Chronic Renal Failure (CSPCRF), *Clin Endocrinol (Oxf)* 39:27-33, 1993.
107. Lim VS, Henriquez C, Sievertsen G, Frohman LA: Ovarian function in chronic renal failure: evidence suggesting hypothalamic anovulation, *Ann Intern Med* 93:21-27, 1980.
108. Ferraris JR, Domene HM, Escobar ME, Caletti MG, et al: Hormonal profile in pubertal females with chronic renal failure: before and under haemodialysis and after renal transplantation, *Acta Endocrinol (Copenh)* 115:289-96, 1987.
109. Schärer K, Schaefer F, Trott M: Pubertal development in children with chronic renal failure. In Schärer K, editor: *Growth and endocrine changes in children and adolescents with chronic renal failure*, Basel, 1989, Karger, pp 151-68.
110. Schaefer F, Seidel C, Mitchell R, Scharer K, Robertson WR: Pulsatile immunoreactive and bioactive luteinizing hormone secretion in adolescents with chronic renal failure. The Cooperative Study

Group on Pubertal Development in Chronic Renal Failure (CSPCRF), *Pediatr Nephrol* 5:566-71, 1991.
111. Veldhuis JD, Carlson ML, Johnson ML: The pituitary gland secretes in bursts: appraising the nature of glandular secretory impulses by simultaneous multiple-parameter deconvolution of plasma hormone concentrations, *Proc Natl Acad Sci U S A* 84:7686-90, 1987.
112. Schaefer F, Veldhuis JD, Robertson WR, Dunger D, Scharer K: Immunoreactive and bioactive luteinizing hormone in pubertal patients with chronic renal failure. Cooperative Study Group on Pubertal Development in Chronic Renal Failure, *Kidney Int* 45:1465-76, 1994.
113. Schaefer F, Daschner M, Veldhuis JD, Oh J, et al: In vivo alterations in the gonadotropin-releasing hormone pulse generator and the secretion and clearance of luteinizing hormone in the uremic castrate rat, *Neuroendocrinology* 59:285-96, 1994.
114. Dong QH, Handelsman DJ: Regulation of pulsatile luteinizing hormone secretion in experimental uremia, *Endocrinology* 128:1218-22, 1991.
115. Wibullaksanakul S, Handelsman DJ: Regulation of hypothalamic gonadotropin-releasing hormone secretion in experimental uremia: in vitro studies, *Neuroendocrinology* 54:353-58, 1991.
116. Schaefer F, Vogel M, Kerkhoff G, Woitzik J, et al: Experimental uremia affects hypothalamic amino acid neurotransmitter milieu, *J Am Soc Nephrol* 12:1218-27, 2001.
117. Daschner M, Philippin B, Nguyen T, et al: Circulating inhibitor of gonadotropin releasing hormone secretion by hypothalamic neurons in uremia, *Kidney Int* 62:1582-90, 2002.
118. Mitchell R, Bauerfeld C, Schaefer F, Scharer K, Robertson WR: Less acidic forms of luteinizing hormone are associated with lower testosterone secretion in men on haemodialysis treatment, *Clin Endocrinol (Oxf)* 41:65-73, 1994.
119. Ramirez G, O'Neill WM, Bloomer HA, Jubiz W: Abnormalities in the regulation of growth hormone in chronic renal failure, *Arch Intern Med* 138:267-71, 1978.
120. Johnson V, Maack T: Renal extraction, filtration, absorption, and catabolism of growth hormone, *Am J Physiol* 233:F185-96, 1977.
121. Haffner D, Schaefer F, Girard J, Ritz E, Mehls O: Metabolic clearance of recombinant human growth hormone in health and chronic renal failure, *J Clin Invest* 93:1163-71, 1994.
122. Schaefer F, Baumann G, Haffner D, et al: Multifactorial control of the elimination kinetics of unbound (free) growth hormone (GH) in the human: regulation by age, adiposity, renal function, and steady state concentrations of GH in plasma, *J Clin Endocrinol Metab* 81:22-31, 1996.
123. Tönshoff B, Veldhuis JD, Heinrich U, Mehls O: Deconvolution analysis of spontaneous nocturnal growth hormone secretion in prepubertal children with preterminal chronic renal failure and with end-stage renal disease, *Pediatr Res* 37:86-93, 1995.
124. Veldhuis JD, Iranmanesh A, Wilkowski MJ, Samojlik E: Neuroendocrine alterations in the somatotropic and lactotropic axes in uremic men, *Eur J Endocrinol* 131:489-98, 1994.
125. Schaefer F, Veldhuis JD, Stanhope R, Jones J, Scharer K: Alterations in growth hormone secretion and clearance in peripubertal boys with chronic renal failure and after renal transplantation. Cooperative Study Group of Pubertal development in Chronic Renal Failure, *J Clin Endocrinol Metab* 78:1298-306, 1994.
126. Schaefer F, Chen Y, Tsao T, Nouri P, Rabkin R: Impaired JAK-STAT signal transduction contributes to growth hormone resistance in chronic uremia, *J Clin Invest* 108:467-75, 2001.
127. Chan W, Valerie KC, Chan JC: Expression of insulin-like growth factor-1 in uremic rats: growth hormone resistance and nutritional intake, *Kidney Int* 43:790-95, 1993.
128. Postel-Vinay MC, Tar A, Crosnier H, et al: Plasma growth hormone-binding activity is low in uraemic children, *Pediatr Nephrol* 5:545-47, 1991.
129. Tönshoff B, Cronin MJ, Reichert M, et al: Reduced concentration of serum growth hormone (GH)-binding protein in children with chronic renal failure: correlation with GH insensitivity. The European Study Group for Nutritional Treatment of Chronic Renal Failure in Childhood. The German Study Group for Growth Hormone Treatment in Chronic Renal Failure, *J Clin Endocrinol Metab* 82:1007-13, 1997.
130. Tönshoff B, Eden S, Weiser E, et al: Reduced hepatic growth hormone (GH) receptor gene expression and increased plasma GH binding protein in experimental uremia, *Kidney Int* 45:1085-92, 1994.
131. Villares SM, Goujon L, Maniar S, et al: Reduced food intake is the main cause of low growth hormone receptor expression in uremic rats, *Mol Cell Endocrinol* 106:51-56, 1994.
132. Martinez V, Balbin M, Ordonez FA, et al: Hepatic expression of growth hormone receptor/binding protein and insulin-like growth factor I genes in uremic rats. Influence of nutritional deficit, *Growth Horm IGF Res* 9:61-68, 1999.
133. Edmondson SR, Baker NL, Oh J, Kovacs G, et al: Growth hormone receptor abundance in tibial growth plates of uremic rats: GH/IGF-I treatment, *Kidney Int* 58:62-70, 2000.
134. Rabkin R, Sun DF, Chen Y, Tan J, Schaefer F: Growth hormone resistance in uremia, a role for impaired JAK/STAT signaling, *Pediatr Nephrol* 20:313-18, 2005.
135. Powell DR, Liu F, Baker BK, et al: Modulation of growth factors by growth hormone in children with chronic renal failure. The Southwest Pediatric Nephrology Study Group, *Kidney Int* 51:1970-79, 1997.
136. Ding H, Gao XL, Hirschberg R, Vadgama JV, Kopple JD: Impaired actions of insulin-like growth factor 1 on protein synthesis and degradation in skeletal muscle of rats with chronic renal failure. Evidence for a postreceptor defect, *J Clin Invest* 97:1064-75, 1996.
137. Phillips LS, Kopple JD: Circulating somatomedin activity and sulfate levels in adults with normal and impaired kidney function, *Metabolism* 30:1091-95, 1981.
138. Fouque D: Insulin-like growth factor 1 resistance in chronic renal failure, *Miner Electrolyte Metab* 22:133-37, 1996.
139. Fouque D, Peng SC, Kopple JD: Impaired metabolic response to recombinant insulin-like growth factor-1 in dialysis patients, *Kidney Int* 47:876-83, 1995.
140. Green H, Morikawa M, Nixon T: A dual effector theory of growth-hormone action, *Differentiation* 29:195-98, 1985.
141. Tönshoff B, Blum WF, Wingen AM, Mehls O: Serum insulin-like growth factors (IGFs) and IGF binding proteins 1, 2, and 3 in children with chronic renal failure: relationship to height and glomerular filtration rate. The European Study Group for Nutritional Treatment of Chronic Renal Failure in Childhood, *J Clin Endocrinol Metab* 80:2684-91, 1995.
142. Phillips LS, Fusco AC, Unterman TG, del GF: Somatomedin inhibitor in uremia, *J Clin Endocrinol Metab* 59:764-72, 1984.
143. Blum WF, Ranke MB, Kietzmann K, Tonshoff B, Mehls O: Growth hormone resistance and inhibition of somatomedin activity by excess of insulin-like growth factor binding protein in uraemia, *Pediatr Nephrol* 5:539-44, 1991.
144. Blum WF, Ranke MB, Kietzmann K: Excess of IGF-binding proteins in chronic renal failure: evidence for relative GH resistance and inhibition of somatomedin activity. In Drop SLS, Hintz RL, editors: *Insulin-like growth factor binding proteins*, Amsterdam, 1989, Elsevier Science, pp 93-99.
145. Lee PD, Hintz RL, Sperry JB, Baxter RC, Powell DR: IGF binding proteins in growth-retarded children with chronic renal failure, *Pediatr Res* 26:308-15, 1989.
146. Powell DR, Liu F, Baker BK, et al: Insulin-like growth factor-binding protein-6 levels are elevated in serum of children with chronic renal failure: a report of the Southwest Pediatric Nephrology Study Group, *J Clin Endocrinol Metab* 82:2978-84, 1997.
147. Powell DR, Durham SK, Brewer ED, et al: Effects of chronic renal failure and growth hormone on serum levels of insulin-like growth factor-binding protein-4 (IGFBP-4) and IGFBP-5 in children: a report of the Southwest Pediatric Nephrology Study Group, *J Clin Endocrinol Metab* 84:596-601, 1999.
148. Powell DR, Liu F, Baker BK, et al: Effect of chronic renal failure and growth hormone therapy on the insulin-like growth factors and their binding proteins, *Pediatr Nephrol* 14:579-83, 2000.
149. Ulinski T, Mohan S, Kiepe D, et al: Serum insulin-like growth factor binding protein (IGFBP)-4 and IGFBP-5 in children with chronic renal failure: relationship to growth and glomerular filtration rate. The European Study Group for Nutritional Treatment of Chronic Renal Failure in Childhood. German Study Group for

Growth Hormone Treatment in Chronic Renal Failure, *Pediatr Nephrol* 14:589-97, 2000.
150. Liu F, Powell DR, Hintz RL: Characterization of insulin-like growth factor-binding proteins in human serum from patients with chronic renal failure, *J Clin Endocrinol Metab* 70:620-28, 1990.
151. Lee DY, Park SK, Yorgin PD, Cohen P, et al: Alteration in insulin-like growth factor-binding proteins (IGFBPs) and IGFBP-3 protease activity in serum and urine from acute and chronic renal failure, *J Clin Endocrinol Metab* 79:1376-82, 1994.
152. Kiepe D, Ulinski T, Powell DR, Durham SK, et al: Differential effects of insulin-like growth factor binding proteins-1, -2, -3, and -6 on cultured growth plate chondrocytes, *Kidney Int* 62:1591-600, 2002.
153. Tönshoff B, Kiepe D, Ciarmatori S: Growth hormone/insulin-like growth factor system in children with chronic renal failure, *Pediatr Nephrol* 20:279-89, 2005.
154. Tönshoff B, Powell DR, Zhao D, et al: Decreased hepatic insulin-like growth factor (IGF)-I and increased IGF binding protein-1 and -2 gene expression in experimental uremia, *Endocrinology* 138:938-46, 1997.
155. Tsao T, Fervenza F, Friedlaender M, Chen Y, Rabkin R: Effect of prolonged uremia on insulin-like growth factor-I receptor autophosphorylation and tyrosine kinase activity in kidney and muscle, *Exp Nephrol* 10:285-92, 2002.
156. Pennisi AJ, Costin G, Phillips LS, et al: Somatomedin and growth hormone studies in pediatric renal allograft recipients who receive daily prednisone, *Am J Dis Child* 133:950-54, 1979.
157. Wehrenberg WB, Janowski BA, Piering AW, Culler F, Jones KL: Glucocorticoids: potent inhibitors and stimulators of growth hormone secretion, *Endocrinology* 126:3200-03, 1990.
158. Luo JM, Murphy LJ: Dexamethasone inhibits growth hormone induction of insulin-like growth factor-I (IGF-I) messenger ribonucleic acid (mRNA) in hypophysectomized rats and reduces IGF-I mRNA abundance in the intact rat, *Endocrinology* 125:165-71, 1989.
159. Gabrielsson BG, Carmignac DF, Flavell DM, Robinson IC: Steroid regulation of growth hormone (GH) receptor and GH-binding protein messenger ribonucleic acids in the rat, *Endocrinology* 136:209-17, 1995.
160. Baron J, Klein KO, Colli MJ, et al: Catch-up growth after glucocorticoid excess: a mechanism intrinsic to the growth plate, *Endocrinology* 135:1367-71, 1994.
161. Silbermann M, Maor G: Mechanisms of glucocorticoid-induced growth retardation: impairment of cartilage mineralization, *Acta Anat (Basel)* 101:140-49, 1978.
162. Jux C, Leiber K, Hugel U, et al: Dexamethasone impairs growth hormone (GH)-stimulated growth by suppression of local insulin-like growth factor (IGF)-I production and expression of GH- and IGF-I-receptor in cultured rat chondrocytes, *Endocrinology* 139:3296-305, 1998.
163. Smink JJ, Koedam JA, Koster JG, van Buul-Offers SC: Dexamethasone-induced growth inhibition of porcine growth plate chondrocytes is accompanied by changes in levels of IGF axis components, *J Endocrinol* 174:343-52, 2002.
164. Kiepe D, Ciarmatori S, Hoeflich A, Wolf E, Tonshoff B: Insulin-like growth factor (IGF)-I stimulates cell proliferation and induces IGF binding protein (IGFBP)-3 and IGFBP-5 gene expression in cultured growth plate chondrocytes via distinct signaling pathways, *Endocrinology* 146:3096-104, 2005.
165. Kiepe D, Ciarmatori S, Haarmann A, Tonshoff B: Differential expression of IGF system components in proliferating vs. differentiating growth plate chondrocytes: the functional role of IGFBP-5, *Am J Physiol Endocrinol Metab* 290:E363-71, 2006.
166. Ramage IJ, Geary DF, Harvey E, Secker DJ, et al: Efficacy of gastrostomy feeding in infants and older children receiving chronic peritoneal dialysis, *Perit Dial Int* 19:231-36, 1999.
167. Van DM, Bilem N, Proesmans W: Conservative treatment for chronic renal failure from birth: a 3-year follow-up study, *Pediatr Nephrol* 13:865-69, 1999.
168. Rodriguez-Soriano J, Arant BS, Brodehl J, Norman ME: Fluid and electrolyte imbalances in children with chronic renal failure, *Am J Kidney Dis* 7:268-74, 1986.
169. Parekh RS, Flynn JT, Smoyer WE, et al: Improved growth in young children with severe chronic renal insufficiency who use specified nutritional therapy, *J Am Soc Nephrol* 12:2418-26, 2001.
170. Trachtman H, Hackney P, Tejani A: Pediatric hemodialysis: a decade's (1974-1984) perspective, *Kidney Int Suppl* 19:S15-22, 1986.
171. Fennell RS III, Orak JK, Hudson T, et al: Growth in children with various therapies for end-stage renal disease, *Am J Dis Child* 138:28-31, 1984.
172. Chantler C, Donckerwolcke RA, Brunner FP, et al: Combined report on regular dialysis and transplantation of children in Europe, 1976, *Proc Eur Dial Transplant Assoc* 14:70-112, 1977.
173. Neu AM, Bedinger M, Fivush BA, et al: Growth in adolescent hemodialysis patients: data from the Centers for Medicare & Medicaid Services ESRD Clinical Performance Measures Project, *Pediatr Nephrol* 20:1156-60, 2005.
174. Shroff R, Wright E, Ledermann S, Hutchinson C, Rees L: Chronic hemodialysis in infants and children under 2 years of age, *Pediatr Nephrol* 18:378-83, 2003.
175. Chadha V, Blowey DL, Warady BA: Is growth a valid outcome measure of dialysis clearance in children undergoing peritoneal dialysis?, *Perit Dial Int* 21 Suppl 3:S179-84, 2001.
176. Schaefer F, Klaus G, Mehls O: Peritoneal transport properties and dialysis dose affect growth and nutritional status in children on chronic peritoneal dialysis. Mid-European Pediatric Peritoneal Dialysis Study Group, *J Am Soc Nephrol* 10:1786-92, 1999.
177. Heaf J: High transport and malnutrition-inflammation-atherosclerosis (MIA) syndrome, *Perit Dial Int* 23:109-10, 2003.
178. Tom A, McCauley L, Bell L, et al: Growth during maintenance hemodialysis: impact of enhanced nutrition and clearance, *J Pediatr* 134:464-71, 1999.
179. Fischbach M, Terzic J, Laugel V, et al: Daily on-line haemodiafiltration: a pilot trial in children, *Nephrol Dial Transplant* 19:2360-67, 2004.
180. Saenger P, Wiedemann E, Schwartz E, et al: Somatomedin and growth after renal transplantation, *Pediatr Res* 8:163-9, 1974.
181. Kleinknecht C, Broyer M, Gagnadoux MF, et al: Growth in children treated with long-term dialysis. A study of 76 patients, *Adv Nephrol Necker Hosp* 9:133-63, 1980.
182. Tejani A, Butt KM, Rajpoot D, et al: Strategies for optimizing growth in children with kidney transplants, *Transplantation* 47:229-33, 1989.
183. Hokken-Koelega AC, van Zaal MA, de Ridder MA, et al: Growth after renal transplantation in prepubertal children: impact of various treatment modalities, *Pediatr Res* 35:367-71, 1994.
184. Ellis D: Clinical use of tacrolimus (FK-506) in infants and children with renal transplants, *Pediatr Nephrol* 9:487-94, 1995.
185. Kohaut EC, Tejani A: The 1994 annual report of the North American Pediatric Renal Transplant Cooperative Study, *Pediatr Nephrol* 10:422-34, 1996.
186. Tejani A, Cortes L, Sullivan EK: A longitudinal study of the natural history of growth post-transplantation, *Kidney Int Suppl* 53:103-08, 1996.
187. Vester U, Schaefer A, Kranz B, et al: Development of growth and body mass index after pediatric renal transplantation, *Pediatr Transplant* 9:445-49, 2005.
188. Sarna S, Hoppu K, Neuvonen PJ, Laine J, Holmberg C: Methylprednisolone exposure, rather than dose, predicts adrenal suppression and growth inhibition in children with liver and renal transplants, *J Clin Endocrinol Metab* 82:75-77, 1997.
189. Seikku P, Raivio T, Janne OA, Neuvonen PJ, Holmberg C: Methylprednisolone exposure in pediatric renal transplant patients, *Am J Transplant* 6:1451-8, 2006.
190. Feldhoff C, Goldman AI, Najarian JS, Mauer SM: A comparison of alternate day and daily steroid therapy in children following renal transplantation, *Int J Pediatr Nephrol* 5:11-14, 1984.
191. Kaiser BA, Polinsky MS, Palmer JA, et al: Growth after conversion to alternate-day corticosteroids in children with renal transplants: a single-center study, *Pediatr Nephrol* 8:320-25, 1994.
192. Jabs K, Sullivan EK, Avner ED, Harmon WE: Alternate-day steroid dosing improves growth without adversely affecting graft survival or long-term graft function. A report of the North American Pedi-

atric Renal Transplant Cooperative Study, *Transplantation* 61:31-36, 1996.
193. Broyer M, Guest G, Gagnadoux MF: Growth rate in children receiving alternate-day corticosteroid treatment after kidney transplantation, *J Pediatr* 120:721-25, 1992.
194. Ingulli E, Tejani AH: Steroid withdrawal after renal transplantation. In Tejani AH, Fine RN, editors: *Pediatric renal transplantation,* New York, 2006, Wiley Liss, pp 221-38.
195. Tönshoff B, Hocker B, Weber LT: Steroid withdrawal in pediatric and adult renal transplant recipients, *Pediatr Nephrol* 20:409-17, 2005.
196. Höcken B, John U, Plank C, et al: Successful withdrawal of steroids in pediatric renal transplant recipients receiving cyclosporine A and mycophenolate mofetil treatment: results after four years, *Transplantation* 78:228-34, 2004.
197. Vidhun JR, Sarwal MM: Corticosteroid avoidance in pediatric renal transplantation, *Pediatr Nephrol* 20:418-26, 2005.
198. Pape L, Ehrich JH, Zivicnjak M, Offner G: Growth in children after kidney transplantation with living related donor graft or cadaveric graft, *Lancet* 366:151-53, 2005.
199. Waller S, Ledermann S, Trompeter R, van't HW, et al: Catch-up growth with normal parathyroid hormone levels in chronic renal failure, *Pediatr Nephrol* 18:1236-41, 2003.
200. Mehls O, Ritz E: Skeletal growth in experimental uremia, *Kidney Int Suppl* 15:S53-62, 1983.
201. Mehls O, Ritz E, Hunziker EB, Eggli P, et al: Improvement of growth and food utilization by human recombinant growth hormone in uremia, *Kidney Int* 33:45-52, 1988.
202. Kovacs G, Fine RN, Worgall S, et al: Growth hormone prevents steroid-induced growth depression in health and uremia, *Kidney Int* 40:1032-40, 1991.
203. Powell DR, Durham SK, Liu F, et al: The insulin-like growth factor axis and growth in children with chronic renal failure: a report of the Southwest Pediatric Nephrology Study Group, *J Clin Endocrinol Metab* 83:1654-61, 1998.
204. Bereket A, Lang CH, Blethen SL, Kaskel FJ, et al: Growth hormone treatment in growth retarded children with end stage renal failure: effect on free/dissociable IGF-I levels, *J Pediatr Endocrinol Metab* 10:197-202, 1997.
205. Koch VH, Lippe BM, Nelson PA, Boechat MI, et al: Accelerated growth after recombinant human growth hormone treatment of children with chronic renal failure, *J Pediatr* 115:365-71, 1989.
206. Rees L, Rigden SP, Ward G, Preece MA: Treatment of short stature in renal disease with recombinant human growth hormone, *Arch Dis Child* 65:856-60, 1990.
207. Tönshoff B, Dietz M, Haffner D, Tonshoff C, et al: Effects of two years of growth hormone treatment in short children with renal disease. The German Study Group for Growth Hormone Treatment in Chronic Renal Failure, *Acta Paediatr Scand Suppl* 379:33-41, 1991.
208. Hokken-Koelega AC, Stijnen T, de Muinck Keizer-Schrama SM, et al: Placebo-controlled, double-blind, cross-over trial of growth hormone treatment in prepubertal children with chronic renal failure, *Lancet* 338:585-90, 1991.
209. Fine RN, Kohaut EC, Brown D, Perlman AJ: Growth after recombinant human growth hormone treatment in children with chronic renal failure: report of a multicenter randomized double-blind placebo-controlled study. Genentech Cooperative Study Group, *J Pediatr* 124:374-82, 1994.
210. Haffner D, Wuhl E, Schaefer F, Nissel R, et al: Factors predictive of the short- and long-term efficacy of growth hormone treatment in prepubertal children with chronic renal failure. The German Study Group for Growth Hormone Treatment in Chronic Renal Failure, *J Am Soc Nephrol* 9:1899-907, 1998.
211. Fine RN, Kohaut E, Brown D, Kuntze J, Attie KM: Long-term treatment of growth retarded children with chronic renal insufficiency, with recombinant human growth hormone, *Kidney Int* 49:781-85, 1996.
212. Hokken-Koelega AC, Mulder P, De JR, Lilien M, et al: Long-term effects of growth hormone treatment on growth and puberty in patients with chronic renal insufficiency, *Pediatr Nephrol* 14:701-06, 2000.
213. Wühl E, Haffner D, Nissel R, Schaefer F, Mehls O: Short dialyzed children respond less to growth hormone than patients prior to dialysis. German Study Group for Growth Hormone Treatment in Chronic Renal Failure, *Pediatr Nephrol* 10:294-98, 1996.
214. Berard E, Crosnier H, Six-Beneton A, Chevallier T, et al: Recombinant human growth hormone treatment of children on hemodialysis. French Society of Pediatric Nephrology, *Pediatr Nephrol* 12:304-10, 1998.
215. Schaefer F, Wuhl E, Haffner D, Mehls O: Stimulation of growth by recombinant human growth hormone in children undergoing peritoneal or hemodialysis treatment. German Study Group for Growth Hormone Treatment in Chronic Renal Failure, *Adv Perit Dial* 10:321-26, 1994.
216. Wühl E, Haffner D, Gretz N, et al: Treatment with recombinant human growth hormone in short children with nephropathic cystinosis: no evidence for increased deterioration rate of renal function. The European Study Group on Growth Hormone Treatment in Short Children with Nephropathic Cystinosis, *Pediatr Res* 43:484-88, 1998.
217. Fine RN, Attie KM, Kuntze J, Brown DF, Kohaut EC: Recombinant human growth hormone in infants and young children with chronic renal insufficiency. Genentech Collaborative Study Group, *Pediatr Nephrol* 9:451-57, 1995.
218. Maxwell H, Rees L: Recombinant human growth hormone treatment in infants with chronic renal failure, *Arch Dis Child* 74:40-43, 1996.
219. Johansson G, Sietnieks A, Janssens F, et al: Recombinant human growth hormone treatment in short children with chronic renal disease, before transplantation or with functioning renal transplants: an interim report on five European studies, *Acta Paediatr Scand Suppl* 370:36-42, 1990.
220. Fine RN, Yadin O, Nelson PA, et al: Recombinant human growth hormone treatment of children following renal transplantation, *Pediatr Nephrol* 5:147-51, 1991.
221. Bartosh S, Kaiser B, Rezvani I, et al: Effects of growth hormone administration in pediatric renal allograft recipients, *Pediatr Nephrol* 6:68-73, 1992.
222. Van DC, Jabs KL, Donohoue PA, Bock GH, et al: Accelerated growth rates in children treated with growth hormone after renal transplantation, *J Pediatr* 120:244-50, 1992.
223. Benfield MR, Parker KL, Waldo FB, Overstreet SL, Kohaut EC: Treatment of growth failure in children after renal transplantation, *Transplantation* 55:305-08, 1993.
224. Jabs K, Van DC, Harmon WE: Growth hormone treatment of growth failure among children with renal transplants, *Kidney Int Suppl* 43:S71-75, 1993.
225. Janssen F, Van Damme-Lombaerts R, Van DM, et al: Effects of recombinant human growth hormone on graft function in renal-transplanted children and adolescents: the three-year experience of a Belgian study group, *Transplant Proc* 25:1049-50, 1993.
226. Tönshoff B, Haffner D, Mehls O, et al: Efficacy and safety of growth hormone treatment in short children with renal allografts: three year experience. Members of the German Study Group for Growth Hormone Treatment in Children with Renal Allografts, *Kidney Int* 44:199-207, 1993.
227. Wühl E, Haffner D, Tonshoff B, Mehls O: Predictors of growth response to rhGH in short children before and after renal transplantation. German Study Group for Growth Hormone Treatment in Chronic Renal Failure, *Kidney Int Suppl* 43:S76-82, 1993.
228. Hokken-Koelega AC, Stijnen T, de Jong RC, et al: A placebo-controlled, double-blind trial of growth hormone treatment in prepubertal children after renal transplant, *Kidney Int Suppl* 53:S128-34, 1996.
229. Maxwell H, Dalton RN, Nair DR, et al: Effects of recombinant human growth hormone on renal function in children with renal transplants, *J Pediatr* 128:177-83, 1996.
230. Janssen F, Van Damme-Lombaerts R, Van DM, et al: Impact of growth hormone treatment on a Belgian population of short children with renal allografts, *Pediatr Transplant* 1:190-96, 1997.
231. Guest G, Berard E, Crosnier H, Chevallier T, et al: Effects of growth hormone in short children after renal transplantation. French Society of Pediatric Nephrology, *Pediatr Nephrol* 12:437-46, 1998.

232. Maxwell H, Rees L: Randomised controlled trial of recombinant human growth hormone in prepubertal and pubertal renal transplant recipients. British Association for Pediatric Nephrology, *Arch Dis Child* 79:481-87, 1998.
233. Fine RN, Stablein D, Cohen AH, Tejani A, Kohaut E: Recombinant human growth hormone post-renal transplantation in children: a randomized controlled study of the NAPRTCS, *Kidney Int* 62:688-96, 2002.
234. Hokken-Koelega AC, Stijnen T, de Ridder MA, et al: Growth hormone treatment in growth-retarded adolescents after renal transplant, *Lancet* 343:1313-17, 1994.
235. Mehls O, Berg U, Broyer M: Chronic renal failure and growth hormone treatment: review of the literature and experience in KIGS. In Ranke MB, Wilton P, editors: *Growth hormone therapy in K-10 years experience*, Heidelberg, Germany, 1999, Barth, pp 327-40.
236. Fine RN, Sullivan EK, Tejani A: The impact of recombinant human growth hormone treatment on final adult height, *Pediatr Nephrol* 14:679-81, 2000.
237. Rees L, Ward G, Rigden SP: Growth over 10 years following a 1-year trial of growth hormone therapy, *Pediatr Nephrol* 14:309-14, 2000.
238. Hokken-Koelega AC, Nauta J, Lilien M, Ploos van Amstel J, Levcenko N: Long-term growth hormone treatment in children with chronic renal failure, *Pediatr Nephrol* 19:C38(S04.3), 2004.
239. Fine RN, Stablein D: Long-term use of recombinant human growth hormone in pediatric allograft recipients: a report of the NAPRTCS Transplant Registry, *Pediatr Nephrol* 20:404-08, 2005.
240. Nissel R, Ucur E, Mehls O, Haffner D: Final height after long-term treatment with recombinant human growth hormone (rhGH) in children with uremic growth failure, *Nephrol Dial Transplant* 21(Suppl 4):367-68, 2006.
241. Fine RN, Pyke-Grimm K, Nelson PA, et al: Recombinant human growth hormone treatment of children with chronic renal failure: long-term (1- to 3-year) outcome, *Pediatr Nephrol* 5:477-81, 1991.
242. Hokken-Koelega AC, Stijnen T, de Jong MC, et al: Double blind trial comparing the effects of two doses of growth hormone in prepubertal patients with chronic renal insufficiency, *J Clin Endocrinol Metab* 79:1185-90, 1994.
243. Fine RN, Brown DF, Kuntze J, Wooster P, Kohaut EE: Growth after discontinuation of recombinant human growth hormone therapy in children with chronic renal insufficiency. The Genentech Cooperative Study Group, *J Pediatr* 129:883-91, 1996.
244. Fine RN, Ho M, Tejani A, Blethen S: Adverse events with rhGH treatment of patients with chronic renal insufficiency and end-stage renal disease, *J Pediatr* 142:539-45, 2003.
245. Koller EA, Stadel BV, Malozowski SN: Papilledema in 15 renally compromised patients treated with growth hormone, *Pediatr Nephrol* 11:451-54, 1997.
246. Haffner D, Nissel R, Wuhl E, et al: Metabolic effects of long-term growth hormone treatment in prepubertal children with chronic renal failure and after kidney transplantation. The German Study Group for Growth Hormone Treatment in Chronic Renal Failure, *Pediatr Res* 43:209-15, 1998.
247. Kaufman DB: Growth hormone and renal osteodystrophy: a case report, *Pediatr Nephrol* 12:157-59, 1998.
248. Picca S, Cappa M, Rizzoni G: Hyperparathyroidism during growth hormone treatment: a role for puberty?, *Pediatr Nephrol* 14:56-58, 2000.
249. Mentser M, Breen TJ, Sullivan EK, Fine RN: Growth-hormone treatment of renal transplant recipients: the National Cooperative Growth Study experience—a report of the National Cooperative Growth Study and the North American Pediatric Renal Transplant Cooperative Study, *J Pediatr* 131:S20-24, 1997.

CHAPTER

47 Neurodevelopmental Issues in Chronic Renal Disease

Debbie S. Gipson and Stephen Hooper

NEURODEVELOPMENTAL PROCESSES IN CHILDREN AND ADOLESCENTS

Nephrologists must contend with a large array of variables when working with individuals with kidney disease. Issues of severity, progression, treatment options, and the timing of the implementation of these treatment options, to mention just a few of these variables, are all critical when working with patients with this condition. For the pediatric nephrologist, issues pertinent to development also enter into the clinical conceptualization of any specific case. For example, the age of onset, the chronicity of the illness, and factors related to family, school, and social functioning also must be considered for the clinical care for a child. For the pediatric nephrologist, this will entail a multidisciplinary management team that includes other childhood professionals such as psychologists, social workers, psychiatrists, and teachers as well as a working knowledge of how the kidney disease may affect a variety of neurodevelopmental processes. Unfortunately, the study of neurodevelopmental processes likely is not a primary area of academic or clinical investigation for most pediatric nephrologists.

It is important to recognize that there are significant differences between child and adult brain functioning. Early work pointed to the notion that early brain insults to a child would cause a lesser degree of sequelae as compared with the same insult incurred by an adult (i.e., the Kennard Principle); however, more contemporary efforts actually have documented the opposite finding, with children who have sustained early neurologic insults showing more pervasive and, perhaps, severe effects from these insults. Furthermore, Dennis[1] has suggested that the degree and severity of insult are likely related to when the insult occurs during the neurodevelopmental sequence and to the available cognitive reserve of the individual.

In general, brain development is quite rapid during early childhood, with ongoing changes and growth being more subtle. In addition, expectations of developmental attainment and general cognitive performance change as the child ages. All of these factors pertain to pediatric kidney disease and the importance of the pediatric nephrologist having a working knowledge of basic neurodevelopment. In fact, it could be asserted that one of the basic premises of this chapter is that the neurodevelopmental status should always be taken into account when working with children with kidney dysfunction.

A Brief Neurodevelopmental Primer

Brain development begins at conception with the birth of neurons and the subsequent unfolding of the neural tube. These critical processes are followed by three major phases of brain development: cell migration, cell differentiation, and cell death/pruning.[2] At birth, these processes have created a brain that is approximately one fourth of its final weight. Postnatal growth is characterized by further neural differentiation that involves dendritic branching and axonal myelination which, in turn, contribute to increased brain weight and the clearer differentiation of the various sulci and gyri.[3] In addition, these neurodevelopmental processes continue to refine the connections between neurons and to evolve neural pathways in an effort to improve the efficiency of brain functions via a process called *pruning*. The pruning process actually minimizes the number of inefficient connections and maximizes the overall efficiency of the remaining connections, with this process continuing to occur throughout childhood.[4] These neurodevelopmental processes ultimately contribute to the evolution of the primary sensory regions of the brain (i.e., those that deal with major sensory information), then to the secondary brain regions (i.e., those that deal with perceptual functions and sensory integration), and, finally, to tertiary regions, where some of the most critical human functions arguably occur. A disruption of any of these basic neurodevelopmental processes by kidney disease will likely affect the brain-based functioning of any child. Linking these processes to the mechanisms involved in kidney disease may prove to be quite illuminating in terms of what cognitive functions may be affected and vulnerable as a child ages.

Luria's Theoretic Model

Although it is beyond the scope of this chapter to provide a comprehensive description of brain anatomy and related functions, there are heuristic models of brain functioning that may facilitate the integration of neurodevelopmental processes with kidney dysfunction mechanisms. One of those models is Luria's theory of the working brain.

Luria[5] provided one of the first models for understanding how complex human behaviors were processed in the neural network, and his work continues as one of the more influential conceptualizations to this day. For example, Luria noted that most complex human functions were not localized to specific brain regions but rather that they were intricately conducted via interdependent neural connections called *functional systems*. These functional systems provided an avenue for understanding how various brain systems worked together as well as what might happen when one of the components became dysfunctional.

With respect to the development of these functional systems, Luria described the hierarchic organization of various brain regions. The primary zones receive information from afferent subcortical structures, and they are geographically located in the occipital, temporal, and parietal lobules, which correspond with basic visual, auditory, and somatosensory sensations, respectively. The primary zones are uniquely unimodal, and they provide signals to the secondary zones (or the association cortex), where the information continues to be unimodal but where the beginning stages of perception begin. From a neurodevelopmental perspective, the primary zones are present and functional shortly after birth, whereas the secondary zones become functional around 12 months of age and continue to evolve through the ages of 5 to 6 years. The tertiary zones provide the cortical regions, where information from the secondary zones is integrated, organized, and comprehended. The tertiary cortex is multimodal in nature; it slowly begins its developmental unfolding early during the preschool years, and this extends into young adulthood. It is because of this prolonged unfolding in cortical regions such as the frontal lobes, where ongoing development can occur into the second and third decades of life (particularly in females), that an injury to such regions can lie "silent" until environmental demands are placed on these higher-order functions. It remains unclear how this developmental trajectory will be affected by kidney disease.

Finally, Luria integrated these zones of proximal development into three functional brain units. Unit I comprises the brain stem and the associated reticular activating system, and it is responsible for general arousal and core regulatory functions. Disruption to this functional unit will likely manifest as problems with the behavioral regulation of the sleep-wake cycle, under- or overarousal, and general cortical tone. Unit II is comprised of the occipital, parietal, and temporal lobes, and it is generally responsible for information input. Unit II is where information from the auditory, visual, and somatosensory cortices is encoded, analyzed, and stored for use. Disruptions to any part of unit II will create problems with information processing (e.g., receptive language disorder, visual-spatial deficits). Finally, unit III comprises the entire frontal lobe, and it is responsible for many higher-order functions, such as organizing, planning, and general information output. Disruptions to this unit can create specific or generalized problems with organization, inhibition, initiation, shifting from one task to another, and attention regulation. In accordance with the zones of proximal development, these functional units develop in a sequential fashion. Unit I is operational at birth; unit II is in place around 12 months of age and continues to evolve through the preschool years; and unit III begins its development during the preschool years, and this continues into young adulthood. More generally, it is important to note that damage or disruption to one functional unit likely will affect the other functional units, because they are interdependent on one another for information input and output. Luria's proposed units of the brain and the suspected developmental sequence of these brain regions can be seen in Figure 47-1.

On the basis of Luria's model of brain development, the functional units and associated zones of proximal development contribute to the operation of a number of critical brain functions, including motor, sensory, attention, language, visual-spatial, memory, and executive functions.[6] Table 47-1 provides a listing of these brain functions, their subcompo-

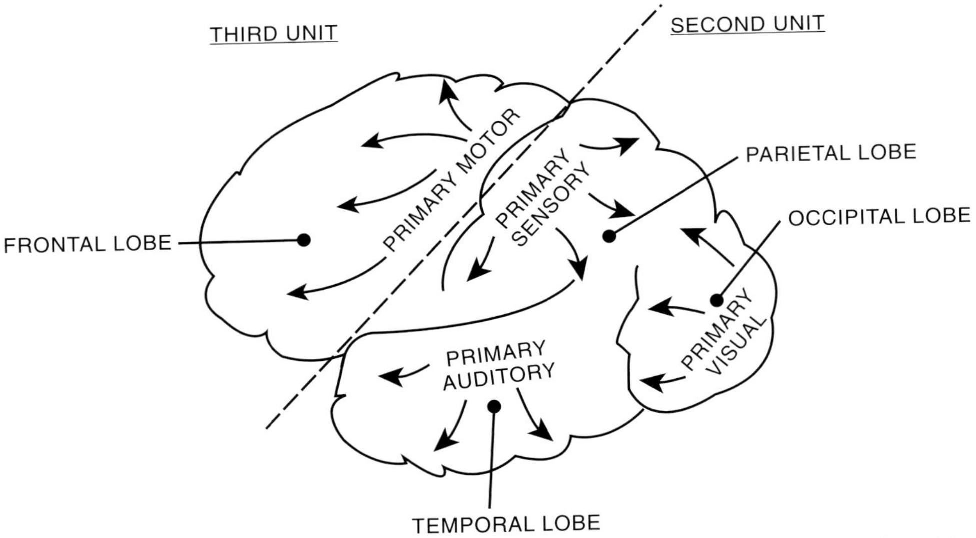

Figure 47-1 Brain units and the developmental sequence of the brain regions according to Luria's model.

TABLE 47-1 Basic Brain Functions, Subcomponents, and Examples of Assessments for the Measurement of Children and Adolescents

Basic Brain Functions	Subcomponents	Assessment Examples*
Motor	Fine motor, gross motor	Peabody Motor Scale
Sensory	Visual, auditory, tactile, gustatory, smell	Dean-Woodcock Sensory-Motor Battery
Attention	Encoding, selective, sustained	Conners Continuous Performance Test II; digit span and digit cancellation tasks
Language	Receptive, expressive, pragmatic	Clinical Evaluation of Language Fundamentals IV
Visual-spatial	Visual discrimination, visual-spatial, visual-constructive	Benton Form Recognition Test; Benton Judgment of Line Orientation Test; Developmental Test of Visual-Motor Integration
Memory	Short term versus long term, procedural versus declarative	Wide Range Assessment of Memory and Learning 2; Children's Memory Scale
Executive	Initiation, sustaining, set shifting, inhibition, working memory	Delis-Kaplan Executive Function System; Wechsler Intelligence Scale for Children IV Working Memory Composite; Woodcock-Johnson III Working Memory Composite

* These examples are provided for latency-aged children and adolescents. Similar measures can be selected for infants, preschoolers, younger school-aged children, older adolescents, and young adults.

nents, and examples of the assessment tasks that could be employed to measure these functions. Although many of these types of measures typically would be administered by a psychologist, a neuropsychologist, or another trained professional (e.g., a speech and language pathologist, a physical therapist, an occupational therapist), it is important for the pediatric nephrologist to have a working knowledge of why it may be necessary to obtain such assessments for the clinical care and management of a child with kidney disease. Findings from such evaluations should prove useful for detailing the relative strengths and weaknesses of cognitive functioning that may be present; they should also assist with the securing of necessary school programming and services, guide how best to interact with the client with regard to medical needs and compliance issues, and suggest cognitive functions (e.g., attention regulation, memory) that may require closer monitoring as kidney disease progresses and/or different treatments are implemented. As will be discussed later in this chapter, the neurocognitive functioning of children and adolescents with kidney disease is beginning to receive closer attention.[7] Given the apparent risks that kidney dysfunction can directly and indirectly impose on an individual's cognitive abilities, a working knowledge of neurodevelopmental processes and associated neurocognitive functions on the part of the pediatric nephrologist will be useful for identifying such concerns at an earlier time point in the treatment of kidney disease.

CENTRAL NERVOUS SYSTEM STRUCTURE

Given these typical neurodevelopmental processes and associated brain functions, the examination of brain morphology and functions is also of strong interest in the structure-function continuum. In fact, seminal brain imaging studies of the early 1980s found several cortical abnormalities in children with end-stage renal disease (ESRD). Computed tomography scanning and magnetic resonance imaging have been used to verify neuroanatomic abnormalities such as cerebral atrophy and infarcts in children with ESRD.[8-11] Cerebral atrophy has been documented in children with chronic kidney failure at a frequency that is higher than expected for age and for the general population[9] (Figure 47-2). Research has focused on certain disease populations who are at greater risk for central nervous system (CNS) dysfunction than the general chronic kidney disease (CKD) population. In a cohort of pediatric transplant recipients with congenital nephrotic syndrome as the majority diagnosis, 18 out of 33 (54%) patients had chronic infarct lesions, mostly within the periventricular white matter, and cerebral atrophy was found in 5 out of 33 (15%) patients.[10,12] Evidence of white matter lesions in this sample of patients with congenital nephrotic syndrome was highly correlated with transplantation at a later age ($p < .05$), a longer duration of dialysis ($p < .02$), and a history of hemodynamic crisis ($p < .03$).[12] Pediatric patients with cystinosis also showed that 10 out of 11 (91%) patients had cortical atrophy.[13] Case studies of the CNS and renal involvement of patients with Lowe syndrome have also suggested the presence of cerebral atrophy and seizure disorders.[14] In summary, children with CKD are at risk for CNS structural abnormalities of atrophy and infarcts. These lesions may be observed with greater frequency in populations who are at risk for coagulation disorders (i.e., patients with congenital nephrotic syndrome and anticardiolipin syndrome) and among those with a history of vascular insults that may be acute (e.g., hypertensive crisis) or chronic (e.g., prolonged dialysis dependence).

DEVELOPMENTAL STATUS IN CHRONIC KIDNEY DISEASE

The neurodevelopmental function of the developing child can be assessed through neuropsychologic testing and educational

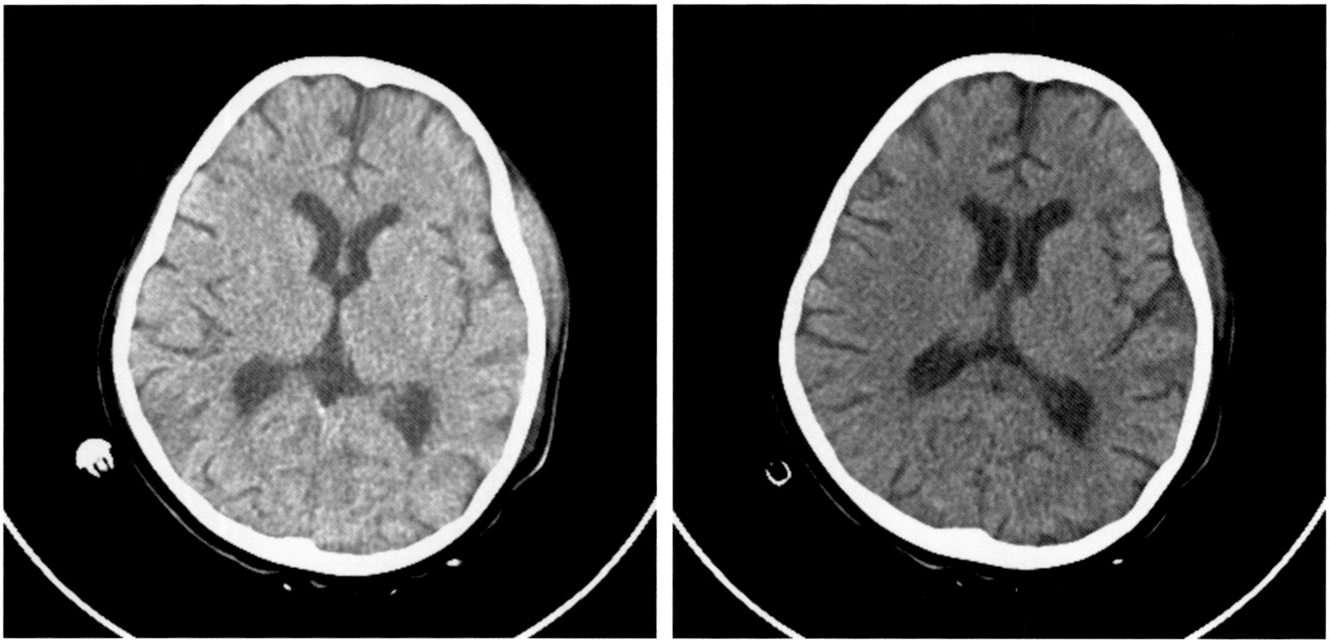

Figure 47-2 **A** and **B,** Computed tomography images of a preschool-aged child with cortical atrophy associated with end-stage kidney disease.

achievement. A multitude of studies over the past three decades has documented delays in neurocognitive development in children with CKD. Consistent with Dennis' theory of brain impairment is that the developmental impact of renal failure has been noted, especially when the disease onset is early during childhood[15,16] and when CKD is severe.[17-20] In addition, there are a multitude of other factors that can influence the cognitive and academic potential of all children, including environment, opportunity, school absenteeism, parental education status, and personal motivation. Given these global factors, the neurodevelopmental status of a child with a chronic health condition will rely on disease-specific risk factors as well as the global influences of the home and family environment.

The assessment of these neurodevelopmental or neuropsychologic functions typically has employed the cognitive domains of general intelligence, attention, executive function, language, visual-spatial abilities, and memory (see Table 47-1). Although infants from the ages of birth to 2 years will require different kinds of assessment strategies to measure these functions, these functions appear to be rather robust across the age span.

Cognitive Functioning

Preschool Age

Considering the vulnerability of the developing brain in infants and young children, one would expect a significant loss of neurodevelopmental progress among preschoolers with CKD. Indeed, several studies have evaluated the general development of children younger than 5 years old using the developmental quotient and the intelligence quotient (IQ). The findings of delayed general, motor, and mental neurodevelopmental testing have been documented in dialysis-dependent children as compared with children with renal insufficiency or the normal population.[21-23] In two separate studies of dialysis-dependent infants, 21% to 25% of infants showed a low average to an impaired range of general development.[23] In a 5-year longitudinal evaluation, full-scale IQ was reported to be within the low or the low-normal range for 21% of transplant recipients who had ESRD from infancy, with 28% showing a low verbal IQ and 44% showing a low nonverbal IQ.[23] Taken together, these studies suggest that approximately 20% to 25% of very young children with ESRD show general developmental delays, and neurodevelopmental impairment appears to be greater with the most severe kidney disease. These developmental concerns appear to persist after a successful kidney transplant, when the insults of CKD begin at the earliest and perhaps the most vulnerable stage of postnatal neurodevelopment. According to Luria's theory, the primary and secondary brain regions could be disrupted in this regard, and these disruptions could put the tertiary brain regions (i.e., the prefrontal regions) at increased risk for an altered developmental trajectory.

School Age

For school-aged children and adolescents with CKD, formal measures of intelligence, IQ, and specific cognitive domains can be obtained. In general, school-aged children with CKD show an IQ distribution that is shifted downward as compared with the normal population.[10,19,21,24,25] The children with ESRD have lower total, verbal, and performance IQs as compared with siblings or healthy control groups.[20,26] When comparing IQs among children treated with different modalities of ESRD therapy, transplant recipients tend to have higher IQs, especially for nonverbal abilities, as compared with dialysis-dependent children or when individual cases are compared at pretransplant versus posttransplant time points.[19,25,27] Conversely, one cross-sectional study found no significant differences in the intellectual functioning of a transplant group as compared with a dialysis-dependent group.[20]

Specific Neurocognitive Functioning

Language The assessment of language typically involves the evaluation of expressive and receptive language, with pragmatic language abilities becoming important to assess with advancing age. Two published studies have evaluated language abilities in children with CKD. Fennell and colleagues[29] found deficits in the verbal abstraction abilities of a cohort of 56 children with CKD as compared with a matched control group. By contrast, Qvist and colleagues[10] documented no deficits in language in their group of 33 pediatric transplant recipients as compared with the normative population, with only 6% of children having problems on language tasks. Furthermore, among children with CKD, the prevalence of hearing loss has been reported to be approximately 8%.[28] Unrecognized or uncorrected hearing loss may impair the development of language skills in young children and the full functioning of the reception of auditory stimuli. The unrecognized or delayed diagnosis of hearing impairment may impede language development independent of the impact of CKD. Research addressing language assessment in children may exclude those with known hearing loss; thus, the language functioning of children with CKD may not be fully represented in published documents.[24] More research is needed within this cognitive domain to determine whether language abilities are an area of concern for preschool- and school-aged children with CKD, particularly with respect to potential delays that may result from hearing impairment. In addition, the assessment of auditory acuity should be a mandatory component of pediatric CKD management to maximize language development.

Visual-Spatial Abilities The perception and construction of two- and three-dimensional forms are fundamental cognitive functions. In patients with CKD, these functions are diminished as a result of renal insufficiency and renal failure. Fennell and colleagues[29] documented deficits in visual-motor abilities in a cohort of 56 children with CKD as compared with a matched typical sample. Similarly, Bawden and colleagues[26] showed that their group of children with ESRD demonstrated significantly lower visual-constructive abilities as compared with sibling controls. By contrast, Qvist and colleagues[10] documented no overall group deficits in the visual-spatial abilities of their sample of transplant recipients as compared with the normative population; however, nearly a quarter of their sample did show visual-spatial deficits. The presence of significant visual disturbances will prevent an accurate assessment of visual-spatial functioning. Visual disturbances have been described in 8% of the Dutch cohort of pediatric transplant recipients collected over a 20-year period.[28] The current literature supports a concern that visual-spatial abilities are diminished in children with CKD with a greater frequency than what is expected in the normative population.

Memory The characterization of memory can be defined in a global way or via different components (e.g., procedural versus declarative; short term versus long term). Children with CKD have been described as experiencing a variety of memory deficits. In a heterogeneous sample of children with CKD, Fennell and colleagues[29] documented lower memory abilities for children with CKD as compared with controls. The memory skills deteriorated over a 1-year period, regardless of treatment modality, which gives rise to concerns about a gradual loss of function as a child survives with CKD. More recently, using a nontransplant sample of children with CKD, Gipson and colleagues[30] showed significantly lower memory abilities in children with CKD as compared with healthy, age-matched children. Specifically, the CKD group demonstrated poorer short-term visual memory, short-term verbal memory, and new learning, with specific concerns for the integrity of working memory functions. In transplant recipients, 20% of a cohort of 33 patients displayed general memory deficits.[10] In a within-patient study of 9 children, mean working memory improved after successful kidney transplantation.[19] A deficit in memory can impair a child or adolescent in the educational and medical environments, particularly with respect to learning, retention, and retrieval of facts and problem solving. The communication of information may require repetition, different types of information presentations (e.g., verbal versus written forms), and the more frequent assessment of retention for successful educational attainment and self-management as the child matures.

Attention and Executive Functions The attention and executive functions are multidimensional, but they involve a number of strongly interrelated abilities. Attention, for example is comprised of a variety of abilities that relate to the encoding of information, selective attention, and sustained attention. Each of these attention abilities may be critical to how a child performs on a specific task or in the classroom environment. Qvist and colleagues[10] reported no group deficits of attention in a renal transplant sample as compared with the normative population; however, 24% of their sample showed generalized attention deficits. Attention abilities have also been compared in children with severe CKD both before and after transplantation in a small study of 9 patients.[19] In this study, improvements in sustained attention and mental processing speed were observed 1 year after transplant.

Similarly, executive functions are multidimensional and comprise higher-order brain processes that include problem solving, set shifting, self-monitoring, planning, and working memory. Denckla[31] has proposed a model of executive functions that includes the following: initiation (i.e., the planning phase and the beginning of a complex task); sustaining (i.e., the continuation of the task over time); set shifting (i.e., changing from one task or problem-solving set to another); and inhibiting (i.e., the regulation of output in an adaptive fashion). Children with stages 2 through 5 CKD (i.e., glomerular filtration rates of <90 ml/min/1.73 m^2) have shown difficulties with problem solving as compared with a typically developing comparison group.[30] The 20 patients with CKD who were studied had difficulty with the initiation and sustaining functions, even after controlling for IQ. The processes involved in set shifting and inhibition were preserved, which may represent the ease with which an activity can be stopped when the child's attention is already waning. These findings set CKD apart from other disorders with which either pervasive or other specific executive function patterns may be present (e.g., fragile X syndrome, autism). The present literature suggests that children with CKD have deficits in attention and executive function that may improve—but not fully abate—with transplantation. Further, in accordance with Luria's neurodevelopmental theory, these findings also suggest disruption in the development of selected prefrontal brain regions that involve initiation and sustaining behaviors.

Summary Across these specific domains of cognition, the findings clearly point to significant concerns for the neuropsychologic integrity of children with CKD, even after successful kidney transplantation. Although several of these domains require more scientific inquiry (e.g., language, visual-spatial function), the frequency of poor cognitive performance with regard to attention, executive function, and memory have stood the test of reproducibility. The contemporary findings across both the intellectual and neurocognitive domains would suggest the need for developmental surveillance by the pediatric nephrologist and developmental specialists beginning well before the onset of ESRD. Partnering with school and developmental specialists can then allow for early intervention when cognitive deficits are identified.

SOCIAL-BEHAVIORAL FUNCTIONING

The extant literature provides no direct links between the neurodevelopmental effects of childhood CKD and later social and emotional functioning. When given quality-of-life questionnaires, both transplant and dialysis-dependent children have reported difficulty with social functioning, self-esteem, and lower general health perception as compared with a healthy control group.[32] In cross-sectional comparison, self- and parent perception of quality of life is best in the healthy controls; it diminishes in transplant recipients, and it is poorest in dialysis-dependent patients.[33] Social milestones are often delayed with chronic illness, and this finding has been confirmed in the ESRD population specifically.[34] Young-adult survivors of childhood-onset ESRD have fewer friends, are less likely to participate in extracurricular activities, and are less likely to establish intimate relationships as compared with their healthy peers.[34]

Psychiatric challenges including depression and anxiety have been reported in children with CKD. Early literature described a high frequency of depression in children with ESRD, including 5 out of 8 pediatric dialysis-dependent children in a single North American report and 17 out of 26 children in a Japanese study.[35,36] More recent data have shown no difference in depressive symptoms across all modalities of therapy in 73 adolescents with CKD.[37] Depression is a frequent psychiatric problem that is found in adult patients with ESRD,[38] and it has been linked to health outcomes such as peritonitis rates and dialysis withdrawal.[39,40] Interestingly, adult patients with ESRD since childhood report having an overall better mental health perception than patients with adult-onset ESRD.[32] Anxiety is observed in increased rates among children with chronic renal insufficiency as compared with the general population.[35,36] Similarly, parents of children with CKD are at risk for anxiety and stress, because the burden of a chronic health condition is often significant. The recognition of the early signs and symptoms of common psychiatric disorders such as depression and anxiety in children and adolescents with CKD and early referral for therapy for affected individuals and families should be a routine part of the management program. Ultimately, the collection of population-based data for depression with links to health outcome and response to intervention would be a significant step forward for this disease population.

COMORBIDITIES AND RISK FACTORS FOR DEVELOPMENTAL DYSFUNCTION

The complications of CKD including anemia, hypertension, cerebral vascular accidents, and adverse effects of therapy may contribute to neurodevelopmental disturbances. The relationship between anemia and cognitive dysfunction has been established in the general pediatrics community[41,42] and in adults with ESRD.[43,44] The findings of slowed CNS response to stimuli, poor attention, and poor cognitive performance have been improved by the restoration of normal or near-normal hemoglobin values with iron and erythropoietin agonists.[45] Rather than attributing all of the improvement to hemoglobin increases alone, accumulating literature supports a role of normalizing iron stores with a direct impact on neurotransmitters as a source of at least some of the observed improvement in cognitive function with the management of iron deficiency and anemia.[46]

Hypertensive emergencies with symptoms of acute encephalopathy and the risk for CNS infarcts are recognized risks for children with acute kidney disease and CKD. Qvist and colleagues[10] have documented overt and silent infarcts in a pediatric population of kidney transplant recipients; the children with infarcts were more likely to require special education services than those without such lesions.

Therapies for CKD may have side effects that affect CNS function. The example of aluminum neurotoxicity is perhaps the most extreme. The exposure of children and adults to high volumes of water through dialysis therapies and to aluminum-containing phosphorus binders has led to aluminum deposition in the CNS, which results in symptoms of cognitive deterioration. This toxicity was recognized during the 1970s, and modifications to water-treatment systems and the avoidance of aluminum-containing medications has profoundly reduced this source of neurotoxicity.

Antihypertensive agents may also have CNS effects. Agents such as clonidine may be used for the dual purpose of blood pressure and attention-deficit disorder control. Conversely, the side effect of somnolence of this agent may not completely reverse over time, and it may contribute to diminished cognitive performance.[47] Other agents (e.g., beta-blockers) may cause diminished working memory, and they may worsen affective disorders such as depression, which reverses with the discontinuation of the medication.[48]

Comorbidities associated with renal disease include many syndromes with CNS structural or functional abnormalities. These problems may be congenital, such as those seen in patients with Joubert syndrome (i.e., global developmental delay, cerebellar malformations, hypotonia) and Down syndrome (i.e., generalized developmental delays). Prematurity alone is a risk factor for neurodevelopmental impairment, which may be compounded by the onset of CKD.[49] Acquired difficulties may occur with disorders that predispose individuals to CNS thrombotic events, such as nephrotic syndrome, complex cardiac lesions, and coagulation disorders. These coexistent conditions are seen in part of the population of children receiving nephrology care. The recognition of these additional risk factors for CNS structural and functional challenges and referral for neurodevelopmental services is often a shared responsibility among the entire management team for these complex children.

EDUCATION OF THE CHILD WITH CHRONIC KIDNEY DISEASE

The vast majority of children with CKD attend full-time school in a traditional setting.[10,23] On the basis of the neurodevelopmental challenges that accompany CKD,[18] one might expect a significant need for special educational services. In North America, an estimated 10% to 15% of school-aged children with CKD receive special education services not related to visual or hearing impairments, which is similar to that seen in the general US population.[50] This figure may represent an ability to perform better than expected as a result of adaptive abilities. Just as one can find a means of performing at peer level with a physical disability, the adaptive capabilities of a child may allow school functioning beyond the predicted level based on neuropsychologic testing. Alternatively, individual educators may assume an academic leniency toward a child with chronic illness, thus making the academic progress appear greater than it is in reality.[51]

When reviewing the cognitive functions summarized previously, one may expect limitations in math and language skills on the basis of difficulties with executive functioning and memory domains. In general, the available studies suggest that dialysis-dependent children have difficulties with the broad academic areas of math, reading, and language and that performance in these areas may improve in the successful transplant recipient.[25] Comparisons of matched patient and sibling performance with regard to these academic achievement scores are not consistent. Brouhard and colleagues[20] reported findings that showed that the combined ESRD group (transplant and dialysis) had lower achievement scores than their sibling controls in math, reading, and spelling. By contrast, Bawden and colleagues[26] demonstrated that children with ESRD showed no group differences on various measures of math, basic reading, reading comprehension, phonologic processing, and spelling as compared with their sibling controls. In data from the Chapel Hill cohort, children with significant renal dysfunction (estimate glomerular filtration rate of <30 ml/min/1.73 m^2) have diminished performance in the academic areas of math and reading as compared with healthy, age-matched controls.[52]

Although work continues to find an optimal means of quantifying academic progress across all children with CKD, long-term educational accomplishments have been documented.

LATE EFFECTS OF CHILDHOOD CHRONIC KIDNEY DISEASE

The question of adult outcomes moves from early wondering and concerns on the part of parents during the infant, toddler, preschool, and elementary school years to bona fide worries during the adolescent and adult transition years. Furthermore, neuropsychologic impairment beginning in children with CKD has been shown to persist into adulthood,[26,53] thus suggesting that these problems are more likely neurodevelopmental in origin and that they will manifest throughout life. A Dutch cohort study found that adult survivors of childhood-onset ESRD have a full-scale IQ that is 10.4 points lower than that of controls ($p < 0.0001$), with similar deficits on the verbal and performance subscales.[53] Educational attainment is also lower for adult survivors of childhood-onset ESRD as compared with the general population.[53] A French retrospective study of transplant recipients demonstrated that only 31.2% of these patients had a high-school diploma.[54] In the Dutch transplant cohort, 57% of adult survivors of childhood-onset ESRD were in the lowest educational strata as compared with 27% of the general population.[28] With the burden of a chronic health condition, diminished cognitive function, and lower levels of education, lower rates of employment and low occupational level have been observed in dialysis-dependent and transplant-dependent patients who have survived childhood-onset ESRD.[55] These rates vary by country, with one French report showing employment rates to be similar to those of the general population.[54]

ASSESSMENT AND MANAGEMENT

A targeted approach to the assessment of CNS structure and function begins with the onset of CKD and may include CNS imaging as indicated by a history of poor cranial growth, hemodynamic instability, or prolonged dialysis dependence. Visual and auditory screening should be a part of routine pediatric practice. These results need to be confirmed or newly documented for this vulnerable population. The early assessment of neurodevelopment and/or neurocognitive function for all children with significant impairment of glomerular filtration and for those who have undergone a transplant is recommended. A specific threshold of kidney dysfunction that affects neurodevelopment has not yet been identified, but the onset of problems clearly precedes ESRD.[18,30] This assessment should include a general assessment of neurodevelopmental and/or cognitive abilities using age-appropriate developmental or intelligence measures. Preschool evaluation also includes fine and gross motor skills with anticipatory intervention for infants who are at significant risk of delay. On the basis of the available literature, additional testing for specific abnormalities in the domains of memory, attention, and executive function should be considered for school-aged children. For children who receive a kidney transplant, an evaluation of neurocognitive functions should be conducted both before and after the procedure. This assessment process should be required, and it should prove useful for identifying remaining deficits and for restructuring specific intervention plans. Furthermore, developmental intervention for preschool-aged children and educational support for school-aged children, adolescents, and even adult learners through individual educational plans, tutoring, or special classes will likely optimize the developmental and educational outcomes of individuals with CKD.

CONCLUSIONS

For more than 40 years, the medical literature has documented neurodevelopmental deficits in children and adult survivors of childhood-onset CKD. The progressive maturation of the CNS through young adulthood suggests a vulnerability to developmental deficits across the entire age spectrum of pediatric nephrology care. Although significant work remains, the current literature provides a rationale for routine neurodevelopmental surveillance at regular intervals, an increased use of an interdisciplinary management model, and early intervention for children with CKD. Such procedures should provide additional input into the clinical care and management of children with CKD, particularly with respect to the potential effects of deteriorating kidney functioning on cognitive, adaptive, and social-behavioral abilities. How these neuropsychologic assets and deficits may affect a patient's life course, educational status, and vocational choices remains to be determined, particularly because such factors may also be influenced by socioeconomic status and other family variables.

REFERENCES

1. Dennis M: Childhood medical disorders and cognitive impairment: biological risk, time, development, and reserve. In Yeates KO, Ris MD, Taylor HG, editors: *Pediatric neuropsychology: research, theory and practice*, New York, 2000, Guilford Press, pp 3-24.
2. Kolb B, Fantie B: Development of the child's brain and behavior. In Reynolds CR, Fletcher-Janzen E, editors: *Handbook of clinical child neuropsychology*, ed 2, New York, 1997, Plenum Press, pp 17-41.
3. Majovski LV: Development of higher brain functions in children: neural, cognitive, and behavioral perspectives. In Reynolds CR, Fletcher-Janzen E, editors: *Handbook of clinical child neuropsychology*, ed 2, New York, 1997, Plenum Press, pp 63-101.
4. Whitaker HA, Bub D, Leventer S: Neurolinguistic aspects of language acquisition and bilingualism, *Ann N Y Acad Sci* 379:59-74, 1981.
5. Luria AR: *The working brain: an introduction to neuropsychology*, New York, 1973, Basic Books.
6. Luria AR: *Higher cortical functions in man*, ed 2, New York, 1980, Basic Books.
7. Gipson DS, Hooper SR, Wetherington CE, Duquette PJ, Stellwagen K: Memory function in pediatric chronic renal failure: preliminary findings, *J Am Soc Nephrol* 14:538A, 2003.
8. Schnaper HW, Cole BR, Hodges FJ, Robson AM: Cerebral cortical atrophy in pediatric patients with end-stage renal disease, *Am J Kidney Dis* 2(6):645-50, 1983.
9. Elzouki A, Carroll J, Butinar D, Moosa A: Improved neurological outcome in children with chronic renal disease from infancy, *Pediatr Nephrol* 8(2):205-10, 1994.
10. Qvist E, Pihko H, Fagerudd P, et al: Neurodevelopmental outcome in high-risk patients after renal transplantation in early childhood, *Pediatr Transplant* 6(1):53-62, 2002.
11. Steinberg A, Efrat R, Pomeranz A, Drukker A: Computerized tomography of the brain in children with chronic renal failure, *Int J Pediatr Nephrol* 6(2):121-26, 1985.
12. Valanne L, Qvist E, Jalanko H, Holmberg C, Pihko H: Neuroradiologic findings in children with renal transplantation under 5 years of age, *Pediatr Transplant* 8(1):44-51, 2004.
13. Nichols SL, Press GA, Schneider JA, Trauner DA: Cortical atrophy and cognitive performance in infantile nephropathic cystinosis, *Pediatr Neurol* 6(6):379-81, 1990.
14. Pueschel SM, Brem AS, Nittoli P: Central nervous system and renal investigations in patients with Lowe syndrome, *Childs Nerv Syst* 8(1):45-48, 1992.
15. Polinsky MS, Kaiser BA, Stover JB: Neurologic development of children with severe chronic renal failure from infancy, *Pediatr Nephrol* 1(2):157-65, 1987.
16. Warady BA, Fivush BA, Alexander SR: Peritoneal dialysis. In Barratt TM, Avner ED, Harmon WE, editors: *Pediatric nephrology*, Baltimore, 1999, Lippincott Williams & Wilkins, pp 1251-65.
17. Fennell RS, Fennell EB, Carter RL, Mings EL, et al: Correlations between performance on neuropsychological tests in children with chronic renal failure, *Child Nephrol Urol* 10(4):199-204, 1990.
18. Fennell RS, Fennell EB, Carter RL, Mings EL, et al: A longitudinal study of the cognitive function of children with renal failure, *Pediatr Nephrol* 4(1):11-15, 1990.
19. Mendley SR, Zelko FA: Improvement in specific aspects of neurocognitive performance in children after renal transplantation, *Kidney Int* 56(1):318-23, 1999.
20. Brouhard BH, Donaldson LA, Lawry KW, et al: Cognitive functioning in children on dialysis and post-transplantation, *Pediatr Transplant* 4(4):261-67, 2000.
21. Hulstijn-Dirkmaat GM, Damhuis IH, Jetten ML, Koster AM, Schroder CH: The cognitive development of pre-school children treated for chronic renal failure, *Pediatr Nephrol* 9(4):464-69, 1995.
22. Ledermann SE, Scanes ME, Fernando ON, Duffy PG, et al: Long-term outcome of peritoneal dialysis in infants, *J Pediatr* 136(1):24-29, 2000.
23. Warady BA, Belden B, Kohaut E: Neurodevelopmental outcome of children initiating peritoneal dialysis in early infancy, *Pediatr Nephrol* 13(9):759-65, 1999.
24. Madden SJ, Ledermann SE, Guerrero-Blanco M, Bruce M, Trompeter RS: Cognitive and psychosocial outcome of infants dialysed in infancy, *Child Care Health Dev* 29(1):55-61, 2003.
25. Lawry KW, Brouhard BH, Cunningham RJ: Cognitive functioning and school performance in children with renal failure, *Pediatr Nephrol* 8(3):326-29, 1994.
26. Bawden HN, Acott P, Carter J, et al: Neuropsychological functioning in end-stage renal disease, *Arch Dis Child* 89(7):644-47, 2004.
27. Kuyer JM, Hulstijn-Dirkmaat GM, van Aken MA: [Effects of kidney transplantation on cognitive functioning of children], *Tijdschr Kindergeneeskd* 58(3):83-89, 1990.
28. Groothoff JW, Cransberg K, Offringa M, et al: Long-term follow-up of renal transplantation in children: a Dutch cohort study, *Transplantation* 78(3):453-60, 2004.
29. Fennell R, Fennell E, Carter R, Mings E, Klausner A: Association between renal function and cognition in childhood chronic renal failure, *Pediatr Nephrol* 4:16-20, 1990.
30. Gipson DS, Hooper SR, Duquette PJ, Wetherington CE, et al: Memory and executive functions in pediatric chronic kidney disease, *Child Neuropsychol* 12(6):391-405, 2006.
31. Denckla MB: Research on executive function in a neurodevelopmental context: application of clinical measures, *Dev Neuropsychol* 12(1):5-15, 1996.
32. Groothoff JW, Grootenhuis MA, Offringa M, Gruppen MP, et al: Quality of life in adults with end-stage renal disease since childhood is only partially impaired, *Nephrol Dial Transplant* 18(2):310-17, 2003.
33. Goldstein SL, Graham N, Burwinkle T, Warady B, et al: Health-related quality of life in pediatric patients with ESRD, *Pediatr Nephrol* 21(6):846-50, 2006.
34. Stam H, Hartman EE, Deurloo JA, Groothoff J, Grootenhuis MA: Young adult patients with a history of pediatric disease: impact on course of life and transition into adulthood, *J Adolesc Health* 39(1):4-13, 2006.

35. Eisenhauer GL, Arnold WC, Livingston RL: Identifying psychiatric disorders in children with renal disease, *South Med J* 81(5):572-76, 1988.
36. Fukunishi I, Kudo H: Psychiatric problems of pediatric end-stage renal failure, *Gen Hosp Psychiatry* 17(1):32-36, 1995.
37. Brownbridge G, Fielding DM: Psychosocial adjustment to end-stage renal failure: comparing haemodialysis, continuous ambulatory peritoneal dialysis and transplantation, *Pediatr Nephrol* 5(5):612-16, 1991.
38. Fabrazzo M, De Santo RM: Depression in chronic kidney disease, *Semin Nephrol* 26(1):56-60, 2006.
39. McDade-Montez EA, Christensen AJ, Cvengros JA, Lawton WJ: The role of depression symptoms in dialysis withdrawal, *Health Psychol* 25(2):198-204, 2006.
40. Troidle L, Watnick S, Wuerth DB, Gorban-Brennan N, et al: Depression and its association with peritonitis in long-term peritoneal dialysis patients, *Am J Kidney Dis* 42(2):350-54, 2003.
41. Sungthong R, Mo-suwan L, Chongsuvivatwong V: Effects of haemoglobin and serum ferritin on cognitive function in school children, *Asia Pac J Clin Nutr* 11(2):117-22, 2002.
42. Oski FA, Honig AS: The effects of therapy on the developmental scores of iron-deficient infants, *J Pediatr* 92(1):21-25, 1978.
43. Stivelman JC: Benefits of anaemia treatment on cognitive function, *Nephrol Dial Transplant* 15 Suppl 3:29-35, 2000.
44. Pickett JL, Theberge DC, Brown WS, Schweitzer SU, Nissenson AR: Normalizing hematocrit in dialysis patients improves brain function, *Am J Kidney Dis* 33(6):1122-30, 1999.
45. Marsh JT, Brown WS, Wolcott D, et al: rHuEPO treatment improves brain and cognitive function of anemic dialysis patients, *Kidney Int* 39(1):155-63, 1991.
46. Beard JL, Connor JR: Iron status and neural functioning, *Annu Rev Nutr* 23:41-58, 2003.
47. Tiplady B, Bowness E, Stien L, Drummond G: Selective effects of clonidine and temazepam on attention and memory, *J Psychopharmacol* 19(3):259-65, 2005.
48. Muller U, Mottweiler E, Bublak P: Noradrenergic blockade and numeric working memory in humans, *J Psychopharmacol* 19(1):21-28, 2005.
49. Bhutta AT, Cleves MA, Casey PH, Cradock MM, Anand KJ: Cognitive and behavioral outcomes of school-aged children who were born preterm: a meta-analysis, *JAMA* 288(6):728-37, 2002.
50. US Department of Education: *Digest of education statistics, 2003*, Washington, DC, 2004, National Center for Education Statistics.
51. Gipson DS, Wetherington CE, Duquette PJ, Hooper SR: The nervous system and chronic kidney disease in children, *Pediatr Nephrol* 19(8):832-39, 2004.
52. Duquette PJ, Gipson DS, Hooper SR, et al: *Intellectual functioning and academic achievement in pediatric chronic kidney disease*, NASP Annual Meeting, 2005.
53. Groothoff JW, Grootenhuis M, Dommerholt A, Gruppen MP, et al: Impaired cognition and schooling in adults with end stage renal disease since childhood, *Arch Dis Child* 87(5):380-85, 2002.
54. Broyer M, Le BC, Charbit M, et al: Long-term social outcome of children after kidney transplantation, *Transplantation* 77(7):1033-37, 2004.
55. Bartosh SM, Leverson G, Robillard D, Sollinger HW: Long-term outcomes in pediatric renal transplant recipients who survive into adulthood, *Transplantation* 76(8):1195-200, 2003.

CHAPTER

48 Nutritional Challenges in Pediatric Chronic Kidney Disease

Donna Secker and Robert Mak

INTRODUCTION

The importance of nutritional status has been emphasized in numerous clinical practice guidelines addressing the care of patients with chronic kidney disease (CKD). However, most of these guidelines are based on opinion rather than evidence.[1] Nutritional status is a complex concept that is difficult to define. Adequate nutritional status can perhaps be best defined as the maintenance of a normal pattern of growth and a normal body composition by the consumption of appropriate amounts and types of food. Significant challenges in the nutritional management of children with CKD remain.

CACHEXIA VERSUS MALNUTRITION IN CHRONIC KIDNEY DISEASE

The loss of protein stores, which presents clinically as wasting, is reported to have a prevalence of 30% and to be an important risk factor for mortality in patients with CKD. There is a debate regarding whether the nutritional state in patients with CKD represents malnutrition or cachexia. Cachexia differs from malnutrition in several key ways. First, despite the fact that the cachectic person is "starving," he or she is also anorexic. Second, in normal starvation, the metabolic rate decreases as a protective mechanism. This protective reduction in metabolic rate is not observed in patients with cachexia. Resting energy expenditure is high in patients with cachexia from renal failure. Third, in simple starvation, fats are preferentially lost, and there is a preservation of lean body mass. In cachexia, lean tissues are wasted, and fats are relatively underused. Finally, the abnormalities of malnutrition can usually be overcome simply by supplying more food or altering the composition of the diet. To date, this approach has not proven to be successful in cachectic patients. There are fundamental metabolic abnormalities in cachectic patients that prevent them from using dietary nutrients effectively. Normal individuals characteristically respond to the restriction of dietary protein by progressively decreasing the irreversible destruction of amino acids and, consequently, the production of urea from the nitrogen of amino acids. At the limits of this adaptive response, another mechanism is activated that leads to a decrease in the degradation of protein and at least some stimulation of protein synthesis. These adaptive responses act to maintain protein balance, and, unless there is severe dietary restriction, they usually suffice to prevent the loss of body proteins. Fortunately, patients with uncomplicated kidney disease, including nephrotic subjects, can activate the same adaptations to dietary protein restriction and maintain protein balance and lean body mass for long periods while they are eating protein-restricted diets. However, when dialysis becomes necessary, the amounts of protein and energy required for protein balance increase sharply, and it is not known whether these adaptive responses occur in patients with end stage renal disease (ESRD) or how effective they are for preventing excessive catabolism.[2-5]

Anorexia, which is defined as the loss of appetite and early satiety, often accompanies cachexia, and it has been suggested to play a role in the loss of body weight. However, the loss of skeletal muscle is not prominent in primary anorexic states, because the brain adapts to using ketone bodies derived from the metabolism of fat, thereby reducing the requirement for gluconeogenesis from amino acids derived from muscle proteins. This suggests that the metabolic changes in anorexia and cachexia are different. Anorexia can arise from the following: (1) decreased taste and smell of food; (2) early satiety; (3) dysfunctional hypothalamic membrane adenylate cyclase; (4) increased brain tryptophan; and (5) cytokine production. The causes of anorexia in cachetic states is not well understood. Gastrointestinal symptoms such as nausea, vomiting, and gastroesophageal reflux are common in patients with CKD (especially infants) and should be treated accordingly before the further consideration of nutritional intervention. Patients with CKD who have anorexia regain their appetites soon after starting dialysis treatment, presumably because of the removal of one or more toxic factors that suppress the appetite. Fractions in the middle molecule weight range that have been isolated from normal urine and uremic plasma ultrafiltrate act in the splanchnic region and the brain to inhibit food intake. Cytokines such as interleukin 6 and tumor necrosis factor α may also cause anorexia.[4-8] Anorexia is associated with higher concentrations of proinflammatory cytokines, higher levels of erythropoietin hyporesponsiveness, poor clinical outcomes (including a fourfold increase in mortality), greater hospitalization rates, and a poorer quality of life in maintenance hemodialysis patients. Depression, which is the most common psychologic disorder among patients with ESRD, is commonly associated with poor oral intake, and it can aggravate poor nutrition in chronic dialysis patients.[9]

Energy expenditure is increased in cachetic patients with CKD, and it is related to inflammation. Resting energy expenditure correlated with surrogate markers of inflammation such as C-reactive protein, and the treatment of infection and the subsequent resolution of elevated C-reactive protein levels was associated with the normalization of elevated resting energy expenditure in patients with CKD. Furthermore, elevated resting energy expenditure was associated with increased mortality and cardiovascular death in patients on peritoneal dialysis, which was related to its close correlations with cachexia and inflammation in these patients. The underlying mechanism of the elevated resting metabolic rate may involve several pathways, such as the increased activity of mitochondrial uncoupling proteins, which promote futile metabolic cycles (i.e., the burning of energy without generating adenosine triphosphate).[3,10]

NUTRITIONAL ASSESSMENT

The Kidney Disease Outcome Quality Initiative (K/DOQI) Clinical Practice Guidelines for Nutrition in Chronic Renal Failure addressed the evaluation of the protein-energy nutritional status of children receiving maintenance dialysis only.[1] No guidelines for pediatric patients with CKD before the onset of ESRD are available. The dialysis guidelines emphasize that no single measure provides a complete picture of nutritional status; consequently, many different measures are recommended, with the implication that the treating team will integrate the results into a cogent assessment of nutritional status. The recommended measures include the assessment of dietary intake, serum albumin, height or length (and standard deviation score), estimated dry weight, weight-to-height index, skinfold thickness (sites not specified), mid-arm circumference and muscle circumference or area, and head circumference for children less than 3 years old. For children who are maintained on hemodialysis, the K/DOQI guidelines also suggest the measurement of the protein equivalent of nitrogen appearance to estimate protein intake.[11] Measurements of nutritional parameters are confounded in CKD as a result of salt and water imbalance and the potential inappropriateness of using age-matched controls in a population that is short and delayed in puberty. It has been suggested that it is more appropriate to express measures relative to height age and/or pubertal stage.[12,13]

Anthropometric Measures

The most commonly used assessment is height, weight, and head circumference plotted on percentile charts. These values are often expressed as standard deviation scores (number of standard deviations from the mean for a normal population of the same age). Another assessment is the body mass index (BMI; weight/height^2), which can be prognostic, because extremes are associated with increased mortality and morbidity. Wong and colleagues[14] demonstrated that the adjusted relative mortality risk of children with ESRD is 60% higher at BMI standard deviations of −2.5 and +2.5 as compared with an ideal BMI standard deviation of 0.5. However, BMI does not distinguish between differences in fat mass and lean body mass. Thus, an appropriate BMI for age does not indicate ideal body composition. Indeed, there is recent evidence that there is excess fat mass despite a loss of lean body mass in children with CKD.[15] Skinfold thickness is a measure of subcutaneous fat, and mid-arm circumference is a measure of muscle mass. Decreased values have been found in children with CKD. However, both are unreliable tools, because values are confounded by edema, regional fat distribution, and age-related variations.[12,13]

Dietary Assessment

This is recommended at monthly intervals for infants, every 3 to 4 months for older children on dialysis, and every 6 months and every 3 to 4 months for children with moderate and severe CKD, respectively.[1] Prospective diaries kept for 3 days and retrospective recall are the most commonly used methods. Protein intake can also be calculated using protein catabolic rate formulae.

Serum Albumin

Serum albumin is a surrogate marker for nutritional status in children with ESRD.[1] Indeed, it is an independent biomarker for increased mortality and morbidity.[16] Hypoalbuminemia may be the result of fluid overload; therefore, postdialysis levels should be measured. It has been shown that hypoalbuminemia is related to inflammation rather than decreased dietary intake in adult hemodialysis patients.[17] However, patients on peritoneal dialysis (PD) have significant protein and amino acid losses in the dialysate, which is related to surface area. Infants on PD have almost double the protein loss as compared with older children. Such severe protein losses in these infants may impair growth.[13]

Body Composition Measures

Dual energy x-ray absorptiometry scanning can be used to estimate fat mass, lean body mass, and bone mineral density. However, lean body mass assessment from this type of scanning is often confounded by fluid overload in patients with CKD.[13] Bioelectrical impedance, total body potassium, and in vivo neutron activation are alternative methodologies that are mostly used as research tools.

NUTRITIONAL MANAGEMENT

There is no such thing as a standard renal diet. Dietary modifications, especially restrictions, are imposed only when they are clearly needed and should be individualized according to the child's age, development, and food preferences. Needed changes may include alterations to calorie, protein, fat, phosphorus, calcium, sodium, potassium, and/or fluid intakes. Restrictions are kept as liberal as possible to help meet energy needs and to encourage adherence. Depending on the response in the relevant parameter, the restriction can be liberalized or tightened. The nutrition care plan requires frequent monitoring and adjustments in response to changes in the child's nutritional status, age, development, anthropometrics, food preferences, residual renal function, biochemistries, renal replacement therapy, medications, and psychosocial status. Close collaboration with a social worker is invaluable for helping families deal with financial burdens that interfere with their ability to follow recommended dietary changes.

Diet instructions should begin with a simple explanation of the role of the nutrient in the body, the rationale for the diet modification, the desired outcomes to be achieved (e.g., normal blood pressure, specific amount of weight gain), and what happens if the child eats too much (or too little) of the nutrient. Guidelines for change should be practical, individualized to the patient's and the family's lifestyle and eating habits, and positive in that they emphasize the foods that the child can eat to replace those that need to be limited or avoided. Cultural food preferences play a major role in a child's ability to adhere to dietary changes. Dietary instructions should be tailored to help families modify—but not eliminate—cultural food preferences, such as salty sauces and seasonings, tropical fruits, greens, dried beans, legumes, and lentils. Background information about cultural diets and translated versions of renal diets and food lists are available.[18,19] Food models, pictures of foods from supermarket advertisements, and actual food containers and their labels make teaching sessions more interesting and hands on. During follow up, food records can be reviewed to assess the child's accomplishments, to identify problems that the child or family may be having with modifying dietary intake, and to trigger additional suggestions for maintaining dietary changes. Nutritional counselling is recommended on an ongoing basis because of the dynamic nature of a child's development, food preferences, residual renal function, and medical condition.

Messages provided by team members about the importance of nutrition magnify caregivers' attention to food intake. This can add to parental stress and increase the risk for eating problems (e.g., food refusal, self-induced vomiting, misbehavior at mealtime). Parents feeling frustrated or anxious about feeding their infants or children may pressure them to eat or give inappropriate attention (e.g., verbal prompts to eat, playful interaction, attempts to console) to undesired behaviors (e.g., gagging, turning the head away) while at the same time rewarding desired behaviors (e.g., accepting food, swallowing, sitting quietly) with only very brief and minimal interaction. Parents require anticipatory guidance to minimize these behaviors; in reality, undesired behavior should be ignored and desired behavior reinforced (e.g., verbal praise, playful interaction). The consistency of the parental response to the child's behavior is essential. As infants progress from commercial jarred foods to homemade foods, parents require additional dietary teaching, and, as children begin to eat outside of the home and have more autonomy with regard to food choices, they too require dietary teaching and reinforcement. Adopting and maintaining changes to eating habits is easier if the whole family makes similar changes or at least avoids eating restricted foods in front of the child. In addition, caregivers outside of the immediate family (e.g., grandparents, nursery school staff, babysitters, public school teachers) should be aware of diet modifications and asked to provide consistency of care with helping the child follow his or her diet. Adolescents can be empowered to make better food choices at the school cafeteria or at fast-food restaurants if they are given nutrient content information from their favorite eating places.

ENERGY

Requirements

Meeting caloric requirements is important not only for weight gain and growth but also to avoid using protein as an energy source through gluconeogenesis. The energy requirements of children with CKD have not been shown to differ from healthy children[20] nor is there evidence that children with CKD will grow better if their intake exceeds recommended amounts for healthy children. As a result, the prescribed caloric intake for children with CKD should initially be based on national recommendations for chronologic age and then adjusted according to the child's response and/or his or her need for additional calories to allow for catchup growth.[1,20,21]

The early anticipation and correction of energy malnutrition, especially in infants, is important to avoid the loss of growth potential. Initial studies demonstrated that the growth of infants and toddlers with CKD is compromised when energy intake falls below 80% of recommendations for healthy children,[22] and subsequent studies have shown that the average caloric intake of children with various stages of CKD is below 80% of the recommended daily allowance (RDA).[23-27] Increasing energy intake to 100% of the RDA using oral supplements or nasogastric or gastrostomy tube feeding can increase weight gain and stabilize growth rates in all ages and achieve catchup growth in infants who are treated before they reach 2 years of age.[28-32] Improving energy intake has also been associated with a decrease in the number of days of hospitalization and a reduction in peritonitis rates.[33] The RDA values have since been replaced by the 2002 dietary reference intakes (DRIs), which include predictive equations for normal and overweight children and which include physical activity factors for children 3 years old and older. It is important to note that the DRIs for energy are approximately 10 kcal/kg (15% to 20%) lower for infants and toddlers and similar or slightly higher for school-aged children and adolescents; hence, adverse effects on growth may occur if the caloric intake of infants or toddlers is below 90% to 95% of the newer DRI.

Appetite Stimulants

The stimulation of nutritional intake in cancer patients with megestrol acetate (MA) fails to restore the loss of lean body mass, and weight gain achieved is the result of an accumulation of adipose tissue and water. Few studies have been conducted in patients on hemodialysis (HD). After the administration of a moderate dose of MA (≥320 mg/day) to a patient on chronic HD, a fat mass increase (by 163%) and a fat-free mass decrease (by 10.6%) as consequences of improvement of reported appetite and increases of energy and protein intakes have been observed.[34] The long-term administration of MA in 17 patients on HD and in 3 of these patients for 5 to 6 months improved appetite, and an increase in dry weight was reported.[35] In 10 hypoalbuminemic dialysis patients, Rammohan and colleagues[36] demonstrated that the daily administration of 400 mg of MA solution for 16 weeks improved appetite, protein and energy intake, and quality of life. Williams and colleagues[37] conducted a double-blind crossover study in 24 patients on HD with poor appetite and serum albumin levels of less than 4 g/dL who received MA (160 mg/day) or placebo for 3 months and then switched to the other therapy. Of these patients, 4 withdrew because of diarrhea, and 2 died as a result of comorbid conditions. Of the 18 patients who completed the study, no significant increase in albumin or lean body mass was observed. It is well known that MA can induce many side effects, such as headaches, dizziness, confusion, diarrhea, hyperglycemia, thromboembolic phenomena, breakthrough uterine bleeding, peripheral edema, hypertension, adrenal suppression, and adrenal insufficiency.[37] On the basis of these considerations, it seems that the use of MA in clinical practice cannot be recommended. Large, randomized, controlled trials are warranted to really define the exact role of MA in the prevention and treatment of anorexia in patients on HD. There are few data regarding children with CKD.[38]

The stimulatory effects of the gut hormone ghrelin on food intake and meal appreciation suggest that it could be an effective treatment for anorexic patients. The potential use of ghrelin for the treatment of anorexia in CKD patients was demonstrated in a recent report. Wynne and colleagues[39] have tested the effects of subcutaneous ghrelin administration on patients with CKD with mild to moderate malnutrition. The single-dose (3.6 nmol/kg) subcutaneous ghrelin administration significantly increased the mean absolute energy intake in patients with CKD as compared with those patients receiving saline placebo. When expressed as a proportional energy increase for each individual patient, ghrelin administration resulted in an immediate doubling of energy intake. However, the increase in energy intake in those patients was not followed by increased total energy intake over the following 24 hours. Multiple daily dosing of ghrelin or the administration of long-acting ghrelin mimetics holds the promise of improving appetite and nutrition in patients with CKD and ESRD.

Recent experimental data show that elevated circulating levels of cytokines such as leptin may be an important cause of uremia-associated cachexia via signalling through the central melanocortin system. Melanocortin receptor antagonism holds the therapeutic promise of preventing anorexia and cachexia in patients with CKD.[5,9]

Nutritional Supplementation

When voluntary intake is low, calories can be maximized by adding concentrated sources of carbohydrate and/or fat to feedings, choosing calorie-rich foods, and avoiding calorie-free foods and fluids such as water. Infant formulas such as Good Start and Similac PM 60/40 contain lesser amounts of phosphorus and potassium, and they may be required by some infants to maintain normal serum levels. To meet requirements, commercial carbohydrate and/or fat products can be added to infant feedings to increase their standard energy density (20 kcal/oz, 0.67 kcal/ml) as high as 60 kcal/oz (2 kcal/ml) without significantly increasing electrolyte and mineral content.[40,41] The choice to add a carbohydrate module (e.g., Moducal, Polycose, Scandical), fat, or a combination of both (both types of modules; Duocal) should be made after considering serum glucose and lipid profiles, the presence or absence of malabsorption or respiratory distress (carbohydrate metabolism increases carbon dioxide production), and the cost to the caregivers. When making more than two or three increases in energy density, the distribution of calories from carbohydrate and fat should be kept similar to the base feeding. Unless fat malabsorption is present, a "heart-healthy" oil such as corn or canola oil is a good, low-cost choice, especially for infants on PD who have hypertriglyceridemia from absorbing additional glucose from the dialysate. Increasing the caloric density of formula by concentration (i.e., adding more formula powder or liquid concentrate and less water) is typically not an option because of the accompanying increase in sodium, potassium, and phosphorus content. Gradual, stepwise increases in energy density of 2 to 4 kcal/oz theoretically improve tolerance. A recent study demonstrated that infants less than 1 year old with failure to thrive tolerated high-energy infant formula (30 kcal/oz or 1.0 kcal/ml) when it was started at full strength[42]; however, the authors suggested that younger infants (<12 weeks old) may benefit from a graded introduction to avoid increased bowel frequency.

Glucose absorption from peritoneal dialysate solutions provides an additional 8 to 26 kcal/kg for children on PD,[1] and, although some guidelines recommend including these calories when assessing caloric intake,[1] many practitioners consider them to be "bonus" calories for underweight children and agree with recommendations that they be considered specifically for infants and children who become overweight on PD.[20]

Calories can be added to foods using heart-healthy margarines or oils, cream and other fats, sugars, syrups, or commercial carbohydrate modules. Commercial calorie supplements such as milkshakes or energy bars may be useful; however, their phosphorus and potassium content may be too high. Nonrenal enteral supplements designed for children older than 1 year (e.g., Compleat Pediatric, Kindercal, Nutren Junior, PediaSure, Resource Just for Kids) have fairly high calcium and phosphorus content to support bone growth. These products are contraindicated in children with hyperphosphatemia and/or hyperkalemia. In the absence of a pediatric renal feeding, adult renal products (e.g., Magnacal Renal, Nepro, NovaSource Renal, NutraRenal, Renalcal, Suplena), which are available in normal and lower protein content and designed to be calorically dense and low in minerals and electrolytes, are recommended for children who are more than 4 years old, but they have also been used successfully at diluted strength in children less than 1 year old.[42a] Serum magnesium levels require monitoring when transitioning from an infant feed to one of these products, because their magnesium content is significantly higher than breast milk or infant formula. The acceptance of these products can be improved by mixing them with nondairy creamers, flavored soda, fruit, sherbet, and/or ice to make shakes or slush-type drinks.

When energy intake remains low despite the use of diet manipulations and oral supplements, enteral feedings are recommended.[1,20,21]

Tube Feeding

Nasogastric, gastrostomy, gastrojejunostomy, and jejunostomy tubes have all been used successfully to provide additional nutrition, fluids, and/or medications by intermittent bolus or continuous infusion. Indications for tube feeding include recurrent emesis, an oral intake that is less than recommended, and poor weight gain and growth. Tube feeding helps to minimize the risk of force feeding, and, despite caregivers' initial reluctance to agree to their insertion, tube feeding helps to relieve the stress that can accompany the meeting of nutritional requirements. Oral stimulation and nonnutritive sucking should be provided to infants who are totally dependent on tube feeding to help smooth their transition to oral feeding after successful transplantation. Using a multidisciplinary approach, several centers have reported transitioning all of their patients over to complete oral feedings within 2 to 6 months after successful transplantation,[43-45] thereby illustrating that tube feeding need not preclude the development of normal oral feeding skills.

The choices of formula and feeding are guided by age, biochemistries, gastrointestinal function, fluid allowance, and, where possible, the consideration of monetary costs to the caregivers. Feedings are initiated and advanced according to pediatric guidelines[46] and tolerance. Volumes and rates that are based on body weight help to avoid intolerance in patients who are underweight or small for their age (Table 48-1). Whenever possible, the volume of feeds should be minimized to optimize tolerance and keep the hours of feeding manageable within the child's daily schedule. Infants are preferentially given intermittent bolus feeds to maintain normal blood sugars. Continuous overnight feeds are generally avoided for infants as a result of an increased risk of vomiting and gastroesophageal reflux associated with uremia and the potential for aspiration; continuous feedings may be required if the patient's gastrointestinal tolerance of bolus feedings is poor. Continuous overnight feeds are generally preferred for children and adolescents to facilitate daytime hunger and oral intake.

Reported complications include emesis, obstruction, exit-site infection, tube displacement, and peritonitis.[47-49] When vomiting and gastroesophageal reflux are not responsive to medical therapy, jejunal (gastrojejunostomy or jejunostomy) feeding or a fundoplication may be warranted.[1] To decrease the risk of peritonitis, the placement of gastrostomy, gastrojejunostomy, and jejunostomy tubes should occur before or concomitant with insertion of a PD catheter, whenever possible.[49-51] In particular, percutaneous endoscopic gastrostomy insertion after PD initiation carries a high risk for fungal peritonitis and potential PD failure. Suggested precautions for lowering the risk of peritonitis include antibiotic and antifungal prophylaxis, withholding PD for 2 to 3 days, and gastrostomy placement by an experienced endoscopy team.[51]

Parenteral Nutrition

Published guidelines for administering parenteral nutrition (PN) in children with acute or chronic kidney failure are limited. Concentrated solutions of amino acids, dextrose, and lipids are required when fluids are restricted. Unless otherwise indicated, energy requirements during PN are 10% lower than enteral requirements, because there is no thermal effect of feeding. Standard amino acid solutions (i.e., both essential and nonessential amino acids) are generally used and provided according to (enteral) protein recommendations specific to the child's age and renal replacement therapy. Amino acids, dextrose, and lipids can be advanced according

TABLE 48-1 **Guidelines for Initiating and Advancing Tube Feedings**

Age	Initial Hourly Infusion	Daily Increases	Goal
Continuous Feedings			
0 to 1 year	10 to 20 ml/h or 1 to 2 ml/kg/h	5 to 10 ml/8 h or 1 ml/kg/h	21 to 54 ml/h or 6 ml/kg/h
1 to 6 years	20 to 30 ml/h or 2 to 3 ml/kg/h	10 to 15 ml/8 h or 1 ml/kg/h	71 to 92 ml/h or 4 to 5 ml/kg/h
6 to 14 years	30 to 40 ml/h or 1 ml/kg/h	15 to 20 ml/8 h or 0.5 ml/kg/h	108 to 130 ml/h or 3 to 4 ml/kg/h
>14 years	50 ml/h or 0.5 to 1 ml/kg/h	25 ml/8 h or 0.4 to 0.5 ml/kg/h	125 ml/h
Bolus Feedings			
Age	**Initial Hourly Infusion**	**Daily Increases**	**Goal**
0 to 1 year	60 to 80 ml every 4 h or 10 to 15 ml/kg/feed	20 to 40 ml every 4 h	80 to 240 ml every 4 h or 20 to 30 ml/kg/feed
1 to 6 years	80 to 120 ml every 4 h or 5 to 10 ml/kg/feed	40 to 60 ml every 4 h	280 to 375 ml every 4 h or 15 to 20 ml/kg/feed
6 to 14 years	120 to 160 ml every 4 h or 3 to 5 ml/kg/feed	60 to 80 ml every 4 h	430 to 520 ml every 4 h or 10 to 20 ml/kg/feed
>14 years	200 ml every 4 h or 3 ml/kg/feed	100 ml every 4 h	500 ml every 4 h or 10 ml/kg/feed

Note: Rates expressed per kg of body weight are useful for small-for-age patients
From Wilson SE: Pediatric enteral feeding. In Grand RJ, Sutphen JL, et al, editors: *Pediatric nutrition, theory and practice,* Toronto, Ontario, 1987, Butterworth.

to normal pediatric PN guidelines and serum urea, glucose, and triglyceride (or intralipid) concentrations. Mineral and electrolyte content should be adjusted to maintain acceptable serum concentrations, and acetate and chloride content should be adjusted to maintain the acid-base balance. Standard pediatric dosages of parenteral multivitamins and trace elements can be used; the risk of toxicity, especially for vitamin A, is minimal with a daily injectable multivitamin provided that the child has no other exogenous source of vitamin A (i.e., oral diet is minimal).

Intradialytic Parenteral Nutrition

The administration of parenteral amino acids, dextrose, and lipids during hemodialysis sessions has been used to reverse weight loss and increase weight and body mass index and/or percentage of ideal body weight in small groups of malnourished children and adolescents who are unable to be supplemented enterally.[52-54] Intradialytic PN has been used to provide 27 to 53 kcal/kg,[52] 0.5 to 1.5 g protein/kg,[52-54] and 0.4 to 0.6 g fat/kg[52-54] per 3- to 4-hour treatment. Reported maximum infusion rates were 0.2 to 0.3 g fat/kg/hr for lipids[52-54] and 9 mg dextrose/kg/min for carbohydrates.[54] Adverse events (i.e., hypophosphatemia, transient hyperglycemia, lipid intolerance, mildly elevated liver function tests) have been minor. Intradialytic PN is costly and should only be used for children who are unable to meet nutritional requirements enterally.

Limiting Energy Intake

Big appetites and excessive energy intake are most often seen in children on high-dose glucocorticosteroid therapy (e.g., nephrotic syndrome, vasculitis, after transplantation). Children and caregivers should receive early education about the potential for overweight and obesity and given strategies for controlling caloric intake and increasing physical activity to maintain a healthy weight. Overweight is sometimes seen in infants and children on PD as a result of significant dialysate glucose resorption, which is usually greater in young infants because of the enhanced permeability of their peritoneal membranes for small molecules. To help control weight gain in these patients, dialysate calories should be considered when estimating energy intake, and icodextrin dialysate, which contains a poorly absorbed, high-molecular-weight, starch-derived glucose polymer to provide the osmotic force for ultrafiltration, can be used to lower the caloric load.

PROTEIN

Requirements

Children need to be in positive nitrogen balance to support growth. Optimal protein requirements for children with CKD stages I through V have not been determined but begin with requirements for healthy children (e.g., RDAs) and are increased by proteinuria, glucocorticosteroids, acidosis, losses through dialysis, peritonitis, and catabolism. Although low-protein diets have been recommended for slowing the progression of renal failure for many years, there is no convincing or conclusive evidence in adults or children that long-term protein restriction is efficacious.[20,55,56] In a small randomized controlled trial,[57] reducing dietary protein intake to the World Health Organization's recommendations for minimal intake did not decrease the progression of CKD in children and is therefore not currently recommended.

Limited data are available regarding the amount of protein required by children on dialysis. To allow for losses of protein through the dialysis process, the K/DOQI Nutrition Guidelines[1] recommend adding 0.4 g protein/kg/d to the RDA to compensate for protein losses on HD and 0.7 to 0.8 g/kg/d for losses on PD. Like the energy recommendations, the RDAs have been replaced with the 2002 DRIs, which, for protein, are lower than the RDAs across all age groups. The Caring for Australasians with Renal Impairment (CARI) guidelines[20] suggest adding similar increments of 0.4 g/kg/d for children on HD and 0.5 to 1.0 g/kg/d for children on PD to protein recommendations from the Food and Agriculture Organization of the United Nations (FAO) and the World Health Organization.[58] Requirements on PD are highest on a g/kg basis for infants and toddlers, because protein losses are inversely related to body weight and peritoneal surface area (e.g., 220 to 280 mg/kg/d for children who are less than 6 years old versus 90 to 190 mg/kg/d for older children).[59] Losses are similar for all modes of PD (i.e., continuous ambulatory peritoneal dialysis, continuous cycling peritoneal dialysis, tidal) but vary widely among individuals.

During the immediate posttransplant period, protein needs are thought to be increased by approximately 50% in association with surgical stress and the catabolic effects of steroids, but they are decreased back to normal recommendations around 3 months after transplantation.

Modifying Dietary Protein Intake

Despite anorexia and poor appetites, voluntary protein intake usually exceeds recommendations,[23,24,57] which is acceptable as long as serum urea and phosphate levels are within acceptable limits. To minimize uremia, excessive protein intake (i.e., >150% to 175% of requirements) should be avoided, and protein of high biologic value should be encouraged to minimize urea production through the reuse of circulating nonessential amino acids for protein maintenance. Edefonti and colleagues[26] performed nitrogen balance studies in children on PD and found that nitrogen balance was adequate to meet the nitrogen requirements for growth and all of the metabolic needs of uremic children (i.e., estimated to be ≥+50 mg/kg/d) in only 50% of the studies. In 36% of the studies, results were considered relatively satisfactory (i.e., 0 to 50 mg/kg/d), and, in 14% of the studies, children were in negative nitrogen balance. Children who had been on dialysis for more than 1 year had lower energy and protein intakes and poorer nitrogen balance results.

Occasionally, protein intake may be inadequate as a result of anorexia, chewing problems, low meat intake, or a low phosphorus diet that limits protein-rich dairy foods. Persistently low urea levels (i.e., <50 mg/dL or <18 mmol/L) may be a sign of overall inadequate protein and caloric intake. Powdered protein modules (e.g., Resource Instant Protein Powder) can be added to expressed breast milk, infant formula, beverages, pureed foods, cereals, or other moist foods to boost their protein content, and minced or chopped meat, chicken, fish, egg, tofu, or skim milk powder can be added to soups, pasta, or casseroles. Milk, milk products, and eggs can be substituted if meat is disliked; however, their high phosphorus content must be considered.

Intraperitoneal Amino Acids

Peritoneal dialysate solutions containing a mixture of essential and nonessential amino acids instead of glucose as the osmotic agent have been used to improve protein malnutrition and nitrogen balance in children who are unable to meet protein requirements enterally.[60,61] Most often, one exchange per day is replaced with the amino acid dialysate, with 50% to 90% of infused amino acids being absorbed. To avoid using the amino acids for energy, the solution is typically given during the day, when meals and snacks provide a source of calories; however, giving the amino acids overnight via a cycler coupled with standard glucose dialysate as an energy source has also been used with good effect.[60] Potassium supplementation is often needed. Amino-acid-containing dialysates are not used routinely, because they are not available universally, and their cost is higher.

Protein Catabolic Rate and Protein Nitrogen Appearance

In adults, the calculation of the protein catabolic rate (PCR), which is also called the *protein equivalent of nitrogen appearance,* is commonly used to estimate dietary protein intake in dialysis patients who are in a steady state. Because protein breakdown under fasting conditions and dietary protein requirements are directly influenced by body mass, PCR is normalized to body weight (i.e., normalized PCR [nPCR]) and expressed in g/kg per day.[1] PCR is estimated from interdialytic changes in urea nitrogen concentration in serum and the urea nitrogen losses in dialysate (for PD patients) and urine (for patients with residual renal function), and it is theoretically more accurate than food diaries and recall. Because PCR fluctuates on a daily basis on the basis of what is eaten, a single PCR value does not give a good picture of usual or average protein intake; thus, monthly measurements are more informative.

Differences between metabolic activity and body composition in children and adults have led to a more cautious use of nPCR in pediatrics. Specific questions include whether the contribution of urea and nonurea nitrogen to total nitrogen appearance differs by age and how accurately nPCR approximates dietary protein intake in growing children, who should be in positive nitrogen balance (and therefore are not in a steady state).[62] In 2000, the K/DOQI nutrition guidelines stated that there was insufficient evidence to recommend its routine use in pediatric patients.[1] Since then, pediatric studies of nPCR relative to hemodialysis adequacy and outcomes have fostered increasing interest in and recommendations for its use in children on HD.[11,63,63a] The assessment of dietary protein intake (i.e., nPCR) is an integral part of assessing dialysis adequacy, because a child with a low predialysis urea level could be a well-nourished patient who is adequately dialyzed, but he or she could also be a patient with a low protein intake that masks inadequate dialysis.[64] For adolescents on HD, nPCR values below 1.0 to 1.2 g/kg/d have been associated with weight loss,[53,65] thereby suggesting a target level similar to that of adults (i.e., ≥1.0 to 1.2 g/kg/d). Target values for children and infants on HD have not yet been delineated, but they would theoretically be higher than for adolescents. The estimation of PCR can be performed using published regression equations[64] or urea kinetic modeling software programs that also calculate nPCR,[66] as described in Chapter 57.

Although PCR has been used to estimate dietary protein intake in children on PD,[62,67-69] associated outcome measures have not been evaluated, and there are no recommendations for the determination of PCR in this population.[11]

CARBOHYDRATE

There are no guidelines regarding the carbohydrate content of the diet for children with CKD. After transplantation, glucocorticosteroids and immunosuppressive agents such as tacrolimus cause impaired glucose tolerance, glycosuria, and a relative resistance to insulin that lead to diabetes in approximately 5% to 20% of children.[70] The management of children with diabetes should follow the recommendations provided by national diabetes associations (e.g., the American Diabetes Association[71]), including the avoidance of simple carbohydrates, weight control, and physical exercise.[72]

Fiber

Children with constipation or hypercholesterolemia may benefit from an increase in dietary fiber. Many high-fiber foods are restricted in the renal diet as a result of their high phosphorus and/or potassium content. If these foods are included more often, dosages of phosphate or potassium binders or the potassium content of the dialysate may need to be adjusted.[73] The fiber, potassium, and phosphorus content of selected high-fiber foods is available elsewhere.[73] Small amounts of several high-fiber foods throughout the day (e.g., homemade applesauce made from unpeeled apples, dried cranberries as snacks or added to cereal or cookies, shredded cabbage added to salad) may be easier to consume than one large portion of a single high-fiber item. Natural fiber can also be included in the diet in the form of a commercial tasteless powder added to meals (e.g., Metamucil, UniFiber, HyFiber)[73]; some of these products contain 30 to 60 mg (0.8 to 1.6 mmol) of potassium per dose. These products do not interfere with the absorption of medications or vitamins. High-fiber diets require additional fluid intake, which may be difficult for fluid-restricted children.

FAT

Requirements

Fats are an important source of calories for growing children. There are no guidelines for the amount of fat required by children with CKD.

Modifying Dietary Fat Intake

Caregivers are instructed to offer high-fat foods and to add fats to feedings as a concentrated source of calories (9 kcal/g fat) for children with poor weight gain. Hyperlipidemia is present in many children with CKD as well as in children who have undergone transplants,[74,75] and cardiovascular disease is reported to be either the first or second most common cause of death in children on chronic dialysis.[73] For these reasons, "heart-healthy" fats (e.g. margarines and oils made from canola, corn, safflower, soy, olives, and peanuts) should be used. Tube feeding can provide an appropriate energy intake with a balanced fat and carbohydrate profile that does not adversely affect serum lipids.[76]

There is a shortage of studies of dyslipidemias in children in the CKD population; hence, the K/DOQI dyslipidemia and cardiovascular guidelines[72,73] recommended that prepubertal children be managed according to existing national guidelines for children in the general population (e.g., the National Cholesterol Education Program[77]) and that pubertal and postpubertal children and adolescents be managed according to the K/DOQI guidelines for adults.[73] Therapeutic lifestyle changes for children are similar to those recommended for adults,[73] and they focus on decreasing the intake of saturated fatty acids, total fat, and cholesterol and on controlling the intake of calories and increasing physical activity to reach or maintain a healthy body weight. Studies in the general pediatric population have shown no adverse effects of dietary fat restriction on growth, development, or nutritional status; however, diet and lifestyle recommendations should be used with caution or not at all in children who are malnourished.[73] If, after 6 months, dietary changes fail to improve lipid concentrations and potential secondary causes of dyslipidemia have been ruled out, drug therapy should be considered.[73] The phosphate-binding agent sevelamer hydrochloride also acts as a bile acid sequestrant, and it has been shown to lower total and low-density lipoprotein cholesterol in patients with CKD.

Plant Sterols

Plant sterols and stanols block the absorption of endogenous and dietary cholesterol from the small intestine by entering into micelles, which are needed for cholesterol to dissolve. As a result, cholesterol becomes insoluble, and it is excreted in the stool. Studies in the general population have shown that 2 to 3 g of plant sterols per day lowers low-density lipoprotein cholesterol by 6% to 15% in hypercholesterolemic children and adults.[73] There is no contraindication to the use of commercial products containing plant sterols (e.g., Benecol or Take Control margarines) in patients with CKD.[73]

Soy

The meta-analysis of studies in the general adult population examining the effect of soy protein on dyslipidemias concluded that 25 g or more of soy protein daily reduces serum cholesterol by 9.3%, low-density lipoprotein cholesterol by 12.9%, and triglycerides by 10.5%.[78] Studies in the CKD population have not been performed, and the K/DOQI dyslipidemia guidelines made no recommendations regarding the use of soy protein. Families who wish to increase their child's soy intake may need additional counselling to help incorporate these products into the child's diet, because they are generally higher in sodium, potassium, and/or phosphorus content. Soy products have become increasing available in the marketplace, thereby making it easier to achieve an intake of 25 g/day.

Omega-3 Fatty Acids

Omega-3 fatty acids have beneficial effects on several risk factors that have a role in the development of cardiovascular disease (i.e., systemic inflammation, thrombotic tendency, lipid profiles, endothelial function, proinflammatory responses, cardiac rhythm, hypertension).[72] On the basis of recommendations for the general population[79] and available evidence regarding the potential benefits of omega-3 fatty acids on cardiovascular risk and outcomes in adult patients with CKD, the K/DOQI cardiovascular guidelines[72] state that it would seem beneficial for well-nourished, stable dialysis patients with or without evidence of cardiovascular disease to include food sources of omega-3 fatty acids (e.g., cold-water fish, canola oil, soybeans, walnuts, flaxseeds and their products) in their diet at least twice a week. Studies of and recommendations for the use of omega-3 fatty acids for children with CKD are limited. Therapeutic doses (3 to 8 g/d) in the form of fish oil supplements significantly reduced serum triglyceride concentrations and improved atherogenic serum lipoprotein profiles in 16 children on dialysis.[80]

Because deficiencies of essential fatty acids have been detected in patients with immunoglobulin A nephropathy, omega-3 fatty acid supplementation has been proposed as a therapeutic intervention to slow the progression to ESRD in this population. Two meta-analyses of studies of adults have been performed, both of which concluded that a clear beneficial effect could not be demonstrated.[20] Recently, neither omega-3 fatty acids (4 g/d) nor alternate-day prednisone showed benefit over placebo for slowing the progression of renal failure in children with immunoglobulin A nephropathy.[81]

Further studies of the safety and efficacy of using therapeutic doses of omega-3 fatty acid in children with CKD are needed before they can be used with confidence.

VITAMINS, MINERALS, AND TRACE ELEMENTS

Requirements

The optimum intake of vitamins and micronutrients for children with various stages of CKD has not been studied. The risk of micronutrient deficiency is increased by anorexia, dietary restrictions, drug-nutrient interactions, increased needs, and losses of water-soluble nutrients through the dialysis process. Several small studies in children on dialysis have shown that the dietary intake of most water-soluble vitamins[82-84] is lower than healthy recommendations but that the dietary intake and serum concentrations of some vitamins exceed normal ranges when multivitamin supplementation occurs. Children in these studies were supplemented with an adult renal multivitamin, which may in part explain their higher serum concentrations. The dietary intake of fat-soluble vitamins meets recommendations, and there is no loss of these vitamins through dialysis. Serum concentrations of vitamins A and E are normal or high without supplementation.[82-85] Hypervitaminosis A, which is reported in children on dialysis,[86] can aggravate anemia, hyperlipidemias, hypercalcemia, and bone disease and cause headache, anorexia, nausea, vomiting, and alopecia.[87] Vitamin K deficiency is possible, especially for those who have poor dietary intakes and who receive antibiotics frequently. Vitamin K plays a role in bone health and therefore has been a focus of limited study in adults with ESRD.[88-90] No studies of vitamin K deficiency or supplementation in children with CKD have been performed.

Hyperhomocysteinemia is associated with an increased risk of thrombosis and vascular disease, is found in children with CKD, and is associated with a low folate status.[91,92] Folic acid supplementation increases serum folate and red cell folate concentrations, and it decreases hyperhomocysteinemia to values that are comparable with those of controls[93-95]; however, whether this leads to a decrease in cardiovascular and thrombotic risk has not been established. Farid and colleagues[96] affected a decrease in hyperhomocysteinemia concentrations with combined folic acid and vitamin B12 supplementation but not with folic acid supplements alone. Folic acid supplementation should be considered for children with hyperhomocysteinemia.[91,93,95,96]

Trace elements are important components of many enzymatic pathways and proteins, and deficiencies of these micronutrients may have major adverse effects in growing children. Low dietary intakes of zinc and copper in small numbers of children on dialysis have been reported.[23,85] Esfahani and colleagues[97] reported low serum zinc concentrations in children on HD as compared with children on conservative management and controls and observed an inverse relationship between the length of time on dialysis and the serum zinc concentration. Warady and colleagues[98] found low serum copper and ceruloplasmin concentrations in 14 of 17 (82%) children receiving thrice-weekly HD. Three children with the lowest copper values had recombinant-human-erythropoietin-resistant anemia that responded to copper supplementation. A possible association between the use of sevelamer hydrochloride and copper deficiency was suggested, because 13 of 14 (93%) copper-deficient children had been taking sevelamer for a mean of 331 ± 294 days.

Modifying Micronutrient Intake

Recommendations regarding micronutrient supplementation for children with CKD are mixed. There are no pediatric guidelines for vitamin supplementation in children who are not on dialysis. For adults following protein-restricted diets, guidelines suggest supplementation with vitamins B1 (>1 mg/d), B2 (1 to 2 mg/d), and B6 (1.5 to 2 mg/d).[99]

Vitamin D supplementation should be provided for all exclusively breastfed infants, especially those at highest risk for vitamin-D-deficiency rickets (i.e., infants born to vitamin-D-deficient mothers, who have limited exposure to sunlight, or who are dark skinned).[100] A vitamin D metabolite or analog is required for all children to facilitate calcium and phosphorus homeostasis and to treat or prevent renal osteodystrophy. In children with CKD stages II to IV, an active vitamin D sterol (e.g., calcitriol) as well as supplemental vitamin D_3 (cholecalciferol) should be started when serum levels of 25-hydroxyvitamin D [25 (OH)D] are <30 ng/ml (<75 nmol/L) and when serum levels of parathyroid hormone (PTH) are above the target range for the CKD stage[101] (see Chapter 50). After successful renal transplantation, multivitamin therapy is rarely needed, because dietary restrictions are lifted and appetite and intake significantly improve. During the early posttransplant period, supplements of magnesium, phosphorus, and vitamin D may be required.[102]

For children on dialysis, the 2000 K/DOQI nutrition guidelines recommended supplementing water-soluble vitamins, zinc, and copper when intake is below recommended levels or when monitoring reveals laboratory or clinical evidence of deficiency.[1] More recently, the 2005 K/DOQI cardiac guidelines stated that current opinion and evidence suggest that it is prudent to supplement rather than risk deficiency, especially when supplementation is safe at the recommended levels.[72] These guidelines recommend a daily vitamin supplement that provides the recommended published vitamin profile for dialysis patients, with special attention paid to folic acid and vitamins B2, B6, and B12. The CARI guidelines suggest supplementing water-soluble vitamins for dialysis patients who are not receiving nutritional supplements.[102a] There is good agreement that the routine supplementation of fat-soluble vitamins A, E, and K be avoided throughout all stages of CKD,[1,20] although they may individually or collectively be required by some children (e.g., those with concomitant liver disease and/or fat malabsorption).

In the absence of a pediatric product, an adult renal B and C vitamin is used; it is crushed and dissolved in water for infants and children who are unable to swallow tablets, or it is given in liquid form, where available (e.g., Nephronex). These preparations contain no more than 60 to 100 mg of vitamin C to avoid complications of the retention of oxalate, a metabolite of vitamin C for which the kidney is the only route of excretion. Commonly, infants and toddlers are prescribed half a tablet daily, and children are given 1 tablet daily. In some instances, a regular liquid B and C vitamin can be used, if available. A pediatric renal multivitamin has recently been developed in the United Kingdom, but it is not yet widely available. Some renal vitamin supplements also contain one or more micronutrients (e.g., zinc).

Supplemental oral or intravenous iron is usually required by children of all ages on erythropoietin-stimulating agents to avoid storage iron depletion, to prevent iron-deficient erythropoiesis, and to achieve and maintain target hemoglobin concentrations between 11 and 13 g/dl (110 to 130 g/L).[103] There is insufficient evidence to recommend the use of vitamin C or L-carnitine for the management of anemia in children with CKD.[103]

BALANCING CALCIUM AND PHOSPHORUS INTAKE

Metabolic bone diseases are common in children with CKD, because the kidney plays important roles in the body's balance of calcium, phosphorus, and magnesium and is responsible for the final step in the formation of calcitriol (the active form of vitamin D) and the degradation of PTH. Vitamin D is important, because it inhibits production and release of PTH from the parathyroid glands and increases serum calcium levels by stimulating calcium absorption from the gut. Hypocalcemia and hyperphosphatemia begin to appear at an early stage in renal disease, about the time that 50% of kidney function is lost.[101] Both contribute to renal osteodystrophy (ROD), which is composed of a wide range of skeletal disorders that are associated with kidney disease. The incidence of ROD is higher in children as compared with adults as a result of high bone turnover in the growing skeleton. ROD may impair linear growth; therefore, the maintenance of normal calcium, phosphorus, calcium-phosphorus product, and PTH levels is critical.

A low-phosphorus diet (Table 48-2) in combination with phosphate binders and vitamin D treatment is an essential part of therapy for the prevention of hyperphosphatemia, hypocalcemia, ROD, and poor growth. Even during the early stages of CKD, when serum phosphorus concentrations remain normal, dietary phosphorus should be decreased to general recommendations for age (e.g., DRI)[104] when the serum PTH concentration is above the recommended target range for the stage of CKD.[101] When dietary modifications are unsuccessful for controlling serum phosphorus concentrations within the target range, calcium-containing phosphate binders should be prescribed.[101] Doses of binders are usually established empirically; however, tables have been provided for estimating the initial prescription that are based on average phosphorus intake and absorption, average dialysis clearance, and binding potential for available binders.[101] Hypophosphatemia found in children with renal tubular phosphate wasting or other causes should be corrected using a high-phosphorus diet, enteral phosphorus supplementation, or a reduction of any phosphate binders.

TABLE 48-2 Strategies for Lowering Dietary Phosphorus Intake and/or Absorption in Nonbreastfed Infants and Children

- Use a low-phosphorus formula (e.g., Similac PM 60/40, Good Start), and consider continuing it beyond 1 year of age to delay the introduction of phosphorus-rich cow's milk.
- Fresh or frozen breast milk can be safely pretreated with sevelamer to markedly reduce its phosphorus content without significantly changing its content, with the exception of calcium and protein.[130]
- Limit foods that are naturally high in phosphorus, such as milk, yogurt, cheese, organ meats, dried beans and peas, nuts and nut butters, chocolate, quick breads, and whole-grain or bran products.
- Read labels to avoid foods and drinks in which phosphate salts have been added by the manufacturer for nonnutritive reasons, such as "enhanced" products (i.e., fresh meat that is marinated in a solution of sodium, phosphate, and water to increase its shelf life and improve tenderness), carbonated beverages (colas), and canned ice tea or juice drinks that contain phosphoric acid.
- Choose lower-phosphorus foods such as liquid nondairy creamers, nondairy milk substitutes, and sherbet.
- Not all children eat three meals per day; the timing of the administration of phosphorus binders needs to reflect when during the day and/or night the largest amounts of phosphorus are taken (e.g., with overnight tube feeding).
- Children and caregivers can be taught to adjust binders according to the phosphate content of meals.

Important limitations of vitamin D therapy include hypercalcemia and worsening hyperphosphatemia as a result of the stimulation of their absorption from the gut and the oversuppression of PTH levels. Recent awareness of the adverse effects of hypercalcemia and a high serum calcium-phosphorus level on metastatic calcification and vascular disease has caused clinicians to carefully evaluate calcium loads from diet and phosphate binders and to seek alternate types of phosphorus binders and vitamin-D-type supplements. To prevent or control ROD and to decrease the risk of calcification, the 2005 K/DOQI bone guidelines for children with CKD[101] have made recommendations for the strict control of both serum PTH levels and the calcium-phosphorus product (Table 48-3) and for closely monitoring maximum dietary phosphorus intake and the intake of calcium from calcium-containing phosphorus binders and the diet (Table 48-4). A variety of noncalcium-containing phosphorus binders (including the short-term use of aluminum-based binders or the long-term use of sevelamer hydrochloride/Renagel), synthetic vitamin D analogues (which have less calcemic activity; e.g., paricalcitriol/Zemplar, doxercalciferol/Hectorol), and calcimimetics (which lower PTH levels by increasing the sensitivity of the calcium-sensing receptor sites to extracellular calcium; e.g., cinacalcet hydrochloride/Sensipar) are available for the treatment of hypercalcemia.[101]

Restricting dietary phosphorus complicates efforts to achieve adequate protein intake, because both nutrients are often found in the same foods. The lowest amount of phosphorus in proportion to the quantity and quality of protein comes from animal flesh proteins (average: 11 mg phosphorus/gram protein), whereas eggs, dairy products, legumes, and lentils have higher phosphorus-to-protein ratios (average: 20 mg phosphorus/gram protein).[101]

After transplantation, glucocorticosteroid therapy can induce osteoporosis; therefore, calcium supplementation may be needed for children who are unable to meet general recommendations for calcium (e.g., DRI).[104] A high intake of phosphorus-rich foods and fluids is encouraged during the early transplantation period to manage hypophosphatemia as a result of transient impaired renal phosphate reabsorption.[102]

MODIFYING SODIUM INTAKE

Sodium is directly linked to fluid balance; therefore, the need for sodium supplementation or restriction varies with the primary kidney disease and the volume of urine output. CKD

TABLE 48-3 Recommended Target Ranges for Serum Parathyroid Hormone and Calcium-Phosphorus Product

	Chronic Kidney Disease Stage			
Target Range	II	III	IV	V
Serum parathyroid hormone level	35 to 70 pg/ml	35 to 70 pg/ml	70 to 110 pg/ml	200 to 300 pg/ml
Calcium-phosphus product level	Age ≤12 years: <65 mg^2/dl^2 (5.25 $mmol^2/L^2$) Age >12 years: <55 mg^2/dl^2 (4.4 $mmol^2/L^2$)			

From the National Kidney Foundation: K/DOQI clinical practice guidelines for bone metabolism and disease in children with chronic kidney disease, *Am J Kidney Dis* 46(4 Suppl 1):S1-121, 2005.

TABLE 48-4 **Recommendations for Maximum Phosphorus and Calcium Intake for Children with Hyperphosphatemia**

	Dietary Phosphorus Intake (mg/d)*		Calcium Intake (mg/d)†	
Age (Years)	High Parathyroid Hormone, Normal Phosphorus	High Parathyroid Hormone, High Phosphorus	From Calcium-Containing Phosphorus Binders	Total (Diet Plus Binders)
0 to 0.5	≤100	≤80	≤420	≤2500
0.5 to 1.0	≤275	≤220	≤540	≤2500
1 to 3	≤460	≤370	≤1000	≤2500
4 to 8	≤500	≤400	≤1600	≤2500
9 to 18	≤1250	≤1000	≤2500	≤2500

From the National Kidney Foundation: K/DOQI clinical practice guidelines for bone metabolism and disease in children with chronic kidney disease, *Am J Kidney Dis* 46(4 Suppl 1):S1-121, 2005, and Institute of Medicine: *Dietary reference intakes for calcium, phosphorous, magnesium, vitamin D, and fluoride,* Washington, National Academy of Sciences, 1997.
*To convert mg to mmol, divide by 31.
†To convert mg to mmol, divide by 40.

during infancy is often caused by polyuric salt-wasting conditions such as obstructive uropathy, renal dysplasia, tubular disease, or polycystic kidney disease. Urinary sodium losses in these infants often exceeds sodium intake from breast milk or formula; therefore, salt supplementation is required to prevent sodium depletion, a decrease in extracellular volume, and impaired growth.[105,106] Supplementation with 4 to 7 mmol/kg/d of sodium chloride may be required in children with CKD and renal dysplasia[20,106]; supplements may be given separately or added to breast milk or infant formula, provided that the infant reliably receives the full volume of breast milk or formula.

Children with glomerular disease or those with oliguria or anuria typically need sodium and fluid restrictions for fluid balance and the control of hypertension. Serum sodium concentration reflects water balance rather than total body sodium; therefore, it is not a good indicator of the need for sodium restriction or supplementation. Sodium and fluid restrictions are more liberal for children on PD than HD. One month after transplantation, almost 80% of children are hypertensive as a result of the effects of immunosuppressive medications and thus they require sodium restriction.[102] Restaurant meals and salt added by manufacturers provide 75% of the daily sodium intake of most North Americans.[107] For children who require sodium restriction, K/DOQI guidelines recommend limiting sodium intake to less than 2000 mg/d[72] to 2500 mg/d (90 to 110 mmol/d).[108] The most recent Dietary Guidelines for Americans[79,109] recommend that hypertensive individuals who are more than 2 years old consume no more than 1500 mg (65 mmol) of sodium per day. For infants and young children, sodium intakes of 1500 to 2500 mg/d would be too generous on a mmol/kg basis; guidelines commonly used in clinical practice for this population are closer to 1 to 3 mmol/kg/d.[110]

ADJUSTING FLUID INTAKE

Fluid intake should be adjusted on the basis of the child's clinical state, taking into account the volume of urine output, the glomerular filtration rate, and the presence of edema and hypertension.[20] Infants and children who need to eliminate their daily osmotic load (e.g., those with nephrogenic diabetes insipidus) or those with a salt-losing nephropathy typically have high obligatory fluid output and require high fluid intakes to prevent chronic dehydration, malaise, and poor growth. High fluid intakes may also be part of the management of children with nephrolithiasis or urinary tract infections.[20] As these children lose renal function, they and their caregivers may have difficulty understanding the reversal of fluid management. After transplantation, high fluid intakes are also prescribed to maintain good perfusion of the transplanted kidney and to avoid immunosuppressant toxicity, which can occur with dehydration.[102] To prevent steroid-induced hyperglycemia and excessive weight gain, water and calorie-free fluids are encouraged.

During CKD stages I through IV, fluid restriction is rarely needed. After urine output decreases and edema occurs, a limit on fluid intake is required; without restriction, fluid overload, hypertension, and subsequent cardiac, cerebrovascular, renal, and respiratory complications may occur. Children on PD seldom need fluid restrictions, because higher glucose concentration dialysates can be used to increase ultrafiltration. Fluid limits are more often needed for patients on HD to limit interdialytic (fluid) weight gain to less than 5% of dry weight between dialysis sessions.[63] The prescribed total fluid intake is based on insensible fluid losses, 24-hour urine output, ultrafiltration capacity for children on dialysis, other losses (e.g., vomiting, diarrhea, gastrointestinal drains, burns, fever), and, if necessary, an amount to be deficited. Through education, children and their caregivers should follow a reduced fluid intake regimen (Table 48-5) in combination with a reduced sodium intake (Table 48-6). Reducing salt intake can have the secondary benefits of reducing thirst and water demand as well as improving edema and hypertension control.[11,20,63] Many fruits and vegetables contain significant amounts of water (e.g., grapefruit, watermelon, lettuce, cucumbers), and, depending on an individual's diet, fluid from solid foods can contribute up to 800 to 1000 ml/d. The frequency of dialysis should be increased if a fluid restriction is adversely affecting a child's nutritional status.[63]

TABLE 48-5 Discussion Points to Help Children Cope with Their Fluid Restrictions

- Talk about the reason for restricting fluids and the consequences of excessive or inadequate fluid intake.
- Let them know that fluids include water, soup, milk, juice, and soda.
- Be sure they are aware that foods made from fluids (e.g., ice, popsicles, freezies, ice cream, Jello, pudding, yogurt, gravy) also count as fluid.
- Drain liquids from canned fruit.
- Tell children to drink only when they are thirsty and to have just enough to quench their thirst.
- Have children avoid salty or very sweet foods or drinks, because they increase thirst.
- Know how much glasses and cups contain; have children drink from the same small glass.
- For a visual reminder of how much fluid is left for the day, suggest filling a container with the amount of water equal to the daily fluid allowance. Each time a liquid is used, pour out and discard that amount from the container.
- Spread out the child's fluid intake evenly throughout the day.
- Have the child take medications with applesauce, baby fruit, or mealtime liquids.
- Help minimize the child's dry mouth and lips by having the child use lip balms or moisturized lipsticks, gargle with mouthwash with a low alcohol content, and brush the teeth often.
- To decrease thirst, have the child suck on ice, lemon wedges, hard sour candy, or sugarless mints; chew thirst-quenching or sugarless gum; rinse with cold water or mouthwash; use breath spray; or eat cold or frozen low-potassium fruits such as grapes or strawberries.

TABLE 48-6 Discussion Points to Help Children Lower Their Sodium Intake

- Prepare homemade baby foods without salt or salty foods.
- Transition infants to low-sodium finger foods.
- Cook with a small amount of salt, but do not add salt at the table.
- Rely on fresh rather than processed foods.
- Read ingredient lists and nutrient content tables on food labels to avoid salty foods.
- Salty foods are defined as having more than 140 to 200 mg (6 to 9 mmol) of sodium per serving.
- Salt substitutes replace sodium chloride with potassium chloride and are not suitable for children with hyperkalemia.
- Add flavor to foods using spices, herbs, lemon juice, and vinegar.
- Modify recipes to lower the sodium content, or look for renal or low-sodium cookbooks.
- Do not drink or use water from a water-softening system that replaces hard minerals with sodium.
- Eat out less often, especially at fast-food restaurants.
- Obtain nutrient content information from fast-food restaurants to choose lower sodium foods.
- Plan ahead for special occasions; pack low-salt snacks for outings.
- Avoid foods that are high in sodium, including these popular ones: soy sauce, luncheon meat, ham, bacon, sausage, pepperoni, hot dogs, processed cheese slices, string cheese, cheese spreads, Kraft dinners, pickles, ketchup, salted crackers, potato chips, nacho chips, other salted snack foods, and dried soup mixes.
- Choose foods that are lower in sodium, such as fresh meats and poultry, homemade hamburgers, hard or "block" cheeses, cream cheese, salt-free crackers, homemade macaroni and cheese, unsalted chips, peanuts, and popcorn.

TABLE 48-7 Discussion Points to Help Children Lower Their Potassium Intake

- When possible, feed an infant breast milk or an infant formula with a lower potassium content.
- If necessary, pretreat infant formula or enteral feedings with a potassium binder to lower the potassium content by approximately 50%.
- The potassium content of commercial baby foods differs from the equivalent table food (e.g., jarred, strained bananas versus fresh bananas).
- A food is defined as being high in potassium if it contains more than 200 mg (5 mmol) per serving.
- Potassium in food cannot be tasted, and its content is infrequently listed on food labels.
- Many fruits and vegetables are high in potassium.
- Fruit drinks, beverages, punches, and soft drinks contain little or no potassium as compared with juices.
- Peeling, cutting into smaller pieces, and presoaking potassium-rich vegetables such as potatoes lowers their potassium content.
- Cooking vegetables in water (i.e., boiling) lowers their potassium content, whereas other methods of cooking (i.e., microwaving, steaming, deep frying, baking, roasting) do not.
- Do not drink or use water from a water-softening system that replaces hard minerals with potassium.
- Review serving sizes, because eating a large serving can turn a low-potassium food into a high source of potassium.
- Avoid salt substitutes, because they contain potassium in place of sodium.
- Avoid foods that are high in potassium, including these popular ones: bananas, oranges and orange juice, mangoes, papayas, dried fruits, baked potatoes, french fries, potato chips, tomato products, and chocolate.
- Choose foods that are lower in potassium, such as apples, grapes, cherries, berries, cranberry juice, boiled or mashed potatoes, white rice, onion rings, popcorn, pretzels, corn chips, cream sauces, and sugar candies without chocolate, nuts, or raisins.

LIMITING POTASSIUM INTAKE

Potassium is directly linked to nerve and muscle function, and elevated serum concentrations can produce cardiac arrhythmias and arrest. Hyperkalemia is often asymptomatic, particularly in children who develop a gradual tolerance to higher and higher levels. The restriction of dietary potassium (Table 48-7) is dictated by serum concentrations, and it is usually not necessary until the glomerular filtration rate falls to less than 10% of normal. Children started on an angiotensin-converting enzyme inhibitor may require restriction earlier. Because PD occurs daily, children on PD seldom need dietary potassium restriction after they reach full maintenance dialysate exchange volumes (i.e., 1.1 L/m^2). Occasionally a child on PD may require potassium supplementation to maintain normal serum concentrations. Depending on residual renal function, most children on standard HD need to follow a low-potassium diet, whereas those on daily HD typically do not. No evidence-based guidelines or recommendations exist regarding the level of potassium restriction for children of different ages. Common practice has been to limit intake to 1 to 3 mmol/kg/d (39 to 117 mg/kg/d) for infants and toddlers and to 2 to 4 g/day (51 to 102 mmol/d) for children and adolescents. During the early posttransplant period, hyperkalemia may result from cyclosporine or tacrolimus therapy, especially when blood concentrations are above the target range.

If necessary, infant formulas, enteral feedings, and drinks can be pretreated with an ion exchange resin (e.g., sodium polystyrene sulfonate, calcium polystyrene sulfonate) to lower their potassium content.[111-113] When these binders are mixed with a formula or drink, the insoluble resin exchanges sodium or calcium with potassium and then settles to the bottom of the container. After approximately 30 to 60 minutes, the potassium-depleted formula is decanted from the sediment on the bottom and administered orally or via a feeding tube (with flushes of at least 10 ml of water before and after). Many fruits and vegetables are high in potassium, and children and caregivers should be advised to avoid fruit juices (with the exception of cranberry juice) and to choose fruit drinks, beverages, punches, or soft drinks instead. The prescription of potassium exchange resins may be necessary if dietary potassium restriction does not normalize serum concentrations. Calcium-based resins should be considered rather than sodium-based resins for the child with moderate to severe hypertension. Not all hyperkalemia is related to the diet. When a dietary source of hyperkalemia cannot be identified, nondietary causes should also be investigated, including hemolysis; acidosis; constipation; hyperglycemia; medications such as penicillin, beta-blockers, angiotensin-converting enzyme inhibitors, nonsteroidal anti-inflammatory drugs (e.g., indomethacin), steroids, cyclosporine, and tacrolimus; tissue destruction as a result of chemotherapy, infection, surgery, or catabolism; inadequate dialysis; and the use of a HD dialysate with too high a potassium concentration.[114] Serum bicarbonate should be corrected when levels are below 22 mmol/L.[1,20]

OTHER NUTRITIONAL ISSUES

Complementary Medicine

In hopes of preventing or reversing the progression of a child's kidney disease, caregivers may turn to a variety of naturopathic products that target various renal ailments (e.g., hypertension, urinary tract infection). Some complementary medicines are nephrotoxic (and their toxicity may be greater in the presence of existing renal impairment),[20] whereas some have immunostimulant effects that can cause kidney allograft dysfunction or rejection. Other complementary agents have potentially harmful effects on drug action, urinary retention, diuresis, blood pressure, serum concentrations of potassium or oxalates, and clotting. Because they are not prescribed, caregivers often consider these products harmless or not important, and they may not mention their use. Practitioners should therefore probe for use of herbal products and alternative/complementary medications when taking a dietary history. A number of resources are available to help the practitioner assess potentially harmful products[20,115-117]; these products are described in detail in Chapter 66.

Eating During Hemodialysis Treatment

Food intake during hemodialysis may contribute to poor dialysis tolerance by redistributing some of the circulating blood to splanchnic organs and decreasing the blood volume of the large vessels.[118] The effect of eating during hemodialysis treatments has not been studied in the pediatric population; however, research in adults has shown that eating during hemodialysis can cause low blood pressure, cramping or other gastrointestinal symptoms, and poor tolerance of fluid removal.[118,119] By extrapolation, many pediatric dialysis centers do not allow eating or drinking during dialysis, or they limit intake to small snacks, especially for children who are experiencing low blood pressure or cramps during dialysis.

Nephrotic Syndrome

A low-sodium, controlled-calorie diet that limits the intake of simple carbohydrates (i.e., sugars) and total and saturated fats and that promotes the selection of heart-healthy fats is commonly used to manage the edema, weight gain, and hyperlipidemia seen in children with nephrotic syndrome.[120,121] The management of hyperlipidemia is controversial, and it may play more of a role if the nephrotic state is prolonged. Fluid restriction is not usually required unless edema is severe. Except for children with congenital nephrotic syndrome of the Finnish type who require a very high protein intake (i.e., 3 to 4 g/kg),[122,123] manipulations to increase or reduce dietary protein intake to try to compensate for proteinuria and hypoalbuminemia are not indicated.[123]

Physical Activity

Despite the correction of renal anemia with erythropoietin, many children remain physically inactive and have poorer exercise capacities than healthy children.[124,125] Physical inactivity results in weakness, stiffness, muscle wasting, and negative nitrogen balance, and, in adults, it is associated with increased mortality risk.[126] Weight gain in children who are on supplemental tube feeding is frequently suspected to be caused by increased fat mass rather than lean mass. In adults, exercise intervention has been shown to improve strength, endurance, and physical functioning, whereas aerobic exercise training has improved blood pressure control, lipid profiles, and self-reported quality of life.[127] Minimal experience with exercise programs in children with CKD has been reported; however, a recent study showed that after 3 months, a moderate-intensity, twice-weekly, hour-long exercise program during HD led to significant improvements in children's endurance and upper and lower body strength to levels that were similar to those of healthy children.[125] Routine counselling and encouragement to increase physical activity should be part of standard care.[128] Regular participation in school gym classes and community sport and exercise programs should be promoted, and parents should be encouraged to get their children moving by involving the whole family in games or active play (e.g., walking, dancing, biking, rollerblading, bowling, skating, badminton, tennis, hiking, cross-country skiing). Nephrology team members can promote fitness by organizing games and sports at annual kidney get-togethers, encouraging children to attend kidney camps, and raising awareness of the National Kidney Foundation's US Transplant Games.

Transplantation

During the pretransplant evaluation, the assessment of the child's nutritional status provides the opportunity to identify and correct deficits and to educate the child and family about dietary changes that will occur after transplantation. Post-

TABLE 48-8 Suggestions for Healthy Eating after a Transplant

- To avoid contracting a foodborne illness, be especially careful when handling, preparing, and consuming foods.
- Focus on a combination of heart-healthy eating habits and physical activity to achieve and maintain a healthy weight and appropriate cholesterol, blood pressure, and blood glucose levels.
- Choose and prepare foods with little or no salt and sugar.
- Choose sugar-free and calorie-free beverages.
- Eat a diet that is rich in vegetables, fruits, and whole-grain, high-fiber foods.
- Limit intake of saturated fat, trans fat, and cholesterol by choosing lean meats, vegetable/soy alternatives, and fat-free (skim) and low-fat (1% fat) dairy products. Minimize intake of partially hydrogenated fats.
- Eat fish at least twice a week, especially those that are relatively high in omega-3 fatty acids (e.g., salmon, trout, herring). Avoid mercury-contaminated fish (e.g., shark, swordfish, king mackerel, tilefish).
- Pay attention to portion size.
- Aim for a minimum of 30 minutes of physical activity each day. Reduce sedentary activities such as watching television and playing computer games.

transplant diet modifications aid in the management of the side effects of multidrug immunosuppressive therapy, including appetite stimulation and weight gain, protein catabolism, hypertension, hyperglycemia, hyperkalemia, dyslipidemias, hypophosphatemia, hypomagnesemia, and gastrointestinal disturbances. These modifications emphasize lifestyle changes that include heart-healthy eating habits and physical activity (Table 48-8). Weight control and high daily fluid intakes become new challenges for children who have previously struggled to gain weight and adhere to fluid restrictions. Grapefruit juice and other grapefruit products should be avoided, because they can alter the absorption of certain medications, including some immunosuppressants (e.g., cyclosporine) and calcium-channel blockers.

Vegetarianism

Populations that commonly follow a vegetarian diet include Hindus, Buddhists, Muslims, Jains, and Seventh-Day Adventists. Some adolescents or families follow a vegetarian diet for health reasons or beliefs about animal rights, and some children dislike the taste or texture of meat and inadvertently assume a vegetarian style of eating. Health benefits of vegetarianism, especially for patients with CKD stages I through IV, include improved lipid profiles, less proteinuria, and a reduced postprandial glomerular filtration rate. Vegetable protein can be consumed in larger amounts as compared with animal proteins and have similar effects on urea. Therefore, modifying the source of protein rather than restricting the amount may be an effective diet strategy for progressive renal disease.

Vegetarians (especially vegans) and children on PD may require specific dietary counselling to meet their protein requirements within other dietary restrictions. Plant sources of protein alone can provide adequate amounts of essential amino acids if a variety of plant foods are consumed daily and energy needs are met. Adequate caloric intake is essential to promote positive nitrogen balance. Although the bioavailability of plant protein phosphorus is lower than animal protein sources (50% to 60% versus 70% or more), the higher ratio of phosphorus to protein in plant protein sources (i.e., nuts, seeds, legumes) often means that the vegetarian child requires more phosphorus binders to control hyperphosphatemia and meet dietary protein recommendations. The selection of low-potassium fruits and vegetables is necessary to accommodate the high-potassium contributions of soy, nuts, legumes, and seeds. Potassium-binding resins (e.g., Kayexalate) and/or low-potassium baths for HD patients may be needed. Processed plant protein sources (e.g., veggie burgers and wieners, marinated tofu) are typically high in sodium, as are savory snacks and meals in cups; reading labels can help with the avoidance of these products and the identification of better choices.

SUMMARY

The significance of nutritional management in children with CKD is underscored by its association with outcomes. Surrogate markers of poor nutrition such as serum albumin and growth retardation correlate with mortality and morbidity in children with ESRD. Children on dialysis with a height standard deviation score of less than 2.5 have a threefold higher risk of death as compared with those with normal height standard deviations.[129] Nutritional challenges in children with CKD remain as a result of the paucity of evidence-based recommendations. Well-designed and adequately powered clinical trials are urgently needed to define practice guidelines. Molecular studies into the pathophysiology of uremic cachexia hold the promise of novel therapies to treat this potentially fatal complication of CKD.

REFERENCES

1. National Kidney Foundation Dialysis Outcome Quality Initiative: Clinical practice guidelines for nutrition in chronic renal failure, *Am J Kidney Dis* 35(6 Suppl 2):S105-36, 2000.
2. Mak R, Cheung W, Cone R, Marks D: Orexigenic and anorexigenic mechanisms in the control of nutrition in chronic kidney disease, *Pediatr Nephrol* 20:427-31, 2005.
3. Mak RH, Cheung W: Energy homeostasis and cachexia in chronic kidney disease, *Pediatr Nephrol* 21:1807-14, 2006.
4. Mak R, Cheung W, Cone R, Marks D: Cytokine and adipokine signaling in uremic cachexia, *Nature Clin Pract Nephrol* 2:529-34, 2006.
5. Mak R, Cheung W, Cone R, Marks D: Leptin and inflammation-associated cachexia in chronic kidney disease, *Kidney Int* 69:794-97, 2006.
6. Mak R, Cheung W: Adipokines and gut hormones in end-stage renal disease, *Perit Dial Int* (in press).
7. Mak R, Cheung W, Purnell J: Ghrelin in chronic kidney disease: too much or too little?, *Perit Dial Int* 27:51-55, 2007.
8. Cheung W, Marks D, Yu X, Cone R, Mak R: The role of leptin and melanocortin signaling in uremia-associated cachexia, *J Clin Invest* 115:1659-65, 2005.
9. Kalantar-Zadeh K, Block G, McAllister C, Humphreys M, Kopple J: Appetite and inflammation, nutrition, anemia, and clinical outcome in hemodialysis patients, *Am J Clin Nutr* 80:299-307, 2004.
10. Wang S, Sea M, Tang N, et al: Resting energy expenditure and subsequent mortality risk in peritoneal dialysis patients, *J Am Soc Nephrol* 15:3134-43, 2004.

11. National Kidney Foundation: KDOQI clinical practice guidelines and clinical practice recommendations for hemodialysis adequacy, peritoneal dialysis adequacy, and vascular access, update 2006. *Am J Kidney Dis* 48(1 Suppl 1):S1-322, 2006.
12. Foster B, Leonard M: Measuring nutritional status in children with chronic kidney disease, *Am J Clin Nutr* 80:801-14, 2004.
13. Rees L, Shaw V: Nutrition in children with CRF and on dialysis, *Pediatr Nephrol* 22:1689-702, 2007.
14. Wong CS, Gipson DS, Gillen DL, Emerson S, et al: Anthropometric measures and risk of death in children with end-stage renal disease, *Am J Kidney Dis* 36:811-19, 2000.
15. Rashid R, Neill E, Smith W, King D, et al: Body composition and nutritional intake in children with chronic kidney disease, *Pediatr Nephrol* 21:1730-38, 2006.
16. Wong C, Hingorani S, Gillen D, Sherrard D, et al: Hypoalbuminemia and risk of death in pediatric patients with end-stage renal disease, *Kidney Int* 61:630-37, 2002.
17. Kaysen G, Dubin J, Muller H, et al: Inflammation and reduced albumin synthesis associated with stable decline in serum albumin in hemodialysis patients, *Kidney Int* 65:1408-15, 2004.
18. Patel C, Denny M: *Cultural foods & renal diets for the clinical RD*, ed 2, San Mateo, CA, 1997, CRN Northern California/Northern Nevada and National Kidney Foundation.
19. Patel C, Denny M: *Cultural foods & renal diets for the renal patient*, ed 2, San Mateo, CA, 1997, CRN Northern California/Northern Nevada and National Kidney Foundation.
20. Pollock C, Voss D, Hodson E, Crompton C: The CARI guidelines. Nutrition and growth in kidney disease, *Nephrology* 10(Suppl 5): S177-230, 2005.
21. Coleman J, Edefonti A, Watson A, for the European Paediatric Peritoneal Dialysis Working Group: Guidelines by an ad hoc European committee on the assessment of growth and nutritional status in children on chronic peritoneal dialysis. *Perit Dial Int* 21:323, 2001.
22. Betts P, Magrath G: Growth pattern and dietary intake of children with chronic renal insufficiency, *BMJ* 2:189-93, 1974.
23. Ratsch I, Catassi C, Verrina E, Gusmano R, et al: Energy and nutrient intake of patients with mild-to-moderate chronic renal failure compared with healthy children: an Italian multicentre study, *Eur J Pediatr* 151:701-05, 1992.
24. Foreman JW, Abitol CL, Trachtman H, Garin EH, et al: Nutritional intake in children with renal insufficiency: a report of the growth failure in children with renal diseases study, *J Am Coll Nutr* 15(6):579-85, 1996.
25. Canepa A, Perfumo F, Carrea A, Menoni S, et al: Protein and calorie intake, nitrogen losses, and nitrogen balance in children undergoing chronic peritoneal dialysis, *Adv Perit Dial* 12:326-29, 1996.
26. Edefonti A, Picca M, Damiani B, Loi S, et al: Dietary prescription based on estimated nitrogen balance during peritoneal dialysis, *Pediatr Nephrol* 13:253-58, 1999.
27. Food and Nutrition Board: *Recommended dietary allowances*, ed 10, Washington, DC, 1989, National Research Council.
28. Reed EE, Roy LP, Gaskin KJ, Knight JF: Nutritional intervention and growth in children with chronic renal failure, *J Ren Nutr* 8:122-26, 1998.
29. Van Dyck M, Bilem N, Proesmans W: Conservative treatment for chronic renal failure from birth: a 3-year follow-up study, *Pediatr Nephrol* 13:865-69, 1999.
30. Ledermann SE, Shaw V, Trompeter RS: Long-term enteral nutrition in infants and young children with chronic renal failure, *Pediatr Nephrol* 13:870-75, 1999.
31. Coleman JE, Watson AR, Rance CH, Moore E: Gastrostomy buttons for nutritional support on chronic dialysis, *Nephrol Dial Transplant* 13:2041-46, 1998.
32. Norman LJ, MacLean WC, Watson AR: Optimising nutrition in chronic renal sufficiency—growth, *Pediatr Nephrol* 19:1245-52, 2004.
33. Dabbagh S, Fassinger N, Clement K: The effect of aggressive nutrition on infection rates in patients maintained on peritoneal dialysis, *Adv Perit Dial* 7:161-64, 1991.
34. Burrows J, Bluestone P, Wang J, et al: The effects of moderate dose of megestrol acetate on nutritional status and body composition in a hemodialysis patient, *J Ren Nutr* 9:89-94, 1999.
35. Boccanfuso J, Hutton M, McAllister B: The effects of megestrol acetate on nutritional parameters in a dialysis population, *J Ren Nutr* 10:36-43, 2000.
36. Rammohan M, Kalantar-Zadeh K, Liang A, Ghossein C: Megestrol acetate in a moderate dose for the treatment of malnutrition-inflammation complex, *J Ren Nutr* 15:345-55, 2005.
37. Williams J, Perius M, Humble A, et al: Effect of megestrol acetate on the nutritional status of malnourished hemodialysis patients, *J Ren Nutr* 7:231, 1997.
38. Bossola M, Tazza L, Giungi S, Luciani G: Anorexia in hemodialysis patients: an update, *Kidney Int* 70:417-22, 2006.
39. Wynne K, Giannitsopoulou K, Small C, et al: Subcutaneous ghrelin enhances acute food intake in malnourished patients who receive maintenance peritoneal dialysis: a randomized placebo-controlled trial, *J Am Soc Nephrol* 16:2111-18, 2005.
40. Spinozzi NS, Nelson PA: Nutrition support in the newborn intensive care unit, *J Ren Nutr* 6(4):188-97, 1996.
41. Yiu VW, Harmon WE, Spinozzi N, Jonas M, Kim MS: High-calorie nutrition for infants with chronic renal disease, *J Ren Nutr* 6:203-06, 1996.
42. Evans S, Twaissi H, Daly A, Davies P, MacDonald A: Should high-energy infant formula be given at full strength from its first day of usage?, *J Hum Nutr Diet* 19:191-97, 2006.
42a. Gast T, Bunchman T, Barletta GM: Nutritional management of infants with CKD/ESRD with use of "adult" renal-based formulas, *Perit Dial Int* 27(Suppl 1):534, 2007.
43. Dello Strologo L, Principato F, Sinibaldi D, Appiani AC, et al: Feeding dysfunction in infants with severe chronic renal failure after long-term nasogastric tube feeding, *Pediatr Nephrol* 11(1):84-86, 1997.
44. Coleman JE, Watson AR: Growth posttransplantation in children previously treated with chronic dialysis and gastrostomy feeding, *Adv Perit Dial* 14:269-73, 1998.
45. Kari JA, Gonzalez C, Ledermann SE, Shaw V, Rees L: Outcome and growth of infants with severe chronic renal failure, *Kidney Int* 57(4):1681-87, 2000.
46. Wilson S: Pediatric enteral feeding. In Grand R, Sutphen J, et al, editors: *Pediatric nutrition, theory and practice*, Toronto, Ontario, 1987, Butterworth.
47. Wood E, Bunchman T, Khurana R, Fleming S, Lynch R: Complications of nasogastric and gastrostomy tube feedings in children with end stage renal disease, *Adv Perit Dial* 6:262-64, 1990.
48. O'Regan S, Garel L: Percutaneous gastrojejunostomy for caloric supplementation in children on peritoneal dialysis, *Adv Perit Dial* 6:273-75, 1990.
49. Ramage IJ, Harvey E, Geary DF, Hebert D, et al: Complications of gastrostomy feeding in children receiving peritoneal dialysis, *Pediatr Nephrol* 13(3):249-52, 1999.
50. Ledermann SE, Spitz L, Moloney J: Gastrostomy feeding in infants and children on peritoneal dialysis, *Pediatr Nephrol* 17:246-50, 2002.
51. von Schnakenburg C, Feneberg R, Plank C, Zimmering M, et al: Percutaneous endoscopic gastrostomy in children on peritoneal dialysis, *Perit Dial Int* 26:69-77, 2006.
52. Krause I, Shamir R, Davidovits M, Frishman S, et al: Intradialytic parenteral nutrition in malnourished children treated with hemodialysis, *J Ren Nutr* 12(1):55-59, 2002.
53. Goldstein SL, Baronette S, Vital Gambrell T, Currier H, Brewer ED: nPCR assessment and IDPN treatment of malnutrition in pediatric hemodialysis patients, *Pediatr Nephrol* 17:531-34, 2002.
54. Orellana P, Juarez-Congelosi M, Goldstein S: Intradialytic parenteral nutrition and biochemical marker assessment for malnutrition in adolescent maintenance hemodialysis patients, *J Ren Nutr* 15(3):312-17, 2005.
55. Norman LJ, Macdonald IA, Watson AR: Optimising nutrition in chronic renal insufficiency—progression of disease, *Pediatr Nephrol* 19:1253-61, 2004.
56. Wingen AM, Mehls O: Nutrition in children with preterminal chronic renal failure. Myth or important therapeutic aid?, *Pediatr Nephrol* 17(2):111-20, 2002.
57. Wingen AM, Fabian-Bach C, Schaefer F, Mehls O, for the European Study Group for Nutritional Treatment of Chronic Renal Failure in Childhood: Randomised multicentre study of a low-protein diet

on the progression of chronic renal failure in children, *Lancet* 349(9059):1117-23, 1997.
58. Food and Agriculture Organization/World Health Organization: *Energy and protein requirements. Report of Joint FAO/WHO Expert Committee. WHO Technical Report Series no. 724*, Geneva, 1985, World Health Organization.
59. Broyer M, Niaudet P, Champion G, Chopin JG, et al: Nutritional and metabolic studies in children on continuous ambulatory peritoneal dialysis, *Kidney Int* Suppl 15:S106-10, 1983.
60. Canepa A, Verrina E, Perfumo F, Carrea A, et al: Value of intraperitoneal amino acids in children treated with chronic peritoneal dialysis, *Perit Dial Int* 18(Suppl 2):S435-40, 1999.
61. Qamar I, Secker D, Levin L, Balfe J, et al: Effects of amino acid dialysis compared to dextrose dialysis in children on continuous cycling peritoneal dialysis, *Perit Dial Int* 19:237-47, 1999.
62. Schaefer F, Wolf S, Klaus G, Langenbeck O, Mehls O, Mid-European CPO Study Group (MPCS): Higher KT/V urea associated with greater protein catabolic rate and dietary protein intake in children treated with CCPD compared to CAPD, *Adv Perit Dial* 10:310-14, 1994.
63. Fischbach M, Edefonti A, Schroder C, Watson A, for The European Pediatric Dialysis Working Group: Hemodialysis in children: general practical guidelines, *Pediatr Nephrol* 20:1054-66, 2005.
63a. National Kidney Foundation Dialysis Outcome Quality Initiative: Clinical practice guidelines for hemodialysis adequacy, *Am J Kidney Dis* 48(Suppl 1):S2-S90, 2006.
64. Goldstein S: Prescribing and monitoring hemodialysis. In Warady B, Fine A, Schaefer F, Alexander S, editors: *Pediatric dialysis*, Dordrecht, Germany, 2004, Kluwer Academic Publishers, pp 135-45.
65. Juarez-Congelosi M, Orellana P, Goldstein R: nPCR and sAlb as nutrition status markers in pediatric hemodialysis patients, *Hemodial Int* 10(1):129, 2006.
66. *KT/V dialysis adequacy*. Available at: http://www.kt-v.net. Accessed September 17, 2007.
67. Schaefer F, Klaus G, Mehls O: Peritoneal transport properties and dialysis dose affect growth and nutritional status in children on chronic peritoneal dialysis, *J Am Soc Nephrol* 10(8):1786-92, 1999.
68. Cano F, Marin V, Azocar M, Delucchi M, et al: Adequacy and nutrition in pediatric peritoneal dialysis, *Adv Perit Dial* 19:273-78, 2003.
69. Cano F, Azocar M, Cavada G, Delucchi A, et al: Kt/V and nPNA in pediatric peritoneal dialysis: a clinical or a mathematical association?, *Pediatr Nephrol* 21:114-18, 2006.
70. Greenspan L, Gitelman S, Leung M, Glidden D, Mathias R: Increased incidence in post-transplant diabetes mellitus in children: a case-control analysis, *Pediatr Nephrol* 17:1-5, 2002.
71. American Diabetes Association: Standards of medical care in diabetes, *Diabetes Care* 27(Suppl 1):S15-35, 2004.
72. National Kidney Foundation: K/DOQI clinical practice guidelines for cardiovascular disease in dialysis patients, *Am J Kidney Dis* 45(4 Suppl 3):S1-154, 2005.
73. National Kidney Foundation: K/DOQI clinical practice guidelines for managing dyslipidemias in chronic kidney disease, *Am J Kidney Dis* 41(Suppl 3):S1-92, 2003.
74. Querfeld U: Disturbance of lipid metabolism in children with chronic renal failure, *Pediatr Nephrol* 7:749-57, 1993.
75. Querfeld U, Salusky IB, Nelson P, Foley J, Fine RN: Hyperlipidemia in pediatric patients undergoing peritoneal dialysis, *Pediatr Nephrol* 2:447-52, 1988.
76. Kari JA, Shaw V, Vallance DT, Rees L: Effect of enteral feeding on lipid subfractions in children with chronic renal failure, *Pediatr Nephrol* 12(5):401-04, 1998.
77. National Cholesterol Education Program: Report of the expert panel on blood cholesterol levels in children and adolescents, *Pediatrics* 89:495-584, 1992.
78. Anderson MA, Dewey KG, Frongillo E, Garza C, et al: An evaluation of infant growth: the use and interpretation of anthropometrics in infants, *Bull World Health Organ* 73:165-74, 1995.
79. Lichtenstein AH, Appel LJ, Brands M, Carnethon M, et al: Diet and lifestyle recommendations revision 2006. A scientific statement from the American Heart Association Nutrition Committee, *Circulation* 114:82-96, 2006.
80. Goren A, Stankiewicz H, Goldstein R, Drukker A: Fish oil treatment of hyperlipidemia in children and adolescents receiving renal replacement therapy, *Pediatrics* 88(2):265-68, 1991.
81. Hogg RJ, Lee J, Nardelli N, Julian BA, et al: Clinical trial to evaluate omega-3 fatty acids and alternate day prednisone in patients with IgA nephropathy: report from the Southwest Pediatric Nephrology Study Group, *Clin J Am Soc Nephrol* 1(3):467-74, 2006.
82. Kriley M, Warady BA: Vitamin status of pediatric patients receiving long-term peritoneal dialysis, *Am J Clin Nutr* 53:1476-79, 1991.
83. Warady BA, Kriley M, Alon U: Vitamin status of infants receiving long-term peritoneal dialysis, *Pediatr Nephrol* 8:354-56, 1994.
84. Pereira A, Hamani N, Nogueira P, Carvalhaes J: Oral vitamin intake in children receiving long-term dialysis, *J Ren Nutr* 10(1):24-29, 2000.
85. Coleman J, Watson A: Vitamin, mineral and trace element supplementation of children on chronic peritoneal dialysis, *J Hum Nutr Diet* 4:13-17, 1991.
86. Norman L, Coleman JE, Watson A, Wardell J, Evans J: Nutritional supplements and elevated serum vitamin A levels in children on chronic dialysis, *J Hum Nutr Diet* 9:257-62, 1996.
87. Muth I: Implication of hypervitaminosis A in chronic renal failure, *J Ren Nutr* 1(1):2-8, 1991.
88. Nakashima A, Yorioka N, Doi S, Masaki T, Ito T, Harada S: Effects of vitamin K2 in hemodialysis patients with low serum parathyroid hormone levels, *Bone* 34(3):579-83, 2004.
89. Chazot C, Kopple JD: Vitamin metabolism and requirements in renal disease and renal failure. In Kopple J, Massry S, editors: *Nutritional management of renal disease*, Baltimore, 1997, Williams & Wilkins, pp 415-77.
90. Kohlmeier M, Saupe J, Shearer M, Schaefer K, Asmus G: Bone health of adult hemodialysis patients is related to vitamin K status, *Kidney Int* 51:1218-21, 1997.
91. Merouani A, Lambert M, Delvin EE, Genest J Jr, et al: Plasma homocysteine concentration in children with chronic renal failure, *Pediatr Nephrol* 16(10):805-11, 2001.
92. Litwin M, Abuauba M, Wawer ZT, Grenda R, et al: Folate, vitamin B12, and sulfur amino acid levels in patients with renal failure, *Pediatr Nephrol* 16(2):127-32, 2001.
93. Kang H, Lee B, Hahn H, Lee D, et al: Reduction of plasma homocysteine by folic acid in children with chronic renal failure, *Pediatr Nephrol* 17:511-14, 2002.
94. Bennett-Richards K, Kattenhorn M, Donald A, Oakley G, et al: Does oral folic acid lower total homocysteine levels and improve endothelial function in children with chronic renal failure?, *Circulation* 105(15):1810-15, 2002.
95. Schroder CH, de Boer AW, Giesen AM, Monnens LA, Blom H: Treatment of hyperhomocysteinemia in children on dialysis by folic acid, *Pediatr Nephrol* 13(7):583-85, 1999.
96. Farid F, Faheem M, Heshmat N, Shaheen K, Saad S: Study of the homocysteine status in children with chronic renal failure, *Am J Nephrol* 24:289-95, 2004.
97. Esfahani S, Hamidian M, Madani A, Ataei N, et al: Serum zinc and copper levels in children with chronic renal failure, *Pediatr Nephrol* 21:1153-56, 2006.
98. Warady B, Nelms C, Jennings J, Johnson S: Copper deficiency: a common cause of erythropoietin (rHuEPO) resistant anemia in children on hemodialysis (HD)?, *Hemodial Int* 9(1):99, 2005.
99. Harris D, Thomas M, Johnson D, Nicholls K, Gillin A: Caring for Australasians with Renal Impairment (CARI). The CARI guidelines. Prevention of progression of kidney disease, *Nephrology* 11(Suppl 1):S2-197, 2006.
100. American Academy of Pediatrics Section on Breastfeeding: Breastfeeding and the use of human milk. Policy statement, *Pediatrics* 115(2):496-506, 2005.
101. National Kidney Foundation: K/DOQI clinical practice guidelines for bone metabolism and disease in children with chronic kidney disease, *Am J Kid Dis* 46(4 Suppl 1):S1-121, 2005.
102. Kasiske BL, Vazquez MA, Harmon WE, Brown RS, et al: Recommendations for the outpatient surveillance of renal transplant recipients, *J Am Soc Nephrol* 11(Suppl 15):S1-86, 2000.

102a. Hudson E: Caring for Australasions with renal impairment (CARI), the CARI guidelines. Micronutrient intake in children, *Nephrology* 10(Suppl 5):S213-14, 2005.
103. National Kidney Foundation: KDOQI clinical practice guidelines and clinical practice recommendations for anemia in chronic kidney disease, *Am J Kidney Dis* 47(5 Suppl 3):S1-145, 2006.
104. Institute of Medicine: *Dietary reference intakes for calcium, phosphorous, magnesium, vitamin D, and fluoride,* Washington, 1997, National Academy of Sciences.
105. Rodriguez-Soriano J, Arant BS: Fluid and electrolyte imbalances in children with chronic renal failure, *Am J Kidney Dis* 7:268-74, 1986.
106. Parekh RS, Flynn JT, Smoyer WE, Milne JL, et al: Improved growth in young children with severe chronic renal insufficiency who use specified nutritional therapy, *J Am Soc Nephrol* 12(11): 2418-26, 2001.
107. Mattes RD, Donnelly D: Relative contributions of dietary sodium sources, *J Am Coll Nutr* 10(4):383-93, 1991.
108. National Kidney Foundation: K/DOQI clinical practice guidelines on hypertension and antihypertensive agents in chronic kidney disease, *Am J Kidney Dis* 43(5 Suppl 1):S1-290, 2004.
109. United States Department of Health and Human Services and the Department of Agriculture: *Dietary Guidelines for Americans, 2005.*
110. Rock J, Secker D: Nutrition management of chronic kidney disease in the pediatric patient. In Byham-Gray L, Wiesen K, editors: *A clinical guide to nutrition care in kidney disease,* ed 1, Chicago, 2004, Renal Dietitians Dietetic Practice Group of the American Dietetic Association and the Council on Renal Nutrition of the National Kidney Foundation, pp 127-49.
111. Bunchman TE, Wood EG, Schenck MH, Weaver KA, et al: Pretreatment of formula with sodium polystyrene sulfonate to reduce dietary potassium intake, *Pediatr Nephrol* 5:29-32, 1991.
112. Rivard AL, Raup SM, Beilman GJ: Sodium polystyrene sulfonate used to reduce the potassium content of a high-protein enteral formula: a quantitative analysis, *JPEN J Parenter Enteral Nutr* 28(2):76-78, 2004.
113. Schroder C, van den Berg A, Willems J, Monnens L: Reduction of potassium in drinks by pre-treatment with calcium polystyrene sulphonate, *Eur J Pediatr* 152:263-64, 1993.
114. Beto J, Bansal VK: Hyperkalemia: evaluating dietary and nondietary etiology, *J Ren Nutr* 2(1):28-29, 1992.
115. Medical Education Institute: *Alternative treatments*. Available at: www.kidneyschool.org. Accessed September 17, 2007.
116. Cooke J: Practical aspects of herbal supplement use in chronic kidney disease, *J Ren Nutr* 14(1):e1-4, 2004.
117. Dahl N: Herbs and supplements in dialysis patients: panacea or poison?, *Semin Dial* 14(3):186-92, 2001.
118. Strong J, Burgett M, Buss ML, Carver M, et al: Effects of calorie and fluid intake on adverse events during hemodialysis, *J Ren Nutr* 11(2):97-100, 2001.
119. Shibagaka Y, Takaichi K: Significant reduction of the large-vessel blood volume by food intake during hemodialysis, *Clin Nephrol* 49:49-54, 1998.
120. Watson A, Coleman JE: Dietary management in nephrotic syndrome, *Arch Dis Child* 69(2):179-80, 1993.
121. Roth K, Amaker B, Chan J: Nephrotic syndrome: pathogenesis and management, *Pediatr Rev* 23:237-48, 2002.
122. Holmberg C, Antikainen M, Ronnholm K, Ala-Houhala M, Jalanko H: Management of congenital nephrotic syndrome of the Finnish type, *Pediatr Nephrol* 9:87-93, 1995.
123. Royle J, Postlethwaite R: What protein intake is recommended for nephrotic syndrome?, *Pediatr Nephrol* 5(5):581, 1991.
124. Pattaragarn A, Warady B, Sabath R: Exercise capacity in pediatric patients with end-stage renal disease, *Perit Dial Int* 24(3):274-80, 2004.
125. Montgomery L, Parker T, MacDougall K, Goldstein S: Effect of twice weekly exercise for pediatric hemodialysis patients, *Hemodial Int* 10(1):129-30, 2006.
126. Stack A, Molony D, Rives T, Tyson J, Murthy B: Association of physical activity with mortality in the US dialysis population, *Am J Kid Dis* 45(4):690-701, 2005.
127. Painter P: Physical functioning in end-stage renal disease patients: update 2005, *Hemodial Int* 9(3):218-35, 2005.
128. Painter P, Johansen K: Improving physical functioning: time to be a part of routine care, *Am J Kidney Dis* 48(1):167-70, 2006.
129. Furth SL, Hwang W, Yang C, Neu AM, et al: Growth failure, risk of hospitalization and death for children with end-stage renal disease, *Pediatr Nephrol* 17:450-55, 2002.
130. Ferrara E, Lemire J, Reznik V, Grimm P: Dietary phosphorus reduction by pretreatment of human breast milk with sevelamer, *Pediatr Nephrol* 19:775-79, 2004.

CHAPTER 49

Anemia in Chronic Renal Disease

Larry A. Greenbaum

INTRODUCTION

Anemia is one of the most common problems in children with chronic kidney disease (CKD); it is almost universal in children with CKD stage V. The development of recombinant human erythropoietin (rHuEPO) revolutionized the treatment of anemia in CKD, but anemia management remains challenging. Many management issues remain uncertain, including the ideal target hemoglobin (Hb) level. There are European and American consensus guidelines for the management of anemia in patients with CKD.[1,2]

PATHOPHYSIOLOGY OF ANEMIA

A variety of factors contribute to anemia in patients with CKD (Table 49-1). The principal cause is the decreased production of erythropoietin by the kidneys. However, many children are still anemic despite the availability of rHuEPO, which emphasizes the multifactorial cause of anemia in children with CKD.

Erythropoietin Deficiency

The kidneys produce erythropoietin, and kidney damage leads to decreased erythropoietin production. In children with CKD, erythropoietin levels are inappropriately low for the degree of anemia.[3] The degree of erythropoietin deficiency generally worsens as the glomerular filtration rate (GFR) decreases, but the level of GFR at which inadequate erythropoietin causes anemia varies among patients, partially as a result of the nature of the underlying kidney disease. Some studies suggest that significant anemia caused by erythropoietin deficiency in children with CKD only develops when the GFR falls below 20 to 35 ml/min/1.73 m^2.[3,4]

Blood Loss

Excessive blood loss may directly cause anemia, or it may lead to iron deficiency (described later). Causes of blood loss in children with CKD include phlebotomy, blood lost in the dialyzer and tubing during hemodialysis (HD),[5] gastrointestinal losses,[5] and increased menstrual bleeding as a result of the acquired platelet function defect of CKD. Children receiving HD have increased intestinal blood loss as compared with other children with CKD.[5]

Decreased Red Blood Cell Survival

Red blood cells in children with CKD have a decreased lifespan.[5] This may be partially the result of carnitine deficiency (described later),[6] and it may be a direct consequence of erythropoietin deficiency, because red cell survival increases in CKD patients after they are started on rHuEPO.[7] Red blood cells in patients receiving HD have an increased osmotic fragility. Hemolytic anemia may occur as a result of a child's primary disease (e.g., systemic lupus erythematosus) or as a complication of a medication (e.g., hemolytic uremic syndrome caused by cyclosporine).

Bone Marrow Suppression

In an in vitro assay, serum from children with CKD directly suppresses red blood cell production.[3] The specific inhibitory substances have not yet been identified, but dialysis appears to effectively remove some of these molecules, thereby allowing for decreased doses of rHuEPO.[8] In a study of teenagers receiving HD, the children with Hb levels of less than 11 g/dl had a slightly lower Kt/V_{urea} level (1.53 versus 1.46). However, dialysis adequacy did not predict anemia in the multiple regression analysis, perhaps as a result of the high overall Kt/V_{urea} level in this patient population.[9] Severe bone marrow suppression may occur in children after renal transplantation as a result of medications[10] or infections, especially parvovirus B19.[11]

Iron Deficiency

Iron deficiency is a significant cause of anemia in patients with CKD, and it is multifactorial (Table 49-2). In one study of older children, a serum transferrin saturation (TSAT) level of less than 20% was an independent predictor of anemia.[9] However, serum ferritin was not predictive of anemia, perhaps because ferritin is often elevated in patients with CKD with concurrent inflammation, which may inhibit red cell synthesis (described later). Iron deficiency often develops after the initiation of rHuEPO therapy, because the increase in red blood cell synthesis depletes iron stores.

Inadequate Dialysis

In adults who are receiving dialysis, there is evidence that anemia is associated with inadequate dialysis. An increase in the dialysis dose leads to an improvement in Hb. In addition,

TABLE 49-1 Causes of Anemia in Chronic Kidney Disease

Erythropoietin deficiency
Blood loss
Hemolysis
Bone marrow suppression
Iron deficiency
Inadequate dialysis
Malnutrition
Chronic or acute inflammation
Infection
Hyperparathyroidism
B12 or folate deficiency
Aluminum toxicity
Carnitine deficiency
Medications (e.g., angiotensin-converting enzyme inhibitors)
Systemic disease • Hemoglobinopathy • Hypothyroidism • Systemic lupus erythematosus • Malignancy

TABLE 49-2 Causes of Iron Deficiency in Children with Chronic Kidney Disease

Blood loss • Phlebotomy • Hemodialysis • Menses • Gastrointestinal
Dietary iron deficiency
Poor absorption of enteral iron
Iron depletion during recombinant human erythropoietin therapy

there is an inverse relationship between Kt/V_{urea} and rHuEPO dose. There is no evidence for a direct relationship between Kt/V_{urea} and anemia in children receiving dialysis, perhaps because of the low numbers of children who receive inadequate dialysis. Children receiving HD with a central venous catheter have a lower Kt/V_{urea} level, a lower Hb level, and a lower albumin level than children who receive dialysis with a fistula.[12] The exact role of the dialysis dose in this observation is not yet clear.

Malnutrition

Malnutrition may be another factor that contributes to anemia in patients with CKD. In one pediatric study, a low albumin level was one predictor of anemia.[9] There are many possible explanations for the relationship between malnutrition and anemia. Generalized malnutrition may be a marker for nutritional iron deficiency or for a deficiency of other nutrients that influence red cell production or survival. Another possible explanation for this observation is the relationship between markers of malnutrition and markers of inflammation.[13] As described later in this chapter, inflammation is another mechanism of resistance to rHuEPO. It is possible that inflammation causes malnutrition and that this directly causes resistance to rHuEPO. An alternative explanation is that inflammation directly causes rHuEPO resistance and that malnutrition is a surrogate marker of inflammation.

Inflammation and Infection

Acute and chronic inflammation are well-known causes of decreased red blood cell synthesis. Inflammation is one of the mechanisms of the anemia of chronic disease and of the decreased erythropoiesis that occurs during infections. Inflammation and decreased red blood cell synthesis also occur after surgical procedures.

Interleukin-6 appears to be the most important inflammatory mediator of the anemia of chronic disease. Interleukin-6 increases liver production of hepcidin, which directly inhibits the release of iron from macrophages. The consequent decrease in serum iron prevents adequate red cell production. Hepcidin also appears to impair intestinal iron absorption.[14]

Markers of inflammation are commonly increased in patients with CKD, and there are a variety of putative mechanisms. Surgical procedures and acute infections are more common in patients with CKD, especially those who are receiving dialysis or who have had a kidney transplant. The impaired immune system in patients with uremia may lead to an increase in nonspecific inflammation.[15] Patients with CKD may have underlying systemic diseases, such as systemic lupus erythematosus or Wegener's granulomatosis. HD may induce inflammation via complement activation, the direct activation of inflammatory cells by the dialysis membrane, and the diffusion of endotoxin into the patient from the dialysate.

In adult patients with CKD, there is an inverse relationship between the rHuEPO dose and markers of inflammation.[16] One postulated mechanism for the effect of inflammation on red cell production is an inflammatory block, which is a condition in which body stores of iron are adequate but there is an ineffective delivery of iron to the bone marrow. Inflammation may cause an inflammatory block via the sequestration of iron in ferritin, which increases during inflammation. In addition, inflammation activates the reticuloendothelial system, thereby leading to the uptake of iron. Findings during inflammatory blockade may include elevated C-reactive protein (CRP) levels, resistance to rHuEPO, high serum ferritin levels, and low levels of serum iron and TSAT.[16] This mechanism is common to the anemia of many chronic diseases.

In addition to an inflammatory block, the enteral absorption of iron decreases in patients with CKD and increased markers of inflammation. Furthermore, cytokines produced during inflammation directly inhibit red cell synthesis in the bone marrow. Finally, as described previously, inflammation is associated with malnutrition, which may also contribute to anemia.

Hyperparathyroidism

Hyperparathyroidism may decrease bone marrow production of red blood cells.[17] The treatment of hyperparathyroidism via parathyroidectomy may lead to an increase in the Hb level.

Vitamin B12 or Folate Deficiency

Patients with CKD may rarely develop a megaloblastic anemia as a result of folate or vitamin B12 deficiency. Poor nutritional intake in combination with dialytic losses may predispose patients with CKD to deficiencies of these water-soluble vitamins. There is some evidence that routine folate supplementation improves the response to rHuEPO, even in the absence of low serum levels of folic acid.[18]

Aluminum Toxicity

Aluminum overload may cause a microcytic anemia in patients with CKD.[19] Currently, aluminum overload is an uncommon cause of anemia as a result of the recognition of the dangers of aluminum-containing phosphate binders.

Carnitine Deficiency

Carnitine deficiency may occur in patients with CKD, principally as a result of the removal of carnitine by dialysis, although decreased dietary intake and endogenous synthesis may also contribute.[6] Renal losses of carnitine are significant in children with Fanconi syndrome. Carnitine deficiency may decrease red blood cell survival by reducing the strength of the red cell membrane.[6] Intravenous carnitine may reduce rHuEPO dose requirements in adults receiving HD, but there is disagreement regarding the strength of the evidence; carnitine should not be used routinely (if at all) outside of a research setting.[1,2,6,20]

Medications

A variety of medications can inhibit erythropoiesis, especially certain medications that are used in renal transplant recipients.[10] Angiotensin-converting enzyme inhibitors and angiotensin receptor blockers, which decrease the response to rHuEPO, are especially pertinent in patients with CKD because of their widespread use.[21]

Summary

Erythropoietin deficiency and iron deficiency are the most common causes of anemia in children with CKD. The interrelated effects of malnutrition and inflammation are important causes of refractory anemia, but the precise pathogenesis remains unclear.

EPIDEMIOLOGY OF ANEMIA IN PEDIATRIC CHRONIC KIDNEY DISEASE

For patients receiving peritoneal dialysis (PD) and HD in the United States, an Hb level below 11 g/dl is more common in children than in adult patients. Nevertheless, pediatric HD patients are less likely to receive intravenous iron.[22]

Among HD patients less than 18 years old in the United States, the mean Hb level was 11.2 g/dl, with a standard deviation of 1.6 g/dl. Thirty-eight percent of the patients had a mean Hb level below 11 g/dl, despite 97% of the patients receiving rHuEPO. The percentage of patients with a mean Hb level below 11 g/dl has decreased, possibly reflecting an increase in prescribed rHuEPO dose and the percentage of patients prescribed intravenous iron. In univariate analysis, risk factors for an Hb level below 11 g/dl were dialysis for less than 6 months, mean Kt/V_{urea} level of less than 1.2, a low serum albumin level, and the use of a catheter for vascular access.[23] In another study of children receiving HD or PD, risk factors for anemia included increasing age, dialysis for less than 6 months, and treatment with PD. Adolescents receiving PD were especially likely to be anemic, thus suggesting a possible role of nonadherence.[24]

Anemia is common in children after kidney transplantation, and it appears to be increasing.[25] The principal cause of anemia is allograft dysfunction, although modern immunosuppressive medications may be responsible for the increased prevalence of anemia in these patients. Iron deficiency is common among children who are anemic after renal transplantation.

CLINICAL EFFECTS OF ANEMIA

There are a wide range of clinical consequences from anemia in patients with CKD (Table 49-3). In adults, there is evidence that anemia increases mortality, possibly via its deleterious cardiovascular effects. The correction of anemia ameliorates a wide range of symptoms in adults and children. In addition, the correction of anemia may slow the progression of predialysis CKD to end-stage renal disease.

Mortality

Studies in adult dialysis patients have shown an association between anemia and increased mortality and hospitalization rates. In an analysis of pediatric patients, anemia 30 days after the initiation of dialysis was associated with a significant increase in mortality and hospitalization rates.[26] However, a randomized study in adults did not show any benefit of targeting a higher hematocrit level.[27] No randomized study has shown a significant benefit of a higher target Hb level.

Cardiovascular Disease

Cardiovascular disease is the leading cause of death in adults and children receiving dialysis. The correction of anemia has beneficial effects in adults with CKD, and there are a few

TABLE 49-3 Clinical Effects of Anemia

Cardiovascular • Left ventricular hypertrophy
Systemic
• Fatigue • Depression • Decreased quality of life • Sleep disturbances • Decreased exercise tolerance • Impaired cognitive function • Loss of appetite

pediatric studies that address this issue. In a group of children receiving dialysis, the treatment of anemia with rHuEPO partially corrected the elevated cardiac index after 6 months and produced a significant reduction in left ventricular mass index by 12 months.[28] In a study by Mitsnefes and colleagues,[29] children with severe left ventricular hypertrophy (LVH) had significantly lower Hb values than children without LVH. However, anemia did not predict LVH in the final multiple regression model.

Systemic Symptoms

Anemia may cause a variety of symptoms, including fatigue, depression, sleep disturbances, decreased exercise tolerance, loss of appetite, and impaired cognitive function. The correction of anemia with rHuEPO in adults with CKD causes improvement in many systemic symptoms, including functional ability, cognitive function, sleep and eating behaviors, energy and activity levels, health psychologic affect, libido, and distance walked during a stress test.

There is clear evidence of the deleterious effects of anemia on child development. There is an association in children with CKD between anemia and lower scores of health-related quality of life.[30] Studies of the effect of rHuEPO in children with CKD have shown improvements in quality of life, exercise tolerance, appetite, peak oxygen consumption, treadmill time during exercise testing, Wechsler intelligence score, and ventilatory aerobic threshold.[31-33] There does not appear to be a beneficial effect of anemia correction on the growth retardation associated with CKD.[34]

CLINICAL EVALUATION OF ANEMIA

Initial Evaluation

Most children with CKD are anemic as a result of inadequate erythropoietin production, and they are treated empirically with an erythropoiesis-stimulating agent (ESA; either rHuEPO or darbepoetin-α), unless there are specific findings that suggest an alternative cause (Table 49-4).

The initial evaluation of children with CKD and anemia should include a complete blood count, a reticulocyte count, a ferritin level, an iron level, total iron binding capacity, and a TSAT. The TSAT is calculated by dividing the serum iron by the total iron binding capacity. A cost-effectiveness analysis in adults argues against routine screening for aluminum overload or deficiencies of folate or B12.[35] Erythropoietin deficiency causes a normocytic anemia; macrocytosis or microcytosis should lead to the consideration of other causes (see Table 49-4). A low mean corpuscular volume (MCV) occurs with iron deficiency, thalassemia, and in up to 50% of patients with anemia of chronic disease. A high MCV suggests the possibility of B12 or folate deficiency. The concomitant depression of white blood cells or platelets raises the specter of malignancy, although an isolated low white blood cell count may be the result of a transient viral infection or a medication. Systemic lupus erythematosus may cause depression of the white blood cell count and platelet count as well as autoimmune Coombs'-positive hemolytic anemia. Erythropoietin deficiency causes an inappropriately low reticulocyte count, and the presence of an adequate reticulocytosis suggests alternative explanations, such as blood loss or hemolysis.

Iron deficiency is common among children with CKD, even before they start taking an ESA. There are a variety of explanations for iron deficiency in children with CKD (see Table 49-2). All children with CKD should be asked about gastrointestinal blood loss and, when appropriate, menstrual losses. A more aggressive workup (e.g., testing stool for occult blood, endoscopy) is appropriate in children with significant unexplained iron deficiency before they are started on ESA therapy. Along with low serum ferritin and TSAT, children with iron deficiency typically have a low MCV. Because it is a marker of inflammation, serum ferritin may be misleadingly normal in children with CKD despite iron deficiency.

The evaluation of the ferritin and TSAT establishes a baseline, because iron deficiency is likely to develop during ESA treatment. In addition, although all patients starting an ESA should receive oral iron supplementation unless iron overload is present, iron deficiency before starting ESA therapy may significantly attenuate the response to therapy. Such patients are candidates for intravenous iron.

Chronic Monitoring

Routine monitoring in children with anemia caused by CKD includes the periodic assessment of Hb, MCV, and iron stores. The development of macrocytosis in a patient after starting an ESA is usually a result of the expected reticulocytosis; an increasing Hb level, which argues against a nutritional deficiency anemia, supports this explanation. Iron overload may

TABLE 49-4 **Indications for Additional Evaluation in Children with Chronic Kidney Disease and Anemia**

Indication	Response
Macrocytosis	Consider B12 or folate deficiency (unless brisk reticulocytosis is present)
Decreased platelets and/or white blood cells	Consider malignancy, acute infection, systemic lupus erythematosus, or medications
History of using aluminum-containing phosphate binders or other symptoms of aluminum overload	Consider aluminum toxicity
Anemia despite adequate reticulocytosis	Consider excessive blood loss or hemolysis
Microcytosis	Consider iron deficiency, hemoglobinopathy, or inflammation
Iron deficiency before starting recombinant human erythropoietin	Consider causes of iron deficiency (see Table 49-2)

also cause an increased MCV.[36] Microcytosis is usually caused by iron deficiency.

A decrease in the Hb level and an increase in ESA dose requirements are expected during acute infections[37] or after surgical procedures.[38] Dose requirements increase after blood loss that causes a fall in Hb; this persists until the Hb returns to the target range. Depleted iron stores are the usual explanation for a poor response to ESA therapy. As discussed later in this chapter, some children have a functional iron deficiency and may respond to intravenous iron, although the ferritin and TSAT levels may not be low. Additional evaluation is indicated in children who have an unexplained increase in the ESA dose requirement, who need unexpectedly large doses of ESA, or who have a decreasing Hb level.

A reticulocyte count is the usual first step in evaluating unexplained anemia or an excessive ESA requirement. An appropriately elevated reticulocyte count (corrected for the degree of anemia) argues that the patient is anemic as a result of blood loss or hemolysis. Blood loss is also suggested by a minimal increase in ferritin and TSAT despite the use of multiple doses of intravenous iron. The child should then have stool tested for occult blood; an evaluation for hemolysis may also be appropriate. Inadequate reticulocytosis suggests that there is a defect in red cell production. This may be caused by poor adherence or technique failure in a patient receiving home ESA. There may be a readily identifiable explanation, such as severe secondary hyperparathyroidism. Alternatively, additional testing may be necessary. A serum aluminum level is an appropriate test in the child with a history of using aluminum-containing phosphate binders. One of the most common causes of a poor response to ESA is an inflammatory block as a result of acute or chronic inflammation; an elevated CRP level supports this diagnosis.[15] Other testing, depending on the patient, may include a serum carnitine level and serum levels of folate and B12. A hematologist should evaluate refractory anemia with no identifiable explanation.[1,2]

TREATMENT OF ANEMIA

Treatment with an ESA is necessary in many children with CKD, including children with chronic allograft dysfunction.[39] Almost all children receiving dialysis are treated with an ESA. In addition, almost all treated patients require oral or intravenous iron. When possible, other underlying causes of anemia should be corrected (see Table 49-1). Blood transfusions should be reserved for children with symptomatic anemia or with worsening anemia caused by blood loss, hemolysis, or unresponsiveness to ESA.[1,2]

There are no data regarding the ideal target Hb level for children (or whether the target should be adjusted on the basis of age and gender). The adult literature is also inconclusive regarding the ideal target Hb level. Current guidelines suggest a target Hb level of more than 11 g/dl, but the optimal upper limit is controversial, with the National Kidney Foundation's Kidney Disease Outcomes Quality Initiative (K/DOQI) and the European guidelines recommending an upper limit of 13 g/dl and 14 g/dl, respectively. However, both guidelines recognize clinical situations that require different target Hb values. For example, there are clearly children who require a higher target Hb level (e.g., a child with underlying cyanotic heart disease) or a lower target level (e.g., a child with sickle cell disease).

Hemoglobin Monitoring

Hb monitoring is preferred over hematocrit monitoring, because Hb measurements are more standardized and consistent. For patients receiving HD, the K/DOQI guidelines recommend that blood samples should be taken immediately before dialysis.[2] This may lead to a falsely low Hb value as a result of hemodilution from fluid gain between dialysis sessions. Hence, this should be considered in children with significant interdialytic weight gain. It is reasonable to measure the Hb level before an HD session after a short interdialytic period (2 days), because the effect of hemodilution on Hb is generally less significant.

The frequency of monitoring varies, depending on the patient. Children who are being given a stable dose of ESA and who are within their target Hb range can have an Hb level performed as infrequently as monthly if they are receiving dialysis and even less often if they have not yet started dialysis. After the initiation of ESA or after a dosing change, an Hb level should generally be obtained every 1 to 2 weeks until it has stabilized within the target range.

Recombinant Human Erythropoietin

Multiple studies in adult patients demonstrated the efficacy of intravenous and subcutaneously administered rHuEPO for correcting the anemia of CKD. A placebo-controlled trial demonstrated that rHuEPO is effective in children with CKD,[33] and many other observational studies have confirmed this finding.

Pharmacokinetics

The pharmacokinetics of rHuEPO in CKD have been studied in both children and adults. There are clear differences that are based on the route of administration; there is less complete absorption with subcutaneous rHuEPO, but it produces a significantly longer half-life as compared with intravenous administration. In studies of children with CKD, the measured mean half-life of rHuEPO is 5.6 to 7.5 hours for intravenous dosing and 14.2 to 25.2 hours for subcutaneous dosing. For intravenous dosing, there is evidence in adults that the half-life of rHuEPO increases as the dose increases.

Dosing

There are dramatic differences in the dosing needs of children with CKD who are receiving rHuEPO, even when the doses are adjusted for patient size.[23,40] A variety of variables influence the dosing needs of patients (Table 49-5), but it remains difficult to predict the dosing needs of an individual patient. Factors affecting the necessary dose per kilogram of rHuEPO in children with CKD include the stage of CKD (higher in stage V), the mode of dialysis (higher in HD as a result of increased blood loss),[41] the age of the patient (higher in younger patients),[23,40] the route of administration (higher with intravenous versus subcutaneous),[23] and the dosing frequency (higher with less-frequent dosing regimens). Concurrent causes of poor response to rHuEPO (e.g., iron deficiency,

TABLE 49-5 Factors That Influence Erythropoietin Dosing

Route of administration
Mode of dialysis
Initial and target hemoglobin levels
Endogenous erythropoietin
Patient age
Dosing frequency
Presence of other causes of anemia (see Table 49-1)

inflammation, hyperparathyroidism) often result in higher doses. Blood loss as a result of HD, blood draws, and other sources increases the need for rHuEPO. Blood draws can be especially problematic in the youngest patients, because these patients often require more frequent monitoring, and the relative losses per kilogram of body weight tend to be higher. Finally, the residual renal production of EPO can decrease the need for rHuEPO.

In children who are receiving PD or in predialysis patients, an appropriate starting dose for subcutaneous rHuEPO is 100 units/kg/week divided into two doses. However, once-weekly dosing may be appropriate for a child with mild anemia. Children who are less than 5 years old are likely to require a higher dose, and a starting dose of 150 units/kg/week may be appropriate in such patients, especially if severe anemia (Hb level of <8 g/dl) is present. For children receiving HD and intravenous rHuEPO dosing, a starting dose of 150 units/kg/week divided into three doses is reasonable, again with the caveat that higher doses are likely necessary in children who are less than 5 years old. A starting dose of 200 to 300 units/kg/week may be more appropriate in such patients, especially if there is concomitant severe anemia.

The majority of children receiving chronic subcutaneous dosing of rHuEPO can be maintained on weekly dosing to minimize the number of painful injections. However, some patients require more frequent injections; a minority of patients receive less-frequent injections.

When children receive intravenous dosing during HD, it is important to inject rHuEPO via the bloodlines. The use of the venous drip chamber may result in reduced drug delivery as a result of the "trapping" of rHuEPO, although this appears to be somewhat machine dependent.

For children receiving subcutaneous dosing, the site of injection should be rotated. The discomfort of subcutaneous dosing can be reduced by using a multidose vial, which contains the local anesthetic benzyl alcohol as a preservative. In children who are using a single-use vial, adding bacteriostatic saline that contains benzyl alcohol to the rHuEPO in a 1 : 1 ratio can decrease injection site pain.

Frequent dose adjustments are typically necessary for patients who are receiving rHuEPO. This is probably the result of variations in the factors that cause anemia (see Table 49-1) and that influence rHuEPO dosing (see Table 49-5). In addition, more active erythropoiesis is needed to increase a patient's Hb level. Hence, the dose that patients need to increase their Hb level into the target range is often more than the dose needed to maintain a stable Hb. Patients may need higher doses of rHuEPO at the start of therapy or after a decrease in Hb as a result of blood loss or a transient illness.

When HD is initiated in most children, they are converted to the intravenous dosing of rHuEPO, which should then almost always be given thrice weekly. According to the results of adult studies, the total weekly dose of rHuEPO should be increased by 50% when a patient changes from subcutaneous to intravenous dosing. Similarly, patients changing from intravenous dosing to subcutaneous dosing should have their weekly dose decreased by 33%. However, most pediatric patients who convert between intravenous and subcutaneous dosing are also changing dialysis modality. Given the higher needs for rHuEPO in children on HD,[40] patients changing to intravenous dosing because they are initiating HD may require an additional increase in their dose. In children who are less than 10 years old and certainly in those less than 5 years old, rHuEPO dosing requirements during HD are very high.[23] This suggests that these patients may require an increase in their rHuEPO dose after beginning HD, irrespective of any change in the route of administration. Young children should have careful monitoring of the Hb level when HD is initiated, with the dose of rHuEPO increased further, if necessary. Even in older children there is extreme variability in the dose requirements when converting to intravenous dosing; dose requirements may increase or decrease. The ability to more aggressively treat iron deficiency in children receiving HD (described later) may result in a decrease in rHuEPO requirements.

The goal of rHuEPO therapy is to maintain the patient's Hb level within a desired target range. Overly rapid increases in Hb can be associated with hypertension and should be avoided. In patients with an Hb level that is below the target, the goal is to increase the Hb by 1 to 2 g/dl per month. The dose of rHuEPO should be increased by 25% if the patient is below the target Hb level and has not increased at least 1g/dl during the previous month. The dose should be reduced by 25% if the Hb level is greater than the target or if the Hb has increased by more than 2 g/dl during the previous month. The rHuEPO should be temporarily held if the Hb level is more than 1 g/dl over the target or if the Hb has increased by more than 2 g/dl during the previous month and is above the target Hb.

Complications

An increase in blood pressure after starting rHuEPO therapy may occur in children.[33,42] This appears to be more common in children who receive higher doses of rHuEPO and who, consequently, have a more rapid increase in Hb.[43] Hence, rapid increases in Hb should be avoided. Although the increase in red cell mass appears to be one mechanism of the hypertension, there also appears to be a direct effect of rHuEPO on the vasculature.

A possible increase in vascular access clotting after rHuEPO treatment has been attributed to the increase in Hb. There may also be a small negative effect on dialytic clearance, but this is not clinically significant.

Iron deficiency may develop in children who are treated with rHuEPO.[33,42] This is the result of iron use for red blood cell synthesis. Consequently, unless iron overload is present, all patients treated with rHuEPO should receive iron supplementation and be screened for iron deficiency before and during therapy.

A rare complication of rHuEPO is the development of antierythropoietin antibodies.[44] These antibodies neutralize both endogenous erythropoietin and rHuEPO, which results in red cell aplasia. Immunosuppressive therapy, including renal transplantation, results in hematologic recovery in many patients.[45] Patients with undetectable antierythropoietin antibodies may subsequently respond to rHuEPO.[45]

Darbepoetin-α

Although rHuEPO is effective for correcting the anemia of end-stage renal disease, the need for frequent injections is taxing for children and their parents. Darbepoetin-α (Aranesp) is a genetically engineered molecule with a longer half-life than rHuEPO, thus permitting less-frequent administration. The longer half-life of darbepoetin-α is the result of two additional N-glycosylation sites.

Efficacy

Studies in adults demonstrate the comparable efficacy of rHuEPO and darbepoetin-α despite less-frequent dosing of darbepoetin-α.[46,47] One study has shown that many CKD patients do well when receiving darbepoetin-α subcutaneously as infrequently as once every 3 to 4 weeks.[48]

In a prospective study, children receiving rHuEPO were randomized to rHuEPO or darbepoetin-α at a less-frequent dosing interval (0.84 μg of darbepoetin-α per week for each 200 units per week of rHuEPO). There was no significant difference in the Hb level or the side effects between the groups at the end of the 20-week study (B. Warady, personal communication). A small prospective study evaluated the response to converting 7 children receiving HD from thrice-weekly rHuEPO to once-weekly darbepoetin-α (1 mcg of darbepoetin-α per week for each 200 units per week of rHuEPO). There were problems initially with elevated Hb levels and associated hypertension, especially in the younger children who were receiving high doses of rHuEPO. This was corrected by reducing the dose of darbepoetin-α, thus suggesting that this dose-conversion ratio may be inappropriate in younger children and that careful monitoring of the initial response is necessary when converting to darbepoetin-α. The mean steady-state dose of darbepoetin-α after 3 months was 0.51 mcg/kg/week.[49]

In a larger prospective study, children with CKD and anemia were given darbepoetin-α at a starting dose of 0.45 μg/kg/week. There was a significant improvement in the Hb level, and it was sustained during the 28 weeks of the study. By the end of the study, slightly more than half of the patients were receiving darbepoetin-α at dosing intervals of at least 2 weeks.[50] A small study has described the successful use of darbepoetin-α in infants, with a starting dose of 0.5 μg/kg/week.[51] The dose was able to be reduced, and the dosing interval was increased to 3 to 4 weeks in some of the infants.[51]

Pharmacokinetics

One study evaluated the half-life of darbepoetin-α in 12 pediatric patients with CKD.[52] Nine of the patients were receiving HD, but one patient was receiving PD, and two were not yet receiving dialysis. Each patient received one dose of darbepoetin-α (0.5 mcg/kg) intravenously and subcutaneously. The half-life of darbepoetin-α with intravenous administration was 22.1 hours (standard deviation, 4.5 hours). The half-life was 42.8 hours (standard deviation, 4.8 hours) with subcutaneous administration. The pharmacokinetics were comparable to a similarly designed study in adults except for increased bioavailability (54% versus 37%) and an earlier time to maximum plasma concentration (36 hours versus 54 hours) in the pediatric patients when darbepoetin-α was administered subcutaneously.[52,53] Hence, darbepoetin-α may be absorbed more rapidly in pediatric patients.[52] More rapid absorption was also seen in pediatric studies of rHuEPO.[54]

Dosing

On the basis of protein mass, 1 mcg of darbepoetin-α is equivalent to 200 units of rHuEPO. Nevertheless, the manufacturer's recommended darbepoetin-α dose when converting patients from rHuEPO to darbepoetin-α is not a direct conversion based on a ratio of 1 mcg of darbepoetin-α to 200 units of rHuEPO (Table 49-6). The recommended conversion ratios are based on an analysis of the dose-conversion clinical trials.[55] This analysis indicates that proportionally less darbepoetin-α was needed in patients who began the trial on higher doses of rHuEPO.[55] The explanation for this observation is unclear. It is possible that the efficacy of darbepoetin-α increases at higher doses. Alternatively, there may simply be a "regression to the mean" in those patients who were on very high doses of rHuEPO. These patients may have had a transient reason (e.g., inflammation) that led to high ESA dose requirements that subsequently resolved, thereby allowing for the lowering of the darbepoetin-α dose during the study.

One challenge with darbepoetin-α administration in children is the lack of a multidose vial. First, many small pediatric patients are likely to need less than 25 μg, which is the smallest available single-dose vial in the United States; this results in wasting of the unused medication. Second, pediat-

TABLE 49-6 **Starting Dose of Darbepoetin-α on the Basis of Previous Dosing of Recombinant Human Erythropoietin**

Previous Weekly Recombinant Human Erythropoietin Dose (units/week)	Weekly Darbepoetin-α Dose (mcg/week)
<2500	6.25
2500 to 4999	12.5
5000 to 10,999	25
11,000 to 17,999	40
18,000 to 33,999	60
34,000 to 89,999	100
≥90,000	200

Table based on recommendations of manufacturer (Amgen: Thousand Oaks, CA).

TABLE 49-7 **Available Preparations of Darbepoetin-α (Single-Use Vials in the United States)**

25 mcg†	40 mcg†	60 mcg†	100 mcg†	150 mcg†	200 mcg†	300 mcg†	500 mcg

†Preparations that are available in low-volume, prefilled syringes (0.3 to 0.6 mL, depending on the dose).

ric patients may not tolerate the discomfort of 1-ml injections, or they may require multiple injections to tolerate the full 1-ml volume of the single-dose vials. A useful alternative is to use darbepoetin-α in more concentrated, single-dose, prefilled syringes. Thus, the dosing of darbepoetin-α necessitates knowledge of the available preparations (Table 49-7), and it requires creative adjustments of doses and dosing intervals to minimize the wasting of medication.

Recommendations for converting patients from rHuEPO to darbepoetin-α that are based on adult data are available (see Table 49-6). The one pediatric study used a conversion ratio of 0.84 μg/kg/week of darbepoetin-α for each 200 units/kg/week of rHuEPO. Patients who are receiving rHuEPO twice or thrice weekly should receive darbepoetin-α weekly, and patients who are receiving weekly rHuEPO should receive darbepoetin-α every other week.

On the basis of the pediatric literature, a reasonable starting dose of darbepoetin-α in ESA-naïve patients is approximately 0.5 mcg/kg given weekly. Alternatively, the same total dose could be given every 2 weeks (i.e., 1 mcg/kg every 2 weeks). Every 2-week dosing at initiation should be reserved for patients with an Hb level that is only mildly below the target. Close monitoring of the Hb level is essential for all patients as a result of the variable response to darbepoetin-α.

As with rHuEPO, frequent dose adjustments of darbepoetin-α are often necessary.[46] Because darbepoetin-α has a long half-life, it is important to not increase the dose too quickly to avoid overshooting the target Hb. Many patients require lower doses after their Hb level reaches the target range. When adjusting darbepoetin-α dosing, it is desirable to round doses on the basis of the available preparations (see Table 49-7) to avoid excessive wasting of the medication. Nevertheless, excessive rounding is not appropriate; some patients will need to discard some of their medication. Table 49-8 presents one system for dose adjustment. It is unclear whether the darbepoetin-α is evenly distributed in the prefilled syringes. Hence, gentle mixing of the medication and transfer to a 1-ml syringe have been recommended for patients who do not require a full dose.[51]

The dose frequency of darbepoetin-α can be gradually reduced from weekly to every other week to every 3 weeks and then to every 4 weeks. Not all patients will tolerate decreased dose frequency, especially beyond every 3 weeks. The dose frequency can be reduced whenever the patient has an Hb level that would normally mandate decreasing the dose. Alternatively, the dose frequency can be reduced in patients who are receiving a stable darbepoetin-α dose and who have an Hb level that is in the target range. The total weekly dose should remain the same. For patients receiving darbepoetin-α less often than weekly, consideration should be given to increasing the dose frequency if a patient requires more than one dose increase, especially if the total weekly dose is relatively high.

TABLE 49-8 **Dose Adjustment Table for Darbepoetin-α**

6.25	10	15	20	30	40	50	60	80	100	130	150	200

Doses are given in micrograms. The dose to the left of the current dose should be used for dose decreases, and the dose to the right of the current dose should be used for dose increases.

Complications

Side-effect profiles have been similar in studies comparing intravenous darbepoetin-α with intravenous rHuEPO.[46,47] In one study, there was a statistically significant increase in pruritus in the darbepoetin-α group.[47] Injection site pain appears to be more common with darbepoetin-α, and there have been cases of antibodies developing to darbepoetin-α that have resulted in pure red cell aplasia.

MONITORING IRON STORES

Serum ferritin and TSAT are currently the most widely used tests for monitoring iron stores. A variety of other tests (e.g., soluble transferrin receptor, percentage of hypochromic red blood cells, erythrocyte zinc protoporphyrin) have been evaluated, but none of these is readily available or well studied in pediatric patients. In all children with CKD, TSAT and serum ferritin should be measured at initiation of ESA. Subsequent monitoring should be at least every 3 months. Children who are initiating HD should have iron studies every 1 to 2 months until the Hb level is in the target range. More frequent monitoring is also appropriate in a variety of other clinical situations, including a patient with a poor response to ESA therapy, after a course of intravenous iron, or during the administration of chronic intravenous iron therapy. Children receiving intravenous iron doses of more than 1.5 mg/kg or of more than 100 mg should have a delay of at least 1 week before serum iron parameters are checked.

Diagnosis of Iron Deficiency

The gold standard for diagnosing iron deficiency in patients with CKD is the bone marrow assessment of iron stores, a test that is impractical on a routine basis. An alternative definition is the response to intravenous iron. An increase in the Hb level or a decrease in the ESA dose after receiving intravenous iron suggests that the patient was iron deficient. This definition is not perfect (the response to intravenous iron may be coincidental or the patient may not respond for other reasons), but it has been widely used in clinical research and clinical practice.

The traditional criteria for iron deficiency—the combination of a low serum ferritin and a low TSAT—are not applicable in patients with CKD. The serum ferritin level is especially problematic because ferritin is an acute phase reactant, and it is therefore often elevated in patients with CKD as a result of infection and nonspecific inflammation. Moreover, treatment with an ESA can induce functional iron deficiency. This occurs because the high rate of red blood cell synthesis depletes the readily available iron, although total body iron stores may be adequate. Patients with functional iron deficiency as a result of rapid erythropoiesis may have a normal ferritin level but a low TSAT. Often the ferritin level decreases in these patients but remains in the normal range, and it is therefore not as useful of a predictor of iron deficiency as the TSAT.

Although a normal or elevated serum ferritin level does not exclude iron deficiency,[56,57] a low serum ferritin level is a specific predictor of iron deficiency in children with CKD.[58,59] K/DOQI recommends treating patients with a serum ferritin level of less than 100 ng/ml (or of less than 200 ng/ml in adult patients receiving HD) for iron deficiency.[2] There is concern that this goal for ferritin may be inappropriately high for infants with CKD.[51]

A TSAT of less than 20% has been widely used as a criterion for iron deficiency in patients with CKD. In one pediatric study, it was highly specific for identifying iron deficiency.[57] K/DOQI advises treating patients with a TSAT of less than 20% for iron deficiency but not routinely using intravenous iron if the ferritin level is greater than 500 ng/ml.[2]

A TSAT below 20% and a serum ferritin level above 100 ng/ml suggest functional iron deficiency, as described previously. This same scenario can also occur with an inflammatory block, a condition in which inflammation prevents the effective delivery of iron for erythropoiesis. Clinical signs of infection, a low serum iron level, an elevated CRP, an increasing ferritin level, and a poor response to intravenous iron support a diagnosis of an inflammatory block.

IRON THERAPY

After erythropoietin deficiency, iron deficiency is the leading cause of anemia in children with CKD. The treatment of iron deficiency often allows the achievement of the target Hb level with a lower dose of ESA. Iron therapy should not be given to patients who have iron overload, which is commonly defined as a ferritin level of more than 800 ng/ml or a TSAT of more than 50%.

Oral Iron

Only a small percentage of iron taken orally is absorbed, thereby limiting its efficacy in patients who have high iron requirements as a result of blood loss (e.g., children receiving HD).[5] Adherence to therapy may be problematic as a result of problems with gastric irritation and constipation.

There is an upregulation in oral iron absorption in dialysis patients who have a low serum ferritin level or decreased marrow iron stores. However, HD patients demonstrate decreased absorption of oral iron as compared with normal controls; inflammation as measured by CRP levels may further decrease iron absorption.

Oral iron absorption improves if it is not given with food, so iron should be given either 1 hour before or 2 hours after a meal. Calcium carbonate and calcium acetate decrease iron absorption; oral iron should not be given at the same time as these phosphate binders. Sevelamer seems to have little effect on oral iron absorption.[60] H_2-receptor antagonists and proton pump inhibitors may also adversely affect iron absorption.

Children should receive a dose of 3 to 5 mg/kg/day of elemental iron (maximum dose, 150 to 300 mg/day). Oral iron may be adequate therapy in many children who are not receiving HD. In children who are receiving HD, oral iron is often not sufficient to correct absolute or functional iron deficiency.[56,57] Children receiving intravenous iron should not receive oral iron.

Intravenous Iron

Given the limitations of oral iron and the high incidence of iron deficiency in dialysis patients, intravenous iron is frequently used in children with CKD. During a 3-month period, 68% of children in the United States receiving HD were prescribed intravenous iron.[23] However, 35% of patients with a TSAT of less than 20% and a ferritin level of less than 100 ng/ml did not receive any intravenous iron.[23]

There are currently three intravenous iron preparations available in the United States: (1) iron dextran (INFeD); sodium ferric gluconate conjugate in sucrose, hence referred to as *iron gluconate* (Ferrlecit); and iron sucrose (Venofer). The European Pediatric PD Working Group recommends not using iron dextran as a result of concerns about life-threatening anaphylactic reactions.[20] Studies in children, including a meta-analysis,[61] have shown the efficacy of intravenous iron for correcting iron deficiency, improving Hb levels, and reducing rHuEPO dose requirements.[56,57,62-65]

Acute Dosing

Acute doses of intravenous iron are given when the patient has a TSAT below 20% or a ferritin level below 100 ng/ml (200 ng/ml in adult HD patients). Intravenous iron should not be given when the TSAT is greater than 50% or the serum ferritin level is more than 500 ng/ml. The goal of acute intravenous iron dosing is to normalize the serum ferritin and the TSAT. In some cases, an acute dose may be used as a trial of intravenous iron in a patient with normal iron studies but a poor response to ESA. In these patients, the goal of acute intravenous iron is a reduction in ESA dose or the correction of resistant anemia. In adult HD patients, studies suggest that a total dose of 1000 mg of iron divided over multiple consecutive dialysis sessions is appropriate, because smaller doses are not as effective.[66] A total dose of 1000 mg given as 100-mg doses over 10 dialysis sessions has been used in older children with good results.[57] A randomized study of children receiving HD compared two acute dosing regimens of iron gluconate (1.5 mg/kg/dose and 3.0 mg/kg/dose; maximum dose, 125 mg/dose) given during eight consecutive HD sessions. The patients had a TSAT of less than 20% and/or a ferritin level of less than 100 ng/ml at baseline. Both doses led to an increase in the Hb level and the normalization of iron indices. Because there was no difference in the response, the authors recommended a dose of 1.5 mg/kg/dose with a maximum of 125 mg/dose.[64] Iron gluconate and iron sucrose are provided in 62.5- and 50-mg vials. Hence, the dose per dialysis session can be adjusted to minimize the wasting of the drug as long as the maximum single dose is not exceeded. On the basis of the available evidence, the total dose for acute pediatric dosing should be between 12 and 25 mg/kg (1000 mg maximum) divided over 8 to 12 HD sessions.

Chronic Dosing

Acute dosing is effective for correcting iron deficiency, but, especially in HD patients, there is a risk of ongoing episodes of iron deficiency as a result of continued blood loss. Transient iron deficiency may lead to decreased red blood cell synthesis; this has led to more frequent chronic intravenous iron use. In one pediatric study, 1 mg/kg of iron gluconate for 12 weeks led to a significant increase in the Hb level.[56] In another pediatric study, chronic intravenous iron sucrose (2 mg/kg [maximum, 200 mg] weekly) produced a reduction in the rHuEPO dose.[63]

A randomized 16-week study of children receiving HD compared maintenance intravenous iron dextran (doses of 25, 50, or 100 mg/week based on weight; doses therefore ranged from 1.25 to 2.5 mg/kg/week) with oral iron (4 to 6 mg/kg/day). The patients receiving intravenous iron had a significant increase in ferritin as compared with the oral iron group. There was a trend toward a reduction in the rHuEPO dose in the intravenous iron group as compared with the oral iron group.[65] Another study randomized children receiving HD to intermittent intravenous iron or maintenance intravenous iron. There was a higher rate of iron overload in the children receiving intermittent intravenous iron.[67] This observation may be the result of a decreased ability to use stored iron in children receiving HD as a result of an inflammatory block. The low doses of maintenance intravenous iron are immediately employed for red cell synthesis, thus avoiding an excessive accumulation of stored iron. This contrasts with intermittent intravenous iron; the high doses cannot all be used immediately, thereby increasing the risk of eventual iron overload.

One pediatric study prospectively followed children who were started on a maintenance dose of 1 mg/kg/week of iron gluconate and then adjusted the dose of iron gluconate on the basis of iron studies. The majority of the patients completing the study required a dose of 1.5 mg/kg to maintain adequate iron stores.[68]

Maintenance intravenous iron in children receiving HD should be started at about 1 mg/kg/week, usually given as a once-weekly dose. The maintenance dose is titrated to keep the TSAT above 20% and the ferritin level above 100 ng/ml; intravenous iron should be held if the TSAT is greater than 50% or the ferritin level is greater than 500 ng/ml.

For children receiving PD or who have not yet started dialysis, the goal is usually to minimize the need for intravenous line placement by maximizing the dose given during a single infusion. In adults, iron gluconate doses of 250 mg over 60 or 90 minutes were well tolerated.[69] In children, one study reported the administration of doses ranging from 1.5 to 8.8 mg/kg, with the child receiving the highest dose having a significant adverse event.[62] Thus, acute doses of iron gluconate should not exceed 4 mg/kg (250 mg if the child weighs >60 kg), which should be given over at least 90 minutes.

In adults, iron sucrose doses of 300 mg given over 1.5 to 2 hours, appear to be well tolerated. Alternatively, iron sucrose doses of 200 mg can be given over 2 minutes in adults, although there is a small risk of symptoms of acute iron overload, especially among smaller patients.[70] Doses of iron sucrose as high as 500 mg have been given, but the infusion time must be extended to avoid side effects.[71] In children, one study reported the administration of doses of 7 mg/kg of iron sucrose, with a maximum dose of 200 mg.[63]

Complications

There are some complications of intravenous iron that are specific to the particular preparation. Iron dextran may cause an acute anaphylactic reaction that is potentially fatal.[72] Iron sucrose[73] and iron gluconate[66] have safer side-effect profiles. Children who have had anaphylactic reactions to iron dextran have tolerated other iron preparations.[62] High doses of iron dextran may cause patients to develop arthralgias and myalgias.[74]

There are reports of laboratory findings and clinical symptoms that may be the result of acute iron toxicity during the use of iron sucrose and iron gluconate. This effect is related to the dose and infusion rate, and it is presumably the result of the rapid release of free iron. Symptoms with iron gluconate have included loin pain, hypotension, emesis, and paresthesias.[75] Iron sucrose side effects have included rash, flushing, and hypotension, which were rapidly reversible.[76] These side effects limit the maximum single dose of these compounds as compared with iron dextran, which releases free iron at a slower rate.

Iron overload is a potential complication of intravenous iron therapy; 14% of US pediatric HD patients had a ferritin concentration of more than 800 ng/ml in 2001.[23] There is concern that current intravenous iron protocols may lead to more problems with iron overload, which has been seen in children receiving acute or maintenance intravenous iron.[63,67]

Intravenous iron may increase the risk of infection. However, a multivariate analysis did not find a relationship between intravenous iron and infection, although there was a trend toward more infections among those patients who received large amounts of intravenous iron as compared with those who received lower doses.[77] Given this potential complication, intravenous iron should be held in patients with acute infections.

REFERENCES

1. Locatelli F, Aljama P, Barany P, et al: Revised European best practice guidelines for the management of anaemia in patients with chronic renal failure, *Nephrol Dial Transplant* 19 Suppl 2:ii1-47, 2004.
2. National Kidney Foundation: KDOQI clinical practice guidelines and clinical practice recommendations for anemia in chronic kidney disease, *Am J Kidney Dis* 47:S1-145, 2006.
3. McGonigle RJ, Boineau FG, Beckman B, et al: Erythropoietin and inhibitors of in vitro erythropoiesis in the development of anemia in children with renal disease, *J Lab Clin Med* 105:449-58, 1985.
4. Chandra M, Clemons GK, McVicar MI: Relation of serum erythropoietin levels to renal excretory function: evidence for lowered set point for erythropoietin production in chronic renal failure, *J Pediatr* 113:1015-21, 1988.
5. Muller-Wiefel DE, Sinn H, Gilli G, Scharer K: Hemolysis and blood loss in children with chronic renal failure, *Clin Nephrol* 8:481-86, 1977.
6. Eknoyan G, Latos D, Lindberg J: Practice recommendations for the use of L-carnitine in dialysis-related carnitine disorder. National Kidney Foundation Carnitine Consensus Conference, *Am J Kidney Dis* 41:868-76, 2003.
7. Polenakovic M, Sikole A: Is erythropoietin a survival factor for red blood cells?, *J Am Soc Nephrol* 7:1178-82, 1996.
8. Richardson D, Lindley E, Bartlett C, Will E: A randomized, controlled study of the consequences of hemodialysis membrane composition on erythropoietic response, *Am J Kidney Dis* 42:551-60, 2003.
9. Frankenfield DL, Neu AM, Warady BA, Fivush BA, et al: Anemia in pediatric hemodialysis patients: Results from the 2001 ESRD Clinical Performance Measures Project, *Kidney Int* 64:1120-24, 2003.
10. Arbeiter K, Greenbaum L, Balzar E, et al: Reproducible erythroid aplasia caused by mycophenolate mofetil, *Pediatr Nephrol* 14:195-97, 2000.
11. Subtirelu MM, Flynn JT, Schechner RS, Pullman JM, et al: Acute renal failure in a pediatric kidney allograft recipient treated with intravenous immunoglobulin for parvovirus B19 induced pure red cell aplasia, *Pediatr Transplant* 9:801-04, 2005.
12. Chand DH, Brier M, Strife CF: Comparison of vascular access type in pediatric hemodialysis patients with respect to urea clearance, anemia management, and serum albumin concentration, *Am J Kidney Dis* 45:303-08, 2005.
13. Kalantar-Zadeh K, Ikizler TA, Block G, Avram M, Kopple J: Malnutrition-inflammation complex syndrome in dialysis patients: causes and consequences, *Am J Kidney Dis* 42:864-81, 2003.
14. Ganz T: Molecular pathogenesis of anemia of chronic disease, *Pediatr Blood Cancer* 46:554-57, 2006.
15. Barany P: Inflammation, serum C-reactive protein, and erythropoietin resistance, *Nephrol Dial Transplant* 16:224-27, 2001.
16. Barany P, Divino Filho JC, Bergstrom J: High C-reactive protein is a strong predictor of resistance to erythropoietin in hemodialysis patients, *Am J Kidney Dis* 29:565-68, 1997.
17. Rao DS, Shih MS, Mohini R: Effect of serum parathyroid hormone and bone marrow fibrosis on the response to erythropoietin in uremia, *N Engl J Med* 328:171-75, 1993.
18. Pronai W, Riegler-Keil M, Silberbauer K, Stockenhuber F: Folic acid supplementation improves erythropoietin response, *Nephron* 71:395-400, 1995.
19. Kaiser L, Schwartz KA: Aluminum-induced anemia, *Am J Kidney Dis* 6:348-52, 1985.
20. Schroder CH: European Pediatric Peritoneal Dialysis Working Group: The management of anemia in pediatric peritoneal dialysis patients. Guidelines by an ad hoc European committee, *Pediatr Nephrol* 18:805-09, 2003.
21. Erturk S, Nergizoglu G, Ates K, et al: The impact of withdrawing ACE inhibitors on erythropoietin responsiveness and left ventricular hypertrophy in haemodialysis patients, *Nephrol Dial Transplant* 14:1912-16, 1999.
22. Chavers BM, Roberts TL, Herzog CA, Collins AJ, St Peter WL: Prevalence of anemia in erythropoietin-treated pediatric as compared to adult chronic dialysis patients, *Kidney Int* 65:266-73, 2004.
23. Centers for Medicare and Medicaid Services: 2002 annual report, end stage renal disease clinical performance measures project, *Am J Kidney Dis* 42:S1-96, 2003.
24. Fadrowski JJ, Furth SL, Fivush BA: Anemia in pediatric dialysis patients in end-stage renal disease network 5, *Pediatr Nephrol* 19:1029-34, 2004.
25. Mitsnefes MM, Subat-Dezulovic M, Khoury PR, Goebel J, Strife CF: Increasing incidence of post-kidney transplant anemia in children, *Am J Transplant* 5:1713-18, 2005.
26. Warady BA, Ho M: Morbidity and mortality in children with anemia at initiation of dialysis, *Pediatr Nephrol* 18:1055-62, 2003.
27. Besarab A, Bolton WK, Browne JK, et al: The effects of normal as compared with low hematocrit values in patients with cardiac disease who are receiving hemodialysis and epoetin, *N Engl J Med* 339:584-90, 1998.
28. Morris KP, Skinner JR, Hunter S, Coulthard MG: Cardiovascular abnormalities in end stage renal failure: the effect of anaemia or uraemia?, *Arch Dis Child* 71:119-22, 1994.
29. Mitsnefes MM, Daniels SR, Schwartz SM, Meyer RA, et al: Severe left ventricular hypertrophy in pediatric dialysis: prevalence and predictors, *Pediatr Nephrol* 14:898-902, 2000.
30. Gerson A, Hwang W, Fiorenza J, et al: Anemia and health-related quality of life in adolescents with chronic kidney disease, *Am J Kidney Dis* 44:1017-23, 2004.
31. Montini G, Zacchello G, Baraldi E, et al: Benefits and risks of anemia correction with recombinant human erythropoietin in children maintained by hemodialysis, *J Pediatr* 117:556-60, 1990.
32. Burke JR: Low-dose subcutaneous recombinant erythropoietin in children with chronic renal failure. Australian and New Zealand Paediatric Nephrology Association, *Pediatr Nephrol* 9:558-61, 1995.
33. Jabs K, Alexander S, McCabe D, Lerner G, Harmon W: Primary results from the U.S. multicenter pediatric recombinant erythropoietin (EPO) study, *J Am Soc Nephrol* 5:546, 1994.
34. Jabs K: The effects of recombinant human erythropoietin on growth and nutritional status, *Pediatr Nephrol* 10:324-27, 1996.
35. Hutchinson FN, Jones WJ: A cost-effectiveness analysis of anemia screening before erythropoietin in patients with end-stage renal disease, *Am J Kidney Dis* 29:651-57, 1997.
36. Gokal R, Weatherall DJ, Bunch C: Iron induced increase in red cell size in haemodialysis patients, *Q J Med* 48:393-401, 1979.
37. Hymes LC, Hawthorne SM, Clowers BM: Impaired response to recombinant erythropoietin therapy in children with peritonitis, *Dial Transplant* 23:462-63, 1994.
38. van Iperen CE, Kraaijenhagen RJ, Biesma DH, Beguin Y, et al: Iron metabolism and erythropoiesis after surgery, *Br J Surg* 85:41-45, 1998.
39. Aufricht C, Balzar E, Steger H, et al: Subcutaneous recombinant human erythropoietin in children with renal anemia on continuous ambulatory peritoneal dialysis, *Acta Paediatr* 82:959-62, 1993.
40. Ho M, Stablein DM: *North American Pediatric Renal Transplant Cooperative Study (NAPRTCS) annual report*, Rockville, MD, 2003, The Emmes Corporation.
41. Sieniawska M, Roszkowska-Blaim M: Recombinant human erythropoietin dosage in children undergoing hemodialysis and continuous ambulatory peritoneal dialysis, *Pediatr Nephrol* 11:628-30, 1997.
42. Brandt JR, Avner ED, Hickman RO, Watkins SL: Safety and efficacy of erythropoietin in children with chronic renal failure, *Pediatr Nephrol* 13:143-47, 1999.
43. Yalcinkaya F, Tumer N, Cakar N, Ozkaya N: Low-dose erythropoietin is effective and safe in children on continuous ambulatory peritoneal dialysis, *Pediatr Nephrol* 11:350-52, 1997.
44. Casadevall N, Nataf J, Viron B, et al: Pure red-cell aplasia and antierythropoietin antibodies in patients treated with recombinant erythropoietin, *N Engl J Med* 346:469-75, 2002.
45. Bennett CL, Cournoyer D, Carson KR, et al: Long-term outcome of individuals with pure red cell aplasia and antierythropoietin antibodies in patients treated with recombinant epoetin: a follow-up report from the Research on Adverse Drug Events and Reports (RADAR) Project, *Blood* 106:3343-47, 2005.

46. Nissenson AR, Swan SK, Lindberg JS, et al: Randomized, controlled trial of darbepoetin alfa for the treatment of anemia in hemodialysis patients, *Am J Kidney Dis* 40:110-18, 2002.
47. Vanrenterghem Y, Barany P, Mann JF, et al: Randomized trial of darbepoetin alfa for treatment of renal anemia at a reduced dose frequency compared with rHuEPO in dialysis patients, *Kidney Int* 62:2167-75, 2002.
48. Walker R: *Aranesp (darbepoetin alfa) administered at a reduced frequency of once every 4 weeks (Q4W) maintains hemoglobin levels in patients with chronic kidney disease (CKD) receiving dialysis*, National Kidney Foundation Clinical Nephrology Meeting, Chicago, 2002.
49. De Palo T, Giordano M, Palumbo F, et al: Clinical experience with darbepoetin alfa (NESP) in children undergoing hemodialysis, *Pediatr Nephrol* 19:337-40, 2004.
50. Geary DF, Keating LE, Vigneux A, Stephens D, et al: Darbepoetin alfa (Aranesp) in children with chronic renal failure, *Kidney Int* 68:1759-65, 2005.
51. Durkan AM, Keating LE, Vigneux A, Geary DF: The use of darbepoetin in infants with chronic renal impairment, *Pediatr Nephrol* 21:694-97, 2006.
52. Lerner G, Kale AS, Warady BA, et al: Pharmacokinetics of darbepoetin alfa in pediatric patients with chronic kidney disease, *Pediatr Nephrol* 17:933-7, 2002.
53. Macdougall IC, Gray SJ, Elston O, et al: Pharmacokinetics of novel erythropoiesis stimulating protein compared with epoetin alfa in dialysis patients, *J Am Soc Nephrol* 10:2392-95, 1999.
54. Evans JH, Brocklebank JT, Bowmer CJ, Ng PC: Pharmacokinetics of recombinant human erythropoietin in children with renal failure, *Nephrol Dial Transplant* 6:709-14, 1991.
55. Scott SD: Dose conversion from recombinant human erythropoietin to darbepoetin alfa: recommendations from clinical studies, *Pharmacotherapy* 22:160S-5S, 2002.
56. Tenbrock K, Muller-Berghaus J, Michalk D, Querfeld U: Intravenous iron treatment of renal anemia in children on hemodialysis, *Pediatr Nephrol* 13:580-82, 1999.
57. Greenbaum LA, Pan CG, Caley C, Nelson T, Sheth KJ: Intravenous iron dextran and erythropoietin use in pediatric hemodialysis patients, *Pediatr Nephrol* 14:908-11, 2000.
58. Campos A, Garin EH: Therapy of renal anemia in children and adolescents with recombinant human erythropoietin (rHuEPO), *Clin Pediatr (Phila)* 31:94-99, 1992.
59. Morris KP, Watson S, Reid MM, Hamilton PJ, Coulthard MG: Assessing iron status in children with chronic renal failure on erythropoietin: which measurements should we use?, *Pediatr Nephrol* 8:51-56, 1994.
60. Pruchnicki MC, Coyle JD, Hoshaw-Woodard S, Bay WH: Effect of phosphate binders on supplemental iron absorption in healthy subjects, *J Clin Pharmacol* 42:1171-76, 2002
61. Gillespie RS, Wolf FM: Intravenous iron therapy in pediatric hemodialysis patients: a meta-analysis, *Pediatr Nephrol* 19:662-66, 2004.
62. Yorgin PD, Belson A, Sarwal M, Alexander SR: Sodium ferric gluconate therapy in renal transplant and renal failure patients, *Pediatr Nephrol* 15:171-75, 2000.
63. Morgan HE, Gautam M, Geary DF: Maintenance intravenous iron therapy in pediatric hemodialysis patients, *Pediatr Nephrol* 16:779-83, 2001.
64. Warady BA, Zobrist RH, Wu J, Finan E; Ferrlecit Pediatric Study Group: Sodium ferric gluconate complex therapy in anemic children on hemodialysis, *Pediatr Nephrol* 20:1320-27, 2005.
65. Warady BA, Kausz A, Lerner G, et al: Iron therapy in the pediatric hemodialysis population, *Pediatr Nephrol* 19:655-61, 2004.
66. Nissenson AR, Lindsay RM, Swan S, Seligman P, Strobos J: Sodium ferric gluconate complex in sucrose is safe and effective in hemodialysis patients: North American Clinical Trial, *Am J Kidney Dis* 33:471-82, 1999.
67. Ruiz-Jaramillo Mde L, Guizar-Mendoza JM, Gutierrez-Navarro Mde J, Dubey-Ortega LA, Amador-Licona N: Intermittent versus maintenance iron therapy in children on hemodialysis: a randomized study, *Pediatr Nephrol* 19:77-81, 2004.
68. Warady BA, Zobrist RH, Finan E; Ferrlecit Pediatric Study Group: Sodium ferric gluconate complex maintenance therapy in children on hemodialysis, *Pediatr Nephrol* 21:553-60, 2006.
69. Folkert VW, Michael B, Agarwal R, et al: Chronic use of sodium ferric gluconate complex in hemodialysis patients: safety of higher-dose (> or = 250 mg) administration, *Am J Kidney Dis* 41:651-57, 2003.
70. Macdougall IC, Roche A: Administration of intravenous iron sucrose as a 2-minute push to CKD patients: a prospective evaluation of 2,297 injections, *Am J Kidney Dis* 46:283-89, 2005.
71. Chandler G, Harchowal J, Macdougall IC: Intravenous iron sucrose: establishing a safe dose, *Am J Kidney Dis* 38:988-91, 2001.
72. Fletes R, Lazarus JM, Gage J, Chertow GM: Suspected iron dextran-related adverse drug events in hemodialysis patients, *Am J Kidney Dis* 37:743-49, 2001.
73. Coyne DW, Adkinson NF, Nissenson AR, et al: Sodium ferric gluconate complex in hemodialysis patients. II. Adverse reactions in iron dextran-sensitive and dextran-tolerant patients, *Kidney Int* 63:217-24, 2003.
74. Auerbach M, Chaudhry M, Goldman H, Ballard H: Value of methylprednisolone in prevention of the arthralgia-myalgia syndrome associated with the total dose infusion of iron dextran: a double blind randomized trial, *J Lab Clin Med* 131:257-60, 1998.
75. Pascual J, Teruel JL, Liano F, Sureda A, Ortuno J: Serious adverse reactions after intravenous ferric gluconate, *Nephrol Dial Transplant* 7:271-72, 1992.
76. Hoigne R, Breymann C, Kunzi UP, Brunner F: Parenteral iron therapy: problems and possible solutions, *Schweiz Med Wochenschr* 128:528-35, 1998.
77. Hoen B, Paul-Dauphin A, Kessler M: Intravenous iron administration does not significantly increase the risk of bacteremia in chronic hemodialysis patients, *Clin Nephrol* 57:457-61, 2002.

CHAPTER

50 Disorders of Bone Mineral Metabolism in Chronic Kidney Disease

Claus P. Schmitt and Otto Mehls

INTRODUCTION

Disturbances of bone and mineral metabolism almost inevitably develop in the course of chronic kidney disease (CKD). These comprise altered calcium, phosphate and magnesium homeostasis, abnormal synthesis and secretion of parathyroid hormone (PTH) and vitamin D, and alterations in bone metabolism and function. If not treated appropriately, severe and sometimes disabling complications may occur.

Only recently it has become apparent that alterations of bone and mineral metabolism originating in childhood contribute not only to degenerative bone disease but to vascular morbidity and mortality in adult life. Hence, adequate control of bone and mineral metabolism is one of the major challenges in the treatment of pediatric patients with chronic renal failure.

EPIDEMIOLOGY

As early as in CKD stage II, that is, a glomerular filtration rate (GFR) of 60 to 90 ml/min * 1.73 m², $1,25(OH)_2D_3$ plasma concentrations decline and iPTH and fibroblast growth factor 23 (FGF-23) levels start to increase (Figure 50-1). When end-stage renal disease (ESRD) is reached, two thirds of pediatric and adult patients have abnormal histologic bone findings. The specific features of bone disease depend on the degree of hyperparathyroidism and the therapeutic measures taken to control the disease, whereas the mode of dialysis therapy does not appear to play a major role.[1] Adynamic bone disease has a high prevalence, being observed in 40% to 50 % of adult and almost 30% of pediatric ESRD patients[1-3] (Figure 50-2).

PATHOGENESIS

Bone and mineral homeostasis is regulated in a complex network of local and systemic factors. Patients with CKD develop major disturbances in calcium, $1,25(OH)_2D_3$, and phosphate homeostasis and subsequently abnormal parathyroid gland function—which ultimately drives the course of the disease (Figure 50-3).

Disorders of Calcium Homeostasis

In healthy individuals, 99% of total body calcium is stored in the bone, 0.975% is stored in soft tissues, and only 0.025% is circulating in blood. Plasma ionized calcium levels are tightly controlled by PTH and $1,25(OH)_2D_3$. The parathyroid gland senses changes in ionized calcium by a G-protein–coupled membrane receptor. Acute hypocalcemia is counteracted by an instantaneous and marked increase in PTH release from storage vesicles (rapidly normalizing plasma calcium levels) and by an increased PTH gene transcription and synthesis rate, an adaptive response that takes several hours to occur.

In addition, hypocalcemia stabilizes PTH mRNA by increased binding of a cytosolic adenosine-uridine–rich protein (AUF1) in the 3′ untranslated region of the PTH mRNA.[4] A subsequent increase in $1,25(OH)_2D_3$ synthesis further stabilizes plasma calcium levels via stimulation of gastrointestinal calcium absorption. In CKD, reduced $1,25(OH)_2D_3$ synthesis impairs intestinal calcium resorption—resulting in an activation of the regulatory circuits described previously and a resetting of ionized calcium at low or low-normal levels.

The calcemic response of bone to PTH is reduced. Higher PTH levels are required to maintain calcium homeostasis and bone turnover. Uremic toxins, low levels of $1,25(OH)_2D_3$, accumulation of PTH fragments and osteoprotegerin, and altered PTH receptor expression have been implicated in the skeletal resistance to PTH—providing yet another mechanism contributing to the development of hyperparathyroidism[4] (Figure 50-3).

Plasma ionized calcium is the major regulator of the parathyroids at the level of gene expression, secretion, and cell proliferation. Induction of hypocalcemia stimulates PTH release and PTH peptide synthesis via stabilization of PTH mRNA. If this is sustained, profound parathyroid cell proliferation may be induced.[5,6] Hypocalcemia appears to be a more important regulator of the parathyroid than vitamin D, as suggested by the efficient control of hyperparathyroidism in vitamin-D–receptor knockout mice by a selective increase in dietary calcium content.[7] Moreover, calcimimetic agents suppress PTH by as much as 80% independently of plasma phosphate and $1,25(OH)_2D_3$ levels.

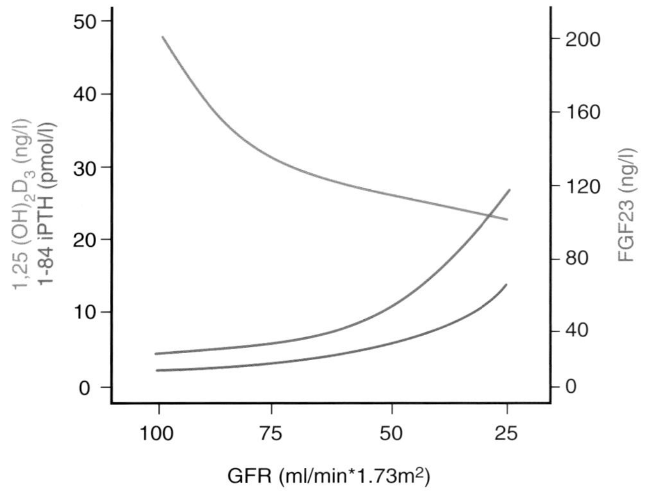

Figure 50-1 Mean plasma intact PTH, $1,25(OH)_2D_3$ (left y-axis), and FGF-23 concentrations (right Y axis) in patients with different degrees of CKD. Individual values may vary considerably, especially in patients with advanced renal failure. (Adapted from Reichel H, Deibert B, Schmidt-Gayk H, Ritz E: Calcium metabolism in early chronic renal failure: Implications for the pathogenesis of hyperparathyroidism, *Nephrol Dial Transplant* 6(3):162-69, 1991; and adapted from Shigematsu T, Kazama JJ, Yamashita T, Fukumoto S, Hosoya T, Gejyo F, et al.: Possible involvement of circulating fibroblast growth factor 23 in the development of secondary hyperparathyroidism associated with renal insufficiency, *Am J Kidney Dis* 44(2):250-56, 2004.)

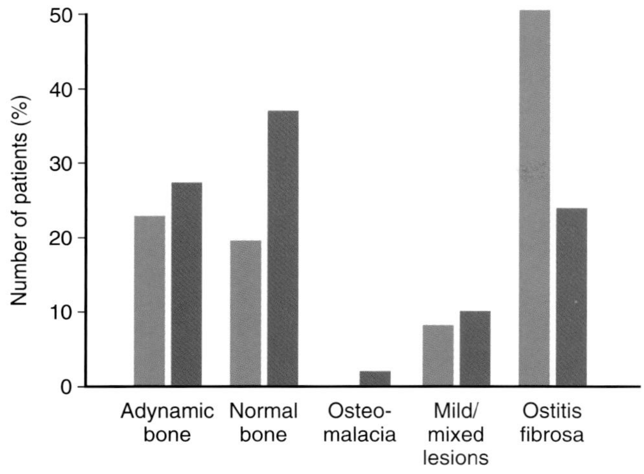

Figure 50-2 Spectrum of renal osteodystrophy in children with CKD stage V diagnosed in the United States in the early 1990s and in Poland in the late 1990s. (*Hatched bars* adapted from Salusky IB, Ramirez JA, Oppenheim W, Gales B, Segre GV, Goodman WG: Biochemical markers of renal osteodystrophy in pediatric patients undergoing CAPD/CCPD, *Kidney Int* 45(1):253-58, 1994. Filled bars adapted from Ziolkowska H, Paniczyk-Tomaszewska M, Debinski A, Polowiec Z, Sawicki A, Sieniawska M: Bone biopsy results and serum bone turnover parameters in uremic children, *Acta Paediatr* 89(6):666-71, 2000.)

Abnormalities of $1,25(OH)_2D_3$ Metabolism in CKD

$25(OH)_2D_3$ is converted to the systemically active $1,25(OH)_2D_3$ by the renal enzyme 1-alpha hydroxylase. Progressive loss of intact renal parenchyma, low $25(OH)_2D_3$ levels, and increased FGF-23 release from the bone result in low circulating $1,25(OH)_2D_3$ levels and thus in reduced intestinal calcium absorption and hypocalcemia. Subsequently, PTH plasma levels increase to maintain calcium homeostasis and to stimulate 1-alpha hydroxylase. Hence, in the presence of hyperparathyroidism even normal levels of $1,25(OH)_2D_3$ must be considered inappropriately low.

$1,25(OH)_2D_3$ controls parathyroid gland function not only by modulating plasma ionized calcium but directly by suppressing PTH gene transcription[8] and by upregulating its own receptor in parathyroid cells. Moreover, $1,25(OH)_2D_3$ binds to a response element in the promoter region of the calcium receptor—resulting in increased calcium receptor abundance and increased sensitivity of the parathyroid gland to ionized calcium.[9] Hypocalcemia, on the other hand, compromises vitamin D action by upregulating calreticulin (a repressor of the vitamin response element in the parathyroid).[10] In addition, $1,25(OH)_2D_3$ regulates parathyroid cell proliferation—with low levels promoting parathyroid gland hyperplasia.

$1,25(OH)_2D_3$ has numerous additional important functions outside the bone and parathyroid. It is an important regulator of the immune system and affects the contractility, growth, and migration of vascular smooth muscle cells (VSMCs) and the evolution of vascular calcifications. Both endothelial and VSMCs express high-affinity vitamin D3 receptors. $1,25(OH)_2D_3$ deficiency may contribute to cardiovascular disease by unrepressed production of proteins (such as bone morphogenetic protein-2[11,12]) involved in arterial calcification or by suppressed production of local inhibitors of mineralization (e.g., matrix GLA protein).[13]

On the other hand, high doses of $1,25(OH)_2D_3$ promote vascular calcification via an increased calcium phosphate product and transition of VSMCs to an osteoblast-like phenotype. Of note in this context, $1,25(OH)_2D_3$ is not just an endocrine factor exclusively secreted by the kidney. Extrarenal 1-α-hydroxylase expression has been demonstrated in various tissues such as bone, smooth muscle cells, and parathyroid glands,[14,15] suggesting an additional paracrine mode of action independent of renal conversion.

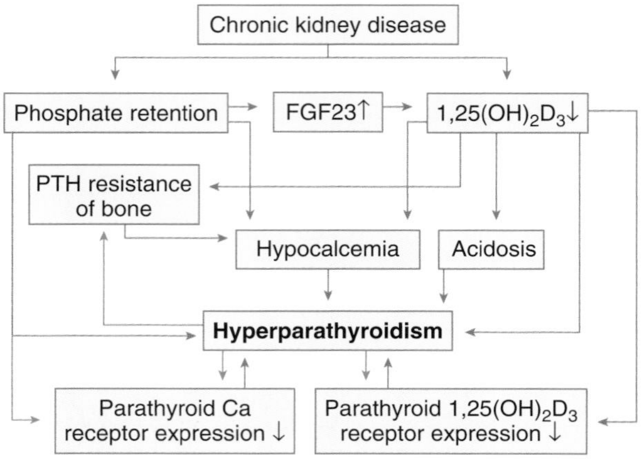

Figure 50-3 Pathophysiology of secondary hyperparathyroidism.

Vitamin D25 Deficiency

Recent investigations have demonstrated that $25(OH)_2D_3$ deficiency, as defined by 25-OH-D-levels below 30 to 40 ng/ml, is frequent in CKD—probably due to dietary restrictions and a sedentary lifestyle with reduced sun exposure. Low $25(OH)_2D_3$ levels result in muscle weakness[16] and bone pain, and aggravate renal bone disease.[17,18] Bone histomorphologic changes are correlated with plasma $25(OH)_2D_3$ levels.[19] In vitro, a concentration of 40 ng/ml $25(OH)_2D_3$ is as efficient in suppressing PTH as calcitriol at a maximally PTH-suppressive dose.

Abnormalities of Phosphate Metabolism

Phosphate excretion declines with failing renal function. Increased plasma phosphate levels are, however, usually not observed before severe renal insufficiency has developed because the kidney has a phosphate secretory reserve stimulated by FGF-23 and PTH. FGF-23 is synthesized in bone and increases renal phosphate excretion by reducing the expression of the type IIa Na+/Pi co-transporter in proximal tubular cells. In early CKD, the circulating level of the phosphaturic hormone FGF-23 rises to prevent hyperphosphatemia. At the same time, FGF-23 reduces 1-alpha hydroxylase—thereby stimulating PTH release[20,21] (Figures 50-1 and 50-3).

Hyperphosphatemia has multiple deleterious effects. Hyperphosphatemia contributes to hyperparathyroidism independently of plasma calcium and $1,25(OH)_2D_3$[22,23] via increasing PTH gene transcription, PTH peptide secretion, and parathyroid cell proliferation. Furthermore, hyperphosphatemia reduces renal $1,25(OH)_2D_3$ synthesis, inhibits the suppressive action of $1,25(OH)_2D_3$ on the parathyroid glands, and promotes resistance of bone to PTH. Another indirect mechanism by which high phosphate drives hyperparathyroidism is via physicochemical precipitation of calcium-phosphate salts, a process that aggravates hypocalcemia.

Secondary Hyperparathyroidism

The multiple effects of $1,25(OH)_2D_3$ deficiency, hypocalcemia, and hyperphosphatemia in CKD converge in the development of *secondary hyperparathyroidism*—with a progressive demineralization of the bone. Pre–pro-PTH gene transcription rate, mRNA stability, protein synthesis, and secretion of the mature protein are increased. Persistent hyperparathyroidism induces distinct changes in parathyroid gland morphology and function. Parathyroid cell proliferation results in diffuse and polyclonal and eventually monoclonal cell growth associated with the formation of adenoma.

Regulatory systems include endothelin, transforming growth factor (TGF)-alpha, epidermal growth factor receptor, and the cell cycle inhibitor p21.[24-27] Monoclonal parathyroid cell growth is the result of an array of genetic aberrations that includes gene deletions, loss of heterozygosity, clonal rearrangement and/or oncogene overexpression, and tumor suppressor gene inactivation. Polymorphisms in the PTH, vitamin D receptor, and calcium receptor genes may also be involved and may explain some of the clinical variability of the disease.[28] Reduced expression of the parathyroid calcium-sensing receptor and of the vitamin D receptor leads to a progressive escape from the two key physiologic control mechanisms and ultimately to parathyroid gland autonomy (Figure 50-4).

The reduced sensitivity of the parathyroid to calcium ions has often been described as a change in the calcium "set point." It is usually defined as the serum calcium concentration at mid-range between the maximal and minimal PTH concentration induced by stepwise changes of serum calcium levels. This static concept has been challenged.[29] Minute-by-minute analyses of PTH secretion revealed distinct alterations of the dynamics of oscillatory PTH release in uremic patients, including a markedly reduced secretory capacity to counteract changes in ionized calcium by modulation of the frequency and mass of PTH secretory bursts.[30]

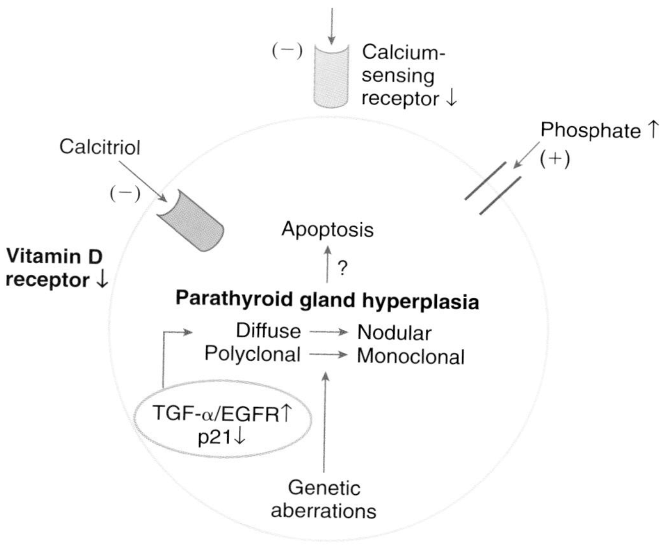

Figure 50-4 Cellular alterations of parathyroid gland function.

Apoptosis is a rare event in normal parathyroid tissue. Although uremia is associated with increased apoptosis of parathyroid cells, this mechanism is insufficient to counterbalance enhanced proliferation.[31] Whether an inversion of this imbalance (i.e., regression of parathyroid hyperplasia) can ever occur in uremic patients, or after correction of uremia, remains controversial.

The Impact of Metabolic Acidosis

Metabolic acidosis, an almost inevitable covariate in patients with failing renal function, has a number of untoward effects on bone. These include physicochemical dissolution of bone with net calcium efflux, inhibition of osteoblast, and activation of osteoclast activity. This is associated with impaired bone mineralization and an increased incidence of osteomalacia, which can be improved by correction of metabolic acidosis.[32] Moreover, some evidence suggests that metabolic acidosis increases PTH levels in CKD patients and enhances the peripheral actions of PTH on bone by increasing the expression and ligand affinity of the PTH receptor.[33] However, the quantitative contribution of metabolic acidosis to bone disease in CKD patients remains uncertain.

PTH Fragments

The transcriptional product of the PTH gene encodes the 84 amino acids of the mature peptide, a "pre" signal sequence of 25 amino acids and a "pro" hexapeptide. This single-chain 115-amino-acid peptide, called pre-pro-PTH, is rapidly converted to PTH by cleavage. The signal sequence is required for proper PTH processing and secretion. Mutations within this segment can cause hypoparathyroidism.[34] The remaining peptide is processed to 1-84 PTH and a mixture of fragments, which were at one time considered biologically inactive.

It is now apparent, however, that PTH metabolism is regulated—most notably by variation in blood ionized calcium concentration—and that certain *N*-terminally truncated fragments, including 7-84 PTH, offset the classic biologic actions of PTH.[35] They are present in blood and accumulate appreciably in end-stage kidney disease.[36,37] 7-84 PTH internalizes the PTH type-1 receptor without prior activation. This may be one explanation for the reduced PTH1R abundance in uremia, the resistance of bone to PTH, and the dissociation of phosphorus and calcium homeostasis in CKD patients. Alternatively, PTH fragments may also signal via receptors distinct from the PTH1R, for example, through a putative C-terminal PTH receptor[38] and by this impact on bone. The clinical relevance of the circulating PTH fragments is still unclear.

Bone Morphogenetic Protein-7

The kidney and bone interaction is not confined to the homeostasis of calcium phosphate and 1,25$(OH)_2D_3$ synthesis. CKD can impair bone remodeling. Bone morphogenetic protein-7 (BMP-7), which is widely expressed throughout embryonic development and critically involved in the development of many organ systems (including the bones), is produced and secreted in postnatal life mainly by renal collecting tubule cells. CKD is associated with a marked deficiency of circulating BMP-7, most likely due to reduced renal synthesis. In the uremic rat model, adynamic bone disease develops if serum calcium, phosphate, vitamin D, and PTH levels are maintained in the normal range.

This observation has led to the hypothesis that the variable histopathologic appearance of uremic bone may reflect the net balance of hyperparathyroidism, inducing a high turnover and BMP-7 deficiency that cause a low-turnover state. At least in the uremic rat, exogenous administration of BMP-7 can reverse both adynamic and high-turnover bone disease by improving osteoblast number and bone formation activity.[39,40] Moreover, BMP-7 reduces vascular calcifications in uremic animals, possibly by increasing the skeletal deposition of phosphorus and calcium.[41]

HISTOLOGIC FINDINGS

The term *renal osteodystrophy* is reserved for the total spectrum of histologic changes in CKD-associated bone disease. The type of renal osteodystrophy in an individual patient depends on the therapeutic interventions taken to counteract an otherwise progressive disease. Whereas in untreated children with CKD histologic signs of fibrosis and demineralization prevail, aggressive long-term treatment with calcium and vitamin D is associated with low bone turnover (Figure 50-5). At present, an adequate balance with normal or mild alterations in bone morphology is achieved only in about a third of children.[1] Table 50-1 provides a histologic classification of renal osteodystrophy, and Figure 50-6 shows respective histopathologies.

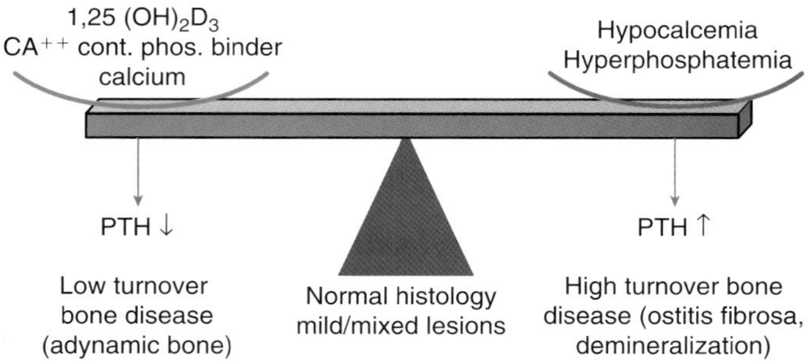

Figure 50-5 The type of renal bone disease depends on therapeutic interventions.

TABLE 50-1 Histologic Classification of Renal Osteodystrophy

Type	Etiology	Description	Comments
High-turnover bone disease (ostitis fibrosa)	Hyperparathyroidism	• Increased bone formation, resorption, and osteoid deposition/seams • Disorganized collagen (woven bone), marrow fibrosis	• Common in untreated patients • Skeletal deformities, bone pain, epiphysiolysis
Low-turnover: I adynamic bone	• Relatively low PTH • Ca^{++} load, vitamin D metabolites • Uremic toxins • Altered cytokines/growth factors	• Low bone formation and resorption rate • Decreased osteoid deposition	• Most common type • Increased fracture risk (?) • Extraosseus calcifications
II osteomalacia	• Aluminium • Unknown factors	• Accumulation of osteoid • Inhibition of the mineralization process	• Incidence decreased with adequate dialysate purification and withdrawal of aluminium cont. phosphate binders
Mixed disease	• Hyperparathyroidism • Aluminium • Unknown factors	• Increased remodeling, resorption, and osteoid • Areas of low bone formation	

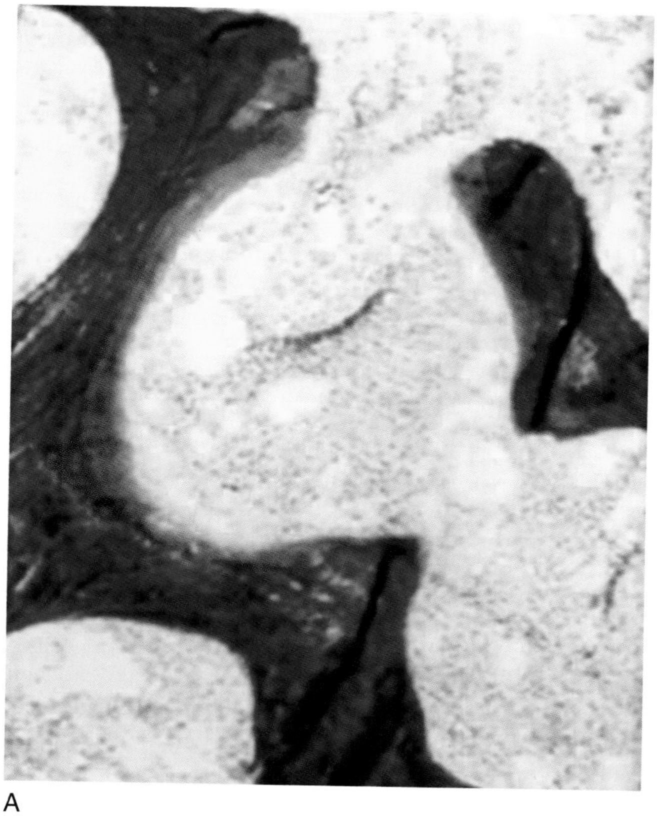

A

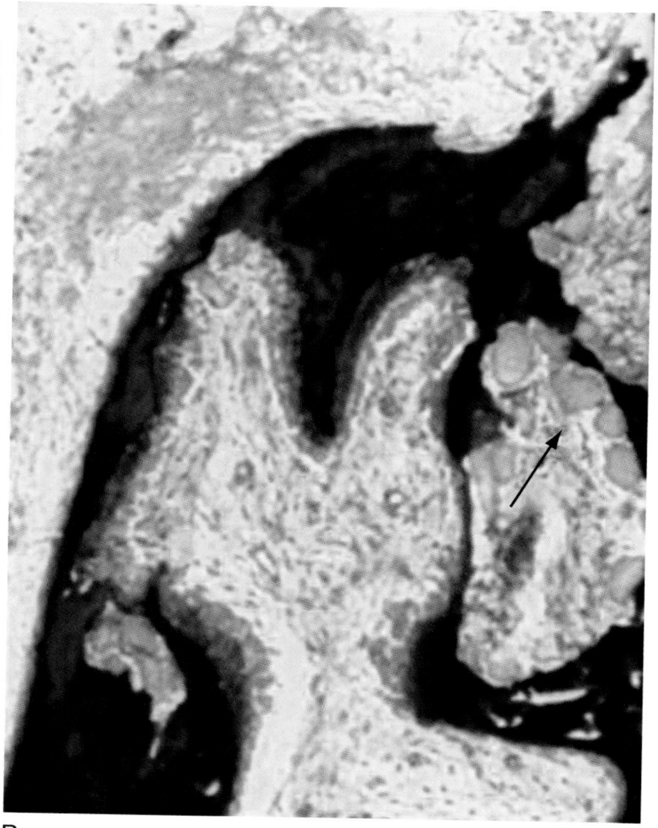

B

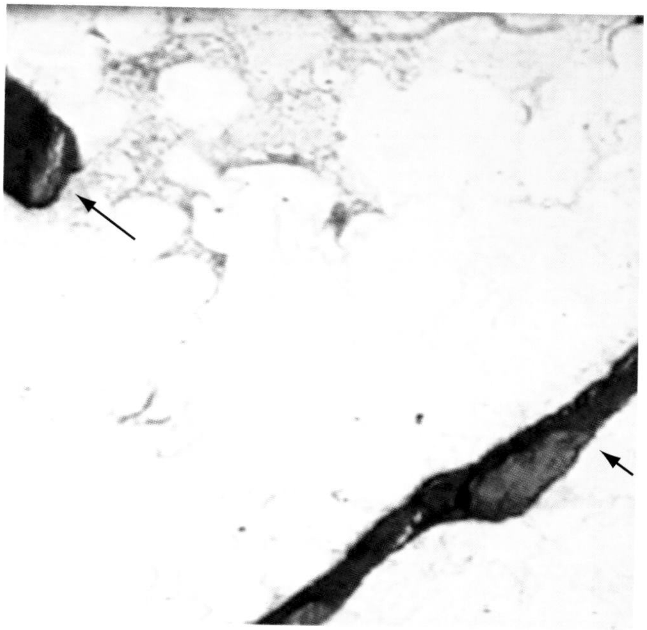

C

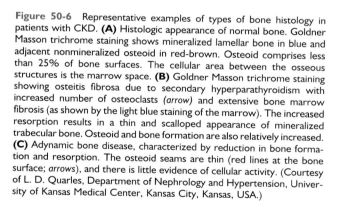

Figure 50-6 Representative examples of types of bone histology in patients with CKD. **(A)** Histologic appearance of normal bone. Goldner Masson trichrome staining shows mineralized lamellar bone in blue and adjacent nonmineralized osteoid in red-brown. Osteoid comprises less than 25% of bone surfaces. The cellular area between the osseous structures is the marrow space. **(B)** Goldner Masson trichrome staining showing osteitis fibrosa due to secondary hyperparathyroidism with increased number of osteoclasts *(arrow)* and extensive bone marrow fibrosis (as shown by the light blue staining of the marrow). The increased resorption results in a thin and scalloped appearance of mineralized trabecular bone. Osteoid and bone formation are also relatively increased. **(C)** Adynamic bone disease, characterized by reduction in bone formation and resorption. The osteoid seams are thin (red lines at the bone surface; *arrows*), and there is little evidence of cellular activity. (Courtesy of L. D. Quarles, Department of Nephrology and Hypertension, University of Kansas Medical Center, Kansas City, Kansas, USA.)

BONE MINERAL ACCRETION AND PEAK BONE MASS

Bone mass is genetically determined,[42] but exogenous factors also play a major role. Bone mass markedly increases during childhood, reaching a peak when final height is reached. Skeletal calcium increases from 25 g in newborns to 900 and 1200 g in adult females and males, respectively. Increased $1,25(OH)_2D_3$ levels coincide with an increased rate of skeletal calcium accumulation during puberty.[43]

In healthy adolescents, approximately 25% of total skeletal mass is laid down during the 2-year interval of peak height velocity. It has been hypothesized that an optimal bone mass accretion in childhood and adolescence is crucial in buffering bone loss in later life. It may also prevent fractures.[44] This concept must be doubted today. First, the calcium content per bone volume does not change with age.[45] Second, radiologic determinations of bone mineral density (BMD) are not a measure of bone strength.

Third, bone mass depends on bone and body size, bone geometry, and muscle strength. Thus, taller persons have higher bone mass but not necessarily higher bone strength than shorter persons. Moreover, a high skeletal mass and bone strength obtained by athletic training will decrease with decreasing sporting activity.[46] The focus of bone researchers has shifted away from bone mass to bone geometry or bone strength. Both are altered in children with uremic bone disease, depending on the degree of hyperparathyroidism, disturbed vitamin D metabolism, and therapeutic counteractions taken to control the disease.

CLINICAL MANIFESTATIONS

Symptoms of renal osteodystrophy can develop early, especially in children with congenital CKD. Initial signs are often vague and specific and may not come to the attention of caregivers. Young infants, in particular, require meticulous monitoring because their high growth velocity and enhanced pressure load to joints with increasing mobility can rapidly lead to severe deformations.

Bone Pain

Bone pain is a common manifestation in children with CKD. Initial symptoms may be difficult to distinguish from other causes of pain, but they become more specific with progressive disease and localize to the weight-bearing joints (e.g., knees, ankles, and hips). Because symptoms vary considerably among individual patients, they do not allow for conclusions regarding the type and severity of an underlying bone disease. Limping, bone deformities, and axial displacement require a prompt and thorough diagnostic process including biochemical and radiographic studies.

Myopathy

Patients with severe bone disease may also show muscular symptoms such as muscular weakness and wasting, exercise limitation, and waddling gait. The pathogenesis seems to be complex. One major cause of such symptoms is vitamin D deficiency.[47] Inefficient clearance of uremic toxins, insulin resistance, carnitine deficiency,[48] malnutrition, and anemia[49] also contribute. Recent studies indicate an abnormal oxygen conductance from the muscular microcirculation to the normally functioning mitochondria.[50] Myopathy may further deteriorate bone strength.[46]

Skeletal Deformities

Bone deformities include bowing of the weight-bearing bones, with genua valga being most frequent. Genua vara, coxa vara, ulnar deviation, and ankle deformations may also be seen—whereas avascular necrosis rarely occurs unless glucocorticoids are given. In infants, skeletal abnormalities often resemble vitamin-D–deficient rickets. Widening of the metaphyseal regions may develop in all long bones. The degree is dependent on the severity of metabolic bone disease and on metaphyseal growth, which vary with age.

Particular attention has to be paid to deformations in small children, when they start to put weight on their limbs, to scramble and finally walk around. Physical examination should always include a detailed bone status, followed in case of suspicious findings by radiologic studies. To prevent and treat skeletal deformities, tight control of secondary hyperparathyroidism, correction of vitamin D deficiency, and maintenance of mineral salt and acid–base homeostasis is mandatory. Unfortunately, corrective orthopedic procedures are still required in up to 25% of children. It should be kept in mind, however, that deformities acquired in early life may be completely corrected in the course of the growth process.[51]

Slipped Epiphyses

Pronounced secondary hyperparathyroidism, hypocalcemia, and severe osteitis fibrosa promote the disintegration of the growth plate and increase the risk of epiphysiolysis. Fibrotic alterations develop in the region connecting the epiphysis and the metaphysis. The growth cartilage columns are disorganized and are partly substituted by fibrous tissue predisposed to local displacement with shear stress. Slipped epiphyses are more common in children with severe hyperparathyroidism, especially when insufficiently controlled for an extended period.[51]

The most frequent localization is the proximal femur, followed by the distal radius, ulna, distal femur, humerus, tibia, and fibula—often depending on the mechanical stress put on the joints. Virtually any epiphysis may be involved (Figures 50-7 and 50-8). Because epiphyseal slipping is a potentially severe and eventually incapacitating complication resulting in osteonecrosis, severe deformities, and degenerative joint disease, one should always be aware of the characteristic clinical symptoms. These include pain, limping, waddling gait, inability to walk, and limited range of motion. In infants, deformities may develop within a few weeks. Diagnosis is established by radiography. Treatment includes correction of factors involved in the metabolic bone disease, in particular control of secondary hyperparathyroidism, reduced weight bearing, and conservative orthopedic measures. If these measures are not successful, surgical intervention for stabilization may be required. Surgery should only be performed after control of secondary hyperparathyroidism has been achieved,

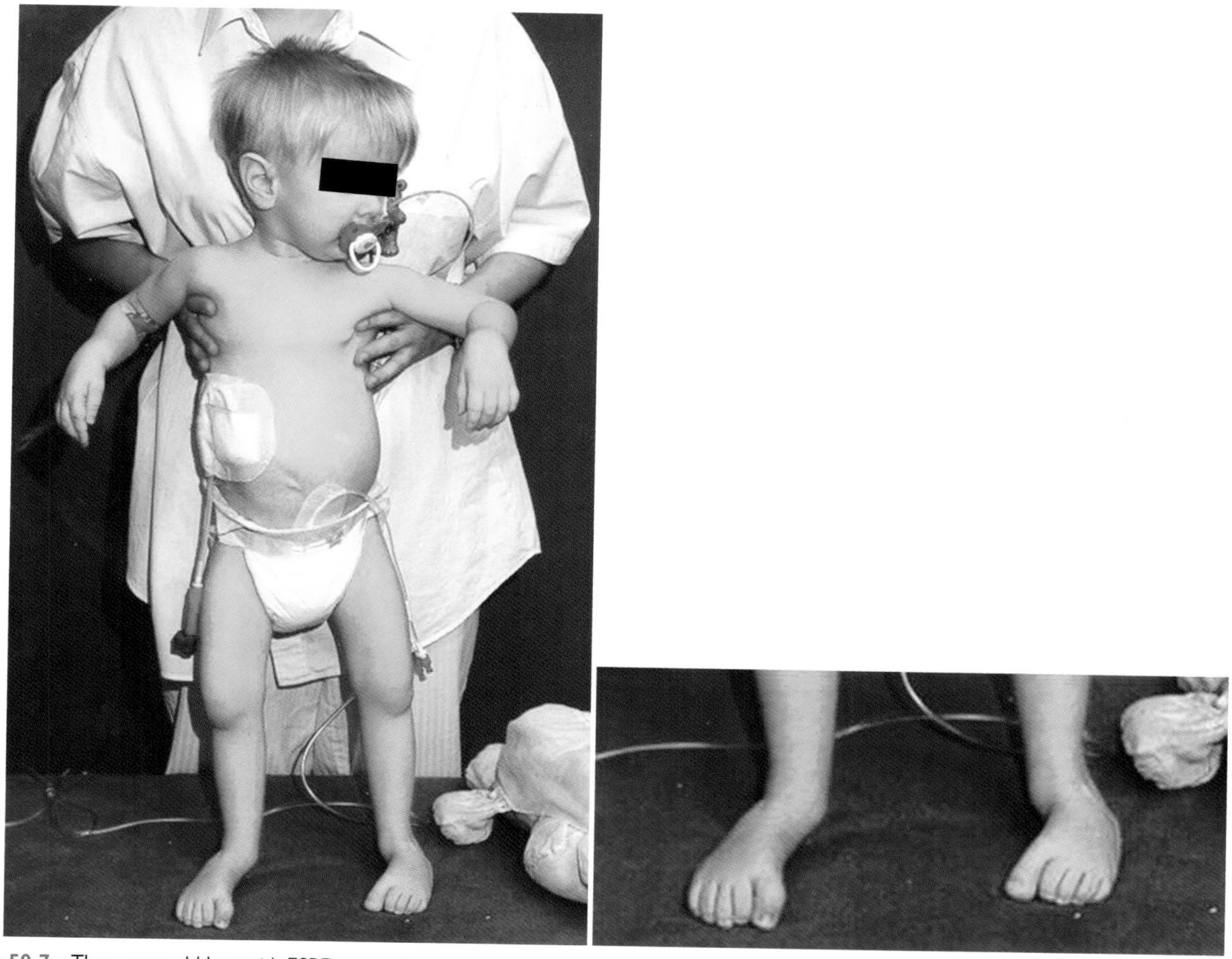

Figure 50-7 Three-year-old boy with ESRD at age 1 year due to prune belly syndrome. He rapidly developed severe renal osteodystrophy with epiphyseal slipping of multiple joints after nonadherence to calcitriol therapy.

if necessary by parathyroidectomy. Even though prospective studies are missing, a failure of orthopedic corrective measures has been documented in patients with uncontrolled high-turnover bone disease.

Fractures

Healthy children have an incidence of 14 fractures per 1000 person years. These are mainly localized to the limbs.[52] In CKD children, fracture risk is increased—although precise data on the fracture incidence have not been reported. Hyperparathyroidism and reduced plasma $1,25(OH)_2D_3$ levels result in high bone turnover, which compromises bone dimension and bone strength. Bone deformities, slipped epiphyses, and microfractures are more common than complete bone fractures.

Whereas microfractures may be rapidly repaired by high bone turnover, macrofractures might result from exceptionally low bone turnover. However, this concept has not consistently been proven.[53] The fracture risk of adult dialysis patients is increased severalfold,[54] which has been correlated with plasma iPTH in a U-shaped manner—with the lowest risk observed at average PTH levels of about 300 pg/ml.[55] After pediatric renal transplantation, the incidence of fractures is increased to 76 fractures per 1000 patient-years, two thirds of which are located at the vertebra.[52]

Growth Retardation

Growth failure, a regular feature of children with CKD, is mainly due to endogenous growth hormone and IGF1 resistance, malnutrition (especially in infants), and metabolic acidosis. The effects of altered vitamin D and PTH metabolism on growth are not entirely clear.

In animal studies, vitamin D deficiency and low levels of $1,25(OH)_2D_3$ result in a reduced growth rate—which can be improved by substitution.[56] In children with CKD, a short-term improvement of growth rate has been reported with $1,25(OH)_2\text{-}D_3$ treatment. However, this was not confirmed in long-term observations.[57,58] Excessive vitamin D treatment may even result in adynamic bone disease and growth retardation.[59] In vitro, calcitropic and somatotropic hormones interact with the proliferation of growth plate chondrocytes.[60,61] PTH-rP, which acts via the type I PTH receptor, is an important local inhibitor of growth plate chondrocyte

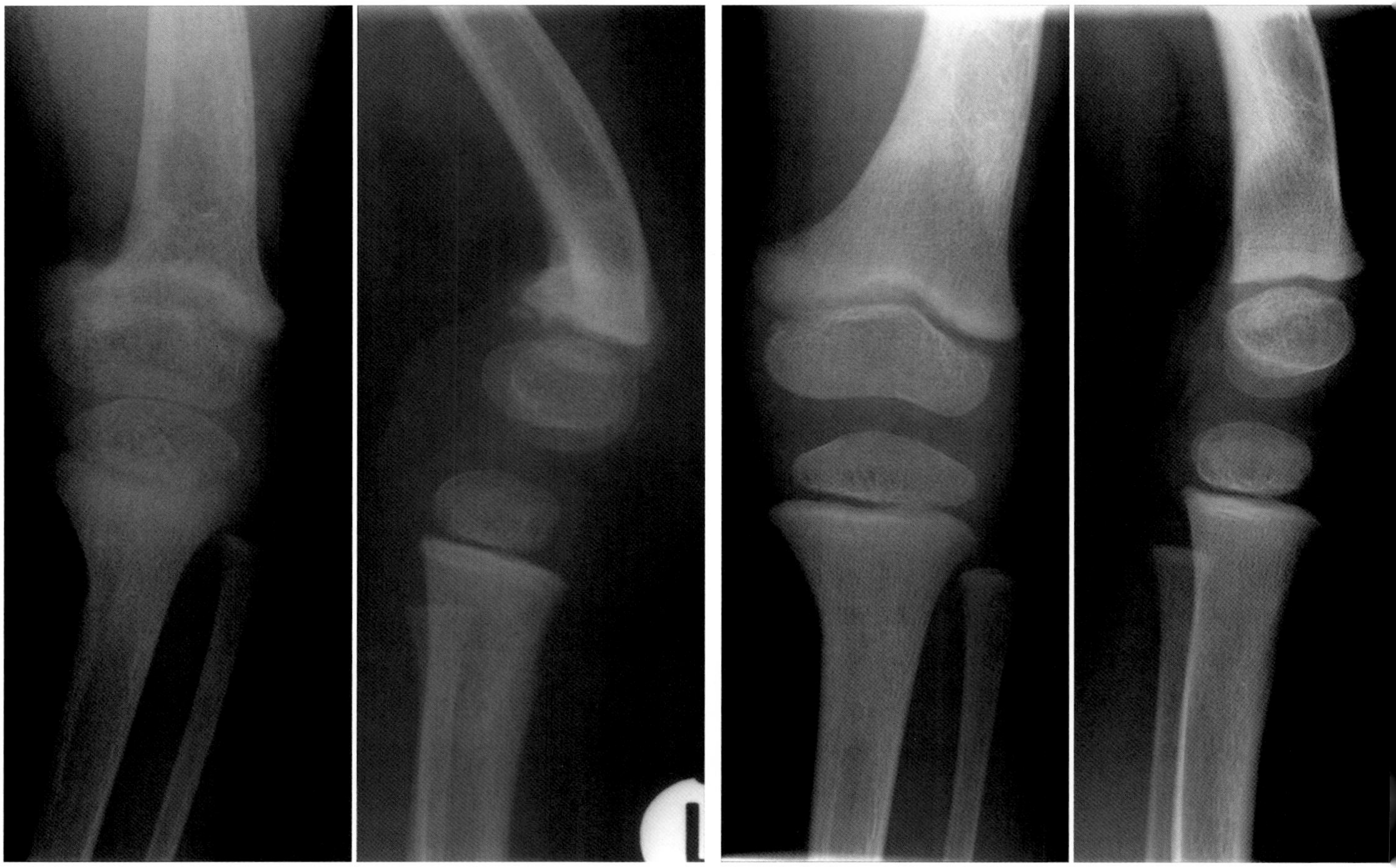

Figure 50-8 X-rays of the left knee of the same boy shown in Figure 50-7. **(A)** Prior to therapy. **(B)** After one year of treatment with calcitriol and calcium i.v. and i.p. and parathyroidectomy with autotransplantation of parathyroid tissue. The severe deformities have substantially improved. Surgical intervention was not required.

maturation.[62] In rats, intermittent bolus injection of PTH increases growth rate—whereas this is not seen with continuous PTH infusion.[63]

From clinical observation, it is not clear which PTH levels are optimal for growth. A positive correlation between mean plasma PTH levels and growth has been observed in two studies, suggesting that higher PTH levels promote growth.[59,64] Others reported a normal growth rate in children with CKD stages II through IV, with PTH levels in the normal range. A normal growth rate was also observed in children with CKD stage V, with mean plasma PTH concentrations only 50% above the upper limit of normal. In these children, particular attention was paid to adequate nutritional support and a strict control of serum phosphate levels within the normal range. Whether normal bone turnover is maintained with this strategy is unclear because bone biopsies were not performed.[65,66] With intensified daily dialysis, serum phosphate can be normalized and PTH maintained slightly above the upper-normal level. In addition, catch-up growth is observed with this treatment.[67]

Cardiovascular Calcifications

Cardiovascular mortality is dramatically increased in uremic patients. Excessive vascular calcification is one of the main mechanisms underlying this most important limitation to renal replacement therapy. More than 90% of young adults with childhood onset of CKD already have significant coronary artery calcifications. Alterations of the morphologic and functional properties of arteries can already be observed as early as in the second decade of life.[68]

There is a strong correlation between abnormalities of bone and mineral metabolism and the development of vascular calcifications. Vascular calcifications are directly related to hyperphosphatemia, the average calcium/phosphate product over time, intake of calcium-containing phosphate binders, and plasma PTH levels.[69,70] In a postmortem analysis of 120 children with CKD, soft-tissue and vascular calcifications were associated with the use of active vitamin D and calcium-containing phosphate binders.[71]

Calcium load is often high in children with advanced CKD treated with active vitamin D and calcium-containing phos-

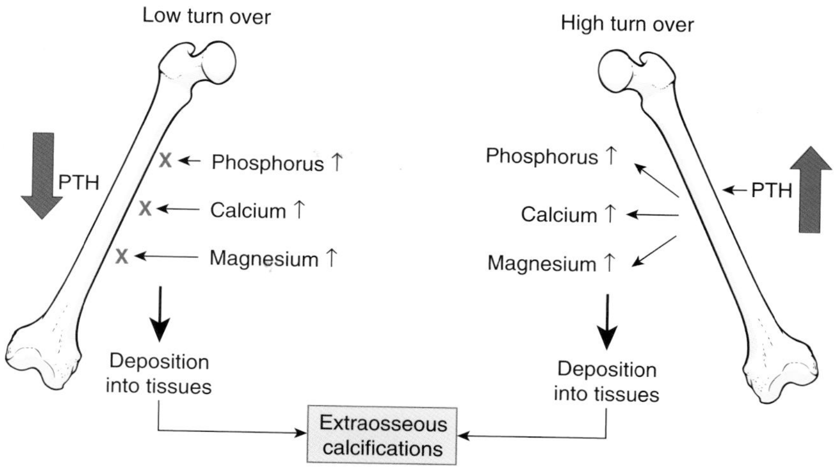

Figure 50-9 Bone disease and soft-tissue calcification. Low PTH levels (low-turnover bone disease) prevent mineral deposition into bone. High PTH levels result in mineral release from bone. Excessive minerals precipitate in soft tissues.

phate binders. In addition, dialysis solutions usually contain unphysiologically high calcium levels. On the other hand, the calcium-buffering capacity of bone is reduced in patients with low-turnover and high-turnover bone disease (Figure 50-9). Of note, calcifications are not merely a passive process of precipitation. They are triggered by oxidative stress and advanced glycation end products and are regulated by locally and systemically acting proteins. The plasma protein fetuin is significantly reduced in CKD patients and correlates with cardiovascular mortality.[72]

Calcifications may also occur in sites other than the vascular wall, such as the lung and periarticular areas. Calciphylaxis, a severe form of extraskeletal calcifications, has been described in children with tertiary hyperparathyroidism.[73] It is characterized by painful nodules that become mottled or violaceous, indurated, and ultimately ulcerated. Accurate diagnosis and optimal treatment of disturbance in bone and mineral metabolism may be crucial in preventing these life-limiting sequelae in children with CKD.

Posttransplant Bone Disease

Successful renal transplantation should reverse all pathologic conditions that result in metabolic bone disease. However, immunosuppressive treatment (in particular, glucocorticoids) interferes with bone metabolism. In addition, any degree of CKD may develop in the posttransplant course. Persistent hypophosphatemia is a common finding in renal allograft recipients, especially within the first months postsurgery. Precise pediatric data have not yet been reported. Tubular dysfunction secondary to any toxicity, persistent HPT, and increased plasma FGF-23 levels are considered the main causes of exaggerated renal phosphate secretion after transplantation.

Of note, plasma phosphate levels can be normal despite reduced total body phosphate content. In these patients, increased skeletal phosphate removal due to increased PTH and inappropriately low calcitriol levels may counterbalance the phosphatonin (FGF-23)-induced persistent renal phosphate loss.[74,75] In children undergoing successful transplantation, skeletal lesions improve but do not resolve completely in the majority.[76] Assessment of BMD by means of dual-energy x-ray absorptiometry (DEXA) shows conflicting results, possibly due to inadequate standardization and a failure to correct for height and muscular mass. Recent peripheral quantitative computer tomography (pQCT) results demonstrate nearly normal BMD for height and muscle mass, whereas cortical thickness is reduced.[77]

The fracture risk is increased after renal transplantation.[52] Avascular necrosis is reported to develop in 4% of children after organ transplantation, most often in the femoral head. However, it may also develop in the talus, the humeral neck, and other skeletal sites.[78] Avascular necrosis has become less common in recent years, due to steroid sparing with newer immunosuppressive protocols.

ASSESSMENT OF RENAL BONE DISEASE

Apart from thorough physical examination, the diagnosis of the uremic bone mineral metabolic disorder is mainly based on repeated biochemical and radiographic analyses (Table 50-2). Bone biopsies are rarely needed for the clinical management of patients.

Biochemistry

Serum Calcium

Measurement of total calcium is the most common method of assessing serum calcium levels. However, normal total serum calcium may not indicate normal serum ionized calcium levels and should be corrected for serum albumin concentration if this is low. Serum calcium is usually normal or low in untreated patients with advanced CKD, with the maintenance of calcium homeostasis being exerted mainly by a compensatory increase in PTH. Once treatment with active vitamin D and calcium-containing phosphate binders is initiated, serum calcium levels increase and PTH declines.

Hypercalcemia is still rare in calcitriol-treated children with stage IV CKD,[64] but is seen in about 6% of measurements in children on peritoneal dialysis treated with calcitriol, calcium-containing phosphate binders, and peritoneal dialysis (PD) solutions with ionized calcium concentrations of 1.75 mmol/L.[79] Children with low-turnover bone disease and children with tertiary hyperparathyroidism treated with

TABLE 50-2 **Guidelines for the Frequency of Measurements for Biochemical and Radiologic Markers of Renal Osteodystrophy***

CKD Stage	GFR (ml/min × 1.73 m²)	Calcium/Ca^{++}, Serum Bicarbonate, Phosphate, AP, PTH	Serum 25(OH)$_2$D$_3$	Left Hand and Wrist X-Ray
2	60-89	At least annually	At least annually	
3	30-59	At least every 6 months	At least annually	In the case of abnormal biochemical findings
4	15-29	At least every 3 months	At least annually	In the case of abnormal biochemical findings
5	<15, dialysis	At least monthly	At least annually	Every 6-12 months

* More frequent measurements may be required in young children, in patients treated with severe renal osteodystrophy, noncompliant patients, and after renal transplantation.
Sources: Adapted from NKF K/DOQI: Clinical practice guidelines for bone metabolism and disease in children with chronic kidney disease, *Am J Kidney Dis* 46(1):S1-S100, 2005; and Klaus G, Watson A, Edefonti A, Fischbach M, Rönnholm K, Schaefer F, et al: European Pediatric Dialysis Working Group (EPDWG). Prevention and treatment of renal osteodystrophy in children on chronic renal failure: European guidelines, *Pediatr Nephrol* 21(2):151-59, 2006.

calcitriol are particularly prone to hypercalcemia because the calcium-buffering capacity of bone is reduced. An important differential diagnosis of hypercalcemia in children on dialysis is volume depletion. This condition is usually characterized by a high total but normal ionized calcium concentration. Alternative causes of hypercalcemia to consider include immobilization and, rarely, paraneoplastic release of PTHrP and extrarenal calcitriol production in granulomatous diseases such as tuberculosis and sarcoidosis.

Serum Phosphate

Dietary phosphate intake usually exceeds renal phosphate removal if GFR drops below 40 ml/min/1.73 m², but hyperphosphatemia may be noted earlier if phosphate intake is high. The serum concentration of phosphate should be kept in the normal range. Of note, renal phosphate threshold[80] and serum phosphate concentrations are age dependent—with an upper limit of normal of 2.4 mmol/L in small infants, 2.1 and 1.9 in preschool and school children, and 1.44 to 1.9 mmol/L in adolescents (according to various reference tables).[81,82]

The physiologic range depends on whether a child is growing or is postpubertal. In nonfasting adolescents, serum phosphate is subject to significant circadian variations that follow an M-shaped curve—with peaks at 4 P.M. and 3:30 A.M. and a maximal diurnal amplitude of 1 mmol/L.[83] However, these fluctuations largely disappear with advancing CKD and are not related to food intake in ESRD patients.[84]

Parathyroid Hormone

Plasma PTH levels are a key element in the diagnosis and therapeutic monitoring of renal osteodystrophy. These levels should be measured together with calcium, phosphate, alkaline phosphatase, and blood bicarbonate at least every 6 months when GFR drops below 60, every 3 months at a GFR below 30 ml/min * 1.73 m², and every month when ESRD is reached (Tables 50-2 and 50-3).

PTH measurements, however, have significant limitations. Early assays cross-reacted with C-terminal PTH fragments, which accumulate in CKD, of different and largely unknown function. To circumvent this problem, two-site immunoassays for detecting "intact" iPTH were developed. The first generation of these assays recognizes an epitope between residues 7 and 34, thus still cross-reacting with PTH fragments lacking portions of the *N*-terminus (e.g., 7-84 PTH).[85] 7-84 PTH is secreted by the parathyroid glands and counteracts biologic actions of 1-84 PTH. Accumulation occurs in renal failure with great interindividual variability (Figure 50-10). Accordingly, the predictability of the underlying histologic type of bone disease based on repeated iPTH measurements using a first-generation PTH assay is weak. In children with CKD stage V, values of iPTH below 200 pg/ml suggest adynamic bone disease and values above 500 pg/ml suggest osteitis fibrosa. However, considerable overlap exists.[3,86]

Second-generation PTH assays using an antibody binding to the *N*-terminus measure whole 1-84 PTH more specifically.[87] The difference of PTH levels as measured by first- and second-generation assays is used to estimate the plasma concentration of *N*-terminally truncated fragments. Given the paucity of clinical studies correlating plasma PTH concentrations to bone histology, it may still be premature to generally

TABLE 50-3 **Target iPTH Range in Children with CKD 2 to 5***

CKD Stage	GFR (ml/min × 1.73 m²)	Target iPTH Range
2	60-89	35-70 pg/ml
3	30-59	35-70 pg/ml
4	15-29	70-110 pg/ml
5	<15, dialysis	200-300 pg/ml

* Recommendations for CKD stage 2-4 are opinion based; stage 5 recommendations are evidence based. Second-generation PTH assays provide values which are only 50%-60% values obtained with iPTH assays; this however may vary considerably.
Sources: Adapted from NKF K/DOQI: Clinical practice guidelines for bone metabolism and disease in children with chronic kidney disease, *Am J Kidney Dis* 46(1):S1-S100, 2005; and Klaus G, Watson A, Edefonti A, Fischbach M, Rönnholm K, Schaefer F, et al: European Pediatric Dialysis Working Group (EPDWG). Prevention and treatment of renal osteodystrophy in children on chronic renal failure: European guidelines, *Pediatr Nephrol* 21(2):151-59, 2006.

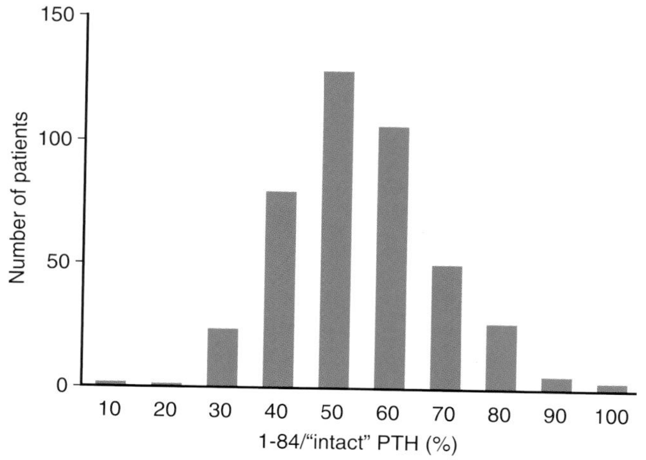

Figure 50-10 Relative amount of 1-84 PTH in relation to "intact" PTH in patients with ESRD. First-generation intact PTH assays measure both 1-84 PTH and a C-terminal fragment, presumably 7-84 PTH. 7-84 PTH antagonizes 1-84 PTH effects. (Adapted from Gao P, Scheibel S, D'Amour P, John MR, Rao SD, Schmidt-Gayk H, et al: Development of a novel immunoradiometric assay exclusively for biologically active whole parathyroid hormone 1-84: Implications for improvement of accurate assessment of parathyroid function, *Bone Miner Res* 16(4):605-14, 2001.)

recommend second-generation PTH assays to distinguish different types of bone disease and to ascribe a role for *N*-terminally truncated peptides such as 7-84 PTH in the pathogenesis of renal osteodystrophy. Notably, a correlation of the various PTH peptides with longitudinal growth could not be demonstrated in children with CKD.[65] A weak correlation of the 1.84 PTH to C-terminal fragment ratio was observed.

Alkaline Phosphatase

Measurements of serum total alkaline phosphatase (AP), a marker of osteoblast activity, can be helpful in predicting bone turnover in conjunction with PTH.[88] Values are strongly age dependent, with higher activity present during periods of rapid growth. Bone-specific alkaline phosphatase may further increase predictability of bone turnover and may be advantageous in subgroups of patients (e.g., those with hepatic diseases) to exclude measurement of nonskeletal enzyme. The potential benefits have to be weighed against the considerably higher costs.

$25(OH)_2D_3$ and $1,25(OH)_2D_3$

Serum levels of $25(OH)_2D_3$ provide an estimate of vitamin D body stores. These levels should be greater than 30 to 40 ng/ml. The upper range of normal in healthy children is 70 ng/ml, but this has not been validated for patients with CKD. Low levels indicate vitamin D deficiency, whereas normal levels during $25(OH)_2D_3$ therapy do not necessarily reflect repleted vitamin D stores. Because $25(OH)_2D_3$ has a variety of physiologic functions, vitamin D deficiency must be avoided at all stages of CKD.

$25(OH)_2D_3$ serum levels should be measured if serum PTH increases above the target range, and according to current opinion-based recommendations should be measured annually in patients with $25(OH)_2D_3$ in the target range[81] (Table 50-2). However, considering the increasing evidence of a high incidence of vitamin D deficiency and substantial beneficial effects of $25(OH)_2D_3$ in CKD more frequent determinations may be justified. The serum half-life of $25(OH)_2D_3$ is 3 weeks.[89] We routinely measure $25(OH)_2D_3$ twice a year in CKD stage V, and more frequently when higher doses are given to replete stores.

Determinations of plasma $1,25(OH)_2D_3$ concentration are expensive, and the information obtained is limited. $1,25(OH)_2D_3$ plasma concentrations have not yet been correlated with the incidence of hypercalcemia or vascular calcifications in CKD patients. Plasma measurements may occasionally be helpful to demonstrate or rule out nonadherence to calcitriol treatment. Oral $1,25(OH)_2D_3$ is rapidly absorbed, and peak plasma levels are reached within 3 hours in children with CKD.[90]

Additional Serum Markers of Bone Turnover

Biomarkers of bone formation (e.g., osteocalcin and procollagen type I carboxyl terminal peptides) and of bone resorption (e.g., type I collagen cross-linked telopeptide and pyridinoline) have not been studied widely to date in children with CKD. Most of them are eliminated via the kidney and accumulate with reduced renal function. Tartrate-resistant acid phosphatase (TRAP)-5b and osteoprotegerin may prove useful indicators of bone metabolism based on the central role of receptor activator of nuclear factor κB (RANK) ligand and osteoprotegerin in bone metabolism.[91] Further studies correlating the circulating levels of these potential biomarkers to bone histology, growth, and established biochemical markers will be required to determine their usefulness in the monitoring of uremic bone disease.

Aluminium

The use of aluminium-containing phosphate binders is not recommended in children. In addition, dialysis water purification has generally improved. Therefore, aluminium-related bone disease and encephalopathy should not develop under these conditions—eliminating the need to determine plasma aluminium levels on a regular basis. Exposure to aluminium, however, may still occur in some countries.[92] In such cases, plasma aluminium levels need to be monitored.

Imaging

Radiography of the Skeleton

Although radiographs of the skeleton are relatively insensitive in detecting renal bone disease, hand and wrist x-rays are routinely performed to screen for clinically important signs of bone disease and to estimate skeletal maturation. In children with CKD stages III and IV, a hand x-ray should be performed when clinical or biochemical findings suggest bone disease. In CKD stage V, radiographies should be repeated at least every 12 months. In children with severe hyperparathyroidism, more frequent x-rays of the skeleton (including sites other than the hand) may be required.

Severe hyperparathyroidism induces hyperosteoclasia and osteitis fibrosa, which can be radiologically detected as subperiostal resorption zones (Figure 50-11). Subperiostal erosions of the phalanges may be the most sensitive sign of secondary hyperparathyroidism, correlating with serum PTH

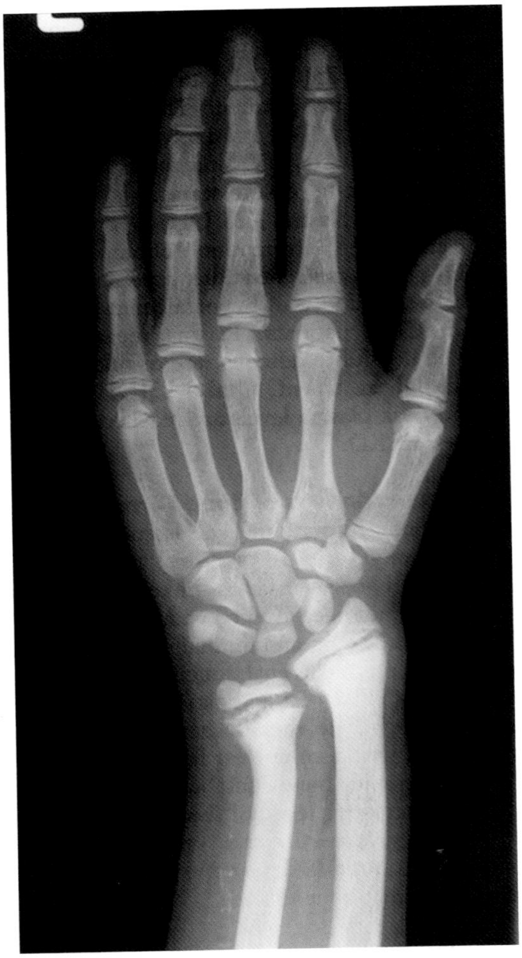

Figure 50-11 X-ray of left hand of 16-year-old boy with signs of severe renal bone disease: subperiostal erosions (especially of the middle phalanges), brown tumor in the second digit, "ricket-like" lesions, and vascular calcifications at the forearm. (Courtesy of J. Troeger, University Hospital for Paediatric and Adolescent Medicine, Heidelberg, Germany.)

levels.[93] They have also been seen as acroosteolyses at the end phalanges and at sites of ligament endings such as clavicles, ischium, pubes, femoral heads, and the inner side of upper tibia diaphysis.

In the skull, hyperparathyroidism results in a ground-glass or granular appearance, focal radiolucencies, and sclerotic areas. In children with CKD, widened radiolucent areas of the growth zones also indicate accumulation of fibrous tissue—in contrast to nutritional rickets, in which the radiolucent areas are mainly due to accumulation of unmineralized growth cartilage. Brown tumors also present with an accumulation of hyperosteoclastic tissue. They are typically seen at the metaphyses of long bones, but are found at other skeletal sites such as the jaw.[94]

In contrast to signs in hyperosteoclastic patients, there are no specific signs of osteomalacia. In renal patients, widened growth zones and deformities are more likely induced by lesions of high bone turnover than by osteomalacia. Even Looser zones (straight, wide radiolucent bands within the cortex) can represent (in addition to fibrous tissue) osteomalacic lesions. In patients with low growth rates, radiologic signs of metabolic bone disease are less pronounced. Signs may become apparent during periods of increased growth, for example, during growth hormone treatment.

Measurements of Bone Mineral Density

Measurements of BMD are not routinely used in the monitoring of CKD-associated bone disease, but must still be considered investigational. Prospective interventional studies are lacking, and problems in interpreting results are common. DEXA is the most widely used method of measuring bone mineral content and BMD. BMD (g/cm^2) is often falsely taken as a surrogate parameter of bone strength and fracture risk.

BMD increases physiologically in childhood with age, but is more closely correlated with measures of body size (such as height and weight). As a consequence, measurements must not be normalized to age but to body height, bone size, or muscle function.[46] The interpretation of DEXA measurements is further complicated by the lack of a distinction made between cortical and cancellous bone.

pQCT is an alternative technology that permits resolution of cancellous and cortical bone. In children with renal osteodystrophy, pQCT revealed slightly reduced cortical bone density. This novel technique also holds some promise in unmasking differences in total bone density between patients with high-turnover and adynamic bone disease.[95]

Bone Biopsy

Micromorphometric analysis of the bone is the gold standard for characterization and quantification of renal bone disease. The biopsy procedure is safe and is well tolerated by most children. It provides information on the current histologic status, and, if double tetracycline staining is performed, on the dynamics of bone formation and mineralization. Bone biopsies are not needed for the routine diagnosis and treatment of renal osteodystrophy. There are only a few clinical situations in which bone biopsy may be considered, such as in the decision making for parathyroidectomy and to diagnose aluminium osteopathy. Bone biopsies also retain a role in clinical trials for which the effects of therapeutic interventions require definitive verification.

Imaging of the Parathyroid Glands

In children with severe secondary hyperparathyroidism, sonography of the parathyroid glands should be performed. Parathyroid glands usually cannot be detected by ultrasound unless they are enlarged. Tc-99m methoxyisobutyl isonitrile MIBI scan and magnetic resonance imaging (MRI) may provide additional information in cases for which parathyroidectomy is considered. However, the indication of advanced imaging procedures in patients with refractory hyperparathyroidism is controversial. One justification for extensive diagnostics is the need to screen for an ectopic gland, especially prior to reexploration of unsuccessful parathyroidectomies. Preoperative imaging by ultrasound, and even by MIBI scan or MRI, may fail to detect adenomas. Therefore, a negative result should not prevent thorough surgical exploration if it is clinically indicated.

Imaging of Vascular Alterations

The intima media thickness (IMT) of the common carotid artery as assessed by high-resolution sonography is a sensitive marker of early vascular lesions. In children with CKD, carotid IMT has been correlated with the time-averaged serum calcium and P product, the cumulative dose of calcium-based phosphate binders, and the mean calcitriol dose.[68,96] In experienced hands, repetitive sonographic IMT assessments can be a valuable diagnostic tool of vasculopathy secondary to altered bone and mineral metabolism.

In cases of severely disturbed bone and mineral metabolism, plain x-rays may be performed to screen for vascular and soft-tissue calcifications (Figure 50-11). Coronary artery calcifications can be assessed quantitatively by electron-beam or echocardiogram-gated computer tomography.

TREATMENT

General Guidelines

Many of the factors contributory to the development of secondary hyperparathyroidism and renal osteodystrophy are present early in the course of renal disease. Because patients are usually asymptomatic, insufficient attention is often paid to progressive alterations in bone and mineral homeostasis. With advancing renal failure, parathyroid glands become hyperplastic and less sensitive to therapeutic interventions. Therefore, *prevention* should always be the primary objective in children with CKD—with the aim of delaying its development and its osseous and cardiovascular sequelae.

Optimal control of serum *phosphate* levels is probably the crucial element of preventive management. Hyperphosphatemia is an independent risk factor for secondary hyperparathyroidism, renal osteodystrophy, and vascular calcifications. As early as in CKD stage II, regular dietary counseling should be performed, and drug therapy may already be considered. On the other hand, hypophosphatemia (as commonly seen in children with associated tubulopathies even in CKD stages II through IV or after renal transplantation) may induce hypophosphatemic osteomalacia and should also be avoided.

Serum *calcium* should be maintained in the normal range, taking care of maintaining a normal serum calcium phosphorus ion product. The upper limit for the serum calcium × phosphorus ion product recommended in adults (55 mg^2/dl^2) is applicable to adolescents, whereas the upper-normal limit is higher in children below 12 years of age (65 mg^2/dl^2) and even higher in infants. In CKD stage V, even serum calcium levels in the upper-normal range should be avoided.[81,97] In dialyzed patients, dialysis fluids with 1.2 to 1.3 mmol/L Ca^{2+} content should be used. In the case of hypercalcemia, all calcium-containing phosphate binders must be withheld, vitamin D therapy stopped, and, if hypercalcemia persists, low-calcium dialysis fluid administered.

The sensitivity of the skeleton to PTH effects decreases with declining renal function. Therefore, an increasing PTH target level has been suggested. These target levels are outlined in Table 50-3. For CKD stages II through IV, target PTH recommendations only reflect expert opinion. For patients with CKD stage V, there is some biopsy-derived evidence for the indicated target ranges. However, these data have been challenged by recent studies.[65,66] If plasma PTH levels are below the target range and serum calcium levels are increased, vitamin D therapy and calcium-containing phosphate binders should be reduced or even discontinued. In addition, a reduction in dialysate calcium concentration may be justified. A scheme summarizing the treatment in patients with established hyperparathyroidism is shown in Figure 50-12. Of note, growth hormone should not be given to patients with uncontrolled hyperparathyroidism, symptomatic high-turnover bone disease, or slipped epiphysis.

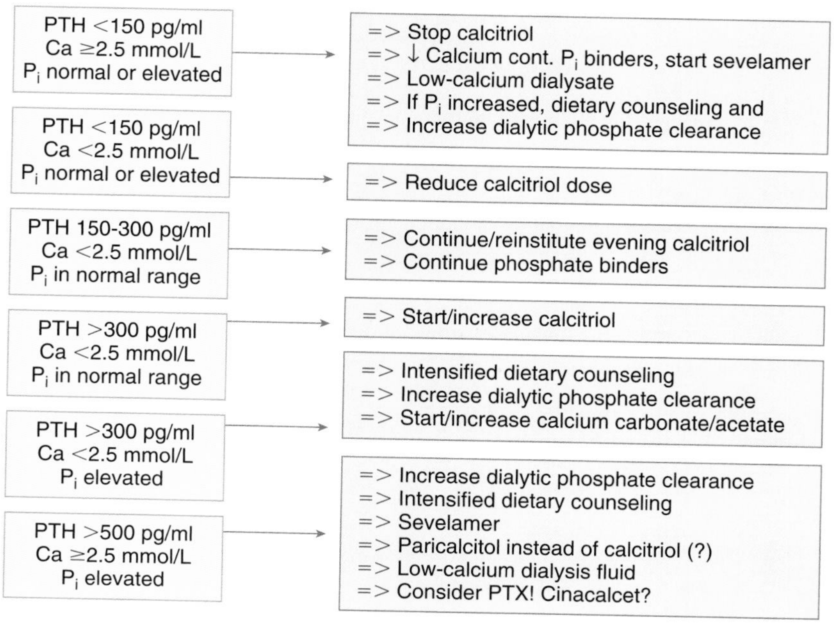

Figure 50-12 Therapeutic algorithm for secondary hyperparathyroidism.

Diet

For detailed dietary recommendations regarding dietary calcium and phosphorus intake, see Chapter 48.

Dialysis

The efficacy of dialysis in removing excess phosphate is limited (e.g., an anuric child of 20 kg body weight and a daily protein intake of 1.4 g/kg ingests 430 mg phosphate per day). Concomitant intake of calcitriol and phosphate binders will result in absorption of roughly 50% of phosphate (215 mg/d). This amount of phosphate is the maximum that can be eliminated by conventional dialysis. At a protein intake of 2 g/kg * d, the phosphate balance will be positive by more than 60 mg per day on a conventional PD or hemodialysis schedule. A weekly creatinine clearance of more than 80 L/1.73m² would be required to compensate for the dietary phosphate load. This efficacy can only be achieved by frequent[98] or long nocturnal hemodialysis.[99] Slow-flow nocturnal hemodialysis performed over 6 to 9 hours per night five to six times per week dramatically improves phosphate clearance and may even require phosphate supplementation per as or in the dialysis bath to prevent phosphate depletion and aggravation of bone disease.[100] If such intensified hemodialysis is not available or not feasible, repeated dietary counseling and optimized oral phosphate binder management are essential (see material following). In children receiving automated PD, total PD fluid turnover should be maximized using maximally tolerable fill volumes, maximally acceptable cycler times, and additional daytime exchanges.

Phosphate Binders

Restriction of phosphorus intake may be sufficient in early stages of CKD. However, normophosphatemia may only be maintained at the expense of increased PTH and FGF-23 plasma levels—both of which decrease tubular phosphate reabsorption. As renal function deteriorates, dietary control of phosphate becomes more difficult and overt hyperphosphatemia usually develops. Oral phosphate binding agents must be added.

Calcium salts are used as first-line phosphate binders. They have limited phosphate binding capacity (Figure 50-13). The dose required depends on the oral phosphorus intake, and often reaches several grams per day. Although in hypocalcemic and rapidly growing children the additional calcium load still is beneficial, most patients tend to develop hypercalcemia with prolonged administration. Significantly more calcium is absorbed and little phosphorus retained when calcium-containing phosphate binders are not given with meals.[101]

Twenty-five percent of calcium acetate consists of elemental calcium, whereas 40% of calcium carbonate consists of elemental calcium. Calcium acetate binds more phosphorus per unit of calcium content and thus allows for higher doses and improved phosphate control. If given at similar doses, calcium acetate results in a reduced incidence of hypercalcemia compared to calcium carbonate (Table 50-4). On the

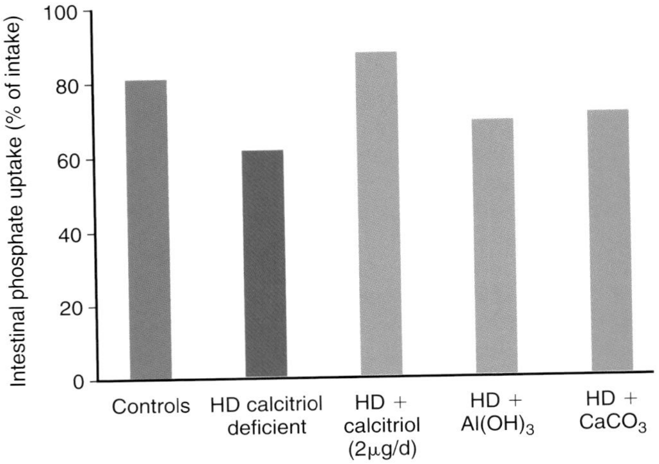

Figure 50-13 Effect of calcitriol and oral phosphate binders on intestinal phosphate uptake. Calcitriol significantly increases phosphate uptake in hemodialysis patients. $Al(OH)_3$ and $CaCO_3$, each given at a dose of 75 mEq prior to a standardized meal, reduce phosphate uptake to a similar degree. $CaCO_3$, however, increases oral calcium intake by 1.4g compared to placebo. The intestinal calcium uptake increases to 28% of the ingested amount compared to 14% with placebo. (Adapted from Ramirez JA, Emmett M, White MG, Fathi N, Santa Ana CA, Morawski SG, et al.: The absorption of dietary phosphorus and calcium in hemodialysis patients, *Kidney Int* 30(5):753-59, 1986.)

TABLE 50-4 Phosphate Binding Agents

Compound	Calcium Content (%)	Calcium Absorbed (%)	Phosphate Bound per g Compound	Phosphate Bound per Ca^{++} Absorbed	Comment
Calcium carbonate	40	20-30	39 mg/g	≈1 mg / 8 mg	High Ca^{++} load, inexpensive, GI side effects
Calcium acetate	25	22 (between meals, 40)	45 mg/g	≈1 mg / 3 mg	GI side effects, less Ca^{++} load than $CaCO_3$, inexpensive
Mg + Ca carbonate	Variable	20-30 of Ca	NA	≈1 mg / 2.3 mg	Less Ca^{++} load, GI side effects, long-term effects?
Sevelamer HCL	0	0	NA	NA	Ca^{++} and Al^{+++} free, cholesterol ↓, costs ↑, acidosis ↑
Aluminium cont. binders	0	0	Similar to calcium acetate	NA	Effective but toxic, not recommended

NA, Not applicable or no data.

other hand, fewer gastrointestinal side effects have been reported with calcium carbonate. An individual choice is required to ensure optimal patient compliance and control of calcium and phosphate uptake. Calcium citrate is also effective, but citrate increases aluminium resorption and should therefore be avoided.

Aluminium-containing phosphate binders are efficient phosphate absorbers but may result in aluminium intoxication. Their administration is not recommended in children. If their use cannot be avoided (e.g., in the case of a severely increased calcium phosphate product not manageable otherwise), dosage should be limited to 30 mg/kg * d. Aluminium-containing binders should only be given if other calcium-free alternatives (see material following) are not available, and if given should be restricted to a regimen of 4 weeks maximum. If hyperphosphatemia persists, parathyroidectomy needs to be considered.

Magnesium salts reduce the calcium load but also have less intestinal phosphate binding activity. Therefore, higher doses are required. Diarrhea, hyperkalemia, and hypermagnesemia frequently develop. The long-term effects of an increased magnesium load are not clear. An inverse relationship between serum Mg and hyperparathyroidism and vascular calcification has been demonstrated in adult dialysis patients, and thus potential benefits have been attributed to magnesium salts.[102] At present, magnesium-containing phosphate binders may be given as adjuncts to calcium-containing binders. Adjustments in dialysate magnesium concentrations may be required.[103]

Calcium-Free and Aluminium-Free Phosphate Binders

Growing evidence for a role of the oral calcium load in the progression of cardiovascular calcifications urged the development of calcium-free phosphate binders, which can be given routinely. They are especially indicated in patients with a calcium intake exceeding twice the recommended daily intake (of 210 mg/d in the first 6 months of life to 1250 mg/d in adolescents), reduced PTH levels (as adynamic bone disease is likely), hypercalcemia, or emerging soft-tissue calcifications.

Sevelamer hydrochloride is a hydrogel of polyallylamine, which is resistant to digestive degradation and therefore not absorbed. It binds dietary phosphate and releases hydrochloric acid. This may reduce plasma bicarbonate levels.[104,105] Intestinal binding of bile acids significantly lowers LDL cholesterol.[104] The major advantage of sevelamer is that in contrast to calcium-containing phosphate binders sevelamer reduces serum phosphate without increasing serum calcium levels. Hypercalcemia occurs less frequently.[104,106] One prospective randomized trial, however, demonstrated less efficient reduction in serum phosphate compared to calcium acetate.[105] Of note, there is evidence for reduced progression of coronary artery calcifications[107] and improved survival[108] in adult dialysis patients receiving sevelamer compared to patients receiving calcium salts. The long-term beneficial effects associated with sevelamer use should therefore outweigh the increased treatment costs.

Lanthanum carbonate binds intestinal phosphate more effectively than calcium carbonate and sevelamer. However, patients on extended treatment show increased lanthanum serum levels. Significant tissue accumulation has been demonstrated in rats.[109] In light of the past experience with aluminium toxicity, lanthanum-containing phosphate binders are currently not recommended in children with CKD.

$25(OH)_2D_3$ Vitamin D3

Oral treatment with ergocalciferol or cholecalciferol is mandatory when serum $25(OH)_2D_3$ concentrations are below 30 to 40 ng/ml in order to prevent muscular weakness, secondary hyperparathyroidism, and osteomalacia. At least in early stages of CKD, supplementation of cholecalciferol can prevent or reduce hyperparathyroidism and should be given before calcitriol is considered.

Whereas a daily dose of 1000 to 2000 units of cholecalciferol may be given to prevent deficiency, higher doses are needed to replete stores. In adults, daily preventive doses of up to 4000 units per day have been recommended. However, the risk of intoxication with extended treatment has not been evaluated to date. The risk will increase considerably as soon as the $25(OH)_2D_3$ body stores are repleted. Repletion may escape the measurements of plasma $25(OH)_2D_3$ levels if performed infrequently. We use 2000 to 3000 units per day for repletion, checking plasma levels every 4 weeks until a level above 40 mg/ml has been reached.

Active Vitamin D3 Sterols

If plasma PTH levels remain elevated despite normal serum $25(OH)_2D_3$ and phosphate levels, treatment with calcitriol or analogues is required. *Calcitriol* and 1-α hydroxyvitamin D are most often used in children to compensate for reduced renal 1-α hydroxylase activity and to prevent and control secondary hyperparathyroidism. The dose of calcitriol depends on initial PTH, calcium, and phosphate values. An initial dose of 5 to 10 ng/kg * d is effective and safe in most children with CKD.[64]

The frequency of calcium, phosphate, and PTH monitoring should be adapted to the dose of vitamin D administered. Clinical evidence suggests that calcitriol binds to plastic materials and should therefore not be given via nasogastric tubes. A liquid formulation is available that can be given orally. Calcitriol efficiently controls secondary hyperparathyroidism. However, with prolonged treatment a substantial number of children develop adynamic bone disease—which has been associated with a reduced growth rate and frequent episodes of hypercalcemia.[59,64]

A second consequence to consider with active vitamin D treatment is the increase not only of intestinal absorption of calcium but of phosphate. Calcitriol increases intestinal phosphate absorption from about 60% to about 90%.[110,111] Calcitriol use is often limited by aggravated hyperphosphatemia and hypercalcemia. Calcitriol, hypercalcemia, and hyperphosphatemia contribute to extraosseus tissue calcifications and decreased survival in children with ESRD.[68,69] Deterioration of renal function is not accelerated by calcitriol, at least if administered at moderate doses that do not result in an increased calcium and phosphate product.[112,113]

The mode of calcitriol administration is of minor importance. Some studies (including bone biopsies) suggested a strong effect of calcitriol on bone metabolism with intermittent oral, intravenous, and intraperitoneal administration. These studies, however, were not controlled against a daily administration mode.[79,114] Direct comparison of intermittent versus daily calcitriol in adult patients with CKD stage V demonstrated that the intermittent administration of calcitriol is only slightly superior in lowering serum PTH levels[115] and bone AP.[116]

Prospective randomized studies comparing daily versus intermittent oral calcitriol in healthy children and children with CKD stages II through IV did not reveal any differences in PTH suppression, nor in intestinal calcium absorption, the incidence of hypercalcemia and hyperphosphatemia, or longitudinal growth rates.[64,90,117] Overall, the response to calcitriol depends less on the mode of administration than on the degree of secondary hyperparathyroidism and hyperphosphatemia and on the degree of parathyroid gland autonomy. Circadian rhythms of calcitriol pharmacodynamics, however, are of clinical relevance. Experimental and clinical studies demonstrated a reduced calcimic action of calcitriol with similar PTH suppression when administered in the evening and not in the morning.[118,119]

Synthetic vitamin D analogues have been developed to reduce intestinal calcium and phosphate absorption at equipotent PTH suppressive action. Three different sterols have been approved: 22-oxacalcitriol, 19-nor-1,25 dihydroxy vitamin D2 (paricalcitol), and 1α-hydroxyvitamin D2 (doxercalciferol). No pediatric treatment experience has been published for any of these compounds. In adult hemodialysis patients, paricalcitol treatment is associated with a more rapid achievement of PTH control and fewer episodes of sustained hypercalcemia and increased calcium and P product than calcitriol therapy.[120] Retrospective analyses even suggest improved patient survival with paricalcitol compared to calcitriol.[121] The preliminary evidence for a superior efficacy-safety profile of the synthetic vitamin D analogues must be balanced against their high costs.

There is also observational evidence for a survival benefit associated with the use of vitamin D sterols in general.[122] This finding, which awaits confirmation in prospective trials, may reflect a plethora of beneficial immunologic and cardiovascular effects of active vitamin D compounds.[123] In summary, active vitamin D sterols are indispensable therapeutic agents in the management of CKD but should always be used with caution and with awareness of their limited therapeutic window—beyond which major untoward effects to the bone, cardiovascular, and potentially other systems may occur.

Calcimimetic Agents

Calcimimetics are a new class of compounds that bind to the parathyroid calcium sensing receptor, increase its sensitivity to ionized calcium by allosteric modification, and dose dependently decrease plasma PTH levels by up to 80%. The effect is largely independent of baseline PTH and phosphate levels and thus allows for control of parathyroid gland function even in patients with otherwise refractory hyperparathyroidism. Cinacalcet is the only currently approved calcimimetic agent. Cinacalcet also reduces serum calcium and phosphate levels,[124] possibly via increased mineral deposition into bone. Whether calcimimetic agents significantly improve clinically relevant end points such as bone and cardiovascular morbidity is currently under investigation. Main side effects are nausea and vomiting (which can be attenuated by evening administration) and hypocalcemia. No studies in children have been performed so far. The calcium-sensing receptor is expressed on epiphyseal chondrocytes. Moreover, calcimimetics reduce serum testosterone levels by 30%. Hence, an impact on longitudinal growth and pubertal development cannot be ruled out. Although animal studies do not indicate an impact of cinacalcet on longitudinal growth,[125] clinical trials are required before general use of cinacalcet can be recommended in children with CKD.

Parathyroidectomy

Despite intensive vitamin D and phosphate binder treatment, some children with CKD may develop refractory hyperparathyroidism—particularly when renal transplantation cannot be performed for an extended period. In adult CKD patients less than 45 years of age, the incidence of parathyroidectomy is more than 2 per 100 patient-years.[126] In our experience, the incidence of parathyroidectomy in children is at least similar to that of adults. Urgent indications for parathyroidectomy are persistent and recurrent hypercalcemia and progressive extraosseus calcifications (Table 50-5). Whether adequate $25(OH)_2D_3$ treatment and/or calcimimetics reduce the need for parathyroidectomy is still unknown.

Total parathyroidectomy and autotransplantation of tissue fragments in the abdominal subcutaneous layer are preferred to subtotal parathyroidectomy because the remaining tissue tends to grow again and the transplant is easier to access for diagnostic and curative purposes. Total parathyroidectomy without autotransplantation may result in difficulties in controlling calcium homeostasis, in particular after kidney transplantation. Ablation of parathyroid tissue by ethanol injection has been suggested as an alternative to surgery. However, no pediatric experience is available. Some centers give active vitamin D 72 hours prior to surgery to lessen postoperative hypocalcemia. However, this should only be done if calcium and phosphate values are not markedly increased.

Postoperatively, serum ionized calcium needs to be monitored closely because most of the children develop "hungry bone" syndrome. Due to the rapid decline of PTH, skeletal calcium uptake increases markedly. In most children, calcium infusions are required within a few hours after operation—especially in children with high preoperative PTH and alkaline phosphatase levels. Calcium infusion can be started at a rate of 0.05 mmol/kg * h (2 mg/kg * h) of elemental calcium, but must be continuously adapted according to the changes in serum ionized calcium levels. Calcium infusion is often required for several days, and subsequent oral calcium admin-

TABLE 50-5 Indications for Parathyroidectomy

Severe hyperparathyroidism combined with:
- Persistent or recurrent hypercalcemia
- Persistent hyperphosphatemia
- Unresponsiveness to calcitriol and calcium
- Progressive and debilitating bone disease
- Evidence of metastatic calcifications, calciphylaxis
- Otherwise refractory pruritus

istration for many weeks. In addition, patients should be given high doses of calcitriol (up to 2 μg/d) and be dialyzed with a high dialysate calcium concentration. Serum phosphate levels also decline. However, administration of phosphate may aggravate hypocalcemia and should only be initiated at serum phosphate concentrations below normal.

Success rate is high. Parathyroid tissue fragments autotransplanted subcutaneously usually start to secret PTH soon.[127] Plasma levels, however, often remain below the target range. The clinical implication of this is not known, in particular because calcium and phosphate values usually remain in the target range for an extended period. Symptomatic hypocalcemia may develop in children not adhering to the medication. Irreversible recurrent nerve palsy is rare.

Treatment of Children after Renal Transplantation

Children receiving a renal allograft are at risk for multifactorial progressive bone disease. Persistent hyperparathyroidism, hypophosphatemia, and glucocorticoid use require close monitoring of bone metabolism even if transplant function is normal. Serum calcium, phosphate, and bicarbonate should be measured weekly within the first 2 months, and at least monthly during the following months. Subsequent determinations also have to be adapted to renal function.

PTH should be checked initially, and 1 month posttransplantation. If plasma PTH remains elevated, further controls and therapeutic measures are required. If renal function is reduced, the frequency of determinations should accord with the stage of CKD (Table 50-2). Subsequent treatment strategies should follow the guidelines for CKD (Table 50-3). Hypophosphatemia needs to be treated appropriately. Glucocorticoids should be given at the lowest dose possible, and may be withdrawn in patients with stable transplant function. Calcium and active vitamin D therapy lessen glucocorticoid-induced bone loss in adults and have been recommended. However, no pediatric data have been provided to date.

The Future of Therapy

Bisphosphonates, selectively blocking osteoclasts and thus bone resorption, appear to be safe and effective at all stages of CKD. These agents may have beneficial effects in patients experiencing fracturing, and are recommended for adult high-risk transplant patients on glucocorticoids.[128] A cause of concern is their long-lasting action and the risk of hypocalcemia associated with overdosing. Dose reduction is probably required in CKD stage V, at least based on pharmacokinetic studies. However, more scientific data are mandatory before their use in growing children with CKD or glucocorticoid-induced osteoporosis can be considered.

BMP-7 has been used successfully in animal models of renal osteodystrophy and vascular calcification. Human data are currently limited to orthopedic interventions, where it has been employed successfully to induce the healing of pathologic fractures.[129]

PROGNOSIS

Despite an increasing number of therapeutic options, the management of mineral metabolism remains difficult. More than one third of adults with pediatric-onset CKD have clinical symptoms of bone disease, and almost one out of five patients is disabled by bone disease.[130] The CKD-associated alterations of bone mineral metabolism disorders and their treatment during childhood years substantially contribute to the development of uremic arteriopathy, and probably to the excessive cardiovascular mortality in early adult life.[69] Barriers to success are limited patient compliance;[131] the inefficacy of prescribed measures; the prohibitive costs of novel, more efficacious therapies; and the progressive development of parathyroid autonomy.

Still, there is hope that the increased use of calcium-free phosphate binders, the prevention of $25(OH)_2D_3$ deficiency, and the employment of new vitamin D analogues and calcimimetics may substantially improve the prognosis of mineral disorder and vasculopathy in children with CKD. Moreover, the attention to clinical practice guidelines with defined target values, the establishment of patient registries monitoring achievement of these targets, and the fostering of prospective randomized trials evaluating clinical outcome parameters should result in more favorable long-term outcomes of children with CKD currently treated in pediatric units.

REFERENCES

1. Ziolkowska H, Paniczyk-Tomaszewska M, Debinski A, Polowiec Z, Sawicki A, Sieniawska M: Bone biopsy results and serum bone turnover parameters in uremic children, *Acta Paediatr* 89(6):666-71, 2000.
2. Spasovski GB, Bervoets AR, Behets GJ, Ivanovski N, Sikole A, Dams G, et al: Spectrum of renal bone disease in end-stage renal failure patients not yet on dialysis, *Nephrol Dial Transplant* 18(6):1159-66, 2003.
3. Salusky IB, Ramirez JA, Oppenheim W, Gales B, Segre GV, Goodman WG: Biochemical markers of renal osteodystrophy in pediatric patients undergoing CAPD/CCPD, *Kidney Int* 45(1):253-58, 1994.
4. Moallem E, Kilav R, Silver J, Naveh-Many T: RNA-protein binding and post-transcriptional regulation of parathyroid hormone gene expression by calcium and phosphate, *J Biol Chem* 273(9):5253-59, 1998.
5. Iwasaki Y, Yamato H, Nii-Kono T, Fujieda A, Uchida M, Hosokawa A, et al: Insufficiency of PTH action on bone in uremia, *Kidney Int Suppl* 102:S34-S36, 2006.
6. Naveh-Many T, Rahamimov R, Livni N, Silver J: Parathyroid cell proliferation in normal and chronic renal failure rats: The effects of calcium, phosphate, and vitamin D, *J Clin Invest* 96(4):1786-93, 1995.
7. Li YC, Amling M, Pirro AE, Priemel M, Meuse J, Baron R, et al: Normalization of mineral ion homeostasis by dietary means prevents hyperparathyroidism, rickets, and osteomalacia, but not alopecia in vitamin D receptor-ablated mice, *Endocrinology* 139(10):4391-96, 1998.
8. Silver J, Naveh-Many T, Mayer H, Schmelzer HJ, Popovtzer MM: Regulation by vitamin D metabolites of parathyroid hormone gene transcription in vivo in the rat, *J Clin Invest* 78(5):1296-1301, 1986.
9. Canaff L, Hendy GN: Human calcium-sensing receptor gene: Vitamin D response elements in promoters P1 and P2 confer transcriptional responsiveness to 1,25-dihydroxyvitamin D, *J Biol Chem* 277(33):30337-50, 2002.
10. Sela-Brown A, Russell J, Koszewski NJ, Michalak M, Naveh-Many T, Silver J: Calreticulin inhibits vitamin D's action on the PTH gene

in vitro and may prevent vitamin D's effect in vivo in hypocalcemic rats, *Mol Endocrinol* 12(8):1193-1200, 1998.

11. Drissi H, Pouliot A, Koolloos C, Stein JL, Lian JB, Stein GS, van Wijnen AJ: 1,25-(OH)2-vitamin D3 suppresses the bone-related Runx2/Cbfa1 gene promoter, *Exp Cell Res* 274(2):323-33, 2002.
12. Virdi AS, Cook LJ, Oreffo RO, Triffitt JT: Modulation of bone morphogenetic protein-2 and bone morphogenetic protein-4 gene expression in osteoblastic cell lines, *Cell Mol Biol* 44(8):1237-46, 1998.
13. Fraser JD, Otawara Y, Price PA: 1,25-Dihydroxyvitamin D3 stimulates the synthesis of matrix gamma-carboxyglutamic acid protein by osteosarcoma cells: Mutually exclusive expression of vitamin K-dependent bone proteins by clonal osteoblastic cell lines, *J Biol Chem* 263(2):911-16, 1988.
14. Segersten U, Correa P, Hewison M, Hellman P, Dralle H, Carling T, et al: 25-hydroxyvitamin D(3)-1alpha-hydroxylase expression in normal and pathological parathyroid glands, *J Clin Endocrinol Metab* 87(6):2967-72, 2002.
15. Somjen D, Weisman Y, Kohen F, Gayer B, Limor R, Sharon O, et al: 25-hydroxyvitamin D3-1alpha-hydroxylase is expressed in human VSMCs and is upregulated by parathyroid hormone and estrogenic compounds, *Circulation* 111(13):1666-71, 2005.
16. Schott GD, Wills MR: Muscle weakness in osteomalacia, *Lancet* 1(7960):626-29, 1976.
17. Shah N, Bernardini J, Piraino B: Prevalence and correction of 25(OH) vitamin D deficiency in peritoneal dialysis patients, *Perit Dial Int* 25(4):362-66, 2005.
18. Mucsi I, Almasi C, Deak G, Marton A, Ambrus C, Berta K, et al: Serum 25(OH)-vitamin D levels and bone metabolism in patients on maintenance hemodialysis, *Clin Nephrol* 64(4):288-94, 2005.
19. Coen G, Mantella D, Manni M, Balducci A, Nofroni I, Sardella D, et al: 25-hydroxyvitamin D levels and bone histomorphometry in hemodialysis renal osteodystrophy, *Kidney Int* 68(4):1840-48, 2005.
20. Larsson T, Nisbeth U, Ljunggren O, Juppner H, Jonsson KB: Circulating concentration of FGF-23 increases as renal function declines in patients with chronic kidney disease, but does not change in response to variation in phosphate intake in healthy volunteers, *Kidney Int* 64(6):2272-79, 2003.
21. Shigematsu T, Kazama JJ, Yamashita T, Fukumoto S, Hosoya T, Gejyo F, et al: Possible involvement of circulating fibroblast growth factor 23 in the development of secondary hyperparathyroidism associated with renal insufficiency, *Am J Kidney Dis* 44(2):250-56, 2004.
22. Slatopolsky E, Finch J, Denda M, Ritter C, Zhong M, Dusso A, et al: Phosphorus restriction prevents parathyroid gland growth. High phosphorus directly stimulates PTH secretion in vitro, *J Clin Invest* 97(11):2534-40, 1996.
23. Almaden Y, Canalejo A, Hernandez A, Ballesteros E, Garcia-Navarro S, Torres A, et al: Direct effect of phosphorus on PTH secretion from whole rat parathyroid glands in vitro, *J Bone Miner Res* 11(7):970-76, 1996.
24. Kanesaka Y, Tokunaga H, Iwashita K, Fujimura S, Naomi S: Endothelin receptor antagonist prevents parathyroid cell proliferation of low calcium diet-induced hyperparathyroidism in rats, *Endocrinology* 142(1):407-13, 2001.
25. Gogusev J, Duchambon P, Stoermann-Chopard C, Giovannini M, Sarfati E, Drueke TB: De novo expression of transforming growth factor-alpha in parathyroid gland tissue of patients with primary or secondary uraemic hyperparathyroidism, *Nephrol Dial Transplant* 11(11):2155-62, 1996.
26. Cozzolino M, Lu Y, Sato T, Yang J, Suarez IG, Brancaccio D, et al: A critical role for enhanced TGF-alpha and EGFR expression in the initiation of parathyroid hyperplasia in experimental kidney disease, *Am J Physiol Renal Physiol* 289(5):F1096-F1102, 2005.
27. Cozzolino M, Lu Y, Finch J, Slatopolsky E, Dusso AS: p21WAF1 and TGF-alpha mediate parathyroid growth arrest by vitamin D and high calcium, *Kidney Int* 60(6):2109-17, 2001.
28. Aucella F, Morrone L, Stallone C, Gesualdo L: The genetic background of uremic secondary hyperparathyroidism, *J Nephrol* 18(5):537-47, 2005.
29. Schmitt CP, Schaefer F: Calcium sensitivity of the parathyroid in renal failure: another look with new methodology, *Nephrol Dial Transplant* 14(12):2815-18, 1999.
30. Schmitt CP, Huber D, Mehls O, Maiwald J, Stein G, Veldhuis JD, et al: Altered instantaneous and calcium-modulated oscillatory PTH secretion patterns in patients with secondary hyperparathyroidism, *J Am Soc Nephrol* 9(10):1832-44, 1998.
31. Zhang P, Duchambon P, Gogusev J, Nabarra B, Sarfati E, Bourdeau A, et al: Apoptosis in parathyroid hyperplasia of patients with primary or secondary uremic hyperparathyroidism, *Kidney Int* 57(2):437-45, 2000.
32. Cochran M, Wilkinson R: Effect of correction of metabolic acidosis on bone mineralisation rates in patients with renal osteomalacia, *Nephron* 15(2):98-110, 1975.
33. Disthabanchong S, Martin KJ, McConkey CL, et al: Metabolic acidosis up-regulates PTH/PTHrP receptors in UMR 106-01 osteoblast-like cells, *Kidney Int* 62(4):1171-77, 2002.
34. Arnold A, Horst SA, Gardella TJ, Baba H, Levine MA, Kronenberg HM: Mutation of the signal peptide-encoding region of the preproparathyroid hormone gene in familial isolated hypoparathyroidism, *J Clin Invest* 86(4):1084-87, 1990.
35. Slatopolsky E, Finch J, Clay P, Martin D, Sicard G, Singer G, et al: A novel mechanism for skeletal resistance in uremia, *Kidney Int* 58(2):753-61, 2000.
36. Lepage R, Roy L, Brossard JH, Rousseau L, Dorais C, Lazure C, et al: A non-(1-84) circulating parathyroid hormone (PTH) fragment interferes significantly with intact PTH commercial assay measurements in uremic samples, *Clin Chem* 44(4):805-09, 1998.
37. Waller S, Ridout D, Cantor T, Rees L: Differences between "intact" PTH and 1-84 PTH assays in chronic renal failure and dialysis, *Pediatr Nephrol* 20(2):197-99, 2005.
38. Divieti P, Geller AI, Suliman G, Juppner H, Bringhurst FR: Receptors specific for the carboxyl-terminal region of parathyroid hormone on bone-derived cells: Determinants of ligand binding and bioactivity, *Endocrinology* 146(4):1863-70, 2005.
39. Lund RJ, Davies MR, Brown AJ, Hruska KA: Successful treatment of an adynamic bone disorder with bone morphogenetic protein-7 in a renal ablation model, *J Am Soc Nephrol* 15(2):359-69, 2004.
40. Gonzalez EA, Lund RJ, Martin KJ, McCartney JE, Tondravi MM, Sampath TK, et al: Treatment of a murine model of high-turnover renal osteodystrophy by exogenous BMP-7, *Kidney Int* 61(4):1322-31, 2002.
41. Davies MR, Lund RJ, Hruska KA: BMP-7 is an efficacious treatment of vascular calcification in a murine model of atherosclerosis and chronic renal failure, *J Am Soc Nephrol* 14(6):1559-67, 2003.
42. Langman CB: Genetic regulation of bone mass: From bone density to bone strength, *Pediatr Nephrol* 20(3):352-55, 2005.
43. Aksnes L, Aarskog D: Plasma concentrations of vitamin D metabolites in puberty: Effect of sexual maturation and implications for growth, *J Clin Endocrinol Metab* 55(1):94-101, 1982.
44. Goulding A, Jones IE, Taylor RW, Williams SM, Manning PJ: Bone mineral density and body composition in boys with distal forearm fractures: a dual-energy x-ray absorptiometry study, *J Pediatr* 139(4):509-15, 2001.
45. Wong SY, Kariks J, Evans RA, Dunstan CR, Hills E: The effect of age on bone composition and viability in the femoral head, *J Bone Joint Surg Am* 67(2):274-83, 1985.
46. Schonau E: The peak bone mass concept: is it still relevant? *Pediatr Nephrol* 19(8):825-831, 2004.
47. Ritz E, Boland R, Kreusser W: Effects of vitamin D and parathyroid hormone on muscle: Potential role in uremic myopathy, *Am J Clin Nutr* 33(7):1522-29, 1980.
48. Ahmad S, Robertson HT, Golper TA, Wolfson M, Kurtin P, Katz LA, et al: Multicenter trial of L-carnitine in maintenance hemodialysis patients: II. Clinical and biochemical effects, *Kidney Int* 38(5):912-18, 1990.
49. Marrades RM, Roca J, Campistol JM, Diaz O, Barbera JA, Torregrosa JV, et al: Effects of erythropoietin on muscle O2 transport during exercise in patients with chronic renal failure, *J Clin Invest* 97(9):2092-100, 1996.
50. Sala E, Noyszewski EA, Campistol JM, Marrades RM, Dreha S, Torregrossa JV, et al: Impaired muscle oxygen transfer in patients with chronic renal failure, *Am J Physiol Regul Integr Comp Physiol* 280(4):R1240-R1248, 2001.

51. Mehls O, Ritz E, Kreusser W, Krempien B: Renal osteodystrophy in uraemic children, *Clin Endocrinol Metab* 9(1):151-76, 1980.
52. Helenius I, Remes V, Salminen S, Valta H, Makitie O, Holmberg C, et al: Incidence and predictors of fractures in children after solid organ transplantation: A 5-year prospective, population-based study, *J Bone Miner Res* 21(3):380-87, 2006.
53. Parfitt AM: Renal bone disease: A new conceptual framework for the interpretation of bone histomorphometry, *Curr Opin Nephrol Hypertens* 12(4):387-403, 2003.
54. Alem AM, Sherrard DJ, Gillen DL, Weiss NS, Beresford SA, Heckbert SR, et al: Increased risk of hip fracture among patients with end-stage renal disease, *Kidney Int* 58(1):396-99, 2000.
55. Danese MD, Kim J, Doan QV, Dylan M, Griffiths R, Chertow GM: PTH and the risks for hip, vertebral, and pelvic fractures among patients on dialysis, *Am J Kidney Dis* 47(1):149-56, 2006.
56. Mehls O, Ritz E, Gilli G, Wangdak T, Krempien B: Effect of vitamin D on growth in experimental uremia, *Am J Clin Nutr* 31(10):1927-31, 1978.
57. Chesney RW, Moorthy AV, Eisman JA, Jax DK, Mazess RB, DeLuca HF: Increased growth after long-term oral 1alpha,25-vitamin D3 in childhood renal osteodystrophy, *N Engl J Med* 298(5):238-42, 1982.
58. Chan JC, McEnery PT, Chinchilli VM, Abitbol CL, Boineau FG, Friedman AL, et al: A prospective, double-blind study of growth failure in children with chronic renal insufficiency and the effectiveness of treatment with calcitriol versus dihydrotachysterol: The Growth Failure in Children with Renal Diseases Investigators, *J Pediatr* 124(4):520-28, 1994.
59. Kuizon BD, Goodman WG, Juppner H, Boechat I, Nelson P, Gales B, et al: Diminished linear growth during intermittent calcitriol therapy in children undergoing CCPD, *Kidney Int* 53(1):205-11, 1998.
60. Klaus G, Weber L, Rodriguez J, Fernandez P, Klein T, Grulich-Henn J, et al: Interaction of IGF-I and 1 alpha, 25(OH)2D3 on receptor expression and growth stimulation in rat growth plate chondrocytes, *Kidney Int* 53(5):1152-56, 1998.
61. Green J, Goldberg R, Maor G: PTH ameliorates acidosis-induced adverse effects in skeletal growth centers: The PTH-IGF-I axis, *Kidney Int* 63(2):487-500, 2003.
62. Vortkamp A, Lee K, Lanske B, Segre GV, Kronenberg HM, Tabin CJ: Regulation of rate of cartilage differentiation by Indian hedgehog and PTH-related protein, *Science* 273:613-22, 1996.
63. Schmitt CP, Hessing S, Oh J, Weber L, Ochlich P, Mehls O: Intermittent administration of parathyroid hormone (1-37) improves growth and bone mineral density in uremic rats, *Kidney Int* 57(4):1484-492, 2000.
64. Schmitt CP, Ardissino G, Testa S, Claris-Appiani A, Mehls O: Growth in children with chronic renal failure on intermittent versus daily calcitriol, *Pediatr Nephrol* 18(5):440-44, 2003.
65. Waller SC, Ridout D, Cantor T, Rees L: Parathyroid hormone and growth in children with chronic renal failure, *Kidney Int* 67(6):2338-45, 2005.
66. Cansick J, Waller S, Ridout D, Rees L: Growth and PTH in prepubertal children on long-term dialysis, *Pediatr Nephrol* 22:1349-54, 2007.
67. Fischbach M, Terzic J, Menouer S, Dheu C, Soskin S, Helmstetter A, et al: Intensified and daily hemodialysis in children might improve statural growth, *Pediatr Nephrol* 21(11):1746-52, 2006.
68. Litwin M, Wuhl E, Jourdan C, Trelewicz J, Niemirska A, Fahr K, et al: Altered morphologic properties of large arteries in children with chronic renal failure and after renal transplantation, *J Am Soc Nephrol* 16(5):1494-500, 2005.
69. Oh J, Wunsch R, Turzer M, Bahner M, Raggi P, Querfeld U, et al: Advanced coronary and carotid arteriopathy in young adults with childhood-onset chronic renal failure, *Circulation* 106(1):100-05, 2002.
70. Goodman WG, Goldin J, Kuizon BD, Yoon C, Gales B, Sider D, et al: Coronary-artery calcification in young adults with end-stage renal disease who are undergoing dialysis, *N Engl J Med* 342(20):1478-83, 2000.
71. Milliner DS, Zinsmeister AR, Lieberman E, Landing B: Soft tissue calcification in pediatric patients with end-stage renal disease, *Kidney Int* 38(5):931-36, 1990.
72. Ketteler M, Bongartz P, Westenfeld R, Wildberger JE, Mahnken AH, Bohm R, et al: Association of low fetuin-A (AHSG) concentrations in serum with cardiovascular mortality in patients on dialysis: A cross-sectional study, *Lancet* 361(9360):827-33, 2003.
73. Zouboulis CC, Blume-Peytavi U, Lennert T, Stavropoulos PG, Schwarz A, Runkel N, et al: Fulminant metastatic calcinosis with cutaneous necrosis in a child with end-stage renal disease and tertiary hyperparathyroidism, *Br J Dermatol* 135(4):617-22, 1996.
74. Bhan I, Shah A, Holmes J, Isakova T, Gutierrez O, Burnett SA, et al: Post-transplant hypophosphatemia: Tertiary "Hyper-Phosphatoninism"? *Kidney Int* 70(8):1486-94, 2006.
75. Cayco AV, Wysolmerski J, Simpson C, Mitnick MA, Gundberg C, Kliger A, et al: Posttransplant bone disease: Evidence for a high bone resorption state, *Transplantation* 70(12):1722-28, 2000.
76. Sanchez CP, Salusky IB, Kuizon BD, Ramirez JA, Gales B, Ettenger RB, et al: Bone disease in children and adolescents undergoing successful renal transplantation, *Kidney Int* 53(5):1358-64, 1998.
77. Ruth EM, Weber LT, Schoenau E, Wunsch R, Seibel MJ, Feneberg R, et al: Analysis of the functional muscle-bone unit of the forearm in pediatric renal transplant recipients, *Kidney Int* 66(4):1694-1706, 2004.
78. Helenius I, Jalanko H, Remes V, Tervahartiala P, Salminen S, Sairanen H, et al: Avascular bone necrosis of the hip joint after solid organ transplantation in childhood: A clinical and MRI analysis, *Transplantation* 81(12):1621-27, 2006.
79. Salusky IB, Kuizon BD, Belin TR, Ramirez JA, Gales B, Segre GV, et al: Intermittent calcitriol therapy in secondary hyperparathyroidism: A comparison between oral and intraperitoneal administration, *Kidney Int* 54(3):907-14, 1998.
80. Kruse K, Kracht U, Gopfert G: Renal threshold phosphate concentration (TmPO4/GFR), *Arch Dis Child* 57(3):217-23, 1982.
81. NKF K/DOQI: Clinical practice guidelines for bone metabolism and disease in children with chronic kidney disease, *Am J Kidney Disease* 46(1):S1-S100, 2005.
82. European Society for Paediatric Nephrology: *ESPN handbook*. 1st ed. Lyon, France: ESPN 2002:461.
83. Markowitz ME, Rosen JF, Laxminarayan S, Mizruchi M: Circadian rhythms of blood minerals during adolescence, *Pediatr Res* 18(5):456-62, 1984.
84. Trivedi H, Moore H, Atalla J: Lack of significant circadian and post-prandial variation in phosphate levels in subjects receiving chronic hemodialysis therapy, *J Nephrol* 18(4):417-22, 2005.
85. Brossard JH, Cloutier M, Roy L, Lepage R, Gascon-Barre M, D'Amour P: Accumulation of a non-(1-84) molecular form of parathyroid hormone (PTH) detected by intact PTH assay in renal failure: Importance in the interpretation of PTH values, *J Clin Endocrinol Metab* 81(11):3923-29, 1996.
86. Gal-Moscovici A, Popovtzer MM: New worldwide trends in presentation of renal osteodystrophy and its relationship to parathyroid hormone levels, *Clin Nephrol* 63(4):284-89, 2005.
87. John MR, Goodman WG, Gao P, Cantor TL, Salusky IB, Juppner H: A novel immunoradiometric assay detects full-length human PTH but not amino-terminally truncated fragments: Implications for PTH measurements in renal failure, *J Clin Endocrinol Metab* 84(11):4287-90, 1999.
88. Urena P, Hruby M, Ferreira A, Ang KS, de Vernejoul MC: Plasma total versus bone alkaline phosphatase as markers of bone turnover in hemodialysis patients, *J Am Soc Nephrol* 7(3):506-12, 1996.
89. Batchelor AJ, Compston JE: Reduced plasma half-life of radio-labelled 25-hydroxyvitamin D3 in subjects receiving a high-fibre diet, *Br J Nutr* 49(2):213-16, 1983.
90. Ardissino G, Schmitt CP, Bianchi ML, Dacco V, Claris-Appiani A, Mehls O: No difference in intestinal strontium absorption after oral or IV calcitriol in children with secondary hyperparathyroidism: The European Study Group on Vitamin D in Children with Renal Failure, *Kidney Int* 58(3):981-88, 2000.
91. Kazama JJ: Osteoprotegerin and bone mineral metabolism in renal failure, *Curr Opin Nephrol Hypertens* 13(4):411-15, 2004.
92. Diaz López JB, Jorgetti V, Carosi H, et al: Epidemiology of renal osteodystrophy in iberoamerica, *Nephrol Dial Transplant* 13(3):41-45, 1998.

93. Andress DL, Endres DB, Maloney NA, Kopp JB, Coburn JW, Sherrard DJ: Comparison of parathyroid hormone assays with bone histomorphometry in renal osteodystrophy, *J Clin Endocrinol Metab* 63(5):1163-69, 1986.
94. Mehls O, Ritz E, Krempien B, Willich E, Bommer J, Scharer K: Roentgenological signs in the skeleton of uremic children: An analysis of the anatomical principles underlying the roentgenological changes, *Pediatr Radiol* 1(3):183-90, 1973.
95. Chesney RW: Bone mineral density in chronic renal insufficiency and end-stage renal disease: How to interpret the scans, *J Pediatr Endocrinol Metab* 17(4):1327-32, 2004.
96. Jourdan C, Wuhl E, Litwin M, Fahr K, Trelewicz J, Jobs K, et al: Normative values for intima-media thickness and distensibility of large arteries in healthy adolescents, *J Hypertens* 23(9):1707-15, 2005.
97. Klaus G, Watson A, Edefonti A, Fischbach M, Rönnholm K, Schaefer F, et al: European Pediatric Dialysis Working Group (EPDWG). Prevention and treatment of renal osteodystrophy in children on chronic renal failure: European guidelines, *Pediatr Nephrol* 21(2):151-59, 2006.
98. Fischbach M, Terzic J, Laugel V, Dheu C, Menouer S, Helms P, et al: Daily on-line haemodiafiltration: A pilot trial in children, *Nephrol Dial Transplant* 19(9):2360-67, 2004.
99. Geary DF, Piva E, Tyrrell J, Gajaria MJ, Picone G, Keating LE, et al: Home nocturnal hemodialysis in children, *J Pediatr* 147(3):383-87, 2005.
100. Hothi DK, Harvey E, Piva E, Keating L, Secker D, Geary DF: Calcium and phosphate balance in adolescents on home nocturnal haemodialysis, *Pediatr Nephrol* 21(6):835-41, 2006.
101. Sechet A, Hardy P, Hottelart C, Rasombololona M, Abighanem O, Oualim Z, et al: A role of calcium carbonate administration timing in relation to food intake on its efficiency in controlling hyperphosphatemia in patients on maintenance dialysis, *Artif Organs* 22(7):564-68, 1998.
102. Wei M, Esbaei K, Bargman J, Oreopoulos DG: Relationship between serum magnesium, parathyroid hormone, and vascular calcification in patients on dialysis: A literature review, *Perit Dial Int* 26(3):366-73, 2006.
103. Guillot AP, Hood VL, Runge CF, Gennari FJ: The use of magnesium-containing phosphate binders in patients with end-stage renal disease on maintenance hemodialysis, *Nephron* 30(2):114-17, 1982.
104. Pieper AK, Haffner D, Hoppe B, Dittrich K, Offner G, Bonzel KE, et al: A randomized crossover trial comparing sevelamer with calcium acetate in children with CKD, *Am J Kidney Dis* 47(4):625-35, 2006.
105. Qunibi WY, Hootkins RE, McDowell LL, Meyer MS, Simon M, Garza RO, et al: Treatment of hyperphosphatemia in hemodialysis patients: The Calcium Acetate Renagel Evaluation (CARE) study, *Kidney Int* 65(5):1914-26, 2004.
106. Salusky IB, Goodman WG, Sahney S, Gales B, Perilloux A, Wang HJ, et al: Sevelamer controls parathyroid hormone-induced bone disease as efficiently as calcium carbonate without increasing serum calcium levels during therapy with active vitamin D sterols, *J Am Soc Nephrol* 16(8):2501-08, 2005.
107. Chertow GM, Burke SK, Raggi P: Treat to Goal Working Group: Sevelamer attenuates the progression of coronary and aortic calcification in hemodialysis patients, *Kidney Int* 62(1):245-52, 2002.
108. Block GA, Raggi P, Bellasi A, Kooienga L, Spiegel DM: Mortality effect of coronary calcification and phosphate binder choice in incident hemodialysis patients, *Kidney Int* 71(5):438-41, 2007.
109. Lacour B, Lucas A, Auchere D, Ruellan N, de Serre Patey NM, Drueke TB: Chronic renal failure is associated with increased tissue deposition of lanthanum after 28-day oral administration, *Kidney Int* 67(3):1062-69, 2005.
110. Brickman AS, Coburn JW, Friedman GR, Okamura WH, Massry SG, Norman AW: Comparison of effects of 1 alpha-hydroxy-vitamin D3 and 1,25-dihydroxy-vitamin D3 in man, *J Clin Invest* 57(6):1540-47, 1976.
111. Ramirez JA, Emmett M, White MG, Fathi N, Santa Ana CA, Morawski SG, et al: The absorption of dietary phosphorus and calcium in hemodialysis patients, *Kidney Int* 30(5):753-59, 1986.
112. Nordal KP, Dahl E: Low dose calcitriol versus placebo in patients with predialysis chronic renal failure, *J Clin Endocrinol Metab* 67(5):929-36, 1988.
113. Bianchi ML, Colantonio G, Campanini F, Rossi R, Valenti G, Ortolani S, et al: Calcitriol and calcium carbonate therapy in early chronic renal failure, *Nephrol Dial Transplant* 9(11):1595-99, 1994.
114. Andress DL, Norris KC, Coburn JW, Slatopolsky EA, Sherrard DJ: Intravenous calcitriol in the treatment of refractory osteitis fibrosa of chronic renal failure, *N Engl J Med* 321(5):274-79, 1989.
115. Caravaca F, Cubero JJ, Jimenez F, Lopez JM, Aparicio A, Cid MC, et al: Effect of the mode of calcitriol administration on PTH-ionized calcium relationship in uraemic patients with secondary hyperparathyroidism, *Nephrol Dial Transplant* 10(5):665-70, 1995.
116. Indridason OS, Quarles LD: Comparison of treatments for mild secondary hyperparathyroidism in hemodialysis patients: Durham Renal Osteodystrophy Study Group, *Kidney Int* 57(1):282-92, 2000.
117. Ardissino G, Schmitt CP, Testa S, Claris-Appiani A, Mehls O: Calcitriol pulse therapy is not more effective than daily calcitriol therapy in controlling secondary hyperparathyroidism in children with chronic renal failure: European Study Group on Vitamin D in Children with Renal Failure, *Pediatr Nephrol* 14(7):664-68, 2000.
118. Tsuruoka S, Nishiki K, Sugimoto K, Fujimura A: Time of day improves efficacy and reduces adverse reactions of vitamin D3 in 5/6 nephrectomized rat, *Life Sci* 71(15):1809-20, 2002.
119. Tsuruoka S, Wakaumi M, Sugimoto K, Saito T, Fujimura A: Chronotherapy of high-dose active vitamin D3 in haemodialysis patients with secondary hyperparathyroidsm: a repeated dosing study, *Br J Clin Pharmacol* 55(6):531-37, 2003.
120. Sprague SM, Llach F, Amdahl M, Taccetta C, Batlle D: Paricalcitol versus calcitriol in the treatment of secondary hyperparathyroidism, *Kidney Int* 63(4):1483-90, 2003.
121. Teng M, Wolf M, Lowrie E, Ofsthun N, Lazarus JM, Thadhani R: Survival of patients undergoing hemodialysis with paricalcitol or calcitriol therapy, *N Engl J Med* 349(5):446-56, 2003.
122. Teng M, Wolf M, Ofsthun MN, Lazarus JM, Hernan MA, Camargo CA Jr., et al: Activated injectable vitamin D and hemodialysis survival: A historical cohort study, *J Am Soc Nephrol* 16(4):1115-25, 2005.
123. Andress DL: Vitamin D in chronic kidney disease: a systemic role for selective vitamin D receptor activation, *Kidney Int* 69(1):33-43, 2006.
124. Strippoli GF, Tong A, Palmer SC, Elder G, Craig JC: Calcimimetics for secondary hyperparathyroidism in chronic kidney disease patients, *Cochrane Database Syst Rev* 18(4):CD006254, 2006.
125. Nakagawa K, Geldyyev A, Oh J, Gross ML, Santos F, Schaefer F, et al: Calcimimetics do not alter epiphyseal growth in healthy and uremic rats, *J Am Soc Nephrol* 17:132A, 2006.
126. Foley RN, Li S, Liu J, Gilbertson DT, Chen SC, Collins AJ: The fall and rise of parathyroidectomy in U.S. hemodialysis patients, 1992 to 2002, *J Am Soc Nephrol* 16(1):210-18, 2005.
127. Schmitt CP, Locken S, Mehls O, Veldhuis JD, Lehnert T, Ritz E, et al: PTH pulsatility but not calcium sensitivity is restored after total parathyroidectomy with heterotopic autotransplantation, *J Am Soc Nephrol* 14(2):407-14, 2003.
128. EBPG Expert Group on Renal Transplantation: European best practice guidelines for renal transplantation: Section IV, long-term management of the transplant recipient. IV.8. Bone disease, *Nephrol Dial Transplant* 17(4):43-48, 2002.
129. Dimitriou R, Dahabreh Z, Katsoulis E, Matthews SJ, Branfoot T, Giannoudis PV: Application of recombinant BMP-7 on persistent upper and lower limb non-unions, *Injury* 36(4):S51-S59, 2005.
130. Groothoff JW, Offringa M, Van Eck-Smit BL, Gruppen MP, Van De Kar NJ, Wolff ED, et al: Severe bone disease and low bone mineral density after juvenile renal failure, *Kidney Int* 63(1):266-75, 2003.
131. Cochat P, De Geest S, Ritz E: Drug holiday: A challenging child-adult interface in kidney transplantation, *Nephrol Dial Transplant* 15(12):1924-27, 2000.

CHAPTER 51

Cardiovascular Disease in Pediatric Chronic Kidney Disease

Uwe Querfeld and Mark Mitsnefes

EPIDEMIOLOGY

Cardiovascular Disease and Cardiac Events

Although cardiovascular disease (CVD) is exceptional in children and young adults in the general population, it is the leading cause of death in children and adolescents on renal replacement therapy (RRT). In young adult patients with end-stage renal disease (ESRD) aged 25 to 34 years, the comparative CVD mortality is excessively high—with a 500-fold increased incidence that resembles the CVD mortality of elderly patients aged 75 and older in the general population.[1]

The risk for CVD seems increased even with incipient renal failure. Pooled data from large community-based studies (Atherosclerosis Risk in Communities Study, Cardiovascular Health Study, Framingham Heart Study, and Framingham Offspring Study) show that moderate renal insufficiency is associated with a 19% excess risk for cardiovascular complications.[2] Adult patients with CKD are at much greater risk of developing congestive heart failure and cardiovascular death than of progressing to dialysis.[3] Although data on the prevalence of CVD in earlier stages of CKD in young patients is limited,[4] mortality of children in the United States on maintenance dialysis is mainly due to CVD.

Chavers and colleagues[5] have performed a retrospective assessment of CVD in a large pediatric dialysis population of 1454 children observed during 1991 through 1996. Of these, 452 (31.3%) had a cardiac-related event. The percentage was close to 25% in patients aged 0 to 14 years, but 36.9% in patients aged 15 to 19 years. Arrhythmia was the most frequent cardiac event, followed by valvular disease, cardiomyopathy, and cardiac arrest. This study clearly demonstrated that cardiac events (including death from CVD) can be observed in all age groups of children and adolescents on dialysis. Altogether, 38% of the total death rate (7.4%) was due to cardiac complications.

Similarly, cardiac death is the leading cause of death after transplantation. Cross-sectional studies of young adults with childhood-onset ESRD have found a cardiac death rate of 35% in U.S. children transplanted at ages 0 to 19 years.[6] In a study by the Hannover group of 150 German children transplanted between 1970 and 1993, patient mortality from CVD was 23%—almost 10 times as high as the occurrence of malignancies.[7] In studies including both dialyzed and transplanted young adults with childhood-onset ESRD, mortality was due to CVD in respectively 32% (Charité Berlin[8]) and 50% (University of Heidelberg[9]) of the total mortality.

In a retrospective Dutch national survey, cardiac death was the most prevalent form of death 10 years after successful renal transplantation (with a rate of 33%).[10] A 40-year retrospective analysis of long-term survival from the Australia and New Zealand Dialysis and Transplant Registry[11] of all children and adolescents who were under 20 years of age when RRT commenced showed mortality rates 30 times higher than in age-matched controls in the general population. CVD was the most common cause of death (45%).

Death from CVD was further analyzed in a large retrospective survey of children treated with dialysis and transplantation during 1990 through 1996 in the United States.[12] Altogether, 1380 deaths were observed among patients who started ESRD therapy as children and died before 30 years of age. Cardiovascular death accounted for 23% of deaths. Black patients carried a significantly higher risk of cardiac death than white patients among all age groups. Transplant recipients had a significantly lower risk (by an average of 78%) of cardiac death than dialysis patients. Thus, among black patients the cardiac death rate was 21.4 per 1000 patient-years on dialysis and 2.1 per 1000 patient-years after transplantation. Among white patients, it was 20.5 per 1000 patient-years on dialysis and 1.3 per 1000 patient-years after transplantation.

Taken together, these data show that CVD is worldwide the largest obstacle to long-term survival of children and adolescents with CKD. Mortality is excessively high on dialysis, and continues to be a threat after renal transplantation.

Young versus Elderly

Importantly, the term *cardiac death* may include several diagnostic categories, such as cardiac arrest, arrhythmia, myocardial infarction, valvular heart disease, cardiomyopathy, and so on. Although it is common to group these diagnoses, this may obscure the issue. The diagnosis of arrhythmia could be due to hyperkalemia (possibly due to noncompliance, dietary mistakes, acidosis, insufficient dialysis, and the like) or to coronary artery disease or other causes. Therefore, diagnostic categories do not necessarily permit conclusions regarding the pathogenesis of CVD events.

In a detailed analysis of death from any cause ($n = 326$) over a 5-year period among European children aged less than 15 years treated with dialysis or transplantation, 16.9% were cardiac deaths. An additional 7.4% of deaths were attributed to "cardiac arrest, cause unknown," and 9.5% were attributed to vascular mortality (mainly cerebrovascular). Of note, only 2 of the 326 patients died of confirmed myocardial infarction, whereas cardiac death in the majority was associated with hyperkalemia, fluid overload, hypertensive cardiac failure, or other causes.[13] Even if some cases of cardiac arrest of unknown cause were due to myocardial infarction, this diagnosis seems to apply to only a small subgroup of young patients in mortality statistics.

Using the United States Renal Data System (USRDS) database, Parekh et al.[12] performed a detailed cross-sectional analysis to evaluate the causes of cardiac death in children and young adults aged 0 to 30 years. Of the specific categories of cardiovascular deaths, cardiac arrest was the most common cause in each of the age groups—followed by arrhythmia and cardiomyopathy. The incidence of cardiac arrest in the youngest age group (0-4 years) was 5 to 10 times higher than in other age groups. This was, as noted by the authors, perhaps a reflection of the difficulty of ascertaining the true cause of death in young children. Some of these young children might have died from other comorbid conditions, such as congenital disorders not included in the USRDS database.

The high rate of sudden death in children, especially in infants with ESRD, is poorly understood and warrants further investigation. In adults, sudden death is often a result of fatal arrhythmias due to acute ischemia of preexisting atherosclerotic disease. It is believed that arrhythmias are also the likely cause of most cases of sudden cardiac death (SCD) in children. However, the origin of acquired malignant arrhythmias in children is unlikely to be an atherosclerotic lesion. Dilated hypertrophic cardiomyopathies in particular are a leading cause of SCD in children.[14]

The macroscopic and microscopic structural abnormalities in cardiomyopathies involve fibrosis and cellular hypertrophy and predispose to an electrical instability with resultant arrhythmias. Ischemia of small coronary vessels secondary to medial hypertrophy might result in dispersion of repolarization properties and arrhythmia from reentrant or autonomic mechanisms. As we discuss in more detail further in this chapter, many children with CKD develop left ventricular hypertrophy (LVH)—which is frequently severe, especially in children on prolonged dialysis therapy.[15,16]

It is currently unknown if LVH in young patients with CKD is characterized by structural abnormalities similar to familial or idiopathic hypertrophic cardiomyopathies associated with SCD. To what extent LVH can contribute to an increased risk for SCD in children with CKD is also not known. Deadly arrhythmias in children with ESRD could also be evoked by acute changes in the cardiac extracellular or intracellular ionic milieu, especially involving abnormalities of sodium- and potassium-based repolarization currents.

In contrast, ischemic heart disease is a major cause of death in adult dialysis patients, with 22% of cardiac deaths attributed to acute myocardial infarction.[17] The average age of dialysis patients in the United States is currently 58.2 years (www.usrds.org). The high prevalence of death from CVD in this population, especially in patients with diabetes,[18] clearly indicates advanced cardiac and vascular disease. In a retrospective survey (1977-1995) of the USRDS database, there were 34,189 dialysis patients with acute myocardial infarction. The rate of in-hospital death was 26%. The all-cause mortality was 59% at 1 year and 73% at 2 years. The 1- and 2-year cardiac mortality was 41% and 52%, respectively.[17] Therefore, ischemic heart disease and myocardial infarction are typical complications of CVD in elderly patients with CKD and carry a dismal prognosis. In contrast, young patients as a rule have no symptoms of ischemic heart disease (such as angina pectoris) and no myocardial infarction. Instead, they remain asymptomatic.

Could this imply that ischemic heart disease is silent and therefore underdiagnosed? Silent myocardial ischemia is frequently found in patients with CKD, especially during dialysis.[19] Myocardial infarction may also be disguised, as has been noted in younger women (who may have significantly different symptoms at initial presentation).[20] There is a paucity of studies regarding electrocardiogram monitoring in children with CKD, but circadian rhythms of blood pressure and heart rate are altered in children with hypertensive chronic renal failure.[21] There are no systematic autopsy studies in young patients with CKD focusing on vascular and coronary pathology. Therefore, the lack of symptomatic ischemic heart disease in young patients and paucity of cardiac deaths due to confirmed myocardial infarction remains an important observation. However, it is presently unknown whether absence of symptoms truly implies absence of advanced vascular and cardiac disease.

The Heart/Kidney Connection

Recent epidemiologic studies in adult patients have demonstrated that with a decrease in glomerular filtration rate (GFR) there is an incremental increase in the standardized rate for CVD events, hospitalizations, and death from any cause. These data, collected from more than a million ambulatory visits of adult patients, showed that the age-adjusted death rate from CVD events was almost 20 times higher in patients with a GFR below 15 than with a GFR greater than 60. Hospitalization rates were 10 times higher, and the rate of death from any cause was 15 times higher.[22]

Although these data were based on serum-creatinine–based GFR estimations, the use of cystatin-C–based formulas may be an equal or better predictor of CVD risk[23] (especially in the elderly).[24] Thus, renal disease in all age groups seems to be an important risk factor for the development of CVD, and (analogous to the linear and continuous relationship of serum cholesterol levels and coronary artery disease) the serum creatinine level has been termed the "cholesterol of the twenty-first century." Altogether, these epidemiologic data suggest that there is a "heart/kidney connection" or "cardiorenal syndrome."

The link has been further strengthened by recent data showing the influence of proteinuria on CVD and on all-cause mortality. In a study of the Japanese general population involving almost 100,000 participants aged 40 to 79 years participating in annual health checkups, proteinuria was an independent predictor of CVD and all-cause mortality. For individuals with proteinuria and reduced GFR, the risk for CVD death was twofold higher in men and fourfold to sixfold higher in women.[25]

Finally, it now appears possible that de novo heart and kidney disease result from similar risk factors. Researchers involved in the Framingham study have recently found that the presence of the traditional risk factors (for atherosclerosis) actually predicts new-onset kidney disease in this community-based population survey. In a longitudinal cohort study involving 2585 participants (who attended both a baseline examination during 1978 through 1982 and a follow-up examination during 1998 through 2001 and who were free of kidney disease at baseline), traditional risk factors for CVD (i.e., age, male sex, baseline GFR, body mass index, smoking, diabetes) at baseline examination were indeed significant predictors of new-onset kidney disease during follow-up.

In addition, hypertension, cholesterol, and impaired fasting glucose tolerance were significant individual predictors. However, these were not included in the multivariate model.[26] Interestingly, the number of risk factors at baseline had a cumulative effect on the risk for CKD. In a separate study, the glycemic status as assessed by an oral glucose tolerance test was predictive in an incremental manner for the development of CKD during a follow-up of 7 years.[27] These data have led to a renewed appreciation of classical risk factors as the driving force for the development of de novo heart and kidney disease.

RISK FACTORS

In the general population, CVD in most patients is the result of atherosclerosis. Atherosclerosis is a multifactorial disease affecting the heart and large and medium-size arteries, with a focal distribution and with the characteristic appearance of lipid-rich plaques in the intima of the arterial wall. Clinical manifestations include coronary heart disease, cerebrovascular disease, aortic aneurysm, and peripheral arterial occlusive disease.

This disease is slowly progressive over several decades. Atherosclerosis has a multifactorial pathogenesis, but the occurrence of the disease is associated with typical risk factors: dyslipidemia, hypertension, smoking, male gender, diabetes, abdominal obesity, and lack of physical activity. This rule seems almost universal, as recently documented in the Interheart study—a case-control study of acute myocardial infarction in 52 countries. Remarkably, these traditional risk factors (in combination with psychosocial factors, consumption of fruits, vegetables, and alcohol) accounted for 90% of the attributable risk in men and 94% in women—indicating their worldwide predictive value irrespective of gender, race, or region.[28]

CKD has been appropriately described as a "vasculopathic state"[29] because of the extraordinary risk indicated by the accumulation of numerous risk factors. The occurrence and prevalence of these risk factors have been exhaustively described.[30-32] Traditional risk factors (for atherosclerosis), nontraditional (uremic) risk factors, and cardiomyopathy (a risk factor in itself) most likely act synergistically—resulting in altered vascular and cardiac structure and function in CKD.[33]

The question remains: What risk factors have the most clinical relevance for patients with CKD? Obviously, the answer can only come from prospective cohort studies. In adults, the respective role of traditional and novel risk factors for CVD in patients with CKD has been recently examined.[34] A total of 5808 persons aged 65 years or older participated in the Cardiovascular Health Study cohort. The average length of follow-up was 8.6 years. The cardiovascular mortality risk rate was 32 deaths per 1000 person-years among those with chronic kidney disease versus 16 per 1000 person-years among those without.

In multivariate analyses, diabetes, systolic hypertension, smoking, low physical activity, nonuse of alcohol, and LVH were predictors of cardiovascular mortality in persons with chronic kidney disease. Among the novel risk factors, only C-reactive protein and interleukin 6 were significantly associated with outcome—and the inclusion of novel risk factors in a multivariate model added almost no predictive value. Thus, in these elderly patients with CKD traditional risk factors had much stronger associations with cardiovascular mortality than novel risk factors.

Risk Factor Principles and Caveats

The introduction of the concept of risk factors for CVD in the 1960s was an important advance in epidemiology. As a public health principle, risk factors are established causes of a disease (at a given level predictive of a disease). If they are reduced, disease outcome can be modified. Recently, these principles have been somewhat diluted in that any association with the occurrence of CVD found in observational studies has been called a risk factor. At one time, a total of 246 risk factors were thus collected.[35]

This abundance of risk factors may actually pose a problem for the clinician. Which are truly important and which should or can be treated? Moreover, there is often lack of evidence of a predictive value for disease outcome—and moreover for modifying disease outcome with treatment of the risk factor. For example, hyperhomocysteinemia is a prevalent nontraditional risk factor independently associated with CVD in dialysis patients.[36] However, no trials have yet demonstrated a beneficial effect of lowering homocysteine values on cardiac mortality or surrogate end points for CVD. Although these trials may have been underpowered (necessitating large-scale prospective multicenter studies),[37] treatment failure may have many other explanations—including patient variability and comorbidity, drug pharmacology, target blood levels, and the like. However, the relationship between elevated plasma homocysteine levels and mortality from CVD may have to be reexamined.[38]

To make things more complicated, many risk factors with clearly established predictive value in the general population have been observed to behave differently in special populations (e.g., patients with congestive heart failure, with advanced age, malignancy, or CKD). Studies in these groups showed changes in the normal relation between risk factors and clinical outcomes, varying from major alterations from the relations found in the general population to a complete mirror-image reversal. The phenomenon has been termed *risk factor reversal* or *reverse epidemiology*.[39]

As an example of the phenomenon, octogenarians were found to have high circulating Lp(a) levels. Patients with congestive heart failure had better survival with a higher body mass index. Among dialysis patients, obesity, hypercholesterolemia, and hypertension appear to be protective (i.e., associated with a longer survival).[38] The phenomenon of reverse epidemiology is presently not fully explained, but it has been hypothesized that the combination of protein-energy malnutrition, chronic inflammatory state, and oxidative stress could be responsible.[40] The clinical implications from these findings are wide ranging. Optimal blood pressure, body weight, and serum concentrations of risk factors (as well as target levels for interventional studies) may need to be redefined in patients with CKD.

It is presently unclear if these arguments apply to subgroups (e.g., patients with confirmed presence of the malnutrition-inflammation complex) or to these special populations as a whole. Nevertheless, therapeutic studies are probably affected at large by reverse epidemiology or other risk factor interactions that are as yet unknown. The recent 4-D study may serve as an example. In this randomized double-blind prospective study of 1255 subjects with type 2 diabetes mellitus receiving maintenance hemodialysis, patients were randomly assigned to receive 20 mg of atorvastatin per day or placebo. The composite primary end point of this study was cardiovascular death, nonfatal myocardial infarction, and stroke. For all of these end points, statins have a beneficial class effect in the general population.[41]

Unexpectedly, atorvastatin had no statistically significant effect on the composite primary end point.[18] The failure of statins to reduce cardiovascular mortality in diabetic hemodialysis patients has been attributed to the timing of the intervention (i.e., at a too advanced stage of established CVD).[18] The average age of patients in the study was 65 years. Significant comorbidity is present in this age group, even at the initiation of dialysis treatment.[1] As exemplified by this study, it is unknown whether medical interventions (such as statins, lipid-lowering or antioxidant therapy, folate substitution, or other therapeutic trials) might be more successful in younger populations. Although such patients (under age 40) constitute a minority in most hemodialysis units, they might indeed have the greatest survival benefit.

Children and adolescents with CKD harbor a multitude of risk factors for CVD that at this age seems without parallel.[42] The overall effect of these risk factors and their relative contribution to morbidity and mortality in young patients is yet unknown. Prospective studies with "hard" end points (cardiac and vascular events) in this age group are difficult if not impossible to perform. On the other hand, the analysis of risk factors in elderly patients may be obscured by comorbid conditions such as diabetes, preexisting atherosclerosis, or reverse epidemiology. In this respect, studies in young patients may provide a diagnostic window to the evolution of CVD in uremia.

Noninvasive Studies of CVD in Young Adults with Childhood-Onset ESRD

Cross-sectional studies (of young adults with childhood-onset CKD) evaluating cardiac and vascular properties (structures and functions) with noninvasive methods have provided important insights into the prevalence and clinical significance of risk factors for CVD in young patients. The major limitations of these studies are their retrospective nature and a variable exposure time to CKD/ESRD and to different forms of RRT (dialysis, transplantation).

TABLE 51-1 Carotid Intimal-Medial Thickness in Young ESRD Patients

Author	Year	*n* Patients (D/TX)	Age (Years)
Oh[9]	2002	39 (13/26)	19-39
Groothoff[43]	2002	130 (29/101)	21-41
Mitsnefes[46]	2005	60 (44 CKD, 16 D)	6-21
Litwin[45]	2005	126 (55 CKD, 37 D, 34 TX)	10-20
Briese[8]	2005	40 (9/31)	18-39

Vascular and Cardiac Parameters

In a Holland nationwide study, Groothoff and colleagues[43] were the first to systematically collect data on vascular and cardiac abnormalities in a population with a mean age of 29.0 (20.7 to 40.6) years. Compared with controls, patients (n = 130) had no significant changes in intima-medial thickness (IMT) (Table 51-1) but did have reduced parameters of arterial elasticity of the carotid artery—such as mean arterial wall distensibility, increased stiffness parameter beta, and increased elastic incremental [E(inc)] modulus.

In 140 patients in the same study, left ventricular mass index (LVMI) exceeded 150 g/m^2 in 47% of all male patients and 120 g/m^2 in 39% of all female patients—both consistent with LVH. Diastolic dysfunction [low ratio of maximal early (E wave) and late (A wave) diastolic flow velocities (E/A)] was found in 18 (13%) patients. Twenty-seven patients (19%) had aortic valve calcification. A high LVMI was associated with a current high blood pressure and male gender, and a low E/A ratio was associated with aging and a lower GFR (<25 ml/min/1.73 m^2). Aortic valve calcification was associated with prolonged peritoneal dialysis.[44]

In a study of 39 young adults (mean age of 27 years) treated in Heidelberg, Oh et al.[9] found a significantly increased IMT associated with cumulative dialysis and ESRD time and the cumulative serum calcium and phosphate product. The Berlin Group studied arterial and cardiac changes in 40 young adults (mean age 23.6 years) and analyzed associations with risk factors and prescribed medications.[8] Although the IMT was not significantly different from controls, postischemic blood flow as measured by venous occlusion plethysmography of the lower extremity was reduced by a mean of 40% (Figure 51-1).

LVH was present in 25 patients (62.5%), left ventricular diastolic dysfunction was present in 22.5%, and systolic function was normal in all but one patient. In this study, morphologic alterations of the heart and arteries were significantly correlated with the duration of ESRD and dialysis time, and with the cumulative intake of calcium-containing phosphate binders and active vitamin D preparations. Functional changes

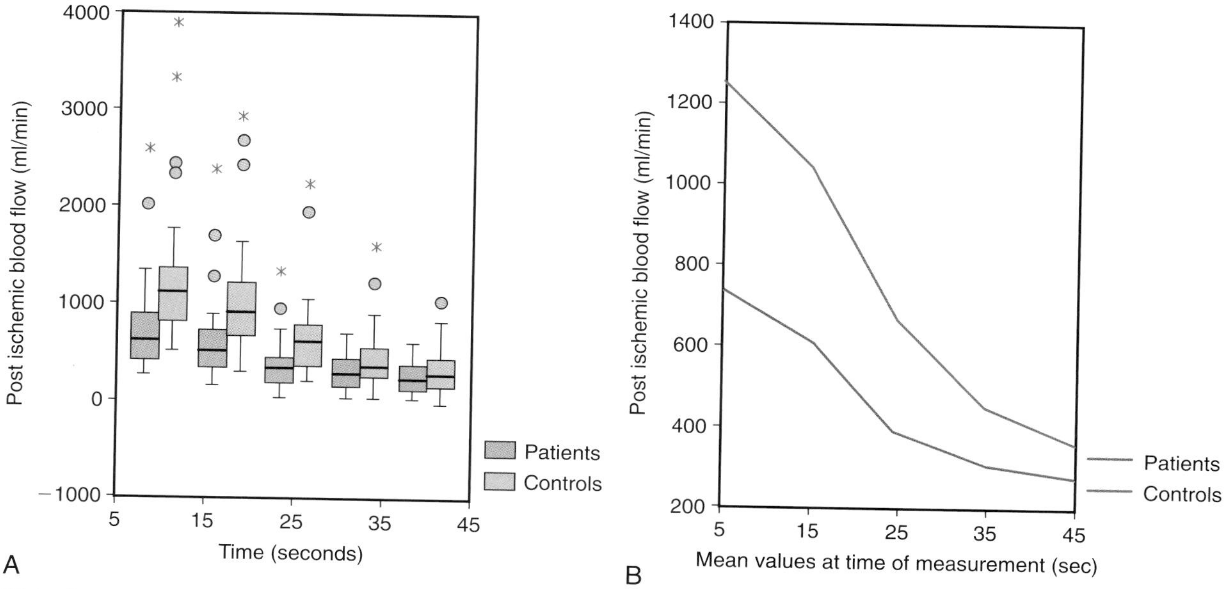

Figure 51-1 Postischemic vascular reactivity. **A,** Box plots of measurements of postischemic blood flow in the right leg, measured by venous occlusion plethysmography. Time period (1-5) corresponding to 10-second intervals after release of the cuff. Patients and controls showed significant differences in blood flow at all time points ($p = 0.0001$). **B,** Mean postischemic blood flow curves, constructed from original data (plot A). Height ($p = 0.00003$) and slope ($p = 0.0021$) of the curves show significant differences in patients and controls. (From Briese S, Wiesner S, Will JC, et al: Arterial and cardiac disease in young adults with childhood-onset end-stage renal disease-impact of calcium and vitamin D therapy, *Nephrol Dial Transplant* 21(7):1906-14, 2006.)

(vascular reactivity) were correlated with the duration of ESRD and with nontraditional risk factors.

Litwin et al.[45] measured carotid and femoral IMT in 55 children with stages II through IV CKD (37 children on dialysis and 34 after renal transplantation). Both carotid and femoral IMT were significantly increased in all patient groups, and most markedly abnormal in dialysis patients. Carotid IMT correlated with mean past serum calcium phosphorus (Ca × P) product, the cumulative dose of calcium-based phosphate binders, and the time-averaged mean calcitriol dose.

Mitsnefes et al.[46] also showed that children with mild to moderate CKD and on dialysis had greater carotid IMT than the controls. In their study, children on dialysis had greater IMT and arterial stiffness [E(inc)] than CKD patients and controls. Calcium-phosphorus product predicted increased IMT, and increased serum phosphorus and iPTH predicted increased arterial stiffness.

Taken together, these studies have revealed several important clues to the evolution of vascular and cardiac changes in ESRD: (1) the presence of early systemic CVD involving conduit arteries (aorta, carotid artery; IMT), muscular arteries (femoral artery; IMT), peripheral resistance vessels (venous occlusion plethysmography), and the heart (echocardiography); (2) a profound decrease in postischemic vascular reactivity and evidence for vascular stiffness; (3) the occurrence of calcifications in coronary arteries (see material following) and heart valves; (4) no association of vascular and cardiac abnormalities with classical risk factors except hypertension; and (5) significant correlations of these changes with disturbances of calcium and phosphorus metabolism and therapeutic interventions (specifically, the cumulative intake of calcium-containing phosphate binders and vitamin D preparations).

Coronary Artery Calcifications

Following the groundbreaking study of Braun et al.,[47] which demonstrated progressive coronary artery calcification (CAC) in adult dialysis patients, six studies have investigated coronary calcifications by EBCT (electron beam computed tomography) and spiral CT specifically in young patients with childhood-onset CKD[8,9,48-51] (Table 51-2). Although the percentage of patients with calcifications was quite variable (10%, 15%, 36%, 46%, 47%, and 92%), some of the calcium scores were remarkably high. In the study by Goodman et al.,[48] calcifications were associated with the calcium intake from phosphate binders, the calcium-phosphorus product, age, and the mean duration of dialysis.

In the Heidelberg study,[9] 92% of patients had CAC and 19% valve calcifications. Coronary calcium scores were strongly correlated with C-reactive protein (CRP) and *Chlamydia pneumoniae* seropositivity, time-averaged mean serum parathyroid hormone (PTH), and plasma homocysteine. In the Berlin study,[8] patients with CAC were older, had longer treatment times with dialysis, and a twofold to threefold higher intake of calcium and of active vitamin D metabolites than patients without CAC. Civilibal et al.[51] screened 53 patients (mean age 15.7 years) with ESRD for the presence and predisposing factors of CAC. CAC was present in 15% of patients (three hemodialysis patients, three peritoneal dialysis patients, and two renal transplant recipients). The patients with CAC had longer duration of total dialysis and higher time-integrated serum phosphorus levels, calcium-phosphate product, intact parathyroid hormone, vitamin B12 levels, and amount of cumulative dose of calcium-containing oral phosphate binders.

These studies indicate a varying prevalence of vascular calcifications in young adults with ESRD and a correlation

TABLE 51-2 **Coronary Artery Calcifications in Young ESRD Patients**

Author	Year of Publication	*n* (Patients) (D/TX)	Age (Years)	Method	Result (Positive)
Eifinger[49]	2000	16 (4/12)	14-39	EBCT	6/13 (46%)
Goodman[48]	2000	39 (39/0)	7-30	EBCT	14/39 (36%)
Oh[9]	2002	39 (13/26)	19-39	Spiral CT	37/39 (92%)
Ishitani[50]	2005	19 (0/19)	21-48	EBCT	9/19 (47%)
Briese[8]	2006	40 (9/31)	18-39	EBCT	10/40 (10%)
Civilibal[51]	2006	53 (39/14)	11-21	Spiral CT	8/53 (15%)

with the presence of nontraditional risk factors (e.g., a high calcium-phosphorus product, high PTH levels, and markers of inflammation/infection). They also suggested that the current treatment of renal osteodystrophy in children with calcium-containing phosphate binders and active vitamin D preparations is associated in a dose-dependent manner with CAC—a surrogate marker for advanced CVD.[52] The clinical suspicion that massive calcium deposits in the coronary artery may carry a grave prognosis has been confirmed by a prospective study of 110 adult hemodialysis patients. The presence and extent of vascular calcifications were strong predictors of cardiovascular and all-cause mortality.[53] However, it is yet unknown to what extent the finding of CAC translates into cardiac morbidity and mortality in young patients.

The presence of such a significant amount of calcium in coronary artery lesions is extremely unusual in young patients. In the natural history of atherosclerosis, the occurrence of arterial calcification as a major part of arterial lesions is a "late event" in the general population. We know from autopsy studies of young subjects (under the age of 40) with accidental death that calcium deposits emerge as granules of microscopic size in advanced lesions (type IV), which are only present in a minority of these subjects. Advanced lesions containing large amounts of calcium do not appear until the fifth decade of life.[54] This should be taken as further evidence of a uremia-related specific form of (coronary) arteriopathy.[33]

In adult patients with CKD, the presence of CAC has also been associated with age and measures of arterial stiffness.[53,55] Arterial stiffness, measured at the common carotid artery[56] or the aorta,[57] is a marker of the extent of coronary artery disease and an independent predictor of survival in adult dialysis patients.[58] Although prospective studies linking vascular function to survival in children have not been performed, it may be safe to say that the presence of CAC in young patients (being regarded as a marker of advanced CVD in adult CKD patients) indicates severe vascular involvement resembling advanced vascular aging. Such patients should be closely monitored for progression, and efforts should be made to lower exposure to CVD risk factors. Recent studies in adults indicate that patients with CAC may benefit from treatment with calcium-free phosphate binders.[59,60]

In the study by Oh et al.,[9] the presence of CAC was closely correlated with CRP. In a multivariate analysis, CRP and plasma homocysteine levels remained as independent predictors in a model (together with iPTH and the calcium-phosphate product), explaining 75% of the variation in CAC. This indicates that inflammatory processes play a major role in the pathogenesis of these vascular changes. CRP levels are significant predictors of mortality in adult hemodialysis patients.[61]

Interestingly, a recent study in 312 adult hemodialysis patients has identified a potential link between inflammation and calcification. Ketteler et al.[62] demonstrated a significant association of survival on dialysis with fetuin-A serum concentrations. Fetuin is a circulating inhibitor of calcification in vivo and is downregulated during the acute phase response. It is conceivable that persistently low concentrations of this glycoprotein during chronic low-grade inflammation in uremic patients could facilitate calcification, and this notion is further supported by the observation of an impaired ex vivo capacity (of sera from patients with low fetuin concentrations) to inhibit calcium phosphate precipitation.[62] Further studies are needed to clarify the role of fetuin among the multiple pathways leading to vascular damage by inflammatory mechanisms in uremia.[63]

Whether arterial calcifications can regress is an unresolved issue. Studies investigating the physicochemical properties of calcified arteries have found that calcium (in human atherosclerotic lesions and in experimental models of uremic animals with calcitriol- and hyperphosphatemia-induced calcifications) is mainly deposited in the form of hydroxyapatite.[64] This process occurs also in biologic mineralization, such as in bone formation. A recent study in rats (with normal renal function) indicates the potential reversibility of medial calcifications induced by calcitriol treatment.[65]

Regression of atherosclerotic calcifications, however, has not been demonstrated thus far in humans. In animal experiments with monkeys fed a high-cholesterol atherogenic diet for several years (resulting in advanced intima lesions) followed by years of a low-cholesterol diet, regression of lesions was observed—with disappearance of macrophages and lipid and foam cells but not of calcium.[54] Clinical studies with EBCT follow-up have shown that progression of CAC may be attenuated (in patients treated with calcium-free phosphate binders), but have not shown regression.[66]

One should be reminded that calcifications may not be confined to the coronary arteries. In 1990, Milliner et al.[67] published the first systematic study on the prevalence and distribution of soft-tissue calcifications in pediatric patients with ESRD. These authors retrospectively reviewed clinical, biochemical, and autopsy data of 120 patients treated between 1960 and 1983. Soft-tissue calcifications were found in 72 of 120 patients (60%), and most frequently involved blood vessels, lung, kidney, myocardium, coronary arteries, central nervous system, and gastric mucosa. This report revealed for the first time the extent of organ involvement (and especially cardiovascular damage caused by calcifications) at a young age in patients with ESRD.

Thus, disturbances in calcium and phosphorus metabolism (hypercalcemia, hyperphosphatemia, elevations in the Ca-x-P product, and PTH levels) and the treatment of renal osteodystrophy with phosphate binders and vitamin D preparations have emerged as major risk factors for CVD in children and adolescents—showing much stronger associations with calcifications and other surrogate markers of CVD than conventional risk factors in young patients. For this reason, it is worth considering potential mechanisms explaining these associations.

CVD AND TREATMENT OF RENAL OSTEODYSTROPHY

Calcium

Urinary calcium excretion in normal adults is about 200 mg/day (5 mmol/day). Fecal excretion varies depending on dietary intake, but calcium balance is positive in healthy subjects <35 years of age. Calcium excretion diminishes with deterioration of GFR. Adults with ESRD, with a calculated intake of dietary calcium of 1000 mg/d (25 mmol/day), have a positive calcium balance of about 250 mg (6.25 mmol)/week.[68] If this is extrapolated to pediatric patients, who have a much higher intake of dietary calcium from food (and higher calcium requirements for bone growth), the net positive balance in ESRD might be much higher—assuming similar calcium absorption.

In the absence of firm data on the physiologic requirements of calcium in uremic children, it is difficult to estimate the true positive calcium balance. In addition, calcium intake from phosphate binders is comparatively higher in children. On a milligram-per-kilogram basis, the recommended dose for adults (calcium carbonate) is about 40 to 80 mg/kg (1-2 mmol/kg). In children, it is 50 to 200 mg/kg (1.25-5 mmol/kg). In clinical studies, adults have received about 70 mg/kg/day (1.75 mmol/kg/day) of calcium carbonate or acetate.[69] Children have received 110 mg/kg/day (range 10-340) or 2.75 mmol/kg/day (range 0.25-8.5).[70]

Depending on the dialysate used, calcium balance is also positive on maintenance dialysis—ranging from 52 to 536 mg/day (1.3-13.4 mmol/day) in adult hemodialysis patients and from 32 to 208 mg/day (0.8-5.2 mmol/day) in peritoneal dialysis patients, respectively.[68] In addition, hypercalcemic episodes (which occur with an overall incidence of 3.5 per 100 patient-months in children with calcium carbonate treatment[70]) should be considered periods of high positive calcium balance. It is of interest that in a retrospective study concerning the safety and efficacy of calcium carbonate these hypercalcemic episodes were associated with a reversible decline in GFR in 62% of patients.[70]

A high calcium-phosphorus product in animal models is associated with calcifications in the kidney and deterioration of GFR.[71] Finally, one has to consider the additive effect of vitamin D metabolites. It is well known that intestinal calcium resorption is regulated by active vitamin D. It can be expected that the concomitant use of vitamin D preparations dramatically increases calcium absorption in uremic patients, although studies of calcium balance in children with ESRD are lacking.

Phosphorus

Normal levels of Ca and P are higher in healthy infants and young children, and the "physiologic" range of Ca × P at a given age in patients with CKD is unknown. Nevertheless, both the observed increase in PTH levels accompanying a decrease in GFR and (vice versa) the decrease of PTH levels with dietary phosphorus restriction observed in children with moderate renal failure[72] permit the conclusion that a positive P balance and/or hyperphosphatemia is one of the driving forces of the development of secondary hyperparathyroidism and renal osteodystrophy.

Seventy percent of adult patients have elevated phosphorus levels on dialysis, and mortality increases linearly with increasing serum phosphorus levels.[73] The overall positive phosphorus balance, assuming 800 to 1000 mg/day (32.3 mmol/day) of dietary intake of phosphorus, has been calculated as 1200 mg/week (39 mmol/week) in hemodialysis patients.[68] The problem of hyperphosphatemia in clinical practice is likely to be even more pronounced in pediatric patients. In young children, the recommended P intake is much higher per kilogram of body weight than in adolescents or adults because protein requirements are higher and nutrition is mainly provided by milk or milk-based formulas and dairy products. Because most pediatric CKD patients also have to be treated with active vitamin D preparations to prevent rickets and severe renal osteodystrophy in the growing skeleton, the positive P balance is probably further increased because of upregulated intestinal P resorption. However, this remains to be proven.

Hyperphosphatemia has been shown to contribute to the pathogenesis of CVD by various mechanisms. One is by driving secondary *hyperparathyroidism*. The hyperparathyroid state contributes to CVD by noxious effects on blood pressure, cardiac contractility, cardiomyocyte functioning, and cardiac remodeling and by enhancing various pro-atherosclerotic mechanisms.[74] Another mechanism increases the risk of arterial *calcifications* via elevations in the Ca × P product by *direct effects* on cells in the arterial wall.

In vitro studies have shown that increased phosphorus concentrations in the culture medium can produce a change of vascular smooth muscle cells toward an osteoblastic phenotype, giving these cells the potential of osteoid formation.[75] Proteins involved in bone mineralization were also detected in calcified and uncalcified areas of arteries of uremic patients.[76] In view of the importance of calcium and phosphorus concentrations in blood, the regulatory role of vitamin D on these minerals deserves special consideration.

Vitamin D

In clinical practice, vascular calcifications are probably occurring in two types of situations: in periods of a *high calcium-phosphorus product in serum* [e.g., severe hyperparathyroidism with mobilization of calcium and phosphate from bone (high bone turnover)], often accompanied by the attempt to control the PTH secretion with high doses of calcitriol (enhancing at the same time calcium and phosphate resorption), and (2) periods of low bone turnover, largely induced by *oversuppression of PTH secretion* with active vitamin D metabolites and accompanied by hypercalcemia. It is conceivable that in these situations the arterial wall is taking up calcium that is either mobilized from bone or cannot be metabolized by bone.

Active vitamin D metabolites (e.g., calcitriol) could promote vascular calcifications not only by increasing intestinal calcium and phosphorus absorption, or by arresting calcium delivery to bone (low bone turnover), but by having direct effects on the vascular wall. Indeed, it has been shown in animal experiments (5/6 nephrectomized rats) that treatment with calcitriol for 6 weeks induced systemic CVD—including severe arterial calcifications in the absence of hypercalcemia or an elevated Ca × P product.[77]

Recent studies have shown that the process of mineralization is highly regulated in smooth muscle cells, the main cell type of the media. It seems that this process results from the balance of many factors either promoting or preventing mineralization, and under normal conditions is essentially inhibited.[78] Under calcifying conditions, however, vascular smooth muscle cells can undergo a phenotypic transition to osteoblast-like cells—expressing several genes involved in osteogenesis. With transition, these cells express the core binding factor alpha 1 (Cbfa1)—an osteoblast-specific transcription factor regulating the expression of multiple genes in the osteoblast.[79] In vitro, an increase in extracellular phosphorus[80] and uremic serum[81] is able to induce calcium deposition, increased expression of Cbfa1, and an osteoblast phenotype. This could lead the way to the secretion of an osteoid-like extracellular matrix (i.e., bone formation in the arterial wall).

Vascular smooth muscle cells express the vitamin D receptor and upregulate the receptor if excessive doses of calcitriol are administered to animals. In vitro, calcitriol increases expression of alkaline phosphatase (an enzyme involved in osteogenesis) and calcium deposition in these cells.[80] However, calcitriol does not seem to promote calcification by upregulation of Cbfa1 but by modulating secretion of PTH-RP[80] or by other yet unknown mechanisms (e.g., upregulation of other promoters or downregulation of inhibitors). In addition, calcitriol promotes migration of rat aortic smooth muscle cells in vitro—a further potential mechanism contributing to vascular remodeling.[82]

Endothelial Dysfunction

Endothelial dysfunction (ED) is characterized by a reduced bioavailability of vasodilators [in particular, nitric oxide (NO)], whereas endothelium-derived contracting factors are increased—leading to impaired endothelium-dependent vasodilatation. Disturbed endothelial functions are a hallmark of CKD and may be a common final pathway of various disturbances in metabolic, hormonal, and cell signaling (Figure 51-2)—leading to the acquisition of a proinflammatory, prothrombogenic, and proatherogenic endothelial cell phenotype.[83]

This attractive hypothesis regards ED as an "integrated index of all atherogenic and atheroprotective factors" and as the "ultimate risk of the risk factors"[84] and proposes the endothelium as a promising target for medical interventions. However, clinical assessment of patients remains unsatisfactory—reflecting the lack of well-established criteria for the diagnosis of ED. Hypertension, macro- and microvasculopathy, impaired synthesis of protective plasmatic factors (e.g., von Willebrand factor), vascular inflammatory changes,

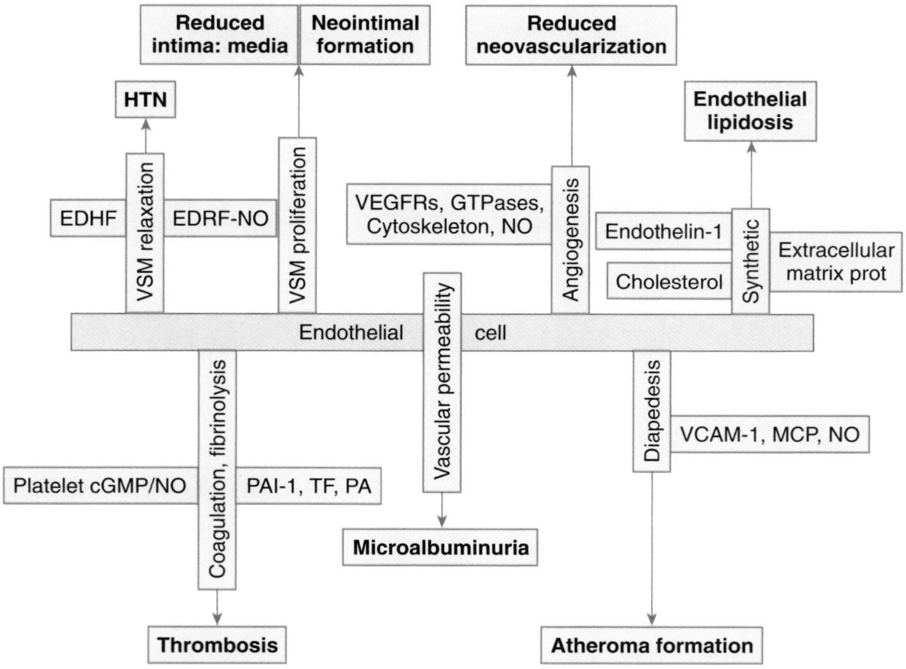

Figure 51-2 Endothelial dysfunction as a hypothetical common final pathway in CVD. (From Moe SM, Duan D, Doehle BP, O'Neill KD, Chen NX: Uremia induces the osteoblast differentiation factor Cbfa1 in human blood vessels, *Kidney Int* 63(3):1003-11, 2003.)

increased vascular permeability manifesting as microalbuminuria, and other syndromes may all be caused by (or reflect the presence of) ED.[83]

In clinical practice, endothelial function has been measured mainly by endothelium-dependent vasodilatation at the brachial artery. Although this method (reflecting vasodilatation of conduit arteries) has found widespread use, it is highly observer dependent and has limited reproducibility[85] and large within-subject variability.[86] Other methods include postischemic reactive hyperemia measured at the forearm[87] or the lower extremity[8] (reflecting vascular reactivity of resistance vessels) and laser Doppler flowmetry assessment of cutaneous blood flow, reflecting cutaneous microvascular function.[88] Severely diminished responses to ischemia can be demonstrated with all methods in patients with CKD.

ED is also associated with arterial stiffness.[89] In the general population, arterial stiffness is closely related to aging and is an independent predictor of mortality. It is regulated by a number of factors, including vascular smooth muscle tone. Recent studies have shown an association of endothelial function (flow-mediated dilatation of the brachial artery) with measurements of arterial stiffness (i.e., pulse pressure, pulse wave velocity, and augmentation index) in healthy individuals.[90] These methods have been widely applied in the evaluation of adults with ESRD and have clearly demonstrated the presence of increased arterial stiffness as a principal disturbance[91] with a high predictive value for survival in hemodialysis patients.[92] Similar studies in children have not been performed. Further studies are needed to clarify the differential involvement of particular endothelial functions as reflected by these measurements and to assess their usefulness as surrogate end points in therapeutic trials.

THE HEART IN PEDIATRIC CKD

Cardiac Remodeling

Cardiac remodeling is a chronic and progressive process resulting in genome expression—molecular, cellular, and interstitial transformations that manifest as changes in the size, shape, and function of the heart after cardiac injury.[93] The triggers that initiate cardiac injury are diverse. In the case of CKD, mechanical or hemodynamic overload is the initial stimulus—although hormones and cytokines may play an important role in its maintenance (Figure 51-3). The first response to imposed pressure or volume overload is the hypertrophy of cardiomyocytes.

Myocyte hypertrophy is likely an adaptive mechanism designed to improve pump function by expanding the number of contractile units in the myocardium while simultaneously reducing wall stress by increasing wall thickness. The transduction of mechanical stress occurs through the integrin proteins—transmembrane receptors that couple extracellular matrix components directly to the intracellular cytoskeleton and nucleus. A signal for hypertrophy is mediated by a complex cascade of signaling systems within cardiomyocytes, resulting in gene reprogramming. Activated hypertrophy-

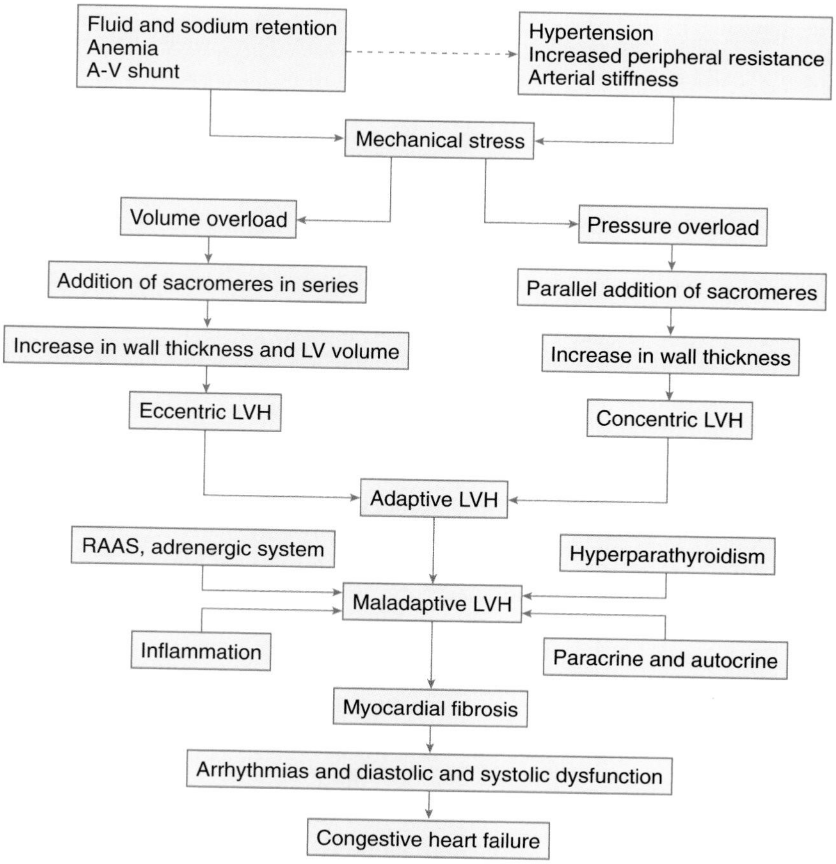

Figure 51-3 Pathophysiologic mechanisms of LVH.

related genes induce the synthesis of new contractile proteins, which are organized into new sarcomeres.

The patterns of sarcomere formation induced by pressure or volume overload are distinct. Pressure-induced hypertrophy, concentric LVH, is characterized by a parallel addition of sarcomeres that results in the increase of the cross-sectional area and diameter of the myocytes. Concentric LVH is closely associated with systolic or pulse pressure. From a physiologic point of view, increased systolic blood pressure and pulse pressure due to increased peripheral resistance and arterial stiffness are the principal factors opposing LV ejection and leading to increased LV workload.

With volume-induced hypertrophy (eccentric LVH), the addition of sarcomeres occurs in series—resulting in longitudinal cell growth with secondary addition of new sarcomeres in parallel. Myocyte diameter and length are proportionally increased, resulting in a balanced increase in overall wall thickness and LV volume. In the transition to maladaptive LVH, LV dilatation becomes disproportional to wall thickness—with myocytes elongated without an increase in diameter. In patients with CKD, the principal features of volume-induced LV enlargement are volume and sodium retention, anemia, and arteriovenous shunt.

Experimental models of cardiac hypertrophy support the theory that mechanical stress due to either pressure or volume overload is a trigger for activation of multiple other mechanisms leading to myocardial remodeling.[94] These factors include a local overexpression of the renin-angiotensin-aldosterone system (RAAS), the adrenergic system, inflammatory cytokines, and other autocrine and paracrine mechanisms. In patients with CKD, these mechanisms might be activated independently of hemodynamic overload because uremia per se is associated with alteration in multiple humoral factors.[95,96] Based on multiple clinical data, angiotensin-converting enzyme (ACE) inhibition and beta-receptor blockade is currently the standard of care for the vast majority of patients at risk for heart failure.

The "cytokine hypothesis" implies the role of inflammatory cytokines in the cardiac remodeling.[97] Among them, TNF-α has been studied most as a factor associated with the progression of cardiac failure. Other important cytokines involved in the process of cardiac remodeling include IL-6 and IL-1β. Unlike ACE inhibitors or beta blockers, the anti–TNF-α therapy showed no benefits and potential harmful effect in two multicenter clinical trials in adults with chronic heart failure (CHF).[98] The role of TNF-α blockade in the prevention of CHF has not been investigated. Other humoral factors (hyperparathyroidism, hyperhomocysteinemia, hyperinsulinemia) have been shown to be associated with LVH. Whether these factors are simply markers of LVH or are factors leading to the development of LVH has yet to be determined.

Initially, LVH is beneficial. It optimizes ejection performance by normalizing systolic wall stress and reducing tension among greater number of sarcomeres. Sustained overload is associated with progression to a maladaptive phase of LVH. Unlike in direct cardiac injury (e.g., acute ischemia), in which both necrosis and apoptosis produce cell death, chronic remodeling and transition to overt CHF have been associated primarily with an elevated degree of apoptosis. However, it is not clear whether apoptosis is a cause or consequence of CHF. With time, capillary density, coronary reserve, and subendocardial perfusion decrease—resulting in myocardial fibrosis.[99] Intermyocardiocyte fibrosis is a unique feature of uremic heart disease. Experimental uremic models showed selective increase in cardiac interstitial cells and nuclear volume but not in endothelial cell volume.[100] During this phase, patients present with arrhythmias and diastolic and systolic dysfunction—ultimately transitioning to overt CHF.

Early Markers of Cardiomyopathy

Because symptomatic CVD is very rare in children, the focus of research has been on identifying in children with CKD early markers or intermediate CV outcomes. Over the last two decades, echocardiographically detected abnormalities of the LV (such as LVH and LV dysfunction) have been accepted as early markers of cardiomyopathy. These abnormalities constitute strong independent predictors of coronary artery disease, CHF, and cardiac mortality in the general population and in adults with hypertension and CKD.

LVH is present in one third of adults with preterminal CKD,[101-105] and its frequency increases with worsening of kidney function—reaching 74% at the time of initiation of dialysis.[106,107] In 1989, Silberberg et al.[108] showed that adult patients on chronic dialysis who were diagnosed with LVH had a 52% higher 5-year mortality rate than patients without LVH. Foley et al.[109] determined that LV dilatation and systolic dysfunction at the start of dialysis were independently associated with mortality. The results of these studies triggered an investigation of cardiac structure and function in pediatric patients with CKD. Recent studies have proven that abnormalities of LV are also present in children with CKD.

Evaluation of LVM in Children

M-mode echocardiographic measurement is currently the most commonly used imaging modality in assessing LVM. The LVM is calculated according to recommendations from the American Society of Echocardiography.[110] This method applies measurements of LV end-diastolic cavity (LVED) and septal (IVS) and posterior wall (PW) thicknesses and accurately predicts LVM through the equation $0.8\ [1.04\{[LVED + PW + IVS]^3 - LVED^3\}] + 0.6$. Adjusting the calculated LVM to account for differences in age, height, and weight is the next step in establishing uniform reference values and criteria for LVH. Unfortunately, there is no uniform definition of LVH in children.

The most ideal indexing parameter is lean body mass, but this is difficult to measure. Indexing LVM by patient height raised to approximately cubic exponential power has been shown to produce the greatest reduction in LVM variability in normal subjects, in particular to detect differences between normal and obese subjects.[111] This indexing also correlates most closely to indexing by lean body mass.[112] However, in children dispersion of residual variation of LVM/height$^{2.7}$ increases with either increasing height or age—suggesting that other variables affect ventricular growth in children.

Although further investigation is needed to determine the most ideal indexing parameter, dividing LVM by height$^{2.7}$ (g/m$^{2.7}$) seems to work well for older children and adolescents.[113] For children older than 9 years, the value of the LVM index 95th percentile is relatively stable and is 38 to 42 g/$m^{2.7}$. The fourth report on blood pressure in children recommends an LVM index value of 51g/$m^{2.7}$ as a conservative cutoff point for the presence of LVH.[114] This value is above the 99th percentile for children and adolescents and is associated with up to a fourfold increase in cardiovascular morbidity in adults with hypertension.[113]

The use of this value to define LVH in children younger than 5 years is problematic because the normative values for LVM index (g/$m^{2.7}$) in this age range are significantly higher than in older children. In fact, the value of 51 g/$m^{2.7}$ represents the normal LVM index for children 1 to 5 years of age—as shown in the study of 2704 healthy children with a body mass index less than the 95th percentile.[115] The authors determined that the use of LVM indexed to height raised in quadratic exponential power (g/m^2) might be a good choice for defining LVH cutoff points in young children because the values for this index are relatively unchanged in children younger than 9 years.

In addition to measurement of LVM, M-mode echocardiography can be used to define LV geometric patterns. LV geometry is evaluated based on the 95th percentiles for LVM index and relative wall thickness (RWT) (Figure 51-4). RWT is calculated from measurements made at end diastole as the ratio of the PW thickness plus IVS thickness over the LVED.

Normal geometry is defined as LVM index and RWT below the 95th percentile. Concentric remodeling is defined as LVM index below the 95th percentile with RWT greater than the 95th percentile. Eccentric LVH is defined as LVM index greater than the 95th percentile and RWT below the 95th percentile. Concentric LVH is defined as both LVM index and RWT greater than the 95th percentile. As in the case of the LVM index, the 95th percentile values for RWT are not uniform and vary from 0.375 to 0.41. Thus, the frequencies of different geometric patterns may differ depending on the cutoff points used in the study.

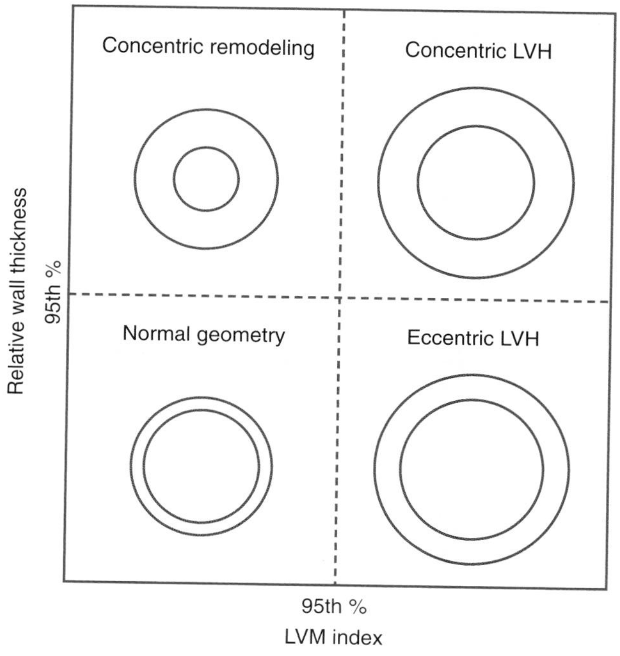

Figure 51-4 LV geometry.

Studies of LVH in Children with CKD

As in adults, LVH develops when renal insufficiency is mild or moderate in children and progresses as renal function deteriorates. About one third of children with CKD have an increased LVM index.[116-118] The Effect of Strict Blood Pressure Control and ACE Inhibition on the Progression of CRI in Pediatric Patients (ESCAPE) trial analyzed cross-sectional echocardiographic data from 156 children aged 3 to 18 years with stages II through IV CKD.[118] In this study, concentric LVH was observed in 12.1% and eccentric LVH in 21% of patients. Also in this study, patients with CKD stage IV had significantly higher LVM index than patients with CKD stage III or stage II (Figure 51-5).

In a 2-year prospective longitudinal study of 31 pediatric subjects with CKD stages II through IV, Mitsnefes et al.[119] showed that a substantial proportion of children had a significant increase in LVM index—with many of the children developing LVH. Indeed, 32% of patients who initially had normal LVM index developed incident LVH.

At initiation of maintenance dialysis, 69% to 82% of pediatric patients had evidence of LVH.[120,121] LVH persists (40%-75%) during long-term dialysis.[15,116,122-125] Both concentric and eccentric geometric patterns of LVH are present in these patients. Children on hemodialysis appear to have higher LVM index and LVH prevalence (82%) than children on peritoneal dialysis (68%),[15] possibly due to poorer blood pressure control in hemodialyzed children. Postmortem studies have shown that more than 50% of children with ESRD have evidence of LVH.[126] Small retrospective studies also suggest that with better blood pressure and volume control LVH regression might be achieved in young patients on dialysis.[120,121] On the other hand, a recent retrospective study demonstrated that LVH remains very prevalent and severe in a selected group of children who remained on maintenance dialysis for at least 2 years.[16]

As in children prior to transplantation, most pediatric studies indicate that LVH remains common posttransplant. Johnstone et al.[116] found LVH in 63% of pediatric patients. Matteucci et al.[127] reported that 82% (23 of 28) of transplanted children had LVM index greater than the 95th percentile. In a study by Morgan et al.,[128] the prevalence of LVH was 72% before transplantation and 54% posttransplant. Another study comparing the changes in LVM index in children who had initial evaluation while on dialysis and a follow-up study after transplantation showed no significant difference in the prevalence of LVH while on dialysis (52%) or after transplantation (56%).[129]

In the largest pediatric renal transplant study, El-Husseini et al.[130] studied 73 patients aged 17 years or less at 4.6 years (median) after transplantation. The prevalence of LVH was 48%. The significant factors associated with LVH were pretransplant dialysis, posttransplant hypertension, and anemia. A longitudinal study by Kitzmueller et al.[131] analyzed 20 repeated pairs of echocardiographic measurements made after a mean of 2 years of follow-up. In their study, no change in the LVM index or in the incidence of LVH (60% at base-

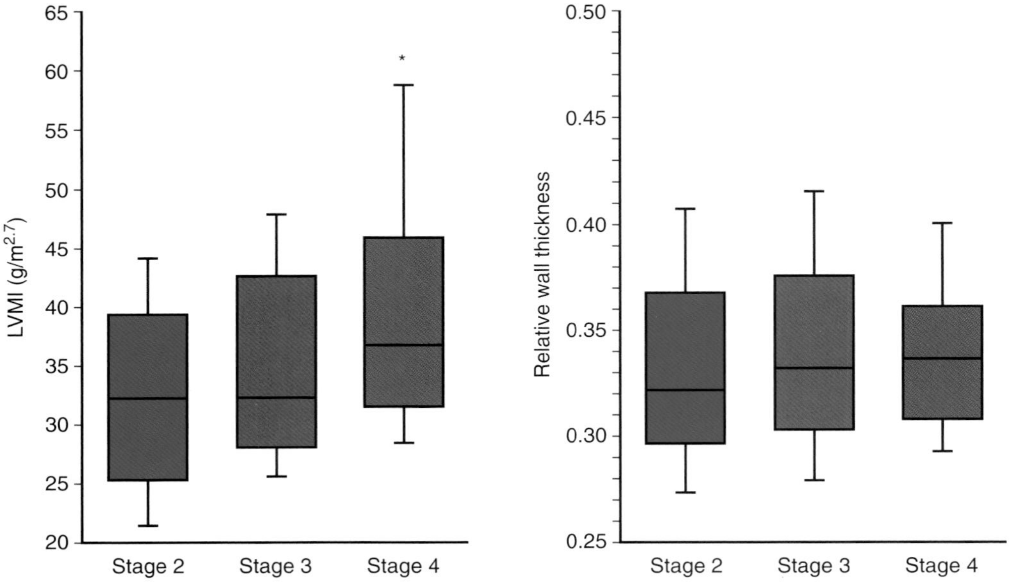

Figure 51-5 Distribution of left ventricular mass index and relative wall thickness according to chronic kidney disease stage. Central line indicates median, lower, and upper box borders of the 25th and 75th distribution percentiles, and extension borders the 10th and 90th distribution percentiles. The symbol * indicates significant difference to stage II and stage III ($p < 0.05$). (From Matteucci MC, Wuhl E, Picca S, et al: Left ventricular geometry in children with mild to moderate chronic renal insufficiency, *J Am Soc Nephrol* 17(1):218-26, 2006.)

line and 70% at follow-up) after renal transplantation was observed.

In contrast to the previously cited studies, a significantly lower frequency of LVH was found in a study by Englund et al.[132]—who reported the results of a longitudinal analysis of children who received renal transplants 10 to 20 years previously. Of 53 children who received a renal transplant between 1981 and 1991, 47 survived and were observed for 10 to 20 years. Before primary transplant, 51% of the 53 children were prescribed antihypertensive treatment. Echocardiography was performed every other year during the later part of this follow-up period.

At the 10-year follow-up, echocardiography showed minor LVH in only two children with hypertension. No child without hypertension at 10 years showed LVH. Progressive aortic insufficiency was discovered in two children, one of whom had a supravalvular aortic aneurysm requiring surgical repair 10 years after transplant. Carotid ultrasound performed once in 22 children (median 11.7 ± 2.5 years after transplant) did not reveal any stenoses or plaque formations despite abnormal plasma cholesterol values in more than 50% of the children.

The factors associated with cardiac hypertrophy in children are similar to those in adults with CKD. As in adults, most pediatric studies of patients with preterminal and terminal renal failure found a significant relationship between low hemoglobin and increased LVM index.[15,118,119] However, recent adult studies questioned the effect of correction of anemia on the reduction of LVH. The Multicenter Canadian Trial evaluated the impact of hemoglobin normalization on cardiac outcomes in dialysis patients with asymptomatic cardiomyopathy.[133] In this study, the achievement of normal hemoglobin did not significantly reduce either LVM or volume compared to lower hemoglobin. Indeed, maintaining subnormal hemoglobin concentration in dialysis patients was enough to obtain a regression of LVH provided adequate blood pressure control and a reduction in pulse pressure were achieved by means of angiotensin-converting enzyme inhibitors.[134]

Levin et al.[135] conducted a clinical trial of 147 patients with mild to moderate CKD who were randomly assigned to the treatment group receiving erythropoietin to maintain or achieve hemoglobin level targets of 12.0 to 14.0 g/dl and a control/delayed treatment group with hemoglobin levels of 9.0 +/− 0.5 g/dl and target level of 9.0 to 10.5 g/dl. In their study, there was no statistically significant difference between groups for mean change in LVM index from baseline to 24 months. The authors concluded that the association between hemoglobin level and LVM index likely is not causal.

Similar negative results of the effect of hemoglobin control on LVH regression or progression were demonstrated in two other studies of adults with CKD stages III and IV.[136,137] Of note, the previously cited studies enrolled subjects with relatively mild degrees of baseline anemia and could not answer the question whether treatment of patients with initially significantly decreased hemoglobin levels might lead to reduction of LVM. In contrast, Morris et al.[138] observed a significant reduction in LVM index with correction of severe anemia in seven children on chronic dialysis.

A significant relationship between PTH and LVH is found in the general population,[139] and in patients with primary hyperparathyroidism.[140] There are several studies on the association between PTH and LVH in adults with CKD.[141,142] In children, elevated PTH was associated with progression of LVH in stages II through IV CKD.[119,143] In a study by Hara et al.,[142] there was a regression of LVH and improvement in cardiac contraction after parathyroidectomy in 10 patients on maintenance hemodialysis. In contrast, Harnett et al.[144] showed no effect of PTH level on the development of LVH in dialyzed adults.

The mechanisms of PTH-induced cardiac hypertrophy may be different in patients with primary and secondary hyperparathyroidism. Elevated serum calcium is attributed to LVH development in patients with primary hyperparathyroidism. The possible mechanisms of parathyroid-induced cardiac hypertrophy in secondary hyperparathyroidism of CKD include a direct effect of PTH on cardiomyocytes and an indirect effect via elevated blood pressure.[74] Support for a causal relationship comes from in vitro studies showing that PTH appears to have chronotropic, inotropic, and hypertrophic effects on cardiomyocytes.[145,146]

In adults with CKD, hypertension is directly linked to the development of LVH.[147] The relationships between blood pressure and LVH in pediatric CKD are unclear. Consistent correlations of LVM and blood pressure are limited to children with ESRD.[15,124] A detailed cross-sectional analysis of blood pressure characteristics by ambulatory blood pressure monitoring (ABPM) in children from the ESCAPE trial did not demonstrate any relationship between office blood pressure or ABPM parameters and LVM, suggesting only a minor role of hypertension in the pathogenesis of LVH in early CRI.[118] However, analysis of longitudinal data suggests that ABPM might be an important tool in assessing the risk of development of LVH in children with CKD.[119] In this study, the authors determined that increase in nighttime systolic blood pressure load (number of blood pressure measurements above the 95th percentile for blood pressure value) was independently associated with the increase in LVM index over time—arguing that persistent and chronic elevation of blood pressure might be important in the development of LVH.

Left Ventricular Function and Pediatric CKD

In contrast to adults, in whom systolic dysfunction is frequently associated with early cardiac failure and decreased survival, in children with CKD systolic LV function is usually preserved.[116,148,149] The majority of pediatric studies have examined LV systolic performance using indices of performance that are dependent on loading conditions. This presents a major problem in patients with CRI or on dialysis because they may have substantial alteration of preload and afterload.

A load-independent index of contractility can be determined based on the relation between heart-rate–corrected velocity of circumferential fiber shortening (VCF) and end-systolic wall stress (WS) by calculation of the difference between measured and predicted VCF for the calculated WS.[150] Using this index, Mitsnefes et al.[117] showed that children with CRI or on maintenance dialysis had increased LV contractility at rest. However, patients on dialysis had decreased contractile reserve during exercise—which might herald the development of a maladaptive stage of LVH. The mechanism of increased contractility in pediatric patients with CKD is not clear. The combination of increased heart rate, cardiac output, and hypertension in these patients is consistent with a hyperdynamic circulation and suggests the possible role of sympathetic overactivity.

A recent study from the ESCAPE trial argues that subclinical systolic dysfunction is already present in predialysis children.[151] The authors analyzed LV shortening at the midwall level [midwall shortening (mS)], which has been shown to more accurately reflect the contractile force independent of pathologic changes in LV geometry.[152,153] Using this index, the study determined that the prevalence of subclinical systolic dysfunction as defined by impaired mS was more than fivefold higher in patients with CKD compared with control subjects (24.6 versus 4.5%; $p < 0.001$). Systolic dysfunction was most common (48%) in patients with concentric hypertrophy and was associated with lower hemoglobin levels. The authors concluded that the combination of concentric LV geometry with midwall dysfunction might represent a cardiac phenotype designating an increased risk for the development of overt CVD.

Very few studies have assessed LV diastolic function in pediatric patients with chronic renal failure. Doppler measurement of mitral inflow velocity has been the most widely used method for assessing LV diastolic function. Using this method, Goren et al.[149] showed that LV relaxation (E/A ratio) was impaired in dialyzed children compared with controls. Johnstone et al.[116] also found a reduction in the E/A ratio in children on chronic peritoneal dialysis and with preterminal renal failure, although none of these patients had an E/A ratio <1.0—which is considered abnormal. Unfortunately, the transmitral Doppler velocities (and therefore the E/A ratio) are affected by several factors, including left atrial pressure and preload.

This is particularly important for patients with advanced chronic renal failure because many of them are hypervolemic. Recently, new indices were introduced to evaluate diastolic function using tissue Doppler imaging (TDI). In contrast to E/A, the TDI indices may be less load dependent and provide a more accurate measure of diastolic function. Recent studies employing TDI determined that children with CKD have abnormal diastolic function.[154,155] In these studies, children on chronic dialysis had significantly worse diastolic function than children with mild to moderate CRI or posttransplant.

Poor diastolic function in patients on dialysis was associated with anemia, hyperphosphatemia, increased calcium-phosphorus ion product, and LVH. The clinical significance of diastolic dysfunction in pediatric patients with CKD is not known. Longitudinal studies are necessary to determine if abnormal diastolic function predicts the development of systolic dysfunction and congestive heart failure in these patients.

THE FUTURE

At present, therapeutic options of preventing CVD in children and adolescents with CKD are limited to the treatment of modifiable risk factors (i.e., hypertension, hyperhomocysteinemia, and the like).[156] In clinical practice, the most difficult problem will be to find improvements for the current treatment of renal osteodystrophy. Serum levels of calcium and phosphorus previously considered safe have been questioned,[157] and revised guidelines (KDOQI) for the clinical management of the Ca × P product have now been established for adults[158] and children.[159,160] These goals, however, are often difficult to achieve in practice.

It can be hoped that treatment with new vitamin D analogues[161] and/or concomitant treatment with calcimimetic drugs[162] will facilitate management of disturbances in calcium, phosphorus, and PTH. However, the safety of calcimimetic drugs for children remains to be clarified. The use of new calcium-free phosphate binders[163] is a promising option, and pediatric studies with sevelamer[164,165] have demonstrated the feasibility and safety of this approach. However, a liquid preparation of sevelamer will be required if this drug is to be prescribed for small children.

Noninvasive measurements of vascular and cardiac structure and function could serve as surrogate end points in future studies evaluating therapeutic interventions for CVD. One such parameter is IMT of the carotid artery, where normative data have been collected in children. In addition, partial reversibility of increased IMT in patients with ESRD has been observed after successful renal transplantation.[45] Another parameter is echocardiographic evaluation for the presence of LVH. The K/DOQI Clinical Practice Guidelines for Cardiovascular Disease in Dialysis Patients[147] recommend that "children commencing dialysis should be evaluated for the presence of cardiac disease (cardiomyopathy and valvular disease) using echocardiography once the patient has achieved dry weight (ideally within 3 months of the initiation of dialysis therapy)."

Unfortunately, these guidelines do not provide recommendations for echocardiographic evaluation for children prior to dialysis or after kidney transplantation. The fourth report on blood pressure control in children[114] recommends echocardiographic evaluation for the presence of LVH in children with comorbid conditions (diabetes and kidney disease) and blood pressure between the 90th and 95th percentile, and in all children with blood pressure above the 95th percentile. Based on these recommendations, it seems appropriate to perform echocardiography in children with CRI and in renal transplant recipients who have abnormal blood pressure. Echocardiography should also be considered in children with anemia. If LVH is diagnosed, periodic follow-up echocardiographic monitoring is suggested. Finally, considering the long-term risk of CVD in young patients the introduction of extended forms of dialysis (e.g., nocturnal dialysis[166] or daily dialysis[167]) needs to be seriously considered for children and adolescents with CKD—especially when rapid transplantation is not possible.

REFERENCES

1. Foley RN, Parfrey PS, Sarnak MJ: Clinical epidemiology of cardiovascular disease in chronic renal disease, *Am J Kidney Dis* 32(5/3): S112-S119, 1998.
2. Weiner DE, Tighiouart H, Amin MG, et al: Chronic kidney disease as a risk factor for cardiovascular disease and all-cause mortality: A pooled analysis of community-based studies, *J Am Soc Nephrol* 15(5):1307-315, 2004.
3. Foley RN, Murray AM, Li S, et al: Chronic kidney disease and the risk for cardiovascular disease, renal replacement, and death in the United States Medicare population, 1998 to 1999, *J Am Soc Nephrol* 16(2):489-95, 2005.
4. Chavers BM, Herzog CA: The spectrum of cardiovascular disease in children with predialysis chronic kidney disease, *Adv Chronic Kidney Dis* 11(3):319-27, 2004.
5. Chavers BM, Li S, Collins AJ, Herzog CA: Cardiovascular disease in pediatric chronic dialysis patients, *Kidney Int* 62(2):648-53, 2002.
6. U.S. Renal Data System. USRDS 2000 Annual Data Report, 2000. Bethesda: The National Institutes of Health, National Institute of Diabetes and Digestive and Kidney Diseases 2000.
7. Offner G, Latta K, Hoyer PF, et al: Kidney transplanted children come of age, *Kidney Int* 55(4):1509-17, 1999.
8. Briese S, Wiesner S, Will JC, et al: Arterial and cardiac disease in young adults with childhood-onset end-stage renal disease-impact of calcium and vitamin D therapy, *Nephrol Dial Transplant* 21(7):1906-14, 2006.
9. Oh J, Wunsch R, Turzer M, et al: Advanced coronary and carotid arteriopathy in young adults with childhood-onset chronic renal failure, *Circulation* 106(1):100-05, 2002.
10. Groothoff JW, Gruppen MP, Offringa M, et al: Mortality and causes of death of end-stage renal disease in children: A Dutch cohort study, *Kidney Int* 61(2):621-29, 2002.
11. McDonald SP, Craig JC: Long-term survival of children with end-stage renal disease, *N Engl J Med* 350(26):2654-62, 2004.
12. Parekh RS, Carroll CE, Wolfe RA, Port FK: Cardiovascular mortality in children and young adults with end-stage kidney disease, *J Pediatr* 141(2):191-97, 2002.
13. Brunner FP, Fassbinder W, Broyer M, et al: Survival on renal replacement therapy: data from the EDTA Registry, *Nephrol Dial Transplant* 3(2):109-22, 1988.
14. Maron BJ: Sudden death in young athletes, *N Engl J Med* 349(11):1064-75, 2003.
15. Mitsnefes MM, Daniels SR, Schwartz SM, Meyer RA, Khoury P, Strife CF: Severe left ventricular hypertrophy in pediatric dialysis: Prevalence and predictors, *Pediatr Nephrol* 14(10-11):898-902, 2000.
16. Mitsnefes MM, Barletta GM, Dresner IG, et al: Severe cardiac hypertrophy and long-term dialysis: The Midwest Pediatric Nephrology Consortium study, *Pediatr Nephrol* 21(8):1167-70, 2006.
17. Herzog CA: Acute myocardial infarction in patients with end-stage renal disease, *Kidney Int Suppl* 71:S130-S133, 1999.
18. Wanner C, Krane V, Marz W, et al: Atorvastatin in patients with type 2 diabetes mellitus undergoing hemodialysis, *N Engl J Med* 353(3):238-48, 2005.
19. Nakamura S, Uzu T, Inenaga T, Kimura G: Prediction of coronary artery disease and cardiac events using electrocardiographic changes during hemodialysis, *Am J Kidney Dis* 36(3):592-99, 2000.
20. Shaw LJ, Bairey Merz CN, Pepine CJ, et al: Insights from the NHLBI-Sponsored Women's Ischemia Syndrome Evaluation (WISE) Study: Part I, gender differences in traditional and novel risk factors, symptom evaluation, and gender-optimized diagnostic strategies, *J Am Coll Cardiol* 47(3):S4-S20, 2006.
21. Portaluppi F, Montanari L, Ferlini M, Gilli P: Altered circadian rhythms of blood pressure and heart rate in non-hemodialysis chronic renal failure, *Chronobiol Int* 7(4):321-27, 1990.
22. Go AS, Chertow GM, Fan D, McCulloch CE, Hsu CY: Chronic kidney disease and the risks of death, cardiovascular events, and hospitalization, *N Engl J Med* 351(13):1296-305, 2004.
23. Fried LF, Katz R, Sarnak MJ, et al: Kidney function as a predictor of noncardiovascular mortality, *J Am Soc Nephrol* 16(12):3728-35, 2005.
24. Shlipak MG, Sarnak MJ, Katz R, et al: Cystatin C and the risk of death and cardiovascular events among elderly persons, *N Engl J Med* 352(20):2049-60, 2005.
25. Irie F, Iso H, Sairenchi T, et al: The relationships of proteinuria, serum creatinine, glomerular filtration rate with cardiovascular disease mortality in Japanese general population, *Kidney Int* 69(7):1264-71, 2006.
26. Fox CS, Larson MG, Leip EP, Culleton B, Wilson PW, Levy D: Predictors of new-onset kidney disease in a community-based population, *JAMA* 291(7):844-50, 2004.
27. Fox CS, Larson MG, Leip EP, Meigs JB, Wilson PW, Levy D: Glycemic status and development of kidney disease: The Framingham Heart Study, *Diabetes Care* 28(10):2436-40, 2005.

28. Yusuf S, Hawken S, Ounpuu S, et al: Effect of potentially modifiable risk factors associated with myocardial infarction in 52 countries (the INTERHEART study): case-control study, *Lancet* 364(9438):937-52, 2004.
29. Luke RG: Chronic renal failure: A vasculopathic state, *N Engl J Med* 339(12):841-43, 1998.
30. Muntner P, He J, Astor BC, Folsom AR, Coresh J: Traditional and nontraditional risk factors predict coronary heart disease in chronic kidney disease: Results from the atherosclerosis risk in communities study, *J Am Soc Nephrol* 16(2):529-38, 2005.
31. Zoccali C: Traditional and emerging cardiovascular and renal risk factors: An epidemiologic perspective, *Kidney Int* 70(1):26-33, 2006.
32. Zoccali C, Tripepi G, Cambareri F, et al: Adipose tissue cytokines, insulin sensitivity, inflammation, and cardiovascular outcomes in end-stage renal disease patients, *J Ren Nutr* 15(1):125-30, 2005.
33. Querfeld U: The clinical significance of vascular calcification in young patients with end-stage renal disease, *Pediatr Nephrol* 19(5):478-84, 2004.
34. Shlipak MG, Fried LF, Cushman M, et al: Cardiovascular mortality risk in chronic kidney disease: Comparison of traditional and novel risk factors, *JAMA* 293(14):1737-45, 2005.
35. Hopkins PN, Williams RR: A survey of 246 suggested coronary risk factors, *Atherosclerosis* 40(1):1-52, 1981.
36. Bostom AG, Shemin D, Verhoef P, et al: Elevated fasting total plasma homocysteine levels and cardiovascular disease outcomes in maintenance dialysis patients: A prospective study, *Arterioscler Thromb Vasc Biol* 17(11):2554-58, 1997.
37. Bostom AG, Carpenter MA, Kusek JW, et al: Rationale and design of the Folic Acid for Vascular Outcome Reduction In Transplantation (FAVORIT) trial, *Am Heart J* 152(3):448, e1-e7, 2006.
38. Kalantar-Zadeh K, Block G, Humphreys MH, McAllister CJ, Kopple JD: A low, rather than a high, total plasma homocysteine is an indicator of poor outcome in hemodialysis patients, *J Am Soc Nephrol* 15(2):442-53, 2004.
39. Kalantar-Zadeh K, Block G, Humphreys MH, Kopple JD: Reverse epidemiology of cardiovascular risk factors in maintenance dialysis patients, *Kidney Int* 63(3):793-808, 2003.
40. Kalantar-Zadeh K, Kopple JD: Relative contributions of nutrition and inflammation to clinical outcome in dialysis patients, *Am J Kidney Dis* 38(6):1343-50, 2001.
41. Eto M, Luscher TF: The cardioprotective effects of statins, *Coron Artery Dis* 15(5):243-45, 2004.
42. Querfeld U: Cardiovascular considerations of pediatric ESRD. In B Warady, F Schaefer, R Fine, S Alexander (eds.), *Pediatric dialysis*. Dordrecht/Boston/London: Kluwer Academic Publishers 2004: 353-67.
43. Groothoff JW, Gruppen MP, Offringa M, et al: Increased arterial stiffness in young adults with end-stage renal disease since childhood, *J Am Soc Nephrol* 13(12):2953-61, 2002.
44. Gruppen MP, Groothoff JW, Prins M, et al: Cardiac disease in young adult patients with end-stage renal disease since childhood: A Dutch cohort study, *Kidney Int* 63(3):1058-65, 2003.
45. Litwin M, Wuhl E, Jourdan C, et al: Altered morphologic properties of large arteries in children with chronic renal failure and after renal transplantation, *J Am Soc Nephrol* 16(5):1494-500, 2005.
46. Mitsnefes MM, Kimball TR, Kartal J, et al: Cardiac and vascular adaptation in pediatric patients with chronic kidney disease: Role of calcium-phosphorus metabolism, *J Am Soc Nephrol* 16(9):2796-803, 2005.
47. Braun J, Oldendorf M, Moshage W, Heidler R, Zeitler E, Luft FC: Electron beam computed tomography in the evaluation of cardiac calcification in chronic dialysis patients, *Am J Kidney Dis* 27(3):394-401, 1996.
48. Goodman WG, Goldin J, Kuizon BD, et al: Coronary-artery calcification in young adults with end-stage renal disease who are undergoing dialysis, *N Engl J Med* 342(20):1478-83, 2000.
49. Eifinger F, Wahn F, Querfeld U, et al: Coronary artery calcifications in children and young adults treated with renal replacement therapy, *Nephrol Dial Transplant* 15(11):1892-94, 2000.
50. Ishitani MB, Milliner DS, Kim DY, et al: Early subclinical coronary artery calcification in young adults who were pediatric kidney transplant recipients, *Am J Transplant* 5(7):1689-93, 2005.
51. Civilibal M, Caliskan S, Adaletli I, et al: Coronary artery calcifications in children with end-stage renal disease, *Pediatr Nephrol* 21(10):1426-33, 2006.
52. Haydar AA, Hujairi NM, Covic AA, Pereira D, Rubens M, Goldsmith DJ: Coronary artery calcification is related to coronary atherosclerosis in chronic renal disease patients: A study comparing EBCT-generated coronary artery calcium scores and coronary angiography, *Nephrol Dial Transplant* 19(9):2307-12, 2004.
53. Blacher J, Guerin AP, Pannier B, Marchais SJ, London GM: Arterial calcifications, arterial stiffness, and cardiovascular risk in end-stage renal disease, *Hypertension* 38(4):938-42, 2001.
54. Stary HC: Natural history of calcium deposits in atherosclerosis progression and regression, *Z Kardiol* 89(2):28-35, 2000.
55. Haydar AA, Covic A, Colhoun H, Rubens M, Goldsmith DJ: Coronary artery calcification and aortic pulse wave velocity in chronic kidney disease patients, *Kidney Int* 65(5):1790-94, 2004.
56. Blacher J, Pannier B, Guerin AP, Marchais SJ, Safar ME, London GM: Carotid arterial stiffness as a predictor of cardiovascular and all-cause mortality in end-stage renal disease, *Hypertension* 32(3):570-74, 1998.
57. Blacher J, Safar ME, Guerin AP, Pannier B, Marchais SJ, London GM: Aortic pulse wave velocity index and mortality in end-stage renal disease, *Kidney Int* 63(5):1852-60, 2003.
58. Blacher J, Guerin AP, Pannier B, Marchais SJ, Safar ME, London GM: Impact of aortic stiffness on survival in end-stage renal disease, *Circulation* 99(18):2434-39, 1999.
59. Asmus HG, Braun J, Krause R, et al: Two year comparison of sevelamer and calcium carbonate effects on cardiovascular calcification and bone density, *Nephrol Dial Transplant* 20(8):1653-61, 2005.
60. Block GA, Spiegel DM, Ehrlich J, et al: Effects of sevelamer and calcium on coronary artery calcification in patients new to hemodialysis, *Kidney Int* 68(4):1815-24, 2005.
61. deFilippi C, Wasserman S, Rosanio S, et al: Cardiac troponin T and C-reactive protein for predicting prognosis, coronary atherosclerosis, and cardiomyopathy in patients undergoing long-term hemodialysis, *JAMA* 290(3):353-59, 2003.
62. Ketteler M, Bongartz P, Westenfeld R, et al: Association of low fetuin-A (AHSG) concentrations in serum with cardiovascular mortality in patients on dialysis: A cross-sectional study, *Lancet* 361(9360):827-33, 2003.
63. Ketteler M, Wanner C, Metzger T, et al: Deficiencies of calcium-regulatory proteins in dialysis patients: A novel concept of cardiovascular calcification in uremia, *Kidney Int Suppl* 2003(84): S84-S87.
64. Verberckmoes SC, Persy V, Behets GJ, et al: Uremia-related vascular calcification: More than apatite deposition, *Kidney Int* 71(4):298-303, 2006.
65. Bas A, Lopez I, Perez J, Rodriguez M, Aguilera-Tejero E: Reversibility of calcitriol-induced medial artery calcification in rats with intact renal function, *J Bone Miner Res* 21(3):484-90, 2006.
66. Chertow GM, Burke SK, Raggi P: Sevelamer attenuates the progression of coronary and aortic calcification in hemodialysis patients, *Kidney Int* 62(1):245-52, 2002.
67. Milliner DS, Zinsmeister AR, Lieberman E, Landing B: Soft tissue calcification in pediatric patients with end-stage renal disease, *Kidney Int* 38(5):931-36, 1990.
68. Hsu CH: Are we mismanaging calcium and phosphate metabolism in renal failure? *Am J Kidney Dis* 29(4):641-49, 1997.
69. Bleyer AJ: Phosphate binder usage in kidney failure patients, *Expert Opin Pharmacother* 4(6):941-47, 2003.
70. Clark AG, Oner A, Ward G, et al: Safety and efficacy of calcium carbonate in children with chronic renal failure, *Nephrol Dial Transplant* 4(6):539-44, 1989.
71. Cozzolino M, Dusso AS, Liapis H, et al: The effects of sevelamer hydrochloride and calcium carbonate on kidney calcification in uremic rats, *J Am Soc Nephrol* 13(9):2299-308, 2002.
72. Portale AA, Booth BE, Halloran BP, Morris RC Jr.: Effect of dietary phosphorus on circulating concentrations of 1,25-dihydroxyvitamin D and immunoreactive parathyroid hormone in children with moderate renal insufficiency, *J Clin Invest* 73(6):1580-89, 1984.
73. Block GA, Hulbert-Shearon TE, Levin NW, Port FK: Association of serum phosphorus and calcium x phosphate product with mor-

tality risk in chronic hemodialysis patients: a national study, *Am J Kidney Dis* 31(4):607-17, 1998.
74. Rostand SG, Drueke TB: Parathyroid hormone, vitamin D, and cardiovascular disease in chronic renal failure, *Kidney Int* 56(2):383-92, 1999.
75. Steitz SA, Speer MY, Curinga G, et al: Smooth muscle cell phenotypic transition associated with calcification: Upregulation of Cbfa1 and downregulation of smooth muscle lineage markers, *Circ Res* 89(12):1147-54, 2001.
76. Moe SM, O'Neill KD, Duan D, et al: Medial artery calcification in ESRD patients is associated with deposition of bone matrix proteins, *Kidney Int* 61(2):638-47, 2002.
77. Haffner D, Hocher B, Muller D, et al: Systemic cardiovascular disease in uremic rats induced by 1,25(OH)2D3, *J Hypertens* 23(5):1067-75, 2005.
78. Tintut Y, Demer LL: Recent advances in multifactorial regulation of vascular calcification, *Curr Opin Lipidol* 12(5):555-60, 2001.
79. Jono S, McKee MD, Murry CE, et al: Phosphate regulation of vascular smooth muscle cell calcification, *Circ Res* 87(7):E10-E17, 2000.
80. Jono S, Nishizawa Y, Shioi A, Morii H: 1,25-Dihydroxyvitamin D3 increases in vitro vascular calcification by modulating secretion of endogenous parathyroid hormone-related peptide, *Circulation* 98(13):1302-06, 1998.
81. Moe SM, Duan D, Doehle BP, O'Neill KD, Chen NX: Uremia induces the osteoblast differentiation factor Cbfa1 in human blood vessels, *Kidney Int* 63(3):1003-11, 2003.
82. Rebsamen MC, Sun J, Norman AW, Liao JK: 1alpha,25-dihydroxyvitamin D3 induces vascular smooth muscle cell migration via activation of phosphatidylinositol 3-kinase, *Circ Res* 91(1):17-24, 2002.
83. Goligorsky MS: Endothelial cell dysfunction: can't live with it, how to live without it, *Am J Physiol Renal Physiol* 288(5):F871-F880, 2005.
84. Bonetti PO, Lerman LO, Lerman A: Endothelial dysfunction: a marker of atherosclerotic risk, *Arterioscler Thromb Vasc Biol* 23(2):168-75, 2003.
85. Jarvisalo MJ, Jartti L, Marniemi J, et al: Determinants of short-term variation in arterial flow-mediated dilatation in healthy young men, *Clin Sci (Lond)* 110(4):475-82, 2006.
86. De Roos NM, Bots ML, Schouten EG, Katan MB: Within-subject variability of flow-mediated vasodilation of the brachial artery in healthy men and women: Implications for experimental studies, *Ultrasound Med Biol* 29(3):401-06, 2003.
87. London GM, Pannier B, Agharazii M, Guerin AP, Verbeke FH, Marchais SJ: Forearm reactive hyperemia and mortality in end-stage renal disease, *Kidney Int* 65(2):700-04, 2004.
88. Kruger A, Stewart J, Sahityani R, et al: Laser Doppler flowmetry detection of endothelial dysfunction in end-stage renal disease patients: correlation with cardiovascular risk, *Kidney Int* 70(1):157-64, 2006.
89. Wilkinson IB, Hall IR, MacCallum H, et al: Pulse-wave analysis: Clinical evaluation of a noninvasive, widely applicable method for assessing endothelial function, *Arterioscler Thromb Vasc Biol* 22(1):147-52, 2002.
90. McEniery CM, Wallace S, Mackenzie IS, et al: Endothelial function is associated with pulse pressure, pulse wave velocity, and augmentation index in healthy humans, *Hypertension* 48(4):602-08, 2006.
91. Wang MC, Tsai WC, Chen JY, Huang JJ: Stepwise increase in arterial stiffness corresponding with the stages of chronic kidney disease, *Am J Kidney Dis* 45(3):494-501, 2005.
92. London GM, Cohn JN: Prognostic application of arterial stiffness: Task forces, *Am J Hypertens* 15(8):754-58, 2002.
93. Cohn JN, Ferrari R, Sharpe N for the International Forum on Cardiac Remodeling: Cardiac remodeling: Concepts and clinical implications. A consensus paper from an international forum on cardiac remodeling, *J Am Coll Cardiol* 35(3):569-82, 2000.
94. Swynghedauw B: Molecular mechanisms of myocardial remodeling, *Physiol Rev* 79(1):215-62, 1999.
95. London GM, Parfrey PS: Cardiac disease in chronic uremia: Pathogenesis, *Adv Ren Replace Ther* 4(3):194-211, 1997.
96. Guerin AP, Adda H, London GM, Marchais SJ: Cardiovascular disease in renal failure, *Minerva Urol Nefrol* 56(3):279-88, 2004.
97. Seta Y, Shan K, Bozkurt B, Oral H, Mann DL: Basic mechanisms in heart failure: the cytokine hypothesis, *J Card Fail* 2(3):243-49, 1996.
98. Krum H: Tumor necrosis factor-alpha blockade as a therapeutic strategy in heart failure (RENEWAL and ATTACH): unsuccessful, to be specific, *J Card Fail* 8(6):365-68, 2002.
99. Amann K, Wiest G, Zimmer G, Gretz N, Ritz E, Mall G: Reduced capillary density in the myocardium of uremic rats: A stereological study, *Kidney Int* 42(5):1079-85, 1992.
100. Tyralla K, Amann K: Morphology of the heart and arteries in renal failure, *Kidney Int Suppl* 84:S80-S83, 2003.
101. Greaves SC, Gamble GD, Collins JF, Whalley GA, Sharpe DN: Determinants of left ventricular hypertrophy and systolic dysfunction in chronic renal failure, *Am J Kidney Dis* 24(5):768-76, 1994.
102. Levin A, Singer J, Thompson CR, Ross H, Lewis M: Prevalent left ventricular hypertrophy in the predialysis population: Identifying opportunities for intervention, *Am J Kidney Dis* 27(3):347-54, 1996.
103. Levin A, Thompson CR, Ethier J, et al: Left ventricular mass index increase in early renal disease: Impact of decline in hemoglobin, *Am J Kidney Dis* 34(1):125-34, 1999.
104. Tucker B, Fabbian F, Giles M, Johnston A, Baker LR: Reduction of left ventricular mass index with blood pressure reduction in chronic renal failure, *Clin Nephrol* 52(6):377-82, 1999.
105. Tucker B, Fabbian F, Giles M, Thuraisingham RC, Raine AE, Baker LR: Left ventricular hypertrophy and ambulatory blood pressure monitoring in chronic renal failure, *Nephrol Dial Transplant* 12(4):724-28, 1997.
106. Foley RN, Parfrey PS, Harnett JD, et al: Clinical and echocardiographic disease in patients starting end-stage renal disease therapy, *Kidney Int* 47(1):186-92, 1995.
107. Paoletti E, Bellino D, Cassottana P, Rolla D, Cannella G: Left ventricular hypertrophy in nondiabetic predialysis CKD, *Am J Kidney Dis* 46(2):320-27, 2005.
108. Silberberg JS, Barre PE, Prichard SS, Sniderman AD: Impact of left ventricular hypertrophy on survival in end-stage renal disease, *Kidney Int* 36(2):286-90, 1989.
109. Foley RN, Parfrey PS, Harnett JD, Kent GM, Murray DC, Barre PE: The prognostic importance of left ventricular geometry in uremic cardiomyopathy, *J Am Soc Nephrol* 5(12):2024-31, 1995.
110. Devereux RB, Reichek N: Echocardiographic determination of left ventricular mass in man: Anatomic validation of the method, *Circulation* 55(4):613-18, 1977.
111. de Simone G, Daniels SR, Devereux RB, et al: Left ventricular mass and body size in normotensive children and adults: Assessment of allometric relations and impact of overweight, *J Am Coll Cardiol* 20(5):1251-60, 1992.
112. Daniels SR, Meyer RA, Liang YC, Bove KE: Echocardiographically determined left ventricular mass index in normal children, adolescents and young adults, *J Am Coll Cardiol* 12(3):703-08, 1988.
113. de Simone G, Devereux RB, Daniels SR, Koren MJ, Meyer RA, Laragh JH: Effect of growth on variability of left ventricular mass: Assessment of allometric signals in adults and children and their capacity to predict cardiovascular risk, *J Am Coll Cardiol* 25(5):1056-62, 1995.
114. National High Blood Pressure Education Program Working Group on High Blood Pressure in Children and Adolescents: The fourth report on the diagnosis, evaluation, and treatment of high blood pressure in children and adolescents, *Pediatrics* 114(2):555-76, 2004.
115. Khoury PR DS, Gidding SS and Kimball TR: Left ventricular mass index in children: What is the right index? *J Am Soc Echo* 17:555, 2004.
116. Johnstone LM, Jones CL, Grigg LE, Wilkinson JL, Walker RG, Powell HR: Left ventricular abnormalities in children, adolescents and young adults with renal disease, *Kidney Int* 50(3):998-1006, 1996.
117. Mitsnefes MM, Kimball TR, Witt SA, Glascock BJ, Khoury PR, Daniels SR: Left ventricular mass and systolic performance in pedi-

atric patients with chronic renal failure, *Circulation* 107(6):864-68, 2003.
118. Matteucci MC, Wuhl E, Picca S, et al: Left ventricular geometry in children with mild to moderate chronic renal insufficiency, *J Am Soc Nephrol* 17(1):218-26, 2006.
119. Mitsnefes MM, Kimball TR, Kartal J, et al: Progression of left ventricular hypertrophy in children with early chronic kidney disease: 2-year follow-up study, *J Pediatr* 149(5):671-75, 2006.
120. Mitsnefes MM, Daniels SR, Schwartz SM, Khoury P, Strife CF: Changes in left ventricular mass in children and adolescents during chronic dialysis, *Pediatr Nephrol* 16(4):318-23, 2001.
121. Ulinski T, Genty J, Viau C, Tillous-Borde I, Deschenes G: Reduction of left ventricular hypertrophy in children undergoing hemodialysis, *Pediatr Nephrol* 21(8):1171-78, 2006.
122. Morris KP, Skinner JR, Wren C, Hunter S, Coulthard MG: Cardiac abnormalities in end stage renal failure and anaemia, *Arch Dis Child* 68(5):637-43, 1993.
123. O'Regan S, Matina D, Ducharme G, Davignon A: Echocardiographic assessment of cardiac function in children with chronic renal failure, *Kidney Int Suppl* 15:S77-S82, 1983.
124. Palcoux JB, Palcoux MC, Jouan JP, Gourgand JM, Cassagnes J, Malpuech G: Echocardiographic patterns in infants and children with chronic renal failure, *Int J Pediatr Nephrol* 3(4):311-14, 1982.
125. Drukker A, Urbach J, Glaser J: Hypertrophic cardiomyopathy in children with end-stage renal disease and hypertension, *Proc Eur Dial Transplant Assoc* 18:542-47, 1981.
126. Litwin M, Grenda R, Prokurat S, et al: Patient survival and causes of death on hemodialysis and peritoneal dialysis: Single-center study, *Pediatr Nephrol* 16(12):996-1001, 2001.
127. Matteucci MC, Giordano U, Calzolari A, Turchetta A, Santilli A, Rizzoni G: Left ventricular hypertrophy, treadmill tests, and 24-hour blood pressure in pediatric transplant patients, *Kidney Int* 56(4):1566-70, 1999.
128. Morgan H, Khan I, Hashmi A, Hebert D, McCrindle BW, Balfe JW: Ambulatory blood pressure monitoring after renal transplantation in children, *Pediatr Nephrol* 16(11):843-47, 2001.
129. Mitsnefes MM, Schwartz SM, Daniels SR, Kimball TR, Khoury P, Strife CF: Changes in left ventricular mass index in children and adolescents after renal transplantation, *Pediatr Transplant* 5(4):279-84, 2001.
130. El-Husseini AA, Sheashaa HA, Hassan NA, El-Demerdash FM, Sobh MA, Ghoneim MA: Echocardiographic changes and risk factors for left ventricular hypertrophy in children and adolescents after renal transplantation, *Pediatr Transplant* 8(3):249-54, 2004.
131. Kitzmueller E, Vecsei A, Pichler J, et al: Changes of blood pressure and left ventricular mass in pediatric renal transplantation, *Pediatr Nephrol* 19(12):1385-89, 2004.
132. Englund M, Berg U, Tyden G: A longitudinal study of children who received renal transplants 10-20 years ago, *Transplantation* 76(2):311-18, 2003.
133. Foley RN, Parfrey PS, Morgan J, et al: Effect of hemoglobin levels in hemodialysis patients with asymptomatic cardiomyopathy, *Kidney Int* 58(3):1325-35, 2000.
134. Paoletti E, Cassottana P, Bellino D, Specchia C, Messa P, Cannella G: Left ventricular geometry and adverse cardiovascular events in chronic hemodialysis patients on prolonged therapy with ACE inhibitors, *Am J Kidney Dis* 40(4):728-36, 2002.
135. Levin A, Djurdjev O, Thompson C, et al: Canadian randomized trial of hemoglobin maintenance to prevent or delay left ventricular mass growth in patients with CKD, *Am J Kidney Dis* 46(5):799-811, 2005.
136. McMahon LP, Roger SD, Levin A: Development, prevention, and potential reversal of left ventricular hypertrophy in chronic kidney disease, *J Am Soc Nephrol* 15(6):1640-47, 2004.
137. Roger SD, McMahon LP, Clarkson A, et al: Effects of early and late intervention with epoetin alpha on left ventricular mass among patients with chronic kidney disease (stage 3 or 4): Results of a randomized clinical trial, *J Am Soc Nephrol* 15(1):148-56, 2004.
138. Morris KP, Skinner JR, Hunter S, Coulthard MG: Cardiovascular abnormalities in end stage renal failure: The effect of anaemia or uraemia? *Arch Dis Child* 71(2):119-22, 1994.
139. Saleh FN, Schirmer H, Sundsfjord J, Jorde R: Parathyroid hormone and left ventricular hypertrophy, *Eur Heart J* 24(22):2054-60, 2003.
140. Stefenelli T, Abela C, Frank H, et al: Cardiac abnormalities in patients with primary hyperparathyroidism: implications for follow-up, *J Clin Endocrinol Metab* 82(1):106-12, 1997.
141. London GM, De Vernejoul MC, Fabiani F, et al: Secondary hyperparathyroidism and cardiac hypertrophy in hemodialysis patients, *Kidney Int* 32(6):900-07, 1987.
142. Hara S, Ubara Y, Arizono K, et al: Relation between parathyroid hormone and cardiac function in long-term hemodialysis patients, *Miner Electrolyte Metab* 21(1-3):72-76, 1995.
143. Mitsnefes MM KJ, Khoury PR, Daniels SR: Adiponectin in children with chronic kidney disease: Role of adiposity and kidney dysfunction, *CJASN* 2(1):46-51, 2007.
144. Harnett JD, Kent GM, Barre PE, Taylor R, Parfrey PS: Risk factors for the development of left ventricular hypertrophy in a prospectively followed cohort of dialysis patients, *J Am Soc Nephrol* 4(7):1486-90, 1994.
145. Bogin E, Massry SG, Harary I: Effect of parathyroid hormone on rat heart cells, *J Clin Invest* 67(4):1215-27, 1981.
146. Katoh Y, Klein KL, Kaplan RA, Sanborn WG, Kurokawa K: Parathyroid hormone has a positive inotropic action in the rat, *Endocrinology* 109(6):2252-54, 1981.
147. K/DOQI: Clinical practice guidelines for cardiovascular disease in dialysis patients, *Am J Kidney Dis* 45(4/3):S1-S153, 2005.
148. Colan SD, Sanders SP, Ingelfinger JR, Harmon W: Left ventricular mechanics and contractile state in children and young adults with end-stage renal disease: Effect of dialysis and renal transplantation, *J Am Coll Cardiol* 10(5):1085-94, 1987.
149. Goren A, Glaser J, Drukker A: Diastolic function in children and adolescents on dialysis and after kidney transplantation: An echocardiographic assessment, *Pediatr Nephrol* 7(6):725-28, 1993.
150. Colan SD, Borow KM, Neumann A: Left ventricular end-systolic wall stress-velocity of fiber shortening relation: A load-independent index of myocardial contractility, *J Am Coll Cardiol* 4(4):715-24, 1984.
151. Chinali M, de Simone G, Matteucci MC, et al: Reduced systolic myocardial function in children with chronic renal insufficiency, *J Am Soc Nephrol* 18(2):593-98, 2007.
152. de Simone G, Devereux RB, Roman MJ, et al: Assessment of left ventricular function by the midwall fractional shortening/end-systolic stress relation in human hypertension, *J Am Coll Cardiol* 23(6):1444-51, 1994.
153. de Simone G, Devereux RB, Celentano A, Roman MJ: Left ventricular chamber and wall mechanics in the presence of concentric geometry, *J Hypertens* 17(7):1001-06, 1999.
154. Mitsnefes MM, Kimball TR, Border WL, et al: Impaired left ventricular diastolic function in children with chronic renal failure, *Kidney Int* 65(4):1461-66, 2004.
155. Mitsnefes MM, Kimball TR, Border WL, et al: Abnormal cardiac function in children after renal transplantation, *Am J Kidney Dis* 43(4):721-26, 2004.
156. Parekh RS, Gidding SS: Cardiovascular complications in pediatric end-stage renal disease, *Pediatr Nephrol* 20(2):125-31, 2005.
157. Block GA: Prevalence and clinical consequences of elevated Ca × P product in hemodialysis patients, *Clin Nephrol* 54(4):318-24, 2000.
158. K/DOQI. Clinical practice guidelines for bone metabolism and disease in chronic kidney disease, *Am J Kidney Dis* 42(4/3):S1-S201, 2004.
159. Hogg RJ, Furth S, Lemley KV, et al: National Kidney Foundation's Kidney Disease Outcomes Quality Initiative clinical practice guidelines for chronic kidney disease in children and adolescents: Evaluation, classification, and stratification, *Pediatrics* 111(6/1):1416-21, 2003.
160. Klaus G, Watson A, Edefonti A, et al: Prevention and treatment of renal osteodystrophy in children on chronic renal failure: European guidelines, *Pediatr Nephrol* 21(2):151-59, 2006.
161. Martin KJ, Gonzalez EA: Vitamin D analogues for the management of secondary hyperparathyroidism, *Am J Kidney Dis* 38(5/5):S34-S40, 2001.

162. Lopez I, Aguilera-Tejero E, Mendoza FJ, et al: Calcimimetic R-568 decreases extraosseous calcifications in uremic rats treated with calcitriol, *J Am Soc Nephrol* 17(3):795-804, 2006.
163. Querfeld U: The therapeutic potential of novel phosphate binders, *Pediatr Nephrol* 20(3):389-92, 2005.
164. Pieper AK, Haffner D, Hoppe B, et al: A randomized crossover trial comparing sevelamer with calcium acetate in children with CKD, *Am J Kidney Dis* 47(4):625-35, 2006.
165. Salusky IB, Goodman WG, Sahney S, et al: Sevelamer controls parathyroid hormone-induced bone disease as efficiently as calcium carbonate without increasing serum calcium levels during therapy with active vitamin D sterols, *J Am Soc Nephrol* 16(8):2501-08, 2005.
166. Geary DF, Piva E, Gajaria M, Tyrrel J, Picone G, Harvey E: Development of a nocturnal home hemodialysis (NHHD) program for children, *Semin Dial* 17(2):115-17, 2004.
167. Fischbach M, Terzic J, Laugel V, et al: Daily on-line haemodiafiltration: A pilot trial in children, *Nephrol Dial Transplant* 19(9):2360-67, 2004.

CHAPTER 52

Psychosocial and Ethical Issues in Children with Chronic Kidney Disease

Arlene C. Gerson, Christine Harrison, and Susan L. Furth

INTRODUCTION

Medical advances have resulted in considerable improvements in life expectancies for children with chronic kidney disease (CKD).[1-3] As it is now the norm for infants and young children with CKD to survive childhood, there is increased attention to the psychosocial outcomes of these youth as they become adults. Some of the interest is motivated by an effort to determine the relative value of available treatment options, whereas other interest seems to be stimulated by a desire to improve psychosocial outcomes of this vulnerable group.[4] This chapter reviews research pertaining to psychosocial outcomes of children with CKD, provides recommendations for including systematic assessment of psychosocial status in research studies and in clinical practice, and briefly examines some ethical issues associated with the treatment of children with CKD.

Unfortunately, there are no prospective longitudinal studies and no cross-cultural comparisons of the psychosocial issues common to children with CKD. Furthermore, generalization of the available study results is hindered by a variety of methodologic issues—including the lack of uniform assessment tools, small sample sizes, and the analysis of heterogenous patient samples. Fortunately, there has been increased recognition of the importance of obtaining standardized assessments of psychosocial outcomes in children with kidney disease and increased funding to support large-scale prospective multi-institutional research.[5-7]

Although reliable information about psychosocial outcomes can be assessed using standardized psychological instruments and structured psychiatric survey tools that have been validated regionally, pediatric nephrologists are increasingly recommending the use of generic quality-of-life surveys to assess the functional outcomes of their pediatric patients.[8,9] Most of the available multidimensional quality-of-life surveys that have been validated for use with children who have CKD assess well-being across multiple areas of life. In addition to the assessment of physical health and well-being, social, psychological, and educational/occupational well-being are also queried in most generic quality-of-life surveys.[10-12] A conceptual definition of quality of life is illustrated schematically in Figure 52-1. The illustration highlights the interdependent nature of the domains of quality of life and the importance of multidimensional assessment in understanding the full range of manifestations of health and illness that ultimately impact psychosocial outcomes.

Recently published research provides strong evidence of the feasibility and utility of administering short, easy-to-complete, and easy-to-score quality-of-life survey tools in busy pediatric nephrology clinics.[9,13-15] The most comprehensive evaluation of the child's functioning can be obtained by querying both the caregiver and the youth with CKD. Moderate differences in impairment ratings between children and caregivers are not uncommon and should be explored.[9,10,16]

In the event that significant problems in physical, social, emotional, educational functioning are observed, nephrologists can refer children for further evaluation to a psychologist, psychiatrist, or clinical social worker who is experienced in working with children with health problems. It may be that early (<8 years old) and periodic (yearly) assessment of psychosocial adjustment will allow for earlier detection of health-related quality-of-life problems, earlier intervention, and improved positive outcomes in the areas of vocational, educational, and social functioning.[17] Economic benefit may also be realized if successful early intervention is achieved.[18,19]

PSYCHOLOGICAL AND BEHAVIORAL ADJUSTMENT

The psychological and behavioral adjustment of children with CKD has been evaluated by a number of research groups in an attempt to better understand the differential impact of various treatments and the risk factors for poor long-term health outcomes. In a series of studies completed in Manchester, England, with a group of patients who received dialysis during childhood, increased psychiatric morbidity of a minor nature was observed in a subset of children.[20-25]

Moreover, parents and youth report that the problems did not have any serious impact on the child's emotional state or quality of life.[21,24] This research team also observed that although the renal group described more psychological problems when they were less than 17 years old (when compared to a healthy age and socioeconomic status (SES)-matched control group) they did not have evidence of significantly higher rates of psychiatric disorders in adulthood, had lower

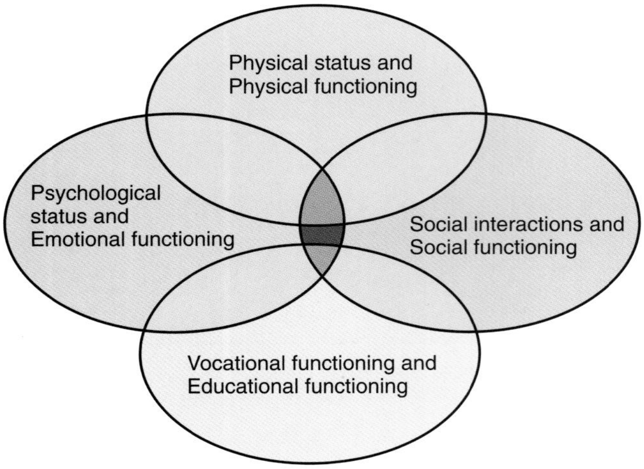

Figure 52-1 Conceptual diagram of quality-of-life construct.

rates of use of drugs and alcohol, and as a majority were generally satisfied with their life circumstances.[20]

Similar findings were observed by Fukunishi and Kudo, who evaluated the prevalence of psychiatric problems in a group of 53 Japanese children with end-stage renal disease (ESRD); 26 children receiving continuous ambulatory peritoneal dialysis (CAPD), 27 children with kidney transplants compared to an age-, gender-, and SES-matched group of 27 healthy youth, using a semistructured psychiatric interview (Diagnostic Interview for Children and Adolescents). Fukunishi and Kudo observed 65% of the CAPD group, 18% of the transplant group, and 4% of the control group to have separation anxiety disorder. Fifteen percent of the CAPD group, 4% of the transplant group, and 0% of the control group had generalized anxiety disorder. In addition, 4% of the CAPD group and 33% of the transplant group met the criteria for diagnosis of adjustment disorder.[26] The prevalence of other serious psychiatric disorders (such as major depression, conduct disorder, and oppositional defiant disorder) was not found to be higher in children with ESRD than in their matched control group of healthy children.[26]

In a recent cross-sectional study comparing 111 French children and adolescents who had received kidney or liver transplants with healthy youth, parents of the transplant recipients reported that 15% had problems in psychological functioning of a minor nature (lack of independence, refusal to mature).[27] In addition, parents reported anxiety problems in 12% of the transplant recipients.[27]

A recent study by Soliday et al. in the United States of 41 children with steroid sensitive nephrotic syndrome, chronic renal insufficiency, or kidney transplant using the Achenbach Child Behavior Checklist (CBCL) similarly failed to find significant differences in the prevalence of child behavior problems in the CKD group compared to a control group of healthy children of similar age, SES, education, and ethnicity.[28] Soliday et al. note that less than 15% of their CKD group had scores on the CBCL suggesting clinically significant behavior problems.

In addition to evaluating the prevalence of mental health and behavioral problems, several researchers have focused on trying to understand specific risk factors associated with psychiatric morbidity. Fielding and Brownbridge, in their assessment of psychological functioning and adjustment of 60 children and adolescents undergoing dialysis, observed that ESRD children who had greater functional impairment (i.e., feeling tired, having aches and pains, feeling ill, trouble sleeping, trouble walking independently, trouble running) as a result of their illness were more likely to be more depressed and more anxious and to show more behavioral disturbance than ESRD children with less functional impairment.[29] In addition, they observed that younger children on dialysis demonstrate greater adverse behavioral problems than older children.[29] Several researchers have concluded that the observed adjustment problems in youth with CKD may be related to poor relationships with peers at school rather than directly resulting from the experience of having kidney disease.[26,29]

EDUCATIONAL AND OCCUPATIONAL FUNCTIONING

CKD does unfortunately appear to have a negative impact on long-term educational attainment and occupational functioning of children. In a recent study evaluating 64 Canadian children with CKD, with a mean age of 13, McKenna et al. found 40% to be receiving special education and 85% to be attending school full time.[9] In comparison with a group of healthy children, the children with CKD studied by McKenna et al. reported more problems with school functioning. Roscoe et al. reported on the educational and occupational functional outcomes (defined by educational level, ability to care for oneself, and employment) in 118 Canadian adolescents who were 11 to 19 years old when dialysis was initiated and who had a mean age of 22 years at the time they were evaluated. They found that 13% were neither enrolled in an educational program nor employed.[30]

Similarly, poor educational outcomes were observed in a European sample.[31] Ehrich et al. analyzed data from the European Dialysis and Transplant Association registry of 617 patients who started renal replacement therapy (RRT) as children and were 21 to 35 years of age when the study was undertaken. Ehrich et al. found that 56% had completed secondary school, 16% were in a school for the handicapped, and 56% were employed. In comparison to the "healthy" population of the same age, employment was somewhat lower.[31] Morton et al. reported on the educational outcome of a British group of 45 young adult survivors of CKD compared to a normal age-matched control group of similar socioeconomic status. Morton et al. observed that more of the renal patients were unemployed (31%) than were the healthy subjects (12%) and that lack of educational qualifications and unemployment were more common in the renal groups than in the control group.[20]

In a recent cross-sectional study comparing the quality of life of 111 French children and adolescents who had received kidney or liver transplants to healthy youth, self-reported quality of life was generally good and was comparable to healthy youth—although transplant recipients reported less happiness at school.[27] Manificat et al. also observed that in comparison to healthy youth transplant recipients reported less happiness engaging in sports and when moving (running, jumping). Further information on the employment status of transplant patients was presented in the single-center experience of 150 German children transplanted between 1970 and 1993 reported by Offner et al.[32] Notably, 9% of patients with functioning grafts and 29% of patients on dialysis after graft failure were unemployed.[32]

A study evaluating the prevalence of academic problems (defined as falling grades or significant underachievement in a child with adequate intellectual ability) in Japanese children with ESRD also observed a high prevalence of school maladjustment.[33] Fukunishi and Honda (1995), who compared 35 kidney transplant recipients and 30 children receiving CAPD (mean age 9.7 years) to 33 healthy children, observed academic problems in 36% of the CAPD group, 40% of the transplant group, and 3% of the control group.[33]

Rosenkranz et al. undertook a large-scale multicenter study of 479 German children and adolescents with childhood-onset CKD and found that school attendance was in general satisfactory, with 22% of the youth attending schools for disabled or handicapped. However, only 14 of 53 adolescents (26%) over 16 years had graduated from school. Occupational functioning was evaluated in the 49 adult patients in their sample and only 21 (43%) were in some form of employment.[34] In a more recent evaluation of education and occupational functioning of a group of 39 young adults with childhood-onset CKD, Rosenkranz et al. observed some improvement in educational and occupational attainments (i.e., 58% "graduated" from high school and 67% were in paid employment).[35]

SOCIAL ADJUSTMENT

Children with CKD do unfortunately seem to have long-term social adjustment difficulties. A recently published study comparing 62 Canadian youth with CKD with healthy controls indicated that social functioning was more frequently impaired and more seriously impaired in the CKD group.[9] Similarly, Roscoe et al. reported on the social outcomes (marital status, achievement of parenthood) of 118 Canadian adolescents who were 11 to 19 years old when dialysis was initiated between 1966 and 1986.[30] With mean age of 22 years and mean follow-up of 8 years, Roscoe found that almost 70% of patients were living with family members—with only 28.9% living on their own or with a spouse.

Similarly, high rates of non-independent living (61%) were observed by Ehrich et al.—who analyzed data from the European Dialysis and Transplant Association registry of 617 patients who started RRT as children.[31] Morton et al. also observed in their sample of young adult survivors of CKD in the United Kingdom that living with parents and lack of experience of close relationships were more common in the renal groups than in their age- and SES-matched control group. Roesenkranz et al. (1992) observed a similarly prevalent lack of age-appropriate independence in a German sample, with a large proportion (86%) of patients over 17 years continuing to live with their parents or other persons taking care of them.[34] In a more recent evaluation of a young adult sample of German youth with childhood-onset kidney disease, Rosenkranz et al. observed an increase in the prevalence of age-appropriate independent living (i.e., 49%).[35]

MEDIATORS OF PSYCHOSOCIAL MORBIDITY

Fortunately, there do appear to be some factors that mediate negative psychosocial outcomes. Social support, for example, appears to provide some degree of protection to both the individual with CKD and the family. Fielding and Brownbridge found that parents who received more social support from outside immediate family reported fewer treatment-related problems, were less depressed, and were less likely to rate their children as disturbed than parents of CKD children who had limited extrafamilial social support.[29] Similarly, lack of social support seems to be a mediator of psychosocial morbidity in children with CKD.[29,36] In addition, interfamily support also appears to reduce the risk of psychosocial morbidity.[28,36]

Cross-sectional and longitudinal research comparing psychosocial status of youth on dialysis and youth after transplantation has frequently reported better psychosocial functioning in children with CKD who have received a kidney transplant.[13,14,24] For example, Reynolds et al. reported that children evaluated after transplantation perceived improvement in mood and self-concept and parents perceived improvements in general physical and psychological health after transplantation.[24] Similarly, Gerson et al. reported on 21 adolescents on dialysis compared to 39 adolescents with chronic renal insufficiency (CRI), and 53 adolescent transplant recipients, and observed adolescents on dialysis had more limitations in physical activity and greater physical impairment. Conversely, McKenna et al.[9] did not observe youth undergoing dialysis to have greater physical impairment than transplant recipients or youth with CRI.

ETHICAL ISSUES AND CONSIDERATIONS IN THE TREATMENT OF CHILDREN WITH CKD

A host of ethical issues arise for health care providers who care for infants, children, and young adults with chronic kidney disease. As children are embedded within families, and often are unable to make decisions for themselves, health care practitioners must collaborate with parents or legal guardians in order to make decisions in children's best interests—and pediatric health care organizations should promote family-centered care.[37]

For these reasons, an approach relying solely on the principles of autonomy (patient self-determination), beneficence (evaluating whether the proposed treatment preserves life and offers benefit over harm), and justice is inadequate for resolving the ethical issues that confront nephrologists. Rather, a relational ethic that includes consideration of these principles but emphasizes the context of the child and family and relationships among the child-family-healthcare provider triad provides a better basic framework for resolving the ethical dilemmas facing pediatric nephrologists.[38-40]

The notion that the nurturing, enhancement, and preservation of relationships should motivate ethical decision making in health care grew from the discomfort expressed by some bioethicists that the traditional moral theories and principles were detached from the real problems faced by patients, families, and health care practitioners. Pediatrics is a "relationship-rich" subspecialty in light of the variety of relationships between parents and children, between siblings, among individuals representing the wide range of health care disciplines typically represented on the health care team, and between the team and family itself.

THE BEST INTERESTS STANDARD AND SURROGATE DECISION MAKERS

It is generally agreed that the most appropriate surrogate decision makers for young children are their parents, unless they are acting in such a way that the child may be harmed.[41,42] When pediatric nephrologists are unable to resolve situations in which parents appear to be making decisions that are not in a child's best interests, it may be necessary to contact child protection authorities or other locally available child advocacy services. Otherwise, decisions are best made by parents and the child's health care providers working together and sharing information. Decisions should be made in the child's best interests, considering both benefits and burdens of treatment.[43-46]

The most common ethical dilemma discussed by pediatric nephrologists is when to initiate or withdraw dialysis.[47] When dialysis was first introduced as a viable treatment option, there was much debate about whether it was fair to expose children to a treatment that had so many unknown long-term risks.[48-50] Once dialysis was established as a relatively safe treatment with life-prolonging potential, ethical discussions about when to discontinue dialysis became more frequent.[51] In addition, considerable debate has occurred about the benefits of initiating dialysis in infants who have multiorgan complications and a poor chance of good recovery.[45,47]

While there seems to be some interest in developing guidelines for dialysis initiation and discontinuation, efforts to obtain a consensus have been challenging.[52,53] Therefore, as the debate continues regarding specific guidelines for pediatric dialysis treatment general guidelines pertaining to medical treatment of children have been developed that can assist pediatric nephrologists in making difficult decisions pertaining to the initiation and discontinuation of dialysis.[44-46]

THE CHILD'S ROLE IN DECISION MAKING

There has been a growing discussion about the role children and adolescents should have in decisions regarding dialysis initiation and discontinuation,[54-57] and in treatment decisions generally.[40] It is respectful of children and adolescents to provide them with developmentally appropriate information and to include them in decisions as appropriate and when it is their wish to have a say about their treatment.[58] Different jurisdictions may address children's and adolescents' legal right to give their own informed consent in different ways.

Sometimes a child's right to make his or her own health care decisions will rest on an age of consent, sometimes on the age of majority. Sometimes an individual's right to make his or her own decisions will rest on the mental capacity to do so, regardless of their age. As there may be considerable variability in these matters, health care providers are advised to be aware of local policy and law. Although some older children and adolescents may wish to make their own decisions, some may not—and it is reasonable to encourage decision making as a family or to support a child's wish to have his or her parents make decisions.

KIDNEY TRANSPLANTATION

When kidney transplantation became available to children, ethical debate initially revolved around whether it was fair to subject children to a medical treatment that had many potential risks. As pediatric kidney transplantation became safer, ethical dialogue expanded to discussions of who should be recommended for transplantation, when kidney transplantation should be recommended, and who should be allowed to donate a kidney. Ethical concerns are not uncommon when nonadherence with dialysis is observed and when suboptimal social support is suspected. Health care providers struggle with questions such as the following.

- Under what circumstances should a child with little family support to promote adherence to medical regimens be recommended for kidney transplantation?[59]
- Is it fair to deny a potentially life-saving treatment to a child because of the actions of his or her parents?

A child's right to donate a kidney to a sibling[60] or to a parent has also been ethically evaluated,[61,62] as has the appropriateness of allowing a developmentally delayed child to be a kidney donor.[63,64] In an environment where the need for organs far exceeds their availability, clinicians may find themselves discussing the ethics of resource allocation—and may be challenged by the tension between their roles as social agents and care providers.

When faced with questions such as "Should a developmentally delayed child be recommended for kidney transplantation?"[65-67] or "Should a child with severe conduct problems be recommended for kidney transplantation?,"[68] clinicians might consider predictions of the potential societal benefit a recipient might make versus the duty of society to protect those who are particularly vulnerable. Different theories of justice will determine the conclusions reached, although the potential for the child to benefit from a transplant should be a primary consideration.

ADDRESSING CONFLICT

There is general endorsement of the importance of involving parents in the process of resolving ethically challenging dilemmas.[45,47,52,69,70] Especially in difficult situations, where the relative burden of the underlying illness and its associated treatment is determined to have uncertain treatment benefit, parental preferences are appropriately granted great weight.[71] Although the relative weight given to parental opinions may differ by country or social and medical circumstances of the child, a collaborative approach to decision making is favored—with health care providers and parents working together to decide the child's best interests.

The utility of multidisciplinary input in clinical situations that are ethically complicated is well documented.[45] The goal of multidisciplinary ethics discussions is to encourage candid debate that results in clarification of what course of action will serve the best interest of the child. A number of excellent articles have been written that provide in-depth discussion and guidance concerning commonly encountered dilemmas within pediatric nephrology practice.[2,47,63] The use of published discourse and local resources should provide clinicians with support that empowers the development of ethical relationships and solutions in caring for children with kidney disease. When parents and health care teams disagree, conflict resolution may be assisted by ethics committees and ethics consultants. Although the ultimate resolution of ethical situations is likely to vary across health care providers, the process of determining a course of action should follow a format similar to that outlined in Table 52-1.

TABLE 52-1 Suggested Format for Consideration of Ethical Issues

1. Members of the health care team should reach consensus about a medical recommendation.
2. The patient and family should be given information, time, and opportunity to reflect and ask questions, as well as the opportunity to consult with others.
3. The best interests of the child should guide decision making, with consideration of the interests of parents and other family members.
4. Children and adolescents should be increasingly involved in decision making as they mature.
5. Ethics committees and consultants may be helpful in resolving conflicts.

SUMMARY AND RECOMMENDATIONS

Advances in medical treatment for children with CKD have resulted in increased numbers of youth surviving childhood and an increased interest in their psychosocial outcome as adults. Although serious psychological and behavioral problems do not appear to be the norm for youth with childhood-onset kidney disease, educational problems and social functioning difficulties are commonly observed in adults who had childhood-onset kidney disease. To better understand the risk factors for poor psychosocial outcomes and to develop interventions to improve outcomes, there is a need for multicenter prospective longitudinal evaluation of children with kidney disease.

Medical advances have also led to increased ethical debate about the appropriateness of particular treatments and the appropriateness of the withdrawal of treatment in children with CKD. Nephrologists are encouraged to familiarize themselves with published discourse and to use local resources (ethics committees and consultants) for assistance in addressing ethically challenging dilemmas.

REFERENCES

1. NAPRTCS. North American Pediatric Renal Transplant Cooperative Study 2005 Annual Report. https://web.emmes.com/study/ped/annlrept/annlrept.html, 2005.
2. Broyer M, Chantler C, Donckerwolcke R, Ehrich JHH, Rizzoni G, Scharer K: The paediatric registry of the European Dialysis and Transplant Association: 20 years experience, *Pediatr Nephrol* 7:758-68, 1993.
3. Reiss U, Wingen AM, Scharer K: Mortality trends in pediatric patients with chronic renal failure, *Pediatr Nephrol* 10:41-45, 1993.
4. Furth SL, Gerson AC, Neu AM, Fivush BA: The impact of dialysis and transplantation on children, *Adv Ren Replace Ther* 8:206-23, 2001.
5. Chesney RW, Brewer E, Moxey-Mims M, Watkins S, Furth SL, Harmon WE, et al: Report of an NIH task force on research priorities in chronic kidney disease in children, *Pediatr Nephrol* 1:14-25, 2006.
6. Neu A: Special issues in pediatric kidney transplantation, *Advances in Chronic Kidney Disease* 13:62-69, 2006.
7. Furth SL, Cole SR, Moxey-Mims M, Kaskel F, Mak R, Schwartz G, et al: Design and methods in the chronic kidney disease in children (CKiD) prospective cohort study, *CJASN* 1:1006-15, 2006.
8. Goldstein SL, Graham N, Burwinkle T, Warady B, Farrah R, Varni JW: Health related quality of life in pediatric patients with ESRD, *Pediatr Nephrol* 21:846-50, 2006.
9. McKenna AM, Keating LE, Vigneaux A, Stevens S, Williams A, Geary DF: Quality of life in children with chronic kidney disease: Patient and caregiver assessments, *Nephrol Dial Tranplant* 21(7):1899-905, 2006.
10. Varni JW, Seid M, Kurtin PS: PedsQL 4.0: Reliability and validity of the pediatric quality of life inventory version 4.0 generic core scales in healthy and patient populations, *Med Care* 39:800-12, 2001.
11. Starfield B, Riley AW, Green B, Ensminger M, Ryan SA, Kelleher K, et al: The adolescent child health and illness profile: A popluation-based measure of health, *Med Care* 33:553-66, 1995.
12. Landgraf JM, Abetz LN, Ware JE: *The CHQ user's manual, second edition*, Boston: Health Act 1996.
13. Goldstein SL, Graham N, Burwinkle T, Warady B, Farrah R, Varni JW: Health related quality of life in pediatric patients with ESRD, *Pediatr Nephrol* 21:846-50, 2006.
14. Gerson AC, Fivush BA, Pham N, Fiorenza J, Robertson J, Weiss R, et al: Assessing health status and health care utilization in adolescents with chronic kidney disease, *JASN* 16:1427-32, 2005.
15. Gerson AC, Fiorenza J, Barth K, Hwang W, Fivush BA, Furth SL: The effect of anemia on quality of life in adolescents with chronic illness, *AJKD* 44:1017-23, 2004.
16. Eiser C, Morse R: The measurement of quality of life in children: Past and future prespectives, *J Dev Behav Pediatr* 22:248-56, 2001.
17. Armstrong FD: Neurodevelopment and chronic illness: Mechanisms of disease and treatment, *MRDDRR* 12:168-73, 2006.
18. Seid M, Varni JW, Segall D, Kurtin PS: Health-related quality of life as a predictor of pediatric healthcare costs: A two year prospective cohort analysis, *Health and Quality of Life Outcomes* 2:48, 2004.
19. Varni JW, Burwinkle T, Seid M: The PedsQL 4.0 as a school population health measure: Feasibility, reliability, and validity, *Quality of Life Research* 15:203-15, 2006.
20. Morton MJS, Reynolds JM, Garralda ME, Postlethwaite RJ, Goh D: Psychiatric adjustment in end-stage renal disease: A follow up study of former paediatric patients, *J Psychosom Res* 38:296-303, 1994.
21. Postlethwaite RJ, Garralda ME, Eminson DM, Reynolds J: Lessons from psychosocial studies of chronic renal failure, *Arch Dis Child* 75:455-58, 1996.
22. Reynolds JM, Garralda ME, Jameson RA, Postlethwaite RJ: Living with renal failure, *Child Care Health Dev* 12:401-07, 1986.
23. Reynolds JM, Garralda ME, Jameson RA, Postlethwaite RJ: How parents and families coped with renal failure, *Arch Dis Child* 63:821-26, 1988.
24. Reynolds JM, Garralda ME, Postlethwaite RJ, Goh D: Changes in psychosocial adjustment after renal transplantation, *Arch Dis Child* 66:508-13, 1991.
25. Reynolds JM, Morton MJS, Garralda ME, Postlethwaite RJ, Goh D: Psychosocial adjustment of adult survivors of a paediatric dialysis and transplant programme, *Arch Dis Child* 68:110, 1993.

26. Fukunishi I, Kudo H: Psychiatric problems of pediatric end-stage renal failure, *General Hospital Psychiatry* 17:32-36, 1995.
27. Manificat S, Dazord A, Cochat P, Morin D, Plainguet F, Debray D: Quality of life of children and adolescents after kidney or liver transplantation: Child, parents and caregiver's point of view, *Pediatr Transplant* 7:228-35, 2003.
28. Soliday E, Kool E, Lande MB: Psychosocial adjustment in children with kidney disease, *J Pediatr Psychol* 25:93-103, 2000.
29. Fielding D, Brownbridge G: Factors related to psychosocial adjustment in children with end-stage renal failure, *Pediatr Nephrol* 13:766-70, 1999.
30. Roscoe JM, Smith LF, Williams EA, Stein M, Morton AR, Balfe JW, et al: Medical and social outcome in adolescents with end-stage renal failure, *Kidney Int* 40:948-53, 1991.
31. Ehrich JHH, Rizzoni G, Broyer M, Brunner FP, Brynger H, Fassbinder W, et al: Rehabilitation of young adults during renal replacement therapy in Europe. 2. Schooling, employment, and social situation, *Nephrol Dial Transplant* 7:579-86, 1992.
32. Offner G, Latta K, Hoyer PF: Kidney transplanted children come of age, *Kidney Int* 55:1509-17, 1999.
33. Fukunishi I, Honda M: School adjustment of children with end-stage renal disease, *Pediatr Nephrol* 9:553-57, 1995.
34. Rosenkranz J, Bonzel K-E, Bulla M, Michalk D, Offner G, Reichwald-Klugger E, et al: Psychosocial adaptation of children and adolescents with chronic renal failure, *Pediatr Nephrol* 6:459-63, 1992.
35. Rosenkranz J, Reicwald-Klugger E, Oh J, Turzer M, Mehls O, Schafer F: Psychosocial rehabilitation and satisfaction with life in adults with childhood-onset of end-stage renal disease, *Pediatr Nephrol* 20:1288-94, 2005.
36. Christensen AJ, Turner CW, Slaughter JR, Holman JM Jr.: Perceived family support as a mediator of psychological well-being in end-stage renal disease, *J Behav Med* 12:249-65, 1989.
37. Rauch-Percelay J, Zipes D: Introduction to pediatric hospital medicine, *Pediatr Clin North Am* 52:963-67, 2005.
38. Bergum V, Dossetor J: *Relational ethics: The full meaning of respect*. Hagarstown: University Publishing Group 2005.
39. Nelson H, Nelson J: *The patient in the family: An ethics of medicine and families*. New York: Routledge 1995.
40. Harrison C, Kenny N, Sidarous M, Rowell M: Bioethics for clinicians: Involving children in medical decision making, *Can Med Assoc* 156:825-28, 1997.
41. Diekema D: Parental refusal of medical treatment: The harm principle as threshold for state intervention, *Theoretical Medicine* 25:243-64, 2004.
42. Rhodes R, Holzman I: The not unreasonable standard for assessment of surrogates and surrogate decisions, *Theoretical Medicine* 25:367-85, 2004.
43. Office of the United Nations High Commissioner for Human Rights: United Nations convention on the rights of the child. http://www.unhchr.ch/html/menu3/b/k2crc.htm, 1989.
44. British Medical Association: Ethics, children, parental responsibility. http://www.bma.org.uk/ap.nsf/Content/Parental, 2006.
45. American Academy of Pediatrics Committee on Bioethics: Ethics and the care of critically ill infants and children, *Pediatrics* 98:149-52, 1996.
46. Canadian Paediatric Society Bioethics Committee: Treatment decisions regarding infants, children and adolescents, *Paediatrics and Child Health* 9:99-103, 2004.
47. Shooter M, Watson A: The ethics of withholding and withdrawing dialysis therapy in infants, *Pediatr Nephrol* 14:347-51, 2000.
48. Cohen C: Ethical and legal considerations in the care of the infant with end-stage renal disease whose parents elect conservative therapy: An American perspective, *Pediatr Nephrol* 1:166-71, 1987.
49. Fine RN, Salusky IB, Ettenger RB: The therapeutic approach to the infant, child, and adolescent with end-stage renal disease, *Pediatr Clin North Am* 34:789-801, 1987.
50. Warady B: Neurodevelopment of infants with end-stage renal disease: Is it improving? *Pediatr Transplant* 6:5-7, 2002.
51. Fauriel I, Moutel G, Moutard ML, Montuclard L, Duchange N, Callies I, et al: Decisions concerning potentially life-sustaining treatments in paediatric nephrology: A multicentre study in French-speaking countries, *Nephrol Dial Transplant* 19:1252-57, 2004.
52. Galla JH: Clinical practice guideline on shared decision-making in appropriate initiation of and withdrawal from dialysis, *J Am Soc Nephrol* 11:1340-42, 2000.
53. Riano I, Malaga S, Callis L, Loris C, Martin-Govantes J, Navarro M, et al: Towards guidelines for dialysis in children with end-stage renal disease, *Pediatr Nephrol* 15:157-62, 2000.
54. Doyal L, Henning P: Stopping treatment for end-stage renal failure: the rights of children and adolescents, *Pediatr Nephrol* 8:768-71, 1994.
55. Spencer GE: Children's competency to consent: An ethical dilemma, *J Child Health Care* 4:117-22, 2000.
56. Gabbai N, Rauch-Elnekav H, Spitz M, Weissman I: Treatment decisions in paediatric dialysis: Children's versus parental rights, *Edtna Erca J* 25:39-41, 1999.
57. Kunin H: Ethical issues in pediatric life threatening illness: Dilemmas, consent, assent and communication, *Ethics Behav* 7:43-57, 1997.
58. UNESCO: Universal declaration on bioethics and human rights. http://portal.unesco.org/en/ev.php-URL_ID=31058&URL_DO=DO_TOPIC&URL_SECTION=201.html, 2005.
59. Furth SL, Hwang W, Neu AM, Fivush BA, Powe NR: Effects of patient compliance, parental education and race on nephrologists' recommendations for kidney transplantation in children, *Am J Transplant* 3:28-34, 2003.
60. Delmonico FL, Harmon WE: The use of a minor as a live kidney donor, *Am J Transplant* 2:333-36, 2002.
61. Ross LF: Justice for children: The child as organ donor, *Bioethics* 8:105-26, 1994.
62. Spital A: Should children ever donate kidneys?: Views of U.S. transplant centers, *Transplantation* 64:232-36, 1997.
63. Steinberg D: Kidney transplants from young children and the mentally retarded, *Theor Med Bioeth* 25:229-41, 2004.
64. Martens MA, Jones L, Reiss S: Organ transplantation, organ donation and mental retardation, *Pediatr Transplantation* 10:658-64, 2006.
65. Ohta T, Motoyama O, Takahashi K, Hattori M, Shishido S, Wada N, et al: Kidney transplantation in pediatric recipients with mental retardation: Clinical results of a multicenter experience in Japan, *Am J Kidney Dis* 47:518-27, 2006.
66. EBPG Expert Group on Renal Transplantation: European best practice guidelines for renal transplantation. Section IV: Long-term management of the transplant recipient. IV.11 Paediatrics (specific problems), *Nephrol Dial Transplant* 17:55-58, 2002.
67. Orr R, Johnston J, Ashwal S, Bailey L: Should children with severe cognitive impairment recieve solid organ transplants? *The Journal of Clinical Ethics* 11:219-29, 2006.
68. Reinhart JB, Kemph JP: Renal transplantation for children: Another view, *JAMA* 260:3327-28, 1988.
69. Lelie A: Decision-making in nephrology: shared decision making? *Patient Educ Couns* 39:81-89, 2000.
70. Sharman M, Meert KL, Sarnaik AP: What influences parents' decisions to limit or withdraw life support? *Pediatr Crit Care Med* 6:513-18, 2005.
71. Solomon MZ, Sellers DE, Heller KS, Dokken DL, Levetown M, Ruston C, et al: New and lingering controversies in pediatric end-of-life care, *Pediatrics* 116:872-83, 2005.

CHAPTER 53

Dialysis Modality Choice and Initiation in Children

Cornelis H. Schröder and Denis F. Geary

INDICATIONS FOR INITIATION OF DIALYSIS

Determination of the optimal or precise time to start renal replacement therapy for children is seldom straightforward except in extreme circumstances, such as following bilateral nephrectomies. Both clinical and laboratory parameters contribute to the decision to start renal replacement therapy. If preemptive renal transplantation is selected, preparations can be made well in advance. However, when one of the different dialysis modalities is chosen the timing is more critical.

Fortunately, there are currently several recent pediatric guidelines available, which are based on experience and expert opinion of pediatric nephrologists as well as the Kidney Disease Outcomes Quality Initiative (K/DOQI) guidelines for adult patients.[1-5] The decision to start dialysis should include the considerations discussed in the sections that follow.

Severity of Renal Dysfunction

According to the K-DOQI guidelines,[1] initiation of dialysis should be considered when the glomerular filtration rate (GFR) falls below 14 ml/min/1.73 m^2 body surface area (BSA) and is strongly recommended when the GFR is <8 ml/min/1.73 m^2. However, use of these figures raises the question of how GFR should be measured. Inulin clearance, although the gold standard for determination of GFR, is rarely performed in daily clinical practice.

Radionuclide GFR measurements (chromium^{51}-EDTA, ^{125}I iothalamate sodium, technetium^{99}-DTPA), although reliable, are used infrequently in children with renal failure because they are expensive and inconvenient for routine clinical practice. As a result, most institutions apply either the Schwartz formula[6] (based on serum creatinine and body height) or the creatinine clearance (based on the determination of creatinine in a 24-hour urine collection). The standard creatinine clearance is calculated from a 24-hour urine collection and a blood sample as

$$Cr_{Cl} = \frac{U_{vol} \times U_{cr} \times 1.73}{1440 \times S_{cr} \times BSA} \text{ ml/min/1.73m}^2$$

where U_{vol} = 24-hour urine volume, U_{cr} = urinary creatinine concentration, S_{cr} = serum creatinine concentration, and BSA = body surface area in m^2. The constants 1.73 and 1440 are for the standardized adult body surface area and the number of minutes in a day. Because the collection of a 24-hour specimen may be difficult particularly in children, the Schwartz equation is widely applied:

$$GFR = \frac{H \times k}{S_{cr}} \text{ ml/min/1.73m}^2$$

Here, H = height of the patient in cm, S_{cr} = serum creatinine concentration (mg/dl), and k is an age-dependent constant: 0.55 (49) for boys 2 to 12 years of age and girls 2 to 21 years, 0.70 (62) for boys 13 to 18 years, 0.45 (40) for term infants <1 year old, and 0.33 (29) for low birth weight infants <1 year old. The numbers in brackets are the k values if the creatinine is measured in µmol/L.

Both latter methods may seriously overestimate GFR because of active tubular creatinine excretion, particularly if GFR is in the lower range.[7] If GFR is decreasing and tubular secretion of creatinine remains relatively stable, the secretion component contributes significantly to the calculation of GFR. At very low GFR levels, glomerular filtration and tubular secretion of creatinine may be equal. To improve the accuracy of GFR estimation, two methods may be used.

- One method is determination of the GFR after blocking tubular creatinine secretion with cimetidine.[8] Although infrequently used in clinical practice, the protocol is relatively simple and should be applied on a larger scale. Cimetidine should be administered in two daily doses for the two days prior to the collection of urine. Dosage is dependent on the estimated renal clearance: 20 mg/kg/day > 75 ml/min/1.73 m^2 with a dose reduction to 80% if clearance is 50 to 75 ml/min/1.73 m^2, 70% if 30 to 50 ml/min/1.73 m^2, 60% if 20 to 30 ml/min/1.73 m^2, and 50% if <20 ml/min/1.73 m^2. Using this protocol, creatinine clearance very closely related to inulin clearance can be determined.
- Alternatively, endogenous solutes may be used to measure GFR by defining GFR as the arithmetic mean of urea and creatinine clearance.[1] Because urea undergoes some tubular reabsorption as well as glomerular filtration, this arithmetic mean essentially corrects for secretion of creatinine.

GFR (ml/min) = (kidney urea clearance + kidney creatinine clearance/2)

This is then corrected to 1.73 m^2 body surface area (as outlined previously). Because there is insufficient evidence on the preferred method for determination of GFR in children, the published guidelines do not dictate what method is preferable.

Clinical Factors

The clinical well-being of the patient is more important than the determination of GFR as a basis for deciding when dialysis should be started. The presence of fluid overload and hypertension, gastrointestinal symptoms (such as nausea and vomiting, malnutrition, and growth retardation), and neurological consequences of uremia will accelerate the decision to initiate dialysis.

Symptoms such as lethargy, nausea, and anorexia may be subtle and difficult to elucidate—particularly when their onset is insidious. Detailed history or questionnaires may be required to determine the impact of progressive renal dysfunction on the child's quality of life. Families may minimize or fail to appreciate symptoms because of their common desire to delay dialysis.

Biochemical Factors

In addition to the clinical symptoms outlined previously, laboratory abnormalities such as hyperkalemia, hyperphosphatemia, and acidosis substantially influence the decision to start dialysis. Hyperkalemia generally does not occur until GFR is less than 20 to 30 ml/min/1.73 m^2. It should be treated by dietary potassium restriction and the oral administration of potassium-binding resins such as sodium polystyrene sulfonate and calcium polystyrene sulfonate.

Hyperphosphatemia may also be a serious problem as the GFR drops below 30 ml/min/1.73 m^2. It is treated by a dietary restriction of phosphate intake as well as by phosphate-binding medication (calcium carbonate, calcium acetate, or sevelamer). Metabolic acidosis, which is common in children with congenital urological disorders, becomes more prominent when GFR falls below 20 ml/min/m^2—and may be treated by oral sodium bicarbonate or sodium citrate.

As children progress from chronic kidney disease stage III (estimated GFR 30-60 ml/min/1.73 m^2) to IV and then V (estimated GFR <15 ml/min/1.73 m^2), their requirement for medical oversight increases. A schedule for evaluation of children with chronic renal failure proposed by Greenbaum and Schaefer[4] is outlined in Table 53-1.

The most important determinant concerning the start of dialysis is the comfort and well-being of the patient. Dialysis should be started before the clinical condition deteriorates so that postinitiation significant clinical improvement should not be observed. It is no longer appropriate to delay dialysis until the patient's predialysis morbidity is substantial. Although this sounds quite simple and obvious, the determination of the moment to start dialysis is not straightforward.

Early initiation of dialysis may be beneficial for the nutritional status and well-being of the patient. On the other hand, there is a risk of complications from dialysis therapy. Some of the benefits and potential drawbacks of early dialysis initiation are outlined in Table 53-2 and discussed in the material following.

TABLE 53-1 Evaluation Schedule for Children with Chronic Renal Failure*

Timing	Evaluation
At least every 3 months	Height, weight, head circumference in infants, blood pressure, acid-base status, electrolytes, creatinine, BUN, CBC, albumin, PTH, estimation of GFR
Every 6 to 12 months	Echocardiography, ABPM, hand X-ray, neurodevelopmental assessment in infants

* From Greenbaum L, Schaefer FS: The decision to initiate dialysis in children and adolescents. In BA Warady, FS Schaefer, RN Fine, SR Alexander (eds.), *Pediatric dialysis.* Dordrecht, The Netherlands: Kluwer Academic Publishers 2004:177-196.

BUN, Blood urea nitrogen; *CBC*, complete blood count; *PTH*, parathyroid hormone; *ABPM*, ambulatory blood pressure monitoring.

TABLE 53-2 Advantages and Disadvantages of Early Dialysis Initiation

Advantages	Disadvantages
Improved general well being	Psychosocial impact on patient
Improved biochemical values	Psychosocial impact on family
Closer medical follow-up	Increased cost to family
Improved nutrition	Increased cost to health care system
Improved fluid balance and blood pressure	—

In children, who have a longer life expectancy than adults, the choice of dialysis modality requires careful consideration. Every peritonitis episode may damage the peritoneal membrane, and similarly every fistula failure will seriously damage a blood vessel that might be needed in the future. Such considerations are important even if a very short course of dialysis is anticipated because of prearranged living donor transplant.

For example, attempts to preserve vessels for future fistula formation, by insertion of temporary central venous catheters either in a subclavian or femoral location, may cause permanent stenosis or thrombosis of major vessels—which may compromise use of those vessels for future permanent vascular access or even transplantation. Therefore, extreme care is warranted because lifelong function of the first kidney graft is unlikely in children.

INSTITUTIONAL REQUIREMENTS

Minimal Patient Numbers

Dialysis in children should only be performed in experienced centers, where a multidisciplinary team is available for the treatment and guidance of both children and parents.[2] Centers should have experience with, and preferably provide, both hemodialysis and peritoneal dialysis so that the advantages and disadvantages of each modality can be clearly explained to the patients in an unbiased manner.

Because the incidence and prevalence of end-stage renal disease in children are low (5.8 and 38.7 per million of the child population <16 years of age),[9] a population of several million people is needed to provide a critical mass of patients to ensure continued maintenance of expertise by a staff. Although it is difficult to estimate a minimum number of children required for the staff of a dialysis unit to maintain their expertise, a number of approximately 10 dialysis patients seems reasonable. However, in countries where geographic distances between centers are large and populations are small a program may have to function with smaller patient numbers.

Staff Requirements

The pediatric dialysis unit and staff should be embedded in a large tertiary pediatric department, and close cooperation with a center for nephrology in adults is desirable. In addition to pediatric nephrologists, specialized pediatric dialysis nurses should be available—as well as a dedicated social worker, pediatric dietitian, and whenever possible a pediatric psychologist. Play therapists may be of great value, and schoolteachers must be available for the children on hemodialysis. If either home peritoneal or hemodialysis is contemplated, a home visit by a dialysis nurse and possibly a social worker is needed.[2]

The number of nurses required in providing care for home peritoneal, home hemodialysis, and in-center hemodialysis has not been standardized. Therefore, estimates of these requirements must be based on experience as well as extrapolation from adult dialysis centers. In the Toronto adult dialysis units, one nurse is intended to support 20 home dialysis patients. In addition, these positions must be covered during times primary support nurses are on vacation or involved in training a new dialysis patient.

There are no firm guidelines for the numbers of such staff for children. Therefore, by extrapolation from the adult experience and recognizing the much greater intensity of labor required for children on dialysis we try to ensure that one full-time nurse supports approximately half the number of home dialysis children (i.e., about 10) a nurse would support in an adult unit. Finally, nurse versus patient ratios for in-center hemodialysis in children are much smaller than the ratio found in adult units. In the dialysis unit at the Hospital for Sick Children, nurses are not scheduled to care for more than two stable adolescent patients, and for younger (or clinically unwell) children a 1 : 1 nurse-to-patient ratio may be required. As well as a pediatric nephrologist, a pediatric dialysis nurse should be available for patient/parent consultation at all times.

It is recommended in the KDOQI Nutrition Guidelines that for adults one full-time dietitian is recommended to provide ongoing nutritional support for 100 maintenance dialysis patients.[10] However, because of the intrinsic importance of optimal nutrition to promote growth in children with end-stage renal disease and the complexity of care required to optimize nutrition in infants or children with specialized feeding requirements (e.g., tube feeds) a pediatric renal dietitian cannot hope to support the same number of patients as his or her adult colleagues. Details of the dietary support provided for children on home peritoneal dialysis (PD) have been described by Coleman et al., who report that an overall mean of 4.2 patient contacts is required monthly—with a greater number for children undergoing tube feeds.[11] This intrinsic difference between adult and pediatric nephrology dietitians must be considered when dietetic staffing is planned.

A dialysis technologist is required to ensure maintenance of equipment according to manufacturers' recommendations. The technologist is also responsible for ensuring that appropriate standards for water treatment are maintained. Finally, the availability of an in-house expert in dialysis technology is a great support for doctors and nurses less technologically skilled.

Specialized surgical expertise must be available to provide access for both hemodialysis (HD) and PD, as well as for ongoing support. It has been proven that results are superior if an interested senior surgeon is responsible for both PD[12] and HD[13] access programs, particularly if microsurgical techniques are applied.[13] These surgeons usually, though not necessarily, are also involved in planning and preparation of the child for transplantation. Preferably, renal transplantation is performed in the same hospital where the dialysis unit is located. This ensures consistent treatment by the same team members, adding both medical benefits and feelings of security for patients and parents.

Interventional radiology should be readily available for assistance with diagnosis and treatment of access-related problems. The role of the interventional radiologist in pediatric nephrology is outlined in Chapter 69.

Patient Education

The dialysis unit staff should include nurses whose primary role is to train patients for home PD, and if appropriate for HD. Standards for home PD training are not consistent, and the time required to complete training is ill defined and individualized.[2] In an international survey of 317 PD nurses in adult units, the reported time devoted to patient training varied from 6 to 96 hours.[14] In this survey, the incidence of peritonitis in the dialysis unit did not appear to be related to the duration of patient training. However, results of a similar survey of 76 pediatric nephrology centers providing home PD for a total of 597 children were more concerning.[15]

The peritonitis rate was significantly lower in programs with larger patient numbers and longer training time dedicated to theory and practical/technical skills. Therefore, while acknowledging that practice will vary from one unit to another it is our opinion that home PD training should include at least 5 uninterrupted days of family/patient education by the nurse trainer.

There is less experience with training requirements for home HD in children. In our unit, this training extends over a 6-week period and occurs during the patient's in-center dialysis sessions (usually three times weekly). At the end of 6 weeks, the patient or his or her caregiver must perform their own dialysis safely in the hospital unit on at least three occasions before transfer to the home.[16]

Space Allocation

Each hospital caring for children on dialysis must have appropriate space devoted solely to this patient population. Two panels of Canadian experts have suggested that 12 m^2 (130 square feet) of space is required to care for each dialysis bed/chair.[17,18] This is separate from the nursing station, supplies and storage rooms, staff offices, and technologist work space. In addition, space may be required for the teaching and recreational therapy of children—with storage for the necessary books and equipment. Teaching areas for home PD should be separate, whereas teaching space for home HD will make use of the regular in-center dialysis space but should be in a private area large enough to incorporate teaching.

The pediatric dialysis unit should have a clearly defined protocol for the transition of patients on dialysis to the departments of nephrology in adult dialysis units. Because a pediatric unit generally collaborates with many units for adults, the development and maintenance of such a protocol should be the responsibility of the pediatric unit.

MODALITY SELECTION

Of the dialysis modalities, peritoneal dialysis is the preferred initial renal replacement therapy for children (particularly for younger children). For technical reasons, PD is indicated in almost all children under the age of 2—and for 80% aged less than 5 years.[19] PD is also used as the primary modality in large numbers of older children. In a multicenter European study, 73% of 189 children were older than 5 years at initiation of PD.[20] Factors ranked according to priority for choice of therapy included age of the child (30%), parent choice (27%), distance from unit (14%), patient choice (11%), social conditions (7%), and inability to perform another modality (6%).

For older children, HD is applied for dropouts from the PD program, if there are medical (rare) or psychosocial (more often) reasons for not performing PD, and less commonly as the first choice.[19] Important psychosocial reasons for elective choice of HD include inability or unwillingness of the family to accept responsibility for care of the child's dialysis at home and inadequate home space or living conditions.

The main advantage of PD (and less commonly, home HD) is also the main drawback: relative independence from the hospital. The treatment is performed at home, generally by the parents, and outpatient clinic visits generally occur on a monthly basis. This gives the child and family the opportunity to live a relatively normal life, in their natural surroundings (school, playing grounds) most of the time. For PD patients, holidays may be more easily planned than with HD.

An additional advantage of PD is the fact that residual renal function is better preserved than with HD.[21] However, for all home dialysis therapies the primary responsibility for provision of dialysis and other medical care falls on the parents—causing an immense burden on them despite the 24-hour availability of advice from the dialysis unit. This burden may give rise to severe burnout symptoms, depression, and familial dysfunction. The factors discussed in the sections that follow, outlined in Table 53-3, play a role in the decision whether to choose PD or HD.

TABLE 53-3 Factors Contributing to the Choice of Dialysis Modality in Children

- Age
- Geographic location
- Medical
- Family composition
- Social support
- Compliance
- Native kidney function
- Other factors

Patient Age

As mentioned previously, the age of the child is an important determinant. In infants, the creation of a functioning arteriovenous fistula for HD is almost impossible—and indwelling venous catheters carry the risk of infection, thrombosis, and malfunction. Cardiovascular instability may also hamper effective HD treatment. These drawbacks of HD provide strong reasons in favor of PD in the young age group. The lowest age at which extended HD may be comfortably performed is dependent on the skills of both access surgeons and dialysis team.

In some countries, use of maintenance HD is very rare before age 2 years. Nonetheless, maintenance HD has been reported in children less than 10 kg[22] and is the initial modality in 20% of North American children aged less than 2 years[19]—although outcomes are worse than in older children.[22] At the other end of the age spectrum, teenagers and young adolescents may have significant concerns about a bloated abdomen and the peritoneal catheter because this affects their body image and emotional/sexual development. This may be a relative contraindication to maintenance PD.

Geographic Location

Because pediatric dialysis units are not as ubiquitously available as their counterparts for adults, distances between the dialysis unit and the patient's home may be considerable. In some countries, this may be an important component of the decision-making process for the selection of dialysis modality. Generally, patients who live a long distance from the hospital will be best suited to PD—although recent revival of interest in home HD suggests that this may be a feasible alternative.[23,24]

Medical

Medical factors may also play a role in modality selection. The presence of multiple intraabdominal adhesions due to infections or repeated surgery may preclude the performance of PD, as will the presence of gastroschesis. The same holds true for the existence of pleuroperitoneal fistulae, which generally only become manifest after the start of treatment. Intestinal or urinary stomata may form relative contraindications, mainly depending on their localization on the body.

Nonetheless, the presence of skin diversions or gastrostomy tubes is relatively common in young children for whom PD is the dialysis of choice.[25,26] In such cases, a high presternal placement of the PD catheter (or more commonly an abdominal exit site placement as far as possible from the ostomy) should be considered.

The presence of a ventriculo-peritoneal (V-P) shunt for treatment of hydrocephalus is a concern when considering institution of PD. The inherent risk of peritonitis has the potential to imperil the function and survival of the V-P shunt. Nonetheless, it has been demonstrated that maintenance PD can be successful in this circumstance. Grunberg reviewed nine children on PD with meningomyeloceles, six of whom had functioning V-P shunts. None developed ventriculitis or V-P shunt dysfunction, even though four had PD-related peritonitis. One child presented with a massive PD-related hydrothorax.[27]

Family Composition

The composition of the family is an important determinant for the success of home dialysis. The burden of the treatment is additional to other normal family care responsibilities and perhaps busy jobs of one or both parents. Therefore, factors such as the presence of other young children in the family and/or a single-parent situation may be relative contraindications for PD. The importance of age-appropriate involvement of siblings in educational sessions about dialysis and renal failure, to prevent their potential alienation and reduce their anxieties, has been emphasized by Batte and colleagues.[28]

Social Support

The individual situation of caregivers is obviously also dependent on many other psychosocial and economic factors. The financial situation, social network, and relations with other members of the family (grandparents) and with friends are important contributors to the level of burden the family will suffer. It is important that sometimes there is someone available for taking over the tasks of the parents and provide parent relief.

Additional home supervision may be necessary if there are concerns about the educational level or emotional stability of the parent/caregiver. The school is an additional organization to be considered, and must be encouraged to express a positive attitude toward a PD patient in its classrooms. In our experience, this support is usually ensured if communication between the dialysis unit staff and educators with the schoolteachers and administrators is appropriate.

Patient Compliance

Concerns about noncompliance with the dialysis regimen, particularly for those children who demonstrated nonadherence to medical therapy prior to dialysis, have been minimized with the introduction of devices that monitor home cycler PD treatments (e.g., Pro Card, Baxter Healthcare). Similarly, we have recommended that prior noncompliance is actually a positive indication for home nocturnal HD because the treatment of our patients is remotely monitored and documented via modem or PC.[16]

Residual Renal Function

It is widely accepted in the adult literature that residual renal function is better preserved in patients on PD compared with those on HD. It has been similarly reported by Fischbach et al. that native kidney urine output is better preserved in children on PD.[21] Preservation of residual renal function may greatly impact quality of life by enhancing solute clearance and thus permitting a less restricted diet.

Other Factors

Other factors that influence the choice of dialysis modality include the basic understanding and attitude of the caregivers toward their child's treatment and disease. This attitude may be influenced by many cultural factors, including information from the press and from patient associations and other environmental factors. Finally, ethical decisions often arise concerning the appropriateness of starting dialysis for treatment—particularly of smaller children with severe developmental or additional physical handicaps.

Although these considerations are discussed in detail in Chapter 52, it is accepted that the underlying principle guiding these decisions is that they should primarily be based on what is in the best interests of the child. It is clear that many (largely nonmedical) factors play a role in the choice of dialysis modality. The pediatric nephrologist or other individual who has cared for and knows the predialysis patient best may not have the best insight into all of these factors. Therefore, in The Netherlands we have developed an information-decision circuit that includes separate information-sharing meetings among pediatric nephrologist, pediatric dialysis nurse, social worker, and parents—and depending on age and maturity including the child.

During these meetings, information is exchanged about all items previously discussed—and a picture of the dialysis treatment for this individual is created for the family and the dialysis team. If hurdles are anticipated by one of the parties, additional professionals (pediatric psychologist, play therapist, teacher) may be consulted. After these meetings, a second joint appointment will be made after a period of 1 to 2 weeks. This interval allows the family and the dialysis team to make up their minds and come to a conclusion. At the second meeting, the goal is to come to a final decision with respect to the choice of dialysis modality. Using this practice, it is very rare to find after a few months that the wrong modality was chosen. Similar multidisciplinary groups should be involved in all institutions.

The choice of in-center HD for children has the important advantage of placing the responsibility for dialysis (and for most other aspects of medical care) where this responsibility more naturally lies (i.e., with the nurses and the physicians of the dialysis unit). The treatment is carried out by professionals, and the caregivers only have to provide for the appropriate administration of diet and medication. Although this can also be a major burden, the treatment itself is not usually performed at home.

There are few medical contraindications for intermittent HD. As described previously, vascular access may be problematic—especially in younger age groups. The presence of significant coagulation disorders, which potentially lead to recurrent vascular access clotting, will also impact the decision to choose HD as the primary modality.

Because the classic dialysis schedule consists of about three weekly sessions of about 4 hours, the child will be absent from school and social environment for a considerable amount of time. This problem is exaggerated if more time is spent in the dialysis unit, which may become more common based on the excellent short-term clinical outcomes reported by Tom et al. and Fischbach et al. using 5 hours' HD thrice weekly or daily hemodiafiltration.[29,30] Therefore, the dialysis center has to provide an appropriate amount of schooling and other entertainment during dialysis hours. As a consequence of these frequent and longstanding visits to the dialysis unit, symptoms of hospitalization will always occur in these children—sometimes leading to a dependent attitude and compounding the difficulty of transition to an adult unit.

In adult patients, there is accumulating experience with adapted HD schedules in the home situation (nightly dialysis, short daily dialysis). Although spectacular results are reported using these techniques, it should be emphasized that the burden placed on the family is even greater than with the PD modalities. In children, experience with these new HD schedules is positive—although still very limited.[23,24]

There is general consensus that renal transplantation offers much better opportunities for a near normal life for children than does dialysis, irrespective of which modality is chosen. Transplantation may allow the patient to maintain normal activity, and may reduce contact with the hospital to a minimum. The dialysis team has a great opportunity to advocate for transplantation in families reluctant to proceed with this treatment option. Because of their close contact with patients and their families, the dialysis team should play an important role in educating them about transplantation.

Finally, the dialysis staff is in a unique situation to anticipate potential problems, such as nonadherence to medications likely to be administered posttransplant to specific individuals. However, as detailed in Chapter 58 by Cochat and Hebert, there are still many limitations to transplantation—and a persisting shortage of deceased donors in many countries. Therefore, it is important (even if advocating for preemptive transplantation) that the role and value of dialysis not be diminished. It must also be emphasized that for every child with end-stage renal disease dialysis may be unavoidable and is an acceptable treatment option.

REFERENCES

1. National Kidney Foundation: K/DOQI clinical practice guidelines for pediatric peritoneal dialysis, *Am J Kidney Dis* 48(1):S98-S130, 2006.
2. Watson A, Gartland C for the European Paediatric Peritoneal Dialysis Working Group: Guidelines by an ad hoc European committee for elective chronic peritoneal dialysis in pediatric patients, *Perit Dial Int* 21:240-44, 2001.
3. Fischbach M, Edefonti A, Schröder C, Watson A for the European Pediatric Dialysis Working Group: Hemodialysis in children: General practice guidelines, *Pediatr Nephrol* 20:1054-66, 2005.
4. Greenbaum L, Schaefer FS: The decision to initiate dialysis in children and adolescents. In BA Warady, FS Schaefer, RN Fine, SR Alexander (eds.), *Pediatric dialysis*. Dordrecht, The Netherlands: Kluwer Academic Publishers 2004:177-96.
5. National Kidney Foundation: K-DOQI clinical practice guidelines for hemodialysis adequacy, *Am J Kidney Dis* 48(1):S2-S91, 2006.
6. Schwarts GJ, Brion LP, Spitzer A: The use of plasma creatinine concentration for estimating glomerular filtration rate in infants, children, and adolescents, *Pediatr Clin N Am* 34:571-91, 1987.
7. Shemesh O, Golbetz H, Kriss JP, Myers BD: Limitations of creatinine as a filtration marker in glomerulopathic patients, *Kidney Int* 28:830-38, 1985.
8. Hellerstein S, Erwin P, Warady BA: The cimetidine protocol: A convenient, accurate, and inexpensive way to measure glomerular filtration rate, *Pediatr Nephrol* 18:71-72, 2003.
9. Miklovicova D, Cornelissen M, Cransberg K, Groothoff JW, Dedik L, Schröder CH: Etiology and epidemiology of end-stage renal disease in Dutch children 1987-2001, *Pediatr Nephrol* 20:1136-42, 2005.
10. National Kidney Foundation: K-DOQI clinical practice guidelines for nutrition in chronic renal failure: Appendix IV (role of the renal dietitian), *Am J Kidney Dis* 35(6/2):S17-S105, 2000.
11. Coleman JE, Norman IJ, Watson AR: Provision of dietetic care in children on peritoneal dialysis, *J Renal Nutr* 9(3):145-48, 1999.
12. Harvey EA: Peritoneal access in children, *Perit Dial Int* 21(3):S218-S222, 2001.
13. Bourquelot P, Cussenot O, Corbi P, Pillion G, Gagnadoux MF, Bensman A, et al: Microsurgical creation and follow up of arteriovenous fistulae for chronic hemodialysis in children, *Pediatr Nephrol* 4:156-59, 1990.
14. Bernardini J, Price V, Figueiredo A, Riemann A, Leung D: International survey of peritoneal dialysis training programs, *Perit Dial Int* 26(6):658-63, 2006.
15. Holloway M, Mujais S, Kandert M, Warady BA: Pediatric peritoneal dialysis training: Characteristics and impact on peritonitis rates, *Perit Dial Int* 21(4):401-04, 2001.
16. Geary DF, Piva E, Gajaria M, Tyrrel J, Picone G, Harvey E: Development of a nocturnal home hemodialysis (NHHD) program for children, *Semin Dial* 17(2):115-17, 2004.
17. Health and Welfare Canada: *End-stage renal disease program guidelines*. Ottawa: Health Canada, 1986.
18. Hollomby D, Goldstein M, Keaney C, McCready W for the College of Physicians and Surgeons of Ontario: *Clinical practice parameters and facility standards for hemodialysis, second edition*. Toronto: The College of Physicians and Surgeons of Ontario, chapter 6, p 25, 2001.
19. Leonard MB, Donaldson LA, Ho M, Geary DF: A prospective cohort study of incident maintenance dialysis in children: A NAPRTC study, *Kidney Int* 63(2):744-55, 2003.
20. Watson AR, Thurlby D, Schröder C, Fischbach M, Schaefer F, Edefonti A, et al: Choice of end stage renal failure therapy in eight European centres, *Pediatr Nephrol* 15:C38, 2000.
21. Fischbach M, Terzic J, Menouer S, Soulami K, Dangelser C, Helmstetter A, et al: Effects of automated peritoneal dialysis on residual daily urinary volume in children, *Adv Perit Dial* 17:269-73, 2001.
22. Al-Hermi BE, Al-Saran K, Secker D, Geary DF: Hemodialysis for end-stage renal disease in children weighing less than 10 kg, *Ped Nephrol* 13(5):401-03, 1999.
23. Simonsen O: Slow nocturnal dialysis as a rescue treatment for children and young patients with end-stage renal failure, *J Am Soc Nephrol* 11:327A, 2000.
24. Geary DF, Piva E, Tyrrell J, Gajaria MJ, Picone G, Keating LE, et al: Home nocturnal hemodialysis in children, *J Ped* 147(3):383-87, 2005.
25. Ramage I, Geary DF, Harvey E, Secker DJ, Balfe JA, Balfe JW: Efficacy of gastrostomy feeding in infants and older children receiving chronic peritoneal dialysis, *Perit Dial Int* 19(3):231-36, 1999.
26. Watson AR: Gastrostomy feeding in children on chronic peritoneal dialysis, *Perit Dial Int* 26(1):41-42, 2006.
27. Grunberg J, Rebori A, Verocay MC: Peritoneal dialysis in children with spina bifida and ventriculoperitoneal shunt: One center's experience and review of the literature, *Perit Dial Int* 23(5):481-86, 2003.
28. Batte S, Watson AR, Amess K: The effects of chronic renal failure on siblings, *Ped Nephrol* 21(2):246-50, 2006.
29. Fischbach M, Terzic J, Laugel V, Dheu C, Menouer S, Helms P, et al: Daily on line hemodiafiltration: A pilot trial in children, *Nephrol Dial Transplant* 19:2360-67, 2004.
30. Tom A, McCauley L, Bell L, Rodd C, Espinosa P, Yu G, et al: Growth during maintenance hemodialysis: Impact of enhanced nutrition and clearance, *J Ped* 134(4):464-71, 1999.

CHAPTER

54 Peritoneal Dialysis Access

Bradley A. Warady and Walter S. Andrews

PERITONEAL DIALYSIS ACCESS

Peritoneal dialysis (PD) is the predominant initial dialytic modality for children with end-stage renal disease (ESRD). This is especially true for children who have acquired ESRD during their first decade of life.[1] Data from the North American Pediatric Renal Trials and Collaborative Studies (NAPRTCS) reveals that of the 5639 dialysis initiations entered into the dialysis registry between 1992 and 2005 more than 60% were for PD.[2] Reasons for the preferential selection of PD in children have included its ability to greatly reduce the need for dietary restrictions, its simplicity of operation, the lack of a need for routine blood access, and the ability of the child to attend school on a regular basis.

However, for there to be successful PD there must be a successful peritoneal catheter. Ideally, the catheter provides reliable and rapid dialysate flow rates without leaks or infections. The first description of placement of a chronic indwelling catheter for PD was in 1968 by Tenckhoff, and the Tenckhoff catheter remains the one most often used.[3,4]

Although significant improvements have occurred with the access device over time, the catheter has continued to be characterized on occasion as the Achilles' heel of PD because of the catheter-related complications that occur. This chapter explores the key characteristics of catheters, the primary surgical techniques for placement, and the most common catheter-related complications in children. It is hoped that this information will result in an increased likelihood of a problem-free PD access for the pediatric patient.

ACCESS TYPES

The catheters commonly used for chronic PD are constructed of soft material, such as silicone rubber or polyurethane. The key elements of the catheters are the unique intraperitoneal configurations (curled or straight), number of Dacron cuffs (one or two), and subcutaneous tunnel configuration (straight or "swan-neck").[5,6] If one includes the orientation of the catheter exit site on the abdomen as yet another variable, more than 13 different combinations of catheter characteristics are actually possible—as documented in the 2006 annual report of the NAPRTCS.[2] As noted previously, the most common catheter with these characteristics used by pediatric patients is the Tenckhoff catheter.

A review of the NAPRTCS registry catheter data by vintage for those placed at the time of dialysis initiation between 1992 and 2005 reveals that most were of the Tenckhoff curled (62.8%) or Tenckhoff straight (28.7%) variety[2] (Table 54-1). Among all 3842 catheters recorded, those with curled intraperitoneal configurations were used twice as often as those with straight intraperitoneal segments[2] (Table 54-2). The curled Tenckhoff catheter was also previously reported as being the most commonly used pediatric catheter (88% usage) in the 1995 survey of the Pediatric Peritoneal Dialysis Study Consortium (PPDSC).[7]

The presumed advantages of the curled catheter over the original straight catheter include (1) better separation between the abdominal wall and the bowel, (2) more catheter side holes available for inflow and outflow, (3) less inflow pain, (4) less of a tendency for migration out of the pelvis, (5) less prone to omental wrapping, and (6) potentially less trauma to bowel.[5] In contrast to the NAPRTCS data, the Italian PD registry reflects a predominance of straight catheters.[4] This mitigates definitive data supporting the advantages of the curled versus the straight catheter. In addition, conclusions that curled catheters are in all cases more advantageous have recently been challenged.[4,8,9] Noteworthy is the fact that neither the NAPRTCS data nor a formal review of the available prospective studies provides evidence of any association between the intraperitoneal configuration and the development of peritonitis or exit-site/tunnel infection.[2,10]

The next catheter characteristic to consider is the number of Dacron cuffs on the catheter. If a single-cuff catheter is used, it is generally recommended that the cuff be positioned between the rectus sheaths in the rectus muscle (not in a superficial position). In one series, this decreased the incidence of subsequent peritonitis by nearly 37% compared to subcutaneous placement of the cuff. When a second cuff was added as a means of securing the catheter's position and potentially helping prevent bacterial migration, there were initial reports of problems with cutaneous extrusion of the second cuff.[11,12] This was likely secondary to excess torque being placed on the catheter at the time of placement as a result of the angle between the exit site and the abdominal wall portion of the catheter. It also proved most likely to occur if the outer cuff was less than 2.0 cm from the exit site.[5] Cuff extrusion often resulted in the development of an exit-site infection and the occasional need for shaving of the

TABLE 54-1 Peritoneal Access Data by Vintage

	Straight (%)	Curled (%)	Toronto (%)	Presternal (%)	Other (%)
Dialysis Initiated					
1992	36.8	57.1	1.4	4.7	—
1993	33.3	57.2	1.0	8.4	—
1994	29.4	64.9	0.8	4.9	—
1995	34.7	57.6	0.2	7.2	0.2
1996	26.3	62.9	1.5	9.0	0.2
1997	22.4	67.8	1.6	7.4	0.8
1998	28.8	58.9	—	11.3	1.0
1999	21.7	68.4	0.3	9.5	—
2000	23.0	66.4	—	10.6	—
2001	26.3	65.6	—	7.3	0.8
2002	16.2	73.9	1.4	4.1	4.5
2003	25.3	64.6	—	1.1	9.0
2004	27.4	65.6	—	—	7.0
2005	22.9	59.0	—	—	18.1

Source: NAPRTCS. North American Pediatric Renal Trials & Collaborative Studies (NAPRTCS) 2005 Annual Report, Rockville, MD: EMMES Corporation 2006.

TABLE 54-2 Characteristics of Peritoneal Dialysis Accesses

Catheter	Cuffs	Tunnel	Exit Site	*n* (3842)	% (100)
Curled	One	Straight	Lateral	566	14.7
Curled	Two	Swan-neck/curved	Down	328	8.5
Curled	Two	Straight	Lateral	306	8.0
Straight	One	Straight	Lateral	283	7.4
Curled	Two	Straight	Down	266	6.9
Curled	One	Straight	Down	245	6.4
Curled	One	Straight	Up	192	5.0
Straight	One	Straight	Up	127	3.3
Presternal	Two	Swan-neck/curved	Down	122	3.2
Straight	Two	Straight	Lateral	99	2.6
Curled	Two	Swan-neck/curved	Lateral	106	2.8
Straight	One	Swan-neck/curved	Lateral	98	2.6
Straight	One	Straight	Unknown	118	3.1
Other combinations*	—	—	—	986	25.7

Source: NAPRTCS. North American Pediatric Renal Trials & Collaborative Studies (NAPRTCS) 2006 Annual Report, Rockville, MD: EMMES Corporation, 2007.
* Includes all combinations <2.5%

cuff from the catheter.[13-15] Although there are very few reports describing the incidence of distal cuff extrusion with double-cuff catheters in children, two series from 1986 and 2004 reported outer cuff extrusion rates of 8% and 4.8%, respectively.[4,16] It may in part be for this reason that 56% of the catheters in the NAPRTCS database are single cuff.[2]

There is, however, some data to suggest that single-cuff catheters are associated with a higher incidence of exit-site infections and peritonitis. Lewis et al. compared the incidence of catheter-related infections in children with single- and double-cuff peritoneal catheters and found a significantly lower incidence of infections in the double-cuff group.[17] The National CAPD Registry also documented that double-cuff

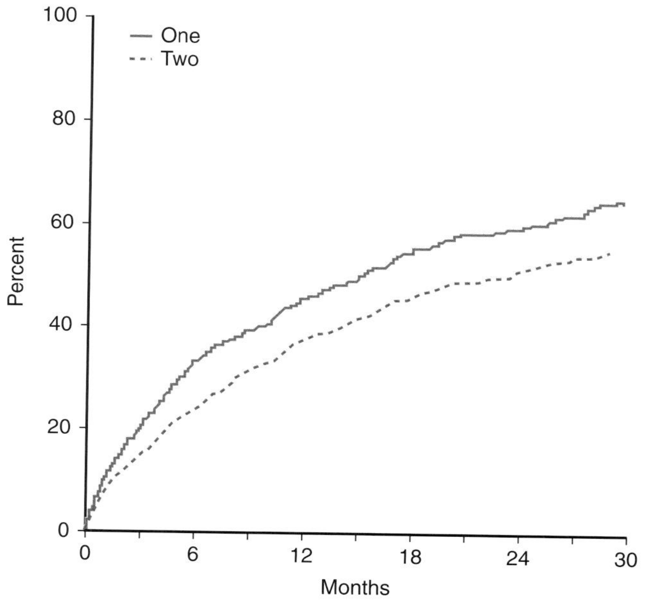

Figure 54-1 Comparison between one-cuff and two-cuff catheters and the time to the first episode of peritonitis. (Adapted from North American Pediatric Renal Transplant Cooperative Study (NAPRTCS), 2005 Annual Report, Rockville MD, EMMES Corp.)

catheters were less likely to require removal secondary to an exit-site infection.[18]

A similar conclusion can be drawn from the NAPRTCS registry data that reports a significantly lower incidence of peritonitis in association with double-cuff catheters (1/19.7 patient-months) compared to single-cuff catheters (1/15.0 patient-months).[2] In addition, the NAPRTCS data show a longer time to first peritonitis episode in the double-cuff catheter group[2] (Figure 54-1). Unfortunately, there has only been a single prospective randomized trial in adults addressing the issue of single- versus double-cuff catheters, and this study showed no significant difference in the risk of peritonitis or exit-site/tunnel infection.[19]

The shape of the extraperitoneal portion of the catheter is variable and can be straight or can have a preformed angle (e.g., swan-neck configuration) in which there is an inverted U-shaped arc (170-180 degrees) between the deep and the superficial cuffs. The latter configuration was originally described by Twardowski, et al. and has been recommended by many pediatric programs as a significant improvement in catheter design.[20] Although the cumulative NAPRTCS data report a swan-neck/curved tunnel in only 28% of catheters, identical to the results of the North American survey by Washburn et al., data recently collected by the International Pediatric Peritonitis Registry (IPPR) revealed that >45% of the catheters were of the swan-neck variety or had a downward-pointed exit site (B. Warady, personal communication).[21]

The purpose of the catheter arc is to allow the catheter to exit the skin in a downward-pointing direction and to allow the distal end of the catheter to enter the peritoneal cavity in an unstressed condition (i.e., without too much torque because of the synthetic material's memory)—thereby decreasing the chance for its migration out of the pelvis and the development of early drainage failure. Most studies have found this positive outcome to be true.[22-24] A modification of this catheter type is the swan-neck presternal catheter. The major difference between the swan-neck presternal catheter and the standard swan-neck catheter is that the presternal catheter has a very long subcutaneous portion and the catheter typically exits over the anterior chest wall. This catheter has been utilized when it is necessary to make the exit site remote from the abdomen, such as in patients with stomas. Whereas the most extensive work with this catheter has been conducted by Twardowski with adult patients, Warchol et al. initially noted that the use of this type of catheter resulted in an exit-site infection rate of 1/162 patient-months in children compared to the reported pediatric PD catheter exit-site infection rates of 1/25 to 1/71 patient-months.[25,26] A more recent report by Warchol et al. documented an exit-site infection rate of 1/70.2 patient-months with the presternal catheter.[27]

As previously mentioned, a presumed advantage of the swan-neck catheter is that it allows a downward-pointing exit site, which may be associated with a decreased likelihood for the accumulation of dirt and debris within the catheter tunnel prompting the development of a tunnel infection/peritonitis. An upward-facing exit site emerged as an independent risk factor for peritonitis in an analysis by Furth et al. of the 1992 through 1997 NAPRTCS data.[28] More recently, the 2006 NAPRTCS data found that a straight catheter tunnel was associated with a peritonitis rate of 1/15.4 patient-months, whereas the rate associated with a swan-neck/curved tunnel was only 1/21.1 patient-months.[2] Likewise, the peritonitis rates associated with an upward- or downward-oriented exit site were 1/13.8 patient-months and 1/20.0 patient-months, respectively.[2]

A study from Network 9 in the United States has also highlighted a significantly lower peritonitis rate with permanently bent catheters. With a downward-pointing exit site, Golper et al. noted a 38% decrease in the incidence of peritonitis associated with an exit-site and/or tunnel infection.[29] It is of interest, however, that exit-site orientation does not appear to influence time to first peritonitis episode in infants enrolled in the NAPRTCS registry—despite their presumed high-risk status for infection because of the presence of diapers (Table 54-3). Finally, whereas some studies have found the use of the swan-neck catheter to be associated with less frequent cuff extrusion, lower exit-site irritation, and fewer exit-site/tunnel infections other studies were unable to confirm these results.[30-32]

In summary, the lack of prospective studies designed to evaluate PD catheter characteristics makes it impossible to conclude that one catheter characteristic is superior to another based on definitive evidence. However, quite convincing is the NAPRTCS registry data that points out that the time to first peritonitis episode is longer with catheters characterized by the following.

- Two cuffs compared to one
- Swan-neck tunnels compared to straight tunnels
- Downward-pointing exit sites compared to lateral and upward exit sites

The annualized rate of peritonitis is lowest with the aforementioned combination of characteristics (Figure 54-2).[2] This information has prompted an increase in the percentage

TABLE 54-3 Kaplan-Meier Estimates of Time to First Peritonitis Episode for Patients Ages 0 to 1 Year at Dialysis Initiation

	DOWN EXIT SITE		UP EXIT SITE	
Time (Months)	*n*	% with Peritonitis	*n*	% with Peritonitis
0	214	0.0	142	0.0
6	172	4.5	115	5.4
12	135	11.7	94	13.3
18	94	24.3	59	34.5
24	69	35.5	52	41.2
30	56	44.1	39	48.5
36	44	53.2	32	55.2
42	33	61.1	24	62.6
48	22	72.2	21	65.8

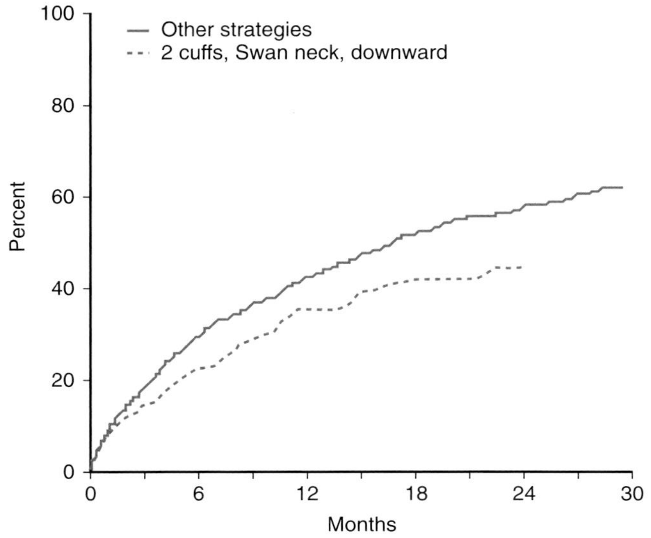

Figure 54-2 A comparison of time to first episode of peritonitis between a catheter that has a downward-facing exit site, a swan-neck shape, and two cuffs versus all other strategies. (Adapted from North American Pediatric Renal Transplant Cooperative Study (NAPRTCS), 2005 Annual Report, Rockville MD, EMMES Corp.)

of NAPRTCS patients using the double-cuff/swan-neck/downward-pointed exit-site configuration—from 5% in 1992 through 1995 to 17.4% since then. This is a change that has not, however, been experienced worldwide.[2,4] The continued collection of this type of information, and ultimately the performance of prospective trials, is mandatory if the optimal catheter characteristics are to be determined.

PREOPERATIVE EVALUATION AND PREPARATION

All patients who are going to undergo PD catheter placement require careful preoperative evaluation. One factor that has been repeatedly cited in the literature as being associated with an increased risk for postplacement PD catheter migration is constipation.[33] Constipation is common in patients with chronic kidney disease (CKD), and must be addressed preoperatively with the use of either laxatives or an enema. If an enema is used, attention to its phosphorus content is imperative.

A careful physical examination is required to determine if the patient has any evidence of a hernia. In children who receive PD, the incidence of hernias is inversely proportional to age—with an overall frequency of 11.8% to 53.0%.[34-36] The highest frequency of inguinal hernias occurs within the first year of life. They are often bilateral, and most require surgical correction. Umbilical hernias can worsen as a result of the increase in intraabdominal pressure generated by the dialysis fluid. As a result, some have advocated peritoneography or laparoscopic inspection for hernias at the time of catheter placement.[37,38] The hernias can, in turn, be fixed either prior to or at the time of insertion of the PD catheter.[39-41] When available, forehand knowledge of the need for hernia repair will allow the surgeon to allot the appropriate operative time to perform this additional procedure.

A critical portion of the catheter placement procedure is deciding the most appropriate location of the exit site. In babies, the exit site of the catheter is typically placed outside the diaper area to help prevent contamination—and in older children it should be either above or below the belt line (an issue ideally discussed with the patient in the preoperative setting). The presence of a vesicostomy, ureterostomy, colostomy, or gastrostomy will also influence the exit-site location. The exit site must be planned so that it is on the opposite side of the abdomen from the stoma sites. If this is not possible, the catheter may need to exit on the chest in order to get as much distance as possible between the stoma and the exit site. Placement of the exit site on the chest wall with a downward orientation has successfully limited the number of infections in such high-risk situations in children and adults.[25-27,42]

Preoperative antibiotic use has been shown in several studies to decrease the incidence of peritonitis after the placement of a PD catheter in children and adults. Interestingly, these studies have shown that any class of antibiotic will be associated with this reduction in peritonitis.[10,43-47] Currently, we utilize a first- or second-generation cephalosporin unless the patient is known to be colonized with methicillin-resistant *Staphylococcus* aureus—as has been recommended in the pediatric and adult guidelines of the International Society of Peritoneal Dialysis (ISPD), as well as in the European guidelines.[45,48-50]

Routine prophylaxis with vancomycin is not recommended in order to try to avoid the development of vancomycin-resistant organisms, despite the finding in an adult experience of superior results with prophylactic vancomycin versus a cephalosporin.[51] If the child has a lower gastrointestinal stoma, we often add a single dose of an aminoglycoside antibiotic. Some programs, including our own, will also screen the patient for *S. aureus* nasal carriage prior to catheter placement. If positive, a course of intranasal mupirocin (twice daily for 5 days) is recommended.[50]

OMENTECTOMY

The data on the use of omentectomy to prevent PD catheter occlusion is fairly convincing.[52,53] If an omentectomy is performed, the incidence of catheter occlusion is about 5% compared to an occlusion rate of 10% to 22.7% in patients without an omentectomy.[40,54] A survey conducted by the PPDSC found that an omentectomy was routinely performed in 53% of centers at the time of catheter placement, similar to the 59% figure from a survey of North American surgeons.[7,21] An omentectomy was performed with the insertion of 82.4% of catheters in the Italian PD registry.[4]

One group of investigators, however, interpreted their own data related to the issue of omentectomy somewhat differently.[54] Even though they noted a 20% decrease in the incidence of catheter blockage when an omentectomy was performed, they calculated that eleven omentectomies would be required to prevent two omental PD catheter blockages. Therefore, they felt that nine patients would undergo an unnecessary omentectomy. In their hands, a secondary omentectomy was not difficult—resulting in their conclusion that omentectomies should only be carried out after a blockage occurs. We feel, however, that an omentectomy is a fairly simple procedure that can be carried out at the initial operation with little morbidity and should be strongly considered in all cases.

FIBRIN SEALANT

Fibrin glue has been used in a variety of surgical specialties for its ability to be an effective sealant. The use of fibrin glue in PD has been reported to be both effective in treating established leaks and, when used at the time of catheter implantation, may help prevent the development of initial peritoneal leaks.[55-57] Our experience with fibrin glue would support both of these assertions. Typically, the application of only 2 cc of fibrin glue is adequate to provide coverage around the internal cuff and down the tunnel between the inner and outer cuffs.

SURGICAL TECHNIQUE

Since Moncrief and Popovich first reported the use of continuous ambulatory PD (CAPD), there have been a number of modifications of the technique for the implantation of the PD catheter.[21,58,59] The complications of dialysate leakage, dislocation of the catheter, erosion/extrusion of the cuffs, exit-site infection, tunnel infection, and peritonitis have in one way or another influenced the surgical technique. To decrease the incidence of these complications, emphasis needs to be placed on careful surgical technique and on the surgical skill of the operator.

The best results will be obtained if the catheters are inserted by surgeons who have developed an interest and an expertise in the procedure. The two most common PD catheter insertion techniques are open and laparoscopic. Other approaches include blind placement using the Tenckhoff trocar, blind placement using a guidewire (Seldinger technique), and the minitrocar peritoneoscopy placement technique.[33]

OPEN TECHNIQUE

As previously mentioned, the insertion site of the PD catheter in our hands is generally determined such that the exit site is downward facing and is either above the belt line or diaper area (infants). In very large children, it is below the belt line. If the patient has the potential for having a gastrostomy in the future, the catheter exit site is positioned on the right-hand side of the abdomen. Otherwise, the catheter is placed on the left-hand side of the abdomen to avoid any interference with the future transplant incision. The most frequent open technique utilizes an incision over the rectus muscle.

The rectus muscle is split in the direction of its fibers and the posterior sheath is then opened longitudinally. The catheter is threaded over a stiffening wire to allow its placement deep in the pelvis, a few degrees to the right of midline to help prevent obstruction to flow in the setting of a full rectum. The posterior sheath is closed and the inner cuff is fixed to the posterior sheath as part of this closure. The inner cuff is positioned within the rectus muscle and the anterior sheath is then closed tightly around the catheter with a second purse string suture around the cuff of the catheter at the level of the anterior rectus sheath.

The lateral fascial opening through which the catheter is tunneled should be kept small to decrease the risk of dialysate leakage. The catheter is then tunneled out to the skin, and the outer cuff is situated 2.0 cm from the catheter exit site. Shorter distances between the exit site and outer cuff predispose to cuff extrusion, whereas greater distances lead to formation of a deep sinus tract, granulation tissue formation, and an increased risk for the development of a tunnel infection.[33,41]

A lateral insertion through the rectus is generally deemed preferable to the midline because of the thinness of the abdominal wall in children and a decreased propensity for postoperative leakage in children when inserted in this location.[41] However, the few prospective trials conducted in adults have not demonstrated any superiority of one approach versus the other in terms of infection risk. The laterally placed catheter is more difficult to remove, and a midline approach has actually been associated with a significant reduction in the risk for complications associated with catheter removal or replacement in one adult trial.[10]

The advantage of the open technique is the ability to directly visualize the placement of the catheter into the pelvis. This is particularly beneficial in those patients who have previously undergone pelvic surgery. In addition, the open technique easily allows an omentectomy to be performed at the same time. The major problem with this technique is the necessity for a significant incision in the peritoneum. In turn, for optimal dialysis performance and a decreased likelihood of postoperative leakage of dialysis fluid this technique usually requires a 2-week rest period between the time of catheter insertion and the initiation of dialysis.[50,60] This approach allows for healing of the peritoneal incision and for incorporation of the cuff into the peritoneum and posterior sheath.

LAPAROSCOPIC TECHNIQUE

With the development of laparoscopy, techniques have been developed that allow the percutaneous placement of a PD catheter under direct vision.[61] An additional advantage of the laparoscopic technique, which we believe is the operative technique of choice in those patients with enough adipose tissue to create a seal around trocar sites, is that it allows the use of much smaller peritoneal incisions and thereby decreases the chance for dialysate leakage. We currently use a modification of the technique first described by Daschner et al.[62]

Under general anesthesia, a vertical incision is made in the umbilicus and the umbilical fascia is sharply incised. Using blunt dissection, the peritoneum is entered and (depending on the size of the child) a 3-mm or 5-mm port is placed. A corresponding 3-mm or 5-mm laparoscope is then inserted and the abdomen is insufflated. As with the open technique, the catheter insertion site is chosen with consideration of the patient's size, exit-site orientation, and gastrostomy usage.

The peritoneal entrance site is positioned so that the inner catheter cuff will be located between both sheaths of the rectus muscle. At this point, a 3-mm or 5-mm instrument is inserted through a stab wound at the marked catheter exit site. If an omentectomy is to be performed, a second 3- to 5-mm port is inserted at the marked entrance site of the catheter. The omentum can then be removed by the use of electrocautery and/or clips. We feel that a complete omentectomy is not absolutely necessary as long as the majority of the omentum is removed.

After the omentectomy has been performed, a guidewire is inserted into the abdomen via the entrance site port. The port is then removed and the skin incision enlarged to approximately 1 cm. Using a peel-away sheath technique, a number 20 French sheath is then inserted into the abdomen over the guidewire (Figure 54-4). The PD catheter is then placed on a stiffener and inserted into the pelvis under direct vision. The pneumoperitoneum is maintained by pushing the proximal cuff of the PD catheter into the sheath, thereby preventing gas loss. Once the catheter has been positioned into the pelvis, the sheath is removed (Figure 54-5).

As the sheath is being removed, the inner cuff is positioned to lie between the anterior and posterior portions of the rectus sheath. The inner cuff is then fixed to the anterior rectus sheath with a purse string suture of 3-0 Polydioxanone (PDS). Care is taken to make sure that the innermost portion of the cuff does not project into the peritoneum (Figure 54-6). The peritoneum is also carefully inspected for evidence

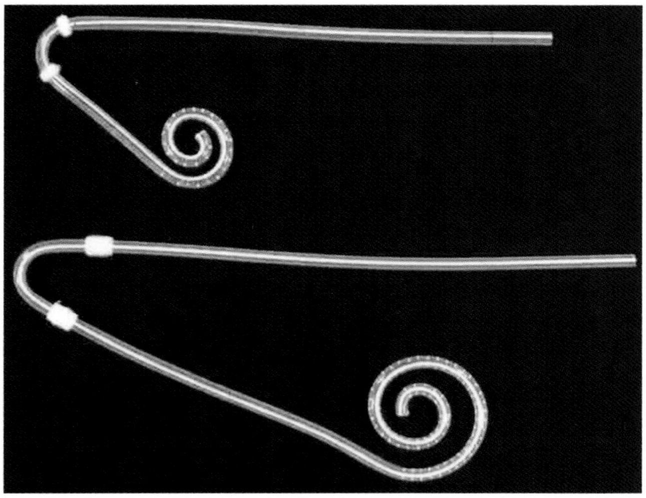

Figure 54-3 Tenckhoff curled catheter with double cuff and swan-neck bend. (Courtesy of Dr. Bradley Warady.)

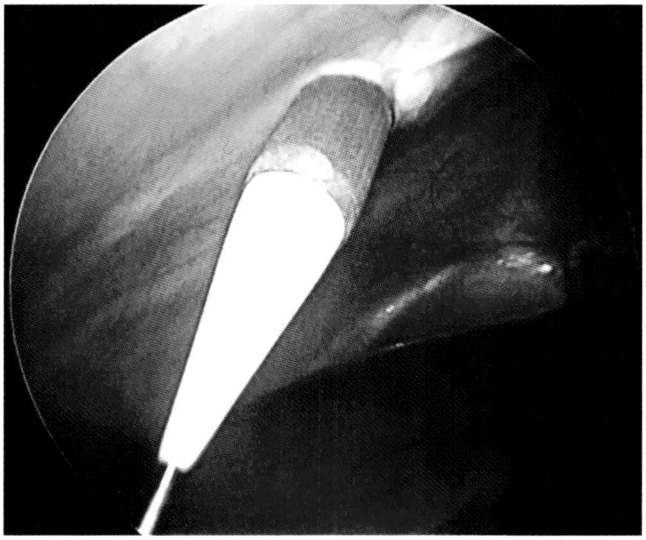

Figure 54-4 A laparoscopic view of the number 20 French peel-away sheath being inserted into the peritoneum over a guidewire. (From Andrews WS: Surgical issues in pediatric peritoneal dialysis. In AR Nissenson, RN Fine (eds.), *Clinical dialysis, fourth edition.* New York: McGraw-Hill 2005.)

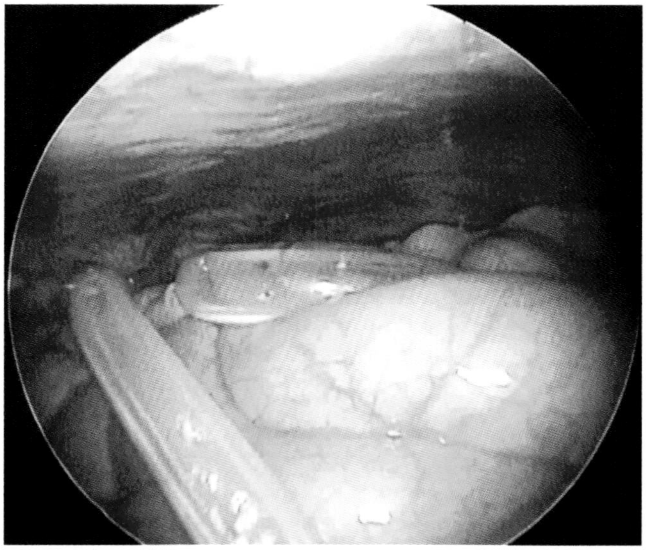

Figure 54-5 A laparoscopic view of a PD catheter, which lies positioned in the pelvis. The catheter is sitting between the bowel and the anterior abdominal wall. (From Andrews WS: Surgical issues in pediatric peritoneal dialysis. In AR Nissenson, RN Fine (eds.), *Clinical dialysis, fourth edition.* New York: McGraw-Hill 2005.)

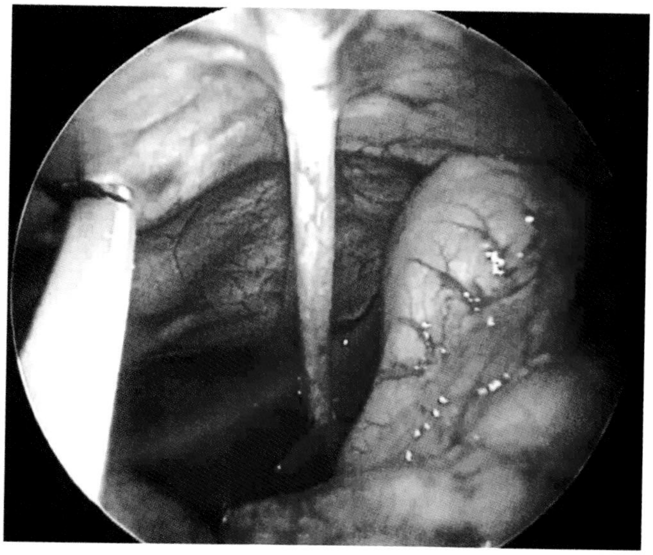

Figure 54-6 A laparoscopic view of a PD catheter *(left)* showing it leaving the peritoneal cavity. Note that the inner cuff is not visible within the peritoneal cavity. (From Andrews WS: Surgical issues in pediatric peritoneal dialysis. In AR Nissenson, RN Fine (eds.), *Clinical dialysis, fourth edition*. New York: McGraw-Hill 2005.)

of any indirect hernias, as noted previously. If these are identified, they are fixed after completion of the PD catheter insertion. The camera and all ports are then removed and the umbilical fascia is repaired.

At the previously marked catheter exit site, a deep subcutaneous tunnel is created between the catheter exit site and the catheter entrance site using a number 20 French sheath dilator or a tendon passer. The catheter is then pulled through the tunnel, positioning the outer cuff so that it is approximately 2.0 cm from the exit site. At this point, fibrin sealant is injected around the outer cuff site at the level of the anterior rectus sheath and down the tunnel between the outer and inner cuffs. We feel that this helps ensure a leak-free closure. The entrance site of the catheter is then closed in two layers. The exit site of the catheter is dressed and the catheter is secured to prevent local trauma, but no fixation suture is used at the exit site. The use of suture is contraindicated because of an associated risk for infection and poor exit-site healing.[45]

POSTIMPLANTATION CARE

Because it is not occlusive, the exit site of the catheter is a major potential site of infection after PD catheter placement. In an attempt to address this issue, Moncrief has suggested that the external portion of the catheter should initially remain buried beneath the skin in a subcutaneous pocket for 4 to 6 weeks.[63] With this technique, the exterior component of the catheter is exteriorized and the exit site is created when both cuffs have had an opportunity to undergo tissue incorporation.

Although successful in its application, prospective trials in which standard insertion with resting was compared to implantation and subcutaneous burial of the catheter for 6 weeks have not demonstrated a significant difference in the rate of peritonitis or exit-site infections or in long-term catheter survival.[47,64,65] Twardowski et al., on the other hand, have merely recommended that initially the exit site should be covered with several layers of sterile gauze and kept dry.[66,67] Some oozing from the exit site is common, and the gauze can wick this away from the skin.

An occlusive dressing should *not* be used. Occlusive dressings tend to trap fluid at the exit site, predisposing to bacterial growth and subsequent infection. Trauma to the exit site, usually from repeated catheter motion, needs to be minimized. Therefore, the catheter must be securely fixed with a dressing—and dressing changes should not routinely occur more often than once per week until the exit site is healed.

Ideally, specially trained staff should conduct the dressing changes, which allows a consistent aseptic technique to be followed and a decreased risk for bacterial colonization of the access.[68,69] Submersion of the exit site should be avoided to prevent colonization with waterborne organisms. This is the approach used in our program—one that has helped prevent the development of early exit-site infections as a complication of catheter implantation in virtually all cases.[68]

TIMING OF CATHETER USE

Some controversy exists as to whether the catheter should be used immediately after placement or whether a timed period (i.e., break-in period) should elapse prior to its use to facilitate healing and help prevent the development of complications such as leakage and infection. The 1998 ISPD catheter guidelines recommend a dialysis-free period of 10 to 15 days after catheter insertion, and the European guidelines recommend at least 2 weeks, whenever possible—in each case discouraging routine peritoneal flushing to check for catheter patency and function.[5,50]

The recommendation regarding catheter initiation is in part supported by a study conducted by Patel et al. in which immediate versus delayed (an average of 20 days) catheter use was compared.[70] Although the authors noted an increased incidence of dialysate leakage in the immediate-use group, the study also revealed a disconcerting increase in exit-site infections, tunnel infections, and peritonitis in the delayed catheter use group. In a retrospective review of NAPRTCS data, Rahim et al. found that early (<14 days) versus late onset of usage was associated with an increased risk of leakage. However, there was no difference found in the risk of infection.[60]

Finally, the Italian PD registry did not reveal any difference in the incidence of leakage or catheter survival when comparing catheters used early (<7 days) versus late.[4] Accordingly, although the available data might suggest a preference for delayed catheter usage without regular flushing of the catheter (a practice followed in our center irrespective of patient age), there is no definitive evidence for any particular break in period and a prospective randomized trial is clearly needed to address this issue.[8] Of course, when early usage is necessary, efforts should be made to minimize any increase in the intraperitoneal pressure by using small exchange volumes—possibly in the supine position with a cycling device.

CHRONIC EXIT-SITE CARE

The goal of exit-site care is to prevent the development of exit-site infections. As suggested by Twardowski and Prowant, exit-site care consists of assessing the exit site, cleansing the exit site, immobilizing the catheter, and protecting the exit site and tunnel from trauma.[66,71,72] At present, there is no optimal approach to chronic care. It is, however, agreed that a noncytotoxic cleansing agent should be used (e.g., 20% poloxamer 188, soap) and that a dressing may be associated with fewer infections in the pediatric patient.[50]

A recent survey of exit-site care practices in 22 pediatric sites and 125 adults sites found that significantly fewer pediatric programs compared to adult programs conducted daily care and used tap water or antibacterial soap, whereas a greater percentage "air dried" the cleaned exit site and used a semipermeable dressing over an absorbent layer compared to adult programs (B. Prowant, personal communication). In our center, we conduct exit-site care daily in which the exit site is cleansed with chlorhexidine (4%), air dried, and then covered with a semipermeable dressing.

In addition to direct exit-site care, data in children and adults support the use of prophylactic antibiotic agents to decrease *S. aureus* infections. Although early recommendations suggested the need to assess patients/caregivers for *S. aureus* nasal carriage status, some centers now prescribe the therapy to all patients—with recognition of the risk for the emergence of antibiotic resistance.[46,73-75] Mupirocin and gentamicin creams have both been shown to be efficacious.[76,77]

MECHANICAL COMPLICATIONS

Mechanical complications are generally felt to be the second most common reason (after infection) for catheter failure. The mechanical complications include obstruction of the catheter by omentum, migration of the catheter out of the pelvis, and blockage of the catheter by fibrin or clots. The issue of obstruction by omentum has been previously reviewed and as previously mentioned can usually can be prevented by conducting a partial omentectomy at the time of catheter insertion. When omental blockage does occur, laparoscopic removal of the involved omentum can typically be easily accomplished.

Migration of the catheter out of the pelvis can lead to poor dialysate inflow or outflow or to pain with dialysis. One approach to repositioning the catheter is through the use of interventional radiology techniques, in which a guidewire is used to move the catheter back to a workable position in the abdomen. Using this technique, Savader et al. reported that in patients who underwent multiple manipulations a durable patency rate of 50% was achieved in those patients who had an early (less than 30 days) catheter malposition—whereas the durable patency rate was 82% in patients with late (greater than 30 days) malpositions.[78] The complication rate was low (3%), with only a single episode of peritonitis. Comparison of success rates from multiple reports is somewhat difficult due to differences in the techniques used and the period of follow-up.[79,80]

Our center has used a laparoscopic approach to reposition catheters. In patients who have had no previous abdominal procedures besides the peritoneal catheter placement, we create a pneumoperitoneum by insufflating through the malpositioned PD catheter. Once a pneumoperitoneum is achieved, a 3-mm port is placed in the left upper quadrant and a 3-mm laparoscope is inserted. A stab wound is then made in the right upper quadrant and a 3-mm grasper is inserted. The catheter is then manipulated under direct vision and is repositioned back into the pelvis. Any adhesions encountered during the repositioning of the catheter are lysed at the same time. In addition, we have used this technique to free catheters that have become encased in adhesions. This technique avoids a large incision in the peritoneum—thus allowing a rapid return to dialysis.

For catheters that are functioning poorly but have not migrated out of the pelvis per radiologic evaluation, occlusion by fibrin or blood clot is common and tissue plasminogen activator (TPA) has been shown to be very effective in unblocking these catheters. Two mg of TPA is reconstituted in 40 cc of normal saline and is instilled in the catheter for 1 hour. This has resulted in the restoration of patency in 57% of the catheters.[81-83]

EXIT-SITE INFECTION, TUNNEL INFECTION, AND PERITONITIS

Catheter exit-site/tunnel infections and peritonitis are a significant cause of catheter failure. In a review of the NAPRTCS data from 1992 to 1997, the incidence of exit-site/tunnel infections increased from 11% at 30 days post catheter insertion to 30% by 1 year after catheter insertion.[28] The Italian PD registry documented catheter infections as the most common catheter-related complication, with a prevalence of 73.2% and an incidence of 1 episode per 27.4 patient-months.[4]

Whereas the goal in all cases should be the prevention of catheter related infection by following published recommendations and by regular monitoring with the use of an exit-site scoring system (Table 54-4), medical management is typically successful when infections arise.[49,84] One approach to the treatment of exit-site tunnel infections in children is outlined in Table 54-5.[85] In situations in which antibiotic

TABLE 54-4 Exit-Site Scoring System*

	0 Points	1 Point	2 Points
Swelling	No	Exit only (<0.5 cm)	Including part of or entire tunnel
Crust	No	<0.5 cm	>0.5 cm
Redness	No	<0.5 cm	>0.5 cm
Pain on pressure	No	Slight	Severe
Secretion	No	Serous	Purulent

* Infection should be assumed with a cumulative exit-site score of 4 or greater.

TABLE 54-5 **Management of Exit-Site/Tunnel Infections***

Therapeutics	
0 Hours • Obtain culture and Gram stain of exudate and/or perform drainage. • If clinical appearance mandates immediate therapy prior to culture result, initiate empiric therapy with first-generation cephalosporin or ciprofloxacin PO.	
Gram-Positive Organism	**Gram-Negative Organism**
Penicillinase-resistant penicillin PO or first-generation cephalosporin PO	Ciprofloxacin 20 mg/kg/day PO in divided doses (>12 years; maximum 1.0 gm/day) or Ceftazidime load: 250 mg/L IP; maintenance: 125 mg/L IP in each bag
Adjust antibiotics to culture and sensitivity (ISPD pediatric recommendations)	Adjust antibiotics to culture and sensitivity (ISPD pediatric recommendations)
If no improvement after 48 to 72 hours, add rifampin 20 mg/kg/day PO in divided doses (maximum 600 mg/day)	If pseudomonas and receiving ciprofloxacin without improvement after 48 to 72 hours, consider adding ceftazidime load: 250 mg/L IP; maintenance: 125 mg/L IP in each bag
2 Weeks: Reevaluate	
Infection resolved: Stop therapy	
Infection improved: Continue therapy for 2 weeks and reevaluate	
After adequate and prolonged antibiotic treatment, if no improvement: consider catheter revision (cuff shaving) or removal	

* Glycopeptides (e.g., vancomycin or teicoplanin) should be avoided for the routine treatment of exit-site infections secondary to *Staphylococcus* species due to concerns of emerging bacterial resistance.

Source: Warady BA, Alexander SR, Firanek C, et al: *Peritoneal dialysis catheter and complications management for children.* Deerfield, IL: Baxter Healthcare Corporation 2001.

therapy of an exit-site/tunnel infection was unsuccessful, surgical salvage by unroofing and cuff shaving has been conducted.[13-15]

In an additional report, Wu et al. has described a technique in which the authors were able to preserve the intraperitoneal portion of the dialysis catheter and simply excise the external infected portion of the catheter.[86] This was accomplished by cutting down on the entrance site of the catheter into the peritoneum. At this point, the catheter is divided just above the internal cuff—and a new external portion with a new external cuff is then glued to the internal portion of the old catheter and passed out to the skin via a separate tunnel. The infected external portion of the catheter is then removed. They reported 26 catheter revisions in 23 patients with 100% resolution of the infection without interruption of PD. To date, we have not had to utilize this technique, but it is intriguing to consider it for those patients in whom interruption of PD would be extraordinarily difficult.

The more standard surgical intervention for infection would be complete removal of the catheter when there is refractory peritonitis, fungal peritonitis, or a refractory catheter exit-site/tunnel infection.[4,49] Preservation of the peritoneum should always take precedence over preservation of the catheter. In those patients in whom the infection is caused by a gram-positive organism and the dialysate white blood cell count is <100/mm^3, catheter removal and replacement can occur as a single procedure under antibiotic coverage.[4,87-89] In contrast, refractory peritonitis, fungal peritonitis, and gram-negative infections mandate that there be at least a 2- to 3-week interval between catheter removal and reinsertion.

PD CATHETER CARE POST KIDNEY TRANSPLANTATION

It has been recommended that dressing care occur weekly during the posttransplant period. In most cases, catheters are removed 4 to 8 weeks following successful renal transplantation. Routine PD cultures should not be obtained. Although two studies noted the absence of a significant early increase in catheter infections after kidney transplantation if the PD catheters were left in place but not used, one of the studies did find an increased incidence of catheter infections after the first posttransplant month.[90,91] They also noted that the majority of complications that would require the use of the catheter occurred within the first month. For this reason, they advocate (with which we agree) that the peritoneal catheter can be safely left in place for 1 month without scheduled flushing—after which time it should be removed if it is no longer needed.

COMPLICATIONS WITH PD CATHETER REMOVAL

An interesting short report by Korzets et al. makes the case that the removal of a PD catheter can be associated with significant complications.[92] In their series of 40 catheter removals, 10 (25%) of the procedures were associated with complications (and 8 of these required further surgical intervention). Half of their complications were related to bleeding. Their usual technique was to remove the PD catheters under local anesthesia, which they felt contributed significantly to their complication rate.

This experience also makes a strong case against using traction as the removal technique because of the complications of a retained cuff and subsequent infection. The surgeon removing the catheter must be aware of the device type and implant procedure and recognize that the more complex the catheter design the more difficult the removal. In summary, the removal of a PD catheter is a real operation that requires strict attention to detail to prevent annoying but potentially significant complications that could require a return to the operating room.

SUMMARY

The peritoneal catheter is the lifeline for the patient receiving PD. Attention to detail is, in turn, necessary for everything from the selection of the best location for the exit site to the prophylactic measures used to hopefully prevent infectious complications. The establishment of a catheter "team" and the regular evaluation of treatment results are initiatives designed to optimize the function of this important component of PD.

REFERENCES

1. Warady BA, Bunchman TE: An update on peritoneal dialysis and hemodialysis in the pediatric population, *Curr Opin Pediatr* 8:135-40, 1996.
2. NAPRTCS. *North American Pediatric Renal Trials & Collaborative Studies (NAPRTCS) 2006 Annual Report*. Rockville, MD: EMMES Corporation 2007.
3. Tenckhoff H, Schecter H: A bacteriologically safe peritoneal access device, *Trans Am Soc Artif Intern Organs* 14:181-86, 1966.
4. Rinaldi S, Sera F, Verrina E, et al: Chronic peritoneal dialysis catheters in children: A fifteen-year experience of the Italian Registry of Pediatric Chronic Peritoneal Dialysis, *Perit Dial Int* 24:481-86, 2004.
5. Gokal R, Alexander SR, Chen TW, et al: Peritoneal catheters and exit site practices: Toward optimum peritoneal access, 1998 update, *Pediatr Dial Int* 18:11-13, 1998.
6. Twardowski ZJ: Peritoneal access: The past, present, and the future, *Contrib Nephrol* 150:195-201, 2006.
7. Neu AM, Kohaut EC, Warady BA: Current approach to peritoneal access in North American children: A report of the pediatric peritoneal dialysis study consortium, *Adv Perit Dial* 11:289-92, 1995.
8. Dönmez O, Durmaz O, Ediz B, et al: Catheter-related complications in children on chronic peritoneal dialysis. In A Khanna (ed.), *Advances in peritoneal dialysis*. Toronto: Multimed 2005.
9. Stegmayr BG, Wikdahl AM, Bergstrom M, et al: A randomized clinical trial comparing the function of straight and coiled Tenckhoff catheters for peritoneal dialysis, *Perit Dial Int* 25:85-88, 2005.
10. Strippoli GF, Tong A, Johnson D, et al: Catheter type, placement and insertion techniques for preventing peritonitis in peritoneal dialysis patients, *Cochrane Database Syst Rev* CD004680, 2004.
11. Alexander SR, Tank ES: Surgical aspects of continuous ambulatory peritoneal dialysis in infants, children and adolescents, *J Urol* 127:501-04, 1982.
12. Vigneaux A, Hardy BE, Balfe JA: Chronic peritoneal catheter in children: One or two dacron cuffs? *Perit Dial Bull* 1:151, 1981.
13. Scalamogna A, De Vecchi A, Maccario M, et al: Cuff-shaving procedure: A rescue treatment for exit-site infection unresponsive to medical therapy, *Nephrol Dial Transplant* 10:2325-27, 1995.
14. Yoshino A, Honda M, Ikeda M, et al: Merit of the cuff-shaving procedure in children with chronic infection, *Pediatr Nephrol* 19:1267-72, 2004.
15. Crabtree JH, Burchette RJ: Surgical salvage of peritoneal dialysis catheters from chronic exit-site and tunnel infections, *Am J Surg* 190:4-8, 2005.
16. Stone MM, Fonkalsrud EW, Salusky IB, et al: Surgical management of peritoneal dialysis catheters in children: Five-year experience with 1,800 patient-month follow-up, *J Pediatr Surg* 21:1177-1181, 1986.
17. Lewis MA, Smith T, Postlethwaite RJ, et al: A comparison of double-cuffed with single-cuffed Tenckhoff catheters in the prevention of infection in pediatric patients, *Adv Perit Dial* 13:274-76, 1997.
18. Lindblad AS, Novak JW, Nolph KD, et al: The 1987 USA National CAPD Registry report, *ASAIO Trans* 34:150-56, 1988.
19. Eklund B, Honkanen E, Kyllonen L, et al: Peritoneal dialysis access: Prospective randomized comparison of single-cuff and double-cuff straight Tenckhoff catheters, *Nephrol Dial Transplant* 12:2664-66, 1997.
20. Twardowski ZJ, Prowant BF, Nichols WK, et al: Six-year experience with swan neck catheters, *Perit Dial Int* 12:384-89, 1992.
21. Washburn KK, Currier H, Salter KJ, et al: Surgical technique for peritoneal dialysis catheter placement in the pediatric patient: A North American survey, *Adv Perit Dial* 20:218-21, 2004.
22. Gadallah MF, Mignone J, Torres C, et al: The role of peritoneal dialysis catheter configuration in preventing catheter tip migration, *Adv Perit Dial* 16:47-50, 2000.
23. Moreiras PM, Cuina L, Goyanes GR, et al: Mechanical complications in chronic peritoneal dialysis, *Clin Nephrol* 52:124-30, 1999.
24. Lye WC, Kour NW, van der Straaten JC, et al: A prospective randomized comparison of the swan neck, coiled, and straight Tenckhoff catheters in patients on CAPD, *Perit Dial Int* 16(1):S333-S335, 1996.
25. Twardowski ZJ: Presternal peritoneal catheter, *Adv Ren Replace Ther* 9:125-32, 2002.
26. Warchol S, Roszkowska-Blaim M, Sieniawska M: Swan neck presternal peritoneal dialysis catheter: Five-year experience in children, *Perit Dial Int* 18:183-87, 1998.
27. Warchol S, Ziolkowska H, Roszkowska-Blaim M: Exit-site infection in children on peritoneal dialysis: Comparison of two types of peritoneal catheters, *Perit Dial Int* 23:169-73, 2003.
28. Furth SL, Donaldson LA, Sullivan EK, et al: Peritoneal dialysis catheter infections and peritonitis in children: A report of the North American Pediatric Renal Transplant Cooperative Study, *Pediatr Nephrol* 15:179-82, 2000.
29. Golper TA, Brier ME, Bunke M, et al. for the Academic Subcommittee of the Steering Committee of the Network 9 Peritonitis and Catheter Survival Studies: Risk factors for peritonitis in long-term peritoneal dialysis: The Network 9 peritonitis and catheter survival studies, *Am J Kidney Dis* 28:428-36, 1996.
30. Eklund BH, Honkanen EO, Kala AR, et al: Catheter configuration and outcome in patients on continuous ambulatory peritoneal dialysis: A prospective comparison of two catheters, *Perit Dial Int* 14:70-74, 1994.
31. Eklund BH, Honkanen EO, Kala AR, Kyllonen LE: Peritoneal dialysis access: Prospective randomized comparison of the swan neck and Tenckhoff catheters, *Perit Dial Int* 15:189-92, 1995.
32. Lo WK, Lui SL, Li FK, et al: A prospective randomized study on three different peritoneal dialysis catheters, *Perit Dial Int* 23:S127-S131, 2003.
33. Flanigan M, Gokal R: Peritoneal catheters and exit-site practices toward optimum peritoneal access: A review of current developments, *Perit Dial Int* 25:132-39, 2005.
34. von Lilien T, Salusky IB, Yap HK, et al: Hernias: A frequent complication in children treated with continuous peritoneal dialysis, *Am J Kidney Dis* 10:356-60, 1987.
35. van Asseldonk JP, Schroder CH, Severijnen RS, et al: Infectious and surgical complications of childhood continuous ambulatory peritoneal dialysis, *Eur J Pediatr* 151:377-80, 1992.
36. Holtta TM, Ronnholm KA, Jalanko H, et al: Peritoneal dialysis in children under 5 years of age, *Perit Dial Int* 17:573-80, 1997.
37. Khoury AE, Charendoff J, Balfe JW, et al: Hernias associated with CAPD in children, *Adv Perit Dial* 7:279-82, 1991.
38. Tank ES, Hatch DA: Hernias complicating chronic ambulatory peritoneal dialysis in children, *J Pediatr Surg* 21:41-42, 1986.

39. Remes J, Peeters J, Coosemans W, et al: Five years of surgical experience with peritoneal dialysis, *Acta Chir Belg* 98:66-70, 1998.
40. Conlin MJ, Tank ES: Minimizing surgical problems of peritoneal dialysis in children, *J Urol* 154:917-19, 1992.
41. Brandt ML, Brewer ED: Peritoneal dialysis access in children. In BA Warady, F Schaefer, RN Fine, et al. (eds.), *Pediatric dialysis*. Dordrecht, The Netherlands: Kluwer Academic Publishers 2004.
42. Chadha V, Jones LL, Ramirez ZD, et al: Chest wall peritoneal dialysis catheter placement in infants with a colostomy, *Adv Perit Dial* 16:318-20, 2000.
43. Sardegna K, Beck AM, Strife CF: Evaluation of perioperative antibiotics at the time of dialysis catheter placement, *Pediatr Nephrol* 12:149-52, 1998.
44. Harvey EA: Peritoneal access in children, *Perit Dial Int* 21(3):S218-S222, 2001.
45. Piraino B, Bailie GR, Bernardini J, et al: Peritoneal dialysis-related infections recommendations: 2005 update, *Perit Dial Int* 25:107-31, 2005.
46. Bonifati C, Pansini F, Torres DD, et al: Antimicrobial agents and catheter-related interventions to prevent peritonitis in peritoneal dialysis: Using evidence in the context of clinical practice, *Int J Artif Organs* 29:41-49, 2006.
47. Strippoli GF, Tong A, Johnson D, et al: Catheter-related interventions to prevent peritonitis in peritoneal dialysis: A systematic review of randomized, controlled trials, *J Am Soc Nephrol* 15:2735-46, 2004.
48. Warady BA: Peritoneal dialysis catheter related infections in children, *Pediatr Infect Dis J* 17:1165-66, 1998.
49. Warady BA, Schaefer F, Alexander S, et al: Consensus guidelines for the treatment of peritonitis in pediatric patients receiving peritoneal dialysis, *Perit Dial Int* 20:610-24, 2000.
50. Dombros N, Dratwa M, Feriani M, et al: European best practice guidelines for peritoneal dialysis 3: Peritoneal access, *Nephrol Dial Transplant* 20:ix8-ix12, 2005.
51. Gadallah MF, Ramdeen G, Mignone J, et al: Role of preoperative antibiotic prophylaxis in preventing postoperative peritonitis in newly placed peritoneal dialysis catheters, *Am J Kidney Dis* 36:1014-19, 2000.
52. Reissman P, Lyass S, Shiloni E, et al: Placement of a peritoneal dialysis catheter with routine omentectomy: Does it prevent obstruction of the catheter? *Eur J Surg* 164:703-07, 1998.
53. Pumford N, Cassey J, Uttley WS: Omentectomy with peritoneal catheter placement in acute renal failure, *Nephron* 68:327-28, 1994.
54. Lewis M, Webb N, Smith T, et al: Routine omentectomy is not required in children undergoing chronic peritoneal dialysis, *Adv Perit Dial* 11:293-95, 1995.
55. Sojo E, Bisigniano L, Turconi A, et al: Is fibrin glue useful in preventing dialysate leakage in children on CAPD? Preliminary results of a prospective randomized study, *Adv Perit Dial* 13:277-80, 1997.
56. Sojo E, Grosman MD, Monteverde ML, et al: Fibrin glue is useful in preventing early dialysate leakage in children on chronic peritoneal dialysis, *Perit Dial Int* 24:186-90, 2004.
57. Rusthoven E, van de Kar NA, Monnens LA, et al: Fibrin glue used successfully in peritoneal dialysis catheter leakage in children, *Perit Dial Int* 24:287-89, 2004.
58. Popovich RP, Moncrief JW, Decherd JW, et al: The definition of a novel wearable/portable equilibrium peritoneal dialysis technique, *Trans Am Soc Artif Intern Organs* 5:64, 1976.
59. Gadallah MF, Pervez A, el Shahawy MA, et al: Peritoneoscopic versus surgical placement of peritoneal dialysis catheters: A prospective randomized study on outcome, *Am J Kidney Dis* 33:118-22, 1999.
60. Rahim KA, Seidel K, McDonald RA: Risk factors for catheter-related complications in pediatric peritoneal dialysis, *Pediatr Nephrol* 19:1021-28, 2004.
61. Wang JY, Chen FM, Huang TJ, et al: Laparoscopic assisted placement of peritoneal dialysis catheters for selected patients with previous abdominal operation, *J Invest Surg* 18:59-62, 2005.
62. Daschner M, Gfrörer S, Zachariou Z, et al: Laparoscopic tenckhoff catheter implantation in children, *Perit Dial Int* 22:22-26, 2002.
63. Moncrief JW, Popovich RP: Moncrief-Popovich catheter: Implantation technique and clinical results, *Perit Dial Int* 14(3):S56-S58, 1994.
64. Danielsson A, Blohme L, Tranaeus A, et al: A prospective randomized study of the effect of a subcutaneously "buried" peritoneal dialysis catheter technique versus standard technique on the incidence of peritonitis and exit-site infection, *Perit Dial Int* 22:211-19, 2002.
65. Esson ML, Quinn MJ, Hudson EL, et al: Subcutaneously tunneled peritoneal dialysis catheters with delayed externalization: Long-term follow-up, *Adv Perit Dial* 16:123-28, 2000.
66. Twardowski ZJ, Prowant BF: Exit-site healing post catheter implantation, *Perit Dial Int* 16(3):S51-S70, 1996.
67. Twardowski ZJ, Prowant BF: Exit-site study methods and results, *Perit Dial Int* 16(3):S6-S31, 1996.
68. Jones LL, Tweedy L, Warady BA: The impact of exit-site care and catheter design on the incidence of catheter-related infections, *Adv Perit Dial* 11:302-05, 1995.
69. Prowant BF, Warady BA, Nolph KD: Peritoneal dialysis catheter exit-site care: Results of an international survey, *Perit Dial Int* 13:149-54, 1993.
70. Patel UD, Mottes TA, Flynn JT: Delayed compared with immediate use of peritoneal catheter in pediatric peritoneal dialysis, *Adv Perit Dial* 17:253-59, 2001.
71. Twardowski ZJ, Prowant BF: Exit-site study methods and results, *Perit Dial Int* 16:S6-S31, 1996.
72. Twardowski ZJ, Prowant BF: Classification of normal and diseased exit sites, *Perit Dial Int* 16(3):S32-S50, 1996.
73. Mupirocin Study Group: Nasal mupirocin prevents *Staphylococcus aureus* exit-site infection during peritoneal dialysis, *J Am Soc Nephrol* 7:2403-08, 1996.
74. Lobbedez T, Gardam M, Dedier H, et al: Routine use of mupirocin at the peritoneal catheter exit site and mupirocin resistance: Still low after 7 years, *Nephrol Dial Transplant* 19:3140-43, 2004.
75. Perez-Fontan M, Rosales M, Rodriguez-Carmona A, et al: Mupirocin resistance after long-term use for *Staphylococcus aureus* colonization in patients undergoing chronic peritoneal dialysis, *Am J Kidney Dis* 39:337-41, 2002.
76. Wong SS, Chu K, Cheuk A, et al: Prophylaxis against gram-positive organisms causing exit-site infection and peritonitis in continuous ambulatory peritoneal dialysis patients by applying mupirocin ointment at the catheter exit-site, *Perit Dial Int* 23:153-58, 2003.
77. Bernardini J, Bender F, Florio T, et al: Randomized, double-blind trial of antibiotic exit site cream for prevention of exit site infection in peritoneal dialysis patients, *J Am Soc Nephrol* 16:539-45, 2005.
78. Savader SJ, Lund G, Scheel PJ, et al: Guide wire directed manipulation of malfunctioning peritoneal dialysis catheters: A critical analysis, *J Vasc Interv Radiol* 8:957-63, 1997.
79. Rutherford RB, Becker GJ: Standards for evaluation and reporting the results of surgical and percutaneous therapy for peripheral artery disease, *JVIR* 2:169-74, 1991.
80. Siegel RL, Nosher JL, Gesner LR: Peritoneal dialysis catheters: Repositioning with new fluoroscopic technique, *Radiology* 190:899-901, 1994.
81. Shea M, Hmiel SP, Beck AM: Use of tissue plasminogen activator for thrombolysis in occluded peritoneal dialysis catheters in children, *Adv Perit Dial* 17:249-52, 2001.
82. Sakarcan A, Stallworth JR: Tissue plasminogen activator for occluded peritoneal dialysis catheter, *Pediatr Nephrol* 17:155-56, 2002.
83. Krishnan RG, Moghal NE: Tissue plasminogen activator for blocked peritoneal dialysis catheters, *Pediatr Nephrol* 21:300, 2006.
84. Schaefer F, Klaus G, Muller-Wiefel DE, et al: Intermittent versus continuous intraperitoneal glycopeptide/ceftazidime treatment in children with peritoneal dialysis-associated peritonitis, *J Am Soc Nephrol* 10:136-45, 1999.
85. Warady BA, Alexander SR, Firanek C, et al: *Peritoneal dialysis catheter and complications management for children*. Deerfield, IL, Baxter Healthcare Corporation 2001.
86. Wu YM, Tsai MK, Chao SH, et al: Surgical management of refractory exit-site/tunnel infection of Tenckhoff catheter: Technical innovations of partial replantation, *Perit Dial Int* 19:451-54, 1999.

87. Swartz RD, Messana JM: Simultaneous catheter removal and replacement in peritoneal dialysis infections: Update and current recommendations, *Adv Perit Dial* 15:205-08, 1999.
88. Schroder CH, Severijnen RS, de Jong MC, et al: Chronic tunnel infections in children: Removal and replacement of the continuous ambulatory peritoneal dialysis catheter in a single operation, *Perit Dial Int* 13:198-200, 1993.
89. Majkowski NL, Mendley SR: Simultaneous removal and replacement of infected peritoneal dialysis catheters, *Am J Kidney Dis* 29:706-11, 1997.
90. Andreetta B, Verrina E, Sorino P, et al: Complications linked to chronic peritoneal dialysis in children after kidney transplantation: Experience of the Italian Registry of Pediatric Chronic Peritoneal Dialysis, *Perit Dial Int* 16(1):S570-S573, 1996.
91. Arbeiter K, Pichler A, Muerwald G, et al: Timing of peritoneal dialysis catheter removal after pediatric renal transplantation, *Perit Dial Int* 21:467-70, 2001.
92. Korzets Z, Hasdan G, Bulkan G, et al: Early postoperative complications of removal of Tenckhoff peritoneal dialysis catheter, *Perit Dial Int* 20:789-91, 2000.

CHAPTER

55 Pediatric Peritoneal Dialysis Prescription

Enrico Eugenio Verrina and Francesco Perfumo

INTRODUCTION

A basic knowledge of the anatomy and physiology of the peritoneal cavity is helpful to understand the mechanics of peritoneal dialysis (PD) and the kinetics of solute and fluid transport.[1] The PD system has three major components.

- *Peritoneal microcirculation:* Peritoneal capillary blood flow has been suggested to vary between 50 and 100 ml/minute. However, the effective amount of this flow that is involved in peritoneal exchanges is unknown, and it could be much lower.
- *Peritoneal membrane* (Figure 55-1): Represents the barrier that solutes and water have to cross. This consists of the following.
    - *Capillary wall:* Peritoneal capillaries are mainly of the continuous type, with less than 2% of fenestrated capillaries.[2] Endothelial cells are linked to each other by tight junctions and surrounded by a basement membrane. The endothelium plays a central role in the control of vascular permeability.[3]
    - *Interstitium:* Consists of extracellular matrix, containing a limited number of cells (fibroblasts, mononuclear cells) and some lymphatic vessels. Hyaluronan, a major component of the extracellular matrix, was reported to be an important determinant of the resistance to fluid and solute transport.[4]
    - *Layer of lubricated mesothelial cells:* Forms a system of tight and gap junctions, microvillous projections at the free surface, and several organelles in their cytoplasm. Mesothelial cells were reported to participate in glucose transport and regulation of water and solute fluxes through tight junction modulation, but their actual role as a rate-limiting barrier is still debated.[4,5]
- *Dialysis fluid compartment:* Includes the composition of the solution and the modalities of delivery. Dialysis fluid is infused in the peritoneal cavity in an amount scaled to patient body size and clinical conditions. Standard dialysis solutions contain an osmotic agent to produce the osmotic gradient required to obtain ultrafiltration (UF), and a buffer to correct the patient's metabolic acidosis, calcium, magnesium, and electrolytes.

The driving forces of solute and water exchange across the peritoneal membrane, between the dialysis solution and the capillary blood and surrounding tissues,[6] are represented by the following.

- *Diffusion:* Consists of a solute exchange between two solutions (blood and dialysis fluid) separated by a semipermeable membrane (peritoneal membrane). Main factors affecting the rate of solute diffusion are represented by the following.
    - *Concentration gradient between blood and dialysate:* Because blood flow through the peritoneal membrane is relatively stable (and apparently well preserved even in unstable patients who are moderately hypotensive), concentration gradient is best maintained by changing the dialysate in the abdomen as often as is feasible.
    - *Molecular weight:* Because diffusion is a size-selective process, small molecules (urea, creatinine) diffuse more rapidly than larger molecules (vitamin B12, "middle molecules").
    - *Effective surface area and permeability of peritoneal membrane:* The vascular surface area available for dialytic exchange can be determined using the so-called three-pore permeability model,[7] and can be influenced by fill volume, patient posture, and PD fluid composition.[8,9] Permeability of the tissue between the capillary lumen and the peritoneal space can be altered by disease. It increases during acute peritonitis, whereas it can be progressively impaired by peritoneal fibrosis.
- *UF:* The bulk movement of water along with permeable solutes across the peritoneal membrane. In PD the driving force for UF is primarily represented by the osmotic pressure of dialysis fluid exerted by glucose or other osmotic agents. The effects of hydrostatic pressure gradient are usually of minor importance in PD unless exceedingly high levels of intraperitoneal pressure (IPP) are reached.[10] Other factors that can affect UF are membrane surface area and hydraulic permeability. The flux of water (J_F) across the membrane can be expressed by the following equation.[11]

$$J_F = K_f\,([P_c + s_f] - [p_c + P_f])$$

Here, K_f is the peritoneal membrane permeability coefficient, P_c is the hydraulic pressure in the capillary, s_f is the osmotic pressure of the peritoneal fluid, p_c is the oncotic pressure in the capillary, and P_f is the hydraulic pressure of the fluid

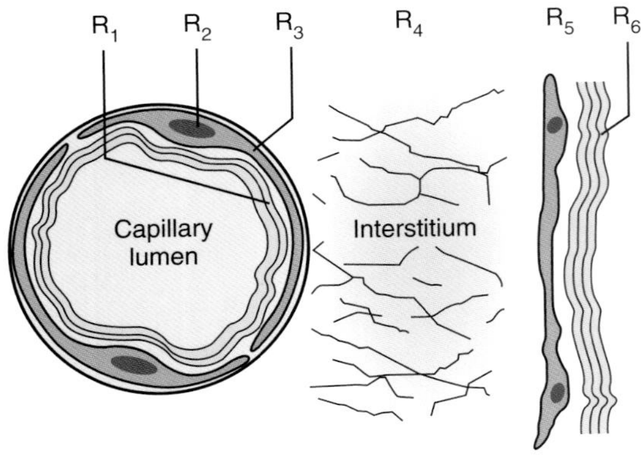

Figure 55-1 Components of the peritoneal transport barrier. Six anatomic sites of resistance to solute transport are illustrated: R_1, blood film along capillary wall; R_2, capillary endothelium; R_3, capillary basement membrane; R_4, interstitium; R_5, mesothelial cells; R_6, peritoneal fluid film along mesothelial cell layer.

under flux. A significant amount of fluid and solutes is also absorbed into the lymphatics. The rate of lymphatic absorption has been reported to be higher in children than in adults.[12] Net UF results from the balance between osmotic UF drawing fluid into the peritoneal cavity and lymphatic and capillary absorption of peritoneal fluid. Increased lymphatic absorption may play a role in some patients in whom net UF is reduced, as well as in the absorption of a significant amount of macromolecules.

- *Convective solute transport:* As water moves from capillaries to peritoneal cavity on a pressure gradient, the dissolved molecules are dragged along (solvent drag). The convective transport of a solute depends on the rate of UF and on membrane permeability, which can be expressed by the sieving coefficient and calculated by dividing the concentration of solute in ultrafiltrate by its concentration in plasma water (in the absence of a concentration gradient).

ASSESSMENT OF PERITONEAL MEMBRANE TRANSPORT CHARACTERISTICS

Because peritoneal solute and fluid transport varies considerably from patient to patient, peritoneal transport characteristics should be assessed at the beginning of PD treatment (one month after catheter implantation). These characteristics should then be monitored on a routine basis (two to four times per year) and in the case of clinical events that may cause changes in transport capacity (e.g., recurrent and/or particularly severe peritonitis episodes).[13,14]

Peritoneal membrane function tests constitute the first step of the process of tailoring PD prescription on individual patient needs and characteristics. Their application to the pediatric patient population has long been hampered by differences in peritoneal membrane properties between children and adults. More recently, the significance of these differences has been called into question as studies on larger numbers of patients have developed standardized methods of evaluating the parameters of peritoneal transport in children.[15,16]

Appropriate scaling for body size plays a central role in the standardization of the procedure of equilibration tests and in the calculation of membrane function parameters. Because peritoneal surface area correlates better with body surface area (BSA) than with body weight (BW), and because this relationship is constant and age independent, scaling the exchange volume by BSA enables us to compare peritoneal transport properties in adults and children of different age groups.[15-18] BSA can be calculated by use of mathematical formulae from a patient's BW and body height (BH).

Peritoneal Equilibration Test

The peritoneal equilibration test (PET) measures the rate at which solutes [usually creatinine (Cr), urea, and glucose) come to equilibration between the blood and the dialysate. To reach a satisfactory level of reproducibility of PET results, a standard PET in children can be performed with a dwell volume of 1100 ml/m^2 BSA—which approximates the standard 2000 ml/1.73 m^2 volume supplied to adults[19] using a 2.5% dextrose PD solution. A 4.25% dextrose solution can be used to obtain a more accurate assessment of UF and of sodium sieving.[20]

Dialysate to plasma (D/P) ratio of Cr and dialysate glucose concentration to initial dialysate glucose concentration at time 0 (D/D0) are calculated at 2 and 4 hours of the test. A serum sample is obtained at time 2 hours. Dialysate Cr concentration must be corrected for the interference of the high glucose levels in the dialysate by the following formula.

$$\text{Corrected Cr (mg/dl)} = \text{measured Cr (mg/dl)} - \text{correction factor} \times \text{dialysate glucose (mg/dl)}$$

The correction factor should be determined in the laboratory of each dialysis center by dividing measured Cr of a fresh PD solution by glucose concentration. Urea and creatinine D/P ratios, and glucose D/D0 ratio, can be compared to the results from a large pediatric study in which the same standard pediatric PET was adopted[16] to characterize patients as having a high, high average, low average, or low solute transport[19] (Figures 55-2 and 55-3). High transport for Cr (and/or urea) implies its fast removal from blood, whereas high transport for glucose denotes its fast elimination from dialysate—thus dissipating the osmotic gradient required for UF.

Mass Transfer Area Coefficient

The mass transfer area coefficient (MTAC) parameter is an expression of the diffusive permeability of the peritoneal membrane of each patient, and describes the maximal clearance theoretically achievable at a constantly maximal gradient for diffusion (i.e., dialysate solute concentration = 0). Determination of MTAC, which is independent of dialysate volume and glucose concentration, helps to model both long- and short-dwell dialysis and to individualize dialysis prescription.

Computer technology gives reliable results in the calculation of MTAC even in pediatric patients.[21] Whereas MTAC values are largely independent of age when normalized to BSA,[16,21] relatively greater solute clearances might be expected in infants due to higher peritoneal permeability or larger effective surface area of the peritoneal membrane.[16]

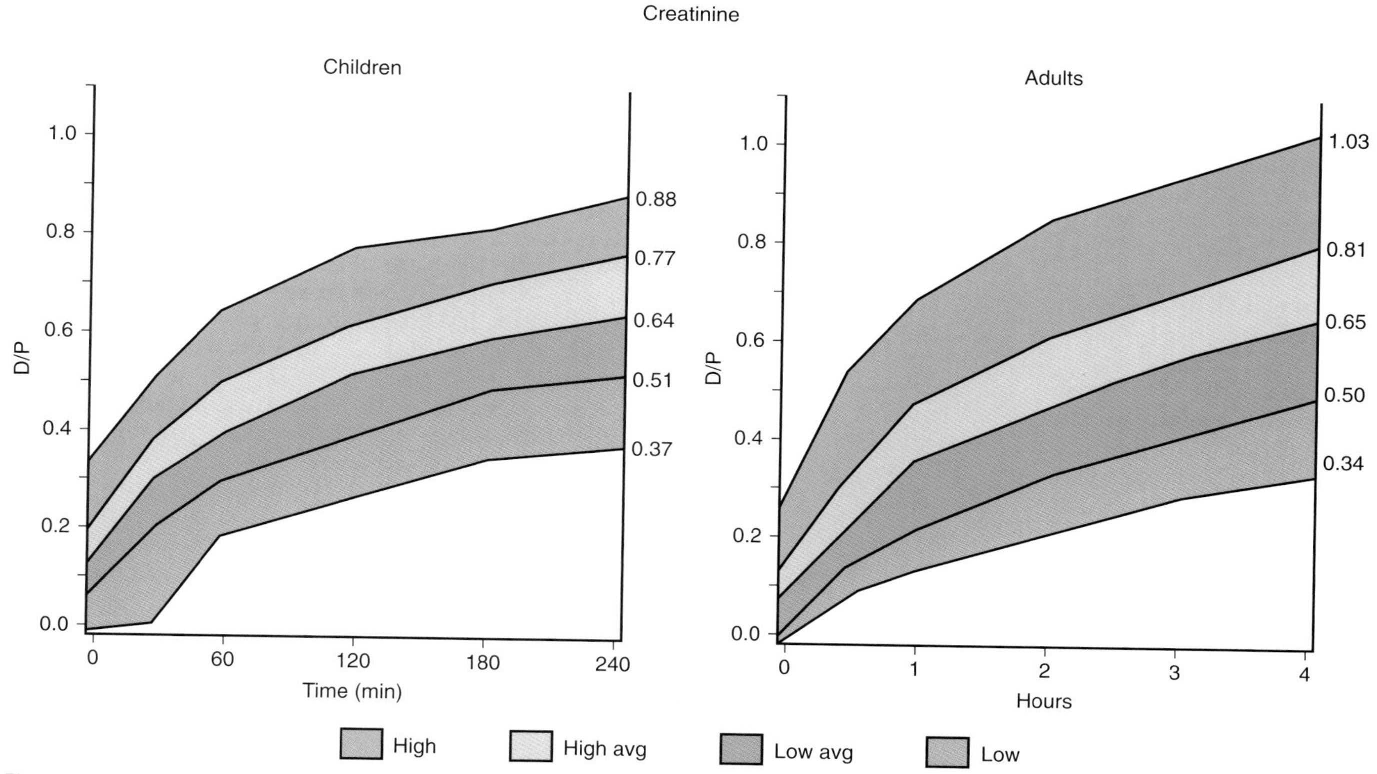

Figure 55-2 Peritoneal equilibration test results for creatinine in pediatric and adult patients. The four categories of peritoneal transport (colored areas) are bordered by the maximal, mean + 1 standard deviation (SD), mean, mean − 1 SD, and minimal values for pediatric and adult study population. *D/P*, Dialysate to plasma ratio. Data adapted from Warady BA, Alexander SR, Hossli S, Vonesh E, Geary D, Watkins S, et al: Peritoneal membrane transport function in children receiving long-term dialysis, *J Am Soc Nephrol* 7:2385-91, 1996.

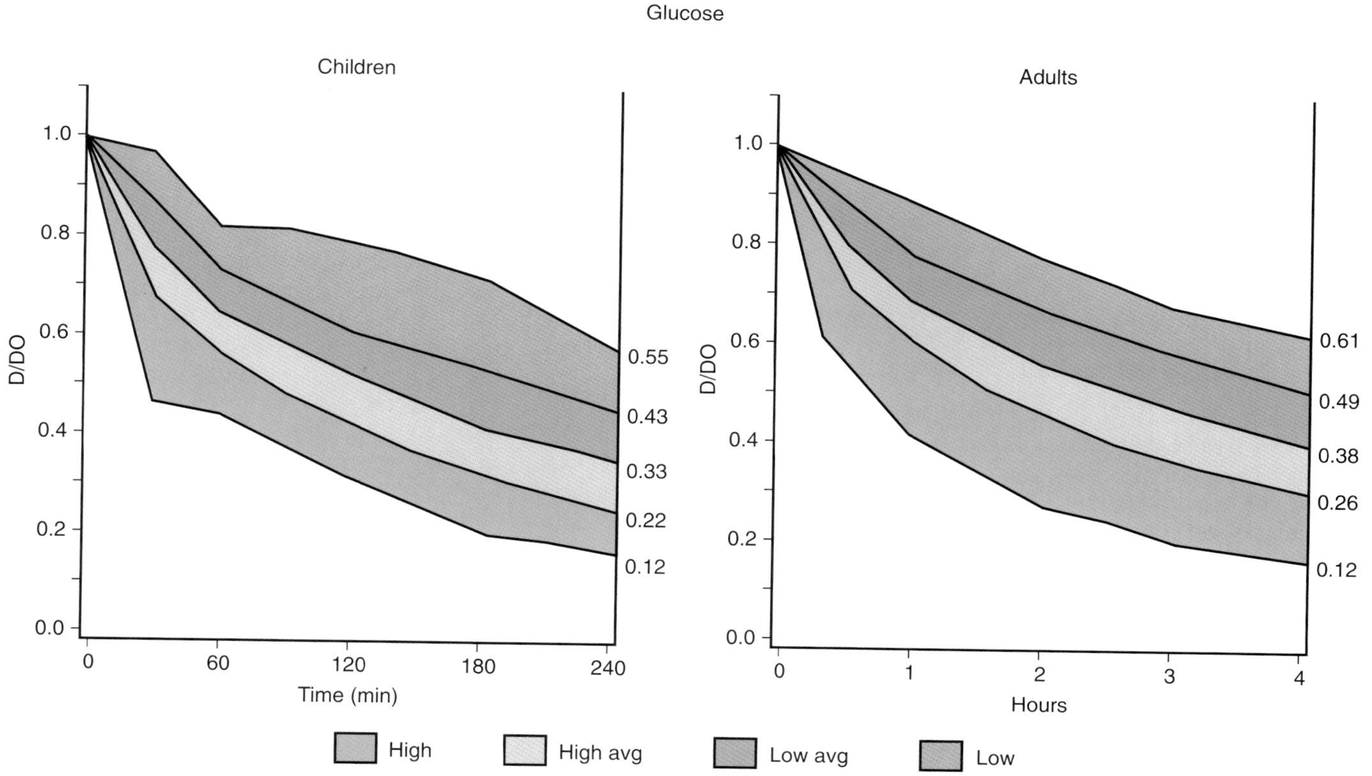

Figure 55-3 Peritoneal equilibration test results for glucose in pediatric and adult patients. The four categories of peritoneal transport (colored areas) are bordered by the maximal, mean + 1 standard deviation (SD), mean, mean − 1 SD, and minimal values for pediatric and adult study population. *D/DO*, Dialysate glucose to initial dialysate glucose concentration ratio. Data adapted from Warady BA, Alexander SR, Hossli S, Vonesh E, Geary D, Watkins S, et al: Peritoneal membrane transport function in children receiving long-term dialysis, *J Am Soc Nephrol* 7:2385-91, 1996.

Standard Permeability Analysis

Standard permeability analysis (SPA) can be considered an adaptation of PET, where the addition of poly-disperse dextran 70 to the test solution allows for simultaneous measurement of transcapillary UF, marker clearance, and intraperitoneal volume (IPV). By using a test volume of 1200 ml/m² BSA and 1.36% glucose or 3.86% glucose as a test solution, comparable results of SPA were obtained in adult and pediatric patients.[22,23]

Peritoneal Dialysis Capacity Test

The peritoneal dialysis capacity (PDC) test, as described by Haraldsson,[7] is based on the three-pore model of solute and fluid transport across the peritoneal membrane.[24,25] According to this model, the peritoneum is characterized as a heteroporous three-pore membrane with few (~1%-2%) water-exclusive ultrasmall pores (aquaporins) [radius 2-4 angstrom (Å)], a small percentage (~5%) of large pores (radius 200-300 Å), and a majority (~90%-95%) of small pores (radius 40-60 Å).

Small hydrophilic solute transport occurs primarily by diffusion across the small pores, although convection also plays a role. The movement of proteins and other macromolecules occurs by convection across the large pores. Fluid transport can occur across all three pathways and is determined by crystalloid and colloid osmotic pressures. The PDC test is used to calculate the following three parameters: (1) the effective peritoneal surface area, or unrestricted pore area over diffusion distance ($A_0/\Delta X$), corresponding to the diffusion capacity for solutes; (2) absorption (i.e., the final rate of fluid reabsorption from the abdominal cavity); and (3) the large pore volume flow, which represents the rate of protein-rich fluid passing through the large pores from blood to dialysate.

The PDC can be performed following a protocol of five exchanges in 24 hours using different dwell times and two glucose solutions, or a simplified protocol for patients on automated PD (APD).[26] The PDC was successfully applied in children to model individual peritoneal membrane function,[26] and in one pediatric study D/P or D/D0 ratios derived from PET analysis were used to estimate $A_0/\Delta X$ by using a specific computer program.[8]

DETERMINATION OF INTRAPERITONEAL FILL VOLUME

Whereas peritoneal membrane surface area per unit (kg) of BW is twice as large in infants as that in adults, the relationship between BSA (m²) and peritoneal membrane surface area is constant and age independent.[27] If IPV is scaled by BW, infants and young children will receive a small exchange volume in proportion to the surface area of their peritoneal membrane. On the contrary, scaling IPV by BSA maintains the ratio of dwell volume to peritoneal surface area constant across patient age groups—thus avoiding the false perception of peritoneal hyperpermeability in infants and small children while performing peritoneal function tests.[28] This has become a standard in pediatric PD prescription.[13,27]

Both IPV and patient posture are factors that can dynamically affect the recruitment of effective peritoneal membrane area available for dialytic exchange, which corresponds to the unrestricted pore area over diffusion distance ($A_0/\Delta X$) as determined using the three-pore model.[7,8] The peritoneal vascular surface area is maximized as IPV is raised from 800 to 1400 ml/m² BSA.[8] An excessive IPV may cause patients discomfort, as well as a series of complications—such as pain, dyspnea, hydrothorax, hernia, and loss of UF due to an increased lymphatic drainage.

Measurement of the hydrostatic IPP can help determine the fill volume tolerance of the individual patient.[10] The maximum tolerable IPV was defined as the volume causing an IPP of 18 cm H_2O in the supine position. At and above this limit, abdominal pain and/or a decrease in respiratory vital capacity may occur.[29,30] Although IPP is influenced by factors such as gender and ponderosity and gradually adapts to a given IPV, the level of IPP in general is a reproducible patient-characteristic parameter.[27,31]

In conclusion, an IPV of 1400 ml/m² BSA seems optimal in ensuring maximum recruitment of vascular pore area in children. However, this should be considered a maximal limit—the safety of which (e.g., with respect to the risk of hernia formation) has not been validated in children. In clinical practice, the initial fill volume prescription can be 600 to 800 ml/m² during daytime and 800 to 1000 ml/m² overnight. As PD treatment goes on, fill volume can be increased in steps (according to patient tolerance and IPP measurement) to help maintain the desired targets of depuration adequacy for each patient.[13]

PERITONEAL DIALYSIS SOLUTIONS

The composition of PD solutions is aimed at facilitating removal of water and waste products, and at helping to maintain electrolyte and calcium homeostasis and acid/base balance. For this purpose, standard PD solutions contain an osmotic agent that produces the osmotic gradient required for UF, a buffer to correct metabolic acidosis, calcium, magnesium, and electrolytes (Table 55-1). Different types of commercially available PD solutions can be employed to meet individual peritoneal transport characteristics, metabolic and clinical needs (malnutrition, UF failure), and the situation of PD complications (peritonitis).

Moreover, during the past decade the increasing knowledge of the harmful effects that prolonged exposure to standard PD solutions with high glucose and lactate concentration, low pH, high osmolarity, and high level of glucose degradation products (GDPs) may have on the peritoneal membrane (Figure 55-2) has led to the development of more biocompatible PD solutions. The material following briefly reviews the characteristics of PD solutions that may help in PD prescription,[32] in accordance with clinical and experimental experience achieved in pediatric patients.[33]

OSMOTIC AGENTS

Throughout the history of PD, glucose has been utilized almost exclusively as an osmotic agent. A number of alternatives have been proposed over time, but only two of these (icodextrin and amino acids) are commercially available at present.

TABLE 55-1 **Components of Peritoneal Dialysis Solutions (Range of Concentrations in Standard Commercially Available PD Solutions)**

1. Osmotic agent • Glucose (dextrose) • Icodextrin • Amino acids	 1.36-3.86 (1.5-4.5) g/dl 7.5 g/dl 1.1 g/dl
2. Buffer • Lactate • Bicarbonate • Lactate/bicarbonate	 35-40 mmol/L* 34 mmol/L† 15/25 mmol/L‡
3. Sodium	132-134 mmol/L
4. Calcium	1.25-1.75 mmol/L
5. Magnesium	0.25-0.75 mmol/L
6. Chloride	95-103.5 mmol/L

* pH = 5.5-6.5.
† pH = 7.4.
‡ pH = 7.0-7.4.

TABLE 55-2 **Toxic Effects of Conventional PD Solutions on Membrane Integrity (High Glucose Concentration and/or Low pH)**

High Glucose Concentration and/or Low pH
• Hyperosmolar stress
• Glycation of structural proteins
• Formation of highly reactive: • GDPs • AGE • Amadori adducts
• Effects on peritoneal cells metabolism through: • Polyol pathway • Protein kinase activation • Gene induction
• Local release of cytokines and growth factors: • Inflammatory state • Fibrogenic processes • Neoangiogenesis • Peritoneal fibrosis
Impairment of: • Mesothelial cell integrity • Peritoneal macrophage function • Intraperitoneal host defense • Membrane permeability

AGE, Advanced glycation end products; *GDPs*, glucose degradation products.

Glucose

The crystalloid osmotic effect of glucose is exerted through the system of ultrasmall pores (aquaporins), and can be enhanced by increasing glucose concentration from 1.36% to 2.27% and 3.86% (or 1.5%, 2.5%, and 4.25%, as dextrose). The absorption of glucose [molecular weight (MW), 180 daltons (Da)] from dialysis fluid leads to a quite rapid dissipation of the osmotic gradient. Although the rate of absorption varies considerably among patients, glucose is usually unsuitable for maintenance of UF during a long dwell. Adverse effects of glucose-based PD solutions[34,35] include the following (Table 55-2).

- *Systemic metabolic effects:* The caloric load due to glucose absorption can worsen the hyperinsulinemia and dyslipidemia associated with the uremic condition;
- *Structural and functional damage:* To the peritoneal membrane, caused by such factors as hyperosmolar stress and the presence of highly reactive GDPs—leading to glycation of structural proteins, the formation of Amadori adducts and advanced glycosylation end products (AGEs), and effects on peritoneal cell metabolism via the polyol pathway, protein kinase activation, and gene induction.

Reduced GDP formation has been obtained by the separation of glucose from the other constituents in two-chamber bag systems, which permit glucose sterilization at a lower pH than is possible in single-chamber bags.[35,36] In summary, although glucose is effective in UF induction along short dwells the lowest glucose concentration of PD solution should be employed in daily practice while still being compatible with a patient's clinical needs.[33]

Polyglucose

Icodextrin, the commercially available polyglucose solution, consists of a family of glucose polymers with an average molecular weight of 16,200 Da. Disappearance of these macromolecules from the peritoneal cavity mainly occurs by absorption into the lymphatic system at a rather low rate. Thus, a 7.5% icodextrin solution (ICO) produces sustained UF over a long dwell by means of colloid osmotic pressure. Over a 12- to 14-hour dwell, net UF obtained with ICO is similar to that obtained with a 3.86% glucose solution and is significantly greater than that reached with a 1.36% glucose solution in adult and in pediatric patients.[37-39]

The UF profile obtained by using ICO during a 14-hour daytime dwell in seven pediatric patients (median age 9.2 years, range 2.7 to 13.4 years) is presented in Figure 55-4. At 14 hours of the dwell, mean net UF corresponded to 17% of the infused volume.[40] Use of ICO in pediatric patients helps to significantly increase solute removal.[38] Because icodextrin generates water transport through the small-pore system, it does not induce sodium sieving.[41] Therefore, sodium removal is usually greater than that achieved with glucose-based solutions.

Over a 14-hour dwell, icodextrin absorption rate was reported to be as high as 45% in children.[40] Icodextrin is metabolized by amylase to maltose and a number of oligosaccharides. Their serum levels usually reach a steady-state level within 2 weeks from the start of treatment, whereas they are no longer detectable 2 weeks after discontinuation of the use of ICO.[38] Sterile peritonitis was reported in some patients treated with ICO, and was caused by peptidoglycan contamination of dialysate by thermophilic acidophilic bacteria.[42]

Hypersensitivity reactions, mainly manifesting in a mild to moderate skin rash, may be observed at the beginning of the treatment with ICO. They usually resolve without any sequelae after ICO discontinuation.[38] In vitro and ex vivo studies have shown that ICO is more biocompatible with the peritoneal membrane than glucose-based solutions, possibly due to its isoosmolar property, lack of glucose, and lower GDP content.[43] However, it has recently been reported that

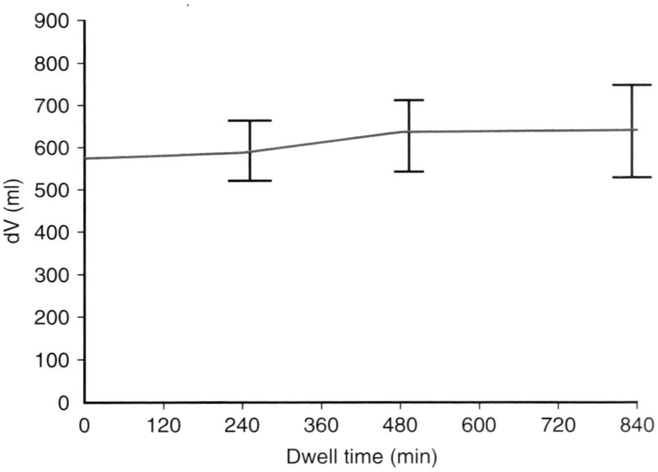

Figure 55-4 Intraperitoneal volume (IPV) versus time curve obtained in seven children during a 14-hour daytime dwell with 7.5% icodextrin PD solution. IPV was evaluated by direct drained volume (dV) measurement at each time point of the curve.

ICO may also restrain the normal process of mesothelial cell repopulation and induce repair by means of connective tissue.[44] The situations in which ICO can be employed to increase UF and solute removal are summarized in Table 55-3.[33,37,38] The use of ICO is recommended in not more than one dwell per day.

Amino Acids

In children on continuous ambulatory PD (CAPD), the effect on nutritional status of using an amino acid (AA) solution in a long dwell was controversial. Increases of blood urea nitrogen and worsening of acidosis have been observed.[45] On the other hand, combined intraperitoneal infusion of AA and glucose during a nocturnal APD session promoted utilization of AA for protein synthesis.[46] This schedule was reported to improve anthropometric parameters in children on APD,[47] and to positively influence muscle protein turnover in adult patients.[48] In summary, the use of AA solution in children on APD may be indicated in order to:

- Improve treatment biocompatibility, due to lack of glucose and a less acidic composition (pH 6.2 to 6.7)
- Prevent AA loss in dialysate
- Supply AA in malnourished patients

BUFFERS

Lactate

This metabolic precursor of bicarbonate has been traditionally employed as a buffer because PD solutions containing a mixture of bicarbonate, calcium, magnesium, and glucose are difficult to prepare, sterilize, and store. In fact, calcium and magnesium precipitate as carbonate salts during autoclaving—and glucose caramelizes at physiologic pH. Lactate is absorbed from dialysis fluid along its concentration gradient. Therefore, its absorption can be increased by rapid exchanges and high dialysate volume. Lactate is metabolized to bicarbonate in the liver. Use of acidic (pH 5.5 to 6.5) lactate-buffered PD solutions is associated with several drawbacks:

- During a dwell with lactate, bicarbonate back-diffuses in dialysate.
- Some patients experience pain during inflow.
- Lactate may induce local release of growth factors that stimulate fibrogenic processes and neoangiogenesis, thus contributing to peritoneal fibrosis and to the impairment of peritoneal membrane transport function (see Table 55-2).

Bicarbonate

A growing body of evidence from both in vitro and clinical studies suggests that the use of multicompartment bag systems is associated with better biocompatibility than conventional lactate-based solutions.[49] In particular, bicarbonate-based solutions with neutral pH (7.0 to 7.4) have shown a series of improvements in biocompatibility parameters—such as increased concentration of cancer antigen 125 (Ca 125)—that may reflect mesothelial cell mass, decreased hyaluronan concentration (an indicator of inflammation), and better preservation of macrophage and mesothelial cell function.[50-53]

Bicarbonate solutions are also associated with a lower incidence of infusion pain, a problem that can be related to irritation of the peritoneum by GDPs and the acidity of lactate-based solutions.[9,53] In children on APD, neutral-pH bicarbonate-buffered PD fluid provided more effective correction of acidosis and better preservation of peritoneal cell mass than conventional lactate-based PD fluids.[52] Schmitt and colleagues[54] found that peritoneal mass transfer kinetics were similar with bicarbonate and lactate for water and most solutes, except for slightly lower phosphate and creatinine transport rates at 1-hour dwell time with bicarbonate solution.

These more physiologic PD fluids have been shown to prevent hyperperfusion, and to reduce the loss of proteins into dialysate. Their use was associated with lower IPP, but also with a reduction of the vascular exchange area—which may impact dialysis adequacy.[9] PD solutions containing 34 mmol/L of bicarbonate or 25 mmol/L of bicarbonate plus 15 mmol/L of lactate are commercially available.[33]

SODIUM

Commercially available PD solutions most frequently have a sodium concentration of 132 to 134 mmol/L (see Table 55-1); that is, slightly lower than plasma sodium concentration. Therefore, diffusion of sodium is usually less important than convection transport that can be accomplished by transcapillary UF, colloid-osmosis–induced backfiltration, and absorption into the lymphatic system. Sodium sieving

TABLE 55-3 **Indications for the Use of 7.5% Icodextrin PD Solution**
• Long nighttime dwell in CAPD patients
• Long daytime dwell in nocturnal APD patients
• Type I UF failure
• Peritonitis-associated UF failure

CAPD, Continuous ambulatory peritoneal dialysis; *APD*, automated peritoneal dialysis; *UF*, ultrafiltration.

associated with the transcellular water transport through ultrasmall pores can contribute to a reduction of the dialysate concentration of sodium during the initial phase of the dwell (the sodium sieving coefficient is 0.75).

Although this mechanism has almost no clinical consequences during CAPD, much more water than sodium may be removed with short-dwell APD. Therefore, dialysis solutions with lower sodium concentration may be employed in APD patients where they cannot be in CAPD patients—especially when a large amount of high-glucose solution is prescribed. Such solutions are currently being studied in clinical trials. The process of colloid osmosis generated by icodextrin does not lead to sodium sieving, and higher sodium removal can be expected with icodextrin-based PD fluids.[41]

CALCIUM

Diffusion and convective transport are involved in calcium transfer across the peritoneal membrane. Accordingly, calcium peritoneal flux is dependent on:

- Serum ultrafiltrable calcium concentration
- PD solution calcium concentration
- Duration of the dwell
- Rate of UF

Standard PD solutions contain:

- *1.75 mmol/L of calcium:* Ionized calcium of these solutions is higher than the ionized calcium level normally present in blood, and diffusion of calcium from dialysate to blood would lead to a positive calcium balance.
- *1.25 mmol/L:* These solutions are frequently employed with the goal of reducing the incidence of hypercalcemia, especially in children receiving calcium carbonate or calcium acetate (as a phosphate binder) and vitamin D analogues.[7]

To avoid hypercalcemia and/or a high calcium × phosphate product, attention should be paid to the risk of inducing vascular and soft-tissue calcification. The use of non–calcium-containing phosphate binders (sevelamer) would be indicated in these cases. On the other hand, in children maintenance of a slightly positive calcium balance may be useful to ensure adequate mineralization of the growing skeleton.

CHOICE OF PD MODALITY AND PRESCRIPTION

Chronic PD can be performed manually (CAPD) or by utilizing a device (automated PD, APD). The PD regimen is continuous (with dialysis solution present in the peritoneal cavity evenly throughout 24 hours) or intermittent (with empty abdomen for part of the day, usually during daytime).

The utilization of APD has rapidly expanded during the past 15 years because it allows individualized PD prescription and better quality of life.[55] Among children, APD has become the PD method of choice and has largely replaced CAPD[56,57] in those countries where APD use is not limited by cost constraints.

CAPD

CAPD is performed by three to five daily exchanges (typically four), including three to four of approximately equal length during the daytime and a nighttime exchange of 8 to 12 hours. As a continuous procedure, CAPD allows complete equilibration of small solutes and a certain removal of middle molecules. However, a large volume of intraperitoneal fluid during the daytime may be associated with patient discomfort, occurrence of abdominal hernias (particularly in young infants), and problems of body image (particularly in adolescents). In addition, continuous absorption of glucose from the dialysate compromises appetite and aggravates uremic dyslipidemia.

CAPD is usually effective in children with residual renal function, but purification should be closely monitored. According to the guidelines of the European Paediatric Peritoneal Dialysis Working Group on the adequacy of pediatric PD prescription,[13] initial fill volume can be 600 to 800 ml/m^2 during the day and 800 to 1000 ml/m^2 overnight. If an increase of the dialysis dose is indicated, these volumes can be gradually enhanced according to patient tolerance and the prevailing IPP.[29-31] Fill volume can at first be increased in only part of the exchanges, and then in all four exchanges if targets are not met. As a next step, the number of exchanges can be increased to five per day.

If there is inadequate UF overnight due to rapid glucose absorption, icodextrin PD solution can be employed. Increasing the number of exchanges to obtain adequate UF and solute removal may represent an excessive burden on families. In this case, a shift to an APD modality should be considered.

APD

APD is performed at night with the help of a device (cycler) that delivers PD fluid to the patient. The reasons for the preference for APD in the treatment of pediatric patients on chronic PD are psychosocial and clinical.

- Performed at nighttime, APD enables children to attend school full time and reduces the impact of dialysis treatment on the daily lives of patients and their families—thus providing a higher level of psychological and social rehabilitation of end-stage renal failure (ESRF) children compared with other forms of chronic dialysis.
- Nighttime dialysis in the supine position allows for large fill volumes, thus ensuring a more effective contact between dialysate and the peritoneal membrane—with maximum recruitment of peritoneal vascular area available for solute transport. Small-solute diffusive transport coefficients have been reported to be higher in the supine position than during the ambulatory upright position.[8,27,28]
- The wide range of treatment options available with APD enables the dialysis prescription to be tailored to the individual patient age, body size, clinical condition, growth-related metabolic needs, and peritoneal transport status.

APD regimens may be continuous (if an IPV of dialysis fluid is constantly present) or intermittent, if a patient's abdomen is empty during a certain period of the day (usually daytime; Figure 55-5). The variants of APD discussed later in this chapter are commonly practiced.

Nightly Intermittent PD

Nightly intermittent PD (NIPD) consists of a series of short nocturnal cycles without a daytime dialysate dwell. As dis-

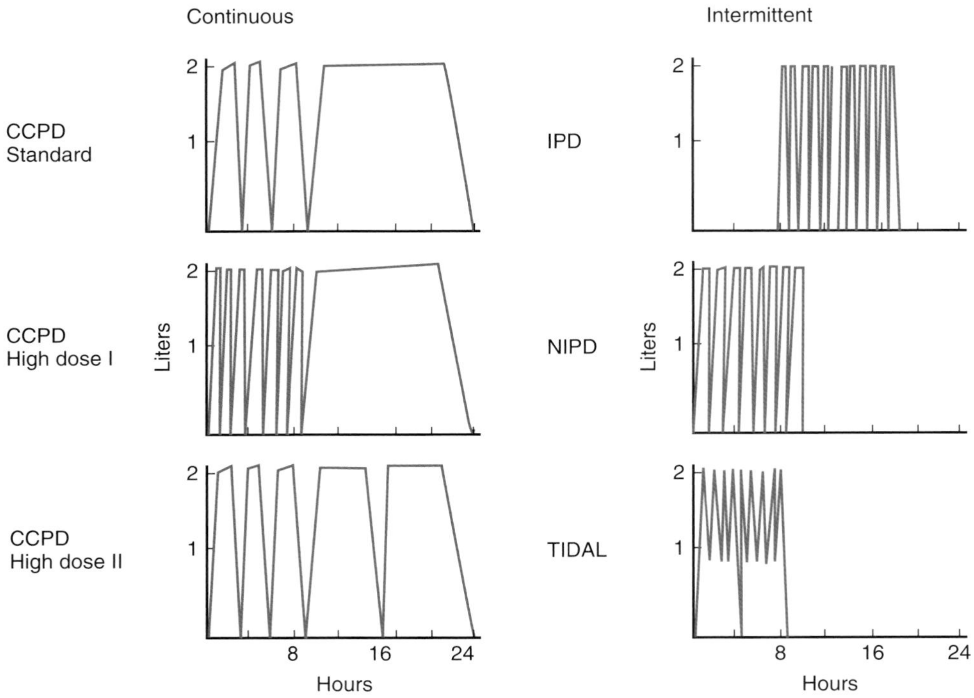

Figure 55-5 Continuous *(left side)* and intermittent *(right side)* regimens of automated peritoneal dialysis (APD). *CCPD*, Continuous cycling peritoneal dialysis (PD); *IPD*, intermittent peritoneal PD; *NIPD*, nightly intermittent PD.

TABLE 55-4 Potential Advantages and Limitations of Nightly Intermittent Peritoneal Dialysis

Advantages	Limitations
• No daytime glucose absorption	• Reduced small solute clearance in patients with low and low-average transporter status
• No risk of daytime net fluid resorption	• Reduced middle molecule clearance
• Normal daytime IPP	• No flush of catheter and lines at the start of the night session
• Preservation of body image	
• Reduced loss of proteins and amino acids	
• Better long-term preservation of the peritoneal membrane	

IPP, intraperitoneal pressure.

cussed previously, maintaining a dry peritoneal cavity during the daytime hours has a number of advantages that may be particularly beneficial to the pediatric population. These are summarized in Table 55-4. At the same time, the absence of a daytime dwell is associated with some limitations of NIPD compared to continuous PD modalities (Table 55-4) and makes this modality not suitable for functionally anuric patients.

The delivery of a small volume of PD fluid at the end of the night session may allow for a "drain before fill" phase, thus reducing the chance of peritoneal infection due to touch contamination. The assessment of peritoneal transport status is important when selecting patients for NIPD because this is primarily indicated in patients with a high-transport peritoneal membrane and who show rapid equilibration of solute concentrations and adequate UF only with rapid exchanges. NIPD may represent the initial APD regimen for children who have a significant residual diuresis,[13] with a typical initial prescription characterized by the following.

- Nine to 12 hours of total treatment time.
- A fill volume of 800 to 1000 ml/m^2 exchanged 5 to 10 times (young infants frequently require more cycles).
- Dialysis solution should contain 1.36% glucose or higher concentrations, depending on UF requirements. Solutions with different concentrations can be mixed by the cycler to titrate tonicity of the infused solution according to a patient's individual needs.

Along the course of treatment, NIPD prescription can evolve according to clearance and UF requirements—which are mainly dictated by the decline of residual urine volume. During this phase, maintenance of fluid balance is of crucial importance to treatment outcomes.[58-60] The efficiency of NIPD can be improved by the following measures, usually applied in the order listed.

- Maximizing the fill volume (according to patient tolerance and IPP limits) up to 1200 ml/m^2.
- Increasing the number of exchanges in high and high-average transporters. This can be done up to a point,

beyond which clearance and UF may decrease because the proportion of treatment time without efficient dialysis due to the fill and drain phases becomes more relevant than the benefit of increasing dialysate volume.

- Increasing the total treatment time (as patient compliance and social life allows). The number of exchanges can be kept constant in low and low-average transport patients.
- Increasing the tonicity of PD solution to enhance UF rate.

If these adjustments of NIPD prescription do not sufficiently enhance solute and water removal, the patient may be at risk of inadequate dialysis and should be considered for a different APD regimen.

Continuous Cycling PD

In continuous cycling PD (CCPD), a fresh exchange of PD solution ranging in volume from 50% to 100% of the fill volume applied at night is left in the abdomen at the end of the nocturnal APD session. Daytime exchange can be drained at bedtime, when the cycler is reconnected—reducing patient involvement, as with NIPD, to one session for preparation of the equipment and connection to the cycler and one short disconnection in the morning. Because glucose is largely absorbed during the long daytime dwell, ICO can be employed to obtain sustained UF and solute removal during this exchange.[38,39]

Over a long dwell exchange, complete saturation of dialysate with small solutes is often achieved. Therefore, clearances obtained during a daytime dwell are also influenced by the convective transport of solutes that is associated with net UF. The daytime dwell is effective in improving solute clearance. In particular, removal of middle-size uremic toxins is poorly accomplished by short cycles of APD and is more a function of total dialysis time.[61]

Phosphate removal by PD is almost never sufficient to adequately control hyperphosphatemia, and there is a continued need for dietary restriction and phosphate binder administration. However, phosphate clearance can be improved by increasing dwell volume[27] and by optimizing the duration of exchanges through the calculation of the phosphate purification dwell time (PPT) from a PET.[62] CCPD is indicated in NIPD patients when desired targets of solute and fluid removal have become difficult to achieve, especially if residual renal function is rapidly declining, and in patients with high-average peritoneal transport. As a further step, in CCPD patients who

- require higher solute clearances,
- have insufficient UF due to a high glucose absorption rate, or
- have a low-average transport status,

one or two exchanges of dialysate can be performed at midday or in the afternoon using the cycler in a disconnectable manner. More patient involvement is required by this modality, but it allows one to achieve small-solute D/P equilibration during each of the daytime exchanges and to optimize the UF profile.[61]

Tidal PD

Tidal PD (TPD) is a variant of APD in which an initial infusion of solution into the peritoneal cavity is followed, after a usually short dwell time, by only partial dialysate drainage—leaving an intraabdominal volume. The drained "tidal" volume is replaced with fresh dialysis fluid to restore the initial IPV at each cycle. The entire dialysate volume is drained only at the end of the APD session. The amount of ultrafiltrate expected to be generated during each cycle must be estimated and added to the drain volume to prevent overfilling of the peritoneal cavity.

TABLE 55-5 **Indications for the Use of Tidal Peritoneal Dialysis (TPD)**
• Increase solute clearance
• Improve PD mechanics efficiency
• Avoid repeated cycler alarms of incomplete drainage
• Reduce pain on drainage

The rationale of TPD use (Table 55-5) is to increase clearances (as a result of the continuous contact between dialysate and peritoneal membrane, which maintains a sustained diffusion of solutes), to improve the efficiency of the dialysis modality by reducing inflow and outflow dead times (particularly when high dialysate flow rates are adopted), to avoid repeated cycler alarms of low flow rate in case of peritoneal adhesions and catheter malfunction, and to reduce pain occurring during the drainage phase.

The major determinants of TPD efficiency are total volume of delivered PD fluid and individual peritoneal transport. Only high-transport patients can reach adequate solute clearances with intermittent nightly TPD (NTPD), whereas high-average transport patients would benefit from one or more daytime dwells—thus undergoing a continuous form of TPD (CTPD). In pediatric patients, TPD efficiency was equal to or higher than that of standard APD. However, larger total session volumes were required.[63,64]

Optimization of TPD may be obtained by adapting the tidal volume to the individual drainage profile, thus reducing the fill and drain dead times to a minimum.[65] The fluid drainage profile is not linear (Figure 55-6). A high flow rate is only maintained until a critical IPV is reached. After this breakpoint, the flow rate drops and the final part of the drainage can last more than twice the time of the previous segment. During this slow-flow portion of the drainage phase, the peritoneal cavity is almost empty and solute clearance is greatly reduced.[66] Because the critical IPV is an individual characteristic, tailoring the tidal volume to the drainage profile of each patient may improve the overall efficiency of the system. This optimization can be particularly useful in patients with problems in catheter function.

Continuous Flow Peritoneal Dialysis

Continuous-flow PD (CFPD) is an old concept and represents one of the first PD techniques applied but soon abandoned owing to various technical problems and high costs.[67] In adult patients, CFPD relies on a 2- to 3-liter dwell volume and a continuous dialysate flow at 100 to 300 ml/min. This high flow rate requires a highly efficient dual-lumen peritoneal catheter, or two catheters with endings separated as distantly as possible. Moreover, CFPD requires the facility to generate or regenerate large volumes of PD fluid.

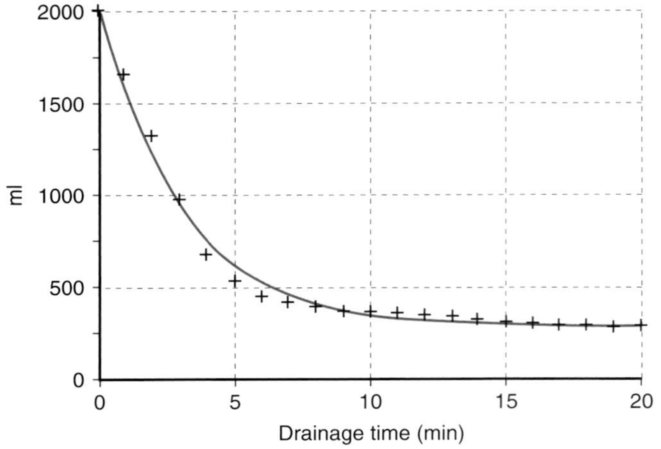

Figure 55-6 Example of volume-versus-time curve describing intraperitoneal fluid drainage through the peritoneal catheter. In this case, the flow rate dropped after the first 5 minutes and a residual volume was still present after 20 minutes of drainage (record from the memory card of the cycler).

The theoretical key advantages of CFPD are an enhanced small-solute clearance and UF permitting shorter dialysis sessions and intermittent treatment, the use of reduced dialysate glucose concentration and bicarbonate solutions, and a reduction in protein loss (in that proteins that accumulate in the dialysate are returned to the patient). Online preparation of PD fluids would allow individualization of compositions with respect to glucose, buffer, sodium, and calcium content.[68]

Very recently, new technologies have been developed that permit accurate fluid handling, reliable monitoring of pressures and flows in the circuit, and online generation or regeneration of PD fluid using a modified hemodialysis system. Moreover, a dual-lumen catheter with adequate flow characteristics has been developed.[69] Potential problems and disadvantages that will require consideration in the further development of CFPD include the unknown effects of high dialysate flow rate on peritoneal cells, the unknown effects of exposure of PD fluid to hemodialysis membranes, the risks of peritoneal infection associated with the procedure (multiple connections), the potential for abdominal overdistension, and the cost of equipment and disposables. Moreover, UF control and a means of accurately balancing transperitoneal with external UF still constitute technical challenges.[69]

CFPD holds promise to become an attractive modality for daily home dialysis in the future, provided the remaining technical problems can be solved and the technology offered at an affordable price.

APPLICATION OF SOFTWARE PROGRAMS TO APD PRESCRIPTION

There are several possibilities for modifying dialysis prescription in APD in order to meet the needs of the individual patient. This represents an advantage compared to CAPD, for which the only possible adaptations of prescription consist of adding one more bag and increasing fill volume. Conversely, APD prescription is complicated by the multitude of prescription parameters that can be modified simultaneously. Kinetic modeling can facilitate the prescription process by enabling the clinician to estimate the consequences of different APD regimens to solute and fluid removal, taking into account the patient's individual clinical and biochemical conditions and peritoneal membrane transport characteristics.[70] Omitting the conventional "trial and error" approach, mathematical simulation of APD schedules is a time-saving way of optimizing dialysis prescription.

Several kinetic modeling software programs have been developed to cope with the underlying mathematical complexity, each based on specific membrane transport models and using data from a peritoneal function assessment for data entry. Two of these software programs have been validated and applied to pediatric patients.[21,26,71] The accuracy of these mathematical models is good with respect to predicting solute removal, whereas UF prediction is less satisfactory. The limited performance with respect to UF prediction may be related to the inability of kinetic modeling to account for changes in residual dialysate volumes, the marked day-to-day variability of UF, the large variability of daily fluid intake, and the confounding effects of residual diuresis in nonanuric patients. Moreover, mathematical modeling refers to perfect and virtually uneventful APD sessions (no alarms, no delay in the drain and fill phases).

In conclusion, computer-assisted kinetic models can be regarded as useful tools for the calculation and normalization of kinetic indices, and for mathematical simulation of the various APD regimens. They are helpful in selecting the optimal dose of dialysis for a given patient, but application control by direct measurement of actual solute clearances and UF rate remains mandatory.

ASSESSMENT OF PD ADEQUACY

Small-Solute Clearance and Dialysis Adequacy

The correlation between the delivered dialysis dose and the adequacy of dialysis treatment was first analyzed in hemodialysis patients by studies mainly based on urea kinetics evaluation. The resultant concept of "adequate" dialysis was originally created to define a minimum hemodialysis dose below which a clinically unacceptable rate of negative outcome might occur (patient hospitalization, morbidity, mortality). During the 1990s, the influence of small-solute clearance on the outcome of patients on PD was a major focus of interest.

Observational studies in adult CAPD patients suggested that better patient survival and lower morbidity were associated with higher clearances of small molecules, such as urea and creatinine.[72,73] As a consequence, small-solute clearance was considered the key criterion of PD adequacy in clinical practice guidelines such as those of the Kidney Disease Outcomes Quality Initiative (K/DOQI).[74] The year 2000 K/DOQI recommendations on the minimally adequate PD proposed the following targets of total (peritoneal plus renal) clearances.

- For adult patients on CAPD, a Kt/V urea of at least 2.0 per week and a total creatinine clearance (CrCl) of at least 60 liters/week/1.73 m^2 BSA for patients with high and high-average peritoneal membrane transport, and 50 liters/week/1.73 m^2 for those with low and low-average transport

- For adult patients on NIPD, a Kt/V urea of at least 2.2 and a total CrCl of at least 66 liters/week/1.73 m^2
- For adult patients on CCPD, a Kt/V urea of at least 2.1 and a total CrCl of at least 63 liters/week/1.73 m^2

Differences in adequacy targets of different PD regimens were based on the theoretical assumption that there is an 8% difference in clearance between CAPD and NIPD, and the required dose of CCPD would be intermediate between those for CAPD and NIPD. It should be noted that weekly dose recommendations for CAPD patients were reported as evidence based, whereas those for NIPD and CCPD patients were opinion based.

In the absence of definitive outcome data in pediatrics to indicate that any measure of dialysis adequacy is predictive of well-being, morbidity, or mortality, K/DOQI guidelines stated that by clinical judgment the target doses of PD for children should meet or exceed the adult ones. This would be particularly true for infants, who have high protein requirements.

Some of the assumptions included in the K/DOQI guideline have later been challenged, and some recommendations proved difficult to be fully applicable in clinical practice—especially among pediatric patients. For instance, it is generally accepted that a CrCl of more than 63 liters/week/1.73 m^2 is not easy to achieve, especially in anuric patients—even when exchange volume is maximized and the frequency of the exchanges is individualized and adjusted to the peritoneal membrane transport characteristics.[75-77] A discrepancy between urea and creatinine PD adequacy parameters is often noted,[78,79] especially in patients on APD and in children.[13]

- Urea clearance is for the most part related to dialysate volume and number of exchanges.
- CrCl is predominantly affected by the duration of the dwell time, and by the presence of residual renal function.
- Scaling of Kt/V to BW and CrCl to BSA may differently influence values obtained in the calculation of these parameters in infants and small children as a result of a higher ratio of BSA to weight.[13]

Neither urea clearance nor CrCl is the perfect index for predicting outcome in PD patients. However, they can be considered two potentially complementary measurements of dialysis dose.[79] An essential component of peritoneal adequacy measurement is the contribution of residual renal function (RRF) to small-solute clearance.

K/DOQI recommendations were based on the assumption that renal and peritoneal clearances were equivalent. Subsequently, several studies (including a reanalysis of the data from the Canusa study[80]) showed that RRF is a much stronger predictor of patient survival than peritoneal clearance. Accordingly, prospective randomized interventional studies[81,82] were unable to demonstrate any clear survival advantage with increases in peritoneal small-solute clearances. Speculative explanations for failure of increased PD dose for improving outcomes include the following:

- Higher IPP associated with larger exchange volume
- Failure to increase clearance of middle molecules
- Increased exposure to glucose-based dialysate[83]

In light of the results of interventional studies,[81,82] the minimally acceptable small-solute clearance has been lowered to a Kt/V urea of at least 1.7/week in the latest revision of the K/DOQI guidelines. In the presence of RRF, the contribution of renal and peritoneal clearance may be added for practical reasons. However, RRF should be monitored regularly in order to be able to adjust PD prescription in a timely fashion.

In summary, renal clearance and peritoneal clearance have different effects on patient survival—and preservation of RRF should be a primary objective in PD. Nephrotoxic drugs should be avoided, and the use of potentially renoprotective agents such as ACE inhibitors and angiotensin receptor blockers should be considered. Small-solute clearance targets, as defined by currently available guidelines, should be considered part of global patient care—and the failure to achieve them should not necessarily call for PD abandonment if all other aspects of patient care are successfully addressed by PD as currently performed.

Fluid Balance and Ultrafiltration

Continuous adjustment of the PD prescription to achieve and maintain fluid balance is extremely important. PD has been considered an optimal approach in reaching this therapeutic result because of its continuous nature, which avoids fluctuations of volume status and offers better homeostatic stability than intermittent therapies. Nevertheless, PD population surveys show a high prevalence of hypertension and cardiovascular mortality—and UF proved a significant predictor of survival in two recent studies on anuric adult patients.[60,84] The routine monitoring and evaluation of volume status are therefore essential in the process of attaining adequate PD, and can be performed according to the International Society for Peritoneal Dialysis recommendations on evaluation and management of UF problems in PD[85] (with some adaptations to the pediatric patient).

In the absence of validated and readily applicable indicators of volume status, the assessment of patient "target weight" mainly relies on clinical judgment. In clinical practice, the desirable target weight of a PD patient could be reasonably approximated to that weight at which the patient is edema free and normotensive (with minimal need for antihypertensive medications). Because fluctuations in patient weight secondary to growth and to changes of nutritional status may occur, reevaluation of target weight at regular intervals is mandatory. Factors affecting the maintenance of patient fluid balance and related recommended interventions are reported in Table 55-6. To increase the efficacy of PD prescription to attain an adequate UF rate, the following parameters should be considered:

- *Peritoneal membrane transport characteristics:* These affect net fluid removal at a given dwell time by determining the osmotic gradient time curve. A modification of the standard PET utilizing 4.25% dextrose solution can be employed to evaluate UF kinetics.[85,86]
- *Dwell time:* The osmotic gradient dissipates over time, and continued lymphatic absorption occurs at an almost constant rate.
- *PD solution tonicity:* An increase of dextrose tonicity is associated with an increase in UF.

These parameters are interrelated and should be considered jointly. For instance, low dialysate dextrose concentration and prolonged dwell time will inevitably lead to inadequate fluid

TABLE 55-6 Factors Affecting the Maintenance of Patient Fluid Balance, and Related Recommended Interventions

Factor Influencing Fluid Balance	Recommended Intervention
• Salt and water intake	• Dietary counseling
• Amount of residual diuresis	• Protection of RRF • Use of loop diuretics
• Peritoneal transport characteristics	• Peritoneal equilibration tests (basal + follow-up)
• PD prescription	• Tailoring on: • Peritoneal function • Patient needs
• Malfunction of PD catheter	• PD prescription adaptation • Correction of malfunction
• Compliance to PD prescription	• Patient/partner education

TABLE 55-7 Strategies for Improving Ultrafiltration Rate

Short Dwells	Long Dwells
• Increase: • Number of cycles • Glucose concentration • Overall treatment time • Fill volume	• Utilize icodextrin solution • Replace single long exchange with two exchanges • Increase glucose concentration

removal in high-transport patients.[85] Dextrose solutions are indicated for short dwells, whereas for the nighttime dwell in CAPD and the daytime dwell in APD ICO may be more appropriate. Icodextrin is also effective in maintaining adequate UF rate during peritonitis episodes.[87]

APD solution with a neutral pH combined with a reduced lactate concentration, partially replaced by bicarbonate, significantly increased UF in a group of adult PD patients—conceivably by causing less peritoneal vasodilation than conventional acidic lactate-based PD solutions.[88] In practice, strategies for improving UF rate might be summarized as outlined in Table 55-7.[89] A potentially useful rule of thumb in defining the optimal dwell duration in children on APD according to peritoneal transport characteristics is the accelerated peritoneal examination (APEX) time during a PET. This is the time point at which the D/P urea and the D/D0 glucose equilibration curves cross.[62] APD cycle length should be equivalent to the APEX time.

Clearance of Middle Molecules

One of the possible explanations for the lacking effect of increased dialysis dose on survival may be the failure to improve clearance of middle molecules, ranging from 300 to 5000 Da in molecular weight.[83] Small-solute and middle-molecule clearances respond differently to changes in PD prescription. Whereas the former is mainly determined by the frequency and volume of dialysate dwell, the latter depends more on the duration of contact of the peritoneum with dialysate.[90,91]

Removal of middle molecules and low-molecular-weight proteins, such as β_2-microglobulin and leptin, mainly depends on RRF.[92,93] Moreover, an increase of the restriction coefficient for macromolecules was reported in relation to time on PD—which is associated with an increased size selectivity and a reduced peritoneal permeability for higher-molecular-weight solutes.[23] Hence, particular attention should be paid to middle-molecule clearance—especially in children on NIPD and as RRF is declining. Increased β_2-microglobulin and leptin clearance have been reported in patients receiving a long dwell with ICO.[94]

Clinical Correlates of PD Adequacy in Pediatric Patients

Large-scale prospective outcome studies on PD patients are lacking owing to the small number of patients per center, and to the relatively short period of time on PD prior to renal transplantation. Nevertheless, some pediatric studies have effectively addressed the issue of the correlation between PD dose and selected clinical aspects.

Growth is a potentially valuable outcome measure specific to pediatrics. Multivariate analysis of the data of a multicenter study showed a weak positive correlation of height standard deviation score (SDS) with dialytic creatinine clearance, and a negative correlation with peritoneal transport status (i.e., children with high transport on PET had a lower change in height SDS).[95] Hölttä and colleagues[75] reported accelerated height velocity in 62% of the patients who met or exceeded DOQI target clearances. Chadha and colleagues[96] presented data showing that growth correlates with renal solute clearance, but not with peritoneal clearance. Similar to adult studies, these data may suggest that peritoneal and residual renal small-solute clearances are not equivalent.

Nutrition is an issue of particular interest in pediatric PD because it can significantly affect growth and development of children. Dietary protein intake is inconsistently correlated with delivered Kt/V urea.[97-99] However, the relationship between Kt/V urea and the normalized protein equivalent of nitrogen appearance (nPNA) has often been criticized as merely being the result of mathematical coupling. Finally, a higher Kt/V was associated with a lower serum albumin level in children.[100] Pediatric nutrition guidelines have been developed by DOQI.[101]

A study in 18 children on PD showed that increasing weekly Kt/V and CrCl was positively correlated with cardiac function and inversely with left ventricular mass.[102]

Solute Removal Index

An alternative measure of PD dose, other than Kt/V urea and CrCl, may be represented by the solute removal index (SRI)—which normalizes removal to the solute content of the body at the beginning of treatment so that the ratio between net urea removal and predialysis urea body pool is calculated. SRI enables one to compare different dialytic treatments, or the results of the same treatment in patients differing in body size.[103]

In conclusion, in children (even more than in adult patients) adequacy of PD treatment is far from being defined by targets of solute and fluid removal. Clinical assessment of

TABLE 55-8 Clinical Assessment of PD Treatment Adequacy in Pediatric Patients

- Clinical and laboratory results
- Peritoneal and renal clearances
- Hydration status
- Nutritional status
- Dietary intake of energy, proteins, salts, and trace elements
- Electrolyte and acid/base balance
- Calcium phosphate homeostasis
- Control of anemia
- Blood pressure control
- Growth and mental development
- Level of psychosocial rehabilitation

adequacy of PD treatment in pediatric patients should comprehensively take into consideration a series of clinical, metabolic, and psychosocial aspects (summarized in Table 55-8). In any case, the expected benefit of increasing PD dose should be balanced against its potential negative effect on a patient's lifestyle.

SCHEDULE OF PD TREATMENT MONITORING

Regular assessment of the delivered dialysis dose can be performed following the NKF-DOQI clinical practice guidelines,[74] with some adaptations to specific problems of childhood. This assessment is fundamentally based on direct measurement of dialytic and renal clearance through a 24-hour collection of dialysate and urine.[89] For practical reasons, peritoneal and renal clearance can be added to determine total clearance—even if they have a different impact on a patient's outcome. All dialysate discharged during 24 hours should be accurately collected (including daytime exchange, if present), total volume precisely measured, and a sample obtained after mixing effluent thoroughly.

The same attention should be paid in performing a complete 24-hour urine collection. Urine collection requires a preservative, such as thymol, to be added to the collection or refrigeration to inhibit the growth of bacteria that can degrade urea. Dialysate does not require refrigeration or preservative.

Urea clearance is usually expressed as Kt/V urea and is normalized for urea distribution volume, which is assumed equal to total body water (TBW). Gold-standard isotope dilution techniques for determining TBW are laborious and costly and are hence not applicable in clinical practice. Therefore, anthropometric prediction equations based on height and weight are commonly used to estimate TBW. Because equations derived from healthy children[104] systematically overpredicted TBW and were less precise in children on PD, a new set of anthropometric TBW prediction equations validated in this patient population has been developed.[105]

- Boys: $TBW = 0.10 \times (HtWt)^{0.68} - 0.37 \times \text{weight}$
- Girls: $TBW = 0.14 \times (HtWt)^{0.65} - 0.35 \times \text{weight}$

Here, HtWt represents the new anthropometric parameter "height times weight," which correlates linearly with TBW when both values are log transformed. Weekly peritoneal Kt/V urea can be calculated with the following formula:[89]

$$(\text{24-hour D/P urea} \times \text{24-hour dialysate volume} \times 7) : V,$$

where D/P represents the dialysate-to-plasma concentration ratio and V is volume. In patients with RRF, renal Kt/V corresponds to:

$$(\text{ml/min urea clearance} \times 1440\ \text{min/day} \times 7) : (1000\ \text{ml} \times V)$$

CrCl calculation is normalized to BSA, which can be calculated from weight and height by use of the Haycock formula.[106]

$$\text{BSA } (m^2) = (\text{weight, kg})^{0.5378} \times (\text{height, cm})^{0.3964} \times 0.024265$$

This can also be calculated via the Gehan and George formula.[107]

$$\text{BSA } (m^2) = 0.0235 \times (\text{height, cm})^{0.42246} \times (\text{weight, kg})^{0.51456}$$

The following formula can be employed to calculate dialytic CrCl per week.[89]

$$(\text{24-hour D/P Cr} \times \text{24-hour dialysate volume} \times 7 \times 1.73\ m^2) : \text{BSA } (m^2)$$

Residual renal clearance is better expressed as the average of CrCl and urea clearance, each of which can be calculated by the following standard formula.

$$\text{Solute clearance (ml/min)} = (\text{24-hour urine volume in ml} \times \text{urine solute concentration}) : (1440\ \text{min/day} \times \text{serum solute concentration})$$

This calculation is then normalized to a patient's BSA. A calculator program for pediatric dialytic and renal small solute clearances is available at www.pedpd.org, the website of the International Pediatric PD Network (IPPN).

PD dose assessment should be coupled with an evaluation of nutritional status, including anthropometric measurements (skin fold thickness, mid-arm circumference), a 3-day dietary record (to be evaluated by a renal dietitian), and the determination of normalized protein equivalent of nitrogen appearance nPNA—taking dialysate protein losses into account. Body composition of children on PD can be evaluated by means of bioelectric impedance analysis (BIA). Specific equations for predicting free fat mass (FFM) and TBW from BIA data have been established:[108]

$$\text{FFM [kg]} = 0.65 \times (\text{height}^2/\text{impedance}) [\text{ohms/cm}^2] + 0.68 \times \text{age (years)} + 0.15$$

$$\text{TBW [liter]} = 0.144 \times (\text{impedance/height}^2) [\text{ohms/cm}^2] + 40 \times \text{weight [kg]} + 1.99$$

The first measurement of PD dose can be obtained as early as 1 week after the patient is stabilized on a defined PD prescription, when a PET can also be performed. Subsequently, PD dose measurements can be completed every 4 months, and in the event of any significant change in clinical status and/or in the amount of residual diuresis. PET can be repeated every 12 months, or earlier in case of unexpected changes in delivered PD dose or if any clinical condition occurs that could permanently affect the peritoneal transport properties (e.g., recurrent or persistent peritonitis). Routine

TABLE 55-9 **Schedule of Routine Outcome Evaluations in Pediatric Patients on Stable Chronic PD**

Parameters to Be Evaluated	Frequency
• Growth • Weight gain • Head circumference (in infants) • Blood pressure • Serum creatinine and urea • Serum electrolytes • Acid/base status • Hemoglobin/hematocrit • Serum albumin • Record of daily urine volume and UF	Monthly
• Serum ferritin • Serum iron • Total iron binding capacity	Every 2 months
• Alkaline phosphatase • Intact parathyroid hormone	Every 3 months
• CrCl and Kt/V urea from 24-hour dialysate and urine collection	Every 4 months
• Neurodevelopment assessment	Every 6 months
• Ambulatory blood pressure monitoring • Echocardiography • Hand and wrist x-ray for bone age	Every 12 months

TABLE 55-10 **Signs and Symptoms Prompting a Timely Assessment of Dialysis Adequacy and Prescription**

- Clinical manifestations of overt uremia (uremic pericarditis, pleuritis)
- Clinical and/or biochemical signs of malnutrition
- Arterial hypertension
- Hyperkalemic episodes
- Hyperphosphatemia (excessive serum calcium x phosphate product)
- Kt/V urea and/or CrCl below minimal recommended targets
- Clues of patient/family noncompliance

outcome evaluations in pediatric patients on chronic PD can be organized as indicated in Table 55-9.[89]

In the course of PD treatment, attention should be paid by parents, dialysis nurses, and physicians to potential manifestations of inadequate dialysis. In practice, the signs and/or symptoms that should be punctually recorded and evaluated are listed in Table 55-10:

Two fundamental concepts should be stressed once again:

- Numerical targets of small-solute removal should be interpreted cautiously and in the context of patient clinical assessment. Failure to reach these targets should be regarded as a warning sign, leading to careful reevaluation of each constituent of the therapeutic program.
- Contribution of RRF to the adequacy of PD treatment is extremely important and tends to deteriorate with time on chronic dialysis, albeit at a slower rate in PD than in HD patients.[109,110] Therefore, RRF should be regularly measured—although this may be difficult to do accurately in children, requiring good cooperation by caregivers. While RRF is declining, adaptation of PD prescription by increasing the dialysis component should be performed in a timely manner to anticipate the occurrence of signs and/or symptoms of inadequate treatment.

METHODS OF MONITORING THE MECHANICS OF APD AND PATIENT COMPLIANCE

Machines for APD (Cyclers)

Over the last 10 to 15 years, APD has experienced a rapid evolution closely linked to the development of new automatic machines.[111] Because APD is a home-based therapy performed by the patient or his or her caregiver, cyclers for APD should fulfill the following basic requirements.

- Small size, light in weight, and easy portability (component miniaturization)
- Simple interface with unequivocal messages (touch screen)
- Safe, accurate, and reliable functioning

Access to the prescription and control level of the cycler is usually protected by a password known only by authorized personnel, whereas data of the ongoing treatment can be easily visualized on the display of the cycler. The following technology advances have been recently incorporated in APD cyclers.

- Pressure monitors for assessing IPP
- Online warming of dialysate
- Gravity-assisted roller or diaphragm pumps for dialysate infusion and drainage
- Cassette receptacle for the tubing set to simplify the procedure and to minimize the risk of operator error and contamination
- Bar code readers for matching the prescription with the solution selected by the patient
- Automated connecting devices for facilitating the connection between the bags and the tubing manifold
- Ad hoc connectors for performing one exchange of dialysate during the day

In particular, cyclers to be used for treatment of children should have a specific pediatric mode designed to:

- Accurately deliver even small volumes of dialysate
- Have a low recirculation volume for low-fill-volume PD regimens
- Allow dialysate drainage at low flow rates (physiological for infants and small children) without alarming
- Allow programming of individualized minimum drain volume and minimum drain time for each patient according to PD schedule and peritoneal catheter function

In more general terms, future cyclers for APD should be designed not only to individualize PD prescription but to:

- Measure delivered dialysis dose and UF
- Monitor patient compliance with the prescribed therapy
- Detect catheter malfunction
- Detect excessive increases in IPP

As a future goal, the ideal APD cycler should not only be able to perform all treatment schedules in an accurate and safe way but to optimize the performance of the selected PD regimen.[111] The cycler could use the recorded information of the patient response to a given treatment schedule to suggest, or even automatically attempt, an improved regimen. The following are examples.

- Dialysate inflow and outflow time could be adjusted on the basis of the flow rate that has been registered during the previous exchange.
- Online detection of UF related to fluid osmolarity, dwell time, and fill volume could serve as automatic feedback for PD fluid composition in the next cycle. Bedside production of dialysis solution could individualize PD treatment with respect to osmotic agent and calcium and to buffer and sodium content.[68,111]

Registration and Transmission of PD Treatment Data

The introduction of microchips and computer technology in the new APD cyclers has led to the possibility of capturing on an electronic device the patient's prescription, medical history, and treatment events. This system provides information on the home dialysis PD treatment and serves a means of monitoring patient compliance, thus creating a database of therapy information. The cycler system usually includes a data card that can store up to 60 to 90 days of actual treatment data. Data stored in the memory card can be downloaded when the patient comes to the dialysis unit, or retrieved via modem as often as needed.

For instance, the pattern of the peritoneal catheter's flow during each treatment cycle can be evaluated with the help of graphs and charts (Figure 55-6)—and any catheter malfunction can be detected (even if it has not yet been the cause of cycler alarms or of clinical symptoms). Thus, PD prescription can be adapted to the drainage profile of each individual patient/catheter in order to minimize fill and drain dead times. An example of the application of this adaptation process is represented by optimization of tidal volume to individual drainage profile, thus eliminating the flow rate drop occurring beyond the breakpoint.[65,66]

The recording of a PD session may also reveal an excessive incidence of cycler alarms during the nightly treatment, resulting in sleep deprivation and a loss of quality of life for patients and parents.[112] Tube kinking and catheter malfunction are the more frequent causes of drain alarms. In some cases, unsuitable setting of alarm limits (such as leaving the default setting) may generate the occurrence of an excessive number of useless and disturbing alarms.

Through comparison of the prescribed versus the actually delivered therapy, the system is able to identify if a patient has made changes in the prescribed dialysis schedule on his/her initiative (Table 55-11). Noncompliance is an important obstacle to achieving an adequate dialysis dose, and is a significant cause of morbidity, patient hospitalization, and technique failure.[112-114] Several methods of assessing patient adherence to PD prescription have been proposed, based on:

- Comparison of measured versus predicted creatinine excretion[113]
- Home visits to check dialysis solution supply inventories[115]
- Patient self-report confidential questionnaires[116]
- Comparison of self-reports of compliance with the rate of predicted versus measured Kt/V urea and CrCl[117]

However, none of these methods provides a complete assessment of noncompliance in patients on home PD—and they should be used in an integrated way. On the other hand, recording and transmitting PD session data through an electronic device on a regular basis:

- represent an objective method of assessing patient compliance
- can enhance patient adherence to PD prescription because the awareness of the recording makes the patient feel more confident about treatment control and renders doctor/patient communication more explicit
- can enhance dialysis staff ability to understand the reasons for inadequate depuration, and accordingly change PD prescription

Cycler data cards can be easily reprogrammed by the physician or the dialysis nurse to address patient prescription changes. Therefore, the use of these electronic devices eliminates the need for patients to program and manually record APD treatment data—thus shortening training time and simplifying data collection and management by the team of the dialysis unit.

The possibility of a modem connection of the home cycler and the dialysis unit makes teledialysis possible. APD treatment data can be visualized and monitored by the staff in the dialysis unit online (while the treatment is being administered at a patient's home) or offline in the morning after the end of the nighttime APD session. Alternatively, data are transferred through the modem connection from the cycler memory card to the personal computer of the dialysis unit on a regular basis (e.g., every 7 to 10 days)—or when there is any problem observed by the patient or the caregiver or any doubt about the cycler or peritoneal catheter function.

Information stored in the file of each patient is examined and evaluated by the physician and dialysis nurse according to a scheduled program. Data can be organized in charts and graphs, and elaborated statistically. Modem connection allows for early detection of therapy problems and may reduce the feeling of isolation and detachment the patient and family may experience in the course of long-term home PD—especially if they live far from the dialysis center.

The results reported on the use of telemedicine in a pediatric PD program[112] (as well as our unpublished personal experience) show that "telePD" allows one to identify and successfully address clinical and psychosocial problems, as well as to increase patient and family satisfaction with home PD treatment. Whether telePD is able to significantly reduce the need for patient hospitalization or the incidence of technique failure in a population of home APD children should be evaluated in large-scale studies. As a further evaluation,

TABLE 55-11 Most Common Changes Made in APD Schedule by Noncompliant Patients and/or Caregivers

Noncompliant patient/caregiver may:
• Skip treatment cycles
• Shorten treatment time
• Manually change treatment parameters
• Bypass therapy phases or cycles
• Reduce fill volume by performing manual drains

the teledialysis system can be integrated by a digital camera and an ISDN line to provide private videoconferencing and video capture of images. Thus, the dialysis and exit-site care procedures can be followed by the dialysis center server or by the physician's personal computer.

APPROACH FOR INCREASING PATIENT COMPLIANCE WITH PD PRESCRIPTION

Interventions aimed at increasing adherence to the prescribed PD schedule should be considered an essential component of the prescription process and a key factor in achieving the expected therapeutic results. They are targeted to patient, family, and dialysis staff, and should be accomplished through a comprehensive structured program.

Patient- and family-targeted interventions are mainly based on active involvement by patient and family in the choice of dialysis modality and on their education in performing home dialysis treatment. Patient selection should include the action points reported in Table 55-12. Patient and family preparation for home PD[118] should:

- Start well before dialysis initiation
- Involve a multidisciplinary team: nephrologist, renal nurse, renal dietitian, psychologist, social worker, school teacher, play staff
- Make use of appropriate written information and other teaching aids
- Encourage contacts with similar-aged children on home dialysis
- Include a home visit and a liaison with the nursery/school/college and the family doctor

Training for home PD procedures should involve two family members and may be completed in the home environment. Ultimate goals of patient and family education are:

- To achieve an adequate level of knowledge, understanding, and participation in PD modality and in the process of PD prescription
- To reduce patient and family anxiety and stress by increasing awareness of the disease process and treatment options
- To convince the patient and family of the appropriateness and beneficial effects of the prescribed treatment, and of the fact that compliance with prescription will improve outcome

Once PD treatment has started, regular telephone contact and support for the family should be planned. Moreover, acquired knowledge and skills of performing home PD should be assessed at regular intervals. Interventions targeted at dialysis staff in addressing the issue of patient compliance should enhance staff ability to:

- Individualize PD prescription and evaluate its results
- Explain the reasons for prescription changes
- Manage treatment complications as much as possible on an outpatient basis
- Test and recognize signs of patient noncompliance

Dialysis staff education about compliance should be monitored and regularly updated.

TABLE 55-12 Action Points of Patient/Family Selection for Home PD Treatment

- Early patient/family referral to dialysis staff
- Evaluation of patient's clinical needs and patient and family lifestyle
- Structured, unbiased information on modalities
- Evaluation of physical and psychological ability of the caregiver(s) to perform dialysis tasks
- Assessment of patient home environment

CONCLUSIONS

A major issue in the field of pediatric PD treatment is represented by that of the individualization of prescription in a patient population in which body size, dietary intake, metabolic needs, growth rate, risk of clinical and technical complications, and psychosocial rehabilitation expectancy are extremely variable. The wide-ranging treatment options offered by APD provide the possibility of tailoring the treatment schedule to the individual patient's needs and requests. However, the prescription process requires a good and updated knowledge of:

- The pathophysiology of peritoneal membrane structure and function
- Existing clinical practice guidelines and recognized treatment standards
- APD solutions, machines, and technical devices
- Available prescription tools (software programs based on kinetic models)

The biocompatibility of PD solutions and material should be improved in order to:

- Optimize the efficiency of exchanges in terms of solute and fluid removal
- Reduce the incidence of treatment reactions and complications
- Achieve long-term preservation of peritoneal membrane function

Prospective randomized trials of dialysis adequacy and observational studies in adult patients have confirmed the strong association between the presence of RRF and a reduction of mortality. Moreover, the benefit from RRF exceeds the clearance of small solutes and fluid removal and includes clearance of middle molecules and small proteins; production of erythropoietin; activation of vitamin D_3, and other incompletely defined metabolic functions. Therefore, regular evaluation and careful preservation of RRF represent key factors in the success of PD treatment.

Regular assessment of the results of a prescribed PD schedule should be performed in accordance with a well-structured program, taking into account all parameters involved in the definition of adequacy of dialysis treatment in childhood (not simply numerical targets of small-solute depuration). From this point of view, outcome-based measures of dialysis adequacy need to be developed in children because prospective randomized pediatric dialysis patient outcome trials are lacking.

At the same time, outcome studies reaching cohort sizes similar to those in adult patient trials are structurally impossible to perform in the pediatric field owing to small patient numbers and short dialysis times prior to kidney transplantation. Nevertheless, there is enough clinical and research experience and knowledge in the pediatric PD scientific literature to allow the achievement of a satisfactory level of treatment adequacy by using the available parameters and tools in an integrated fashion.

Between the extremes of a minimally effective PD dose (the amount of dialysis below which there is an increase in morbidity and mortality) and the maximal effective dose (the dose above which there are no further benefits) for each child on PD we should aim to define a patient's optimal PD dose; that is, the amount of dialysis above which the expected additional benefit does not justify the increase of the treatment-associated burden on patient and family.

ACKNOWLEDGMENT

The authors wish to thank Daniela Accerbis for manuscript preparation.

REFERENCES

1. Nolph KD, Twardowski ZJ: The peritoneal dialysis system. In KD Nolph (ed.), *Peritoneal dialysis.* Dordrecht: Martinus Nijhof 1985:23.
2. Gotloib L, Shostak A, Bar-Sella P, Eiali V: Fenestrated capillaries in human parietal and rabbit diaphragmatic peritoneum, *Nephron* 41:200-2, 1985.
3. Pecoits-Filho R: The peritoneal cavity: A room with a view to the endothelium, *Perit Dial Int* 25:432-34, 2005.
4. Krediet RT, Lindholm B, Rippe B: Pathophysiology of peritoneal membrane failure, *Perit Dial Int* 20(4):22-42, 2000.
5. Flessner M, Henegar J, Bigler S, Genous L: Is the peritoneum a significant barrier in peritoneal dialysis? *Perit Dial Int* 23:542-49, 2003.
6. Krediet RT: The physiology of peritoneal transport and ultrafiltration. In R Gokal, R Khanna, RT Krediet, K Nolph (eds.), *Textbook of peritoneal dialysis.* Dordrecht, The Netherlands: Kluwer Academic Publishers 2000:135-73.
7. Haraldsson B: Assessing the individual peritoneal dialysis capacities of individual patients: A clinical tool based on the three pore model, *Kidney Int* 47:1187-98, 1995.
8. Fischbach M, Haraldsson B: Dynamic changes of total pore area available for peritoneal exchange in children, *J Am Soc Nephrol* 12:1524-29, 2001.
9. Fischbach M, Terzic J, Chauvé S, Laugel V, Muller A, Haraldsson B: Effect of peritoneal dialysis fluid composition on peritoneal area available for exchange in children, *Nephrol Dial Transplant* 19:925-32, 2004.
10. Fischbach M, Terzic J, Laugel V, Escande B, Dangelser C, Helmstetter A: Measurement of hydrostatic intraperitoneal pressure: A useful tool for the improvement of dialysis dose prescription, *Pediatr Nephrol* 18:976-80, 2003.
11. Ahmad S: Peritoneal dialysis. In S Ahmad (ed.), *Manual of clinical dialysis.* London: Science Press 1999:65-68.
12. Mactier RA, Khanna R, Moore H, Russ J, Nolph K, Groshong T: Kinetics of peritoneal dialysis in children: Role of lymphatics, *Kidney Int* 34:82-88, 1998.
13. Fischbach M, Stefanidis CJ, Watson AR: Guidelines by an ad hoc European committee on adequacy of the pediatric peritoneal dialysis prescription, *Nephrol Dial Transplant* 17:380-85, 2002.
14. Morgenstern B: Peritoneal dialysis and prescription monitoring. In BA Warady, FS Schaefer, RN Fine, SR Alexander (eds.), *Pediatric dialysis.* Dordrecht, The Netherlands: Kluwer Academic Publishers 2004:147-61.
15. Morgenstern BZ: Peritoneal equilibration in children, *Perit Dial Int* 16(1):532-39, 1996.
16. Warady BA, Alexander SR, Hossli S Vonesh E, Geary D, Watkins S, et al: Peritoneal membrane transport function in children receiving long-term dialysis, *J Am Soc Nephrol* 7:2385-91, 1996.
17. Schaefer F, Langebeck D, Heckert KH, Scharer K, Mehls O: Evaluation of peritoneal solute transfer by the peritoneal equilibration test in children. In R Khanna, KD Nolph, B Prowant, ZJ Twardowski, D Oreopoulos (eds.), *Advances in peritoneal dialysis.* Seattle: Toronto Press 1992:410-15.
18. Warady BA, Alexander SR, Hossli S, Vonesh E, Geary D, Kohaut E: The relationship between intraperitoneal volume and solute transport in pediatric patients, *J Am Soc Nephrol* 5:1935-39, 1995.
19. Twardowski ZJ, Nolph KD, Khanna R, Prowant BF, Ryan LP, Moore HL: Peritoneal equilibration test, *Perit Dial Bull* 7:138-47, 1987.
20. Pride ET, Gustafson J, Graham A, Spoinhour L, Mauck V, Brown P, et al: Comparison of a 2.5% and a 4.25% dextrose peritoneal equilibration test, *Perit Dial Int* 22:365-70, 2002.
21. Verrina E, Amici G, Perfumo F, Trivelli A, Canepa A, Gusmano R: The use of PD Adequest mathematical model in pediatric patients on chronic peritoneal dialysis, *Perit Dial Int* 18:322-28, 1998.
22. Reddingius RE; Schröder CH, Willems JL, Lelivelt M, Kohler BEM, Krediet RT, Monnens LAH: Measurement of peritoneal fluid handling in children on continuous ambulatory peritoneal dialysis using dextran 70, *Nephrol Dial Transplant* 10:866-70, 1995.
23. Bouts AHM, Davin JC, Groothoff JW, Ploos van Amstel S, Zweers MM, Krediet RT: Standard peritoneal permeability analysis in children, *J Am Soc Nephrol* 11:943-50, 2000.
24. Rippe B, Stelin G: Simulations of peritoneal solute transport during CAPD: Application of two-pore formalism, *Kidney Int* 35:1234-44, 1989.
25. Rippe B, Stelin G, Haraldsson B: Computer simulation of peritoneal fluid transport in CAPD, *Kidney Int* 40:315-25, 1991.
26. Schaefer F, Haraldsson B, Haas S, Simkova E, Feber J, Mehls O: Estimation of peritoneal mass transport by three-pore model in children, *Kidney Int* 54:1372-79, 1998.
27. Fischbach M, Terzic J, Menouer S, Haraldsson B: Optimal volume prescription for children on peritoneal dialysis, *Perit Dial Int* 20:603-06, 2000.
28. Kohaut EC, Waldo FB, Brienfeld M: The effects of changes in dialysate volume on glucose and urea equilibration, *Perit Dial Int* 14:236-39, 1994.
29. Durand P-Y, Chanliau J, Gamberoni J, Hestin D, Kessler M: Measurement of hydrostatic intraperitoneal pressure: A necessary routine test in peritoneal dialysis, *Perit Dial Int* 16(1):S84-S87, 1996.
30. Fischbach M, Terzic J, Becmeur F, Lahlou A, Desprez P, Battouche D: Relationship between intraperitoneal hydrostatic pressure and dialysate volume in children on PD, *Adv Perit Dial* 12:330-34, 1996.
31. Fischbach M, Terzic J, Provot E, Weiss L, Bergere V, Menouer S, et al: Intraperitoneal pressure in children: Fill-volume related and impacted by body mass index, *Perit Dial Int* 23:391-94, 2003.
32. Verrina E, Perfumo F: Technical aspects of the peritoneal dialysis procedure. In BA Warady, FS Schaefer, RN Fine, SR Alexander (eds.), *Pediatric dialysis.* Dordrecht, The Netherlands: Kluwer Academic Publishers 2004:113-34.
33. Schröder CH: The choice of dialysis solutions in pediatric chronic peritoneal dialysis: Guidelines by an ad hoc European Committee, *Perit Dial Int* 21:568-74, 2001.
34. Holmes CJ, Shockley TR: Strategies to reduce glucose exposure in peritoneal dialysis, *Perit Dial Int* 20:S37-S41, 2000.
35. Sitter T, Sauter M: Impact of glucose in peritoneal dialysis: Saint or sinner? *Perit Dial Int* 25:415-25, 2005.
36. Williams JD, Topley N, Craig KJ, Mackenzic RK, Pischetsrieder M, Lage C, et al: The Euro-Balance Trial: The effect of a new biocompatible peritoneal dialysis fluid (balance) on the peritoneal membrane, *Kidney Int* 66:408-18, 2004.

37. Posthuma N, ter Wee PM, Donker AJM, Oe PL, Peers EM, Verbrugh HA: Assessment of the effectiveness, safety, and biocompatibility of icodextrin in automated peritoneal dialysis, *Perit Dial Int* 20(2):S106-S113, 2000.
38. De Boer AW, Schröder CH, Van Vliet R, Willems JL, Monnens LAH: Clinical experience with icodextrin in children: Ultrafiltration profiles and metabolism, *Pediatr Nephrol* 15:21-24, 2000.
39. Rusthoven E, Krediet RT, Willems HL, Monnens LAH, Schröder CH: Peritoneal transport characteristics with glucose polymer-based dialysis fluid in children, *J Am Soc Nephrol* 15:2940-47, 2004.
40. Verrina E, Amici G, Perfumo F, Trivelli A: Evaluation of icodextrin absorption and ultrafiltration (UF) curve over a long day dwell in children on continuous cycling peritoneal dialysis, *Perit Dial Int* 21(1):S93, 2001.
41. Rusthoven E, Krediet RT, Willems HL, Monnens LA, Schröder CH: Sodium sieving in children, *Perit Dial Int* 25(3):S141-S142, 2005.
42. Martis L, Patel M, Giertych J, Mongoven J, Taminne M, Perrier MA, et al: Aseptic peritonitis due to peptidoglycan contamination of pharmacopoeia standard dialysis solution, *Lancet* 365(9459):588-94, 2005.
43. Cooker LA, Holmes CJ, Hoff CM: Biocompatibility of icodextrin, *Kidney Int* 62(81):S34-S45, 2002.
44. Gotloib L, Wajsbrot V, Shostak A: Osmotic agents hamper mesothelial repopulation as seen in the doughnut in vivo model, *Perit Dial Int* 25(3):S26-S30, 2005.
45. Canepa A, Perfumo F, Carrea A, Giallongo F, Verrina E, Cantalupi A, et al: Long-term effect of amino-acid dialysis solution in children on continuous ambulatory peritoneal dialysis, *Pediatr Nephrol* 5(2):215-19, 1991.
46. Canepa A, Carrea A, Menoni S, Verrina E, Trivelli A, Gusmano R, et al: Acute effects of simultaneous intraperitoneal infusion of glucose and amino acids, *Kidney Int* 59:1967-73, 2001.
47. Canepa A, Verrina E, Perfumo F, Carrea A, Menoni S, Delucchi P, et al: Value of intraperitoneal amino acids in children treated with chronic peritoneal dialysis, *Perit Dial Int* 19(2):S435-S440, 1999.
48. Garibotto G, Sofia A, Canepa A, Saffioti S, Sacco P, Sala MR, et al: Acute effects of peritoneal dialysis with dialysate containing dextrose or dextrose and amino acids on muscle protein turnover in patients on chronic renal failure, *J Am Soc Nephrol* 12:557-67, 2001.
49. Witowski J, Jorres A: Effects of peritoneal dialysis solutions on the peritoneal membrane: Clinical consequences, *Perit Dial Int* 25(3): S31-S33, 2005.
50. Jones S, Holmes CJ, Krediet RT, Mackenzie R, Faict D, Tranaeus A, et al: Bicarbonate/lactate-based peritoneal dialysis solution increases cancer antigen 125 and decreases hyaluronic acid levels, *Kidney Int* 59:1529-38, 2001.
51. Jones S, Holmes CJ, Mackenzie R, Stead R, Coles GA, Williams JD, et al: Continuous dialysis with bicarbonate/lactate-buffered peritoneal dialysis fluids results in a long-term improvement in ex vivo peritoneal macrophage function, *J Am Soc Nephrol* 13:S97-S103, 2002.
52. Haas S, Schmitt CP, Arbeiter K, Bonzel KE, Fischbach M, John U, et al: Improved acidosis correction and recovery of mesothelial cells mass with neutral–pH bicarbonate dialysis solution among children undergoing automated peritoneal dialysis, *J Am Soc Nephrol* 14:2632-38, 2003.
53. Fusshoeller A, Plail M, Grabensee B, Plum J: Biocompatibility pattern of a bicarbonate/lactate-buffered peritoneal dialysis fluid in APD: A prospective, randomized study, *Nephrol Dial Transplant* 19:2101-06, 2004.
54. Schmitt CP, Haraldsson B, Doetschmann R, Zimmering M, Greiner C, Böswald M, et al: Effects of pH-neutral, bicarbonate-buffered dialysis fluid on peritoneal transport in children, *Kidney Int* 61:1527-36, 2002.
55. Brunkhorst RR: Individualized PD prescription: APD versus CAPD, *Perit Dial Int* 25(3):S92-S94, 2005.
56. Fine RN, Ho M: The role of APD in the management of pediatric patients: A report of the North American Pediatric Renal Transplant Cooperative Study, *Seminars in Dialysis* 15(6):427-29, 2002.
57. Verrina E, Edefonti A, Gianoglio B, Rinaldi S, Sorino P, Zacchello G, et al: A multicenter experience on patient and technique survival in children on chronic dialysis, *Pediatr Nephrol* 19:82-90, 2004.
58. Mujais S, Nolph K, Gokal R, Blake P, Burkart J, Coles G, et al: Evaluation and management of ultrafiltration problems in peritoneal dialysis, *Perit Dial Int* 20(4):S5-S21, 2000.
59. Abu-Alfa AK, Burkart J, Piraino B, Pullian J, Mujais S: Approach to fluid management in peritoneal dialysis: A practical algorithm, *Kidney Int* 62(81):S8-S16, 2002.
60. Jansen MAM, Termorshuizen F, Korevaar JC, Dekker FW, Boeschoten E, Krediet RT: Predictors of survival in anuric peritoneal dialysis patients, *Kidney Int* 68:1199-205, 2005.
61. Freida P, Issad B: Continuous cyclic peritoneal dialysis prescription and power. In C Ronco, G Amici, M Feriani, G Virga (eds), *Automated peritoneal dialysis*. Basel: Karger 1999:99-108.
62. Fischbach M, Lahlou A, Eyer D, Desprez P, Geisert J: Determination of individual ultrafiltration time (APEX) and purification phosphate time by peritoneal equilibration test: Application to individual peritoneal dialysis modality prescription in children, *Perit Dial Int* 16(1):S557-S560, 1996.
63. Edefonti A, Consalvo G, Picca M, Giani M, Damiani B, Ghio L, et al: Dialysis delivery in children in nightly intermittent and tidal peritoneal dialysis, *Pediatr Nephrol* 9:329-32, 1995.
64. Hölltä T, Rönnholm K, Holmerg C: Adequacy of dialysis with tidal and continuous cycling peritoneal dialysis in children, *Nephrol Dial Transplant* 15:1438-42, 2000.
65. Amici G: Continuous tidal peritoneal dialysis: Prescription and power. In C Ronco, G Amici, M Feriani, G Virga (eds), *Automated peritoneal dialysis*. Basel: Karger 1999:134-41.
66. Brandes JC, Packard WJ, Watters SK, Fritsche C: Optimization of dialysate flow and mass transfer during automated peritoneal dialysis, *Am J Kidney Dis* 25:603-10, 1998.
67. Ronco C, Dell'Aquila R: Continuous flow peritoneal dialysis, *Perit Dial Int* 21(3):S138-S143, 2001.
68. Brunkhorst R, Fromm S, Wrenger E, Berke A, Petersen R, Riede G, et al: Automated peritoneal dialysis with "online" prepared bicarbonate-buffered dialysate: Technique and first clinical experiences, *Nephrol Dial Transplant* 13:3189-92, 1998.
69. Ronco C, Amerling R: Continuous flow peritoneal dialysis: Current state-of-the-art and obstacles to further development, *Contrib Nephrol* 150:310-20, 2006.
70. Vonesh EF: Membrane transport models and computerized kinetic modeling applied to automated peritoneal dialysis. In C Ronco, G Amici, M Feriani, G Virga (eds), *Automated peritoneal dialysis*. Basel: Karger 1999:15-34.
71. Warady BA, Watkins SL, Fivush BA, Andreoli SP, Salusky I, Kohaut EC, et al: Validation of PD Adequest 2.0 for pediatric dialysis patients, *Pediatr Nephrol* 16:205-11, 2001.
72. Maiorca R, Brunori G, Zubani R, Cancarini GC, Manili L, Camerini E, et al: Predictive value of dialysis adequacy and nutritional indices for mortality and morbidity in CAPD and HD patients: A longitudinal study, *Nephrol Dial Transplant* 10:2295-305, 1995.
73. Churchill DN, Taylor DW, Keshaviah PK, Thorpe KE, Beecroft ML: Adequacy of dialysis and nutrition in continuous peritoneal dialysis: Association with clinical outcomes. Canada-USA Peritoneal Dialysis Study Group, *J Am Soc Nephrol* 7:198-207, 1996.
74. National Kidney Foundation: K/DOQI Clinical Practice Guidelines for Peritoneal Dialysis Adequacy, 2000, *Am J Kidney Dis* 37(1): S65-S136, 2001.
75. Höltta T, Ronholm K, Jalanko H, Holberg C: Clinical outcome of pediatric patients on peritoneal dialysis under adequacy control, *Ped Nephrol* 14:889-97, 2000.
76. van der Voort JH, Harvey EA, Braj B, Geary DF: Can the DOQI guidelines be met by peritoneal dialysis alone in pediatric patients? *Ped Nephrol* 14:717-19, 2000.
77. Chada V, Warady BA: What are the clinical correlates of adequate peritoneal dialysis? *Semin Nephrol* 21:480-89, 2001.
78. Malhotra C, Murata GH, Tzamaloukas AH: Creatinine clearance and urea clearance in PD: What to do in case of discrepancy, *Perit Dial Int* 17:532-35, 1997.
79. Blake PG: Creatinine is the best molecule to target adequacy of peritoneal dialysis, *Perit Dial Int* 20(2):S65-S69, 2000.

80. Bargman JM, Thorpe KE, Churchill DN: Relative contribution of residual renal function and peritoneal clearance to adequacy of dialysis: A reanalysis of the CANUSA study, *J Am Soc Nephrol* 12:2158-62, 2001.
81. Paniagua R, Amato D, Vonesh E, Correa-Rotter R, Ramos A, Moran J, et al: Effects of increased peritoneal clearances on mortality rates in peritoneal dialysis: ADEMEX, a prospective randomized controlled trial, *J Am Soc Nephrol* 13:1307-20, 2002.
82. Lo W-K, Ho Y-W, Li C-C, Wong K-S, Chan T-M, Yu W-Y: Effect of Kt/V survival and clinical outcome in CAPD patients in a prospective randomized trial, *Kidney Int* 64:649-56, 2003.
83. Churchill DN: Impact of peritoneal dialysis dose guidelines on clinical outcome, *Perit Dial Int* 25(3):S95-S98, 2005.
84. Brown EA, Davies SJ, Ruthford P, Meeus F, Borras M, Divino Filho J, et al: Survival of functionally anuric patients on automated peritoneal dialysis: The European APD Outcome Study, *J Am Soc Nephrol* 14:2948-57, 2003.
85. Mujais S, Nolph K, Blake P, Burkart J, Coles G, Kawaguchi Y, et al: Evaluation and management of ultrafiltation problems in peritoneal dialysis, *Perit Dial Int* 20:(4):S5-S21, 2000.
86. Ho-dac-Pannekeet MM, Atasever B, Strujik DG, Krediet RT: Analysis of ultrafiltration failure in peritoneal dialysis patients by means of standard peritoneal permeability analysis, *Perit Dial Int* 17:144-50, 1997.
87. Posthuma N, ter Wee PM, Donker AJM, Peers EM, Oe PL, Verbrugh HA: Icodextrin use in CCPD patients during peritonitis: Ultrafiltration and serum disaccharide concentrations, *Nephrol Dial Transplant* 13:2341-44, 1998.
88. Simonsen O, Sterner G, Carlson O, Wieslander A, Rippe B: Improvement of peritoneal ultrafiltration with peritoneal dialysis solution buffered with bicarbonate/lactate mixture, *Perit Dial Int* 26:353-59, 2006.
89. Warady B, Schaefer F, Alexander SR, Firanek C, Mujais S: *Care of the pediatric patient on peritoneal dialysis: Clinical process for optimal outcomes*. Baxter Healthcare Corporation, 2004.
90. Kim DJ, DO JH, Huh WS, Kim YG, Oh HY: Dissociation between clearances of small and middle molecules in incremental peritoneal dialysis, *Perit Dial Int* 21:462-66, 2001.
91. Paniagua R, Ventura MJ, Rodriguez E, Sil J, Galindo T, Hurtado ME, et al: Impact of fill volume on peritoneal clearances and cytokine appearance in peritoneal dialysis, *Perit Dial Int* 24:156-62, 2004.
92. Montini G, Amici G, Milan S, Mussap M, Naturale M, Ratsch I-M, et al: Middle molecule and small protein removal in children on peritoneal dialysis, *Kidney Int* 61:1153-59, 2002.
93. Bammens B, Evenpoel P, Verbecke K, Vanrenterghem Y: Removal of middle molecules and protein-bound solutes by peritoneal dialysis and relation with uremic symptoms, *Kidney Int* 64:2238-43, 2003.
94. Opatrna S, Opatrny K, Racek J, Sefrna F: Effect of icodextrin-based dialysis solution on peritoneal leptin clearance, *Perit Dial Int* 23:89-91, 2003.
95. Schaefer F, Klaus G, Mehls O: Peritoneal transport properties and dialysis dose affect growth and nutritional status in children on chronic peritoneal dialysis, *J Am Soc Nephrol* 10:1786-92, 1999.
96. Chada V, Blowey DL, Warady BA: Is growth a valid outcome measure of dialysis clearance in children undergoing peritoneal dialysis? *Perit Dial Int* 21(3):S179-S184, 2001.
97. Schaefer F, Wolf S, Klaus G, Langenbeck D, Mehls O: Higher Kt/V urea associated with greater protein catabolic rate and dietary protein intake in children treated with CCPD compared to CAPD, *Adv Perit Dial* 10:310-14, 1994.
98. Aranda RA, Pecoits-Filho RFS, Romao JE Jr., Kakehashi E, Sabbaga E, Marcondes M, et al: Kt/V in children on CAPD: How much is enough? *Perit Dial Int* 19:588-89, 1999.
99. Fischbach M, Terzic J, Lahlou A, Berger MC, Eyer D, Desprez P, et al: Nutritional effects of Kt/V in children on peritoneal dialysis: Are there benefits from larger dialysis doses? *Adv Perit Dial* 11:306-8, 1995.
100. Brem AS, Lambert C, Hill C, Kitsen J, Shemin DG: Outcome data on pediatric dialysis from the end-stage renal disease clinical indicators project, *Am J Kidney Dis* 36:310-17, 2000.
101. K/DOQI Nutrition Work Group: Clinical practice guidelines for nutrition in chronic renal failure, *Am J Kidney Dis* 35(2):S1-S140, 2000.
102. Bakkaloglu SA, Ekim M, Kocak G, Atalay S, Tumer N: Impact of dialysis adequacy on cardiac function in pediatric CAPD patients, *Perit Dial Int* 21:395-400, 2001.
103. Verrina E, Brendolan A, Gusmano R, Ronco C: Chronic replacement therapy in children: Which index is best for adequacy? *Kidney Int* 54:1690-96, 1998.
104. Mellits ED, Cheek DB: The assessment of body water and fatness from infancy to adulthood, *Monogr Soc Res Child Dev* 35(140):12-26, 1970.
105. Morgenstern BZ, Wühl E, Sreekumaran Nair K, Warady B, Schaefer F: Anthropometric prediction of total body water in children who are on pediatric peritoneal dialysis, *J Am Soc Nephrol* 17:285-93, 2006.
106. Haycock GB, Schwartz GJ, Wisotsky DH: Geometric method for measuring body surface area: A height-weight formula validated in infants, children, and adults, *J Pediatr* 93:62-6, 1978.
107. Gehan E, George SL: Estimation of human body surface area from height and weight, *Cancer Chemoter Rep* 54:225-35, 1970.
108. Schaefer F, Wühl E, Feneberg R, Mehls O, Scharer K: Assessment of body composition in children with chronic renal failure, *Pediatr Nephrol* 14:673-78, 2000.
109. Feber J, Scharer K, Schaefer F, Mikova M, Janda J: Residual renal function in children on hemodialysis and peritoneal dialysis therapy, *Ped Nephrol* 8:579-83, 1994.
110. Fischbach M, Terzic J, Menouer S, Soulami K, Dangelser C, Helmstetter A, et al: Effects of automated peritoneal dialysis on residual urinary volume in children, *Adv Perit Dial* 17:269-73, 2001.
111. Ronco C, Amerling R, Dell'Aquila R, Rodighiero MP, Di Loreto P: Evolution of technology for automated peritoneal dialysis, *Contrib Nephrol* 150:291-309, 2006.
112. Edefonti A, Boccola S, Picca M, Paglialonga F, Ardissino G, Marra G, et al: Treatment data during pediatric home peritoneal dialysis, *Ped Nephrol* 18:560-64, 2003.
113. Nolph KD, Twardowski ZJ, Khanna R, Moore HL, Prowant BF: Predicted and measured daily creatinine production in CAPD: Identifying non-compliance, *Perit Dial Int* 15:22-25, 1995.
114. Blake PG: Noncompliance in peritoneal dialysis patients, *Perit Dial Int* 17:330-32, 1997.
115. Bernardini J Nagy M, Piraino B: Pattern of non compliance with dialysis exchanges in peritoneal dialysis patients, *Am J Kidney Dis* 35:1104-10, 2000.
116. Blake PG, Korbert SM, Blake R, Bargman JM, Burkasts M, Delano BG, et al: A multicenter study of non compliance with continuous ambulatory peritoneal dialysis exchanges in US and Canadian patients, *Am J Kidney Dis* 35:506-14, 2000.
117. Amici G, Viglino G, Gandolfo C, Da Rin G, Bocci C, Cavalli PL: Compliance study in peritoneal dialysis using PD Adequest software, *Perit Dial Int* 16(1):S176-S178, 1996.
118. Watson AR, Gartland C: Guidelines by an ad hoc European committee for elective chronic peritoneal dialysis in pediatric patients, *Perit Dial Int* 21:240-44, 2001.

CHAPTER

56 Hemodialysis Vascular Access: Complications and Outcomes

Deepa H. Chand and Ian John Ramage

Pediatric end-stage renal failure programs across the developed world have evolved over the past three decades. Technological advances in vascular access, dialysis membranes, and hemodialysis machines have been part of the improved package of care that has facilitated the provision of chronic renal replacement therapy in children and adolescents of all ages. Although renal transplantation is accepted as the treatment of choice, more than three fourths of children with end-stage renal disease (ESRD) will require dialysis as their initial mode of renal replacement therapy upon entry into the end stage—with almost half of all children receiving hemodialysis initially.[1]

The prevalence of ESRD and the modality of renal replacement show marked variation around the world, with the prevalence of hemodialysis reported as between 27% and 100% of pediatric and adolescent patients and with an over-representation of non-Caucasian hemodialysis patients in U.K. registry data.[1,2] According to the most recent United States Renal Data System (USRDS) report, approximately 7200 children in the United States initiated therapy for ESRD, with hemodialysis being the initial therapy in approximately 50%.[1]

Dialysis delivery in all patient groups is dependent on the provision of adequate access, with specific problems in the pediatric population arising from the technical difficulties imposed by the smaller vascular diameter and lower arterial flow rates. The recognition that the requirement for hemodialysis vascular access is life-long provides the surgeon, nephrologist, dialysis nursing team, and interventional radiologist with a considerable challenge in optimizing vascular access during childhood.

Increased use of peritoneal dialysis, shortened time spent on dialysis, perceived difficulties in creating and using native arteriovenous fistulae (AVF) and autologous venous grafts (AVGs) in small children, and improvement in central venous catheter (CVC) technology have contributed to the increasing use of vascular catheters as permanent hemodialysis access in children and adolescents at initiation and throughout the course of dialysis therapy. However, older children and adolescents (most notably males) are more likely to utilize permanent vascular access in the form of AVF or AVGs.[1,3-5]

The development of reliable vascular access for the provision of chronic hemodialysis in the adult population was first achieved using the "Scribner shunt" consisting of two cannulae inserted respectively into the radial artery and the cephalic vein.[6] This form of access was not without problems, with 50% reported as needing at least one revision and 31% requiring multiple revisions.[7] The Scribner shunt had a reported average life span of 113 days, with 40% requiring removal for clotting or infection.[8] Nonetheless, the reliability of this technique and its subsequent modification for children provided the first form of chronic vascular access for hemodialysis.[9]

The Brescia-Cimino AVF, first described in 1966, has emerged as the gold standard for vascular access in both adults and children with regard to complication rates and longevity.[5,10,11] The size of the pediatric vasculature poses problems for the surgeon in creating AVF, and may explain the higher rate of primary nonfunction in this patient group compared with adolescents.[5] The use of microsurgical techniques has permitted the use of this technique in younger children, with results in experienced centers comparable to fistula formation in older children. The use of other vascular sites is discussed later in this chapter, but preference should be given to creating upper limb access on the nondominant side.

The formation of AVG has been advocated following the failure of a native fistula, although this is by no means universally accepted.[12] Historically, bovine carotid heterografts and saphenous vein autografts have been used to create vascular access. However, there is little published data on their use in pediatrics. Historical reports from predominantly adult-based series describing saphenous vein autografts report an increased incidence of vessel dilatation and aneurysm formation with resulting fistula, potentially causing high-output cardiac failure.[13,14] The literature relating to bovine carotid heterografts is not encouraging. Applebaum compared bovine carotid heterografts with synthetic grafts and found a complication rate of 69%, with almost 50% thrombosing. Other complications include aneurysm formation, with a long-term patency of 31%.[15]

The most commonly used vascular access across all ages and genders is the cuffed CVC, providing reliable access for long-term dialysis.[1] These catheters were developed from acute access devices used for the short-term treatment of acute renal failure in both adults and children. The development of softer silastic rubber catheters for long-term vascular access and the delivery of parenteral nutrition have led to the use of these catheters in acute and chronic renal replacement therapy.[16,17] They provide immediately usable vascular access in a patient population in whom the challenges of permanent vascular access creation are well recognized.

The choice of vascular access is often dictated by the time between presentation to the nephrologist and the requirement for dialysis. Although the majority of pediatric patients initiating hemodialysis do not present acutely, those with an immediate need for dialysis almost exclusively have their initial dialysis session undertaken via a CVC.[5] Excluding this population, it has been shown that children and adolescents who remain on hemodialysis long term are more commonly dialyzed via central venous lines—with a median time to permanent vascular access formation of 1653 days (CI 1516-1836) and with only 5% of patients undergoing permanent dialysis access formation after 1 year of hemodialysis (with figures of 13.5% and 25.1% reported at 2 and 3 years, respectively).[18] Although native AVF have demonstrated superior survival in comparison to other access types in children and adolescents, the choice of vascular access in pediatric patients requiring hemodialysis will inevitably be influenced by local expertise. However, several other factors may influence the choice of access type.[5,19]

As mentioned previously, hemodialysis is transient for the majority of children with ESRD, acting as a bridge to transplantation or the initiation of peritoneal dialysis. In such cases, the need for permanent vascular access is often deemed unnecessary. The technical difficulties associated with permanent vascular access creation in smaller children are well documented. As such, in preference to the risk of sacrificing permanent vascular access as a consequence of failed surgery in early childhood cuffed CVCs are often chosen—although these too are not without long-term complications.[4]

Similarly, in this age group there is a perception that younger children do not tolerate vascular access cannulation—although the evidence appears to suggest the contrary.[5,20] The etiology of end-stage renal failure may also influence the choice of vascular access because the nephrotic syndrome has been shown to limit vascular access survival and consequently cuffed CVCs may be used in preference (although this again is likely to be influenced by local expertise).[5,19]

ARTERIOVENOUS FISTULA

The ideal hemodialysis access is one that provides for maximal blood flows with the ability to be accessed repeatedly with the fewest complications. For chronic hemodialysis, three types of access are currently available: AVF, arteriovenous graft (AVG), and CVCs. In 2003, approximately 70% of children in France were dialyzed through an AVF, whereas only 24% were dialyzed with a CVC.[21] In contrast, 77% of all children are dialyzed with a CVC in the United States—whereas only 11% were dialyzed with AVF and 12% with AVG.[21]

AVF remain the preferred hemodialysis access for all patients, including pediatric patients. The National Kidney Foundation Kidney Disease Outcomes Quality Initiative (NKF/K-DOQI) guidelines recommend a prevalent AVF rate of 40% and incident rate of 50% in hemodialysis patients.[22] Published data, however, demonstrate that this is not the case in both the adult and pediatric population—with continued use of tunneled CVCs at initiation of dialysis and at day 60.[5,23] The guidelines also recommend that distal sites in the nondominant arm be utilized first, then moving proximally with subsequent access placements as warranted. A schematic of common and rare AV access sites is depicted in Figure 56-1.

The earliest AVF placed was a peripheral Brescia-Cimino fistula utilizing the radial artery and cephalic vein at the wrist. The first successful radial-cephalic fistula was placed in a pediatric patient in 1970.[24] The typical technique used for placement involves dissection of the vessels, dilatation of the vessels, and an end-to-side anastomosis of the artery and vein. There are notable differences in children that can be considered as the surgeon approaches placement of a radial-cephalic AVF. Due to the smaller caliber of the vessels, a finer suture is often utilized in children. The key to a successful surgical outcome involves a well-approximated anastomosis without distortion of the vessels. Minimally accepted size parameters for the vessels are approximately 1.5 to 2.0 mm

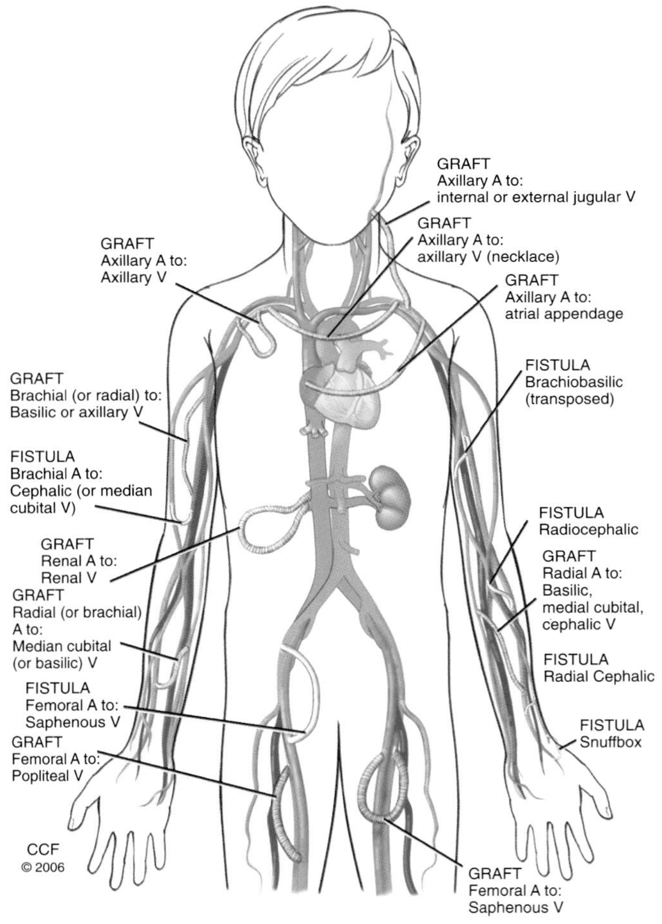

Figure 56-1 AV access sites. (Copyright © 2006, Cleveland Clinic Foundation.)

for the radial artery, 2.5 mm for the forearm cephalic vein, and 3.0 mm for the basilic or upper arm cephalic vein. These allow a dilator to pass and a side-to-end anastomosis to be created.[25]

If a radial-cephalic AVF is not feasible due to vessel size or other precluding factors, a brachial artery-cephalic vein AVF in the upper arm provides an alternative site—albeit a more proximal one. In this type of autologous fistula, the brachial artery in the upper arm is anastomosed to the cephalic vein in the upper arm. A subsequent option for AVF placement is the transposed brachial artery-basilic vein fistula. First described in 1976 by Dagher and colleagues, this technique has gained popularity over the past decade due to the need for alternative sites in patients who are not optimal candidates for radial-cephalic or brachial-cephalic AVF. Initial patency rates have been reported as high as 92%, and 1-year patency rates range from 47% to 92%. Although patency rates are not as high as for other types of AVF, they are significantly better than those reported for AVG.[26,27] Of note, steal syndrome has been reported more frequently in transposed brachial-basilic AVF than for other AVF—most likely due to the larger diameter of the arterialized vein.

An alternative technique for AVF creation is the proximal radial artery native AVF, which can be utilized in the patient in which creation of an AVF is extremely difficult.[28] These patients include those with diabetes, those with small or obliterated vessels due to multiple prior venipunctures, those with compromised vascular inflow, obese patients, or those with multiple prior failed accesses. In the pediatric patient, this may include patients with severe renal osteodystrophy with bony deformities. In this approach, the lower forearm proximal radial artery is connected to the medial antebrachial vein to create an AVF in those in whom a radial-cephalic AVF is not possible. This procedure often requires the use of valvutomes to ablate venous valves. This type of AVF allows the utility of the lower forearm (with less surrounding adipose tissue), avoiding the need to use the upper arm—thereby allowing for quicker maturation and decreased incidence of steal phenomenon. Patency rates up to 91% have been reported with this technique.[29]

There are distinguishing factors in children that need to be considered in the creation of an AVF. Preoperative management should always include a thorough history and physical examination with focus on the vascular status. This includes evaluation of vessel length, determination of elasticity of the veins after applying venostasis, and the checking for signs of venous obstruction. However, if the anatomy is questionable as to vessel caliber, route, and so on, imaging techniques should be utilized. This can include duplex ultrasound, magnetic resonance angiography, or venography. In addition, some children have a high degree of spasticity of both the arterial and venous vessels. Options for overcoming the spasms can include use of papaverine or the gradual use of coronary dilators intraoperatively.

Postoperatively, one can consider the use of a peripherally acting vasodilator such as a calcium channel blocker while the access matures to decrease the degree of vasospasm, thereby reducing the risk of thrombosis. If there is a history of prior thrombus or suspicion of a hypercoagulable state, a comprehensive evaluation for an underlying etiology should be undertaken. Although antiplatelet agents have not been shown to prevent rethrombosis, they have been shown to decrease the incidence of thrombosis in a new access (relative risk of 0.35 versus placebo).[30] Although warfarin and low-molecular-weight heparin are not usually used in pediatric patients with a hypercoagulable state, repeated thromboses may require their use. It is recommended that these agents be administered with consultation from a hematologist or vascular medicine specialist.

Furthermore, surgical adjuncts such as loupe magnification, inflatable tourniquet, or operating microscope to enhance visualization should be considered.[31] Creation of successful AVF (with the aid of an operating microscope) in children as small as 5 kg in size has been reported in the literature.[32] When an operating microscope is used, failure to mature approximates 5% to 10%, with no significant differences in long-term survival rates.[33] Postoperatively, patients should be educated regarding care of the access—such as avoidance of blood pressure measurements in the extremity.

Major complications associated with the use of AVF include primary failure of maturation. Typical primary failure rates of radial-cephalic fistulae approximate 30%, brachial-cephalic approximate 10%, and brachial-basilic approximate 30%.[34] An AVF may mature as quickly as 4 weeks after placement. However, maturation may take up to 6 months. Risks of primary failure are increased in obese patients or those with vascular compromise. In obese patients, a two-stage approach may be utilized in which a fistula is created and then several weeks later elevated to allow for cannulation. Physical examination of the fistula should be the primary determinant of time to usage, as opposed to time period after placement. However, once a fistula has matured the secondary failure rate is very low—with most radial-cephalic fistulae having a patency rate of approximately 50% 10 years post initial maturation.[34]

The most common long-term complication of a fistula is thrombosis (Figure 56-2), which is often secondary to stenosis (venous or arterial). Risk factors for the development of thrombosis include shear vascular stress from turbulent blood flow, leading to endothelial cell injury and resulting in myointimal proliferation and fibromuscular hyperplasia. Pseudoaneurysm formation occurs in up to 5% of fistulae and is most likely due to trauma of the vessel wall created by multiple punctures at the same site. Rotation of cannulation sites or the use of the buttonhole technique can help prevent aneurysm/pseudoaneurysm formation. The buttonhole technique employs the creation of a track through which the fistula is cannulated at each session. This track minimizes trauma to the vessel wall, resulting in fewer infiltrations, fewer missed attempts, and minimization of pain to the patient. Other complications include steal phenomenon, venous hypertension, and infection—all of which are rare in children with less than 5% cumulative incidence.

A common misconception among providers is that children avoid AVF due to cannulation discomfort. In fact, a survey conducted by Brittenger and colleagues in 75 pediatric hemodialysis patients showed that 39% felt almost no discomfort, 39% felt tolerable discomfort, and 22% felt great discomfort.[35] Upon answering if the patient would prefer to return to a CV, 93% responded no, 4% said yes, and 3% said

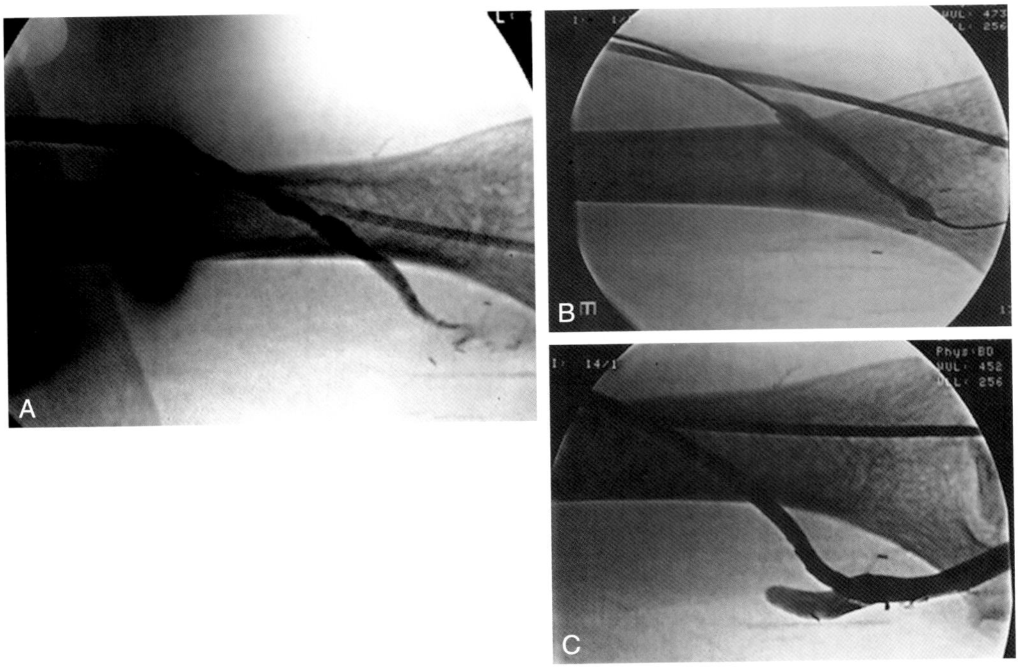

Figure 56-2 Vascular thrombosis. **A,** Pretherapy, **B,** During angioplasty. **C,** Postangioplasty.

they didn't know. No patient in the study was converted to a CVC due to pain.[35]

Cosmetic reasons are sited for not placing an AVF in children. This is especially true with a radial-cephalic AVF, which may become excessively dilated. Rotation of cannulation sites can help prevent overdilatation. Nonetheless, patients need to be educated in advance regarding the cosmetic features of AVF/AVG use. Consideration should also be given to the fewer activity restrictions with an AVF or AVG such as the ability to shower, swim, and so on.

ARTERIOVENOUS GRAFTS

An AVG utilizes the principle of a native fistula, with insertion of a synthetic conduit to connect the artery and vein. Synthetic materials available include saphenous vein, bovine, umbilical, Dacron, polyurethane, cryopreserved femoral vein, and polytetrafluoroethylene (PTFE). The PTFE is the most commonly utilized due to the fewest complication rates. The graft can be straight or looped (whichever allows for the greatest surface area for cannulation) and ranges between 4 and 8 mm in diameter. Common locations for placement include radial-cephalic, brachial-cephalic, brachial-axillary, and axillary-axillary.

Leg grafts are also common in children. Advantages of an AVG include shorter time to maturation (many can be used in approximately 2 weeks from placement), large surface area for cannulation, and lower primary failure rates. Primary failure rates have been reported as low as 0% to 13% with an AVG, which is substantially less than an AVF. However, the disadvantages long term make AVG a less desirable form of permanent access. Disadvantages compared to AVF include a greater risk of thrombosis and infection. The Dialysis Outcomes and Practice Patterns Study (DOPPS) in adults found that grafts were nearly four times more likely to require a thrombectomy than an AVF. In addition, graft infection rates approximate 10% (compared to <2% to 5% for AVF).[36,37] Because the graft material is synthetic, infection often requires surgical intervention—with possible resection of the graft. No separate pediatric data exist.

MONITORING OF AVF AND AVG

Routine access monitoring is recommended using a combination of physical inspection, review of access pressures and dialysis blood flow rates, measurement of recirculation, and venous pressure monitoring and/or ultrasound dilution. Ideally, a combination of all of these surveillance tools should be utilized—although Chand and colleagues reported that static venous pressure monitoring does not accurately predict access failure in pediatric hemodialysis patients.[38] Goldstein and colleagues have published reports of the benefits of ultrasound dilution for access monitoring in children.[39]

The device costs may be prohibitive. However, collaboration with an adult dialysis facility may allow for use of such a machine. If routine surveillance is suspicious for thrombosis or stenosis, a fistulagram should be obtained to determine the etiology. Based on the NKF-K/DOQI guidelines, if stenosis is >50% of the access diameter and associated with prior access thrombosis, elevated venous pressures, abnormal urea kinetics, recirculation, or abnormal physical examination percutaneous transluminal angioplasty or surgical exploration should be performed.

This can be performed by an experienced interventional radiologist, or by a surgeon. Success rates in adults are as high as 80% with regard to correction of the stenosis.[22] If angio-

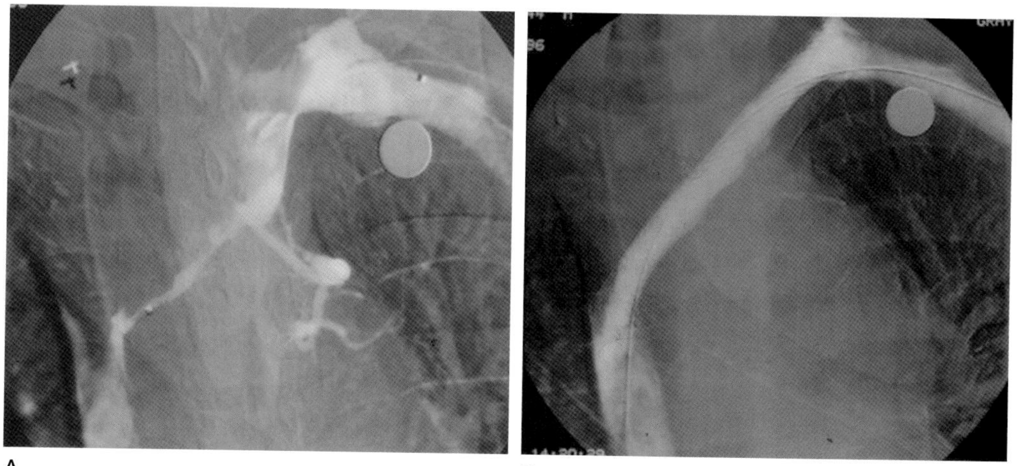

A B

Figure 56-3 Vessel stenosis. **A,** Preangioplasty. **B,** Postangioplasty.

plasty needs to be performed more than two times in 3 months, referral for surgical revision should be considered if the patient has alternative sites available. Stenting should be considered in select circumstances if the patient does not have alternative access sites or demonstrates contraindication to surgery. If an access is modified, it is important to continue routine surveillance because the rate of stenosis recurrence can be as high as 70% within 1 year. Results of angioplasty can be verified postprocedure (Figure 56-3).

CENTRAL VENOUS CATHETERS

CVCs were first used as hemodialysis access in the mid 1970s.[40] The NKF/K-DOQI guidelines recommend a catheter prevalence rate of <10% for chronic hemodialysis patients. Catheters are acceptable if needed in an emergency, if dialysis access is maturing, or if all other permanent access options have been exhausted. If needed for longer than 3 weeks, a cuffed tunneled catheter should be used. For chronic dialysis, soft blunt-tipped dual-lumen catheters are placed and advanced into the vein. The preferred site for CVC placement is the right internal jugular vein, with the tip at the caval atrial junction or in the right atrium.

Blood flow rates have been shown to be approximately 40% higher in the right internal jugular vein compared to the left internal jugular catheters.[41] In addition, compared to femoral vein catheters (which are commonly used for acute dialysis treatments) right atrial catheters have been shown to exhibit significantly less recirculation due to cardiac output flows.[42] Alternative sites (in order of preference) are the right external jugular vein, the left internal and external jugular veins, subclavian veins, femoral veins, and translumbar access to the inferior vena cava. Catheters should be placed by an experienced surgeon, interventional radiologist, or interventional nephrologist. Of note, the CVC should not be placed on the same side as a maturing AV access. The largest bore of catheter possible should be used to maximize blood flow rates. Several types of chronic CVCs are available for use in children, although no catheter has been proven to be superior to another (Figure 56-4). They are most commonly made of polyurethane, silicone, or carbothane. However, alternative materials used to manufacture CVC in the past include polyethylene and Teflon. Polyethylene catheters are rigid and are therefore more commonly used for acute rather than chronic treatments. Teflon is not used any longer due to its rigidity. Polyurethane is the most commonly used material for chronic catheters due to its strength. It allows for rigidity to keep vessels patent while being thin enough to allow for maximum lumen diameter.

However, caution must be used with polyurethane catheters because povidone-iodine–containing or polyethylene-glycol–containing ointments (such as mupirocin) can weaken the catheter. Carbothane catheters are made of a polyurethane/polycarbonate polymer and offer the advantages of polyurethane with regard to rigidity, but are significantly thinner. Another advantage of carbothane is its resistance to degradation by iodine, peroxide, and alcohols. Silicone catheters are very flexible. However, they must be thicker in construction to avoid lumen collapse and/or kinking. Although it is compatible with most antibiotic ointments, it is weakened by iodine and caution must be used. Dialock Hemodialysis System (Biolink Inc., Norwell, MA, USA) and the LifeSite Hemodialysis Access System (Vasca, Inc., Tewksbury, MA, USA) catheters are made of silicone.

The first dual-lumen catheter used for chronic dialysis was the Quinton Permcath, which is a single catheter with a Dacron cuff that is inserted through a split sheath. The cuff fixes the catheter into place within the subcutaneous tract and limits the level at which a fibrin sheath develops along the catheter. This catheter remains in use today.

The Tesio catheter, in which two single-lumen catheters are placed side by side through the vein, is a cuffed catheter with side holes arranged in a spiral around the tip of the catheter. Due to the arrangement of the side holes, the advantage of this type of catheter system is that it allows for a higher blood flow through the catheter and less chance for catheter occlusion. Theoretically, there should be a decrease in recirculation as well due to the increased distance between

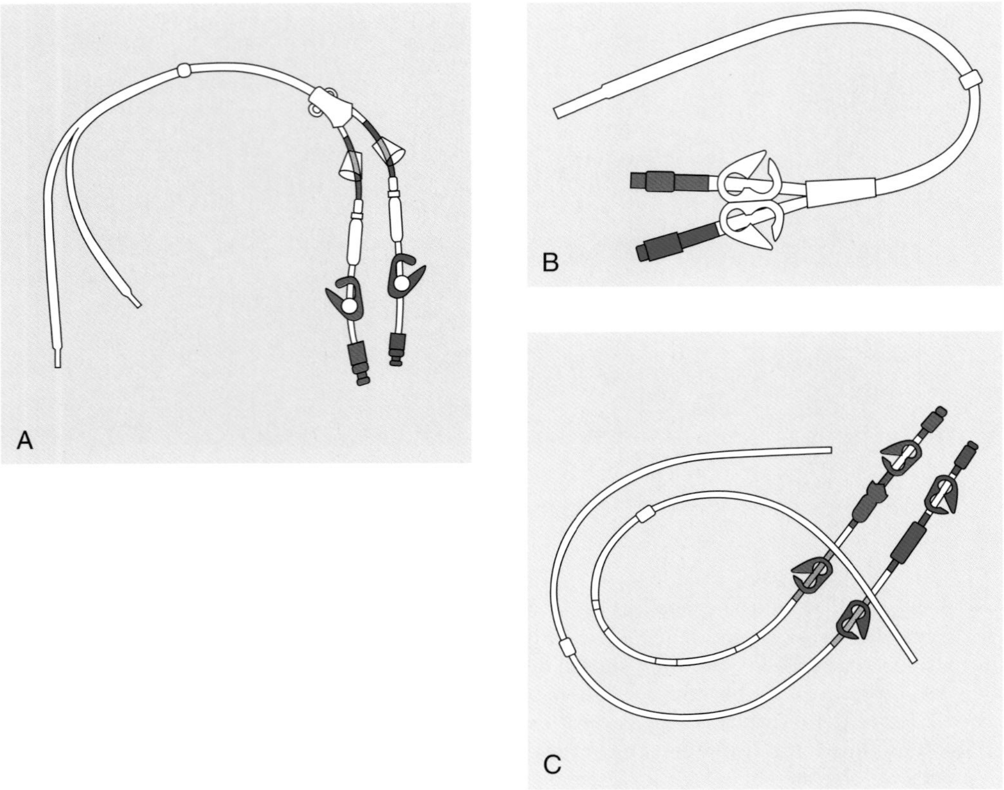

Figure 56-4 Types of CVC. **A,** Split Cath. **B,** Permcath. **C,** Tesio.

the arterial and venous lumens. A study performed in the pediatric hemodialysis population by Sheth and colleagues showed a significant difference in line survival when a Tesio catheter was used as opposed to a dual-lumen catheter (46% versus 0% at 1 year).[43] However, there was no significant difference noted in clearances as measured by Kt/V or infection rates with the Tesio catheter as opposed to the dual-lumen catheter.

The Split Cath catheter is a dual-lumen cuffed catheter with a D-shaped configuration in the midshaft, which separates into two distal tips—each with circumferential side holes. This allows for the insertion of only one catheter, but yet offers the advantage of side holes on all sides. There is also a step down in diameter at the tip of each of the lines, causing a decrease in luminal pressure at the end of the catheter—maximizing the blood flow through the side ports. Adult studies have shown higher blood flows and less recirculation than with other dual-lumen catheters, with function similar to that of the Tesio catheters.[40,44]

Immediate complications of CVC include arterial puncture, pneumothorax, hemothorax, hemomediastinum, dysrhythmias, air embolism, vessel perforation, cerebral infarct, and pericardial tamponade (Figures 56-5 and 56-6). Common long-term complications include central vein stenosis, thrombosis, infection, fibrin sheath formation, and nerve trauma. Central vein stenosis is most commonly associated with subclavian vein catheters, and thus avoidance of the subclavian vein is recommended. Reports have confirmed an up to 40% incidence of vessel stenosis upon CVC removal, regardless of cause for removal.[45]

Similarly, fibrin sheath formation has been reported in up to 50% of catheters (Figure 56-7).[46] Fibrin sheath formation typically originates at the site of catheter insertion and migrates to block the intake and outflow holes of the catheter. Because the sheath is in the vessel itself rather than the catheter, reinsertion of the catheter at the same site may result in the fibrin sheath covering the new catheter—resulting in continued catheter dysfunction. Options for removal of fibrin sheath include injection of a thrombolytic agent such as tissue plasminogen activator, urokinase, or streptokinase; fibrin sheath stripping; and mechanical disruption of the sheath at the time of catheter replacement.

Thrombolytic agents may be infused continuously or instilled into the catheter as a "lock." Unfortunately, this treatment can be expensive and often is not successful. Fibrin sheath stripping involves manually stripping off the sheath by looping the catheter with a snare. This approach requires a femoral approach, increasing the risk of complications. Manual disruption involves the use of a balloon at the time of catheter replacement to disrupt the fibrin sheath, allowing for time before another sheath reforms.

Infection remains a common complication of CVC. Exit-site infections manifested by drainage or erythema at the skin site of the CVC can often be prevented with proper hygiene and dressing care. If an exit-site infection develops, topical, oral, or intravenous antibiotics are often successful for treat-

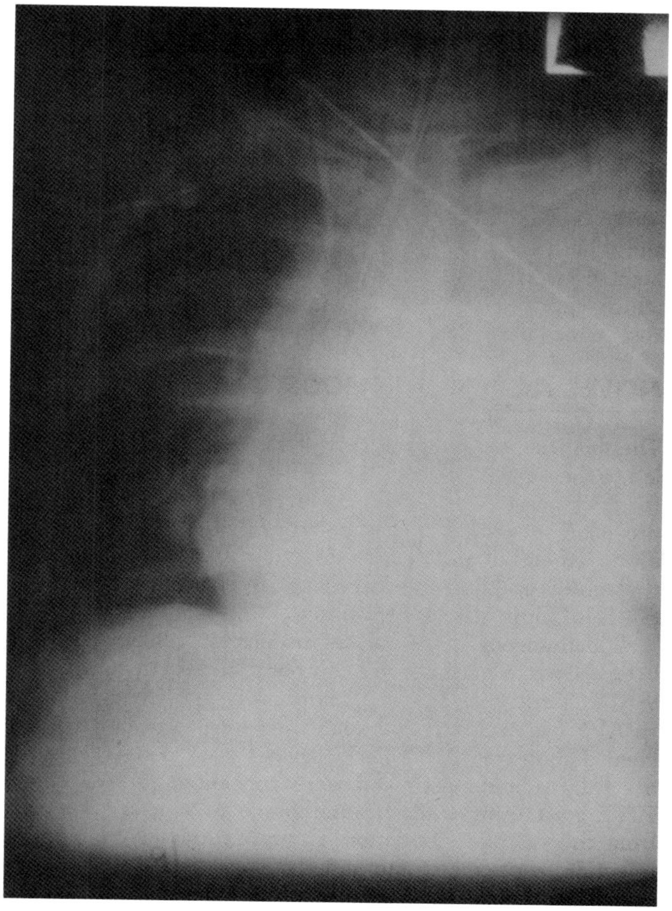

Figure 56-5 Hemothorax following CVC placement.

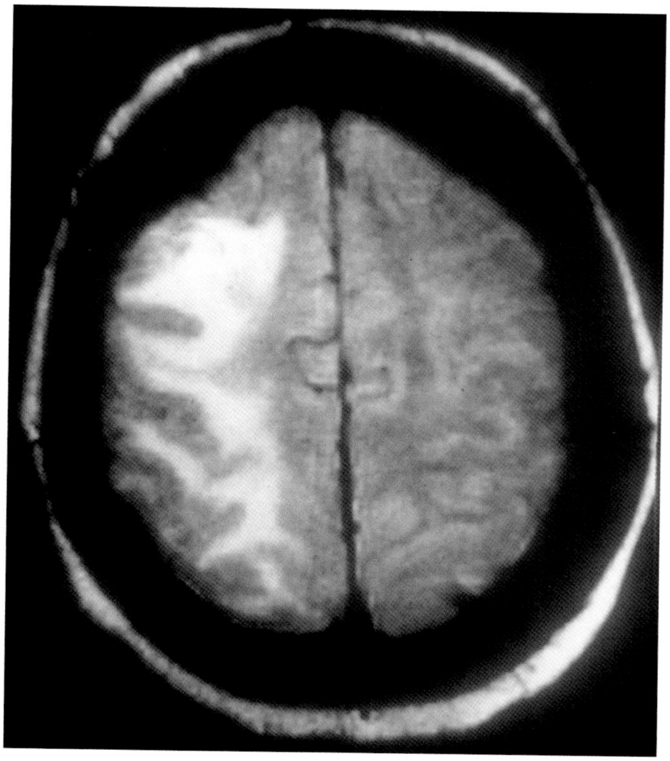

Figure 56-6 Cerebral infarct after central line placement.

ment. However, if the infection involves the catheter tract it may not be possible to treat the infection without catheter removal and this should be considered early in the treatment course. The CVC should not be replaced at the same site until the infection has resolved for at least 48 to 72 hours. Furthermore, a CVC infection with serious systemic signs of fever, sepsis, and so on should also be removed immediately and not reinserted in the same location for at least 48 to 72 hours. Potential complications of untreated infections include osteomyelitis, endocarditis, and epidural abscess.

COMPARISON OF ACCESS TYPES BY OUTCOMES

In pediatric hemodialysis patients, hospitalization rates for all reasons approximate 200 per 1000 patient-years at risk, with infection related to a vascular device being the primary indication for hospitalization. In those patients with a CVC, the risk of infection approximates 1.2 per patient-year at risk compared to <0.5 per patient-year at risk for a patient dialyzed with AVF or AVG in the United States.[1] In fact, approximately 46% of pediatric hemodialysis patients are admitted within the first 3 years of initiation of dialysis—largely for infectious reasons.

Similarly, mortality rates are highest for pediatric hemodialysis patients in the United States, with 5-year survival rates for hemodialysis and peritoneal dialysis patients approximating 81% compared to 92% for transplant recipients. Although cardiovascular complications are the predominant cause of mortality in transplant recipients, infection remains the predominant cause in dialysis patients. Given that infection rates are significantly higher for CVC than AVG or AVF, the data compel the use of AVF or AVG when possible.

Furthermore, in a recent study of 140 pediatric hemodialysis patients Chand and colleagues found that clinical outcome parameters were significantly better for those children dialyzed with an AVF or AVG as opposed to CVC when adjusting for variables such as time on dialysis, dialysis vintage, blood flow rates, and so on.[47] Specifically, when comparing clearances as measured by urea reduction rates (URR) URR rates were significantly better for patients who dialyzed with AVF or AVG compared to CVC. Kt/V was not found to be significantly different. Hemoglobin concentrations were higher for those dialyzed with AVF compared to AVG and CVC.

Similarly, recombinant human erythropoietin (rHuEPO) doses were significantly lower in those with an AVF compared to AVG or CVC. Of note, those dialyzed with an AVG still required less rHuEPO compared to those dialyzed with CVC. Serum albumin levels were significantly higher in those dialyzed with an AVF or AVG compared to a CVC, also suggesting that chronic inflammation may be more pronounced with CVC as opposed to AVF or AVG. This could also contribute to the need for higher rHuEPO doses in these patients, contributing to higher costs of dialysis. Leavey and colleagues found similar results in adult hemodialysis patients.[48]

Ramage and colleagues conducted a 20-year retrospective study in 114 patients to determine the long-term vascular access survival in pediatric hemodialysis patients. Primary access failure occurred in 23% of AVFs, 60% of AVG, and 4% of CVC. Confounding variables associated with primary failure included hypoalbuminemia and number of prior access procedures. Median survival times were approximately 3.1 years for AVF and 0.6 year for CVC.[5]

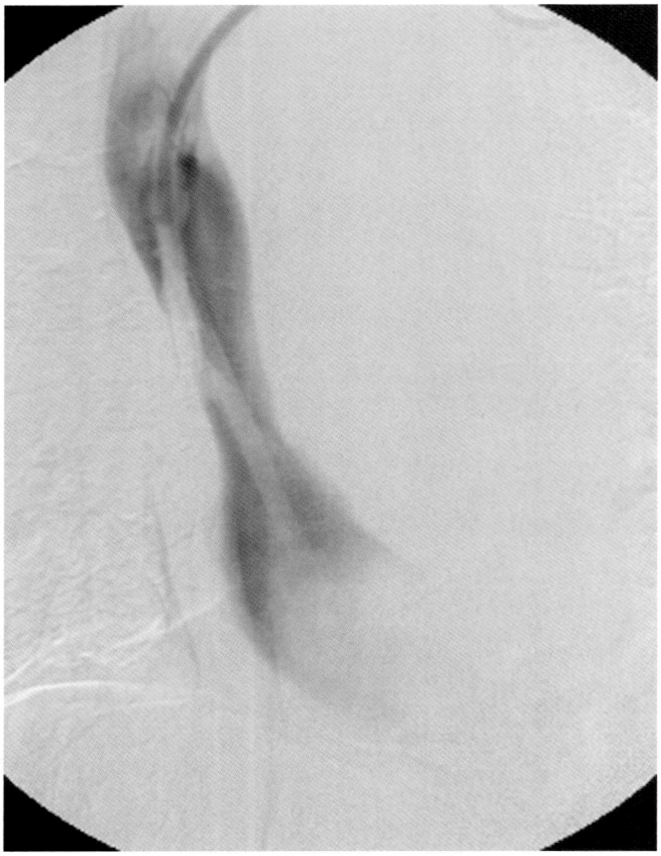

Figure 56-7 Fibrin sheath surrounding CVC.

Goldstein and colleagues reported 1-year survival rates for cuffed catheters in pediatric hemodialysis patients to be 27%, with the most common causes for removal being infection (36%), kinking (14%), elective removal (9%), trauma (9%), and other (9%).[49] According to the 2005 USRDS report, the highest insertion costs among vascular types is for CVC—which approximates $11,700 (compared to AVF insertion cost, which approximates $5000 per procedure).[1]

NOVEL ACCESS METHODS

The financial and personal cost of vascular access failure has led to the suggestion from the NKF-DOQI that a goal of 50% for AVF placement should be targeted for chronic dialysis provision in adults.[22] The limitations of CVCs have been discussed earlier and include infection, low blood flow rates, thrombosis and occlusion secondary to changes in body position, and fibrin sheath deposition.

Subcutaneous hemodialysis vascular access devices have been shown to have a lower complication rate in comparison to CVCs and may be used temporarily until maturation of an AVF has occurred, although their long-term use has also been demonstrated.[50-52] Early devices used ports that were not fully subcutaneous and were connected to a synthetic PTFE graft using a silastic membrane to separate the port from the vascular circulation. Complications in the form of infection, septicemia, and vascular stenosis and thrombosis precluded their generalized use. Newer devices, such as the Dialock Hemodialysis System (Biolink Inc., Norwell, MA, USA) and the LifeSite Hemodialysis Access System (Vasca, Inc., Tewksbury, MA, USA) (Figure 56-8), are completely subcutaneous and have differences in design.

The Dialock system consists of a single titanium port connected to two number 11 French catheters placed in the right atrium. On the opposite side of the port to the catheters are

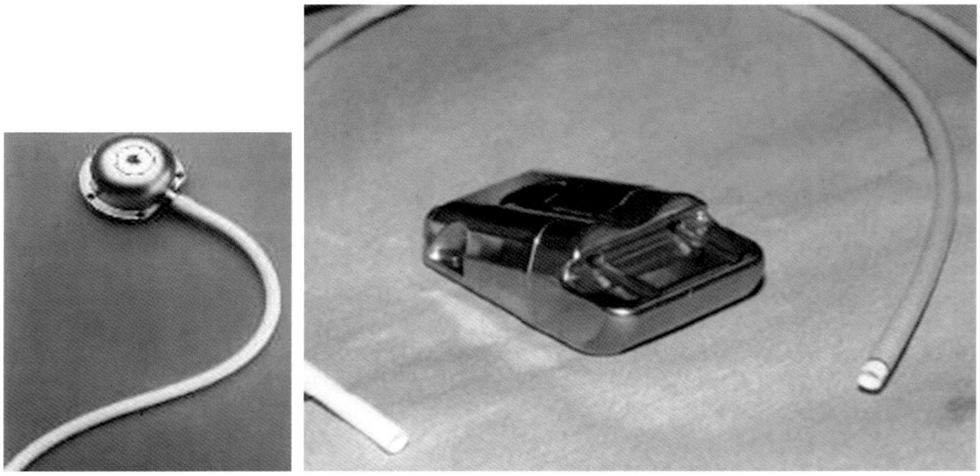

A B

Figure 56-8 Implantable vascular devices. **A,** Lifesite. **B,** Dialock.

two grooves designed to direct the two needles required to puncture the septum valve and facilitate dialysis access. The LifeSite system consists of two distinct stainless steel and titanium ports connected to number 12 French catheters placed in the right atrium, with the return (venous) catheter placed distally.

Randomized clinical trial data are available for the LifeSite system compared to the Tesio-Cath system and demonstrate adequate clearance as measured by a Kt/V of 1.5 L, higher blood flow rates, and fewer thrombotic and bacteremic episodes (with a further reduction in the latter noted with the use of 70% isopropyl alcohol as an antimicrobial agent instilled into the port).[53-55] Although there are no randomized clinical trials of the Dialock system to date, preliminary studies report adequate Kt/V clearances (1.48), sufficient blood flow rates, and acceptable thrombotic and infectious complications.[54,55] The benefits of these devices in the dialysis population are apparent, and with future development of a reduction in size would be available to the pediatric population.

ACUTE VASCULAR ACCESS

Although native AVF or AVG should be considered the access of choice for children with ESRD, temporary vascular access for the treatment of acute renal failure or fluid overload is a frequent requirement for infants and children requiring intensive care. However, temporary vascular access is often required for children with isolated acute renal failure, in children with end-stage renal failure requiring acute dialysis while awaiting maturation of their primary dialysis access (peritoneal or vascular), and in children with acute access dysfunction who require temporary access until revision of the permanent vascular access can occur.

The choice of access site will be influenced by specific clinical circumstances (e.g., previous vascular access for angiography, ascites, abdominal mass, or abnormal abdominal vasculature may preclude the use of the most common acute vascular access site in the pediatric intensive care setting, the femoral veins). In such cases, and in the majority of cases of acute renal failure outside intensive care, the most common site for both acute and chronic vascular access is the right internal jugular.

Femoral vein catheterization is less difficult and has fewer risks associated with insertion. However, while the catheter is in place, the child must remain bedbound, and the catheter is more likely to become infected than when in other sites. In addition, because blood flow is reduced in the lower inferior vena cava compared with the superior vena cava, there is an increased risk of thrombosis. Catheterization of the internal jugular vein is used most commonly in patients with isolated acute renal failure and has largely replaced temporary catheterization of the subclavian vessels because of the increased risk of complications at the time of insertion. There is also increased recognition that cannulation of the subclavian vessels is associated with a higher incidence of vascular trauma and subsequent stenosis than is cannulation of the jugular vessels. The consequence of even minor stenosis of the subclavian vein may be the failure of future forearm AVF in the ipsilateral arm.

The choice of catheter is made on the basis of patient size and local preference. Insertion is made using the Seldinger technique, with the majority being uncuffed polyurethane catheters that are rigid at room temperature (facilitating insertion) but more malleable at body temperature (minimizing vascular trauma). The catheter should be the smallest possible (minimizing vascular trauma) yet large enough to deliver the desired blood flow (approximately 50 to 150 ml/minute required for continuous therapies in comparison to 300 ml/minute for intermittent or chronic hemodialysis delivery).

The complications related to catheter insertion are related to the site of catheter insertion and include arterial puncture, local bleeding, air embolism, and nerve injury. Complications specific to jugular catheters are pneumothorax, hemothorax, air embolism, arrhythmias and pericardial tamponade. Complications specific to femoral catheters include retroperitoneal bleeding. The use of a portable ultrasound device has been shown to decrease the failure rate and incidence of local complications compared to the traditional use of anatomic landmarks—with one study in an adult population using the Site-Rite II device reporting an increase in successful jugular cannulation from 36% to 83% and a decrease in accidental carotid puncture from 8% to 0%.[56]

As with CVC use in chronic hemodialysis patients, infection in uncuffed catheters may occur locally around the exit site or within the tunnel created by the catheter. It may also be associated with systemic infection. Exit-site infection may be treated successfully with antibiotic therapy. However, if symptoms persist catheter removal is warranted. Tunnel infections usually manifest as pain and discoloration around the catheter tract, with local exudation of pus. This requires catheter replacement and antibiotic therapy, and occasionally deroofing of the tract. In the presence of systemic infection, the possibility of catheter-related sepsis must be considered.

In those with an alternative source of infection, continued therapy against this source should be commenced (with the catheter remaining in situ). In the absence of an alternate source of infection, blood cultures should be taken from a peripheral site and from the line itself. The catheter should be removed. Following removal, the catheter tip should be sent for culture—and once blood cultures are negative for a period of 48 hours a new catheter may be inserted.

Specific problems exist with the use of small-gauge catheters in infants and smaller children. In this population, catheter malfunction is more likely to be due to kinking of the catheter (necessitating catheter replacement).[49] This patient group presents a greater technical challenge in catheter placement, and very small infants may require the insertion of two separate venous catheters to permit continuous therapies. The use of a single-lumen catheter for intermittent hemodialysis has been shown to deliver adequate blood flows and may have a place in the management of the smaller infant requiring hemodialysis.[57]

SUMMARY

Although renal transplantation remains the ideal choice for renal replacement therapy in children, hemodialysis remains a necessity. Given that hemodialysis is the most commonly used form of initial renal replacement therapy and that many children will resume hemodialysis after graft failure, it is imperative that dialysis providers optimize vascular access. Preservation of future sites is essential in preventing morbidity and mortality in children with ESRD. As such, the options of vascular access should be discussed among dialysis caregivers: vascular access surgeons, pediatric nephrologists, dialysis nurses, and interventional radiologists.

A multidisciplinary approach to patient education should also be employed, with utilization of recreational therapists and child life professionals to assist in patient understanding. This multidisciplinary approach can help overcome many of the perceived barriers to autologous dialysis access in children. Permanent access should be placed by an experienced surgeon, whether this is a pediatric general surgeon, transplant surgeon, or vascular access surgeon. Ideally, this should be done in a pediatric center. However, experience should supersede if outcomes are superior.

Communication between the dialysis team and surgeon is critical to successful outcomes. The role of the interventional radiologist has emerged over the past decade, and can be extremely useful for preoperative evaluation and for salvage of poorly functioning AVF or AVG. Establishment of protocols may allow for streamlining of communication among all parties involved.

Whenever possible, an AVF should be used as the initial choice—with the mantra remaining "distal before proximal." If the AVF can be placed prior to the need for dialysis, a CVC can be avoided. However, this is not always possible—and a CVC may be essential as short-term access (especially if an AVF or AVG is maturing). In those patients in the process of living donor transplant evaluation, an AVG could be considered over an AVF due to shorter maturation times. Alternatively, if a patient is being evaluated for a deceased donor renal transplant placement, an AVF or AVG should be considered in the interim.

If failure of the access occurs, the patient should be reassessed with regard to vascular access options. If the access is potentially viable, angioplasty should be considered. If not, alternative sites for autologous AVF should be explored first. If an AVF is not a viable option, consideration should be given to a synthetic AVG. Venography may be helpful in defining options for access placement. CVC should remain a last resort for permanent dialysis access in children.

ACKNOWLEDGMENTS

The authors would like to thank Mark J. Sands, MD, and Beth Halasz for their imaging and illustrative contributions, respectively.

REFERENCES

1. U.S. Renal Data System: *USRDS 2005 Annual Data Report: Atlas of End-Stage Renal Disease in the United States*. Bethesda, MD: National Institutes of Health, National Institute of Diabetes and Digestive and Kidney Diseases 2005.
2. *U.K. Renal Registry Report 2005*. Bristol, UK: UK Renal Registry, 2005.
3. Warady BA, Sullivan EK, Alexander SR: Lessons from the peritoneal dialysis patient database: A report of the North American Pediatric Renal Transplant Cooperative Study, *Kidney Int Suppl* 53:S68-S71, 1996.
4. Beanes SR, Kling KM, Fonkalsrud EW, et al: Surgical aspects of dialysis in newborns and infants weighing less than ten kilograms, *J Ped Surg* 35:1543-48, 2000.
5. Ramage IJ, Bailie A, Tyerman KS, McColl JH, Pollard SG, Fitzpatrick MM: Vascular access survival in children and young adults receiving long-term hemodialysis, *Am J Kidney Dis* 45:708-14, 2005.
6. Quinton W, Dillard D, Scribner BH: Cannulation of blood vessels for prolonged hemodialysis, *Trans An Soc Artif Int Organs* 6:104-13, 1960.
7. Franzone AJ, Tucker BL, Brennan LP, Fine RN, Stiles QR: Hemodialysis in children: Experience with arteriovenous shunts, *Arch Surg* 102:592-93, 1971.
8. Idriss FS, Nikaidoh H, King LR, Swenson O: Arteriovenous shunts for hemodialysis in infants and children, *J Pediatr Surg* 6:639-44, 1971.
9. Buselmeier F, Kjellstrand CM, Ratazzi CC, Simons RL, Najarian JS: A new subcutaneous prosthetic A-V shunt: Advantages over the standard Quinton-Scribner shunt and A-V fistula, *Proc Clin Dial Transplant Forum* 2:67-75, 1972.
10. Brescia MJ, Cimino JE, Appel K, Hurwich BJ: Chronic hemodialysis using venepuncture and a surgically created arteriovenous fistula, *N Engl J Med* 275:1089-92, 1966.
11. Juan A, Armadans L, Eugenio F: The function of permanent vascular access, *Nephrol Dial Transplant* 15:402-8, 2000.
12. Lumsden AB, MacDonald J, Allen RC, Dodson TF: Hemodialysis access in the pediatric patient population, *Am J Surg* 168:197-201, 1994.
13. Bourquelot P, Cussenot O, Corbi P, Pillion G, Gagnadoux MF, Bensman A, et al: Microsurgical creation and follow-up of arteriovenous fistulae for chronic hemodialysis in children, *Pediatr Nephrol* 4:156-59, 1990.
14. D'Apuzzo VG, Grushkin CM, Brennan LP, Stiles QR, Fine RN: Saphenous vein autograft arteriovenous fistula for extended hemodialysis in children, *Acta Paediatr Scand* 62:28-32, 1973.
15. Applebaum H, Shashikumar VL, Somers LA, Gruskin AB, Grossman M, McGarvey MJ, et al: Improved hemodialysis access in children, *J Pediatr Surg* 15:764-69, 1980.
16. Hickman RO, Buchner CD, Clift RA, Sanders JE, Stewart P, Thomas ED: A modified right atrial catheter for access to the venous system in marrow transplant patients, *Am J Surg* 140:791-96, 1980.
17. Broviac JW, Cole JJ, Scribner BH: Silicone rubber atrial catheter for prolonged parenteral nutrition, *Surg Gynecol Obstet* 136:602-6, 1973.
18. Neu AM, Ho PL, McDonald R, Warady BA: Chronic dialysis in children and adolescents: The 2001 NAPRTCS Annual Report, *Pediatr Nephrol* 17:656-63, 2002.
19. Sheth RD, Brandt ML, Brewer ED, Nuchtern JG, Kale AS, Goldstein SL: Permanent hemodialysis vascular access survival in children and adolescents with end-stage renal disease, *Kidney Int* 62:1864-69, 2002.
20. Arbus GS, Sniderman S, Trusler GA: Long-term experience with fistulas in children on hemodialysis, *Clin Nephrol* 2:68-72, 1974.
21. Bourquelot P, Raynaud F, Pirozzi N: Microsurgery in children for creation of arteriovenous fistulas in renal and non-renal diseases, *Ther Apher Dial* 7(6):498-503, 2003.
22. National Kidney Foundation: *NKF-K/DOQI clinical practice guidelines for vascular access: Update 2000*. National Kidney Foundation–Kidney Disease Outcomes Quality Initiative, *Am J Kid Dis* 37: S137-S181, 2001.
23. USRDS: Excerpts from United States Renal Data System 1997 Annual Data Report, *Am J Kid Dis* 30:S1-S213, 1997.
24. Wander JV, Moore ES, Jonasson O: Internal arteriovenous fistulae for dialysis in children, *J Pediatr Surg* 5:533-38, 1970.
25. Gradman WS, Lerner G, Mentser M, Rodriguez H, Kamil ES: Experience with autogenous arteriovenous access for hemodialysis in children and adolescents, *Ann Vasc Surg* 19:609-12, 2005.

26. Segal JH, Kayler LK, Henke P, Merion RM, Leavey S, Campbell DA: Vascular access outcomes using the transposed basilic vein arteriovenous fisula, *Am J Kidney Dis* 42(1):151-57, 2003.
27. Taghizadeh A, Dasgupta P, Khan MS, Taylor J, Koffman G: Long-term outcomes of brachiobasilic transposition fistula for haemodialysis, *Eur J Vasc Endovasc Surg* 26(6):670-72, 2003.
28. Jennings WC: Creating arteriovenous fistulas in 132 consecutive patients, Arch Surg 141(1):27-32, 2006.
29. Roberts JK, Sideman MJ, Jennings WC: The difficult hemodialysis access extremity: Proximal radial arteriovenous fistulas and the role of angioscopy and valvutomes, *Am J Surg* 190:869-73, 2005.
30. Sreedhara R, Himmelfarb J, Lazarus M, Hakim R: Anti-platelet therapy in graft thrombosis: Results of a prospective, randomized double-blind study, *Kidney Int* 45:1477, 1994.
31. Pieptu D, Luchian S: Loupes-only microsurgery, *Microsurgery* 23:181-88, 2003.
32. Bourquelot P, Wolfeler L, Lamy L: Microsurgery for hemodialysis distal arteriovenous fistula in children weight less than 10 kg, *Proc Eur Dial Transplant Assoc* 18:537-41, 1981.
33. Bagolan P, Spagnoli A, Ciprandi G, Picca S, Leozappa G, Nahom A, et al: A ten-year experience of Brescia-Cimino arteriovenous fistula in children: technical evolution and refinements, *J Vasc Surg* 27:640-44, 1998.
34. Oliver, MJ: Chronic hemodialysis vascular access: Types and placement. *www.uptodate.com* 2006.
35. Brittinger WD, Walker G, Twittenhoff WED, Konrad N: Vascular access for hemodialysis in children, *Pediatr Nephrol* 11:87-95, 1997.
36. Robbin ML, Oser RF, Allon M: Hemodialysis access graft stenosis: US detection, *Radiology* 208:655, 1998.
37. Swedberg SH, Brown BG, Rigley R: Intimal fibromuscular hyperplasia at the venous anastamosis of PTFE grafts in hemodialysis patients: Clinical, immunocytochemical, light and electron microscopic assessment, *Circulation* 80:1726, 1989.
38. Chand DH, Poe SA, Strife CF: Venous pressure monitoring does not accurately predict access failure in children, *Pediatr Nephrol* 17(9):765-69, 2002.
39. Goldstein SL, Allsteadt A, Smith CM, Currier H: Proactive monitoring of pediatric hemodialysis vascular access: Effects of ultrasound dilution on thrombosis rates, *Kidney Int* 62(1):272-75, 2002.
40. Schwab SJ, Beathard G: The hemodialysis conundrum: Hate living with them, but can't live without them, *Kidney Int* 56:1-17, 1999.
41. Oliver MJ, Edwards LJ, Treleaven DJ: Randomized study of temporary hemodialysis catheters, *Int J Artif Organs* 25:40-44, 2002.
42. Cortez AJ, Paulson WD, Schwab SJ: Vascular access as a determinant of adequacy of dialysis, *Semin Nephrol* 25:96-101, 2005.
43. Sheth RD, Kale AS, Brewer ED, Brandt ML, Nuchtern JG, Goldstein SL: Successful use of Tesio catheters in pediatric patients receiving chronic hemodialysis, *Am J Kid Dis* 38(3):553-59, 2001.
44. Trerotola SO, Shah H, Johnson M, Namyslowski J, Moresko K, Patel N, et al: Randomized comparison of high-flow versus conventional hemodialysis catheters, *JVIR* 10:1032-38, 1999.
45. Schon D, Whittman D: Managing the complications of long-term tunneled dialysis catheters, *Semin Dial* 16(4):314-22, 2003.
46. Hoshal VJ, Ause RG, Hoskins PA: Fibrin sleeve formation on indwelling subclavian central venous catheters, *Arch Surg* 102:353-58, 1971.
47. Chand DH, Brier M, Strife CF: Comparison of vascular access type in pediatric hemodialysis patients with respect to urea clearance, anemia management, and serum albumin concentration, *Am J Kidney Dis* 45(2):303-8, 2005.
48. Leavey SF, Strawderman RL, Young EW: Cross sectional and longitudinal predictors of serum albumin in hemodialysis patients, *Kidney Int* 58:2119-28, 2000.
49. Goldstein SL: Hemodialysis catheter survival and complications in children and adolescents, *Pediatr Nephrol* 11(1):74-77, 1997.
50. Beathard GA, Posen GA: Initial clinical results with the LifeSite hemodialysis access system, *Kidney Int* 58:2221-27, 2000.
51. Canuad B, Levin N, Ing T, My H, Dubrow AJ, Polaschegg HD, et al: Dialock: Pilot trial of a new vascular port access device for hemodialysis, *Semin Dial* 12:382-88, 1999.
52. Moran J: Use of LifeSite hemodialysis access system improves blood flow and access patency. In Zwischenberger MD (editor), *ASIO Journal*. New York: American Society for Artificial Internal Organs (ASAIO) 2001.
53. Sands JJ: Increasing AV fistulas: re-visiting a time tested solution, *Semin Dial* 13:351-53, 2000.
54. Moran J: Subcutaneous vascular access devices, *Semin Dial* 14(6):452-57, 2001
55. Canaud B, My H, Morena M, Lamy-Lacavalerie B, Leray-Moragues H, Bosc JY, et al: Dialock: A new vascular access device for extracorporeal renal replacement therapy: Preliminary clinical results, *Nephrol Dial Transplant* 14:692-98, 1999.
56. Farrell J, Gellens M: Ultrasound-guided cannulation versus the landmark-guided technique for acute haemodialysis access, *Nephrol Dial Transplant* 12:1234-37, 1997.
57. Coulthard MG, Sharp J: Haemodialysing infants: Theoretical limitations, and single versus double lumen lines, *Pediatr Nephrol* 16:332-34, 2001.

CHAPTER

57 Pediatric Hemodialysis Prescription, Efficacy, and Outcome

Daljit K. Hothi and Denis F. Geary

EVOLUTION OF PEDIATRIC HEMODIALYSIS

Hemodialysis (HD) was introduced as a practical treatment for uremia by Willem Kolff at the end of the Second World War.[1] It was a decade later that Mateer and colleagues reported the first experience using HD to treat uremic children. These authors described HD in five children, aged 15 to 17 years, using a 50-foot (15.2 meters) cellophane tubing and a 32-liter dialysis bath (Figure 57-1). The duration of each procedure was as much as 13 hours, which improved the metabolic status of their patients and permitted satisfactory ultrafiltration (UF). The authors alluded to problems with heparinization of the circuit, and to potential adverse consequences related to changes in plasma calcium and potassium levels.[2]

They achieved blood access through cannulae placed in the radial artery, with blood return to the saphenous vein, for each procedure. This method of blood access was not suited to extended use, thereby preventing the use of maintenance HD as a practical therapeutic option on a sustained basis for children with chronic renal failure. This problem was overcome by Scribner and colleagues[3] by the development of silastic arteriovenous cannula inserted in the forearm vessels, which could be used for repeated blood access. What followed was the report by Dr. Fine and colleagues[4] describing the use of HD for maintenance treatment of end-stage renal disease (ESRD) in five adolescents.

Each of these children was dialyzed three times weekly for 7 to 8 hours each session, using a concentrated dialysis solution mixed with tap water to provide a physiologic solution. Blood flows averaged 160 ml/min, and produced mean urea clearances of 45 ml/min. This resulted in an average decrease of blood urea nitrogen (BUN) by 48% of the predialysis levels during each 7- to 8-hour dialysis session. It was now clearly possible to consider HD as a realistic option for maintenance treatment of children with chronic renal failure. However, difficulties persisted with this treatment in small children, and the need for prolonged treatment (as much as 20 hours per week) meant that these children spent long periods of time in the hospital.

In 1971, Kjellstrand and colleagues addressed some of these issues—reporting their experience treating 10 children who weighed less than 15 kg.[5] Based on the experience of adult dialysis, which commonly achieved 100 to 140 ml/min clearance of urea (approximately 2 ml/min/kg for a 50- to 70-kg adult), the authors suggested that the same principles should be applied to children and that urea clearance should be related to body weight. They recommended that a urea clearance of 2 to 3 ml/min/kg should be the goal for urea removal during a dialysis session. Multiplying this by the number of hours on dialysis ((Figure 57-2) allowed prediction of the expected fall in urea during that session. This formula established a standard for dialysis urea clearance in children, which is used in many dialysis units to the present day.

Despite the success of the Scribner shunt (allowing repeated blood access), it became apparent with experience that clotting and infection of these shunts were common problems. The introduction of arterovenous fistulae for blood access overcame this problem, and remains the gold standard for dialysis access. However, creation of fistulae in small children requires great surgical skill—as well as a critical mass of patients to maintain expertise, which is not readily available in many centers.

Because of these problems, and to avoid repeated needle punctures for small children, Mahan and colleagues described the use of a Hickman central venous catheter for prolonged HD vascular access in 26 small children.[6] Central venous catheters have rendered the Scribner shunt almost obsolete, and have become the most widely used HD access. Whereas these catheters have allowed many children to obtain puncture-free HD, and have been particularly useful in small infants, they have a high rate of clotting and infection and in our opinion should only be used for long-term access when it is not possible to create a suitable fistula.

The advances outlined previously have made HD available to many children. However, dialysis-related symptoms such as hypotension, nausea, and cramps as a result of imprecise fluid or solute removal persisted as prominent causes of morbidity. Improvements in dialysis equipment and processes (in particular the introduction of volumetric dialysis machines, sodium and UF profiles, and blood volume monitors) have greatly improved the accuracy of UF and solute clearance.[7,8] Despite this, it is still not uncommon for children on HD to

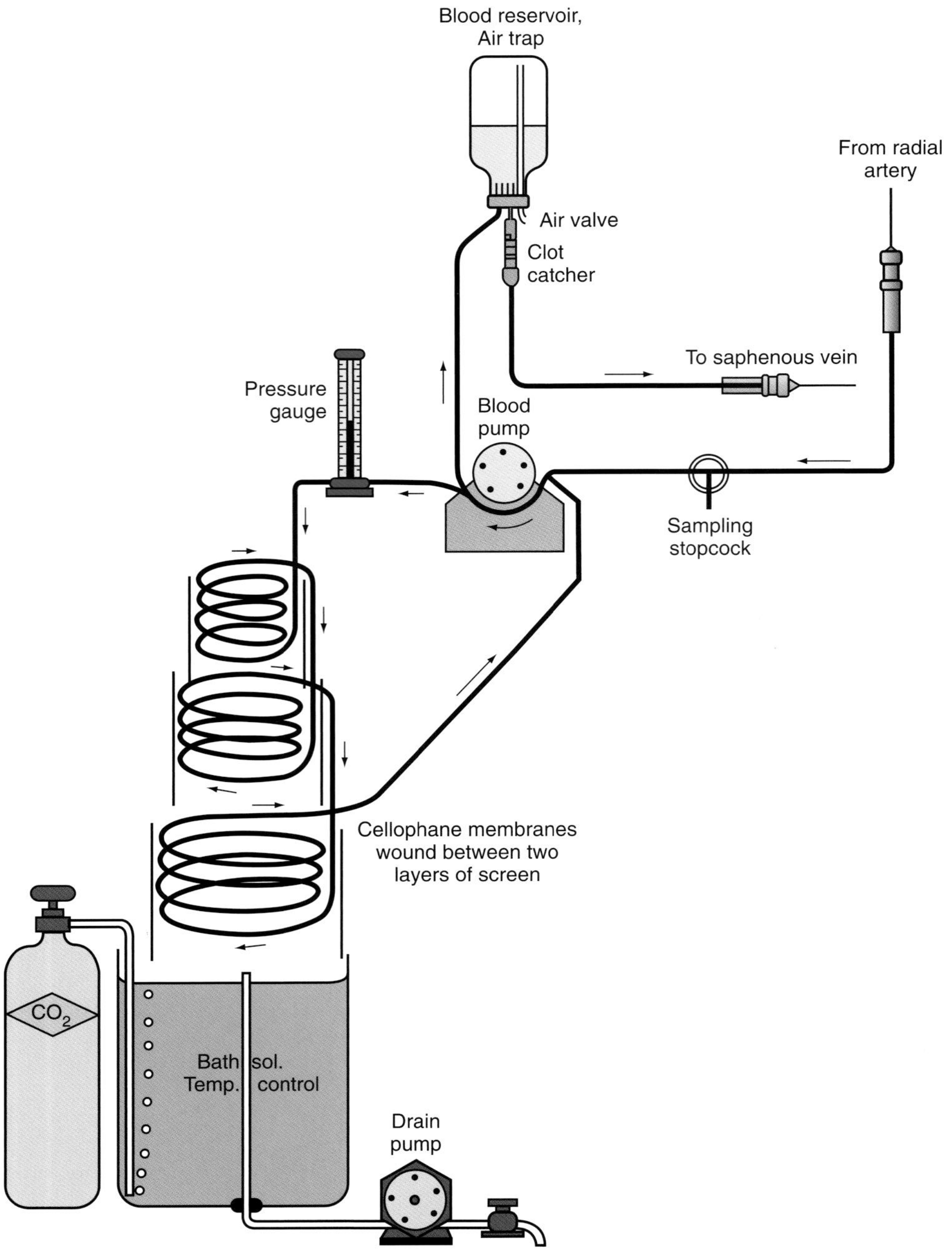

Figure 57-1 Diagrammatic representation of the artificial kidney used in these studies. The dialyzing membrane consists of 50 feet (15.2 m) of cellophane tubing flattened between cylinders of perforated stainless steel. (From Mateer FM, Greenman L, Danowski TS: Hemodialysis of the uremic child, *AMA Am J Dis Child* 89(6):645-55, 1955.)

experience headaches, nausea, hypotension, and muscle cramps.

Further technological improvements will continue to improve the HD experience, but it is unlikely that symptoms will be eliminated until the intermittent nature of HD is altered. In this regard, the major recent change in HD prescription has been the introduction of short daily or nocturnal dialysis—which improves well-being and mortality in adults.[9] Initial experiences with frequent or nocturnal HD, involving small numbers of children, described by Fischbach and colleagues[10] and by ourselves,[11] are very positive—although widespread application of this or similar methodology in children remains futuristic.

PRESCRIBING HEMODIALYSIS

Research in HD is dominated by adult data, with little data in pediatrics. In theory, the principles are universal and appli-

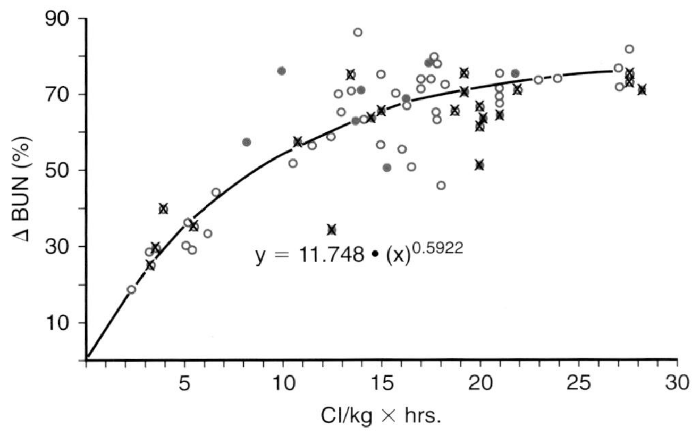

Curve	Correlation r	Correlation P
All observations	0.7933	<0.001
Dialysis <3 hr. (x)	0.7883	<0.001
BUN >50 mg% (o)	0.9016	<0.001
BUN <50 mg% (•)	0.2085	N.S.

Figure 57-2 Cl/Kg × Hrs related to Δ BUN (%). *Δ BUN (%)*, Fall in BUN with dialysis, expressed as a percentage of predialysis BUN; *Cl*, clearance of BUN across dialyzer during actual dialysis; *Kg*, patient's weight; *hrs*, length of dialysis. *BUN <50 mg%* and *BUN >50 mg%* relate to predialysis values. (From Kjellstrand CM, Shideman JR, Santiago EA, et al: Technical advances in hemodialysis of very small pediatric patients, *Proc Clin Dial Transplant Forum* 1:124-32, 1971.)

cable to children. However, adjustments are required to accommodate the spectrum of age, weight, and physiologic development specific to children.

ESTIMATION OF DRY WEIGHT

One of the primary objectives of HD is UF to a target estimated dry weight. Dry weight is most commonly defined as the post-HD weight at which the patient is as close to euvolemia without experiencing symptoms indicative of overhydration or underhydration at or after the end of HD. Overestimation of the dry weight places the patient at risk of developing volume-dependent hypertension, left ventricular hypertrophy, and congestive heart failure. An underestimation increases the risk of symptoms from intradialytic volume depletion. In children, growth and changes in lean body mass and body habitus necessitate regular and frequent reevaluation of the dry weight to detect subtle differences in the ratio of TBW to body mass. Therefore, tests for evaluating dry weight have to be easily accessible, reproducible, and ideally noninvasive.

Clinical Assessment

A clinical examination is the most widely used test for volume status. However, at best it only provides a crude assessment of volume status. Of greater concern, in the presence of ESRD and its comorbidities, even the most sensitive signs are rendered imprecise. For example, in dialysis patients as fluid is being removed there are a number of factors that can result in hypotension—and thus changes in orthostatic vital signs are not diagnostic of true hypovolemia. In the assessment of central venous pressure in adults, jugular venous distension is the only sign that has been found to be consistently useful, provided heart failure is absent.[12]

Biochemical Markers

Raised plasma atrial natriuretic peptide (ANP) levels correlate with increased plasma volume in renal failure.[13] However, levels can also remain elevated in volume-contracted individuals and hence it lacks the ability to detect volume depletion. Its second messenger [cyclic GMP (cGMP)] is more stable in serum at room temperature but offers no advantage over ANP and lacks specificity, particularly in patients with cardiac or valvular dysfunction. Brain natriuretic peptide (BNP) plasma concentrations are also elevated in patients who are volume overloaded and appears to be superior to ANP in predicting left ventricular hypertrophy and dysfunction and therefore provides useful prognostic information. However, in the context of defining dry weight results have been variable.[14]

Inferior Vena Cava Diameter

Ultrasound-guided supine inferior vena cava (IVC) diameter measurements and their decrease upon deep inspiration, better known as the collapse index (CI; formulated as follows) have been shown to correlate with right atrial pressure and circulating blood volume.

$$CI = [(\text{end expiratory IVC diameter} - \text{end inspiratory IVC diameter})/\text{end expiratory IVC diameter}] \times 100$$

Hypervolemia (defined as a mean right atrial pressure greater than 7 mm Hg) correlated with an IVC diameter greater than 11.5 mm/m^2 and a CI greater than 0.75 (i.e., decrease in IVC diameter during inspiration less than 25% of the baseline diameter during expiration). Conversely, hypovolemia (defined as mean right atrial pressure less than 3 mm Hg) correlated with an IVC diameter of less than 8.0 mm/m^2 and a CI less than 0.4 (i.e., decrease in IVC diameter greater than 60% of baseline).[15]

However, a wide interpatient variability of the normal values is reported in the literature, and no normal standards for children exist. Results are also influenced by the timing of the measurement after dialysis and are difficult to interpret in patients with heart failure or tricuspid regurgitation. As a result of these limitations, although it is a noninvasive test that could conceivably become available at most centers it cannot predict dry weight in children.

Bioelectric Impedance

Bioelectric impedance technology offers the potential to directly assess extracellular volume (ECV), intracellular volume (ICV), and total body water (TBW) by detecting differences in the degree of resistance (impedance) as electric currents pass through each compartment. At low frequencies, current cannot cross cell membranes and hence will only flow through ECV. At higher frequencies, it flows through both the ICV and ECV. Values can also be normalized using resistive indices accounting for differences in patients' lean body mass and bone mineral density, measured by dual-energy x-ray absorptiometry.[16] Three methods for assessing dry weight are currently in practice.

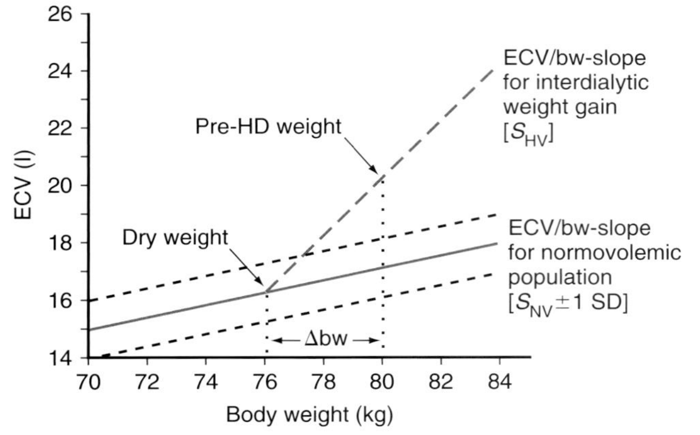

Figure 57-3 The normovolemia/hypervolemia slope model for prediction of dry weight from prehemodialysis *(HD)* extracellular volume *(ECV)* and body weight *(bw)*. At normal hydration state in healthy individuals, a linear relation exists between body weight and ECV (S_{NV} slope). During interdialytic weight gain (Δbw), ECV increases in a 1 : 1 relation with body weight (S_{HV} slope). Dry weight is defined as the weight at which the S_{NV} and S_{HV} slopes intersect. Model developed by Chamney and colleagues. (From Kuhlmann MK, Zhu F, Seibert E, Levin NW: Bioimpedance, dry weight and blood pressure control: New methods and consequences, *Curr Opin Nephrol Hypertens* 14:543-49, 2005.)

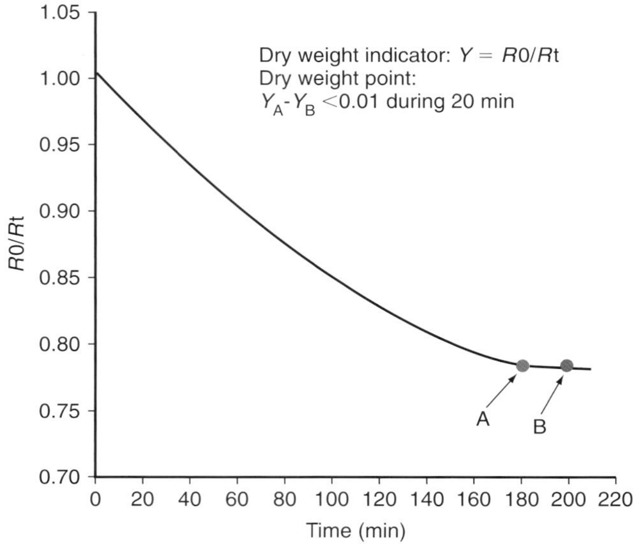

Figure 57-4 The R0/Rt curve reflects changes in calf extracellular volume *(ECV)* during ultrafiltration. Flattening of the curve occurs when all excess ECV has been removed from the calf and calf resistance remains stable for a defined time span (here, 20 minutes) despite ongoing ultrafiltration. The body weight at A is considered the individual dry weight. *(A)* beginning of curve flattening. *(B)* Twenty minutes after beginning of curve flattening. (From Kuhlmann MK, Zhu F, Seibert E, Levin NW: Bioimpedance, dry weight and blood pressure control: new methods and consequences, *Curr Opin Nephrol Hypertens* 14:543-49, 2005.)

The normovolemia/hypervolemia slope method uses whole-body multifrequency bioimpedance spectroscopy[17] to measure the ECV. It can predict the absolute dry weight by direct correlation of predialysis weight versus measured ECV to standard values from the normal adult population (Figure 57-3). Its use is limited because standard values for body weight versus ECV values are not available across the pediatric age range. In addition, inaccuracies are common because the standard values are derived from the normal population (not patients with ESRD) and because of the inherent underestimation of TBW with multifrequency bioimpedance methods.

The resistance-reactance graph method uses whole-body single-frequency bioimpedance analysis.[18] This simple technique is valid for TBW but is unable to separate ECV from ICV and therefore unable to differentiate between excessive body water and true weight gain. The continuous intradialytic calf bioimpedance method uses segmental Multi-frequency bioimpedance spectroscopy (MF-BIS).[19] Calf BIS (c-BIS) is recorded continuously during HD, and changes in extracellular resistance are displayed in real time in the form of a c-BIS curve. As excess ECV is removed, the slope of the c-BIS curve declines and eventually flattens. This is said to represent the point at which all excess ECV has been removed from the calf, and thus dry weight has been achieved (Figure 57-4). Premature flattening of the curve may occur in the presence of venous thrombosis or lymphatic edema. Changes in electrolyte, red cell, and protein concentrations and in patient temperature that commonly occur during HD are all known to influence bioimpedance. Finally, its applicability in pediatrics is unknown.

Noninvasive Blood Volume Monitors

Online noninvasive volume monitoring (NIVM) provides information on individual patients' intradialytic blood volume changes and vascular refilling rates. The magnitude of blood volume changes differs between patients and dialysis sessions. However, if NIVM is combined with postdialytic vascular compartment refilling rates a method of assessing dry weight is established. When refill is likely to occur, for the vast majority it will become evident within the first 10 minutes after stopping UF. This is seen as an increase in the relative blood volume (RBV), which can continue for up to 60 minutes. Reported experience with NIVM reports the ability to divide patients into the following four groups.

- Absence of postdialysis refilling, with no symptoms suggestive of intradialytic hypovolemia (nausea, vomiting, dizziness, cramps, hypotension, malaise) or postdialytic fatigue. The patient is likely to be at his or her dry weight.
- Postdialysis refill, lack of a substantial change in the RBV during HD, and no intradialytic or postdialytic symptoms. This is indicative of extracellular fluid expansion and the need to lower the patient's dry weight.
- Absence of postdialysis refill, intradialytic and/or postdialytic symptoms. This is indicative of hypovolemia and the need to increase the dry weight.
- Postdialysis refill but intradialytic symptoms of hypovolemia. This is indicative of slow vascular refilling rates, but ECV expansion at the end of dialysis. This suggests that the dry weight needs to be reduced incrementally and slowly following changes to the dialysis prescription to increase the UF potential.

Using these principles, Michael and colleagues reported the success of NIVM in determining the dry weight in pediatric HD patients.[20]

Evaluating a patient's dry weight can be a challenge. The limitations and benefits of the available tests for estimating

TABLE 57-1 **Summary of Methods for Assessing Dry Weight**

Modality	Pros	Cons
Biochemical markers	Ease of use; noninvasive	Wide variability; poor correlation with volume depletion; not available in most clinical laboratories; difficult to assess in patients with CHF
IVC diameter	Strong correlation with right heart catheterization, reflecting intravascular volume; noninvasive	Best timing after HD not defined; no normative values for children; *must train skilled technicians; cost; limited availability
Bioimpedance	Measures ECFV and ICFV, thus estimates fluid shifts from various compartments; strongly correlates with ultrafiltration volume in HD	Underestimates volume shifts from trunk; best timing after HD not defined; limited normative values for children*; cost
Blood volume monitoring	Easy to use and interpret; real-time monitoring; decreases intradialytic hypotensive events in chronic HD patients; application and value validated in children*	No standardization; requires active interventions by HD nurses; only measures shifts from intravascular space and its refilling rate; cost

CHF, Congestive heart failure; *HD*, hemodialysis; *ECFV*, extracellular fluid volume; *ICFV*, intracellular fluid volume.
* Comments added to original by Hothi and Geary.
Source: Ishibe S, Peixoto AJ: Methods of assessment of volume status and intercompartmental fluid shifts in hemodialysis patients: Implications in clinical practice, *Semin Dial* 17(1):37-43, 2004.

dry weight are summarized in Table 57-1. As of yet, no gold standard has been defined—and for the majority the applicability of estimating dry weight in pediatrics has not been validated. We recommend the use of blood volume monitoring (BVM) combined with clinical assessment.

BLOOD FLOW RATE

Blood flow rate is a major determinant of solute clearance on dialysis. With increased blood flow, more solute is delivered to the dialyzer—resulting in higher dialyzer clearance ("flow-limited clearance"). However, the clearance achieved is also determined by the membrane's permeability to the solute ("membrane-limited clearance"). Therefore, with poorly permeable solutes, increasing the blood flow will only produce a mild increase in clearance (Figure 57-5). The dialyzer flow clearance is limited and starts leveling off at blood flows of 250 to 300 ml/min, and therefore some adult dialysis units have set this as their maximum blood flow rate.

More so in pediatrics than in adults the effective blood flow rate is largely determined by the vascular access. For chronic HD, we would recommend a blood flow rate equivalent to 4 to 6 ml/kg/min urea clearance obtained from dialyzer urea clearance estimates provided by the manufacturers. In infants, this should be a minimum of 20 ml/min to avoid the risk of clotting the circuit. Effective blood flows are often lower than those prescribed due to factors such as partially occlusive pumps, malposition of the vascular access needle, access failure, tubing diameter changes, and shear effects.

Efficacy of dialysis is also reduced by recirculation effects, which are more pronounced with higher dialyzer blood flow, vascular access inflows lower than dialyzer blood flow, stenosis at the access outflow, single-lumen access (particularly with small stroke volumes), increased length of blood lines, and small needle and tubing diameter.[21,22] This places infants with blood flows determined by small high-resistance double-lumen central venous catheters or single-lumen catheters with high recirculation rates at the highest risk of inadequate dialysis with conventional dialysis regimens. This can be improved by increasing the dialysis time, which in our experience is best tolerated by increasing the frequency (*not* duration) of treatment.

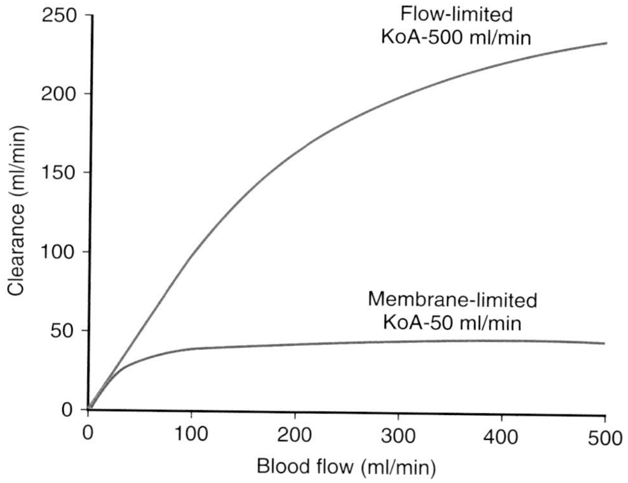

Figure 57-5 Effect of dialyzer blood flow on clearance. When solute permeability, expressed as the mass transfer coefficient (KoA), is high, clearance is highly dependent on blood flow (as shown in the upper curve). When permeability is low, as shown in the lower curve, the dependency on flow disappears. (From Depner TA: *Prescribing hemodialysis: A guide to urea modeling*. Boston: Kluwer Academic Publishers 44:186, 1991.)

EXTRACORPOREAL CIRCUIT

During pediatric dialysis, the total volume of the extracorporeal circuit volume is an important consideration. If this is greater than 10% of the estimated total blood volume (TBV), a circuit prime with 5% albumin or blood is recommended. Even though traditionally blood is preferred, we must remind ourselves that these recommendations come from an era when severe anemia was the rule for children with chronic renal failure. The TBV is approximately equal to 100 ml/kg body weight in neonates (less than 1 month of age) and 80 ml/kg body weight for infants and children up to 16 years of age.

As a general rule, we use blood primes if the patient is anemic. To avoid the risk of clotting the circuit, we suggest priming with packed red blood cells diluted with normal saline to achieve a final hematocrit of 30% to 35%. The potassium load to the patient can be minimized by using fresh blood, and once priming is completed by recirculating the blood through the dialyzer for 10 minutes without connecting to the patient. At the end of dialysis, we do not recommend retransfusing the blood back into the infant. However, if a blood transfusion is required, this should be given as undiluted packed red blood cells during the dialysis session—infused through a peripheral line or via a Y-connection at the venous return site to reduce the possibility of clotting the circuit.

DIALYSIS FLOW RATE

Typically, rates of 300 to 500 ml/min are employed during dialysis. During infant dialysis, even with such blood flow rates the practice within our unit is to start with a dialysate flow rate of 300 ml/min. If clearance is inadequate, increasing the dialysate flow rate can produce improvements. However, the additional benefit eventually plateaus. The Hemodialysis (HEMO) Study provided in vivo confirmation of increased hemodialyzer mass transfer area coefficients (KoA) for urea at high dialysate flow rates.[23] A subsequent study showed that the relative gains in Kt/V (single pool) for increasing the dialysate flow rate from 300 to 500 ml/min and 500 to 800 ml/min were shown to be 11.7% ± 8.7% and 9.9% ± 5.1%, respectively.[24]

DIALYSATE TEMPERATURE

By modifying skin blood flow, we can control heat exchange between the body and the environment. This is mediated by two sympathetic nervous system effects: an adrenergic vasoconstrictor and a less well understood sympathetic vasodilator. During times of increased body core temperature, tonic sympathetic vasoconstriction is relaxed, active vasodilatation is initiated,[25] and the skin blood flow rate can increase from a baseline of 5% to 10% of the total body cardiac output to approximately 60% of cardiac output.[26,27]

Traditionally, dialysate temperatures have been set at ≥37° C based on presumed physiologic normal values and to compensate for losses of heat in the extracorporeal circuit. Both of these assumptions have in fact been found to be untrue. In a study of HD patients, 62.5% of 128 HD adult patients had a predialysis body temperature below 36.5° C, with marked interindividual and intraindividual differences.[28] There is growing evidence in both adults and children of a net gain rather than loss of heat during dialysis. This is the result of higher resting energy expenditure in HD patients compared to the normal population, especially in those with residual renal function.[29]

Second, UF activates sympathetic vasoconstriction, thereby reducing skin blood flow and heat exchange, with a direct correlation between UF volume and net heat gain.[30] If the accumulation of heat causes an increase in body core temperature, UF-induced vasoconstriction is overridden by active vasodilatation. Blood is redistributed to the skin[31] and the peripheral vascular resistance falls, causing decreased cardiac refilling and hypotension. Fine and Penner[28] showed that dialysis patients with subnormal body temperature (below 36° C) dialyzed against a 37° C dialysate had a 15.9% incidence of symptomatic hypotensive episodes, which fell to 3.4% with 35° C dialysate.

The hemodynamic advantage of "cool" HD has been documented but may be uncomfortable for patients and adversely affect urea clearance as a result of compartmental dysequilibrium. Application of thermoneutral (no gain or removal of thermal energy from the extracorporeal circuit) and isothermic (patient temperature is kept constant) dialysis is technically possible, but the dialysis circuit has to be adapted to accommodate a feedback control circuit. A more practical option is to individualize the dialysate temperature based on the patient's predialysis temperature. Even then, efforts may be hampered by the current standards of the Association for the Advancement of Medical Instrumentation (AAMI)—which require that the dialysate temperature at the dialyzer be maintained only within ±1.5° C of its set point value.

Given their increased susceptibility to hypothermia, infants are typically dialyzed against higher dialysate temperatures of 37.5° C to 38° C in combination with external warming strategies. The impact this has on thermal balance and cardiovascular stability has not been studied. From a theoretical stand point it is conceivable that dialysis efficacy, and quality may be improved by using more physiologic dialysate temperatures with the use of external warming methods prior to the dialysate temperatures to maintain normothermia.

ANTICOAGULATION

Anticoagulation of the extracorporeal circuit is not essential but often necessary to prevent clotting of the circuit, which in turn results in blood loss and reduced dialysis efficacy. In pediatrics, unfractionated heparin (UFH) is primarily used to provide systemic anticoagulation. However, in adults the use of other agents [such as low-molecular-weight heparin (LMWH) and citrate] is gaining popularity.

Unfractionated Heparin

UFH consists of a mixture of polyanionic branched glycosaminoglycans with a high affinity for antithrombin that induces a structural change that converts it from a slowly to a very rapidly (1000 times) acting inhibitor of thrombin. In addition, UFH inhibits fibrin formation and thrombin-induced platelet activation and increases vessel wall permeability. Its polyanionic property allows it to bind nonselectively to other proteins and cell membranes, thus mediating many undesired actions (such as activation of lipoprotein lipase causing increased generation of free fatty acids, inducing platelet aggregation at high doses, and with prolonged treatment osteoporotic fractures due to bone loss).[32,33]

UFH prescription is through an intravenous route, but a bolus injection is necessary to saturate the the nonspecific receptors that bind with plasma proteins. Failure to administer this injection can reduce the anticoagulatory bioavailability to approximately 30%. Following this initial bolus, the dose-response relationship is almost linear. Heparin is metabolized by the liver, and the kidney is responsible for clearing the desulfated end products. However, there is a marked interindividual sensitivity to heparin and therefore it is essential to individualize heparin requirements during dialysis and repeatedly review dosing needs.

There is no agreed concensus on the level of anticoagulation required for optimal anticoagulation of the extracorporeal circuit and practices vary from 25% to 300% above baseline. The final decision rests on an evalution of the risk of bleeding against that of clotting. The risk of clotting is inversely related to the dialysis blood flow rate and is higher in less biocompatible dialyzers (such as cuprophane membranes) because they are associated with increased platelet activation. The consequences of bleeding are greater in infants, and the risks are higher in children with comorbidities such as synthetic liver disease, hypersplenism associated with pancytopenia, and bleeding disorders. In our unit, we use an activated clotting time (ACT) 50% above the baseline and achieve adequate anticoagulation for the majority of patients. Our standard prescription consists of a bolus dose of 15 to 20 u/kg of heparin at the start of dialysis, followed by a continuous infusion of 15 to 20 u/kg/hour (which is stopped 30 minutes before the end of dialysis).

Heparin-Induced Thrombocytopenia

Heparin-induced thrombocytopenia (HIT) is uncommon in children but is a diagnosis that should be considered in children with deteriorating platelet counts. It is an antibody-mediated activation of platelets that causes platelet activation and subsequent risk of thromboembolic events. It is characterized by markedly increased thrombin levels, heparin-dependent IgG antibodies, and thrombocytopenia. In the presence of HIT, an alternative method of anticoagulation is necessary. Several alternatives are commercially available but only danaparoid sodium use has been reported in pediatric HD, with stabilization of both the thrombocytopenia and thromboembolic events.[34]

However, owing to a 30% cross-reactivity with platelet-heparin antibodies the net benefit can be limited.[35] Hirudin, a direct thrombin inhibitor, provides effective anticoagulation but has a prolonged half-life in renal failure and can be associated with anaphylactic reactions.[36,37] The most promising agent is argatroban, a synthetic direct thrombin inhibitor that has a rapid onset of action, a half-life ranging from 39 to 51 minutes, and hepatic metabolism. Argatroban therefore requires no dose adjustment in dialysis patients and only a 20% systemic clearance is seen even with high-flux dialyzers.

Citrate

Citrate exerts its anticoagulant effect by chelating ionized calcium ions, thus preventing activation of calcium-dependent procoagulants. It is unique in its ability to provide "regional anticoagulation," which is anticoagulation of the extracorporeal circuit without systemic effects. This is achieved by infusing citrate solution through the arterial limb of the circuit, citrate clearance during dialysis, and neutralization of any remaining citrate by infusing ionized calcium into the venous limb of the circuit. This makes it a very attractive option for patients with a bleeding risk.

Citrate is a small molecule and is dialyzable, with an extraction coefficient similar to that of urea. Any citrate that escapes into the systemic circulation is rapidly cleared by the tricarboxylic acid pathway in liver and skeletal muscle. Ineffective clearance during dialysis or poor hepatic metabolism can result in citrate toxicity and is diagnosed biochemically by an increased anion gap acidosis and high total plasma calcium combined with low plasma ionized calcium. Citrate dialysis can also be complicated by hypocalcemia, causing arrhythmias and paresthesias, hypernatremia and volume expansion, and metabolic alkalosis (one molecule of trisodium citrate is metabolized to three molecules of bicarbonate).

The use of citrate as an anticoagulant in HD is not a novel therapy but is not widely employed as a routine therapy because it is technically very demanding. However, in light of recent evidence reporting its antimicrobial and antiinflammatory effects[38] it is very difficult to dismiss it outright. Expertise of citrate use in pediatrics is growing through its application in plasmapharesis and continuous renal replacement therapy. Nonetheless, until protocols are simplified and validated in children it cannot presently be seen as an alternative to heparin for routine dialysis therapy.

Low-Molecular-Weight Heparin

LMWH are smaller molecules prepared from UFH through enzymatic or chemical depolymerization. They differ from heparin in the fact that their main anticoagulatory action is through the inhibition of factor Xa, with a variable degree of thrombin inactivation. Again, differences in interindividual sensitivity exist. Therefore, fixed dosing is inappropriate despite the fact that bioavailability following a single subcutaneous injection reaches 100%. Furthermore, LMWH clearance is principally by the kidney, and therefore in ESRD the drug's pharmacokinetics become unpredictable.

LMWH can achieve a sustained intradialytic anticoagulation following a single bolus at the start of dialysis and therefore represents an extremely simple method of anticoagulation. In addition, the negative charge of the LMWH complexes make them impermeable across dialysis membranes and therefore in spite of their low molecular weight clearance by HD or hemofiltration is insignificant.[39,40] One metaanalysis comparing the safety and efficacy of LMWH with UFH found no differences in the incidence of extracorporeal thrombosis and reported a comparable risk of bleeding.[41]

The convenience of single-bolus administration of LMWHs makes them an attractive option in busy large-numbered adult dialysis units. However, in children concerns of their prolonged half-life and lack of a commercially available antidote are restricting their use. Therefore, without the evidence of an anticoagulation advantage over UFH and the lack of pediatric safety data we cannot presently advocate routine use of LMWHs in children.

Infants

In children weighing less than 10 kg, the increased likelihood of clotting has to be weighted against the detrimental effects of a bleed. Tighter control of the degree of anticoagulation can be achieved with lower ACT target ranges using tight heparin regimens[42] (Figure 57-6).

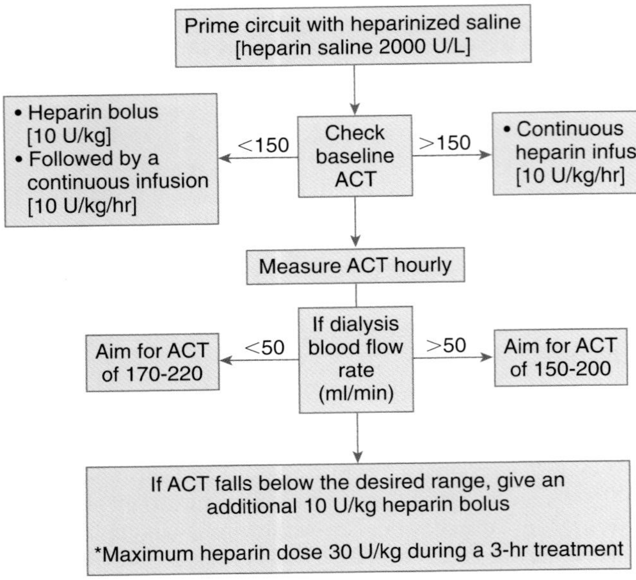

Figure 57-6 Tight heparin regimen.

Bleeding Tendency

In high-risk groups there is a 10% to 30% risk of bleeding with UFH. Alternative options include regional anticoagulation with citrate, use of prostacyclin infusion, high–flow-rate HD, and modification of the standard heparin regimen. In our experience, low-dose heparin or heparin-free dialysis combined with regular intermittent saline flushes has been effective in providing adequate anticoagulation of the extracorporeal circuit without causing bleeding complications.[42]

The choice of dialyzer can also influence the anticoagulatory requirement of the circuit. Use of more biocompatible circuits causes less platelet activation and can reduce the risk of clotting. Alternatively, new dialyzer membranes that provide a source of anticoagulant within the circuit are now available, such as the modified AN69 polyacrylonitrile membrane that binds UFH. We have no personal experience with such dialyzers.

DIALYSATE COMPOSITION

Dialysate content may be adjusted to address specific therapeutic needs.

Sodium

Following a sodium load, even in the presence of renal failure the mechanisms responsible for preserving plasma tonicity will maintain plasma sodium within narrow limits by changing the plasma volume. During HD, dialysate sodium generates a crystalloid osmotic pressure and thus influences fluid shift between the various body compartments. However, it also permeates the dialysis membrane and thus has the potential for becoming a sodium load.

One of the primary objectives of HD is the removal of the sodium and fluid gained in the interdialytic period. Sodium is predominantly cleared by convection with the excess water. Pure UF has approximately the same sodium concentration as plasma and therefore there is no net change in a patient's plasma sodium concentration. Diffusive sodium transport is proportional to the difference in sodium activity between blood and dialysate compartments. Dialysate sodium activity is approximately equal to 97% of the measured sodium concentration, but varies with changes in dialysate temperature, pH, and the presence of additional ions.

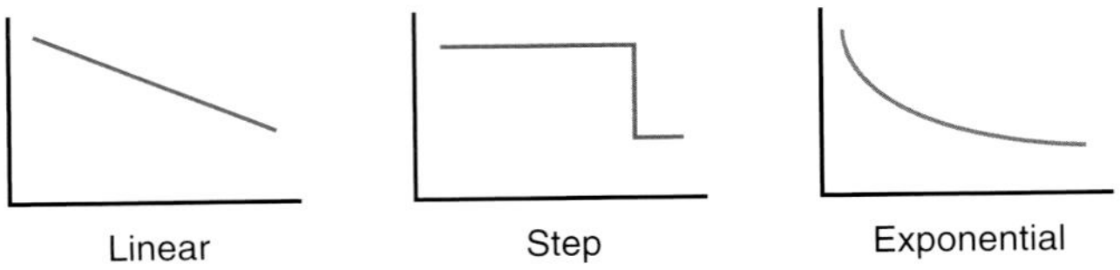

Figure 57-7 Sodium profiling methods.

The concentration of free sodium ions in plasma water, unbound to protein and other anions, can be measured by direct ionometry. This sodium value will be higher than the plasma sodium values from most clinical laboratories. Clinical laboratories report sodium as a concentration in total plasma, rather than plasma water, which makes up only 94% of total plasma. Plasma sodium activity is influenced by the Donnan effect: negatively charged proteins (mainly albumin) produce a small electrical potential difference across the membrane (negative on the plasma side) that prevents movement of the positively charged sodium ions. Concentration differences between interstitium and plasma also stem from the Donnan effect. In the absence of UF, we can approximate the concentration of dialysate sodium to achieve isotonic dialysis by correcting the blood sodium measured by direct ionometry for a Donnan factor of 0.967. However, for plasma sodium values reported from clinical laboratories (which are lower than those by direct ionometry because of dilution in whole plasma) a value of dialysate sodium approximately equal to the plasma value will correct for the Donnan effect, and provide isonatric dialysis.[45]

Hyponatric dialysis causes osmotic fluid shift from the extracellular to intracellular compartment, contributing to dialysis disequilibrium disorder and intradialytic hypotension. Hypernatric dialysis transfers sodium to the patient, causing interstitial edema, interdialytic thirst, increased interdialytic weight gain, and worsening hypertension. A therapeutic advantage can be gained by manipulating the dialysate sodium concentration throughout dialysis. This is referred to as sodium profiling, and typically utilizes a sodium concen-tration that falls in a step, linear, or exponential fashion (Figure 57-7).

The higher dialysate sodium at the start allows a diffusive sodium influx to counterbalance the rapid decline in plasma osmolarity due to clearance of urea and other low-molecular-weight solutes. Low dialysate sodium at the end aids diffusive clearance of the sodium load and minimizes hypertonicity. Compared to a constant dialysate sodium bath, modeling has been shown to increase stability of intradialytic blood volume and to reduce intradialytic cramps and interdialytic fatigue in children[43] and adults.[44] Outcomes have been better with the linear and step profiles compared with exponential. Step profiles are most effective at attenuating postdialytic hypotension and early intradialytic hypotension. Linear profiles best reduce cramps and late intradialytic hypotension. Sodium profiling is also indicated in the prevention of dialysis dysequilibrium.

The difficulty with sodium profiling is finding the concentration gradient that offers the benefits of cardiovascular stability without exposing the patient to a small but repeated sodium load. A net sodium gain of 1 mmol/L will result in a 1.3% expansion of the extracellular space. If there are concerns about inducing hypervolemia, neutral sodium balance profiles may be preferred using isonatic dialysate. Reported benefits are similar to those described with sodium profiling, but with a significant decrease in the interdialytic weight gain and thirst score.[46,47] This difference is likely due to an improvement of sodium balance. Nonetheless, monitoring for changes in interdialytic weight gain and blood pressure is still recommended.

Potassium

Patients are typically dialyzed against a potassium bath of 1 to 2 mmol/L. In severe hyperkalemia, a lower dialysate potassium concentration of 0 to 1 mmol/L is necessary—and if predialysis serum potassium levels are normal a potassium bath of 3 to 4 mmol/L may be required. Potassium clearance is influenced by a number of factors, including acid/base status, tonicity, glucose, insulin concentration, and catecholamine activity.[48] As a consequence, there is a wide variability in the total amount removed.

The rate of potassium removal is high at the start of dialysis, which then declines as the plasma potassium falls. The risks of arrhythmia, QT dispersion,[49] and ventricular ectopic beats are increased with hypokalemia. This risk is further increased if the rate of decline is rapid early in dialysis, even if the actual plasma potassium levels are normal. Conversely, failure to normalize serum potassium levels is also arrhythmogenic.[50] The use of potassium profiles for a slow gradual reduction of plasma potassium to within the normal range has been used in adult patients with underlying heart conditions. Profiles have been successful for reducing the number of premature ventricular complexes per hour by 36% without an adverse effect on predialysis serum potassium levels.[51] However, this did not translate into an overall survival advantage. Potassium profiles are not readily available and the potential benefits have not been demonstrated in children.

There is weak evidence linking hypokalemia with rebound hypertension. Comparing concentrations of dialysate potassium, there was an increased risk of intradialytic hypertension with 1- and 2-mmol/L baths but not with the 3-mmol/L potassium bath.[52] Thus, gentler potassium clearance may be useful in those prone to intradialytic hypertension.

Acetate versus Bicarbonate

Acetate was originally used as the buffer in dialysate because it was inexpensive, offered equimolar conversion to HCO_3, and was bacteriostatic. However, 10% of patients (especially women) are poor metabolizers of acetate. The high plasma acetate levels led to impaired lipid and ketone acid metabolism, vasodilatation, depressed left ventricular function, intradialytic hypotension, and hypoxemia—particularly in the first hour.[53] Consequently, most centers switched to sodium bicarbonate.

The preparation of bicarbonate-based dialysate requires a second proportioning pump that mixes solution or dry powder bicarbonate with water, and an "acid" compartment containing a small amount of acetate or lactate, sodium, potassium, calcium, magnesium, chloride, and glucose. During the mixing procedure, the acid in the acid concentrate reacts with an equimolar amount of bicarbonate to generate carbonic acid and carbon dioxide. The generation of carbon dioxide causes the final solution pH to fall to approximately 7 to 7.4. It is this lower pH with the lower concentrations of calcium and magnesium that prevents precipitation from occurring in the final solution. Often, cartridge systems containing pure dry sodium bicarbonate powder are preferred because they are less conducive to bacterial growth and because liquid bicarbonate has to be used within 8 hours of opening the container to avoid significant bicarbonate loss.

Ordinarily, dialysis corrects the metabolic acidosis of ESRD by the removal of organic anions and restoration of the bicarbonate deficit. Plasma bicarbonate levels rise by 4 to 5 mmol/L and then fall to predialysis levels by 48 hours. The adjusted survival of HD patients decreases with predialysis serum bicarbonate levels less than 18 mmol/L and greater than 24 mmol/L,[54] suggesting a U-shaped correlation with mortality. The severity of metabolic acidosis also correlates with bone disease,[55] muscle wasting,[56] and beta-2 microglobulin levels in chronic renal failure.[57]

With standard dialysate bicarbonate concentrations of 35 mmol/L, the HEMO study showed that 25% of patients had predialysis levels below 19 mmol/L.[58] Furthermore with increasing sevelamer use, these figures may underestimate the number of untreated patients. Increasing the dialysate bicarbonate concentration to 39 to 40 mmol/L will improve predialysis bicarbonate levels, but in some may result in a transient alkalosis. This has a hypothetical risk of facilitating calcific uremic arteriolopathy and intradialytic vascular instability by causing a sudden drop in plasma potassium and calcium levels.

A lower bicarbonate concentration may be required in patients with concurrent respiratory disease if they present with a mixed metabolic acidosis and respiratory alkalosis (high pH, low pCO_2). With the use of a standard bicarbonate dialysate solution, the transfer of bicarbonate will correct the metabolic acidosis and cause an acute rise in serum pH. This may induce cardiac arrhythmias and an encephalopathy from decreased cerebral perfusion.

The dialysate bicarbonate can be adjusted to help manage other biochemical abnormalities. Alkalosis has been shown to increase phosphate clearance, and in patients with dangerously high serum potassium levels this can result in a rapid fall in potassium levels. Acidosis results in a slower rate of decline in potassium levels but offers the benefit of a reduced rebound effect.[59]

Finally, on a more experimental level the use of citric acid in place of acetic acid in the dialysate acid concentrate was shown to improve acidosis and delivered dose of dialysis.[60] The role of citrate is expanding in the dialysis community. However, caution is advised because it increases aluminium absorption and therefore plasma aluminum levels must be monitored.

Calcium

Owing to fear of inducing extraskeletal calcium deposition, the K/DOQI guidelines suggest maintaining plasma calcium levels in the low normal range. Using a dialysate calcium concentation of 1.25 mmol/L permits higher doses of vitamin-D–based and calcium-based phosphate binders in the management of hyperparathyroidism. In a proportion of patients, this can lead to hypocalcemia and become the stimulus for worsening hyperparathyroidism.[61]

Hypocalcemia also depresses myocardial contractility and reduced vascular reactivity,[62] and thus increases the risk of intradialytic hypotension. These are both indications for the short-term use of a higher-calcium bath. In our experience, the only situation requiring routine use of 1.5-mmol/L calcium baths is with nocturnal HD patients due to reduced need for calcium-containing phosphate binders and increased calcium clearance.[63]

Phosphate

The factors that limit the removal of excessive phosphate are dialysis clearance and the kinetics of phosphate distribution within the body. Phosphate is the major anion in the intracellular compartment, and the steep gradient between the intracellular and extracellular compartments is maintained by active carrier systems. During dialysis, plasma phosphate levels initially fall but thereafter plateau or increase—with a postdialysis rebound effect persisting for up to 4 hours.[64] The implication is slow mobilization of phosphate from bone and intracellular stores and the generation of phosphate triggered by falling extracellular[65] or intracellular levels.[66] The point at which phosphate generation is initiated appears to correlate with predialysis phosphate levels. There is also evidence of a "switching on" effect to protect against critically low intracellular phosphate levels.

In spite of these challenges, phosphate purification can be improved with higher bicarbonate dialysis and by quotidian dialysis. We have shown a significant reduction in the predialysis phosphate level in four adolescents on home nocturnal HD (five to six times per week; 6 to 8 hours per session), allowing complete freedom of dietary restrictions and phosphate binders.[63] In all the patients, similar to experiences in adults,[9] it was necessary to add phosphate to the dialysate to prevent hypophosphatemia. A good source of phosphate is fleet enema (CB Fleet Co., Lynchburg, VA), which contains 43 mg/ml phosphorous and 37 mg/ml Na. To avoid calcium phosphate precipitation, this must be added to the bicarbonate component of a dual proportioning system.[63] The other situation when phosphate may be required is in severely malnourished children who develop hypophosphatemia secondary to refeeding syndrome.

Magnesium

Typically, the concentration of magnesium in dialysate is 0.5 to 1 mmol/L. If magnesium-containing phosphate binders are used, a lower concentration may be required to avoid hypermagnesemia. Conversely, low magnesium levels can result in cramping and arrhythmias—and therefore higher magnesium baths may help to improve cardiovascular stability and intradialytic symptoms.

Glucose

Glucose concentration of dialysate usually approximates 100 to 200 mg/dl (6-11 mmol/L). This level of glucose should ensure that patients remain normoglycemic unless hyperglycemic or hypoglycemic at the start. If hyperglycemic, a dialysate glucose in the recommended range will remove glucose—and if the patient is hypoglycemic the dialysate will provide supplemental glucose. There is a theoretical risk of inducing hypertriglyceridemia by addition of glucose to dialysate, but this should not be significant with dialysate values of 100 to 200 mg/dl. If the patient is hyperkalemic, less potassium might be removed if the dialysate glucose is elevated as a result of hyperinsulinemia, which pushes potassium into cells. Again, as a general rule, this should not be a problem with the dialysate glucose levels recommended.

INTRADIALYTIC NUTRITION

During fluid removal from the vascular compartment, a number of compensatory mechanisms maintain the central blood volume. Venoconstriction of the splanchnic bed[67] (and possibly the splenic[68] vascular bed) mobilizes blood, forcing it centrally toward the heart to maintain cardiac refilling; this is counterproductive, and therefore food consumption may need to be limited. If food is consumed during dialysis, blood is diverted to the splanchnic circulation. In patients prone to intradialytic hypotension, this is counterproductive and should be limited. In addition, fluids ingested have to be included in the gross UF to be removed. However, for the majority eating during dialysis offers an opportunity to consume restricted foods. Anecdotally, these controlled treats help to improve overall adherence to dietary restrictions.

Intradialytic total parenteral nutrition (TPN) is an alternative method of providing calories and protein to undernourished patients during HD via venous access. For further details, we refer the reader to the chapter on nutrition. This impacts the dialysis treatment because it also increases the gross UF volume. In our experience, the UF goal is best achieved by utilizing a constant UF rate because it parallels the infusion of TPN into the vascular space.

DIALYSATE QUALITY

National quality standards for the water used to prepare dialysate and the effluent dialysate have been set, but the criteria are different around the world (Table 57-2). Dialysate contaminants can be both chemical and biologic in nature, and can cause significant morbidity (Table 57-3). It is therefore imperative that each dialysis unit ensures that disinfection practices are in place to achieve these standards, combined with regular surveillance to ensure that they are sustained.

In recent years, the emphasis has been drifting toward the use of ultrapure dialysate. Dialysate quality is known to be an important component of the biocompatibility of the HD procedure and is therefore a contributor to the chronic inflammation of dialysis.[69] In vitro studies have shown that bacterial products can cross both high-flux and low-flux dialysis membranes and stimulate synthesis of inflammatory mediators such as cytokines within the blood compartment.[70,71] The degree of cytokine stimulation is related to the concentration of endotoxin and other "cytokine-induced substances" in the dialysate compartment[72,73] and to the permeability of the dialysis membranes to these substances.

TABLE 57-2 Upper Limits for Bacteria and Endotoxin in Water and Dialysate Used for Hemodialysis

	WATER		DIALYSATE	
	Bacteria (CFU/ml)	Endotoxin (EU/ml)	Bacteria (CFU/ml)	Endotoxin (EU/ml)
AAMI, RDF:1981	200	NS	2000	NS
AAMI, RD62:2001	200	2	NS	NS
AAMI, proposed	NS	NS	200	2
ERA-EDTA, best practice guidelines	100	0.25	100*	0.25*
European pharmacopoeia	100	0.25	NS	NS
Swedish pharmacopoeia	100	0.25	100	0.25
Ultrapure	0.1	0.3	0.1	0.3

AAMI, Association for Advancement of Medical Instrumentation; *NS*, not specified.
* Implied.
Source: Ward RA: Ultrapure dialysate, *Semin Dial* 17(6):489-97, 2004.

TABLE 57-3 Water Contaminants and Associated Complications*

Dissolved Organic Material	Complications
Contaminants	
Pesticides, herbicides	• No documentation during dialysis
Chloramines, chlorine compounds	• Severe hemolytic anemia
Bacteria and pyrogens	
Bacteria	• Bacteremia or septicemia • Fever, chills, shaking • Hypotension and death
Pyrogens	• Pyrogenic reaction-fever • Chills, uncontrollable • Shaking, vomiting, hypotension

* Not exhaustive.
Source: Fischbach M, Edefonti A, Schroder C, Watson A for the European Pediatric Dialysis Working Group: Hemodialysis in children: General practical guidelines, *Pediatr Nephrol* 20(8):1054-66, 2005.

TABLE 57-4 Dialysis Membranes: Practical Parameters of Choice

Membrane surface area to match body surface area of patient: Influences priming blood volume requirement
Type of membrane: Biocompatibility toward complement system
Solute permeability: Maximum clearance for urea and the other uremic toxins (e.g., phosphate, related to potential patient osmotic risk)
Hydraulic permeability: Possibility of use for HF or HDF procedure, but because of back filtration risk, ultrapure pure dialysate recommended for high flux membranes
Adsorption capacity on to the membrane (a characteristic of synthetic membranes)
Mode of sterilization: reduced allergic reactions with steam sterilization/gamma irradiation compared with ethylene oxide
Cost

Source: Adapted from Fischbach M, Edefonti A, Schroder C, Watson A for the European Pediatric Dialysis Working Group: Hemodialysis in children: General practical guidelines, *Pediatr Nephrol* 20(8):1054-66, 2005.

In general, polysulfone- and polyamide-based membranes are effective barriers to endotoxins because of their high adsorptive properties[72]—whereas high-flux and low-flux cellulose-based membranes are less protective.[74,75] Cuprophan membranes have the highest permeability to endotoxins and other cytokine-inducing substances.[75] In addition, even though in vivo studies have reported increased plasma markers of inflammation such as CRP and IL-6 with contaminated dialysate data demonstrating the superiority of ultrapure dialysate in reducing the production of proinflammatory cytokines has been conflicting[76-78] except with the use of highly permeable membranes.[75,79]

Several small adult prospective studies have investigated the benefits of ultrapure dialysate on clinical outcomes. The most commonly researched parameters have been nutrition,[80] responsiveness to erythropoietin,[81] preservation of residual renal function,[77,82] and occurrence of beta-2-microglobulin amyloidosis.[82,83] Collectively, the results suggest an improvement in all four clinical outcomes and an increased responsiveness to vaccines[84] and reduced cardiovascular morbidity.[85,86]

Therefore, in conclusion there is evidence supporting a link between dialysate bacterial and endotoxin contamination and chronic inflammation. However, the impact is dependent on the permeability of the dialysis membrane. In our opinion, the question of whether ultrapure dialysate provides a survival and morbidity advantage (especially in children) has not been answered. Therefore, at present we cannot justify the additional resource and financial burden that will be incurred with implementation of ultrapure dialysate for routine pediatric HDs. However, its use is necessary for hemodiafiltration practices and should be considered in treatments associated with a significant risk of backfiltration and those using cuprophan membranes.

CHOICE OF HEMODIALYZER

When selecting a dialyzer for chronic HD, several membrane characteristics need to be taken into consideration (Table 57-4).

Surface Area

To improve efficacy, dialyzers are designed to maximize the surface area available for diffusion. Two designs have dominated the industry; namely, hollow-fiber and parallel plate dialyzers. In the latter, parallel layers of membranes are separated by flat supporting structures. Their greatest disadvantage is their high compliance and thus large filling and priming volumes. In children, therefore, they have largely been replaced by hollow-fiber dialyzers—which consist of a bundle of capillaries potted with sealing material at both ends into a plastic tubular housing unit. They have virtually no compliance and lower priming volumes, but the sealing materials are at risk of releasing solvents or ethylene oxide after gas sterilization—thus producing anaphylactic reactions. As a guide, the dialyzer membrane surface area should be approximately equal to the patient's body surface area.

Biocompatibility

The dialysis membrane is in direct contact with the patient's blood and can initiate leucocyte and complement activation. The extent of the inflammatory response characterizes the biocompatibility of the material used for the dialyzer. In broad terms, three membrane types are presently available: unmodified cellulose, modified/regenerated cellulose, and synthetic.

Unmodified cellulose membranes, such as cuprophan, are relatively inexpensive but also the most bioincompatible. The modified cellulose membranes (such as those made of cellulose acetate or hemophan) have some or all of the hydroxyl groups esterified to make them more biocompatible. However, such modifications may result in increased activation of the coagulation cascade and thus increase the anticoagulation requirement of the HD circuit.

Synthetic membranes are made from polysulfone, polycarbonate, polyamide, or polyacryl-polyamide acrylate (PMNA). These membranes are generally relatively biocompatible, except for the negatively charged AN69 polyacrylonitrile membranes. They are known to cause hypotension, inflammatory hyperemia, edema, and pain secondary to a bradykinin-mediated reaction. Dialysis patients most at risk are infants requiring a blood to prime their HD circuit[87] and children concurrently taking ACE inhibitors[88] or angiotensin II receptor antagonists.[89] Synthetic membranes are generally more hydrophobic than cellulose membranes and therefore have higher adsorption properties.[90] Their increased ability to bind proteins may be partly responsible for their improved biocompatibility, which also makes them the membrane of choice for therapies such as albumin dialysis or in the treatment of acute toxicities where the undesired plasma toxin is highly protein bound.

Hydraulic Permeability

A useful measure of the hydraulic permeability of a membrane is the K_{UF}, the UF coefficient. This is defined as the volume of ultrafiltrate produced per hour per mm Hg transmembranous pressure, determined at a blood flow of 200 ml/min. K_{UF} is most directly influenced by the membrane's mean pore size. In turn, the mean pore size influences the solute sieving coefficient and molecular weight cutoff for a membrane. High-flux dialyzers with larger mean pore sizes have a higher molecular weight cutoff and are most efficient in clearing larger uremic compounds.

UF rate and the dialyzer membrane's sieving coefficient are the most important determinants of convective solute removal.[91] Therefore, in consideration of predominantly convective therapies such as hemofiltration or hemodiafiltration (HDF) high-flux dialyzers are required.

Solute Permeability

Membrane solute permeability refers to the clearance of middle-molecular-weight molecules, and is assessed by measuring the rate of beta-2-microglobulin clearance. It is determined by the number of pores, the size of the pores, and membrane wall thickness. A highly permeable membrane is one that is thin, with a high pore density and large-diameter pores. Efficiency, represented as KoA (mass transfer coefficient of urea), is a measure of urea clearance—a surrogate marker of small-molecule clearance.

Traditionally, membranes are characterized as low flux or high flux according to their solute permeability. High-flux membranes are highly permeable membranes that can permit convective solute clearance of molecules weighing between 5000 and 25,000 Daltons (Table 57-5), but urea clearance rates vary. Highly efficient membranes have high urea clearance rates but differ in their hydraulic permeability, and thus may be limited in their ability to clear middle molecules.

Effect of Dialyzer Membrane on Clinical Outcomes

Several small adult studies have shown that modified cellulose and synthetic membranes reduce uremia-related amyloidosis; preserve residual renal function; improve lipid profiles, plasma

TABLE 57-5 **Dialyzer Classification**

Class	Surface Area	K_{UF} (ml/hr/mm Hg)	Urea Clearance	β2M Clearance
Conventional	<1.5 m^2	<12	Moderate	Negligible
High Efficiency	>1.5 m^2	>12	High (*KoA > 600 ml/min)	Negligible
Mid-flux	Variable	12-30	Variable	Moderate
High-flux	Variable	>30	Variable	High (>20 ml/min*)

* Comments added to original by Hothi and Geary.
Source: Clark WR, Ronco C: Determinants of haemodialyser performance and the potential effect on clinical outcome, *Nephrol Dial Transplant* 16(5):56-60, 2001.

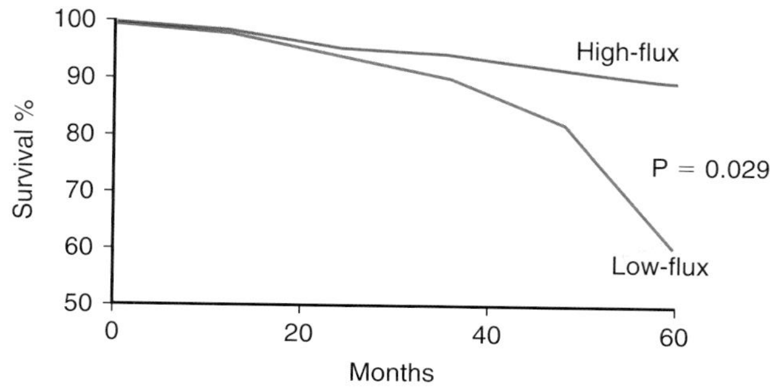

Figure 57-8 Kaplan-Meier analysis of the effect of membrane flux on survival in chronic hemodialysis patients. (From Woods HF, Nandakumar M: Improved outcome for haemodialysis patients treated with high-flux membranes, *Nephrol Dial Transplant* 15(1):36-42, 2000.)

albumin, and protein catabolic rate; improve responsiveness to erythropoietin; and reduce inflammation and infective episodes.[92] However, others have reported no difference.[92,93]

In a historical prospective analysis of the USRDS database, Bloembergen and colleagues demonstrated a 20% decrease in the relative risk of death for modified cellulose and synthetic membranes compared with cellulose membranes.[94] In a retrospective analysis of 715 patients, Woods and colleagues[95] compared mortality in a group treated exclusively with low-flux polysulfone dialyzers with another treated for at least 3 months with high-flux polysulfone dialyzers. In a Cox proportional analysis, the high-flux group had a significant 65% reduction in the risk of death compared with the low-flux group. A Kaplan-Meier analysis suggested a higher 5-year survival in the high-flux group, but a statistically significant difference was only seen after 4 years of dialysis (Figure 57-8).

In conclusion, epidemiologic studies suggest improved morbidity and mortality in dialysis patients treated with modified cellulose or synthetic membranes. However, few have been able to demonstrate whether the effects were due to differences in flux, biocompatibility, or middle-molecule clearance.

OPTIMIZING ULTRAFILTRATION POTENTIAL

During HD, the objective is to remove the sodium and water that accumulates in the interdialytic period within the few hours of treatment time. The major barrier to achieving this goal is the development of hemodynamic instability, manifesting as hypovolemia-related symptoms or intradialytic hypotension. This occurs on average in 20% to 30% of treatments, and can result in underdialysis because of treatment interruptions and leave the patient volume overloaded. Frequent hypotensive episodes may accelerate decline in residual renal function and potentially lead to serious vascular complications such as cerebral, cardiac, and mesenteric ischemia.

In children, the UF goal is often higher because of prescribed liquid nutritional supplements or poor adherence to fluid restrictions. Children may also be unable to verbalize complaints during dialysis, and this places a greater reliance on monitors. In this section, we discuss the pathophysiology of intradialytic hypotension, the value of BVM both as an objective measure of plasma refilling and in a predictive role for impending intradialytic hypotension, and the various therapeutic interventions that may facilitate UF potential.

PATHOPHYSIOLOGY: INTRADIALYTIC HYPOTENSION

During dialysis, as fluid is being removed plasma refilling, passive venoconstriction, and active increases in heart rate, heart contractility, and arterial tone are working simultaneously to preserve the effective plasma volume. As a result, even with a UF volume equal to the entire plasma volume the measured blood volume only changes by 10% to 20%. Impaired compensatory responses cause hypotension in the face of TBW expansion.

Most of the plasma volume resides in the veins, with a marked difference in the venous capacitance between organs. During UF, the ability to mobilize blood from the splanchnic venous pool is vital in preserving the central blood volume. Venous tone is affected by vasoactive hormones, the sympathetic nervous system, and upstream filling pressures. The De-Jager Krogh phenomenon refers to the transmission of upstream arterial pressure through the capillaries to the veins, causing venous distension and altered venous capacitance. During arteriolar constriction, the distending pressure to the vein is reduced and blood is extruded centrally toward the heart to maintain cardiac refilling.

Conversely, factors that cause arterial dilatation (such as antihypertensives) increase venous capacitance, reduce cardiac filling pressures, and through transmission of increased hydrostatic pressure to the capillary bed inhibit vascular refilling. Adenosine is thought to augment splanchnic blood pooling through an inhibitory effect on norepinephrine release and by causing regional vasodilatation. It is hypothesized that during a sudden but not gradual intradialytic hypotension episode ischemia prevails, resulting in increased consumption of adenosine triphosphate (ATP) and generation of adenosine.[96] In fact, pretreating hypotensive-prone patients with caffeine (an adenosine receptor antagonist) was shown to lower the number of hypotensive episodes.[97]

The sympathetic nervous system is the principal control mechanism of arteriolar tone and therefore of central blood pressure. Patients with ESRD show an increased basal level of peripheral sympathetic activity.[98] In HD patients prone to hypotension, a paradoxical decrease in sympathetic activity is seen at the time of a hypotensive episode[98]—which results in a rapid decline in the peripheral vascular resistance and increased vascular bed capacitance. Problems with sympathetic end-organ responsiveness and the efferent parasympathetic baroreceptor pathway have also been reported, but the underlying mechanism remains unexplained.

Some believe this may be a heightened manifestation of the Bezold-Jarisch reflex, a cardiodepressor reflex resulting in a sudden loss of symphathetic tone that causes abrupt severe hypotension accompanied by bradycardia. It is postulated that conditions associated with reduced cardiac refilling pressures (such as left ventricular hypertrophy, diastolic dysfunction, and structural heart defects) stimulate cardiac stretch receptors and thus maladaptively trigger a variant of the Bezold-Jarisch reflex (resulting in hypotension).

The final and interconnecting component relating to intradialytic hypotension is plasma refilling. This refers to the movement of fluid from the extravascular to the vascular compartment under the influences of hydraulic, osmotic, and oncotic pressure gradients at the capillary wall. If UF rates exceed refilling rates, the intravascular volume will fall. Arterial vasoconstriction decreases hydrostatic pressures in the capillary bed, facilitating vascular refilling. The oncotic pressure, which is effectively the plasma protein concentration, promotes refilling. Plasma sodium and glucose mobilize fluid from the intracellular space as a result of increased plasma tonicity.[99]

Plasma hematocrit level correlates with refilling rates, but the mechanism is unknown. Finally, refilling is facilitated by greater tissue hydration and occurs at a faster rate when the interstitial space is overloaded. Hypovolemia within the uremic milieu can augment ineffective venoconstriction, inadequate cardiac refilling, reduced plasma refilling, and activation of the sympaticoinhibitory Bezold-Jarisch reflex—leading to sudden hypotension.

BLOOD VOLUME MONITORING

Online NIVM makes it feasible to indirectly measure blood volume, in real time and continuously throughout dialysis. This is based on the principle of mass conservation: the concentration of measured blood constituents (hemoglobin/hematocrit/plasma protein) confined to the vascular space changes in proportion to changes in the vascular volume. NIVMs differ by the intrinsic sensing technique used for monitoring.

- *Optical:* Measures the optical absorbance of monochromatic light, via an optoprobe in the arterial line. The optical density of whole blood is really a measure of red blood cell (RBC) concentration; that is, the hematocrit rather than the hemoglobin content. Scattering of light from the surface of RBC yields a nonlinear relationship between the measured optical density and hematocrit. The Crit-line (In-Line Diagnostics, Riverdale, Utah), a standalone device, is designed to correct for this—whereas the Hemoscan (Hospal-Dasco, Medolla, Italy), a component of the dialysis machine, adjusts the optical density for variations in oxygen saturation.
- *Blood density:* Blood density is dependent on the total protein concentration (plasma protein concentration + mean cellular hemoglobin concentration). The Blood Volume Monitor (BVM, Fresenius AG, Bad Homburg, Germany) measures the velocity of sound through blood, as a reflection of blood density, by means of a cell inserted in the pre-pump segment of the arterial line. This is adjusted for temperature, a factor known to impact sound velocity and blood density.
- *Electrical conductance:* Conductivity of blood depends on hematocrit, temperature, plasma electrolytes, and nonelectrolyte concentrations. The difference between high- and low-frequency conductivity is a measure of hematocrit. The extracorporeal plasmatic impedance meter (IPEC, Laboratoire Eugedia, Chambly, France) translates changes in conductivity into relative changes in plasma volume.

All three methods report results as a percentage change in RBV, and in some these are displayed graphically. NIVM devices have an inherent degree of inaccuracy because they function on the assumption that there is uniform mixing of red cells and plasma throughout the circulation. We know this to be untrue in dialysis because posture, redistribution of blood during UF, intradialytic administration of blood products, consumption of food, and hydration status can alter RBC volume and induce RBC shifts with regional blood flow.

Each device is fitted with computer software that converts measured changes to percentage RBV based on internal calibration reference points. These may differ between machines, and therefore an absolute RBV value on one device may not read the same on another. Schneditz and colleagues demonstrated a 2% difference in RBV change (BVM 2% less reduction in blood volume compared to Crit-line) between the Crit-line and BVM, which developed approximately 1 hour into dialysis and persisted thereafter.[100] An awareness of these limitations is important before routine application of these devices in practice.

Despite the aforementioned limitations, BVM is a very useful tool in measuring the change in blood volume as fluid is being removed during UF. It also provides insight into an individual patient's vascular refilling ability. Theoretically, this could allow the UF rate to be individualized based on observed RBV changes. If fluid removal is too rapid, as detected by a steep declining slope on the NIVM monitor, the UF rate could be decreased before hypotension occurs. If fluid removal is too slow, as suggested by a flat slope, the UF rate could be safely increased. Steuer and colleagues achieved a twofold reduction in intradialytic symptoms using NIVM in six hypotension-prone adults without reducing the UF volume or treatment times.[101]

Others have shown an increase in the UF potential, lowering of the dry weight, improved patient well-being, and reduced hospitalization due to fluid overload. Access to information on blood volume status can be particularly helpful in the pediatric HD setting because the prevalence of intradialytic and interdialytic morbidity may be higher because children often do not verbalize early warning symptoms. Such information can also help differentiate between symptoms caused by etiologies other than hypovolemia. Jain and colleagues showed reduced dialysis-associated morbidity with NIVM, with the greatest impact on children weighing less than 35 kg.[102] Michael observed improved targeting of the dry weight in children, which reduced the requirement for antihypertensive medication.[20]

Using a constant dialysate sodium concentration of 140 mmol/L, Jain and colleagues also defined a safe UF rate as an RBV change of <8% per hour in the first 90 minutes and <4% thereafter, with no more than a 12% net RBV change per dialysis session.[102] They are the only group to introduce the idea of a predictive role of RBV levels of impending intradialytic symptoms or hypotension in pediatrics. Adult literature has been more comprehensive and reports conflicting data. Kim showed[103] that if RBV fell below a given threshold arterial hypotension appeared. Subsequently, larger observational studies demonstrated that critical maximal RBV reduction had no predictive power. However, these studies found that irregularity of the RBV course and switching from an exponential to a linear decrease of the RBV were the most powerful predictors of intradialytic hypotension.[104,105]

In conclusion, there is clearly an interindividual and intra-individual variation in the pattern of RBV change during dialysis. Although ultrafiltration pays a central role in the determination of intra-HD hypotension, the etiology of intradialytic hypotension is multifactorial. This will manifest as a variable predisposition to hypotension using the same UF rate. In our opinion, combining our knowledge of the pathophysiology of intradialytic hypotension we can use NIVM to give more information on RBV reduction relative to different intradialytic interventions but not as an absolute predictor of hypotension or total UF volume tolerance.

STRATEGIES FOR OPTIMIZING ULTRAFILTRATION

Preventing Intradialytic Hypotension

As we have already discussed, hemodynamic stability during dialysis is improved by withholding antihypertensives on dialysis days; avoiding food during dialysis; cooling dialysate, bicarbonate buffers, and high sodium dialysate; and treating intradialytic hypocalcemia. In a select number of patients, in spite of hypervolemia marked intradialytic hypotension results in premature discontinuation of therapy. In these cases, the intradialytic blood pressure can be artificially maintained by pharmacologic measures. One study demonstrated that prophylactic caffeine administration, an adenosine antagonist, reduced the occurrence of sudden intradialytic hypotensive episodes.[97]

A more widely used alternative is midodrine, a prodrug of the a-1 adrenergic receptor agonist desglymidodrine. It maintains intradialytic blood pressure by mediating constriction of both arterial and venous capacitance vessels and preventing venous pooling while increasing the central blood pressure. It is administered through the oral route, achieves peak levels at 1 hour, and has a half-life of 3 hours. We have used it in children with success, with starting doses of 2.5 mg incrementally increased to 10 mg. A systematic review of nine trials, using midodrine doses of 2.5 to 10 mg given 15 to 30 minutes before dialysis, reported a benefit in six trials (with attenuation of the drop in blood pressure during dialysis) and a decrease in the number of hypovolemia-related symptoms. No serious adverse events were described, but minor reactions (e.g., scalp paresthesia, heartburn, flushing, headache, weakness, and neck soreness) were reported.[106]

ULTRAFILTRATION PROFILES

Modifying the UF rate throughout dialysis to allow adequate vascular refilling has the potential to increase the UF potential. This is the rationale behind UF profiles. The plasma refilling capacity increases proportionately with interstitial volume expansion. Decreasing stepwise or linear profiles starts with high UF rates at the time of maximal tissue hydration, progressively reducing the rate in line with decreasing interstitial hydration in the hope of maintaining the crucial balance between fluid removal and vascular refilling. Intermittent profiles aim to provide periods of active mobilization of interstitial fluid into the vascular space when UF rates are low, thereby making it amenable to removal during periods of high UF rates (Figure 57-9).

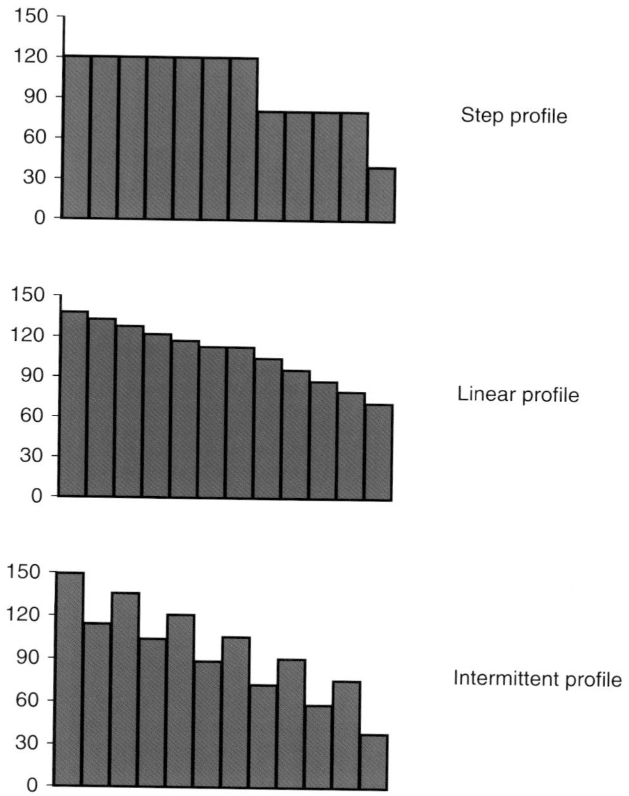

Figure 57-9 UF profiles.

Donauer and colleagues reported less symptomatic hypotension with the decreasing profiles, but the intermittent profile was associated with an increased incidence of symptomatic hypotension and postdialysis fatigue.[107] The incidence of intradialytic hypotension was highest with UF rates greater than 1.5 times the average. Ronco and colleagues observed hypotension at a rate of 6.7 per 100 treatments when the UF rate was 0.3 ml/min/kg, increasing to 15.8 at a UF rate of 0.4 ml/min/kg, 25.6 at a rate of 0.5 ml/min/kg, and 67.4 at a rate of 0.6 ml/min/kg.[108] In children, application of these figures would suggest that hypotension may occur in 25% of patients if a UF rate of 30 ml/kg/hour (300 ml/hour in a 10-kg child) is exceeded. These data have not been validated in children, but in our experience increasing the UF rate certainly increases the likelihood of intradialytic morbidity. UF profiles will inevitably result in a higher UF rate for part of the treatment, and the maximal UF rate has to be factored in when considering the most appropriate profile for a patient.

Combining UF profiles with sodium profiles can induce plasma hypertonicity, through utilization of a high UF rate during a high-sodium period, and thus provide a greater driving force for plasma refilling. It has been shown to be superior to either sodium or UF profiles alone in attenuating intradialytic symptoms and cardiovascular instability. Ebel and colleagues compared three regimens: (1) constant dialysate sodium of 138 mmol/L, (2) UF profile of 40% of the total UF goal in the first hour, 30% in the second hour, 30% in the subsequent 90 minutes, and none in the last 30 minutes, and (3) combined UF profile with a sodium profile with a dialysate sodium 10% higher than the predialysis plasma sodium, decreased in five steps to 138 in the last hour.

The standalone UF and sodium profiles showed evidence of intracellular fluid shift and intravascular hypovolemia. The combined profiles showed higher refilling rates and net removal of fluid from the interstitium and reduced renin, aldosterone, epinephrine, and norepinephrine levels[109]—possibly reflecting improved vascular stability. Song and colleagues selected adult patients prone to intradialytic hypotension. They showed that sodium-positive profiles (time-averaged dialysate Na concentration of 143 mEq/L) improved UF performance (ability to achieve the UF goal, premature discontinuation of treatment), but at the expense of gradual sodium and water expansion.

Sodium-neutral profiles (time-averaged dialysate Na concentration of 138 mEq/L) achieved better hemodynamic stability without the additional sodium burden, but were only moderately successful for UF performance. The combination of a sodium-neutral profile and UF profile achieved both good UF performance and reduced intradialytic and interdialytic symptoms, as well as a postdialysis weight closer to the dry weight.[47]

BIOFEEDBACK

The kidneys' unique ability to maintain homeostasis is achieved by continuously adjusting purification in response to a complex system of sensing and feedback mechanisms. Until now we have been unable to simulate this because traditional HD prescriptions are based on information from previous observations. Recently introduced biofeedback systems adjust the treatment prescription based on real-time repeated observations from an online monitoring system using a negative feedback system designed to return the deviating factor to a preset nominal value.

A linear relationship exists between conductivity and sodium content of dialysate. Conductivity feedback systems allow prediction of final plasma water conductivity when the dialysate conductivity is known, and of the dialysate conductivity required to obtain the final plasma water conductivity. Conductivity kinetic models have been shown to have a level of imprecision of <0.14 mS/cm, roughly equivalent to 1.4 mmol/L in terms of ionized plasma water sodium concentration and 56 mmol in terms of sodium balance.[110] It is hoped that through achievement of negative or neutral sodium balance with these systems that over time fluid balance will improve and the UF requirement per dialysis session will lessen. Preliminary trials report a benefit in UF potential combined with improved cardiovascular stability, but no pediatric efficacy data are available.

Blood-volume–controlled feedback systems respond to RBV changes.[111] At the start of therapy, treatment duration, UF goal, and a target for a maximum decline in blood volume are set. The blood volume control system will then adjust the UF rate and (when using the Hemocontrol module) dialysate conductivity to maintain RBV along this preset target. Initial results report a reduced incidence of intradialytic hypotensive episodes and attenuation of postdialysis symptoms,[112] perhaps through improved RBV preservation[111,113] or by avoiding rapid RBV fluctuations or prolonged periods of linear RBV decreases. Studies in hypotension-prone patients demonstrate a partial response, with a substantial number of nonresponders.[114,115]

A randomized controlled study comparing sodium profiling, conductivity, and blood-volume–controlled systems to standard HD reported a significant increase in predialytic plasma sodium during the sodium profile but not with the two feedback systems. Despite these differences, the predialytic blood pressure and interdialytic weight gain did not differ among the treatment modalities. Overall, the incidence of symptomatic intradialytic hypotension was lowest in the blood-volume–controlled system.[116] These novel biofeedback systems are attractive on paper, but they are not widely available and have only very limited anecdotal experience in children.

CONVECTIVE MODALITIES

Traditional methods of isoosmotic fluid removal during sequential dialysis techniques (pure UF followed by dialysis) are used to achieve higher UF rates without inducing hemodynamic instability. Isolated UF can be performed by placing the HD machine in bypass or UF mode. However, because the patient is no longer being warmed by the dialysate hypothermia can develop. This concern of temperature regulation combined with reduced clearance efficacy limits the time that can be spent on isolated UF.

The increased application of convective techniques within dialysis prescriptions has evolved to HDF. Conventional HDF consists of a standard HD circuit with the addition of a substitution fluid circuit placed before (predilution mode) or after (postdilution mode) the hemofilter. Predilution mode is often used because it helps overcome the limitations of blood flow and reduces the risk of the circuit clotting by limiting the rise in blood viscosity with UF. A high-flux synthetic membrane is a prerequisite because the hemofilter has to be able to tolerate high transmembrane pressures while retaining its high permeability to achieve the high UF rates necessary to obtain sufficient clearance.

Ultrapure dialysate is recommended to limit the inflammatory response induced by backfiltration of dialysate across the dialysis membrane. During online HDF this is all the more important because substitution fluid is produced from the ultrapure dialysate. Fischbach and colleagues report safety and efficacy data with predilutional HDF in children, prescribed six times per week for 3 hours using the Fresenius 4008 and FX 6 polysulfone dialyzers. Blood flow rate was 180 ± 50 ml/min and fixed dialysate flow rate was 500 ml/min. The substitution fluid rate was 0.65 to 1.0 times the blood flow rate (limited to a maximum of 200 ml/min), and the UF rate was limited to 1.5% ± 0.5% body weight. They observed increased predialysis hemoglobin levels, decreased predialysis phosphatemia, slow reduction of the mean predialysis beta-2-microglobulin levels, withdrawal of antihypertensives in most of the children, and improved left ventricular function.[10] These results are comparable to data emerging from the adult literature.

More pertinent to our discussion of UF performance is the recurring association of HDF with improved cardiovascular tolerance to sodium and water removal compared to conventional HD.[117] Even though the reasons for this remain unclear, many possibilities arise. During HD, the peripheral vascular resistance falls. With HDF, however, it is maintained[118]—and therefore for an equivalent blood volume loss there is a significantly smaller decline in systolic blood pressure.[117] During HDF, there is significant cooling within the extracorporeal circuit—which counteracts the heat generated during dialysis and prevents the increase in core temperature and subsequent peripheral vasodilatation. Finally, it has been proposed that the improved hemodynamic stability is secondary to decreased sodium clearance.[119] With HDF, there are clear advantages in hemodynamic stability. However, with routine use cases of worsening hypertension have been reported. Therefore, close monitoring of blood pressure is recommended—with an immediate return to HD in the presence of any deterioration.

QUOTIDIAN HEMODIALYSIS

Conversion to frequent HD has been shown to reduce intradialytic and interdialytic hemodynamic instability and improved fluid balance.[120] These may simply be the result of gentler and more gradual fluid removal, improving the balance between UF and vascular refilling. However, there is growing evidence indicating an improvement in a number of uremic cardiovascular comorbidities in association with superior toxin clearance.

A variety of regimens fall under the concept of frequent dialysis. The two most commonly practiced in pediatrics are short daily HD (SDHD)—defined as hemodialysis for 2 to 3 hours per session, prescribed 5 to 6 times per week and nocturnal hemodialysis (NHD) for 6 to 8 hours per session prescribed 5 to 6 times per week during sleep. SDHD can be accomplished using the conventional HD prescription over a shorter time period, implemented in-center. With NHD, however, some modifications are required—and it is only really suited for home use. We have successfully implemented NHD in teenagers using reduced dialysate flow rates of 200 to 300 ml/min and blood flow rates of 150 to 200 ml/min to avoid rapid overclearance. We have observed the need for a higher dialysate calcium concentration of 1.5 mmol/L to prevent hypocalcemia, as well as phosphate supplementation in the dialysate.[11]

SPECIFIC CONSIDERATIONS RELATED TO DIALYSIS HYPERTENSION

Hypertension is endemic in HD patients. The North American Pediatric Renal Transplant Cooperative Study (NAPTRTCS) database reported that 64% of HD patients required antihypertensive medication at the initiation of dialysis, and 40% still required medication at 2 years. Dialysis-related hypertension is predominantly caused by chronic volume overload. In a significant proportion, the blood pressure can be normalized with improved salt and fluid balance.

One of the difficulties in managing hypertension relates to the challenges of diagnosis. Different methods for measuring blood pressure are now accessible in most units. Current normative values are based on mercury sphygmomanometer measurements.[121] However, owing to convenience for the assessor (be it a nurse or parent), casual blood pressure (CBP) measurements are being increasingly measured using automatic and semiautomatic blood pressure devices. Recent comparisons of the mercury sphygmomanometer and the dinamap, an oscillometric device, showed that dinamap readings were higher (the systolic by 10 mm Hg and diastolic by 5 mm Hg).[122] In the hospital setting, CBP measurements taken in the HD units are often inaccurate.

There is a recognized heightened white coat effect due to the anticipatory anxiety associated with cannulation of a fistula or graft or related to the dialysis treatment. The presence of a functioning dialysis access can limit the measurement of blood pressure to the other arm (or in the presence of two fistulae the lower limb). No normative lower limb blood pressure data are available, but Frauman and colleagues showed that systolic leg pressures were on average 15 mm Hg higher than arm pressures—whereas no differences in diastolic blood pressure were observed.[122] Furthermore, in contrast to patients with essential hypertension HD can exhibit significant variability of blood pressure—depending on the time of measurement (namely, predialytic, postdialytic, or interdialytic).

In adults, the average interdialytic blood pressure is higher on the second day compared to the first day. However, such a variation is not consistently seen in children with chronic hypertension.[123,124] Based on these concerns, ambulatory blood pressure monitoring (ABPM) is gaining favor owing to increased reproducibility compared to CBP readings and to superior correlation with end-organ damage.[125,126] However, application is limited by age—with very few studies including children <6 years of age. It clearly has a diagnostic role, but due to its demands on time and resources it is not suitable for monitoring blood pressure on a frequent basis. In children, home blood pressure most reliably predicted ambulatory blood pressure. In children, the current consensus recommends diagnosing hypertension using predialysis blood pressure measurements in combination with home CBP readings—with a move toward routine use of ABPM.

Hypertension is defined as a blood pressure greater than the 95th percentile corrected for age, height, and sex (as defined by the Working Group Update in 2004).[127] Additional parameters that influence the decision to treat include a wide pulse pressure, blood pressure load (percentage of readings above the 95th percentile of target values), and nondippers (sleep blood pressure decrease less than 10% of daytime baseline readings). These have all been shown to be more potent predictors of total mortality than systolic or diastolic blood pressure.[128]

For a full discussion of treatment, we refer you to the section on hypertension, but we would like to draw your attention to some specific dialysis-related issues. The dialysis procedure can lend itself to treatment with the use of a lower-sodium dialysate, sodium profiles, or quotidian dialysis.[129,130] ACE inhibitor and angiotensin II receptor blocker (ARB) therapies decrease aortic pulse wave velocity and aortic systolic pressure, with a simultaneous antiinflammatory effect associated with the lowering of plasma CRP levels. However, anaphylactic reactions (which are especially severe in the presence of acidic blood primes) have been observed during HD in patients dialyzed with the AN69 membrane and who are concurrently taking ACE inhibitors.

ARBs result in significant reduction of systolic blood pressure in HD patients,[131] without further reducing low diastolic blood pressure. Therefore they will best suit patients with isolated hypertension. In addition, adult data reporting the use of carvedilol as an antihypertensive also found it beneficial in reducing dialysis-related ventricular arrhythmias and that it proved effective in improving left ventricular dysfunction in patients with dilated cardiomyopathy.[132]

Shorter-acting ACE inhibitors (such as enalapril and captopril) are cleared by HD, but fosinopril is not. The beta-blockers atenolol and metoprolol are removed during HD, but clearance of propanolol is insignificant. Minoxidil and methyldopa are cleared by HD, but no data exists for doxazocin. Neither amlodipine nor ARBs (such as losartan) have significant clearance during HD.

DIALYSIS DYSEQUILIBRIUM SYNDROME

Dialysis discomfort and dysequilibrium due to cellular osmotic distress occur as a result of changes in osmolarity, inducing water shifts from the extracellular to the intracellular compartment across the highly permeable blood/brain membrane. Dialysis dysequilibrium syndrome (DDS) was first described in 1962. It manifests during or immediately after HD as a self-limiting entity, but recovery can take several days. Symptoms typically include nausea, vomiting, headache, blurred vision, muscular twitching, disorientation, hypertension, tremors, seizures, and coma. Other symptoms (such as muscular cramps, anorexia, restlessness, and dizziness) have been reported. One of the greatest challenges associated with DDS resides in the fact that the diagnosis is essentially one of exclusion.

The exact pathophysiology of DDS remains unclear, and two mechanisms have been proposed. The first, named the reverse urea effect, believes that urea clearance from plasma occurs more rapidly than from brain tissue. This results in a transient osmotic gradient and net movement of water from plasma to brain, causing cerebral edema. The second theory suggests the development of a paradoxical acidemia of cerebrospinal fluid and cerebral cortical grey matter in patients and animals treated with rapid HD. This is accompanied by increased brain osmole activity due to displacement of sodium and potassium ions and enhanced organic acid production. The increased intracellular osmolarity induces fluid shifts, with subsequent cytotoxic edema. Both mechanisms allude to rapid changes in brain volume. This is thought to destroy the blood/brain barrier and disrupt cerebral autoregulation (Table 57-6).

Treatment options are both preventative and therapeutic. The dialysis prescription can be adjusted to reduce the rate of plasma urea clearance by downgrading the surface area of the dialyzer, by decreasing the blood flow rate, or by switching to SDHD. Intradialytic osmotic shifts can be minimized with the use of sodium profiles or higher dialysate sodium concentrations, the substitution of bicarbonate for acetate in the dialysate, or treatment using sequential HD with an initial period of UF alone followed by conventional dialysis in the case that a patient is grossly fluid overloaded. Adult centers more commonly prescribe prophylactic phenytoin to reduce neurologic excitability and the risk of seizures, but this has no effect on the underlying cerebral edema.

TABLE 57-6 **Patients Identified as High Risk for Developing DDS**

Pediatric age group
Preexisting neurologic disease
Severe metabolic acidosis
New patients just starting HD, particularly in the presence of a high predialysis urea
Patients with a high UF goal
Clinical situations associated with cerebral edema, such as rapid rehydration therapy, hyponatremia, malignant hypertension, diabetes mellitus, and hypoglycemia

Mannitol is more commonly used in pediatrics, both in a preventative and therapeutic role. Mannitol is an osmotically active solute, and can therefore artificially increase plasma osmolarity at the time of rapid urea clearance. Therapeutically, it rapidly lowers intracranial hypertension within minutes of administration—with a maximal effect at 20 to 40 minutes. A maximal intradialytic dose of 1 g/kg is recommended once a week in high-risk patients. If more frequent dosing is required, a smaller dose of 0.5 g/kg is advised because mannitol accumulates in renal failure (half-life of 36 hours) and can cause a rebound rise in the intracranial pressure—especially in the face of acidosis. Other adverse effects include nausea, vomiting, lower limb edema, thrombophlebitis, headaches, and chest pain. An alternative to mannitol in the treatment of DDS is 3% to 5% sodium chloride infusion or higher-dialysate sodium bath. Concurrent antiepileptic therapy is required with both therapies if the patient is seizing.

MALNUTRITION, INFLAMMATION, AND ATHEROSCLEROSIS

Malnutrition and inflammation have been reported to be strong predictors of mortality in dialysis patients, but cardiovascular disease is the most commonly documented cause of mortality. The causes of cardiovascular disease include traditional Framingham risk factors (such as hypertension) and nontraditional risk factors, such as inflammation, oxidative stress, and vascular calcification.[133] C-reactive protein (CRP), an acute-phase protein, is a recognized marker of inflammation. It is also reported to be predictive of cardiovascular disease and cardiovascular events, including mortality and cardiovascular structural changes such as cardiac hypertrophy and higher coronary calcification score. Recent data have also implicated CRP in the pathogenesis of vascular inflammation and atherosclerosis.[134]

Plasma CRP levels increase with declining kidney function, and then continue to rise after initiation of HD—with levels correlating with the length of the dialysis session.[135] It has been postulated that an interaction of circulating monocytes with bioincompatible membranes, blood contact with nonsterile dialysate solution, and/or "back-leaking" of dialysate across the membrane results in a chronic inflammatory state. However, because there is a high incidence of predialytic inflammation,[136] a significant proportion of dialysis patients with normal CRP levels, and conflicting data on cytokine induction during or after dialysis.[137] Therefore, the dialysis procedure is unlikely to be the only factor instigating the inflammatory event. Monitoring CRP levels is useful because it is responsive to intercurrent clinical events and because acute rises suggest the presence of an acute inflammatory stimulus.[138]

Both acute and chronic inflammation in dialysis patients require assessment and may be amenable to treatment. The dialysis prescription can be modified to become less inflammatory by using ultrapure dialysate and synthetic biocompatible membranes. Both ACE inhibitors and statins, more commonly recognized for their respective roles in treating hypertension and hypercholesterolemia, have been reported to have antiinflammatory actions.[139,140] Finally, antiinflammatory initiatives may include lifestyle changes (Table 57-7).

METABOLICS

Dialysis-Related Carnitine Disorder

Levocarnitine (L-carnitine) facilitates the transport of fatty acids across the inner mitochondrial membrane and is thus a critical cofactor for normal energy production in cardiac and skeletal muscle. Skeletal muscle contains the greatest proportion of the body's carnitine pool (98%), and the remainder resides in organs such as the liver, kidney, and heart. L-carnitine exists unbound to plasma proteins and is freely filtered in the glomerulus. Under normal conditions, extensive tubular reabsorption results in a renal clearance of 1 to 3 ml/min. During periods of carnitine deficiency, tubular reabsorption of free carnitine increases—accompanied by a selective excretion of short-chain carnitine esters. This serves to maintain a normal ratio of acylcarnitine to free carnitine of <0.25.

TABLE 57-7 Lifestyle and Dietary Modifications That May Have Antiinflammatory Effects

Soy (phytoestrogen)
Fiber-rich food
Fish (eicosapentenoic acid)
Nuts and seeds (γ-tocopherol)
Diets rich in antioxidants (living food)
Probiotics (living microorganisms)
Diets low in advanced glycation end products
Weight reduction
Exercise training

Source: Stenvinkel P, Lindholm B, Heimburger O: Novel approaches in an integrated history of inflammatory-associated wasting in end-stage renal disease, *Semin Dial* 17(6):505-15, 2004

There is growing evidence of reduced plasma free-carnitine levels in chronic HD patients, with an inverse relationship between muscle carnitine and duration on dialysis.[141] This is postulated to be the result of reduced dietary intake and bioavailability of dietary sources, impaired biosynthesis or transport of L-carnitine from sources of biosynthesis into the general circulation, and dialysis losses. Within a single dialysis session, clearance is approximately 7.8l per hour (or 130 ml/min), which is 30 times greater than the expected renal clearance of L-carnitine in a healthy individual.[142]

Dialysis clearance selectivity results in a rise in the protein-bound acylcarnitine fraction and continued decrease in plasma free-carnitine levels. The subsequent functional carnitine deficiency, recognized as dialysis-related carnitine disorder (DCD), manifests as anemia that is hyporesponsive to erythropoietin, intradialytic hypotension, cardiomyopathy, and skeletal muscle dysfunction causing generalized fatigability, weakness, asthenia, intradialytic muscle cramping, and reduced exercise tolerance.[143]

The National Kidney Foundation Interdisciplinary Consensus Panel recommends L-carnitine[144] supplementation for those patients with a clinical presentation of DCD even in the absence of biochemical findings of a low plasma free-carnitine or elevated ratio of acyl to free carnitine. This stipulation is based on the observation that plasma free-carnitine levels only represent a small fraction of the carnitine pool and are therefore not representative of the total-body carnitine status, demonstrate a lack of association with patient symptoms, and are poor predictors of response to treatment. Timing of the sample relative to dialysis also interferes with interpretation because postdialysis levels gradually return to the predialysis level. This is not entirely caused by a rebound phenomenon but also secondary to dietary intake and biosynthesis, and the two effects are impossible to separate.

The aim of L-carnitine supplementation is to produce clinical improvement and restore the total-body carnitine pool. The challenge is finding a method for monitoring treatment because the most reliable indicator, skeletal muscle L-carnitine concentrations, is unacceptable in the pediatric setting. Therefore, at present less than ideal alternatives (such as plasma free-carnitine levels, the ratio of acyl to free carnitine, and clinical evaluation) are being used. The National Kidney Foundation has even advocated a trial of therapy with three monthly clinical evaluations, discontinuing treatment at 9 to 12 months if no benefits are observed.[144]

It has been suggested that supraphysiologic plasma levels are required to drive L-carnitine from the plasma to skeletal muscle cells. A variety of doses have been reported in the literature, but repeated doses of 20 mg/kg intravenous at the end of dialysis appear to result in a new steady-state plasma carnitine concentration in 6 to 8 weeks, with continuing treatment for 6 to 12 months to replenish the carnitine pool. Oral carnitine supplementation is not recommended in ESRD due to concerns of toxicity from L-carnitine metabolites, which accumulate in renal failure.

Hyperhomocysteinemia

Homocysteine is a non–protein-forming sulfhydryl-containing amino acid that results from methionine metabolism. Only

1% to 2% of total homocysteine circulates in blood in a free reduced form (70% to 90% is protein bound, and the rest exists in oxidized forms). Sulphur amino acid metabolism acts via three pathways: transmethylation, remethylation, and transsulphuration. ESRD results in hyperhomocysteinemia from a decreased whole-body remethylation and transmethylation rate with impaired homocysteine clearance through transsulphuration. In fact, many studies have shown that plasma homocysteine concentrations start rising in CRF and are inversely related to glomerular filtration rate.

There is conflicting evidence on the impact of hyperhomocysteinemia in dialysis patients. A metaanalysis reported a positive association between hyperhomocysteinemia and atherosclerosis, ischemic heart disease, stroke, and thrombosis.[145] Conversely, some recent studies have found no significant (or even an inverse) association between plasma homocysteine level and cardiovascular events and mortality in ESRD patients.[146] The controversy extends further, with differences in opinions on whether the high homocysteine levels or the metabolic dysregulation resulting from hyperhomocysteinemia is responsible for the associated negative effects.

Treatment involves utilization of the cofactors (folate and B12) in the remethylation pathway, but supranormal plasma levels are often required. In a proportion of patients, this is due to a single-nucleotide polymorphism in the 5,10-methylenetetrahydrofolate reductase (MTHFR) gene C677T (TT and CT genotypes)—where the elevated homocysteine can be normalized with folate supplementation (but higher doses are required).[147] A lower dose of folic acid can be as effective if combined with vitamin B12 and vitamin B6. In addition, *N*-acetylcysteine, in the context of lowering plasma homocysteine, has been tested in renal patients but is only effective if administered intravenously.[148]

An alternative therapeutic strategy for managing hyperhomocystemia is through manipulation of the HD prescription. High-flux dialyzers achieve greater clearance but have no impact on predialysis plasma concentrations.[149] However, a single report of dialyzing with extremely high-flux or adsorptive properties for 12 weeks described a significant reduction of predialysis total homocysteine by 33% compared to 15.6% with polysulfon high-flux dialyzers.[150] This is likely due to increased albumin clearance and thus the ability to remove protein-bound homocysteine.

With current therapeutic options, plasma homocysteine levels improve—but normalization is uncommon. Even in the presence of normal levels, markers of homocysteine metabolic dysregulation (such as impaired global DNA methylation) are only mildly improved. The only prospective trial testing the benefit of therapy randomized ESRD patients to 1, 5, or 15 mg of folic acid daily (but no placebo arm was included). After a mean follow-up of 2 years, there was no significant difference in mortality or cardiovascular events among the three groups.[151] However, vitamin therapy has been shown to improve hyperhomocysteinemia-induced endothelial dysfunction.[152] Despite the continuing debate of whether homocysteine is harmful or not, we believe there is a case for folate, vitamin B12, and vitamin B6 therapy in dialysis patients because they have the potential to improve cardiovascular morbidity both by lowering plasma homocysteine levels and by neutralizing elevated oxidative stress.

ADEQUACY

Whereas HD has always been prescribed to achieve solute clearance, UF, correction of metabolic disturbances, and restoration of hemodynamic stability, it was the publication of the National Cooperative Dialysis Study in 1981[54] that focused attention on how dialysis might best be employed to reduce patient morbidity and mortality. This study compared morbidity and mortality in four groups of patients, with high or low timed-average-concentration of urea (TAC-urea) and with either long (4.5-5 hours) or short (2.5-3.5 hours) dialysis. Only degenerated cellulose or cuprophan membranes were used. Dietary protein intake in all patients was estimated from the daily protein catabolic rate and was maintained at values of 0.8 to 1.4 grams per kilo per day. The results showed that the TAC-urea was the most important determinant of patient morbidity and hospitalization, as well as of medically indicated patient study withdrawal.

In a subsequent analysis of the NCDS Study using a single-pool variable-volume urea kinetic model to describe urea metabolism mathematically, Gotch and Sargent argued persuasively for the use of Kt/V_{urea} to measure the adequacy of dialysis.[153] This unitless measure, Kt/V_{urea}, is an estimate of the clearance of urea from the blood during a dialysis session—standardized by TBW, which reflects the urea distribution volume. Since then, Kt/V_{urea} has become accepted as the standard measure of delivered dialysis dose used to assess the adequacy of dialysis. Various methods for calculation of Kt/V have been proposed. These are discussed in the sections that follow, including their advantages and disadvantages.

Urea Kinetic Modeling

Each of these techniques requires sophisticated computer modeling programs, which may not be available in many pediatric dialysis units. However, some readily available internet websites [including Hypertension Dialysis and Clinical Nephrology (*www.hdcn.com*) and *www.Kt-v.net*] provide programs for calculation of single- and double-pool Kt/V measurements. The HDCN program has been employed in pediatric studies.[154]

- *Double-pool Kt/V:* This method recognizes that postdialysis rebound of plasma urea values may be substantial. Hence, a 60-minute postdialysis blood urea sample is required to avoid overestimation of urea removal. This method is probably the most accurate estimate of Kt/V, but the need for a delayed postdialysis blood sample and lack of studies validating it as a predictor of morbidity have limited its use.
- *Single-pool Kt/V:* This method has been validated in major adult studies to predict morbidity. Because it assumes that urea is removed from a single pool, a delayed postdialysis sample is not required. This is clearly a great practical advantage. However, it overestimates urea removal from the body because this method ignores urea rebound postdialysis—which occurs as a result of access and cardiopul-

monary recirculation (70%) and tissue redistribution (30%). Access recirculation diminishes and is insignificant within 15 to 20 seconds if blood flows are less than 50 to 80 ml/min. Cardiopulmonary recirculation only occurs with arteriovenous access and is not a factor with central venous blood line access as it results from a portion of the blood flow returning to the dialyzer after circuiting the heart and lungs, without passing through the other tissues. This rebound ceases 1 to 2 minutes after slowing blood flow. Tissue rebound postdialysis continues over a longer period, and occurs because blood flow to muscle is reduced in dialysis (although this tissue has particularly high urea content).[155] Urea rebound is minimized if the "stop dialysate flow"[156] technique is used with concomitant reduced blood flow reduction below 100 ml/min for the postdialysis blood sample. The recommendations in the literature for timing and methodology of the postdialysis blood sample are inconsistent, and thus we accept the KDOQI recommendations that suggest either of the following two methods.

- Slow blood flow method.
  a. At end of dialysis, turn off dialysate flow and decrease UF as much as possible.
  b. Decrease blood flow below 100 ml/min for 15 seconds.
  c. Obtain a sample.
- Stop dialysate method.
  a. At end of dialysis, stop dialysate flow and decrease UF as much as possible.
  b. Maintain blood flow at a normal rate for 3 minutes.
  c. Obtain a sample.

The major advantage of kinetically modeled methods for estimating Kt/V_{urea} is that they also provide an estimate of urea generation rate, from which normalized protein catabolic rate (nPCR, an estimate of dietary protein intake in the clinically stable patient) can be estimated. However, several potential inaccuracies are intrinsic to the measurement of kinetically derived Kt/V_{urea}. Urea clearance (K) for individual dialyzers is derived from manufacturers' specifications, which does not account for possible blood recirculation or reductions in the efficacy of dialyzers due to clotting of dialysis fibers and does not account for periods of blood flow disturbance due to kinked lines. In addition, determination of urea distribution volume (V) may be imprecise—particularly in children.

Kt/V Simplified Equations

Because of the potential intrinsic inaccuracies of modeled measures of Kt/V_{urea} outlined previously, and more importantly because these computer models may not be readily available in all dialysis units, more simplified equations for calculation of Kt/V_{urea} have been proposed.[157]

$$Kt/V = -\text{Log}\ n\ (R - 0.008t) + (4 - 3.5\ R)\ UF/BW$$

In this simplified equation, to estimate single-pool $spKt/V_{urea}$ R is the ratio of predialysis urea to postdialysis urea, t is the time of dialysis in hours, and BW is body weight in kilograms. This relatively simple calculation has been shown to vary by only 6% from formal urea kinetic modeling in children (Figure 57-10).[154] To correct for postdialysis urea rebound,

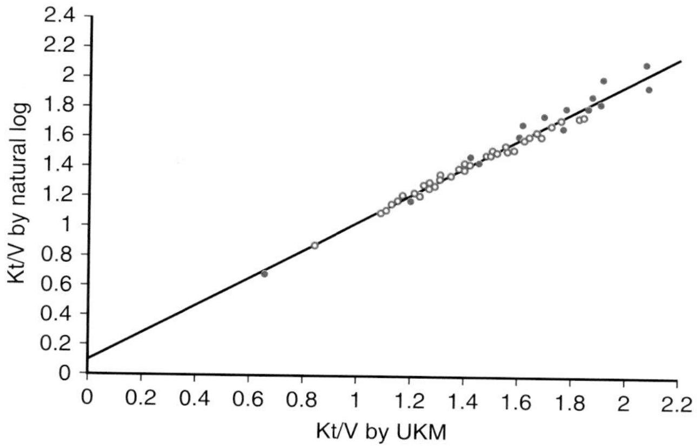

Figure 57-10 Relationship between Kt/V_{urea} derived via urea-kinetics and natural log formula. (From Goldstein SL, Sorof JM, Brewer ED: Natural logarithmic estimates of Kt/V in the pediatric hemodialysis population, *Am J Kidney Dis* 33(3):518-22, 1999.)

the following formulae may be used to calculate equilibrated eKt/V_{urea}.

- For patients with arteriovenous access, $eKt/V = spKt/V - (0.6 \times spKt/V/T) + 0.03$.
- For patients with venovenous access, $eKt/V = spKt/V - (0.47 \times spKt/V/T) + 0.02$.

Urea Reduction Ratio

Another measure of urea removal during dialysis that has been proposed is the urea reduction ratio (URR), which measures the percentage of reduction in blood urea values during a dialysis procedure.

$$\text{Urea reduction ratio percentage} = (1 - Ct/Co \times 100)$$

URR as a marker of dialysis adequacy was evaluated retrospectively in 13,473 patients, and the mortality rate increased by 28% when URR values of <60% were obtained.[158] However, despite the simplicity of this equation and its validation as a measure of morbidity URR is not recommended as the primary measure of dialysis adequacy because significant variations of Kt/V_{urea} may be obtained with each URR value—particularly when URR is greater than 65%. In addition, with increasing UF URR underestimates urea removal. Nonetheless, it is a useful and simple calculation of urea removal—which may be of value in patients with symptoms suggestive of dialysis dysequilibrium.

Measurement of Normalized Protein Catabolic Rate

Although not a direct estimate of dialysis adequacy, nPCR is an indirect measure of daily protein intake in stable dialysis patients. Because protein malnutrition commonly occurs in underdialyzed patients, nPCR is a useful adjunct to be included in decisions concerning appropriate dialysis needs for individual patients. The clinical value of nPCR measurement from single-pool urea kinetic modeling has been confirmed by Goldstein and colleagues,[159] who demonstrated a substantial increase in nPCR associated with improvement in nutritional status of three adolescents treated with intradialytic total parenteral nutrition.

However, Van Hoek and colleagues in a comparison of protein intake from dietary records kept by children—with an estimated nPCR calculated using an online urea monitor—showed significant variation, and PCR significantly underestimated the prescribed and recorded protein intake.[160] These authors concluded that use of their online urea kinetic monitor is therefore not recommended for estimation of nPCR. In addition, as reported by Grupe and colleagues[161] nPCR may be significantly affected by factors other than nutrient intake in as many as 25% of patients. Measurement of nPCR has traditionally relied on the availability of formal urea kinetic modeling and is included with the web-based programs *www.hdcn.com* and *www.Kt-v.net*. Goldstein, however, has demonstrated strong agreement between nPCR calculated from urea kinetic modeling and that provided from the following more simplified algebraic formula.[162]

$$nPCR = 5.43 \times G/V + 0.17$$

In this formula, the urea generation rate (G) is calculated as follows.

$$G\ (mg/min) = (\text{predialysis BUN} \times \text{predialysis V}) - (\text{postdialysis BUN} \times \text{postdialysis V})/T$$

Here, V is TBW estimated from 0.58 × body weight, and T is time in minutes from the end of the dialysis treatment to the beginning of the next dialysis treatment. Validation of this formula has eliminated the need for complicated computer modeling in order to measure nPCR and estimate daily protein intake.

Although the National Cooperative Dialysis Study focused attention on the need for reduction of urea values, a relationship was also observed between an increased risk of hospitalization and a shorter duration of dialysis in a subset of patients with high TAC-urea. This importance of dialysis duration was confirmed by Held and colleagues, who reviewed data on 600 HD patients from 300 dialysis units and found that mortality was reduced in those whose dialysis treatments lasted longer than 3.5 hours.

For those patients who had been on HD for at least 5 years, the relative mortality risk if they were dialyzed for less than 3.5 hours was 2.18 compared to patients who underwent longer dialysis sessions.[163] Similarly, patients receiving 8 hours of dialysis three times weekly in France have a much higher survival than conventionally dialyzed patients in the United States and the United Kingdom. This survival benefit is in part attributed to the duration of each dialysis procedure.[164,165] Finally, from a pediatric perspective it is of interest that catch-up growth has been described in children on HD in Montreal who underwent approximately 5 hours of dialysis three times weekly with intensive nutritional support. These results are superior to any other group of children dialyzed conventionally for 3 to 4 hours who do not receive growth hormone.[166]

The important message from these studies is that the prescribed dialysis dose for an individual patient should be based on more than a simple estimate of urea removal. Overall clinical evaluation of the patient [including growth, nutritional status, presence of cardiovascular disease (including hypertension), calcium phosphate balance, and evidence of renal osteodystrophy] should all be considered when estimating the patient's dialysis needs.

Another concern related to dialysis prescription based primarily on urea removal and current recommendations is that no upper limit for Kt/V_{urea} has been suggested. In our experience, this can lead to an increase in dialysis dysequilibrium symptoms related to excessive urea removal in a 3- to 4-hour dialysis.

In 2000, the KDOQI guidelines recommended that a delivered dose of HD in both adults and children should be measured using formal urea kinetic modeling employing a single-pool variable volume model for quantitation of urea removal during dialysis. The dialysis should provide a single-pool Kt/V_{urea} of at least 1.2. In 2002, the HEMO Study randomized 1846 patients on conventional thrice-weekly HD to a standard or high dose of dialysis as well as to a low-flux or high-flux dialyzer. In high-dose patients, the urea reduction ratio achieved was 75% and the single-pool Kt/V was 1.71—compared with standard-dose patients, whose Kt/V was 1.32 and urea reduction ratio 66%. The high-flux and low-flux dialyzer groups had beta-2-microglobulin clearances of 34 ml/min and 3 ml/min, respectively. Neither dialysis dose nor flux affected the relative risk of death, and the authors concluded that there was no major benefit from a higher dialysis dose than recommended by KDOQI or from the use of high-flux dialysis membranes.[167] A caveat to the HEMO Study acknowledged that their recommendations applied to patients receiving thrice-weekly HD, and might not be applicable to patients undergoing more frequent or prolonged HD sessions.

The KDOQI Clinical Practice Guidelines for HD adequacy were revised in 2005. They recommended a measurement of single-pool Kt/V_{urea} of 1.2 per dialysis as being minimally adequate. The target dose of dialysis they recommend is spKt/V of 1.4 per dialysis or a URR of 70%. The rationale for the minimally adequate dose of dialysis is principally based on the results of the HEMO Study, whereas the target values also took into consideration the European Guidelines for Hemodialysis—which recommended an equilibrated Kt/V of ≥1.2, which corresponds to a single-pool Kt/V of approximately 1.4 to 1.5.[168]

No large-scale studies of HD adequacy have been undertaken in children, and recommendations are therefore based on a number of small observational studies and extrapolations from the adult literature. Buur and colleagues evaluated two different urea kinetic modeling methods and compared them with direct quantification of urea removal by partial dialysate collection. They found that although each method produced different results correlation between these methods was very high.[169] The authors commented that for practical purposes, and to limit blood sampling, one of the direct single-pool methods of urea kinetic modeling should be used.

More recently, a study of eight children aged 8 to 18 years compared an online urea monitor measurement of Kt/V_{urea} (UM 1000, Baxter Healthcare) with single- and double-pool formulas derived by Daugirdas.[170] They also studied the same Kt/V_{urea} measurements on 12 occasions, using single-needle dialysis. They found considerable differences in Kt/V_{urea} between single- and double-pool formulae, and that use of

TABLE 57-8 Published Guidelines for Hemodialysis Adequacy

Source	Urea Clearance	Other
KDOQI, adults	Minimal spKt/V ≈ 1.2 Target spKt/V ≈ 1.4	URR ≈ 65% URR ≈ 70%
KDOQI, children	spKt/V > 1.4	Assess nutrition (nPCR) Optimize ultrafiltration
European, adults	eKt/V > 1.2 spKt/V ≈ 1.4	Double-pool urea kinetics preferred
European, children	eKt/V ≥ 1.2-1.4	Assess nutrition (nPCR) Monitor growth and cardiac function

the online urea monitor method was inaccurate during single-needle dialysis.

Despite the limited data in children, expert working groups have developed guidelines for HD in children both in Europe and North America,[171] together with European adult guidelines.[168] These are summarized in Table 57-8.

SUMMARY AND RECOMMENDATIONS

Complete clinical assessment of the patient (including general symptomatology, height and weight gain, cardiac and blood pressure status, bone health, and some estimate of quality of life) should be routinely performed. Monthly measurement of dialysis adequacy should use single-pool estimation of Kt/V_{urea}. This may be achieved using either formal urea kinetic modeling (*www.hdcn.com* or *www.Kt-v.net*) or using the simplified formula of Daugirdas.

$$Kt/V = -\text{Log } n\ (R - 0.008t) + (4 - 3.5R)\ UF/BW$$

Maintain $spKt/V_{urea}$ between 1.4 and 1.8 for children dialyzed for 3 to 4 hours per session. Monthly estimation of nPCR should be derived from urea kinetic modeling programs or using the Goldstein formula.

$$nPCR = 5.43 \times G/V + 0.17$$

Although nPCR values are a useful guide to protein intake, because nPCR values may be influenced by factors other than nutrient intake these values should be interpreted in conjunction with a review of weight gain and accurate dietary history. With these limitations, maintain nPCR values in the appropriate range for age as outlined in Chapter 48.

REFERENCES

1. Kolff WJ, Burke HTJ: Artificial kidney: Dialyzer with great area, *Acta Medica Scandinav* 117:121-34, 1944.
2. Mateer FM, Greenman L, Danowski TS: Hemodialysis of the uremic child, *AMA Am J Dis Child* 89(6):645-55, 1995.
3. Scribner EH, Buri R, Caner JEZ, Hegstrom R, Burnell JM: The treatment of chronic uremia by means of intermittent dialysis: Preliminary report, *Trans Am Soc Artif Int Organs* 6:114, 1960.
4. Fine RN, De Palma JR, Lieberman E, Donnell GN, Gordon A, Maxwell MH: Hemodialysis in children with chronic renal failure, *Pediatrics* 73(5):705-13, 1985.
5. Kjellstrand CM, Shideman JR, Santiago EA, Mauer M, Simmons RL, Buselmeier TJ: Technical advances in hemodialysis of very small pediatric patients, *Proc Clin Dial Transplant Forum* 1:124-32, 1971.
6. Mahan JD, Mauer M, Nevins TE: The Hickman Catheter: A new hemodialysis access device for infants and small children, *Kidney Int* 24(5):694-97, 1983.
7. Sadowski RH, Allred E, Jabs K: Sodium modeling ameliorates intradialytic and interdialytic symptoms in young hemodialysis patients, *J Am Soc Nephrol* 4(5):1192-98, 1993.
8. Goldstein SL, Smith CM, Currier H: Noninvasive interventions to decrease hospitalization and associated costs for pediatric patients receiving hemodialysis, *J Am Soc Nephrol* 14:2127-31, 2003.
9. Pierratos A: Daily nocturnal hemodialysis, *Kidney Int* 65:1975-86, 2004.
10. Fischbach M, Terzic J, Laugel V, Dheu C, Menouer S, Helms P, et al: Daily on-line haemodiafiltration: A pilot trial in children, *Nephrology Dialysis Transplantation* 19(9):2360-67, 2004.
11. Geary DF, Piva E, Tyrrell J, Gajaria MJ, Picone G, Keating LE, et al: Home nocturnal hemodialysis in children, *J Pediatr* 147(3):383-87, 2005.
12. Ishibe S, Peixoto AJ: Methods of assessment of volume status and intercompartmental fluid shifts in hemodialysis patients: Implications in clinical practice, *Seminars in Dialysis* 17(1):37-43, 2004.
13. Kouw PM, Kooman JP, Cheriex EC, Olthof CG, de Vries PM, Leunissen KM: Assessment of postdialysis dry weight: A comparison of techniques, *J Am Soc Nephrol* 4:98-104, 1993.
14. Nishikimi T, Futoo Y, Tamano K, Takahashi M, Suzuki T, Minami J, et al: Plasma brain natriuretic peptide levels in chronic hemodialysis patients: Influence of coronary artery disease, *Am J Kidney Dis* 37:1201-8, 2001.
15. Cheriex EC, Leunissen KM, Janssen JH, Mooy JM, van Hooff JP: Echography of the inferior vena cava is a simple and reliable tool for estimation of "dry weight" in haemodialysis patients, *Nephrol Dial Transplant* 4:563-68, 1989.
16. Cox-Reijven PL, Kooman JP, Soeters PB, van der Sande FM, Leunissen KM: Role of bioimpedance spectroscopy in assessment of body water compartments in hemodialysis patients, *Am J Kidney Dis* 38:832-38, 2001.
17. Chamney PW, Kramer M, Rode C, Kleinekofort W, Wizemann V: A new technique for establishing dry weight in hemodialysis patients via whole body bioimpedance, *Kidney Int* 61(6):2250-58, 2002.
18. Piccoli A, Rossi B, Pillon L, Bucciante G: New method for monitoring body fluid variation by bioimpedance analysis: The RXc graph, *Kidney Int* 46(2):534-39, 1994.
19. Zhu F, Kuhlmann MK, Sarkar S, Kaitwatcharachai C, Khilnani R, Leonard EF, et al: Adjustment of dry weight in hemodialysis patients using intradialytic continuous multifrequency bioimpedance of the calf, *Int J Artif Organs* 27(2):104-9, 2004.
20. Michael M, Brewer ED, Goldstein SL: Blood volume monitoring to achieve target weight in pediatric hemodialysis patients, *Pediatr Nephrol* 19(4):432-37, 2004.
21. Depner TA: *Prescribing hemodialysis: A guide to urea modeling*, Boston: Kluwer Academic Publishers 1991:44,186.
22. Vanholder RC, Ringoir SM: Adequacy of dialysis: A critical analysis, *Kidney Int* 42(3):540-58, 1992.
23. Leypoldt JK, Cheung AK, Agodoa LY, Daugirdas JT, Greene T, Keshaviah PR for The Hemodialysis (HEMO) Study: Hemodialyzer mass transfer-area coefficients for urea increase at high dialysate flow rates, *Kidney Int* 51:2013-18, 1997.
24. Schneditz D, Kaufman AM, Polaschegg HD, Levin NW, Daugirdas JT: Cardiopulmonary recirculation during hemodialysis, *Kidney Int* 42:1450-56, 1992.
25. Van Someren EJ, Raymann RJ, Scherder EJ, Daanen HA, Swaab DF: Circadian and age-related modulation of thermoreception and temperature regulation: Mechanisms and functional implications, *Ageing Res Rev* 1(4):721-78, 2002.

26. Bennett LA, Johnson JM, Stephens DP, Saad AR, Kellogg DL Jr.: Evidence for a role for vasoactive intestinal peptide in active vasodilatation in the cutaneous vasculature of humans, *J Physiol* 552(1):223-32, 2003.
27. Johnson JM, Proppe DW: Section 4: Environmental physiology. In MJ Fregly, CM Blatteis (eds.), *Handbook of physiology*. Vol. 1, New York: Oxford University Press 1996:215-43.
28. Fine A, Penner B: The protective effect of cool dialysate is dependent on patients' predialysis temperature, *Am J Kidney Dis* 28(2):262-65, 1996.
29. Ikizler TA, Wingard RL, Sun M, Harvell J, Parker RA, Hakim RM: Increased energy expenditure in hemodialysis patients, *J Am Soc Nephrol* 7(12):2646-53, 1996.
30. Rosales LM, Schneditz D, Chmielnicki H, Shaw K, Levin NW: Exercise and extracorporeal blood cooling during hemodialysis, *ASAIO J* 44(5):M574-M578, 1998.
31. Maggiore Q, Dattolo P, Piacenti M, Morales MA, Pelosi G, Pizzarelli F, et al: Thermal balance and dialysis hypotension, *Int J Artif Organs* 18:518-25, 1995.
32. Nelson-Piercy C: Hazards of heparin: allergy, heparin-induced thrombocytopenia and osteoporosis, *Baillieres Clin Obstet Gynaecol* 11(3):489-509, 1997.
33. Greer IA: Exploring the role of low-molecular-weight heparins in pregnancy, *Semin Thromb Hemost* 28(3):25-31, 2002.
34. Evenepoel P, Maes B, Vanwalleghem J, Kuypers D, Messiaen T, Vanrenterghem Y: Regional citrate anticoagulation for hemodialysis using a conventional calcium-containing dialysate, *Am J Kidney Dis* 39(2):315-23, 2002.
35. Koster A, Meyer O, Hausmann H, Kuppe H, Hetzer R, Mertzlufft F: In vitro cross-reactivity of danaparoid sodium in patients with heparin-induced thrombocytopenia type II undergoing cardiovascular surgery, *J Clin Anesth* 12(4):324-27, 2000.
36. Fischer KG: Hirudin in renal insufficiency, *Semin Thromb Hemost* 28(5):467-82, 2002.
37. Greinacher A, Lubenow N, Eichler P: Anaphylactic and anaphylactoid reactions associated with lepirudin in patients with heparin-induced thrombocytopenia, *Circulation* 108(17):2062-65, 2003.
38. Bohler J, Schollmeyer P, Dressel B, Dobos G, Horl WH: Reduction of granulocyte activation during hemodialysis with regional citrate anticoagulation: Dissociation of complement activation and neutropenia from neutrophil degranulation, *J Am Soc Nephrol* 7(2):234-41, 1996.
39. Ljungberg B, Jacobson SH, Lins LE, Pejler G: Effective anticoagulation by a low molecular weight heparin (Fragmin) in hemodialysis with a highly permeable polysulfone membrane, *Clin Nephrol* 38(2):97-100, 1992.
40. Klingel R, Schwarting A, Lotz J, Eckert M, Hohmann V, Hafner G: Safety and efficacy of single bolus anticoagulation with enoxaparin for chronic hemodialysis: Results of an open-label post-certification study, *Kidney Blood Press Res* 27(4):211-17, 2004.
41. Lim W, Cook DJ, Crowther MA: Safety and efficacy of low molecular weight heparins for hemodialysis in patients with end-stage renal failure: A meta-analysis of randomized trials, *J Am Soc Nephrol* 15(12):3192-206, 2004.
42. Geary DF, Gajaria M, Fryer-Keene S, Willumsen J: Low-dose and heparin-free hemodialysis in children, *Pediatr Nephrol* 5(2):220-24, 1991.
43. Moret K, Aalten J, van den Wall Bake W, Gerlag P, Beerenhout C, et al: The effect of sodium profiling and feedback technologies on plasma conductivity and ionic mass balance: A study in hypotension-prone dialysis patients, *Nephrol Dial Transplant* 21(1):138-44, 2006.
44. Sadowski RH, Allred EN, Jabs K: Sodium modeling ameliorates intradialytic and interdialytic symptoms in young hemodialysis patients, *J Am Soc Nephrol* 4(5):1192-98, 1993.
45. Song JH, Lee SW, Suh CK, Kim MJ: Time-averaged concentration of dialysate sodium relates with sodium load and interdialytic weight gain during sodium-profiling hemodialysis, *Am J Kidney Dis* 40(2):291-301, 2002. Erratum in: *Am J Kidney Dis* 40(6):1357, 2002.
46. de Paula FM, Peixoto AJ, Pinto LV, Dorigo D, Patricio PJ, Santos SF: Clinical consequences of an individualized dialysate sodium prescription in hemodialysis patients, *Kidney Int* 66(3):1232-38, 2004.
47. Song JH, Park GH, Lee SY, Lee SW, Lee SW, Kim MJ: Effect of sodium balance and the combination of ultrafiltration profile during sodium profiling hemodialysis on the maintenance of the quality of dialysis and sodium and fluid balances, *J Am Soc Nephrol* 16(1):237-46, 2005.
48. Redaelli B: Hydroelectrolytic equilibrium change in dialysis, *J Nephrol* 14(4):S7-S11, 2001.
49. Covic A, Diaconita M, Gusbeth-Tatomir P, Covic M, Botezan A, Ungureanu G, et al: Haemodialysis increases QT(c) interval but not QT(c) dispersion in ESRD patients without manifest cardiac disease, *Nephrol Dial Transplant* 17(12):2170-77, 2002.
50. Ichikawa H, Nagake Y, Makino H: Signal averaged electrocardiography (SAECG) in patients on hemodialysis, *J Med* 28(3/4):229-43, 1997.
51. Redaelli B, Locatelli F, Limido D, Andrulli S, Signorini MG, Sforzini S, et al: Effect of a new model of hemodialysis potassium removal on the control of ventricular arrhythmias, *Kidney Int* 50(2):609-17, 1996.
52. Dolson GM, Ellis KJ, Bernardo MV, Prakash R, Adrogue HJ: Acute decreases in serum potassium augment blood pressure, *Am J Kidney Dis* 26(2):321-26, 1995.
53. Dolan MJ, Whipp BJ, Davidson WD, Weitzman RE, Wasserman K: Hypopnea associated with acetate hemodialysis: Carbon dioxide-flow-dependent ventilation, *N Engl J Med* 305(2):72-75, 1981.
54. Lowrie EG, Lew NL: Commonly measured laboratory variables in hemodialysis patients: Relationships among them and to death risk, *Semin Nephrol* 2(3):276-83, 1992.
55. Kraut JA: Disturbances of acid-base balance and bone disease in end-stage renal disease, *Semin Dial* 13(4):261-66, 2000.
56. Mehrotra R, Kopple JD, Wolfson M: Metabolic acidosis in maintenance dialysis patients: Clinical considerations, *Kidney Int Suppl* 88:S13-S25, 2003.
57. Sonikian M, Gogusev J, Zingraff J, Loric S, Quednau B, Bessou G, et al: Potential effect of metabolic acidosis on beta 2-microglobulin generation: in vivo and in vitro studies, *J Am Soc Nephrol* 7(2):350-56, 1996.
58. Uribarri J, Levin NW, Delmez J, Depner TA, Ornt D, Owen W, et al: Association of acidosis and nutritional parameters in hemodialysis patients, *Am J Kidney Dis* 34(3):493-99, 1999.
59. Heguilen RM, Sciurano C, Bellusci AD, Fried P, Mittelman G, Rosa Diez G, et al: The faster potassium-lowering effect of high dialysate bicarbonate concentrations in chronic haemodialysis patients, *Nephrol Dial Transplant* 20(3):591-97, 2005.
60. Ahmad S, Callan R, Cole JJ, Blagg CR: Dialysate made from dry chemicals using citric acid increases dialysis dose, *Am J Kidney Dis* 35(3):493-99, 2000.
61. Fernandez E, Borras M, Pais B, Montoliu J: Low-calcium dialysate stimulates parathormone secretion and its long-term use worsens secondary hyperparathyroidism, *J Am Soc Nephrol* 6(1):132-35, 1995.
62. Fellner SK, Lang RM, Neumann A, Spencer KT, Bushinsky DA, Borow KM: Physiological mechanisms for calcium-induced changes in systemic arterial pressure in stable dialysis patients, *Hypertension* 13(3):213-18, 1989.
63. Hothi DK, Piva E, Keating L, Secker D, Harvey E, Geary D: Calcium and phosphate balance in children on home nocturnal hemodialysis, *Pediatric Nephrology* 21(6):835-41, 2006.
64. Fischbach M, Boudailliez B, Foulard M: Phosphate end dialysis value: A misleading parameter of hemodialysis efficiency, *Pediatr Nephrol* 11:193-95, 1997.
65. Pogglitsch H, Estelberger W, Petek W, Zitta S, Ziak E: Relationship between generation and plasma concentration of inorganic phosphorous: In vivo studies in dialysis patients and in vitro studies on erythrocytes, *Int J Artif Organs* 12:524-32, 1989.
66. Spalding EM, Chamney PW, Farrington K: Phosphate kinetics during haemodialysis: Evidence for biphasic regulation, *Kidney Int* 61:655-67, 2002.
67. Yu A, Nawab Z, Barnes W, et al: Splanchnic erythrocyte content decreases during hemodialysis: A new compensatory mechanism for hypovolemia, *Kidney Int* 51:1986-90, 1997.

68. Jacob S, Ruokonen E, Vuolteenaho O, Lampianen E, Takala J: Splanchnic perfusion during hemodialysis: Evidence for marginal tissue perfusion, *Crit Care Med* 29:1393-98, 2001.
69. Ward RA: Ultrapure dialysate, *Semin Dial* 17(6):489-97, 2004.
70. Laude-Sharp M, Caroff M, Simard L, Pusineri C, Kazatchkine MD, Haeffner-Cavaillon N: Induction of IL-1 during hemodialysis: Transmembrane passage of intact endotoxins (LPS), *Kidney Int* 38(6):1089-94, 1990.
71. Urena P, Herbelin A, Zingraff J, Lair M, Man NK, Descamps-Latscha B, et al: Permeability of cellulosic and non-cellulosic membranes to endotoxin subunits and cytokine production during in-vitro haemodialysis, *Nephrol Dial Transplant* 7(1):16-28, 1992.
72. Lonnemann G, Sereni L, Lemke HD, Tetta C: Pyrogen retention by highly permeable synthetic membranes during in vitro dialysis, *Artif Organs* 25(12):951-60, 2001.
73. Jaber BL, Gonski JA, Cendoroglo M, Balakrishnan VS, Razeghi P, Dinarello CA, et al: New polyether sulfone dialyzers attenuate passage of cytokine-inducing substances from *Pseudomonas aeruginosa* contaminated dialysate, *Blood Purif* 16(4):210-19, 1998.
74. Lonnemann G, Behme TC, Lenzner B, Floege J, Schulze M, Colton CK, et al: Permeability of dialyzer membranes to TNF alpha-inducing substances derived from water bacteria, *Kidney Int* 42(1):61-68, 1992.
75. Schindler R, Krautzig S, Lufft V, Lonnemann G, Mahiout A, Marra MN, et al: Induction of interleukin-1 and interleukin-1 receptor antagonist during contaminated in-vitro dialysis with whole blood, *Nephrol Dial Transplant* 11(1):101-8, 1996.
76. Spittle MA: Chronic inflammation and water quality in hemodialysis patients, *Nephrol News Issues* 15(6):24-26, 28, 2001.
77. Lonnemann G: The quality of dialysate: An integrated approach, *Kidney Int Suppl* 76:S112-S119, 2000.
78. Schouten WE, Grooteman MP, van Houte AJ, Schoorl M, van Limbeek J, Nube MJ: Effects of dialyser and dialysate on the acute phase reaction in clinical bicarbonate dialysis, *Nephrol Dial Transplant* 15(3):379-84, 2000.
79. Schindler R, Lonnemann G, Schaffer J, Shaldon S, Koch KM, Krautzig S: The effect of ultrafiltered dialysate on the cellular content of interleukin-1 receptor antagonist in patients on chronic hemodialysis, *Nephron* 68(2):229-33, 1994.
80. Schiffl H, Lang SM, Stratakis D, Fischer R: Effects of ultrapure dialysis fluid on nutritional status and inflammatory parameters, *Nephrol Dial Transplant* 16(9):1863-69, 2001.
81. Matsuhashi N, Yoshioka T: Endotoxin-free dialysate improves response to erythropoietin in hemodialysis patients, *Nephron* 92(3):601-4, 2002.
82. McKane W, Chandna SM, Tattersall JE, Greenwood RN, Farrington K: Identical decline of residual renal function in high-flux biocompatible hemodialysis and CAPD, *Kidney Int* 61(1):256-65, 2002.
83. Baz M, Durand C, Ragon A, Jaber K, Andrieu D, Merzouk T, et al: Using ultrapure water in hemodialysis delays carpal tunnel syndrome, *Int J Artif Organs* 14(11):681-85, 1991.
84. Schiffl H, Wendinger H, Lang SM: Ultrapure dialysis fluid and response to hepatitis B vaccine, *Nephron* 91(3):530-31, 2002.
85. Lederer SR, Schiffl H: Ultrapure dialysis fluid lowers the cardiovascular morbidity in patients on maintenance hemodialysis by reducing continuous microinflammation, *Nephron* 91(3):452-55, 2002.
86. Kiellstrand CM, Blagg CR, Twardowski ZJ, Bower J: Blood access and daily hemodialysis: Clinical experience and review of the literature, *ASAIO J* 49(6):645-49, 2003.
87. Lacour F, Maheut H: AN 69 membrane and conversion enzyme inhibitors: prevention of anaphylactic shock by alkaline rinsing? *Nephrologie* 13(3):135-36, 1992.
88. Kammerl MC, Schaefer RM, Schweda F, Schreiber M, Riegger GA, Kramer BK: Extracorporal therapy with AN69 membranes in combination with ACE inhibition causing severe anaphylactoid reactions: Still a current problem? *Clin Nephrol* 53(6):486-88, 2000.
89. John B, Anijeet HK, Ahmad R: Anaphylactic reaction during haemodialysis on AN69 membrane in a patient receiving angiotensin II receptor antagonist, *Nephrol Dial Transplant* 16(9):1955-56, 2001.
90. Clark WR, Macias WL, Molitoris BA, Wang NH: Plasma protein adsorption to highly permeable hemodialysis membranes, *Kidney Int* 48(2):481-88, 1995.
91. Henderson L: Biophysics of ultrafiltration and hemofiltration. In C Jacobs, C Kjellstrand, K Koch, J Winchester (eds.), *Replacement of Renal Function By Dialysis, Fourth Edition*. Dortrecht, The Netherlands: Kluwer Academic Publishers 1996:114-45.
92. Locatelli F, Manzoni C: Treatment modalities in comparison: When do clinical differences emerge? *Nephrol Dial Transplant* 15(1):29-35, 2000.
93. Locatelli F, Mastrangelo F, Redaelli B, Ronco C, Marcelli D, La Greca G, Orlandini G: Effects of different membranes and dialysis technologies on patient treatment tolerance and nutritional parameters: The Italian Cooperative Dialysis Study Group, *Kidney Int* 50(4):1293-302, 1996.
94. Bloembergen WE, Hakim RM, Stannard DC, Held PJ, Wolfe RA, Agodoa LY, et al: Relationship of dialysis membrane and cause-specific mortality, *Am J Kidney Dis* 33(1):1-10, 1999.
95. Woods HF, Nandakumar M: Improved outcome for haemodialysis patients treated with high-flux membranes, *Nephrol Dial Transplant* 15(1):36-42, 2000.
96. Woolliscroft JO, Fox IH: Increased body fluid purine levels during hypotensive events: Evidence for ATP degradation, *Am J Med* 81(3):472-78, 1986.
97. Shinzato T, Miwa M, Nakai S, Morita H, Odani H, Inoue I, et al: Role of adenosine in dialysis-induced hypotension, *J Am Soc Nephrol* 4(12):1987-94, 1994.
98. Converse RL Jr., Jacobsen TN, Jost CM, Toto RD, Grayburn PA, Obregon TM, et al: Paradoxical withdrawal of reflex vasoconstriction as a cause of hemodialysis-induced hypotension, *J Clin Invest* 90(5):1657-65, 1992.
99. Ligtenberg G, Barnas MG, Koomans HA: Intradialytic hypotension: New insights into the mechanism of vasovagal syncope, *Nephrol Dial Transplant* 13:2745-47, 1998.
100. Schneditz D, Roob JM, Vaclavik M, Holzer H, Kenner T: Noninvasive measurement of blood volume in hemodialysis patients, *J Am Soc Nephrol* 7(8):1241-44, 1996.
101. Steuer RR, Leypoldt JK, Cheung AK, Harris DH, Conis JM: Hematocrit as an indicator of blood volume and a predictor of intradialytic morbid events, *ASAIO J* 40(3):M691-M696, 1994.
102. Jain SR, Smith L, Brewer ED, Goldstein SL: Non-invasive intravascular monitoring in the pediatric hemodialysis population, *Pediatr Nephrol* 16(1):15-18, 2001.
103. Kim K, Neff M, Kohen B, et al: Blood volume changes and hypotension during hemodialysis, *ASAIO Trans* 16:508-13, 1970.
104. Andrulli S, Colzani S, Mascia F, et al: The role of blood volume reduction in the genesis of intradialytic hypotension, *Am J Kidney Dis* 40:1244-54, 2002.
105. Mitra S, Chamney P, Greenwood R, Farrington K: Linear decay of relative blood volume during ultrafiltration predicts hemodynamic instability, *Am J Kidney Dis* 40:556-65, 2002.
106. Prakash S, Garg AX, Heidenheim AP, House AA: Midodrine appears to be safe and effective for dialysis-induced hypotension: A systematic review, *Nephrol Dial Transplant* 19(10):2553-58, 2004.
107. Donauer J, Kolblin D, Bek M, Krause A, Bohler J: Ultrafiltration profiling and measurement of relative blood volume as strategies to reduce hemodialysis-related side effects, *Am J Kidney Dis* 36(1):115-23, 2000.
108. Ronco C, Feriani M, Chiaramonte S, Conz P, Brendolan L, Bragantini M, et al: Impact of high blood flows on vascular stability in haemodialysis, *Nephrol Dial Transplant* 5(1):109-11, 1990.
109. Ebel H, Laage C, Keuchel M, Dittmar A, Saure B, Ehlenz K, et al: Impact of profile haemodialysis on intra-/extracellular fluid shifts and the release of vasoactive hormones in elderly patients on regular dialysis treatment, *Nephron* 75(3):264-71, 1997.
110. Locatelli F, Di Filippo S, Manzoni C, Corti M, Andrulli S, Pontoriero G: Monitoring sodium removal and delivered dialysis by conductivity, *Int J Artif Organs* 18(11):716-21, 1995.
111. Santoro A, Mancini E, Paolini F, Spongano M, Zucchelli P: Automatic control of blood volume trends during hemodialysis, *ASAIO J* 40:M419-M422, 1994.

112. Dasselaar JJ, Huisman RM, de Jong PE, Franssen CF: Measurement of relative blood volume changes during haemodialysis: Merits and limitations, *Nephrol Dial Transplant* 20(10):2043-49, 2005.
113. Santoro A, Mancini E, Paolini F, et al: Blood volume regulation during hemodialysis, *Am J Kidney Dis* 32:739-48, 1998.
114. Locatelli F, Buoncristiani U, Canaud B, Kohler H, Petitclerc T, Zucchelli P: Haemodialysis with on-line monitoring equipment: tools or toys? *Nephrol Dial Transplant* 20(1):22-33, 2005.
115. Santoro A, Mancini E, Basile C, et al: Blood volume controlled hemodialysis in hypotension-prone patients: A randomized, multicenter controlled trial, *Kidney Int* 62:1034-45, 2002.
116. Moret K, Aalten J, van den Wall-Bake W, Gerlag P, Beerenhout C, van der Sande F, et al: The effect of sodium profiling and feedback technologies on plasma conductivity and ionic mass balance: A study in hypotension-prone dialysis patients, *Nephrol Dial Transplant* 21(1):138-44, 2006.
117. Santoro A, Mancini E, Zucchelli P: The impact of haemofiltration on the systemic cardiovascular response, *Nephrol Dial Transplant* 15(2):49-54, 2000.
118. Fox SD, Henderson LW: Cardiovascular response during hemodialysis and hemofiltration: Thermal, membrane, and catecholamine influences, *Blood Purif* 11(4):224-36, 1993.
119. van der Sande FM, Gladziwa U, Kooman JP, Bocker G, Leunissen KM: Energy transfer is the single most important factor for the difference in vascular response between isolated ultrafiltration and hemodialysis, *J Am Soc Nephrol* 11(8):1512-17, 2000.
120. Saad E, Charra B, Raj DS: Hypertension control with daily dialysis, *Semin Dial* 17:295-98, 2004.
121. Frauman AC, Lansing LM, Fennell RS: Indirect blood pressure measurement in children undergoing hemodialysis: A comparison of brachial and dorsalis pedis auscultatory sites, *AANNT J* 11(1):19-21, 1984.
122. Park MK, Menard SW, Yuan C: Comparison of auscultatory and oscillometric blood pressures, *Arch Pediatr Adolesc Med* 155(1):50-53, 2001.
123. Lingens N, Soergel M, Loirat C, Busch C, Lemmer B, Scharer K: Ambulatory blood pressure monitoring in paediatric patients treated by regular haemodialysis and peritoneal dialysis, *Pediatr Nephrol* 9(2):167-72, 1995.
124. Sherman RA, Daniel A, Cody RP: The effect of interdialytic weight gain on predialysis blood pressure, *Artif Organs* 17(9):770-74, 1993.
125. Portman RJ, Yetman RJ: Clinical uses of ambulatory blood pressure monitoring, *Pediatr Nephrol* 8(3):367-76, 1994.
126. Gavrilovici C, Goldsmith DJ, Reid C, Gubeth-Tatomir P, Covic A: What is the role of ambulatory BP monitoring in pediatric nephrology? *J Nephrol* 17(5):642-52, 2004.
127. National High Blood Pressure Education Program Working Group on High Blood Pressure in Children and Adolescents. The fourth report on the diagnosis, evaluation, and treatment of high blood pressure in children and adolescents, *Pediatrics* 114(2, 4th Report):555-76, 2004.
128. Tozawa M, Iseki K, Iseki C, Takishita S: Pulse pressure and risk of total mortality and cardiovascular events in patients on chronic hemodialysis, *Kidney Int* 61:717-26, 2002.
129. Woods JD, Port FK, Orzol S, Buoncristiani U, Young E, Wolfe RA, et al: Clinical and biochemical correlates of starting "daily" hemodialysis, *Kidney Int* 55:2467-76, 1999.
130. Pierratos A, Ouwendyk M, Francoeur R, Vas S, Raj DS, Ecclestone AM, et al: Nocturnal hemodialysis: three-year experience, *J Am Soc Nephrol* 9:859-68, 1998.
131. Tepel M, van der Giet M, Zidek W: Efficacy and tolerability of angiotensin II type 1 receptor antagonists in dialysis patients using AN69 dialysis membrane, *Kidney Blood Press Res* 24:71-74, 2001.
132. Cice G, Ferrara L, Di Benedetto A, Russo PE, Marinelli G, Pavese F, et al: Dilated cardiomyopathy in dialysis patients: A double-blind, placebo-controlled trial, *J Am Coll Cardiol* 37:407-11, 2001.
133. Foley RN, Parfrey PS, Sarnak MJ: Clinical epidemiology of cardiovascular disease in chronic renal disease, *Am J Kidney Dis* 32: S112-S119, 1998.
134. Calabro P, Willerson JT, Yeh ET: Inflammatory cytokines stimulated C-reactive protein production by human coronary artery smooth muscle cells, *Circulation* 108:1930-32, 2003.
135. Docci D, Bilancioni R, Buscaroli A, Baldrati L, Capponcini C, Mengozzi S, et al: Elevated serum levels of C-reactive protein in hemodialysis patients, *Nephron* 56:364-67, 1990.
136. Panichi V, Migliori M, De Pietro S, Taccola D, Bianchi AM, Giovannini L, et al: C-reactive protein and interleukin-6 levels are related to renal function in predialytic chronic renal failure, *Nephron* 91:594-600, 2002.
137. McIntyre C, Harper I, Macdougall IC, Raine AE, Williams A, Baker LR: Serum C-reactive protein as a marker for infection and inflammation in regular dialysis patients, *Clin Nephrol* 48:371-74, 1997.
138. Sezer S, Kulah E, Ozdemir FN, Tutal E, Arat Z, Haberal M: Clinical consequences of intermittent elevation of C-reactive protein levels in hemodialysis patients, *Transplant Proc* 36:38-40, 2004.
139. Chang JW, Yang WS, Min WK, Lee SK, Park JS, Kim SB: Effects of simvastatin on high-sensitivity C-reactive protein and serum albumin in hemodialysis patients, *Am J Kidney Dis* 39:1213-17, 2002.
140. Vernaglione L, Cristofano C, Muscogiuri P, Chimienti S: Does atorvastatin influence serum C-reactive protein levels in patients on long-term hemodialysis? *Am J Kidney Dis* 43:471-78, 2004.
141. Evans AM, Faull RJ, Nation RL, Prasad S, Elias T, Reuter SE, et al: Impact of hemodialysis on endogenous plasma and muscle carnitine levels in patients with end-stage renal disease, *Kidney Int* 66(4):1527-34, 2004.
142. Evans A: Dialysis-related carnitine disorder and levocarnitine pharmacology, *Am J Kidney Dis* 41(4/4):S13-S26, 2003.
143. Miller B, Ahmad S: A review of the impact of L-carnitine therapy on patient functionality in maintenance hemodialysis, *Am J Kidney Dis* 41(4/4):S44-S48, 2003.
144. Eknoyan G, Latos DL, Lindberg J for the National Kidney Foundation Carnitine Consensus Conference: Practice recommendations for the use of L-carnitine in dialysis-related carnitine disorder, *Am J Kidney Dis* 41(4):868-76, 2003.
145. Wald DS, Law M, Morris JK: Homocysteine and cardiovascular disease: Evidence on causality from a metaanalysis, *Br Med J* 325:1202, 2002.
146. van Guldener C: Why is homocysteine elevated in renal failure and what can be expected from homocysteine-lowering? *NDT Advance Access* 20 Feb. 2006.
147. Ashfield-Watt PA, Pullin CH, Whiting JM, Clark ZE, Moat SJ, Newcombe RG, et al: Methylenetetrahydrofolate reductase 677C → T genotype modulates homocysteine responses to a folate-rich diet or a low-dose folic acid supplement: a randomized controlled trial, *Am J Clin Nutr* 76(1):180-86, 2002.
148. Scholze A, Rinder C, Beige J, Riezler R, Zidek W, Tepel M: Acetylcysteine reduces plasma homocysteine concentration and improves pulse pressure and endothelial function in patients with end-stage renal failure, *Circulation* 109:369-74, 2004.
149. House AA, Wells GA, Donnelly JG, Nadler SP, Hebert PC: Randomized trial of high-flux vs low-flux haemodialysis: Effects on homocysteine and lipids, *Nephrol Dial Transplant* 15(7):1029-34, 2000.
150. Van Tellingen A, Grooteman MP, Bartels PC, Van Limbeek J, Van Guldener C, Wee PM, et al: Long-term reduction of plasma homocysteine levels by super-flux dialyzers in hemodialysis patients, *Kidney Int* 59(1):342-47, 2001.
151. Wrone EM, Hornberger JM, Zehnder JL, McCann LM, Coplon NS, Fortmann SP: Randomized trial of folic acid for prevention of cardiovascular events in end-stage renal disease, *J Am Soc Nephrol* 15:420-26, 2004.
152. Bayes B, Pastor MC, Bonal J, Junca J, Romero R: Homocysteine and lipid peroxidation in haemodialysis: Role of folinic acid and vitamin E, *Nephrol Dial Transplant* 16(11):2172-75, 2001.
153. Gotch FA, Sargent JA: A mechanistic analysis of the National Cooperative Dialysis Study (NCDS), *Kidney Int* 28:526-34, 1985.
154. Goldstein SL, Sorof JM, Brewer ED: Natural logarithmic estimates of Kt/V in the pediatric hemodialysis population, *American Journal of Kidney Diseases* 33(3):518-22, 1999.

155. Daugirdas JT: Simplified equations for monitoring Kt/V, PCRn, eKt/V, and ePCRn, *Advances in Renal Replacement Therapy* 2(4):295-304, 1995.
156. Geddes CC, Traynor J, Walbaum D, Fox JG, Mactier RA: A new method of post dialysis blood urea sampling; the stop dialysate flow method, *Nephrol Dial Transplant* 15:517-23, 2000.
157. Daugirdas JT: Second generation logarithmic estimates of single-pool variable volume Kt/V: An analysis of error, *J Am Soc Nephrol* 4:1205-13, 1993.
158. Owen WF, Lew NL, Liu Y, Lowrie EG, Lazarus JM: The urea reduction ratio and serum albumin concentration as predictors of mortality in patients undergoing hemodialysis, *NEJM* 329:1001-6, 1993.
159. Goldstein SL, Baronette S, Gambress TV, Currier H, Brewer ED: nPCR assessment and IDPN treatment of malnutrition in pediatric hemodialysis patients, *Pediatr Nephrol* 17:531-34, 2002.
160. Van Hoek KJM, Lilien MR, Brinkman DC, Schroeder CH: Comparing a urea kinetic monitor with Daugirdas formula and dietary records in children, *Pediatr Nephrol* 14:280-83, 2000.
161. Grupe WE, Harmon WE, Spinozzi NS: Protein and energy requirements in children receiving chronic hemodialysis, *Kidney Int* 15(1): S6-S10, 1983.
162. Goldstein, SL: Hemodialysis in the pediatric patient, *Advances in Renal Replacement Therapy* 8(3):73-179, 2001.
163. Held PJ, Levin NW, Bovejerg RR, Pauly MV, Diamond LH: Mortality and duration of hemodialysis treatment, *JAMA* 265:871-75, 1991.
164. Laurent G, Charra B: The results of an 8 h thrice weekly haemodialysis schedule, *Nephrol Dial Transplant* 13(6):125-31, 1998.
165. Innes A, Charra B, Burden RP, Morgan AG, Laurent G: The effect of long, slow haemodialysis on patient survival, *Nephrol Dial Transplant* 14(4):919-22, 1999.
166. Tom A, McCauley L, Bell L, Rodd C, Espinosa P, Yu G, et al: Growth during maintenance hemodialysis: impact of enhanced nutrition and clearance, *J Pediatr* 134(4):464-71, 1999.
167. Eknoyan G, Beck GJ, Chung AK, et al: Effective dialysis dose and membrane flux in maintenance hemodialysis, *NEJM* 347(25):2010-19, 2002.
168. European best practices guidelines for hemodialysis [Part 1]. Section II: Hemodialysis adequacy, *Nephrol Dial Transplant* 17(Suppl 7):17-20, 2002.
169. Buur T, Bradbury MG, Smye SW, Brocklebank JT: Reliability of hemodialysis urea kinetic modeling in children, *Pediatr Nephrol* 8:574-78, 1994.
170. Van Hoek KJM, Lilien MR, Brinkman DC, Schroeder CH: Comparing a urea kinetic monitor with Daugirdas formula and dietary records in children, *Pediatr Nephrol* 14:280-83, 2000.
171. Fischbach M, Edefonti A, Schroder C, Watson A for the European Pediatric Dialysis Working Group: Hemodialysis in children: General practical guidelines, *Pediatr Nephrol* 20(8):1054-66, 2005.

CHAPTER 58

Demographics of Pediatric Renal Transplantation

Pierre Cochat and Diane Hébert

INTRODUCTION

Kidney transplantation (Tx) has become the treatment of choice for end-stage renal disease (ESRD) in children. European best practice guidelines for renal Tx, including pediatric-specific issues, have been available since 2002.[1] The upper age limit for pediatric renal care differs among countries [e.g., 15 (Norway) to 21 years (Croatia, United States)], and the average pediatric Tx activity is 4% to 5% of the combined adult and pediatric activity.[2]

CULTURAL AND ETHICAL ISSUES

Access to Transplantation

The access to Tx depends entirely on economic resources, ranging from no access to Tx in many developing countries (Haiti, Gabon, Sudan, Ethiopia, Bangladesh, Nigeria, Paraguay) to a wide but still insufficient access in most developed areas (Europe, North America, Australia, Japan). Organ Tx is a very expensive procedure and may therefore be regarded as a public health challenge.

The use of living donors (LDs) is less expensive than the development of a national network for organ allocation based on deceased donors (DDs). It is therefore logical to accept that countries that initiate a Tx program need to start their experience with LDs and then progressively move to both LDs and DDs, provided an ethical framework for DDs has been established. Twin cooperation between developing and developed countries/centers should be encouraged in order to provide assistance to developing countries.

However, different Tx practices are encountered among developing countries based on economic, religious, political, and cultural backgrounds. Some countries (Morocco) choose to refer selected patients to developed countries for Tx. Other countries (Turkey, Malaysia) have started a Tx program using for the most part related LDs. Still other countries (Egypt, Middle East, India) have a limited Tx activity based on paid unrelated LDs, and finally some countries (Brazil, South Africa) have developed a well-organized Tx network allowing adequate use of both DDs and LDs.

In addition, in many developing countries access to Tx may depend on familial resources (absence of national health care system versus private insurance systems), age at ESRD (treatment withdrawal may be applied for infants and young children, sometimes up to 10 years of age), type of primary disease when identified (inherited inborn error of metabolism), Tx procedure (need for a combined liver and kidney Tx), associated morbidities (mental retardation), and even sometimes gender.[3]

Economic Issues

The risk versus benefit ratio of transplantation is often challenging because Tx is very costly. Successful Tx requires a very specialized environment with high technical expertise: specialized surgery, immunosuppressive drug prescription and monitoring, tissue typing laboratory, microbiologic investigation, adequate diagnostic imaging systems, pathology techniques, access to dialysis and intensive care, and so on. A medical economic evaluation should be performed prior to initiating a new Tx program. For example, in Pakistan the average income per capita approximates $500 U.S. per month and the average cost of generic cyclosporin A + azathioprine is approximately $1500 U.S. and $3000 U.S. for cyclosporin A + mycophenolate mofetil.

Ethical Issues

Tx Tourism

Tx tourism is a growing concern in many countries and can occur in different ways. In this scenario, children with ESRD go to a developed country with transplant resources to receive a transplant or a potential recipient travels to a developing country to purchase a kidney. Another frequent option is for a recipient to organize a trip to a developed country with his potential donor.

All of these practices should be submitted to international supervision in order to avoid unethical practices and to continue to regard Tx as a tribute to human cooperation. The World Health Organization adopted a resolution in 2004 addressing all forms of transplant tourism and organ trafficking, but many of these practices have continued.[4] Many of the national and international professional transplantation societies are developing policies addressing this issue.

Handicapped Children

Kidney Tx in handicapped children should occur when there is optimal medical care, a cooperative family environment, and expected benefit for the patient. Renal transplantation of the severely retarded infant/child/adolescent may pose specific problems: difficulty with performing procedures or cooperating with medical orders, difficulty in taking drugs, the need for a long-term caregiver, and the use of extra hospital and community resources. On the other hand, the care of the severely retarded infant/child/adolescent is less complex than the care required for a child on dialysis. There is very little information available pertaining to the long-term effects on the caregiver of a retarded transplanted infant/child/adolescent. A small number of short-term studies have shown that mental retardation is not associated with poorer graft outcome.[5]

Enrollment of Children in Clinical Trials

The legal limitation for trials of new drugs in children and the need to offer them the benefit of innovative therapies constitute a paradox. The challenge of research in children is to provide both protection and access. Pilot trials are therefore of major interest in pediatric Tx research, and their design should be based on both experience and collaboration among pediatric transplantation health care providers, clinical researchers, the pharmaceutical industry, and the various government bodies responsible for the studies of novel drugs.

ALLOCATION PRACTICES

Pediatric Kidney Allocation in Europe

The use of LDs ranges from 0% to 83% among countries (Figure 58-1). Most of them are genetically or emotionally related. However, due to organ shortage unrelated unpaid LDs are used in some developed countries (Germany, Israel, Norway, Poland, Sweden, the United Kingdom)—and there is growing interest to consider altruistic donation (the United Kingdom, the Netherlands).

Regarding the use of DDs in Europe, most countries have established an upper age limit that ranges from 30 years of age in France and Switzerland to 65 years in Turkey (with no limit in Germany). Few countries recommend a lower age limit for DDs (e.g., 2 years of age in France, 3 years in Spain, and 5 years in the United Kingdom).[2,6,7] In France, only 3.65% of DDs were less than 16 years of age (but these were designated for recipients under 16 years of age).

In 2004, the average waiting time for DD kidney Tx in children varied from 1.5 to 73.3 months (Figure 58-2)—and there was a concomitant growing trend to perform preemptive Tx in Europe and the United States using DDs and LDs (Figure 58-3).[2,8] Pediatric allocation rules depend on national facilities. A scoring system is used in Italy, the Netherlands, Germany, Croatia, Lithuania, the United Kingdom, and Poland. There is an upper age limit for pediatric allocation of 15 years in Italy and Spain; of 16 years in the Netherlands, Germany, and Poland; and of 18 years in the United Kingdom and France.

Human leukocyte antigen (HLA) matching is a major criterion in most countries, and high panel-reactive antibody (PRA) level (PRA > 80%) is an additional priority in France, the United Kingdom, Poland, Serbia, and Spain. Duration of dialysis waiting time represents a priority in Italy, Germany, Switzerland, Croatia, and Spain.[2,6] Other parameters (such as age group, distance from home to dialysis center, and the number of prior Tx) may be included as allocation criteria. In Europe, there are different criteria for placement on a waiting list (Table 58-1).[2] Kidney Tx is indicated in children with:

- Irreversible renal failure
- A minimal age, ranging from 6 to 12 months
- A minimal body weight, ranging from 5 to 10 kg

The following are relative contraindications:

- ABO incompatibility
- Anti-HLA antibodies against donor antigens
- Malignancy within the previous 2 years
- Active viral infection (HIV, VHB, VHC, EBV, CMV)
- Active systemic disease (hemolytic uremic syndrome, systemic lupus erythematosus, rapidly progressive glomerulonephritis)
- Multiorgan failure
- Severe brain damage[1]

Suggested priorities for kidney allocation in children therefore include highly sensitized patients (PRA > 80%; mainly

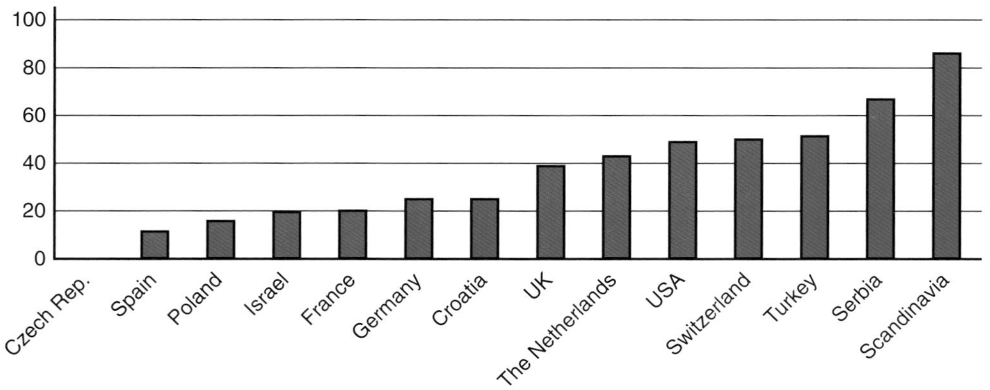

Figure 58-1 Percentage of living (related) donors for pediatric kidney transplantation according to country, 2004.

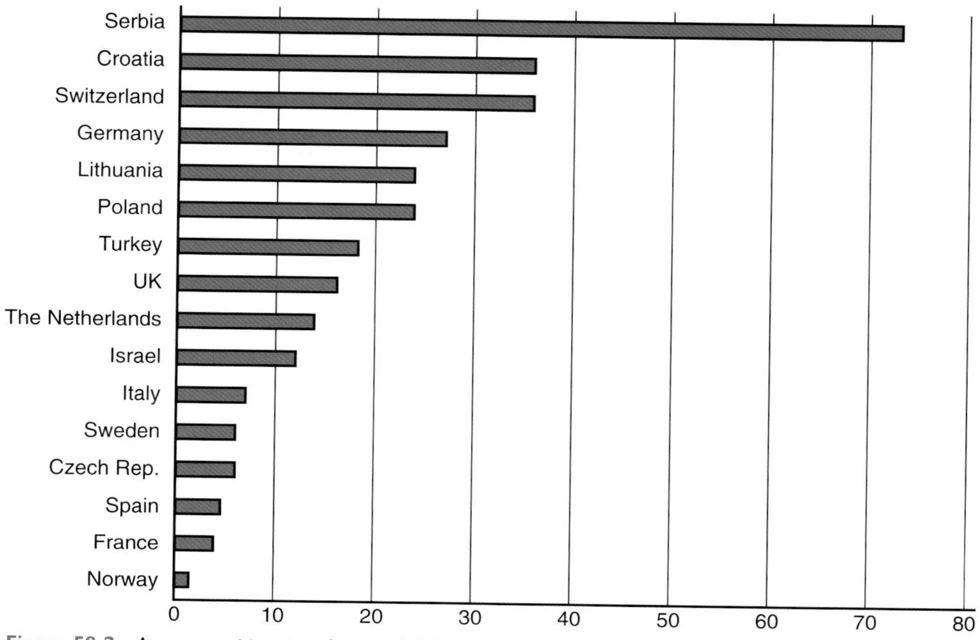

Figure 58-2 Average waiting time (in months) for cadaver kidney transplantation in European children, 2004.

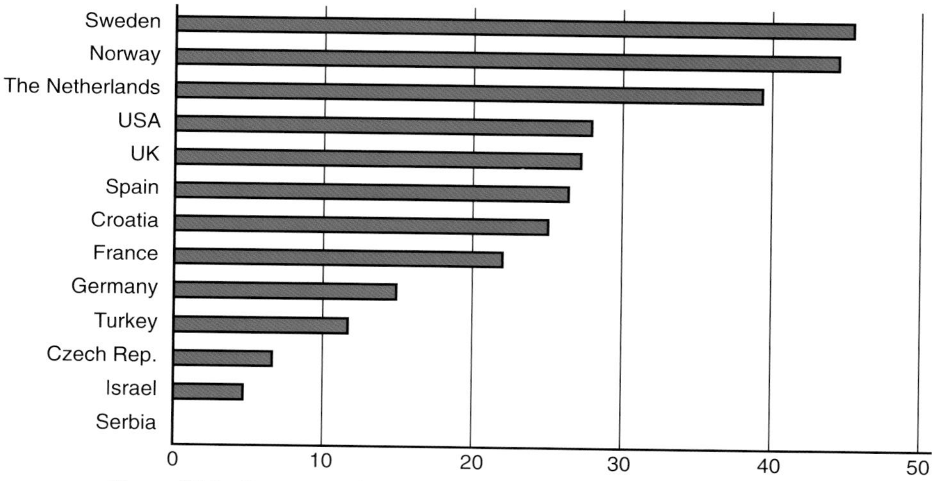

Figure 58-3 Percentage of preemptive kidney transplantation in children, 2004.

those with rare blood groups), zero-HLA/DR mismatch, unavailability of hemodialysis (HD) or peritoneal dialysis (PD) access, and waiting for combined multiorgan Tx. Preemptive transplantation should be recommended in most of these cases.

Organ Allocation in North America

Europe and North America have similar allocation practices. The shortage of DDs has led to increased use of living-unrelated donors in North America.[9] Since 1987, the rate of LD transplantation has risen to about 60% of pediatric Tx, with the highest rate in the younger children. In the United States, allocation of DD Tx is based on a point system that includes the following.

1. Age
2. Sensitization rate
3. HLA matching and waiting times

Since 2006, kidneys from DDs aged less than 35 years have been preferentially allocated to pediatric recipients. In Canada, different allocation schemes are used in the various provincial jurisdictions—but all use a combination of factors, including waiting times, HLA matching, and high PRA.

TABLE 58-1 Criteria for Acceptance on the DD Waiting List in Europe, 2004

	ITA	TUR	NL	SWE	GER	NOR	FRA	CRO	CZE	LIT	UK	POL	SPA
To be on dialysis	+	—	—	—	—	—	—	—	—	+	—	—	+
GFR if preemptive Tx (ml/min/1.73m²)	—	<20	No limit	<10	<25	—	<15	—	No limit	—	<15	—	—
Minimal age (months)	—	24	36	—	6	9	6	60	10	—	21	—	12
Minimal BW (kg)	6	10	12	8	6	9	5	16	—	—	10	8	9
Acceptable HLA mismatch program	—	—	+	—	—	—	+	—	—	—	+	—	—

BW, Body weight; *CRO*, Croatia; *CZE*, Czech Republic; *FRA*, France; *GER*, Germany; *GFR*, glomerular filtration rate; *ITA*, Italy; *LIT*, Lithuania; *NL*, The Netherlands; *NOR*, Norway; *POL*, Poland; *SPA*, Spain; *SWE*, Sweden; *Tx*, transplantation; *TUR*, Turkey; *UK*, United Kingdom; +, yes; –, no.

Kidneys from younger donors are preferentially offered to pediatric recipients.

Organ Allocation in Other Countries

In Australia, the proportion of children receiving an LD kidney has increased from 35% in the 1983-to-1992 decade to 64% in the 1993-to-2002 decade.[10] In Australia, DD kidneys are allocated by state-based algorithms using a ranking and scoring system. This includes mechanisms in which children and adolescents less than 18 years of age and who commenced dialysis before 15 years of age and have been on dialysis for at least 1 year are allocated 30 years' dialysis time to improve their priority score—leading to improved access to DD kidneys for pediatric patients.

In Japan, the majority of pediatric renal transplants are from LD sources because the availability of deceased organ donors is very low. To expand the pool of available LD transplants, ABO-incompatible transplants have been used in children and adolescents more frequently than anywhere else in the world (with improving results).[11]

In India, the majority of pediatric renal transplants are from LD sources. The availability of DDs is limited and varies in different parts of the country.[12,13]

FACTORS AFFECTING OUTCOMES OF TRANSPLANTATION

To ensure current relevance, the data analysis of factors affecting outcomes of kidney Tx in children is limited to papers published during the last 10 years.

Patient and Graft Survival

North American and French 2004 reports on pediatric Tx activity are summarized in Table 58-2.[8,14] Causes of graft failure and death in North America are listed in Tables 58-3 and 58-4.[8]

Short-Term Data

From most recent series in children, 1-, 3-, and 5-year graft survivals are respectively 91% to 95%, 83% to 87%, and 80% to 85% for LD recipients. For DD recipients these figures are respectively 83% to 92%, 71% to 75%, and 65% to 74%.[8,15] Current Tx strategies have brought the short-term graft survival of DD Tx close to that of LD Tx. Interestingly, from two series of 68 and 45 high-risk 15-kg or smaller infant recipients the graft survival was excellent (i.e., respectively 92% at 1 year and 85% at 5 and 10 years[16] and 100% at 2 years and 89.6% at 8 years[17]).

Long-Term Data

The current overall half-life of kidney Tx is 19 to 20 years.[7] There are few long-term studies in children. Offner and colleagues reported a 25-year actuarial survival of 81% for patients and of 31% for the first graft—with best results with living-related donors, preemptive transplantation, and immunosuppression with cyclosporin A.[18]

Estimation of Graft Function

Another way to assess pediatric renal transplant outcome may be based on simple surrogate markers [i.e., estimation of glomerular filtration rate (GFR) from serum creatinine concentration, Schwartz formula, or cystatin C].[19,20]

Determinants of Patient and Graft Survival

Recipient Age

Recipient age at Tx is an important predictor of outcome. In the past, the prognosis of kidney Tx in young children was reported as poor in national databases.[6,21-24] However, these data depended on early study periods and on limited local experience at specialized centers. Current results are comparable to other age groups.[7,14,16,17,25] On the other hand, adolescents now have a worse transplant outcome than other pediatric and adult recipients—most likely secondarily to increased risk of graft loss, late acute rejection, and incomplete rejection reversal largely due to poor compliance with immunosuppressive drugs and medical follow-up.[22,23,26]

Recipient Race

In most North American series, both in children and in adults, the risk of graft failure is increased by 1.57 to 1.90 in African Americans—even after adjustment for matching and rejection. This suggests that non-HLA or socioeconomic events may contribute to racial differences in transplant outcomes.[24,26,27]

Type of Donor

Independent of the selection procedure, both graft and patient survival are better with LD[7,15,26]—although the margin

TABLE 58-2 North American and French 2004 Registry Reports

	France (%)	North America (%)
Primary Diagnosis		
Glomerulonephritis	25.6	24.8
Malformation	25.6	34.1
Inherited renal disease	16.7	13.5
Chronic tubulointerstitial nephritis	18.8	7.0
Vascular disease	2.2	4.4
Other/unknown	11.1	16.2
Recipient Age		
0-2 years	6.2	5.3
2-10 years	43.2	35.6
11-15 years	46.9	31.3
>16 years	3.7	23.7
Recipient Gender		
Male	51.9	59.4
Female	48.1	40.6
Number of Transplants		
Primary transplant	95.1	82.3
Repeat transplant	4.9	17.7
Preemptive Transplantation	22.0	24.6
Type of Donor		
LD	19.8	52.0
DD	80.2	48.0
Donor Age (DD)		
0-2 years	0	1.6
2-10 years	19.8	20.0
11-15 years	37.0	15.6
16-29 years	22.2	30.0
>30 years	21.0	32.8
Graft Survival		
1 year	LD + DD: 92.8	LD: 94.8 – DD: 91.7
5 years	LD + DD: 82.9	LD: 85.0 – DD: 74.2

Data from Agence de la Biomédecine. Rapport d'activité 2004, http://www.efg.sante.fr/fr/index.asp; and from North American Pediatric Renal Transplant Cooperative Study (NAPRTCS). Annual report 2005, *https://web.emmes.com/study/ped/annlrept/annlrept.html*.
LD, Living donor; *DD*, deceased donor.

of difference continues to shrink. Most registry databases include both adult and pediatric DD data, and it is important to consider graft survival and graft function. Adult-size kidneys adapt to pediatric recipients during the first months post-Tx, but graft function does not improve thereafter (along with the increase in body size of the recipient). On the other hand, the absolute GFR of children receiving pediatric grafts increases along with body growth—leading to a stable long-term GFR.[28,29]

The poor results reported with young pediatric DD Tx are usually due to vascular thrombosis,[6,25] which can usually be effectively prevented by anticoagulation—allowing a more appropriate use of donors less than 6 years of age. Promising results have been reported by using en-bloc kidneys from donors younger than 4 years.[21] On the other hand, the use of adult-size kidneys gives excellent long-term graft survival when transplanted into infants and small children—provided acute tubular necrosis (ATN) has been prevented by adequate fluid management in order to improve renal artery blood flow.[30-32]

The use of unrelated LD has grown in Europe and in North America, but the results in early studies are inferior to those with living-related donors.[9] Poorer graft outcome with female donor gender has been reported in adult organ Tx, but this has no significant influence on graft outcome in children. One explanation may come from the smaller nephron dose in adult female donors, which may be adequate for pediatric recipients.[26,33]

Ischemia Time

Independent of the type of donor, cold ischemia damage has a permanent detrimental effect on graft function and survival—mainly when it exceeds 24 hours.[34]

Immunologic Factors

Immunologic factors (HLA mismatch and PRA) have a decreasing adverse effect on renal graft survival. However, significant differences in graft survival are observed mainly with HLA-B and DR mismatch—especially with DD Tx.[7,8]

Pre-Tx Blood Transfusion

A limited number of pretransplant blood transfusions (i.e., 1 to 5) may decrease the risk of acute rejection, but multiple blood transfusions (>5) appear to be a risk factor for graft failure.[35] Therefore, blood transfusions have been omitted from many Tx protocols due to potential viral and immunologic risks together with limited benefit on overall graft survival.

Pre-Tx Dialysis

Preemptive Tx not only increases quality of life and social rehabilitation but provides better graft survival.[7,21,26,36-38] In patients with pre-Tx dialysis, the use of PD can reduce the incidence and severity of delayed graft function (DGF)—independently of cold ischemia time and fluid status.[39] However, the overall graft survival rates of PD and HD patients are similar.[38]

Center Volume Effect

The experience and training of a pediatric Tx team may be linked to improved graft survival because of their expertise with highly specific activities, such as Tx in infants, combined liver and kidney Tx, retransplantation of patients with recurrent diseases, Tx of patients with severe urinary tract problems, and the like.[16,17,31] The risk of DD graft thrombosis has been reported to be increased, as has the occurrence of ATN, in centers reporting fewer than 50 patients. This resulted in lower graft survival at 3 months post-Tx, after which the effect disappeared.[40] However, the center volume effect is limited for most Tx patients—provided children are transplanted in a pediatric center.[1]

Delayed Graft Function

In most papers, DGF is defined as the need for dialysis during the first post-Tx week—which is more frequent with DD Tx than with LD Tx. Its incidence depends on local facilities and national allocation rules, which may influence ischemia time and HLA-DR matching. DGF may be difficult to diagnose with the current definition in children undergoing preemptive Tx, and may be underreported. DGF appears to be an important risk for graft failure, independent of rejection rate.[41] The intraoperative management of young children with adult-size kidneys requires aggressive intravascular volume maintenance in order to maintain optimum aortic blood flow and avoid ATN, vascular thrombosis, and primary nonfunction.[31] Experienced postoperative pediatric intensive care management should be available to all pediatric recipients.[42]

Graft Vascular Thrombosis

Graft thrombosis is responsible for 8% to 12% of graft losses in the pediatric population. The incidence of graft thrombosis has decreased because of better pre-Tx screening for thrombophilia (protein S, protein C, factor V Leiden, and so on) and extended use of anticoagulation prophylaxis in the perioperative period.[43] However, the risk of thrombosis is still elevated in children with specific identified coagulation abnormalities, technically difficult vascular anastomosis, and pre-Tx PD.[38,44] The risk of vascular thrombosis is particularly a cause of graft failure when the recipient and/or the donor is under 6 years of age, and careful attention should be paid to this age group.[25]

Arterial Hypertension

Post-Tx arterial hypertension is found in 56% to 78% of pediatric recipients.[45,46] Causes are multifactorial, including chronic allograft dysfunction, immunosuppression therapy, and renal vascular disorders. Early post-Tx systolic hypertension strongly and independently predicts poor long-term graft survival in pediatric patients.[7,47] In addition, the development of late arterial hypertension is also part of the vicious cycle leading to progressive graft impairment.[18,46] Ambulatory 24-hour blood pressure (BP) patterns are indeed often abnormal after renal Tx in children (mainly in boys), often including elevated load values and nondipping sleep BP—and sometimes sleep BP exceeding awake BP.[45] In addition to decreased graft survival, such abnormal BP is associated with a greater risk for morbid cardiovascular events.

Recurrence of the Primary Disease

Graft failure due to recurrence of the original kidney disease is responsible for 6.9% of graft failure,[8] mainly in patients with focal segmental glomerulosclerosis, atypical hemolytic uremic syndrome, and membranoproliferative and membranous glomerulonephritis. These diseases may require specific pre- and post-Tx interventions in order to limit graft loss to recurrence of primary disease.

TABLE 58-3 Causes of Graft Failure among Pediatric Kidney Tx Recipients in North America

Cause of Graft Failure	Graft Failures (%)
Chronic rejection	33.6
Acute rejection	13.1
Vascular thrombosis	10.6
Death with functioning graft	9.2
Recurrence of primary disease	6.9
Patient discontinued medication	4.4
Primary nonfunction	2.2
Bacterial/viral infection	1.8
Accelerated acute rejection	1.7
Other technical	1.3
Malignancy	1.2
Hyperacute rejection	0.7
Renal artery stenosis	0.6
Cyclosporin toxicity	0.4
De novo kidney disease	0.4
Other/unknown	11.9

Data from North American Pediatric Renal Transplant Cooperative Study (NAPRTCS). Annual report 2005, https://web.emmes.com/study/ped/annlrept/annlrept.html.

TABLE 58-4 Causes of Death among Pediatric Kidney Tx Recipients in North America

Cause of Death	Deaths (%)
Cardiopulmonary	15.4
Bacterial infection	12.9
Cancer/malignancy	11.1
Viral infection	8.5
Other infection	7.9
Hemorrhage	6.7
Dialysis-related complication	2.8
Disease recurrence	1.6
Other	24.4
Unknown	8.7

Data from North American Pediatric Renal Transplant Cooperative Study (NAPRTCS). Annual report 2005, https://web.emmes.com/study/ped/annlrept/annlrept.html.

Acute Rejection

Acute rejection is responsible for 13% to 21% of graft failure in children.[8,21] The number, the severity, and the response to corticosteroids of acute allograft rejection episodes during the first 6 months post-Tx are a major determinant of long-term graft function and survival.[21,26,48,49] However, the use of new immunosuppressive regimens has significantly decreased the rate of initial episodes of rejection.[15] Early acute rejection may also increase the risk of patient death, due to opportunistic infections during aggressive antirejection therapy.[50] The risk of acute rejection by the end of the first year post-Tx is lower with LD Tx.[15]

Infections

Urinary tract infections and vesicoureteric reflux are frequent in Tx children with extravesical urinary anastomosis. This may lead to parenchymal scarring, but there is no evidence of further consequences for long-term renal function.[51,52] Cytomegalovirus (CMV) is the most important opportunistic infection in renal Tx recipients and is associated with an increased risk of rejection, morbidity, and even mortality. Infection can be acquired from the transplanted organ or from reactivation of latent disease. In children, seasonal community CMV coinfection after exposure to an infected donor may promote progression from CMV infection to CMV disease.[53] CMV prophylaxis may be associated with better graft survival, but there is no consensus on the optimal prophylactic treatment.[7,54] However, the widespread and prolonged use of antiviral drugs has changed the natural course and drug resistance of CMV disease.[55]

Polyomavirus (mainly BK virus, BKV)-associated nephropathy is an emerging cause of kidney Tx failure in 1% to 10% of adult patients—mainly among those with intense immunosuppression, often including tacrolimus and/or mycophenolate mofetil plus corticosteroids.[56] An incidence of 3.5% of BKV-associated nephropathy has been reported in children at a median of 15 months post-Tx (positive histology, viruria, and viremia), mainly in seronegative recipients.[57]

Human herpesvirus-6 (HHV-6) infection occurs in approximately 20% of solid-organ Tx recipients early post-transplant, and may lead to the development of fever, skin rash, pneumonia, bone marrow suppression, and rejection.[58] HHV-7 may act as a cofactor for CMV disease. HHV-8 may be associated with Kaposi's sarcoma and acute bone marrow failure in Tx patients.[59]

Pediatric transplant recipients with no immunity to varicella are at high risk of developing serious varicella-related complications. Vaccination is recommended early, prior to transplant, and is usually well tolerated.[60] Further details concerning immunization of renal transplant patients can be found in Chapter 61.

Epstein-Barr virus (EBV) is a ubiquitous herpesvirus that can establish both lytic and latent infection in the host. EBV infection is associated with significant morbidity and mortality in allograft recipients, including post-Tx lymphoproliferative disorder (PTLD). EBV-induced PTLD is a B-cell growth abnormality ranging from hyperplasia to invasive malignancy. The increased incidence of EBV-related disease after Tx is the result of inhibition of the normal antiviral immune response by immunosuppression. Pediatric kidney Tx recipients who are seronegative at the time of transplant are at increased risk of developing EBV-induced complications.

Cancer

The risk of cancer increases with the age at Tx,[8] the duration of posttransplant follow-up, and the use of new immunosuppressive drugs. The incidence of malignant diseases in children was less than 5% after an average follow-up of 13.1 years, as reported in 1999.[18] This has increased with the use of new immunosuppressive drugs: 0.96% in the period 1987 to 1991, 2.0% in the period 1992 to 1995, and 3.1% in the period 1996 to 2005. An increase in PTLD is largely responsible for the higher rate of malignancy post-Tx in recent years.[8]

Chronic Allograft Nephropathy

Chronic allograft nephropathy (CAN) leads to graft failure in 28% to 33% of patients.[8,21] Many factors contribute to CAN, such as subclinical immunologic damage, calcineurin inhibitor nephrotoxicity, noncompliance, arterial hypertension, calcium-phosphate abnormalities, and so on. Angiotensin-converting enzyme inhibition and angiotensin-receptor blocker therapy are well tolerated and are associated with a trend of slowing the progression of renal insufficiency, as well as with a significant benefit for graft and patient survival.[61]

Cardiovascular Disorders

The use of corticosteroids and an abnormal GFR may affect body composition. Most children experience a significant increase in fat mass and a decrease in lean mass during the early post-Tx period.[62] This can be limited by adequate diet, a corticosteroid-sparing regimen, and physical exercise. In the long term, the cumulative risks of obesity, hyperlipidemia, and arterial hypertension lead to increased risk of cardiovascular morbidity and mortality.[63,64] The adjusted relative risk of death in obese children aged 6 to 12 years compared to nonobese transplant patients in North America is 3.65 for LD Tx and 2.94 for DD Tx.[63]

Noncompliance and Transition to Adult Unit

Graft survival may be affected by noncompliance with medication and medical follow-up most frequently in adolescents. The poor graft outcome in adolescents is thought to be largely due to noncompliance. Noncompliance among all causes of graft failure is reported as 7% in nine publications.[65] The average estimated level of drug adherence after renal Tx is only 40% to 50%, which can be improved by ongoing education and individual support.[65]

Additional broader categories of compliance, which are less well documented, include the degree to which patients follow more general recommendations—such as smoking discontinuation, losing weight, and increasing the amount of daily physical exercise.[66] Psychological factors frequently associated with noncompliance are insufficient family support, low self-awareness caused by poor cognitive abilities, and denial. Such problems may be triggered at the time of transfer from pediatric to adult transplant unit, and the rate of graft failure due to noncompliance may be increased during the initial period after the transfer.[67] A close follow-up should therefore be established between the patient and both pediatric and adult units.

Determinants of Post-Tx Rehabilitation and Quality of Life

The aim of kidney Tx in children is to restore their potential for normal growth, development, and quality of life in order to reach mature adulthood.

Growth and Bone and Body Composition

Longitudinal growth in children with ESRD and kidney Tx has improved over the past decade. However, renal Tx induces only moderate catch-up growth during the prepubertal period and final height is reduced in about a third of patients due to the reduced pubertal height gain and preexisting height deficit at the time of Tx.[18,68] Treatment advances mainly include improved nutrition, minimal steroid dosage, and administration of recombinant human growth hormone (rhGH) to the most growth-retarded patients.[69]

Long-term use of rhGH is safe and effective in pediatric allograft recipients. Better results are observed in rhGH recipients less than 10 years old, and final height is increased.[70] In addition, improved growth has been reported with preemptive Tx and by using LDs.[42] The risk-to-benefit ratio of steroid withdrawal/avoidance in pediatric kidney Tx is still under investigation, but encouraging results have been reported.[71] Attainment of adult height, not just growth velocity, needs to be further investigated—together with the optimal drug regimen for preserving transplant GFR and allowing normal longitudinal growth.

The main cause of secondary hyperparathyroidism in ESRD will disappear after a successful renal Tx, provided the GFR is good. However, post-Tx regression of parathyroid hyperfunction may take a long time. Children who have had preemptive Tx achieve normal PTH levels sooner than dialyzed children.[72] Due to differences within the methods of analysis, longitudinal changes in bone mineral density (BMD) after Tx are still controversial.[73] In addition, the investigation of the muscle-bone unit by peripheral quantitative computed tomography is better suited to children than is BMD alone because the reduction in muscular force may contribute to a risk of fracture.[74]

Anemia

Anemia is found in 60% to 80% of pediatric patients from 1 to 5 years post renal Tx, which is more frequent than in adults.[75] It has been mainly attributed to the level of GFR, immunosuppressive drugs, iron deficiency, and bone disease. When required, its treatment with iron therapy and/or erythropoietin may improve quality of life, physical activities, and cognitive performance.

Cognitive Development

Recent data show that children with kidney Tx are currently able to achieve a level of cognitive development near to or at the level of healthy children. The use of cognitive ability testing shows that mental processing speed, reaction time, discrimination sensitivity, and working memory significantly improve after renal Tx.[76] Interestingly, such good neurodevelopmental outcomes have been shown in high-risk patients after renal Tx in early childhood. Most risk factors for impaired development occur prior to Tx (i.e., sensorineural deafness, premature birth, perinatal problems, hypertensive crises, and seizures during dialysis).[77]

Psychosocial Development

Renal Tx in children is associated with better psychological outcomes and rehabilitation than PD or HD. However, transplanted children continue to experience delayed social development, maladaptive problems, and increased psychiatric problems. Measures of communication, daily living skills, and socialization are below healthy norms. The physical effects of illness and treatments contribute to low self-esteem, which is a major factor in noncompliance with both medications and medical follow-up. In addition, the degree of medical adherence often correlates with the degree of psychological distress, family dynamics, and the psychological side effects of immunosuppressive drugs.

In a series of children in Germany with a mean follow-up of 13.1 years after transplantation, 27% suffered from additional disabilities and 14% of adults were unemployed.[18] In another series in France with an average 11.9 year follow-up post-Tx,[78] final height was 156.6 cm for males and 147.4 cm for females—both of which are below the 3rd percentile. The distribution of educational level was lower than the normal population: 27.4% were at the lowest level versus 3% of the general population. However, activity was comparable to the general population: 73% had paid employment, 6.5% were unemployed, and 18.9% were disabled. Twenty-seven percent of males were married, and 8.3% had children—whereas 50% of females were married and 27% had at least one child. Forty-six percent of all such adult patients lived with parents, and 54% were independent. Multivariate analysis showed a significant correlation among education, employment, marital life, independent housing, and final height.

SPECIAL ISSUES IN DEVELOPING COUNTRIES

The outcomes of Tx in developing countries depend on the medical expertise and the economic resources available. In Lucknow (India), the 1-year patient and graft survival was 89% and the 3-year was 70%. The actuarial graft survival at 5 years was 50%.[3] In another series from Johannesburg (South Africa), overall 1-, 5-, and 10-year survival rates were respectively 82%, 44%, and 23% for grafts (i.e., an average graft survival of 4.38 years) and 97%, 84%, and 68% for patients.[79]

Special issues are known to affect the outcome of Tx in developing countries. The primary diagnosis is often unidentified, but may include complex conditions such as urologic problems (urinary tract malformations, reflux nephropathy, neurogenic bladder), postinfectious glomerulonephritis, recurrent disease (focal segmental glomerulosclerosis, membranoproliferative glomerulonephritis, primary hyperoxaluria), lupus nephritis, and unidentified inherited disease. Most Tx are performed from LD, but donor assessments may be limited—sometimes leading to poor outcomes in recipient and donor.

However, DD organ-based programs have been widely developed in several developing places in the world (e.g., South Africa, Brazil, and Taiwan). Due to less than adequate immunosuppression and limited biologic follow-up, acute and chronic rejection are rather frequent and are difficult to manage. This problem is increased by noncompliance due to insufficient knowledge of kidney Tx, distance from home to Tx center, poor acceptance of side effects of drugs, variable drug supply and availability, and the like.[3] The incidence of infectious complications is high due to insufficient or inadequate prophylaxis and to specific problems due to poor hygiene.[3] Patient survival may be influenced by life-threatening complications such as septicemia, invasive fungal infections, cancers, and PTLD.

Most developing countries lack national kidney foundations and insurance systems, and although renal Tx is more cost effective than dialysis only a limited number of political strategies are in favor of promoting Tx. Any type of disease prevention should therefore be regarded as a priority, including health education (to fight unhygienic habits) and the use of traditional medicines (some of which are nephrotoxic). Screening for renal diseases among schoolchildren might identify patients early in the disease course and maximize appropriate intervention.

SUMMARY

Tx is currently the best option for children with ESRD. Surgery and modern immunosuppression have demonstrated excellent results, provided the children are managed in a pediatric center with experience in the management of all aspects of pediatric renal transplantation. However, such a therapeutic option is not accessible to all children in the world because of political, religious, economic, and cultural issues in developing countries.

REFERENCES

1. Cochat P, Offner G: European best practice guidelines for renal transplantation (Part 2): Pediatrics (Specific problems), *Nephrol Dial Transplant* 17(4):55-58, 2002.
2. Cochat P: Pediatric renal allograft allocation practices in Europe (collaborative survey). 39th Annual Meeting of the European Society for Paediatric Nephrology, Istanbul, September 10-13, 2005 (personal communication).
3. Gulati S, Kumar A, Kumar Sharma R, et al: Outcome of pediatric renal transplants in a developing country, *Pediatr Nephrol* 19:96-100, 2004.
4. Bulletin of the World Health Organization. 82:715, 2004, *http://www.who.int/bulletin/volumes/82/9/feature0904/en/index.html*.
5. Martens MS, Jones L, Reiss S: Organ transplantation, organ donation and mental retardation, *Pediatr Transplant* 10:658-64, 2006.
6. Postlethwaite RJ, Johnson RJ, Armstrong S, et al: The outcome of pediatric cadaveric renal transplantation in the UK and Eire, *Pediatr Transplant* 6:367-77, 2002.
7. Collaborative Transplant Study 2006, *http://www.ctstransplant.org*.
8. North American Pediatric Renal Transplant Cooperative Study (NAPRTCS). Annual report 2005, *https://web.emmes.com/study/ped/annlrept/annlrept.html*.
9. Al-Uzri A, Sullivan EK, Fine RN, Harmon WE: Living-unrelated renal transplantation in children: A report of the North American Pediatric Renal Transplant Cooperative Study, *Pediatr Transplant* 2:139-44, 1998.
10. McDonald SP, Craig JC: Australian and Paediatric Nephrology Association: Long-term survival of children with end-stage renal disease, *New Engl J Med* 350:2654-62, 2004.
11. Saito K, Takahashi K: ABO-compatible kidney transplantation in Japan, *International Congress Series* 1292:35-41, 2006.
12. Phadke K, Iyengar A, Karthik S, et al: Pediatric renal transplantation: The Bangalore experience, *Indian Pediatrics* 43:44-48, 2006.
13. Gulati S, Kumar A, Sharma AK, et al: Outcome of pediatric transplants in a developing country, *Pediatr Nephrol* 19:96-100, 2004.
14. Agence de la Biomédecine. Rapport d'activité 2004, *http://www.efg.sante.fr/fr/index.asp*.
15. Seikaly M, Ho PL, Emmett L, Tejani A: The 12th annual report of the North American Pediatric Renal Transplant Cooperative Study: Renal transplantation from 1987 through 1998, *Pediatr Transplant* 5:215-31, 2001.
16. Neipp M, Offner G, Lück R, et al: Kidney transplantation in children weighing less than 15 kg: Donor selection and technical considerations, *Transplantation* 73:409-16, 2002.
17. Millan MT, Sarwal MM, Lemley KV, et al: A 100% 2-year graft survival can be attained in high-risk 15 kg or smaller infant recipients of kidney allografts, *Arch Surg* 135:1063-69, 2000.
18. Offner G, Latta K, Hoyer PF, et al: Kidney transplanted children come of age, *Kidney Int* 55:1509-17, 1999.
19. Bökenkamp A, Ozden N, Dieterich C, et al: Cystatin C and creatinine after successful kidney transplantation in children, *Clin Nephrol* 52:371-76, 1999.
20. Sorof JM, Goldstein SL, Brewer ED, et al: Serial estimation of glomerular filtration rate in children after renal transplantation, *Pediatr Nephrol* 13:737-41, 1999.
21. Cransberg K, van Gool JD, Davin JC, et al: Pediatric renal transplantation in the Netherlands, *Pediatr Transplant* 4:72-81, 2000.
22. Smith JM, Ho PL, McDonald RA, et al: Renal transplant outcomes in adolescents: A report of the North American Pediatric Transplant Cooperative Study, *Pediatr Transplant* 6:493-99, 2002.
23. Maxwell H, Johnson R, O'Neill J, et al: Five-year outcome after paediatric renal transplantation in the UK, *Transplantation* 82(Suppl 3):102, 2006.
24. McDonald R, Donaldson L, Emmett L, et al: A decade of living donor transplantation in North American children: The 1998 annual report of the North American Pediatric Transplant Cooperative Study, *Pediatr Transplant* 4:221-34, 2000.
25. Dall'Amico R, Ginevri F, Ghio L, et al: Successful renal transplantation in children under 6 years of age, *Pediatr Nephrol* 16:1-7, 2001.
26. Ishitani M, Isaacs R, Norwood V, et al: Predictors of graft survival in pediatric living-related kidney transplant recipients, *Transplantation* 70:288-92, 2000.
27. Isaacs RB, Nock SL, Spencer CE, et al: Racial disparities in renal transplant outcomes, *Am J Kidney Dis* 34:706-12, 1999.
28. Berg U, Bohlin AB, Tyden G: Influence of donor and recipient ages and sex on graft function after pediatric renal transplantation, *Transplantation* 64:1424-28, 1997.
29. Dubourg L, Cochat P, Hadj-Aïssa A, et al: Better long-term functional adaptation to the child's size with pediatric compared to adult kidney donor, *Kidney Int* 62:1454-60, 2002.
30. Healey PJ, McDonald R, Waldhausen JHT, et al: Transplantation of adult living donor kidneys into infants and small children, *Arch Surg* 135:1035-41, 2000.
31. Salvatierra O, Singh T, Shifrin R, et al: Successful transplantation of adult-sized kidneys into infants requires maintenance of high aortic blood flow, *Transplantation* 66:819-23, 1998.
32. Sarwal MM, Cecka JM, Millan MT, Salvatierra O: Adult-size kidneys without acute tubular necrosis provide exceedingly superior long-term graft outcomes for infants and small children, *Transplantation* 70:1728-36, 2000.
33. Zeier M, Döhler B, Opelz G, Ritz E: The effect of donor gender on graft survival, *J Am Soc Nephrol* 13:2570-76, 2002.
34. Smits JMA, van Houwelingen HC, de Meester J, et al: Permanent detrimental effect of nonimmunological factors on long-term renal graft survival, *Transplantation* 70:317-23, 2000.
35. Chavers BM, Sullivan EK, Tejani A, et al: Pre-transplant blood transfusion and renal allograft outcome: A report of the North American

Pediatric Transplant Cooperative Study, *Pediatr Transplant* 1:22-28, 1997.
36. Mahmoud A, Saïd MH, Dawahra M, et al: Outcome of preemptive renal transplantation and pretransplantation dialysis in children, *Pediatr Nephrol* 11:537-541, 1997 [erratum in *Pediatr Nephrol* 11:777, 1997].
37. Mange KC, Joffe MM, Feldman HI: Effect of the use or non-use of the long-term dialysis on the subsequent survival of renal transplants from living donors, *N Engl J Med* 344:726-31, 2001.
38. Vats AN, Donaldson L, Fine RN, et al: Pretransplantation dialysis status and outcome of renal transplantation in North American children: A NAPRTCS study, *Transplantation* 69:1414-19, 2000.
39. van Biesen W, Vanholder A, van Loo A, et al: Peritoneal dialysis favorably influences early graft function after renal transplantation compared to hemodialysis, *Transplantation* 69:508-14, 2000.
40. Schurman SJ, Stablein D, Perlman SA, Warady BA: Center volume effect in pediatric renal transplantation, *Pediatr Nephrol* 13:373-78, 1999.
41. Tejani AH, Sullivan EK, Alexander SR, et al: Predictive factors for delayed graft function and its impact on renal graft survival in children: A report of the North American Pediatric Renal Transplant Cooperative Study, *Pediatr Transplant* 3:293-300, 1999.
42. Pape L, Ehrich JH, Zivicnjak M, Offner G: Growth in children after kidney transplantation with living related donor graft or cadaveric graft, *Lancet* 366:151-53, 2005.
43. Robertson AJ, Nargund V, Gray DWR, Morris PJ: Low-dose aspirin as prophylaxis against renal-vein thrombosis in renal-transplant recipients, *Nephrol Dial Transplant* 15:1865-68, 2000.
44. McDonald RA, Smith JM, Stablein D, et al: Pretransplant peritoneal dialysis and graft thrombosis following pediatric kidney transplantation: A NAPRTCS report, *Pediatr Transplant* 7:204-8, 2003.
45. Sorof JM, Poffenbarger T, Portman R: Abnormal 24-hour blood pressure patterns in children after renal transplantation, *Am J Kidney Dis* 35:681-86, 2000.
46. Nagasako SS, Koch Nogueira PC, Goulart-Pinheiro Machado P, Medina Pestana JM: Arterial hypertension following renal transplantation in children: A short term study, *Pediatr Nephrol* 18:1270-74, 2003.
47. Mitsnefes MM, Khoury PR, McEnery PT: Early posttransplantation hypertension and poor long-term renal allograft survival in pediatric patients, *J Pediatr* 143:98-103, 2003.
48. Guyot C, Nguyen JM, Cochat P, et al: Risk factors for chronic rejection in pediatric renal allograft recipients, *Pediatr Nephrol* 10:723-27, 1996.
49. Humar A, Hassoun A, Kandaswamy R, et al: Immunological factors: The major risk for decreased long-term renal allograft survival, *Transplantation* 68:1842-46, 1999.
50. Munoz R, Romero B, Medeiros M, et al: Renal survival in children with early acute rejection, *Pediatr Transplant* 2:294-98, 1998.
51. Howie AJ, Buist LJ, Coulthard MG: Reflux nephropathy in transplants, *Pediatr Nephrol* 17:485-90, 2002.
52. Ranchin B, Chapuis F, Dawahra M, et al: Vesicoureteral reflux after kidney transplantation in children, *Nephrol Dial Transplant* 15:1852-58, 2000.
53. Robinson LG, Hilinski J, Hymes GF, et al: Predictors of cytomegalovirus disease among pediatric transplant recipients within one year of renal transplantation, *Pediatr Transplant* 6:111-18, 2002.
54. Bock GH, Sullivan EK, Miller D, et al: Cytomegalovirus infections following renal transplantation effects of antiviral prophylaxis: A report of the North American Pediatric Transplant Cooperative Study, *Pediatr Nephrol* 11:665-71, 1997.
55. Rowshani AT, Bemelman FJ, van Leeuwen EMM, et al: Clinical and immunologic aspects of cytomegalovirus infection in solid organ transplant recipients, *Transplantation* 79:381-86, 2005.
56. Hirsch HH, Brennan DC, Drachenberg CB, et al: Polyomavirus-associated nephropathy in renal transplantation: Interdisciplinary analyses and recommendations, *Transplantation* 79:1277-86, 2005.
57. Smith JM, McDonald RA, Finn LS, et al: Polyomavirus nephropathy in pediatric kidney transplant recipients, *Am J Transplant* 4:2109-17, 2004.
58. Yoshikawa T: Human herpesvirus-6 and -7 infections in transplantation, *Pediatr Transplant* 7:11-17, 2003.
59. Allen UD: Human herpesvirus type 8 infections among solid organ transplant recipients, *Pediatr Transplant* 6:187-92, 2002.
60. Furth SL, Hogg RJ, Tarver J, et al: Varicella vaccination in children with chronic renal failure: A report from the Southwest Pediatric Nephrology Study Group, *Pediatr Nephrol* 18:33-38, 2003.
61. Lin J, Valeri AM, Markowitz GS, et al: Angiotensin converting enzyme inhibition in chronic allograft nephropathy, *Transplantation* 73:783-88, 2002.
62. Feber J, Braillon P, David L, Cochat P: Body composition in children after renal transplantation, *Am J Kidney Dis* 38:366-70, 2001.
63. Havenold CD, Ho PL, Talley L, Mitsnefes MM: Obesity and renal transplant outcome: A report of the North American Pediatric Renal Transplant Cooperative Study, *Pediatrics* 115:352-56, 2005.
64. Ishitani MB, Milliner DS, Kim DY, et al: Early subclinical coronary artery calcification in young adults who were pediatric kidney transplant recipients, *Am J Transplant* 5:1689-93, 2005.
65. Wolff G, Strecker K, Vester U, et al: Non-compliance following renal transplantation in children and adolescents, *Pediatr Nephrol* 12:703-08, 1998.
66. Nevins T: Non-compliance and its management in teenagers, *Pediatr Transplant* 6:475-79, 2002.
67. Watson A: Non-compliance and transfer from paediatric to adult transplant unit, *Pediatr Nephrol* 14:468-72, 2000.
68. Nissel R, Brazda I, Feneberg R, et al: Effect of renal transplantation in childhood on longitudinal growth and adult height, *Kidney Int* 66:792-800, 2004.
69. Ulinski T, Cochat P: Longitudinal growth in children following kidney transplantation: From conservative to pharmacological strategies, *Pediatr Nephrol* 21:903-9, 2006.
70. Fine RN, Stablein D: Long term use of recombinant human growth hormone in pediatric allograft recipients: A report of the NAPRTCS Transplant Registry, *Pediatr Nephrol* 20:404-8, 2005.
71. Ellis D: Growth and renal function after steroid-free tacrolimus-based immunosuppression in children with renal transplants, *Pediatr Nephrol* 14:689-94, 2000.
72. Koch Nogueira P, Rey N, Saïd MH, Cochat P: Evolution of hyperparathyroidism after renal transplantation in children: Effect of preemptive transplantation and duration of dialysis, *Nephrol Dial Transplant* 12:984-87, 1997.
73. Feber J, Filler G, Cochat P: Is decreased bone mineral density in pediatric transplant recipients really a problem? *Pediatr Transplant* 7:342-44, 2003.
74. Leonard MB: Assessment of bone mass following renal transplantation in children, *Pediatr Nephrol* 20:360-67, 2005.
75. Yorgin PD, Belson A, Sanchez J, et al: Unexpected high prevalence of posttransplant anemia in pediatric and young adult renal transplantation recipients, *Am J Kidney Dis* 40:1306-18, 2002.
76. Mendley SR, Zelko FA: Improvement in specific aspects of neurocognitive performance in children after renal transplantation, *Kidney Int* 56:318-23, 1999.
77. Qvist E, Pikho H, Fagerudd P, et al: Neurodevelopmental outcome in high-risk patients after renal transplantation in early infancy, *Pediatr Transplant* 6:53-62, 2002.
78. Broyer M, Le Bihan C, Charbit M, et al: Long-term outcome of children after kidney transplantation, *Transplantation* 77:1033-37, 2004.
79. Pichter GJ, Beale PG, Bowley DM, et al: Pediatric renal transplantation in a South African teaching hospital: A 20-year perspective, *Pediatr Transplant* 10:441-48, 2006.

CHAPTER

59 Immunosuppression in Pediatric Kidney Transplantation

Burkhard Tönshoff and Anette Melk

INTRODUCTION

Ideally, a host would accept a renal transplant by induction of antigen-specific nonresponsiveness (immunologic tolerance). It is not currently possible to induce specific tolerance, and transplantation requires immunosuppressive therapies. The current goal is to use immunosuppressive agents that are potent, selective, and reversible—with reliable delivery and long-term safety. Most therapies alter immune response mechanisms but are not immunologically specific, and a careful balance is required to find the dose that prevents rejection of the graft while minimizing the risks of oversuppression that lead to the development of infection and certain types of cancer.

Current immunosuppressive agents reduce acute rejection, but do not induce tolerance. It is true that a few patients with organ transplants can successfully withdraw their immunosuppression without rejecting their grafts for long periods. Nevertheless, they are rare exceptions and may eventually reject—even after years. Even though antigen-specific T cells with reactivity to the foreign antigen persist in the host indefinitely, some graft and host adaptation must occur because the level of immunosuppression required long term is very low compared to the levels required within the first weeks.

This adaptation makes long-term immunosuppression possible. However, the long-term risk of cancer in the immunosuppressed patient remains increased. Thus, the distinction between immunosuppression and induction of tolerance is partly artificial. All immunosuppression involves some apparent antigen-specific adaptation, a downregulation of the host response to the graft—and many tolerance protocols involve some nonspecific immunosuppression.

The common immunosuppressive agents used in pediatric renal transplantation include the glucocorticoids, azathioprine, mycophenolate mofetil (MMF), the calcineurin inhibitors (CNIs) cyclosporine and tacrolimus, and antibodies to cell surface antigens on lymphocytes [antilymphocyte globulin (ALG, monoclonal anti-CD3 (OKT3), anti-CD25, and others]. Newer agents are inhibitors of the mammalian target of rapamycin (mTOR; sirolimus/rapamycin and everolimus) and alemtuzumab, a humanized anti-CD52 panlymphocytic monoclonal antibody. The structures of some immunosuppressives are shown in Figure 59-1. Our discussion focuses on these agents and how they inhibit the immune response.

THE IMMUNE RESPONSE

By the time transplant surgery is completed, the graft has experienced acute injury—leading to an increased expression of major histocompatibility complex (MHC) molecules by cells within the graft that are either constitutively expressed (class I, human leukocyte antigen-A [HLA-A], and HLA-B) inducible (class II, HLA-DR) antigens. Injury recruits lymphocytes and antigen-presenting cells (APCs; typically monocytes, macrophages, and dendritic cells) from the host. These injury-related events may influence the probability of rejection and may contribute to the superior outcome in transplants from live donors (with less injury) versus those from cadaveric donors.

Allorecognition of donor MHC molecules may occur either by the direct route (host T cells recognize donor MHC on donor cells) or indirectly (host T cells recognize donor MHC as peptides in the MHC groove of host APCs). T cell receptors (TCRs) engaging MHC-peptide complexes provide signal 1. Costimulatory signals from the APC engaging receptors on the T cells provide signal 2 (Figure 59-2). The major costimulatory molecules of the APC are B7-1/B7-2, which bind CD28 on the T cells. Activated T cells express CD40L that can activate the APC by engaging CD40 on the APC, and Fas ligand (FasL)—which binds Fas on other lymphocytes or other cells to induce apoptosis in the Fas-bearing cell.

Activation of signals 1 and 2 is followed by T cell activation with production of many cytokines. Cytokines, such as interleukin 2 (IL–2), engage other specific receptors on the T cells to provide signal 3—the signal for cell division and clonal expansion. The engagement of CD40 by CD40L and the cytokines and growth factors from T cells regulate the T cell response, recruit and activate inflammatory cells, and alter adhesion molecules to cause mononuclear cells to accumulate in the graft. Depending on the type and degree of signaling, full activation of the T cell may occur—or T cells may undergo partial activation, apoptosis, anergy, or neglect (ignoring the antigen). T cells also bind via CD40L to CD40 on the B cell, thereby directing the switch from IgM to IgG

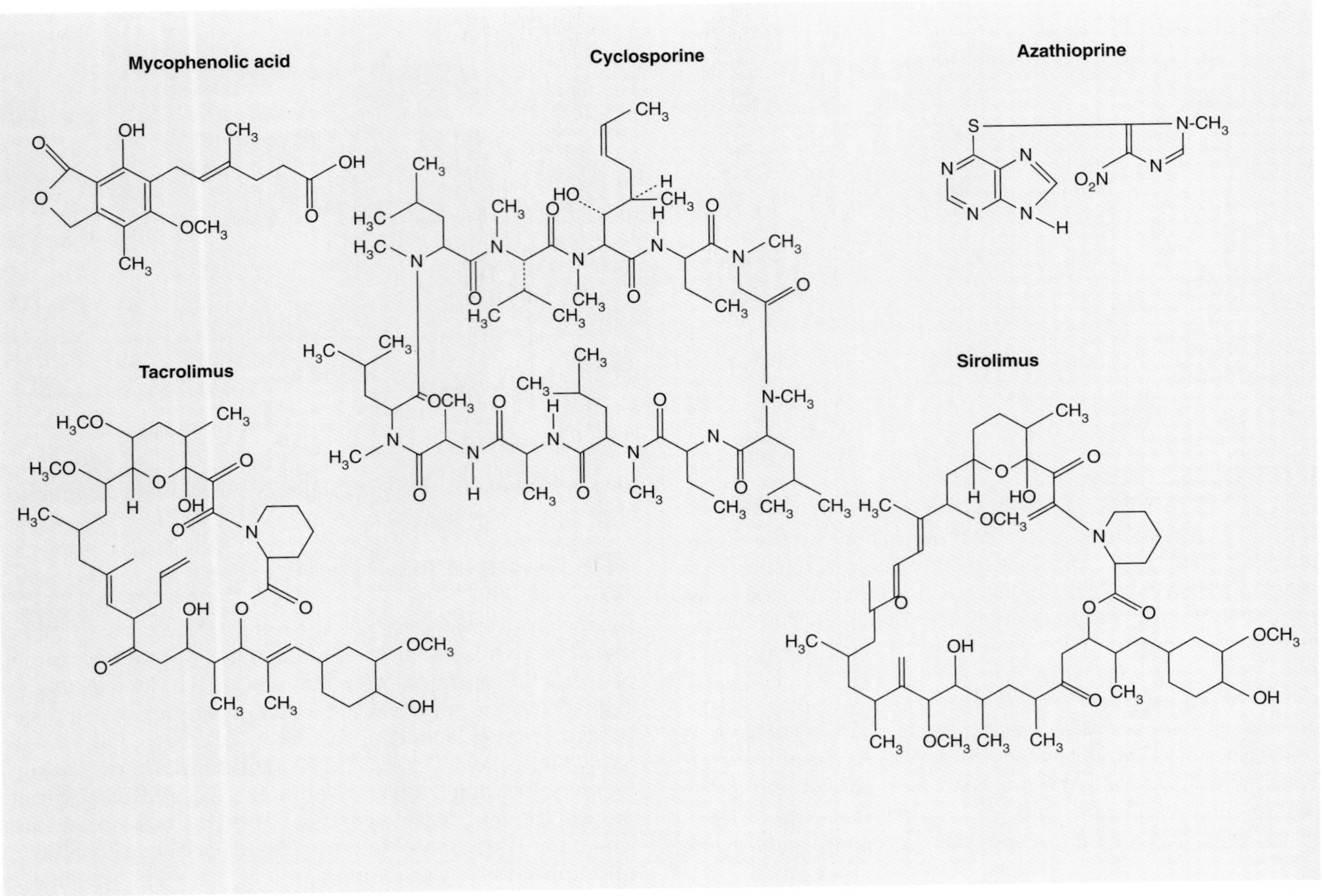

Figure 59-1 Structure of mycophenolic acid, cyclosporine, azathioprine, tacrolimus, and sirolimus. These are all small molecules with molecular weights of 320, 1203, 277, 804, and 914, respectively. (From Johnson RJ, Feehally J (eds.): *Comprehensive clinical nephrology, Second edition*. Philadelphia: Elsevier 2003:1058.)

production by the B cell and promoting the maturation of IgG-producing B cells.

Chemotactic factors (chemokines) and expression of adhesion proteins and foreign (MHC) antigens mediate localization (homing) of the T (CD4 and CD8) cells to the graft endothelium. Lymphocyte recirculation depends on the ability to enter and leave lymphoid tissue. CD8 T cells that recognize peptide in the groove of class I MHC become cytotoxic T cells (CTLs). Graft rejection is associated with infiltration by cytotoxic (CD8) lymphocytes. Delayed-type hypersensitivity may also be involved in T-cell–mediated damage. Antibody-mediated injury may also occur and cause damage to endothelium. A summary of the effects of immunosuppressive drugs is presented in Figure 59-3.

INDUCTION IMMUNOSUPPRESSIVE THERAPY

Induction refers to the administration of an intensive immunosuppressive regimen during the perioperative period. The rationale behind this approach is that the risk of acute rejection is greatest in the first weeks or months after transplantation. Induction therapies often involve the use of polyclonal or monoclonal antibodies to achieve rapid and profound early immunosuppression. Polyclonal antibodies used for this purpose include those against thymocytes (e.g., commercially available rabbit or equine preparations). Monoclonal antibodies include basiliximab (a chimeric human–murine anti-CD25 or anti–interleukin-2 receptor antibody), daclizumab (a humanized anti–interleukin-2 receptor antibody), OKT3 (muromonab-CD3, a mouse anti-CD3 antibody), and alemtuzumab (an anti-CD52 antibody targeting both B and T cells).

A number of trials have been and are being conducted in adult and pediatric renal transplant recipients to look at the effects of the different prophylactic antibody induction therapies. Evaluation of these trials or of any induction protocol requires consideration of the following factors: incidence and severity of delayed allograft function or primary nonfunction, including the requirement for and duration of dialysis following transplantation; incidence of acute rejection; incidence, type, and severity of associated infections; long-term allograft survival and function; mortality and morbidity, including length of hospitalization, and cost; and incidence and type of malignancy during long-term follow-up.

Several studies from single centers and registries, as well as metaanalyses, have found that induction with antibodies may be superior to non antibody-based regimens, even in

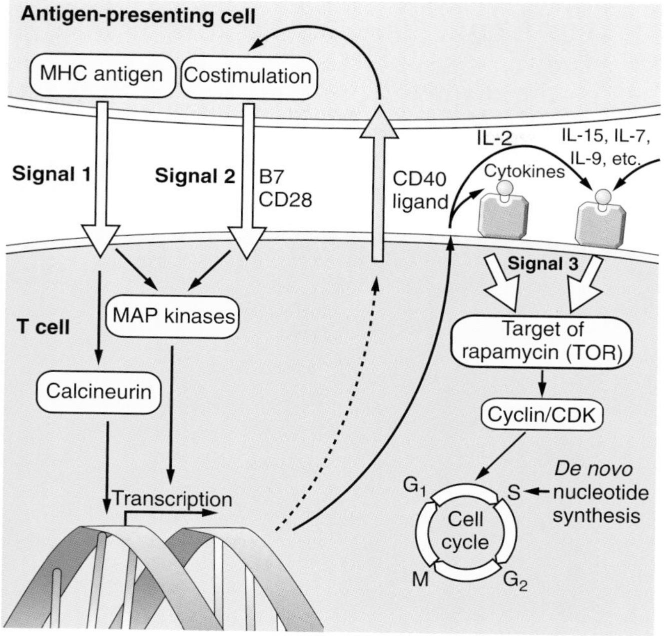

Figure 59-2 The three events in T-cell activation. Engagement of the T-cell receptor with the antigenic peptide in the context of self–MHC class II molecule leads to the activation of the calcineurin pathway and results in the induction of cytokine genes (e.g., IL–2; signal 1). Signal 2, the costimulatory signal, involves the engagement of CD28 with members of the B7 family. This synergizes with signal 1 to induce cytokine production. Interaction between cytokine production and its corresponding receptor leads to induction of cell division, probably through the target of rapamycin (TOR) pathway. This constitutes signal 3. (From Feehally J, Floege J, Johnson RJ (eds.): *Comprehensive clinical nephrology, Third edition*. Philadelphia: Mosby 2007:1035.)

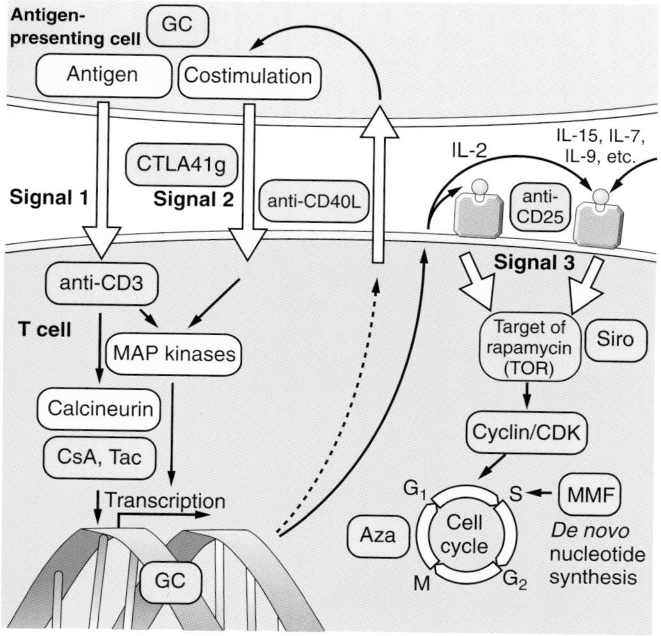

Figure 59-3 Effects of various immunosuppressive drugs on T-cell signaling. (From Feehally J, Floege J, Johnson RJ (eds.): *Comprehensive clinical nephrology, Third edition*. Philadelphia: Mosby 2007:1036.)

low-risk groups.[1] Unfortunately, most (if not all) published studies have addressed only some of the previously cited issues. As a result, although each protocol may have its own advantages and/or disadvantages in a particular patient population none is yet proven to be superior when the previously cited factors are considered. The optimal prophylactic induction immunosuppressive therapy for preventing renal transplant rejection therefore remains controversial.

Figure 59-4 presents the induction antibody use from 1996 to 2005, as reported in the NAPRTCS 2006 Annual Report.[2] The frequency of use of the different immunosuppressive antilymphocyte regimens for induction therapy has varied markedly over the last 15 years. In 2005, 33.1% of pediatric patients did not receive induction antibody therapy, 32.6% received basiliximab, 22.7% received daclizumab, and 11.6% received antithymocyte globulin (ATG) or ALG.

Lymphocyte-depleting Antibodies

Polyclonal Antibodies

Because of the redundancy of the immune system, polyclonal antibodies (which have a broad specificity) should theoretically be more effective in induction therapy than monoclonal antilymphocyte agents such as OKT3. ATGAM is a purified gamma globulin solution obtained by immunization of horses with human thymocytes. It contains antibodies to a wide variety of human T-cell surface antigens, including the MHC antigens. Thymoglobulin is a polyclonal antibody preparation derived from the rabbit. It is approved for the treatment of rejection by the Federal Drug Administration (FDA) of the United States. As for ATGAM, thymoglobulin contains antibodies to a wide variety of T-cell antigens and MHC antigens.

Polyclonal antibodies act in three ways: by activating or altering the function of lymphocytes, by lysing lymphoid cells, and by altering the traffic of lymphoid cells and sequestering them. These antibodies are potently immunosuppressive, but often produce side effects. By triggering T cells, they generate significant first-dose effects—with the release of tumor necrosis factor alpha (TNFα), interferon-γ (IFN-γ), and other cytokines, causing a first-dose reaction (flu-like syndrome, fever, and chills).

Efficacy and Safety

Few studies have compared the relative efficacy of thymoglobulin and ATGAM for induction therapy. In one study in adult renal transplant recipients, 72 patients were randomly assigned in a double-blind 2 : 1 fashion to receive thymoglobulin at 1.5 mg/kg intravenously or ATGAM at 15 mg/kg intravenously, intraoperatively, and then daily for at least 6 days.[3] The delayed graft function rate was only 1% for both groups. At 1 year, the group administered thymoglobulin had a significantly lower acute rejection rate (4% versus 25%, respectively) and higher allograft survival (98% versus 83%, respectively).

The lower rejection rate was thought to be due in part to a more sustained lymphopenia with thymoglobulin, whereas the exceptionally low delayed graft function rate seen in both groups may have been due to the intraoperative use of the ATGs. Both antibodies have the ability to block a number of adhesion molecules, cytokines, chemokines, and their receptors, which may contribute to ischemia reperfusion injury and delayed graft function. At 5 years, allograft survival was significantly better in the thymoglobulin arm (77% versus 57% percent, respectively).[4] Two cases of posttransplant lymphoproliferative disorder developed with ATGAM, whereas none were observed with thymoglobulin. The mean 5-year serum creatinine concentration was similar in both groups.

In pediatric renal transplant recipients, a historical cohort study compared the rates of survival, rejection, and infection in patients who received induction therapy with ATGAM ($n = 127$) or thymoglobulin ($n = 71$).[5] Maintenance immunosuppression included cyclosporine, azathioprine or MMF, and prednisone. Mean follow-up was 90 ± 25 months for ATGAM recipients and 32 ± 15 months for thymoglobulin recipients. Overall, the incidence of acute rejection was lower in thymoglobulin recipients versus ATGAM recipients (33% versus 50%, respectively; $p = 0.02$).

Epstein-Barr virus (EBV) infection was higher in thymoglobulin recipients versus ATGAM recipients (8% versus 3%, respectively; $p = 0.002$). However, the two groups did not significantly differ in patient and graft survival rates, incidence of chronic rejection, EBV lymphoma, or other infections. The authors concluded that thymoglobulin induction was associated with a decreased incidence of acute rejection and an increased incidence of EBV infection in pediatric renal transplant recipients.

Monoclonal Antibodies (OKT3)

Monoclonal antibodies have also been produced to different T-cell surface receptors. The first antibody used in clinical transplantation was the anti-CD3 antibody, OKT3, which binds to the delta chain of the T-cell receptor and is a potent inhibitor of almost all T-cell functions. Although OKT3 is extremely effective, its use is limited in part by the formation of anti-OKT3 antibodies. Such antibodies are common among children. Among 40 children receiving OKT3 as prophylactic therapy, for example, 71% developed antiidiotypic antibodies after one course of therapy.[6]

The most serious side effect of OKT3 is the "first-dose reaction," which occurs in more than two thirds of patients after the first dose of OKT3. It consists of fever, chills, headache, vomiting, diarrhea, hypotension, and occasionally pulmonary edema (particularly in fluid overloaded patients). These symptoms are related to the activation of T cells and the release of several cytokines. They are partially prevented by the administration of corticosteroids, pentoxifylline, or anti-TNF monoclonal antibodies.

Efficacy and Safety

One randomized trial in 287 pediatric renal transplant recipients compared the use of OKT3 in one arm and intravenous cyclosporine in another arm.[7] Maintenance therapy consisted of cyclosporine A together with prednisone and either azathioprine or MMF. Morbidity, mortality, rejection rates, and adverse reactions in the two study arms were similar. Through 4 years, graft failure was 27% in OKT3-treated patients and 19% in cyclosporine-treated patients ($p = 0.15$).

One-year graft survival was 89.1% in OKT3-treated patients and 89.2% in cyclosporine-treated patients. In multivariate analysis, OKT3-treated patients had a numerically

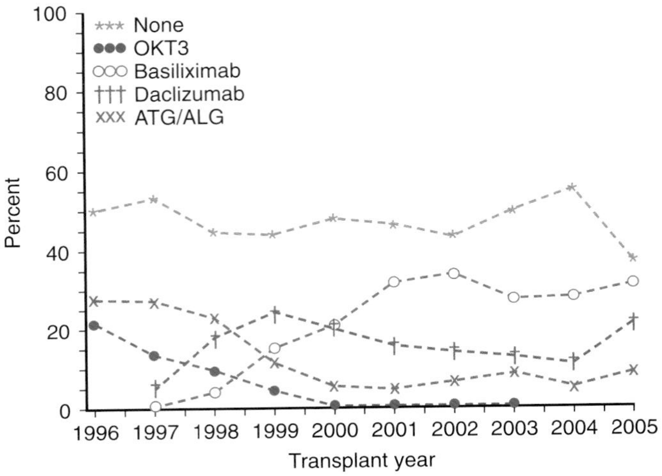

Figure 59-4 Induction antibody use in pediatric renal transplant recipients by year of renal transplantation. (From the NAPRTCS 2006 Annual Report. *https://web.emmes.com/study/ped/index.htm*.)

inferior graft survival (RR = 1.4, CI 0.8-2.2, $p = 0.22$). With OKT3, graft survival was inferior for children aged 6 years or younger. This trial demonstrated that the incidence of acute rejection or graft failure in pediatric patients is not improved by OKT3 induction therapy relative to cyclosporine induction. Due to the results of this trial and other experiences, the use of OKT3 for induction therapy in renal transplant recipients has been almost completely abandoned in recent years (Figure 59-1).

Interleukin-2 Receptor Antibodies

Full T-cell activation leads to the calcineurin-mediated stimulation of the transcription, translation, and secretion of interleukin-2 (IL-2), a key autocrine growth factor that induces T-cell proliferation. Thus, an attractive therapeutic option is abrogation of IL-2 activity via the administration of anti–IL-2 receptor antibodies. Two monoclonal anti–IL-2 receptor antibodies have been approved by the FDA for use in renal transplantation in adults and pediatric patients: daclizumab (a humanized monoclonal antibody) and basiliximab, a chimeric monoclonal antibody.

Both antibodies are directed against CD25, the IL-2 receptor 55 kDa α-chain (Figure 59-5). The IL-2 receptor consists of three transmembrane protein chains: CD25, CD122, and CD132. CD25 is present on nearly all activated T cells, but not on resting T cells. IL-2 induces clonal expansion of activated T cells. Although CD25 does not transduce the signal, it is responsible for the association of IL-2 with the β- and γ-chains, which triggers the activated T cell to undergo rapid proliferation. These antibodies bind to activated T cells and render them resistant to IL-2 by blocking, shedding, or internalizing the receptor. They may also deplete and sequester some activated T cells. However, IL-2 receptor functions are partially redundant because other cytokine receptors have overlapping functions (e.g., IL-15 receptors). Therefore, saturating IL-2 receptors produces stable but relatively mild immunosuppression and is only effective in combination with other immunosuppressives.

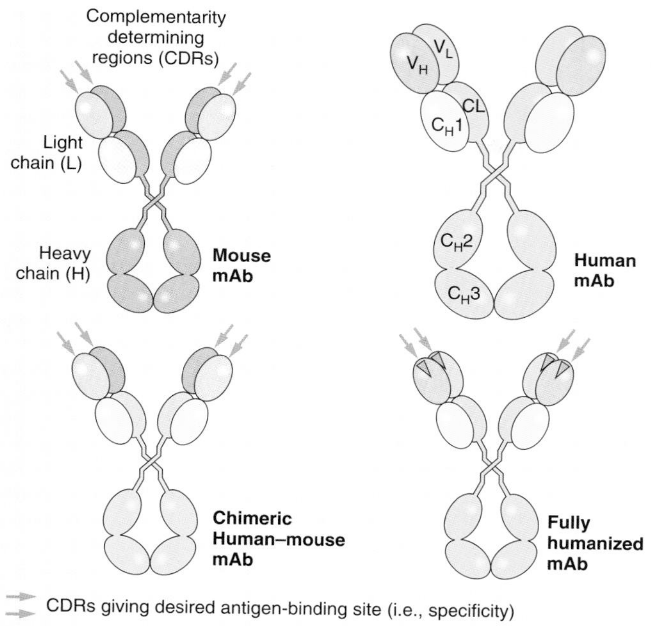

Figure 59-5 Chimeric versus humanized monoclonal antibodies. (From Feehally J, Floege J, Johnson RJ (eds.): *Comprehensive clinical nephrology, Third edition*. Philadelphia: Mosby 2007:1044.)

Efficacy and Safety

A 2004 metaanalysis in adult renal transplant recipients involving 38 trials that enrolled nearly 5000 patients assessed the effect of IL-2 receptor antibodies on allograft loss and rejection rate.[8] Data were derived from published trials and abstracts of completed and ongoing trials. From these 38 trials, 14 trials enrolling 2,410 patients compared IL-2 receptor antagonists with placebo for at least one outcome. Compared with placebo, IL-2 receptor antagonists reduced acute rejection rates at 6 months (RR 0.66, CI 0.59-0.74) and 1 year (RR 0.67, CI 0.60-0.75). However, the incidence of graft loss was the same.

Only nine trials with a total enrollment of 778 patients examined the efficacy of IL-2 receptor antagonists versus other antibody therapy. Among these studies, other antibody therapies were associated with lower rates of biopsy-proven acute rejection, combined end point of graft loss and death, all-cause mortality, and delayed graft function. However, significantly fewer adverse effects were observed with IL-2 receptor antagonists. Rarely, episodes of severe acute hypersensitivity have been described among patients either initially exposed to basiliximab and/or following reexposure after several months.[9]

Recently, the efficacy and safety of basiliximab has been evaluated in two randomized trials in pediatric renal transplant recipients. In a 6-month multicenter randomized controlled open-label parallel-group trial, the efficacy and safety of adding basiliximab to a standard tacrolimus-based regimen was assessed.[10] Patients received tacrolimus, azathioprine, and steroids ($n = 93$) or tacrolimus, azathioprine, steroids, and basiliximab ($n = 99$). Basiliximab was administered at 10 mg (patients <40 kg) or 20 mg (patients ≥40 kg) within 4 hours of reperfusion. The same dose was repeated on day 4. Biopsy-proven acute rejection rates were 20.4% without basiliximab and 19.2% with basiliximab. Steroid-resistant acute rejection rates were 3.2% and 3.0%, respectively. Patient survival was 100%, and graft survival rates were 95% in both arms. The nature and incidence of adverse events were similar in both arms except for toxic nephropathy and abdominal pain, which were significantly higher in the basiliximab arm. Median serum creatinine concentrations at 6 months and glomerular filtration rates (GFRs) were comparable. The authors concluded that adding basiliximab to a tacrolimus-based regimen is safe in pediatric patients but does not improve clinical efficacy.

A second multicenter prospective trial, this time placebo-controlled and double blind, evaluated the efficacy and safety of basiliximab in 202 pediatric patients on maintenance therapy with cyclosporine, MMF, and steroids.[11] Cyclosporine was adjusted to target trough levels of 150 to 250 ng/ml for the first 3 months and 100 to 200 ng/ml thereafter. A protocol biopsy was performed at month 6. The incidence of biopsy-proven acute rejection Banff grades I through III at month 6 was 11.0% on basiliximab compared to 16.1% on placebo (NS). Five patients in each group had presumptive rejection. Antibody therapy for steroid-resistant rejection was given in three patients on basiliximab and five patients on placebo. Two graft losses, one in each group, were observed. Two deaths occurred in the basiliximab group during the first 6 months. The overall incidence of adverse events was similar in both groups. Two patients on basiliximab and five patients on placebo developed posttransplant lymphoproliferative disease (PTLD). The authors from this study concluded that the incidence of biopsy-proven acute rejection episodes was numerically but not significantly lower on basiliximab. Whether basiliximab has an effect on long-term results needs to be the subject of future evaluations.

Comparison with Thymoglobulin

Few studies have compared the use of different induction immunosuppressive regimens. In one prospective randomized international study, short courses of antithymocyte globulin and basiliximab were compared in adult patients at high risk for acute rejection or delayed graft function who received a renal transplant from a deceased donor.[12] Patients taking cyclosporine, MMF, and prednisone were randomly assigned to receive either rabbit antithymocyte globulin (1.5 mg per kilogram of body weight daily, 141 patients) during transplantation (day 0) and on days 1 through 4 or basiliximab (20 mg, 137 patients) on days 0 and 4.

The primary end point was a composite of acute rejection, delayed graft function, graft loss, and death. At 12 months, the incidence of the composite end point was similar in the two groups ($p = 0.34$). The antithymocyte globulin group, compared to the basiliximab group, had lower incidences of acute rejection (15.6% versus 25.5%, respectively; $p = 0.02$) and of acute rejection that required treatment with antibody (1.4% versus 8.0%, respectively; $p = 0.005$). The antithymocyte globulin group and the basiliximab group had similar incidences of graft loss (9.2% and 10.2%, respectively), delayed graft function (40.4% and 44.5%, respectively), and death (4.3% and 4.4%, respectively).

Although the incidences of all adverse events, serious adverse events, and cancers were also similar between the two groups, patients receiving antithymocyte globulin had a greater incidence of infection (85.8% versus 75.2%, respectively; $p = 0.03$) but a lower incidence of cytomegalovirus disease (7.8% versus 17.5%, respectively; $p = 0.02$). The authors concluded that among patients at high risk for acute rejection or delayed graft function who received a renal transplant from a deceased donor induction therapy consisting of a 5-day course of antithymocyte globulin, compared to basiliximab, reduced the incidence and severity of acute rejection but not the incidence of delayed graft function. Patient and graft survival were similar in the two groups.

One long-term study compared the results of monoclonal anti–IL-2 receptor antibody versus polyclonal antilymphocyte antibodies as induction therapy in renal transplantation.[13] The influence of induction therapy on 5-year patient and graft survival as well as on renal function in 100 kidney graft recipients at low immunologic risk treated with ALG ($n = 50$) versus anti–IL-2 receptor monoclonal antibody ($n = 50$) was compared in a prospective multicenter study. Long-term immunosuppressive treatment included cyclosporine, MMF, and a short course of steroids in all patients. Five-year graft (86% versus 86%) and patient (94% versus 94%) survivals were identical in both study arms. Moreover, neither serum creatinine nor proteinuria were significantly different between the two groups. These results show that the choice of the induction therapy does not seem to have a major impact on long-term outcomes among renal recipients at low immunologic risk.

Alemtuzumab

Alemtuzumab (Campath-1H) is a humanized anti-CD52 panlymphocytic (both B and T cells) monoclonal antibody approved for treatment of chronic lymphocytic leukemia. It is important to mention that alemtuzumab is currently not approved for organ transplantation and that with its off-label use patients must be informed about its evolving experimental nature. The dose and frequency of administration of aleumtuzumab, and the optimal maintenance immunosuppressive regimen to be utilized with this agent, remain to be determined.

Although alemtuzumab is increasingly being used for induction therapy after renal transplantation, only two small randomized controlled trials have been performed in kidney transplant recipients.[14-16] In the larger of the two studies, the administration of alemtuzumab permitted less intense maintenance immunosuppressive therapy in some transplant recipients—including very low-dose cyclosporine, sirolimus, or tacrolimus alone, or steroid-free regimens.[15] Ninety renal transplant recipients were randomly assigned to thymoglobulin (group A), alemtuzumab (group B), or daclizumab (group C). All three arms subsequently received tacrolimus and MMF, but maintenance steroid therapy was only given to patients in groups A and C. Target levels for tacrolimus and mycophenolate were also lower in group B. At a median period of 15 months, patient and allograft survival rates and acute rejection rates were similar in all groups.

A number of observational studies have also been performed in pediatric patients. Some potential benefits of using alemtuzumab in pediatric transplant recipients are the possible avoidance of corticosteroids and use of low-dosage maintenance immunosuppression. Bartosh and colleagues[17] reported four high-risk pediatric kidney transplant recipients who received alemtuzumab for unique indications. Three patients experienced acute rejection, two of which were positive for complement degradation product C4d (a diagnostic marker of humoral alloresponse). Another experienced recurrence of focal segmental glomerulosclerosis. They conclude that alemtuzumab did not prevent recurrence of underlying kidney disease or the risk of antibody-mediated rejection.

Recently, the Pittsburgh experience with antilymphoid antibody preconditioning and tacrolimus monotherapy for pediatric kidney transplantation was reported.[18] Lymphoid depletion in 17 unselected pediatric recipients of live ($n = 14$) or deceased donor kidneys ($n = 3$) was accomplished with ATG ($n = 8$) or alemtuzumab ($n = 9$). Tacrolimus was begun posttransplantation, with subsequent lengthening of intervals between doses (spaced weaning). Steroids were added temporarily to treat rejection in two patients (both ATG subgroup) and to treat hemolytic anemia in two others. After 16 to 31 months (mean 22), patient and graft survival were respectively 100% and 94%.

The only graft loss was in a nonweaned noncompliant recipient. In the other 16, serum creatinine was 0.85 ± 0.35 mg/dl and creatinine clearance was 90.8 ± 22.1 ml/min per 1.73 m^2. All 16 patients are on monotherapy (15 tacrolimus, 1 sirolimus), and 14 receive doses every other day or three times per week. There were no wounds or other infections. Two patients developed insulin-dependent diabetes. The authors from this study concluded that the strategy of lymphoid depletion and minimum posttransplant immunosuppression appears safe and effective for pediatric kidney recipients.[18]

Induction Therapy and Long-term Outcome

With acute rejection rates now routinely less than 20%, comparisons of immunosuppressive agents are increasingly focused on long-term outcomes. Improving outcomes requires a sensitive balance between achieving effective rejection prophylaxis and avoiding complications such as infection or malignancy that impact on mortality. Clinical trials, however, rarely include adequate patient numbers to detect significant differences in graft survival rates or malignancy and do not generally provide extended follow-up.

A recent analysis used data from the United Network of Organ Sharing registry on all kidney transplants performed between 1987 and 2003.[19] There were 539 cases of PTLD among 84,907 kidney transplant recipients who received either polyclonal antibody induction or no induction therapy. In an adjusted analysis, the relative risk for PTLD development versus no induction was significantly higher with use of equine antithymocytic globulin (adjusted relative risk = 1.61, $p = 0.0003$) or antilymphocytic globulin (adjusted relative risk = 1.35, $p = 0.0055$) but not with rabbit antithymocytic globulin (adjusted relative risk = 1.17, $p = 0.29$, NS).

Median follow-up times were significantly shorter in the rabbit antithymocytic globulin cohort than the antilymphocytic globulin or equine antithymocytic globulin cohort (median 368 versus 1433 and 2055 days). However, in an analysis restricted to pediatric recipients (in which median times to PTLD are less than 200 days) only equine antithymocytic globulin was associated with a higher adjusted relative risk for PTLD (2.16, $p = 0.0078$)—whereas rabbit antithymocytic globulin and antilymphocytic globulin were not. This difference may only partially be explained by shorter follow-up time and may represent differential hazard for PTLD among the agents.

Slightly different results were reported from the Collaborative Transplant Study (CTS) database, in which graft survival and non-Hodgkin lymphoma at 3 years were evaluated according to type of induction in 112,122 patients receiving a deceased donor renal transplant during 1985 to 2004.[20] Antibody induction with thymoglobulin or IL-2 receptor antibodies was associated with a significant and equivalent improvement in 3-year renal allograft survival. However, the risk of non-Hodgkin lymphoma was strikingly higher with thymoglobulin, ATGAM, and OKT3—whereas there was no increase in lymphoma risk with IL-2 receptor antibodies or ATG-Fresenius (Figure 59-6). The prevalence of lymphoma was approximately ninefold higher in renal transplant patients 3 years after transplantation than in a nontransplant population over the same period. The appropriate use of induction therapy seems to represent one strategy for reducing the risk of PTLD in the future.

Recommendations

There is at present no consensus for immunosuppressive induction therapy following renal transplantation in children. According to recent results from two prospective randomized controlled trials in pediatric patients, induction therapy with basiliximab in pediatric patients with low or normal immunologic risk on maintenance therapy with either tacrolimus in conjunction with azathioprine or cyclosporine in conjunction with MMF did not lead to a statistically significant reduction in the incidence of acute rejection episodes.[10,11]

Ongoing studies in the United States and Europe are currently investigating the potential of IL-2 receptor antibodies in replacement of corticosteroids. Another potential application is delayed graft function when the use of CNIs should be avoided. At the present time, there is no consistent evidence that induction therapy is beneficial or cost effective in low-risk patients on triple therapy with CNIs in conventional doses, MMF, and glucocorticoids.

Induction therapy produces the greatest benefits in groups at high risk for allograft rejection. These high-risk groups include African Americans, recipients of kidneys with prolonged cold ischemia time, and those at high immunologic risk—particularly individuals who are presensitized. The sequential induction regimen of thymoglobulin or IL-2 receptor-blocking antibodies followed by cyclosporine or tacrolimus is recommended in these high-risk groups.

MAINTENANCE IMMUNOSUPPRESSIVE THERAPY

Maintenance immunosuppressive therapy is administered to renal transplant recipients to help prevent acute rejection. Although an adequate level of immunosuppression is required to dampen the immune response to the allograft, the level of chronic immunosuppression is slowly decreased over time to help lower the overall risk of infection and malignancy. These risks directly correlate with the degree of overall immunosuppression. The type of immunosuppression may also be varied to decrease the risk of developing chronic allograft nephropathy, the most common underlying long-term cause of allograft loss (see Chapter 60).

Conventional maintenance regimens consist of a combination of immunosuppressive agents that differ in their mechanism of action. This strategy minimizes morbidity and

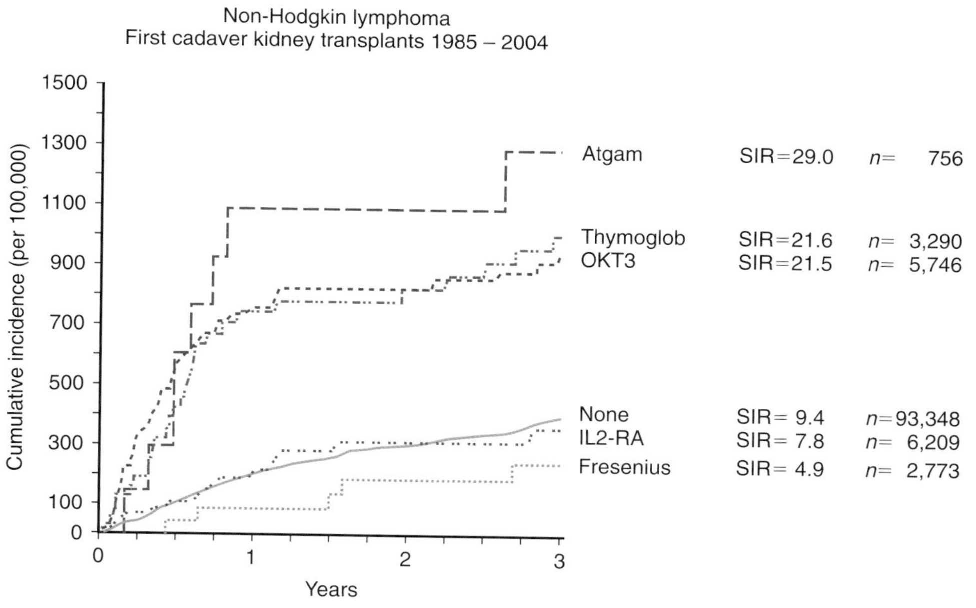

Figure 59-6 Cumulative incidence of non-Hodgkin lymphoma (NHL) after renal transplantation from a deceased donor according to type of induction therapy for patients receiving a transplant during 1985 to 2004. Standardized incidence ratio (SIR) values compare the observed risk of lymphoma versus the estimated risk in the nontransplant control population matched for age, sex, and geographic origin. (From Opelz G, Naujokat C, Daniel V, Terness P, Dohler B: Disassociation between risk of graft loss and risk of non-Hodgkin lymphoma with induction agents in renal transplant recipients, *Transplant* 81:1227-33, 2006.)

mortality associated with each class of agent while maximizing overall effectiveness. Such regimens may vary by transplant center and geographic area. There are a number of important issues to consider when deciding the immunosuppressive protocol to administer in a particular patient. The risk for acute rejection and allograft loss is highest in the first 3 months after transplantation.

As a result, immunosuppression should be at its highest during this period. The occurrence of the most serious side effects of immunosuppressive therapy, infections and malignancy, correlate with the total amount of immunosuppression. It is therefore essential that immunosuppression be tapered slowly to a maintenance level by 6 to 12 months posttransplantation.

Allograft survival rates vary among the various immunosuppressive agents due to patient-specific clinical characteristics such as age, obesity, ethnicity, hyperlipidemia, and/or delayed allograft function. Immunosuppressive agents should therefore be chosen in part based on specific patient characteristics. Other issues that must be taken into account are related to the immunologic history of the patient. Is the patient sensitized? Is this the first kidney transplant or a retransplant? How many acute rejection episodes has the patient had? What is the degree of HLA matching or mismatching?

The optimal maintenance immunosuppressive therapy in pediatric renal transplantation is not established. The major immunosuppressive agents currently being used in various combination regimens are corticosteroids (primarily oral prednisone or methylprednisolone), azathioprine, MMF, cyclosporine (in standard form or microemulsion), tacrolimus, and sirolimus. We and most transplant centers currently utilize a maintenance regimen consisting of triple immunosuppression therapy with a CNI (tacrolimus or cyclosporine), an antimetabolite (MMF or azathioprine), and methylprednisolone. Sirolimus is also used by some transplant centers in triple therapy regimens, often in place of the CNI or the antimetabolite.

Within the NAPRTCS registry, marked changes in the type of maintenance immunosuppression and dosing strategies have been observed in the past years.[2] These are substantially caused by the introduction of new drugs such as MMF and tacrolimus (Table 59-1). The use of a combination therapy consisting of cyclosporine, prednisone, and azathioprine at day 30 posttransplant has declined since 1996 through 1997 from 27% of living donor and 24% of deceased donor organ recipients to 1% in each group in 2000 through 2004. The regimen of prednisone, tacrolimus, and MMF has become more popular. It was used in 48% of living donor and 53% of deceased donor organ transplants in 2000 through 2005, compared to about 12% of all transplants in 1996 through 1997.

Approximately 80% of patients receive triple drug therapy at 6 months posttransplant, with MMF replacing azathioprine in recent cohorts. Among transplanted grafts with ≥30 days function that have occurred since 1996, the observed drug utilization rates are outlined in Table 59-1. Substantial increases in tacrolimus, MMF, and sirolimus usage are observed—with a significant decrease in azathioprine usage. Azathioprine usage has decreased sharply, from 34% in 1997 to 2% in 2005. The majority of sirolimus therapy (90%) was initiated within the first 2 days posttransplant. Cyclosporine was used in 78% of the 1997 transplants at day 30, and it continues to show a decline in utilization (to 8.7% in 2004). Of cyclosporine recipients since 1996 with a documented formulation, 84% reported the use of Neoral.

Glucocorticoids

Glucocorticoids, developed in the early 1950s, represent one of the principal types of agent used for both maintenance immunosuppression and treatment of acute rejection.

Mechanism of Action

Glucocorticoids have both antiinflammatory and immunosuppressive actions.[21] Lymphopenia and monocytopenia occur with the inhibition of lymphocyte proliferation, survival, activation, homing, and effector functions. Glucocorticoids suppress production of numerous cytokines and vasoactive substances, including IL-1, TNFα, IL-2, MHC class II, chemokines, prostaglandins (via inhibition of phospholipase A2), and proteases. Glucocorticoids also cause neutrophilia (often with a left shift), but neutrophil chemotaxis and adhesion are inhibited. They also affect nonhematopoietic cells.

Glucocorticoids exert their effect by binding to glucocorticoid receptors (GRs), which belong to a family of ligand-

TABLE 59-1 Observed Drug Utilization Rates in Pediatric Renal Transplant Recipients Among Transplanted Grafts with ≥30 Days' Function That Have Occurred Since 1996

	PERCENT DRUG UTILIZATION: DAY 20 POSTTRANSPLANT								
	1997 (*n* = 593)	1998 (*n* = 542)	1999 (*n* = 553)	2000 (*n* = 541)	2001 (*n* = 491)	2002 (*n* = 445)	2003 (*n* = 378)	2004 (*n* = 345)	2005 (*n* = 174)
Cyclosporine	77.7	71.2	66.9	56.3	46.8	27.0	15.3	8.7	11.5
Tacrolimus	14.5	22.0	23.3	33.5	40.9	57.3	59.8	71.0	63.2
Mycophenolate	44.0	65.7	66.0	63.0	53.2	57.3	55.8	64.1	64.9
Azathioprine	33.9	19.7	15.2	13.3	12.8	1.8	4.2	3.5	1.7
Sirolimus	—	0.2	0.4	5.8	15.5	20.5	18.5	11.0	7.5

From the NAPRTCS 2006 Annual Report. *https://web.emmes.com/study/ped/index.htm*. Used by permission.

regulated transcription factors called nuclear receptors. GRs are normally present in the cytoplasm in an inactive complex with heat shock proteins (hsp90, hsp70, and hsp56). The binding of glucocorticoids to the GR dissociates hsp from the GR and forms the active glucocorticoids–GR complex, which migrates to the nucleus and dimerizes on palindromic DNA sequences in many genes [called the glucocorticoid response element (GRE)]. The binding of GRs in the promoter region of the target genes can lead to induction or suppression of gene transcription (e.g., of cytokines).

GRs also exert effects by interacting directly with other transcription factors independent of DNA binding. One principal effect of glucocorticoids on immune and inflammatory responses may be attributable to their ability to affect gene transcription by regulating key transcription factors involved in immune regulation: activator protein-1 (AP-1) and nuclear factor-kappa B (NF-κB). The regulation of NF-κB by steroids may operate by induction of IkB, the inhibitor of NF-κB (Figure 59-7). Other effects of glucocorticoids are mediated through the release of a regulatory protein, lipocortin, which inhibits phospholipase A2—thereby inhibiting the production of leukotrienes and prostaglandins. The total immunosuppressive effect of glucocorticoids is complex, reflecting effects on cytokines, adhesion molecules, and apoptosis and activation of inflammatory cells.

Pharmacokinetics and Drug Interactions

The major glucocorticoids used are prednisone or prednisolone (given orally with comparable efficacy) and methylprednisolone (given orally or intravenously with 25% more potency). These agents are rapidly absorbed and have short plasma half-lives (60-180 minutes) but long biologic half-lives (18-36 hours).

The effect of prednisone (dose/weight) is greater in the setting of renal failure or hypoalbuminemia, in women, and in the elderly—whereas less prednisone effect is observed in children. Certain drugs can decrease steroid efficacy by increasing metabolism: rifampin (rifampicin), phenytoin, phenobarbital (phenobarbitone), and carbamazepine. In contrast, increased steroid effects may be observed in patients receiving oral contraceptives, estrogens, ketoconazole, and erythromycin.

Administration

In many transplant centers, the initial dose of corticosteroids is usually administered during surgery as intravenous methylprednisolone, at doses between 2 and 10 mg/kg body weight. The oral dose of corticosteroids used for maintenance therapy varies between 15 and 60 mg/m^2 per day (0.5 to 2 mg/kg body weight per day), which is gradually tapered over time to approximately 4 to 5 mg prednisone per m^2 surface area—usually taken as a single morning dose. Some clinicians use alternate-day therapy after 6 or 12 months posttransplant, whereas others administer continuous low-dose steroid treatment.

Side Effects

Corticosteroids have multiple side effects in children, including growth impairment, susceptibility to infections, cushingoid appearance, body disfigurement, acne, cardiovascular complications, arterial hypertension, hyperglycemia, aseptic bone necrosis, osteopenia, cataracts, poor wound healing, and psychological effects (Table 59-2). The risk for infection is excessive if high-dose pulse therapy is prolonged (typically >3 g per 1.73 m^2). Glucocorticoid dosage should, therefore, be decreased gradually during rejection treatment even if

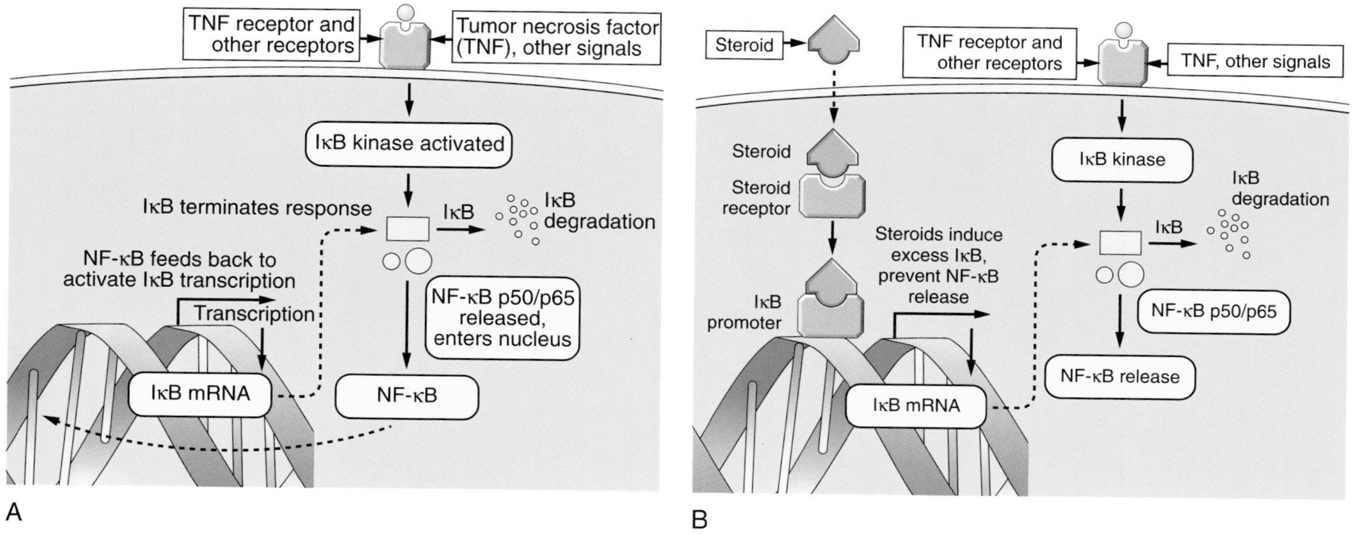

Figure 59-7 Corticosteroids and regulation of transcription factors. **A,** The mechanism of NF–κB and its regulation by induction of synthesis of its inhibitor IB. Activation of IκB kinase leads to IκB degradation. Released NF–κB enters the nucleus and activates IκB transcription. Synthesis of IκB feeds back to terminate the cycle. **B,** The mechanism of corticosteroid immunosuppression by inhibition of NF–κB. The corticosteroid–corticosteroid receptor complex migrates to the nucleus and interacts with the promoter of the IκB gene to induce the synthesis of excess IκB, the natural inhibitor of NF–κB. IκB in excess prevents the release of NF–κB to the nucleus upon stimulation by cytokines such as tumor necrosis factor (TNF). (From Feehally J, Floege J, Johnson RJ (eds.): *Comprehensive clinical nephrology, Third edition*. Philadelphia: Mosby 2007:1039.)

TABLE 59-2 Semiquantitative Comparison of Safety Profiles of Current Primary Immunosuppressive Compounds

	Glucocorticoids	Sirolimus	Cyclosporine	Tacrolimus	Mycophenolate mofetil
Nephrotoxicity*	—	+	+++	++(+)	—
Hyperlipidemia	++	+++	++	+(+)	—
Arterial hypertension	+	—	+++	++	—
Neurotoxicity	+	—	+++	+++	—
Posttransplant diabetes mellitus	++	—	++	+++	—
Bone marrow suppression	—	++	—	—	++
Gastrointestinal adverse effects†	—	+	+	+	+++
Hepatotoxicity	—	+	+	+	—
Esthetic changes	++	—	++	+	—
Wound healing problems‡	+	++	—	—	+
Pulmonary toxicity	—	+	—	—	—
Fetal toxicity	—	NA	+	+	?
Osteoporosis	++	?	+	+	—
Inhibition of longitudinal growth	+++	?	—	—	—

* Sirolimus without calcineurin inhibitor.
† Gastrointestinal disorders: diarrhea, abdominal pain, nausea and vomiting, ileus, rectal disorders, and mucosal ulcerations.
‡ Wound healing problems, including lymphocele formation.
—, Drug has no effect on this adverse effect; +, mild; ++, moderate; +++, severe; *?*, clinical data available but insufficient to provide conclusions; *NA*, no information available.

serum creatinine fails to improve. Interestingly, glucocorticoids are not associated with increased risk for malignancy. One of the most important reasons for stopping corticosteroids or switching to alternate-day therapy is statural growth impairment, which is frequently observed in those on continuous treatment.

Steroid Withdrawal or Avoidance

The long-term dose of corticosteroids varies among transplant centers. Some teams stop corticosteroids after 6 to 12 months. Complete steroid withdrawal has been previously associated with an increased incidence of acute rejection in many studies. However, protocols using combinations with newer immunosuppressive agents show promise for this approach. Data both in adult and pediatric renal transplant recipients indicate that the introduction of tacrolimus or a cyclosporine/MMF-based immunosuppressive maintenance therapy and the initiation of steroid withdrawal late (i.e., >6 months) after renal transplantation has significantly increased the safety of this strategy.[22-24]

In our experience, there is an obvious long-term benefit and a very small risk in patients with stable graft function withdrawn from small doses of steroids 1 year posttransplant. This case-control study (covering a mean follow-up period of 46 ± 2.3 months and involving 40 pediatric renal transplant recipients aged 11.4 ± 4.9 years) analyzed the safety and efficacy of steroid withdrawal in patients receiving cyclosporine microemulsion, MMF, and low-dose prednisone treatment.[25] Steroid withdrawal in all 20 pediatric renal transplant recipients on cyclosporine and MMF was successful and was not associated with an acute rejection episode. None of the 20 patients undergoing steroid withdrawal experienced an acute rejection episode throughout the study period. Moreover, graft function as assessed by creatinine clearance remained stable in patients off steroids.

It was suggested that these favorable results (compared to previous reports in patients on cyclosporine and azathioprine) can be ascribed to the higher immunosuppressive potency of MMF than that of azathioprine. In addition, increased exposure to mycophenolic acid (MPA, the active compound of MMF) in response to steroid withdrawal might have compensated (at least in part) for the lower immunosuppressive level achieved with the remaining therapy with cyclosporine and MMF.

Increased MPA exposure after steroid withdrawal has been ascribed to reduced MPA metabolism as a consequence of a decreased activity of the hepatic enzyme UDP-glucuronosyltransferase (mainly involved in the metabolism of MPA). Hence, late steroid withdrawal in selected pediatric renal transplant recipients under an immunosuppressive maintenance therapy with cyclosporine and MMF appears to be safe at least over the mean observation period of 4 years. Methods of identifying candidates who will suffer adverse renal consequences from steroid withdrawal will hopefully be available in the future and may facilitate this strategy.

An alternative approach to facilitating steroid withdrawal in pediatric renal transplant recipients is a tacrolimus-based immunosuppressive regimen. In one study from Pittsburgh,[22] for example, steroid withdrawal was possible in 70% of their patients—with 5-year actuarial patient and graft survival rates of respectively 96% and 82%, a 39% incidence of rejection, and a mean serum creatinine level of 1.2 ± 0.5 mg/dl. In children who were withdrawn from steroids, the mean height standard deviation score at the time of transplantation and at 1 and 4 years was respectively −2.3 ± 2.0, −1.7 ± 1.0, and 0.36 ± 1.5.[22] Of successfully transplanted patients, 86% did not take antihypertensive medications. However, the incidence of PTLD in this report (4%-17%) appears to be higher than observed in children on a cyclosporine/MMF-based immunosuppressive regimen (1%).[26]

Steroid avoidance may eventually be found to provide the best overall risk-to-benefit ratio with maintenance immunosuppressive therapy in renal transplantation. Steroid avoidance protocols have been used successfully and are presently undergoing extensive evaluation in the United States and in Europe. However, many of these protocols have chosen low-risk individuals and utilized aggressive induction therapy with extended daclizumab induction therapy, tacrolimus, and MMF.[27] Steroid withdrawal has the advantage over steroid avoidance that immunologic high-risk patients and those with unstable graft function can easily be identified beforehand and be excluded from steroid-free immunosuppression. Nevertheless, steroid withdrawal or avoidance following renal transplantation remains a controversial issue.

Calcineurin Inhibitors

Cyclosporine (a lipophilic cyclic peptide of 11 amino acid residues) and tacrolimus (a macrolide antibiotic) are drugs with similar mechanisms of action that have become major maintenance immunosuppressive agents used in transplantation.

Mechanism of Action

Cyclosporine and tacrolimus act by inhibiting the calcium-dependent serine phosphatase calcineurin, which is normally rate limiting in T-cell activation (Figure 59-8). Calcineurin is activated by the engagement of the T-cell receptor, activation of tyrosine kinases and of phospholipase C-γ1, release of inositol triphosphate, release of calcium stored in the endoplasmic reticulum, and opening of membrane calcium channels. Calcineurin provides an essential step for transducing signal 1 to permit cytokine and CD40L transcription.

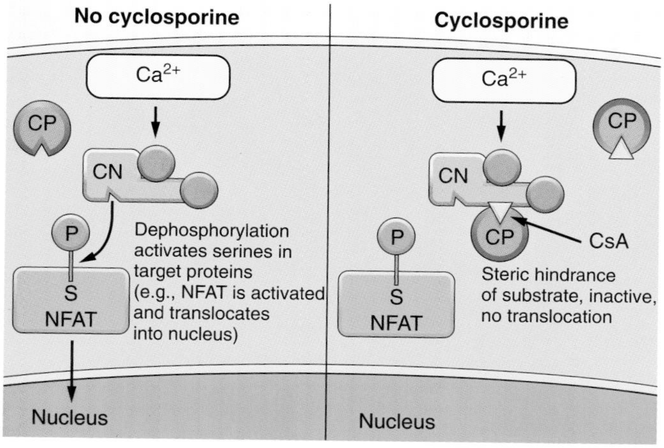

Figure 59-8 Calcineurin inhibition prevents nuclear factors (NFAT) dephosphorylation, activation, and translocation. In the absence of cyclosporine, calcium activates calcineurin by exposing its phosphatase site—which in turn activates its target protein (e.g., the transcription factor NFAT). Cyclosporine forms a complex with cyclophilin (CN), which binds to calcineurin (CN) and sterically hinders the phosphatase site. (From Feehally J, Floege J, Johnson RJ (eds.): *Comprehensive clinical nephrology, Third edition.* Philadelphia: Mosby 2007:1040.)

A high cytoplasmic calcium concentration activates calcineurin, which then dephosphorylates regulatory sites in key transcription factors—the nuclear factors of activated T lymphocytes ($NFAT_p$ and $NFAT_c$). This causes the NFAT proteins to translocate (with calcineurin) into the nucleus and bind to their DNA target sequences in the promoters of cytokine genes. Calcineurin has been implicated in the dephosphorylation of transcription factor Elk-1, and indirectly in the activation of Jun/AP-1 and NF-kB.

Cyclosporine and tacrolimus cross cell membranes freely and bind to immunophilins [cyclophilin and FK-binding protein 12 (FKBP12), respectively], which are ubiquitous and abundant intracellular proteins with isomerase activity. The active complex then binds to a site on calcineurin and blocks its interactions with key substrates. The inactivity of calcineurin bound to cyclosporine–cyclophilin or tacrolimus–FKBP12 is the key to the immunosuppressive effect and some of the toxic effects of these drugs. Although inhibition of calcineurin has many effects on the T cell, the best studied is the blocking of the translocation (movement) of NFAT proteins from the cytoplasm into the nucleus.

Cyclosporine and tacrolimus partially inhibit the calcineurin pathway at therapeutic blood levels (e.g., trough levels of 200 μg/L cyclosporine or 5-20 μg/L tacrolimus).[28] However, even partial inhibition of calcineurin reduces the transcription of many genes associated with T-cell activation [e.g., IL-2, interferon-γ (IFN-γ), granulocyte–macrophage colony-stimulating factor (GM-CSF), TNF-α, IL-4, and CD40L]. Therefore, the functional consequence of partial calcineurin inhibition is probably a quantitative limitation in cytokine production, CD40L expression, and lymphocyte proliferation. The effect of cyclosporine and tacrolimus on calcineurin in vivo is rapidly reversible, emphasizing the importance of patient compliance, drug monitoring, and reliable formulations for delivery. The effects on non T cells could also be clinically significant.

Pharmacokinetics and Drug Interactions

Cyclosporine and tacrolimus are both variably absorbed and are metabolized extensively by the liver (via the cytochrome P450 system). Cyclosporine is excreted primarily by the biliary system. The absorption of some cyclosporine preparations may be bile dependent and therefore may be reduced in the presence of cholestatic liver disease. The absorption of the microemulsion formulation of cyclosporine or of tacrolimus is bile independent. Neither cyclosporine nor tacrolimus is affected by alterations in renal function.

Both cyclosporine and tacrolimus bind to cells and to plasma components (primarily lipoproteins for cyclosporine and albumin for tacrolimus) in the blood. Consequently, they must be assayed in whole blood. Many drugs and agents can affect cyclosporine and tacrolimus levels through effects on their absorption or metabolism (see Chapter 60). The absorption of cyclosporine is decreased, and its metabolism is increased, in children compared to adults. The required dosages are therefore comparably higher. Cyclosporine is usually administered initially as 8 to 15 mg/kg daily in divided doses (or intravenously using one third the oral dose over a 24-hour period) during the induction phase, with target trough blood levels of 150 to 300 mg/L for the first 3 to 6 months posttransplant.

Doses are reduced after 3 to 6 months (typically 4-6 mg/kg daily). Long-term target trough blood levels of 75 to 125 mg/L appear to provide comparable patient and graft survival as higher blood levels but with less risk of malignancy.[29] A microemulsion form of cyclosporine (Neoral) has been developed that gives more reliable and slightly higher absorption and may require a slightly lower dose. Generic forms of cyclosporine are becoming available. Oral formulations of cyclosporine may not be equivalent and readily interchangeable, and knowledge of the characteristics of the oral formulations is necessary before switching between them.

Tacrolimus is 20- to 30-fold more potent than cyclosporine and is therefore administered at a 20-fold lower dose. Initial dosing is usually 0.2 to 0.3 mg/kg daily in two divided doses orally (or 0.05-0.1 mg/kg daily intravenously over 24 hours), and target trough levels are 5 to 15 mg/L. Because tacrolimus is more water-soluble than cyclosporine, it is not as dependent on bile salts for absorption. However, food intake can reduce the absorption of tacrolimus by as much as to 40%. Thus, it is recommended that this agent be taken on an empty stomach.[30] In addition, tacrolimus is best absorbed in the morning—and some evidence in adults suggests that this agent can be given once a day.[31]

Efficacy: Comparison of Cyclosporine and Tacrolimus

To help assess the relative efficacy of tacrolimus and cyclosporine, a 2005 metaanalysis and metaregression was performed based on 30 trials consisting of 4102 adult patients.[32] Tacrolimus was associated with a significantly lower risk of allograft loss at 6 months (RR of 0.56, CI 95%, 0.36 to 0.86), which was independent of cyclosporine formulation or concentration but was diminished with increased doses of tacrolimus. Although not always statistically significant, allograft loss at later time points also favored tacrolimus [RR of 0.77 (CI of 0.58 to 1.02) at one year, 0.74 (CI of 0.46 to 1.21) at two years, and 0.71 (CI of 0.52 to 0.96) at three years].

In addition, a relatively decreased acute rejection risk at 1 year was noted with tacrolimus (RR of 0.66, CI 95%, 0.60 to 0.79). However, no difference in allograft survival rates was observed with these two agents in a retrospective study of adult nondiabetic patients.[33] Based on data from the United States Renal Data System (USRDS) during the years 1996 to 2000, allograft survival rates were similar among those who received either cyclosporine or tacrolimus (hazard ratio of 1.031). In addition, a retrospective study from the USRDS database found that a regimen of cyclosporine, mycophenolate, and prednisone was associated with a lower risk for allograft failure than tacrolimus, mycophenolate, and prednisone.[34]

Despite this variability between studies, the overall conclusion from data in adults is that tacrolimus-based immunosuppression is associated with decreased acute rejection rates, a superior long-term renal function, and more favorable cardiovascular risk profile than cyclosporine microemulsion-based immunosuppression. This translates into improved long-term renal allograft survival. This statement is supported by the recently published results of the SYMPHONY trial, which compared standard immunosuppression versus three regimens with low-dose or no CNI in de novo single-organ renal transplant patients over 1 year.[35]

In this prospective randomized open study with four parallel arms, 1645 adult patients in 15 countries were randomized to standard immunosuppression with normal-dose cyclosporine (target trough level 150-300 ng/ml for 3 months and 100-200 ng/ml thereafter), to MMF 1 g bid and corticosteroids, or to one of three regimens consisting of daclizumab induction (2 mg/kg followed by 4×1 mg/kg every 2 weeks), of MMF (1-g bid) and corticosteroids potentiated by a low dose of cyclosporine (50-100 ng/ml) or tacrolimus (3-7 ng/ml), or of sirolimus (4-8 ng/ml).

The low-dose tacrolimus group was significantly superior to all other groups with respect to GFR and biopsy-proven acute rejection (BPAR) ($p < 0.01$), and to normal-dose cyclosporine and low-dose sirolimus for graft survival (pairwise $p < 0.05$). The authors concluded that immunosuppression consisting of daclizumab induction, MMF, low-dose tacrolimus, and corticosteroids provides the most optimal balance between efficacy (control of acute rejection) and toxicity (preserving graft function and graft survival).[35]

In pediatric patients, the efficacy and safety of tacrolimus and cyclosporine were compared in one multicenter trial in 196 patients, who were randomly assigned to receive either tacrolimus or cyclosporine microemulsion administered concomitantly with azathioprine and corticosteroids.[36] Tacrolimus therapy resulted in a significantly lower incidence of acute rejection (36.9%) compared to cyclosporine therapy (59.1%) ($p = 0.003$). The incidence of corticosteroid-resistant rejection was also significantly lower in the tacrolimus group compared to the cyclosporine group (7.8% versus 25.8%, respectively; $p = 0.001$). The difference was also significant for biopsy-confirmed acute rejection (16.5% versus 39.8%, respectively; $p < 0.001$).

At 1 year, patient survival was similar (96.1% versus 96.6%, respectively). Ten grafts were lost in the tacrolimus group compared to 17 graft losses in the cyclosporine group ($p = 0.06$). At 1 year, the tacrolimus group had a significantly better GFR calculated according to the Schwartz formula. The authors concluded that tacrolimus is significantly more effective than cyclosporine microemulsion in preventing acute rejection after renal transplantation in the pediatric population. A follow-up study at 4 years showed that patient survival was similar (94% versus 92%, respectively; $p = 0.86$). However, graft survival significantly favored tacrolimus (86% versus 69%, respectively; $p = 0.025$).[37]

At 4 years posttransplant, the mean GFR according to the Schwartz formula was 71.5 ± 22.9 ml/min/1.73 m^2 ($n = 51$) versus 53.0 ± 21.6 ml/min/1.73 m^2 ($n = 44$, $p = 0.0001$) for tacrolimus versus cyclosporine, respectively. Cholesterol remained significantly higher with cyclosporine throughout follow-up. Three patients in each arm developed PTLD. Incidence of insulin-dependent diabetes mellitus was not different. The authors concluded that tacrolimus was significantly more effective than cyclosporine in preventing acute rejection in pediatric renal recipients. Renal function and graft survival were also superior with tacrolimus.

A retrospective study of the NAPRTCS database of 986 pediatric renal transplant recipients treated with cyclosporine, MMF, and steroids ($n = 766$) or with tacrolimus, MMF, and steroids ($n = 220$) revealed that tacrolimus and cyclosporine in combination with MMF and steroids produce similar rejection rates and graft survival in pediatric renal transplant recipients.[38] However, tacrolimus was associated with improved graft function at 1 and 2 years posttransplant (Figure 59-9). There was no difference in time to first rejection, risk for rejection, and risk for graft failure or graft survival at the first year posttransplant or at 2 years posttransplant. Tacrolimus-treated patients were significantly less likely to require antihypertensive medication at 1 and 2 years posttransplant.

At 1 year posttransplant, tacrolimus-treated patients enjoyed a higher mean GFR at both 1 year (98.6 ml/min/1.73 m^2 versus 78.0 ml/min/1.73 m^2, $p = 0.0003$) and 2 years posttransplant (96.7 ml/min/1.73 m^2 versus 73.2 ml/min/1.73 m^2, $p < 0.0001$). There is therefore evidence that tacrolimus is superior to cyclosporine (conventional or microemulsion form) in preventing acute rejection after renal transplantation in adults and pediatric populations when used as part of triple therapy in conjunction with azathioprine and corticosteroids. It also seems more effective in improving long-term graft survival in adults. Further follow-up studies are required to see if tacrolimus improves long-term survival of kidney grafts in children.

Side Effects

Cyclosporine and tacrolimus have similarities and differences in their toxicity profiles (Table 59-2). Both can cause nephrotoxicity, hyperkalemia, hyperuricemia with occasional gouty attacks, hypomagnesemia secondary to urinary loss, arterial hypertension, diabetes mellitus, and neurotoxicity (especially tremor). In the European pediatric study, the incidence of hypomagnesemia was significantly higher in the tacrolimus-treated group (34%) compared to the cyclosporine-treated group (12.9%).[36]

Similarly, diarrhea was more frequent in tacrolimus-treated patients (13.6% versus 3.2%). Hypertrichosis, gum hyperplasia, and flu syndrome were reported only in cyclosporin-treated patients—and tremor was reported only in tacrolimus-treated patients.[36] These results are similar to adults, for whom tremor is consistently more common with tacrolimus and hirsutism and gum disease more common with cyclosporine.[39] Arterial hypertension and hyperlipidemia are more commonly observed with cyclosporine. In the NAPRTC study, in which CNIs were used in combination with MMF and steroids, tacrolimus-treated patients were significantly less likely to require antihypertensive medications at 1 and 2 years posttransplant.[36]

This is similar to adults, for whom a lower systemic blood pressure was reported in the tacrolimus-treated patients in several studies.[39] In the European pediatric study, mean total cholesterol levels were reported to decrease in the tacrolimus group and increase in the cyclosporine group at the end of 6 months.[36] Similarly in adults, several studies have shown that lipid levels are much lower in tacrolimus-treated recipients

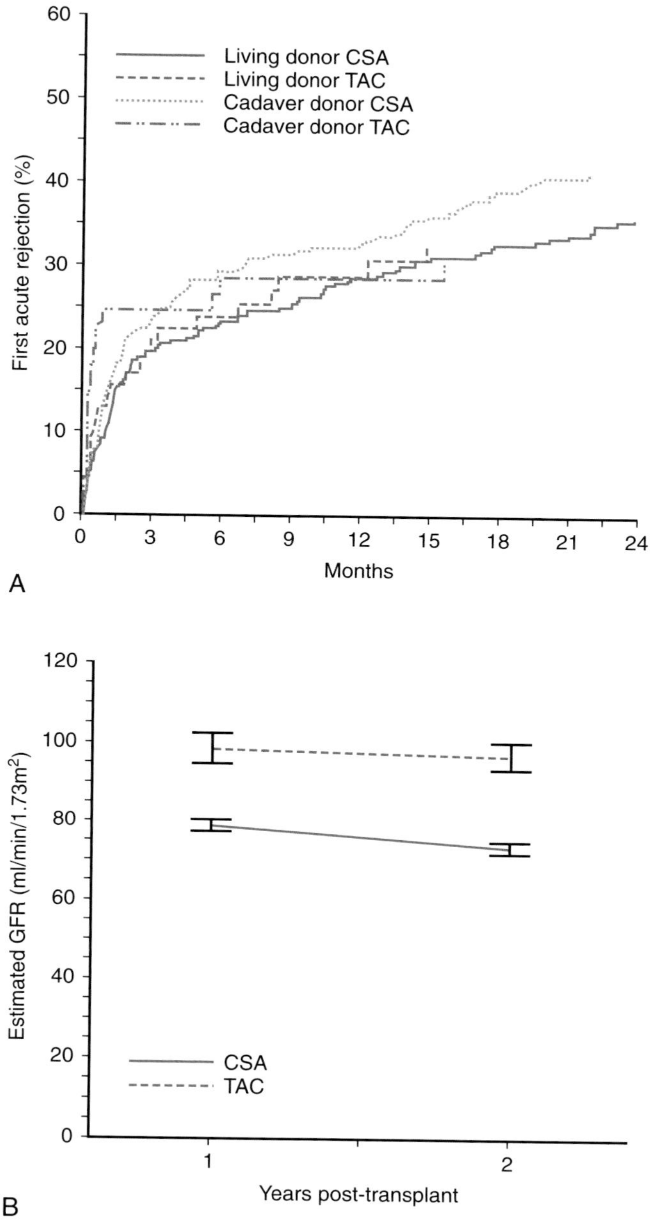

Figure 59-9 **A,** Kaplan–Meier estimates of the percentage of patients experiencing a first acute rejection in the first 2 years posttransplant by treatment group [tacrolimus (TAC), mycophenolate mofetil (MMF), and steroids versus cyclosporine (CSA), MMF, and steroids] and donor source (CAD, LD). Patients were included in this analysis if they were transplanted between 1997 and 1999 and had 2 years of follow-up in the database. **B,** Mean estimated GFR as calculated by the Schwartz formula at 1 and 2 years posttransplant in patients treated with TAC, MMF, and steroids or with CSA, MMF, and prednisone. (From Neu AM, Ho PL, Fine RN, Furth SL, Fivush BA: Tacrolimus vs. cyclosporine A as primary immunosuppression in pediatric renal transplantation: A NAPRTCS study, *Pediatr Transplant* 7:217-22, 2003.)

than in cyclosporine-treated patients.[39] The improved lipid profiles on tacrolimus may contribute to a better long-term outcome with less cardiovascular morbidity.

On the other hand, tremor and glucose intolerance are more common with tacrolimus. In the pediatric multicenter

European study, there was no difference in the incidence of new-onset insulin-dependent diabetes mellitus between tacrolimus-treated (3%) and cyclosporin-treated (2.2%) patients.[19] Although in early clinical trials of tacrolimus a significantly higher incidence of diabetes mellitus was reported in tacrolimus-treated adult patients than in cyclosporine-treated recipients, the incidence of diabetes mellitus with tacrolimus immunosuppression has become less frequent in recent randomized trials comparing these two CNIs.[39] Posttransplant diabetes regresses after dose reduction in some but not all patients. Both reduction of corticosteroids dosage and the low target trough tacrolimus concentrations contribute to the recent marked reduction of the incidence of diabetes mellitus under tacrolimus immunosuppression in both adults and children.[37,39]

Cyclosporine may also be associated with coarsening of facial features, especially in children. Bone pain that is responsive to calcium channel inhibitors may also occur with cyclosporine use, and sometimes may require changing to tacrolimus. The most common serious problem with the CNIs is nephrotoxicity, with both a reversible vasomotor component and an irreversible component. Both cyclosporine and tacrolimus can cause acute elevations in serum creatinine that reverse with reduction of the dose, apparently caused by renal vasoconstriction that itself may be mediated by calcineurin inhibition. Chronically, cyclosporine and tacrolimus can induce a tubular atrophy and interstitial fibrosis with characteristic hyalinosis of the afferent arteriole.[40]

This lesion appears to result from long-standing renal vasoconstriction, perhaps mediated in part by an increase in local vasoconstrictors (angiotensin II, endothelin-1, thromboxane, and sympathetic nerve transmitters) and an inadequate vasodilatory response (impaired nitric oxide formation). The importance of this lesion is apparent from studies in cardiac and liver transplant recipients in which cyclosporine or tacrolimus use is associated with progression to ESRD in many patients.[41]

This problem was more acute at a time when higher doses of cyclosporine were administered for longer periods. Currently, cyclosporine and tacrolimus toxicity is associated with only mild to moderate declines in renal function. However, as the number of patients with long-standing nonrenal transplants increases there is increasing concern about future ESRD in this population. It is important to make the diagnosis of CNI toxicity by renal biopsy and to reduce or stop the CNI if possible.[42]

Experimentally, cyclosporine nephropathy is exacerbated in the presence of salt restriction and volume depletion and is lessened by treatment with angiotensin-converting enzyme (ACE) inhibitors, calcium channel antagonists, vasodilators (hydralazine), and glucocorticoids. Cyclosporine and tacrolimus can cause the hemolytic-uremic syndrome, probably through endothelial dysfunction. This complication, which is usually associated with elevated drug levels, may respond to temporary withdrawal of cyclosporine or tacrolimus, plasma exchange, switching to another CNI, or switching to another class of immunosuppressive drug.

There is no difference in the incidence of PTLD between tacrolimus-treated and cyclosporine-microemulsion–treated recipients when used in combination with azathioprine and steroids [1% (1/103) versus 2.1% (2/93)][36] or when used in conjunction with MMF/steroids (1.4% versus 2%).[38] This is similar to adults, for whom recent large randomized studies could not show any difference in the incidence of malignancy between patients treated with tacrolimus or cyclosporine.[39]

Therapeutic Drug Monitoring

Cyclosporine is a drug with a narrow therapeutic index and broad intraindividual and interindividual pharmacokinetic variability. Serious clinical consequences may occur because of underdosing or overdosing. Hence, individualization of cyclosporine dosage by therapeutic drug monitoring is required. The traditional monitoring strategy for cyclosporine is based on predose trough level measurements (C_0). However, C_0 shows a relatively poor correlation with cyclosporine exposure [area under the concentration-time curve (AUC)] and with clinical outcome.[43]

Studies on the pharmacokinetic and pharmacodynamic relationship of cyclosporine have shown that cyclosporine induces a partial inhibition of calcineurin activity, the rate-limiting step in the activation of primary human T lymphocytes, and the target of the cyclosporine/cyclophilin complex.[44] The greatest calcineurin inhibition and the maximum inhibition of IL-2 production occur in the first 1 to 2 hours after dosing. Calcineurin is only partially inhibited in patients, which can result in rejection even when cyclosporine blood concentrations are in the putative therapeutic range.

From these observations, it was hypothesized that the cyclosporine AUC_{0-4} (absorption profile) or the C_2 concentration (sample 2 hours postinsertion) may be a better predictor of immunosuppressive efficacy than the cyclosporine AUC_{0-12}. However, a prospective randomized study in adult renal transplant recipients did not show any advantage of C_2 monitoring in the early posttransplant period compared to a C_0 monitoring strategy. It did lead, however, to significantly higher cyclosporine doses and blood levels than C_0 monitoring.[45] In a large study in pediatric renal transplant recipients, cyclosporine absorption profiles predicted the risk of acute rejection—whereas the single pharmacokinetic parameters C_0 and C_2 did not.[46]

A disadvantage of C_2 monitoring is the fact that it requires a timed blood sample within a narrow time window (±15 minutes) of C_2 that necessitates further organizational requirements for physicians and nursing staff—which may be judged differently between transplant centers. In our center, we routinely monitor cyclosporine therapy by 12-hour predose trough concentrations. We aim for the following trough levels in conjunction with MMF therapy and prednisone (measured by the immunoassay enzyme multiplied immunoassay technique [EMIT]): months 0 to 3 posttransplant (120-200 mg/L) and thereafter (80-160 ng/ml). We feel that a monitoring strategy based on cyclosporine C_2 concentrations in the stable period posttransplant is an additional tool in preventing chronic cyclosporine-induced nephrotoxicity. In patients with low or normal immunologic risk who are on additional maintenance therapy with MMF, we aim for cylosporine C_2 concentrations between 300 and 600 mg/L beyond the first year posttransplant. C_2 concentrations are monitored every 3 to 6 months.

When tacrolimus is utilized, a monitoring strategy based on trough levels is in general sufficient because trough levels are good indicators of systemic exposure. In most transplant centers, doses are adjusted to attain target whole-blood trough concentrations of 10 to 15 ng/ml during the first 3 months posttransplantation, between 5 and 10 ng/ml during months 4 to 12, and 3 to 8 ng/ml thereafter.[47] It must be emphasized that these target ranges are dependent on the concomitant immunosuppressive therapy. In the SYMPHONY trial, for example, low tacrolimus exposure (trough levels between 3 and 7 ng/ml) in the first year posttransplant in conjunction with MMF, prednisone, and daclizumab induction was associated with excellent efficacy and little tacrolimus-associated toxicity.[35]

Antimetabolic Agents: Azathioprine

Azathioprine, developed by Nobel Prize laureates Elion and Hitchings in the1950s, has been widely used in renal transplantation for four decades. Azathioprine is a purine analog derived from 6-mercaptopurine (6-MP).

Mechanism of Action

Azathioprine is metabolized in the liver to 6-MP and further converted to the active metabolite thioinosinic acid (TIMP) by the enzyme hypoxanthine–guanine phosphoribosyltransferase. Some of the immunosuppressive activity of azathioprine is attributable to 6-MP. Azathioprine acts mainly as an antiproliferative agent by interfering with normal purine pathways, by inhibiting DNA synthesis, and by being incorporated itself into DNA—thereby affecting the synthesis of DNA and RNA.[48]

TIMP interferes with the synthesis of guanylic and adenylic acids from inosinic acid by inhibiting several enzymes. TIMP is also converted to thioguanylic acid, a precursor for thiodeoxyguanosine triphosphate, which is incorporated into the developing strands of DNA and interferes with the DNA synthesis. TIMP also interferes with the induction of a number of coenzymes, such as that produced by nicotinamide mononucleotide-adenylyl transferase. By inhibiting the synthesis of DNA and RNA, azathioprine suppresses the proliferation of activated B and T lymphocytes.

In addition, azathioprine has been shown to reduce the number of circulating monocytes by arresting the cell cycle of promyelocytes in the bone marrow. The antiproliferative action of azathioprine probably explains much of its observed effects on the immune system and its toxicity. Azathioprine shows some selectivity in its effects on certain cell types and different types of immune reaction.[48] For instance, it has been shown that the primary immune responses are more susceptible to azathioprine than the secondary responses despite the fact that there is a more rapid proliferation of lymphocytes during a secondary response.

Pharmacokinetics and Drug Interactions

Azathioprine is adminstered orally at 1.5 mg/kg per day in conjunction with CNIs, and 2.5 mg/kg per day when used without CNIs. Higher initial doses (5 mg/kg per day) combined with monitoring of 6-thioguanine nucleotide levels in red blood cells are associated with an approximately 20% reduction in the acute rejection rate compared to lower doses.[49] It is metabolized in the liver to 6-MP and further converted to the active metabolite TIMP.

Because 6-MP is degraded by xanthine oxidase, allopurinol (a xanthine oxidase inhibitor) will increase the levels of TIMP. Severe leukopenia can occur if allopurinol (used for the treatment of hyperuricemia and gout) is given with azathioprine. Thus, allopurinol should generally be avoided in patients treated with azathioprine. If, however, the patient has severe gout and allopurinol must be used azathioprine doses must be reduced by about two thirds and the white blood cell count must be carefully monitored. Azathioprine eventually has to be discontinued in many such patients. A possible alternative is switching from azathioprine to MMF, which does not interact with allopurinol.

Side Effects

The major side effect of azathioprine is bone marrow suppression. All three hematopoietic cell lines can be affected, leading to leukopenia, thrombocytopenia, and anemia. The hematologic side effects are dose related and can occur late in the course of therapy. They are usually reversible upon dose reduction or temporary discontinuation of the drug. Azathioprine should be temporarily withheld if the white cell count falls below 3,000/mm^3 or if the count drops by 50% between blood draws. Recovery usually occurs within 1 to 2 weeks.

The drug can then be restarted at a lower dose and increased gradually to the usual maintenance dose while monitoring the white cell count. Occasionally, azathioprine has to be discontinued because of recurrent or persistent leukopenia. The mean cell volume is commonly increased in patients on full-dose azathioprine, and red cell aplasia can eventually result. Interactions between azathioprine and ACE inhibitors have been reported, causing anemia and leukopenia.

Another potentially serious side effect of azathioprine, which requires decreasing the dose or even stopping the drug, is hepatotoxicity. This complication is manifested by abnormal liver function tests, usually showing a cholestatic picture. The diagnosis of azathioprine-induced liver disease is one of exclusion, and the patient should be evaluated for other more serious causes of hepatic dysfunction. Azathioprine has also been linked to the development of skin cancer, the most common malignancy in renal transplant patients. As a result, patients taking azathioprine for a prolonged period should be instructed to avoid direct exposure to sunlight or to use heavy sun screens when exposed. Other side effects include increased susceptibility to infection and hair loss.

Antimetabolic Agents: Mycophenolate Mofetil

MMF impairs lymphocyte function by blocking purine biosynthesis via inhibition of the enzyme inosine monophosphate dehydrogenase (IMPDH). MMF was developed as a replacement for azathioprine for maintenance immunosuppression. It is not nephrotoxic, and has less bone marrow toxicity than azathioprine. However, gastrointestinal toxicity can occur—usually manifested by gastritis and diarrhea.

Mechanism of Action

Mycophenolic acid (MPA), the active ingredient of the prodrug MMF, acts by blocking de novo purine synthesis in

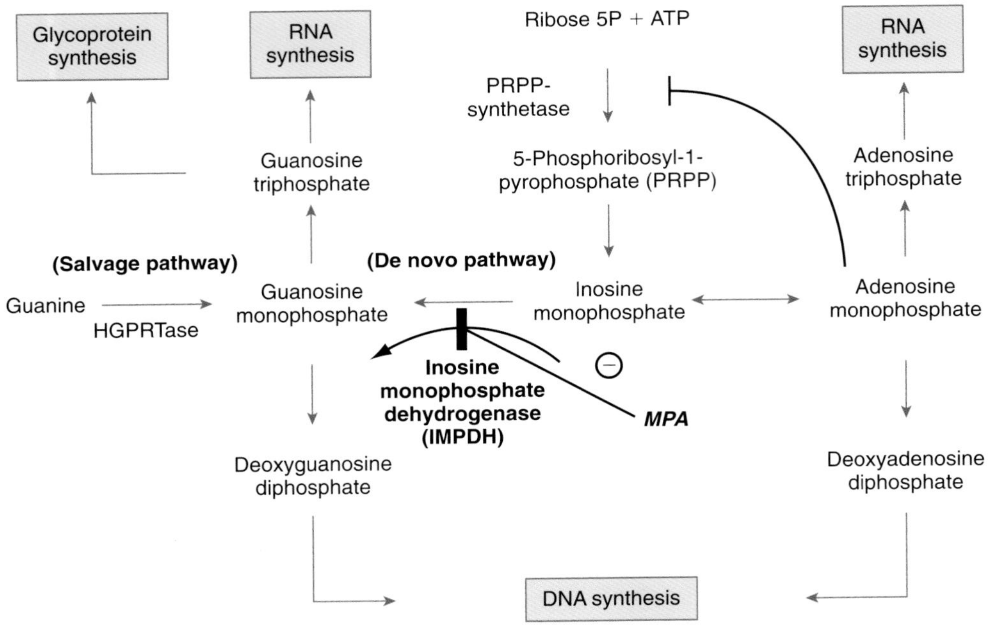

Figure 59-10 Immunosuppressive mechanism of mycophenolic acid. By inhibiting inosine monophosphate dehydrogenase (IMPDH), MPA antagonizes the de novo pathway of purine synthesis on which lymphocytes particularly depend. Accumulation of adenosine monophosphate inhibits 5-phosphoribosyl-1-pyrophosphate (PRPP) activity, thereby diminishing the substrate of IMPDH. Depletion of guanosine phosphates inhibits DNA and RNA synthesis. Lymphocytes lack the salvage pathway of purine synthesis, which depends on the activity of the enzyme hypoxanthine guanosine phosphoribosyl transferase (HGPRTase).

lymphocytes. Purines can be generated either by de novo synthesis or by recycling (salvage pathway). Lymphocytes preferentially use de novo purine synthesis, whereas other tissues (such as brain) use the salvage pathway. MPA uncompetitively inhibits IMPDH, which is the rate-limiting enzyme in the de novo synthesis of guanosine monophosphate (GMP) (Figure 59-10).

Inhibition of IMPDH creates a relative deficiency of GMP and a relative excess of adenosine monophosphate (AMP). GMP and AMP levels act as a control on de novo purine biosynthesis, which is essential for T- and B-lymphocyte proliferation but not for division in other cells. Therefore MMF, by blocking IMPDH, creates a block in de novo purine synthesis that selectively interferes with proliferative responses of T and B lymphocytes—inhibiting clonal expansion and thus inhibiting antibody production, the generation of cytotoxic T cells, and the development of delayed type hypersensitivity.

Furthermore, MPA impairs the ability of dendritic cells to present antigen, suppresses the recruitment of monocyte lineage cells, suppresses the glycosylation of adhesion molecules, inhibits vascular smooth muscle proliferation, improves endothelial function, and inhibits mononuclear cell recruitment into allografts and nephritic kidneys.[50] MPA also decreases cytokine-induced nitric oxide synthesis and prevents the formation of reactive species such as peroxynitrite. Furthermore, MPA exhibits antioxidant effects in experimental nephropathies. These properties of MPA likely augment its immunosuppressive properties by limiting fibrosis and vascular sclerosis after immunologic injury.[51]

Dosage and Pharmacokinetics

MMF, a semisynthetic ethyl ester of MPA, is rapidly and completely absorbed and hydrolyzed by esterases to yield the active drug MPA. The recommended dose in pediatric patients in conjunction with cyclosporine is 1200 mg/m^2 per day in two divided doses. The recommended MMF dose in conjunction with tacrolimus is 800 mg/m^2 per day in two divided doses. However, recent data from a large prospective randomized study in both pediatric and adult renal transplant recipients on fixed dose MMF versus a concentration-controlled regimen (the FDCC study) indicates that a higher initial MMF dose (e.g., 1,800 mg MMF/m^2 per day in conjunction with cyclosporine and 1,200 mf MMF/m^2 per day in conjunction with tacrolimus for the first 2 to 4 weeks posttransplant) is required to achieve adequate MPA exposure in the majority of patients.[52] The MMF dose should be reduced with active cytomegalovirus infection. When MMF is associated with diarrhea (a side effect of MMF; see material following), spreading the dose to three to four doses per day may be effective in controlling it.

The difference in MMF dosing depending on the concomitant CNI is explained by a pharmacokinetic interaction of cyclosporine with the main MPA metabolite 7-O-MPA glucuronide (7-O-MPAG). Cyclosporine inhibits the multidrug-resistant protein-2–mediated transport of 7-O-MPAG into the bile. MPAG is subject to enzymatic and nonenzymatic hydrolysis in bile, and more importantly in the intestine—thereby liberating the unconjugated drug MPA, which is then reabsorbed into the systemic circulation. This enterohepatic circulation is responsible for a secondary MPA peak occurring 6 to 12 hours after administration. The impact of the enterohepatic cycle on the MPA plasma concentration varies within and between individuals due to factors such as meal times or comedication of drugs that interrupt the enterohepatic circulation (e.g., bile acid sequestrants, antibiotics).

These factors should be considered when evaluating MPA concentrations (particularly predose concentrations) in clinical practice. Furthermore, genetic abnormalities and disease can affect enterohepatic cycling and thus the bioavailability of MPA.[53] If cyclosporine doses are tapered, the predose concentrations of MPA significantly increase—and after complete discontinuation of cyclosporine they can reach about twice the values seen in patients still on cyclosporine cotherapy. When using MMF in combination with tacrolimus or sirolimus, lower MMF doses can be used to achieve comparable MPA exposure (guided by therapeutic drug monitoring) to that seen with cyclosporine.[53] However, an uncritical approach used by some centers to reduce the MMF dose generally by 50% when coadministered with tacrolimus or sirolimus is not advisable.

The metabolism of MPA due to glucuronidation can also be affected by drug induction. Corticosteroids are known inducers of UDP-glucuronosyl transferases in vitro, and there is evidence that this may hold true in vivo. In one study, for example, the effect of steroid withdrawal on MPA bioavailability was studied in 26 kidney transplant recipients.[54] Twelve months after transplantation, the time at which steroids were completely withdrawn, a 33% increase in the mean dose-normalized MPA predose concentrations and MPA-AUCs compared with concentrations at 6 months (when the patients were still receiving maintenance doses of steroids) was observed. The relevant drug-drug interactions are summarized in Table 59-3.

An important pharmacokinetic property of MPA is its extensive and tight protein binding, particularly to serum albumin. The free MPA fraction in individuals with conserved renal function ranges from 1% to 3%. Based on in vitro studies, the free MPA fraction is responsible for the pharmacologic activity of the drug. Furthermore, it is an important determinant of the MPA clearance. Of the factors evaluated for their effect on MPA protein binding, serum albumin turned out to be the most important. In patients with delayed graft function or renal impairment, there are many factors that can affect MPA protein binding—resulting in a substantially elevated free MPA concentration accompanied by total MPA concentrations that are not significantly different from those found in patients with relatively preserved renal function.[55]

This is particularly important because such patients are prone to an increased risk for toxicity. In pediatric renal transplant recipients, the free MPA-AUC is a significant risk factor for leukopenia or severe infections at concentrations above 600 μg*L/h.[56] The effect of impaired renal function on plasma protein binding of MPA is most likely caused by accumulation of its major phenolic glucuronide metabolite 7-O-MPAG. This metabolite is primarily excreted through the kidneys and causes competitive displacement of MPA from protein molecules. Displacement is facilitated by hypoalbuminemia and acidosis, which are usually found under this condition.[55] In addition to renal impairment, hyperbilirubinemia can also lead to displacement of MPA from its protein binding sites. Therefore, monitoring of the free MPA-AUC may be advantageous in patients who show the symptoms previously mentioned.

TABLE 59-3 Drug-Drug Interactions Between MMF and Frequently Used Comedications

Drug	Effect	Site of Interaction
Antacids	MPA AUC ↓	Absorption
Cholestyramine	MPA AUC ↓ MPAG AUC ↓	Absorption
Corticosteroids	MPA trough ↓ MPA AUC ↓ MPAG ↑	Glucuronidation
Cyclosporine	MPA trough ↓ MPA AUC ↓	Enterohepatic cycling
Metronidazole	MPA AUC ↓ MPAG AUC ↓	Enterohepatic cycling, suppression of anaerobic bacterial glucuronidase
Norfloxacin	MPA AUC ↓ MPAG AUC ↓	Enterohepatic cycling, suppression of anaerobic bacterial glucuronidase
Phosphate binder	MPA AUC ↓ Cmax ↓	Absorption

Efficacy

Three multicenter clinical trials established the efficacy of MMF in addition to cyclosporine plus glucocorticoids in the primary prevention of renal allograft rejection in clinical renal transplantation in adults compared to treatment with azathioprine or placebo. MMF reduced rejection by about 50%, and reduced the requirement for steroids or OKT3/ATG treatment for acute rejection and graft loss owing to rejection. As with other new immunosuppressives, MMF may be contributing to the improvement in long-term function and graft and patient survival. Triple therapy with MMF, glucocorticoids, and either cyclosporine or tacrolimus has become widespread in the management of transplant recipients. MMF can also be added to cyclosporine or tacrolimus for rescue and in reversing refractory acute rejection in renal transplant patients.[57]

Following the success of the early MMF studies in adults, MMF was investigated in pediatric renal transplant recipients in open-label studies with historical controls—because randomized controlled trials were quite difficult to carry out in light of the relatively small numbers of pediatric kidney transplants performed each year. Because studies in adult renal transplant recipients had previously established the superiority of MMF over azathioprine or placebo in reducing the risk of acute rejection, it was important for the pediatric transplant community to have prompt access to open-label studies. For a summary of selected published studies of MMF used in combination with cyclosporine and steroids in pediatric renal transplantation, see Table 59-4.

Data from three large multicenter studies[60-64] and one smaller study[65] provided support for the safety and efficacy

TABLE 59-4 **Selected Published Studies of Mycophenolate Mofetil in Combination with Cyclosporine and Steroids in Pediatric Renal Transplantation**

Reference	No. of Patients (Study Group/ Controls)	Study Design	No. of Follow-up Years	IMMUNOSUPPRESSIVE REGIMEN: Induction	IMMUNOSUPPRESSIVE REGIMEN: MMF dose	OUTCOMES (INCIDENCE): Acute Rejection	OUTCOMES (INCIDENCE): Patient Survival	OUTCOMES (INCIDENCE): Graft Survival
Ettenger, 1997 (58)	37	Single-center, open label	1	Antithymocite globulin	8–30 mg/kg bid	13%		97%
Benfield 1999 (59)	36/31	Open label, consecutive enrollment in AZA or MMF groups	0,5	OKT3 or intravenous CSA	1000 mg/ m²/day ^	MMF (25%) AZA (39%) $p = 0.3$	MMF (97%) AZA (87%) $p = 0.3$	MMF (89%) AZA (81%) $p = 0.3$
Bunchman, 2001 (60); Hoecker, 2005 (61)	100	Multicenter, open label	1,3	Optional, varied agents	600 mg/m² bid	29%	98%	93%
Staskewitz, 2001 (62); Jungraithmayr, 2003 (63)	65/54 (86)*	Multicenter, open label	1 3	None	600 mg/m² bid	MMF (29%) AZA (59%) $p<0.001$ MMF (44%) AZA (59%) $p<0.05$	MMF (100%) AZA (94%) p = NS MMF(99%) AZA (94%) p = NS	MMF (89%) AZA (83%) p = NR MMF (98%) AZA (80%) $p<0.001$
Cransberg, 2005 (64)	96/207	Multicenter, open label, consecutive enrollment vs. historical controls (AZA)	1	None	600 mg/m² bid	MMF (37%) AZA (72%) $p<0.001$	MMF(100%) AZA (96%) $p = 0.07$	MMF (92%) AZA (73%) $p = 0.001$
Ferraris, 2005 (65)	29/29	Dual-center, open label, historical controls (AZA)	5	None	600 mg/m² bid	MMF (21%) AZA (59%) $p<0.01$	MMF(97%) AZA (93%) p = NS	MMF (90%) AZA (83%) p = NS

* Number of patients in follow-up report indicated in parentheses.

AZA, Azathioprine, bid, twice daily; *CNI*, calcineurin inhibitor; *CsA*, cyclosporine A; *MMF*, mycophenolate mofetil; *NR*, not reported; *NS*, not significant.

of MMF in the pediatric renal transplant population when used with cyclosporine and prednisone (Table 59-4). Induction therapy was optional in one study[60] and not used in the other two studies.[62,64] The incidence of acute rejection within the first 6 months to 1 year for patients receiving MMF in these studies ranged from 28% to 37%.[60,62,64]

Those studies comparing MMF patient groups to historical controls reported significant reductions in the incidence of acute rejection with MMF versus azathioprine.[62,64] There was also a significant improvement in the incidence of acute rejection between patients receiving MMF and those receiving azathioprine at 3 years in a follow-up report to one study.[63] In one large study,[60] there were no differences in the incidence of acute rejection when the results were stratified by age. Long-term (3-year) graft and patient survival were excellent, with a 30% incidence of acute rejection (Table 59-4).[61]

Effects of Mycophenolate Mofetil on Long-Term Renal Allograft Function

MMF is considered to mitigate chronic failure of renal allografts. The major cause of late graft failure is thought to be chronic allograft nephropathy (CAN), a term used to describe the histologic changes that accompany long-term deterioration of graft function: tubular atrophy, interstitial fibrosis, and fibrointimal thickening of arterioles. It has been postulated that this entity may be mediated by pathways involving humoral immunity. The course of CAN may be accelerated by CNI toxicity, which itself can result in progressive interstitial fibrosis of the allograft. It also has been shown in small single-center experiences that antidonor antibody responses can be reduced with tacrolimus and MMF in combination in the case of CAN.[66]

Because humoral responses are felt to be an important accompaniment to CAN, this property of MMF also may contribute to its effects on decreasing long-term graft loss.[57] In fact, MMF is devoid of intrinsic renal, cardiovascular, or metabolic toxicities. A few studies provide information on the impact of MMF on long-term allograft function in pediatric renal transplant recipients. Ferraris and colleagues[65] evaluated renal allograft function at 5 years after transplantation in 29 patients. Although there was no significant difference in the incidence of chronic rejection (10.3% versus 25% for MMF versus azathioprine), patients receiving MMF were significantly more likely to have event-free survival (events included a 20% or greater decline in 1/serum creatinine, death, or graft loss) than those receiving azathioprine (69% versus 17%, respectively; $p < 0.0001$).

The use of MMF in these patients allowed a lower dose of steroids to be used at 5 years posttransplant, resulting in significant growth benefits in patients receiving MMF when compared with those receiving azathioprine.[65] In another

TABLE 59-5 **Adverse Events Leading to MMF Dose Reduction or Interruption in More Than 5% of Patients during the 3-year Study Period of the MMF Suspension Trial in Pediatric Renal Transplant Recipients[61]**

	NUMBER OF ADVERSE EVENTS (AE) BY AGE GROUP			
Specific AE	**<6 Years (*n* = 33)**	**6 to <12 Years (*n* = 34)**	**12 to 18 Years (*n* = 33)**	**All Ages (*n* = 100)**
Any body system	23 (70 %)	17 (50 %)	14 (42 %)	54 (54 %)
Hemic and Lymphatic System				
Leukopenia	13 (39%)*	8 (24%)	4 (12%)	25 (25%)
Anemia	5 (15%)*	2 (6%)	0	7 (7%)
Body as a Whole				
Sepsis	3 (9%)	4 (12%)	3 (9%)	10 (10%)
Fever	4 (12%)	1 (3%)	1 (3%)	6 (6%)
Abdominal pain	2 (6%)	1 (3%)	2 (6%)	5 (5%)
Digestive System				
Diarrhea	9 (27%)*	6 (18%)	1 (3%)	16 (16%)
Skin and Appendages				
Herpes zoster	5 (15%)	1 (3%)	4 (12%)	10 (10%)

* $p < 0.05$ versus the age groups "6 to < 12 years" and "12 to 18 years."
Numbers, with percentages in parentheses, are the result of intent-to-treat analysis.
From Hoecker B, Weber LT, Bunchman T, Rashford M, Toenshoff B for the Tricontinental MMF Suspension Study Group: Mycophenolate mofetil suspension in pediatric renal transplantation: Three-year data from the tricontinental trial, *Pediatr Transplant* 9:504-11, 2005.

study in 36 pediatric renal transplant patients with CAN, MMF was either added to a regimen consisting of cyclosporine or tacrolimus and steroids or was substituted for azathioprine in patients receiving a triple-therapy regimen.[67] A year after conversion, 61% had an improvement in GFR—with 22% remaining stable and only 17% having a further decline in renal function. Taken together, these studies suggest that MMF may improve both early and late allograft outcome in children and adolescents.

Side Effects

The major toxicity of MMF is gastrointestinal, mainly diarrhea, possibly as a result of the high concentrations of acyl-MPAG in the gut. MMF is devoid of intrinsic renal, cardiovascular, or metabolic toxicities but can increase the risk for CMV infections, leukopenia, and perhaps mild anemia (Table 59-2). MPA has been associated with protection from *Pneumocystis carinii* pneumonia (PCP) and may actually have some anti-PCP activity because *Pneumocystis carinii* has IMPDH activity. MMF should not be used in pregnant transplant patients because its safety in pregnancy has not yet been established.

In the MMF suspension trial in pediatric renal transplant recipients, safety of MMF was evaluated based on the occurrence of adverse events—including the development of opportunistic infections and malignancies. Adverse events, which called for MMF dose reduction or interruption of MMF administration in more than 5% of all patients, are listed in Table 59-5. Most frequently noted were hematologic problems (such as leukopenia) and gastrointestinal disorders (such as diarrhea), which occurred in 25% and 16% of all patients, respectively, and were observed more often in the youngest age group. In general, the risk of developing side effects declined with increasing age (Table 59-5).

Therapeutic Drug Monitoring

Patients on standard-dose MMF therapy show considerable interpatient variability in pharmacokinetic parameters. This variability is attributable to factors that influence exposure to MMF, such as patient renal function, serum albumin levels, and concomitant medications (such as cyclosporine) that inhibit enterohepatic recirculation of the active metabolite of MMF, MPA (Table 59-3). This variability is clinically relevant because higher plasma concentrations of MPA are correlated with reduced risk of acute rejection after kidney transplantation.[56,68] These findings have suggested that individualizing the dose regimen of MMF may further improve clinical outcomes compared to a standard-dose regimen.

The potential for therapeutic drug monitoring of patients receiving MMF to improve clinical outcomes was first demonstrated in a randomized concentration-controlled trial in renal transplant patients receiving MMF, cyclosporine, and corticosteroids[69] and in studies in pediatric patients.[56] Recommendations describing MMF therapeutic drug monitoring have been published.[68] After ensuring adequate levels of MPA immediately after transplantation, optimal efficacy may require only a few dose adjustments because intrapatient variability in exposure appears low. Regarding frequency of monitoring and dose adjustments, sampling is suggested on days 3 and 7 and once during days 10 through 14 posttransplant.

Because 4 to 5 days are required for a patient to reach a new steady state after a dose adjustment is made, monitoring more frequently would be of limited additional benefit. A repeat therapeutic drug monitoring analysis may be done 3 to 4 weeks posttransplant, or if the immunosuppressant regimen is changed substantially, or to evaluate a clinical event such as rejection or adverse event. If an MPA level seems aberrant with respect to previously obtained levels, or if an initial level is extremely high or low, a repetition of the therapeutic drug monitoring sample is advised. In general, the MPA-AUC is more strongly correlated with acute rejection than with the predose plasma concentration and is therefore selected as the pharmacokinetic parameter for drug monitoring by most investigators. However, because determination of AUC is impractical to perform in routine clinical practice a limited sampling strategy for monitoring MPA is currently recommended.[68,70]

An algorithm based on three pharmacokinetic (PK) sampling time points during the first 2 hours after MMF dosing (estimated $AUC_{0\text{-}12} = 18.6 + 4.3 \cdot C_0 + 0.54 \cdot C_{0.5} + 2.15 \cdot C_2$) has been validated for the estimation of MPA exposure.[70] For pediatric patients on MMF in conjunction with tacrolimus or no CNI, a different algorithm for the estimation of MPA exposure based on a limited sampling strategy must be used (estimated $AUC_{0\text{-}12} = 10.0 + 3.95 \cdot C_0 + 3.24 \cdot {-}_{0.5} + 1.01 \cdot C_2$).[71] The currently recommended therapeutic window for MPA exposure in conjunction with full-dose CNI therapy is 30 to 60 mg · h/L. However, in view of the cost and effort involved in performing therapeutic drug monitoring, more evidence for the validity of a dose individualization approach is needed.

Controlled trials are required to provide the basis for MPA target concentrations in various combination therapies with conventional and new immunosuppressive drugs. This is particularly important with respect to the development of optimal dosing strategies in the context of steroid and/or CNI sparing protocols because MMF has become the main long-term immunosuppressant in many centers. Furthermore, a critical evaluation of the predictive power of different monitoring approaches—such as serial determination of predose MPA concentrations, estimated AUCs, free MPA concentration, and metabolite concentrations (AcMPAG) and the value of pharmacodynamic measures (IMPDH activity)—should be performed. Furthermore, identification of indicators for the individual immune responsiveness would be helpful in individualizing target levels and in selecting optimal therapeutic regimens.

Target of Rapamycin Inhibitors

Sirolimus (rapamycin) is a macrocyclic triene antibiotic produced by the actinomycete *Streptomyces hygroscopicus*, which was first isolated from soil samples collected from the Via Atari region of Rapa Nui (Easter Island). Sirolimus was approved in September of 1999 by the United States FDA and in December of 2000 by the Committee for Proprietary Medicinal Products (CPMP), the Scientific Advisory Board of the European Medicines Evaluation Agency, for use in adult renal transplant recipients. Everolimus (RAD) is an analog of sirolimus that is still in clinical trials but seems to have similar effectiveness and side effect profile as sirolimus.

Mechanism of Action

Sirolimus displays a novel mechanism of immunosuppressive action, which is distinct from that of the other immunosuppressive drugs. Interaction with at least two intracellular proteins is required to elicit its antiproliferative activity. Sirolimus first binds to the cytosolic immunophilin FK-binding protein 12 (FKBP12) (Figure 59-11). In contrast to the tacrolimus-FKBP12 complex, the complex of sirolimus with FKBP12 does not inhibit calcineurin activity.

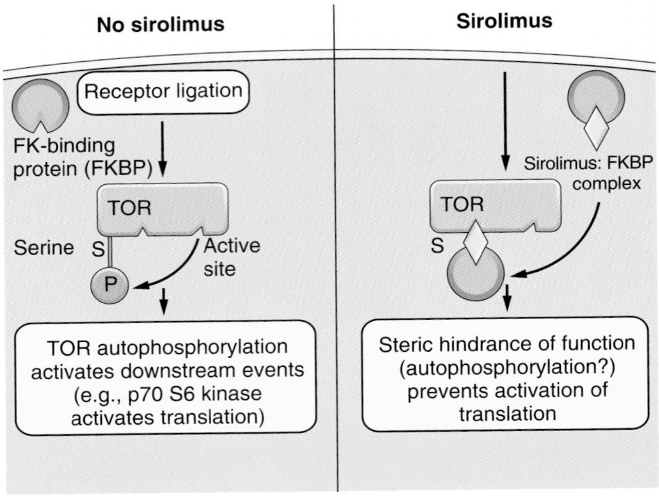

Figure 59-11 Action of sirolimus. In the absence of sirolimus, receptor ligation causes activation of a kinase enzyme called target of rapamycin (TOR). Sirolimus prevents the activation of TOR by binding to FK-binding proteins (FKBP) and preventing autophosphorylation of TOR through steric hindrance. (From Feehally J, Floege J, Johnson RJ (eds.): *Comprehensive clinical nephrology, Third edition*. Philadelphia: Mosby 2007:1043.)

Instead, this complex binds to and inhibits the activation of the mammalian target of rapamycin (mTOR), a key regulatory kinase. This inhibition suppresses cytokine-mediated T-cell proliferation, inhibiting the progression from the G1 phase to the S phase of the cell cycle. Thus, sirolimus acts at a later stage in the cell cycle than do the CNIs cyclosporine and tacrolimus. Sirolimus can, therefore, be used in combination with the CNIs to produce a synergistic effect.[72]

Pharmacokinetics

Sirolimus is available as tablet or oral solution. Information on the pharmacokinetics of sirolimus in pediatric transplant patients is limited.[73] Clinical studies on adult populations indicate a low (ca. 14%) and variable bioavailability.[74] The low bioavailability of sirolimus may be due to extensive intestinal and hepatic metabolism by the cytochrome P450 3A enzyme family and to counter transport by the multidrug efflux pump P-glycoprotein in the intestine. Accordingly, considerable variability in the pharmacokinetics of this compound may be expected. Sirolimus shows a high plasma protein binding.

According to data obtained in adults, the free fraction is only about 8%.[74] After oral intake, maximal concentrations are reached after 1 hour. The drug is more than 90% excreted by the biliary system, but great variations in elimination time have been found—especially prolonged times in patients with hepatic impairment. Sirolimus is widely distributed in tissues, including blood cells.

Preliminary data from a study in pediatric patients with stable chronic renal failure indicate differences in the apparent clearance after oral intake normalized by body weight between young (5-11 years) and older (12-18 years) patients, suggesting that higher doses should be given to the former group.[75] Younger children (4-10 years) may require sirolimus dosing every 12 hours. This seems in line with data from a further small group of stable pediatric renal transplant recipients maintained on a regimen of cyclosporine, prednisone, and sirolimus. When the pharmacokinetic profiles were separated according to age groups, children demonstrated a higher apparent clearance after oral intake (485 ± 199 ml/h/kg) compared with adolescents (376 ± 262 ml/h/kg) and adults (208 ± 95 ml/h/kg).[76]

In a further study with 21 transplanted children treated with sirolimus and tacrolimus, pharmacokinetic profiles were measured in the first week after initiating sirolimus.[73] Again, the mean half-life was markedly shorter for children (11.8 ± 5.5 hours) compared with adults (62.0 ± 16.0 hours). The relationship between trough whole-blood concentrations of sirolimus with the AUC was excellent ($r^2 = 0.98$). This is in line with findings in adult patients in which a good correlation ($r^2 = 0.85 - 0.95$) between C_{min} and AUC was observed.[77] Studies in adult patients also indicated that C_{min} (<5 μg/L) correlated with the severity of acute rejection episodes and was related to adverse effects at sirolimus values above 15 μg/L.[78]

In the posttransplant period, pediatric patients appeared to undergo changes in their pharmacokinetic patterns—with a progressive increase in sirolimus concentrations noted at 2, 4, and 8 weeks posttransplantation.[76] This finding emphasizes the need for a close monitoring of whole-blood sirolimus concentrations in pediatric patients to allow detection of changes in the AUC. In contrast to the findings of Sindhi and colleagues,[73] Ettenger and Grimm[76] reported a substantial scatter in trough levels of pediatric patients and a lower correlation with AUC. Further pharmacokinetic studies are needed to clarify this point.

Interactions have been shown for high-fat meals, and various drug interactions have been described between sirolimus and other drugs. An increased exposure is observed in particular with azole antifungals (e.g., itraconazole, ketoconazole), cyclosporine, erythromycin, nelfinavir, and diltiazem—whereas a decrease of exposure is seen in the presence of rifampin and phenytoin. There is an important interaction with cyclosporine: sirolimus levels are increased by concomitant administration of the microemulsion formulation of cyclosporine, and sirolimus increases cyclosporine levels about twofold through competition for the cytochrome P450 3A4 system. Because of this interaction, cyclosporine levels must be adjusted accordingly.

Clinical Trials

In clinical renal transplantation in adults, sirolimus in combination with cyclosporine efficiently reduces the incidence of acute allograft rejection. Because of the synergistic effect of sirolimus on cyclosporine-induced nephrotoxicity, a prolonged combination of the two drugs inevitably leads to progressive irreversible renal allograft damage. Early elimination of CNI therapy or complete avoidance of the latter by using sirolimus therapy is the optimal strategy for this drug. Prospective randomized phase II and phase III clinical studies have confirmed this approach, at least for recipients with a low to moderate immunologic risk.

For patients with a high immunologic risk or recipients exposed to delayed graft function, sirolimus might not constitute the best therapeutic choice—despite its ability to enable CNI sparing in the latter situation—because of its antiproliferative effects on recovering renal tubular cells. Whether lower doses of sirolimus or a combination with a reduced dose of tacrolimus would be advantageous in these high-risk situations remains to be determined. Taken together, sirolimus has gained a proper place in the present-day immunosuppressive armament used in adult renal transplantation and will contribute to the development of a tailor-made immunosuppressive therapy aimed at fulfilling the requirements outlined by the individual patient profile.[79]

In pediatric patients, sirolimus is used primarily as a rescue agent, particularly in cases of CNI toxicity. Sirolimus may allow the reduction or even the elimination of CNI in the presence or absence of MMF. In a mixed population of transplanted children, it could be demonstrated that sirolimus as a rescue agent lowered tacrolimus requirements by 50% and resulted in significant improvements in measured serum creatinine and in calculated creatinine clearance.[73]

The indications for sirolimus in pediatric renal transplant recipients still remain to be defined. In the setting of chronic CNI-induced nephrotoxicity, whether conversion to sirolimus in a CNI-free regimen is superior to CNI minimization is still under investigation. In one case-control study, for example, the efficacy and safety of a sirolimus-based immunosuppressive regimen plus MMF and corticosteroids was analyzed versus CNI minimization plus MMF and corticosteroids in 19 pediatric recipients with biopsy-proven CNI-induced nephrotoxicity.[80]

In the sirolimus group, an improvement of GFR by 10.3 ± 3.0 ml/min/1.73 m² ($p < 0.05$ versus baseline) 1 year after study entry was observed in 7 of 10 patients, and a stabilization in the remaining three—whereas in the CNI minimization group GFR improved by 17.7 ± 7.1 ml/min/1.73 m² ($p < 0.05$) in six of nine recipients and stabilized in the remaining three (Figure 59-12). No patient in either group experienced an acute rejection episode. The main adverse event under sirolimus therapy was a transient hyperlipidemia in 70% of patients. Hence, in this study in pediatric patients with declining graft function because of CNI-induced nephrotoxicity CNI withdrawal and switch to a sirolimus-based therapy or CNI minimization were associated with a comparable improvement of GFR after 12 months of observation.

Side Effects

Clinically relevant adverse effects of sirolimus that require a specific therapeutic response or can potentially influence short- and long-term patient morbidity and mortality as well as graft survival include hypercholesterolemia, hypertriglyceridemia, infectious and noninfectious pneumonia, anemia, lymphocele formation, and impaired wound healing (Table 59-2). These drug-related adverse effects are important determinants in the choice of a tailor-made immunosuppres-

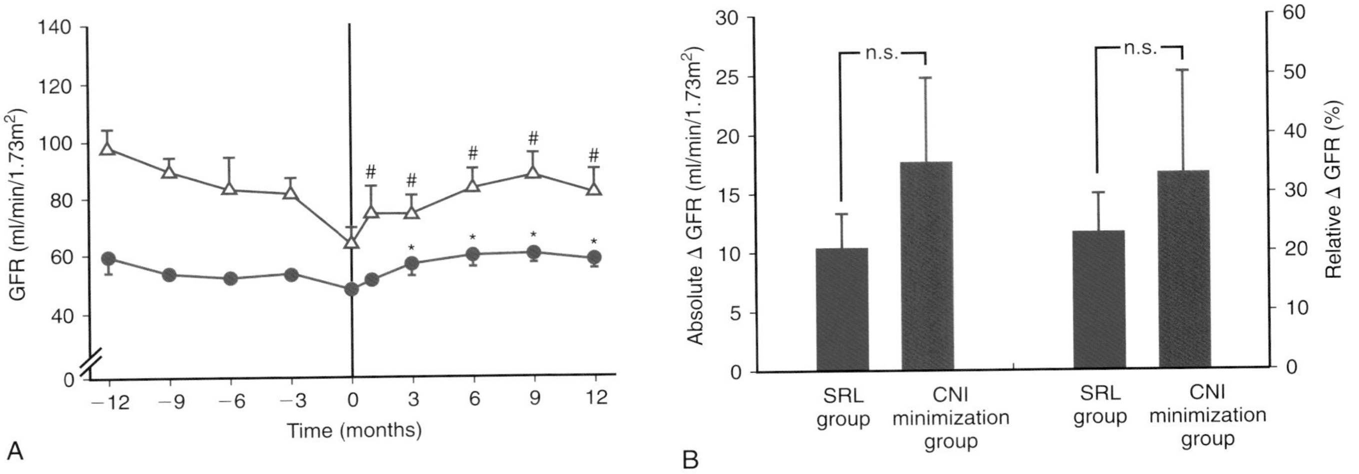

Figure 59-12 **A,** Mean glomerular filtration rate (GFR) in the sirolimus (SRL)-treated cohort (closed symbols) and the calcineurin inhibitor (CNI) minimization cohort (open triangles) 12 months before and after study entry (* $p < 0.05$ versus baseline). **B,** The absolute and the relative gain of GFR in the SRL-treated cohort and the CNI minimization cohort. There was no statistically significant difference. (From Hocker B, Feneberg R, Kopf S, Weber LT, Waldherr R, et al: SRL-based immunosuppression vs. CNI minimization in pediatric renal transplant recipients with chronic CNI nephrotoxicity, *Pediatr Transplant* 10:593-601, 2006.)

sive drug regimen that complies with the individual patient risk profile.

Equally important in the latter decision is the lack of severe intrinsic nephrotoxicity associated with sirolimus and its advantageous effects on arterial hypertension, posttransplantation diabetes mellitus, and esthetic changes induced by CNIs. Mild and transient thrombocytopenia, leukopenia, gastrointestinal adverse effects, and mucosal ulcerations are all minor complications of sirolimus therapy that have less impact on the decision to select this drug as the basis for tailor-made immunosuppressive therapy. In the pilot studies of sirolimus, there was an outbreak of PCP (with some deaths)—and PCP prophylaxis must be used with sirolimus or everolimus, and indeed with all transplant immunosuppressives, at least in the first few months.

An additional side effect in the setting of CNI withdrawal and sirolimus introduction is aggravation of proteinuria in patients with preexisting proteinuria by a still incompletely defined mechanism. The available data are consistent with the hypothesis that the increase of proteinuria is causally related to CNI withdrawal and not because of initiation of sirolimus. On the other hand, it cannot be excluded that sirolimus itself might also affect glomerular permeability in some patients. The potential complication of increased proteinuria, which is an independent risk factor for long-term renal allograft function, should therefore be borne in mind when a conversion of the immunosuppressive regimen from a CNI-based to a sirolimus-based maintenance therapy is considered. Preliminary results show that TOR inhibitor treatment may impair gonadal function after renal transplantation, but the clinical significance of these effects is unknown.

Therapeutic Drug Monitoring

In adult patients, it has been documented that monitoring of sirolimus is essential to avoid underexposure or overexposure with this drug. According to its European label, monitoring is mandatory in the European Union. So far, there is little experience with sirolimus monitoring in pediatric patients where this drug is currently used as a rescue agent—particularly in cases of cyclosporine or tacrolimus toxicity.

Provisional monitoring guidelines for sirolimus are as follows. The trough concentration should be determined in ethylenediaminetetraacetic acid disodium salt (EDTA) whole blood. The therapeutic window currently recommended by Wyeth (European label) for trough sirolimus concentrations in adult de novo renal transplant patients on triple therapy with cyclosporine, corticosteroids, and sirolimus is 4 to 12 μg/L. Sirolimus should be determined by a specific chromatographic procedure such as HPLC-UV or LC/MS-MS. Preliminary recommendations based on experiences in adult kidney transplant recipients requiring conversion to a CNI-free regimen have been published.[80] In such maintenance patients, a sirolimus trough concentration of 5 to 10 μg/L is proposed when sirolimus is used in combination with MMF. These therapeutic ranges may serve as a guide for pediatric renal transplant recipients.

Sirolimus levels should be determined after the loading dose, after a new steady state is reached (constant dosage over at least five half-lives), after a dose change, and in particular after introduction or discontinuation of inhibitors or inducers of cytochrome P450 3A4 and the P-glycoprotein transporter. The frequency for monitoring should be once per week during the first month and every other month thereafter. Monitoring is also necessary after changes in cyclosporine dosing and steady-state concentrations, after changes in the relative timing of sirolimus and cyclosporine, and after changes in the patient's condition (liver disease, hyperlipidemia, leukopenia). It is also necessary if a compliance problem is suspected.

CONCLUSIONS

Transplantation in children carries unique challenges.[81] Although issues such as controlling rejection and minimizing side effects are similar between adults and children, maintenance immunosuppressant regimens that affect developmental processes have a disproportionate impact on children. This is particularly true in the case of corticosteroids, which have many side effects (Table 59-2). Some of these effects can be quite devastating in pediatric patients. In addition, the CNIs, most commonly cyclosporine, induce cosmetic side effects such as gingival hyperplasia and hirsutism (Table 59-2).

These side effects especially affect adolescents, who have been shown to be up to four times more nonadherent with their medications than adults or younger patients—and who have the least successful long-term graft survival of all age groups. Steroid avoidance has been successful in the short term, when MMF is combined with tacrolimus and either extended-dose daclizumab or antithymocyte globulin is added. With the goal of eliminating steroids, the combination of MMF and tacrolimus may strike the correct balance between adequate and overimmunosuppression.

However, there is at present no consensus for immunosuppressive therapy following renal transplantation in children. Clearly, much additional work is needed to define optimal immunosuppressive regimens in pediatric renal transplant patients—particularly with respect to newer and evolving regimens. The safety and efficacy of these protocols, with special emphasis on long-term graft survival and PTLD, need to be established.

REFERENCES

1. Szczech LA, Berlin JA, Aradhye S, et al: Effect of anti-lymphocyte induction therapy on renal allograft survival: A meta-analysis, *J Am Soc Nephrol* 8:1771-77, 1997.
2. The NAPRTCS 2006 Annual Report. *https://web.emmes.com/study/ped/index.htm*.
3. Brennan DC, Flavin K, Lowell JA, et al: A randomized, double-blinded comparison of Thymoglobulin versus ATGAM for induction immunosuppressive therapy in adult renal transplant recipients, *Transplant* 67:1011-18, 1999.
4. Hardinger KL, Schnitzler MA, Miller B, et al: Five-year follow up of thymoglobulin versus ATGAM induction in adult renal transplantation, *Transplant* 78:136-41, 2004.
5. Khositseth S, Matas A, Cook ME, Gillingham KJ, Chavers BM: Thymoglobulin versus ATGAM induction therapy in pediatric kidney transplant recipients: A single-center report, *Transplant* 79:958-63, 2005.
6. Niaudet P, Jean G, Broyer M, Chatenoud L: Anti-OKT3 response following prophylactic treatment in paediatric kidney transplant recipients, *Pediatr Nephrol* 7:263-67, 1993.
7. Benfield MR, Tejani A, Harmon WE, McDonald R, Stablein DM, et al for the CCTPT Study Group: A randomized multicenter trial of OKT3 mAbs induction compared with intravenous cyclosporine in pediatric renal transplantation, *Pediatr Transplant* 9:282-92, 2005.
8. Webster AC, Playford EG, Higgins G, et al: Interleukin 2 receptor antagonists for renal transplant recipients: A meta-analysis of randomized trials, *Transplant* 77:166-76, 2004.
9. Novartis 6 Oct. 2000 "Dear Healthcare Provider" letter.
10. Grenda R, Watson A, Vondrak K, Webb NJ, Beattie J, et al: A prospective, randomized, multicenter trial of tacrolimus-based therapy with or without basiliximab in pediatric renal transplantation, *Am J Transplant* 6:1666-72, 2006.
11. Tönshoff B, Offner G, Höcker B, Pape L, Rascher W, et al: A multicenter, placebo-controlled trial evaluating the efficacy and safety of basiliximab (Simulect) in combination with CsA, MMF and steroids in pediatric renal allograft recipients: 12 months results, *Pediatr Nephrol* 21:1513, 2006.
12. Brennan DC, Daller JA, Lake KD, Cibrik D, Del Castillo D for the Thymoglobulin Induction Study Group: Rabbit antithymocyte globulin versus basiliximab in renal transplantation, *N Engl J Med* 355:1967-77, 2006.
13. Al Najjar A, Etienne I, Le Pogamp P, Bridoux F, Le Meur Y, et al: Long-term results of monoclonal anti-Il2-receptor antibody versus polyclonal antilymphocyte antibodies as induction therapy in renal transplantation, *Transplant Proc* 38:2298-99, 2006.
14. Vathsala A, Ona ET, Tan SY, Suresh S, Lou HX, et al: Randomized trial of alemtuzumab for prevention of graft rejection and preservation of renal function after kidney transplantation, *Transplant* 80:765-74, 2005.
15. Ciancio G, Burke GW, Gaynor JJ, Carreno MR, Cirocco RE, et al: Randomized trial of three renal transplant induction antibodies: Early comparison of tacrolimus, mycophenolate mofetil, and steroid dosing, and newer immune-monitoring, *Transplant* 80:457-65, 2005.
16. Morris PJ, Russell NK: Alemtuzumab (Campath-1H): A systematic review in organ transplantation, *Transplant* 81:1361-67, 2006.
17. Bartosh SM, Knechtle SJ, Sollinger HW: Campath-1H use in pediatric renal transplantation, *Am J Transplant* 5:1569-73, 2005.
18. Shapiro R, Ellis D, Tan HP, Moritz ML, Basu A, et al: Antilymphoid antibody preconditioning and tacrolimus monotherapy for pediatric kidney transplantation, *J Pediatr* 148:813-18, 2006.
19. Dharnidharka VR, Stevens G: Risk for post-transplant lymphoproliferative disorder after polyclonal antibody induction in kidney transplantation, *Pediatr Transplant* 9:622-26, 2005.
20. Opelz G, Naujokat C, Daniel V, Terness P, Dohler B: Disassociation between risk of graft loss and risk of non-Hodgkin lymphoma with induction agents in renal transplant recipients, *Transplant* 81:1227-33, 2006.
21. Franchimont D: Overview of the actions of glucocorticoids on the immune response: A good model to characterize new pathways of immunosuppression for new treatment strategies, *Ann NY Acad Sci* 1024:124-37, 2004.
22. Chakrabarti P, Wong HY, Scantlebury VP, Jordan ML, Vivas C, et al: Outcome after steroid withdrawal in pediatric renal transplant patients receiving tacrolimus-based immunosuppression, *Transplant* 70:760-64, 2000.
23. Töenshoff B, Hoecker B, Weber LT: Steroid withdrawal in pediatric and adult renal transplant recipients, *Pediatr Nephrol* 20:409-17, 2005.
24. Opelz G, Dohler B, Laux G: Collaborative Transplant Study: Long-term prospective study of steroid withdrawal in kidney and heart transplant recipients, *Am J Transplant* 5:720-28, 2005.
25. Hoecker B, John U, Plank C, Wuehl E, Weber LT, et al: Successful withdrawal of steroids in pediatric renal transplant recipients receiving cyclosporine A and mycophenolate mofetil treatment: Results after four years, *Transplant* 78:228-34, 2004.
26. Jungraithmayr T, Staskewitz A, Kirste G, Boswald M, Bulla M, et al for the German Pediatric Renal Transplantation Study Group: Pediatric renal transplantation with mycophenolate mofetil-based immunosuppression without induction: Results after three years, *Transplant* 75:454-61, 2003.
27. Vidhun JR, Sarwal MM: Corticosteroid avoidance in pediatric renal transplantation, *Pediatr Nephrol* 20:418-26, 2005.
28. Batiuk TD, Kung L, Halloran PF: Evidence that calcineurin is rate-limiting for primary human lymphocyte activation, *J Clin Invest* 100:1894-901, 1997.
29. Dantal J, Hourmant M, Cantarovich D, Giral M, Blancho G, et al: Effect of long-term immunosuppression in kidney-graft recipients on cancer incidence: Randomised comparison of two cyclosporin regimens, *Lancet* 351:623-28, 1998.
30. Venkataramanan R, Jain A, Warty VW, Abu-Elmagd K, Furakawa H, et al: Pharmacokinetics of FK 506 following oral administration: A comparison of FK 506 and cyclosporine, *Transplant Proc* 23:931-33, 1991.
31. Hardinger KL, Park JM, Schnitzler MA, Koch MJ, Miller BW, et al: Pharmacokinetics of tacrolimus in kidney transplant recipients:

Twice daily versus once daily dosing, *Am J Transplant* 4:621-25, 2004.
32. Webster AC, Woodroffe RC, Taylor RS, Chapman JR, Craig JC: Tacrolimus versus ciclosporin as primary immunosuppression for kidney transplant recipients: Meta-analysis and meta-regression of randomised trial data, *BMJ* 331:810, 2005.
33. Woodward RS, Kutinova A, Schnitzler MA, Brennan DC: Renal graft survival and calcineurin inhibitor, *Transplant* 80:629-33, 2005.
34. Goldfarb-Rumyantzev AS, Smith L, Shihab FS, et al: Role of maintenance immunosuppressive regimen in kidney transplant outcome, *Clin J Am Soc Nephrol* 1:563, 2006.
35. Tedesco-Silva A, Demirbas S, Vitko B, Nashan A, Gurkan R, et al: Symphony: Comparing standard immunosuppression to low-dose cyclosporine, tacrolimus or sirolimus in combination with MMF, daclizumab and corticosteroids in renal transplantation, *Transplant* 82:83, 2006.
36. Trompeter R, Filler G, Webb NJ, et al: Randomized trial of tacrolimus versus cyclosporin microemulsion in renal transplantation, *Pediatr Nephrol* 7:141-49, 2002.
37. Filler G, Webb NJ, Milford DV, Watson AR, Gellermann J, et al: Four-year data after pediatric renal transplantation: A randomized trial of tacrolimus vs. cyclosporin microemulsion, *Pediatr Transplant* 9:498-503, 2005.
38. Neu AM, Ho PL, Fine RN, Furth SL, Fivush BA: Tacrolimus vs. cyclosporine A as primary immunosuppression in pediatric renal transplantation: A NAPRTCS study, *Pediatr Transplant* 7:217-22, 2003.
39. Tanabe K: Calcineurin inhibitors in renal transplantation: what is the best option? *Drugs* 3:1535-48, 2003.
40. Nankivell BJ, Borrows RJ, Fung CL, O'Connell PJT, Allen RD, et al: The natural history of chronic allograft nephropathy, *N Engl J Med* 349:2326-33, 2003.
41. Ojo AO, Held PJ, Port FK, et al: Chronic renal failure after transplantation of a nonrenal organ, *N Engl J Med* 349:931-40, 2003.
42. Toenshoff B, Hoecker B: Treatment strategies in pediatric solid organ transplant recipients with calcineurin inhibitor-induced nephrotoxicity, *Pediatr Transplant* 10:721-29, 2006.
43. Oellerich M, Armstrong VW: Two-hour cyclosporine concentration determination: An appropriate tool to monitor neoral therapy? *Ther Drug Monit* 24:40-46, 2002.
44. Halloran PF, Helms LM, Kung L, et al: The temporal profile of calcineurin inhibition by cyclosporine in vivo, *Transplant* 68:1356-61, 1999.
45. Kyllonen LE, Salmela KT: Early cyclosporine C0 and C2 monitoring in de novo kidney transplant patients: A prospective randomized single-center pilot study, *Transplant* 81:1010-15, 2006.
46. Weber LT, Armstrong VW, Shipkova M, Feneberg R, Wiesel M, et al for Members of the German Study Group on Pediatric Renal Transplantion: Cyclosporin A absorption profiles in pediatric renal transplant recipients predict the risk of acute rejection, *Ther Drug Monit* 26:415-24, 2004.
47. Gaston RS: Maintenance immunosuppression in the renal transplant recipient: An overview, *Am J Kidney Dis* 38:25-35, 2001.
48. Elion GB: The pharmacology of azathioprine, *Ann NY Acad Sci* 685:400-07, 1993.
49. Bergan S, Rugstad HE, Bentdal O, Sodal G, Hartmann A, et al: Monitored high-dose azathioprine treatment reduces acute rejection episodes after renal transplantation, *Transplant* 66:334-39, 1998.
50. Allison AC, Eugui EM: Mechanisms of action of mycophenolate mofetil in preventing acute and chronic allograft rejection, *Transplant* 80:181-90, 2005.
51. van Leuven SI, Kastelein JJ, Allison AC, Hayden MR, Stroes ES: Mycophenolate mofetil (MMF): Firing at the atherosclerotic plaque from different angles? *Cardiovasc Res* 69:341-47, 2006.
52. van Gelder T, Tedesco Silva H, de Fijter H, Budde K, Kuypers D, et al: A prospective, randomized, open-label, multicenter study comparing fixed-dose versus concentration-controlled mycophenolate mofetil regimens for de novo renal transplant recipients: The Fixed-Dose Concentration-Controlled (FDCC) trial, *Transplantation*, in press.
53. Shipkova M, Armstrong VW, Oellerich M, Wieland E: Mycophenolate mofetil in organ transplantation: Focus on metabolism, safety and tolerability, *Expert Opin Drug Metab Toxicol* 1:505-26, 2005.
54. Cattaneo D, Perico N, Gaspari F, Gotti E, Remuzzi G: Glucocorticoids interfere with mycophenolate mofetil bioavailability in kidney transplantation, *Kidney Int* 62:1060-67, 2002.
55. Weber LT, Shipkova M, Lamersdorf T, et al For the German Study Group on Mycophenolate Mofetil Therapy in Pediatric Renal Transplant Recipients: Pharmacokinetics of mycophenolic acid (MPA) and determinants of MPA free fraction in pediatric and adult renal transplant recipients, *J Am Soc Nephrol* 9:1511-20, 1998.
56. Weber LT, Shipkova M, Armstrong VW, et al: The pharmacokinetic-pharmacodynamic relationship for total and free mycophenolic acid in pediatric renal transplant recipients: A report of the German Study Group on Mycophenolate Mofetil Therapy, *J Am Soc Nephrol* 13:759-68, 2002.
57. Srinivas TR, Kaplan B, Schold JD, Meier-Kriesche HU: The impact of mycophenolate mofetil on long-term outcomes in kidney transplantation, *Transplant* 80:11-20, 2005.
58. Ettenger R, Cohen A, Nast C, et al: Mycophenolate mofetil as maintenance immunosuppression in pediatric renal transplantation, *Transplant Proc* 29:340-41, 1997.
59. Benfield MR, Symons JM, Bynon S, et al: Mycophenolate mofetil in pediatric renal transplantation, *Pediatr Transplant* 3:5-9, 1999.
60. Bunchman T, Navarro M, Broyer M, et al: The use of mycophenolate mofetil suspension in pediatric renal allograft recipients, *Pediatr Nephrol* 16:978-84, 2001.
61. Hoecker B, Weber LT, Bunchman T, Rashford M, Toenshoff B for the Tricontinental MMF Suspension Study Group: Mycophenolate mofetil suspension in pediatric renal transplantation: Three-year data from the tricontinental trial, *Pediatr Transplant* 9:504-11, 2005.
62. Staskewitz A, Kirste G, Tönshoff B, et al for the German Pediatric Renal Transplantation Study Group: Mycophenolate mofetil in pediatric renal transplantation without induction therapy: Results after 12 months of treatment, *Transplant* 71:638-44, 2001.
63. Jungraithmayr T, Staskewitz A, Kirste G, et al: Pediatric renal transplantation with mycophenolate mofetil-based immunosuppression without induction: Results after three years, *Transplant* 75:454-61, 2003.
64. Cransberg K, Marlies Cornelissen EA, Davin JC, et al: Improved outcome of pediatric kidney transplantations in the Netherlands: Effect of the introduction of mycophenolate mofetil? *Pediatr Transplant* 9:104-11, 2005.
65. Ferraris JR, Ghezzi LF, Vallejo G, et al: Improved long-term allograft function in pediatric renal transplantation with mycophenolate mofetil, *Pediatr Transplant* 9:178-82, 2005.
66. Theruvath TP, Saidman SL, Mauiyyedi S, et al: Control of antidonor antibody production with tacrolimus and mycophenolate mofetil in renal allograft recipients with chronic rejection, *Transplant* 72:77-83, 2001.
67. Henne T, Latta K, Strehlau J, et al: Mycophenolate mofetil-induced reversal of glomerular filtration loss in children with chronic allograft nephropathy, *Transplant* 76:1326-30, 2003.
68. Van Gelder T, Meur YL, Shaw LM, et al: Therapeutic drug monitoring of mycophenolate mofetil in transplantation, *Ther Drug Monit* 28:145-54, 2006.
69. Van Gelder T, Hilbrands LB, Vanrenterghem Y, et al: A randomized double-blind, multicenter plasma concentration controlled study of the safety and efficacy of oral mycophenolate mofetil for the prevention of acute rejection after kidney transplantation. *Transplant* 68:261-66, 1999.
70. Weber LT, Hoecker B, Armstrong VW, Oellerich M, Toenshoff B: Validation of an abbreviated pharmacokinetic profile for the estimation of mycophenolic acid exposure in pediatric renal transplant recipients, *Ther Drug Monit* 28:623-31, 2006.
71. Filler G, Mai I: Limited sampling strategy for mycophenolic acid area under the curve, *Ther Drug Monit* 22:169-73, 2000.
72. Kahan BD, Camardo JS: Rapamycin: Clinical results and future opportunities, *Transplant* 72:1181-93, 2001.
73. Sindhi R, Webber S, Venkataramanan R, et al: Sirolimus for rescue and primary immunosuppression in transplanted children receiving tacrolimus, *Transplantation* 72:851-55, 2001.

74. MacDonald A, Scarola J, Burke JT, Zimmerman JJ: Clinical pharmacokinetics and therapeutic drug monitoring of sirolimus, *ClinTher* 22(B):B101-B121, 2000.
75. del Mar Fernandez De Gatta, Santos-Buelga D, Dominguez-Gil A, Garcia MJ: Immunosuppressive therapy for paediatric transplant patients: Pharmacokinetic considerations, *Clin Pharmacokinet* 41:115-35, 2002.
76. Ettenger RB, Grimm EM: Safety and efficacy of TOR inhibitors in pediatric renal transplant recipients, *Am J Kidney Dis* 38:S22-S28, 2001.
77. Mahalati K, Kahan BD: Clinical pharmacokinetics of sirolimus, *Clin Pharmacokinet* 40:573-85, 2001.
78. Kahan BD, Napoli KL, Kelly PA, et al: Therapeutic drug monitoring of sirolimus: Correlations with efficacy and toxicity, *Clin Transplant* 14:97-109, 2000.
79. Kuypers DR: Benefit-risk assessment of sirolimus in renal transplantation, *Drug Saf* 28:153-81, 2005.
80. Hocker B, Feneberg R, Kopf S, Weber LT, Waldherr R, et al: SRL-based immunosuppression vs. CNI minimization in pediatric renal transplant recipients with chronic CNI nephrotoxicity, *Pediatr Transplant* 10:593-601, 2006.
81. Ettenger R, Sarwal MM: Mycophenolate mofetil in pediatric renal transplantation, *Transplant* 80(2):S201-S210, 2005.

CHAPTER

60 Acute Allograft Dysfunction

Anne M. Durkan and Lisa A. Robinson

The mean 5-year survival of renal allografts in children has improved to 80% for living donor grafts and 65% for deceased donor grafts. This is largely due to the advent of newer immunosuppressants, but other factors (such as improved pretransplant care, improved donor selection, and better perioperative care) have also contributed.[1] The use of the newer immunosuppressants has resulted in fewer acute rejection episodes and it is now widely acknowledged that the challenge to further improve graft outcome largely needs to target a reduction in chronic allograft nephropathy.

Indeed, chronic allograft nephropathy is now the principal cause of graft failure in children.[1] However, acute allograft dysfunction (AAD) is still encountered often—and acute dysfunction may directly impact the development and severity of chronic allograft nephropathy.[2-4] AAD can be broadly defined as deterioration in renal function occurring within the first 6 months posttransplant. Causes of AAD in the immediate perioperative period, as well as later, are outlined in Table 60-1 and are discussed in the material following.

Multiple factors (including ischemia, infection, and rejection) have the potential to cause acute damage to the kidney. Dysfunction can occur in the immediate postoperative period, a process termed delayed graft function (DGF). Alternatively, the dysfunction may occur following a period of demonstrable graft function. At the extreme end of the spectrum of DGF is primary nonfunction, whereby the graft never gains adequate function. Adult data from the Organ Procurement and Transplantation Network suggests a rate of 2% to 15%, whereas the pediatric data report that 3.7% of grafts never function due to primary nonfunction, thrombosis, or technical failure.[1] Overall, primary nonfunction accounts for 2.3% of graft losses.[1]

Acute graft dysfunction is seen more frequently in deceased donor organs. Within this group, recipient age of less than 5 years or 13 to 20 years, cold ischemia time of more than 36 hours, Human Leukocyte Antigen (HLA) mismatching, and earlier vintage of transplantation increase the risk of AAD.[5,6] Furthermore, transplanted kidney recipients who are of African American race have worse outcomes. This is probably due to both environmental and genetic factors, much of which is poorly understood.[5,7]

Earlier reports showed infants of less than 2 years to have more AAD and subsequently worse graft survival. More recently, however, there has been a significant improvement, with current 1-year graft survival rates similar or better than those of other pediatric age groups.[7-11] Of course, other factors in the early posttransplant period (such as hypertension and obesity) can also affect the long-term survival and function of the grafted kidney.[12,13]

ALLOGRAFT DYSFUNCTION IN THE IMMEDIATE POSTOPERATIVE PERIOD

Hyperacute Rejection

Hyperacute rejection occurs as the result of preformed antibodies to donor antigen. The reaction between these anti-HLA recipient antibodies and HLA class I, or sometimes class II, antigen on donor endothelial cells leads to arteriolonecrosis and occlusion of vascular lumina within minutes to hours. There is a polymorphonuclear leukocyte infiltrate but usually no lymphocyte invasion of the kidney. It is easily identified when the graft becomes blue and flaccid prior to closure of the abdomen and should always be considered in cases of primary nonfunction. Hyperacute rejection is accompanied by a marked rise in lactate dehydrogenase in the plasma, and on Doppler ultrasound there is no flow to the kidney. There is a classic "dead tree" appearance on angiography. Almost inevitably, allograft nephrectomy is required.

A seminal paper in 1969 by Patel identified recipient antibodies to antigen on the donor white cells as a major risk factor for immediate graft loss or hyperacute rejection.[14] Since that time, complement-dependent cytotoxicity (CDC) cross matching has been performed routinely before all renal transplants. Since the initial description of the CDC cross-match technique, numerous modifications have been applied to increase the sensitivity and specificity of the test. These include the addition of a complement-fixing antihuman globulin before the complement, which allows the detection of low titers of antibodies and those antibodies that do not fix complement in vitro.[15,16]

A further technique is the flow cytometric cross match (FCXM), which is a complement-fixation–independent test whereby recipient serum is incubated with donor lymphocytes that are then labeled with a fluorochrome-conjugated secondary antibody. The surface fluorescence is then detected, allowing a semiquantitation of the antibody. The advantages of this technique are that it is less subjective, it is 1 to 3 logs more sensitive than the antihuman globulin CDC technique, and it allows independent but simultaneous labeling of T and B cells. A positive FCXM with negative CDC cross match is

TABLE 60-1 **Causes of Acute Allograft Dysfunction**

Dehydration: Poor fluid intake Excessive fluid loss (e.g., diarrhea)
Infection: Bacterial (e.g., UTI) Viral (e.g., CMV, BKV)
Obstruction: Blocked catheter Ureteric stenosis Functional (e.g., morphine-induced urinary retention) Incomplete bladder emptying
Drug toxicity: Aminoglycosides Calcineurin inhibitors Antivirals (e.g., acyclovir) Other
Rejection: Hyperacute Acute
Vascular: Thrombosis Stenosis

TABLE 60-2 **Risk Factors for Delayed Graft Function**[28,36-41]

Procurement
Cold ischemia time >24 hours
Preservation fluid
Cold storage preservation
Donor
Marginal donors
Age >55 years
Need for inotropic support
Non–heart-beating
Surgical
Urine leak
Ureteral obstruction
Recipient
African American race
Previous blood transfusions
Native nephrectomies
Hypovolemia
Weight
Previous transplant
Thrombophilic tendency
PRA >50%
Calcineurin toxicity
Non–HLA-matched kidney

associated with an increased risk of graft loss in the first 3 months posttransplant. However, some investigators believe that the FCXM alone is too sensitive and would therefore inappropriately deny some patients a transplant.[17,18]

There are also solid-phase assays available. Enzyme-linked immunosorbent assays (ELISAs) and microparticle-based techniques are superior at detecting class I and II HLA antigens, and many would advocate the use of more than one cross-matching technique to maximize the diagnostic potential.[19-22] The introduction of the cross match has dramatically reduced the risk of hyperacute rejection. However, despite the array of tests available, some patients have a negative lymphocyte cross match and still have early graft loss.[23]

The 2006 North American Renal Trials and Collaborative Studies (NAPRTCS) data report hyperacute rejection as the cause of graft loss in 0.7%. Two somewhat controversial theories are currently put forward for this finding: (1) that antiendothelial antibodies or non-HLA antibodies not detected by the current cross-match techniques are responsible, and (2) that preactivated lymphocytes may be responsible for the rejection. Further complicating matters are the wide-ranging discrepancies between laboratories performing the cross match. Many laboratories are not using the more sensitive tests, and there are significant variations in methodologies used for the established tests.[17]

Delayed Graft Function

DGF is encountered more often following transplantation of a kidney from a deceased donor. The reported incidence of DGF varies immensely (2%-50%) and this is largely because there is no uniformly accepted definition.[3,23-27] The most recent NAPRTCS data (2006) define DGF as the requirement for dialysis in the first week posttransplantation and reports rates of 5.2% for living donor and 17% for deceased donor transplants. Obviously, this definition of DGF excludes those in whom there is significant acute tubular necrosis but sufficient urine output to preclude the need for dialysis. There are some patients who are dialyzed for other reasons, for example, for hyperkalemia. DGF has significant implications for the long-term prognosis of grafts, with a difference in overall 5-year survival of 55% and 73% for kidneys with and without DGF, respectively.[1]

Numerous factors are associated with an increased risk of DGF (Table 60-2) and can involve the donor, the recipient, the procurement of the kidney, and the surgical procedure. Some of these factors are more problematic in the adult population because the shortage of kidneys has resulted in the use of more marginal donors and more non–heart-beating donors. Currently, this practice has not generally been adopted in pediatrics and therefore does not pose the same problems. The NAPRTCS data have demonstrated that the risk of DGF following transplantation from a deceased donor is increased in those of African American ethnicity (22.7%), those receiving more than five blood transfusions pretransplant (27.9%), previous native nephrectomies (23.5%), previous transplant (27.5%), and cold ischemia time greater than 24 hours (24.7%).[1]

Initial reports were cautious regarding the use of laparoscopic nephrectomies for transplant into young children.

However, recent studies suggest that at experienced centers the outcomes are as good as with open nephrectomized kidneys.[29] The impact of a pretransplant mode of dialysis on early graft function is somewhat debatable. There are adult data suggesting that peritoneal dialysis favors a better initial function compared to hemodialysis, but the limited pediatric data found no association between mode of dialysis and initial graft function.[30-34] This difference may be partly due to the increased risk of graft thrombosis in the pediatric transplant population who have previously had peritoneal dialysis.[35]

A further important recipient risk factor is hypovolemia at the time of transplant. If this is a perceived problem, additional fluid boluses should be administered during the procedure. The use of the immunosuppressive agent OKT3 has previously been reported to increase the risk of DGF because it increases the risk of intrarenal thrombosis secondary to activation of tissue factor on endothelial cells. OKT3 is now used only rarely. Postoperative risk factors include urine leak and obstruction (discussed in more detail in material following).

Pathophysiology

DGF is mainly due to ischemia-reperfusion injury, and not surprisingly the most common histologic finding is acute tubular necrosis. Ischemia results in a cascade of inflammatory mediator release. Depleted adenosine triphosphate (ATP) levels result in anaerobic glycolysis with accumulation of cellular lactic acid. This decreases the intracellular pH and causes lysosomal instability with release of lysosomal enzymes. Oxygen free radicals are formed, which further induce nitric oxide production—resulting in the production of more oxidants. Nitric oxide also contributes to the disruption of the actin cytoskeleton, with loss of the tubular barrier and obstruction of the tubules with cellular debris.[42] Cytoprotective mechanisms are subsequently induced to protect from further damage and to encourage cell regeneration.[43,44]

During the reperfusion stage, there is a return to aerobic metabolism. Unfortunately, during this period high concentrations of oxygen free radicals are also generated.[45] Although the host's natural antioxidants are activated, their ability to protect the organ is overwhelmed by the degree of inflammation, leading to cell death by apoptosis.[46] In addition, the effects of ischemia-reperfusion injury stimulate the upregulation of chemokines and cytokines, which attract leukocytes to the damaged organ, further compounding the inflammation.

There is a second burst of chemokine release about 3 hours after the kidney is transplanted. At this time, there is also involvement of the complement system—especially the C5a pathway. Complement activation further attracts leukocytes (particularly neutrophils, monocytes, and natural killer cells) to the kidney. Activated leukocytes roll along the endothelium and adhere via an interaction between the endothelial cell and the leukocyte. Endothelial cells express cell adhesion molecules, such as intercellular cell adhesion molecule-1 (ICAM-1) and vascular cell adhesion molecule-1 (VCAM-1). The ligands for these receptors are integrins, which are expressed on leukocytes. Binding to the adhesion molecule tethers the leukocyte, which then passes through the endothelial wall by diapedesis. The sum of these interactions is a complex pattern of cell injury, release of inflammatory mediators, and cell death.

There are emerging studies assessing the role of genetic makeup in the development of DGF. One study has found that grafts from donors expressing the polymorphism for glutathione-*S*-transferase enzyme GSTM1*B alone or with GSTM1*A have lower risk for DGF.[47] A further group has found that polymorphisms in the IL-1 beta receptor antagonist increase the risk of both DGF and further rejection episodes.[48]

Graft Thrombosis

A further cause of acute graft dysfunction in the early postoperative period is graft thrombosis. About 2% to 3% of all renal grafts in the pediatric population thrombose, and not surprisingly this is seen more frequently in the early posttransplant period.[49,50] Thrombosis is encountered more commonly in younger children, particularly those aged less than 2 years at the time of transplant.[10,49,51] The size of the native vessels is undoubtedly a contributing factor to this, and the frequent discrepancy between donor and recipient vessels increases the surgical difficulty of the anastomosis.

Previously high rates of thrombosis were also seen when very young donors were used, and this is one of the reasons children under the age of 5 to 6 years are now usually excluded from being donors.[35,52] Thrombosis is now the third most common cause of graft loss, accounting for 10.5% of losses between 1987 and 2006. However, as acute rejection rates have fallen, graft thrombosis has contributed an increasing percentage to the total graft loss, and between 1996 and 2001 accounted for 21%.[1,35]

Thrombosis is reported to occur more commonly in grafts from deceased donors, in those with prolonged cold ischemic time beyond 24 hours, and in retransplants.[35,49,51] Furthermore, there are data to suggest that pretransplant peritoneal dialysis increases the risk of thrombosis.[35,53] Interestingly, the most recent NAPRTCS data suggest that the risk factors found previously are not significant and a new finding is that the use of IL-2 receptor blockers more than halves the risk of graft thrombosis.[50] Obviously, further studies are required to establish the true risk factors for this usually devastating complication.

The routine use of prophylactic anticoagulation remains controversial, and the evidence for its use is somewhat patchy. Currently, there are many different protocols in use in different centers, ranging from no anticoagulation to the use of one or more anticoagulants. One study has compared the use of routine unfractionated heparin with historical controls given no anticoagulation and found no reduction in the rate of allograft thrombosis.[49] On the other hand, reduced thrombosis rates with the use of low-molecular-weight heparin have been reported.[54,55]

Further complicating this issue is the apparent higher incidence of thrombophilic risk factors in the end-stage renal failure population. In one study of pediatric pre-transplant patients, 27% were found to have an increased risk of thrombophilia.[56] As an aside, the patients in this study received intensified anticoagulation with heparin and aspirin and at follow-up there were no graft losses due to thrombosis. Until there is a large enough randomized controlled trial, the benefit of anticoagulation will remain undetermined.

Obstruction

Obstruction to the flow of urine from the allograft can occur at any time but is more commonly seen in the early postoperative period. Complete obstruction will result in no urine output, but partial obstruction may only be detected on ultrasound. The scan may show dilatation of the renal pelvis with or without urine in the bladder, depending on the level of the obstruction. The major concerns with obstruction are the increased pressure on the ureteric anastomosis, with the risk of rupture and the long-term effects of increased pressure on the renal parenchyma. There are many reasons for the early increased risk of obstruction, including blood clots, stenosis of the ureter (particularly at the anastomosis site), and external compression or kinking of the ureter.

There is inevitable bleeding at the time of transplant, and it is not unusual for clots to form. The majority of patients posttransplant will have either a urethral or suprapubic catheter in place to drain the bladder, or rarely a urinary diversion. One of these methods should facilitate the passage of clots, although it is possible for clots to block the catheter. Flushing of the catheter is often required in the first few days after the transplant. Inadequate drainage of urine can also be the result of dislodgement of the catheter.

Many centers also routinely place a stent into the ureter of the allograft at the time of transplantation, which generally remains in situ for 6 weeks to minimize the risk of stenosis or effects of external compression. External compression of the ureter may be caused by a hematoma, a urinoma, a lymphocele, feces, or any other mass in the vicinity of the graft. Ultrasound will usually be able to follow the length of the ureter and will detect any mass effect compressing it. Transplant ureters are also at risk of kinking, especially if a large adult donor has been used without appropriate trimming of the ureter. Rarely, further surgical intervention is necessary.

Beyond the early postoperative period, problems with obstruction are more often encountered in patients with known bladder problems and in those with incomplete bladder emptying. Double voiding regimes, clean intermittent catheterization, or indwelling drainage may be necessary in these children to relieve the obstruction.

Urine Leak

This potentially devastating complication is fortunately rare, and the incidence appears to be decreasing. Leakage is usually due to ureteral necrosis around the anastomosis site, which causes urine to collect in the abdomen. If an abdominal drain has been placed at the time of surgery, the drain fluid can easily be tested for the creatinine concentration—which would be comparable to that of the urine rather than the blood. If there is no drain, fine-needle aspiration of the fluid will aid in the diagnosis (nuclear medicine imaging may also be useful). Early surgical intervention is essential, but often the graft is irreversibly damaged. The adult literature has demonstrated poorer wound healing in patients treated with sirolimus and subsequent increased urine leakage.[57]

Investigation of Delayed Graft Function and Perioperative Allograft Dysfunction

If no urine is obtained postoperatively, a systematic approach should be able to identify the cause. Assessment of the patient, ensuring that there is adequate volume replacement to maintain good blood pressure, and central venous pressure are critical. The position of the urinary catheter should be assessed, and it should be checked for any blockage. A Doppler ultrasound will demonstrate the blood flow to the kidney. If the kidney looks well perfused and the patient is well hydrated, the most likely cause of the DGF is acute tubular necrosis. However, most would advocate an early biopsy to rule out hyperacute rejection.

If good urine volumes have been present but then decrease, factors such as inadequate fluid replacement or a blocked catheter should be considered initially. These problems are encountered commonly and are easily resolved. If the patient is assessed to be normovolemic or hypervolemic, a trial of a loop diuretic may be appropriate. If there is still no response, more serious complications (such as urinary leak, graft thrombosis, and hyperacute rejection) will need to be investigated.

A Doppler ultrasound with or without an MAG3/DTPA scan will assess the perfusion of the kidney. Ultrasound will also detect any obstruction to the kidney and will usually pick up any fluid collections around the kidney suggestive of a urine leak or lymphocele. A renal biopsy is required to rule out rejection. In exceptional cases, surgical reexploration is required to assess the viability of the kidney.

Treatment of Delayed Graft Function

By the most commonly used definition, dialysis will be required. Most centers use hemodialysis, and many patients either have an existing dialysis catheter or have had a hemodialysis catheter inserted at the time of transplant. There is no absolute contraindication to peritoneal dialysis in most patients, but many centers do not use this mode of dialysis.

Data from the Organ Procurement Transplant Network in the United States show that 50% recover adequate function by the tenth posttransplant day. The use of calcineurin inhibitors (CNIs) is often minimized or delayed until good graft function is obtained. These patients are often treated with anti-thymocyte globulin (ATG) until graft function improves, or for a maximum of 10 days, as an alternative to CNIs, because there is evidence to suggest less DGF with ATG.[58]

ACUTE GRAFT DYSFUNCTION BEYOND THE EARLY POSTOPERATIVE PERIOD

There are numerous causes for graft dysfunction beyond the early postoperative period, as indicated in Table 60-1. The most common cause of an increase in plasma creatinine is inadequate fluid intake. This is easily amenable to treatment, although compliance with fluid intake in some patients is less than satisfactory. Of course, inadequate fluid intake is exacerbated by episodes of gastrointestinal upset and it is not uncommon for children with acute vomiting and diarrhea to require admission to a hospital for intravenous rehydration. In very young children and in those with learning difficulties, the oral intake of sufficient fluids can remain problematic for some time after the transplant, and additional fluids can be supplemented via a feeding tube—particularly if tube feeds were used pretransplant.

Infection

The use of immunosuppression inevitably increases the risk of developing an infection. In addition, many patients have anatomic abnormalities of their renal tract, which puts them at further risk, particularly for urinary tract infections. A recent study has demonstrated vesicoureteric reflux in 70% of transplant patients, with the majority of these children developing urinary tract infection and subsequent scarring.[59] Furthermore, viral infections cause significant problems in the immunosuppressed posttransplant patient, and there is now increasing awareness of the impact of infections such as cytomegalovirus (CMV), Epstein-Barr virus (EBV), and BK polyoma virus. Posttransplant infectious complications are discussed fully in Chapter 62.

Drug Toxicity

Many drugs are nephrotoxic, and the transplanted kidney may be particularly sensitive to drug effects. CNIs are routinely used in maintenance immunosuppressive regimens. Although these drugs have undoubtedly improved graft survival, they can cause acute allograft dysfunction, particularly when supraoptimal blood levels are achieved and contribute to chronic allograft nephropathy. For this reason, close surveillance of blood levels is required, although toxicity can occur with apparently subtherapeutic levels.

There can often be difficulty differentiating CNI toxicity from acute rejection on clinical grounds alone, and a biopsy is generally required, because obviously the treatment is drastically different for the two conditions. Further problems with fluctuating CNI blood levels may be encountered during periods of gastrointestinal upset and as a result of the concomitant administration of many other drugs (outlined in Table 60-3). Table 60-3 is not comprehensive, and drug interactions with CNIs should always be checked prior to prescribing.

Nephrotoxic drugs such as aminoglycosides, antivirals, and angiotensin-converting enzyme inhibitors may also cause AAD, and caution should be exercised when prescribing any medications—taking into account the renal function and possible drug interactions. Wherever possible, a non-nephrotoxic drug should be used if there is a choice of more than one medication.

Rejection

With the newer immunosuppressive regimes, the risk of acute rejection has fallen dramatically. In the late 1980s, 1-year acute rejection rates of 59% for living-donor kidneys and 73% for deceased-donor kidneys were reported, whereas more recently these same rates are down to 13% and 16%, respectively.[1,60,61] The other major change over time is an increase in the use of renal biopsies to confirm the diagnosis of rejection. Previously, most rejection episodes were diagnosed by the treating physician after excluding other causes of renal dysfunction—whereas now more than 80% of rejection episodes are biopsy proven.[1]

Facilitating uniformity in the diagnosis of rejection has been a goal of the Banff schema, which provides a clear description of the histologic findings in rejection and allows an assessment of the severity of the rejection process. The Banff Working Classification of Renal Allograft Pathology is an international consensus opinion that originated during a meeting in 1991 and was published 2 years later.[62] It has been updated regularly since then, and in 1997 there was a major revision that incorporated the classification used by the National Institutes of Health (the Collaborative Clinical Trials in Transplantation classification).[63]

The classification has been validated in numerous studies and provides a standardized method of reporting allograft pathology, which is important to establishing endpoints in clinical trials and as a basis for alterations in therapy.[64-69] The severity of rejection, as assessed by the classification, also impacts directly on the prognosis of the renal allograft.[70-75] The 1997 revision not only updated the criteria for the diagnosis of rejection but modified the criteria for the adequacy of a renal transplant biopsy specimen.[63] To improve diagnostic ability, a sample of cortex is now only considered adequate if it contains at least 10 glomeruli and at least 2 arteries. This is achievable even in pediatric patients, and a biopsy should be performed whenever rejection is a diagnostic possibility.[76]

The Banff schema is designed to provide a description of the histologic findings rather than grades of pathology. In the revised version, there is more emphasis on the importance of vasculitis because this has been demonstrated to be associated with a poorer response to therapy and a worse long-term

TABLE 60-3 **Drugs Affecting Calcineurin Inhibitor Levels**

Increased CNI Levels	Possibly Increased CNI Levels	Decreased CNI Levels	Increased Risk of Nephrotoxicity
Macrolide antibiotics	Omeprazole	Rifampicin	NSAIDs
Antifungals (e.g., fluconazole)	Danazol	St. John's wort	Aminoglycosides
Calcium channel blockers (e.g., nifedipine)	Antivirals (e.g., atazanavir)	Anti-epileptics (e.g., carbamazepine and phenytoin)	Sulfonamides
Grapefruit juice	Allopurinol	Griseofulvin	Thiazides
Metoclopramide	Amiodarone	Octreotide	Fenofibrate
High-dose methylprednisolone	Estrogens and progestogens	Barbiturates	Melphalan
Other CNI anti-malarials (e.g., chloroquine)	Chloramphenicol	Caspofungin	Acyclovir

TABLE 60-4 **Banff 97 Diagnostic Categories**[63,79]

1. Normal
2. Antibody-mediated rejection ATN-like: C4d+,[a] minimal inflammation Capillary: Margination and/or thromboses, C4d+ Arterial: Transmural inflammation/fibrinoid change, C4d+
3. Borderline changes: Suspicious for acute rejection, with foci of mild tubulitis but no intimal arteritis
4. Acute/active cellular rejection IA. Significant interstitial infiltration (>25% of parenchyma) and foci of moderate tubulitis (>4 mononuclear cells/tubular cross section or group of 10 tubular cells) IB. Significant interstitial infiltration (>25% of parenchyma) and >10 mononuclear cells/tubular cross section or group of 10 tubular cells IIA. Mild to moderate intimal arteritis IIB. Severe intimal arteritis >25% of luminal area Transmural arteritis and/or arterial fibrinoid change and necrosis of medial smooth muscle cells
5. Chronic/sclerosing allograft nephropathy Mild interstitial fibrosis and tubular atrophy without (a) or with (b) specific changes of chronic rejection Moderate interstitial fibrosis and tubular atrophy without (a) or with (b) specific changes of chronic rejection Severe interstitial fibrosis and tubular atrophy without (a) or with (b)

[a] C4d = a component of complement.

prognosis.[64,77,78] The description for antibody-mediated rejection was further modified in 2003.[79] Table 60-4 outlines the various diagnostic categories.

The pathophysiology of rejection is still hotly contended. In the late 1950s, there were those who believed in cell-mediated rejection and those who believed in humoral rejection. The cell-mediated theory gained in popularity and it is only fairly recently that the humoral (antibody-mediated) rejection theory has regained momentum.[80] Because cellular infiltrates are visible on histologic specimens and antibodies are often difficult to detect (see material following), the common teaching has been that cellular rejection is the mechanism involved in acute rejection. It is also possible that some combination of both mechanisms exists. Furthermore, humoral factors are increasingly being implicated in the development of chronic allograft nephropathy.

Acute Cellular Rejection

The transplantation of foreign tissue results in immune activation directed at the donor antigens. The mechanisms involved in this process are described in Chapter 59, but a brief summary follows. The immune response requires the recipient to recognize the alloantigens, which is achieved largely through the genes of the major histocompatibility complex (MHC)—although the "minor" histocompatibility complex may also contribute. The MHC genes code for HLA class I molecules (HLA A, B, and C) and the HLA class II molecules (HLA DP, DQ, and DR), in addition to other proteins responsible for the processing of antigens.

HLA class I molecules are expressed on almost all nucleated cells, whereas class II molecules are expressed mainly on B lymphocytes, macrophages, and dendritic cells (but can also be expressed on activated endothelium, epithelium, and T lymphocytes). In allograft rejection, the exogenous antigen is presented on class II molecules—which are then recognized by CD4+ (i.e., expressing CD4 antigen) T helper cells. Activated T helper cells produce cytokines, which promote T-cell proliferation and differentiation, induce antibody secretion by B cells, and induce cytotoxicity in macrophages, natural killer cells, and cytotoxic T cells.

Antigen specificity is provided by clonally restricted T-cell receptors (TCRs) which recognize a peptide-HLA complex. CD4 acts as a co-receptor, bringing the required proteins for activation into proximity of the TCR complex. Stimulation of the TCR results in phosphorylation of many proteins and activation of second messenger systems. This, together with a rise in intracellular calcium, activates the DNA-binding factors needed for IL-2 transcription and activates calcineurin—which through the modification of the nuclear factor of activated T cells results in the formation of the functional protein that promotes IL-2 gene transcription. For complete recognition and response to alloantigen, at least two signals are required. The most studied and potent costimulatory pathway is the CD28-B7 ligand receptor binding. Without stimulation of both signals, there is immune anergy.[81,82]

The local cytokine milieu and the antigen presented result in the differentiation of naive T helper cells into Th1 or Th2 cell subsets, which secrete different cytokines and hence have different functions.[83] Th1 cells are mainly involved in cell-mediated immunity, whereas Th2 cells are involved in humoral immunity. The recruitment, proliferation, and differentiation of leukocytes in rejection are all dependent on cytokine and chemokine production. Chemokines also facilitate adhesion of the leukocytes to the endothelial wall prior to diapedesis into the tissue, either directly or by activating integrins or adhesion molecules.[84]

Having penetrated the endothelial barrier, cytotoxic T lymphocytes bring about graft destruction by either releasing cytotoxic substances such as perforin and granzyme B or by the induction of apoptosis.[85-88] The mechanism of action of other cells (such as natural killer cells) remains to be fully elucidated, but it does not appear to be affected by current immunosuppressive regimes—suggesting a novel pathway(s).[89]

Antibody-Mediated Rejection

Antibody-mediated hyperacute rejection, as previously described, is a well-accepted phenomenon. Acute humoral rejection, beyond the immediate reperfusion period, can be difficult to diagnose because it may manifest as acute tubular injury with no evidence of circulating antibodies. This is not to say that antibodies are not present but rather that the currently available techniques are not sensitive enough to detect them. Other suggested explanations for the lack of detectable antibodies include that the graft absorbs the antibodies (removing them from the plasma) and that the rejection is caused by factors other than antibodies, such as platelet activation.

In 1993, the first work showing that deposition in the peritubular capillaries of a terminal component of the complement cascade (C4d) was associated with a worse outcome for renal allografts was published.[90] Subsequent studies have confirmed that C4d staining is associated with a poorer outcome, and in 1999 Collins et al. were the first to demonstrate that positive C4d staining was correlated with the presence of a donor-specific antibody.[91-94] Many laboratories will now routinely stain biopsy specimens for C4d, although some authors advocate caution in associating this with humoral rejection only because C4d is not directly implicated in rejection and indeed it may afford some benefit to the graft in the form of accommodation or acquired resistance to humoral injury.[95,96]

Although it is believed that most of the responsible antibodies are donor-specific anti-HLA, there may be other antibodies involved. It is not yet certain that HLA is the only histocompatibility locus, suggesting another possible explanation for the lack of detectable antibodies in some patients. B-cell activation and regulation occur via several mechanisms that are T-cell dependent or independent. B-cell responses against MHC antigens are T-cell dependent and require the involvement of antigen-presenting cells and costimulatory molecules such as CD40 ligand or soluble interleukins. These responses take two to three weeks to develop and lead to immunologic memory, allowing a more efficient antibody response upon repeat stimulation.

Antibodies act on the vascular endothelium. At very high levels, they stimulate a procoagulant state such that the perfusion to the organ is severely compromised—resulting in cell and graft death. However, at lower levels antibodies interact with the endothelium and fix complement. There is subsequent cytolysis, and it has been hypothesized that there may be cycles of injury and repair over time that result in gradual intimal vessel thickening as seen in chronic allograft nephropathy.[79] This theory is supported by data from Lee et al., who demonstrated that all patients lost their grafts at variable time periods after developing antibodies.[97] The control of B-cell function remains incompletely understood, and obviously further work is necessary to optimize immunosuppressive regimens.

Markers of Rejection

As previously mentioned, the gold standard for the diagnosis of rejection is the kidney biopsy. However, this is invasive and not without significant risk. Particularly in children, it often requires sedation or anesthesia. There has been a lot of interest recently in less invasive techniques—particularly in urinary biomarkers and gene profiling of peripheral blood lymphocytes—to aid in the diagnosis of rejection and in the monitoring of treatment response, with some promising results.

Investigation of gene expression in peripheral blood lymphocytes has been helped by the introduction of real-time polymerase chain reaction (RT-PCR), which has increased the sensitivity of PCR. Employing reverse transcriptase PCR, the combined upregulation of the genes for perforin and FasL predicted clinically evident biopsy-proven rejection.[98]

Granulysin expression in peripheral blood lymphocytes was also found to be a marker of acute rejection, but confounding the results was the finding of increased expression in infection.[99] Other studies have shown that increased transcription of granzyme B; Th1 and Th2 cytokines; IL-18, IL-13, and IL-15 together; and IL-4 and TNF-α are additional potential predictors of rejection. However, the effect of concurrent infection on these has not been explored.[100-104]

Detection of urinary gene transcripts from cells excreted into the urine has also been evaluated. Increased levels of granzyme B, perforin, IFN-γ–inducible chemokine IP-10, and the chemokine receptor CXCR3 all correlate with acute rejection.[105,106] More recently, urinary FOXP3 was reported to be associated with rejection.[107] DNA microarray technology is yet another tool that will possibly assist in the deciphering of the molecular signature of acute rejection, but this technique is still in its infancy and is not routinely available.[108]

Investigation of particular gene polymorphisms may offer a further advantage in the stratification of patients to certain immunosuppressive regimes in the future. Of course, there is huge variability in the incidence and outcomes of acute rejection, the progression of chronic nephropathy, and the development of tolerance—suggesting significant redundancy and overlap in immune responses elicited by expressed genes.

A further area of research gaining in momentum is the field of urine proteomics. With the completion of the human genome project, the next obvious step was to identify the proteins expressed by each gene. This is complicated by post-translational modifications to proteins (such as phosphorylation) that may result in more than one protein being expressed by any one gene. There is no universally accepted definition of the proteome, but it is broadly the characterization of the proteins expressed by the cell, tissue, or organism.

The proteome is dynamic and will vary between individuals, between cell types, and in the same cell type under different physiologic and pathologic conditions. Techniques employed to investigate the proteome include mass spectrometry, electrophoresis, and liquid chromatography. Currently, precise urinary protein markers of rejection are not available. However, several groups have identified peaks of interest by mass spectrometry that are being further evaluated.[109-114]

It is hoped that in the future a combination of the previously described techniques will permit much more refined and perhaps individually tailored immunosuppressive regimens, offering the chance to increase immunosuppression when rejection is imminent and decreasing it when there is a stable and quiescent profile.

Treatment of Acute Allograft Rejection

Rejection still remains a significant concern in the early posttransplant period. According to the 2006 NAPRTCS Annual Report,[1] acute rejection accounted for 7.4% of index graft failures since 1 January 2000. The majority of these grafts failed because of chronic rejection (41.3%). Although chronic rejection is known to occur through both immunologic and nonimmunologic mechanisms, acute rejection plays a leading role in this process. In fact, the occurrence of one or more episodes of acute rejection increases the risk of chronic rejection and graft failure by upwards of threefold.[115-119] Thus, effective means of diagnosing and treating acute rejection are absolutely essential to long-term preservation of graft function.

Although different centers have adopted different strategies for the management of acute renal allograft rejection, a reasonable overall approach involves tailoring the initial treatment to the type and degree of rejection present. For cases of mild rejection (Banff I within the fourth category of acute cellular rejection), pulsed corticosteroids (methylprednisolone 5-15 mg/kg daily, for 3 to 5 days) are the mainstay of treatment. Intravenous pulses are followed by an increased dose of maintenance oral corticosteroids, which is gradually tapered back to the previous dose over several weeks.[120-123] Among adult renal transplant patients, steroids have been reported to reverse rejection in 60% to 70% of cases.[115,120,121,123]

After the initial course of pulsed steroids, if there is no response or if severe rejection (Banff III within the fourth category of acute cellular rejection) is present, a second-line agent should be considered. Many centers use an antilymphocyte preparation, generally anti-thymocyte globulin or OKT3. Several studies, including a multicenter randomized trial, have demonstrated the efficacy of these agents in reversing acute rejection.[120,121,124-126] In these studies, success rates ranging from 50% to 90% have been reported.[124-126]

Several unconventional therapies have been used to treat refractory acute allograft rejection in adult recipients. These include mycophenolate mofetil, anti-IL-2 receptor antibodies, intravenous immune globulin, and more recently, alemtuzumab (Campath-1H).[127-133] Although all of these agents have been reported to reverse steroid-resistant rejection, adverse effects associated with heightened immunosuppression (especially serious infection and malignancy) may limit their clinical utility. A closer evaluation of the risks versus benefits of these agents in the treatment of acute rejection needs to be undertaken.

With the advent of new immunosuppressive medications over the last decade, humoral rejection has emerged as an important cause of graft dysfunction in the early posttransplant period. Indeed, graft dysfunction caused by antibody-mediated pathways has been estimated to occur in 3% to 10% of kidney transplants and to be associated with 20% to 30% of episodes of acute rejection.[134] It is not surprising that therapies aimed at decreasing antibody-mediated injury improve the outcome. Plasmapheresis, intravenous immunoglobulin, and rituximab (anti-CD20 antibody) have all been reported to improve humoral rejection—although much controversy exists as to how these therapies should be employed.[135-139]

Following histopathologic confirmation of humoral rejection (including C4d staining), one recommendation would be to immediately institute plasmapheresis with or without intravenous immunoglobulin.[139] Plasmapheresis can be performed until there is clinical improvement, which has been reported to require three to six sessions.[139] Although the optimal dose of intravenous immunoglobulin is not well established, therapeutic benefit has been described with doses from 0.4 to 2.0 g/kg.[138,139]

The timing of administration of rituximab, given as a single intravenous dose (375 mg/m^2), is also controversial.[135] The two most common options involve administration of rituximab at the outset versus reserving this therapy for cases refractory to plasmapheresis and/or intravenous immunoglobulin.[135] In any event, response to treatment should be confirmed using both clinical parameters and repeat renal transplant biopsy with immunostaining for C4d.

An examination of the most recent report of NAPRTCS reveals that among pediatric living-donor graft recipients with acute rejection, 53% had return of serum creatinine to baseline values, whereas 43% had partial reversal of rejection (NAPRTCS 2006 Annual Report, unpublished data). Among recipients of deceased-donor grafts, the outcomes were slightly worse, with 47% undergoing complete reversal and 47% partial reversal of rejection (NAPRTCS 2006 Annual Report, unpublished data). As expected, the likelihood of sustaining complete reversal diminished with subsequent episodes of rejection.

Alterations to Maintenance Immunosuppression after Reversal of Acute Rejection

When a child develops acute renal allograft rejection, the underlying reasons must be carefully evaluated and treatment modified accordingly. Noncompliance with medications is a particularly important cause of rejection in the adolescent population.[140] In such patients, as well as in patients with subtherapeutic levels of immunosuppressive drugs, it is reasonable (after appropriate education and counseling of the patient) to resume therapy with the same agents as those used before rejection developed. For these patients, the dose of steroids should be transiently increased prior to tapering, and careful therapeutic monitoring of drug levels should be performed.

If, however, rejection develops despite therapeutic drug levels, one should give careful consideration to changing the immunosuppressive medications. A common practice involves switching patients taking azathioprine to mycophenolate mofetil, and those on cyclosporine to tacrolimus.[141,142] Some groups would advocate the use of rapamycin either alone or in combination with a CNI, but this practice requires a more systematic evaluation among pediatric kidney transplant recipients.[143,144]

Recurrence of Disease Posttransplantation

Recurrence of the original kidney disease is a common cause of graft dysfunction in the posttransplant period. Recurrence of original disease accounted for 6.4% of failures among index grafts and 9.5% of failures among subsequent grafts.[1] Although both glomerular and metabolic diseases may recur in the transplanted kidney, the majority of recurrences are glomerular in nature. Although every disease may recur at any time posttransplant, certain diseases [such as FSGS, IgA nephropathy, MPGN, hemolytic uremic syndrome (HUS), Henoch-Schönlein purpura (HSP), and oxalosis] tend to recur early after transplantation. Other kidney diseases, such as SLE nephritis and membranous nephropathy, tend to be late recurring (see Chapter 61).

Glomerular Diseases

Focal Segmental Glomerulosclerosis Focal segmental glomerulosclerosis (FSGS) is the most common cause of graft loss secondary to disease recurrence. Of index graft failures occurring since 1 January 2000, 7.9% were due to recurrence of disease.[1] Of these, 45% were due to recurrence of FSGS.[1] When FSGS is the original disease causing renal failure, recurrence has been reported to occur in 14% to 60% of first transplants and in up to 80% of subsequent transplants.[145-156] Compared with the overall transplant population, patients with FSGS have worse short- and long-term allograft survival, with increased incidence of primary nonfunction of the graft and of acute tubular necrosis requiring dialysis.[157,158]

FSGS generally recurs early, with 78% of cases occurring during the first month after transplantation.[153,155] Rarely, recurrence may occur intraoperatively at the time of transplant. Recurrent disease should be suspected if there is significant proteinuria, which is often accompanied by hypoalbuminemia and other features of nephrotic syndrome. The diagnosis is confirmed histologically using renal transplant biopsy. Several risk factors for development of recurrent FSGS have been identified.

- An aggressive clinical course of primary FSGS in the native kidneys, with rapid progression to end-stage renal disease (ESRD) within 3 years of diagnosis.[153,155,156,158]
- There may be a higher incidence of recurrence in the transplanted kidney in children in whom primary disease occurred between the ages of 6 and 15 years.[159]
- Previous recurrence of FSGS in a renal transplant predicts future recurrence in 75% to 100% of subsequent grafts.[160]
- Renal histopathology demonstrating diffuse mesangial proliferation has been associated with a high recurrence rate (80%) and poor outcome, leading to graft failure in 70% of patients.[153]
- The role of race in predicting recurrence of FSGS has been evaluated by several groups. Although African American children tend to have a more aggressive course of initial disease, they appear to be at somewhat lower risk for recurrence posttransplant (9%) compared to white children (23%) and Hispanic children (23%).[156] In another report, Korean children demonstrated a similar rate of recurrence of FSGS to that of non–African American children (41%).[151]

Although the majority of cases of FSGS are sporadic, familial forms of FSGS have been linked to mutations in several genes encoding slit diaphragm proteins—including nephrin, podocin, WT1, alpha-actinin-4, CD2AP, and most recently, TRPC6.[161-163] In this setting, FSGS is presumably due to structural alterations in podocyte proteins of the native kidneys. As such, one would not predict recurrence of disease for these patients.

By and large this seems to be the case. However, there have been recent reports of high rates of recurrent FSGS in patients with a certain *NPHS2* mutation and resultant abnormal expression of podocin.[164-166] In these patients, the rate of recurrence may be comparable to that for idiopathic FSGS.[164-166] These data raise many questions regarding the pathogenic mechanisms that lead to the development of proteinuria and FSGS. Whenever possible, genetic mutations should be identified in FSGS prior to transplantation so that families can be appropriately counseled and staff can anticipate the risks of recurrence.

Optimal management of recurrent FSGS remains a controversial topic. To date, no controlled clinical trials comparing different treatment strategies have been performed, and current management recommendations have been adapted from anecdotal reports and small case series. Because FSGS has been related to a "circulating permeability factor" that increases glomerular permeability to protein, therapies aimed at removing this factor may be beneficial.[167,168]

Several groups have suggested the favorable effects of plasmapheresis on remission of recurrent FSGS and on overall graft survival.[155,167-178] Different plasmapheresis protocols have been reported, with colloid replacement varying from 5% albumin to intravenous gammaglobulin to fresh frozen plasma.[171,175,177] In most reports, plasmapheresis was started early—within 7 days of recognition of nephrotic range proteinuria.[175] Some centers recommend prophylactic use of plasmapheresis even before nephrotic syndrome develops.[173]

The outcome of plasmapheresis in recurrent FSGS may be linked to the number of sessions performed, typically ranging from 5 to 13 treatments.[171,175,177] At our own center, a relatively intensive course of plasmapheresis is initiated when FSGS recurs in a transplanted kidney. Our protocol involves 10 sessions of plasmapheresis within the first 12 days. Thereafter, plasmapheresis is performed every other day for four treatments, and then weekly for four additional treatments. Response to therapy is assessed by measuring urine protein to creatinine ratios as well as by measuring total protein excretion in timed collections. After initiation of plasmapheresis, the time to remission is also highly variable—ranging from 5 to 27 days.[171,175,177]

In several randomized controlled studies, CNIs (most notably cyclosporine) have been shown to be effective in inducing remission in some children with primary steroid-resistant nephrotic syndrome and FSGS. However, the efficacy of cyclosporine in inducing remission of recurrent posttransplant FSGS is quite debatable. Several case reports have suggested benefits of cyclosporine at high doses. In one report, oral cyclosporine (13-35 mg/kg/day) improved nephrotic syndrome in two of six patients with recurrent FSGS.[177]

At 2 years of follow-up, these two patients retained their grafts. In contrast, the four patients who did not receive cyclosporine all lost their grafts.[155,172] In other series, cyclosporine has been administered intravenously at 3 mg/kg/day for up to 3 weeks—followed by maintenance oral cyclosporine.[171,179] In 11 of 14 children who experienced recurrence of FSGS, remission lasted for 3.7 years.[180] In this study, the best outcomes were observed when plasmapheresis was used in combination with high-dose cyclosporine.[180]

Another therapy for recurrent FSGS that could potentially remove any inciting circulating factors is immunoabsorption with protein A columns. However, the efficacy of this treatment is unproven.[170,181,182] Because children with steroid-dependent or frequently relapsing nephrotic syndrome are frequently successfully treated with oral cyclophosphamide, this treatment has also been used to treat FSGS recurrence in allografts. Experience with oral cyclophosphamide in this setting is quite limited, but it has been reported to be well tolerated and to lead to long-term remission in some patients.[147,182] In one series involving pediatric subjects, a cumulative dosage of 115 to 121 mg/kg body weight of cyclophosphamide was used over a 3-month period.[183] As for other states of significant proteinuria, angiotensin-converting enzyme inhibitors may help to diminish protein excretion.[153,171] Hyperlipidemia associated with nephrotic syndrome should be appropriately assessed and managed.

Membranoproliferative Glomerulonephritis Membranoproliferative glomerulonephritis (MPGN) type I accounts for approximately 2% of primary etiologies of renal transplant in children.[1] In a meta-analysis of 11 studies involving 140 transplants, the recurrence rate of type I MPGN in children was 30% and led to graft failure in 33%.[184] In a European study, histologic recurrences occurred in 77% and led to graft failure in 17% of patients.[185] The median time to recurrence is 20 months, and mean graft survival is 40 months once recurrence has occurred.[184] In a recent study from the Australia and New Zealand Dialysis and Transplant Registry (ANZDATA), disease recurred in 10% of patients and resulted in allograft loss in 14%.[186]

MPGN type II represents about 1% of causes of kidney transplant in children (NAPRTCS 2006 Annual Report, unpublished data). Although MPGN type II has a high rate of histopathologic recurrence, significant clinical morbidity (including graft failure) is less common than with MPGN type 1.[160,184,187-189] In one study, however, graft loss occurred in up to 25% of recurrent MPGN type II.[190] Recurrence is often clinically asymptomatic, but proteinuria and hypocomplementemia may be present. With MPGN type I, and especially with MPGN type II, high-dose corticosteroids and plasmapheresis may be helpful.[187,191]

IgA Nephropathy and Henoch-Schönlein Purpura

Recurrence of primary IgA in allografts in children has been reported but not well characterized. The recurrence rate is significantly higher in living-related donor (LRD) transplants (83%) compared to kidneys from deceased donors (14%).[155,192] Clinical symptoms of recurrence include hematuria and proteinuria and are often mild. The overall rate of graft loss due to recurrence is low (3%).[184]

Information regarding recurrence of HSP nephritis in pediatric renal transplant recipients is also quite limited. Disease recurs in 31% to 53% of transplants, with subsequent graft loss in 8% to 22%.[155,184,193-195] HSP is more likely to recur in LRD compared to deceased-donor kidney transplants, and when progression from diagnosis to ESRD in the native kidneys is rapid.[184,194-196] Very few data exist regarding optimal treatment of disease recurrences. At our center, the treatment used for the primary disease is tried initially.

Hemolytic Uremic Syndrome

According to data from a recent NAPRTCS report, HUS recurred in 8.8% of renal transplants.[196] The original disease in the majority of these patients was atypical HUS, not associated with a diarrheal prodrome. In another report, disease recurred only rarely (0.8%) in typical diarrhea-positive HUS compared to 21% with atypical HUS.[197] Among children with atypical HUS, those who had factor H deficiency experienced a particularly high rate of recurrence (45%).[197] Recurrence of HUS occurred early, usually within 1 month after transplantation. It has been suggested that HUS recurrence is triggered by other immunologic inciting factors, such as infection with cytomegalovirus, rejection, or bacterial infection.[198]

Use of CNIs, either cyclosporine or tacrolimus, may also precipitate recurrence of HUS. Clinical symptoms and signs are variable and include decreased urine output and elevated serum creatinine, hematuria, and proteinuria. Hemolysis and thrombocytopenia are not always present. Diagnosis is made by renal transplant biopsy. Recommended management includes stopping the CNI, initiating plasmapheresis, and enhancing antirejection prophylaxis. At our own center, plasmapheresis is often performed daily for at least 7 days.

Once graft function has been restored, the CNI may be restarted. However, disease may recur in 20% to 30% of patients. Some authors report improved outcome when one CNI is substituted for the one used before HUS recurred. Overall outcome is reported to be poor, with 5 of 6 grafts lost following recurrence of HUS in a recent NAPRTCS report.[196] With atypical HUS, disease recurs slightly more often in living related donor kidneys. If a family history of disease is evident, potential donors should undergo genetic testing prior to consideration of transplant.

Metabolic Diseases

Primary Hyperoxaluria Type I (Oxalosis)

The inherent metabolic defect in oxalosis is deficiency of hepatic peroxisomal alanine glyoxalate aminotransferase (AGT), a gene encoded on chromosome 2q37.3.[199] AGT deficiency results in increased synthesis and urinary excretion of oxalate, and in deposition of calcium oxalate crystals in tissues throughout the body—especially in kidney, myocardium, and bone tissue. Renal manifestations of oxalosis include recurrent calcium oxalate urolithiasis, progressive nephrocalcinosis, and ESRD.

Renal transplantation alone does not correct the underlying enzymatic defect, and abnormally high production of oxalate persists. Calcium oxalate crystal deposition often occurs in the transplanted kidney (90%), eventually provoking graft failure.[155,200] Not surprisingly, combined liver and kidney transplantation leads to better outcomes than kidney transplantation alone.[201,202] The transplanted liver can metabolize oxalate stored within tissues, and the transplanted kidney helps to excrete the oxalate load. Long-term follow-up of patients with successful combined liver and kidney transplant has demonstrated normal plasma oxalate concentration and normal urinary excretion of oxalate.[203,204] More recently, 8-year follow-up posttransplantation has shown that adults receiving kidney transplant alone had adjusted graft survival of 47% compared to 76% graft survival for combined liver and kidney transplant.[205]

Whether kidney transplantation is performed alone or in combination with liver transplantation, aggressive attention to fluid management and reduction of oxalate load helps to optimize long-term kidney function. Aggressive long-term hemodialysis pretransplantation may lessen tissue deposition of oxalate and decrease the oxalate load. In the postoperative period, aggressive hydration and urinary dilution are advisable. Adjunctive therapies may include pyridoxine, neutral phosphate, citrate, and noncalciuric diuretics (e.g., thiazides).

Sickle-Cell Anemia

Renal allograft survival in patients with sickle-cell anemia is somewhat decreased compared to patients with other etiologies for ESRD.[206] Although in the short term allograft survival is similar in both groups, long-term survival is somewhat worse.[206] In children, sickle-cell disease is a rare cause of ESRD. Limited reports demonstrate 12- and 24-month graft survival of 89 and 71%, respectively.[207] Kidney transplantation may lead to improved erythropoiesis, which in turn leads to more abnormal red blood cells. This may promote sickle crises within the transplanted kidney. Thus, after kidney transplantation medical management should aim to prevent recurrent crises.[208]

De Novo Disease in Kidney Transplantation

Many glomerular diseases may occur de novo following kidney transplantation, and these should be kept in mind when considering the causes of renal dysfunction, proteinuria, and hematuria posttransplant.[209] In particular, HUS may develop de novo, particularly in patients taking CNIs.

In patients with Alport's syndrome due to presence of the α5 non-collagenous portion of type IV collagen in the graft glomerular basement membrane (GBM), the primary disease does not recur after transplantation. Rarely, however, exposure of this antigen in the GBM of the transplanted kidney to the immune system of the naive host will incite a vigorous immune reaction. The recipient may develop anti-GBM antibodies that then deposit in a linear fashion along the basement membrane. These events may result in rapidly progressive crescentic glomerulonephritis. Plasmapheresis may be attempted when these events occur, but generally graft survival is poor.[160]

REFERENCES

1. North American Pediatric Renal Trials and Collaborative Studies: Annual Report 2006. *www.NAPRTCS.org*.
2. Tejani A, Stablein DM, Donaldson L, et al: Steady improvement in short-term graft survival of pediatric renal transplants: The NAPRTCS experience, *Clin Transpl* 95-110, 1999.
3. Knight RJ, Burrows L, Bodian C: The influence of acute rejection on long-term renal allograft survival: A comparison of living and cadaveric donor transplantation, *Transplantation* 72:69-76, 2001.
4. Ojo AO, Wolfe RA, Held PJ, et al: Delayed graft function: Risk factors and implications for renal allograft survival, *Transplantation* 63:968-74, 1997.
5. Hwang AH, Cho YW, Cicciarelli J, et al: Risk factors for short- and long-term survival of primary cadaveric renal allografts in pediatric recipients: A UNOS analysis, *Transplantation* 80:466-70, 2005.
6. Johnson RW, Webb NJ, Lewis MA, et al: Outcome of pediatric cadaveric renal transplantation: A 10 year study, *Kidney Int Suppl* 53:S72-S76, 1996.
7. Benfield MR, McDonald RA, Bartosh S, et al: Changing trends in pediatric transplantation: 2001 Annual Report of the North American Pediatric Renal Transplant Cooperative Study, *Pediatr Transplant* 7:321-35, 2003.
8. Mickelson JJ, MacNeily AE, Leblanc J, et al: Renal transplantation in children 15 Kg or less: The British Columbia Children's Hospital experience, *J Urol* 176:1797-800, 2006.
9. Ojogho O, Sahney S, Cutler D, et al: Superior long-term results of renal transplantation in children under 5 years of age, *Am Surg* 68:1115-19, 2002.
10. Kari JA, Romagnoli J, Duffy P, et al: Renal transplantation in children under 5 years of age, *Pediatr Nephrol* 13:730-36, 1999.
11. Neipp M, Offner G, Luck R, et al: Kidney transplant in children weighing less than 15 kg: Donor selection and technical considerations, *Transplantation* 73:409-16, 2002.
12. Mitsnefes MM, Omoloja A, McEnery PT: Short-term pediatric renal transplant survival: Blood pressure and allograft function, *Pediatr Transplant* 5:160-65, 2001.
13. Sorof JM, Poffenbarger T, Portman R: Abnormal 24-hour blood pressure patterns in children after renal transplantation, *Am J Kidney Dis* 35:681-86, 2000.
14. Patel R, Terasaki PI: Significance of the positive crossmatch test in kidney transplantation, *N Engl J Med* 280:735-39, 1969.
15. Johnson AH, Rossen RD, Butler WT: Detection of alloantibodies using a sensitive antiglobulin microcytotoxicity test: Identification of low levels of pre-formed antibodies in accelerated allograft rejection, *Tissue Antigens* 2:215-26, 1972.
16. Fuller TC, Fuller AA, Golden M, et al: HLA alloantibodies and the mechanism of the antiglobulin-augmented lymphocytotoxicity procedure, *Hum Immunol* 56:94-105, 1997.
17. Gebel HM, Bray RA, Nickerson P: Pre-transplant assessment of donor-reactive, HLA-specific antibodies in renal transplantation: Contraindication vs. risk, *Am J Transplant* 3:1488-500, 2003.
18. Karpinski M, Rush D, Jeffery J, et al: Flow cytometric crossmatching in primary renal transplant recipients with a negative anti-human globulin enhanced cytotoxicity crossmatch, *J Am Soc Nephrol* 12:2807-14, 2001.
19. Zachary AA, Delaney NL, Lucas DP, et al: Characterization of HLA class I specific antibodies by ELISA using solubilized antigen targets: I. Evaluation of the GTI QuikID assay and analysis of antibody patterns, *Hum Immunol* 62:228-35, 2001.
20. Pei R, Wang G, Tarsitani C, et al: Simultaneous HLA Class I and Class II antibodies screening with flow cytometry, *Hum Immunol* 59:313-22, 1998.
21. Pei R, Lee JH, Shih NJ, et al: Single human leukocyte antigen flow cytometry beads for accurate identification of human leukocyte antigen antibody specificities, *Transplantation* 75:43-49, 2003.
22. Gebel HM, Bray RA: Sensitization and sensitivity: Defining the unsensitized patient, *Transplantation* 69:1370-4, 2000.
23. Iwaki Y, Cook DJ, Terasaki PI, et al: Flow cytometry crossmatching in human cadaver kidney transplantation, *Transplant Proc* 19:764-66, 1987.
24. Gjertson DW: Impact of delayed graft function and acute rejection on kidney graft survival, *Clin Transpl* 467-480, 2000.
25. A randomized clinical trial of cyclosporine in cadaveric renal transplantation: Analysis at three years. The Canadian Multicentre Transplant Study Group, *N Engl J Med* 314:1219-25, 1986.
26. Berber I, Tellioglu G, Yigit B, et al: Pediatric renal transplantation: Clinical analysis of 28 cases, *Transplant Proc* 38:430-31, 2006.
27. Jacobs SC, Cho E, Foster C, et al: Laparoscopic donor nephrectomy: The University of Maryland 6-year experience, *J Urol* 171:47-51, 2004.

28. Koning OH, Ploeg RJ, van Bockel JH, et al: Risk factors for delayed graft function in cadaveric kidney transplantation: A prospective study of renal function and graft survival after preservation with University of Wisconsin solution in multi-organ donors. European Multicenter Study Group, *Transplantation* 63:1620-28, 1997.
29. Singer JS, Ettenger RB, Gore JL, et al: Laparoscopic versus open renal procurement for pediatric recipients of living donor renal transplantation, *Am J Transplant* 5:2514-20, 2005.
30. Fontana I, Santori G, Ginevri F, et al: Preliminary report on impact of pretransplant dialysis on early graft function: Peritoneal versus hemodialysis, *Transplant Proc* 36:453-54, 2004.
31. Snyder JJ, Kasiske BL, Gilbertson DT, et al: A comparison of transplant outcomes in peritoneal and hemodialysis patients, *Kidney Int* 62:1423-30, 2002.
32. Nevins TE, Danielson G: Prior dialysis does not affect the outcome of pediatric renal transplantation, *Pediatr Nephrol* 5:211-14, 1991.
33. Van Biesen W, Veys N, Vanholder R, et al: The impact of the pre-transplant renal replacement modality on outcome after cadaveric kidney transplantation: The Ghent experience, *Contrib Nephrol* 150:254-58, 2006.
34. Maiorca R, Sandrini S, Cancarini GC, et al: Kidney transplantation in peritoneal dialysis patients, *Perit Dial Int* 14(3):S162-S168, 1994.
35. McDonald RA, Smith JM, Stablein D, et al: Pretransplant peritoneal dialysis and graft thrombosis following pediatric kidney transplantation: A NAPRTCS report, *Pediatr Transplant* 7:204-08, 2003.
36. Boom H, Mallat MJ, de Fijter JW, et al: Delayed graft function influences renal function, but not survival, *Kidney Int* 58:859-66, 2000.
37. Tejani AH, Sullivan EK, Alexander SR, et al: Predictive factors for delayed graft function (DGF) and its impact on renal graft survival in children: A report of the North American Pediatric Renal Transplant Cooperative Study (NAPRTCS), *Pediatr Transplant* 3:293-300, 1999.
38. Shoskes DA, Halloran PF: Delayed graft function in renal transplantation: Etiology, management and long-term significance, *J Urol* 155:1831-40, 1996.
39. Dawidson IJ, Sandor ZF, Coorpender L, et al: Intraoperative albumin administration affects the outcome of cadaver renal transplantation, *Transplantation* 53:774-82, 1992.
40. Hernandez A, Light JA, Barhyte DY, et al: Ablating the ischemia-reperfusion injury in non-heart-beating donor kidneys, *Transplantation* 67:200-06, 1999.
41. Agarwal A, Pescovitz MD: Immunosuppression in pediatric solid organ transplantation, *Semin Pediatr Surg* 15:142-52, 2006.
42. Shoskes DA, Xie Y, Gonzalez-Cadavid NF: Nitric oxide synthase activity in renal ischemia-reperfusion injury in the rat: Implications for renal transplantation, *Transplantation* 63:495-500, 1997.
43. Walker LM, Walker PD, Imam SZ, et al: Evidence for peroxynitrite formation in renal ischemia-reperfusion injury: Studies with the inducible nitric oxide synthase inhibitor L-N(6)-(1-Iminoethyl) lysine, *J Pharmacol Exp Ther* 295:417-22, 2000.
44. Emami A, Schwartz JH, Borkan SC: Transient ischemia or heat stress induces a cytoprotectant protein in rat kidney, *Am J Physiol* 260:F479-85, 1991.
45. Haugen E, Nath KA: The involvement of oxidative stress in the progression of renal injury, *Blood Purif* 17:58-65, 1999.
46. Castaneda MP, Swiatecka-Urban A, Mitsnefes MM, et al: Activation of mitochondrial apoptotic pathways in human renal allografts after ischemiareperfusion injury, *Transplantation* 76:50-54, 2003.
47. St Peter SD, Imber CJ, Jones DC, et al: Genetic determinants of delayed graft function after kidney transplantation, *Transplantation* 74:809-13, 2002.
48. Manchanda PK, Bid HK, Kumar A, et al: Genetic association of interleukin-1beta and receptor antagonist (IL-1Ra) gene polymorphism with allograft function in renal transplant patients, *Transpl Immunol* 15:289-96, 2006.
49. Nagra A, Trompeter RS, Fernando ON, et al: The effect of heparin on graft thrombosis in pediatric renal allografts, *Pediatr Nephrol* 19:531-35, 2004.
50. Smith JM, Stablein D, Singh A, et al: Decreased risk of renal allograft thrombosis associated with interleukin-2 receptor antagonists: A report of the NAPRTCS, *Am J Transplant* 6:585-88, 2006.
51. Singh A, Stablein D, Tejani A: Risk factors for vascular thrombosis in pediatric renal transplantation: A special report of the North American Pediatric Renal Transplant Cooperative Study, *Transplantation* 63:1263-67, 1997.
52. Dall'Amico R, Ginevri F, Ghio L, et al: Successful renal transplantation in children under 6 years of age, *Pediatr Nephrol* 16:1-7, 2001.
53. Vats AN, Donaldson L, Fine RN, et al: Pretransplant dialysis status and outcome of renal transplantation in North American children: A NAPRTCS Study. North American Pediatric Renal Transplant Cooperative Study, *Transplantation* 69:1414-19, 2000.
54. Broyer M, Gagnadoux MF, Sierro A, et al: Preventive treatment of vascular thrombosis after kidney transplantation in children with low molecular weight heparin, *Transplant Proc* 23:1384-85, 1991.
55. Alkhunaizi AM, Olyaei AJ, Barry JM, et al: Efficacy and safety of low molecular weight heparin in renal transplantation, *Transplantation* 66:533-34, 1998.
56. Kranz B, Vester U, Nadalin S, et al: Outcome after kidney transplantation in children with thrombotic risk factors, *Pediatr Transplant* 10:788-93, 2006.
57. Valente JF, Hricik D, Weigel K, et al: Comparison of sirolimus vs. mycophenolate mofetil on surgical complications and wound healing in adult kidney transplantation, *Am J Transplant* 3:1128-34, 2003.
58. Goggins WC, Pascual MA, Powelson JA, et al: A prospective, randomized, clinical trial of intraoperative versus postoperative thymoglobulin in adult cadaveric renal transplant recipients, *Transplantation* 76:798-802, 2003.
59. Coulthard MG, Keir MJ: Reflux nephropathy in kidney transplants, demonstrated by dimercaptosuccinic acid scanning, *Transplantation* 82:205-10, 2006.
60. McEnery PT, Alexander SR, Sullivan K, et al: Renal transplantation in children and adolescents: The 1992 annual report of the North American Pediatric Renal Transplant Cooperative Study, *Pediatr Nephrol* 7:711-20, 1993.
61. Seikaly M, Ho PL, Emmett L, et al: The 12th Annual Report of the North American Pediatric Renal Transplant Cooperative Study: Renal transplantation from 1987 through 1998, *Pediatr Transplant* 5:215-31, 2001.
62. Solez K, Axelsen RA, Benediktsson H, et al: International standardization of criteria for the histologic diagnosis of renal allograft rejection: The Banff working classification of kidney transplant pathology, *Kidney Int* 44:411-22, 1993.
63. Racusen LC, Solez K, Colvin RB, et al: The Banff 97 working classification of renal allograft pathology, *Kidney Int* 55:713-23, 1999.
64. Corey HE, Greenstein SM, Tellis V, et al: Renal allograft rejection in children and young adults: The Banff classification, *Pediatr Nephrol* 9:309-12, 1995.
65. Gaber LW, Moore LW, Alloway RR, et al: Correlation between Banff classification, acute renal rejection scores and reversal of rejection, *Kidney Int* 49:481-87, 1996.
66. Dittmer ID, Zwi LJ, Collins JF: Validation of the Banff criteria for acute rejection in renal transplant biopsies, *Aust N Z J Med* 25:681-87, 1995.
67. Croker BP, Clapp WL, Abu Shamat AR, et al: Macrophages and chronic renal allograft nephropathy, *Kidney Int Suppl* 57:S42-S49, 1996.
68. Gough J, Rush D, Jeffery J, et al: Reproducibility of the Banff schema in reporting protocol biopsies of stable renal allografts, *Nephrol Dial Transplant* 17:1081-84, 2002.
69. Rush DN, Jeffery JR, Gough J: Sequential protocol biopsies in renal transplant patients: Repeated inflammation is associated with impaired graft function at 1 year, *Transplant Proc* 27:1017-18, 1995.
70. Mueller A, Schnuelle P, Waldherr R, et al: Impact of the Banff '97 classification for histological diagnosis of rejection on clinical outcome and renal function parameters after kidney transplantation, *Transplantation* 69:1123-27, 2000.
71. Bates WD, Davies DR, Welsh K, et al: An evaluation of the Banff classification of early renal allograft biopsies and correlation with outcome, *Nephrol Dial Transplant* 14:2364-69, 1999.

72. Waiser J, Schreiber M, Budde K, et al: Prognostic value of the Banff classification, *Transpl Int* 13(1):S106-S111, 2000.
73. Nankivell BJ, Fenton-Lee CA, Kuypers DR, et al: Effect of histological damage on long-term kidney transplant outcome, *Transplantation* 71:515-23, 2001.
74. Tanaka T, Kyo M, Kokado Y, et al: Correlation between the Banff 97 classification of renal allograft biopsies and clinical outcome, *Transpl Int* 17:59-64, 2004.
75. Palomar R, Ruiz JC, Zubimendi JA, et al: Is there any correlation between pathologic changes for acute rejection in kidney transplantation (Banff 97) and graft function? *Transplant Proc* 34:349, 2002.
76. Durkan AM, Beattie TJ, Howatson A, et al: Renal transplant biopsy specimen adequacy in a paediatric population, *Pediatr Nephrol* 21:265-69, 2006.
77. Colvin RB, Cohen AH, Saiontz C, et al: Evaluation of pathologic criteria for acute renal allograft rejection: Reproducibility, sensitivity, and clinical correlation, *J Am Soc Nephrol* 8:1930-41, 1997.
78. Nickeleit V, Vamvakas EC, Pascual M, et al: The prognostic significance of specific arterial lesions in acute renal allograft rejection, *J Am Soc Nephrol* 9:1301-08, 1998.
79. Racusen LC, Colvin RB, Solez K, et al: Antibody-mediated rejection criteria, an addition to the Banff 97 classification of renal allograft rejection, *Am J Transplant* 3:708-14, 2003.
80. Terasaki PI: Humoral theory of transplantation, *Am J Transplant* 3:665-73, 2003.
81. Shahinian A, Pfeffer K, Lee KP, et al: Differential T cell costimulatory requirements in CD28-deficient mice, *Science* 261:609-12, 1993.
82. Guinan EC, Gribben JG, Boussiotis VA, et al: Pivotal role of the B7:CD28 pathway in transplantation tolerance and tumor immunity, *Blood* 84:3261-82, 1994.
83. Mosmann TR, Cherwinski H, Bond MW, et al: Two types of murine helper T cell clone. I. Definition according to profiles of lymphokine activities and secreted proteins, *J Immunol* 136:2348-57, 1986.
84. Anderson JA, Lentsch AB, Hadjiminas DJ, et al: The role of cytokines, adhesion molecules, and chemokines in interleukin-2-induced lymphocytic infiltration in C57BL/6 mice, *J Clin Invest* 97:1952-59, 1996.
85. Kagi D, Vignaux F, Ledermann B, et al: Fas and perforin pathways as major mechanisms of T cell-mediated cytotoxicity, *Science* 265:528-30, 1994.
86. Kagi D, Ledermann B, Burki K, et al: Cytotoxicity mediated by T cells and natural killer cells is greatly impaired in perforin-deficient mice, *Nature* 369:31-37, 1994.
87. Heusel JW, Wesselschmidt RL, Shresta S, et al: Cytotoxic lymphocytes require granzyme B for the rapid induction of DNA fragmentation and apoptosis in allogeneic target cells, *Cell* 76:977-87, 1994.
88. Larsen CP, Alexander DZ, Hendrix R, et al: Fas-mediated cytotoxicity: An immunoeffector or immunoregulatory pathway in T cell-mediated immune responses? *Transplantation* 60:221-24, 1995.
89. Vampa ML, Norman PJ, Burnapp L, et al: Natural killer-cell activity after human renal transplantation in relation to killer immunoglobulin-like receptors and human leukocyte antigen mismatch, *Transplantation* 76:1220-28, 2003.
90. Feucht HE, Schneeberger H, Hillebrand G, et al: Capillary deposition of C4d complement fragment and early renal graft loss, *Kidney Int* 43:1333-38, 1993.
91. Collins AB, Schneeberger EE, Pascual MA, et al: Complement activation in acute humoral renal allograft rejection: Diagnostic significance of C4d deposits in peritubular capillaries, *J Am Soc Nephrol* 10:2208-14, 1999.
92. Crespo M, Pascual M, Tolkoff-Rubin N, et al: Acute humoral rejection in renal allograft recipients: I. Incidence, serology and clinical characteristics, *Transplantation* 71:652-58, 2001.
93. Mauiyyedi S, Crespo M, Collins AB, et al: Acute humoral rejection in kidney transplantation: II. Morphology, immunopathology, and pathologic classification, *J Am Soc Nephrol* 13:779-87, 2002.
94. Herzenberg AM, Gill JS, Djurdjev O, et al: C4d deposition in acute rejection: An independent long-term prognostic factor, *J Am Soc Nephrol* 13:234-41, 2002.
95. Cascalho M: B cell tolerance: Lessons from transplantation, *Curr Drug Targets Cardiovasc Haematol Disord* 5:271-5, 2005.
96. Platt JL: C4d and the fate of organ allografts, *J Am Soc Nephrol* 13:2417-19, 2002.
97. Lee PC, Terasaki PI, Takemoto SK, et al: All chronic rejection failures of kidney transplants were preceded by the development of HLA antibodies, *Transplantation* 74:1192-94, 2002.
98. Vasconcellos LM, Schachter AD, Zheng XX, et al: Cytotoxic lymphocyte gene expression in peripheral blood leukocytes correlates with rejecting renal allografts, *Transplantation* 66:562-66, 1998.
99. Sarwal MM, Jani A, Chang S, et al: Granulysin expression is a marker for acute rejection and steroid resistance in human renal transplantation, *Hum Immunol* 62:21-31, 2001.
100. Sabek O, Dorak MT, Kotb M, et al: Quantitative detection of T-cell activation markers by real-time PCR in renal transplant rejection and correlation with histopathologic evaluation, *Transplantation* 74:701-07, 2002.
101. Dugre FJ, Gaudreau S, Belles-Isles M, et al: Cytokine and cytotoxic molecule gene expression determined in peripheral blood mononuclear cells in the diagnosis of acute renal rejection, *Transplantation* 70:1074-80, 2000.
102. Simon T, Opelz G, Wiesel M, et al: Serial peripheral blood interleukin-18 and perforin gene expression measurements for prediction of acute kidney graft rejection, *Transplantation* 77:1589-95, 2004.
103. Tan L, Howell WM, Smith JL, et al: Sequential monitoring of peripheral T-lymphocyte cytokine gene expression in the early post renal allograft period, *Transplantation* 71:751-59, 2001.
104. Gibbs PJ, Tan LC, Sadek SA, et al: Quantitative detection of changes in cytokine gene expression in peripheral blood mononuclear cells correlates with and precedes acute rejection in renal transplant recipients, *Transpl Immunol* 14:99-108, 2005.
105. Li B, Hartono C, Ding R, et al: Noninvasive diagnosis of renal-allograft rejection by measurement of messenger RNA for perforin and granzyme B in urine, *N Engl J Med* 344:947-54, 2001.
106. Tatapudi RR, Muthukumar T, Dadhania D, et al: Noninvasive detection of renal allograft inflammation by measurements of mRNA for IP-10 and CXCR3 in urine, *Kidney Int* 65:2390-97, 2004.
107. Muthukumar T, Dadhania D, Ding R, et al: Messenger RNA for FOXP3 in the urine of renal-allograft recipients, *N Engl J Med* 353:2342-51, 2005.
108. Sarwal M, Chua MS, Kambham N, et al: Molecular heterogeneity in acute renal allograft rejection identified by DNA microarray profiling, *N Engl J Med* 349:125-38, 2003.
109. Clarke W, Zhang Z, Chan DW: The application of clinical proteomics to cancer and other diseases, *Clin Chem Lab Med* 41:1562-70, 2003.
110. Schaub S, Rush D, Wilkins J, et al: Proteomic-based detection of urine proteins associated with acute renal allograft rejection, *J Am Soc Nephrol* 15:219-27, 2004.
111. Schaub S, Wilkins J, Weiler T, et al: Urine protein profiling with surface-enhanced laser-desorption/ionization time-of-flight mass spectrometry, *Kidney Int* 65:323-32, 2004.
112. Schaub S, Wilkins JA, Antonovici M, et al: Proteomic-based identification of cleaved urinary beta2-microglobulin as a potential marker for acute tubular injury in renal allografts, *Am J Transplant* 5:729-38, 2005.
113. Schaub S, Wilkins JA, Nickerson P: Proteomics in renal transplantation: Opportunities and challenges, *Clin Transpl*:253-60, 2004.
114. O'Riordan E, Orlova TN, Mei JJ, et al: Bioinformatic analysis of the urine proteome of acute allograft rejection, *J Am Soc Nephrol* 15:3240-48, 2004.
115. Benfield M: Current status of kidney transplant: Update 2003, *Pediatr Clin N Am* 50:1301-34, 2003.
116. Guyot C, Nguyen J, Cochat P, et al: Risk factors for chronic rejection in pediatric renal allograft recipients, *Pediatr Nephrol* 10:723-27, 1996.
117. Matas A: Impact of acute rejection on development of chronic rejection in pediatric renal transplant recipients, *Pediatr Transplantation* 4:92-99, 2000.
118. Tejani A, Sullivan E: The impact of acute rejection on chronic rejection: A report of the North American Pediatric Renal

Transplant Cooperative Study, *Pediatr Transplantation* 4:107-11, 2000.
119. Tejani A: Chronic rejection in pediatric renal transplantation: Where are we? *Pediatr Transplantation* 4:83-85, 2000.
120. Debray D, Furlan V, Baudoin V, et al: Therapy for acute rejection in pediatric organ transplant recipients, *Pediatr Drugs* 5:81-93, 2003.
121. Marks R, Finke J: Biologics in prevention and treatment of graft rejection, *Springer Semin Immun* 27:457-76, 2006.
122. Mazzucchi E, Lucon A, Nahas W, et al: Histological outcome of acute cellular rejection in kidney transplantation after treatment with methylprednisolone, *Transplantation* 67:430-34, 1999.
123. Shinn C, Malhotra D, Chan L, et al: Time course of response to pulse methylprednisolone therapy in renal transplants with acute allograft rejection, *Am J Kidney Dis* 34:304-07, 1999.
124. Gaber A, First M, Tesi R, et al: Results of the double-blind, randomized, multicenter, phase III clinical trial of thymoglobulin versus ATGAM in the treatment of acute graft rejection episodes after renal transplantation, *Transplantation* 66:29-37, 1998.
125. Mariat C, Alamartine E, Diab N, et al: A randomized prospective study comparing low-dose OKT3 to low-dose ATG for the treatment of acute steroid-resistant rejection episodes in kidney transplant recipients, *Transpl Int* 11:231-36, 2004.
126. Mochon M, Kaiser B, Palmer J, et al: Evaluation of OKT3 monoclonal antibody and anti-thymocyte globulin in the treatment of steroid-resistant acute allograft rejection in pediatric renal transplants, *Pediatr Nephrol* 7:259-62, 1993.
127. Jordan S, Tyan D, Czer L, et al: Immunomodulatory actions of intravenous immunoglobulin (IVIG): Potential applications in solid organ transplant recipients, *Pediatr Transplantation* 2:92-105, 1998.
128. Basu A, Ramkumar M, Tan H, et al: Reversal of acute cellular rejection after renal transplantation with Campath-1H, *Transplant Proc* 37:923-26, 2005.
129. Csapo Z, Benavides-Viveros C, Podder H, et al: Campath-1H as rescue therapy for the treatment of acute rejection in kidney transplant recipients, *Transplant Proc* 37:2032-36, 2005.
130. Goh H, Lye W: Biopsy-proven resolution of steroid-resistant acute rejection with basiliximab therapy in a renal allograft recipient, *Transplant Proc* 33:3213-14, 2001.
131. Morris P, Russell N: Alemtuzumab (Campath-1H): A systematic review in organ transplantation, *Transplantation* 81:1361-67, 2006.
132. Mycophenolate Mofetil Acute Renal Rejection Study Group: Mycophenolate mofetil for the treatment of a first acute renal allograft rejection, *Transplantation* 65:235, 1998.
133. Mycophenolate Mofetil Acute Renal Rejection Study Group: Mycophenolate mofetil for the treatment of a first acute renal allograft rejection, three-year follow-up, *Transplantation* 71:1091, 2001.
134. Watschinger B, Pascual M: Capillary C4d deposition as a marker of humoral immunity in renal allograft rejection, *J Am Soc Nephrol* 13:2420-23, 2002.
135. Becker Y, Becker B, Pirsch J, et al: Rituximab as treatment for refractory kidney transplant rejection, *Am J Transplant* 4:996, 2004.
136. Jordan S, Quartel A, Czer L, et al: Posttransplant therapy using high-dose human immunoglobulin (intravenous gammaglobulin) to control acute humoral rejection in renal and cardiac allograft recipients and potential mechanism of action, *Transplantation* 66:800-05, 1998.
137. Montgomery R, Zachary A, Racusen L, et al: Plasmapheresis and intravenous immune globulin provides rescue therapy for refractory humoral rejection and allows kidneys to be successfully transplanted into cross-match-positive recipients, *Transplantation* 70:887-95, 2000.
138. Pascual M, Saidman S, Tolkoff-Rubin N, et al: Plasma exchange and tacrolimus-mycophenolate rescue for acute humoral rejection in kidney transplantation, *Transplantation* 66:1460-64, 1998.
139. Rocha P, Butterly D, Greenberg A, et al: Beneficial aspect of plasmapheresis and intravenous immunoglobulin on renal allograft survival of patients with acute humoral rejection, *Transplantation* 75:1490-95, 2003.
140. Feinstein S, Keich R, Becer-Cohen R, et al: Is noncompliance among adolescent renal transplant recipients inevitable? *Pediatrics* 115:969-73, 2005.
141. Offerman G: Immunosuppression for long-term maintenance of renal allograft function, *Drugs* 64:1325-38, 2004.
142. Scott L, McKeage K, Keam S, et al: Tacrolimus: A further update of its use in the management of organ transplantation, *Drugs* 63:1247-97, 2003.
143. Ettenger R, Grimm E: Safety and efficacy of TOR inhibitors in pediatric renal transplant recipients, *Am J Kidney Dis* 38(4, Suppl 2):S22-S28, 2001.
144. Kahan B: The potential role of rapamycin in pediatric transplantationas observed from adult studies, *Pediatr Transplantation* 3:175-80, 1999.
145. Artero M, Brava C, Amend W, et al: Recurrent focal glomerulosclerosis: natural history and response to therapy, *Am J Med* 92:375-83, 1992.
146. Cheong H, Han H, Park H, et al: Early recurrent nephrotic syndrome after renal transplantation in children with focal segmental glomerulosclerosis, *Nephrol Dial Transplant* 15:78-81, 2000.
147. Dall'Amico R, Ghiggeri G, Carraro M, et al: Prediction and treatment of recurrent focal segmental glomerulosclerosis after renal transplantation in children, *Am J Kidney Dis* 34:1048-55, 1999.
148. First M: Living-related donor transplant should be performed with caution in patients with focal segmental glomerulosclerosis, *Pediatr Nephrol* 9:S40-S42, 1995.
149. Fujisawa M, Ishimura T, Higuchi A, et al: Long-term outcome of focal segmental glomerulosclerosis after Japanese pediatric renal transplantation, *Pediatr Nephrol* 17:165-68, 2002.
150. Kaplan-Pavlovcic S, Ferluga D, Hvala A, et al: Recurrent focal segmental glomerulosclerosis after renal transplantation: Is early recurrent proteinuria always a surrogate marker for recurrence of the disease? *Transplant Proc* 34:3122-24, 2002.
151. Kim S, Ha J, Jung I, et al: Recurrent focal segmental glomerulosclerosis following renal transplantation in Korean peditric patients, *Pediatr Transplantation* 5:105-11, 2001.
152. Muller T, Sikora P, Offner G, et al: Recurrence of renal disease after kidney transplantation in children: 24 years of experience in a single center, *Clin Nephrol* 49:82-90, 1998.
153. Newstead C: Recurrent disease in renal transplant, *Nephrol Dial Transplant* 18:vi68-vi74, 2003.
154. Schachter A, Harmon W: Single-center analysis of early recurrence of nephrotic syndrome following renal transplantation in children, *Pediatr Transplantation* 5:406-9, 2001.
155. Seikaly M: Recurrence of primary disease in children after renal transplantation: An evidence-based update, *Pediatr Transplantation* 8:113-19, 2004.
156. Tejani A, Stablein D: Recurrence of focal segmental glomerulosclerosis posttransplantation: A special report of the North American Pediatric Renal Transplant Cooperative Study, *J Am Soc Nephrol* 2(12):S258-63, 1992.
157. Kashtan C, McEnery P, Tejani A, et al: Renal allograft survival according to primary diagnosis: A report of the North American Pediatric Renal Transpant Cooperative Study, *Pediatr Nephrol* 9:679-84, 1995.
158. Baum M: Outcomes after renal transplantation for FSGS in children, *Pediatr Transplant* 8:329-33, 2004.
159. Rizzoni G, Ehrich J, Brunner F, et al: Combined report on regular dialysis and transplantation of children in Europe, 1990, *Nephrol Dial Transplant* 6(4):31-42, 1991.
160. Cameron J: Recurrent primary disease and de novo nephritis following renal transplantation, *Pediatr Nephrol* 5:412-21, 1991.
161. Winn M: Approach to the evaluation of heritable diseases and update on familial focal segmental glomerulosclerosis, *Nephrol Dial Transplant* 18(6):vi14-vi20, 2003.
162. Winn M, Conlon P, Lynn K, et al: A mutation in the TRPC6 cation channel causes familial focal segmental glomerulosclerosis, *Science* 308:1801-04, 2005.
163. Pollak M: The genetic basis of FSGS and steroid-resistant nephrosis, *Semin Nephrol* 23:141-46, 2003.
164. Billing H, Mueller D, Ruf R, et al: NPHS2 mutation associated with recurrence of proteinuria after transplantation, *Pediatr Nephrol* 19:561-64, 2004.

165. Bertelli R, Ginevri F, Caridi G, et al: Recurrence of focal segmental glomerulosclerosis after renal transplantation in patients with mutations of podocin, *Am J Kidney Dis* 41:1314-21, 2003.
166. Weber S, Tonshoff B: Recurrence of focal-segmental glomerulosclerosis in children after renal transplantation: Clinical and genetic aspects, *Transplantation* 80:S128-34, 2005.
167. Savin V, Artero M, Sharma R: Risk of recurrence of focal segmental glomerulosclerosis (FSGS) after transplantation can be assessed using an in vitro assay of serum, *J Am Soc Nephrol* 4:125-29, 1993.
168. Benchimol C: Focal segmental glomerulosclerosis: Pathogenesis and treatment, *Curr Opin Pediatr* 15:171-80, 2003.
169. Andresdottir M, Ajubi N, Croockewit S, et al: Recurrent foveal glomerulosclerosis: Natural course and treatment with plasma exchange, *Nephrol Dial Transplant* 14:2650-56, 1999.
170. Belson A, Yorgin P, Al-Uzri A, et al: Long-term plasmapheresis and protein A column treatment of recurrent FSGS, *Pediatr Nephrol* 16:985-89, 2001.
171. Cochat P, Schell M, Ranchin B, et al: Management of recurrent nephrotic syndrome after kidney transplantation in children, *Clin Nephrol* 46:17-20, 1996.
172. Ingulli E, Tejani A: Incidence, treatment and outcome of recurrent focal segmental glomerulosclerosis post-transplantation in 42 allografts in children: A single center experience, *Transplantation* 512:401-05, 1991.
173. Ohta T, Kawaguchi H, Hattori M, et al: Effect of pre- and postoperative plasmapheresis on posttransplant recurrence of focal segmental glomerulosclerosis in children, *Transplantation* 71:628-33, 2001.
174. Ponticelli C, Campise M, Tarantino A: The different patterns response plasmapheresis of recurrent focal and segmental glomerulosclerosis, *Transplant Proc* 34:3069-71, 2002.
175. Pradhan M, Petro J, Palmer J, et al: Early use of plasmapheresis for recurrent post-transplant FSGS, *Pediatr Nephrol* 18:934-38, 2003.
176. Saleem M, Ramanan A, Rees L: Recurrent focal segmental glomerulosclerosis in grafts treated with plasma exchange and increased immunosuppression, *Pediatr Nephrol* 14:361-64, 2000.
177. Shariatmadar S, Noto T: Therapeutic plasma exchange in recurrent focal segmental glomerulosclerosis following transplantation, *J Clin Apheresis* 17:78-83, 2002.
178. Wuhl E, Fydryk J, Wiesel M, et al: Impact of recurrent nephrotic syndrome after renal transplantation in young patients, *Pediatr Nephrol* 12:529-33, 1998.
179. Salomon R, Gagnadoux M-F, Niaudet P: Intravenous cyclosporine therapy in recurrent nephrotic syndrome after renal transplantation in children, *Transplantation* 75:810-14, 2003.
180. Mowry J, Marik J, Cohen A, et al: Treatment of recurrent focal segmental glomerulosclerosis with high-dose cyclosporine A and plasmapheresis, *Transplant Proc* 25:1345-46, 1993.
181. Dantal J, Bigot E, Bogers W, et al: Effect of plasma protein absorption on protein excretion in kidney transplant recipients with recurrent nephrotic syndrome, *N Engl J Med* 330:7-14, 1994.
182. Kershaw D, Sedman A, Jelsch R, et al: Recurrent focal segmental glomerulosclerosis in pediatric renal transplant recipients: successful treatment with oral cyclophosphamide, *Clin Transpl* 8:546-49, 1994.
183. Nathanson S, Cochat P, Andre J-L, et al: Recurrence of nephrotic syndrome after renal transplantation: Influence of increased immunosuppression, *Pediatr Nephrol* 20:1801-04, 2005.
184. Cameron J: Glomerulonephritis in renal transplants, *Transplantation* 34:237-45, 1982.
185. Gagnadoux M-F, Niaudet P, Broyer M: Non-immunological risk factors in pediatric renal transplantation, *Pediatr Nephrol* 7:89-95, 1993.
186. Briganti EM, Russ GR, McNeil JJ, et al: Risk of renal allograft loss from recurrent glomerulonephritis, *New Engl J Med* 347:103-09, 2002.
187. Baqi N, Tejani A: Recurrence of original disease in pediatric renal transplant, *J Nephrol* 10:85-92, 1997.
188. Broyer M, Selwood N, Brunner F: Recurrence of primary renal disease on kidney graft: A European pediatric experience, *J Am Soc Nephrol* 2:S255-S257, 1992.
189. O'Meara Y, Green A, Carmody M, et al: Recurrent glomerulonephritis in renal transplantation: Fourteen years' experience, *Nephrol Dial Transplant* 4:730-34, 1989.
190. Andresdottir MB, Assmann KJM, Hoitsma AJ, et al: Renal transplantation in patients with dense deposit disease: Morphological characteristics of recurrent disease and clinical outcome, *Nephrol Dial Transplant* 14:1723-31, 1999.
191. EBPG Expert Group on Renal Transplantation: European best practice guidelines for renal tranplantation, *Nephrol Dial Transplant* 17(Suppl 4):60-67, 2002.
192. Bachman U, Biava C, Amend W, et al: The clinical course of IgA nephropathy and Henoch-Schonlein purpura following renal transplantation, *Transplantation* 42:511-14, 1986.
193. Hasegawa A, Kawamura T, Ito H: Fate of renal grafts with recurrent Henoch-Schonlein purpura nephritis in children, *Transplant Proc* 21:2130-33, 1989.
194. Habib R, Antignac C, Hinglais N: Glomerular lesion in the transplanted kidney in children, *Am J Kidney Dis* 10:198-207, 1987.
195. Meulders Q, Pirson Y, Cosyns J, et al: Course of Henoch-Schonlein nephritis after renal transplantation: Report on ten patients and review of the literature, *Transplantation* 48:1179-86, 1994.
196. Quan A, Sullivan E, Alexander S: Recurrence of hemolytic uremic syndrome after renal transplantation in children: A report of the North American Pediatric Renal Transplant Cooperative Study, *Transplantation* 72:742-45, 2001.
197. Loirat C, Niaudet P: The risk of recurrence of hemolytic uremic syndrome after renal transplantation in children, *Pediatr Nephrol* 18:1095-101, 2003.
198. Piovesan E, Castilhos C, Pozza R, et al: Hemolytic uremic syndrome after kidney transplantation, *Transplant Proc* 34:2779-80, 2002.
199. Hoppe B, Langman C: A United States survey on diagnosis, treatment and outcome of primary hyperoxaluria, *Pediatr Nephrol* 18:986-91, 2003.
200. Matthew T: Recurrence of disease following renal transplantation, *Am J Kidney Dis* 12:85-96, 1988.
201. Ellis S, Hulton S, McKiernan P, et al: Combined liver-kidney transplantation for primary hyperoxaluria type I in young children, *Nephrol Dial Transplant* 16:348-54, 2001.
202. Gagnadoux M-F, Lacaille F, Niaudet P, et al: Long term results of liver-kidney transplantation in children with primary hyperoxaluria, *Pediatr Nephrol* 16:946-50, 2001.
203. De-Pauw L, Gelin M, Danpure C, et al: Combined liver-kidney transplantation in primary hyperoxaluria type I, *Transplantation* 50:886-87, 1990.
204. McDonald J, Landreneau M, Rohr M, et al: Reversal by liver transplantation of the complications of primary hyperoxaluria as well as the metabolic defect, *N Engl J Med* 321:1100-03, 1989.
205. Cibrik D, Kaplan B, Arndorfer J, et al: Renal allograft survival in patients with oxalosis, *Transplantation* 74:707-10, 2002.
206. Ojo A, Govaerts T, Schmouder R, et al: Renal transplantation in end-stage sickle cell nephropathy, *Transplantation* 67:291-95, 1999.
207. Warady B, Sullivan E: Renal transplantation in children with sickle cell disease: A report of the North American Pediatric Renal Transplant Cooperative Study (NAPRTCS), *Pediatr Transplantation* 2:130-33, 1998.
208. Scheinman J: Sickle cell disease and the kidney, *Semin Nephrol* 23:66-76, 2003.
209. Sorof JM, Goldstein SL, Brewer ED, et al: Use of anti-hypertensive medications and post-transplant renal allograft function in children, *Pediatr Transplant* 4:21-27, 2000.

CHAPTER

61 Chronic Renal Transplant Dysfunction

Nicholas J. A. Webb and Heather Maxwell

INTRODUCTION

In recent times, short-term renal allograft survival has improved significantly in both children and adults. However, the improvement in longer-term graft survival has been less impressive (Figure 61-1). It is not uncommon for the plasma creatinine to drift upward over the years following transplantation, and this is reflected in a steady rate of graft attrition with increasing time posttransplantation. To date, there has been little progress in preventing chronic allograft dysfunction and subsequent loss.

The classification of chronic allograft dysfunction is not ideal. Poor graft function, particularly when present for many years after transplantation, is often referred to as chronic rejection (or indeed simply labeled chronic graft dysfunction). Many of these kidneys are not biopsied, and it is therefore difficult to obtain accurate data on the precise causes of late graft loss. In the 2006 North American Pediatric Renal Trials Cooperative Study (NAPRTCS) report, 34.7% of all graft losses were recorded as due to chronic rejection, 12.9% to acute rejection, 10.5% to vascular thromboses, 9.2% to death with a functioning graft, and 6.8% to recurrence of the original disease (Table 61-1). The remaining losses were due to a variety of other conditions, each causing a small number of graft failures. Ciclosporin toxicity is cited as the cause of graft failure in 0.4% of cases.[1]

However, in reported series where transplant biopsies are routinely performed for late graft dysfunction chronic allograft nephropathy (CAN) is a common finding. Often, no distinction is made between CAN and chronic rejection—although the terms are not synonymous. Understanding and preventing CAN will be an important step toward improving long-term graft survival.

CHRONIC ALLOGRAFT NEPHROPATHY

CAN refers to several pathogenic mechanisms that result in similar appearances upon biopsy. The term was designed to encompass what are initially distinct processes; namely, rejection, calcineurin inhibitor (CNI) toxicity, disease recurrence, and obstruction (which may coexist with more general processes such as ischemia, hypertension, and hyperlipidemia). CAN is the final common response to these processes.

When looking for potential influences on or causes of graft loss, however, the literature does not discriminate well among the various processes contributing to CAN. Thus, preventing and treating this entity remains a challenge. In the literature, CAN is often used interchangeably with the term *chronic allograft dysfunction*—which describes the clinical pattern of gradual, progressive deterioration of graft function at least 3 months after transplantation (commonly associated with proteinuria and de novo or worsening hypertension).

The etiology of CAN is complex, with multiple factors affecting graft histology and function through various pathophysiologic processes. The graft has a limited response to insults, and the result is CAN—with evidence of interstitial fibrosis, tubular atrophy, and less commonly vascular changes and glomerulopathy. A distinct pathologic process may be evident in the early stages, but often there is more than one precipitant (e.g., an elderly donor kidney with established chronic damage and primary nonfunction that then develops an acute rejection episode and later displays CNI toxicity). Furthermore, in the later stages of any of these processes the main histologic changes are those of fibrosis and tubular loss. For these reasons, it can be difficult to tease out all of the individual pathologic processes involved in CAN.

Histologic Diagnosis of CAN

The pathologic changes seen in CAN affect all constituent elements of the kidney; namely, the interstitium, the tubules, the vessels, and the glomeruli. The interstitium shows variable degrees of fibrosis (with focal infiltrates of lymphocytes and plasma cells) together with areas of tubular atrophy and loss (Figure 61-2). Vessel walls show subintimal accumulation of connective tissue, mononuclear cell infiltrates, proliferation of myofibroblasts, and disruption and duplication of the internal elastic lamina (Figure 61-3). Arteriolar hyaline changes (especially nodular changes) are suggestive of CNI toxicity (see material following), whereas widespread endothelial changes with more severe arteritis are more suggestive of chronic rejection.

Transplant glomerulopathy is found in approximately 5% to 15% of cases of CAN. The glomeruli are enlarged, and the capillary walls are thickened with occasional double contours (as seen in membranoproliferative glomerulonephritis) due to mesangial interposition (Figures 61-4 and 61-5). There is usually an increase in mesangial matrix. This is thought to be a response to chronic humoral rejection and is associated with accelerated graft loss.[2] Immunofluorescence may show the presence of granular mesangial IgM (and to a lesser extent

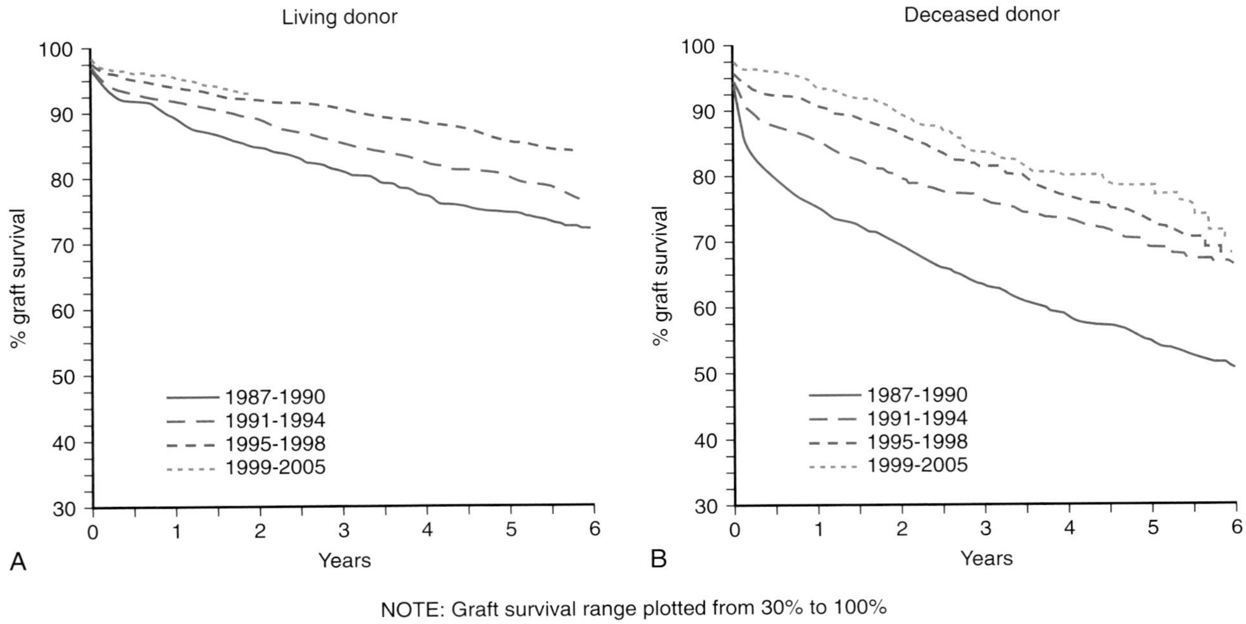

Figure 61-1 Percentage of graft survival for patients transplanted in successive time periods for living and deceased donor transplantation. (From the NAPRCTS Report 2006.)

TABLE 61-1 Causes of Graft Failure in 2551 Patients as Reported in the North American Pediatric Renal Trials and Collaborative Studies Report 2006

	INDEX GRAFT FAILURES		SUBSEQUENT GRAFT FAILURES		ALL GRAFT FAILURES	
	n	%	*n*	%	*n*	%
Total	2251	100	305	100	2556	100
Death with functioning graft	211	9.4	23	7.5	234	9.2
Primary nonfunction	58	2.6	2	0.7	60	2.3
Vascular thrombosis	231	10.3	38	12.5	269	10.5
Other technical	28	1.2	4	1.3	32	1.3
Hyperacute rejection	13	0.6	4	1.4	17	0.7
Accelerated acute rejection	33	1.5	8	2.6	41	1.6
Acute rejection	291	12.9	40	13.1	331	12.9
Chronic rejection	776	34.5	111	36.4	887	34.7
Recurrence of original kidney disease	145	6.4	29	9.5	174	6.8
Renal artery stenosis	15	0.7	0	0.0	15	0.6
Bacterial/viral infection	44	2.0	4	1.3	47	1.8
Ciclosporin toxicity	11	0.5	0	0.0	11	0.4
De novo kidney disease	7	0.3	2	0.7	9	0.4
Patient discontinued medication	104	4.6	8	2.6	112	4.4
Malignancy	30	1.3	2	0.7	32	1.3
Other/unknown	254	11.3	30	9.8	284	11.1

C3 deposition), and electron microscopy the presence of subendothelial accumulation of electron-lucent deposits. There may be peritubular basement membrane splitting and lamination. Glomerular staining for C4d, a complement component, has been reported in transplant glomerulopathy—with some biopsies also showing staining for C4d in the peritubular capillaries.[2]

The Banff classification standardizes reporting of acute and chronic rejection. The original Banff schema was devised in 1991,[3] and has subsequently been updated—with greater

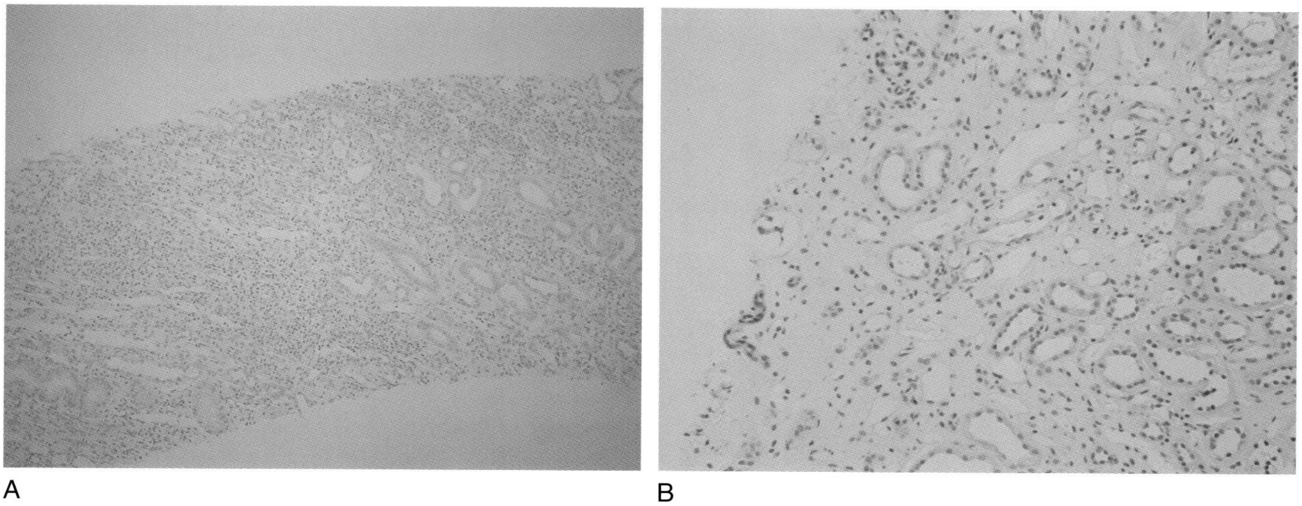

Figure 61-2 H&E stained renal transplant biopsy showing large areas of interstitial fibrosis, a chronic inflammatory cell infiltrate, and tubular atrophy at low power **(A)** and medium power **(B).** (Courtesy of Dawn Penman.)

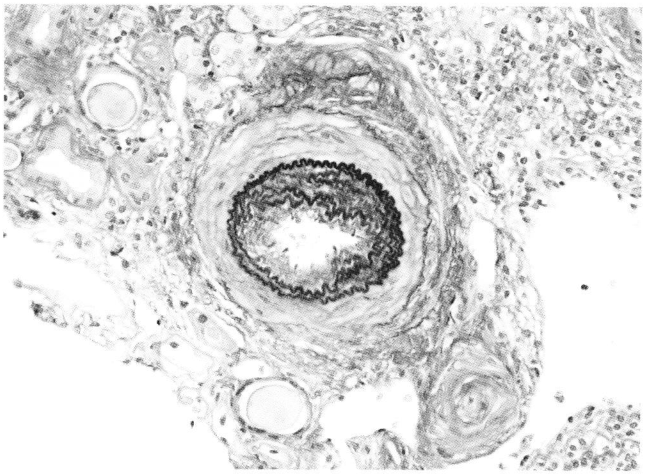

Figure 61-3 EMSB stained renal transplant biopsy showing an artery with thickening of the intima and multiple reduplications of the internal elastic lamina. (Courtesy of Barbara Young.)

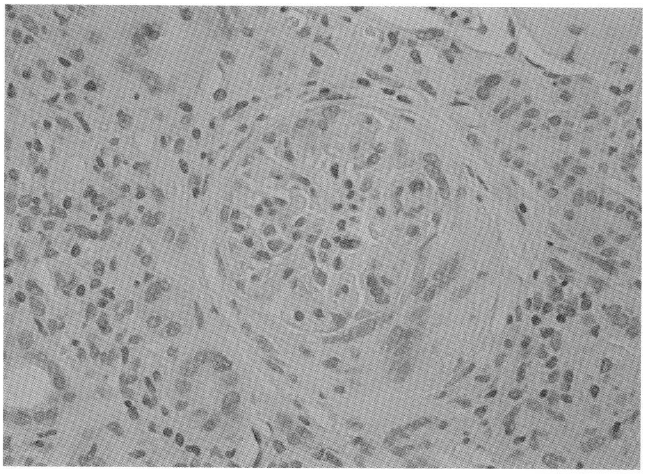

Figure 61-4 H&E stained renal transplant biopsy showing transplant glomerulopathy with increased mesangial matrix and thickening of the glomerular capillary loops. (Courtesy of Dawn Penman.)

emphasis on the type rather than the degree of rejection[4] (Table 61-2). For chronic changes, the Banff classification is based mainly on the degree of interstitial fibrosis and tubular atrophy because these changes are less subject to sampling error—although vascular and glomerular changes (less commonly seen) are more specific to CAN.

The chronic elements can be brought together to determine a CAN score of grades I (mild), II (moderate), and III (severe). The chronic allograft damage index (CADI)[5] is another system that has been used. This is a semiquantitative assessment of a number of chronic and inflammatory indicators that reflect graft outcome. Banff and CADI have been adjusted to be comparable.

The Banff criteria will in the near future be updated,[6] and the emphasis will be on determining recognizable and potentially treatable causes such as viral infection, chronic rejection, and CNI toxicity. In biopsies where there is no discernable cause of changes, the term *sclerosis* will be used instead to reflect the presence of tubular atrophy and interstitial fibrosis with no evidence of specific etiology. These changes to the Banff schema should mean that their use in future studies will allow more useful interpretation of study results, but to date a substantial proportion of the literature refers to the Banff 1993-1995 and 1997 criteria.

Natural History of CAN

Much of our understanding of the natural course of CAN has come about through studies utilizing serial protocol biopsies, where changes may be evident upon biopsy long before there is any clinical indication of a problem—and where a biopsy taken early after transplantation can be compared with samples taken at a later time.

Protocol biopsy studies have shown that chronic changes can be present within the first 1 to 3 months after trans-

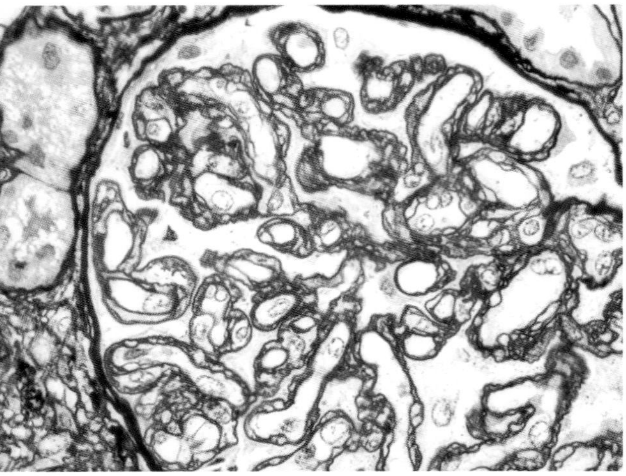

Figure 61-5 High-power view of a glomerulus from a patient with transplant glomerulopathy processed with a silver stain to demonstrate duplication of the basement membrane. (Courtesy of Ian Roberts.)

plantation. One of the most useful series included 119 adult diabetic patients (receiving simultaneous kidney pancreas transplants) who underwent serial protocol biopsies.[7] Because donors for kidney pancreas transplants tend to be young, these kidneys had normal histology prior to transplantation. Biopsies were performed at 0, 1, and 3 months—and again at 1, 3, 5, 7, and 10 years. The first year was characterized by increased Banff scores for chronic interstitial fibrosis and tubular atrophy (Figure 61-6). Grade I CAN occurred at a median of 3 months posttransplantation, and by 1 year was present in 94% of biopsies. Of note, some 1-month biopsy specimens showed the presence of chronic changes.

With time, the number of biopsies with more severe changes gradually increased such that by 10 years 80% of protocol biopsies had moderate (grade II) changes and 50% had severe (grade III) changes. Approximately two thirds of the interstitial fibrosis occurred within the first year, with a slower gradual accumulation thereafter over the next 9 years of the study.

Some biopsies had evidence of acute but subclinical rejection, so called because there is no associated increase in serum creatinine. Biopsies where there was subclinical rejection at one point in time had more interstitial fibrosis on later biopsies.

Thus, it is apparent from studies of early protocol biopsies that histologic changes occur earlier than clinical changes and that by the time the plasma creatinine rises these changes may be irreversible. Furthermore, chronic change on early biopsies has been shown to be predictive of later graft function.[8] Other studies have shown that it is the presence of fibrosis and acute inflammatory cell infiltrate together that is predictive of worse graft dysfunction.[9,10]

This study of kidney-pancreas transplants also reported the almost universal presence of CNI toxicity posttransplantation. Signs of CNI toxicity were often present within the first year, and became almost universal thereafter.[7] CNI toxicity is associated with later CAN. Glomerulosclerosis is seen at a later stage, and is more likely in those with earlier changes of fibrosis and in those who have changes in CNI toxicity.[11]

In a study of 266 patients with protocol biopsies at 6, 12, and 26 weeks posttransplantation, 5% had changes of CAN at 6 weeks and 11% at 12 weeks—and 37% of transplants showed grade I CAN changes at 26 weeks.[12] The strongest risk factor for chronic changes at 6 months was a reduced estimated glomerular filtration rate at 12 weeks, and indeed in this study a lower glomerular filtration rate was already evident at 6 weeks. Other risk factors were acute rejection episodes before 12 weeks, nephrocalcinosis, arterionephrosclerosis, cold ischemia time (ischemia/reperfusion injury), and nonliving donation.

Etiology of CAN

The causes of CAN are many and include immune and nonimmune factors.

Immunologic Factors

There is good evidence that alloimmune processes are important in the development of CAN, and most aspects of the immune response are implicated. Studies in CAN have implicated direct and indirect cellular responses, as well as humoral responses.[13] CAN is more common in those who have had acute rejection episodes,[14] where there is a higher preformed antibody level before transplantation[15] and where there is de novo production of antidonor human leukocyte antigen (HLA).[16] Further indirect evidence of an immunologic role is the association of CAN with underimmunosuppression[17] and the fact that the incidence of CAN is lower in HLA-identical recipients compared with recipients with HLA mismatches.[14]

The role of acute rejection episodes is not entirely straightforward. Acute rejection episodes are associated with an increased risk of graft failure (the half-life in cadaveric grafts was 6.6 years compared to 12.5 years when there was no acute rejection).[18] However, not all acute rejection episodes result in an increased risk of graft failure. Vascular rejection,[19] repeated episodes,[20] episodes that do not resolve,[21] and late acute rejection episodes[22] are those most strongly linked to the development of CAN.

Late acute rejection remains a significant problem in the pediatric population. The 2006 NAPRTCS report records that out of 3897 pediatric kidney recipients who were rejection free at 1 year posttransplantation 827 (21.2%) subsequently experienced an acute rejection episode (i.e., a late first rejection). Treatment of these rejection episodes resulted in complete reversal in 40.6% of cases, and 53.6% were partially reversed. There were 42 (5.1%) graft failures. This complete reversal rate was lower than the overall reversal rate observed after a first rejection episode, which was 61% in living donor recipients and 55% in deceased donor recipients.[1] Earlier data from the same group showed the rate of late first rejection to be higher among 6- to 12-year-olds and 13- to 17-year-olds compared with the younger age groups.[23]

The adolescent group also had significantly lower rates of reversal of rejection (early and late acute rejection combined) than the other age groups combined. Late acute rejection is also a significant cause of graft loss. Analysis of the United

TABLE 61-2 **Banff Classification for Chronic Allograft Nephropathy***

Grade	Histopathologic Findings	Quantitative Criteria for Interstitial Fibrosis (ci)	Quantitative Criteria for Tubular Atrophy (ct)	Quantitative Criteria for Allograft Glomerulopathy (cg)	Quantitative Criteria for Mesangial Matrix Increase (mm)	Quantitative Criteria for Vascular Fibrous Intimal Thickening (cv)
		ci0—Interstitial fibrosis in up to 5% of cortical area	ct0—No tubular atrophy	cg0—No glomerulopathy; double contours in <10% of peripheral capillary loops in the most severely affected glomeruli	mm0—No mesangial matrix increase	cv0—No chronic vascular changes
I (mild)	Mild interstitial fibrosis and tubular atrophy without (a) or with (b) specific changes suggesting chronic rejection	ci1—Interstitial fibrosis in 6% to 25% of cortical area	ct1—Tubular atrophy in up to 25% of the area of cortical tubules	cg1—Double contours affecting up to 25% of peripheral capillary loops in the most severely affected glomeruli	mm1—Up to 25% of nonsclerotic glomeruli affected (at least moderate matrix increase)	cv1—Vascular narrowing of up to 25% luminal area by fibrointimal thickening of arteries + breach of internal elastic lamina or presence of foam cells or mononuclear cells†
II (moderate)	Moderate interstitial fibrosis and tubular atrophy (a) or (b)	ci2—Interstitial fibrosis in 26% to 50% of cortical area	ct2—Tubular atrophy involving 26% to 50% of the area of cortical tubules	cg2—Double contours affecting 26% to 50% of peripheral capillary loops in the most severely affected glomeruli	mm2—26% to 50% of nonsclerotic glomeruli affected (at least moderate matrix increase)	cv2—Increased severity of changes described above with 26% to 50% narrowing of vascular luminal area†
III (severe)	Severe interstitial fibrosis and tubular atrophy and tubular loss (a) or (b)	ci3—Interstitial fibrosis in >50% of cortical area	ct3—Tubular atrophy in >50% of the area of cortical tubules	cg3—Double contours affecting >50% of peripheral capillary loops in the most severely affected glomeruli	mm3—>50% of nonsclerotic glomeruli affected (at least moderate matrix increase)	cv3—Severe vascular changes with >50% narrowing of vascular luminal area†
					The threshold criterion for the moderately increased mm is the expanded mesangial interspace between adjacent capillaries. If the width of interspace exceeds two mesangial cells on average in at least two glomerular lobules, the mm is moderately increased.	

* Glomerular and vascular changes in lesions help define type of chronic nephropathy. Chronic rejection can be diagnosed if typical vascular lesions are seen. An adequate specimen is one with 10 or more glomeruli and at least 2 arteries. The threshold for a minimal sample is 7 glomeruli and 1 artery.
† In the most severely affected vessel.
Adapted from Racusen L, et al: The Banff 97 working classification of renal allograft pathology, *Kidney Int* 55:713-23, 1999.

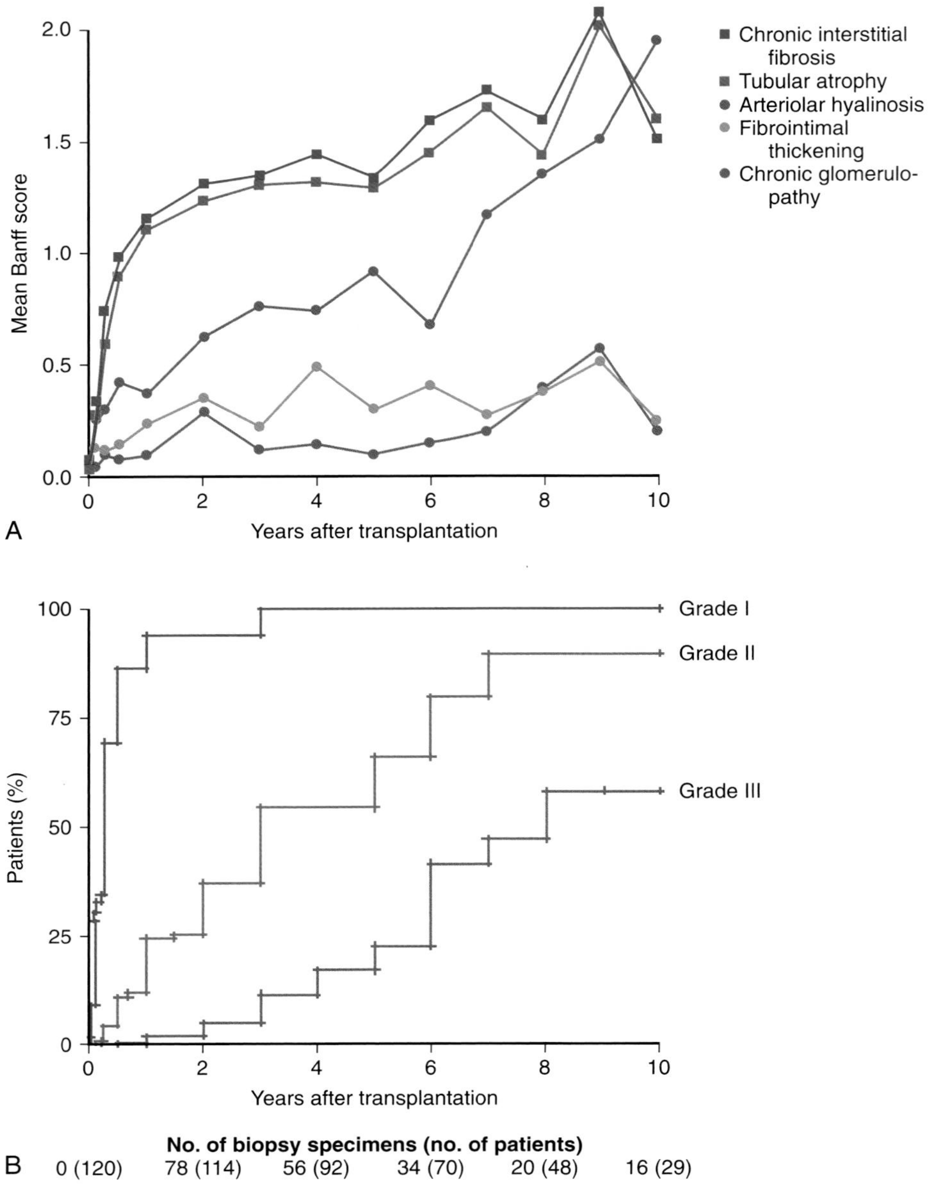

Figure 61-6 **A,** Mean Banff score for each chronic element in protocol renal biopsies taken over 10 years. **B,** Prevalence of mild (CAN I), moderate (CAN II), and severe (CAN III) chronic allograft nephropathy up to 10 years post renal transplantation. (From Nankivell BJ, et al: The natural history of chronic allograft nephropathy, *New Engl J Med* 349:2326, 2003.)

Network for Organ Sharing (UNOS) database has shown late acute rejection to be the cause of graft failure in 14% of adolescents compared with 7% in other age groups. The adolescent group is known to have the poorest long-term graft survival of all age groups (a 5-year graft survival of 77.3% compared with 83.4%, 81.2%, and 81.4%, respectively, in the 6- to 12-, 2- to 5-, and 0- to 1-year age groups for living donor grafts).[23]

A number of causes of late acute rejection have been identified. A small number of cases may occur following attempts on the part of the transplant team to minimize immunosuppression toward reducing long-term adverse effects. Other cases may occur secondarily to viral or other infections. However, nonadherence with immunosuppressive therapy is by far the most significant cause, and some authorities have gone as far as to state that all cases of late acute rejection in children should be considered to be secondary to nonadherence until proved otherwise.

Humoral rejection is increasingly being recognized as important in a subset of patients with CAN. These patients tend to have high preformed antibody levels prior to transplantation, and histology is more likely to show transplant glomerulopathy. C4d staining of the peritubular capillaries is a useful marker in these patients.[24]

Nonimmunologic Factors

Many nonimmunologic factors contribute to CAN, some of which can be distinguished histologically and some of which cannot. Such factors include disease in the donor kidney, ischemia, obstruction, hypertension, recurrence of the original kidney disease, infection (cytomegalovirus [CMV], BK virus), and CNI toxicity. Several studies have examined factors predictive of the development of CAN. Such factors represent stresses to the allograft.

Increased Donor Age Advancing donor age has been shown to be associated with reduced graft survival,[25] which may represent reduced functional renal mass—although other factors (such as donor hypertension or arteriosclerosis) may be important.

Brain Death Brain death, through hemodynamic and neurohormonal changes, reduces the viability of deceased donor kidneys.[26] Deceased donor kidneys are more likely to develop CAN than kidneys from living donors.[27]

Preservation Injury, Cold Ischemia Time, and Delayed Graft Function

Ischemia/reperfusion injury, often associated with brain death, contributes to the incidence of delayed graft function. In some series, delayed graft function is associated with reduced graft survival. Delayed graft function, which is usually associated with acute tubular necrosis, may result in a reduced number of functioning nephrons. Delayed function is more likely with older donors, in whom the number of functional glomeruli is already reduced. With ischemia, there is increased expression of cytokines, adhesion molecules, and HLA-DR molecules—and delayed graft function can be associated with acute rejection episodes. Graft outcome with delayed graft function and acute rejection episodes is worse than with delayed graft function alone.[28]

Hypertension In addition to increasing the risk of cardiovascular events and end-organ damage (including left ventricular hypertrophy), systolic and diastolic hypertension are known to be independently associated with a subsequent gradual deterioration of renal function and graft failure in adult transplant recipients.[29] Hypertension also exacerbates proteinuria, which is also known to be an independent risk factor for progression of renal disease. Known risk factors for posttransplantation hypertension include obesity, renal artery stenosis, the use of corticosteroids and CNIs, acute and chronic graft dysfunction, recurrent or de novo glomerulonephritis, high renin release from native kidneys, and the presence of angiotensin-converting enzyme (ACE) gene polymorphisms.[30]

The incidence of posttransplantation hypertension in children is high, NAPRTCS data on 277 children reporting that 70% required antihypertensive therapy at 1 month posttransplantation compared with 48% pretransplantation (this figure falling to 59% by 2 years posttransplantation).[31] These data are supported by those from recent prospective randomized controlled trials (RCTs) in pediatric renal transplantation. In a large European study comparing tacrolimus, azathioprine, and corticosteroids with ciclosporin, azathioprine, and corticosteroids, 88.3% of the tacrolimus group and 86.2% of the ciclosporin group received, respectively, a mean of 2.3 and 2.2 antihypertensive medications in the first 6 months posttransplantation.[32] Corticosteroid-free regimens are associated with significantly lower incidences of hypertension—Saarwal et al. reporting a rate of hypertension of 14.3% in steroid-free patients at a mean of 20 months posttransplantation, the corresponding figure in steroid-treated patients being 57% ($p = 0.002$).[33]

Hyperlipidemia In addition to the potential benefit of lowering the risk of cardiovascular disease, a reduction in plasma cholesterol levels may reduce the rate of glomerulosclerosis. Lipids are thought to be implicated in the pathogenesis of nephrosclerosis, and the lowering of plasma cholesterol levels might reduce the rate of nephron loss in patients with renal transplants (as has been shown in a number of small trials in patients with progressive renal dysfunction).[34-36]

Calcineurin Inhibitor Toxicity The introduction of ciclosporin in the mid-1980s was associated with a significant reduction in acute rejection and a subsequent marked improvement in short-term graft survival. However, the predicted increase in long-term graft survival that should have followed was not seen. The development of CNI toxicity and subsequent CAN explains much of this phenomenon. Protocol biopsy studies have shown that CNI toxicity can be seen as early as 3 months, and by 5 years it is present in greater than 93% of biopsies.[7]

The two CNIs in common use are ciclosporin and tacrolimus. Both inhibit T-cell activation by reducing the production of Il-2. They also cause dose-dependent acute and reversible afferent arteriolar vasoconstriction, which can cause acute renal dysfunction associated with a reduction in glomerular filtration rate, hyperkalemia, hypertension, renal tubular acidosis, increased reabsorption of sodium, and oliguria.[37] Histologically acute CNI toxicity is diagnosed by isometric tubular vacuolation, endothelial cell swelling, mucoid intimal thickening, eosinophilic globules in the media, and focal medial necrosis. Prolonged therapy results in arterial wall destruction with myointimal necrosis, narrowing of the arterial lumen, and arteriolar hyaline deposits consisting of fibrin, IgM, C3, and C1q (Figure 61-7).

Arteriolar myocyte vacuolization may be seen. Striped fibrosis with tubular atrophy, due to arteriolar spasm, is seen in the interstitium. The fibrosis begins in the medulla and extends to the medullary rays of the cortex. These changes are not dose dependent and are not reversible. The vascular lesions may improve with cessation of the CNI, but the fibrosis is unaltered. The pathophysiology is not entirely clear, but may be due to continuing chronic ischemia (from vasoconstriction). However, there is also evidence in animal models to suggest that the renin-angiotensin system and inhibition of nitric oxide may be involved. Renin-angiotensin system blockade has been shown to be protective in terms of preventing the development of fibrosis, reducing expression of transforming growth factor (TGF-β), and preventing programmed cell death.[38]

That ciclosporin and tacrolimus can cause renal failure is evident from the number of nonrenal organ transplant recipients who develop renal insufficiency when on treatment with CNIs.[39] Renal dysfunction is also seen in patients on ciclosporin for autoimmune disease.[40]

Other Factors Other factors (such as CMV infection, BK virus, and recurrence of the original disease) can result in chronic changes evident upon biopsy, which with time may become indistinguishable from CAN.

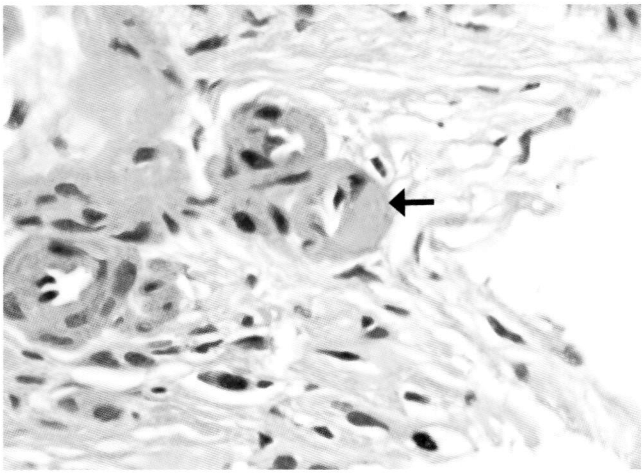

Figure 61-7 H&E stained section showing nodular hyalinosis, indicated by the arrow, in a small arteriole from a patient with ciclosporin toxicity. (Courtesy of Barbara Young.)

TABLE 61-3 Prevention and Management of Early Chronic Allograft Nephropathy

Pretransplant
Avoidance of older/marginal donors
Minimize cold ischemia time
Minimize chances of ATN
Posttransplant
Prevention and prompt treatment of acute rejection +/– the use of protocol biopsies
Reduce, avoid, or stop CNIs
Use or switch to MMF
Maintain blood pressure within range for age
Screening for viral infections
Awareness of compliance/concordance issues

ATN, Acute tubular necrosis; *CNIs*, calcineurin inhibitors; *MMF*, mycophenolate mofetil.

Pathophysiology of CAN

The many and varied factors contributing to CAN cause damage to the graft through a number of pathophysiologic mechanisms. These include ischemic damage to tubules from sclerosed glomeruli, injury to the peritubular capillaries, and ongoing damage as a result of low-grade inflammation from incompletely resolved rejection. Accelerated senescence has also been postulated as a mechanism (e.g., telomere shortening has been seen in transplanted kidneys along with other markers of cell aging).[41] This might explain the worse outcome that is seen with older donor kidneys.

Hyperfiltration, hypertension, and proteinuria may aggravate the damage and cause further sclerosis. The renin-angiotensin system has been implicated. Other possible mechanisms include overproduction of reactive oxygen species and cytokines such as TGF-β and IFN-γ, which are profibrotic. TGF-β has been studied extensively and is associated with matrix production and inhibition of matrix degradation, as well as with the transformation of epithelial cells into myofibroblasts (all of these processes resulting in increased fibrosis).[42] Many other factors, such as angiotensin II and endothelin-1, are implicated in promoting fibrosis and are summarized in a recent review that includes potential treatments for limiting fibrosis.[42] The cytokine genotype of the recipient may be an important modifying factor.[43]

Prevention of CAN

Are there strategies that might prevent the development of CAN? When considering the etiologies and pathophysiology, one would assume that better HLA matching, avoidance of acute rejection, the use of both younger and more living donors, and reduction in cold ischemia time should reduce the occurrence of CAN. It is difficult to study any of these factors in isolation. In addition to addressing donor factors, recipient factors are also important (such as avoidance of hypertension, diabetes, and hyperlipidemia)—and importantly there is the effect of immunosuppression on graft outcome. Table 61-3 summarizes potential management strategies for minimizing CAN.

The long-term course of CAN is such that any intervention studies will require many years of follow-up to determine effect. In the short term, reliance is placed on surrogate markers in looking for change. Renal function and histologic change on early biopsies have been proposed as surrogate markers of CAN.

Treatment of Hypertension

There is much debate regarding the best method for diagnosing hypertension in children following renal transplantation, with many units now adopting ambulatory blood pressure monitoring (ABPM) as routine. However, there are fewer data regarding epidemiology and outcomes using this method. This is well reviewed elsewhere.[44]

A number of antihypertensive agents are routinely used in children following renal transplantation, commonly the calcium channel antagonists in the early posttransplantation period and the ACE inhibitors and/or angiotensin (II) recetor blockers (ARBs) at a later stage once graft function has stabilized. These latter agents are theoretically advantageous given that they are known to be more effective than other antihypertensive agents in slowing the rate of progression of diabetic and nondiabetic proteinuric renal disease[45,46] and have been shown to have other nephroprotective properties.[47]

Although hypertension has been identified as an independent risk factor for deterioration of allograft function, there are no published intervention studies in either adults or children demonstrating that the maintenance of blood pressure within the normal range by the use of antihypertensive agents improves allograft survival. It is at present unclear whether casual blood pressure measurement or ABPM monitoring should be used to detect hypertension and to monitor the efficacy of antihypertensive therapy.

Based on the finding that tight blood pressure control may improve outcomes in native renal disease, many have argued that transplant recipients should have target blood pressures below those set for the general population. Evidence to support this approach is also lacking, and it may be that the additional drug therapy needed to achieve this goal compounds the problems of polypharmacy and its associated adherence issues in the teenage population. Hypertension is associated with progression of renal dysfunction and predisposes to atherosclerosis. It is also associated with graft loss in a dose-dependent fashion. This is discussed further in material following.

Treatment of Subclinical Rejection

Protocol biopsy studies have shown the presence of subclinical acute rejection in patients with stable graft function.[7,48] The presence of subclinical rejection is predictive of a higher serum creatinine at 2 years[48] and of worse outcome.[9] Furthermore, treatment of subclinical rejection has been associated with a better outcome.[48,49] In one study, patients with subclinical rejection on 1-month biopsies were treated with augmented immunosuppression. Treatment was associated with a reduction in chronic changes on later biopsies.[49] Another study randomized patients to undergo protocol biopsies and treatment of subclinical rejection or to have no protocol biopsies.[48]

Those who were biopsied and treated were found to have less tubular atrophy and fibrosis at 6 months, and a lower plasma creatinine at 2 years. A retrospective study in children showed an improved glomerular filtration rate at 18 months posttransplantation in patients who had a protocol biopsy at 3 months (with treatment of subclinical rejection where present with methylprednisolone and augmentation of baseline immunosuppression) compared to a historic control group who did not have a protocol biopsy at 3 months.[50]

Alteration of Immunosuppressive Treatment

Few studies have prospectively assessed the effects of various immunosuppressive regimens on the incidence of CAN. Indeed, most studies report the effect on chronic allograft failure rather than CAN. Chronic allograft failure is a clinical rather than histologic definition, being graft loss beyond 6 months posttransplantation—censored for patient death or graft loss secondary to acute rejection, graft thrombosis, infection, surgical complications, or recurrent disease.

Calcineurin Inhibitors Despite being responsible for significant improvements in short-term graft survival, it is well established that CNIs are associated with chronic nephrotoxicity. Nankivell demonstrated that CNI toxicity was evident in greater than 90% of biopsies by 5 years, and 100% by 10 years.[7] There are 15-year follow-up data showing that adult patients managed on continuous ciclosporin therapy have a worse graft function and survival compared to those randomized to 3 months of ciclosporin followed by azathioprine and prednisolone.[51]

Ciclosporin versus Tacrolimus A RCT in pediatric recipients comparing ciclosporin to tacrolimus reported lower acute rejection rates and superior graft survival and renal function with tacrolimus.[32,52] The beneficial effect of tacrolimus on glomerular filtration rate may be due to the effects of reduced acute rejection episodes or to the fact that it is less nephrotoxic. No histologic data are available from this study.

Protocol biopsy studies show that tacrolimus treatment is associated with less interstitial fibrosis and a lower expression of the fibrotic precursors TGF-β, thrombospondin, and fibronectin than ciclosporin.[53] This RCT showed that there was less CAN in patients treated with tacrolimus than those treated with ciclosporin, although this was not found in the earlier FK506 Kidney Transplant Study Group trial.[54] There is also conflicting evidence of the effect of conversion of ciclosporin to tacrolimus once CAN has developed. One study reported no benefit,[55] whereas a more recent study has shown that conversion to tacrolimus in patients with established CAN is associated with an improvement in serum creatinine at 12 and 36 months—with a continued deterioration seen in those who remained on ciclosporin.[56]

CNI Withdrawal after the Development of CAN The detection of CNI toxicity on biopsy has prompted the withdrawal of CNI therapy. In the azathioprine era, this resulted in an increase in acute rejection episodes and was associated with an increase in chronic rejection and progressive immunologic injury.[57] When mycophenolate mofetil (MMF) has been substituted for ciclosporin, complete withdrawal of ciclosporin has been possible without an increase in acute rejection episodes.[58] This study of adult patients with established CAN reported an improvement in renal function (without acute rejection episodes)—after commencing MMF over 4 weeks and reducing and then stopping ciclosporin over the following 6 weeks—compared with patients who remained on ciclosporin.

It is difficult to know whether the beneficial effects are due to withdrawal of CNI or to addition of MMF, or indeed to both. There are many reports of patients with CAN or chronic allograft dysfunction for whom the dose of CNI has been reduced or stopped after the addition of MMF or sirolimus.[59-61] Most studies report an improvement in plasma creatinine, but none have shown any effect on graft or patient survival (although follow-up has been relatively short). Meta-analysis of studies performed in adults has shown that the late withdrawal of CNIs is associated with a significant increase in the rate of acute rejection [pooled difference 0.11 (95% CI 0.07-0.15)], although the relative risk of graft loss is not increased [RR 1.06 (95% CI 0.81-1.29)].[57] CNI withdrawal in pediatric patients has produced similar results.[62]

Early Withdrawal of CNI Many of the studies of CNI withdrawal have been in patients with chronic allograft dysfunction, where there are already extensive histologic changes on biopsy. Other studies have withdrawn CNI as early as 3 to 4 months posttransplantation. In one study, patients received sirolimus, ciclosporin, and prednisolone for 3 months and then were randomized to either withdrawal or continuation of ciclosporin.[63] Following ciclosporin withdrawal, there was no increase in the incidence of acute rejection episodes—but glomerular filtration rate was improved and biopsy at 3 years showed less CAN than in those who remained on CNI.

CNI Avoidance The results of studies investigating the complete avoidance of CNIs are currently being reported. As discussed further in material following, in adult transplant recipients the incidence of normal biopsies (Banff 0) 2 years posttransplantation was higher in patients treated with basiliximab, sirolimus, MMF, and prednisone than in those receiving basiliximab, ciclosporin, MMF, and prednisone.[64] A similar study comparing sirolimus, MMF, and prednisone with tacrolimus, MMF, and prednisone reported similar Banff chronicity scores at 1 year for interstitial, tubular, and glomerular changes. However, there were fewer chronic vascular changes in the sirolimus group.[65]

Calcineurin-free protocols have been possible using some of the newer immunosuppressive agents (discussed further in material following). These agents require consideration in their own right, as there may be reasons their use is associated with less CAN.

Mycophenolate Mofetil MMF, the prodrug of mycophenolic acid (MPA), is a potent antimetabolite that has a number of other effects that could be of potential benefit in CAN. These have recently been reviewed by Allison and Eugui.[66] MMF inhibits the proliferation of T and B lymphocytes, and decreases the production of antibody by B lymphocytes. It increases T-cell apoptosis and under some conditions eliminates T cells responding to specific antigen and thus could promote tolerance. It suppresses the induction of cytotoxic T cells, thereby reducing rejection. Its actions on B cells theoretically reduce the production of donor-specific antibody, which is increasingly recognized as playing an important role in chronic rejection and CAN.

Furthermore, MPA suppresses the ability of dendritic cells to act as antigen-presenting cells by reducing expression of major histocompatability complex and costimulatory molecules. Perhaps its most interesting role is its ability to reduce recruitment of monocytes into the graft, thereby reducing production of proinflammatory cytokines. It does this through a number of mechanisms, including an effect on the vascular endothelium. MPA can induce apoptosis of monocytes and can affect the type of cytokines they can produce. It can also suppress i-NOS production.

MPA has an antifibrotic effect through decreased production of TNF-α and IL-1, and notably (unlike the CNIs) does not have an effect on TGF-β. MMF has also been shown to suppress smooth-muscle cell proliferation and therefore could have a role in attenuating the proliferative arteriopathy seen in chronic rejection. MMF is able to potentiate the effect of ACE inhibitors and ARBs in reducing proteinuria and monocyte infiltration in the rat remnant kidney.[67]

Has the theory been borne out in practice? When used without a CNI, MMF regimens are associated with a high rate of acute rejection episodes.[68] However, compared to azathioprine or placebo, MMF when used in conjunction with ciclosporin and prednisolone decreased the incidence of early acute rejection—and renal function was superior at all time points during the first year. Graft survival was no different at 1 year, but death-censored graft survival was improved at 3 years compared to placebo.[69] These studies were underpowered to look at graft survival. However, United States Renal Data System (USRDS) registry data have shown that at 4 years patients on MMF have improved survival, improved death-censored graft survival (86 vs. 82%, $p < 0.001$), and reduced cumulative risk for chronic allograft failure compared with patients receiving azathioprine.[70]

The latter was true for patients with and without acute rejection episodes. Even after controlling for acute rejection episodes, the risk of graft loss was reduced by 27%. MMF thus appears to have an effect on CAN that is independent of acute rejection. As these are registry data, it is difficult to interpret the mechanism. In particular, no information is given as to the dose of CNI used or whether it is less than in the patients receiving azathioprine. However, a Spanish study of adult recipients with CAN receiving ciclosporin and prednisolone, with or without azathioprine, had MMF either added to the regimen or substituted for azathioprine.[71] In this group of patients, treatment with MMF reduced the progressive deterioration of renal function (an effect independent of ciclosporin blood levels).

Most studies report the effects of immunosuppressive therapy on graft survival or acute rejection episodes. However, one study has examined the effect of MMF on the incidence of biopsy-proven CAN. In a study of adult patients receiving ciclosporin, steroids, and azathioprine or MMF, the prevalence of CAN in the intention-to-treat analysis at 1 year was lower in protocol biopsies in patients receiving MMF (46% versus 71%).[72]

A nonrandomized study reported the effects of regimens of ciclosporin and azathioprine, ciclosporin and MMF, and tacrolimus and MMF on 1-year chronic interstitial fibrosis and tubular atrophy scores.[11] The lowest scores were seen with tacrolimus and MMF, followed by ciclosporin and MMF and then ciclosporin and azathioprine. The combination of tacrolimus and MMF markedly reduced the incidence of subclinical rejection at 3 months in the same study—subclinical rejection being a risk factor for CAN.

Overall, there would appear to be early evidence that MMF has a role in reducing the incidence of CAN. MMF and tacrolimus appear to be a good combination. Scientific Renal Transplant Registry (SRTR) data suggest that recipients receiving tacrolimus and MMF do better than those receiving ciclosporin and MMF or those on tacrolimus and sirolimus,[73] and the early results of the Symphony Study show that acute rejection, graft function, and graft survival are superior with MMF and tacrolimus compared to standard or low-dose ciclosporin and MMF or to sirolimus and MMF.[74] The combination of tacrolimus and MMF has also been shown to be effective in controlling antibody-mediated rejection.[75]

There are no RCT data of the use of MMF in pediatric renal transplantation, but Henne et al. reported 36 pediatric patients with CAN who had MMF added to their immunosuppressive regimen or substituted for azathioprine.[76] After 1 year, glomerular filtration rate had improved in 61% and remained stable in 22%.

Sirolimus Sirolimus is a potent immunosuppressive antiproliferative drug that acts to reduce Il-2–induced proliferation of lymphocytes by binding to FK binding protein and forming a complex that binds to the protein kinase mTOR. This in turn inactivates signal transduction pathways and causes cell cycle arrest.[77] The antiproliferative effects on cells such as vascular endothelium and fibroblasts offer potential benefits in preventing or reducing CAN, but these same antiproliferative effects are likely to be responsible for poor wound healing, bone marrow suppression, and impairment of renal function.[78]

Sirolimus has minimal nephrotoxicity of its own, but unfortunately has been shown to increase the nephrotoxicity of ciclosporin. It has been used as a means of reducing or avoiding CNI. However, when used without a CNI its potency is in question.[79] When used with a CNI, there are low acute rejection rates but an increase in creatinine and reduction in glomerular filtration rate.[80]

Enhanced CNI toxicity was thought likely to be lower when sirolimus was used with tacrolimus, but this does not appear to be the case.[81] Registry data show reduced patient and graft survival at 3 years with sirolimus and tacrolimus compared to tacrolimus and MMF, with high-risk patients faring the worst.[73] Although there was no difference in acute rejection rate, the graft survival curves diverge with time—which is suggestive of ongoing nephrotoxicity.

A metaanalysis suggests that replacement of CNI in a triple regimen with an mTOR inhibitor does not alter acute rejection rates, and increases calculated glomerular filtration rate at 1 year.[82] There is, however, an increase in the development of lymphoceles, in bone marrow suppression, and in plasma lipid levels. Poor wound healing has been noted. Replacement of an antimetabolite with an mTOR inhibitor in a CNI-based triple regimen reduces acute rejection by about 23% but reduces estimated glomerular filtration rate by approximately 8 ml/min.[82] RCTs have shown poorer graft survival with a combination of sirolimus and CNI compared to withdrawal of the CNI at 2 to 4 months[83] or compared to ciclosporin and MMF.[84]

The studies that withdrew a CNI at 3 months showed that CADI scores improved, but surprisingly even at 3 months significant histologic changes were already present.[63] Studies have examined the avoidance of a CNI altogether. Flechner reported comparable results using basiliximab, MMF, prednisolone, and either sirolimus or ciclosporin.[64] Another approach has been to use tacrolimus rather than ciclosporin, and Larson has recently compared tacrolimus, MMF, and prednisolone with sirolimus, MMF, and prednisolone.[65] In this study, despite one arm having a CNI there was no difference in acute rejection episodes, no difference in glomerular filtration rate at 2 years, and little difference in Banff CAN scores at 1 year—although the chronic vascular component in the tacrolimus group was more marked.

The Symphony Study has compared several immunosuppressive regimens in a multinational study of 1,645 adult patients, and 1-year follow-up data are now available.[74] Standard triple therapy with ciclosporin, MMF, and corticosteroid was compared with daculzimab induction, corticosteroid and either low-dose ciclosporin and MMF, low-dose tacrolimus and MMF, or low-dose sirolimus and MMF. Biopsy-proven acute rejection occurred less often in the tacrolimus and MMF group compared with all other groups, and graft survival was better than standard triple therapy or sirolimus. Glomerular filtration rate (GFR) was better in the tacrolimus group than any of the other groups, including the sirolimus and MMF group. This suggests that low-dose tacrolimus with MMF may be an acceptable combination in terms of nephrotoxicity and CAN. Sirolimus has been used in pediatric transplantation, with low rejection rates and good graft outcomes.[85]

ACE Inhibitors For patients who have established CAN, it may be possible to influence the rate of progression. Graft loss is correlated with the degree of proteinuria and hypertension, both of which are amenable to treatment with ACE inhibition or ARBs and other antihypertensive agents as required. Once CAN is present, hypertension, raised creatinine, and proteinuria are risk factors for graft loss.[86]

Can ACE inhibitors or ARBs prevent CAN? A study of the use of Losartan in the first 2 years posttransplantation is addressing this question and is nearing completion.[87] Unfortunately, preliminary results show no benefit of sustained treatment with losartan (started between the fourth and eighth posttransplantation week) on 2 year graft survival, creatinine, or proteinuria—nor on CAN score.

NONADHERENCE

Nonadherence, defined by the World Health Organization (WHO) as "the degree to which the person's behavior corresponds with the agreed recommendations from a health care provider," is a major risk factor for late acute rejection and CAN. It is a common problem after renal transplantation—systematic review in adult subjects having shown that 22% of organ recipients are nonadherent with treatment and that a median of 36% of graft losses are associated with prior nonadherence (the odds of graft failure increasing sevenfold where nonadherence occurs).

A systematic review of studies investigating nonadherence following solid organ transplantation in children and adolescents showed the prevalence of medication nonadherence to be even higher (32%) for kidney recipients (31% for liver recipients and 16% for heart recipients).[88] Nonadherence was associated with very significant adverse clinical outcomes—being an etiologic factor in graft loss in 14.1% of patients.

No studies were found that directly addressed the relationship between nonadherence and late acute rejection in renal transplant recipients, although 33.2% of late acute rejection episodes in liver recipients and 73.3% of late rejection in heart recipients were associated with medication nonadherence. Analysis of risk factors for nonadherence shows these to be multiple and complex. It has been proposed by the WHO that five distinct categories of risk factor exist.

- Socioeconomic factors
- Patient-related factors
- Condition-related factors
- Treatment-related factors
- Factors related to the health care system and health care team

Significant risk factors include adolescence, low socioeconomic status, ethnicity (increased nonadherence has been reported in African Americans), single-parent families and family instability, poor knowledge of medications and disease, learning difficulties, prior history of nonadherence (e.g., while on dialysis), adverse cosmetic side effects of drugs, and the complexity and duration of drug regimen.[88]

Methods of documenting nonadherence include self-reporting by the patient or their family, physical or biochemical markers (absence of cushingoid features or low measured blood drug levels), adverse events related to nonadherence (acute rejection, graft loss), electronic monitoring, and monitoring of pill usage or dispensing records.

Strategies that have been reported to improve adherence include simplification or modification of the drug regimen whereby the number of drugs and doses is reduced by the increased use of once-daily medications. Drugs should be palatable and not be associated with adverse cosmetic effects. The patient should be educated regarding the purpose of the medicine and the importance of adherence, along with relevant information about adverse effects. Small reward systems may be effective. Many children and adolescents find the use of a dosette box and/or the use of cues (medicines being taken at meal times or at tooth brushing) or alarm systems (digital watches, mobile phones) helpful.

It is important that the family support the child, and many also find peer support groups helpful. Finally, it is important that the transplant team hold regular frank and open discussions about nonadherence with all of their patients—particularly those older children and adolescents in the high-risk age group. It is also important that they arrange for early intervention by a psychologist, psychiatrist, or other appropriate health care professional where significant problems arise.

THE ABNORMALLY FUNCTIONING BLADDER

Transplantation into the dysfunctional lower urinary tract has historically been associated with high complication rates and inferior graft survival.[89,90] The goal of treatment in patients with renal failure secondary to a dysfunctional lower urinary tract is to provide a sterile, compliant, nonrefluxing low-pressure reservoir that is continent and easily emptied. With improvements in the understanding of the importance of bladder function and the introduction of routine urodynamic assessment, anticholinergic therapies, clean intermittent catheterization (CIC), and the surgical technique of augmentation enterocystoplasty (which has in the large majority of patients replaced urinary diversion by means of urinary conduit formation), outcomes have improved.

The largest pediatric series reports 31 transplants in 30 children, 17 of which had augmented bladders, 12 incontinent urinary conduits, and 1 a continent urinary reservoir.[91] Although no details are provided about donor source, graft survival (90% at 1 year, 78% at 5 years, and 60% at 10 years) was comparable to overall NAPRTCS graft survival data from the same time period. Importantly, in all of the 11 cases where the grafts were lost the causes of graft loss were predominantly immunologic (similar to those in children with normal bladders). Although 68% of these children were affected by symptomatic urinary tract infections, it was not felt that these were associated with graft loss. Similar good graft survival data have been reported in other series,[92-95] although urinary tract infection, nephrolithiasis, and metabolic acidosis are commonly reported complications.

Deterioration of renal function in the transplant recipient with an abnormal lower urinary tract should prompt urgent investigation, including culture of the urine to exclude infection, ultrasound examination, and repeat urodynamic assessment where a high-pressure system, incomplete bladder emptying, or other significant abnormality is suspected. The potential for noncompliance with CIC, anticholinergic therapy, or an antibiotic regimen is great and needs to be discussed and appropriately managed at an early stage.

RECURRENT AND DE NOVO GLOMERULAR DISEASE

In adult transplant recipients, recurrent and de novo disease was reported to be detected in 3.4% of patients at a mean period of 678 days posttransplantation.[96] In this series of 4,913 patients reported from the Renal Allograft Disease Register, the mean number of days (and range) to diagnosis of recurrent focal segmental glomerulosclerosis (FSGS), mesangiocapillary glomerulonephritis, membranous nephropathy, and IgA nephropathy was, respectively, 475 (range, 5-2280), 594 (range, 155-1708), 664 (range, 88-2365), and 846 (range, 155-2325) days.

During a mean period of follow-up of 65 months, those patients with recurrent and de novo disease had a significantly higher rate of graft failure than those without recurrent disease (55% versus 25%, $p < 0.001$). With the fall in the incidence of acute rejection, recurrent disease now ranks as the third most common cause of graft loss in adult patients after CAN and death with a functioning graft.[97,98]

No good data exist regarding the incidence of recurrent disease in pediatric transplant recipients. The 2006 NAPRTCS report shows recurrent disease to be the cause of 174 of 2556 (6.8%) graft losses and 8 of 510 (1.6%) deaths. The most commonly recurring diseases were FSGS (78 cases), hemolytic uremic syndrome,[16] mesangiocapillary glomerulonephritis,[16] and oxalosis.[1,10] Only 0.3% of graft losses were secondary to de novo disease.

This section focuses on recurrent and de novo membranous nephropathy and recurrent SLE, both of which occur late posttransplantation in children. Other recurrent glomerular diseases that present early in the posttransplantation period [particularly FSGS and hemolytic uremic syndrome (HUS)[99]] are discussed Chapter 60.

RECURRENT AND DE NOVO MEMBRANOUS NEPHROPATHY

Membranous nephropathy (MN) is a rare cause of end-stage renal failure (ESRF) in children. Of 8990 transplant recipients registered on the NAPRTCS database, only 41 (0.5%) had MN recorded as the cause of their ESRF[1] and only one case is recorded among 1695 (0.06%) children with ESRF in the British Association for Paediatric Nephrology database. The number of cases of recurrent disease is therefore likely to be very small.

Recurrent MN is defined as MN occurring in the transplanted kidney in a patient known to have developed ESRF secondarily to MN. More commonly, MN presents in the transplanted kidney where an alternative disease was the cause of the ESRF (i.e., de novo MN). There is a third group of patients in whom the cause of their ESRF remains unknown and where MN develops in the transplanted kidney. In this situation, it is not possible to determine whether this represents recurrent or de novo disease.

There is marked variation in the reported prevalence of both de novo and recurrent MN in large series of adult patients. Of the 4913 patients reported by the Renal Allograft Disease Registry, 8 had recurrent MN and 8 had de novo MN at a mean of 664 (range, 88-2365) days posttransplantation.[96] In contrast, Schwartz et al. detected de novo MN in 21 of 848 patients undergoing 1029 transplants—this being the second most common cause of nephrotic range proteinuria after CAN.[100]

Elsewhere, the prevalence of de novo MN in adult patients has been reported as 0.4% to 9.2% of all transplant recipients—and that of recurrent MN as high as 29% to 50%.[101] These and other data clearly indicate the higher overall incidence of de novo compared to recurrent disease. The variation in the reported prevalence may be accounted for by differences in duration of follow-up and variation in practice regarding indications for biopsy, including whether routine protocol biopsies are performed.

Attempts to identify risk factors for recurrent and de novo MN have produced inconsistent results, with small numbers generally precluding any form of meaningful analysis. The Renal Allograft Disease Registry report noted an overall preponderance of males among those with all forms of recurrent and de novo disease, although this did not reach statistical significance. Of the 16 patients with MN, 15 (93.8%) were male.[96]

Recurrent and de novo MN present with proteinuria of varying degrees. Renal function is generally preserved in the early stages. In contrast to idiopathic MN in the native kidney, the rate of spontaneous remission is very low. No specific therapy has been shown to be consistently effective, although success in adult patients has been reported with the use of pulse intravenous methylprednisolone.[102] General measures (similar to those for any patient with proteinuria) should include the use of ACE inhibition and angiotensin receptor blockade, meticulous control of blood pressure, and the use of lipid-lowering therapy where indicated.

Whether recurrent or de novo MN results in an increased rate of graft loss remains controversial. Smaller series of adult patients have reported a number of patients who rapidly lost their grafts, particularly those who had nephrotic range proteinuria or impaired renal function at diagnosis.[103] However, the Renal Allograft Disease Registry did not identify recurrent or de novo MN as a risk factor for graft loss ($p = 0.13$). Briganti et al. reported similar findings [unadjusted hazard ratio for allograft loss 1.58 (95% CI 0.71-3.50, $p = 0.26$)].[104] Where graft loss has occurred in the setting of recurrent or de novo MN, the risk of recurrent or de novo disease in a subsequent graft (although reported) is uncommon and retransplantation is not in any way contraindicated.[105]

LUPUS NEPHRITIS

Recurrent lupus nephritis (LN) was previously thought to be uncommon, occurring in 1% to 4% of transplants (although more recent studies have reported a higher incidence). In the largest series from a single center, Stone et al. reported 106 transplants in 97 consecutive patients, of whom 9 developed recurrent disease at a mean of 3.1 years posttransplantation.[106] This resulted in graft loss in 4 cases. A further recent series reported the outcome of 50 adult transplant recipients.[107] Recurrent LN was detected in 15 of 31 who underwent renal biopsy—an overall rate of recurrence of 30%. The higher rate of detection in these recent studies may be in part accounted for by the routine use of immunofluorescence and electron microscopy on biopsy specimens (features of recurrent WHO class II LN may be missed if light microscopy is used in isolation).

The NAPRTCS 2006 report indicates LN to be the cause of ESRF in 141 of 8990 (1.6%) index renal transplants and 199 of 5993 (3.3%) dialysis patients.[1] The only large pediatric series reporting the outcome of transplantation in children with LN comes from the same organization.[108] Of 94 children who underwent 100 transplants, 1 case of disease recurrence resulted in graft loss—although the study was unable to determine the true incidence of recurrent disease because cases that did not result in graft loss were not captured. Overall, the results of transplantation in children with LN were comparable with those of the control group of children with ESRF secondary to other causes. The incidence of recurrent disease as a cause of graft loss in the LN group (3%) was similar to that in the control group (4%).

POLYOMAVIRUS INFECTION

BK virus (BKV) is a human polyomavirus that causes trivial symptoms in the immunocompetent, although it may cause significant pathology in the immunosuppressed transplant recipient. It was named using the initials of the 39-year-old renal transplant recipient in whom the virus was first recognized as a pathogen.[109] (Additional discussion of this topic is found in Chapter 62.)

Infection is common in the normal childhood population, who generally remain asymptomatic. By 3 years of age, 50% will have detectable antibodies to BKV (rising to nearly 100% by 10 years of age). Antibody titers fall thereafter, and 60% to 80% of adult populations in the United States and Europe have serologic evidence of prior infection.[110-113] The virus is believed to be transmitted from human to human, possibly via respiratory secretions. No animal reservoir is known to exist.[114] Following infection, the virus remains latent in renal and uroepithelial cells.

In the renal transplant recipient, infection may be primary (when BKV infects a patient with no previous exposure to the virus) or secondary, when there is either reactivation of latent infection or reinfection of a previously seropositive individual with a new viral strain. Infection may be acquired in the community or transmitted via the donor organ. Primary infection is a greater problem in younger pediatric recipients because they are more likely to be BKV naive at the time of transplantation. Conversely, in adult recipients infection is most commonly secondary due to reactivation of latent infection—often associated with the treatment of acute rejection.[115,116] Following infection, the transplant recipient may remain asymptomatic or may develop clinical symptoms (including mild fever, lethargy, and gastrointestinal upset).

The most significant clinical manifestation of BKV infection in the renal transplant recipient is BKV nephropathy (BKVN). This generally presents clinically with deterioration in renal function, although with increasing use of protocol biopsies an increasing number of early cases are being detected in which there has been no deterioration in renal function. Progressive renal dysfunction resulting in graft loss is reported to occur in 30% to 60% of adult cases of BKVN,[117] which is known to be associated with inferior graft survival.[118] This rate of graft loss may now be falling with increased recognition of the virus, earlier diagnosis, and earlier treatment by reduction of immunosuppressive therapy (see material following). Less often, BKV infection can cause ureteric stenosis[119] and hemorrhagic cystitis—the latter having been reported in a pediatric kidney recipient[120] (although this is a more common manifestation of BKV infection in bone-marrow–transplant recipients).[121,122]

Renal histology remains the gold standard for diagnosing BKVN, although a number of other tests may indicate the presence of BKV infection and hence the need to consider renal biopsy. The urine may contain decoy cells (virus-infected uroepithelial cells; positive predictive value for diagnosing BKVN 20%), and BKV DNA may be detected by polymerase chain reaction (PCR) in urine (positive predictive value 40%) and in plasma (positive predictive value 60%).[117] A single study has shown that the detection of viral VP1 mRNA in urine has a positive and negative predictive value in excess of 90%.[123] Although lacking in specificity, the detection of BKV DNA in plasma and urine is a very sensitive test and has excellent negative predictive value. Furthermore, the tests may be employed to monitor response to reduction of immunosuppressive therapy and to specific anti-BKV therapy (see material following).

It is important to recognize that the detection of BKV in blood and urine does not necessarily indicate the presence of BKVN, and infection with BKV does not necessarily progress to BKVN. A prospective study in adult patients reported that 29.5% of renal transplant recipients developed decoy cells in the urine at a median of 23 weeks (range, 4-73) and that 13.7% developed BK viremia, although only 6.4% developed BKVN at a median of 28 weeks (range, 8-86) posttransplantation.[116] Other adult studies have reported the median time to development of BKVN to be 9 to 14 months.[124-126] In the largest published pediatric series, 6 of 173 (3.5%) children developed histologically confirmed BKVN at a median of 15 months posttransplantation.[127] A further retrospective review of 100 pediatric kidney recipients reported 70% of children to be BKV seropositive at the time of transplantation. Viruria developed in 26%, and viremia in 5%. Similar to the previously cited study,[127] 3% subsequently developed BVKN.[128] The sole prospective pediatric study reported to date detected BK viruria in 20%, and 4.3% developed BKVN.[129]

Histologically, BKVN is characterized by the presence of severe tubular injury with cellular enlargement, marked nuclear atypia, epithelial necrosis, denudation of tubular basement membranes, focal intratubular neutrophilic infiltration, and mononuclear interstitial infiltration—with or without concurrent tubulitis (Figure 61-8). There may be difficulties in distinguishing these changes (particularly tubulitis) from those of acute rejection, although the presence of intranuclear viral inclusions within the tubular and parietal epithelium of Bowman's capsule suggests BKVN.[114] Specific immunohistochemical studies for BKV may be available in some centers. BKVN may sometimes coexist with the histologic changes of acute rejection. Changes may be focal initially, but late disease is characterized by widespread interstitial fibrosis.

Risk factors for the development of BKVN include the use of the newer, more potent, immunosuppressive agents. Studies that have investigated the effects of specific agents (including tacrolimus and mycophenolate mofetil) have produced conflicting results, although it is clear that prior to the mid-1990s (when these agents were introduced) BKVN was a rare occurrence. In the largest published pediatric series, five of the six cases of BKVN had received MMF as initial

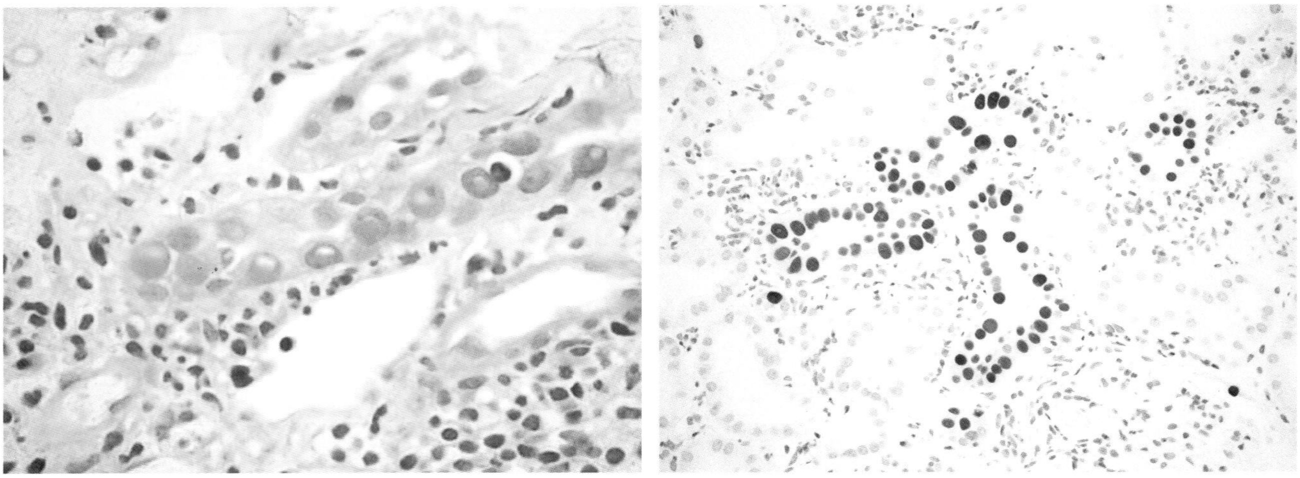

A B

Figure 61-8 **A,** H&E stained section showing characteristic nuclear enlargement of tubular epithelial cells with smudged chromatin and basophilic BKV (polyoma) viral inclusions. **B,** Positive immunohistochemical (peroxidase) staining for SV40, which cross reacts with BKV in tubular epithelial cell nuclei. (Images courtesy of Dr. Ian Roberts and Dr. Lorna McWilliam.)

immunosuppressive therapy and four had developed acute rejection prior to the diagnosis of BKVN.[127]

It is likely to be the overall level of immunosuppression that is important, rather than any particular agent. Increased awareness of the disorder and the availability of diagnostic testing modalities may have in part contributed to the recent apparent rise in disease prevalence. Interestingly, BKVN is very uncommon in the recipients of other solid organs, suggesting that other factors (including graft ischemia) may be of importance.[110] The risk of BKN appears to be greater in pediatric patients among whom a seronegative recipient receives a kidney from a seropositive donor.[127]

There is often a history of recent treatment for acute rejection, and as previously discussed the histologic features of BKVN may be difficult to distinguish from acute rejection. It is likely that the enhanced immunosuppression administered to treat rejection allows enhanced replication of the virus.

Treatment for polyomavirus includes reduction of immunosuppressive therapy, with careful monitoring of the patient to ensure that acute rejection does not ensue. This strategy allows the immune system to regain control over BKV replication and keep latent infection in check. Reported strategies include reduction of CNI dose, reduction in MMF dose, and switching from MMF to azathioprine until viral clearance is achieved. A number of reports have suggested that adopting this approach results in a reduction in the number of cases that progress to graft failure, although both long-term follow-up studies and large RCTs are absent.[130]

Studies in adult patients have shown that a preemptive reduction of immunosuppression following the detection of BK viremia may prevent the development of BKVN.[131] Specific antiviral therapy with cidofovir or leflunomide is known to inibit BKV. Both modalities have been used in the treatment of BKVN,[132-134] although these agents have not been studied in prospective RCTs and experience with their use in children is very limited.[134] Although cidofovir has been clearly shown to reduce viremia, this has also been reported with reduction of immunosuppression alone and trials need to address whether cidofovir should be administered in all patients with BKVN or only in those for whom reduction of immunosuppression has been unsuccessful. Furthermore, cidofovir is known to be nephrotoxic at the dose given for CMV disease. Dose reduction may therefore be indicated.

Retransplantation following graft loss secondary to BKVN has been reported in 15 adult cases, with recurrence occurring in 2. In this situation, it is important to allow enough time following loss of the first graft to mount an antiviral immune response prior to retransplantation—along with removal of the primary allograft if surgically feasible.[135]

RENOVASCULAR LESIONS

Thrombosis

Renal venous and arterial thromboses generally occur early in the posttransplantation period and are discussed in Chapter 60.

Renal Artery Stenosis

Renal artery stenosis (RAS) can present at any time, although it is most commonly detected between 3 months and 2 years posttransplantation. The patient may present with an unexplained deterioration in renal function—where other causes, including rejection, obstruction, and CNI toxicity, have been eliminated—with deteriorating or difficult-to-treat hypertension, or more uncommonly with flash pulmonary edema. Renal function may deteriorate rapidly if intensive diuretic therapy and ACE inhibitors or ARBs are used.

There are few clinical signs of RAS. A bruit may be heard over the graft, although this finding is not specific. Other causes include physiologic vascular turbulence, stenoses in other vessels, and biopsy-induced arteriovenous fistulas. Furthermore, significant RAS has been reported in the absence of an audible bruit.[136]

Series of adult renal transplant recipients report an incidence of RAS of 1% to 23%,[137] with a recent large series reporting an incidence of 4.4%.[138] The reported incidence is likely to vary according to the definition of RAS adopted, the indications for investigation for possible RAS, and the diagnostic modalities employed. In one adult study, the incidence of RAS increased from 2.4% to 12.4% following the introduction of routine Doppler ultrasound examination.[139]

It might be expected that the incidence of RAS in pediatric recipients is somewhat lower, given the lower rate of recipient atherosclerotic disease and the likely lower rate of donor atherosclerotic disease associated with the use of generally younger donors. However, a series from Guy's Hospital, UK, reported the detection of RAS in 30 (8.7%) of 345 pediatric transplants by arteriography—which was performed following the detection of otherwise unexplained deterioration of renal function, difficult-to-control hypertension, or vascular bruit.[140]

Similar incidences of 9.7%, 7.8%, and 4.8% were respectively reported in further large pediatric series from Paris,[141] Los Angeles,[142] and Toronto.[143] Although registry data regarding the overall incidence of RAS are lacking, the NAPRTCS registry has reported that of 2309 grafts lost in North American pediatric recipients 15 (0.65%) were lost to RAS. Fourteen of these were deceased donor grafts.[144]

Stenosis may be detected at the site of the vascular anastamosis. Such lesions are generally related to technical issues, including trauma to the donor vessels during surgery, malpositioning of the kidney, and local endothelial injury from the perfusion catheter tip. These tend to arise early posttransplantation. Preanastamotic and postanastamotic stenoses generally occur later and may be single, multiple, or diffuse. Risk factors identified in adult patients include atherosclerotic disease in either donor or recipient vessels, CMV infection,[145] and the use of deceased donor organs.[146] In pediatric series, RAS was previously shown to be more common with the use of kidneys from donors under four years of age, although this practice is becoming increasingly uncommon.[140,147] There have been a number of series that have suggested that RAS may occur as a result of allograft rejection.[139]

The diagnosis of RAS is made radiologically, and angiography remains the gold standard investigation. Investigation of suspected RAS should commence with the use of color Doppler ultrasound, which is reported to have a sensitivity of 87% to 94% and a specificity of 86% to 100% in adult kidney recipients.[137] The procedure does not involve the use of ionizing radiation and is widely available, although there is significant interoperator variability. Findings suggestive of RAS include the demonstration of a focal segmental region of flow abnormality characterized by an elevated peak systolic velocity (indicating blood flow acceleration at the site of the artery stenosis), turbulent flow, and a decreased resistive index—indicating decreased renal parenchymal perfusion.

In adult patients, a peak systolic velocity of greater than 150 cm/sec and a resistive index of less than 0.50 have been reported to detect (with a sensitivity if 90% to 100% and a specificity of 87% to 100%) a hemodynamically significant (greater than 50%) renal artery stenosis.[148] Where changes suggestive of RAS are detected, formal arteriography is indicated to confirm the diagnosis. Definitive treatment of any lesion detected may be possible as part of this procedure (see material following). Arteriography may be complicated by contrast-medium–induced acute renal failure and hypersensitivity reactions, although the risk of these complications has fallen significantly with the introduction of the newer contrast agents. Other potential complications include bleeding, thromboembolism, groin hematomas, pseudoaneurysms, and traumatic arteriovenous fistulas.[149] An alternative approach is the use of gadolinium-enhanced MR angiography, which has the advantage of being radiation free and is associated with very few other complications.

Mild lesions where renal function is stable and hypertension is the major clinical manifestation may be treated conservatively with the use of ACE inhibitors. Following institution of therapy, it is important that renal function and plasma electrolytes be checked early to ensure that there is no rise in plasma creatinine or hyperkalemia. More significant lesions (narrowing of >50% of the luminal diameter) require definitive treatment because it is recognized that the presence of RAS is associated with inferior graft survival rates.[139]

Percutaneous angioplasty and stenting is a well-established procedure that can be performed at the time of diagnostic angiography and that may restore renal perfusion in up to 70% to 90% of adult cases—with improvement in blood pressure and renal function.[136,137,146] The Guy's Hospital pediatric series from the early 1990s reported 14 technically successful angioplasties in 12 patients, with angiographic improvement in 9 and clinical improvement in 7.[140] In general, the best results are achieved with short linear stenoses distant from the anastamosis.[150]

Complications (including graft thrombosis, intimal flaps, arterial rupture and dissection, and local hematoma) may occur in up to 10%.[136] The reported restenosis rate is about 10%,[146] although this may be reduced by the use of stents—the successful use of which has been reported in children.[151] The newer sirolimus-coated stents, which have been shown to reduce restenosis rates in the coronary arteries, have the potential to reduce this restenosis rate further.

Surgery is reserved for those patients for whom angioplasty is unsuccessful or technically difficult. Methods of surgical correction of RAS include venous bypass of the lesion, patch graft, localized endarterectomy, and resection or revision of the anastamosis. The use of autotransplantation has also been reported. These are all technically challenging procedures with significant rates of complication (including graft loss and ureteric injury) and restenosis rates of about 12%.[136] Although good short-term results have been reported in adult patients following angioplasty and surgery, long-term outcomes are lacking.

REFERENCES

1. North American Pediatric Renal Trials and Collaborative Studies 2006 Annual Report, *www.NAPRTCS.org*.
2. Sijpkens YW, Joosten SA, Wong M-C, et al: Immunological risk factors and glomerular C4d deposits in chronic transplant glomerulopathy, *Kidney Int* 65:2409-18, 2004.
3. Solez K, et al: International standardisation of criteria for the histologic diagnosis of renal allograft rejection: The Banff working classification of kidney transplant pathology, *Kidney Int* 44:411-22, 1993.
4. Racusen L, Solez K, et al: The Banff 97 working classification of renal allograft pathology, *Kidney Int* 55:713-23, 1999.
5. Isoniemi HM, Krogerus L, von Willebrand E, et al: Histopathological findings in well-functioning, long-term renal allografts, *Kidney Int* 41:155-60, 1992.
6. Racusen LC, Solez K, Colvin RB: Fibrosis and atrophy in the renal allograft: Interim report and new directions, *Am J Transplant* 2:203, 2002.
7. Nankivell BJ, Borrows RJ, Fung CL-S, et al: The natural history of chronic allograft nephropathy, *New Engl J Med* 349:2326, 2003.
8. Seron D, Moreso F, Ramon JM, et al: Protocol renal allograft biopsies and the design of clinical trials aimed to prevent or treat chronic allograft nephropathy, *Transplantation* 69:1849-55, 2000.
9. Shishido S, Asanuma H, Nakai H, Mori Y, Satoh H, Kamimaki I, et al: The impact of repeated subclinical acute rejection on the progression of chronic allograft nephropathy, *J Am Soc Nephrol* 14:1046-52, 2003.
10. Oreso F, Iberon M, Goma M, et al: Subclinical rejection associated with chronic allograft nephropathy in protocol biopsies as a risk factor for late graft loss, *Am J Transplant* 6:747-52, 2006.
11. Nankivell BJ, Borrows RJ, Fung CL-S, et al: Evolution and pathophysiology of renal-transplant glomerulosclerosis, *Transplantation* 78:461-68, 2004.
12. Schwartz A, Mengel M, Gwinner W, et al: Risk factors for chronic allograft nephropathy after renal transplantation: A protocol biopsy study, *Kidney Int* 67:341-48, 2005.
13. Poggio ED, Clemente M, Riley J, Roddy M, et al: Alloreactivity in renal transplant recipients with and without chronic allograft nephropathy, *J Am Soc Nephrol* 15:1952-60, 2004.
14. Krieger N, Becker B, Heisey DM, Voss BJ, et al: Chronic allograft nephropathy uniformly affects recipients of cadaveric, non-identical living-related and living-unrelated grafts, *Transplantation* 75:1677-82, 2003.
15. Susal C, Opelz G: Kidney graft failure and presensitisation against HLA class I and class II antigens, *Transplantation* 73:1269-73, 2002.
16. Lee PC, Terasaki P, Takemoto SK, et al: All chronic rejection failures of kidney transplants were preceded by the development of HLA antibodies, *Transplantation* 74:1192-94, 2002.
17. Almond PS, Matas A, Gillingham AK, et al: Risk factors for chronic rejection in renal allograft recipients, *Transplantation* 55:752-56, 1993.
18. Lindholm A, Ohlman S, Albrechtsen D, et al: The impact of acute rejection episodes on long-term graft function and outcome in 1347 primary renal transplants treated by 3 ciclosporin regimens, *Transplantation* 53:307-15, 1993.
19. Van Saase JL, van der Woude FJ, Thorogood J, et al: The relation between acute vascular and interstitial rejection and subsequent chronic rejection, *Transplantation* 59:1280-85, 1995.

20. Humar A, Payne WD, Sutherland DE, et al: Clinical determinants of multiple acute rejection episodes in kidney transplant recipients, *Transplantation* 69:2357-60, 2000.
21. Meier-Kriesche HU, Schold JD, Srinivas TR, et al: Lack of improvement in renal allograft survival despite a marked decrease in acute rejection rates over the most recent era, *Am J Transplant* 4:378-83, 2004.
22. Basadonna GP, Matas AJ, Gillingham KJ, et al: Early versus late acute renal allograft rejection: Impact on chronic rejection, *Transplantation* 55:993, 1993.
23. Smith JM, Ho PL, McDonald RA: Renal transplant outcomes in adolescents: A report of the North American Pediatric Renal Transplant Cooperative Study, *Pediatr Transplant* 6:493-99, 2002.
24. Sijkens YW, Joosten SA, Wong M-C, Dekker FW, et al: Immunological risk factors and glomerular C4d deposits in chronic transplant glomerulopathy, *Kidney Int* 65:2409-18, 2004.
25. Randhawa PS, Minervini MI, Lombardero M, et al: Biopsy of marginal donor kidneys: Correlation of histological findings with graft dysfunction, *Transplantation* 69:1352-57, 2000.
26. Gasser M, Waaga AM, Laskowski IA, et al: The influence of donor brain death on short and long-term outcome of solid organ allografts, *Ann Transplant* 5:61-67, 2000.
27. Humar A, Hassoun A, Kandaswamy R, et al: Immunological factors: The major risk factor for decreased long-term renal allograft survival, *Transplantation* 68:1842-46, 1999.
28. Gjertson DW. The impact of delayed graft function and acute rejection on kidney graft survival. In *Clinical transplants*. Edited by Cecka JM, Terasaki PI. Los Angeles: University of Los Angeles Tissue Typing Laboratory;2000:467-80
29. Opelz G, Wujciak T, Ritz E: Association of chronic kidney graft failure with recipient blood pressure: Collaborative Transplant Study, *Kidney Int* 53:217-22, 1998.
30. Buescher R, Vester U, Wingen A-M, Hoyer PF: Pathomechanisms and the diagnosis of arterial hypertension in pediatric renal allograft recipients, *Pediatr Nephrol* 19:1202-11, 2004.
31. Baluarte HJ, Gruskin AB, Ingelfinger JR, Stablein D, Tejani A: Analysis of hypertension in children post renal transplantation: A report of the North American Pediatric Renal Transplant Cooperative Study (NAPRTCS), *Pediatr Nephrol* 8:570-73, 1994.
32. Trompeter R, Filler G, Webb NJA, Watson AR, Milford DV, Tyden G, et al: Randomized multicenter study comparing tacrolimus with cyclosporin in renal transplantation, *Pediatr Nephrol* 17:141-49, 2002.
33. Saarwal MM, Vidhun JR, Alexander SR, Satterwhite T, Millan M, Salvatierra O Jr.: Continued superior outcomes with modification and lengthened follow-up of a steroid-avoidance pilot with extended daclizumab induction in pediatric renal transplantation, *Transplantation* 76:1331-39, 2003.
34. Kasiske BL: Hyperlipidemia in patients with chronic renal disease, *Am J Kid Dis* 32(3):S142-S156, 1998.
35. Kasiske BL, O'Donnell MP, Cowardin W, Keane WF: Lipids and the kidney, *Hypertension* 15:443-550, 1990.
36. Fried LF, Orchard TJ, Kasiske BL, for the Lipids and Renal Disease Progression Meta-analysis Study Group: Effect of lipid reduction on the progression of renal disease: A meta-analysis, *Kidney Int* 59:260-69, 2001.
37. Remuzzi G, Perico N: Cyclosporine-induced renal dysfunction in experimental animals and humans, *Kidney Int* 52:S70-S74, 1995.
38. Oliyea AJ, de Mattos A, Bennett WM: Immunosuppressant-induced nephropathy: Pathophysiology, incidence and management, *Drug Safety* 21:471-88, 1999.
39. Ojo AO, Held PJ, Port FK, et al: Chronic renal failure after transplantation of a nonrenal organ, *N Eng J Med* 349:931-40, 2003.
40. Ponticelli C: Cyclosporine: from renal transplantation to autoimmune diseases, *Annals of the New York Academy of Sciences* 1051:551-58, 2005.
41. Ferlicot S, Durrbach A, Ba N, et al: The role of replicative senescence in chronic allograft nephropathy, *Hum Pathol* 34:924, 2003.
42. Mannon RB: Therapeutic targets in the treatment of allograft fibrosis, *Am J Transplant* 6:867-75, 2006.
43. Tinckam K, Rush D, Hutchison I, et al: The relative importance of cytokine gene polymorphisms in the development of early and late acute rejection and six-month renal allograft pathology, *Transplantation* 79:836-41, 2005.
44. Buescher R, Vester U, Wingen A-M, Hoyer PF: Pathomechanisms and the diagnosis of arterial hypertension in pediatric renal allograft recipients, *Pediatr Nephrol* 19:1202-11, 2004.
45. Remuzzi G, Navis G, DeZeeuw D, DeJong PE: The Gisen Group: Randomized placebo controlled trial of effect of ramipril on decline in glomerular filtration rate and risk of terminal renal failure in proteinuric non-diabetic nephropathy, *Lancet* 349:1857-63, 1997.
46. Giatras I, Lau J, Levey AS: Effect of angiotensin converting enzyme inhibitors on the progression of non-diabetic renal disease: A meta-analysis of randomized trials, *Ann Intern Med* 127:337-45, 1997.
47. Amuchastegui SC, Azzollini N, Mister M, Pezzotta A, Perico N, Remuzzi G: Chronic allograft nephropathy in the rat is improved by angiotensin II receptor blockade but not by calcium channel antagonism, *J Am Soc Nephrol* 9:1948-55, 1998.
48. Rush D, Nickerson P, Gough J, McKenna R, Grimm P, Cheang M, et al: Beneficial effects of treatment of early subclinical rejection: A randomized study, *J Am Soc Nephrol* 9:2129-34, 1998.
49. Kee T, Chapman JR, O'Connell, et al: Treatment of subclinical rejection diagnosed by protocol biopsy of kidney transplants, *Transplantation* 82:36-42, 2006.
50. Seikku P, Krogerus L, Jalanko H, Holmberg C. Better renal function with enhanced immunosuppression and protocol biopsies after kidney transplantation in children, *Pediatr Transplantation* 9:754-62, 2005.
51. Gallagher MP, Hall B, Craig J, et al: on behalf of the Australian Multicenter Trial of cyclosporine Withdrawal Study group and the ANZ Dialysis and Transplantation Registry: A randomized controlled trial of cyclosporine withdrawal in renal–transplant recipients: 15-year results, *Transplantation* 78:1653-60, 2004.
52. Filler G, Webb NJ, Milford DV, et al: Four-year data after pediatric renal transplantation: A randomized trial of tacrolimus vs. cyclosporine microemulsion, *Pediatr Transplant* 9:498-503, 2005.
53. Baboolal K, Jones GA, Janezic A, Griffiths DR, Jurewicz WA: Molecular and structural consequences of early renal allograft injury, *Kidney Int* 61:686-96, 2002.
54. Solez K, Vincenti F, Filo RS: Histopathologic findings from 2-year protocol biopsies from a U.S. multicenter kidney transplant trial comparing tacrolimus versus cyclosporine: A report of the FK506 Kidney Transplant Study Group, *Transplantation* 66:1736-40, 1998.
55. Stoves J, Newstead CG, Baczkowski AJ, et al: A randomized controlled trial of immunosuppression conversion for the treatment of chronic allograft nephropathy, *Nephrol Dial Transplant* 19:2113-20, 2004.
56. Meier M, Nitschke M, Weidtmann B, Jabs WJ, Wong W, Suefke S, et al: Slowing the progression of chronic allograft nephropathy by conversion from cyclosporin to tacrolimus: A randomized controlled trial, *Transplantation* 81:1035-40, 2006.
57. Kasiske BL, Chakkera HA, Louis TA, et al: A meta-analysis of immunosuppression withdrawal trials in renal transplantation, *J Am Soc Nephrol* 11:1910-17, 2000.
58. Dudley C, Pohanka E, Riad H, Dedochova J, Wijngaard P, Sutter C, et al: Mycophenolate mofitil substitution for ciclosporin A in renal transplant recipients with chronic progressive allograft dysfunction: The Creeping Creatinine Study, *Transplantation* 79:466-75, 2005.
59. Watson CJE, Firth J, Williams PF, et al: A randomized controlled trial of late conversion from CNI-based to sirolimus-based immunosuppression following renal transplantation, *Am J Transplant* 5:2496-2503, 2005.
60. Diekmann F, Campistol JM: Conversion from calcineurin inhibitors to sirolimus in chronic allograft nephropathy: Benefits and risks, *Nephrol Dial Transplant* 21:562-68, 2006.
61. Thervet E, Martinez F, Legendre C: Benefit-risk assessment of ciclosporin withdrawal in renal transplant recipients, *Drug Safety* 27:457-76, 2004.
62. Kerecuk L, Taylor J, Clark G: Chronic allograft nephropathy and mycophenolate mofetil introduction in pediatric renal recipients, *Pediatr Nephrol* 20:1630-35, 2005.
63. Mota A, Arias M, Taskinen EI, et al: Sirolimus-based therapy following early cyclosporine withdrawal provide significantly improved

renal histology and function at 3 years, *Am J Transplant* 4:953-61, 2004.
64. Flechner SM, Kurian SM, Solez K, Cook DJ, et al: De novo kidney transplantation without use of calcineurin inhibitors preserves renal structure and function at two years, *Am J Transplant* 4:1776-85, 2004.
65. Larson TS, Dean PG, Stegali MD, et al: Complete avoidance of calcineurin inhibitors in renal transplantation: A randomized trial comparing sirolimus and tacrolimus, *Am J Transplant* 6:514-22, 2006.
66. Allison AC, Eugui EM: Mechanisms of action of mycophenolate mofitil in preventing acute and chronic allograft rejection, *Transplantation* 80(2):S181-S190, 2005.
67. Remuzzi G, Zoja C, Gagliardini E, et al: Combining an anti-proteinuric approach with mycophenolate mofetil fully suppresses progressive nephropathy of experimental animals, *J Am Soc Nephrol* 10:1542-49, 1999.
68. Vincente F, Ramos E, Brattstrom C, et al: Multicenter trial exploring calcineurin inhibitors avoidance in renal transplantation, *Transplantation* 71:1282-87, 2005.
69. European Mycophenolate Mofetil Cooperative Study Group: Mycophenolate mofetil in renal transplantation: 3-year results from the placebo-controlled trial, *Transplantation* 68:391-96, 1999.
70. Ojo AO, Meier-Kriesche H-U, Hanson JA, et al: Mycophenolate mofetil reduces late graft loss independent of acute rejection, *Transplantation* 69:2405-09, 2000.
71. Molina MG, Seron D, Del Morel RG, et al: Mycophenolate mofetil reduces deterioration of renal function in patients with chronic allograft nephropathy, *Transplantation* 77:215-20, 2004.
72. Merville P, Berge F, Deminiere C, et al: Lower incidence of chronic allograft nephropathy at 1 year posttransplantation in patients treated with mycophenolate mofetil, *Am J Transplant* 4:1769-75, 2004.
73. Meier-Kriesche H-U, Schold JD, Srinivas TR, et al: Sirolimus in combination with tacrolimus is associated with worse renal allograft survival compared to mycophenolate mofetil combined with tacrolimus, *Am J Transplant* 5:2273-90, 2005.
74. Ekberg H, Tedesco-Silva H, Demirbas A, et al: Symphony: Comparing standard immunosuppression to low-dose cyclosporine, tacrolimus or sirolimus in combination with MMF, dacluzimab and corticosteroids in renal transplantation, *Am J Transplant* 6(2):300, 2006.
75. Theruvath TP, Saidman SL, Mauiyyedi S, et al: Control of antidonor antibody production with tacrolimus and mycophenolate mofetil in renal allograft recipients with chronic rejection, *Transplantation* 72:77-83, 2001.
76. Henne T, Latta K, Strehlau J, et al: Mycophenolate mofetil-induced reversal of glomerular filtration loss in children with chronic allograft nephropathy, *Transplantation* 76:1326-30, 2003.
77. Sehgal SN: Sirolimus: Its discovery, biological properties, and mechanisms of action, *Transplant Proc* 35(3):227S-230S, 2003.
78. Akselband Y, Harding MW, Nelson PA: Rapamycin inhibits spontaneous and fibroblast growth factor beta-stimulated proliferation of endothelial cells and fibroblasts, *Transplant Proc* 23:2833-36, 1991.
79. Vincenti F, Ramos E, Brattstrom C, et al: Multicenter trial exploring calcineurin inhibitors avoidance in renal transplantation, *Transplantation* 71:1282-87, 2001.
80. MacDonald AS, Group RGS: A worldwide, phase III, randomized, controlled, safety and efficacy study of a sirolimus/cyclosporine regimen for prevention of acute rejection recipients of primary mismatched renal allografts, *Transplantation* 71:271-80, 2001.
81. Mendez R, Gonwa T, Yang HC, et al: A prospective randomized trial of tacrolimus in combination with sirolimus or mycophenolate mofetil in kidney transplantation: Results at 1 year, *Transplantation* 80:303-09, 2005.
82. Webster A, Lee V, Chapman J, Craig J: Target of rapamycin inhibitors (sirolimus and everolimus) for primary immunosuppression of kidney transplant recipients: A systematic review and meta-analysis of randomized trials, *Transplantation* 81:1234-48, 2006.
83. Oberauer R, Segoloni G, Campistol JM, et al: Early cyclosporine withdrawal from a sirolimus-based regimen results in better renal allograft survival and renal function at 48 months after transplantation, *Transpl Int* 18:22-28, 2005.
84. Meier-Kriesche H-U, Steffen BJ, Chi AH, et al: Sirolimus with Neoral versus mycophenolate mofetil with Neoral is associated with decreased renal allograft survival, *Am J Transplant* 4:2059-66, 2004.
85. Gupta P, Kaufman S, Fishbein TM: Sirolimus for solid organ transplantation in children, *Pediatr Transplant* 9:269-76, 2005.
86. Sijpkens YW, Joosten SA, Wong M-C, et al: Immunological risk factors and glomerular C4d deposits in chronic transplant glomerulopathy, *Kidney Int* 65:2409-18, 2004.
87. Campistol JM, Garcia Del Moral R, Alarcon A, et al: Angiotensin II receptor blocker in kidney transplantation: Design and progress of the Aallograft study, *Transplantation* 82(2):238, 2006.
88. Dobbels F, et al: Growing pains: Non-adherence with the immunosuppressive regimen in adolescent transplant recipients, *Pediatr Transplant* 9:381-90, 2005.
89. Reinberg Y, Gonzalez, Fryd D, et al: The outcome of renal transplantation in children with posterior urethral valves, *J Urol* 140:1491, 1988.
90. Bryant JE, Joseph DB, Kohaut EC, et al: Renal transplantation in children with posterior urethral valves, *J Urol* 146:1585, 1991.
91. Datch DA, Koyle MA, Baskin LS, Zaontz MR, Burns MW, Tarry WF, et al., for the Urology Society for Transplantation and Vascular Surgery: Kidney transplantation in children with urinary diversion or bladder augmentation, *J Urol* 165:2265-68, 2001.
92. Fontaine E, Gagnadoux MF, Niaudet P, et al: Renal transplantation in children with augmentation cystoplasty: Long-term results, *J Urol* 159:2110, 1998.
93. Koo H, Bunchman TE, Flynn JT, et al: Renal transplantation in children with severe lower urinary tract dysfunction, *J Urol* 161:240, 1999.
94. Luke PPW, Herz DB, Bellinger MF, Chakrabarti P, Vivas CA, Scantlebury VP, et al: Long-term results of pediatric renal transplantation into a dysfunctional lower urinary tract, *Transplantation* 76:1578-82, 2003.
95. Hatch DA, Belitsky P, Barry JM, et al: Fate of renal allografts transplanted in patients with urinary diversion, *Transplantation* 56:838, 1993.
96. Hariharan S, Adams MB, Brennan DC, Davis CL, First MR, Johnson CP, et al: Recurrent and de novo glomerular disease after renal transplantation: A report from Renal Allograft Disease Registry (RADR), *Transplantation* 68:635-41, 1999.
97. Hariharan S, Johnson CP, Bresnahan BA, et al: Improved graft survival after renal transplantation in the United States, 1988 to 1996, *N Engl J Med* 342:1837-1838, 2000.
98. Briganti EM, Russ GR, McNeill JJ, et al: Risk of renal allograft loss from recurrent glomerulonephritis, *N Engl J Med* 347:103-09, 2002.
99. Quan A, Sullivan EK, Alexander SR: Recurrence of hemolytic uremic syndrome after renal transplantation in children: A report of the North American Pediatric Renal Transplant Cooperative Study, *Transplantation* 72:742-45, 2001.
100. Schwarz A, Krause PH, Offermann G, et al: Impact of de novo membranous glomerulonephritis on the clinical course after kidney transplantation, *Transplantation* 58:650-54, 1994.
101. Poduval RD, Josephson MA, Javaid B: Treatment of de novo and recurrent membranous nephropathy in renal transplant patients, *Semin Nephrol* 23:392-99, 2003.
102. Johnstin PA, Goode BP, Aparicio SR, et al: Membranous allograft nephropathy: Remission of nephrotic syndrome with pulsed methylprednisolone and high dose alternate-day steroids, *Transplantation* 55:214-16, 1993.
103. Truong L, Gelfand J, D'Agati V, et al: De novo membranous glomerulopathy in renal allografts: A report of ten cases and review of the literature, *Am J Kid Dis* 14:131-44, 1989.
104. Briganti EM, Russ GR, McNeill JJ, et al: Risk of renal allograft loss from recurrent glomerulonephritis, *N Engl J Med* 347:103-09, 2002.
105. Josephson MA, Spargo B, Hollandsworth D, Thistlethwaite JR: The recurrence of recurrent membranous nephropathy in a renal transplant recipient: Case report and literature review, *Am J Kid Dis* 24:873-78, 1994.

106. Stone JH, Millward CL, Olson JL, Amend WJC, Criswell LA: Frequency of recurrent lupus nephritis among ninety seven patients during the cyclosporine era, *Arthritis Theum* 41:678-86, 1998.
107. Goral S, Ynares C, Shappell SB, Snyder D, Feurer ID, Kazancioglu R, et al: Recurrent lupus nephritis in renal transplant recipients revisited: It is not rare, *Transplantation* 75:651-56, 2003.
108. Bartosh SM, Fine RN, Sullivan EK: Outcome after transplantation of young patients with systemic lupus erythematosus a report of the North American Pediatric Renal Transplant Cooperative Study, *Transplantation* 72:973-78, 2001.
109. Gardner SD, Field AM, Coleman DV, Hulme B: New human papovavirus (BK) isolated from urine after renal transplantation, *Lancet* 1:1253-57, 1971.
110. Pahari A, Rees L: BK virus-associated renal problems—clinical implications, *Pediatr Nephrol* 18:743-48, 2003.
111. Shah KV, Daniel RW, Warszawski RM: High prevalence of antibodies to BKV, an SV40-related papovirus, in residents of Maryland, *J Infect Dis* 128:784-87, 1973.
112. Flaegstad T, Ronne K, Filipe AR, Traavik T: Prevalence of anti-BK virus antibody in Portugal and Norway, *Scand J Infect Dis* 21:145-47, 1989.
113. Gardner SD: Prevalence in England of antibody to human polyomavirus (BK), *BMJ* 5876:177-78, 1973.
114. Ling Lin P, Vats AN, Green M: BK virus infection in renal transplant recipients, *Pediatr Transplant* 5:398-405, 2001.
115. Andrews CA, Shah KV, Daniel RW, Hirsch MS, Rubin R: A serological investigation of BK virus and JC virus infections in recipients of renal allografts, *J Infect Dis* 158:176-181, 1988.
116. Hirsch HH, Knowles W, Dickenmann M, et al: Prospective study of polyomavirus type BK replication and nephropathy in renal transplant recipients, *N Engl J Med* 347:488-96, 2002.
117. Hariharan S: BK virus nephritis after renal transplantation, *Kidney Int* 69:655-62, 2006.
118. Ahuja M, Cohen EP, Dayer AM, et al: Polyoma virus infection after renal transplantation: Use of immunostaining as a guide to diagnosis, *Transplantation* 71:896-99, 2001.
119. Coleman DV, Mackenzie EF, Gardner SD, Poulding JM, Amer B, Russell WJ: Human polyomavirus (BK) infection and ureteric stenosis in renal allograft recipients, *J Clin Pathol* 31:338-47, 1978.
120. Herman J, Van Ranst M, Snoeck R, Beuselinck K, Lerut E, Van Damme-Lombaerts R: Polyomavirus infection in pediatric renal transplant recipients: Evaluation using a quantitative real-time PCR technique, *Pediatr Transplant* 8:485-92, 2004.
121. Gupta M, Miller F, Nord EP, Wadwa NK: Delayed renal allograft dysfunction and cystitis associated with human polyomavirus (BK) infection in a renal transplant recipient: A case report and review of the literature, *Clin Nephrol* 60:405-14, 2003.
122. Arthur RR, Shah KV, Baust SJ, Charache PA, Santos GW, Saral R: Association of BK viruria with hemorrhagic cystitis in recipients of bone marrow transplants, *N Engl J Med* 315:230-34, 1986.
123. Ding R, Medeiros M, Dadhania D, et al: Noninvasive diagnosis of BK virus nephritis by measurement of messenger RNA for BK virus VP1 in urine, *Transplantation* 74:987-94, 2002.
124. Nickeleit V, Hirsh HH, Binet IF, et al: Polyomavirus infection of renal allograft recipients: From latent infection to manifest disease, *J Am Soc Nephrol* 10:1080-89, 1999.
125. Pappo O, Demetris AJ, Raikow RB, Randhawa PS: Human polyoma virus infection of renal allografts: histolopathologic diagnosis, clinical significance and literature review, *Modern Pathol* 9:105-09, 1996.
126. Randhawa PS, Finkelstein S, Scatlebury V, et al: Human polyoma virus-associated interstitial nephritis in the allograft kidney, *Transplantation* 67:103-09, 1999.
127. Smith JM, McDonald RA, Finn LS, Healey PJ, Davis CL, Limaye AP: Polyomavirus nephropathy in pediatric kidney transplant receipts, *Am J Transplant* 4:2109-17, 2004.
128. Ginevri F, De Santis R, Comoli P, et al: Polyomavirus BK infection in pediatric renal allograft recipients: A single center analysis of incidence, risk factors and novel therapeutic approaches, *Transplantation* 75:1266-70, 2003.
129. Herman J, Van Ranst M, Snoeck R, Beuselinck K, Lerut E, Van Damme-Lombaerts R: Polyomavirus infection in pediatric renal transplant recipients: Evaluation using a quantitative real-time PCR technique, *Pediatr Transplant* 8:485-92, 2004.
130. Trofe J, Cavallo T, First MR, Weiskittel P, Peddi VR, Roy-Chaudhury P, et al: Polyomavirus in kidney and kidney-pancreas transplantation: a defined protocol for immunosuppression reduction and histologic monitoring, *Transplant Proc* 34:1788-89, 2002.
131. Brennan DC, Agha I, Bohl DL, et al: Incidence of BK with tacrolimus versus cyclosporine and impact of pre-emptive immunosuppression reduction, *Am J Transplant* 5:839, 2005.
132. Kadambi PV, Josephson MA, Williams J, et al: Treatment of refractory BK virus-associated nephropathy with cidofovir, *Am J Transplant* 3:186-91, 2003.
133. Williams JW, Javaid B, Kadambi PV, et al: Leflunomide for polyomavirus type BK nephropathy, *N Engl J Med* 352:1157-58, 2005.
134. Vats A, Shapiro R, Singh RP, et al: Quantitative viral load monitoring and cidofovir therapy for the management of BK virus: Associated nephropathy in children and adults, *Transplantation* 75:105-12, 2003.
135. Hirsch HH, Ramos E: Retransplantation after polyomavirus-associated nephropathy: Just do it? *Am J Transplant* 6:7-9, 2006.
136. Fervenza FC, Lafayette RA, Alfrey EJ, Peterson J: Renal artery stenosis in kidney transplants, *Am J Kid Dis* 31:142-48, 1998.
137. Bruno S, Remuzzi G, Ruggenenti P: Transplant renal artery stenosis, *J Am Soc Nephrol* 15:134-141, 2004.
138. Voiculescu A, Schmitz M, Hollenbeck M, Braasch S, Luther B, Sandmann W, et al: Management of arterial stenosis affecting kidney graft perfusion: A single center study in 53 patients, *Am J Transplant* 5:1731-38, 2005.
139. Wong W, Fynn SP, Higgins RM, Walters H, Evans S, Deane C, et al: Transplant renal artery stenosis in 77 patients: Does it have an immunological cause? *Transplantation* 61:215-19, 1996.
140. McMullin ND, Reidy JF, Koffman CG, Rigden SP, Haycock G, Chantler C, et al: The management of renal transplant artery stenosis in children by percutaneous transluminal angioplasty, *Transplantation* 53:559-63, 1992.
141. Fontaine E, Barthelemy Y, Gagnadoux MF, Cuckier J, Broyer M, Beurton D: A review of 72 renal artery stenoses in a series of 715 kidney transplantations in children, *Prog Urol* 4:193-205, 1994.
142. Malekzadeh M, Grushkin CM, Stanley P, Brennan LP, Stiles QR, Lieberman E: Renal artery stenosis in pediatric transplant patients, *Pediatr Nephrol* 1:22-29, 1987.
143. Aliabadi H, McLorie GA, Churchill BM, McMullin N: Percutaneous transluminal angioplasty for transplant renal artery stenosis in children, *J Urol* 143:569-72, 1990.
144. North American Pediatric Renal Trials and Collaborative Studies 2004 Annual Report.
145. Pouria S, State OI, Wong W, Hendry BM: CMV infection is associated with transplant renal artery stenosis, *QJM* 91:185-89, 1998.
146. Patel NH, Jindal RM, Wilkin T, Rose S, Johnson MS, Shah H, et al: Renal arterial stenosis in renal allografts: Retrospective study of predisposing factors and outcome after percutaneous transluminal angioplasty, *Radiology* 219:663-67, 2001.
147. Trompeter RS, Haycock GB, Bewick M, Chantler C: Renal transplantation in very young children, *Lancet* 1:373, 1983.
148. Bruno S, Ferrari S, Remuzzi G, Ruggenenti P: Doppler ultrasonography in posttransplant renal artery stenosis: A reliable tool for assessing effectiveness of revascularization, *Transplantation* 76:147-53, 2003.
149. Hessel SJ, Adams DF, Abrams HL: Complications of angiography, *Radiology* 138:273-81, 1981.
150. Benoit G, Moukarzel M, Hiesse C, Verdelli G, Charpentier B, Fries D: Transplant renal artery stenosis: Experience and comparative results between surgery and angioplasty, *Transplant Int* 3:137-40, 1990.
151. Repetto HA, Rodriguez-Rilo L, Mendaro E, Basso L, Galvez H, Morrone G, et al: Percutaneous treatment of transplant renal artery stenosis in children, *Pediatr Nephrol* 19:1400-03, 2004.

CHAPTER

62 Prevention and Treatment of Infectious Complications in Pediatric Renal Allograft Recipients

Alicia M. Neu and Vikas R. Dharnidharka

INTRODUCTION

Kidney transplantation has made spectacular strides in the last few decades, in both adults and children.[1] Patient and graft survival are now far better than in the 1960s and 1970s. These successes are largely due to more potent immunosuppressive medications, leading to reduction in acute rejection rates.[2] However, the use of more potent medications has led to an increase in the problem of posttransplantation infections. This increase has manifested as an increase in the total frequency of infection,[3] infection becoming the predominant reason for hospitalization posttransplantation in recent years,[4] and the successive emergence of new viral infections in the last few decades.

Specifically, cytomegalovirus (CMV) infections have been prominent in kidney transplant recipients since the 1980s, followed by Ebstein-Barr virus (EBV)-induced posttransplantation lymphoproliferative disorder (PTLD) since the 1990s, and BK-virus–associated allograft nephropathy (BKVAN) in the last 10 years. Infections are not only a significant source of morbidity and hospitalization but an important source of patient mortality and thus graft loss.

Even when adjusting for death, based on the USRDS 2003 report[5] infections as a whole represent an additional risk factor for worse graft survival. Excessive EBV-positive PTLD resulted in the early termination of a large multicenter immunosuppression trial in pediatric kidney transplantation in the United States.[6] Early stoppage of trials prevents the study hypothesis from being validated, wastes large sums of money needed to conduct such trials, and does not advance knowledge or help patients.

SPECIAL CONSIDERATIONS IN PEDIATRIC TRANSPLANTATION

For numerous reasons, organ transplant recipients are at greater risk for infection than immunocompetent persons.[7] The immunosuppressive medications currently in use are all nonselective in nature, suppressing immune responses to alloantigens and to infectious organisms. An organ transplant is a major surgical procedure entailing all of the attendant infection risks of any major surgery.

Chronic kidney failure itself suppresses the immune system to some extent. Further, children are exposed to some unique infection risks. Many of the major viral organisms of importance in kidney transplantation are more severe when occurring as a primary infection. Children are less likely to have been exposed to these viruses from the community before they receive a transplant. These children most commonly receive adult-donor grafts, which may harbor the viruses and lead to a primary infection in a child who is newly exposed to posttransplantation immunosuppression.

Bacterial Infections

Urinary Tract Infection

Urinary tract infection (UTI) is the most common bacterial infection in kidney transplant recipients, in both adults[8,9] and children.[10] The fraction of kidney transplant recipients who will experience a UTI ranges from 20% to 40% in the first year posttransplantation, and 40% to 60% by 3 years posttransplantation.[8-10] UTI is not only a cause of morbidity but is associated with higher rates of graft loss and patient death.[11-12] The urogenital tract is the most common entry point for systemic sepsis.[13] Risk factors for UTI in children include bladder abnormalities, the need for chronic or prolonged bladder catheterizations, and placement of a ureteral stent.[14,15]

UTI risk is highest in the first few months posttransplantation, but some risk remains at later time points. The organisms implicated (such as *Escherichia coli* and *Klebsiella* species) are usually the same as in immunocompetent individuals. A higher percentage of UTIs in transplant patients are due to unusual organisms such as *Pseudomonas* species.[16] Clinical symptoms may include fever, dysuria, graft tenderness, and cloudy urine. In some patients, symptoms may be masked due to external immunosuppression. A rise in serum creatinine may occur, which can mimic acute rejection. UTIs can also precipitate an acute rejection.

The diagnosis of UTI is usually made by urine culture, although patients on sulfamethoxazole/trimethoprim prophylaxis for pneumocystis may not demonstrate positive cultures. In this case, diagnosis may be based on radionuclide scanning or clinical judgment. Treatment is with antimicrobials. Initially, the antimicrobial prescribed should cover the common gram-negative organisms. Once the organism is known, the most specific and cost-effective antimicrobial can be prescribed. Treatment route and total duration vary somewhat by severity of infection, recipient age, and other risk factors present.

Shorter oral courses, such as those used in immunocompetent people, can be used for milder cystitis episodes in older children. In more severe acute pyelonephritis in a younger child recently transplanted, intravenous antimicrobial therapy for 10 to 14 days is preferred. Not all centers prescribe routine prophylaxis for UTI. Sulfamethoxazole/trimethoprim, if given daily, may serve as both UTI and pneumocystis prophylaxis.

Other Bacterial Infections

Other bacterial infections (such as wound infections, line sepsis, and pneumonia) are seen with significant frequency in kidney transplant recipients. Wound infections and line sepsis are commonly due to gram-positive *Staphylococcus* and *Streptococcus*. Pneumonia can be due to multiple etiologies (bacterial, viral, or fungal), but bacterial pathogens are responsible for approximately 44% of cases.[17] In adult transplant recipients, cellulitis and bacterial abscesses are frequent problems—largely due to comorbid diabetes mellitus. In general, children are less likely to develop cellulitis and abscesses and are more likely to develop viral infections than adults. The treatment of these infections is generally no different than standard treatment in immunocompetent hosts, although the duration of therapy may be longer.

Bartonella henselae infection (also known as cat-scratch disease) has been reported in pediatric organ transplant recipients, including kidney transplants.[18] This infection typically presents as fever and lymphadenopathy, and thus may be included in the differential diagnosis for PTLD. However, unlike PTLD this infection is curable with antimicrobial therapy.

Although *Mycobacterium tuberculosis* infection occurs in 1% or less of kidney transplant recipients in North America and Europe, it is much more common in other areas of the world.[19] This infection may present at any time posttransplantation, but is most common in the first posttransplantation year.[20] *Mycobacterium tuberculosis* infection presents with myriad symptoms, including weight loss, cough, fever, and lymphadenopathy—again, acting as a differential diagnosis for PTLD.

The diagnosis of tuberculosis in the transplant recipient is similar to that in other populations, although the tuberculin skin test may be positive in only a third of kidney transplant recipients with tuberculosis.[21] Management of tuberculosis is complex and is evolving. It has long been directed by recommendations developed, updated, and disseminated by expert panels.[22,23] Treatment of the kidney transplant patient with tuberculosis should take into account these recommendations.[19]

Viral Infections

Cytomegalovirus

CMV, a DNA virus of the herpesvirus family, is perhaps the single most important pathogen in solid organ transplantation.[24] Its importance lies in the fact that CMV causes significant morbidity by direct infection and its immunomodulatory effects predispose to other infectious complications.[24] Three patterns of CMV infection may be seen posttransplantation: primary infection, reactivation infection, and superinfection. Primary infection occurs in transplant patients who were CMV seronegative prior to transplantation, most commonly via transmission from a graft from a seropositive donor.[24]

Without preventive therapy, the incidence of symptomatic CMV infection in such recipients is 50% to 65%.[24] Reactivation infection is due to activation of latent virus in seropositive recipients, whereas superinfection is activation of virus from a seropositive donor in a seropositive recipient.[24] Infection with CMV usually presents in the first few months posttransplantation. It can manifest as CMV syndrome (characterized by fever, myalgias, malaise, leukopenia, and thrombocytopenia) or as CMV disease, in which there is clinical evidence of organ involvement by the infection.[24,25]

The transplanted kidney is at higher risk for CMV infection than are the native organs. However, pulmonary, liver, and gastrointestinal tract infection are common, regardless of the organ transplanted.[26-28] As previously stated, in addition to causing direct infection CMV has significant indirect effects—including an increase in the overall state of immunosuppression, leading to increased risk for opportunistic infection.[24] CMV infection also increases the risk of EBV-associated PTLD.[24,29] In addition, CMV and acute rejection are interrelated. CMV infection is a risk factor for acute rejection, whereas rejection leads to release of tumor necrosis factor—triggering the process that ultimately leads to CMV replication.[30]

Prevention of CMV infection can be accomplished with universal prophylaxis (the administration of anti-CMV therapy to all patients except seronegative recipients of a seronegative organ) or preemptive treatment: the administration of anti-CMV therapy to patients at first sign of CMV infection. There is some controversy as to the optimal strategy, as both methods have advantages and disadvantages. Most guidelines recommend universal prophylaxis for high-risk patients (seronegative recipients of seropositive organs or seropositive recipients of seropositive organs in the setting of anti–T-cell antibody immunosuppression), with preemptive therapy reserved for patients at low or intermediate risk.[31-33]

Although several agents are available for prophylaxis, ganciclovir and valganciclovir have largely supplanted oral acyclovir and CMV immune globulin as the recommended treatment for prevention of CMV infection. Many protocols recommend intravenous ganciclovir, followed by oral ganciclovir.[31,33] Oral ganciclovir has poor bioavailability and must be taken in large doses three times daily. Valganciclovir has bioavailability superior to that of oral ganciclovir, with a pharmacokinetic profile similar to intravenous ganciclovir.[34] The standard duration of prophylactic therapy is 100 days, although many centers have extended prophylactic therapy to the first 6 months posttransplantation in reaction to data suggesting significant reduction in late CMV infection with this strategy.[35]

Although prophylactic therapy is expensive, the cost of treating CMV disease and its effects is considerably higher. Several European studies have demonstrated the clinical efficacy and cost advantages of prophylactic treatment with intravenous ganciclovir or oral valacyclovir over preemptive or "wait-and-treat" strategies in kidney transplant recipients.[36-38] These studies did not include the cost of the indirect effects of CMV disease, including the increased risk for graft rejection, PTLD, and opportunistic infection—which would have increased the cost benefit of prophylactic therapy further.[36,37]

For preemptive therapy, intravenous ganciclovir is generally recommended. However, recent studies have demonstrated good results with valganciclovir.[39,40] For preemptive therapy to be successful, frequent monitoring with reliable diagnostic assays must be performed. Table 62-1 summarizes the characteristics of many commonly used assays for the various viral infections.[41] Detection of CMV DNA or RNA by polymerase chain reaction (PCR) and the pp65 antigenemia assay is rapid and has reasonable predictive ability for use in preemptive therapy.[24]

The timing and frequency of screening for CMV viremia are largely center specific and is influenced by donor and recipient CMV serostatus, as well as whether prophylactic or preemptive therapy is employed. Published guidelines for adult patients have recommended monitoring CMV blood PCR every 3 months for the first year in seronegative recipients of a seropositive donor kidney[42] (Table 62-2). However, weekly monitoring for the first 3 months may be indicated for preemptive therapy.[31]

The widespread use of preventive therapy has greatly reduced the incidence of CMV disease, especially in the early posttransplantation period.[43] When CMV disease does occur, treatment with intravenous ganciclovir is the treatment of choice. Some guidelines suggest that valganciclovir, at high doses, may also be used.[33]

Epstein-Barr Virus

EBV is another herpesvirus that causes significant morbidity posttransplantation. Like CMV, this virus commonly infects immunocompetent people sometime in childhood and establishes a prolonged latency in reticuloendothelial cells. Thus, the patterns of infection are identical to CMV: primary infection (often from the graft of a seropositive donor), reactivation, and superinfection. Again, like CMV the primary infection in an immunosuppressed transplant recipient is more virulent. Unlike CMV, EBV infection does not seem to have many indirect effects except for the development of PTLD. PTLD is undoubtedly a major complication and is covered in detail in Chapter 63. This section deals with EBV infection only.

EBV infection can be asymptomatic or present as a nonspecific viral syndrome, similar to CMV infection. Routine PCR monitoring in recent studies suggests that the rate of EBV infection in EBV seronegative pediatric transplant recipients (as defined by systemic viremia) ranges from 50% to 80%.[44-46] EBV viremia, in contrast to PTLD, can be asymptomatic or associated with mild nonspecific viral symptoms. Thus, the diagnosis is almost impossible to make clinically. The diagnosis is made by lab testing performed either as routine surveillance or to investigate the nonspecific illness (Table 62-1).

In the past, the diagnosis was made by documented seroconversion (EBV IgM positive or significant rise in IgG titer). Serologic testing can be performed for antibody against EB nuclear antigen or viral capsid. The former turns positive early, after recent infection. The latter turns positive in more

TABLE 62-1 **Commonly Used Laboratory Methods for Diagnosing Viral Infections (CMV, EBV, or BKV) Following Kidney Transplantation**

Method	Principle	Clinical Use	Comments
Viral culture	Virus isolation	Diagnosis of viral infection and disease pretransplantation	High specificity but poor sensitivity; long turnaround time; virus isolate may be used for phenotypic drug susceptibility
Serology	Antibody detection (IgG, IgM)	Assessment of virus exposure; not as useful for real-time diagnosis of acute disease	IgM suggests acute infection
Antigenemia	pp65 antigen detection (CMV only)	Rapid diagnosis of CMV infection and disease; guide for preemptive therapy; guide for duration of antiviral therapy	More sensitive assay than shell vial assay; lacks standardization (subjective interpretation); operator dependent; requires immediate processing
Nucleic acid detection	Viral nucleic acid (DNA or RNA) detection	Rapid diagnosis of viral infection and disease; guide for antiviral therapy; guide for duration of antiviral therapy	Qualitative assay dose not distinguish latency from active replication; virus quantification can guide duration of antiviral therapy; surrogate marker for antiviral resistance
Immunostaining	SV40 stain for BKV	Diagnosis of BK virus presence in renal allograft tissue	Does not measure degree of inflammation

Adapted with permission from Razonable RR, Paya CV, Smith TF: Role of the laboratory in diagnosis and management of cytomegalovirus infection in hematopoietic stem cell and solid-organ transplant recipients, *J Clin Microbiol* 40:746-52, 2002.

distant infection. More recently, in western countries PCR amplification of viral DNA is the method most commonly used.[47] The reader should note that PCR techniques to detect EBV DNA amplification vary greatly based on the type of sample and laboratory standards. Thus, PCR values from peripheral blood leucocytes and whole blood generally correlate with each other but not with PCR values from plasma.[48,49] As with CMV, posttransplantation screening for EBV is center specific. Published guidelines for adult transplant patients have recommended monitoring EBV PCR from blood every 3 months for the first year in EBV seronegative recipients of a graft from a seropositive donor (Table 62-2).[42]

There is no universally accepted treatment for EBV infection posttransplantation. Reduction in immunosuppression is one modality. The antiviral agents ganciclovir and valganciclovir have activity against EBV. Many centers might use intravenous ganciclovir for initial treatment for acute EBV infection if the patient is hospitalized. If not hospitalized, or if the patient is otherwise well, oral valganciclovir may be adequate. Acyclovir is not effective against EBV. The duration of antiviral treatment is not standardized, but most centers will treat until the EBV PCR has turned negative. Whether all patients with acute EBV seroconversion need reduction in immunosuppression or antiviral treatment is a burning question in pediatric transplantation.[50,51] Children in particular can develop a chronic high load carrier state without ever progressing to PTLD.[52] Nevertheless, the majority of reports indicate that higher EBV PCR values are associated with a greater risk for subsequent PTLD.[53-55]

Oral ganciclovir or valganciclovir is also used for prevention of EBV disease. These agents seem to delay the onset of infection rather than reduce the incidence. Intravenous immunoglobulin (IVIG) does not appear to be of added benefit.[45] An alternative concept is preemptive therapy (i.e., the initiation of antiviral agents at treatment doses as soon as the EBV PCR load exceeds normal). An EBV vaccine, directed against an EBV glycoprotein, is under testing in the United Kingdom. Unlike with CMV, we are not aware of any cost/benefit analysis of EBV monitoring or preventative treatment strategies. Cost effectiveness may change if incidence of the disease changes, as happened in the late 1990s.

Varicella

Varicella-zoster virus (VZV) is the most infectious of the human herpesviruses. Primary infection with VZV results in chickenpox. Following primary infection, the virus remains in the body in a latent state—from which it may be reactivated, resulting in cutaneous herpes zoster (shingles). Most adult kidney transplant recipients have experienced primary infection in childhood and are therefore at risk for reactivation and the development of herpes zoster with the introduction of immunosuppressive medication posttransplantation.[56] Historically, many children were VZV naive at the time of transplantation (and primary infection was a significant cause of morbidity and mortality).[57,58]

With the development of a safe and effective VZV vaccine, routine immunization of pediatric kidney transplant candidates has been documented to reduce the incidence of primary VZV infection posttransplantation.[59] Given these findings, it is recommended that all transplant candidates over 9 to 12 months of age receive immunization with the VZV vaccine.[60] Studies in children with chronic kidney disease and on dialysis suggest that two doses, rather than one, may be necessary to elicit protective antibody levels. It is thus recommended that antibody levels be obtained at least 4 weeks following immunization, and a second dose given if necessary.[60-62]

Although some studies have evaluated the use of this vaccine in posttransplantation patients, both the American Academy of Pediatrics Committee on Infectious Diseases and the Centers for Disease Control and Prevention's (CDC) Advisory Committee on Immunization Practices (ACIP) advise against the use of this live-viral vaccine in immunocompromised patients.[63,64] Thus, it is imperative that immunization be provided and protective antibody levels documented prior to transplantation whenever possible.

Patients who are varicella naive at the time of transplant (i.e., no history of chickenpox or VZV immunization, or failure to develop protective antibody after immunization) and who are exposed to varicella should receive prophylactic therapy. Previous recommendations included the delivery of varicella zoster immune globulin (VZIG). However, this product is no longer being manufactured.[65] In February of 2006, the investigational VZIG product VariZIG (Cangene Corporation, Winnipeg, Canada) became available in North America under an investigational new drug application. The ACIP recommends that use of this product be requested if an immunocompromised patient is exposed to varicella infection.[65] If this product is not available, IVIG (which contains some antivaricella antibody) may be given.[65] Any prophylactic therapy should be given as soon as possible, up to 96 hours after exposure.[65] Patients who develop primary or secondary infection should receive treatment with intravenous acyclovir.[66,67]

TABLE 62-2 **Recommended Schedule for Monitoring for Viral Infections (CMV, EBV, or BKV) Following Kidney Transplantation**

Virus	Population	Screening Test	Frequency
EBV	EBV IgG negative recipient/EBV IgG positive donor	EBV PCR, blood	Every 3 months for first posttransplant year
CMV	CMV IgG negative recipient/CMV IgG positive donor	CMV PCR, blood	Every 3 months for first posttransplant year*
BK	Patients at transplant centers with high rate of BK virus infection	BK PCR, blood and urine	1, 3, 6, 12, and 24 months posttransplant

Adapted from Hariharan S. Recommendations for outpatient monitoring of kidney transplant recipients, *Am J Kidney Dis* 40(2):S22-S36, 2006.
* Weekly monitoring for the first 3 months recommended in preemptive therapy protocols.[31]

BK Virus and BKVAN

BK virus was first isolated from the urine of a kidney transplant recipient in the 1970s[68], but it was not until the late 1990s that this virus emerged as a significant problem in kidney transplantation.[69,70] BKV is a part of the polyoma group of viruses. Although this virus is not from the herpesvirus group, it shares the characteristics of herpesviruses of infecting most immunocompetent people during childhood and establishing a prolonged latency.

Unlike the herpesviruses, the virus does not establish in the reticuloendothelial cells but prefers the uroepithelium. This propensity for the uroepithelium is responsible for the clinical manifestations: hemorrhagic cystitis in bone marrow transplant recipients and allograft nephropathy in kidney transplant recipients. The incidence of BKVAN in pediatric kidney transplantation appears to be the same as in adult kidney transplants (3% to 8%).[71,72] Risk factors include the intensity of immunosuppression,[73,74] recent treatment for acute rejection,[75] and placement of a ureteral stent[76]—although the data implicating specific immunosuppressive agents are conflicting.

BKVAN and BKV infection are two separate entities. Serial PCR surveillance for BKV has shown that urine PCRs turn positive earlier and much more often than peripheral blood PCR. Currently, the diagnosis of BKVAN depends on demonstration of the virus in blood or kidney tissue (by PCR or immunostaining) and on the presence of nephropathy (raised serum creatinine or tissue inflammation). Urine positivity without the other features represents infection without disease, as discussed in the recent guidelines for study monitoring by the American Society of Transplantation.[77]

BKVAN represents a diagnostic challenge because the condition may resemble acute rejection. Symptoms are often minimal or absent. Serum creatinine elevations are found on clinical lab monitoring. Because the treatment of acute rejection (intensifying immunosuppression) is the opposite of the treatment of BKVAN (reduction in immunosuppression), making the correct diagnosis is critical.

Simple BK viremia, without nephropathy, may not need treatment or may be manageable by reduction in immunosuppression. Like the CMV and EBV infections, reduction of immunosuppression is usually the first step in the treatment of full-fledged BKVAN.[70,78,79] However, by the time BKVAN is diagnosed the serum creatinine is significantly raised and subsequent graft survival is worse. Thus, two other concepts are advocated (much like with EBV disease): preemptive monitoring and therapy or simultaneous antiviral therapy while maintaining some immunosuppression.[78] The reader should note that there are virtually no randomized controlled trials to test any of these strategies head to head for any of the viral infections.

Antiviral therapy against BK virus is more complicated than for CMV or EBV because acyclovir, ganciclovir, and their analogues do not have activity against BK virus. Cidofovir is one antiviral drug that has been tried with some success.[80,81] Higher doses of cidofovir can be very nephrotoxic. Probenecid in combination with higher-dose cidofovir or intermediate-dose cidofovir prevents the nephrotoxicity.[82] Some centers convert from mycophenolate mofetil to leflunomide. The latter agent is unique in possessing antiviral and immunosuppressive properties. There is no vaccine against BK virus. Preventive strategies that have been suggested include serial urine BK PCR monitoring and preemptive reduction in immunosuppression (Table 62-2).

Other Infections

Pneumocystis carinii *Pneumonia*

Pneumocystis carinii pneumonia (PCP, but officially renamed *Pneumocystis jiroveci* pneumonia) has fortunately become much rarer with the widespread use of sulfamethoxazole/trimethoprim prophylaxis in the immediate posttransplantation period. Patients typically present with fever, dyspnea and nonproductive cough, interstitial infiltrate on chest x-ray, and hypoxemia. The diagnosis is established by demonstration of *Pneumocystis* in lung secretions obtained from bronchoalveolar lavage or in tissue from lung.[83] Gomori stain or toluidine blue staining will demonstrate the cysts and Giemsa staining will identify the sporozoites.

CMV infection is the major differential diagnosis. Many children may have dual infection, in which CMV infection predisposed to superinfection with PCP. The antimicrobial agents sulfamethoxazole/trimethoprim and pentamidine form the mainstay of treatment. Sulfamethoxazole/trimethoprim may be given either orally or intravenously and is less toxic, whereas pentamidine is only available as a parenteral preparation and has more side effects. Chemoprophylaxis with 3-times-a-week oral sulfamethoxazole/trimethoprim (5 mg/kg trimethoprim component/dose) has reduced the incidence of PCP disease from 3.7% to 0%.[84] This prophylaxis is now recommended in all transplant recipients during the periods of high risk, typically the first 6 months posttransplantation. Some centers also advocate its use after antirejection therapy, particularly with anti–T-cell antibodies. Some centers suggest a lower dose given daily at bedtime.[85]

Parasitic Infections

Although several parasitic infections have been reported in pediatric recipients of solid organ or bone marrow transplantation, there are few reports of such infections in pediatric kidney recipients. Several parasitic infections deserve mention, however, because they have been reported as transmitted by the transplanted graft in adult kidney transplant recipients. *Strongyloides stercoralis* (*S. stercoralis*) is an intestinal nematode that infects tens of millions of people worldwide. It is endemic in tropical and subtropical regions. The highest rate of infection in the United States is in the southeast.[86]

S. stercoralis may remain in the human intestinal tract for decades without symptoms, and then cause disseminated infection with the introduction of immunosuppressive medication posttransplantation.[86] In addition, there are case reports of transmission of strongyloidiasis by kidney transplantation in an adult recipient.[87] Interestingly, cyclosporine (but not tacrolimus) has effects against *S. stercoralis* and may reduce the risk for disseminated strongyloidiasis.[88,89] Active infection typically presents with cutaneous, gastrointestinal, and pulmonary symptoms, as well as with eosinophilia.[90] Disseminated disease, fever, hypotension, and central nervous system symptoms may be present.[90]

In uncomplicated infections, diagnosis is made by detection of larvae in stool, although 25% of infected patients may have negative stool examinations.[91] In disseminated disease, larvae may be found in stool, sputum, bronchoalveolar lavage fluid, and peritoneal and pleural fluid.[86,92] Serologic testing using enzyme-linked immunosorbent assay (ELISA) may also be of value, although this testing may be falsely negative in immunocompromised hosts.[92,93] Thiabendazole, previously the treatment of choice for *S. stercoralis*, has been replaced by ivermectin—with albendazole as an alternative.[94]

Other parasitic infections reported in kidney transplant recipients as transmitted by the transplanted graft include Chagas' disease and posttransplantation malaria.[86,95,96] Chagas' disease is caused by *Trypanosoma cruzi* and is found only in the southern United States, Mexico, and Central and South America. The manifestations of Chagas' disease classically include megaesophagus, megacolon, and cardiac disease, although CNS involvement has been reported in kidney transplant recipients.[95]

Diagnosis is routinely made serologically, and treatment typically consists of benznidazole or nifurtimox. Posttransplantation malaria, transmitted from donors living in high-risk areas, is a commonly reported occurrence.[96] Discussion of these infections is meant to illustrate the potential problem of parasitic infections posttransplantation. Policies for screening potential recipients and donors for these and other para-

TABLE 62-3 Recommended Vaccinations for Pediatric Transplant Candidates and Recipients

Vaccine	Inactivated/Live Attenuated (I/LA)	Recommended before Transplant*/Strength of Recommendation	Recommended after Transplant/Strength of Recommendation	Monitor Vaccine Titers?	Quality of Evidence
Influenza, injected	I	Yes/A	Yes/A	No	II
Hepatitis B	I	Yes/A	Yes†/B	Yes†	II
Hepatitis A	I	Yes/A	Yes/A	Yes	II
Pertussis	I	Yes/A	Yes/A	No	III
Diphtheria	I	Yes/A	Yes/A	No	II
Tetanus	I	Yes/A	Yes/A	No	II
Polio, inactivated	I	Yes/A	Yes/A	No	III
Haemophilus influenzae	I	Yes/A	Yes/A	Yes‡	II
Streptococcus pneumoniae§ conjugated/polysaccharide)	I/I	Yes/A	Yes/A	Yes‡	III
Neisseria meningitidis¶	I	Yes/A	Yes/A	No	III
Rabies**	I	Yes/A	Yes/B	No	III
Varicella	LA	Yes/A	No/D	Yes	II
Measles	LA	Yes/A	No/D	Yes	II
Mumps	LA	Yes/A	No/D	Yes	III
Rubella	LA	Yes/A	No/D	Yes	II
BCG††	LA	Yes/B	No/D	No	III
Smallpox‡‡	LA	No/C	No/D	No	III
Anthrax	I	No/C	No/C	No	III

Adapted from Guidelines for vaccination of solid organ transplant candidates and recipients, *Am J Transplant* 4(10):160-63, 2004.

* Whenever possible, the complete complement of vaccines should be administered before transplantation. Vaccines noted to be safe for administration after transplantation may not be sufficiently immunogenic after transplantation. Some vaccines, such as Pneumovax, should be repeated regularly (every 3 to 5 years) after transplantation.

† Routine vaccine schedule recommended prior to transplant and as early in the course of disease as possible; vaccine poorly immunogenic after transplantation, and accelerated schedules may be less immunogenic. Serial hepatitis B surface antibody titers should be assessed before and after transplantation to assess ongoing immunity.

‡ Serologic assessment recommended if available.

§ Children older than 5 years should receive 23-valent pneumococcal polysaccharide vaccine. Children younger than 2 years should receive conjugated pneumococcal vaccine. Those 2 to 5 years of age should receive vaccination based on age and number of previous immunizations with conjugated pneumococcal vaccine.[97]

¶ Vaccination with conjugated meningococcal vaccine recommended in United States for all children aged 11 to 12 years and adolescents at high school entry or 15 years of age, whichever comes first.[98,99]

** Not routinely administered. Recommended for exposures or potential exposures due to vocation or avocation.

†† The indications for BCG administration in the United States are limited to instances in which exposure to tuberculosis is unavoidable and where the measures to prevent its spread have failed or are not possible.

‡‡ Transplant recipients who are face-to-face contacts of a patient with smallpox should be vaccinated; vaccinia immune globulin may be administered concurrently if available. Those who are less intimate contacts should not be vaccinated.

sitic infections should be based on the presence of risk factors, including residence in or travel to an endemic area.

Fungal Infections

In general, serious invasive fungal infections such as aspergillosis are less common in pediatric kidney transplant recipients than in thoracic organ recipients. *Candida* is the most common organism affecting kidney transplant recipients, as oral thrush, vaginitis, nail infection, or UTI. The diagnosis of thrush is by clinical examination or demonstration of hyphae on a smear. Candidal UTI is diagnosed by urine culture. Treatment for topical *Candida* is by topical nystatin or clotrimazole. Prophylactic measures include nystatin liquid or clotrimazole lozenges. Treatment of invasive disease typically requires amphotericin. Fluconazole may be used for treatment of less severe disease, or for infections that have stabilized after initial therapy with amphotericin.

IMMUNIZATIONS

One of the cornerstones of preventive care in pediatrics is the delivery of routine childhood immunizations. Unfortunately, the complicated medical care required by many children with chronic kidney disease may result in only sporadic delivery of routine well-child care, including immunizations. Given the increased risk for vaccine-preventable disease posttransplantation, complete immunization is especially important in children with end-stage kidney disease as they approach transplantation.

In general, children with chronic kidney disease should receive immunizations according to the recommendations for healthy children in the region. Because they may also be more susceptible to or at risk for more serious infection from pathogens that are not typically problematic in healthy children, candidates for or recipients of kidney transplantation may also benefit from supplemental or additional vaccinations.[62] Table 62-3 provides a list of vaccinations recommended specifically for pediatric transplant candidates and recipients.[60]

Because children with chronic kidney disease on dialysis may have suboptimal response to many immunizations, or lose immunity prior to transplantation, it is important not only to ensure timely delivery of routine childhood immunizations but to monitor antibody titers or levels and revaccinate when indicated. This is especially true of the live-viral vaccines (including for measles, mumps, rubella, and varicella zoster), which are contraindicated in the immunosuppressed patient posttransplantation.

In the posttransplantation period, immunizations may be given after immunosuppressive medications have reached a baseline level (typically 6 to 12 months posttransplantation). Again, live-viral vaccines are generally contraindicated in the posttransplantation period. Because the presence of immunosuppressive medications may impair response to vaccines, maximal protection requires universal immunization of health care workers, family members, and household contacts.[60] In particular, annual immunization with injectable influenza vaccine is required.[60]

SUMMARY

Posttransplantation infections are an extremely important issue in pediatric kidney transplantation. In the recent era, infections have probably become more important than acute rejection because most current immunosuppressive protocols have consistently low rates of acute rejection. The prevention and monitoring of infections are complex but are critical to the ultimate success of the transplantation.

REFERENCES

1. Tejani A, Stablein DM, Donaldson L, Harmon WE, Alexander SR, Kohaut E, et al: Steady improvement in short-term graft survival of pediatric renal transplants: The NAPRTCS experience, *Clin Transpl* 13:95-110, 1999.
2. McDonald R, Ho PL, Stablein DM, Tejani A: Rejection profile of recent pediatric renal transplant recipients compared with historical controls: A report of the North American Pediatric Renal Transplant Cooperative Study (NAPRTCS), *Am J Transplant* 1:55-60, 2001.
3. Dharnidharka VR, Caillard S, Agodoa LY, Abbott KC: Infection frequency and profile in different age groups of kidney transplant recipients, *Transplantation* 81:1662-67, 2006.
4. Dharnidharka VR, Stablein DM, Harmon WE: Posttransplantation infections now exceed acute rejection as cause for hospitalization: A report of the NAPRTCS, *Am J Transplant* 43:384-89, 2004.
5. USRDS 2003 Annual Data Report: Atlas of End-Stage Renal Disease in the United States. Bethesda: U.S. Renal Data System, National Institutes of Health, National Institute of Diabetes and Digestive and Kidney Diseases, 2003.
6. McDonald RA, McIntosh M, Stablein D, Grimm P, Wyatt R, Arar M, et al: Increased incidence of PTLD in pediatric renal transplant recipients enrolled in a randomized controlled trial of steroid withdrawal: A study of the CCTPT, *Am J Transplant* 5(11):418, 2005.
7. Dharnidharka VR, Harmon WE: Management of pediatric postrenal transplantation infections, *Semin Nephrol* 21:521-31, 2001.
8. Maraha B, Bonten H, van Hooff H, Fiolet H, Buiting AG, Stobberingh EE: Infectious complications and antibiotic use in renal transplant recipients during a 1-year follow-up, *Clin Microbiol Infect* 11:619-25, 2001.
9. Martinez-Marcos F, Cisneros J, Gentil M, Algarra G, Pereira P, Aznar J, et al: Prospective study of renal transplant infections in 50 consecutive patients, *Eur J Clin Microbiol Infect Dis* 12:1023-28, 1994.
10. Chavers BM, Gillingham KJ, Matas AJ: Complications by age in primary pediatric renal transplant recipients, *Pediatr Nephrol* 11:399-403, 1997.
11. Abbott KC, Swanson SJ, Richter ER, Bohen EM, Agodoa LY, Peters TG, et al: Late urinary tract infection after renal transplantation in the United States, *Am J Kidney Dis* 44:353-62, 2004.
12. Muller V, Becker G, Delfs M, Albrecht KH, Philipp T, Heemann U: Do urinary tract infections trigger chronic kidney transplant rejection in man? *J Urol* 159:1826-29, 1998.
13. Wagener MM, Yu VL: Bacteremia in transplant recipients: A prospective study of demographics, etiologic agents, risk factors, and outcomes, *Am J Infect Control* 5:239-47, 1992.
14. Chuang P, Parikh CR, Langone A: Urinary tract infections after renal transplantation: A retrospective review at two U.S. transplant centers, *Clin Transplant* 19:230-35, 2000.
15. Takai K, Tollemar J, Wilczek HE, Groth CG: Urinary tract infections following renal transplantation, *Clin Transplant* 12:19-23, 1998.
16. So S, Simmons R: Infections following kidney transplantation in children. In CC Patrick (ed.), *Infections in immunocompromised infants and children*, New York: Churchill Livingstone 1992:215-30.
17. Chang GC, Wu CL, Pan SH, Yang TY, Chin CS, Yang YC, et al: The diagnosis of pneumonia in renal transplant recipients using invasive and noninvasive procedures, *Chest* 12:541-47, 2004.

18. Dharnidharka VR, Richard GA, Neiberger RE, Fennell RS: Cat scratch disease and acute rejection after pediatric renal transplantation, *Pediatr Transplant* 6:327-31, 2002.
19. *Mycobacterium tuberculosis*, *Am J Transplant* 4:37-41, 2004
20. Singh N, Paterson DL: Mycobacterium tuberculosis infection in solid-organ transplant recipients: Impact and implications for management, *Clin Infect Dis* 27:1266-77, 1998.
21. Sakhuja V, Jha V, Varma PP, Joshi K, Chugh KS: The high incidence of tuberculosis among renal transplant recipients in India, *Transplantation* 61:211-15, 1996.
22. API Consensus Expert Committee: API TB Consensus Guidelines 2006: Management of pulmonary tuberculosis, extra-pulmonary tuberculosis and tuberculosis in special situations, *J Assoc Physicians India* 54:219-34, 2006.
23. Taylor Z, Nolan CM, Blumberg HM; American Thoracic Society; Centers for Disease Control and Prevention; Infectious Diseases Society of America: Controlling tuberculosis in the United States: Recommendations from the American Thoracic Society, CDC, and the Infectious Diseases Society of America, *MMWR* 54(45):1161.
24. Pereyra F, Rubin RH: Prevention and treatment of cytomegalovirus infection in solid organ transplant recipients, *Curr Opin Infect Dis* 17:357-61, 2004.
25. Keough WL, Michaels MG: Infectious complications in pediatric solid organ transplantation, *Pediatr Clin N Am* 50:1451-69, 2003.
26. Dummer JS, Hary A, Poorsattar A, Ho M: Early infections in kidney, heart, and liver transplant recipients on cyclosporine, *Transplantation* 36:258-67, 1983.
27. Smyth RL, Scott JP, Borysiewicz LK, Sharples LD, Stewart S, Wreghitt TG, et al: Cytomegalovirus infection in heart-lung transplant recipients: Risk factors, clinical associations, and response to treatment, *J Infect Dis* 164:1045-50, 1991.
28. Bueno J, Green M, Kocoshis S, Furukawa H, Abu-Elmagd K, Yunis E, et al: Cytomegalovirus infection after intestinal transplantation in children, *Clin Infect Dis* 25:1078-83, 1997.
29. Fishman JA, Rubin RH: Infection in organ-transplant recipients, *N Engl J Med* 338:1741-51, 1998.
30. Tokoff-Rubin NE, Fishman JA, Rubin RH: The bidirectional relationship between cytomegalovirus and allograft injury, *Transplant Proc* 33:1773-75, 2001.
31. Preiksaitis JK, Brennan DC, Fishman J, Allen U: Canadian Society of Transplantation consensus workshop on cytomegalovirus management in solid organ transplantation final report, *Am J Transplant* 5:218-27, 2005.
32. Razonable RR, Emery VC: Management of CMV infection and disease in transplant patients, *Herpes* 11:77-86, 2004.
33. Cytomegalovirus, *Am J Transplant* 4:51-58, 2004.
34. Pescovitz MD, Rabkin J, Merion RM, Paya CV, Pirsch J, Freeman RB, et al: Valganciclovir results in improved oral absorption of ganciclovir in liver transplant recipients, *Antimicrob Agents Chemother* 44:2811-15, 2000.
35. Akalin E, Bromberg JS, Sehgal V, Ames S, Murphy B: Decreased incidence of cytomegalovirus infection in thymoglobulin-treated patients with 6 months of valganciclovir prophylaxis, *Am J Transplant* 4:148-49, 2004.
36. Squifflet JP, Legendre C: The economic value of valacyclovir prophylaxis in transplantation, *J Infect Dis* 186(1):S116-S122, 2002.
37. Mauskopf JA, Richter A, Annemans L, Maclaine G: Cost-effectiveness model of cytomegalovirus management strategies in renal transplantation: Comparing valacyclovir prophylaxis with current practice, *Pharmacoeconomics* 3:239-51, 2000.
38. Legendre CM, Norman DJ, Keating MR, Maclaine GD, Grant DM: Valacyclovir prophylaxis of cytomegalovirus infection and disease in renal transplantation: An economic evaluation, *Transplantation* 70:1463-68, 2000.
39. Fishman JA, Doran MT, Volicelli SA, Cosimis AB, Flood JG, Rubin RH: Dosing of intravenous ganciclovir for the prophylaxis and treatment of cytomegalovirus infection in solid organ transplant recipients, *Transplantation* 69:389-94, 2000.
40. Singh N, Wannstedt C, Keyes L, Gayowski T, Wagener MM, Cacciarelli TV: Efficacy of valganciclovir administered as preemptive therapy for cytomegalovirus disease in liver transplant recipients: Impact on viral load and late-onset cytomegalovirus disease, *Transplantation* 79:85-90, 2005.
41. Razonable RR, Paya CV, Smith TF: Role of the laboratory in diagnosis and management of cytomegalovirus infection in hematopoietic stem cell and solid-organ transplant recipients, *J Clin Microbiol* 40:746-52, 2002.
42. Hariharan S: Recommendations for outpatient monitoring of kidney transplant recipients, *Am J Kidney Dis* 4(2):S22-S36, 2006.
43. Paya C, Humar A, Dominguez E, Washburn K, Blumberg E, Alexander B, et al., for the Valganciclovir Solid Organ Transplant Study Group: Efficacy and safety of valganciclovir vs. oral ganciclovir for prevention of cytomegalovirus disease in solid organ transplant recipients, *Am J Transplant* 4:611-20, 2004.
44. Gottschalk S, Rooney CM, Heslop HE: Post transplant lymphoproliferative disorders, *Annu Rev Med* 56:29-44, 2005.
45. Hadou T, Andre JL, Bourquard R, Krier-Coudert MJ, Venard V, Le Faou A: Long-term follow-up of Epstein-Barr virus viremia in pediatric recipients of renal transplants, *Pediatr Nephrol* 20:76-80, 2005.
46. Humar A, Hebert D, Davies HD, Humar A, Stephens D, O'Doherty B, et al: A randomized trial of ganciclovir versus ganciclovir plus immune globulin for prophylaxis against Epstein-Barr virus related posttransplantation lymphoproliferative disorder, *Transplantation* 81:856-61, 2006.
47. Rowe DT, Qu L, Reyes J, Jabbour N, Yunis E, Putnam P, et al: Use of quantitative competitive PCR to measure Epstein-Barr virus genome load in the peripheral blood of pediatric transplant patients with lymphoproliferative disorders, *J Clin Microbiol* 35:1612-15, 1997.
48. Wadowsky RM, Laus S, Green M, Webber SA, Rowe D: Measurement of Epstein-Barr virus DNA loads in whole blood and plasma by TaqMan PCR and in peripheral blood lymphocytes by competitive PCR, *J Clin Microbiol* 41:5245-49, 2003.
49. Hill CE, Harris SB, Culler EE, Zimring JC, Nolte FS, Caliendo AM: Performance characteristics of two real-time PCR assays for the quantification of Epstein-Barr virus DNA, *Am J Clin Pathol* 125:665-71, 2006.
50. Lee TC, Savoldo B, Rooney CM, Heslop HE, Gee AP, Caldwell Y, et al: Quantitative EBV viral loads and immunosuppression alterations can decrease PTLD incidence in pediatric liver transplant recipients, *Am J Transplant* 5:2222-28, 2005.
51. McDiarmid SV, Jordan S, Lee GS, Toyoda M, Goss JA, Vargas JH, et al: Prevention and preemptive therapy of posttransplant lymphoproliferative disease in pediatric liver recipients, *Transplantation* 66:1604-11, 1998.
52. Green M, Webber S: Posttransplantation lymphoproliferative disorders, *Pediatr Clin North Am* 50:1471-91, 2003.
53. Kenagy DN, Schlesinger Y, Weck K, Ritter JH, Gaudreault-Keener MM, Storch GA: Epstein-Barr virus DNA in peripheral blood leukocytes of patients with posttransplantation lymphoproliferative disease, *Transplantation* 60:547-54, 1995.
54. Savoie A, Perpete C, Carpentier L, Joncas J, Alfieri C: Direct correlation between the load of Epstein-Barr virus-infected lymphocytes in the peripheral blood of pediatric transplant patients and risk of lymphoproliferative disease, *Blood* 83:2715-22, 1994.
55. Allen UD, Farkas G, Hebert D, Weitzman S, Stephens D, Petric M, et al: Risk factors for posttransplantation lymphoproliferative disorder in pediatric patients: A case-control study, *Pediatr Transplant* 9:450-55, 2005.
56. Gourishankar S, McDermid JC, Jhangri S, Preiksaitis JK: Herpes zoster infection following solid organ transplantation: Incidence, risk factors and outcomes in the current immunosuppressive era, *Am J Transplant* 4:108-15, 2004.
57. Lynfield R, Jerrin JT, Rubin RH: Varicella in pediatric renal transplant recipients, *Pediatrics* 90:216-20, 1992.
58. Kashtan CE, Cook M, Chavers BM, Mauer SM, Nevins TE: Outcome of chickenpox in 66 pediatric renal transplant recipients, *J Pediatr* 131:874-77, 1997.
59. Broyer M, Tete MJ, Guest G, Gagnadoux MF, Rouzioux C: Varicella and zoster after kidney transplantation: Long term results after kidney transplantation, *Pediatrics* 99:35-39, 1997.
60. Guidelines for vaccination of solid organ transplant candidates and recipients, *Am J Transplant* 4(10):160-63, 2004.
61. Furth SL, Hogg RJ, Tarver J, Moulton LH, Chan C, Fivush BA: Varicella vaccination in children with chronic renal failure: A report

of the Southwest Pediatric Nephrology Study Group, *Pediatr Nephrol* 18:33-38, 2003.
62. Neu AM, Fivush BA: Immunization of children with renal disease. In BS Kaplan, KEC Meyers (eds.), *Pediatric nephrology and urology: The requisites in pediatrics*. Philadelphia: Elsevier Mosby 2004:33-40.
63. American Academy of Pediatrics, Committee on Infectious Diseases: Recommendations for the use of live attenuated varicella vaccine, *Pediatrics* 95:791-96, 1995.
64. Centers for Disease Control and Prevention: Prevention of varicella: Recommendations of the Advisory Committee on Immunization Practices (ACIP), *MMWR Morb Mortal Wkly Rep* 45(RR-11):1-36, 1996.
65. Centers for Disease Control and Prevention: A new product (VariZIG) for postexposure prophylaxis of varicella available under an investigational new drug application expanded access protocol, *MMWR Morb Mortal Wkly Rep* 3(55):209-10, 2006.
66. Nyerges G, Meszner A, Gyarmati E, Kerpel-Frosnius S: Acyclovir prevents dissemination of varicella in immunocompromised children, *J Infect Dis* 157:309-13, 1988.
67. Prober CG, Kirk LE, Keeney RE: Acyclovir therapy of chickenpox in immunosuppressed children—a collaborative study, *J Pediatr* 101:622-25, 1982.
68. Gardner SD, Field AM, Coleman DV, Hulme B: New human papovavirus (B.K.) isolated from urine after renal transplantation, *Lancet* 1:1253-57, 1971.
69. Ramos E, Drachenberg CB, Papadimitriou JC, Hamze O, Fink JC, Klassen DK, et al: Clinical course of polyoma virus nephropathy in 67 renal transplant patients, *J Am Soc Nephrol* 13:2145-51, 2002.
70. Hirsch HH, Steiger J: Polyomavirus BK, *Lancet Infect Dis* 3:611-23, 2003.
71. Smith JM, McDonald RA, Finn LS, Healey PJ, Davis CL, Limaye AP: Polyomavirus nephropathy in pediatric kidney transplant recipients, *Am J Transplant* 4:2109-17, 2004.
72. Vats A: BK virus-associated transplant nephropathy: Need for increased awareness in children, *Pediatr Transplant* 8:421-25, 2004.
73. Mengel M, Marwedel M, Radermacher J, Eden G, Schwarz A, Haller H, et al: Incidence of polyomavirus-nephropathy in renal allografts: Influence of modern immunosuppressive drugs, *Nephrol Dial Transplant* 18:1190-96, 2003.
74. Ginevri F, De Santis R, Comoli P, Pastorino N, Rossi C, Botti G, et al: Polyomavirus BK infection in pediatric kidney-allograft recipients: A single-center analysis of incidence, risk factors, and novel therapeutic approaches, *Transplantation* 75:1266-70, 2003.
75. Nickeleit V, Singh HK, Mihatsch MJ: Polyomavirus nephropathy: Morphology, pathophysiology, and clinical management, *Curr Opin Nephrol Hypertens* 12:599-605, 2003.
76. Brennan DC, Agha I, Bohl DL, Schnitzler MA, Hardinger KL, Lockwood M, et al: Incidence of BK with tacrolimus versus cyclosporine and impact of preemptive immunosuppression reduction, *Am J Transplant* 5:582-94, 2005.
77. Humar A, Michaels M: American Society of Transplantation recommendations for screening, monitoring and reporting of infectious complications in immunosuppression trials in recipients of organ transplantation, *Am J Transplant* 6:262-74, 2006.
78. Randhawa P, Brennan DC: BK virus infection in transplant recipients: An overview and update, *Am J Transplant* 6:2000-05, 2006.
79. Randhawa PS, Demetris AJ: Nephropathy due to polyomavirus type BK, *N Engl J Med* 342:1361-63, 2000.
80. Kadambi PV, Josephson MA, Williams J, Corey L, Jerome KR, Meehan SM, et al: Treatment of refractory BK virus-associated nephropathy with cidofovir, *Am J Transplant* 3:186-91, 2003.
81. Vats A, Shapiro R, Singh Randhawa P, Scantlebury V, Tuzuner A, Saxena M, et al: Quantitative viral load monitoring and cidofovir therapy for the management of BK virus-associated nephropathy in children and adults, *Transplantation* 75:105-12, 2003.
82. Araya CE, Lew JF, Fennell RS, Neiberger RE, Dharnidharka VR: Intermediate-dose cidofovir without probenecid in the treatment of BK virus allograft nephropathy, *Pediatr Transplant* 10:32-37, 2006.
83. Djamin RS, Drent M, Schreurs AJ, Groen EA, Wagenaar SS: Diagnosis of *Pneumocystis carinii* pneumonia in HIV-positive patients: Bronchoalveolar lavage vs. bronchial brushing, *Acta Cytol* 42:933-38, 1998.
84. Elinder CG, Andersson J, Bolinder G, Tyden G: Effectiveness of low-dose cotrimoxazole prophylaxis against *Pneumocystis carinii* pneumonia after renal and/or pancreas transplantation, *Transpl Int* 5:81-84, 1992.
85. Tolkoff-Rubin N, Rubin RH: Infection in the renal transplant patient. In WF Owen, MH Sayegh (eds.), *Dialysis and Transplantation*. Philadelphia: WB Saunders 2000:584-94.
86. Patel R: Infections in recipients of kidney transplants, *Infect Dis Clin N Am* 15:901-52, 2001.
87. Hoy WE, Roberts NJ, Bryson MF, Bowles C, Lee JC, Rivero AJ, et al: Transmission of strongyloidiasis by kidney transplant? Disseminated strongyloidiasis in both recipients of kidney allografts from a single cadaver donor, *JAMA* 246:1937-39, 1981.
88. Nolan TJ, Schad GA: Tacrolimus allows autoinfective development of the parasitic nematode *Strongyloides stercoralis*, *Transplantation* 62:15, 1996.
89. Schad GA: Cyclosporine may eliminate the threat of overwhelming *Strongyloides* in immunosuppressed patients, *J Infect Dis* 153:178, 1986.
90. DeVault GA, King JW, Rohr MS, Landreneau MD, Brown ST III, McDonald JC: Opportunistic infections with *Strongyloides stercoralis* in renal transplantation, *Rev Infect Dis* 12:653-71, 1990.
91. Sato Y, Kobayashi J, Toma H, Shiroma Y: Efficacy of stool examination for detection of Strongyloides infection, *Am J Trop Med Hyg* 53:248-50, 1995.
92. Harris RA Jr., Musher DM, Fainstein V, Young EJ, Clarridge J: Disseminated strongyloidiasis: Diagnosis made by sputum examination, *JAMA* 244:65-66, 1980.
93. Abdalla J, Saad M, Myers JW, Moorman JP: An elderly man with immunosuppression, shortness of breath, and eosinophilia, *Clin Infect Dis* 40:1464, 2005.
94. Drugs for parasitic infections, *Medical Lett Drugs Ther* August 2004.
95. Ferraz AS, Figueiredo JF: Transmission of Chagas' disease through transplanted kidney: Occurrence of the acute form of the disease in two recipients from the same donor, *Rev Med Trop Sao Paulo* 35:461-63, 1993.
96. Türkmen A, Sever MS, Ecder T, Yildiz A, Aydin AE, Erkoç R, et al: Posttransplantation malaria, *Transplantation* 62:1521-23, 1996.
97. American Academy of Pediatrics Committee on Infectious Diseases: Recommendations for the prevention of pneumococcal infections, including the use of pneumococcal conjugate vaccine (Prevnar), pneumococcal polysaccharide vaccine, and antibiotic prophylaxis, *Pediatrics* 106:362-66, 2000.
98. Centers for Disease Control and Prevention: Prevention and control of meningococcal disease recommendations of the Advisory Committee on Immunization Practices (ACIP), *MMWR* 54(RR-7):1-21, 2005.
99. American Academy of Pediatrics Committee on Infectious Diseases: Prevention and control of meningococcal disease: Recommendations for use of meningococcal vaccines in pediatric patients, *Pediatrics* 116:496-505, 2005.

CHAPTER 63

Malignancy after Pediatric Renal Transplantation

Jaap W. Groothoff

INTRODUCTION

For a long time, cancer has been recognized as an emerging threat in adult organ transplant recipients. Although children still have a significantly lower risk of malignancies after transplantation, the incidence has definitely increased over the last decade. More attention given life-threatening cardiovascular comorbidity and the use of more potent immune suppressive agents in transplant recipients are the most probable causes of this development.

According to most studies, posttransplant lymphoproliferative disease (PTLD) accounts for more than 50% of all malignancies in children after solid organ transplantation. In contrast to most other malignancies, PTLD typically presents very soon after transplantation (especially in children)—making it by far the most important type of malignancy pediatric nephrologists may be confronted with. For this reason, we will pay special attention to the diagnostic and therapeutic approach of PTLD in children in this chapter. At the same time, it is good to realize that beyond the age of 18 these patients rapidly become at risk for the more "adult" types of malignancies—especially of skin cancers—at a relatively young age.[1-4]

EPIDEMIOLOGY: INCIDENCE AND TYPES OF CANCER

Cancer in End-Stage Renal Disease

Most data on cancer in patients with end-stage renal disease (ESRD) come from renal graft recipients. Yet, at least in adults, there is evidence that ESRD itself is associated with an increased risk of malignancy. In a large Japanese study among 23,209 dialysis patients, the risk of cancer and the mortality caused by cancer were found to be 1.4 and 1.9 times, respectively, the expected rates in the general population.[5] Combined data of the U.S. Renal Data System (USRDS), the European Dialysis and Transplantation Association (EDTA), and the Australian and New Zealand Dialysis and Transplantation (ANZDT) registry—censored for transplantation—revealed a standardized incidence ratio (SIR) of 1.18 (95% CI 1.17-1.20) for dialysis patients of all age groups.

The risk of cancer was particularly high in young patients. For patients less than 35 years of age, the SIR was 3.68 (95% CI 3.39-3.99).[6] Notably, the overall SIR of the most complete and reliable of the three registries (the ANZDT) was 1.8 (95% CI 1.7-2.0)—suggesting that the combined SIR of all registries of 1.18 is presumably an underestimation. Potential determinants of the increased risk of cancer in dialysis patients are chronic infection, an impaired immune system, nutritional deficiency, former treatment with immunosuppressive drugs of the primary disease, and altered DNA repair.[7] Adult patients who remain on dialysis treatment appear to be especially at risk for renal cell carcinoma (SIR 3.60, 95% CI 3.45-3.76), bladder cancer (SIR 1.5, 95% CI 1.42-1.57), and thyroid or other endocrine organs (SIR 2.28, 95% CI 2.03-2.54).[6]

Cancer after Kidney Transplantation in Adults

The incidence of de novo malignancies in adult recipients of renal transplants is between six and seven times higher than in the general population.[8,9] The cumulative incidence varies from 2.6% to 19.4%.[8-12] This high incidence is thought to be mainly caused by the use of immunosuppressive antirejection therapy. Immunosuppressive agents may directly cause DNA damage and interfere with DNA repair. Moreover, they may increase the susceptibility to oncogenic viruses, such as EBV.[8,9]

Nonmelanoma skin cancer is by far the most frequent malignancy in adult renal graft recipients, followed by Kaposi's sarcoma, PTLD, and renal carcinoma. Kaposi's sarcoma and PTLD are found to be more than twentyfold more common in this group than in the general population. The incidence of kidney cancer is increased fifteenfold. Melanoma, leukemia, hepatocellular or cholangio carcinoma, cervical, and vulvovaginal cancer are increased fivefold. Testicular and bladder cancer are increased threefold.[11] On the contrary, the incidences of carcinomas of the lung, colon, prostate, rectum, and breast (which all occur frequently in the general population) are not increased in transplant recipients.[9,11]

Cancer after ESRD of Childhood

In young adults with renal insufficiency since childhood, cumulative incidences of cancer vary from 0.8% to 17% after

25 years.[1,2] The overall risk of cancer is believed to be tenfold higher than in the general population.[2] According to the USRDS data, renal graft recipients under the age of 18 have a higher relative risk (RR 1.62) of getting a nonskin malignancy and a lower relative risk (RR 0.15) of getting a nonmelanoma skin malignancy compared to patients aged 18 to 34 years.[11] However, these figures most likely underestimate the real burden pediatric transplant recipients may face later in life.

In a Dutch long-term follow-up study [Late Effects of Renal Insufficiency in Children (LERIC)] performed in 1999, we found malignancies in 21 out of 231 renal transplanted patients—with onset of ESRD before the age of 15 years after a mean follow-up of 15.5 years.[2,3] At a longer follow-up (5 years later in 2004), in 15 patients out of the 187 survivors of the first study new malignancies were recorded after a total follow-up time of more than 20 years—making a total of 36 out of 231 renal graft recipients with cancer (15.8%, data not published). The mean age of the survivors at that moment was 35 years (range 25-45). In 23.5% of the new casualties between 1999 and 2004, death was caused by a malignancy (compared to 10% of the original cohort recorded in 1999). Unfortunately, to date very few data on long-term outcome exist to confirm these findings.

Type of Cancer in Pediatric Transplant Recipients

PTLD affects children early after transplantation, and skin cancers become most prevalent 10 to 15 years after transplantation. The pattern of malignancies after transplantation differs in children from that in adults, as has been shown by the data of the Israel Penn (former Cincinnati) Transplant Tumor Registry Study (IPTTRS).[1] They reported on 10,813 types of cancer that occurred in 10,151 organ transplant recipients (data collected between 1968 and 1997), of which 527 were found in 512 pediatric patients (281 kidney transplantations).

According to this report, 60% appeared during childhood. PTLD accounted for 52% of all cancers (compared to 15% in adults). Skin cancers accounted for 20% (38% in adults) of all cancers, and other tumors for 28%.[1] PTLD, sarcoma, renal tumors, brain tumors, and ovarian cancer presented predominantly at childhood. Table 63-1 summarizes the prevalence and outcome of malignancies after pediatric transplantation according to the IPTTRS. Most likely, the IPTTRS underestimates the incidence of skin tumors.[2,4]

TABLE 63-1 **Type of Cancer in Pediatric Renal Recipients**

Malignancy	Median Time of Onset	Relative Frequency	Established Risk Factors Other Than Immunosuppressive Agents	Adverse Outcome
PTLD*: 91% B cell, 8% T cell, 1% Hodgkin's disease or multiple plasmocytoma	Biphasic: early onset (8-360 days, median 6 months); late onset: increasing after 5 years	Very common (50%)*	EBV-naive state/de novo infection, CMV (?), Hepatitis C (?), male gender, Caucasian race	Deceased 48%* (wide range in various reports 0-80% deaths); worse outcome: late onset, T-cell, Burkitt-like
Nonmelanoma skin cancer	Late-onset; mean age 26-28 years	Very common (17%)*	Sun exposure, HPV/warts/actinic keratosis (SCC)	Mostly good, but can be lethal (9%)*
Melanoma	Widespread onset	3%*	Suns exposure, nevi	20% mortality*
Carcinoma vulva/perineum	Late onset	Rare (4%)*	HPV (SCC), condylomata acuminatum	8% mortality*
Kaposi's sarcoma (KS)	Late onset	Rare (3%)*	HHV8 virus, HIV	38% mortality*
Thyroid gland carcinoma	Late onset	Rare (3%)*		Mostly good prognosis
Liver and bile duct carcinoma	Mostly late onset	Rare (3%)*	Hepatitis B (?)	60% mortality
Sarcoma (excl. KS): leiomyosarcoma, rhabdomyosarcoma, fibrosarcoma	Widespread onset, mostly early onset	Rare (3%)*	EBV (leiomyosarcoma)	45% mortality*
Head/neck cancer	Late onset	Rare (2%)*		29% mortality*
Brain tumor (glioblastoma, glioma, neuroectodermal tumor)	Early onset	Rare (1%)*	BK virus	20% mortality (glioblastoma 90-100%)
Renal cell tumor	Widespread onset	Rare (1%)*	BK virus (?)	62% mortality*
Ovarian carcinoma	Widespread onset	Rare (1%)*	Frasier's syndrome (dysgerminoma)	49% mortality*
Uterine cervix carcinoma	Late onset	Rare (1-2%)*		
Leukemia	Mostly late onset	Rare	HLTV-1	67% mortality
Miscellaneous†	Widespread onset	Rare (5%)		

* According the Israel Penn Transplant Tumor Registry: 527 tumors; more long-term follow-up study reveals a higher incidence of skin cancer, being >50% of all cancers.
† Bladder carcinoma, testicular carcinoma, beast cancer, adrenal neuroblastoma, and endometrial carcinoma.

In the Dutch LERIC study, after a follow-up time of 15.5 years, we found 22 cancers in 21 out of 231 pediatric renal transplant recipients. Of these, 13 were skin cancers (59%), 5 were PTLD (23%), 1 was leukemia, 1 was fibrosarcoma, 1 was renal carcinoma, and 1 was leiomyosarcoma[2] Five years later, after 20 years of follow-up, the number of cancers had been increased to 51 in 36 patients of the same cohort. Twenty-two new nonmelanoma skin cancers, 3 melanomas, and 2 cases of late-onset PTLD were diagnosed between 1999 and 2004 (data not published).

The North Italian Transplant program reported on 10 malignancies that had occurred in 454 pediatric renal graft recipients: 6 PTLD, 1 urothelial carcinoma of a native kidney, 1 nephroblastoma of a native kidney, 1 dysgerminoma, and 1 optical glioma of the left eye. All appeared within 25 months after transplantation. The mean follow-up time is not mentioned, but the maximal follow-up was only 12 years.[10]

RISK FACTORS FOR CANCER AFTER KIDNEY TRANSPLANTATION IN CHILDREN

Posttransplant malignancies have several characteristics that distinguish them from sporadic tumors. Most typically, the incidence of nearly all of these malignancies is associated with the combination of high doses of immunosuppressive (IS) therapy and a de novo infection with a certain oncogenic virus. Contrary to the situation in adults, pretransplant malignancies have not proven to be a risk factor for de novo cancer after renal transplantation in children.

Virus Infection

In adults as well as in children, several viruses are associated with the development of cancer. EBV predisposes for PTLD, but also for renal leiomyoma.[13] Herpesvirus 8 is associated with sarcoma, human papillomavirus (HPV), squamous cell skin cancer (type 5), and vulvar and vaginal carcinoma. HTLV-1 virus may cause T-cell leukemia or lymphoma.

BK virus, a human polyomavirus, may cause BK nephropathy after renal transplantation. It is also associated with the posttransplantation appearance of brain cancer, renal carcinoma, and other cancers in humans.[14,15] Reports on the attenuating influence of cytomegalovirus (CMV) and hepatitis C infection on the development of EBV-related PTLD were not confirmed by a recent report of the USRDS, or by a large Australian and New Zealand registry study.[16-19]

Immunosuppressive Therapy

The key role of immunosuppressive therapy in transplant recipients with respect to the increased risk for cancer is beyond the scope of this discussion. Yet, it is difficult to attribute causality to individual agents with respect to cancer risks. The pattern of high incidence of malignancies in times of the use of high doses of immune suppressive agents accounts for all kinds of agents in different sorts of solid organ transplantation. Regimens with antithymocyte globulin (ATG) and OKT3 have especially been associated with an increased risk for cancer,[18,20] but not by all studies.[19]

In an analysis from the United Network of Organ Sharing registry, only equine ATG (and not rabbit ATG or ALG) was associated with increased incidence of PTLD in pediatric renal transplant recipients.[21] In addition, the introduction of the calcineurin inhibitors (i.e., cyclosporine in the mid 1980s and tacrolimus 10 years later) induced a rise in malignancies, especially of PTLD[1,18-20,22] With the reduction of both cyclosporine and tacrolimus dosages, the enhanced influence of both drugs on the development of cancer could no longer be demonstrated.[23]

According to the USRDS database, the use of azathioprine and mycophenolate mofetil (MMF) was associated with a decreased risk of PTLD—whereas the use of ATG and OKT3 increased the risk of PTLD. Patients treated with MMF had a better survival after PTLD. The introduction of IL2-receptor inhibitor in the induction regimens has not increased PTLD risk.[18] Data on the influence of sirolimus are too limited to date to prove its antiproliferative capacities in practice.

Pretransplant Malignancies and Syndromes with Cancer Predisposition

Denys-Drash syndrome (DSS) is characterized by a cancer predisposition as a consequence of genetic mutations occurring at different chromosomal sites. The risk of Wilms' tumor development is related to the presence of a germline mutation in the Wilms' tumor suppressor gene WT1, which is located on chromosome 11p13. In an Italian cohort study, 2 out of 5 patients with DSS developed a de novo cancer after transplantation: 1 PTLD and 1 Wilms' tumor in the left native kidney.[10]

On the other hand, the NAPRTCS reported on 43 Denys-Drash patients out of all registered transplanted children between 1987 and 2002 and found no new malignancies after transplantation in these patients.[24] The same accounted for patients with bilateral Wilms' tumor. According to the NAPRTCS data, out of 37 patients from the period 1992 to 2001 with bilateral Wilms' tumor 10 patients died before transplantation as a result of Wilms' tumor. However, patient survival after transplantation did not differ from patients with other primary diseases.

Only one patient died within 3 years after transplantation as a result of Wilms' tumor.[24] The North Italian Transplant program reported on a 10-year-old girl with Frasier syndrome, who developed a dysgerminoma 25 months after transplantation. She was cured by chemotherapy and surgery. Frasier syndrome is characterized by gonadal dysgenesis, which may lead to a dysgerminoma in 15% to 20%. This represents reason to consider prophylactic gonadectomy in these children.[10,25]

Multinodular Cystic Kidney and Acquired Renal Cystic Disease

Children with *multinodular cystic* kidneys are believed to be at risk for developing a Wilms' tumor. However, a systematic review of all studies on children with conservatively managed unilateral multicystic disease revealed no Wilms' tumor at all. Therefore, in the absence of hypertension nephrectomy is not indicated in these children and long-term follow-up is not mandatory.[26]

In the late 1970s, an association between dialysis-associated *acquired cystic kidney disease* (ACKD) and the development of renal cell carcinoma was reported. In a single-center study, Querfeld and colleagues followed 48 pediatric patients with ESRD (of whom 30% had ACKD). One patient was nephrectomized at 26 years of age because of renal cell carcinoma.[27] Gentle and colleagues reported on a 13-year-old boy with renal cell carcinoma after 9 years of dialysis associated with ACKD.[28] However, a comprehensive review of all adult patients with ACKD revealed no documented increase or renal cell carcinoma compared to patients without ACKD.[29]

Bladder Augmentation by Enterocystoplasty

Bladder augmentation by enterocystoplasty has been a recognized risk factor for bladder cancer for a long time. However, very few data exist on its exact prevalence. Three single-center long-term follow-up studies revealed 3, 7, and 4 cancers out of, respectively, 260, 94, and 186 patients with bladder augmentations.[30,31] Adenocarcinoma of bowel origin and transitional cell carcinoma were the most frequent cancers, usually originating in close proximity to the ureteroenteric anastomosis. Also squamous cell carcinoma may occur in augmented bladders.

Chronic inflammation, stagnant urine, increased mucus production, and bladder stones are potential risk factors of neoplasia. The mean interval time from enteroplasty, performed in children, to cancer occurrence is reported to be 25 years—ranging from 7 to 50 years.[30,31] This very late onset may be the reason for the low number of bladder carcinoma as reported by most outcome studies on cancer in children with ESRD.

Growth Hormone Therapy

In 2000, Tyden and colleagues reported on the development of renal graft cancer in two renal graft recipients treated with recombinant growth hormone (GH).[32] This opened the discussion of the possible oncogenic effect of GH therapy in children with renal disease. GH and IGF-I may transform lymphocytes and induce cell proliferation. The number of IGF-I receptors is increased in neoplastic tissue. However, IGF-expressing transgenic mice showed no enhanced spontaneous tumor formation.

Review of all patients from the Collaborative Transplant Study revealed no increase of renal cell carcinoma in GH-treated patients compared to untreated renal transplant recipients. No cases of renal cell carcinoma have been found in GH-treated patients without renal disease. The preliminary conclusion is that there is no evidence that GH treatment promotes the development of cancer.[33]

POSTTRANSPLANT LYMPHOPROLIFERATIVE DISORDER

PTLD is the most prevalent life-threatening malignancy in renal transplant recipients. In renal transplanted children, it accounts for more than 50% of all malignancies that occur before adulthood.[1] PTLD comprises a group of abnormal lymphoid proliferations (generally of B cells) that may occur in the setting of ineffective T-cell functioning induced by IS. Recent data indicate that it is an increasingly common disease. In pediatric transplantation, incidences ranging from 1.2% to 10% have been reported.[34-36]

The risk of PTLD varies with time. The highest rates are observed within 12 months after transplantation. The median time of early-onset PTLD after transplantation is 6 months. A second peak occurs after 5 to 10 years.[19,37] Early-onset PTLD is associated with EBV infection in 95% of cases and has a better overall prognosis than the late-onset form.[38] The clinical presentation is extremely heterogeneous because any organ may be involved (Table 63-2).

The most common presentation symptoms in kidney graft recipients are unexplained fever, cervical lymphadenopathy, enlarged tonsils, hepatosplenomegaly, allograft dysfunction, graft tenderness, and abdominal pain.[39] Therapeutic options and outcome depend on the type of PTLD and may vary from sole reduction of IS to treatment with rituximab, with or without more aggressive forms of chemotherapy (Table 63-3).

Prevalence and Time of Occurrence of PTLD

PTLD complicates 1% to 10% of all renal transplantations. The risk of PTLD after organ transplantation is about twelvefold higher than in nontransplanted patients.[20] Within the group of renal transplanted patients, the incidence of PTLD in children is 3 to 4 times higher than in adults[40] (Figure 63-1). In a single-center study comprising 1316 transplantations over 8 years, PTLD was found in 10 out of 99 pediatric patients (10.1%) compared to 25 out of 1217 (1.9%) adults.[22]

The time from transplantation to diagnosis may range from 6 weeks to more than 7 years[19,41] and shows a biphasic pattern with a peak during the first year and a second rising incidence after 5 years (Figure 63-2). Young patients are especially at risk for early-onset PTLD, which may occur for more than 2 years after transplantation.[37] In the study of Shapiro and colleagues, the mean time between transplantation and onset of PTLD was 25 ± 24.7 months in adults and 14.4 ± 18.2 months in children.[22] Early-onset PTLD has on average a better prognosis in terms of survival than the late-onset form.[19,22]

PTLD tends to become more prevalent over time (Figure 63-3). The NAPRTCS report showed an increase over time from 254/100,000 years between 1987 and 1991 to 395/100,000 between 1992 and 1996.[34] Given the time between transplantation and onset of PTLD, and the short time of follow-up of the latter group, this figure could be an underestimation of the real increase in incidence.

Pathophysiology of EBV-Associated PTLD

EBV is a lymphotropic herpesvirus. During initial infection, the major envelope glycoprotein gp350 of the virus interacts with CD 21 molecules on the surface of the B-lymphocytes and thus enters the cell. Once the virus has established itself in the host nucleus, it will remain in the body in a state of latency for that individual's lifetime. A small number of B-lymphocytes carry the virus, inducing from time to time low-grade viral replication in the oropharyngeal epithelium.

This latent state is associated with the production of viral proteins, EBNA (EB nuclear antigen), and LMP (latent membrane proteins), which protect the B cell from apoptosis and allow for ongoing viral replication. In healthy persons, the viral replication is kept in check by a cytotoxic T cell (CD8+)-driven EBV-specific immune surveillance.

TABLE 63-2 Clinical Presentation of PTLD

Clinical Signs/Comments	
Unexplained fever, malaise, weight loss	Most common presentation: adenoid and tonsilar enlargement, cervical nodes, hepatosplenomegaly, fever, malaise, abdominal mass, renal involvement; CNS involvement 25%
Abdominal mass, hepato(spleno)megaly, tender (enlarged) graft	
Mass renal graft	
Enlarged tonsils, cervical nodes, CNS manifestations	
Risk Factors/Comments	
EBV seronegativity recipient (+ seropositivity donor)	EBV seronegative 20 times increased risk PTLD compared to seropositive patients; OKT3, equine ATG, high-dose tacrolimus risk factors, MMF/azathioprine associated with reduced risk, controversial data on the influence of CMV and hepatitis C
ATG (?), OKT3	
CMV mismatch (?); hepatitis C (?); male, Caucasian race, young age	
Biologic Predictive Markers and Diagnostic Tools/Comments	
Sharp rise in PCR EBV mononuclear cells, peripheral blood or serum	Predictive values of EBV PCR depend on method of assessment and longitudinal follow-up is warranted
High LDH	Combination of rise in EBV PCR and lack of EBV-specific TLC most predictive for PTLD
Decreased or absent EBV-specific CD8+ T cells	Loss of anti-EBNA in seropositive patients predictive
Lowering/absent anti-EBNA in former seropositive patients	Biopsy suspected tissue (should always be performed)
Ultrasound abdomen, X-thorax, inspection tonsils, CT scan, PET scan	PET scan is very sensitive to PTLD detection
Biopsy suspect tissue	

TABLE 63-3 Therapeutic Options in PTLD

Mononucleosis infectiosa, polymorphic PTLD	1. Reduction IS: PDN, CsA/TAC, MMF/AZA—stop MMF/AZA, ½ CsA/TAC 2. No response: stop CsA/TAC 3. Progressive disease: consider rituximab

Localized monoclonal PTLD:
• Tonsils
• Graft/bowel
	• Tonsils: tonsillectomy and reduction IS
	• Graft/bowl: reduction IS (stop CsA/TAC and MMF/AZA, continuation PDN) and dependent on biopsy:
	  • CD-20^{+}: rituximab (+ CTL infusion)
	  • CD 20^{-}/T-lymphoma: graft removal in case of graft loc., chemotherapy*

Disseminated PTLD	• Early-onset / CD 20^{+}/not severely ill patients, abdominal location, no CNS involvement:
	  1. Reduction IS (stop CsA/TAC and MMF/aza, continuation PDN) and rituximab (and CTL infusion)
	  2. In case of no response: chemotherapy†
	• Disseminated PTLD, ill patients, thoracal and/or CNS location: Stop IS, continuation PDN, rituximab, chemotherapy (+ i.v. and i.th.)† (+ CTL infusion)

CsA, cyclosporin A; *AZA*, azathioprine; *TAC*, tacrolimus; *PDN*, prednisone; *MMF*, mycophenolate mofetil; *CTL*, autologous EBV-specific cytotoxic T- lymphocyte infusions after initial treatment.
* Chemotherapy according to LMB or BFM protocol of particular lymphoma (B cell or T cell).
† rCHOP and mBFM = reduced dosage CHOP modified BFM = dexamethasone 3 g/m^2 days 1 through 6, cyclophosphamide 200 mg/m^2 days 1 through 4, vincristine 1.5 mg/m^2 day 1, etoposide 100 mg/m^2 days 3 and 4, cytarabine 150 mg/m^2 days 3 and 4.

EBV affects the majority of individuals in the western world, so that more than 90% of the adult population has serologic evidence of EBV infection. In immune competent persons, it only causes little significant disease. Impairment of EBV-specific cytotoxic T-cell response induced by the IS is believed to be the essential factor in the development of PTLD. This leads to an uncontrolled viral replication manifested as an increase of virus-carrying B cells in the circulation.

The latently affected cells undergo lytic replication and ultimately B-cell transformation. Cytokine responses, as induced by the immunosuppressive state, allow an uncontrolled monoclonal B-cell proliferation.[42,43] This can ultimately lead to neoplastic PTLD. Malignantly transformed B

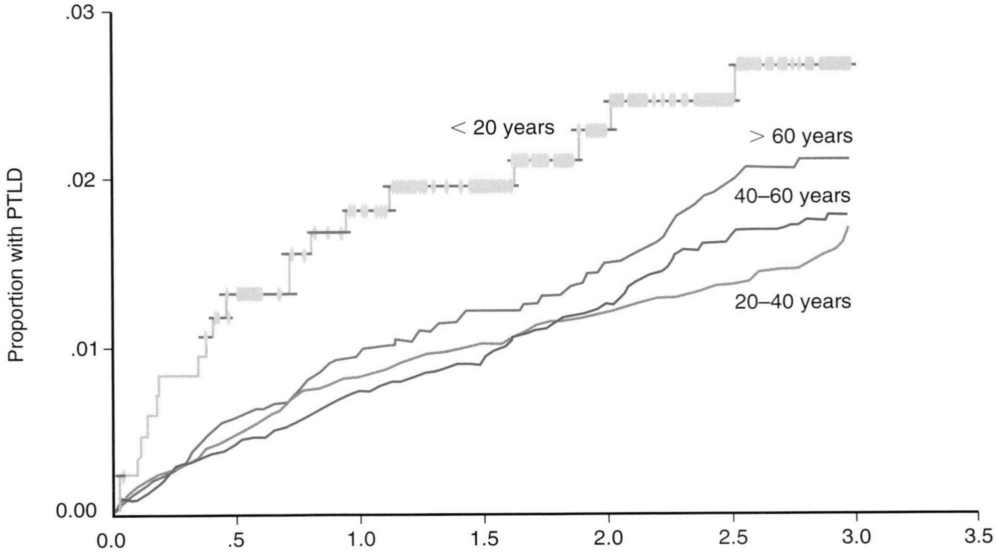

Figure 63-1 Time to diagnosis for PTLD stratified for age: patients <20 years ($n = 855$) versus patients >20 years ($n = 24{,}272$), $p = 0.02$ by log rank test. Data are derived from the USRDS. From Caillard S, Dharnidharka V, Agodoa L, Bohen E, Abbott K: Posttransplant lymphoproliferative disorders after renal transplantation in the United States in era of modern immunosuppression, *Transplantation* 80:1233-43, 2005.

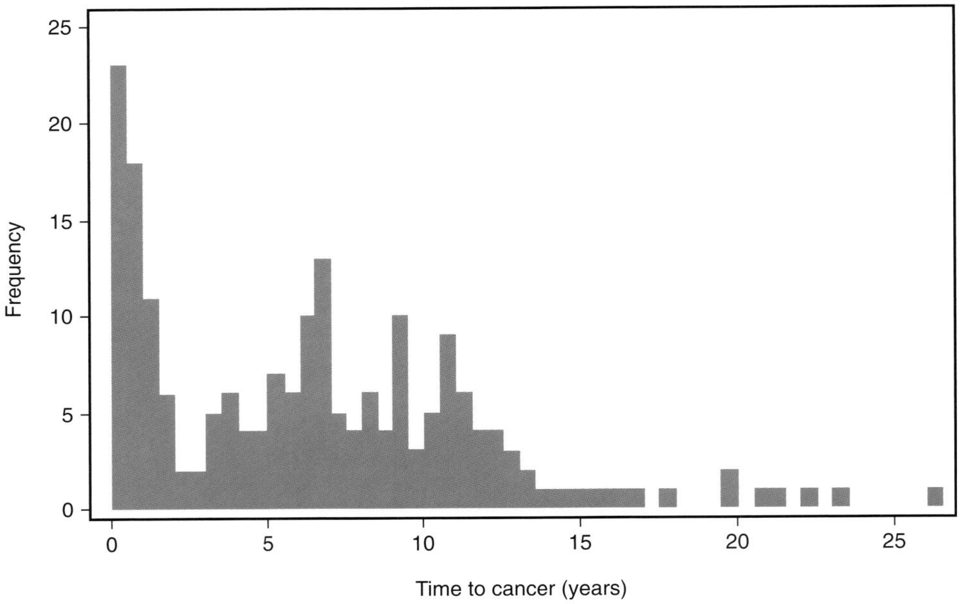

Figure 63-2 Histogram of occurrence of PTLD against time since transplantation. Data from the Australian and New Zealand Dialysis and Transplant Registry. From Faull RJ, Hollett P, MacDonald SP: Lymphoproliferative disease after renal transplantation in Australia and New Zealand, *Transplantation* 80(2):193-19, 2005.

cells are usually from recipient origin. Only in bone marrow transplantation do the abnormal B cells originate from the donor.[38]

Rare Types of PTLD

EBV-Negative PTLD

The rarer types of PTLD often present as late-onset PTLD and may represent sporadic lymphomas arising in immune-compromised patients. Others suggest a "hit and run" role for EBV. Herpesviruses generally persist as episomes in tumor cells. The "hit and run" theory suggests that EBV episomes are lost when there is no selective pressure for their maintenance. In EBV-positive Burkitt's-lymphoma–derived cell lines, it has been shown that some clones lack the viral episomes.

This loss of episomes is not associated with loss of a malignant phenotype. It has been supposed that chromosomal translocations and point mutations may have supplanted EBV as a driving force for proliferation, whereas in others EBV remains essential to the development of a malignant phenotype.[44]

T-Cell PTLD and Leukemia

Only 16 cases of EBV-associated T-cell PTLDs have been reported to date.[45] It has been suggested that EBV may infect

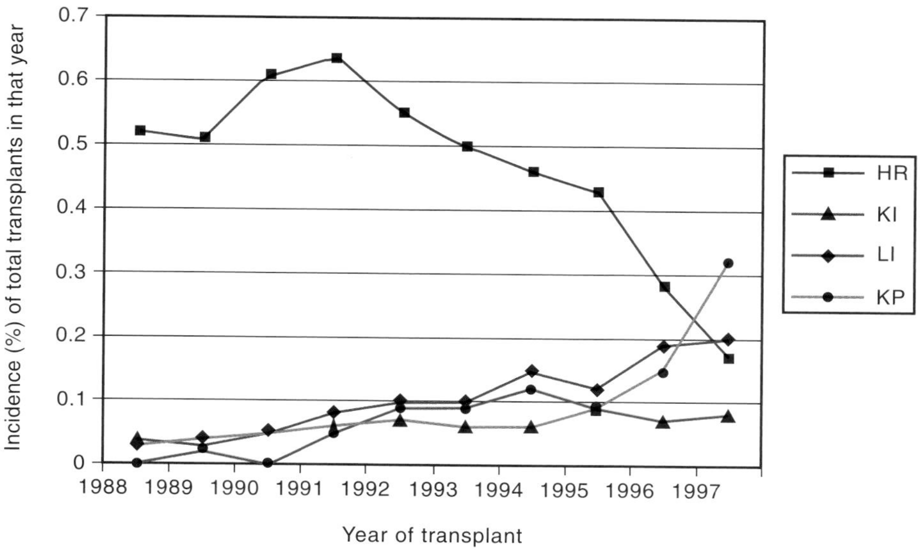

Figure 63-3 Incidence of posttransplant lymphoproliferative disorder (PTLD) by transplant year in different organ systems: Rise per year significant $p < 0.001$ for heart *(HR)*, kidney *(KI)* and liver-pancreas *(LI, KP)*. Heart-lung ($p < 0.005$) and lung transplant data are not shown. Data are derived from the Scientific Registry of the United Network of Organ Sharing (UNOS). From Dharnidharka VR, Tejani AH, Ho PL, Harmon WE: Post-transplant lymphoproliferative disorder in the United States: young Caucasian males are at highest risk, *Am J Transplant* 2:993-98, 2002.

a subset of T cells that express the CD21 receptor. The prognosis is worse than for B-cell PTLD, with a 1-year patient survival of 50%.[46] Levendoglu-Tugal and colleagues reported on an 11-year-old boy with T-cell EBV-negative leukemia.[47] The IPTTRS reported 2% leukemia. In two patients, the leukemia occurred during childhood.[1]

Hodgkin's Disease after Transplantation

Goyal and colleagues reported two patients aged 18 and 19 with EBV-associated Hodgkin's disease. EBV-latent membrane protein-antigen 1 was strongly expressed in the Reed-Sternberg cells. Complete remission was achieved on conventional chemotherapy in both.[48] Dharnidharka and colleagues reported on a 9-year-old girl with Hodgkin's disease after previous B-cell PTLD with classic Reed-Sternberg cells positive for EB RNA.

Complete remission was achieved on discontinuation of IS, except for low-dose prednisone.[49] Axelrod and colleagues reported on an 8-year-old patient with Hodgkin's disease 90 months after transplantation, with EBV-LMP–positive Reed-Sternberg cells but no positive EBV PCR, who responded well to CHOP/ABV chemotherapy.[50]

Risk Factors of PTLD

Virus Infection

EBV seronegativity and the use of potent immunosuppressive drugs are the two most important PTLD risk factors in pediatric recipients. The risk of developing PTLD while being EBV naive has been established in various studies.[34,35,51] The relative risk of PTLD is 20 times increased in the first year after transplantation in EBV-seronegative renal transplant recipients compared to seropositive patients, and about 200 times compared to healthy individuals.[52]

Reports on the influence of CMV and hepatitis C infection on the occurrence of PTLD are conflicting. Earlier studies have revealed a fourfold to sixfold excess risk of PTLD for CMV mismatch to EBV mismatch, as CMV infection could induce a polyclonal B-cell proliferation and attenuate the immune deficiency.[17,53] The same role has been suggested for hepatitis C.[54] However, for both CMV and hepatitis C these reports were not confirmed by a recent report of the USRDS—nor by a large registry study from Australia and New Zealand.[16-19]

Immunosuppressive Therapy

All studies that have longitudinally evaluated the incidence of PTLD show a trend over time toward an increasing incidence and earlier onset of PTLD, in line with the use of more potent immune suppressive agents. The LERIC study comprised 249 Dutch patients (231 transplanted) under the age of 15 years with onset of ESRD. The study was conducted between 1972 and 1992 with a relatively large population that only had been treated with prednisone and azathioprine. Of these, only one patient with early-onset PTLD was found,[2] in contrast to six patients with late-onset PTLD (>10 years after transplantation).

However, data concerning the influence of specific immunosuppressive regimens are as conflicting as in other post-transplant malignancies. Early reports showed an incidence of 13% to 20% with the use of tacrolimus compared to 2% to 3% with the use of cyclosporine maintenance therapy. The USRDS database revealed a 1.5 times increased hazard of PTLD for tacrolimus over cyclosporine.[18] However, it is most likely that the increased risk of PTLD under tacrolimus is dose related—comparable to the outbreak of cancer after the introduction of high doses of cyclosporine.

NAPRTCS reported on 108 cases of PTLD in 6720 pediatric transplant recipients and showed that the tacrolimus association with PTLD was linked to the earlier transplant area from 1987 to 1995 and had disappeared in the most recent era (1996 to 2000), apparently as a result of the dose reduction over time.[23] In a multivariate analysis for time to PTLD in 25,127 kidney transplant recipients of the USRDS database, transplanted between 1996 and 2000, the use of azathioprine and mycophenolate mofetil (MMF) was associated with a decreased risk for PTLD (HR 0.6 and 0.66, respectively, $p < 0.0001$ and $p < 0.02$), whereas the use of ATG and OKT3 increased the risk for PTLD (HR1.55 and 1.36, $p = 0.001$ and $p = 0.01$, respectively). Patients treated with MMF had a better survival after PTLD. The introduction of IL2-receptor inhibitor in the induction regimens has not increased the risk for PTLD.[23]

Cyclophosphamide

Data from the Dutch cohort study revealed that even a low dose of cyclophosphamide as commonly used in frequently relapsing nephrotic syndrome is associated with an increased risk of malignancies. The relative risk was increased 2.5 times at a cumulative dose exceeding 20 mg/kg body weight, and 4.3 times at a dose greater than 100 mg/kg body weight.[2] This implies that with the availability of other, less oncogenic, second-line therapeutic agents the use of cyclophosphamide in nephrotic syndrome should be abolished.

Other Risk Factors

Data of the United Network of Organ Sharing revealed that young Caucasian males were at greatest risk for PTLD.[34,40]

Prevention of PTLD

EBV vaccination is probably the most plausible protective measure for the near future. Until vaccination becomes available, prevention of PTLD consists of EBV surveillance and immunosuppressive drug reduction in the case of primary EBV infection. Reliable information on the beneficial effect of antiviral agents in preventing PTLD is limited. Ganciclovir and, to a lesser extent, acyclovir inhibit lytic EBV replication in vitro. However, they have no effect on the latent state of EBV or on the proliferation of EBV-transformed cells.[38,55]

Two retrospective studies have claimed a beneficial role of the "preemptive" use of antiviral therapy during ATG treatment in solid-organ transplantation.[56,57] A multicenter case-control study comprising data from 20 centers participating in the United Network for Organ Sharing (UNOS) revealed a 38% reduction of PTLD in patients using ganciclovir prophylactic treatment during the first years after transplantation.[58] However, it is difficult to draw conclusions from these data.

The variability of approaches of the various centers was considerable. For more than 40% of patients, no information on the pretransplant EBV status was available. Surprisingly, more pretransplant EBV-positive patients than EBV-negative patients had been treated with prophylactic ganciclovir. Data on dosage were also not available.[58] Well-designed clinical trials are warranted to establish the potential role of antiviral agents in the prevention of PTLD.

Classification and Diagnosis of PTLD

The classification of PTLD remains a matter of debate. PTLD may represent all types of B-cell proliferative disorders, ranging from benign polyclonal conditions to malignant monoclonal B- (and sometimes T-) cell lymphomas. Despite efforts in several consensus meetings, no generally accepted classification system has been established. The latest World Health Organization (WHO) classification divides PTLD into four classes.

- *Early lesions PTLD:* Polyclonal lymphoproliferation, including reactive plasmacytic hyperplasia with normal nodal architecture and infectious mononucleosis-like PTLD. The clinical manifestation is characterized by mononucleosis-like disease and enlargement of tonsils and/or lymph nodes. Oncogenic mutations are not present. This most often occurs within 3 months after transplantation, largely in the context of a primary EBV infection. This type responds well to decreasing IS.
- *Polymorphic PTLD:* Polymorphic proliferation and local invasion of cells with destruction of the nodal architecture. T cells and macrophages are often found. Immunochemistry reveals B cells and T cells. EBV is detected and there are no oncogenic mutations. In most cases, decreasing IS is sufficient, but some warrant more aggressive therapy.
- *Monomorphic PTLD:* Characterized by neoplastic transformation of the tissue, destruction of the underlying lymph node architecture, and invasion of extra-nodal sites by monoclonal cells. This type can be further subclassified according to WHO lymphoma classification and includes diffuse large B-cell lymphoma (the majority), Burkitt's or Burkitt's-like lymphoma, T-cell lymphoma, and plasmacytoma-like lesions. EBV is detected in B-cell lymphoma. T-cell lymphomas are largely EBV positive, and they occur late and have a worse prognosis. Plasmacytoma-like lesions are rare. Treatment ranges from cessation of immunosuppressive treatment and rituximab to chemotherapy and ultimately bone marrow transplantation.
- *Hodgkin lymphoma and Hodgkin-lymphoma–like PTLD.*

Early Detection and Monitoring of Transplanted Patients for PTLD

EBV PCR and EBV-Specific Cytotoxic T Cells

Elevated levels of EBV in mononuclear cells (PBMC) or in plasma by polymerase chain reaction (PCR) is the key to an early detection of PTLD. However, a wide range of methods has been used—all with totally different reference values for EBV load in healthy carriers versus loads in PTLD and non-PTLD transplant recipients.[59] Comparison of real-time quantitative polymerase chain reaction (QR-PCR) of the EB viral load in PBMC and plasma in different populations revealed both higher levels of PBMC-EBV and plasma EBV in PTLD patients compared to transplant recipients with primary or reactivated EBV infection and patients with no signs of EBV infection.[60]

Values of >5000 EBV genomes/μg PBMC DNA were considered diagnostic for PTLD, with a specificity of 0.89 and a sensitivity of 1.0. When plasma was analyzed, a value of >1000 EBV genomes/100 μl plasma had both a sensitivity and specificity of 1.0. However, the small number of patients makes it difficult to assess the predictive value of EBV PCR. Late-onset EBV-associated PTLD may even present in the absence of a positive EBV PCR.[50] In a recent study, EBV-specific T-lymphocytes and EBV PCR were assessed in 45 patients after solid-organ transplantation. A combined low level of EBV-specific T-lymphocytes and high EBV PCR viral load had a 100% positive predictive value.[61]

We found a strong association between spontaneous EBV B-cell transformation (SET) and the inability of making EBV-specific CD8+ T cells in 20 renal transplanted children with EBV reactivation or primary infection. Reduction of IS of SET-positive patients resulted in a negative SET and an increase of EBV-specific CD8+ T cells.[62] In conclusion, EBV PCR is of most value in detecting early-onset PTLD. EBV PCR monitoring should be carried out frequently and should be followed by EBV-specific CD8+ T-cell monitoring in the case of high or increasing levels.

EBV Serology

Anti-EBNA antibodies reflect the immune response on EBV. A reduction of anti-EBNA antibodies in seropositive patients is associated with the development of PTLD and with increased viral load.[63] However, the interpretation of EBV serology can be troublesome in patients with severe immune deficiency.

Positron Emission Tomography

A positron emission tomography (PET) scan using labeled fluor-desoxyglucose (FDG) is a metabolic imaging modality that detects cells with increased glycolytic activity as appears in malignant cells. The PET scan has proven to be able to detect all disease sites in PTLD and may therefore be a very effective diagnostic tool, which can also be used in monitoring the therapeutic effect.[64,65]

Other Markers of Disease

A monoclonal immunoglobulin peak can be detected in 30% after renal transplantation. Persistence of a monoclonal gammopathy for more than 6 months has been associated with an increased incidence of viral infections and PTLD. The prospective value, however, is low. In a series of 200 liver transplantations, two thirds of patients with PTLD presented a monoclonal peak.[66] The β-microglobulin/cystatin C ratio has been shown to be a sensitive and specific marker for PTLD in a small group of children.[67] Lactate dehydrogenase (LDH) is usually raised, and can be used as a nonspecific follow-up marker.

Diagnostic Procedures in PTLD

The diagnostic procedure depends on the clinical presentation. Routine EBV PCR assessment is recommended in all transplanted children, especially in EBV-naive patients. Frequent monitoring is mandatory during periods of high immunosuppression and can be tapered down to three times per month during low-dose maintenance therapy.

In the case of positive EBV PCR, EBV serology and EBV-specific CD8+ T cells should be assessed—and further clinical investigation should include an abdominal ultrasound, x-ray of the thorax, and careful physical examination with special attention given the adenoid and tonsils. Further investigation depends on the presentation. In the case of nodular or extranodular PTLD or more severe disseminated PTLD, a biopsy for histology and a lumbar puncture are mandatory. If possible, a PET scan can be very useful to identify all disease sites.

Location of Disease and Presenting Symptoms of PTLD

The clinical presentation of PTLD is very heterogeneous. The disease can vary from asymptomatic seroconversion to a mononucleosis-like disease and from monoclonal B-cell proliferation with nodal and extranodal tumors to a fulminant disseminated disease. The most common presenting features are fever, malaise, loss of weight, adenoid and tonsillar hypertrophy, abdominal distension, cervical lymphadenopathy, and hepatomegaly and splenomegaly. In 30%, PTLD affects the renal allograft—which may lead to a raised serum creatinine or graft tenderness.[39]

The gut is involved in 25% to 57%, which may lead to abdominal pain and extension, signs of abdominal obstruction, or gastrointestinal bleeding. The central nervous system is affected in about 25%. Presenting symptoms may vary from seizures to ataxia.[10,22,39,41,68] More uncommon presentations involve the lungs, the scalp (thickening), and the intraocular area (PTLD).[39]

Treatment of PTLD

Several regimens for treatment of PTLD have been suggested. Figure 63-4 offers a therapeutic strategy for different clinical situations using one or more of the options discussed in the sections that follow.

Reducing the Dose of Immunosuppressive Therapy

Reducing the dose of IS is the mainstay of treatment in early-onset lesions and polymorphic PTLD. In more severe PTLD, all immunosuppressive agents should be stopped, except for low doses of prednisone. Reduction of IS is only rarely followed by an acute graft rejection, probably as a result of a high state of immune suppression. In theory, the first step should be to lower the tacrolimus or cyclosporine dosage—followed by halving or cessation of mycophenolate mofetil or azathioprine in the case of no response.

However, several strategies of IS reductions have been used and no studies have evaluated the effect of the different regimens on PTLD response. The magnitude of IS reduction is patient specific. The time to response may vary from 1 to 15 weeks.[69] Predictors of no response include a serum LDH > 2.5 times the upper limit of normal, organ dysfunction, and multiple visceral sites of disease. Patients with none of these factors are said to have an 89% response rate, whereas two or more risk factors predict no response.[69] IS reduction may be effective in both EBV-positive and EBV-negative PTLD.[70]

Surgery

The role of surgery is mainly restricted to obtain tissue for the diagnosis. In rare situations, such as localized tumors (adenoid or tonsils) or as debulking in the case of an obstructive bowel tumor, surgery can contribute to the therapy. It should always be combined with IS reduction.

Monoclonal Antibodies: Anti–B-Cell Antibodies

Rituximab (Rituxan, Mabthera), a chimeric monoclonal antibody to CD-20 antigen on the surface of B cells, has proven its important role in PTLD. Its potential mechanisms of action comprise apoptosis, complement activation, and antibody-dependent cell-mediated cytotoxicity. In vitro, the binding of rituximab to the CD-20 antigen leads directly to apoptosis of the targeted lymphocyte. Rituximab is usually administered as slow intravenous infusion of 375 mg/m^2 four times weekly.

It is generally well tolerated. Mild acute side effects include flulike symptoms (fever, chills, rigors, nausea, headache, and rash) and rarely more serious allergic responses such as hypotension, bronchospasm, and angioedema. All of these effects resume after cessation of the administration. Major complications (including tumor lysis syndrome and infusion-related death) have been reported, but appear to be extremely rare. Although B-cell suppression may last for

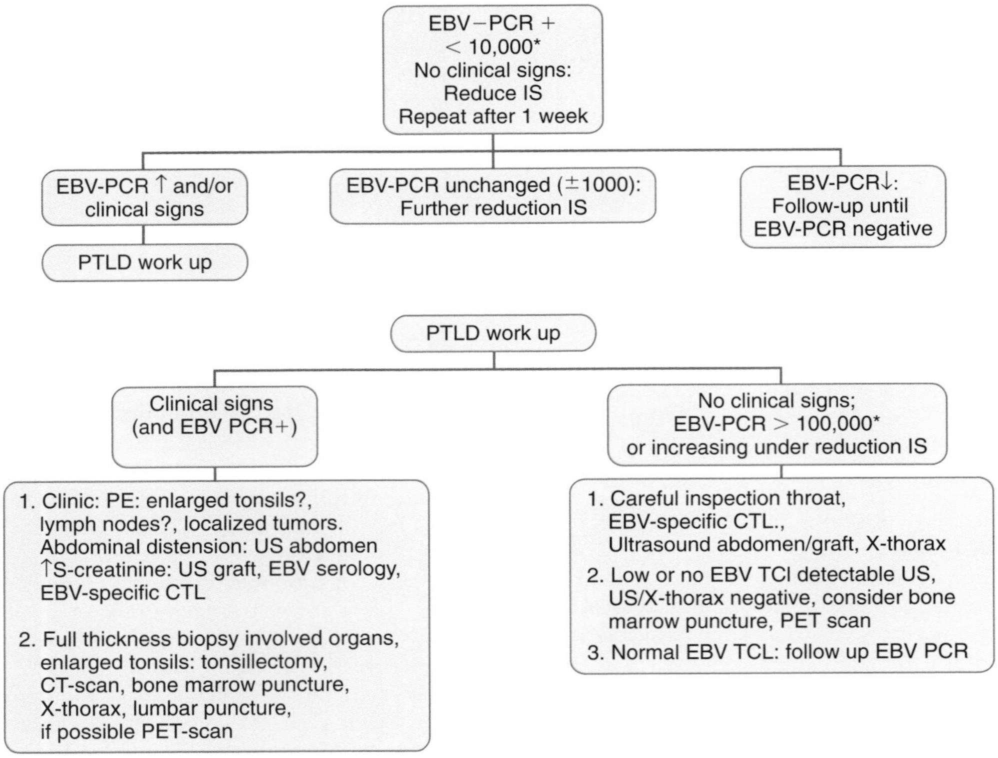

* Absolute level dependent on methodology, i.e., normal values local laboratory

Figure 63-4 Diagnostic work up in case of suspected PTLD.

more than 6 months (some report more than 2 years), no increased infection rate has been reported.[71]

Many case reports, and some larger retrospective reports, on using rituximab in PTLD in various settings have been published. Nearly all patients had concurrent reduction of IS, and some used antiviral medication. Most patients were treated with the usual four doses. Some (intestinal graft) patients, however, have received weekly infusions for 3 to 6 months or longer—with a tapering down to every 3 months after complete remission was achieved. With median follow-up of 8 months (3-30 months), all of these patients remained in complete remission without major infections or other complications.[72]

In a large retrospective trial of 26 pediatric PTLD patients, treatment with rituximab showed a response rate of 85% and a complete remission rate of 69%. Two of the nonresponders were EBV negative, and one presented with a fulminant disease. The same group followed prospectively 14 children with PTLD who did not respond to IS reduction. Out of 12 evaluable patients, 75% achieved complete remission under rituximab. Two patients died; one due to fungal pneumonia and one due to complications after elective surgery.[71] Treatment with only rituximab is not an option for PTLD patients with central nervous system localization because the antibodies do not pass the blood/brain barrier. Other predictors of poor response include multivisceral disease and late-onset PTLD.[73]

Antiviral Therapy

Antiviral drugs have only a very limited role in PTLD. Acyclovir and ganciclovir are not effective in inactivating EBV. In theory, the use of ganciclovir could be indirectly beneficial in preventing CMV infection—hence reducing the chance of EBV activation. The benefits of the prophylactic use of ganciclovir in EBV-naive children undergoing liver transplantation have been reported, but no convincing data in the literature exist to confirm this. Foscarnet, on the other hand, is a direct inhibitor of viral DNA. Treatment has resulted in complete remission in three adult PTLD patients.[74]

Conventional Chemotherapy

Watts and colleagues reported on seven children with Burkitt's-type or diffuse large-cell PTLD with multiple organ involvement after solid-organ transplantation who were treated with tailored chemotherapy according to the pro-MACE/cytaBOM regimen. Two patients died; one of them 10 days after the onset of fulminant disease and the other of concomitant HIV. The other five patients had a complete remission.[75] Comoli and colleagues treated three children with monoclonal B-cell PTLD with modified CHOP and modified BFM chemotherapy in combination with IS reduction, rituximab, and cytotoxic T-cell infusion. All had a complete remission, with graft survival.[68]

T-Cell Therapy

A promising low-toxicity approach in the treatment of PTLD is to restore the viral-specific T-cell immunity by autologous EBV-specific cytotoxic T-lymphocyte (EBV-CTL) infusion. It has been shown to be effective in allogenic stem cell transplant and solid-organ transplant recipients. Khanna and colleagues showed that effective EBV-CTLs even could be generated out of blood obtained in EBV-naive recipients 3 to 4 weeks after seroconversion under full IS.[76] They showed that under infusion of EBV-CTL EBV cytotoxicity increased despite continuation of the IS.

The same group treated EBV-naive patients with PTLD after renal transplantation. In three patients with monoclonal PTLD, immunosuppression was reduced and rituximab as well as a reduced-dosage polychemotherapy was administered. The patients with polyclonal PTLD received only EBV-CTL. All achieved complete remission without loss of the graft, with a median follow-up of 31 months.[77]

Interferon Alpha

There are anecdotal reports of success with interferon alpha, which is supposed to stimulate the host immune system. The risk of rejection is high.[78]

Monitoring of Therapy in PTLD

Clinical follow-up by physical examination and radiologic evaluation should be accompanied by monitoring of the immune response, especially by monitoring EBV-specific CD8+ T cells. Other markers include EBV PCR, EBV serology, and LDH. A decrease of the EBV PCR, increase or appearance of anti-EBNA antibodies, lowering of LDH, and increase or appearance of EBV-specific CD8+ T cells indicate reversal of disease. A decrease of CD69+ T cells, which are high during active PTLD, may indicate a therapeutic response. If available, a PET scan is an elegant tool for monitoring therapeutic response.

SKIN TUMORS

Epidemiology

Skin cancer is the most frequent cancer following renal transplantation in children,[2,4] but it usually becomes manifest only more than 10 to 15 years after transplantation and patients have typically reached young adult age. In the Dutch long-term follow-up study, the risk for nonmelanoma skin cancer was 222-fold higher among pediatric renal transplant recipients than among the general population.[2] The mean age of onset of disease in pediatric renal transplant recipients is about 27 years.[1,2,4] Although rare, onset of disease at childhood has been reported in solid-transplant recipients.

According to IPTTRS data, 16 out of the 101 skin cancers found in pediatric solid-organ transplant recipients presented at childhood[1]—10 of them being squamous cell carcinoma (predominantly of the lower lip) and 6 of them melanomas. The youngest patient was 9 years old. Death from skin cancer occurred in eight patients—five from squamous cell carcinoma and three from melanoma.[1]

Carcinoma

Squamous cell carcinoma (SCC) is by far most prevalent carcinoma, accounting more than 50% of all skin cancers after transplantation. This predominance of SCC over basal cell carcinoma (BCC) is more pronounced in pediatric cases than in adult transplant recipients (SCC/BCC = 2.8 : 1 versus 1.7 : 1).[1] SCC is for the most part found in parts of the body exposed to light (i.e., on the head, neck, hands, and arms).[79] In pediatric transplant recipients, lip cancers account for 23% of all skin cancers.[1]

Skin cancers may appear in the absence of any preexisting skin lesion, but are often preceded by "-type" actinic keratosis, which suggests that HPV may be involved in its pathogenesis. Skin cancers may develop rapidly, and recurrences are common—justifying immediate excision and a careful follow-up.[79]

Melanomas

Melanoma seems to be more prevalent in pediatric than in adult transplantation (12% versus 5%[1]). The absolute figure is low. The IPTTRS counted 12 melanomas on 527 tumors. The Dutch cohort study counted 2 on 21 malignancies.[12] The onset of disease is more disparate. Data from the IPTTRS and the Dutch cohort suggest an earlier onset compared to SCC and BCC. In the IPTTRS, 50% presented during childhood. However, at longer follow-up (20 years) we found three more melanomas in the Dutch cohort (data not published). In the Dutch group, no deaths were reported. The IPTTRS noted 25% of deaths were due to melanoma.[1,2]

Melanocytic nevi, a risk factor for melanoma, may develop in excess after transplantation.[80] In transplantation, melanoma can be transmitted by the donor. Any person with a history of melanoma should be excluded from donation.[79] Human growth hormone may increase the growth rate of melanocytic nevi, but to date no association between growth hormone therapy and the occurrence of melanomas has been found.[81] Sun protection and removal of suspect nevi are the most important preventive measures.

Kaposi's Sarcoma

The IPTTRS reported 2% Kaposi's sarcomas in pediatric transplant recipients, nearly all of which occurred during childhood. Only one child presented with skin cancer. All others had various visceral localizations. The age of occurrence ranged from 5 to 17 years, with, for the most part, the onset occurring within a few months after transplantation.[1] Of eight reported patients, most were renal transplant recipients. In six of them the outcome was fatal. Kaposi's sarcoma is directly associated with HHV8 virus.

Anogenital Cancers

These include cancers of the anus, perinatal skin, perineum, and vulva. In the IPTTRS, they represented 4% of all malignancies.[1] The tumors occurred on average 12 years after transplantation, were more prevalent in females, and often presented multicentric in distribution. Most were associated with preexistent condylomata accuminata, caused by human papillomavirus.[1]

Therapy of skin cancers

The therapy of skin cancers in children is essentially identical to that in adult transplant recipients. Immediate surgical excision is the first step. In CCS and BCC, only multiple recurrences or extensive development requires chemotherapy or radiotherapy. Minimizing immunosuppressive drugs or diversion to drugs with antiproliferative capacities such as rapamycin has been advised in adults.[4]

High dose interferon-alpha has been used successfully in melanoma. Oral retinoids may be beneficial in CCS. In

Kaposi's sarcoma, reduction of the immune suppression is essential and can lead to regression of the lesions. Local radiotherapy, laser treatment, or cryosurgery may be used in progressive skin lesions. Monochemotherapy (vincristine or bleomycine) is required in case of visceral involvement.[79]

Prevention

Removal of suspected skin lesions and sun protection are the most important preventive measures against CCS, BCS and melanomas. Especially in areas with a high UV radiation, strict sun protection has to start as soon as end-stage renal disease is attained. In a Spanish study, adult transplant recipients with occupational sun exposure had a 5-fold higher chance of SCC and BCC as compared with patients with low sun exposure.[82] The cumulative incidence of non-melanoma skin cancers in the high exposure group was 85% after 10 years as compared to 22% in the low exposure group.[82]

OTHER MALIGNANCIES

Sarcomas, excluded Kaposi's sarcoma, are the third most common malignancy in pediatric transplant recipients as reported by the ITPPRS, accounting for 4% of all tumors. Most were leiomyosarcomas, followed by fibrosarcomas.[1]

Renal cell carcinoma accounted for 1% of all malignancies in the IPTTRS, 2% in a report on 208 tumors in 200 pediatric allograft recipients.[1,12] They may present at childhood and are predominantly located in the grafted kidney, contrary to the presentation in adult transplantation. Although renal cell carcinoma may present only 1 year after transplantation, registry studies showed an increased incidence with from 306 per 100,000 patients for the age group 20-30 years to 791 for the age group 41-50 years.[12,32,83,84,85]

Kausman and colleagues reported on a 10-year-old boy with renal graft adenocarcinoma, associated with a recent BK-virus nephropathy.[14] Although they found no BK virus within the tumor, they suggest a "hit and run" mechanism in which the virus temporarily integrates into the host DNA, imposes its oncogenic influence, and disappears out of the tumor as a result of rearrangement and excision. This ability of BK virus has been demonstrated in hamster cells.[86]

Dionne and colleagues reported on a 3-year-old boy with a renal graft leiomyoma with EBV-positive tumor cells. In adults, EBV-associated smooth muscle tumors have been found in several immune deficiencies; 16 pediatric solid organ recipients with EBV smooth muscle tumors have been described[13]. Nocera and colleagues reported on an urothelial carcinoma of the native kidney in a 14-year-old girl who was successfully treated by nephrectomy only.[10]

TABLE 63-4 **Key Messages for the Pediatric Nephrologist**
Malignancies after pediatric renal transplantation are an emerging problem.
The risk of early-onset PTLD in children after renal transplantation is 20 times increased compared to EBV-positive recipients, and 200 times compared to the general population.
Immunosuppressive regimens should be tailored to the individual patient in order to minimize the immune suppression as much as possible. Dose reduction or cessation of calcineurin inhibitors should be considered after 1 year in patients with no history of acute rejection.
Sun-protective measures should be started at the onset of ESRD.
Skin cancer can occur at childhood.
EBV PCR should be monitored frequently in EBV-naive patients, especially during the first years after transplantation.
EBV-specific cytotoxic T cells should be monitored in the case of a (sharply) increasing EBV PCR.
The use of low-dose cyclophosphamide is associated with an increased risk for cancer. Its use in nephrotic syndrome should be avoided.

SUMMARY

Cancer in patients with pediatric onset of ESRD is an emerging problem that pediatric nephrologists should take in account in choosing the therapeutic approach (Table 63-4). Avoidance of high doses of immune suppressive agents after transplantation, and of potentially oncogenic agents such as cyclophosphamide in nephritic and nephrotic syndrome, may decrease the long-term risk of malignancies.

PTLD may occur within weeks after transplantation. EB-naive patients should be monitored after transplantation by regular EBV PCR examinations. Skin malignancies are not harmless and they become highly prevalent at young adulthood in transplanted children. Strict protection against sun exposure should be started at the onset of ESRD in order to reduce the risk of skin cancers. Suspicious nevi should be removed immediately. Any warts and condylomata should be treated vigorously and carefully monitored for malignant degeneration.

ACKNOWLEDGMENTS

The author thanks Marjan van de Wetering, pediatric oncologist, and Jean Claude Davin, pediatric nephrologist, for their very useful comments on the manuscript.

REFERENCES

1. Penn I: De novo malignances in pediatric organ transplant recipients, *Pediatr Transplant* 2(1):56-63, 1998.
2. Coutinho HM, Groothoff JW, Offringa M, Gruppen MP, Heymans HS: De novo malignancy after paediatric renal replacement therapy, *Arch Dis Child* 85(6):478-83, 2001.
3. Groothoff JW, Gruppen MP, Offringa M, Hutten J, Lilien MR, van de Kar NJ, et al: Mortality and causes of death of end-stage renal disease in children: a Dutch cohort study, *Kidney Int* 61(2):621-29, 2002.
4. Euvrard S, Kanitakis J, Cochat P, Claudy A: Skin cancers following pediatric organ transplantation, *Dermatol Surg* 30(4 Pt 2):616-21, 2004.
5. Inamoto H, Ozaki R, Matsuzaki T, Wakui M, Saruta T, Osawa A: Incidence and mortality patterns of malignancy and factors affecting the risk of malignancy in dialysis patients, *Nephron* 59(4):611-17, 1991.
6. Maisonneuve P, Agodoa L, Gellert R, Stewart JH, Buccianti G, Lowenfels AB, et al: Cancer in patients on dialysis for end-stage

renal disease: an international collaborative study, *Lancet* 354(9173):93-99, 1999.
7. Vamvakas S, Bahner U, Heidland A: Cancer in end-stage renal disease: potential factors involved (editorial), *Am J Nephrol* 18(2):89-95, 1998.
8. Gaya SB, Rees AJ, Lechler RI, Williams G, Mason PD: Malignant disease in patients with long-term renal transplants, *Transplantation* 59(12):1705-09, 1995.
9. London NJ, Farmery SM, Will EJ, Davison AM, Lodge JP: Risk of neoplasia in renal transplant patients, *Lancet* 346(8972):403-06, 1995.
10. Nocera A, Ghio L, Dall'Amico R, Fontana I, Cardillo M, Berardinelli L, et al: De novo cancers in paediatric renal transplant recipients: a multicentre analysis within the North Italy Transplant programme (NITp), Italy, *Eur J Cancer* 36(1):80-86, 2000.
11. Kasiske BL, Snyder JJ, Gilbertson DT, Wang C: Cancer after kidney transplantation in the United States, *Am J Transplant* 4(6):905-13, 2004.
12. Agraharkar ML, Cinclair RD, Kuo YF, Daller JA, Shahinian VB: Risk of malignancy with long-term immunosuppression in renal transplant recipients, *Kidney Int* 66(1):383-89, 2004.
13. Dionne JM, Carter JE, Matsell D, MacNeily AE, Morrison KB, de Sa D: Renal leiomyoma associated with Epstein-Barr virus in a pediatric transplant patient, *Am J Kidney Dis* 46(2):351-55, 2005.
14. Kausman JY, Somers GR, Francis DM, Jones CL: Association of renal adenocarcinoma and BK virus nephropathy post transplantation, *Pediatr Nephrol* 19(4):459-62, 2004.
15. White MK, Gordon J, Reiss K, Del VL, Croul S, Giordano A, et al: Human polyomaviruses and brain tumors, *Brain Res Brain Res Rev* 50(1):69-85, 2005.
16. McLaughlin K, Wajstaub S, Marotta P, Adams P, Grant DR, Wall WJ, et al: Increased risk for posttransplant lymphoproliferative disease in recipients of liver transplants with hepatitis C, *Liver Transpl* 6(5):570-74, 2000.
17. Manez R, Breinig MC, Linden P, Wilson J, Torre-Cisneros J, Kusne S, et al: Posttransplant lymphoproliferative disease in primary Epstein-Barr virus infection after liver transplantation: the role of cytomegalovirus disease, *J Infect Dis* 176(6):1462-67, 1997.
18. Caillard S, Dharnidharka V, Agodoa L, Bohen E, Abbott K: Posttransplant lymphoproliferative disorders after renal transplantation in the United States in era of modern immunosuppression, *Transplantation* 80(9):1233-43, 2005.
19. Faull RJ, Hollett P, McDonald SP: Lymphoproliferative disease after renal transplantation in Australia and New Zealand, *Transplantation* 80(2):193-97, 2005.
20. Opelz G, Dohler B: Lymphomas after solid organ transplantation: a collaborative transplant study report, *Am J Transplant* 4(2):222-30, 2004.
21. Dharnidharka VR, Stevens G: Risk for post-transplant lymphoproliferative disorder after polyclonal antibody induction in kidney transplantation, *Pediatr Transplant* 9(5):622-26, 2005.
22. Shapiro R, Nalesnik M, McCauley J, Fedorek S, Jordan ML, Scantlebury VP, et al: Posttransplant lymphoproliferative disorders in adult and pediatric renal transplant patients receiving tacrolimus-based immunosuppression, *Transplantation* 68(12):1851-54, 1999.
23. Dharnidharka VR, Ho PL, Stable in DM, Harmon WE, Tejani AH: Mycophenolate, tacrolimus and post-transplant lymphoproliferative disorder: a report of the North American Pediatric Renal Transplant Cooperative Study, *Pediatr Transplant* 6(5):396-99, 2002.
24. Kist-van Holthe JE, Ho PL, Stablein D, Harmon WE, Baum MA: Outcome of renal transplantation for Wilms' tumor and Denys-Drash syndrome: a report of the North American Pediatric Renal Transplant Cooperative Study, *Pediatr Transplant* 9(3):305-10, 2005.
25. Reznik VM, Mendoza SA, Freidenberg GR: Evaluation of delayed puberty in the female adolescent with chronic renal failure, *Pediatr Nephrol* 7(5):551-53, 1993.
26. Narchi H: Risk of Wilms' tumour with multicystic kidney disease: a systematic review, *Arch Dis Child* 90(2):147-49, 2005.
27. Querfeld U, Schneble F, Wradzidlo W, Waldherr R, Troger J, Scharer K: Acquired cystic kidney disease before and after renal transplantation, *J Pediatr* 121(1):61-64, 1992.
28. Gentle DL, Mandell J, Jennings T: Renal cortical neoplasm in a child with dialysis-acquired cystic kidney disease, *Urology* 47(2):254-55, 1996.
29. Chandhoke PS, Torrence RJ, Clayman RV, Rothstein M: Acquired cystic disease of the kidney: a management dilemma, *J Urol* 147(4):969-74, 1992.
30. Soergel TM, Cain MP, Misseri R, Gardner TA, Koch MO, Rink RC: Transitional cell carcinoma of the bladder following augmentation cystoplasty for the neuropathic bladder, *J Urol* 172(4 Pt 2):1649-51, 2004.
31. Shokeir AA, Shamaa M, el-Mekresh MM, el-Baz M, Ghoneim MA: Late malignancy in bowel segments exposed to urine without fecal stream, *Urology* 46(5):657-61, 1995.
32. Tyden G, Wernersson A, Sandberg J, Berg U: Development of renal cell carcinoma in living donor kidney grafts, *Transplantation* 70(11):1650-56, 2000.
33. Mehls O, Wilton P, Lilien M, Berg U, Broyer M, Rizzoni G, et al: Does growth hormone treatment affect the risk of post-transplant renal cancer? *Pediatr Nephrol* 17(12):984-89, 2002.
34. Dharnidharka VR, Sullivan EK, Stablein DM, Tejani AH, Harmon WE: Risk factors for posttransplant lymphoproliferative disorder (PTLD) in pediatric kidney transplantation: a report of the North American Pediatric Renal Transplant Cooperative Study (NAPRTCS), *Transplantation* 71(8):1065-68, 2001.
35. Funch DP, Brady J, Ko HH, Dreyer NA, Walker AM: Methods and objectives of a large US multicenter case-control study of post-transplant lymphoproliferative disorder in renal transplant patients, *Recent Results Cancer Res* 159:81-88, 2002.
36. Shapiro R, Scantlebury VP, Jordan ML, Vivas C, Ellis D, Lombardozzi-Lane S, et al: Pediatric renal transplantation under tacrolimus-based immunosuppression, *Transplantation* 67(2):299-303, 1999.
37. Smith JM, Rudser K, Gillen D, Kestenbaum B, Seliger S, Weiss N, et al: Risk of lymphoma after renal transplantation varies with time: an analysis of the United States Renal Data System, *Transplantation* 81(2):175-80, 2006.
38. Paya CV, Fung JJ, Nalesnik MA, Kieff E, Green M, Gores G, et al: Epstein-Barr virus-induced posttransplant lymphoproliferative disorders: ASTS/ASTP EBV-PTLD Task Force and The Mayo Clinic Organized International Consensus Development Meeting, *Transplantation* 68(10):1517-25, 1999.
39. Wilde GE, Moore DJ, Bellah RD: Posttransplantation lymphoproliferative disorder in pediatric recipients of solid organ transplants: timing and location of disease, *Am J Roentgenol* 185(5):1335-41, 2005.
40. Dharnidharka VR, Tejani AH, Ho PL, Harmon WE: Post-transplant lymphoproliferative disorder in the United States: young Caucasian males are at highest risk, *Am J Transplant* 2(10):993-98, 2002.
41. Pickhardt PJ, Siegel MJ, Hayashi RJ, Kelly M: Posttransplantation lymphoproliferative disorder in children: clinical, histopathologic, and imaging features, *Radiology* 217(1):16-25, 2000.
42. Tanner JE, Alfieri C: The Epstein-Barr virus and post-transplant lymphoproliferative disease: interplay of immunosuppression, EBV, and the immune system in disease pathogenesis, *Transpl Infect Dis* 3(2):60-69, 2001.
43. Swinnen LJ, Costanzo-Nordin MR, Fisher SG, O'Sullivan EJ, Johnson MR, Heroux AL, et al: Increased incidence of lymphoproliferative disorder after immunosuppression with the monoclonal antibody OKT3 in cardiac-transplant recipients, *N Engl J Med* 323(25):1723-28, 1990.
44. Ambinder RF: Gammaherpesviruses and "Hit-and-Run" oncogenesis, *Am J Pathol* 156(1):1-3, 2000.
45. Dockrell DH, Strickler JG, Paya CV: Epstein-Barr virus-induced T cell lymphoma in solid organ transplant recipients, *Clin Infect Dis* 26(1):180-82, 1998.
46. Pinkerton CR, Hann I, Weston CL, Mapp T, Wotherspoon A, Hobson R, et al: Immunodeficiency-related lymphoproliferative disorders: prospective data from the United Kingdom Children's Cancer Study Group Registry, *Br J Haematol* 118(2):456-61, 2002.
47. Levendoglu-Tugal O, Weiss R, Ozkaynak MF, Sandoval C, Lentzner B, Jayabose S: T-cell acute lymphoblastic leukemia after renal transplantation in childhood, *J Pediatr Hematol Oncol* 20(6):548-51, 1998.
48. Goyal RK, McEvoy L, Wilson DB: Hodgkin disease after renal transplantation in childhood, *J Pediatr Hematol Oncol* 18(4):392-95, 1996.

49. Dharnidharka VR, Douglas VK, Hunger SP, Fennell RS: Hodgkin's lymphoma after post-transplant lymphoproliferative disease in a renal transplant recipient, *Pediatr Transplant* 8(1):87-90, 2004.
50. Axelrod DA, Holmes R, Thomas SE, Magee JC: Limitations of EBV-PCR monitoring to detect EBV associated post-transplant lymphoproliferative disorder, *Pediatr Transplant* 7(3):223-27, 2003.
51. Shroff R, Trompeter R, Cubitt D, Thaker U, Rees L: Epstein-Barr virus monitoring in paediatric renal transplant recipients, *Pediatr Nephrol* 17(9):770-75, 2002.
52. Sokal EM, Antunes H, Beguin C, Bodeus M, Wallemacq P, de Ville de GJ, et al: Early signs and risk factors for the increased incidence of Epstein-Barr virus-related posttransplant lymphoproliferative diseases in pediatric liver transplant recipients treated with tacrolimus, *Transplantation* 64(10):1438-42, 1997.
53. Walker RC, Marshall WF, Strickler JG, Wiesner RH, Velosa JA, Habermann TM, et al: Pretransplantation assessment of the risk of lymphoproliferative disorder, *Clin Infect Dis* 20(5):1346-53, 1995.
54. Buda A, Caforio A, Calabrese F, Fagiuoli S, Pevere S, Livi U, et al: Lymphoproliferative disorders in heart transplant recipients: role of hepatitis C virus (HCV) and Epstein-Barr virus (EBV) infection, *Transpl Int* 13 Suppl 1:S402-S405, 2000.
55. Green M, Reyes J, Webber S, Rowe D: The role of antiviral and immunoglobulin therapy in the prevention of Epstein-Barr virus infection and post-transplant lymphoproliferative disease following solid organ transplantation, *Transpl Infect Dis* 3(2):97-103, 2001.
56. Darenkov IA, Marcarelli MA, Basadonna GP, Friedman AL, Lorber KM, Howe JG, et al: Reduced incidence of Epstein-Barr virus-associated posttransplant lymphoproliferative disorder using preemptive antiviral therapy, *Transplantation* 64(6):848-52, 1997.
57. Davis CL, Harrison KL, McVicar JP, Forg PJ, Bronner MP, Marsh CL: Antiviral prophylaxis and the Epstein Barr virus-related post-transplant lymphoproliferative disorder, *Clin Transplant* 9(1):53-59, 1995.
58. Funch DP, Walker AM, Schneider G, Ziyadeh NJ, Pescovitz MD: Ganciclovir and acyclovir reduce the risk of post-transplant lymphoproliferative disorder in renal transplant recipients, *Am J Transplant* 5(12):2894-900, 2005.
59. Stevens SJ, Verschuuren EA, Verkuujlen SA, Van Den Brule AJ, Meijer CJ, Middeldorp JM: Role of Epstein-Barr virus DNA load monitoring in prevention and early detection of post-transplant lymphoproliferative disease, *Leuk Lymphoma* 43(4):831-40, 2002.
60. Wagner HJ, Wessel M, Jabs W, Smets F, Fischer L, Offner G, et al: Patients at risk for development of posttransplant lymphoproliferative disorder: plasma versus peripheral blood mononuclear cells as material for quantification of Epstein-Barr viral load by using real-time quantitative polymerase chain reaction, *Transplantation* 72(6):1012-19, 2001.
61. Smets F, Latinne D, Bazin H, Reding R, Otte JB, Buts JP, et al: Ratio between Epstein-Barr viral load and anti-Epstein-Barr virus specific T-cell response as a predictive marker of posttransplant lymphoproliferative disease, *Transplantation* 73(10):1603-10, 2002.
62. Vossen MT, Gent MR, Davin JC, Baars PA, Wertheim-van Dillen PM, Weel JF, et al: Spontaneous outgrowth of EBV-transformed B-cells reflects EBV-specific immunity in vivo; a useful tool in the follow-up of EBV-driven immunoproliferative disorders in allograft recipients, *Transpl Int* 17(2):89-96, 2004.
63. Riddler SA, Breinig MC, McKnight JL: Increased levels of circulating Epstein-Barr virus (EBV)-infected lymphocytes and decreased EBV nuclear antigen antibody responses are associated with the development of posttransplant lymphoproliferative disease in solid-organ transplant recipients, *Blood* 84(3):972-84, 1994.
64. O'Conner AR, Franc BL: FDG PET imaging in the evaluation of post-transplant lymphoproliferative disorder following renal transplantation, *Nucl Med Commun* 26(12):1107-11, 2005.
65. Israel O, Keidar Z, Bar-Shalom R: Positron emission tomography in the evaluation of lymphoma, *Semin Nucl Med* 34(3):166-79, 2004.
66. Badley AD, Portela DF, Patel R, Kyle RA, Habermann TM, Strickler JG, et al: Development of monoclonal gammopathy precedes the development of Epstein-Barr virus-induced posttransplant lymphoproliferative disorder, *Liver Transpl Surg* 2(5):375-82, 1996.
67. Bokenkamp A, Grabensee A, Stoffel-Wagner B, Hasan C, Henne T, Offner G, et al: The beta2-microglobulin /cystatin C ratio—a potential marker of post-transplant lymphoproliferative disease, *Clin Nephrol* 58(6):417-22, 2002.
68. Comoli P, Maccario R, Locatelli F, Valente U, Basso S, Garaventa A, et al: Treatment of EBV-related post-renal transplant lymphoproliferative disease with a tailored regimen including EBV-specific T cells, *Am J Transplant* 5(6):1415-22, 2005.
69. Tsai DE, Hardy CL, Tomaszewski JE, Kotloff RM, Oltoff KM, Somer BG, et al: Reduction in immunosuppression as initial therapy for posttransplant lymphoproliferative disorder: analysis of prognostic variables and long-term follow-up of 42 adult patients, *Transplantation* 71(8):1076-88, 2001.
70. Leblond V, Davi F, Charlotte F, Dorent R, Bitker MO, Sutton L, et al: Posttransplant lymphoproliferative disorders not associated with Epstein-Barr virus: a distinct entity? *J Clin Oncol* 16(6):2052-59, 1998.
71. Svoboda J, Kotloff R, Tsai DE: Management of patients with post-transplant lymphoproliferative disorder: the role of rituximab, *Transpl Int* 19(4):259-69, 2006.
72. Berney T, Delis S, Kato T, Nishida S, Mittal NK, Madariaga J, et al: Successful treatment of posttransplant lymphoproliferative disease with prolonged rituximab treatment in intestinal transplant recipients, *Transplantation* 74(7):1000-06, 2002.
73. Benkerrou M, Jais JP, Leblond V, Durandy A, Sutton L, Bordigoni P, et al: Anti-B-cell monoclonal antibody treatment of severe post-transplant B-lymphoproliferative disorder: prognostic factors and long-term outcome, *Blood* 92(9):3137-47, 1998.
74. Oertel SH, Anagnostopoulos I, Hummel MW, Jonas S, Riess HB: Identification of early antigen BZLF1/ZEBRA protein of Epstein-Barr virus can predict the effectiveness of antiviral treatment in patients with post-transplant lymphoproliferative disease, *Br J Haematol* 118(4):1120-23, 2002.
75. Watts RG, Hilliard LM, Berkow RL: Tailored chemotherapy for malignant lymphoma arising in the setting of posttransplant lymphoproliferative disorder after solid organ transplantation, *J Pediatr Hematol Oncol* 24(8):622-26, 2002.
76. Khanna R, Bell S, Sherritt M, Galbraith A, Burrows SR, Rafter L, et al: Activation and adoptive transfer of Epstein-Barr virus-specific cytotoxic T cells in solid organ transplant patients with posttransplant lymphoproliferative disease, *Proc Natl Acad Sci U S A* 96(18):10391-96, 1999.
77. Comoli P, Labirio M, Basso S, Baldanti F, Grossi P, Furione M, et al: Infusion of autologous Epstein-Barr virus (EBV)-specific cytotoxic T cells for prevention of EBV-related lymphoproliferative disorder in solid organ transplant recipients with evidence of active virus replication, *Blood* 99(7):2592-98, 2002.
78. Faro A: Interferon-alpha and its effects on post-transplant lymphoproliferative disorders, *Springer Semin Immunopathol* 20(3-4):425-36, 1998.
79. Dreno B, Mansat E, Legoux B, Litoux P: Skin cancers in transplant patients, *Nephrol Dial Transplant* 13(6):1374-79, 1998.
80. Smith CH, McGregor JM, Barker JN, Morris RW, Rigden SP, MacDonald DM: Excess melanocytic nevi in children with renal allografts, *J Am Acad Dermatol* 28(1):51-55, 1993.
81. Zvulunov A, Wyatt DT, Laud PW, Esterly NB: Lack of effect of growth hormone therapy on the count and density of melanocytic naevi in children, *Br J Dermatol* 137(4):545-48, 1997.
82. Fuente MJ, Sabat M, Roca J, Lauzurica R, Fernandez-Figueras MT, Ferrandiz C: A prospective study of the incidence of skin cancer and its risk factors in a Spanish Mediterranean population of kidney transplant recipients, *Br J Dermatol* 149(6):1221-26, 2003.
83. Claudon M, Panescu V, Le CL, Hubert J, Martin-Bertaux A, Lefevre F, et al: Primary adenocarcinoma of the renal transplant, *Nephrol Dial Transplant* 13(10):2667-70, 1998.
84. Mehls O, Wilton P, Lilien M, Berg U, Broyer M, Rizzoni G, et al: Does growth hormone treatment affect the risk of post-transplant renal cancer? *Pediatr Nephrol* 17(12):984-89, 2002.
85. Greco AJ, Baluarte JH, Meyers KE, Sellers MT, Suchi M, Biegel JA, et al: Chromophobe renal cell carcinoma in a pediatric living-related kidney transplant recipient, *Am J Kidney Dis* 45(6):e105-e108, 2005.
86. Brunner M, di MG, Goldman E: Absence of BK virus sequences in transformed hamster cells transfected by human tumor DNA, *Virus Res* 12(4):315-30, 1989.

CHAPTER 64

Drug Use and Dosage in Renal Failure

Douglas L. Blowey

INTRODUCTION

The optimal use of therapeutic agents is based on an understanding of the characteristics of each patient that determine the relationship between prescribed drug dose and drug effect. Individual differences in drug disposition (pharmacokinetics) and drug response (pharmacodynamics) may greatly influence the anticipated therapeutic effectiveness and adverse effects of a prescribed therapeutic agent. Differences among individuals in drug disposition and response may be due to factors such as age, disease (e.g., kidney failure), genetics, and interactions among therapeutic agents.

Many of the determinants of variation in drug disposition and response are predictable, and successful therapy can be accomplished by anticipating the alterations in drug disposition or response and making the appropriate adjustments to the drug regimen at the onset of therapy. Failure to account for individual differences in drug disposition and response can culminate in therapeutic failure or drug toxicity.

The LADMER system, schematically depicted in Figure 64-1, describes the pathways involved in drug disposition: *l*iberation of drug from the dosage form, *a*bsorption into the systemic circulation, *d*istribution throughout the body, *m*etabolism in various systems, *e*xcretion from the body, and the *r*esponse or effect. Knowledge of the pathways of drug disposition is fundamental to understanding the relationship between the dosage regimen and clinical effect. It also provides a framework for understanding the impact of age, disease, genetics, and drug interactions on the process of delivering the appropriate amount of drug to its intended site of action.

Although complete pharmacologic compendia are available,[1] a comprehensive knowledge of drug distribution and drug response is not necessary to guide most therapeutics in children with kidney failure. Rather, a basic understanding of the fundamental principles of pharmacology and how they apply to the care of the child with kidney failure will suffice in most situations.

KIDNEY-FAILURE–INDUCED ALTERATIONS IN DRUG DISPOSITION

Absorption

Absorption is the passage of drug from its site of administration into the systemic circulation. The amount of drug absorbed into the systemic circulation is primarily affected by the route of administration. When the drug is given intravenously, its absorption is considered complete—with the notable exception of some prodrugs that require metabolic conversion to an active moiety before becoming effective (e.g., fosphenytoin). Most practitioners are familiar with the concept that only a fraction of the total dose administered will be absorbed when administered through the gastrointestinal tract and other extravascular sites (e.g., intramuscular, subcutaneous, rectal, transdermal, and intraperitoneal).

Bioavailability is the term used to describe the fraction of the administered dose that reaches the systemic circulation escaping presystemic metabolism or transport (i.e., first-pass effect). In the setting of extravascular administration (e.g., oral), drug absorption is limited by the drug's ability to pass through the various tissues interfaced between the absorption site and the systemic circulation. The extent of absorption is a function of the anatomic site from which absorption takes place, the physicochemical characteristics of the drug, and the metabolic and transport capacity of tissues the drug must pass through prior to entering the systemic circulation.

Drugs administered by the oral route are absorbed across the intestinal epithelium, a tissue rich in drug-metabolizing enzymes (e.g., cytochromes P-450) and transporters (e.g., P-glycoprotein). After oral administration, most drugs cross the intestinal epithelium by passive diffusion along a concentration gradient. This transport is favored when the therapeutic agent is present in the unbound (free) and nonionized (uncharged) form. The degree of ionization is determined by the physicochemical properties of the drug, such as the pKa (e.g., weak acid, weak base) and the pH of the environment around the drug.

Accordingly, the movement and partitioning of drug across membranes (such as the gastrointestinal epithelium) may be affected by the pH gradient. For example, most NSAIDs are weak acids (e.g., pKa < 4.5) and remain largely nonionized and freely absorbable in the acidic environment of the stomach. Once inside the gastric cell, the more basic pH of the intracellular environment favors the formation of the ionized and poorly diffusible drug species and effectively traps the drug in the gastric epithelium—leading to an accumulation of drug within the gastric epithelium (a possible explanation for the well-known gastric toxicity). Many drugs are well absorbed across the intestinal epithelium but do not

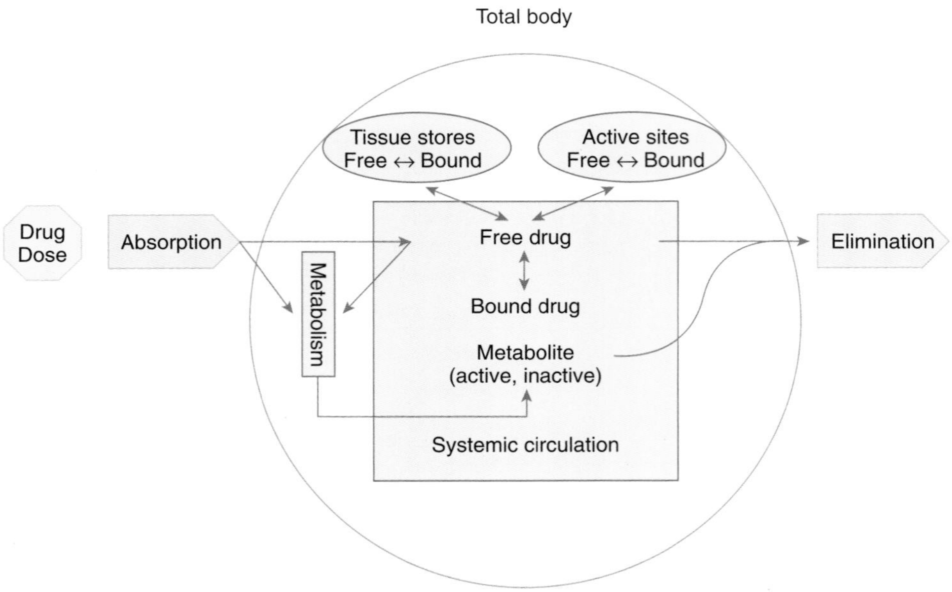

Figure 64-1 Diagram of LADMER system or drug disposition.

reach the systemic circulation due to presystemic metabolism within the intestinal epithelium/liver or recycling of the drug back into the gastrointestinal tract by transporters such as the efflux transporter P-glycoprotein encoded by the multidrug resistance-1 (MDR1) gene[2] (i.e., first-pass effect).

The process of "normal" drug absorption may be altered by a number of mechanisms, including genetic factors (e.g., polymorphisms of drug-metabolizing enzymes or drug transporters), disease-induced changes in the structure and physiology of the absorptive site, and interactions among drugs. Potential changes in drug absorption associated with kidney failure are listed in Table 64-1. Most commonly, the factors impacting drug absorption in kidney failure result in a decrease in the amount of drug absorbed.

Perceived lack of therapeutic efficacy in a child with kidney failure may also result from the patient not receiving the medication as prescribed due to unreported adverse effects, uremic or disease-induced nausea and vomiting, or social factors not specific to the medication. Interaction among concomitant medications is the most familiar and preventable cause of decreased drug absorption in patients with kidney failure. Drug absorption may be limited by binding to other nonabsorbable drugs (e.g., phosphate binders) or food,[3] developmental or drug-induced changes in the physiologic milieu at the absorptive site (e.g., pH, gastric emptying time),[4] or induction of the metabolic capacity of the gastrointestinal epithelium or liver (e.g., increased first-pass effect).

In contrast, the inhibition of intestinal drug-metabolizing enzymes by medications, herbal supplements (e.g., St. John's wort),[5] or dietary substances (e.g., grapefruit juice)[6] can result in a decrease in the first-pass metabolism and an increase in the amount of drug absorbed. For example, the bioavailability of the immunosuppressive agents tacrolimus and cyclosporine is limited by intestinal metabolism via the cytochromes P-450 (CYP) enzymes (mainly CYP3A4/5). The coadminstration of strong CYP3A inhibitors, such as the antifungal agents ketoconazole and itraconazole, can decrease the metabolism of these agents in the gut and increase the amount of active drug reaching the systemic circulation.[7,8]

The enhanced absorption of active drug can result in an increase in blood concentrations and toxicity. In some individuals, a polymorphism in CYP3A5 (e.g., CYP3A5 *1*1) is associated with an extremely high CYP3A5 activity (i.e., "supermetabolizer") that results in an increased tacrolimus metabolism by the intestinal epithelium and an inability to achieve therapeutic systemic levels even with large oral doses.[9,10]

TABLE 64-1 Potential Changes in Drug Disposition with Kidney Failure

	Effect	Mechanism
Absorption	Decreased	• Altered GI pH • Drug interaction: binders, h2 blockers, PPIs • Edema of GI tract, uremic N/V, delayed gastric emptying
Distribution	Increased	• Expansion of body water • Increased free (unbound) drug fraction • Hypoalbuminemia (nephrosis, malnutrition) • Uremic changes in albumin structure • Drug interactions
Metabolism	Decreased	• Inhibition of CYP 450 metabolism • Drug interaction • Direct inhibition by "uremic" milieu
	Increased	• Induced CYP 450 metabolism
Excretion	Decreased	• Decreased GFR • Decreased tubular secretion • Drug interaction • Competition with "uremic" substances

In these individuals, the coadministration of ketoconazole or itraconazole may be of therapeutic benefit due to an inhibition of the intestinal metabolizing enzymes that increases the amount of tacrolimus or cyclosporine absorbed intact and permits the achievement of therapeutic blood levels with reasonable oral doses.[11] Likewise, in developing countries the ketoconazole-tacrolimus interaction has been used to decrease treatment costs associated with immunosuppressive drugs.[12]

Distribution

As a drug enters the systemic circulation, it ultimately disperses into tissue stores and to sites of action (Figure 64-1). The process of partitioning a drug to the various body tissues depends on a number of physiologic factors, including the patient's age, gender, body composition, plasma pH, perfusion of tissue beds, disease states, and the particular physicochemical properties of the drug (such as the drug size, pK_a, drug binding to plasma and tissue constituents, concentration gradients across semipermeable membranes, and lipid solubility). Although some drugs are actively partitioned into certain tissues to the benefit or detriment of the patient, most drugs are not methodically directed to tissue with active sites or receptors but are distributed throughout the body by physical forces.

The distribution volume relates the plasma drug concentration to the amount of drug in the body, and the result (compared to body water) reflects the extent to which a drug is present in the extravascular tissues and not in the plasma. A large volume of distribution implies that the majority of drug present in the body resides outside the vascular space, whereas a small volume of distribution suggests the opposite. The distribution to extravascular sites of drugs that are avidly bound to plasma proteins (e.g., albumin, α_1-acid glycoprotein) is restricted because generally only the protein-unbound (i.e., "free") drug is able to pass through the membranes and interact with receptors at a site of action.

Likewise, highly polar drugs do not easily cross through cell membranes and their distribution is limited. Due to the restricted distribution, highly protein-bound and highly polar drugs are typically characterized by small volumes of distribution. For example, phenytoin is highly protein bound (90%-95%) and has a distribution volume (0.7 L/kg) similar to body water. Likewise, gentamicin (a highly polar compound) has a distribution volume similar to the volume of extracellular fluid (0.45 L/kg in neonates and 0.25 L/kg in adults). From a clinical standpoint, the distribution volume is useful when determining the loading drug dose necessary to achieve instantaneous therapeutic serum drug concentration (formulated as follows).

$$\text{Loading Dose} = (Cp_{des} - Cp_{meas})V_d$$

Here, Cp_{des} is the plasma concentration desired, Cp_{meas} is the plasma concentration measured, and V_d is the distribution volume. The distribution volume also provides some insight into the extent of drug removal that can be anticipated during dialysis. For drugs with a large distribution volume consequent to extensive tissue binding (e.g., digoxin and tricyclic antidepressants), dialysis will generally not result in a significant reduction in the total amount of drug in the body. In contrast, drugs that are largely confined to the extracellular fluid and not extensively bound to plasma proteins (e.g., aminoglycosides) are well removed by dialysis.[13,14]

Kidney failure can dramatically affect the distribution volume of drug, an effect that may result in therapeutic failure or toxicity. Edema, common in kidney failure, expands the distribution volume of agents such as aminoglycosides and vancomycin that preferentially distribute into body water. In these cases, failure to anticipate the expanded distribution volume will lead to underestimating the loading dose—with consequent delay in therapeutic effect. Kidney disease associated with protein loss or poor nutrition may lead to decreased serum albumin and an increase in the free effective fraction of highly protein-bound drugs. This results in an expanded distribution volume and increased concentration of the active drug in the extravascular tissues, exposing the patient to potential toxicity.

Similarly, uremia can induce changes in the albumin structure such that acidic drugs may be bound less avidly. A more common problem in children with decreased plasma protein binding of drugs due to disease-related factors or drug interactions is the misinterpretation of measured concentrations of drug in the plasma. Because most drug assays do not distinguish free drug from bound drug, the reported plasma level reflects the sum of the bound and active unbound species.

As protein binding decreases, the fraction of drug present in the plasma as unbound increases—and for any given plasma concentration there will be more active unbound drug than would be observed in the normal state. For example, 90% to 95% of phenytoin in the plasma is bound to albumin. Small variations in the percentage of phenytoin bound to albumin dramatically affect the amount of free (active) drug. Despite normal or low serum phenytoin levels (free + bound), there is an increased proportion of free drug noted in patients with hypoalbuminemia and renal failure. Failure to recognize the change in the drug distribution may erroneously lead to an increase in dose that may further increase the free (active) drug, resulting in toxicity. Measurement of free rather than total phenytoin permits direct assessment of the problem.

Biotransformation

Biotransformation is the enzymatic conversion of a drug to a new chemical species. The new drug product (i.e., drug metabolite) is usually a less active compound that is more easily eliminated from the body. However, metabolites may be formed that have enhanced or significant pharmacologic activity,[15,16] toxic properties,[17] and a disposition profile different from the parent drug. Most tissues (including the kidney) possess the ability to biotransform drugs through oxidative, hydrolysis, and conjugation reactions. Quantitatively, the liver and gastrointestinal tract are the most important organs of drug metabolism. However, for some drugs (e.g., imipenem) the kidney is the primary site of drug metabolism and kidney disease can impact the biotransformation profile.

Although there are many types of enzymes capable of biotransformation, CYPs are the most important class involved in the metabolism of therapeutic drugs. There is great interindividual variability in the biologic activity of

CYPs as a consequence of genetic, environmental, physiologic, and developmental factors.[18,19] The potential changes in drug metabolism in children with kidney failure are listed in Table 64-1, but for most drugs there is little change in the drug biotransformation profile with kidney disease or kidney failure.

For drugs primarily metabolized by the kidney, a decrease in kidney function can alter the biotransformation profiles and lead to adverse effects. For example, imipenem is a β-lactam antibiotic that is rapidly hydrolyzed by dipeptidases located on the brush border or the proximal renal tubule. Kidney failure impairs the normal metabolism and results in an accumulation of imipenem and an increased risk of seizures.[20] The most common source of altered drug biotransformation in children with kidney failure is the induction or inhibition of drug-metabolizing enzymes resulting from interactions with concomitant medications.

Even when drug metabolism proceeds unaltered, drug metabolites may be formed that are eliminated by the kidney and accumulate in children with kidney failure. For example, the opioid agonist meperidine undergoes hepatic biotransformation to several metabolites [including normeperidine, which is pharmacologically active and causes central nervous system (CNS) excitation—including hallucinations, tremors, and convulsions]. Renal failure significantly increases the plasma half-life of normeperidine, resulting in accumulation and an increased risk of CNS toxicity.[17]

Elimination

Drugs and drug metabolites are eliminated from the body through various excretory pathways, including kidney, biliary, salivary, mammary, sweat, lung, and intestinal. Although some or all of these pathways may be involved in the elimination of a particular drug, the kidney is generally the most important. Any alteration in kidney function can impact the drug's disposition profile (Table 64-1). The final amount of drug or drug metabolite excreted by the kidney is a composite of filtration, tubular secretion, and reabsorption.

Unless limited by size or charge, the unbound component of drug and drug metabolites in the systemic circulation is filtered through the glomeruli at a rate equal to the glomerular filtration rate. For drugs and drug metabolites primarily eliminated by glomerular filtration, the rate of elimination mirrors the kidney's ability to clear other solutes (e.g., creatinine clearance). As such, drug elimination declines as kidney function declines—and drug accumulates in the body if the drug dosing regimen is not adjusted.

The active renal tubular secretion of drugs and drug metabolites by relatively nonspecific anionic and cationic transport systems in the proximal tubule can contribute substantially to the amount of drug eliminated by the kidney. The renal tubular secretion of a drug may be inhibited by other drugs or endogenous substrates that employ the same nonspecific transport systems. One example where this interaction is of clinical importance is the competitive inhibition of penicillin tubular secretion by probenecid.[21]

Reabsorption is the passive diffusion of nonionized (noncharged) drug from the filtrate into the renal tubular cell. Basic urine (e.g., urine pH > 7.5) favors the ionized form of acidic drugs and limits reabsorption, whereas reabsorption of basic drugs is enhanced in basic urine because the nonionized form of the drug is favored. This concept of "ion trapping" is used clinically to enhance the elimination of salicylates in overdose situations.[22]

The clinical significance of decreased kidney function on a drug dosing regimen is a function of the therapeutic index of the drug, the percentage of the total drug elimination due to kidney elimination, and the degree of kidney failure. Often, the most difficult task is obtaining an accurate assessment of kidney function [e.g., glomerular filtration rate (GFR)]. The volume of water and accompanying solute filtered through the glomeruli per unit time is the GFR, the most important measure of kidney function. The GFR is estimated by measuring the rate at which the kidney removes a substance from the blood (e.g., renal clearance).

The measured substance may be an endogenous compound (e.g., creatinine, cystatin C), an exogenous compound that is specifically administered to measure the GFR (e.g., inulin, isotope, iothalamate), or a compound primarily eliminated by glomerular filtration that is administered as part of clinical care (e.g., gentamicin). The clearance of creatinine corrected for body surface area (BSA) is the most common method used to estimate the GFR. Creatinine clearance (C_{cr}), expressed as ml/min/1.73 m^2, is calculated by measuring the amount of creatinine in an accurately timed urine collection and a midcollection plasma creatinine.

$$C_{cr} = \frac{[\text{Urine Cr}(\text{mg/dl}) \times (\text{Urine volume}(\text{ml})/\text{Time}(\text{min}))]}{\text{Plasma Cr}(\text{mg/dl})} \times \frac{1.73\text{m}^2}{\text{BSA}(\text{m}^2)}$$

Creatinine clearance is low at birth and rapidly increases during the first 2 weeks of life, followed by a steady rise until adult values are reached by 8 to 12 months.[23] Although not as accurate as a timed urine collection, creatinine clearance can be quickly estimated by measuring the child's serum creatinine and length.[24]

$$C_{cr} = \frac{\text{Length(cm)} \times \text{“K”}}{\text{Plasma Cr(mg/dl)}}$$

In the previous equation, K represents the creatinine production rate and varies with age: 0.45 (term newborn), 0.55 (child), and 0.7 (adolescent boy). Appropriate K values, if creatinine is measured in μmol/L, are shown in Table 2-4. It is important to understand that the normal relationship among serum creatinine, length, and GFR is altered in disturbances of creatinine biosynthesis (e.g., muscular disease and malnutrition) and in clinical settings where the serum creatinine is rapidly changing (e.g., acute renal failure, recovery from renal failure, and dialysis). In these situations, a timed urine collection is required for an accurate estimate of GFR.

DIALYSIS

The impact of dialysis on drug disposition is determined largely by the extent of drug removal by the dialysis procedure. During dialysis, drug clearance is a composite of ongoing drug removal by renal, hepatic, and other intrinsic clearance pathways and the additional clearance provided by dialysis. In general, drug removal is considered clinically significant when >25% of the administered dose is removed by dialysis. Failure to recognize the extent of drug removal and provide supplemental dosing can result in underdosing and therapeutic compromise.

Drug elimination during dialysis occurs by the processes of diffusion and convection. The contribution of each process to the dialysis clearance of a drug varies among dialysis modalities. Diffusion is the movement of drug across a dialyzer membrane or peritoneal membrane from a higher to lower drug concentration. Convection is the movement of drug across the dialyzer membrane or peritoneal membrane that occurs with the flow of an ultrafiltrate. Only drug present within the systemic circulation in the unbound form is available for removal by dialysis.

Drug cannot be directly removed from tissue stores, and the drug must be redistributed from the tissue sites into the vascular space to be available for elimination by any dialysis procedure. Thus, in general drugs with a large volume of distribution are not efficiently dialyzed. Although drug usually moves in the direction from the blood compartment to dialysis fluid, drug can be absorbed from the dialysis fluid into the blood compartment when the dialysis fluid drug concentration exceeds the serum concentration. Due to the bidirectional movement of drug, therapeutic blood concentrations can be achieved with intraperitoneal administration—as is observed with the intraperitoneal administration of antibiotics during treatment of peritonitis.[25,26]

The efficiency of drug removal is greatest for hemodialysis, followed by continuous renal replacement therapies (CRRTs)—and least by peritoneal dialysis. Although drug removal by CRRT and peritoneal dialysis is less efficient than hemodialysis, the total drug removal may be equivalent because CRRT and peritoneal dialysis are performed for a longer period of time.

GUIDELINES FOR DRUG DOSING IN CHILDREN WITH RENAL FAILURE

The optimal drug prescription for a child with kidney failure considers the multiple factors that impact drug disposition and response and is best achieved by using an individualized approach. Although drug lists and dosing tables can be helpful in organizing those drugs that require attention in children with kidney failure (Table 64-2 at the end of the chapter), such guidelines fall short when it comes to providing dosing recommendations because optimal therapy must be individualized on the basis of the degree of kidney failure, concurrent medications, and developmental factors—all of which can impact the disposition of a drug.

Thus, the provision of safe and effective therapy in children with kidney failure is best accomplished using an individualized systematic approach (as outlined in Figure 64-2). The design of a successful therapeutic regimen begins with an estimate of the child's residual renal function and an estimate of the relative contribution of renal elimination to the total drug elimination obtained from the literature. Reference books such as the *Pediatric Drug Handbook*,[27] *Physicians Desk Reference*, and *Micromedex* are excellent sources for information on drug disposition—and most references are available as electronic documents that can be used on handheld devices for point-of-care therapeutic decisions.

Although children receiving dialysis by definition have very poor renal function, it is inappropriate to assume that there is no renal elimination because many children maintain a significant amount of residual renal function and failure to account for the continued renal elimination of drug may result in insufficient drug dosing and therapeutic failure. If one assumes that drug protein binding, distribution, and metabolism are not altered to a clinically significant degree

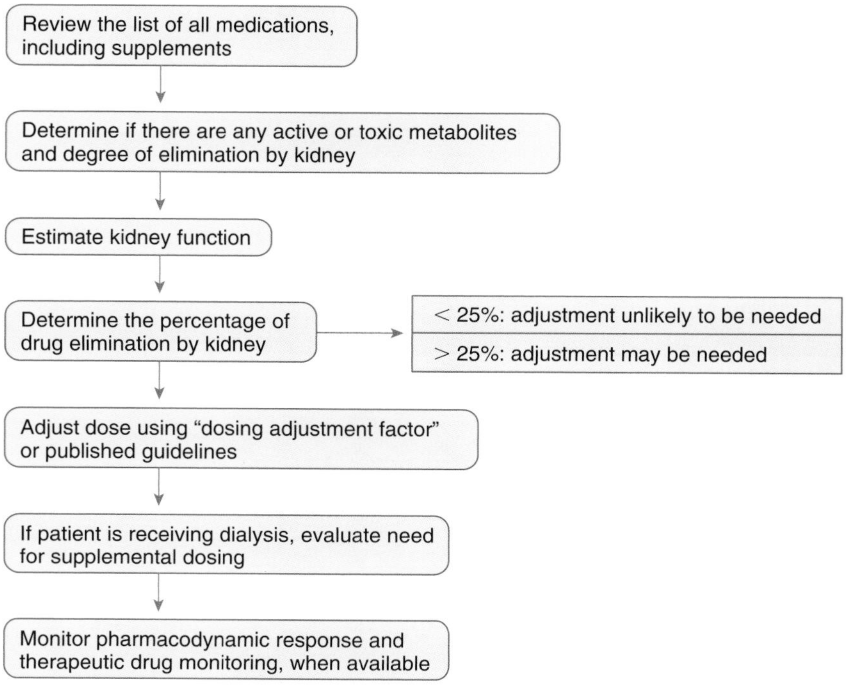

Figure 64-2 Guidelines for drug dosing in children with kidney failure.

in renal failure (an assumption likely true for most drugs), a dosing adjustment factor (Q) can be estimated using the following equation.

$$Q = 1 - \left[\text{Fraction renal elimination} \times \left(1 - \frac{\text{Child's } C_{cr}\,(\text{ml/min/1.73m}^2)}{\text{Normal } C_{cr}\,(\text{ml/min/1.73m}^2)}\right)\right]$$

The appropriate dose amount or dosing interval for a child with reduced kidney function is generated by applying the dosing adjustment factor to either the normal dose amount ($Q \times$ normal dose = adjusted dose) or normal dosing interval (normal dosing interval $\div Q$ = adjusted dosing interval). The dosage adjustment factor estimates the change that occurs in elimination associated with renal failure but does not account for any additional clearance by dialysis. If appropriate, supplemental drug doses may be required to replace the dialysis-related drug losses.

Whether a change is made in the dose amount or dosing interval depends on the therapeutic goal and relationships between drug concentrations and clinical response and toxicity. In general, increasing the dosing interval will increase the variation between peak and trough blood concentration and would be most appropriate for drugs whose effects are based on achieving a certain peak drug level (e.g., aminoglycosides). In contrast, a decrease in variations between peak and trough blood drug concentration will be observed when a normal dosing interval is maintained but the dose amount is decreased. This dosing adjustment would be most appropriate for drugs that should be maintained at a relatively stable blood concentration, such as cephalosporins or blood pressure medications.

Once the prescribed drug dosing schedule has been adjusted for renal failure, a supplemental dose or dosing adjustment may be required for children receiving dialysis when >25% of a drug is removed during the dialysis procedure. Supplemental dosing is given to replace the amount of drug removed by dialysis and may be achieved as a partial or full dose administered after hemodialysis, or an increase in the dosing amount or frequency in children receiving peritoneal dialysis or CRRT. When possible, routine maintenance drugs should be provided after hemodialysis. Guidelines for drug dosing during dialysis are available in selected references.[25,28]

The determinants of drug disposition and action in children with renal failure and those children receiving dialysis are frequently altered such that changes in the dosing regimen are necessary to avoid toxicity or inadequate treatment. In view of the many factors capable of altering both the disposition and action of a given drug, it is important to individualize drug therapy for the known alterations associated with age, kidney failure, and dialysis.

TABLE 64-2 **Drug Dosing Guidelines**

Drug	Adjustment for Renal Failure	SUPPLEMENT FOR DIALYSIS			Comments
		Hemodialysis	CRRT	Peritoneal Dialysis	
Antibiotics and Antiviral and Antifungal Agents					
Acyclovir[29-32]	Yes	Yes	No	No	Neurotoxicity
Amantadine[33-35]	Yes	No	No	No	
Amikacin[36-38]	Yes	Yes	Yes	Yes	TDM
Amoxicillin[39]	Yes	Yes	?	No	
Amphotericin B[40,41]	No	No	No	No	
Ampicillin[42-44]	Yes	Yes	Yes	No	
Azithromycin[35,45]	No	No	No	No	
Cefaclor[46,47]	Yes	Yes	?	No	
Cefazolin[48,49]	Yes	Yes	Yes	Yes	
Cefepime[50-52]	Yes	Yes	Yes	No	Neurotoxicity
Cefixime[53,54]	Yes	No	No	No	
Cefotaxime[42,55,56]	Yes	Yes	Yes	No	
Cefpodoxime[57-59]	Yes	Yes	?	No	
Cefprozil[60]	Yes	Yes	?	?	
Ceftazidime[42,61-63]	Yes	Yes	Yes	No	
Ceftriaxone[42,64,65]	No	No	No	No	
Cefuroxime[42,66,67]	Yes	Yes	Yes	No	
Cephalexin[35]	Yes	Yes	?	No	
Ciprofloxacin[35,68]	Yes	No	No	No	

TABLE 64-2 **Drug Dosing Guidelines—cont'd**

Drug	Adjustment for Renal Failure	SUPPLEMENT FOR DIALYSIS			Comments
		Hemodialysis	CRRT	Peritoneal Dialysis	
Clindamycin[69]	No	No	No	No	
Co-trimoxazole[70,71]	Yes	Yes	?	No	
Erythromycin[35,42,72]	Yes	No	No	No	
Famciclovir[73]	Yes	No	?	No	Dose after hemodialysis
Fluconazole[74,75]	Yes	Yes	Yes	No	
Foscarnet[76]	Yes	Yes	?	?	Nephrotoxicity
Ganciclovir[77,78]	Yes	Yes	Yes	?	Dose after hemodialysis
Gentamicin[13,14,79]	Yes	Yes	Yes	Yes	TDM
Imipenem/Cilastin[42,80,81]	Yes	Yes	Yes	No	Seizures
Isoniazid[82,83]	No	No	No	No	TDM, dose after hemodialysis
Ketoconazole[84]	No	No	No	No	
Loracarbef	Yes	Yes	?	?	
Meropenem[85-87]	Yes	Yes	Yes	?	
Metronidazole[35,42,88]	Yes	No	No	No	Dose after hemodialysis
Oxacillin[89]	No	No	No	No	
Penicillin G[35]	Yes	Yes	Yes	No	
Pentamidine[90,91]	No	No	No	No	
Piperacillin[92-94]	Yes	Yes	Yes	No	
Piperacillin/Tazo	Yes	Yes	?	No	
Rifampin[35,82]	No	No	No	No	
Ticarcillin[95,96]	Yes	Yes	Yes	Yes	
Tobramycin[97,98]	Yes	Yes	Yes	Yes	TDM
Valacyclovir[99,100]	Yes	Yes	No	No	Dose after hemodialysis, neurotoxicity
Valganciclovir[101]	Yes	Yes	?	?	Not recommended for patients on dialysis
Vancomycin[35]	Yes	No	No	No	TDM
Anticonvulsants					
Carbamazepine[102,103]	Yes	No	No	No	TDM
Gabapentin	Yes	No	No	No	Dose after hemodialysis
Lamotrigine[104,105]	Yes	No	?	?	
Phenobarbital[35,106]	Yes	Yes	Yes	Yes	
Phenytoin[35,107] (Fosphenytoin)	No	No	No	No	↓ Protein binding TDM-free levels
Valproic acid[108-110]	No	No	No	No	↓ Protein binding
Cardiovascular Agents					
Amlodipine[111,112]	No	No	?	No	
Atenolol[113,114]	Yes	Yes	?	No	
Captopril[115-118]	Yes	Yes	Yes	No	
Clonidine[119,120]	No	No	?	No	
Digoxin[121-125]	Yes	No	No	No	↓ Vd (adjust loading dose) Avoid K^+ depletion
Enalapril[126,127]	Yes	Yes	Yes	No	
Esmolol[128,129]	No	No	No	No	
Labetalol[130,131]	No	No	No	No	

Continued

TABLE 64-2 **Drug Dosing Guidelines—cont'd**

Drug	Adjustment for Renal Failure	SUPPLEMENT FOR DIALYSIS			Comments
		Hemodialysis	CRRT	Peritoneal Dialysis	
Minoxidil[35,132]	No	No	?	No	
Nifedipine[133,134]	No	No	?	No	
Nadolol[135]	Yes	Yes	?	No	
Metoprolol[35]	No	Yes	?	?	Dose after hemodialysis
Prazosin[136]	No	No	?	No	
Propranolol[137-139]	No	No	No	No	
Immunosuppressive Agents					
Daclizumab	No	?	?	?	
Azathioprine[35]	Yes	Yes	?	?	
Cyclosporine[140,141]	No	No	No	No	TDM, nephrotoxicity
Mycophenolate[142-144]	No	No	No	No	TDM
Prednisone[145]	No	No	No	No	
Sirolimus	No	?	?	?	TDM
Tacrolimus[146]	No	No	No	No	TDM, nephrotoxicity
Miscellaneous Buspirone[147]	Yes	No	?	?	Active metabolites
Cetirizine[148]	Yes	No	?	?	
Codeine[35,149]	Yes	No	?	?	Active metabolites
Diazepam[35]	No	No	?	?	Active metabolites
Enoxaparin[150,151]	Yes	No	?	?	TDM
Famotidine[152-154]	Yes	No	No	No	Active metabolites
Fentanyl[35,155]	Yes	No	?	?	
Fluoxetine[155,156]	No	No	No	No	
Hydromorphone	No	?	?	?	
Imipramine[35,157]	No	No	?	No	
Lansoprazole[158,159]	No	No	?	?	
Lithium[160]	Yes	Yes	?	No	TDM
Loratadine[161]	Yes	No	?	No	
Meperidine[17]	Yes	No	?	?	Seizures, metabolites, not recommended
Methadone[35]	Yes	No	?	?	
Methylphenidate	No	?	?	?	
Midazolam[15]	Yes	?	?	?	Active metabolites
Montelukast	No	?	?	?	
Morphine[16,35,162]	Yes	No	?	?	
Omeprazole[163,164]	No	No	?	?	
Ondansetron	No	?	?	?	
Oxycodone[35]	Yes	?	?	?	Active metabolites
Paroxetine[165]	Yes	No	?	?	
Ranitidine[166-168]	Yes	No	?	No	Dose after hemodialysis
Sufentanil	No	?	?	?	
Warfarin[35]	No	No	?	No	

Modified with permission from Blowey DL. Principles of drug administration in children receiving renal replacement therapy. In: Warady BA, Schaefer FS, Fine RN, Alexander SR, editors. *Pediatric Dialysis.* Great Britain: Kluwer Academic Publishers, 2004: 545-565.

REFERENCES

1. Ritschel W, Kearns GL: *Handbook of basic pharmacokinetics, fifth edition*, Washington, D.C.: American Pharmaceutical Association 1999.
2. Borst P, Elferink RO: Mammalian ABC transporters in health and disease, *Annu Rev Biochem* 71:537-92, 2002.
3. Kays MB, Overholser BR, Mueller BA, Moe SM, Sowinski KM: Effects of sevelamer hydrochloride and calcium acetate on the oral bioavailability of ciprofloxacin, *Am J Kidney Dis* 42(6):1253-59, 2003.
4. Strolin BM, Whomsley R, Baltes EL: Differences in absorption, distribution, metabolism and excretion of xenobiotics between the paediatric and adult populations, *Expert Opin Drug Metab Toxicol* 1(3):447-71, 2005.
5. Holstege CP, Mitchell K, Barlotta K, Furbee RB: Toxicity and drug interactions associated with herbal products: Ephedra and St. John's Wort, *Med Clin North Am* 89(6):1225-57, 2005.
6. Hare JT, Elliott DP: Grapefruit juice and potential drug interactions, *Consult Pharm* 18(5):466-72, 2003.
7. Floren LC, Bekersky I, Benet LZ, et al: Tacrolimus oral bioavailability doubles with coadministration of ketoconazole, *Clin Pharmacol Ther* 62:41-49, 1997.
8. Katari SR, Magnone M, Shapiro R, et al: Clinical features of acute reversible tacrolimus (FK 506) nephrotoxicity in kidney transplant recipients, *Clin Transplant* 11(3):237-42, 1997.
9. Haufroid V, Mourad M, Van KV, et al: The effect of CYP3A5 and MDR1 (ABCB1) polymorphisms on cyclosporine and tacrolimus dose requirements and trough blood levels in stable renal transplant patients, *Pharmacogenetics* 14(3):147-54, 2004.
10. Zhang X, Liu ZH, Zheng JM, et al: Influence of CYP3A5 and MDR1 polymorphisms on tacrolimus concentration in the early stage after renal transplantation, *Clin Transplant* 19(5):638-43, 2005.
11. Berkovitch M, Bitzan M, Matsui D, Finkelstein H, Balfe JW, Koren G: Pediatric clinical use of the ketoconazole/cyclosporin interaction, *Pediatr Nephrol* 8:492-93, 1994.
12. El-Dahshan KF, Bakr MA, Donia AF, Badr A, Sobh MA: Ketoconazole-tacrolimus coadministration in kidney transplant recipients: Two-year results of a prospective randomized study, *Am J Nephrol* 26(3):293-98, 2006.
13. Ernest D, Cutler DJ: Gentamicin clearance during continuous arteriovenous hemodiafiltration, *Crit Care Med* 20(5):586-89, 1992.
14. Hamann SR, Oeltgen PR, Shank WA Jr., Blouin RA, Natarajan L: Evaluation of gentamicin pharmacokinetics during peritoneal dialysis, *Ther Drug Monit* 4(3):297-300, 1982.
15. Bauer TM, Ritz R, Haberthur C, et al: Prolonged sedation due to accumulation of conjugated metabolites of midazolam, *Lancet* 346(8968):145-47, 1995.
16. Ball M, McQuay HJ, Moore RA, Allen MC, Fisher A, Sear J: Renal failure and the use of morphine in intensive care, *Lancet* 1(8432):784-86, 1985.
17. Szeto HH, Inturrisi CE, Houde R, Saal S, Cheigh J, Reidenberg MM: Accumulation of normeperidine, an active metabolite of meperidine, in patients with renal failure of cancer, *Ann Intern Med* 86(6):738-41, 1977.
18. Leeder JS: Drug biotransformation. In W Ritschel, GL Kearns (eds.), *Handbook of basic pharmacokinetics*. Washington, D.C.: American Pharmaceutical Association 1999:134-55.
19. Kearns GL, Abdel-Rahman SM, Alander SW, Blowey DL, Leeder JS, Kauffman RE: Developmental pharmacology: Drug disposition, action, and therapy in infants and children, *N Engl J Med* 349:1157-67, 2003.
20. Calandra G, Lydick E, Carrigan J, Weiss L, Guess H: Factors predisposing to seizures in seriously ill infected patients receiving antibiotics: Experience with imipenem/cilastatin, *Am J Med* 84(5):911-18, 1988.
21. Odugbemi T: An open evaluation study of sulbactam/ampicillin with or without probenecid in the treatment of gonococcal infections in Lagos, *Drugs* 35(7):89-91, 1988.
22. Prescott L, Balali-Mood M, Critchley J, Johnstone A, Proudfoot A: Diuresis or urinary alkalinisation for salicylate poisoning, *Br Med J* 285:1383-86, 1982.
23. Arant BS Jr.: Developmental patterns of renal functional maturation in the human neonate, *J Pediatr* 92(5):705-12, 1978.
24. Schwartz G, Brion LP, Spitzer A: The use of plasma creatinine concentration for estimating glomerular filtration rate in infants, children, and adolescents, *Pediatr Clinics North Am* 34(3):571-90, 1987.
25. Bailie GR, Johnson CA, Mason NA, St Peter WL: *Peritoneal dialysis: A guide to medication use*. Shirley, N.Y.: Nephrology Pharmacy Associates 2005.
26. Warady BA, Schaefer F, Holloway M, et al: Consensus guidelines for the treatment of peritonitis in pediatric patients receiving peritoneal dialysis, *Perit Dial Int* 20(6):610-24, 2000.
27. Taketomo CK, Hodding JH, Kraus DM: *Pediatric Dosage handbook, eleventh edition*. Hudson, OH: Lexi-comp 2004.
28. Veltri MA, Neu AM, Fivush BA, Parekh RS, Furth SL: Drug dosing during intermittent hemodialysis and continuous renal replacement therapy: Special considerations in pediatric patients, *Paediatr Drugs* 6(1):45-65, 2004.
29. Boelaert J, Schurgers M, Daneels R, Van Landuyt HW, Weatherley BC: Multiple dose pharmacokinetics of intravenous acyclovir in patients on continuous ambulatory peritoneal dialysis, *J Antimicrob Chemother* 20(1):69-76, 1987.
30. Laskin OL, Longstreth JA, Whelton A, et al: Effect of renal failure on the pharmacokinetics of acyclovir, *Am J Med* 73(1A):197-201, 1982.
31. Stathoulopoulou F, Almond MK, Dhillon S, Raftery MJ: Clinical pharmacokinetics of oral acyclovir in patients on continuous ambulatory peritoneal dialysis, *Nephron* 74(2):337-41, 1996.
32. Wagstaff AJ, Faulds D, Goa KL: Aciclovir: A reappraisal of its antiviral activity, pharmacokinetic properties and therapeutic efficacy, *Drugs* 47(1):153-205, 1994.
33. Wu MJ, Ing TS, Soung LS, Daugirdas JT, Hano JE, Gandhi VC: Amantadine hydrochloride pharmacokinetics in patients with impaired renal function, *Clin Nephrol* 17(1):19-23, 1982.
34. Bridges CB, Fukuda K, Uyeki TM, Cox NJ, Singleton JA: Prevention and control of influenza: Recommendations of the Advisory Committee on Immunization Practices (ACIP), *MMWR Recomm Rep* 51(RR-3):1-31, 2002.
35. Olyaei AJ, de Mattos A, Bennett W: Prescribing drugs in renal disease. In B Brenner (ed.), *The kidney*. Philadelphia: W. B. Saunders 2000:2606-53.
36. Chow-Tung E, Lau AH, Vidyasagar D, John EG: Effect of peritoneal dialysis on serum concentrations of three drugs commonly used in pediatric patients, *Dev Pharmacol Ther* 8(2):85-95, 1985.
37. Lanao JM, Dominguez-Gil A, Tabernero JM, Macias JF: Influence of type of dialyzer on the pharmacokinetics of amikacin, *Int J Clin Pharmacol Ther Toxicol* 21(4):197-202, 1983.
38. Armendariz E, Chelluri L, Ptachcinski R: Pharmacokinetics of amikacin during continuous veno-venous hemofiltration, *Crit Care Med* 18(6):675-76, 1990.
39. Oe PL, Simonian S, Verhoef J: Pharmacokinetics of the new penicillins. Amoxycillin and flucloxacillin in patients with terminal renal failure undergoing haemodialysis, *Chemotherapy* 19(5):279-88, 1973.
40. Muther RS, Bennett WM: Peritoneal clearance of amphotericin B and 5-fluorocytosine, *West J Med* 133(2):157-60, 1980.
41. Block ER, Bennett JE, Livoti LG, Klein WJ Jr., MacGregor RR, Henderson L: Flucytosine and amphotericin B: Hemodialysis effects on the plasma concentration and clearance, *Ann Intern Med* 80(5):613-17, 1974.
42. Cotterill S: Antimicrobial prescribing in patients on haemofiltration, *J Antimicrob Chemother* 36(5):773-80, 1995.
43. Jusko WJ, Lewis GP, Schmitt GW: Ampicillin and hetacillin pharmacokinetics in normal and anephric subjects, *Clin Pharmacol Ther* 14(1):90-99, 1973.
44. Golper TA, Pulliam J, Bennett WM: Removal of therapeutic drugs by continuous arteriovenous hemofiltration, *Arch Intern Med* 145(9):1651-52, 1985.
45. Kent JR, Almond MK, Dhillon S: Azithromycin: An assessment of its pharmacokinetics and therapeutic potential in CAPD, *Perit Dial Int* 21(4):372-77, 2001.

46. Berman SJ, Boughton WH, Sugihara JG, Wong EG, Sato MM, Siemsen AW: Pharmacokinetics of cefaclor in patients with end stage renal disease and during hemodialysis, *Antimicrob Agents Chemother* 14(3):281-83, 1978.
47. Gartenberg G, Meyers BR, Hirschmann SZ, Srulevitch E: Pharmacokinetics of cefaclor in patients with stable renal impairment, and patients undergoing haemodialysis, *J Antimicrob Chemother* 5(4):465-70, 1979.
48. Marx MA, Frye RF, Matzke GR, Golper TA: Cefazolin as empiric therapy in hemodialysis-related infections: Efficacy and blood concentrations, *Am J Kidney Dis* 32(3):410-14, 1998.
49. Manley HJ, Bailie GR, Asher RD, Eisele G, Frye RF: Pharmacokinetics of intermittent intraperitoneal cefazolin in continuous ambulatory peritoneal dialysis patients, *Perit Dial Int* 19(1):65-70, 1999.
50. Cronqvist J, Nilsson-Ehle I, Oqvist B, Norrby SR: Pharmacokinetics of cefepime dihydrochloride arginine in subjects with renal impairment, *Antimicrob Agents Chemother* 36(12):2676-80, 1992.
51. Wong KM, Chan WK, Chan YH, Li CS: Cefepime-related neurotoxicity in a haemodialysis patient, *Nephrol Dial Transplant* 14(9):2265-66, 1999.
52. Barbhaiya RH, Knupp CA, Pfeffer M, et al: Pharmacokinetics of cefepime in patients undergoing continuous ambulatory peritoneal dialysis, *Antimicrob Agents Chemother* 36(7):1387-91, 1992.
53. Faulkner RD, Yacobi A, Barone JS, Kaplan SA, Silber BM: Pharmacokinetic profile of cefixime in man, *Pediatr Infect Dis J* 6(10):963-70, 1987.
54. Guay DR, Meatherall RC, Harding GK, Brown GR: Pharmacokinetics of cefixime (CL 284,635; FK 027) in healthy subjects and patients with renal insufficiency, *Antimicrob Agents Chemother* 30(3):485-90, 1986.
55. Albin HC, Demotes-Mainard FM, Bouchet JL, Vincon GA, Martin-Dupont C: Pharmacokinetics of intravenous and intraperitoneal cefotaxime in chronic ambulatory peritoneal dialysis, *Clin Pharmacol Ther* 38(3):285-89, 1985.
56. Fillastre JP, Leroy A, Humbert G, Godin M: Pharmacokinetics of cefotaxime in subjects with normal and impaired renal function, *J Antimicrob Chemother* 6(A):103-11, 1980.
57. Hoffler D, Koeppe P, Corcilius M, Przyklinik A: Cefpodoxime proxetil in patients with endstage renal failure on hemodialysis, *Infection* 18(3):157-62, 1990.
58. Borin MT, Hughes GS, Kelloway JS, Shapiro BE, Halstenson CE: Disposition of cefpodoxime proxetil in hemodialysis patients, *J Clin Pharmacol* 32(11):1038-44, 1992.
59. Johnson CA, Ateshkadi A, Zimmerman SW, et al: Pharmacokinetics and ex vivo susceptibility of cefpodoxime proxetil in patients receiving continuous ambulatory peritoneal dialysis, *Antimicrob Agents Chemother* 37(12):2650-55, 1993.
60. Shyu WC, Pittman KA, Wilber RB, Matzke GR, Barbhaiya RH: Pharmacokinetics of cefprozil in healthy subjects and patients with renal impairment, *J Clin Pharmacol* 31(4):362-71, 1991.
61. Welage LS, Schultz RW, Schentag JJ: Pharmacokinetics of ceftazidime in patients with renal insufficiency, *Antimicrob Agents Chemother* 25(2):201-04, 1984.
62. Nikolaidis P, Tourkantonis A: Effect of hemodialysis on ceftazidime pharmacokinetics, *Clin Nephrol* 24(3):142-46, 1985.
63. Kinowski JM, de la Coussaye JE, Bressolle F, et al: Multiple-dose pharmacokinetics of amikacin and ceftazidime in critically ill patients with septic multiple-organ failure during intermittent hemofiltration, *Antimicrob Agents Chemother* 37(3):464-73, 1993.
64. Losno GR, Santivanez V, Battilana CA: Single-dose pharmacokinetics of ceftriaxone in patients with end-stage renal disease and hemodialysis, *Chemotherapy* 34(4):261-66, 1988.
65. Matzke GR, Frye RF, Joy MS, Palevsky PM: Determinants of ceftriaxone clearance by continuous venovenous hemofiltration and hemodialysis, *Pharmacotherapy* 20(6):635-43, 2000.
66. Weiss LG, Cars O, Danielson BG, Grahnen A, Wikstrom B: Pharmacokinetics of intravenous cefuroxime during intermittent and continuous arteriovenous hemofiltration, *Clin Nephrol* 30(5):282-86, 1988.
67. Konishi K, Suzuki H, Hayashi M, Saruta T: Pharmacokinetics of cefuroxime axetil in patients with normal and impaired renal function, *J Antimicrob Chemother* 31(3):413-20, 1993.
68. Singlas E, Taburet AM, Landru I, Albin H, Ryckelinck JP: Pharmacokinetics of ciprofloxacin tablets in renal failure: Influence of haemodialysis, *Eur J Clin Pharmacol* 31(5):589-93, 1987.
69. Roberts AP, Eastwood JB, Gower PE, Fenton CM, Curtis JR: Serum and plasma concentrations of clindamycin following a single intramuscular injection of clindamycin phosphate in maintenance haemodialysis patients and normal subjects, *Eur J Clin Pharmacol* 14(6):435-39, 1978.
70. Nissenson AR, Wilson C, Holazo A: Pharmacokinetics of intravenous trimethoprim-sulfamethoxazole during hemodialysis, *Am J Nephrol* 7(4):270-74, 1987.
71. Paap CM, Nahata MC: Clinical use of trimethoprim/sulfamethoxazole during renal dysfunction, *DICP* 23(9):646-54, 1989.
72. Disse B, Gundert-Remy U, Weber E, Andrassy K, Sietzen W, Lang A: Pharmacokinetics of erythromycin in patients with different degrees of renal impairment, *Int J Clin Pharmacol Ther Toxicol* 24(9):460-64, 1986.
73. Gill KS, Wood MJ: The clinical pharmacokinetics of famciclovir, *Clin Pharmacokinet* 31(1):1-8, 1996.
74. Dudley MN: Clinical pharmacology of fluconazole, *Pharmacotherapy* 10(6/3):141S-145S, 1990.
75. Nicolau DP, Crowe H, Nightingale CH, Quintiliani R: Effect of continuous arteriovenous hemodiafiltration on the pharmacokinetics of fluconazole, *Pharmacotherapy* 14(4):502-05, 1994.
76. Aweeka FT, Jacobson MA, Martin-Munley S, et al: Effect of renal disease and hemodialysis on foscarnet pharmacokinetics and dosing recommendations, *J Acquir Immune Defic Syndr Hum Retrovirol* 20(4):350-57, 1999.
77. Combarnous F, Fouque D, Bernard N, et al: Pharmacokinetics of ganciclovir in a patient undergoing chronic haemodialysis, *Eur J Clin Pharmacol* 46(4):379-81, 1994.
78. Boulieu R, Bastien O, Bleyzac N: Pharmacokinetics of ganciclovir in heart transplant patients undergoing continuous venovenous hemodialysis, *Ther Drug Monit* 15(2):105-07, 1993.
79. Golper TA, Pulliam J, Bennett WM: Removal of therapeutic drugs by continuous arteriovenous hemofiltration, *Arch Intern Med* 145(9):1651-52, 1985.
80. Somani P, Freimer EH, Gross ML, Higgins JT Jr.: Pharmacokinetics of imipenem-cilastatin in patients with renal insufficiency undergoing continuous ambulatory peritoneal dialysis, *Antimicrob Agents Chemother* 32(4):530-34, 1988.
81. Verpooten GA, Verbist L, Buntinx AP, Entwistle LA, Jones KH, De Broe ME: The pharmacokinetics of imipenem (thienamycin-formamidine) and the renal dehydropeptidase inhibitor cilastatin sodium in normal subjects and patients with renal failure, *Br J Clin Pharmacol* 18(2):183-93, 1984.
82. Malone RS, Fish DN, Spiegel DM, Childs JM, Peloquin CA: The effect of hemodialysis on isoniazid, rifampin, pyrazinamide, and ethambutol, *Am J Respir Crit Care Med* 159(5/1):1580-84, 1999.
83. Ellard GA: Chemotherapy of tuberculosis for patients with renal impairment, *Nephron* 64(2):169-81, 1993.
84. Daneshmend TK, Warnock DW: Clinical pharmacokinetics of ketoconazole, *Clin Pharmacokinet* 14(1):13-34, 1988.
85. Tegeder I, Neumann F, Bremer F, Brune K, Lotsch J, Geisslinger G: Pharmacokinetics of meropenem in critically ill patients with acute renal failure undergoing continuous venovenous hemofiltration, *Clin Pharmacol Ther* 65(1):50-57, 1999.
86. Giles LJ, Jennings AC, Thomson AH, Creed G, Beale RJ, McLuckie A: Pharmacokinetics of meropenem in intensive care unit patients receiving continuous veno-venous hemofiltration or hemodiafiltration, *Crit Care Med* 28(3):632-37, 2000.
87. Chimata M, Nagase M, Suzuki Y, Shimomura M, Kakuta S: Pharmacokinetics of meropenem in patients with various degrees of renal function, including patients with end-stage renal disease, *Antimicrob Agents Chemother* 37(2):229-33, 1993.
88. Somogyi AA, Kong CB, Gurr FW, Sabto J, Spicer WJ, McLean AJ: Metronidazole pharmacokinetics in patients with acute renal failure, *J Antimicrob Chemother* 13(2):183-89, 1984.
89. Ruedy J: The effects of peritoneal dialysis on the physiological disposition of oxacillin, ampicillin and tetracycline in patients with renal disease, *Can Med Assoc J* 94(6):257-61, 1966.

90. Conte JE Jr.: Pharmacokinetics of intravenous pentamidine in patients with normal renal function or receiving hemodialysis, *J Infect Dis* 163(1):169-75, 1991.
91. Conte JE Jr., Upton RA, Lin ET: Pentamidine pharmacokinetics in patients with AIDS with impaired renal function, *J Infect Dis* 156(6):885-90, 1987.
92. Thompson MI, Russo ME, Matsen JM, Atkin-Thor E: Piperacillin pharmacokinetics in subjects with chronic renal failure, *Antimicrob Agents Chemother* 19(3):450-53, 1981.
93. Francke EL, Appel GB, Neu HC: Pharmacokinetics of intravenous piperacillin in patients undergoing chronic hemodialysis, *Antimicrob Agents Chemother* 16(6):788-91, 1979.
94. Debruyne D, Ryckelynck JP, Hurault DL, Moulin M: Pharmacokinetics of piperacillin in patients on peritoneal dialysis with and without peritonitis, *J Pharm Sci* 79(2):99-102, 1990.
95. Parry MF, Neu HC: Pharmacokinetics of ticarcillin in patients with abnormal renal function, *J Infect Dis* 133(1):46-49, 1976.
96. Wise R, Reeves DS, Parker AS: Administration of ticarcillin, a new antipseudomonal antibiotic, in patients undergoing dialysis, *Antimicrob Agents Chemother* 5(2):119-20, 1974.
97. Lockwood WR, Bower JD: Tobramycin and gentamicin concentrations in the serum of normal and anephric patients, *Antimicrob Agents Chemother* 3(1):125-29, 1973.
98. Zarowitz BJ, Anandan JV, Dumler F, Jayashankar J, Levin N: Continuous arteriovenous hemofiltration of aminoglycoside antibiotics in critically ill patients, *J Clin Pharmacol* 26(8):686-89, 1986.
99. Izzedine H, Mercadal L, Aymard G, et al: Neurotoxicity of valacyclovir in peritoneal dialysis: A pharmacokinetic study, *Am J Nephrol* 21(2):162-64, 2001.
100. Smiley ML, Murray A, de Miranda P: Valacyclovir HCl (Valtrex): An acyclovir prodrug with improved pharmacokinetics and better efficacy for treatment of zoster, *Adv Exp Med Biol* 394:33-39, 1996.
101. *Valcyte* (product information): Nertley, N.J.: Roche Lab Inc.
102. Kandrotas RJ, Oles KS, Gal P, Love JM: Carbamazepine clearance in hemodialysis and hemoperfusion, *DICP* 23(2):137-40, 1989.
103. Lee CS, Wang LH, Marbury TC, Bruni J, Perchalski RJ: Hemodialysis clearance and total body elimination of carbamazepine during chronic hemodialysis, *Clin Toxicol* 17(3):429-38, 1980.
104. Fillastre JP, Taburet AM, Fialaire A, Etienne I, Bidault R, Singlas E: Pharmacokinetics of lamotrigine in patients with renal impairment: Influence of haemodialysis, *Drugs Exp Clin Res* 19(1):25-32, 1993.
105. Garnett WR: Lamotrigine: Pharmacokinetics, *J Child Neurol* 12(1):S10-S15, 1997.
106. Porto I, John EG, Heilliczer J: Removal of phenobarbital during continuous cycling peritoneal dialysis in a child, *Pharmacotherapy* 17(4):832-35, 1997.
107. Czajka PA, Anderson WH, Christoph RA, Banner W Jr.: A pharmacokinetic evaluation of peritoneal dialysis for phenytoin intoxication, *J Clin Pharmacol* 20(10):565-69, 1980.
108. Lapierre O, Dubreucq JL, Beauchemin MA, Vinet B: Valproic acid intoxication in a patient with bipolar disorder and chronic uremia, *Can J Psychiatry* 44(2):88, 1999.
109. Bruni J, Wang LH, Marbury TC, Lee CS, Wilder BJ: Protein binding of valproic acid in uremic patients, *Neurology* 30(5):557-59, 1980.
110. Orr JM, Farrell K, Abbott FS, Ferguson S, Godolphin WJ: The effects of peritoneal dialysis on the single dose and steady state pharmacokinetics of valproic acid in a uremic epileptic child, *Eur J Clin Pharmacol* 24(3):387-90, 1983.
111. Doyle GD, Donohue J, Carmody M, Laher M, Greb H, Volz M: Pharmacokinetics of amlodipine in renal impairment, *Eur J Clin Pharmacol* 36(2):205-08, 1989.
112. Laher MS, Kelly JG, Doyle GD, et al: Pharmacokinetics of amlodipine in renal impairment, *J Cardiovasc Pharmacol* 12(7):S60-S63, 1988.
113. Wan SH, Koda RT, Maronde RF: Pharmacokinetics, pharmacology of atenolol and effect of renal disease, *Br J Clin Pharmacol* 7(6):569-74, 1979.
114. Flouvat B, Decourt S, Aubert P, et al: Pharmacokinetics of atenolol in patients with terminal renal failure and influence of haemodialysis, *Br J Clin Pharmacol* 9(4):379-85, 1980.
115. Ferguson RK, Rotmensch HH, Vlasses PH: Clinical use of captopril. Illustrative cases, *JAMA* 247(15):2117-19, 1982.
116. Sica DA, Gehr TW, Fernandez A: Risk-benefit ratio of angiotensin antagonists versus ACE inhibitors in end-stage renal disease, *Drug Safety* 22(5):350-60, 2000.
117. Fujimura A, Kajiyama H, Ebihara A, Iwashita K, Nomura Y, Kawahara Y: Pharmacokinetics and pharmacodynamics of captopril in patients undergoing continuous ambulatory peritoneal dialysis, *Nephron* 44(4):324-28, 1986.
118. Duchin KL, Pierides AM, Heald A, Singhvi SM, Rommel AJ: Elimination kinetics of captopril in patients with renal failure, *Kidney Int* 25(6):942-47, 1984.
119. Lowenthal DT, Saris SD, Paran E, Cristal N: The use of transdermal clonidine in the hypertensive patient with chronic renal failure, *Clin Nephrol* 39(1):37-43, 1993.
120. Rosansky SJ, Johnson KL, McConnell J: Use of transdermal clonidine in chronic hemodialysis patients, *Clin Nephrol* 39(1):32-36, 1993.
121. Doherty JE, Flanigan WJ, Perkins WH, Ackerman GL: Studies with tritiated digoxin in anephric human subjects, *Circulation* 35(2):298-303, 1967.
122. Paulson MF, Welling PG: Calculation of serum digoxin levels in patients with normal and impaired renal function, *J Clin Pharmacol* 16(11/12):660-65, 1976.
123. Iisalo E, Forsstrom J: Elimination of digoxin during maintenance haemodialysis, *Ann Clin Res* 6(4):203-06, 1974.
124. Pancorbo S, Comty C: Digoxin pharmacokinetics in continuous peritoneal dialysis, *Ann Intern Med* 93(4):639, 1980.
125. Golper TA, Bennett WM: Drug removal by continuous arteriovenous haemofiltration: A review of the evidence in poisoned patients, *Med Toxicol Adverse Drug Exp* 3(5):341-49, 1988.
126. Sica DA, Cutler RE, Parmer RJ, Ford NF: Comparison of the steady-state pharmacokinetics of fosinopril, lisinopril and enalapril in patients with chronic renal insufficiency, *Clin Pharmacokinet* 20(5):420-27, 1991.
127. Mason NA: Angiotensin-converting enzyme inhibitors and renal function, *DICP* 24(5):496-505, 1990.
128. Lowenthal DT, Porter RS, Saris SD, Bies CM, Slegowski MB, Staudacher A: Clinical pharmacology, pharmacodynamics and interactions with esmolol, *Am J Cardiol* 56(11):14F-18F, 1985.
129. Flaherty JF, Wong B, La Follette G, Warnock DG, Hulse JD, Gambertoglio JG: Pharmacokinetics of esmolol and ASL-8123 in renal failure, *Clin Pharmacol Ther* 45(3):321-27, 1989.
130. Wood AJ, Ferry DG, Bailey RR: Elimination kinetics of labetalol in severe renal failure, *Br J Clin Pharmacol* 13(1):81S-86S, 1982.
131. Halstenson CE, Opsahl JA, Pence TV, et al: The disposition and dynamics of labetalol in patients on dialysis, *Clin Pharmacol Ther* 40(4):462-68, 1986.
132. Halstenson CE, Opsahl JA, Wright CE, et al: Disposition of minoxidil in patients with various degrees of renal function, *J Clin Pharmacol* 29(9):798-802, 1989.
133. Spital A, Scandling JD: Nifedipine in continuous ambulatory peritoneal dialysis, *Arch Intern Med* 143(10):2025, 1983.
134. Kleinbloesem CH, van Brummelen P, Woittiez AJ, Faber H, Breimer DD: Influence of haemodialysis on the pharmacokinetics and haemodynamic effects of nifedipine during continuous intravenous infusion, *Clin Pharmacokinet* 11(4):316-22, 1986.
135. Herrera J, Vukovich RA, Griffith DL: Elimination of nadolol by patients with renal impairment, *Br J Clin Pharmacol* 7(2):227S-231S, 1979.
136. Swan SK, Bennett WM: Drug dosing guidelines in patients with renal failure, *West J Med* 156(6):633-38, 1992.
137. Wood AJ, Vestal RE, Spannuth CL, Stone WJ, Wilkinson GR, Shand DG: Propranolol disposition in renal failure, *Br J Clin Pharmacol* 10(6):561-66, 1980.
138. Lowenthal DT, Briggs WA, Gibson TP, Nelson H, Cirksena WJ: Pharmacokinetics of oral propranolol in chronic renal disease, *Clin Pharmacol Ther* 16(5/1):761-69, 1974.
139. Bianchetti G, Graziani G, Brancaccio D, et al: Pharmacokinetics and effects of propranolol in terminal uraemic patients and in patients undergoing regular dialysis treatment, *Clin Pharmacokinet* 1(5):373-84, 1976.

140. Follath F, Wenk M, Vozeh S, et al: Intravenous cyclosporine kinetics in renal failure, *Clin Pharmacol Ther* 34(5):638-43, 1983.
141. Venkataramanan R, Ptachcinski RJ, Burckart GJ, Yang SL, Starzl TE, Van Theil DH: The clearance of cyclosporine by hemodialysis, *J Clin Pharmacol* 24(11/12):528-31, 1984.
142. Filler G, Grygas R, Mai I, et al: Pharmacokinetics of tacrolimus (FK 506) in children and adolescents with renal transplants, *Nephrol Dial Transplant* 12(8):1668-71, 1997.
143. MacPhee IA, Spreafico S, Bewick M, et al: Pharmacokinetics of mycophenolate mofetil in patients with end-stage renal failure, *Kidney Int* 57(3):1164-68, 2000.
144. Bullingham RE, Nicholls AJ, Kamm BR: Clinical pharmacokinetics of mycophenolate mofetil, *Clin Pharmacokinet* 34(6):429-55, 1998.
145. Frey BM, Frey FJ: Clinical pharmacokinetics of prednisone and prednisolone, *Clin Pharmacokinet* 19(2):126-46, 1990.
146. Venkataramanan R, Jain A, Warty VS, et al: Pharmacokinetics of FK 506 in transplant patients, *Transplant Proc* 23(6):2736-40, 1991.
147. Gammans RE, Mayol RF, LaBudde JA: Metabolism and disposition of buspirone, *Am J Med* 80(3B):41-51, 1986.
148. Awni WM, Yeh J, Halstenson CE, Opsahl JA, Chung M, Matzke GR: Effect of haemodialysis on the pharmacokinetics of cetirizine, *Eur J Clin Pharmacol* 38(1):67-69, 1990.
149. Matzke GR, Chan GL, Abraham PA: Codeine dosage in renal failure, *Clin Pharm* 5(1):15-16, 1986.
150. Buckley MM, Sorkin EM: Enoxaparin: A review of its pharmacology and clinical applications in the prevention and treatment of thromboembolic disorders, *Drugs* 44(3):465-97, 1992.
151. Polkinghorne KR, McMahon LP, Becker GJ: Pharmacokinetic studies of dalteparin (Fragmin), enoxaparin (Clexane), and danaparoid sodium (Orgaran) in stable chronic hemodialysis patients, *Am J Kidney Dis* 40(5):990-95, 2002.
152. Lin JH, Chremos AN, Yeh KC, Antonello J, Hessey GA: Effects of age and chronic renal failure on the urinary excretion kinetics of famotidine in man, *Eur J Clin Pharmacol* 34(1):41-46, 1988.
153. Saima S, Echizen H, Yoshimoto K, Ishizaki T: Hemofiltrability of H2-receptor antagonist, famotidine, in renal failure patients, *J Clin Pharmacol* 30(2):159-62, 1990.
154. Gladziwa U, Klotz U, Krishna DR, Schmitt H, Glockner WM, Mann H: Pharmacokinetics and dynamics of famotidine in patients with renal failure, *Br J Clin Pharmacol* 26(3):315-21, 1988.
155. Aronoff GR, Bergstrom RF, Pottratz ST, Sloan RS, Wolen RL, Lemberger L: Fluoxetine kinetics and protein binding in normal and impaired renal function, *Clin Pharmacol Ther* 36(1):138-44, 1984.
156. Lemberger L, Bergstrom RF, Wolen RL, Farid NA, Enas GG, Aronoff GR: Fluoxetine: Clinical pharmacology and physiologic disposition, *J Clin Psychiatry* 46(3/2):14-19, 1985.
157. Bailey RR, Sharman JR, O'Rourke J, Buttimore AL: Haemodialysis and forced diuresis for tricyclic antidepressant poisoning, *Br Med J* 4(5938):230-31, 1974.
158. Andersson T: Pharmacokinetics, metabolism and interactions of acid pump inhibitors: Focus on omeprazole, lansoprazole and pantoprazole, *Clin Pharmacokinet* 31(1):9-28, 1996.
159. Barradell LB, Faulds D, McTavish D: Lansoprazole: A review of its pharmacodynamic and pharmacokinetic properties and its therapeutic efficacy in acid-related disorders, *Drugs* 44(2):225-50, 1992.
160. Clericetti N, Beretta-Piccoli C: Lithium clearance in patients with chronic renal diseases, *Clin Nephrol* 36(6):281-89, 1991.
161. Matzke GR, Halstenson CE, Opsahl JA, et al: Pharmacokinetics of loratadine in patients with renal insufficiency, *J Clin Pharmacol* 30(4):364-71, 1990.
162. Portenoy RK, Foley KM, Stulman J, et al: Plasma morphine and morphine-6-glucuronide during chronic morphine therapy for cancer pain: Plasma profiles, steady-state concentrations and the consequences of renal failure, *Pain* 47(1):13-19, 1991.
163. Naesdal J, Andersson T, Bodemar G, et al: Pharmacokinetics of [14C]omeprazole in patients with impaired renal function, *Clin Pharmacol Ther* 40(3):344-51, 1986.
164. Howden CW, Payton CD, Meredith PA, et al: Antisecretory effect and oral pharmacokinetics of omeprazole in patients with chronic renal failure, *Eur J Clin Pharmacol* 28(6):637-40, 1985.
165. Doyle GD, Laher M, Kelly JG, Byrne MM, Clarkson A, Zussman BD: The pharmacokinetics of paroxetine in renal impairment, *Acta Psychiatr Scand Suppl* 350:89-90, 1989.
166. McFadyen ML, Folb PI, Miller R, Keeton GR, Marks IN: Pharmacokinetics of ranitidine in patients with chronic renal failure, *Eur J Clin Pharmacol* 25(3):347-51, 1983.
167. Zech PY, Chau NP, Pozet N, Labeeuw M, Hadj-Aissa A: Ranitidine kinetics in chronic renal impairment, *Clin Pharmacol Ther* 34(5):667-72, 1983.
168. Gladziwa U, Krishna DR, Klotz U, et al: Pharmacokinetics of ranitidine in patients undergoing haemofiltration, *Eur J Clin Pharmacol* 35(4):427-30, 1988.
169. Blowey DL: Principles of drug administration in children receiving renal replacement therapy. In: Warady BA, Schaefer FS, Fine RN, Alexander SR, editors, *Pediatric Dialysis.* Great Britain: Kluwer Academic Publishers, 2004:545-565.

CHAPTER 65

Causes and Manifestation of Nephrotoxicity

Vassilios Fanos and Laura Cuzzolin

INTRODUCTION

One of the major functions of the kidney is the concentration of toxic metabolites and drugs. Thus, it is a frequent site of drug toxicity. The glomeruli, tubules, interstitium, and arterioles may be altered. Iatrogenic complications include acute kidney failure (ARF): prerenal, renal, or postrenal (all three of which are often reversible when diagnosed early). Drug-induced kidney disease is frequent in all age groups.[1] In adult patients, nephrotoxicity has been related to 8% to 60% of in-hospital acute kidney injury. The wide range depends on the patient population and the definition of nephrotoxicity.[2] Generally, drug-induced ARF accounts for 20% of all cases of ARF in adult patients.

Moreover, 15% of patients admitted to intensive care units develop drug-induced ARF—the main causes of which are antibiotics.[3] Little is known about the epidemiology of drug-induced disorders in the pediatric kidney. However, the incidence seems lower if compared with adults. Drugs have also been found to be involved in 50% of cases of ARF in premature newborns. Recent data suggest in preterm neonates a significant role for maternal consumption and postnatal administration of nonsteroidal antiinflammatory drugs (NSAIDs) in preterm infants.[4,5]

Many factors make the kidney particularly susceptible and vulnerable to toxic damage[6]: the high renal blood flow (renal blood flow accounts for 25% of cardiac output), the predominantly renal excretion of many drugs, the large capillary surface area, the high degree of specialization of the proximal tubule cells, and the progressive concentration of filtered and secreted compounds in the tubular lumen. Discussion of drug-induced nephrotoxicity must consider the following points.

- A drug may give rise to renal damage in different parts of the nephron, and different drugs can have the same intracellular target.[7,8]
- Many nephrotoxins are taken up by the renal target cell, where they are effectively capable of exerting their damage. The proximal tubule is generally to be regarded as the target structure.[6]
- The nephronic heterogeneity (internephronic, intranephronic, and intrasegmental) influences the type of cell damage. In particular, anatomic, physiologic, and biochemical differences within the nephron may explain the damaging effects of some drugs.[9]
- A number of concurrent pathophysiologic mechanisms often act in unison to effect such things as reduction of renal perfusion, direct tubular toxicity, immunomediated toxicity, and interference with fluids and electrolytes.[1]
- Vulnerability may be related to patient age. In the past, it was suggested that drug-induced kidney damage (especially that caused by aminoglycosides or glycopeptides) is less frequent and severe in newborns than in adults. The main hypotheses in the literature in connection with this are seemingly valid. They comprise: a different ratio of renal volume to corporeal volume (i.e., higher in the neonate), less interception of the drug (i.e., aminoglycoside) by the proximal tubular cells, and less sensitivity of the immature tissue toward the toxins.[8] However, this subject is controversial and indeed neonatal status may itself be a risk factor for drug-induced nephrotoxicity. In fact, it has been confirmed that low birthweight contributes to development of renal disease.[10] The effects of maternally administered drugs on the fetal and neonatal kidney have been well documented and recently reviewed.[11]
- The actual importance of drugs as causes of nephrotoxicity is not easy to define. The drugs are administered to newborns and children who are sick and often seriously ill, and who present hemodynamic abnormalities and/or electrolyte derangements. These situations may be important cofactors in bringing about renal damage.[8]

CORRECT ASSESSMENT AND EARLY DIAGNOSIS OF NEPHROTOXICITY

Adverse effects of drugs on the kidney are silent, especially in early stages, and clinical vigilance is needed. Moreover, early diagnosis of nephrotoxicity is essential because dosage adjustment or discontinuation of renally excreted drugs may prevent further iatrogenic damage because most drug nephrotoxicity is reversible.[2] A take-home message is that drug-induced renal failure is often nonoliguric. Thus, monitoring of renal function is mandatory during potentially nephrotoxic therapies.[2,9,12]

Drug-induced nephrotoxicity specifically due to aminoglycosides (AMGs) has been defined clinically in terms of an increase in serum creatinine (sCr) by more than 20% in relation to baseline values. Later, it was defined in greater detail: increase of 44.2 mmol/L (0.5 mg/dl) in patients with basal sCr no greater than 265 mmol/L (3.0 mg/dl), and increase of 88 mmol/L in patients with basal sCr greater than 265 mmol/L (3.0 mg/dl), were regarded as indicative of a nephrotoxic action of the drug administered. However, traditional laboratory parameters of nephrotoxicity (such as sCr, BUN, and urine analysis) are abnormal only in the presence of substantial renal damage.[13] In particular, sCr does not reflect rapid changes in renal function.[8]

Recently, cystatin C (a marker of glomerular function in the "creatinine blind" period) was evaluated and seems to be more accurate in detecting a reduced glomerular filtration rate (GFR). In fact, in adult patients serum cystatin preceded the increase of sCr during ARF by 1 or 2 days.[14] Urinary biomarkers of nephrotoxicity (microglobulins, enzymes, and growth factors) have been used in clinics for the early noninvasive identification of the renal tubular damage occurring in the course of drug therapy. Moreover, they are helpful in establishing its extent and monitoring its time course.[15,16]

Among urinary microglobulins, alpha-1 microglobulin is preferable because its determination is not affected by the presence of extrarenal factors and/or an acid urinary pH. In the course of tubular functional damage, however, the reabsorbed amount of this low-molecular-weight microglobulin is reduced and the urinary concentration of microglobulins is increased.

Detection of high levels of urinary enzymes [the reference enzyme N-acetyl-beta-D-glucosaminidase (NAG) present in lysosomes, and alanine-aminopeptidase (AAP) present in the brush border of convoluted tubule cells] is a sign of structural tubular damage. In the presence of intact glomerular function, high degrees of AAP and NAG activity in the urine derive exclusively from damage to the renal parenchyma.[17]

Repair of kidney damage is promoted by growth factors. Particularly important is the epidermal growth factor (EGF, molecular weight of 6045 Daltons), produced to a large extent by the cells of Henle's loop and of the distal tubule. Urinary EGF (uEGF) values are reduced in the course of acute and chronic renal failure, and their increase after renal parenchymal damage is a predictive indicator of the rate and extent of renal functional recovery.[18]

Genomic markers may also be helpful in toxic renal injury. In particular, the tissue and urinary expression of kidney injury molecule-1 increases before creatinine and can serve as an early indicator of nephrotoxicity in rats.[19] Similarly, a set of potential biomarkers with a time response and a dose response with respect to the progression of proximal tubular toxicity has been reported.[20]

PATHOPHYSIOLOGIC MECHANISMS

Despite numerous potentially nephrotoxic drugs, only a limited number of patterns (often acting in concert) of renal damage have been described.[2,21]

Direct Tubular Cell Toxicity

This damage is at least in part dose dependent, is generally of surreptitious onset (with symptoms often undetected in the early stages), and is characterized by acute tubular necrosis (with the death of a proportion of the cells of renal proximal tubular cells). The pathologic changes, in severe cases, correspond to a picture of acute tubular necrosis.[22,23] This is typical of the AMGs.

Transient enzymuria and a Fanconi-like syndrome are early signs of proximal tubular damage. These often remain undetected, but may be followed by urine sediment disorders (granular, hyaline, and cellular casts) and renal failure. Other drugs associated with this damage are amphotericin B, calcineurin inhibitors, cisplatin, methotrexate, antivirals (such as foscarnet), cidofovirs, retrovirals, pamidronate, pentamidine, and cocaine.

Immunologically Mediated Renal Toxicity

Immunologic renal toxicity damage is mediated by inflammation of interstitium and tubules. It occurs on an allergic basis in an idiosyncratic dose-independent manner. The onset ranges from a few days (3-5) with a second exposure to up to several weeks after a first exposure.[22] From the histological standpoint, it is characterized by the presence of infiltrates of mononuclear cells, plasma cells, and IgE infiltrates.[23]

The hypersensitivity reaction may be mainly due to a cellular mechanism (more common) resulting in acute tubule-interstitial nephritis or to a humoral mechanism (less common) resulting in focal glomerulonephritis.[23] This damage is typical of antibiotics such as beta-lactams, quinolones (mainly ciprofloxacin), rifampin, macrolides, sulfonamides, tetracyclines,[24,25] most NSAIDs, diuretics (thiazides, loop diuretics, and triamterene), anticonvulsants (phenytoin), cimetidine and ranitidine, allopurinol, and antivirals (acyclovir, indinavir).[26]

Renal Vasoconstriction

This is the main pathophysiologic mechanism of acute nephrotoxicity for calcineurin inhibitors (CI) (CsA: cyclosporin A; tacrolimus: TAC) and vasopressors. Moreover, it contributes to the nephrotoxicity of amphotericin B. CI-induced acute renal toxicity is due to a decrease in renal blood flow and GFR. The main mechanism is a dose-dependent reversible vasoconstriction affecting primarily afferent arterioles (prerenal dysfunction with intact tubular function).[2,12]

Altered Intraglomerular Renal Perfusion

This mechanism is typical of NSAIDs, angiotensin-converting enzyme inhibitors (ACEI), and angiotensin receptor blockers (ARB). Within the kidney, prostaglandins contribute to regulation of renal perfusion and GFR—with their vasodilating properties in opposition to the action of vasoconstrictive substances such as angiotensin II, catecholamines, vasopressin, and endothelin.

Thus, subjects suffering from conditions associated with high levels of vasoconstrictive substances (such as hypovolemia, cardiac failure, sepsis, and hypertension) may develop renal damage when treated with NSAIDs that induce a reduction of prostaglandin synthesis. Renal dysfunction associated with antihypertensive therapy is a result of excessive lowering of blood pressure.[27] Because renal blood flow and renal perfusion are maintained during treatment with ACE inhibitors despite the adverse effect on glomerular function, renal function returns to pretreatment levels when the drug is discontinued.

Crystal Accumulation

The pH-dependent precipitation of crystals in distal tubular lumen is a nephrotoxic mechanism occurring with acyclovir, sulphonamide, methotrexate, indinavir, and triamterene.[28] Crystalluria after fluoroquinolones is rare, and may occur in the condition of dehydration. Among the factors that increase the likelihood of renal crystal deposition, severe volume contraction is the most important. The role of uric acid and calcium phosphate crystals in tumor lysis after chemotherapy for malignancies must also be emphasized.

Alterations of Fluids and Electrolytes

Examples of alteration of fluids and electrolytes are excess of sodium and water removal; metabolic alkalosis and hypokalemia induced by excessive use of diuretics; and hyperkalemia and metabolic acidosis consequent to the state of a pharmacologic hyporeninemic hypoaldosteronism associated with NSAID.[29] A frequent complication of amphotericin B is tubulotoxicity, which includes potassium and magnesium loss in urine, electrolyte alterations, renal tubular acidosis, and loss of urinary concentrating ability.[30]

Glomerular Dysfunction with Nephrotic Syndrome

Drugs involved in glomerular dysfunction with nephritic syndrome include NSAIDs, captopril, interferon, penicillamine, and gold. The most common form is membranous nephropathy. However, minimal-change nephropathy due to NSAIDs has also been described. Resolution can follow discontinuing the drug, although irreversible lesions have also been described.[12]

Thrombotic Microangiopathy

Drug-induced thrombotic microangiopathy is due to several drugs, including cyclosporine, tacrolimus, and chemotherapeutic agents. The main pathologic finding is presence of hyaline thrombi in the microvessels of many organs, including glomerular thrombosis. The manifestations can include fever, hemolytic anemia, thrombocytopenic purpura, renal dysfunction, central nervous system involvement (thrombotic thrombocytopenic purpura, TTP), and predominance of renal failure with anemia and thrombocytopenia (hemolytic uremic syndrome).[12]

Other Mechanisms

Osmotic nephrosis (related mainly to mannitol and immunoglobulins)[22] and rhabdomyolysis have also been described.

DRUG-RELATED RENAL SYNDROMES

Four drug-related renal presentations are possible: ARF, renal tubular dysfunction, nephrotic syndrome, and chronic renal failure. We will briefly focus on ARF (caused by prerenal, intrinsic, and obstructive mechanisms), with practical observation of urinary findings.[12]

Prerenal Acute Renal Failure

Prerenal ARF is related to drugs causing renal vasoconstriction and altered intraglomerular renal perfusion. The urinary sediment is generally without casts, red blood cells, and white blood cells. Urinary sodium is low.

Intrinsic Acute Renal Failure

Intrinsic ARF is determined by acute tubular necrosis, acute allergic interstitial nephritis, and thrombotic microangiopathy. Urine findings show dark granular casts and renal epithelial cell casts, and fractional excretion of sodium is high (2% to 3%, compared to a normal value of <1%) in acute tubular necrosis.

In acute allergic interstitial nephritis, the urinary findings include white blood cells, red blood cells, white cells casts, and mild proteinuria. Eosinophiluria (or eosinophilia) is present in more than 75% of cases, except in cases related to NSAIDs. In thrombotic microangiopathy microscopic hematuria, subnephrotic proteinuria, hyaline casts, and granular casts are present.

Obstructive Acute Renal Failure

Obstructive ARF is related to drugs causing crystal formation. Crystals (needle shaped due to acyclovir and rectangular or rosettes from indinavir), together with red and white cells, are predominant urinary findings.

ANTIBIOTICS

Aminoglycosides

AMGs are still widely employed despite their low therapeutic index.[31,32] The major limitations and concern surrounding the use of AMGs are related to their ability to produce structural and functional renal injury. In fact, approximately 50% of cases of drug-induced hospital-acquired ARF are related to the use of AMGs. Six percent to 26% of patients treated with gentamicin develop ARF. Among antibiotic-induced ARF, 80% are related to the AMGs (60% in single-drug therapy and 20% in combination with cephalosporins).[32]

The AMGs are eliminated without metabolic transformation almost exclusively by the kidneys and via glomerular filtration. A small amount of AMG (5%) after glomerular filtration is transported into the tubular cells in the S1 and S2 segments (first step toward nephrotoxicity). Within the tubular cells, high AMG concentrations occur in the lysosomes. These concentrations then interfere with protein reabsorption, protein synthesis in the endoplasmatic reticulum, mitochondrial respiration, and sodium-potassium pump (second step toward nephrotoxicity)[32] (Figure 65-1).

It has been demonstrated that glycoprotein 330 (gp 330), also called megalin, plays an important role in AMG transport and accumulation.[33] The consequent structural damage may result in cell necrosis associated with corresponding microscopic findings in light (formation of multilaminated membrane structures, myeloid bodies) or electron microscopy. Development of myeloid bodies within tubular cell lysosomes is the most characteristic early cytotoxic effect.

From a clinical point of view, after 1 or 2 days of AMG therapy a conspicuous urinary loss of microglobulins occurs (functional tubular damage). On the third day, a sharp increase in urinary enzymes is observed (structural tubular damage). After 6 days of therapy, cylindruria, proteinuria, polyuria, and reduced urine concentration capacity may be present. In the presence of other risk factors, this may occur earlier.

AMG-induced tubulotoxicity is frequent, but is generally reversible upon discontinuing the drug. The patient is usually

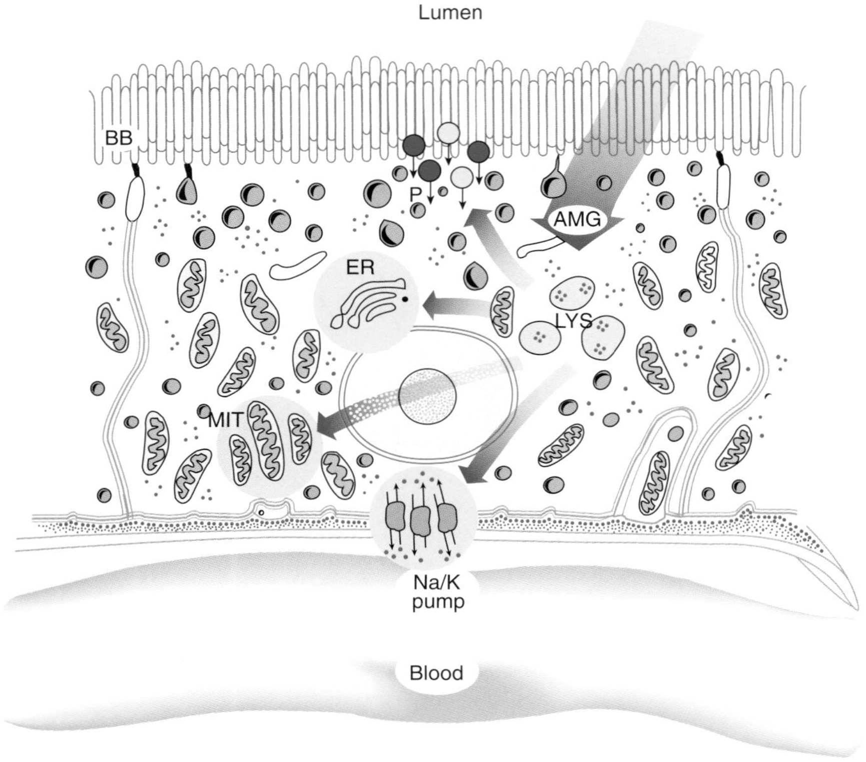

Figure 65-1 Basal mechanism of aminoglycoside nephrotoxicity. Within the proximal tubule, AMG-brush border binding occurs. Once inside the proximal tubule cell, the AMGs are sequestered in the lysosomes *(LYS)*, where they bind to phospholipids. Lysosomal phospholipidosis occurs with lysosomal rupture, impairment of mitochondrial *(MIT)* respiration, alteration of normal protein *(P)* tubular reabsorption, alteration of protein synthesis by endoplasmic reticulum *(ER)*, and depression of Na/K pump. The consequent structural damage may result in cell necrosis. (Redrawn from Fanos V, Cataldi L: Antibacterial-induced nephrotoxicity in the newborn, *Drug Safety* 20(3):245-267, 1999.)

nonoliguric. However, renal damage may alter the pharmacokinetics of the drug—reducing renal excretion and creating a dangerous vicious cycle. The serum creatinine characteristically rises 5 to 10 days after the beginning of therapy, but other less frequent manifestations include an increased urinary excretion of sodium, potassium, magnesium, phosphorus, uric acid, amino acids, and glucose. In selected cases, there may be a full Fanconi syndrome. Acute renal insufficiency may appear only at a later stage.

Numerous factors contribute to the development of AMG nephrotoxicity. Such factors may be related to the antibiotic itself, to the patient and his or her associated pathology, and to the pharmacologic factors presented in the section following.

Factors Contributory to Aminoglycoside Nephrotoxicity

Aminoglycoside Intrinsic Toxicity

AMG-induced nephrotoxicity is graded as follows: gentamicin > tobramycin > amikacin > netilmicin.[34] The superior renal tubular tolerability of netilmicin has been confirmed in newborns by enzymuria measurements.

Aminoglycoside Administration Modalities

Experimentally, the modalities of AMG administration—continuous or intermittent infusion, once-daily administration (ODA), twice-daily administration (TDA), and multiple daily doses (MDD)—condition the renal accumulation kinetics (RAK) of AMGs and thus their nephrotoxicity. Also experimentally, gentamicin and netilmicin present saturable RAK. Tobramycin, on the contrary, presents nonsaturable RAK. In the case of amikacin, RAK is mixed—being saturable at low serum concentrations and nonsaturable at high concentrations.[35]

However, controversial clinical data have been reported on efficacy and safety of ODA with TDA or MDA[36]—although it has been suggested that ODA offers advantages in terms of efficacy and renal safety. In fact, a fivefold difference in gentamicin-related nephrotoxicity was reported in 1250 patients between once-daily and thrice-daily administration.[37]

Nicolau et al. observed a reduction of nephrotoxicity from approximately 4% to 1% in 2,184 patients who received a course of AMGs every 24, 36, or 48 hours determined by estimated creatinine clearance.[38] If sensitive markers of nephrotoxicity are used, these data are further confirmed. Finally, a metaanalysis also confirmed the lower nephrotoxicity of extended interval dosing compared to conventional dosing in children (including newborns).[39]

High Trough and Peak Levels

Therapeutic drug monitoring (TDM) has two major objectives: to ensure therapeutic concentrations and to avoid toxicity. In adult patients, therapeutic efficacy and toxicity correlated well with serum concentrations.[40] Most investigators relate the nephrotoxicity to high trough levels (measured immediately before the next administration of AMG). They should be kept below 10 mg/ml for amikacin and below 2 mg/ml for the other AMGs.

Peak levels (obtained 30 minutes after an IV administration or 60 minutes after an IM administration) of GNT, TBR, and NTM should be maintained at 5 to 8 mg/ml. Peak levels of AMK should be maintained at 15 to 25 mg/ml. Even if the necessity of routine TDM in the first week of life has been questioned,[41,42] neonates (especially in preterm infants) often require TDM and an individually adjusted therapeutic regimen.[43,44] However, AMG nephrotoxicity can occur even with proper TDM.[12]

Other Risk Factors

Prolonged therapy, malnutrition, volume depletion, liver disease, preexisting renal disease, potassium and magnesium depletion, and concomitant exposure to other nephrotoxic drugs (such as amphotericin B, cyclosporin, vancomycin, and NSAIDs) are all risk factors.[12] Clinical conditions commonly observed in the newborn that may amplify AMG nephrotoxicity are neonatal anoxia, respiratory distress syndrome, mechanical ventilation, and hyperbilirubinemia. Sepsis due to gram-negative bacteria is also associated with AMG-induced kidney damage, especially in the presence of renal hypoperfusion, fever, and endotoxinemia.[45]

GLYCOPEPTIDES

The mechanism of vancomycin nephrotoxicity is not clear. The main mechanism is a tubular transport (energy dependent) of the glycopeptide from blood to tubular cell across the basolateral membrane. Similar to some AMGs, saturation of this tubular transport occurs at a particular concentration.[46]

There is an accumulation of vancomycin in the lysosomes of proximal tubular cells, but it is not similar to the behavior of AMG. Nephrotoxicity relates to the combined effect of a large area under the concentration-time curve and duration of therapy. A chronotoxicity of vancomycin has been observed, with morning administration being associated with less toxicity than evening doses.[47]

In most cases, nephrotoxicity associated with vancomycin is reversible even after high doses. Vancomycin nephrotoxicity before 1980 was observed in about 25% of treated adults, and is attributed to impurities present in the old preparations.[48] Nephrotoxicity was seen in 11% of children receiving vancomycin alone.[49]

Risk factors related to vancomycin are high trough values (>10 mg/L) and prolonged therapy periods (>3 weeks).[50] There is no evidence that transient high peak concentrations (>40 mg/L) are associated with toxicity. However, it is not clear whether elevated serum trough levels are the cause or the consequence of renal failure. High baseline serum creatinine concentration, liver disease, neutropenia, and peritonitis are also considered significant risk factors.[47]

An analysis of the literature shows that vancomycin-induced nephrotoxicity in newborns, infants, and children is rare and is often reversible and without clear relation to serum concentration. However, the association AMG-vancomycin should be used with caution when an alternative combination is possible, when TDM of both drugs is impracticable, and in VLBW infants.[51] Compared with vancomycin, teicoplanin is considered less nephrotoxic in pediatrics, but convincing proof by comparative clinical trials is lacking.

BETA LACTAMS

Cephalosporins

The nephrotoxicity of cephalosporins depends principally on two factors: the intracortical concentration of the drug and the intrinsic reactivity of the drug.[52] Depending on the equilibrium created at the tubule cell level among active transport, secretion, and reabsorption, the intracortical concentration of the cephalosporin determines the development of nephrotoxicity (Figure 65-2).

The importance of an antiluminal active organic acid transport is well known. Nephrotoxicity due to cephalosporins is limited by the compounds transported with this system, and prevention of damage is possible by inhibiting this transport (whereas increasing the intracellular uptake of cephalosporin increases toxicity).[24]

The intrinsic reactivity of the cephalosporins indicates their potential negative interaction with the intracellular targets at three levels: lipid peroxidation, acylation and inactivation of tubule proteins, and competitive inhibition of mitochondrial respiration.

Cephaloridine and cephaloglycine are the only cephalosporins capable of causing kidney damage (involving the mitochondria) at therapeutic doses. For all other cephalosporins, the renal damage can occur only at extremely high doses (much greater than routine therapeutic doses).[53] The decreasing nephrotoxicity of cephalosporins in vivo is cephaloglycin > cephaloridine > cefaclor > cephazolin > cephalothin >>> cephalexin > ceftazidime. Generally, third-generation cephalosporins (widely used in pediatrics) give rise to a direct significant increase in serum creatinine in less than 2% of treated cases, with the exception of cefoperazone (5%).[54]

An interesting characteristic of cefotaxime is its low sodium content (about 1/5 and 1/4 of ceftazidime and ceftriaxone, respectively. This could be useful in newborns and children with hypernatremia and/or fluid overload.[55] Cephalosporins (especially cefalexin, cephaletin, cefoxitin, and cefradin) also cause interstitial nephritis.[3] As regards sCr values, it should be recalled that cephalosporins are capable of interfering with the Jaffe reaction—which is the most commonly used technique for assaying creatinine in the blood and in urine.

Penicillins

Reliable statistical data on the frequency of renal complications following the use of penicillins do not exist. None of the penicillins cause toxic nephropathy, but some can cause interstitial nephritis. Acute methicillin-induced acute interstitial nephritis represents the prototype for drug-induced acute interstitial nephritis. It is reported that up to 15% of patients who receive methicillin, continuously for 2 weeks or as intermittent administration (2 or 3 times a week), develop interstitial nephritis.

Acute interstitial nephritis can present with hematuria, alone or in combination with other signs. The triad of fever, rash, and arthralgias occurs in only 10% to 40% of patients, eventually accompanied by eosinophilia or eosinophiluria. Severe cases are uremic and even oliguric. Urinalysis may show proteinuria, white blood cells, or hematuria. No specific tests are disposable for the diagnosis. The discontinuation of the drug causing acute interstitial nephritis leads almost invariably to clinical recovery.[56]

Carbapenems

Carbapenems present a significant potential for nephrotoxicity that is higher than cephalosporins and penicillins. Together

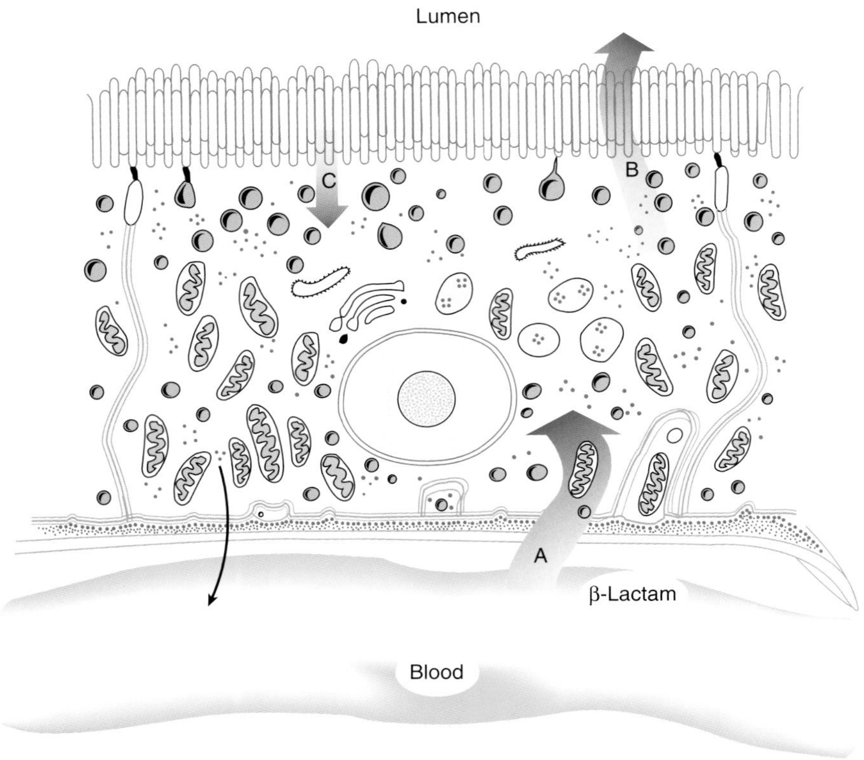

Figure 65-2 Basal mechanism of beta lactams (cephalosporins) nephrotoxicity. Three main processes are involved: (1) an antiluminal active organic acid transport (energy dependent) *(A)*, (2) a tubular secretion by the proximal tubule cells into the lumen *(B)*, and (3) a tubular reabsorption *(C)*. Other processes have low importance. The equilibrium created at the tubule cell level among these three processes is determinant for the development of nephrotoxicity. The intrinsic reactivity of the beta lactam indicates its potential negative interaction with the intracellular targets; namely, a competitive inhibition of mitochondrial respiration. This mechanism could be the common pathway for the amplification of the damage in the case of aminoglycoside therapy combined with cephalosporins. (Redrawn from Fanos V, Cataldi L: Antibacterial-induced nephrotoxicity in the newborn, *Drug Safety* 20(3):245-267, 1999.)

with cephaloridin and cephaloglycin, imipenem and panipenem are the most nephrotoxic beta lactam compounds.[57] Imipenem is hydrolyzed at the renal level by a brush-border enzyme (dehydropeptidase I) giving rise to more toxic and less active metabolites. Consequently, imipenem is administered together with cilastatin (a specific inhibitor of dehydropeptidase I) in a 1 : 1 ratio—which prevents nephrotoxicity. A lower potential for nephrotoxicity was observed with meropenem.

OTHER ANTIMICROBIAL DRUGS

Trimethoprim-sulfamethoxazole may cause renal dysfunction, especially in patients with preexisting renal function. However, this effect is reversible with dose reduction.[58] This antibiotic, often used in the young infant for prophylaxis in urinary tract infections, has received increasing attention as a cause of hyperkalemia by causing antikaliuresis via an amiloride-like blockade of sodium channels in the distal nephron.

Nephrotoxicity due to macrolides must be considered a rare adverse event. It includes glomerulonephritis, interstitial nephritis, and ARF. Similar problems have also been observed with clarithromycin, azithromycin, dirithromycin, and flurithromycin.[8] Nephrotoxic reactions to newer fluoroquinolones[59] appear to be unusual but potentially serious: allergic interstitial nephritis, granulomatous interstitial nephritis, acute tubular necrosis, and ARF (typically nonoliguric).

Crystallization of the antimicrobial may be a contributory factor leading to permanent renal insufficiency and is pH and dose dependent. Strategies for treatment of fluoroquinolone-nephrotoxicity include discontinuation of the drug, maintenance of adequate hydration and urinary pH acidification, steroid use (controversial), and possibly temporary dialysis. Rifampin can cause ARF due to an immunologic reaction.

AMPHOTERICIN B

Amphotericin-B–induced nephrotoxicity is a result of the following processes.[59,60] Amphotericin B has a direct action on the renal tubules mediated by changes in membrane permeability, exerting two major damaging effects; namely, oxidative and ionophoric. This type of damage appears to correlate with the cumulative dose of amphotericin B.[61] Amphotericin-B–induced preglomerular renal vasoconstriction with a consequent reduction in renal blood flow and GFR is another process. Moreover, vehicle-associated nephrotoxicity (deoxycholate, present in conventional amphotericin B) can occur.[59]

ARF is rare. More frequent is tubulotoxicity, which includes potassium and magnesium loss in urine, renal tubular acidosis, and loss of urinary concentrating ability. Risk factors include the amphotericin B cumulative dose, the average daily dose, concomitant diuretics, abnormal baseline creatinine values, and concomitant administration of potentially nephrotoxic drugs.[62]

Information on new lipid formulations of amphotericin B [amphotericin B lipid complex (ABLC), Abelcet, Amphotec, and Ambisome) is limited in children and newborns. Lipid-based preparations share a considerable reduction of nephrotoxicity in adults. Mainly because of cost restraints, the use of such agents is currently limited to those intolerant of or refractory to AmB.[63]

In neonates, unlike other age groups, an increase in sCr values (which may appear after the first few doses) seems unrelated to the total cumulative dose of the drug. Discontinuation of treatment for a few days can lead to recovery. Amphotericin B should be used with caution in newborns receiving other nephrotoxic drugs, such as AMGs.

The concomitant administration of dopamine and/or furosemide has been suggested to prevent injury. However, only salt loading has been clearly shown to ameliorate renal damage in humans. Potassium depletion is seen after weeks of therapy in patients with normal kidneys, and earlier in patients under anticancer treatment. Hypokalemia may be significant and may require aggressive intravenous therapy, with consequent risk of hyperkalemia. Hypomagnesemia may give rise to refractory hypocalcemia.

ANGIOTENSIN-CONVERTING ENZYME INHIBITORS

Adverse effects related to ACE inhibitors have been well documented and include hypotension, oliguria, ARF, and hyperkalemia. The major adverse effect is a reduction in glomerular filtration, particularly in patients with bilateral renal artery stenosis. Because renal blood flow and renal perfusion are maintained during treatment with ACE inhibitors despite the adverse effect on glomerular function, renal function returns to pretreatment levels when the drug is discontinued.[64]

Extreme blood pressure reduction to 60% below pretreatment levels and oliguria have been reported following the administration of captopril doses of 0.3 mg/kg to prematures. Thus, the usual starting dose should be considerably lower, and normotensive blood pressure should be achieved with doses of 0.01 mg/kg to full-term and premature infants.[65] In these patients, other antihypertensive drugs should be used if possible.[66] Moreover, to prevent renal damage treatment with ACE inhibitors should be avoided in the neonatal period when the patient is in critical condition or has a preexisting renal vascular pathology.

In infants, it is necessary to monitor renal function during initiation of therapy with ACE inhibitors—especially if concomitant diuretics are given. In clinical practice, systolic blood pressure may be used to monitor ACE inhibitor therapy. A fall by greater than 15% between 3 and 60 minutes after drug administration indicates a decline in systemic vascular resistance that could compromise renal perfusion.[67]

ACE inhibitors should not be administered during pregnancy because human fetopathies have been seen when these drugs were given after the first trimester of pregnancy,[66] the period of development of fetal kidney. In particular, oligohydramnios, renal tubular dysgenesis, and neonatal anuria were observed. More recently, other authors reported adverse fetal and neonatal renal effects after intrauterine exposure to lisinopril, enalapril, or other ACE inhibitor. In addition, the ACE inhibitor fetopathy syndrome has been associated with reduction of amniotic fluid volume as a consequence of the reduced production of fetal urine.

ACE inhibitors seem to possess renoprotective effects in children. In fact, angiotensin II has emerged as a central mediator of progressive renal injury by virtue of its hemodynamic and nonhemodynamic effects. Renal protection by ACE inhibitors has been demonstrated in adults, and in some pediatric studies involving a small number of subjects. Jankauskiene et al.[68] evaluated the effects of early treatment with enalapril on blood pressure and left ventricular function in 51 children suffering from acute postinfectious glomerulonephritis. Twenty-six patients received enalapril at the dose of 5 to 10 mg t.i.d. for 6 weeks, and 25 served as controls. A good antihypertensive effect and an improvement of echocardiographic parameters were observed in treated children. Moreover, the drug was safe to use because no rise in serum creatinine was observed.

A total of 31 children with hypertension and proteinuria associated with various chronic nephropathies were treated with ramipril for 6 months. Hypertension normalized in 55% of children and proteinuria decreased in 84% of subjects, whereas GFR and serum potassium levels did not change significantly.[69]

On the contrary, of concern was a report by Leversha et al.[70] about serious side effects in 63 infants with heart failure treated with enalapril. Eight patients (12%) developed renal problems requiring discontinuation of the drug, and 3 subjects died in congestive heart failure with renal failure.

DIURETICS

Loop diuretics are the most potent diuretic agents currently available for clinical use.[64]

Furosemide

Furosemide remains the diuretic most widely administered to neonates [25% of neonates admitted to neonatal intensive care unit (NICUs)].[64] This diuretic acts on the luminal side of the renal tubule at the thick ascending limb of the loop of Henle. It inhibits passive reabsorption of sodium, and secondarily of calcium, and must be secreted by the kidney into the tubular fluid to exert its diuretic effect.[64] It is used in congestive heart failure, in nephrotic syndrome, in indomethacin-induced oliguria, in bronchopulmonary dysplasia (BPD), and in respiratory distress syndrome (RDS)—although without the support of clinical trials, or at least systematic review of all available studies.

As regards adverse effects of furosemide on renal function, these are usually associated with chronic drug use or exceptionally large doses. The use of furosemide increased the risk of elevated urea in premature infants born before 30 weeks of gestation. Dehydration is a contraindication to furosemide administration in premature newborns treated with indomethacin for symptomatic patent ductus arteriosus (PDA). Diuretic-induced salt and water depletion can produce a decrease in glomerular filtration that NSAIDs could magnify.[56] The use of furosemide in BPD is associated with some risks because the drug can decrease vascular volume and induce electrolyte deficits.[71] In particular, metabolic alkalosis, hyponatremia, hypokalemia, renal calcifications, and worsening in BPD outcome have been related to long-term administration of furosemide.

In preterm infants, elevated urinary calcium losses may lead to nephrocalcinosis, secondary hyperparathyroidism, bone resorption, and rickets. However, available data are discordant. Ultrasonographic resolution of renal calcification has been well documented after discontinuation of loop diuretics (about 50% of the 13 examined premature infants 5 to 6 months after discontinuation of furosemide). A higher initial calcium-to-creatinine ratio at diagnosis may be a possible predictive factor of the patients who will have persistent nephrocalcinosis.[72] Pope et al. investigated pathophysiologic risk factors associated with nephrocalcinosis in 114 VLBW infants. Among this population, 20 patients (17.5%) developed nephrocalcinosis. However, no difference in furosemide therapy was observed between subjects with or without nephrocalcinosis.

Hydrochlorothiazide

Hydrochlorothiazide is used in combination with beta blockers for treatment of hypertensive children (with digoxin or ACE inhibitors in heart failure, and with indomethacin or amiloride in the treatment of nephrogenic diabetes insipidus to reduce polyuria and avoid dehydration and hypernatremia). As also reported with furosemide, hydrochlorothiazide can decrease vascular volume and induce electrolyte deficits.[71]

The effects of hydrochlorothiazide on renal calcium excretion in 30 children with hypercalciuria were evaluated. It was found that 1 mg/kg/day of the diuretic caused a rapid and long-lasting correction of hypercalciuria and prevented the formation of new urinary stones. Other authors do not recommend hydrochlorothiazide in all children diagnosed with hypercalciuria, suggesting that treatment with thiazides be reserved for those subjects with a markedly increased urine calcium-to-creatinine ratio and family history of urolithiasis.

Spironolactone

Spironolactone, an aldosterone antagonist acting on distal segments of the renal tubule, has a long history of use in pediatrics and has become a standard part of combination diuretic regimens in infants with chronic lung disease (CLD) and heart disease (HD). However, relatively little information has been published to document its efficacy and safety.

The most common adverse effects observed in 100 children treated with spironolactone, given within the recommended range dosage of 1 to 4 mg/kg/day, were alterations in serum potassium concentrations (probably resulting from the combined effects of spironolactone with other diuretics, aspirin, or ACE inhibitors).[73] Hyperkalemia was more common initially, whereas hypokalemia became prevalent during long-term use and required supplementation in about a quarter of the patients.

Mannitol

The routine use of mannitol as osmotic diuretic is not recommended in newborns because it could cause and/or exacerbate renal failure and increase the risk of intraventricular hemorrhage in low-birth-weight infants.

NONSTEROIDAL ANTIINFLAMMATORY DRUGS

NSAIDs are used in the perinatal period as tocolytic agents, to favor closure of PDA and to reduce polyuria in subjects with congenital salt-losing tubulopathies. Moreover, NSAIDs are frequently used in children because of their antipyretic activity—as well as their analgesic and antiinflammatory properties.[27]

The nephrotoxic effects of NSAIDs are related to their mechanism of action. Through blockage of prostaglandin synthesis with inhibition of cyclooxygenase (COX) enzymes, these drugs may provoke renal damage that may result in ARF with or without oliguria, chronic renal failure, significant proteinuria, fluid metabolism alterations, and hyperkalemia. Moreover, interstitial nephritis due to an immunologic reaction could also be responsible for NSAID-associated ARF in children (even if relatively uncommon).[27]

Although the risk of developing ARF is small in healthy young patients, the absolute number of children who may develop ARF is large because the drugs are widely used. Indomethacin has been used for many years as a tocolytic agent to prevent uterine contractions and to treat polyhydramnios. However, its use has been associated with different fetal side effects, including constriction of the ductus arteriosus, renal dysfunction, and oligohydramnios.[27] Several cases of severe and sometimes irreversible renal insufficiency have been described in human neonates exposed to indomethacin, a nonselective COX inhibitor, during fetal life.

Butler-O'Hara and D'Angio (2002) examined retrospectively all neonates admitted to an NICU nursery during a 5-year period and identified 37 preterm newborns whose mothers received indomethacin for tocolysis who were matched with 37 controls. Antenatal indomethacin resulted in a significant prolonged renal insufficiency, with peak creatinine and length of elevation closely correlated. In addition, different case reports reported renal adverse effects (including fatal anuria) related to indomethacin exposure in utero. Other NSAIDs have been given to mothers during pregnancy and similar effects on renal function were observed. Recently, it has been suggested that administration of COX-2–selective inhibitors would not result in perinatal renal impairment. Instead, data from recent studies have shown transient severe oliguria and even permanent renal failure after nimesulide exposure in utero.

For many years, indomethacin has been the drug of choice in the treatment and prophylaxis of PDA in premature neonates. Among its side effects, transient or permanent alterations in renal function have been frequently reported. Reduction of urinary volume and glomerular filtrate are usually reversible within 48 hours by discontinuation of therapy, whereas oliguria may persist for 2 weeks. Strategies for minimizing the renal side effects of indomethacin (such as its association with furosemide or with low doses of dopamine, or the use of prolonged low doses) have not been successful. In every case, indomethacin seems to have no major long-term renal effects. It has been shown that kidney function is restored after as long as 1 month following acute renal impairment.

Ibuprofen has been shown to close successfully the ductus arteriosus in animals and newborns without affecting renal hemodynamics. A prospective randomized study of the effectiveness and the side effects of ibuprofen and indomethacin in the treatment of PDA observed a marked influence of indomethacin on serum creatinine. In another randomized trial involving 5 NICUs in Belgium, the authors[74] confirmed that ibuprofen was significantly less likely to induce oliguria and to increase serum creatinine. This was also observed by other authors after intravenous and oral administration.

Renal failure has been reported as a rare event among children exposed to NSAIDs, and is usually reversible after discontinuation of the drug. However, despite the known mechanism for the potential underlying adverse renal effects NSAIDs are often used as antipyretics even in situations predisposing to ARF (such as in volume-depleted children with diarrhea and/or vomiting).

A number of reports, mainly case reports, have linked ibuprofen and other NSAIDs use to renal complications (such as nonoliguric renal failure or interstitial nephritis documented by renal biopsy) in children. In a randomized trial involving 83,915 children, of whom 55,785 were treated with ibuprofen for fever, no renal impairment was observed.[75]

However, caution should be taken when NSAIDs are administered in association with other potentially nephrotoxic drugs or are given to children with preexisting renal problems and/or situations predisposing to ARF. These situations include diarrhea and/or vomiting, children with cystic fibrosis receiving AMGs, and ibuprofen being administered simultaneously. It was initially hoped that COX-2 inhibitors such as celecoxib and rofecoxib would be less nephrotoxic than conventional NSAIDs, but this has not been confirmed.

CALCINEURIN INHIBITORS

The two drugs of the calcineurin inhibitors (CIs), cyclosporin A (CsA) and tacrolimus (TAC), represent the backbone of current immunosuppressive treatment. Nephrotoxicity is the most common and important side effect of CI therapy and is due to a decrease in renal blood flow and GFR (prerenal dysfunction with intact tubular function). Other renal effects include chronic interstitial fibrosis, thrombotic microangiopathy, salt and water retention, hyperkalemia, and hypomagnesemia.

CsA can injure endothelial and tubular cells. Two well-characterized forms, acute nephrotoxicity (functional renal changes) and chronic nephrotoxicity (structural renal changes), are known. The renin angiotensin aldosterone system plays an important role in the development of CsA-induced toxicity. In fact, CsA induces imbalance in the vasodilator/vasoconstrictor rate at the renal level. On the other hand, endothelial injury can increase vascular permeability and hypovolemia—which activates the sympathetic nervous system.[76]

CsA-induced functional nephrotoxicity consists of a reversible dose-related reduction of renal blood flow (RBF), GFR, and a significant increase in renal vascular resistance (RVR)—with consequent vasoconstriction of the afferent arteriole and direct tubular cell injury. It was demonstrated in rats that direct tubular injury may contribute to CsA nephrotoxicity independently of hemodynamic alterations. However, this was achieved only with a high concentration of CsA (100 μg/ml)—and this effect was dependent on extracellular calcium and magnesium levels. CsA nephrotoxicity seems to be correlated with CsA blood levels, which should be kept within a narrow therapeutic range. Renal tissues may accumulate CsA at levels approximately 20 times greater than blood levels.[77]

The signs of nephrotoxicity appear in the first weeks after therapy, including a transient elevation of the serum creatinine and arterial hypertension in the majority of cases. Both are normalized after reduction or discontinuation of CsA.[78] Renal biopsy is usually without histologic alterations or shows nonspecific changes such as vacuolization or the presence of giant mitochondria in tubular cells. Cyclosporin A has been associated with recurrent or de novo hemolytic-uremic syndrome. Recent studies show that CsA is able to generate reactive oxygen species and lipid peroxidation, which are directly involved in the CsA nephrotoxicity. The use of antioxidants improves the morphologic renal cytoarchitecture, increases antioxidant enzyme content, and reduces lipid peroxidation and reactive oxygen species (ROS).

ANTIVIRAL DRUGS

Nephrotoxicity is the most common adverse clinical effect of antiviral drugs. Tubule cell death is the major cause of toxicity related to the antiviral drugs [acyclovir, foscarnet, interferon (IFN), and cidofovir]. Isolated tubular defects [including Fanconi-like syndrome (cidofovir, tenofovir)], distal tubular acidosis (acyclic nucleotide biphosphonates), and nephrogenic diabetes insipidus (foscarnet) have also been described. Intrarenal obstruction with crystalline deposits has been described in response to acyclovir, gancyclovir, and indinavir therapy.

Intracellular drug concentration is the most common cause of tubular toxicity. The nephrotoxicity of many of these drugs is caused by an increase in intracellular influx through a human organic-anion transporter (hOAT1)–controlled mechanism. A defect in its luminal excretion is caused by a multidrug resistance-associated protein (MRP) type-2–controlled mechanism.

Nephrotoxicity is a well-recognized side effect of intravenous acyclovir, valgancyclovir, and ganciclovir. Seventy to 90% of a dose of acyclovir (ACV) is excreted unchanged in the urine by both glomerular filtration and active tubular secretion. For this reason, its concentration in the tubular fluid can be very high. The coadministration of probenecid reduces renal excretion of acyclovir, suggesting that renal OATs are responsible for tubular secretion of the drug.[79]

ACV is well tolerated at lower and oral doses, but obstructive nephropathy may occur (acyclovir crystals precipitate in renal tubules). The risk of renal failure is increased if the drug is given by rapid intravenous infusion, is given to poorly hydrated patients or those with preexisting renal function alterations, or is given along with other nephrotoxins. Valgancyclovir is an oral prodrug of ganciclovir, with tenfold greater bioavailability than oral ganciclovir. Foscarnet avoids myelosuppressions, but it is associated with significant nephrotoxicity. This includes azotemia, proteinuria, acute tubular necrosis, crystalluria, and interstitial nephritis.

Serum creatinine increases in up to 50% of patients, but renal function returns to normal within a month after stopping therapy. The use of foscarnet should be limited for patients unable to tolerate ganciclovir or with ganciclovir-resistant CMV disease. Foscarnet can affect the vasopressin responsiveness of the collecting duct and interfere with the kidney's ability to concentrate urine, leading to a state of nephrogenic diabetes insipidus (NDI).

Cidofovir, adefovir, and tenofovir are acyclic nucleoside phosphonate analogues, a novel class of antiviral drugs structurally related to natural nucleotides. These drugs are secreted by the kidney and have been shown to be substrates for OAT1 and MPR2. Tanji describes a novel form of nephrotoxicity, mediated by depletion of mDNA from proximal tubular cells through inhibition of mDNA replication. Acute tubular necrosis after treatment is associated with the antiretroviral agent adefovir.[80]

HIV-infected children are at high risk to develop nephrotoxicity such as renal failure, tubular dysfunction, and renal-related biological disorders. In some cases, these abnormalities in renal function are related to antiviral drugs rather than to the disease itself. Infants and children often start antiretrovir therapy at very young ages, and have to use their medication lifelong. The high nephrotoxicity of indinavir (IDV) in adults has been well documented. Its side effects have restricted its use in children.[81]

Indinavir is metabolized by the liver, but 20% of a single oral dose is excreted unchanged in the urine. Ph-dependent crystallization of indinavir may cause kidney stones, flank pain (even without renal stones), interstitial nephritis, elevation of serum creatinine, dysuria, hematuria, crystalluria, and leukocyturia. Indinavir crystals causes an inflammatory response in tubules with sterile leukocyturia and potentially renal failure.[81]

Van Rossum et al. demonstrated that children treated with indinavir have a high cumulative persistent leukocyturia (early marker for the development of renal damage), and frequently an increase in serum creatinine at levels >50% above normal (with younger children at high risk of renal complication). Therefore, children treated with indinavir should be monitored closely. Risk factors include sterile leukocyturia, age <5 to 6 years, an area under the curve of indinavir >19 mg/L/h, and maximal concentration. L-arginine, nifedipine, and magnesium supplementation protect against IDV nephrotoxicity in rats.

CANCER CHEMOTHERAPY

Chemotherapy can cause direct damage to a renal structure (glomerulus, tubules, vessels) or indirect damage following hypoperfusion, hemolytic uremic syndrome (HUS), and tumor lysis syndrome. Moreover, drugs interactions (by decreasing liver metabolism or renal clearance) can increase the serum concentration of antineoplastic agents—causing unexpected nephrotoxicity (even though the correct doses have been prescribed). Nephrotoxicity is relatively common with cisplatin, isofosfamide, mitomicin C, methotrexate at high doses, and interleukin-2. Other drugs (such as dacarbasin and L-asparaginase) can cause hyperazotemia without nephrotoxicity.

Cisplatin

Cisplatin is a highly effective and frequently used drug in the chemotherapy of solid tumors in children. It cannot be replaced by the less nephrotoxic carboplatin or oxaliplatin because of its differential antitumor activity.[81] Cisplatin-induced nephrotoxicity includes polyuria, persistent hypomagnesemia, acute reduction of renal function, chronic renal failure, and occasionally renal salt wasting. More than one of these complications may occur in the same patient.

A large number of patients experience polyuria (the first apparent change in renal function). A reduction in GFR occurs in 20% to 30% of adult patients treated, despite intensive prophylactic hydration and forced diuresis. In addition, electrolyte abnormalities such as hypokalemia are common adverse side effects. Modest amounts of proteinuria (β_2 microglobulin) are likely related to tubular damage, and hemolytic uremic syndrome has been described (especially when cisplatin is combined with bleomycin).

The major site of renal injury is the S3 segment of the proximal tubule, morphologically characterized by tubular necrosis, loss of microvilli, alterations in number and size of lysosomes, and mitochondrial vacuolization. Nephrotoxicity is time and dose dependent. In rats, cisplatin accumulation and cytotoxicity on glomerular and tubular cells depend on urine osmolarity. Low osmolarity increases accumulation and cytotoxicity of cisplatin, whereas isoosmolar and hyperosmolar conditions are protective. This justifies the widely used concurrent infusion of osmotically active substances (a large supply of NaCl and mannitol) during intravenous hydration.

Moreover, functional renal alterations are also correlated to the level of platinum accumulation in the renal tissues. This can be reduced through the use of high hydration.[82] To exert its cytotoxic actions, cisplatin has to enter into the proximal tubular cells. The human organic cation transporter 2 (hOCT2) is the critical transporter for cisplatin nephrotoxicity in isolated human proximal tubules. Organic cations such as cimetidine and verapamil protect against cisplatin nephrotoxicity.[83]

Ifosfamide

Ifosfamide-induced nephrotoxicity is more common in children than in adults. The drug can cause hemorrhagic cystitis, tubular damage (hypophosphatemia, hypomagnesemia, proteinuria, glycosuria, and/or acidosis), and ARF. Risk factors are patient age <5 years, cumulative doses >60 g/m^2, and concurrent administration of cisplatinum. On the contrary, unilateral nephrectomy and the mode of ifosfamide administration are not proven risk factors.[84]

Methotrexate

Methotrexate causes kidney damage by the formation of crystals within the renal tubules. Risk of nephrotoxicity should be decreased by adequate hydration and urine alkalinization.

MANAGEMENT AND PREVENTION

The evolution of drug-induced nephropathies differs from idiopathic nephropathies. It is important for the pediatrician to anticipate and recognize the problem of drug-induced disease because the causative agents are commonly prescribed and because nephrotoxicity is frequent and reversible in

TABLE 65-1 Ten Rules for Prevention of Drug-Induced Renal Damage

1. Do not use nephrotoxic drugs if alternatives are available.
2. Do not use nephrotoxic drugs in high-risk patients.
3. Choose the less nephrotoxic compound.
4. Use correct dosage and therapeutic drug monitoring, if required.
5. Do not use concomitant nephrotoxic drugs.
6. Limit the duration of treatment.
7. Effect early diagnosis of renal damage.
8. Stop the administration of the drug if damage occurs.
9. Use caution in using new drugs in pediatrics.
10. Modify dose and/or interval dosing in renal failure.

many patients.[8,29] Thus, vigilance and early diagnosis are essential for the management of the condition.

The most important first step in treating drug-induced nephropathy is to stop the offending drug. This resolves many cases of prerenal, intrinsic, and obstructive renal failure. In some circumstances (e.g., documented acute interstitial nephritis), oral prednisone 1 to 2 mg/kg/day should be given for 4 to 6 weeks. If renal function does not recover, immunosuppressive agents such as cyclophosphamide can be used.

In obstructive renal failure, volume replacement with intravenous saline and alkalinization of urine may be helpful. However, in selected cases of drug-induced nephrotic syndrome irreversible renal damage has been described. Similarly, renal function does not recover completely in drug-induced TTP-HUS after stopping the drug—although neurologic signs improve with or without plasmapheresis.

Steroid therapy is not beneficial in these cases, and mortality is high. Thus, preventing iatrogenic drug-induced nephrotoxicity is not only possible and desirable but mandatory. How can one avoid nephrotoxicity? Table 65-1 outlines 10 practical rules for prevention.

Rule 1: Alternatives

Do not use nephrotoxic drugs if alternatives are available. The simplest way to prevent drug-induced nephrotoxicity is of course not to administer these drugs. Knowledge of drug safety is a useful element for preventing iatrogenic factor. Lack of nephrotoxicity is one of the parameters to be considered in the choice of drug therapy. Before prescribing a potentially nephrotoxic drug, the risk-to-benefit ratio and the availability of alternative drugs should be considered.

Drugs known to be nephrotoxic should be avoided whenever possible, especially in some situations (such as high-risk surgical patients). Critically ill children are not ideal candidates for potentially nephrotoxic drug treatment, although pediatricians may not have a valid alternative choice (e.g., AMG in patients with life-threatening sepsis). In fact, one must consider two unique pharmacodynamic properties of AMG: postantibiotic effect and concentration-dependent killing. However, aztreonam is a reasonable alternative to AMG therapy in children and low-birth-weight infants with gram-negative infections at risk of nephrotoxicity.[8,87]

Rule 2: High-Risk Patients

Do not use nephrotoxic drugs in high-risk patients. Chronic renal failure and a preexisting renal injury are major risk factors for most nephrotoxins. Diabetes mellitus increases vulnerability to AMG, NSAIDs, and ACE inhibitors. Sepsis itself is a major risk for nephrotoxicity. True intravascular volume depletion is a factor risk for NSAID-induced nephrotoxicity. Volume management is essential for prevention.

Generally, pretreatment hydration can reduce the nephrotoxic potential of many drugs (including amphotericin B, AMG, NSAIDs, cisplatin, and indinavir). A "diuretic holiday" (a period off diuretics before starting ACE) is suggested before starting an ACE inhibitor. Modifiable risk factors should be corrected. In many cases, patients should be prehydrated before the administration of the nephrotoxic drug. In such cases, it is mandatory to accurately monitor urine output and avoid intravascular volume overload.

Rule 3: Choice of Compound

Choose the less nephrotoxic compound. For the kidney, netilmicin is better than gentamicin, teicoplanin is better than vancomicin, and lipid formulations of amphotericin B are better than conventional formulations. Ceftazidime seems the safest cephalosporin for the kidney. Analgesics other than NSAIDs are preferred in children with compromised hemodynamic status or volume depletion.

Rule 4: Dosage and Monitoring

Use correct dosage and therapeutic drug monitoring, if required. The correct drug dosage should be prescribed. For many years, it has been debated whether TDM of AMG and vancomycin will decrease toxicity—especially at the renal level.[87,88] Probably it depends on the patient population, with high-risk patients benefiting more. However, a tailored TDM is generally associated with lower nephrotoxicity.[88,89]

Rule 5: Concomitance

Do not use concomitant nephrotoxic drugs. Specific combinations of drugs (such as cephalosporins and AMG, cephalosporins and acyclovir, and vancomycin and AMG) may result in synergistic nephrotoxicity. The combination AMG-vancomycin is believed to increase the nephrotoxic risk up to sevenfold.

Rule 6: Duration

Limit the duration of treatment. Prolonged duration of treatment has been associated with increased AMG and amphotericin B nephrotoxicity. In adult studies, AMG-related nephrotoxicity may reach approximately 55% of cases according to the duration of the treatment (high risk with duration >10 days). Moreover, repeated courses of AMG therapy a few months apart can enhance nephrotoxicity.

Rule 7: Diagnosis

Seek to diagnose renal damage early. The renal function (and particularly the GFR) should be frequently monitored during the administration of a potentially nephrotoxic drug. Cystatin C, a marker of glomerular function in the "creatinine blind" period, and urinary biomarkers of nephrotoxicity (microglobulins, enzymes, and growth factors) can be used for the early noninvasive identification of renal damage occurring in the course of drug therapy. Moreover, they are helpful in establishing its extent and monitoring its time course.[8]

Rule 8: Damage

Stop the administration of the drug if damage occurs. In many cases, the most important first step in treating drug-induced nephropathy is to stop the offending drug. This is true in many cases, such as for acute interstitial nephritis, nephritic syndrome, drugs associated with TTP-HUS, and obstructive nephropathy.

Rule 9: Pediatric Drugs

Use caution when using new drugs in pediatrics. It is important to be cautious in administering drugs to children prescribed outside the terms indicated in the product license (off-label use as regards dose, age group, route of administration, different indication) or in an unlicensed manner (formulations modified, extemporaneous preparations, imported medicines, chemicals used as drugs).

The lack of approval for pediatric use does not imply a drug is contraindicated or disapproved. It simply means that insufficient data are available to grant approval status and the risks/benefits balance (including nephrotoxicity) cannot be evaluated. This suggestion should be extended to obstetricians because increasing reports of renal damage in newborns are related to drugs administered to the mother.[11]

Rule 10: Renal Failure Dosing

Modify dose and/or interval dosing in renal failure. Normal renal function is important for the excretion and metabolism of many drugs.[90,91] Renal failure alters drug clearance and requires modification in dosage regimens to optimize therapeutic outcome and minimize the risk of toxicity. This is a key point for prevention and is recommended as an essential part of a computer-based system to minimize medical errors and adverse drug events, including drug-induced nephrotoxicity.

REFERENCES

1. Etienne I, Joannides R, Dhib M, Fillastre JP: Drug-induced nephropathies (in French), *Rev Prat* 17(42):2210-16, 1992.
2. Schetz M, Dasta J, Goldstein S, Golper T: Drug-induced acute kidney injury, *Curr Opin Crit Care* 11:555-65, 2005.
3. Hoitsma AJ, Waitzels JFM, Koene R: Drug-induced nephrotoxicity: aetiology, clinical features and management, *Drug Safety* 6(2):131, 1981.
4. Cataldi L, Leone R, Moretti U, De Mitri B, Fanos V, Ruggeri L, et al: Potential risk factors for the development of acute renal failure in preterm newborn infants: A case control study, *Arch Dis Child Fetal Neon Ed* 90:514-19, 2005.
5. Cuzzolin L, Fanos V, Pinna B, di Marzio M, Perin M, Tramontozzi P, et al: Postnatal renal function in preterm newborns: A role of diseases, drugs and therapeutic interventions, *Pediatr Nephrol* 81(7):931-38, 2006.
6. Berndt W: The role of transport in chemical nephrotoxicity, *Toxicol Pathol* 26(1):52-57, 1998.
7. Choundury D, Ahmed Z: Drug-induced nephrotoxicity, *Med Clin North Am* 81:705-17, 1997.
8. Fanos V, Cataldi L: Antibacterial-induced nephrotoxicity in the newborn, *Drug Safety* 20(3):245-67, 1999.
9. Endou H: Recent advances in molecular mechanisms of nephrotoxicity, *Toxicol Letters* 29:102-03, 1998.
10. Lackland DT, Bendall HE, Osmond C: Low birth weights contribute to high rates of early-onset chronic renal failure in the Southeastern United States, *Arch Intern Med* 60(10):1472-76, 2000.
11. Boubred F, Vendemmia M, Garcia-Meric P, Buffat C, Millet V, Simeoni U. Effects of maternally administered drugs on the fetal and neonatal kidney, *Drug Safety* 29(5):397-419, 2006.
12. Guo X, Nzeure C: How to prevent, recognize, and treat drug-induced nephrotoxicity, *Cleveland J Med* 68(4):289-311, 2002.
13. Guder WG, Hofmann W: Markers for the diagnosis and monitoring of renal tubular lesions, *Clin Nephrol* 38(91):93-97, 1992.
14. Herget-Rosenthal S: Early detection of acute renal failure by serum cystatin C, *Kidney Int* 66:1115-22, 2004.
15. Porter GA: Urinary biomarkers and nephrotoxicity, *Miner Electrolyte Metab* 20:181-86, 1994.
16. Scherberich JE: Urinary proteins of tubular origin: Basic immunochemical and clinical aspects, *Am J Nephrol* 10(91):43-51, 1990.
17. Price G: The role of NAG (N-acetyl-Beta-D-glucosaminidase) in the diagnosis of kidney disease including the monitoring of nephrotoxicity, *Clin Nephr* 36(1):14S-19S, 1992.
18. Taira T, Yoshimura A, Lizuka K, et al: Urinary epidermal growth factor levels in patients with acute renal failure, *Am J Kid Disease* 22(5):656-61, 1993.
19. Ichimura T, Hung CC, Yang SA, et al: Kidney injury molecule-1: A tissue and urinary biomarker for nephrotoxicant-induced renal injury, *Am J Physiol Renal Physiol* 286:F552-F563, 2004.
20. Thukral SK, Nordone PJ, Hu R, et al: Prediction of nephrotoxicant action and identification of candidate toxicity related biomarkers, *Toxicol Pathol* 33:343-55, 2005.
21. Koren G: The nephrotoxic potential of drugs and chemicals: Pharmacological basis and clinical relevance, *Med Toxicology* 4:59-72, 1989.
22. Perazella MA: Drug-induced renal failure: Update on new medications and unique mechanisms of nephrotoxicity, *Am J Med Sci* 325(6):349-62, 2003.
23. Pospishil YO, Antonovich MA: Antibiotic associated nephropathy, *Pol J Path* 47(1):13-17, 1996.
24. Kaloyanides GJ: Antibiotic-related nephrotoxicity, *Nephrol Dial Transplant* 9(S4):130-34, 1994.
25. Schwartz A, Perez-Canto A: Nephrotoxicity of antiinfective drugs, *Int J Clin Pharmacol Ther* 36(3):164-67, 1998.
26. Markowitz GS, Perazzella MA: Drug-induced renal failure: A focus on tubulointerstitial disease, *Clin Chim Acta* 351:31-47, 2005.
27. Cuzzolin L, Dal Cerè M, Fanos V: NSAIDs-induced nephrotoxicity from the fetus to the child, *Drug Safety* 24:9-18, 2001.
28. Perazella MA: Crystal-induced acute renal failure, *Am J Med* 106:459-65, 1999.
29. Garella S: Drug-induced renal disease, *Hosp Pract* 15:129, 1993.
30. Springate J: Amphotericin toxicity, *Pediatr Nephrol* 8:632-40,1994.
31. Ford DM: Basic mechanism of aminoglycoside nephrotoxicity, *Pediat Nephrol* 8(5):635-36, 1994.
32. Fanos V, Cataldi L: Renal transport of antibiotics and nephrotoxicity, *J Chemoth* 13(5):461-72, 2001.
33. Moestrup SK, Cui S, Vorum H, et al: Evidence that epithelial glycoprotein 330/megalin mediates uptake of polybasic drugs, *J Clin Invest* 96:1404-13, 1995.
34. Kahlmeter G, Dehlager JI: Aminoglycoside toxicity: A review of clinical studies published between 1975 and 1982, *J Antimicrob Chemother* 135:9-22, 1984.

35. Giuliano RA, Varpoten GA, De Broe ME: The effect of dosing strategy on kidney cortical accumulation of aminoglycosides in rats, *Am J Kidney Dis* 8:297, 1986.
36. Rouger F, Ducher M, Maurin M, Corvaiser S, Claude D, Jeliffe R, et al: Aminoglycoside dosage and nephrotoxicity: Quantitative relationships, *Clin Pharmacokin* 42(5):493-500, 2003.
37. Prins JM, Buller HR, Kuijper EJ, et al: Once versus thrice daily gentamicin in patients with serious infection, *Lancet* 341:335-39, 1993.
38. Nicolau DP, Freeman CD, Belliveau PP, et al: Experience with once-daily aminoglycoside program administered to 2,184 adult patients, *Antimicrob Agents Chemother* 39:650-55, 1995.
39. Contopoulos-Joannides DG, Giotis ND, Baliatsa DV, Ioannidis JP: Extended-interval aminoglycoside administration for children: A meta-analysis, *Pediatrics* 114:e111-e118, 2004.
40. Moore RD, Lietman PS, Smith CR: Clinical response to aminoglycoside therapy: Importance of the ratio of peak concentration to minimal inhibitory concentration, *J Infect Dis* 155:93-99, 1987.
41. de Hoog M, Mouton JW, van der Anker JN: New dosing strategies for antibacterial agents in the neonate, *Seminars in Fetal & Neonatal Medicine* 10(6):185-94, 2005.
42. Best EJ, Palasanthiran P, Gazarian M: Extended-interval aminoglycosides in children: More guidance is needed, *Pediatrics* 115(3):827-28, 2005.
43. Fanos V, Dall'Agnola A: Antibiotics in neonatal infections: A review, *Drugs* 58(3):405-27, 1999.
44. Tom-Revzon C: Strategic use of antibiotics in the neonatal intensive care unit, *J Perinat Neonat Nurs* 18(3):241-58, 2004.
45. Zager RA: Endotoxemia, renal hypoperfusion and fever: interactive risk factors for aminoglycoside and sepsis-associated acute renal failure. *Am J Kidney Dis* 20(3):223-30, 1992.
46. Dufful SB, Begg EJ: Vancomycin toxicity: What is the evidence for dose dependency? *Adverse Drug React Toxicol Rev* 13(2):103-14, 1994.
47. Chow AW, Azar RW: Glycopeptides and nephrotoxicity, *Intens Care Med* 20:523-29, 1994.
48. Faber BT, Modelliring RC: Retrospective study of the toxicity of preparation of vancomycin from 1974 to 1981, *Antimicrob Agents Chemother* 23:138-41, 1985.
49. Dean RP, Wagner DJ, Toplin MD: Vancomycin/aminoglycoside toxicity, *J Pediatr* 106:861-62, 1985.
50. Rybak MJ, Albrecht LS, Boike SC, et al: Nephrotoxicity of vancomycin, alone and with an aminoglycoside, *J Antimicrob Chemother* 25:679-87, 1990.
51. Fanos V, Kacet N, Mosconi G: A review of teicoplanin in the treatment of serious neonatal infections, *Eur J Pediatr* 156:423-27, 1997.
52. Tune BM: Renal tubular transport and nephrotoxicity of beta-lactam antibiotics: Structure-activity relationship, *Miner Eletrol Metab* 20:221-31, 1994.
53. Feketty FR: Safety of parenteral third generation cephalosporins, *Am J Med* 88:38S-44S, 1990.
54. Cunha BA: Third generation cephalosporines: A review, *Clin Ther* 14:616-52, 1992.
55. Kasama R, Sorbello A: Renal and electrolyte complications associated with antibiotic therapy, *Am Family Physician* 53(1):227S-232S, 1996.
56. Hock R, Anderson RJ: Prevention of drug-induced nephrotoxicity in the intensive care unit, *J Critical Care* 10(1):33-43, 1995.
57. Tune BM: Nephrotoxicity of beta-lactam antibiotics: Mechanism and strategies for prevention, *Ped Nephrol* 11(6):768-72, 1997.
58. Trollfors B, Wahl M, Alestig K: Cotrimoxazole, creatinine and renal function, *J Infect* 2:221, 1980.
59. Cuzzolin L, Fanos V: Safety of fluoroquinolones in pediatrics, *Expert Opin Drug Safety* 1(4):319-24, 2002.
60. Fanos V, Cataldi L: Amphotericin B-induced nephrotoxicity: A review, *J Chemoth* 12(6):463-70, 2000.
61. Sawaya B, Briggs J, Schnermann J: Amphotericin B nephrotoxicity: The adverse consequence of altered membrane properties, *J Am Soc Nephrol* 6:156-64, 1995.
62. Fisher MA, Talbot GH, Maislin G: Risk factor for amphotericin B-associated nephrotoxicity, *Am J Med* 87:547-52, 1989.
63. Slain D: Lipid-based amphotericin B for the treatment of fungal infections, *Pharmacotherapy* 19(3):306-23, 1999.
64. Wahlig TM, Thompson TR, Sinaiko A: Drug use in the newborn: Effects on the kidney, *Clin Perinat* 19(1):251-73, 1992.
65. Guignard JP, Gouyon JB, Adelman RD: Arterial hypertension in the newborn infant, *Biol Neonate* 55:77-83, 1989.
66. Odland HH, Thaulow EMD: Heart failure therapy in children, *Exp Rev Cardiovasc Ther* 4(1):33-40, 2006.
67. Buttar HS: An overview of the influence of ACE inhibitors on fetal-placental circulation and perinatal development, *Mol Cell Biochem* 176(1/2):61-71, 1997.
68. Jankauskienè A, Cerniauskienè V, Jakutovic M, Malikenas A: Enalapril influence on blood pressure and echocardiographic parameters in children with acute postinfectious glomerulonephritis, *Medicina (Kaunas)* 41(12):1019-25, 2005.
69. Seeman T, Dusek J, Vondràk K, Flögelovà H, Geier P, Janda J: Ramipril in the treatment of hypertension and proteinuria in children with chronic kidney diseases, *Am J Hypertens* 17:415-20, 2004.
70. Leversha AM, Wilson NJ, Clarkson PM, Calder AL, Ramage MC, Neutze JM: Efficacy and dosage of enalapril in congenital and acquired heart disease, *Arch Dis Child* 70:35-39, 1994.
71. Toth-Heyn P, Drukker A, Guignard JP: The stressed neonatal kidney: From pathophysiology to clinical management of neonatal vasomotor therapy, *Pediatr Nephrol* 14:227-39, 2000.
72. Pope JC, Trusler LA, Klein AM, Walsh WF, Yared A, Brock JW: The natural history of nephrocalcinosis in premature infants treated with loop diuretics, *J Urol* 156:709-12, 1996.
73. Buck ML: Clinical experience with spironolactone in pediatrics, *Ann Pharmacother* 39:823-27, 2005.
74. Van Overmeire B, Smets K, Lecoutere D, Van de Broek H, Weyler J, Degroote K, et al: A comparison of ibuprofen and indomethacin for closure of patent ductus arteriosus, *N Engl J Med* 343:674-81, 2000.
75. Lesko SM, Mitchell AA: An assessment of the safety of pediatric ibuprofen: A practitioner-based randomized clinical trial, *JAMA* 273:929-33, 1995.
76. Morgan BJ, Lyson T, Sherrer U, Victor GR: Cyclosporin causes sympathetically mediated elevation in arterial pressure in rats, *Hypertension* 18(4):458-66, 1990.
77. Carvalho da Costa M, de Castro I, Neto AL, Ferreira AT, Burdman EA, Yu L: Cyclosporin tubular effects contribute to nephrotoxicity: Role for Ca++ and Mg2+ ion, *Nephrol Dial Transl* 18(11):2262-68, 2003.
78. Morales JM, Andres A, Rengel M, Rodicjo GL: Influence of cyclosporine, tacrolimus and rapamycin renal function and arterial hypertension after renal transplantation, *Nephrol Transplant* 16(1):121-24, 2001.
79. Izzedine H, Launay-Vacher V, Deray G: Antiviral drug-induced nephrotoxicity, *American Journal of Kidney Diseases* 45(5):804-17, 2005.
80. Tanji N, Tanji K, Kambham N, Markowitz GS, Bell A, D'Agati V: Adefovir nephrotoxicity: Possible role of mitochondrial DNA depletion, *Human Pathology* 32(7):734-40, 2001.
81. Van Rossum AM, Dieleman JP, Fraaij PLA, Cransberg K, et al: Indinavir associated asymptomatic nephrolithiasis and renal cortex atrophy in two HIV-1 infected children, *AIDS* 15(13):1745-47, 2001.
82. Boulikas T, Vougiouka M: Cisplatin and platinum drugs at the molecular level, *Oncol Rep* 10:1663-82, 2003.
83. Townsend DM, Deng M, Zhang L, Lapus MG, Hanigan MH: Metabolism of cisplatin to a nephrotoxin in proximal tubule cells, *J Am Soc Nephrol* 14:1-10, 2003.
84. Polycarpe E, Arnould L, Schmitt E, Duvillard L, Ferrant E, Isambert N, et al: Low urine osmolarity as a determinant of cisplatin-induced nephrotoxicity, *Int J Cancer* 111(1):131-37, 2004.
85. Ciarimboli G, Ludwig T, Lang D, Pavenstadt H, Koepsell H, Piechota HJ, et al: Cisplatin nephrotoxicity is critically mediated via the human organic cation transporter 2, *Am J Pathol* 167(6):1477-84, 2005.
86. Sawyers CL, Moore RD, Lerner SA, et al: A model for predicting nephrotoxicity in patients treated with aminoglycosides, *J Inf Dis* 153:1062-66, 1986.

87. Bosso JA, Black PG: The use of aztreonam in pediatric patients: A review, *Pharmacotherapy* 11:20-25, 1991.
88. Swan SK: Aminoglycoside nephrotoxicity, *Sem Nephrol* 17:27-33, 1997.
89. Kim MJ, Bertirotno JS Jr., Erb TA, et al: Application of Bayes theorem to aminoglycoside-associated nephrotoxicity: Comparison of extended-interval dosage, individualized monitoring and multiple day dosing, *J Clin Pharmacol* 44:696-707, 2000.
90. Kennedy DL, Goldman SA: Monitoring for adverse drug events, *Am Fam Phys* 56(7):1718, 1997.
91. Hock R, Anderson RJ: Prevention of drug-induced nephrotoxicity in the intensive care unit, *J Crit Care* 10(1):33-43, 1995.

CHAPTER

66 Complementary and Alternative Treatments for Renal Diseases

Gagandeep K. Sandhu and Sunita Vohra

INTRODUCTION

Complementary and alternative medicine (CAM) has been defined as "a broad domain of healing resources that encompass all health systems, modalities, and practices and their accompanying theories and beliefs, other than those intrinsic to the politically dominant health system of a particular society or culture in a given historical period."[1] As such, CAM is a term that encompasses a diverse group of therapies (e.g., homeopathy, chiropractic, acupuncture, etc.) that may be more different from one another than they are from conventional Western medicine.

Boundaries between conventional Western medicine and CAM are not always well defined or fixed. For example, there has been debate whether dietary modifications or vitamins should be considered CAM. In this chapter, we will limit our discussion to the following major CAM modalities: naturopathy, traditional Chinese medicine (TCM), and massage therapy.

Naturopathy is a system that utilizes "natural" treatments for diagnosis, treatment, and health management.[2] The intent is to treat the cause of illness, not just the symptoms. Naturopathy includes exercise therapy, natural health products (NHPs), homeopathy, hydrotherapy, lifestyle modification (including diet), iridology, and spinal manipulation (see Table 66-1).

TCM is an ancient medical system that includes acupressure, acupuncture, breathing exercises, herbs, moxibustion, oriental massage, qi gong, and tai chi[3] (see Table 66-2). An important concept in TCM is qi, a life energy with various mental, physical, and spiritual manifestations. This energy is said to flow throughout the body, along the meridian system, allowing for the integration of internal organs and other body structures. If one's qi is flowing in an orderly fashion, the person is healthy. Disorderly flow causes disease. One of TCM's aims is to restore the orderly flow of qi.

Another important concept is that of yin-yang. Yin and yang represent opposing but complementary qualities.[4] The philosophical and physiologic implications of yin-yang imbalance in TCM theory are complicated and beyond the scope of this chapter. It is confusing, for example, that the term *kidney* in TCM has a very different meaning than it does in conventional western medicine. In TCM theory, it does not imply the physical organ but rather encompasses a number of important TCM concepts. In TCM theory, the kidney's main function is to store Essence—a fluidlike energy that governs conception, growth, development, sexual maturation, reproduction, and pregnancy.[4]

Therapeutic massage involves using pressure to manipulate the body's soft tissues to impact the circulatory, lymphatic, musculoskeletal, and nervous systems to enhance the body's self-healing ability.[5] Massage therapy is sometimes done with essential oils, as in aromatherapy.

The prevalence of CAM use is high in many parts of the world.[6] In 2002, a U.S. survey of more than 31,000 people found that 62% of adults used CAM in the past year when the definition included prayer for health purposes—and 36% of adults used CAM in the past year when prayer was excluded.[7] The same survey found that 19% of adults had used an NHP in the past year. In 2004, an Australian survey of 3015 adults revealed that 52.2% had used CAM in the preceding year.[8]

There is also considerable pediatric CAM use. A 2004 survey of 1800 children in a Canadian pediatric emergency department suggested that 49% had tried at least one CAM therapy in the past year, and 41% had tried an NHP in the past year.[9] This confirmed earlier U.S. data, which suggested 45% of caregivers ($n = 142$) in a pediatric emergency room had given their child at least one herbal remedy in the past year.[10] The prevalence of CAM use is even higher in children suffering from serious, chronic, or recurrent conditions.[11] Despite common use, many pediatricians remain unaware about their patients' CAM use. Less than half of families spontaneously disclose CAM use, and less than half of pediatricians currently inquire about CAM use as part of their routine history taking.[10]

Parents who use CAM are likely to offer CAM to their children. Reasons for use may include dissatisfaction with conventional medicine if it does not offer a cure or causes significant adverse events.[6] Some adults cite lengthy wait times and inadequate time actually spent with their physician as reasons for using CAM. Many CAM users appreciate the longer duration of appointments with CAM practitioners and feel as though they are able to address their concerns more thoroughly.[6] Increased personal control regarding treatment and the perception of CAM therapies as more natural, and

TABLE 66-1 Principles of Selected Naturopathic Therapies

Therapy	General Principles
Homeopathy	The use of substances that cause a particular symptom (e.g., rash) in healthy individuals to treat unwell patients with the same symptom (i.e., "like cures like"), with the belief that progressive dilution of the substance strengthens the remedy.*
Hydrotherapy	The use of water for therapeutic purposes (e.g., immersion in water, exercising in water).†
Iridology	Examination of the iris for diagnostic purposes, based on the belief that particular locations in the iris represent different organs and body areas.*
Spinal manipulation	Manipulation of the spine to treat disease, which is thought to be caused by spinal subluxations.*

* From Ernst E, Pittler MH, Stevinson C, White A (eds.): *The desktop guide to complementary and alternative medicine: An evidence-based approach*. London: Harcourt 2001.
† From Bender T, Karagulle Z, Balint GP, Gutenbrunner C, Balint PV, Sukenik S: Hydrotherapy, balneotherapy, and spa treatment in pain management, *Rheumatol Int* 25(3):220-24, 2005.

TABLE 66-2 Principles of Selected TCM Therapies

Therapy	General Principles
Acupressure	Pressing and/or massaging various acupuncture points (acupoints) across the body.
Acupuncture	The insertion of fine sterile needles into acupoints.
Moxibustion	Moxa sticks, made of *Artemesia vulgaris*, are ignited and held an inch above particular acupoints.*
Oriental massage	Massage involving rolling, kneading, grasping, chopping, rubbing, pinching, pushing and pressing, and so on various acupoints.*
Qi gong	The use of exercises to regulate the mind and breathing to manipulate the flow of qi.*
Tai chi	A system of exercises involving slow movement between specific postures to enhance physical and mental health.†

* From Chung M: Introduction to TCM. 2004 [cited 24 Aug 2006], *URL: http://www.ctcma.bc.ca/intro.asp?id=12#12*.
† From Ernst E, Pittler MH, Stevinson C, White A (eds.): *The desktop guide to complementary and alternative medicine: An evidence-based approach*. London: Harcourt 2001.

therefore more safe, than conventional treatments is another popular reason for its use.[6]

Regulation of CAM practices and products varies considerably within and among countries.[6] For example, within the United States, regulation of CAM providers varies among the states. For example, as of 2002 chiropractors were licensed in all 50 states, non-MD acupuncturists in 42 states, naturopaths in 11 states, and massage therapists in 25 states.[12] Only some states allow acupuncturists to recommend herbal medicine.[12]

Although many U.S. hospitals have started to offer CAM as an ancillary clinical service, different hospitals address issues related to scope of practice, licensure, herb and supplement use, and malpractice liability differently in their models of integrative health care.[13] In some jurisdictions, conventional physicians are largely protected from professional discipline for recommending CAM to their patients.[6] In Canada, naturopaths, acupuncturists, and massage therapists are regulated in some provinces. CAM providers are largely unregulated in the United Kingdom.[6]

There is also significant controversy around the quality of NHPs. Heterogeneity in product quality is common for a variety of reasons. For instance, for any given herbal product (e.g., echinacea) there may be a number of plant species (*Echinacea purpurea, Echinacea pallida, Echinacea augustifolia*) with different phytochemical constituents and different physiologic effects. Differences in growing conditions, time of harvesting, parts used (e.g., aerial versus root), and extraction methods used to prepare the herbal product may vary, compounding differences within and among manufacturers.

Manufacturers have attempted to reconcile this problem by standardizing some herbal products to a marker compound specific to that particular plant. Despite this, there have been problems with the misidentification of plant species used as raw material in the manufacture of some herbal products, leading to serious consequences. In Toronto, a case of neonatal androgenization was reported after a pregnant mother consumed what she thought was Siberian ginseng but actually turned out to be Chinese silk vine.[14] Contamination of herbal products with bacteria, fungi, herbicides, and heavy metals has been reported, as has adulteration with pharmaceutical agents and other materials.

Screening studies have shown that 7% to 23.7% of Chinese herbal medicines have been adulterated.[14] Mislabeling is also a problem with some herbal products, due to the lack of regulation in most countries. A 2003 U.S. study found that 10% (6 of 59) of products marketed as echinacea actually contained no echinacea at all.[15] The same study also reported that only 43% of echinacea preparations marketed as "standardized" met the standard outlined on the label.[14]

Different regulatory approaches have been adopted internationally with regard to NHPs. In the United States, the 1994 Dietary Supplements and Health Education Act reclassified NHPs as dietary supplements (i.e., neither food nor drug), and thereby exempted them from the usual safety and regulatory rules set by the Food and Drug Administration (FDA).[16] The act states that unlike pharmaceutical products dietary supplements can be marketed without proven safety or efficacy. Thus, it is the responsibility of the FDA to demonstrate that a supplement is unsafe, which can be a difficult endeavor. In Canada, Health Canada developed the Natural Health Products Directorate, which has regulatory oversight of NHPs. Although Health Canada has not attempted to standardize NHPs, its regulations demand that manufacturers meet label claims and eliminate contamination and adulteration from products sold in the Canadian marketplace.[17]

A number of legal and ethical considerations surround the use of CAM. A patient's desire to use CAM may delay the use of a known effective conventional treatment for his or her condition. Physicians should always inquire about CAM use and monitor their patients closely for potential interactions with conventional therapies. Those who specialize in dialysis should be especially aware of their patients' use of herbs and dietary supplements so that they can offer appropriate advice. Clinicians may be hesitant to encourage the use of CAM, as it is unfamiliar and has been less extensively researched than conventional therapies.[18]

If a patient expresses interest in using CAM for his or her illness, the physician should review the literature and advise accordingly. If there is sufficient safety and efficacy data, physicians may choose to recommend CAM therapies or refer their patient to a licensed CAM provider and implement an "integrative" approach to health care[18] (see Figure 66-1). Even in such cases, however, the physician should monitor the patient's health closely to optimize patient well-being and to minimize potential harms. Where the efficacy of a CAM therapy is unclear but it has not been proven unsafe, clinicians should caution their patients while continuing to monitor them.

Ideally, the physician would have a discussion with the patient about available options and propose to monitor the patient for a trial period to evaluate the CAM therapy. If the CAM treatment proves to be ineffective or unsafe, the patient should be advised to discontinue its use. To limit liability and promote best practices, physicians should closely monitor their CAM-using patients while continuing to encourage conventional treatment.

In this chapter, we review the best available evidence with regard to naturopathy, TCM, and massage therapy. No relevant data were available concerning iridology, spinal manipulation, and hydrotherapy, which are therefore not discussed further. Where pediatric data were unavailable, adult evidence is included in our discussion. Because limiting research by language can promote bias, a phenomenon exacerbated when reviewing CAM research, our searches were conducted without language restriction.[19]

Of note, the methodologic quality of CAM randomized controlled trials (RCTs) tends to be equal to that of conventional interventions—and CAM systematic reviews tend to be of better quality.[20,21] This should not imply that there is no room for improvement, but should reassure those seeking an evidence-based approach that the quality of CAM evidence is similar to that of conventional medicine. Some problems have emerged in some pockets of CAM evidence, particularly the poor methodologic quality in some Chinese TCM studies.[22]

NEPHROTIC SYNDROME

A variety of complementary approaches have been evaluated in children with nephrotic syndrome, including TCM and dietary modification. In particular, we identified three RCTs and a metaanalysis of Chinese herbal medicines in the treatment of children with nephrotic syndrome. *Tripterygium wilfordii* glycosides, extracted from their wood core, are a traditional Chinese herbal medicine shown to have immunosuppressive and antiinflammatory effects in vitro.[23]

An RCT conducted by Wang et al. analyzed the response of 80 children between the ages of 1 and 13 to *Tripterygium* glycosides plus prednisone ($n = 39$) versus the control treatment of cyclophosphamide plus prednisone ($n = 41$) for the treatment of relapsing primary nephrotic syndrome.[23] Tapering doses of prednisone were administered to both groups over 12 to 18 months. The TCM group was given 1 mg/kg of *Tripterygium* glycosides orally two or three times each day over a period of 3 months.

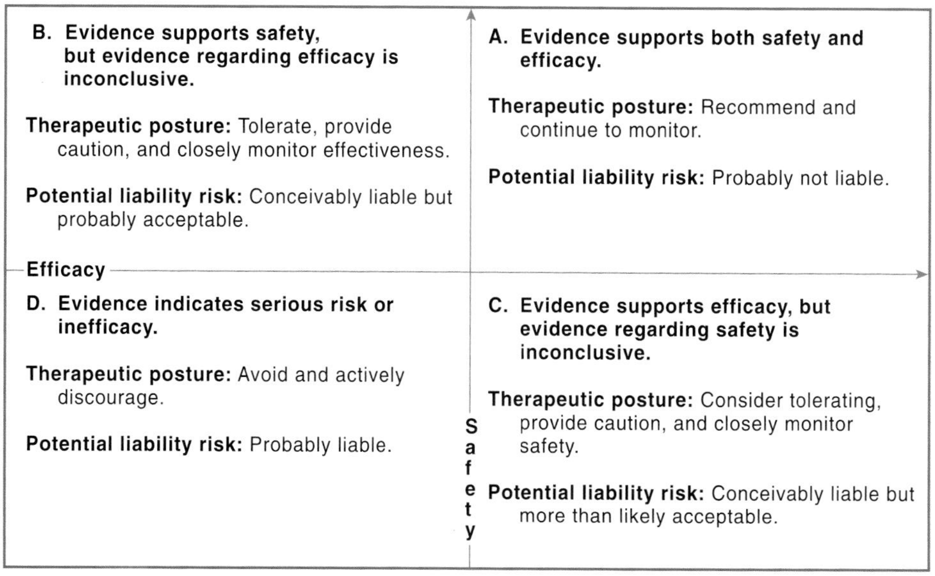

B. Evidence supports safety, but evidence regarding efficacy is inconclusive.
Therapeutic posture: Tolerate, provide caution, and closely monitor effectiveness.
Potential liability risk: Conceivably liable but probably acceptable.
A. Evidence supports both safety and efficacy.
Therapeutic posture: Recommend and continue to monitor.
Potential liability risk: Probably not liable.
Efficacy
D. Evidence indicates serious risk or inefficacy.
Therapeutic posture: Avoid and actively discourage.
Potential liability risk: Probably liable.
C. Evidence supports efficacy, but evidence regarding safety is inconclusive.
Therapeutic posture: Consider tolerating, provide caution, and closely monitor safety.
Potential liability risk: Conceivably liable but more than likely acceptable.
Safety

Figure 66-1 Potential malpractice liability risk associated with complementary and integrative medical therapies. (Used with permission from Cohen MH, Eisenberg DM: Potential physician malpractice liability associated with complementary and integrative medical therapies, *Ann Intern Med* 136(8):596-603, 2002.)

Cyclophosphamide (10 mg/kg/day) was given to the control group by intermittent intravenous pulse over 3 to 6 months. After a follow-up period of 3 to 7 years (mean 4.9 years), the authors found no significant difference between the relapse rates in the two groups ($p > 0.05$). Although the authors concluded that a combination of prednisone and *Tripterygium* glycosides is as effective as prednisone plus cyclophosphamide, methodologically these are not equivalent (i.e., they did not conduct an equivalence trial, which would have required a substantially larger sample size).

Interestingly, this study reported far fewer adverse events in the experimental group than in the control group. There was one case each of transient leukocytopenia and rising guanosine triphosphate (GTP) in the group receiving *Tripterygium* glycosides. In the group receiving conventional treatment, there were 11 cases of alopecia, 6 cases of GI upset, 3 cases of transient leukocytopenia, and 1 case of increasing GTP. In both groups, all symptoms resolved for all cases after treatment was stopped. As safety data regarding *Tripterygium* glycosides beyond this study are unknown, routine clinical use of this extract for nephrotic syndrome demands further study.

Liu conducted an RCT to test the effect of an oral liquid preparation of a combination of 10 Chinese medicinal plants (Chai-Ling-Tang) on 69 children between 5 and 12 years of age with steroid-dependent nephrotic syndrome.[24] Details about its preparation and dosing can be found in the original study. The experimental group ($n = 37$) was given tapering doses of prednisone until they had protein-free urine for 3 weeks. This group was also given consistent doses of Chai-Ling-Tang for 1.5 years. The control group ($n = 32$) was treated with tapering doses of prednisone, along with 2.5 mg/kg/day of cyclophosphamide for 8 weeks. Both groups were monitored for at least 2 years.

Although no significant differences were found between the experimental and control arms with respect to relapse rate, time to absence of proteinuria, amount of prednisone intake, and side effects, there was a trend to improvement in these measures for the TCM arm of the study (these differences were not statistically significant). There were no reports of electrolyte disturbances resulting from long-term treatment with Chai-Ling-Tang in this study. The author concluded that Chai-Ling-Tang's efficacy in treating steroid-dependent nephrotic syndrome is no less than that of cyclophosphamide and suggests that it may serve as a substitute for patients who do not respond to or have severe adverse events from taking cyclophosphamide. As safety information regarding Chai-Ling-Tang outside the context of this trial is unknown, more research is warranted before it can be recommended for routine clinical use in the treatment of nephrotic syndrome.

Li et al. carried out an RCT ($n = 60$) to determine whether tiaojining, a combination product of six principle Chinese medicinal herbs, reduced the risk of infection in children with nephrotic syndrome.[25] The children ranged from age 1 to 13. The experimental group was treated with tiaojining three times a day plus baseline treatment (prednisone) for 8 weeks. Details of how the tiaojining was prepared can be found in the original study. The control group received prednisone alone for 8 weeks. The authors concluded that tiaojining is effective in the prophylaxis of infection in nephrotic children, with a relative risk (RR) of 0.59 (95% CI 0.43 to 0.81, $p = 0.001$). No adverse events were reported. However, the study was of poor methodologic quality. Its methods of randomization, allocation concealment, and blinding were either unstated or unclear. Thus, the evidence for recommending tiaojining for preventing infection in nephrotic children is not strong. Safety data on tiaojining are not available.

Astragalus root is a traditional Chinese medicinal herb, also known as astragalus and Huang qi.[26] A systematic review of 14 RCTs ($n = 524$) was conducted to determine the effect of Radix Astragali combined with conventional treatment for nephrotic syndrome, including prednisone and cyclophosphamide, on nephrotic adults.[26] Metaanalysis showed that Radix Astragali could enhance the therapeutic effect of the conventional therapies [odds ratio (OR) 2.95, 95% CI 2.11 to 4.11, $p < 0.001$] and also reduce the recurrence of primary nephrotic syndrome (OR 0.26, 95% CI 0.13 to 0.54, $p < 0.001$).

Compared with patients who received only conventional treatment, those receiving the experimental treatment had reduced 24-hour proteinuria, increased plasma levels of albumin, and reduced levels of total cholesterol. Only one of the included articles indicated that no adverse events were reported. The remaining articles made no mention of adverse events. Dosages varied among the RCTs, but a reference text recommended dosages of 1 to 4 g of dried root orally three times a day, or a dropperful of tincture orally two or three times a day.[27] The same text urges caution when using astragalus in combination with immunosuppressants, and this use was evaluated in the RCTs cited. The authors of the meta-analysis concluded that although Radix Astragali shows promise as an adjunct therapy for primary nephrotic syndrome in adults its effects need to be confirmed by a large multicenter RCT. As there has been no research done on astragalus in the pediatric population, its use in nephrotic children is premature.

D'Amico et al. tested the effect of a vegetarian soy diet on hyperlipidemia in a prospective crossover trial of 20 adults, aged 17 to 71 (mean age 41) with nephrotic syndrome.[28] After a 2-month baseline period in which the patients ate their usual diets, the patients were changed to the vegetarian soy diet for 2 months—after which they resumed their usual diet for a 2-month washout period. The vegetarian soy diet was rich in monounsaturated and polyunsaturated fatty acids and fiber, low in fat and protein, and free of cholesterol. Details regarding the specific composition of the vegetarian soy diet can be found in the original study.

During the 2-month soy diet period, serum concentrations of total cholesterol, LDL cholesterol, HDL cholesterol, and apolipoproteins A and B were significantly lower than they were during the baseline period—although still not in the normal range. There was also a significant decrease in urinary protein excretion during the soy diet period. All of these values returned toward baseline levels during the washout period, but remained lower than prediet values. The authors note that the decreases in these substances are similar to the result of a 6-week treatment regimen with 40 mg/day lovastatin.

The difference between serum triglyceride levels during the baseline and soy diet periods was not significant. Based on their previous studies, the authors also note that the decrease in urinary protein excretion is unlikely to be a result of quantitatively restricting dietary protein. Instead, they suggest that the quality of protein ingested or perhaps the qualitative and quantitative manipulation of lipid intake as possible reasons for the reduction. The authors concluded that although the results of this study are promising further research is warranted to confirm these effects and to evaluate patient compliance to more long-term dietary restriction.

IgA NEPHROPATHY

There has been considerable research on therapy with omega-3 fatty acids for adults suffering from IgA nephropathy. A metaanalysis conducted in 1997 of five controlled studies ($n = 202$) of fish oil reported that although the mean difference was not statistically significant there was a 75% probability of at least a small beneficial effect.[29] Mixed-effects regression based on three of the studies indicated that this treatment may be more beneficial to more highly proteinuric patients. There was considerable heterogeneity among the five studies, including severity of disease, dosing, treatment duration, and length of follow-up. The authors concluded that additional longer-term research with larger sample sizes is necessary.

The single largest study included in the metaanalysis was a multicenter double-blind RCT of 106 adults with IgA nephropathy.[30] The treatment group ($n = 55$) received 12 g per day of fish oil for 2 years, and the control group ($n = 51$) received placebo. There was a significant difference between the two groups with respect to the primary end point, a 50% or more increase in serum creatinine ($p = 0.02$). The relative risk in the treatment group was 0.18 (95% CI 0.05 to 0.63, $p = 0.002$). The authors concluded that 2 years of fish oil can slow the rate of decline in renal function. No adverse events were reported, but some patients in the treatment group complained of an unpleasant aftertaste after consuming the fish oil capsules. The same authors conducted a study to assess the long-term outcome of the patients enrolled in this experiment, with a mean follow-up time of 6.4 years.[31] After the study, the placebo group had been unblinded and was free to take fish oil. Seventeen patients from the original study switched to fish oil. In the long-term follow-up study, the authors found that patients in the original treatment group were still at significantly less risk of reaching the primary end point than the patients in the original placebo group—including those who had switched to fish oil after the trial's completion ($p = 0.002$). Starting fish oil therapy early seems to offer patients the best clinical outcome.

Since the metaanalysis cited previously, two additional trials have been conducted.[32,33] An RCT compared the effect of low-dose versus high-dose omega-3 fatty acids in 73 patients with severe IgA nephropathy.[32] For 2 years, the low-dose group ($n = 37$) received 1.88 g of eicosapentanoic acid (EPA) and 1.47 g of docosahexanoic acid (DHA) daily. The high-dose group ($n = 36$) received 3.76 g of EPA and 2.94 g of DHA daily. Using a 50% or more increase in serum creatinine as the primary end point, the authors concluded that both dosage regimens were similarly effective in slowing the rate of decline in renal function. More research is warranted to determine the optimal dosage of fish oil.

A second RCT published in 2004 on 28 adults suffering from IgA nephropathy assessed the effect of a low-dose regimen of omega-3 fatty acids.[33] The experimental group ($n = 14$) received 0.85 g of EPA and 0.57 g of DHA twice a day for 4 years. Although the authors state that the control group ($n = 14$) was treated symptomatically, no treatment was specified. In both groups, hypertensive patients were treated with angiotensin-converting enzyme inhibitors, beta blockers, and/or calcium channel blockers.

At the end of the study, significantly fewer patients in the experimental group had a 50% or more increase in their serum creatinine than in the control group ($p < 0.01$). No adverse events were reported. Comparing their results to those of other studies using fish oil to treat IgA nephropathy, the authors suggest that the effect of fish oil may be dose dependent—with higher doses being more beneficial at preventing decline in renal function.

When taken in recommended doses, fish oils are extremely safe for adults.[34] Oral daily amounts exceeding 10 g of fish oil or 3 g of DHA plus EPA are possibly unsafe and may lead to an increased risk of bleeding.[34] Based on known safety and efficacy data, there is promising evidence to warrant the inclusion of fish oil in the treatment of adult IgA nephropathy. Potential use in children warrants further investigation.

UROLITHIASIS

Few studies were found on CAM treatment for urolithiasis. One pilot study assessed the effect of probiotics on oxaluria in six adults with idiopathic calcium oxalate urolithiasis and hyperoxaluria.[35] Probiotics have been defined as "live microorganisms which when administered in adequate amounts confer a health benefit on the host."[36] The six patients received a daily dose of 8×10^{11} freeze-dried lactic acid bacteria for 4 weeks. There was a significant reduction in 24-hour oxalate excretion in all six patients compared to baseline ($p < 0.05$). The mean reduction in oxaluria was 30 g per day. The reduced levels persisted for at least 1 month after treatment was stopped. Although these results are promising, larger studies are warranted before probiotics can be recommended for urolithiasis patients.

Another study evaluated the use of vibration massage therapy (VMT) after extracorporeal shockwave lithotripsy (SWL) in 103 adults with lower caliceal stones.[37] The experimental group ($n = 51$) received SWL and 20- to 25-minute sessions of VMT in 2-day intervals for 2 weeks, whereas the control group ($n = 52$) received SWL alone. The stone-free rates in the experimental and control groups were 80% and 60%, respectively ($p = 0.003$). There was a significantly higher rate of stone recurrence in the control group than in the experimental group ($p = 0.0006$). The mean time to stone recurrence was 16 months in the experimental group versus 11.4 months in the control group ($p = 0.042$). There were more reports of renal colic in the control group ($p = 0.03$). Other complications, such as pyelonephritis and fever, were reported equally in both groups. No studies evaluating VMT in children were identified.

Acupuncture involves the insertion of fine sterile needles into specific acupuncture points on various parts of the body. Lee conducted a randomized trial to evaluate the effect of acupuncture compared to a conventional analgesic (avafortan, which has since been discontinued) in the treatment of 38 adult males with renal colic from urolithiasis.[38] The severity of renal colic was assessed before treatment and 30 minutes following treatment. The mean pain scores were not significantly different between groups prior to treatment. The experimental group ($n = 22$) received acupuncture treatment, and the active control group ($n = 16$) received an intramuscular injection of avafortan. There was no significant difference in the reduction in mean pain score between the two groups, but acupuncture had a significantly faster analgesic onset than avafortan ($p < 0.05$). Although nearly half of the avafortan group experienced side effects (including facial flush, skin rash, drowsiness, and tachycardia), there were no adverse events in the acupuncture group.

A series of studies have demonstrated that adverse events associated with acupuncture are exceedingly rare. In a prospective study including more than 34,000 acupuncture treatments, there were no reports of serious adverse events (i.e., those causing hospital admission, permanent disability, or death).[39] The risk of minor adverse events (such as unacceptable pain, nausea, and fainting) was found to be 1.3 per 1000 treatments. A review by White comments on the avoidable nature of some reported adverse events, such as infection and trauma, through appropriate training/education.[40] Although the adult data are promising, pediatric trials are required before acupuncture may be recommended as a possible alternative treatment for children with renal colic.

URINARY TRACT INFECTIONS

Naturopathic approaches to urinary tract infections (UTI) include use of NHPs, such as probiotics and cranberry juice. The few well-designed trials that evaluate probiotics for the treatment and/or prevention of UTI present conflicting evidence. Many have small sample sizes, and only one is pediatric.

A double-blind RCT conducted by Dani et al. in 12 Italian neonatal intensive care units ($n = 585$) tested whether probiotics could prevent UTI in preterm infants.[41] The authors randomized newborns with a birth weight less than 1500 g or gestational age less than 33 weeks to be given either standard milk feed enriched with 6×10^9 colony-forming units (CFU) of *Lactobacillus GG* ($n = 295$) or standard milk feed supplemented with placebo ($n = 290$) once per day, starting with their first feed and continued until they were discharged. Details regarding the exact preparation of the probiotic-enriched milk feed can be found in the original article. Although the frequency of UTI was less in the probiotic group versus the control group (3.4% versus 5.8%), this difference was not significant. Caution should be applied when giving probiotics to neonates, as they seem to carry a higher risk of serious complications (such as sepsis).[42] Further pediatric evidence is not yet available, but a few studies have been conducted to assess the prevention of UTI by colonizing vaginal flora in adult women. These studies suggest that probiotics may be useful for UTI prevention.[43,44] Reid suggests that a cream or douche applied to the perineum may be a more suitable route of administration for children.[45]

A recent U.S. survey of 117 caregivers of children being treated at a pediatric nephrology clinic reported that 29% of the parents administered cranberry products to their children for therapeutic purposes.[46] Recurrent UTI was reported by 15% of the survey parents as a problem, and the use of cranberry products was 65% among children with recurrent UTI versus 23% among children with other renal problems.

Jepson et al. conducted a systematic review of seven trials ($n = 604$) in men, women, and children to determine the efficacy of cranberry products (particularly cranberry juice) in UTI prophylaxis.[47] A metaanalysis of two of the trials showed that cranberry products (specifically, cranberry concentrate in juice or tablets) significantly decreased 12-month UTI incidence versus either placebo or control in women (RR 0.61, 95% CI 0.41 to 0.91). The difference in UTI incidence between patients given cranberry juice and those given cranberry capsules was not significant (RR 1.11, 95% CI 0.49 to 2.50). The remaining five trials were not included in the metaanalysis due to lack of data or flaws in methodology. Whether cranberry products are effective in preventing UTI in children could not be determined.

The authors note that dropouts were common in many of the studies, implying that cranberry products may not be well tolerated over extended periods. Taste was reported as the main reason children dropped out of trials included in the systematic review. Adults cited the high cost of long-term cranberry juice consumption as one of their reasons for withdrawal. There was one report each of gastroesophogeal reflux, mild nausea, and increased bowel movement frequency. Because the dosing was not uniform among the included studies, the authors were unable to report an optimum dosage.

The authors concluded that although there is some evidence to support the recommendation of cranberry juice to prevent UTI in women larger studies with a longer study period to account for the illness' natural history are necessary to determine the efficacy of cranberry for UTI prophylaxis as well as the optimal dosage and route of administration of cranberry products in susceptible children and adults.

CHRONIC RENAL FAILURE

Several NHPs have been evaluated in chronic renal failure (CRF) including folic acid, l-arginine, rhubarb, and various TCM decoctions. More conventional approaches include evaluation of a low-protein diet. Because one of the leading causes of death among CRF patients is cardiovascular disease, some preliminary research has been done to evaluate the effects of folic acid supplementation on endothelial function and homocysteine levels.

Bennett-Richards et al. conducted a crossover RCT of 23 children with CRF, aged 7 to 17, whereby each subject received 8 weeks of 5 mg/m^2 folic acid per day and 8 weeks of placebo—separated by a washout period of 8 weeks.[48] There was a significant decrease in homocysteine levels during the folic acid phase (10.3 mol/L to 8.6 mol/L, $p = 0.03$), but not during the placebo period. In addition, there was a significant rise in LDL lag times during the folic acid period (58.4 to 68.1 minutes, $p = 0.01$)—leading the authors to postulate that LDLs are less susceptible to oxidation after folic acid supplementation. Based on a significantly improved flow-mediated vessel diameter in the folic acid group, the authors concluded that an 8-week regimen of folic acid can improve endothelial function.

Because folic acid supplementation studies in adults have been largely negative, Bennett-Richards et al. have speculated that this positive finding might be related to timing of treatment—in that atherosclerosis in children is at an earlier stage of its natural history. Although folic acid is extremely safe, studies with clinically relevant outcomes are necessary before folic acid supplementation can be recommended for routine use in children with CRF.

Bennett-Richards et al. conducted a second crossover RCT of 21 children aged 7 to 17 years (mean 11.5 years) with CRF and previously documented endothelial dysfunction to determine the effect of dietary supplementation with oral l-arginine on the response of the endothelium to shear stress.[49] Each child was given a 4-week regimen of 2.5 g/m^2 or 5 g/m^2 of oral l-arginine three times a day, and then a regimen of placebo after a 4-week washout period. Although there was a significant rise in levels of plasma l-arginine after the treatment phase, there was no significant improvement in endothelial function. The authors concluded that dietary supplementation with l-arginine is not useful in the treatment of children with CRF.

Li et al. conducted a systematic review of 18 randomized and quasi-randomized trials ($n = 1322$) to evaluate the use of rhubarb in CRF patients (mean age 39.3 years).[50] The included trials assessed rhubarb versus conventional medicine, as well as rhubarb versus traditional Chinese medicinal herbs. Several forms of rhubarb were used, including tablets and decoctions. The doses and parts of the plant used were not specified. Rhubarb was found to be significantly more effective in treating CRF than conventional medicine alone.

There was no significant difference between the efficacy of rhubarb and that of other traditional Chinese herbs in the treatment of CRF. The review concluded that rhubarb is effective in reducing the symptoms of CRF, but there are too few patients to conclude whether it can slow or stop the long-term progression of the disease. Half the included articles reported that no adverse effects were found. In the remaining half, adverse events were not discussed.

Rhubarb is likely safe when used for short periods (i.e., less than 8 days) and in low doses, but cramps and diarrhea have been reported.[51] Chronic use of rhubarb can lead to numerous adverse effects, including electrolyte depletion, edema, colic, atonic colon, and hyperaldosteronism.[51] Rhubarb leaves contain oxalic acid and are considered toxic if ingested.[51] Patients with renal disorders should be monitored closely when using rhubarb, due to potential electrolyte disturbances.[51] Conclusive dosing information for children is unavailable.

Zhang et al. evaluated TCM in the treatment of CRF in 248 adult patients aged 20 to 60+.[52] For 1 year, the TCM group ($n = 120$) was given conventional drugs (including prednisone and furosemide) in combination with five decoctions of traditional Chinese herbs to treat the primary disease. These herbs were specifically targeted to supplement the kidney (as described by TCM theory) and invigorate blood flow. Patients were dosed and treated individually, based on their specific characteristics. Detailed compositions of the treatments can be found in the original article. Patients in the control group ($n = 128$) were treated with only conventional medicine for 1 year.

Although both groups improved, significant differences were found in improved symptoms (92.5% for TCM versus 49.2% for control group, $p < 0.01$) and in improved creatinine clearance (56 ml/min for TCM versus 37 ml/min for control group, $p < 0.01$) between the two groups. There was no mention of adverse events in this study, and safety information regarding the various traditional Chinese herbs used is unknown. The study findings are intriguing, and further research to replicate the results seems worthwhile.

Wingen et al. conducted a prospective, stratified, multicenter randomized trial in 191 children aged 2 to 18 with CRF from 25 pediatric nephrology centers across Europe to determine whether a low-protein diet could slow disease progression.[53] Patients were divided into three groups according to their primary renal disease, and then stratified based on whether their disease was progressive or nonprogressive. There was random assignment to the control and diet groups.

Protein intake in the diet group was 0.8 to 1.1 g/kg a day, with adjustments made for age. There were no protein intake restrictions in the control group. The study continued in all patients for 2 years, and 112 of the patients agreed to continue for an additional year. Despite reasonable rates of compliance (66%), no statistically significant differences in the decline of creatinine clearance were found. No adverse effects were reported, including no adverse effects on growth from a protein-restricted diet. This study suggests that there is little value in protein restriction in pediatric CRF.

UREMIC PRURITUS

Although no pediatric studies were identified, acupuncture, acupressure, aromatherapy, and homeopathy have been assessed in the treatment of uremic pruritus in adults undergoing dialysis.

Gao et al. conducted an RCT of 68 adults to evaluate the effects of acupuncture for uremic pruritus.[54] Patients in the experimental group ($n = 34$) were treated with acupuncture in 30-minute sessions twice a week for 4 weeks while receiving hemodialysis. The control group ($n = 34$) was treated with 4 mg of Chlor-Trimeton three times daily and a topical dermatitis ointment three times daily for 2 weeks along with hemodialysis. Patients were then observed for the alleviation of pruritus. The effective rate was 95% in the acupuncture group, significantly higher than the effective rate of 70.6% in the control group ($p < 0.01$). Sixteen patients in the acupuncture group maintained this improvement for 3 months, and 18 patients for 1 month. In the control group, all cases experienced recurrence of uremic pruritus immediately once treatment was stopped. Although no pediatric data are available, given promising evidence of efficacy in conjunction with reassuring safety data some clinicians may want to consider including acupuncture for patients with uremic pruritus.

Jedras et al. carried out an RCT to study the effects of acupressure in 60 adults with uremic pruritus.[55] Acupressure is part of TCM and involves pressing and/or massaging various acupuncture points on the body. The treatment group ($n = 30$) received acupressure in 15- to 20-minute sessions three times a week for 5 weeks either immediately before or after dialysis. The control group ($n = 30$) did not receive any treatment other than dialysis. A questionnaire addressing the frequency, intensity, and localization of pruritus (as well as its effects on the patient's well-being) was used to assess pruritus. There were significant differences in mean pruritus scores between the two groups after 6 weeks, 12 weeks, and 18 weeks—with the acupressure group having lower scores ($p < 0.0001$). Acupressure is thought to be even safer than acupuncture, as it avoids needle insertion, and some clinicians may wish to consider it in their patients with uremic pruritus.

Ro et al. studied the effects of aromatherapy with massage in 29 patients aged 26 to 65 (mean age 47.3) with uremic pruritis.[56] The experimental group ($n = 13$) received aromatherapy with massage three times per week for 1 month, along with hemodialysis. Lavender oil and tea tree oil were used in the aromatherapy. The control group ($n = 16$) received only hemodialysis during this period. Pruritus was assessed using a scale that addressed the frequency, severity, and location of pruritus. Pretest scores were not significantly different between the groups, but after the treatment period the pruritus scores were significantly lower in the experimental group versus the control group ($p = 0.01$).

The authors note that larger multicenter studies of longer duration are required to be able to generalize these results and to assess the long-term effects of aromatherapy on such patients. The authors also suggest that the massage component of the aromatherapy may have confounded the results and recommend that control groups in future studies receive massage as well. Headache, nausea, and allergic reactions are possible adverse effects of certain essential oils.[6]

Cavalcanti et al. conducted an RCT to assess the effect of individualized homeopathic treatment on 28 adults with uremic pruritus.[57] Eight patients were withdrawn from the study for reasons that included having a pretreatment pruritus score less than 25% of maximum, being unable to complete forms, and being admitted to a hospital during the treatment phase. One patient in the homeopathy group died before returning for reassessment after prescription. The cause of death was not reported. A homeopath assessed all patients individually. Those in the experimental group received a homeopathic treatment, whereas those in the control group were given placebo.

During the 60-day follow-up period after starting treatment, the homeopath was free to change the prescription based on reassessments of the patients. In total, 40 homeopathic medications were prescribed—with each patient in the experimental group receiving more than one throughout the course of the study. Although there was a significant decrease in pruritus scores in the treatment group, the difference in posttreatment scores was not significant between the two groups at the end of the study ($p = 0.2$). It should also be noted that despite randomization there were some differences between the two groups that may have affected the study's outcome. For example, the experimental group's average age was significantly lower than that of the control group, as was its pretreatment hematocrit level and need for dialysis. The experimental group also tended to have better calcium and phosphorus balance, with lower intact PTH. Owing to the difference in the experimental group with respect to these last two parameters, the possibility of placebo effect cannot be excluded. although the authors concluded that homeopathy may be a valuable alternative in relieving uremic pruritus, the data are not compelling.

Adverse events associated with homeopathy are rare and generally not severe, but can include allergic reactions and symptom aggravation.[58]

END-STAGE RENAL DISEASE

A number of studies have been conducted to evaluate the efficacy of CAM therapies to improve quality of sleep, lessen fatigue and depression, and improve quality of life in adults with end-stage renal disease who receive hemodialysis.[59,60] Their promising results warrant investigation in the pediatric population.

A double-blind RCT by Tsay et al. found that adult patients receiving acupressure along with conventional care reported a better quality of sleep and quality of life than those not receiving any acupressure.[59] Ninety-eight patients experiencing sleep disturbances were randomly assigned to an acupressure group ($n = 35$), a placebo group ($n = 32$), or a control group ($n = 31$). The acupressure group received acupoint massage during hemodialysis three times a week for 4 weeks. The placebo group received sham acupressure, which involves massage on nonacupoints in the same frequency and duration as the acupressure group. The control group received only standard care.

Data collection occurred at baseline and at 1 week posttreatment. Prior to the treatment period, the three groups were equivalent in their sleep quality and quality of life scores. After treatment, sleep quality and quality of life scores were significantly more improved in the acupressure group than in the control group. Of note, subjects who received sham acupressure also had similar improvements—suggesting that this may not have been an appropriate "sham" control. It is extremely difficult to avoid acupuncture points that would produce an effect, because according to TCM theory there are at least 2000 such points both on and off the charted meridians.[61] A longer follow-up period would have been useful in assessing the long-term effects of acupressure. The authors suggest that acupressure could easily be taught to family members of those with end-stage renal disease.

Another RCT assessed the effect of acupressure and massage on fatigue and depression in 58 end-stage renal disease patients receiving hemodialysis.[60] Patients were randomly assigned to either the acupressure group ($n = 28$) or the control group ($n = 30$). The acupressure group received 12 minutes of acupressure plus 3 minutes of lower limb massage three times a week during dialysis for 4 weeks. The control group received only routine care during dialysis. After the 4-week study period, there were significant differences in the perceived fatigue ($p = 0.04$) and feelings of depression ($p = 0.045$) between the two groups. The authors mention that because there was no sham acupressure group a placebo effect cannot be ruled out. However, these promising results merit further investigation.

SUMMARY

Evidence about pediatric CAM exists, including in pediatric renal disease. If the patient and family is interested in CAM, and there is sufficient safety and efficacy data, pediatric health care providers should consider seeking local qualified expertise as appropriate to the family's interests. This chapter examined current data on those CAM interventions that have had formal evaluation, to allow for a more informed discussion among patients, families, and those who care for them.

REFERENCES

1. Zollman C, Vickers A: ABC of complementary medicine: What is complementary medicine? *BMJ* 319:693-96, 1999.
2. Health Professions Regulatory Advisory Council: Advice to the minister of health and long-term care: Naturopathy. 2001 [cited 17 Feb 2006], *http://www.hprac.org/downloads//naturopathy/Naturopathy-ReporttoMinister.pdf*.
3. Health Professions Regulatory Advisory Council: Traditional Chinese medicine and acupuncture: Advice to the minister of health and long-term care. 2001 [cited 17 Feb 2006], *http://www.hprac.org/downloads//tcm/TCM.pdf*.
4. Maciocia G: The foundations of Chinese medicine: A comprehensive text for acupuncturists and herbalists. China: Churchill Livingstone 2004.
5. Freeman J: *Mosby's complementary and alternative medicine: A research-based approach, second edition*, St. Louis: Mosby 2004.
6. Ernst E, Pittler MH, Stevinson C, White A (eds.): *The desktop guide to complementary and alternative medicine: An evidence-based approach*, London: Harcourt 2001.
7. Barnes PM, Powell-Griner E, McFann K, Nahin RL: Complementary and alternative medicine use among adults: United States, 2002, *Adv Data* 27(343):1-19, 2004.
8. MacLennan AH, Myers SP, Taylor AW: The continuing use of complementary and alternative medicine in South Australia: Costs and beliefs in 2004, *Med J Aust* 184(1):27-31, 2006.
9. Goldman RD, Vohra S: Complementary and alternative medicine use by children visiting a pediatric emergency department, *Abstracts from the First Annual Complementary and Alternative Health Care and Paediatrics Forum* 11(2):e247, 2004.
10. Lanski SL, Greenwald M, Perkins A, Simon HK: Herbal therapy use in a pediatric emergency department population: Expect the unexpected, *Pediatrics* 111:981-85, 2003.
11. Ernst E: Prevalence of complementary/alternative medicine for children: A systematic review, *Eur J Pediatr* 158(1):7-11, 1999.
12. Eisenberg DM, Cohen MH, Hrbek A, Grayzel J, Van Rompay MI, Cooper RA. Credentialing complementary and alternative medical providers, *Ann Intern Med* 137(12):965-73, 2002.
13. Cohen MH, Hrbek A, Davis RB, Schachter SC, Kemper KJ, Boyer EW, et al: Emerging credentialing practices, malpractice liability policies, and guidelines governing complementary and alternative medical practices and dietary supplement recommendations: A descriptive study of 19 integrative health care centers in the United States, *Arch Intern Med* 165(3):289-95, 2005.
14. McCutcheon A, Beatty D: Herb quality. In F Chandler (ed.), *Herbs: everyday reference for health professionals*, Ottawa: The Canadian Pharmacists Association and the Canadian Medical Association 2000:25-33.
15. Gilroy CM, Steiner JF, Byers T, Shapiro H, Georgian W: Echinacea and truth in labeling, *Arch Intern Med* 163(6):699-704, 2003.
16. Dietary Supplement Health and Education Act of 1994: Public Law 103-417. 103rd Congress. 1994 [cited 14 Sept 2006], *http://www.fda.gov/opacom/laws/dshea.html*.
17. Natural Health Products Directorate: 2005 [cited 24 Aug 2006], *http://www.hc-sc.gc.ca/ahc-asc/branch-dirgen/hpfb-dgpsa/nhpd-dpsn/index_e.html*.
18. Cohen MH: Legal issues in caring for patients with kidney disease by selectively integrating complementary therapies, *Adv Chronic Kidney Dis* 12(3):300-11, 2005.
19. Pham B, Klassen TP, Lawson ML, Moher D: Language of publication restrictions in systematic reviews gave different results depending on whether the intervention was conventional or complementary, *J Clin Epidemiol* 58(8):769-76, 2005.
20. Klassen TP, Pham B, Lawson ML, Moher D: For randomized controlled trials, the quality of reports of complementary and alternative medicine was as good as reports of conventional medicine, *J Clin Epidemiol* 58(8):763-68, 2005.
21. Lawson ML, Pham B, Klassen TP, Moher D: Systematic reviews involving complementary and alternative medicine interventions had higher quality of reporting than conventional medicine reviews, *J Clin Epidemiol* 58(8):777-84, 2005.
22. Tang JL, Zhan SY, Ernst E: Review of randomised controlled trials of traditional Chinese medicine, *BMJ* 319(7203):160-61, 1999.
23. Wang YP, Liu AM, Dai YW, Yang C, Tang HF. The treatment of relapsing primary nephrotic syndrome in children, *Journal of Zhejiang University Science* 6(7):682-85, 2005.
24. Liu XY. Therapeutic effect of chai-ling-tang (sairei-to) on the steroid-dependent nephrotic syndrome in children, *Am J Chin Med* 23(3/4):255-60, 1995.
25. Li RH, Peng ZP, Wei YL, Liu CH: Clinical observation on Chinese medicinal herbs combined with prednisone for reducing the risks of infection in children with nephrotic syndrome, *Information Journal of Chinese Medicine* 7(10):60-61, 2000.
26. Fan J, Liu L, Li Z, Su B, Guan J: A meta-analysis of Radix Astragali for primary nephrotic syndrome in adults, *Zhong yao xin yao yu lin chuang yao li* 14:62-66, 2003.
27. Fetrow CW, Avila JR: *Professional's handbook of complementary and alternative medicines, third edition*, Philadelphia: Lippincott Williams & Wilkins 2004.
28. D'Amico G, Gentile MG, Manna G, Fellin G, Ciceri R, Cofano F, et al: Effect of vegetarian soy diet on hyperlipidaemia in nephrotic syndrome, *Lancet* 339(8802):1131-34, 1992.
29. Dillon JJ: Fish oil therapy for IgA nephropathy: Efficacy and interstudy variability, *J Am Soc Nephrol* 8(11):1739-44, 1997.
30. Donadio JV, Bergstralh EJ, Offord KP, Spencer DC, Holley KE: A controlled trial of fish oil in IgA nephropathy, *N Engl J Med* 331(18):1194-99, 1994.
31. Donadio JV, Grande JP, Bergstralh EJ, Dart RA, Larson TS, Spencer DC: The long-term outcome of patients with IgA nephropathy treated with fish oil in a controlled trial, *J Am Soc Nephrol* 10(8):1772-77, 1999.
32. Donadio JV, Larson TS, Bergstralh EJ, Grande JP: A randomized trial of high-dose compared with low-dose omega-3 fatty acids in severe IgA nephropathy, *J Am Soc Nephrol* 12:791-99, 2001.
33. Alexopoulos E, Stangou M, Pantzaki A, Kirmizis D, Memmos D: Treatment of severe IgA nephropathy with omega-3 fatty acids: The effect of a "very low dose" regimen, *Ren Fail* 26(4):453-59, 2004.
34. Natural standard monograph. Omega-3 fatty acids, fish oil, alpha-linolenic acid. 2006 [cited 8 Aug 2006], *http://www.naturalstandard.com/monographs/herbssupplements/fishoil.asp*.
35. Campieri C, Campieri M, Bertuzzi V, Swennen E, Matteuzzi D, Stefoni S, et al: Reduction of oxaluria after an oral course of lactic acid bacteria at high concentration, *Kidney Int* 60(3):1097-105, 2001.
36. World Health Organization. Evaluation of health and nutritional properties of probiotics in food including powder milk and live lactic acid bacteria: Food and Agriculture Organization of the United Nations and World Health Organization Expert Consultation Report. 2001 [cited 11 Aug 2006], *http://www.who.int/foodsafety/publications/fs_management/en/probiotics.pdf*.
37. Kosar A, Ozturk A, Serel TA, Akkus S, Unal OS: Effect of vibration massage therapy after extracorporeal shockwave lithotripsy in patients with lower caliceal stones, *J Endourol* 13(10):705-07, 1999.

38. Lee YH, Lee WC, Chen MT, Huang JK, Chung C, Chang LS: Acupuncture in the treatment of renal colic, *J Urol* 147(1):16-18, 1992.
39. MacPherson H, Thomas K, Walters S, Fitter M: A prospective survey of adverse events and treatment reactions following 34,000 consultations with professional acupuncturists, *Acupuncture in Medicine* 19(2):93-102, 2001.
40. White A: A cumulative review of the range and incidence of significant adverse events associated with acupuncture, *Acupuncture in Medicine* 22(3):122-33, 2004.
41. Dani C, Biadaioli R, Bertini G, Martelli E, Rubaltelli FF: Probiotics feeding in prevention of urinary tract infection, bacterial sepsis and necrotizing enterocolitis in preterm infants: A prospective double-blind study, *Biol Neonate* 82(2):103-08, 2002.
42. Land MH, Rouster-Stevens K, Woods CR, Cannon ML, Cnota J, Shetty AK: Lactobacillus sepsis associated with probiotic therapy, *Pediatrics* 115(1):178-81, 2005.
43. Reid G, Bruce AW, Fraser N, Heinemann C, Owen J, Henning B: Oral probiotics can resolve urogenital infections, *FEMS Immunology & Medical Microbiology* 30(1):49-52, 2001.
44. Reid G, Bruce A: Probiotics to prevent urinary tract infections: The rationale and evidence, *World J Urol* 24:28-32, 2006.
45. Reid G: The potential role of probiotics in pediatric urology, *J Urol* 168:1512-17, 2002.
46. Super EA, Kemper KJ, Woods C, Nagaraj S: Cranberry use among pediatric nephrology patients, *Ambul Pediatr* 5(4):249-52, 2005.
47. Jepson RG, Mihaljevic L, Craig J: Cranberries for preventing urinary tract infections, *Cochrane Database Syst Rev* 1:CD001321, 2004.
48. Bennett-Richards K, Kattenhorn M, Donald A, Oakley G, Varghese Z, Rees L, et al: Does oral folic acid lower total homocysteine levels and improve endothelial function in children with chronic renal failure? *Circulation* 105(15):1810-15, 2002.
49. Bennett-Richards KJ, Kattenhorn M, Donald AE, Oakley GR, Varghese Z, Bruckdorfer KR, et al: Oral L-arginine does not improve endothelial dysfunction in children with chronic renal failure, *Kidney Int* 62(4):1372-78, 2002.
50. Li Z, Qing P, Ji L, su B, He L, Fan J: Systematic review of rhubarb for chronic renal failure, *Chin J Evid-Based Med* 4:468-73, 2004.
51. Natural standard monograph. Rhubarb. 2006 [cited 8 Aug 2006], *http://www.naturalstandard.com/naturalstandard/monographs/monoframeset.asp?monograph=/monographs/herbssupplements/rhubarb.asp*.
52. Zhang M, Zhang D, Zhang W, Liu S: Treatment of chronic renal failure by supplementing the kidney and invigorating blood flow, *J Tradit Chin Med* 24(4):247-51, 2004.
53. Wingen AM, Fabian-Bach C, Schaefer F, Mehls O: Randomised multicentre study of a low-protein diet on the progression of chronic renal failure in children: European Study Group of Nutritional Treatment of Chronic Renal Failure in Childhood, *Lancet* 349(9059):1117-23, 1997.
54. Gao H, Zhang W, Wang Y: Acupuncture treatment for 34 cases of uremic cutaneous pruritus, *J Tradit Chin Med* 22(1):29-30, 2002.
55. Jedras M, Bataa O, Gellert R, Ostrowski G, Wojtaszek E, Lange J, et al: Acupressure in the treatment of uremic pruritus, *Dial Transplant* 32(1):8-10, 2003.
56. Ro YJ, Ha HC, Kim CG, Yeom HA: The effects of aromatherapy on pruritus in patients undergoing hemodialysis, *Dermatol Nurs* 14(4):231-34, 2002.
57. Cavalcanti AM, Rocha LM, Carillo R Jr., Lima LU, Lugon JR: Effects of homeopathic treatment on pruritus of haemodialysis patients: A randomised placebo-controlled double-blind trial, *Homeopathy* 92(4):177-81, 2003.
58. Endrizzi C, Rossi E, Crudeli L, Garibaldi D: Harm in homeopathy: Aggravations, adverse drug events or medication errors? *Homeopathy* 94(4):233-40, 2005.
59. Tsay SL, Rong JR, Lin PF: Acupoints massage in improving the quality of sleep and quality of life in patients with end-stage renal disease, *J Adv Nurs* 42(2):134-42, 2003.
60. Cho YC, Tsay SL: The effect of acupressure with massage on fatigue and depression in patients with end-stage renal disease, *J Nurs Res* 12(1):51-59, 2004.
61. Vickers AJ: Placebo controls in randomized trials of acupuncture, *Eval Health Prof* 25(4):421-35, 2002.
62. Cohen MH, Eisenberg DM: Potential physician malpractice liability associated with complementary and integrative medical therapies, *Ann Intern Med* 136(8):596-603, 2002.
63. Bender T, Karagulle Z, Balint GP, Gutenbrunner C, Balint PV, Sukenik S: Hydrotherapy, balneotherapy, and spa treatment in pain management, *Rheumatol Int* 25(3):220-24, 2005.
64. Chung M: Introduction to TCM. 2004 [cited 24 Aug 2006], *http://www.ctcma.bc.ca/intro.asp?id=12#12*.

CHAPTER 67 Nephrotoxicity of Herbal Remedies

Li Yang, Xiaomei Li, and Afroze Ramzan Sherali

PART I: HERB-ASSOCIATED RENAL INJURY

Li Yang and Xiaomei Li

INTRODUCTION

Herbal medicine has been used in health care for thousands of years throughout China and other oriental and Western countries. In recent years, various herbal medicines have been studied using modern pharmacologic or medicinal methods—and many have been found to be extremely useful for the treatment of chronic diseases. It has been reported in Hong Kong that 19.6% of doctor consultations are provided by Chinese medicine practitioners,[1] and about 60% of residents have used Chinese medicines at some point.[2] Although no data are available on its use in the Chinese mainland, nearly every family uses Chinese medications during their lifetimes. Although Chinese herbs in their natural forms, prescribed usually by a qualified practitioner, are probably safe they occasionally cause severe adverse reactions.

Chinese medicines can be briefly categorized into herbal medicines (which exist in nature) and proprietary Chinese medicines, the processed products of herbal medicines. Factors affecting the quality and efficacy of herbal medicines include the species, medicinal component and source of the plant, time of harvesting, processing, compatibility of herbs in a formulation, dosage, method of decoction, and administration. Misuse, erroneous substitutions, quality defects, taking more than the prescribed dose, and allergic reactions are all factors leading to herb-associated toxicity affecting the kidney and other organ systems. Most clinicians are not familiar with herbal nephrotoxicity, which is more common than generally appreciated.

For years, the general public has held the misconception that herbal agents come from "natural" plants and are therefore naturally safe or intrinsically harmless. Many people take herb remedies by self-medication. Thus, it is almost impossible to estimate the prevalence of herb-associated renal impairment. According to literature provided by the Chinese medical journal database from 1991 to 2000, there were about 5000 cases of adverse drug reaction (ADR) induced by herbal medications. More than a hundred types of herbs and proprietary Chinese medicines were incriminated.

Among these reports, the prevalence of renal injury associated with herbal medication is 1.7% to 9.2%.[3] Up to 2006, in the Chinese literature 25 types of herbs involving 13 plant species have been related to renal impairment[4] (Table 67-1). Most of these herb-associated renal injuries presented with acute renal failure after misuse or overdose of herbal medications. The underlying pathology in the majority of cases was toxic acute tubular necrosis, followed in frequency by acute allergic interstitial nephritis.[3] There are also groups of cases that presented as chronic renal failure or slight renal tubular dysfunction.

In recent years, much attention has been focused on aristolochic acid (AA) containing herbal medications of particular importance because they are associated with two severe ADRs: chronic renal failure leading to end-stage renal disease (ESRD) and urothelial transitional cell cancer (TCC). This chapter focuses on the renal injury caused by these types of herbs.

ARISTOLOCHIC ACID NEPHROPATHY

History of Aristolochic Acid Nephropathy

The first case of acute renal failure caused by an overdose of *Caulis aristolochiae manshuriesis* was reported as a rare ADR in 1963 in China.[5] However, the nephrotoxic potential of this herb species was not widely recognized until 1993, when Vanherweghem[6] described two patients who developed rapidly progressive renal failure while taking a weight loss medication containing Chinese herbs. AA rich in *Radix aristolochiae fangchi* was identified as the nephrotoxic ingredient.[7,8] By 1998, more than 100 cases with the same characteristics had been described in Belgium.[9]

Similar cases were consecutively reported in other countries, including Spain,[10] Japan,[11] the United Kingdom,[12] France,[13] Hong Kong,[14] the United States,[15] Korea,[16] mainland China,[17] and Taiwan.[18] All of these cases presented with rapidly progressive renal failure and with renal biopsy specimens showing extensive interstitial fibrosis and severe loss of renal tubules (most prominent in the outer cortex). During the 1990s, the term *Chinese herb nephropathy* (CHN) was used to describe this type of disease because all the cases were related to taking prescriptions containing Chinese herbal medications. Later, AA was identified in all herbal medications as the common component with nephrotoxic and cancerogenic potential. In addition, premutagenic AA-DNA adducts were demonstrated in the kidneys and ureteric tissues of patients with CHN. Rodents given AA alone revealed the typical pathologic features of CHN. For

TABLE 67-1 Medical Herbs Related to Renal Toxicity in the Chinese Literature

Species	Herbal Medicine	Chinese Name	中文名称	ADR Features
Aristolochiaceae Aristolochialinn	Caulis aristolochiae Manshuriesis	Guan-mu-tong	关木通	AKI
	Radix aristolochiae fangchi	Guang-fang-ji	广防己	CRF
	Radix aristolochiae	Qing-mu-xiang	青木香	CRF
	Fructus aristolochiae	Ma-dou-ling	马兜铃	CRF
	Caulis aristolochiae debilis	Tian-xian-teng	天仙藤	CRF
	Herba aristolochiae molissimae	Xun-gu-feng	寻骨风	CRF
	Radix aristolochiae Cinnabarinae	Zhu-sha-lian	朱砂莲	CRF
	Radix aristolochiae Heterophyllae	Hanzhong-fang-ji	汉中防己	CRF
Euphorbiaceae	Fructus crotonis	Ba-dou	巴豆	AKI
	Herba cloxylonis indici	Diu-liao-bang	丢了棒	AKI
Convolvulaceae	Semen pharbitidis	Qian-niu-zi	牵牛子	AKI
Asteraceae	Fructus xanthii	Cang-er-zi	苍耳子	AKI
Orchidaceae	Rhizoma gastrodiae	Tian-ma	天麻	AKI
Loganiaceae	Semen strychni	Ma-qian-zi	马钱子	AKI
Labiatae	Herba leonuri	Yi-mu-cao	益母草	AKI
Ranunculaceae	Radix aconiti kusnezoffii	Cao-wu	草乌	AKI
	Radix aconiti	Chuan-wu	川乌	AKI
	Radix aconiti lateralis preparata	Fu zi	附子	AKI
Simaroubaceae	Fructus bruceae	Ya-dan-zi	鸦胆子	AKI
Meliaceae	Fructus toosendan	Chuan-lian-zi	川楝子	AKI
	Cortex meliae	Ku-lian-pi	苦楝皮	AKI
Leguminosae	Semen abri	Xiang-si-zi	相思子	AKI
Celastraceae	Radix tripterygii	Kunming-shan-hai-tang	昆明山海棠	AKI
	Radix tripterygiiwilfordii	Lei-gong-teng	雷公藤	AKI
Liliaceae	Bulbus iphigeniae indicae	Lijiang-shan-ci-gu	丽江山慈姑	AKI

From Li P, Li X: *Herb related renal injury and herbal medication* [in Chinese]: Ren Min Wei Sheng 2004:391-392.
AKI, Acute kidney injury; *ADR*, adverse drug reaction; *CRF*, chronic renal failure.

these reasons, since 2001 the more appropriate term *aristolochic acid nephropathy* (AAN) has been used instead of CHN.[19]

Today, hundreds of AAN cases have been reported in the literature—especially from China. These Chinese AAN patients primarily inhabit the northern parts of China and a distinct area near the Yangzi River. This specific disease distribution is thought to be attributed to the growth area of AA containing herbs and different medication habits among China's regions. Because the renal injury might not be diagnosed until years after drug withdrawal, AAN cases are still widely seen clinically even though the government has outlawed the use of the predominant incriminated herbs.

Herbs Containing Aristolochic Acids

AA is found primarily in the plant *Aristolochia*, including four species covering about 40 types of herbs (half of which are used as medicinal herbs). AAs containing herbal medicines are usually taken to alleviate gastrointestinal symptoms, cough, and allergies, to lessen menstrual symptoms and symptoms of coronary heart disease, to serve as antirheumatics, to induce weight loss, and to act as diuretics in treating edema. These herbal remedies have shown definite effectiveness, and some of them are still widely used. Table 67-2 lists some of AA-containing herbs in China.

TABLE 67-2 Herbs Containing Aristolochic Acids

Herb	AA-I (%)
Radix aristolochiae fangchi	0.43-3.10
Fructus aristolochiae	0.20-6.10
Caulis aristolochiae manshuriesis	0.18-8.82
Caulis aristolochiae debilis	0.082
Radix aristolochiae	0.49-3.20

Using different methods, AAI has been detected in these herbs in various concentrations (mainly dependent on the source of the plants).[20-37] These herbs can be prescribed in decoction or as processed pills in which the herbs cited in Table 67-2 are the predominant active components. In many developing countries, herbal drugs can also easily be obtained from oriental pharmacies and supermarkets without a doctor's prescription. In some poor areas, herbs can even be bought directly and prepared by the patients themselves for consumption. Therefore, careful attention to the AA-containing herb history of medication in those patients is very important to the diagnosis of AAN.

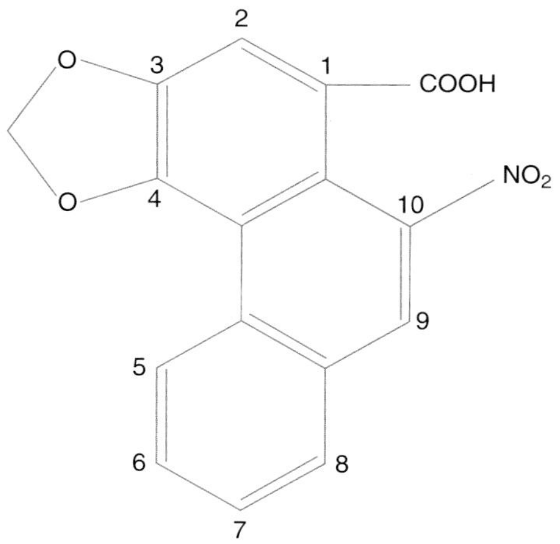

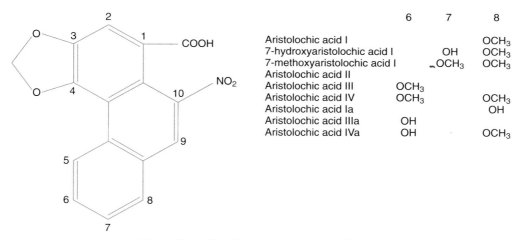

	6	7	8
Aristolochic acid I			OCH_3
7-hydroxyaristolochic acid I		OH	OCH_3
7-methoxyaristolochic acid I		OCH_3	OCH_3
Aristolochic acid II			
Aristolochic acid III	OCH_3		
Aristolochic acid IV	OCH_3		OCH_3
Aristolochic acid Ia			OH
Aristolochic acid IIIa	OH		
Aristolochic acid IVa	OH		OCH_3

Figure 67-1 Chemical structure of aristolochic acids.

Aristolochic Acids

AAs are rarely found in plants. They comprise a group of structurally related nitrophenanthrene carboxylic acids that include 8-methoxy-3,4-methylenedioxy-10-nitro-1-phenanthroic acid (AAI) and 3,4- methylenedioxy-10-nitro-1-phenanthroic acid (AAII)—which differ from each other by one methoxy group (Figure 67-1). Other AAs (such as AAIII, AAIV, AAIa, AAIIIa, and AAIVa), although in minor quantities, exist in the natural botanicals[38-40] (Figure 67-1). In addition to these components, extracts of species of *Aristolochia* also contain aristolactams.[41] Among them, aristolactam I and aristolactam Ia are the main metabolites of AAI in vivo, whereas aristolactam II is the main metabolite of AAII[42] (Figure 67-2).

For a long time, AA had been long known to act as an inhibitor of phospholipase A_2 (PLA_2).[43] In addition, by affecting the arachidonic acid cascade it blocks the production of prostaglandin[44-47] and enhances phagocytosis.[48] During the last century, AA was indeed used for its antiinflammatory, antiviral, antibacterial, and antineoplastic properties.[48-50] However, because AA has been defined as the causal factor of urothelial TCC and AAN the use of this type of chemical has been greatly restricted and research into the mechanism of its carcinogenesis and renal toxicity has intensified.

Clinical Features and Prognosis of AAN

The presentations of AAN described in the literature are diverse, even though the primary manifestation of the disease is recognized as renal tubulointerstitial injury. In particular, Western and native Chinese patients have clinically and pathologically different patterns, a fact thought to be based on different habits of self-medication.

What is now known as typical AAN, mainly reported by Belgian and other Western nephrologists, is characterized by subacute renal failure with rapidly progressive interstitial fibrosis in spite of discontinuation of the offending weight loss medication containing AA. According to Reginster's report, the patients may develop AAN as early as 2 months after exposure to the slimming regimen and as late as 3 years after cessation of the toxic exposure.[51] The clinical manifestations typically include a tubulointerstitial nephropathy with mild tubular proteinuria, a normal urine sediment, normoglycemic glucosuria, anemia out of proportion to the degree of renal dysfunction, mild hypertension,[5,52-54] and in a few cases aseptic leukocyturia.

Asymmetry in kidney size (54%) was more common in AAN than in tubulointerstitial nephropathy due to other causes.[51] The 2-year actuarial renal survival rate only reached 17% in these AAN patients, which was much worse than that of other tubulointerstitial nephropathies (74%).[51] Thus, these AAN patients present with subacute renal injury and an accelerated disease progression to ESRD. The rate of progression of renal failure is related to the duration of the slimming regimen treatment[51] and to the cumulative dose,[55] and is inversely related to the interval between withdrawal of the drugs and diagnosis.[51]

AAN may also present as Fanconi's syndrome, which is for the most part reported in Asian countries. Nearly 20 cases of Fanconi's syndrome have been described in the literature as being associated with AA-containing herbal medicines. These patients usually take Chinese herbal mixtures, and present with proximal tubular dysfunction and decreased glomerular filtration rate of different degrees.[11,56-63] The progression of renal disease varies in this patient group. Some develop progressive renal failure, whereas others maintain stable renal dysfunction. Several cases presented with slightly elevated Scr, with reversal of renal dysfunction after cessation of the causal herbs with or without prednisone therapy.[16,56,58]

AAN patients in China present with three clinical patterns: acute renal failure, chronic renal insufficiency, and renal tubular dysfunction.[16] Patients taking an overdose of AA containing herbal mixtures (up to 10 times the regularly prescribed dosage) usually present with nonoliguric (occasional oliguric) acute renal failure, with obvious tubular dysfunction.[16] The renal pathologic examination shows tubular epithelial cell necrosis, tubular collapse, and denuded tubular basement membranes without signs of regeneration.[16]

In a clinical/pathologic study, five patients with acute renal failure AAN (onset Scr level 120-200 μmol/L) were studied 2 to 6 months after renal biopsy. The Scr levels recovered to normal ranges in two cases (40%), returning to less than 25% of basal level in one case (20%) and no recovery in two cases

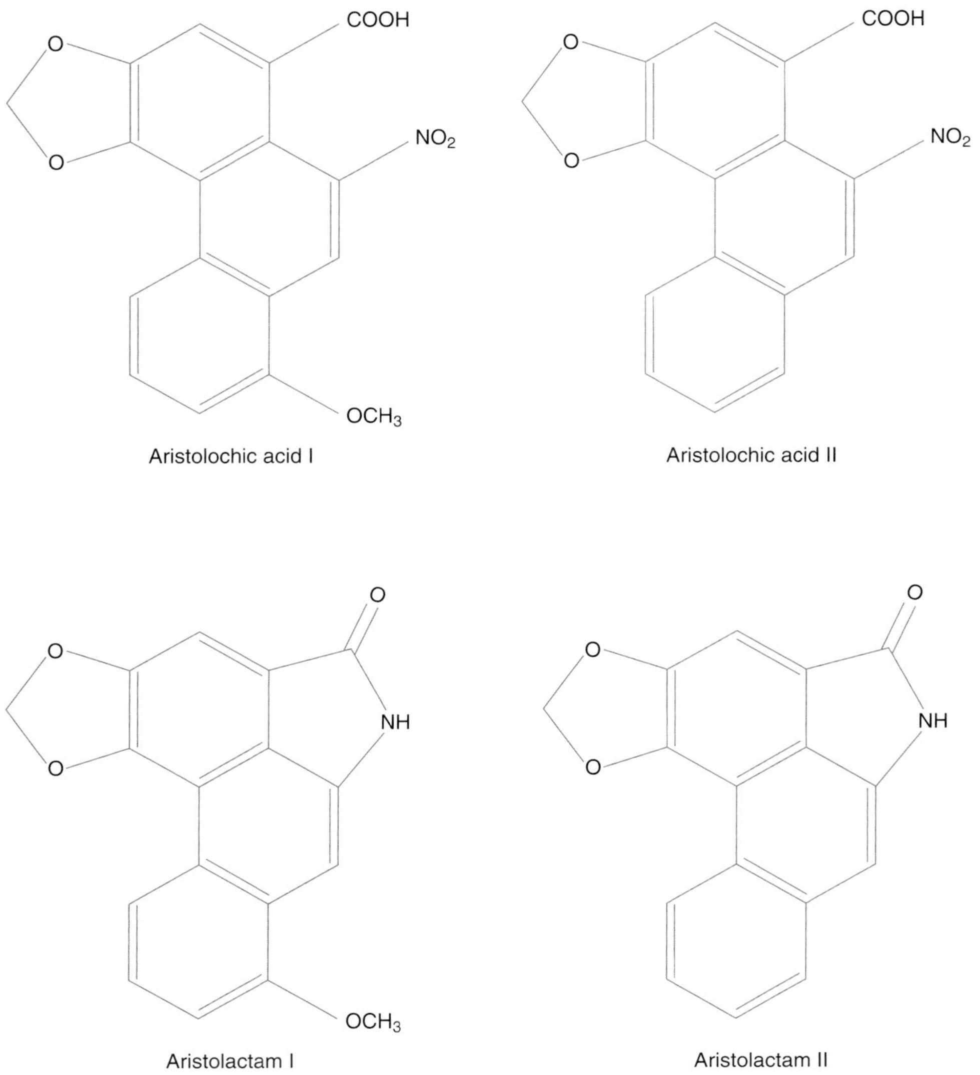

Figure 67-2 Aristolochic acids and aristolactams.

(40%). However, after 2 years one patient had developed ESRD and the other four gradually decreased their renal function—with Scr levels of 300 to 400 μmol/L (Xiaomei Li, unpublished data).

In China, 80% to 90% of patients with AAN present with chronic renal insufficiency. There is chronic tubulointerstitial nephropathy on biopsy, and the clinical history reveals intermittent intake of prescribed pill-form doses of AA for several years.[16] The onset of the disease is quite latent, and thus the majority of patients consult nephrologists after they have entered chronic kidney disease (CKD) stage 3 or even later. With effective therapy for CKD, renal functional decline in this group of patients mainly follows a relatively slow pattern of progression.

The third clinical pattern of AAN in China is renal tubular dysfunction with normal Scr and blood urea nitrogen (BUN).[60] In addition to Fanconi's syndrome, cases of renal tubular acidosis or polyuria have been reported. The clinical course of this tubular dysfunction AAN resembles that of the Fanconi's syndrome patients described previously.

Another possible pattern of AAN is Balkan endemic nephropathy (BEN), which was thought to be a familial type of chronic tubulointerstitial disease with delayed onset of renal failure.[64] Pathologic findings of BEN show hypocellular interstitial fibrosis and rare interstitial infiltrates that resemble the well-defined pathology of AAN.[65] However, the progression of BEN is slower than the typical AAN reported by the Belgian nephrologists. In fact, it more closely resembles the course of chronic AAN in China.

Recent evidence has accumulated that BEN is an environmentally induced disease. An AA-containing plant native to the Balkan region is now thought to contaminate the wheat harvested by local farmers. Over years, the ingestion of small amounts of this plant causes the chronic damage leading to chronic renal disease.[66] Definitive molecular evidence should be accumulated soon to redefine BEN as one form of the AAN disease spectrum.

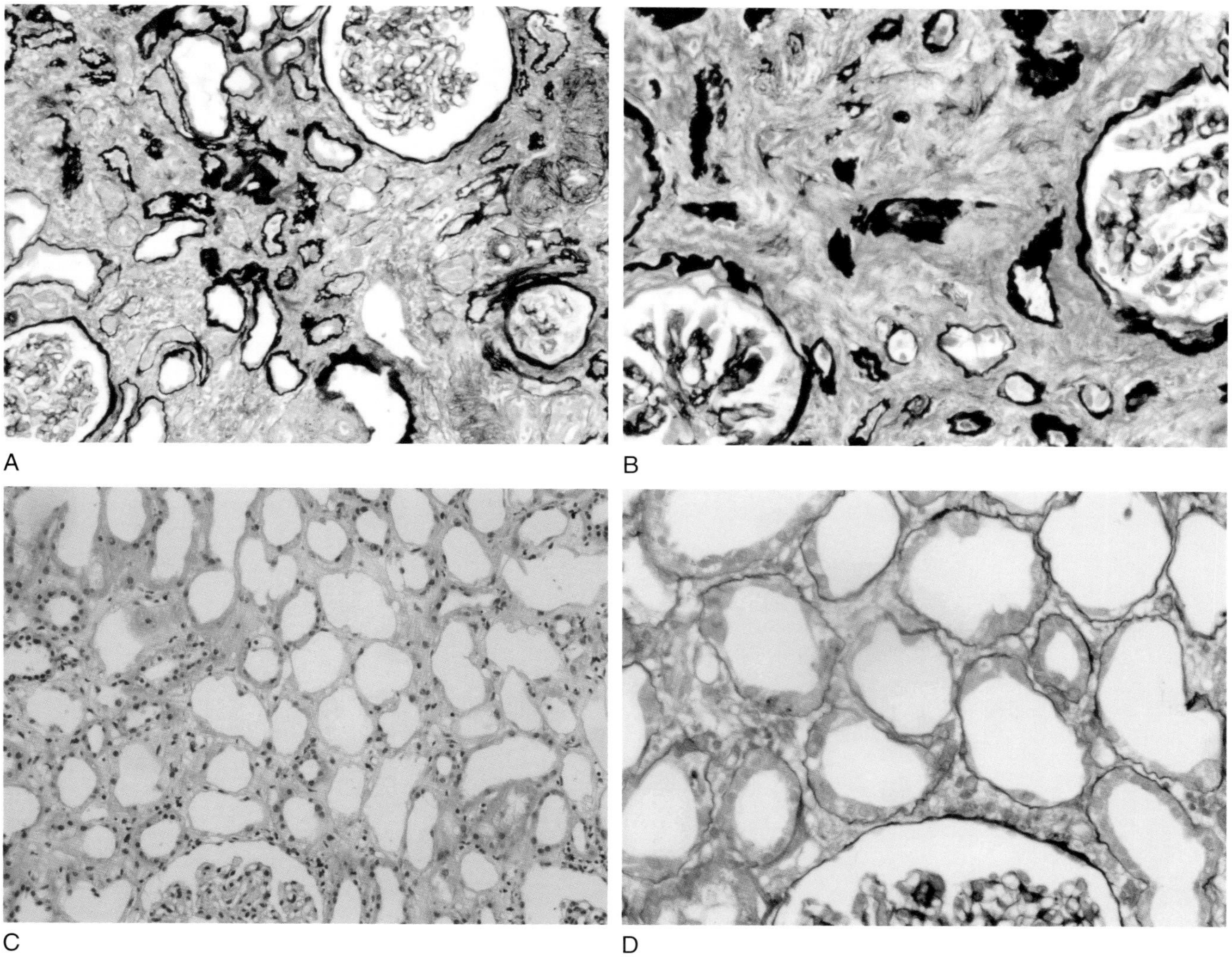

Figure 67-3 Light microscopic features of acute and chronic AAN. **A,** In acute AAN, tubular epithelial cells demonstrate necrosis. They collapse, leaving the tubular basement membrane naked. Signs of regeneration are rarely seen. The interstitium shows edema, with local inflammatory infiltration (HE, ×100). **B,** No obvious fibrosis can be detected in acute AAN (PASM, ×200). **C,** Diffuse tubular atrophy is seen in chronic AAN. The glomeruli demonstrate ischemic shrinkage (PASM, ×100). **D,** Obvious interstitial fibrosis exists in chronic AAN (PASM, ×200).

Histopathology of AAN

The typical pathologic findings of AAN reported in Western countries are extensive hypocellular renal interstitial fibrosis, tubular atrophy, and complete tubular disappearance. Few lymphocytes or monocytes can be found infiltrating between the tubules (Figure 67-3, *A, B*). The intensity decreases from most severe in the outer cortex to less involvement in the inner cortex and medulla.[67]

Glomeruli are relatively spared compared to the severity of tubulointerstitial fibrosis, except for ischemic changes such as glomerular basement membrane (GBM) shrinking and global sclerosis in some cases. Thickening of the walls of interlobular and afferent arterioles is common in these cases. Immunofluorescent staining is almost always negative.[67,68] Electron microscopy shows fibroblast proliferation and collagen deposition in the interstitium. The chronic renal insufficiency type of AAN in China shows the same histologic features.

The Fanconi's syndrome and tubular dysfunction types of AAN in China present much lighter renal pathologic findings, including different degrees of degeneration and atrophy of tubular epithelial cells. Slight edema or focal fibrosis can be detected in some cases in the interstitium.

The pathologic examination of the acute renal failure type of AAN in China generally correlates with overdose toxicity. It exhibits the typical features of acute tubular necrosis (ATN) with epithelial necrosis, tubular collapse, and denudement of the tubular basement membrane (Figure 67-3, C, *D*). However, this type of tubular necrosis has two major features quite different from the classic ATN caused by ischemia or Western medicines. The first is severe epithelial exfoliation that leaves tubular basement membrane (TBM) naked in most cases. The second feature is lack of epithelial regeneration. The same clinical and pathologic features have been seen in an experimental rat model involving AA administration.[69,70]

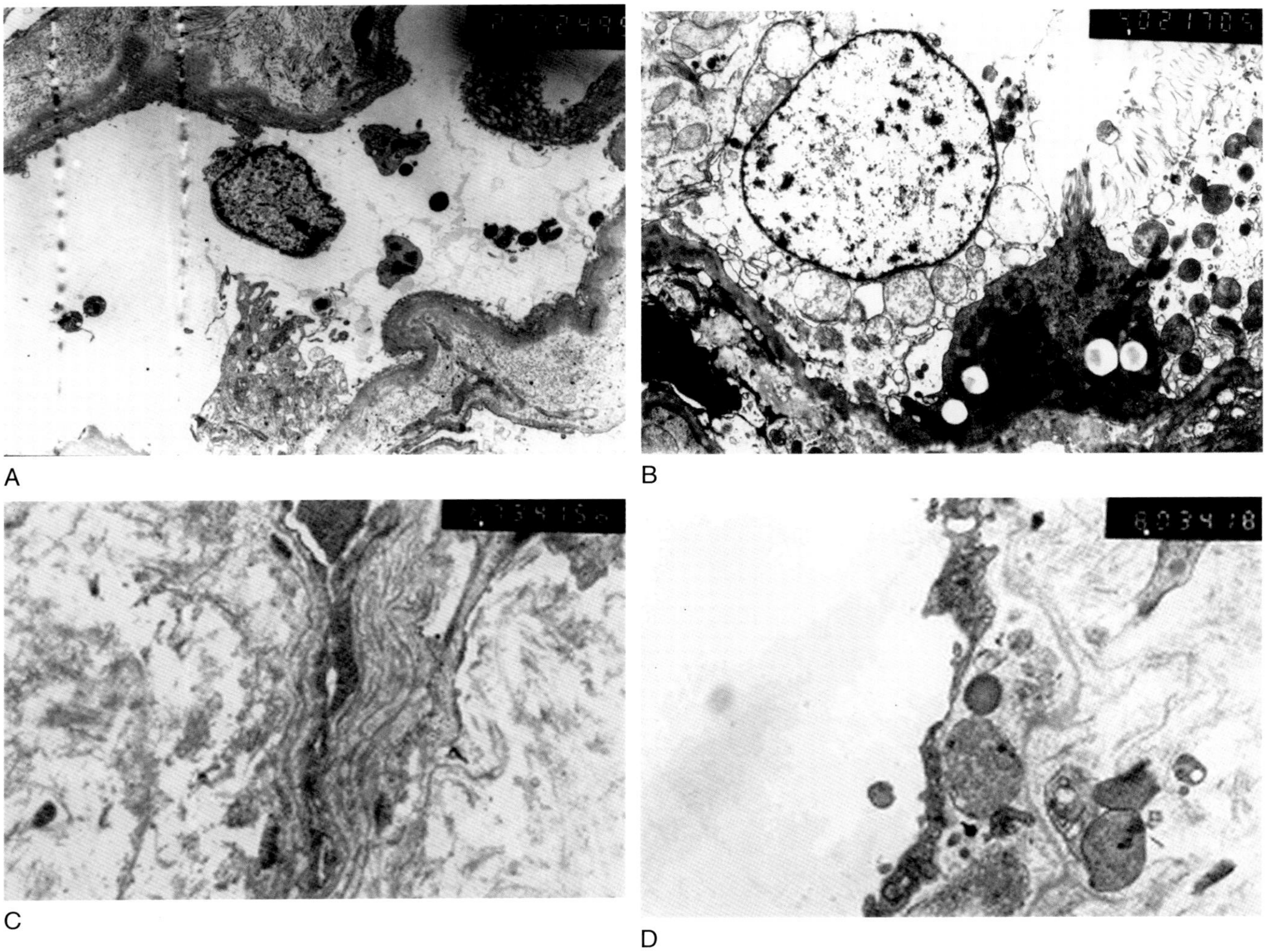

Figure 67-4 Electron microscopic features of acute AAN. **A,** Disruption of the tubular brush border and shedding of the microvilli. In some tubular cells collapsing and shedding are observed. Denuded TBM is seen (EM, ×2000). **B,** Swelling of the mitochondria and endoplasmic reticulum is prominent. Mitochondrial cristae are ruptured and the number of lysosomes is remarkably increased (EM, ×4000). **C,** The basement membrane of PTC (peritubular capillaries) is shrunk and thickened, with multilayers in some parts (EM, ×5000). **D,** The endothelial cells of peritubular capillaries exhibit swelling, with a number of vacuoles and granules occurring in the cell cytoplasm (EM ×8000).

Although no visible fibrosis can be seen on light microscopic examination, early fibroblast proliferation and collagen deposition can be detected by electron microscopy. The endothelial cells of peritubular capillaries exhibit swelling, with a number of vacuoles and granules occurring in the cell cytoplasm. The basement membrane of peritubular capillaries is shrunk and thickened, with multilayers in some parts. The endothelial cells may be detached from the basement membrane (Figure 67-4).

Pathogenesis of AAN

The nephrotoxic effects of AAs have been demonstrated in rodents and rabbits. Administration of AA can result in acute tubular necrosis or induce hypocellular interstitial fibrosis.[71-74] Feeding rats with AA-containing herbs, such as *Caulis aristolochiae manshuriesis* or *Radix aristolochiae fangchi*, can also induce renal impairment resembling that caused by AA.[75,76]

The direct toxicity of AA to the proximal tubule was experimentally confirmed in OK cells (opossum kidney proximal tubule cell line), LLCPK cells (pig proximal tubule cell line), and HK-2 cells (human proximal tubule cell line).[75-77] In HK-2 cells, AA induces epithelial-mesanchymal transdifferentiation (EMT)—which may contribute to the striking interstitial fibrosis.[75,78] Another mechanism that might be involved in the pathogenesis of AAN is microvascular ischemia. In the acute tubular necrosis AAN type, both in patients and rat models, peritubular capillaries are shrunk and diminished[79,80]—likely leading to local ischemia and hypoxia and thereby contributing to the progressive chronic fibrosis.

Although AAN is characterized by hypocellular fibrosis, there still is infiltration of an inflammatory cell—and some authors believe that these cells may also contribute to the fibrosing process.[81,82] Finally, the presence of AA-DNA adducts in the renal tissue of AAN patients and animal models (as well as in OK cells treated with AA) suggests that a modification of DNA might be involved in chronic damage.[75,76,83]

Treatment of AAN

Although AAN has now been recognized for more than 10 years, an effective treatment method is still elusive. The current protocol includes the routine components of treatment for CKD, including control of blood pressure and anemia, maintenance of electrolyte and acid-base balance, and diet modifications including low-protein diets.

Studies are ongoing to find alternative treatments. In a pilot study, 12 AAN patients were treated with corticosteroids. Their progression to end-stage renal failure was slowed.[84] Renin-angiotensin system blockade therapy has provided inconsistent results.[40,85] There are also several pilot studies using traditional Chinese medications for treatment, which showed improvement of renal function in animal models of AAN.[86-88] Randomized placebo-controlled and double-blinded studies are urgently needed to validate treatment methods for AAN.

AA-Associated Urothelial Cancer

In the early 1980s, two independent studies showed that AA was a potent carcinogen in rodents.[72,89] Subsequently, AA was found to be associated with cancers of the kidney, bladder, stomach, lung, and lymphoma in rodents.[90] In humans, AA is also associated with cancers of the bladder, ureter, and renal pelvis.[91] Studies reveal that the carcinogenic effects are associated with the formation of AA-DNA adducts,[92] which can cause mutagenic actions.[93-96]

The occurrence of urothelial cancer in AAN patients ranges from 20% to 40% among reporters.[97-99] A survey conducted by Peking University First Hospital in 283 maintenance dialysis patients revealed that 66 cases (23.3%) had a history of taking AA-containing medications. Twenty-two (33.3%) of the 66 cases developed TCC. The percentage was much higher than that in patients without AA medications (2/198 cases, 1.0%, $p < 0.001$).

The time between the beginning of drug administration and the onset of TCC was approximately 10 years. Of these patients, 44.4% developed TCC after the beginning of dialysis.[99] This phenomenon suggests that the latent period of TCC could be quite long, and AAN patients should be monitored with continued vigilance for a lengthy period. This transitional-cell carcinoma is typically multifocal, has a high-grade development, and has a high rate of recurrence.

AAN in Children

Only a few AAN cases have been reported in pediatrics. Danhua et al.[100] described that three neonates taking a Chinese herbal decoction containing Caulis aristolochiae manshuriesis (Guan-mu-tong) to treat jaundice developed acute renal failure—with obvious acidosis, glucosuria, and mild proteinuria. After supplementary and supportive therapy, all three neonates improved their renal function over the course of several weeks. The acidosis and proteinuria were in remission after several months, with decreased glucosuria. In another three reports,[101-103] four children (ages 4 to 12 years) were reported to suffer renal impairment after long-term (from 1.5 to 8 years) intake of herbal decoctions containing Mutong.

One child had already developed ESRD when she was referred to a nephrologist. Another two presented with Fanconi's syndrome and progressive renal failure. Only one child, with a clinical/pathologic diagnosis of chronic tubulointerstitial nephropathy, achieved partial remission after prednisone therapy. These cases present features resembling those of adult AAN patients, and suggest that AAN is a hazard to children's health meriting greater attention.

PART I REFERENCES

1. Census and Statistics Department, HKSAR. Thematic Household Survey Report No.12.
2. The Chinese Medicinal Material Research Centre of the Chinese University of Hong Kong (January 1991). Report on the Utilization of Traditional Chinese Medicine in Hong Kong.
3. Xiaomei LI: Chinese herbal medicine associated acute renal failure. In W Haiyan (ed.), *Renal failure* [in Chinese]. Shanghai: Shanghai Scientific & Technology 2003:160-71.
4. Ping LI, Xiaomei LI: *Herb related renal injury and herbal medication* [in Chinese]. Beijing: Ren Min Wei Sheng 2004:391-92.
5. Songhan WU: Two cases of acute renal failure caused by Mutong [in Chinese], *Jiang Xi Zhong Yi* 10:12-14, 1963.
6. Vanherweghem JL, Depierreux M, Tielemans C, et al: Rapidly progressive interstitial renal fibrosis in young women: Association with slimming regimen including Chinese herbs, *Lancet* 341:387-91, 1993.
7. Vanhaelen M, Vanhaelen-Fastre R, But PP, Vanherweghem JL: Identification of aristolochic acid in Chinese herbs, *Lancet* 343:174, 1994.
8. But PP: Need for correct identification of herbs in herbal poisoning, *Lancet* 341:637, 1993.
9. Vanherweghem LJ: Misuse of herbal remedies: The case of an outbreak of terminal renal failure in Belgium, *J Altern Complement Med* 4:9-13, 1998.
10. Pena JM, Borras M, Ramos J, Montoliu J: Rapidly progressive interstitial renal fibrosis due to a chronic intake of a herb (Aristolochia pistolochia) infusion, *Nephrol Dial Transplant* 11:1359-60, 1996.
11. Tanaka A, Nishida R, Sawai K, Nagae T, Shinkai S, Ishikawa M, et al: Traditional remedy-induced Chinese herbs nephropathy showing rapid deterioration of renal function [in Japanese], *Nippon Jinzo Gakkai Shi* 39:794-97, 1997.
12. Lord GM, Tagore R, Cook T, Gower P, Pusey CD: Nephropathy caused by Chinese herbs in the UK, *Lancet* 354:481-82, 1999.
13. Stengel B, Jones E: End-stage renal insufficiency with Chinese herbal consumption in France [in French], *Nephrologie* 19:20-25, 1998.
14. Stanley Hok-King Lo, Ka-Leung Mo, Kin-Shing Wong, et al: Aristolochic acid nephropathy complicating a patient with focal segmental glomerulosclerosis, *Nephrol Dial Transplant* 19:1913-15, 2004.
15. Meyer MM, Chen TP, Bennett WM: Chinese herb nephropathy, *Proc Bayl Univ Med Cen* 13:334-37, 2000.
16. Lee S, Lee T, Lee B, et al: Fanconi's syndrome and subsequent progressive renal failure caused by a Chinese herb containing aristolochic acid, *Nephrology* 9:126-33, 2004.
17. Xiaomei LI, Yang L, Yang YU, et al: An analysis of the clinical and pathological characteristics of Mu-Tong (a Chinese herb) induced tubulointerstitial nephropathy [in Chinese], *Chin J Intern Med* 40:681-87, 2001.
18. Lin C-H, Yang C-S: Chinese herb nephropathy [in Chinese], *J Intern Med Taiwan* 13:276-81, 2002.
19. Gillerot G, Jadoul M, Arlt VM, et al: Aristolochic acid nephropathy in a Chinese patient: Time to abandon the term *Chinese herb nephropathy*? *Am J Kidney Dis* 38:E26, 2001.

20. Liou Y, Tan H: GC-MS analysis of Radix aristolochiae and Caulis aristolochiae debilis [in Chinese], *Zhong Guo Zhong Yao Za Zhi* 19:34-36, 1994.
21. Liu Y, Wang B: Analysis of aristolochic acid A in Fructus aristolochiae by HPLC [in Chinese], *Zhong Cao Yao* 21:255-56, 1990.
22. Shen J, Dong L, Qi M, et al: Analysis aristolochic acid A in *Fructus aristolochiae* by HPLC [in Chinese], *Shen Yang Yao Ke Da Xue Xue Bao* 13:218-19, 1996.
23. Zhang X, Xu L: Analysis of effective components in herbs IV: Aristolochic acid in Fructus aristolochiae [in Chinese], *Yao Wu Fen Xi Za Zhi* 2:72-74, 1982.
24. Zhang L, Cui X, Yuan Z, et al: Quantitative analysis of aristolochic acid A in herbs by RP-HPLC [in Chinese], *Yao Wu Fen Xi Za Zhi* 23:215-18, 2003.
25. Zhang Y, Xu G, Jin R, et al: Quantitative analysis of aristolochic acid A in Radix aristolochiae by the method of HPLC [in Chinese], *Zhong Guo Yao Ke Da Xue Xue Bao* 24:55-57, 1993.
26. Mohamed OA, Wang Z, Xu G, et al: Comparative analysis of aristolochic acid in Aristolochiae plants from China and Sudan [in Chinese], *Zhong Guo Yao Ke Da Xue Xue Bao* 30:288-90, 1999.
27. Zhao M, Lai J, Bi K: Quantitative analysis of aristolochic acid A in Radix aristolochiae by HPLC [in Chinese], *Shen Yang Yao Ke Da Xue Xue Bao* 18:125-26, 2001.
28. Ong Eng-Shi, Woo Soo-On, Yong Yuk-Lin, et al: Pressurized liquid extraction of berberine and aristolochic acids in medicinal plants, *J Chromatography A* 313:57-64, 2000.
29. Kazunori H, Masami H, Bunsho M, et al: Quantitative analysis of aristolochic acids, toxic compounds, contained in some medicinal plants, *J Ethnopharmacology* 64:185-89, 1999.
30. Chang C, Nie G, Chen H, et al: Quantitative analysis of aristolochic acid in *Radix aristolochiae* [in Chinese], *Zhong Cheng Yao* 22:229-30, 2000.
31. Sheng R, Pan Y. Comparative analysis of aristolochic acid A in the fruit and root of *Fructus aristolochiae* from cultivated and wild plants [in Chinese], *Nan Jing Zhong Yi Xue Yuan Xue Bao* 10:40-41, 1994.
32. Tan S, Yang G, Liang Y, et al: Quantitative analysis of aristolochic acid C in *Radix aristolochiae* by HPLC [in Chinese], *Zhong Guo Zhong Yao Za Zhi* 18:169, 1993.
33. Cui N, Fang Y, Qian J, et al: Quantitative analysis of aristolochic acid C in *Radix aristolochiae* [in Chinese], *Zhong Cheng Yao* 23:147-48, 2001.
34. Zhang L, Che J, Lu Y, et al: Analysis of aristolochic acid C in Radix aristolochiae, *Te Chan Yan Jiu* 20:28-29, 1998.
35. You L, Wang Z, Jiang X, et al: Quantitative analysis of aristolochic acid C in *Radix aristolochiae* collected from different area [in Chinese], *Zhong Guo Zhong Yao Za Zhi* 28:456-57, 2003.
36. Lee T-Y, Wu M-L, Deng J-F, et al: High-performance liquid chromatographic determination for aristolochic acid in medicinal plants and slimming products, *J Chromatography B* 766:169-74, 2001.
37. Chou L, Chen Z, Liang Y, et al: Analysis of aristolochic acid in Radix aristolochiae fangchi [in Chinese], *Zhong Yao Tong Bao* 11:363-65, 1986.
38. Stiborova M, Frei E, Breuer A, et al.: Aristolactam Ia metabolite of aristolochic acid I upon activation forms an adduct found in DNA of patients with Chinese herbs nephropathy, *Exp Toxicol Pathol* 51:421-27, 1999.
39. Pailer M, Belohlav L, Simonitsch E: Zur Konstitution der Aristolochiasäuren [in German], *Monatsh Chem* 86:676-80, 1995.
40. Pailer M, Bergthaller P, Schaden G: Über die Isolierung und Charakterisierung von vier neuen Aristolochiasäuren (aus Aristolochia clematitis L.) [in German], *Monatsh Chem* 96:863-83, 1965.
41. Debelle FED, Nortier JL, Husson CP, et al: The renin-angiotensin system blockade does not prevent renal interstitial fibrosis induced by aristolochic acids, *Kidney International* 66:1815-25, 2004.
42. Krumbiegel G, Hallensleben J, Mennicke WH, et al: Studies on the metabolism of aristolochic acids I and II, *Xenobiotica* 17:981-91, 1987.
43. Vishwanath BS, Kini RM, Gowda TV: Characterization of three edema inducing phospholipase A2 enzymes from Habu (Trimeresurus flavoviridis) venom and their interaction with the alkaloid aristolochic acid, *Toxicon* 25:501-06, 1987.
44. Moreno JJ: Effect of aristolochic acid on arachidonic acid cascade and in vivo models of inflammation, *Immunopharmacology* 26:1-9, 1993.
45. Norman SJ, Poyser NL: Prostaglandin production by guinea-pig placenta and other uterine tissues during mid-pregnancy, *Placenta* 19:631-41, 1998.
46. Pezzuto JM, Swanson SM, Mar W, Che CT, Cordell GA, Fong HH: Evaluation of the mutagenic and cytostatic potential of aristolochic acid (3,4-methylenedioxy-8-methoxy-10-nitrophenanthrene-1-carboxylic acid) and several of its derivatives, *Mutat Res* 206:447-54, 1988.
47. Vishwanath BS, Fawzy AA, Franson RC: Edema-inducing activity of phospholipase A2 purified from human synovial fluid and inhibition by aristolochic acid, *Inflammation* 12:549-61, 1988.
48. Kupchan SM, Doskotch RW: Tumor inhibitors: I. Aristolochic acid, the active principle of Aristolochia indica, *J Med Pharm Chem* 5:657-59, 1962.
49. Möse JR, Porta J: Weitere Studien über Aristolochiasäure [in German], *Drug Res* 24:52-54, 1974.
50. Kluthe R, Vogt A, Batsford S: Doppelblindstudie zur Beeinflussung der Phagozytosefähigkeit von Granulozyten durch Aristolochiasäure [in German], *Drug Res* 32:443-45, 1982.
51. Reginster F, Jadoul M, van Ypersele de Strihou C: Chinese herbs nephropathy presentation, natural history, and fate after transplantation, *Nephrol Dial Transplant* 12:81-86, 1997.
52. van Ypersele de Strihou C, Vanherweghem JL: The tragic paradigm of Chinese herbs nephropathy, *Nephrol Dial Transplant* 10:157-60, 1995.
53. Kabanda A, Jadoul M, Lauwerys R, et al: Low molecular weight proteinuria in Chinese herbs nephropathy, *Kidney Int* 48:1571-76, 1995.
54. Nortier JL, Deschodt-Lanckman MM, Simon S, et al: Proximal tubular injury in Chinese herbs nephropathy: Monitoring by neutral endopeptidase enzymuria, *Kidney Int* 51:288-93, 1997.
55. Martinez MC, Nortier J, Vereerstraeten P, et al: Progression rate of Chinese herb nephropathy: Impact of Aristolochia fangchi ingested dose, *Nephrol Dial Transplant* 17:408-12, 2002.
56. Krumme B, Endmeir R, Vanhaelen M, Walb D: Reversible Fanconi's syndrome after ingestion of a Chinese herbal "remedy" containing aristolochic acid, *Nephrol Dial Transplant* 16:400-02, 2001.
57. Yang SS, Chu P, Lin YF, Chen A, Lin SH: Aristolochic acid-induced Fanconi's syndrome and nephropathy presenting as hypokalemic paralysis, *Am J Kidney Dis* 39:E14, 2002.
58. Tanaka A, Nishida R, Yoshida T, Koshikawa M, Goto M, Kuwahara T: Outbreak of Chinese herb nephropathy in Japan: Are there any differences from Belgium? *Intern Med* 40:296-300, 2001.
59. Tanaka A, Nishida R, Yokoi H, Kuwahara T: The characteristic pattern of aminoaciduria in patients with aristolochic acid-induced Fanconi's syndrome: Could aminoaciduria be the hallmark of this syndrome? *Clin Nephrol* 54:198-202, 2000.
60. Yu Y, Zheng FL, Li H: Chinese herbs-induced renal failure with Fanconi's syndrome [in Chinese], *Zhonghua Nei Ke Za Zhi* 42:110-12, 2003.
61. Lee CT, Wu MS, Lu K, Hsu KT: Renal tubular acidosis, hypokalemic paralysis, rhabdomyolysis and acute renal failure: A rare presentation of Chinese herbal nephropathy, *Ren Fail* 21:227-30, 1999.
62. Tanaka A, Nishida R, Maeda K, Sugawara A, Kuwahara T: Chinese herb nephropathy in Japan presents adult-onset Fanconi syndrome: Could different components of aristolochic acids cause a different type of Chinese herb nephropathy? *Clin Nephrol* 53:301-06, 2000.
63. Izumotani T, Ishimura E, Tsumura K, Goto U, Nishizawa Y, Morii M: An adult case of Fanconi syndrome due to a mixture of Chinese crude drugs, *Nephron* 65:137-40, 1993.
64. Stefanovic V, Toncheva D, Atanasova S, Polenakovic M: Etiology of Balkan endemic nephropathy and associated urothelial cancer, *Am J Nephrol* 26:1-11, 2006.
65. Cosyns JP, Jadoul M, Squiffl JP, et al: Chinese herbs nephropathy: A clue to Balkan endemic nephropathy? *Kidney Int* 45:1680-88, 1994.
66. Ivic M: The problem of etiology of endemic nephropathy, *Acta Fac Med Naiss* 1:29-37, 1970.
67. Depierreux M, Van Damme B, Vanden Houte K, Vanherweghem JL: Pathologic aspects of a newly described nephropathy related to

the prolonged use of Chinese herbs. *Am J Kidney Dis* 24:172-180, 1994.
68. Cosyns JP, Jadoul M, Squifflet JP, et al: Chinese herbs nephropathy: A clue to Balkan endemic nephropathy? *Kidney Int* 45:1680-88, 1994.
69. Mengs U: Acute toxicity of aristolochic acid in rodents, *Arch Toxicol* 59:328-31, 1987.
70. Mengs U, Stotzem CD: Renal toxicity of aristolochic acid in rats as an example of nephrotoxicity testing in routine toxicology, *Arch Toxicol* 67:307-11, 1993.
71. Mengs U: Acute toxicity of aristolochic acid in rodents, *Arch Toxicol* 59:328-31, 1987.
72. Mengs U, Lang W, Poch J-A: The carcinogenic action of aristolochic acid in rats, *Arch Toxicol* 57:107-19, 1982.
73. Mengs U: On the histopathogenesis of rat forestomach carcinoma caused by aristolochic acid, *Arch Toxicol* 52:209-20, 1983.
74. Debelle FD, Nortier JL, De Prez EG, Garbar CH, et al: Aristolochic acids induce chronic renal failure with interstitial fibrosis in salt-depleted rats, *J Am Soc Nephrol* 13:431-36, 2002.
75. Lebeau C, Arlt VM, Schmeiser HH, et al: Aristolochic acid impedes endocytosis and induces DNA adducts in proximal tubule cells, *Kidney Int* 60:1332-42, 2001.
76. Li B, LI X, Zhang C, et al: Cellular mechanism of renal proximal tubular epithelial cell injury induced by aristolochic acid and aristololactam [in Chinese], *J Peking University* 36:36-40, 2004.
77. Gao R, Zheng F, Liu Y, et al: Aristolochic acid I induced apoptosis in LLCPK cells [in Chinese], *Chin J Nephrol* 15:162-65, 1999.
78. Wen X, Zheng F, Gao R, et al: Transdifferentiation of cultured human renal tubular epithelial cells induced by aristolochic acid I [in Chinese], *J Nephrol Dial Transplant* 9:206-09, 2000.
79. Yang L, Li X, Wang H: Possible mechanisms of the tendency towards interstitial fibrosis in aristolochic acid-induced acute tubular necrosis. *Nephrol Dial Transplant* 22(2):445-56, 2006.
80. Wen Y, Qu L, Li X: HIF-1α expression follows ET-1 up-regulation and VEGF down-regulation in rats with acute renal injury induced by aristolochic acids, *ASN Abstract* TH-PO 309, 2005.
81. Wei Z, Jihong W, Yage L, et al: CD4+, CD8+, CD68+ cells infiltrate in the rat AAN model, *Shenyangbuduiyiyao* 18:295-97, 2005.
82. Wu Y, Liu Z, Hu W, et al: Mast cell infiltration associated with tubulointerstitial fibrosis in chronic aristolochic acid nephropathy. *Hum Exp Toxicol* 24:41-47, 2005.
83. Lebeaul C, Debelle FD, Volker M, et al: Early proximal tubule injury in experimental aristolochic acid nephropathy: Functional and histological studies, *Nephrol Dialy Transplant* 20:2321-32, 2005.
84. Vanherweghem JL, Abramowicz D, Tielemans C, et al: Effects of steroids on the progression of renal failure in chronic interstitial renal fibrosis: A pilot study in Chinese herbs nephropathy, *Am J Kidney Dis* 27:209-15, 1996.
85. Zhu S, Liu J, Chen L, Li Y, et al: Prophylactic therapeutic effect of captopril and losartan on interstitial fibrosis of the rat kidney induced by Guanmutong, *Herald of Medicine* 124:112-15, 2005.
86. Wan C, Zhang J: Comparative effects among ligustrazine, prednisone and enazepril on acute renal tubular necrosis induced by aristolochic acid in rats [in Chinese], *Chin J Nehrol* 2006; 22:426-29, 2006.
87. Wang Y, Liu L, Feng J, et al: Nephroprotective effect of folium ginkgo biloba on chronic aristolochic acid nephropathy [in Chinese], *Chin J Hemoth* 16:104-05, 2006.
88. Sun D, Sun L, Wang W, et al: Effects of ginkgo biloba extract on peritubular capillaries in rats of aristolochic acid nephropathy, *Chin J Modern Med* 16:346-53, 2006. (In Chinese)
89. Xing B, Chen L, Zhou L, et al: Experimental study on the carcinogenicity of aristolochic acid [in Chinese], *Guangxi Yixue* 4:118-21, 1982.
90. Mengs U: On the histopathogenesis of rat forestomach carcinoma caused by aristolochic acid, *Arch Toxicol* 52:209-20, 1983.
91. Nortier JL, Martinez MC, Schmeiser HH, et al: Urothelial carcinoma associated with the use of a Chinese herb (*Aristolchia fangchi*), *New Engl J Med* 342:1686-92, 2000.
92. Arlt VM, Wiessler M, Schmeiser HH: Using polymerase arrest to detect DNA binding specificity of aristolochic acid in the mouse H-ras gene, *Carcinogenesis* 21:235-42, 2000.
93. Robisch G, Schimmer O, Göggelmann W: Aristolochic acid is a direct mutagen in Salmonella typhimurium, *Mutat Res* 105:201-04, 1982.
94. Maier P, Schawalder HP, Weibel B, et al: Aristolochic acid induces 6-thioguanine-resistant mutants in an extrahepatic tissue in rats after oral application, *Mutat Res* 143:143-48, 1985.
95. Frei H, Würgler FE, Juon H, et al: Aristolochic acid is mutagenic and recombinogenic in Drosophila genotoxicity test, *Arch Toxicol* 56:158-66, 1985.
96. Schmeiser HH, Pool BL, Wiessler M: Mutagenicity of the two main components of commercially available carcinogenic aristolochic acid in Salmonella typhimurium, *Cancer Lett* 23:97-101, 1984.
97. Cosyns JP, Jadoul M, Squifflet JP, et al: Urothelial lesions in Chinese-herb nephropathy, *Am J Kidney Dis* 33:1011-17, 1999.
98. Nortier JL Martinez MCM, Schmeiser HH, et al: Urothelial carcinoma associated with the use of a Chinese herb *Aristolochia fangchi, N Engl J Med* 342:1686-92, 2000.
99. Li W, Yang L, Su T, et al: Influence of taking aristolochic acid containing Chinese drugs on occurrence of urinary transitional cell cancer in uremic patients undergoing dialysis [in Chinese], *Natl Med J China* 85:2487-91, 2005.
100. Wang D, Shao L, Ding G: Mutong toxic renal injury in neonates [in Chinese], *Chin J Pediatr* 38:392-93, 2000.
101. Hong YT, Fu LS, Chung LH, et al: Fanconi's syndrome, interstitial fibrosis and renal failure by aristolochic acid in Chinese herbs, *Pediatric Nephrology* 21:577-79, 2006.
102. Renal division of Pediatric Hospital of Tianjin. Fanconi's syndrome and severe anemia, *Chin J Pediatr* 37:255-56, 1999.
103. Yang L, Zhou X, Ning P, et al: Clinical analysis of two cases of aristolochic acid nephropathy [in Chinese], *Chin J Pediatr* 41:552-53, 2003.

PART II: NEPHROTOXIC EFFECTS OF HERBAL REMEDIES

Afroze Ramzan Sherali

INTRODUCTION

Plants and herbs have been used for medicinal purposes all over the world for many centuries. According to the World Health Organization (WHO), the primary form of medical health care used by 80% of the world's population is plant-based remedies.[1] In some countries of Asia, herbal medicines form an integral part of their medical system, such as traditional medicine in China, Ayurvedic medicine in India, and Tibb-e-Unani in Pakistan. Herbal medicine has a long history and tradition in Europe and the United States as well. A study of long term trends in the United States has shown that the public use of complementary and alternative medicine (CAM) has increased steadily since the 1950s.[2,3]

In the rural and urban areas of the Indo-Pakistan subcontinent, herbs have been used for various ailments for the past three centuries and are still the medicines of choice, especially in rural areas. This is attributed to their easy availability and low cost in the face of an inadequate public health care system. In developed countries, desire for a natural lifestyle has resulted in an increased use of CAM.[4]

Herbal medicines and homeopathic medicines are often considered by lay people as similar products. Homeopathy is based on the administration of minute doses of remedies that in larger doses would produce symptoms of disease in a healthy person. Many of these remedies come from plants. In contrast, herbal medicines use dried extract of a plant in therapeutic doses to treat the symptoms of a disease, similar to allopathic medicine.

REGULATORY CONTROLS ON HERBAL MEDICINE

The WHO has reviewed the regulatory control of herbal medicines in 50 countries and has noted the wide variation in the approach to regulation among these countries.[5] Not only is the regulation of medicinal herbs different from one country to another, but also the regulatory processes are not always ideal and are under review.

The majority of quality-related problems are associated with unregulated herbal products. There is substantial evidence that many ethnic medicines such as traditional Chinese medicines (TCM) and traditional Asian medicines (Ayurvedic and Unani) lack adequate quality control procedures and so may give rise to serious public health problems. These problems include contamination with toxic substances, differences between labeled and actual contents, or inclusion of prohibited ingredients (e.g., *Aristolochia*). Inadvertent exposure to *Aristolochia* species in unlicensed herbal medicines has resulted in cases of nephrotoxicity and carcinogenicity in China, Japan, Europe, and the United States.

A number of Bulgarian patients have subsequently developed urethral cancer as a result of exposure to the toxic aristolochic acid.[6-8] The widespread substitution of *Aristolochia* species in TCM products available in the UK has been confirmed in a recent Medicines Control Agency (MCA) study.[9]

SELF-TREATMENT WITH HERBAL PRODUCTS

The majority of the herbal products are self-prescribed; therefore, their safety is of particular importance.[10] There are concerns that patients may be exposed to potentially toxic substances either from the herbal ingredients themselves or from contaminants present in the herbal product. In addition, recent evidence suggests that if conventional medicines are taken along with herbal products, the herbal products may compromise the efficacy of the conventional medication through herb–drug interactions.[11]

HERB–DRUG INTERACTIONS

There is limited information available regarding interactions between conventional medicines and herbal products. There is, however, increasing awareness of this issue.[12,13] There are particular concerns with drugs that have a narrow therapeutic margin, such as anticonvulsants (phenytoin), cyclosporine, and digoxin. Herbal diuretics taken for a prolonged period may potentiate existing diuretic therapy, interfere with the therapy for hypertension, and induce hypokalemia.

PREGNANT/BREAST-FEEDING MOTHERS

Generally, no medicine should be taken during pregnancy unless the benefit to the mother outweighs any possible risk to the fetus. This rule also applies to herbal products. In addition, drugs and medicines taken by a breast-feeding mother may be transferred to the baby in significant amounts in breast milk. Very little information is available about herbal ingredients' safety during breast-feeding; therefore, their use is not recommended during lactation.

USE OF HERBAL MEDICINES IN CHILDREN

Herbal medicines have traditionally been used to treat both adults and children, although their suitability needs to be considered with respect to quality, efficacy, and safety. Herbal products should be used with caution in children as they may contain allergens (e.g., chamomile given to babies for teething pains).

HERBAL MEDICINES USED IN KIDNEY DISEASES

A number of kidney diseases, such as urinary tract infections, nocturnal enuresis, acute and chronic inflammatory conditions, and urolithiasis, are treated by herbal products. Some of these products, along with their herbal use and side effects, are described in the following text and summarized in Table 67-3.

Buchu

Herbal Use

Buchu is used as an herbal product because of its urinary antiseptic and diuretic properties. It has been used for cystitis, urethritis, prostatitis, and specifically for acute cystitis.

Side Effects, Toxicity

None documented for buchu. Although the volatile oil in buchu causes gastrointestinal and renal symptoms.

Corn Silk

Herbal Use

Corn silk has stone-reducing properties and is also used as a diuretic. It has been used for cystitis, urethritis, nocturnal enuresis, prostatitis, and specifically for acute or chronic inflammation of the urinary system.

Side Effects, Toxicity

Allergic reactions to corn silk's pollen and starch are known. These include contact dermatitis and urticaria. Corn silk contains an unidentified toxic component and is listed as being capable of producing a cyanogenetic compound.[14,15]

Contraindications, Warnings

Corn silk may cause an allergic reaction in susceptible individuals. Excessive doses may interfere with hypoglycemic drug therapy (in vivo hypoglycemic activity has been documented)[15] or with hypertensive or hypotensive therapy (in vivo hypotensive activity has been reported). Prolonged use may result in hypokalemia because of the diuretic action.

Pregnancy and Lactation

Corn silk may stimulate uterine contractions. Therefore, it should not be taken in excessive amounts during pregnancy or lactation.

TABLE 67-3 Popular Herbs Used in Kidney Diseases

Name of the Herbal Product	Indications
Buchu (*Agathosma betulina*); also known as *Barosma betulina* or round-leaf buchu	Urinary antiseptic and diuretic, used for acute cystitis and urethritis
Corn Silk (*Zea mays*)	Acute and chronic inflammation of the urinary tract, cystitis, urethritis, and nocturnal enuresis
Couchgrass	Diuretic Cystitis, urethritis, and renal calculi
Juniper	Antiseptic and diuretic
Marshmallow	Urinary tract infections and urinary calculi
Cranberry (*Vaccinium oxycoccus*)	Urinary tract infections
Hydrangea (Seven barks)	Diuretic Urinary calculi
Java Tea	Diuretic Hypertension, diabetes, bladder and kidney disorders, gallstones, and rheumatism
Plantain	Diuretic and antihemorrhagic properties Hematuria with cystitis and hemorrhoids with "bleeding"
Saw Palmetto (*Serenoa repens*)	Diuretic and urinary antiseptic Chronic or subacute cystitis, sex hormone disorders, and prostatic enlargement
Parsley Piert	Kidney and bladder calculi, dysuria, and strangury
Stone Root (*Collin sonia*)	Litholytic Urinary calculi
Uva-Ursi (*Bearberry Canadensis*)	Urinary tract infections
Wild Carrot	Urinary calculi and cystitis

Couchgrass

Herbal Use

Couchgrass is stated to possess diuretic properties. It has been used for cystitis, urethritis, and renal calculi.

Side Effects, Toxicity

None documented for couchgrass.

Contraindications, Warnings

Excessive or prolonged use of couchgrass should be avoided as it may result in hypokalemia because of its diuretic actions.

Pregnancy and Lactation

Limited information about its toxicity is available; therefore, couchgrass should not be used during pregnancy and lactation.

Cranberry

Herbal Use

Cranberry juice and crushed cranberries have been used for a long time in the treatment and prevention of urinary tract infections.[16] Traditionally, cranberries have also been used for many problems, such as stomach ailments, anorexia, vomiting, and blood diseases, as well as in wound dressings.[17] A systematic review of cranberry products for the prevention of UTI reported that two good-quality randomized control trials found there is some evidence that cranberry juice may decrease the number of symptomatic UTIs over a 12-month period in women, but the same is not clear about all age groups. Also, the optimum dosage and method of administration (e.g., juice or tablets) is not clear.[19]

Side Effects, Toxicity

There are no serious side effects documented for cranberry. A systematic review of cranberry products for the prevention of UTIs reported that the drop-out rates in the four studies included[18,20,21] were high (20%-55%)[19] because of cranberry's taste.[20] It has been claimed that ingesting large amounts of cranberry juice may cause formation of uric acid or oxalate stones secondary to a constantly acidic urine because of the high oxalate content of cranberry juice.[16] However, it has also been stated that the role of cranberry juice as a urinary acidifier has not been well established.[23] The use of cranberry juice in preventing the formation of stones that develop in alkaline urine, such as those comprising magnesium ammonium phosphate and calcium carbonate, has been described.[22]

Contraindications, Warnings

Sugar-free cranberry juice should be used by patients with diabetes. Patients using cranberry juice should be advised to drink sufficient fluids in order to ensure adequate urine flow.

Pregnancy and Lactation

There are no known problems with the use of cranberry during pregnancy.

Hydrangea

Herbal Use

Hydrangea has diuretic and antilithic properties. Traditionally, it has been used for cystitis, urethritis, prostatitis, and urinary calculi.

Side Effects, Toxicity

Hydrangea has been reported to cause contact dermatitis and may cause gastroenteritis.

Contraindications, Warnings

Overdose of this herb may cause vertigo and respiratory congestion. Do not use this herb long term.

Pregnancy and Lactation

The safety of hydrangea has not been established. Because of the lack of pharmacological and toxicity data, the use of hydrangea during pregnancy and lactation should be avoided.

Java Tea

Herbal Use

Java tea has traditionally been used in Java for the treatment of hypertension and diabetes.[24] It has also been used in folk medicine for bladder and kidney disorders, gallstones, gout, and rheumatism. Java tea is stated to have diuretic properties.

Side Effects, Toxicity

None documented.

Contraindications, Warnings

None known. Adequate fluid intake (2 L or more per day) should be ensured while using Java tea.

Pregnancy and Lactation

There are no data available on the use of Java tea in pregnancy and lactation. Because of the lack of toxicity data, use of Java tea during pregnancy and lactation should be avoided.

Juniper

Herbal Use

Juniper is used as an antiseptic and a diuretic and is applied topically over joints or muscles for rheumatic pains.

Side Effects, Toxicity

The volatile oil is generally nonsensitizing and nonphototoxic, although a slight irritant when applied externally to human and animal skin. Excessive doses of terpinen-4-oil, the diuretic principle in the volatile oil, may cause renal pain. There may be external and internal symptoms of overdose following excessive use of the essential oil. These are described as burning, erythema, and inflammation with blisters and edema. Internal symptoms include pain in the lumber region, strong diuresis, albuminuria, hematuria, purplish urine, tachycardia, hypertension, and, rarely, convulsions, metrorrhagia, and abortion.

Contraindications, Warnings

Juniper is contraindicated in individuals with existing renal disease. Juniper may potentiate existing hypoglycemic and diuretic therapies; prolonged use may result in hypokalemia.

Pregnancy and Lactation

Juniper is contraindicated in pregnancy. It is reputed to be an abortifacient and to affect the menstrual cycle.

Marshmallow

Herbal Use

Traditionally, marshmallow has been used orally for respiratory infection and cough, GI problems, UTIs, and urinary calculi. It can also be used topically for skin infections.

Side Effects, Toxicity

None documented.

Contraindications, Warnings

Marshmallow may interfere with existing hypoglycemic therapy and the absorption of other drugs taken simultaneously.

Pregnancy and Lactation

There are no known problems with the use of marshmallow during pregnancy or lactation.

Plantain

Herbal Use

Plantain is stated to possess diuretic and antihemorrhagic properties. Traditionally, it has been used for hematuria with cystitis, and specifically for hemorrhoids with bleeding.

Side Effects, Toxicity

Allergic contact dermatitis to plantain has been reported.

Contraindications, Warnings

Plantain may cause a contact allergic reaction; it induces the formation of IgE antibodies, which may cross-react to psyllium.[25] Excessive doses may exert a laxative effect and a hypotensive effect.

Pregnancy and Lactation

In vitro uterotonic activity has been documented for plantain. In view of this, excessive use of plantain, which may also exert a laxative effect, should be avoided during pregnancy.

Saw Palmetto

Herbal Use

Saw palmetto is used as a diuretic and a urinary antiseptic. It also has endocrinologic properties. Traditionally, it has been used for chronic or subacute cystitis, sex hormone disorders, and specifically for prostatic enlargement. Modern interest in saw palmetto is focused on its use in the treatment of symptoms of benign prostatic hyperplasia (BPH).

A systematic review and quantitative meta-analysis of the existing evidence regarding the therapeutic efficacy and safety of the saw palmetto plant extract in men with symptomatic BPH was conducted. The evidence suggests that *Serenoa repens* improves urologic symptoms and flow measures. Further research is needed to determine long term effectiveness and ability to prevent BPH complications.[26]

Side Effects, Toxicity

A systematic review and meta-analysis of 18 randomized clinical trials of saw palmetto extracts reported that adverse effects with saw palmetto were generally mild and comparable to those with placebo.[26] Incubation of high concentrations of saw palmetto extract (Permixon; 9.0 mg/ml for 48 hours) inhibited sperm motility compared with control.[27]

Contraindications, Warnings

In view of the reported antiandrogen and estrogenic activities, saw palmetto may affect existing hormonal therapy, including the oral contraceptive pill and hormone replacement therapy.

Pregnancy and Lactation

The safety of saw palmetto has not been established; therefore, the use of saw palmetto during pregnancy and lactation should be avoided.

Parsley Piert

Herbal Use

Traditionally, parsley piert has been used for kidney and bladder calculi, dysuria, and strangury.

Side Effects, Toxicity

None documented.

Contraindications, Warnings

None documented.

Pregnancy and Lactation

Because of the lack of information, the use of parsley piert during pregnancy and lactation should be avoided.

Stone Root

Herbal Use

Stone root is stated to possess antilithic, litholytic, and diuretic properties. Therefore, it has generally been used for the treatment of urinary calculi.

Side Effects, Toxicity

None documented.

Contraindications, Warnings

None documented.

Pregnancy and Lactation

The safety of stone root has not been established. Use during pregnancy and lactation should therefore be avoided.

Uva-Ursi

Herbal Use

Uva-ursi is most commonly used for UTIs, especially for cystitis with dysuria.

Side Effects, Toxicity

There are no reported side effects in therapeutic doses.

Contraindications, Warnings

Excessive use of uva-ursi should be avoided because of the high tannin content. Prolonged use of uva-ursi to treat a UTI is not advisable. Patients in whom symptoms persist for longer than 48 hours should consult their doctor.

Pregnancy and Lactation

Large doses of uva-ursi are reported to be oxytocic, although in vitro studies have reported a lack of utero activity. Because of the potential toxicity of hydroquinone, the use of uva-ursi during pregnancy and lactation should be avoided.

Wild Carrot

Herbal Use

Traditionally, wild carrot is used for urinary calculi and cystitis.

Side Effects, Toxicity

The oil is reported to be nontoxic, nonirritating, and nonsensitizing.

Contraindications, Warnings

Excessive doses of the oil may affect the kidneys because of the terpinen-4-oil content (see Juniper). Excessive doses may affect existing hypotensive, hypertensive, cardiac, and hormone therapies.

Pregnancy and Lactation

The safety of wild carrot has not been established. Therefore, excessive doses of wild carrot during pregnancy and lactation should be avoided.

NEPHROTOXICITY ASSOCIATED WITH HERBAL MEDICINE

Adverse drug reactions account for nearly 6% of all hospital admissions, of which 7% are a result of nephrotoxicity due to medication-related events.[28] Because most compounds are excreted through the kidneys, they are exposed to a high concentration of the drug or its metabolites, which results in toxicity.

Common herbal medication that can adversely affect the kidney and its function are as follows.

Alfalfa

Herbal Use

Commercial preparations including teas, tablets, and capsules are available. Alfalfa is stated to be a source of vitamins A, C, E, and K and of minerals such as calcium, potassium, phosphorus, and iron. It has been used for avitaminosis A, C, E, or K, hypoprothrombinemia, and debility of convalescence.

Side Effects, Toxicity

Both the alfalfa seed and the herb have been reported to induce a systemic lupus erythematosus (SLE)-like syndrome in female monkeys.[29] This activity has been attributed to canavanine, a nonprotein amino acid constituent which has been found to have effects on human immunoregulatory cells in vitro.[30] Reactivation of quiescent SLE in humans has been associated with the ingestion of alfalfa tablets that were found to contain canavanine.[31]

Contraindications, Warnings

Individuals with a history of SLE should avoid ingestion of alfalfa. Excessive doses may interfere with anticoagulant therapy and hormonal therapy, including the oral contraceptive pill and hormone replacement therapy. Alfalfa may affect blood sugar concentrations in diabetic patients because of the manganese content.

Pregnancy and Lactation

Alfalfa seeds are reputed to affect the menstrual cycle and to be lactogenic. Although the safety of the alfalfa herb has not been established, it is probably acceptable for use during pregnancy and lactation provided that doses do not exceed the amounts normally ingested as a food. Supplementary alfalfa seeds should not be ingested during pregnancy or lactation.

Aristolochia (Snakewood)

Herbal Use

Aristolochic acids (AA), present in Aristolochia plants, are the toxin responsible for Chinese herb nephropathy (CHN), a rapidly progressive tubulointerstitial nephritis (TIN).

Side Effects, Toxicity

Concerns were first raised about the effects of products containing aristolochic acid in Belgium, where, since 1993, more than 100 cases of irreversible nephropathy have been reported in young women who attended a slimming clinic. The nephrotoxicity was traced to the inadvertent use of the toxic *Aristolochia fangchi* root in the formulations as a substitute for *Stephania tetrandra*. Subsequently, many cases of CHN have been described worldwide.[32,33]

AA, the toxic components of the *Aristolochia* species, are known to be nephrotoxic, carcinogenic, and mutagenic. A number of the Belgian patients have developed urothelial cancer as a result of exposure to the toxic aristolochic acids.[34]

Aristolochic acid nephropathy (AAN) with Fanconi syndrome presenting as hypokalemic paralysis is rare and may be unrecognized. A case has been described of a 41-year-old man who presented with the inability to ambulate upon awakening in the morning. Physical examination revealed symmetric paralysis of bilateral lower limbs. Laboratory studies showed profound hypokalemia with renal potassium wasting, hyperchloremic metabolic acidosis, hypophosphatemia with hyperphosphaturia, hypouricemia with hyperuricosuria, and glycosuria, consistent with Fanconi syndrome. Mild renal insufficiency was also observed. A meticulous search for underlying causes of Fanconi syndrome was unrevealing. However, a significant amount (AA-1, 7 μg/g) of AA was detected in the Chinese herb mixture he consumed for the treatment of his leg edema for the past 2 months. His hypokalemia, renal insufficiency, and Fanconi syndrome completely resolved 2 months after the withdrawal of the Chinese herb mixture and the supplementation of potassium citrate and active vitamin D_3. AAN with Fanconi syndrome should be considered as a cause of hypokalemia in any patient administered undefined Chinese herbs.[35]

Boldo

Herbal Use

Boldo has been used for mild digestive disturbances, constipation, and cholethithiasis with pain.

Side Effects, Toxicity

Boldo volatile oil is stated to be one of the most toxic oils. Application of the undiluted oil to the hairless backs of mice has an irritant effect.[37] The oil contains irritant terpenes, including terpinen-4-oil, the irritant in juniper oil.

Contraindications, Warnings

Excessive doses of boldo may affect the kidneys because of the volatile oil and should be avoided by individuals with an existing kidney disorder. It should not be used by individuals with liver disease and bile duct obstruction.

Pregnancy and Lactation

The safety of boldo taken during pregnancy has not been established. Because of the volatile oil present in it, the use of boldo during pregnancy should be avoided.

Cat's Claw

Herbal Use

Cat's claw is mostly used for gastrointestinal tract disturbances, arthritis, and various malignant tumors.

Side Effects, Toxicity

There has been a report of acute renal failure in a Peruvian woman with systemic lupus erythematosus who had added a product containing cat's claw to her regimen of prednisone, atenolol, metolazone, frusemide, and nifedipine.[38] She was diagnosed with acute allergic interstitial nephritis with a serum creatinine concentration of 3.6 mg/dl. Upon discontinuation of cat's claw, her renal function improved (serum creatinine 2.7 mg/dl).

Contraindications, Warnings

Cat's claw may interact with immunosuppressive therapy and therefore should be avoided in patients who have received organ transplants, including renal and bone marrow transplants.

Creatine

Herbal Use

Creatine monohydrate is an endogenous compound synthesized by the liver, kidneys, and pancreas from amino acid precursors. It serves as an energy substrate by contributing to the synthesis of adenosine triphosphate. Creatine has proven effective in enhancing muscle performance during brief, high intensity exercise, but has no effect on longer-duration exercise.[39] Much controversy surrounds the use of creatine supplements and their potential to induce renal dysfunction.

Side Effects, Toxicity

Five cases of acute renal failure (ARF) secondary to exercise-induced rhabdomyolysis have been described in men taking performance-enhancing supplements including creatine (5.25 g/day), with or without ephedrine.[40-42] Three patients required dialysis, four developed compartment syndrome, and one died of multiorgan failure within 48 hours of admission.[40] There have been two case reports of direct nephrotoxicity due to creatine. One patient presented with an elevated serum creatinine after 4 weeks of ingesting 5 g of creatine daily. Urinalysis revealed proteinuria, white cell casts, and dysmorphic red cells; in addition, a renal biopsy revealed acute interstitial nephritis, acute tubular necrosis, and focal thickening of the basement membrane with effacement of glomerular foot processes. The patient recovered fully after hydration and discontinuation of the creatine.[43] The second patient had a known nephrotic syndrome with focal segmental glomerulosclerosis (FSGS) and had been in remission for 5 years on cyclosporine.[44] After consuming creatine for 13 weeks, the patient's serum creatinine increased and his GFR decreased significantly. One month after stopping the creatine supplements, the patient's renal function returned to baseline.[44] In contrast to these case reports, several small trials argue against creatine as a nephrotoxic agent.[45-47]

Contraindications, Warnings
Creatine should not be taken by patients suffering from nephrotic syndrome, especially FSGS.

Ground Ivy
Herbal Use
Traditionally, ground ivy has been used for bronchitis, gastritis, and diarrhea.

Side Effects, Toxicity
Ground ivy volatile oil contains many terpenoids and terpene-rich volatile oils, which are an irritant to the gastrointestinal tract and kidneys. However, in comparison with pennyroyal, the overall yield of volatile oil is much less (0.03%-0.06% in ground ivy and 1%-2% in pennyroyal).

Contraindications, Warnings
Excessive doses may be an irritant to the gastrointestinal mucosa and should be avoided by individuals with existing renal disease.

Pregnancy and Lactation
The safety of ground ivy has not been established. In view of the lack of toxicity data and the possible irritant and abortifacient action of the volatile oil, the use of ground ivy during pregnancy and lactation should be avoided.

Horse Chestnut
Herbal Use
Traditionally, horse chestnut has been used for the treatment of varicose veins, hemorrhoids, phlebitis, diarrhea, fever, and enlargement of the prostate gland. The German Commission E approved use of horse chestnut for treatment of chronic venous insufficiency in the legs.

Side Effects, Toxicity
Two incidences of toxic nephropathy have been reported and were stated as probably secondary to the ingestion of high doses of aescin,[48] the main saponin component of horse chestnut. In Japan, where horse chestnut has been used as an antiinflammatory drug after surgery or trauma, hepatic injury has been described in a male patient who received an intramuscular injection of a proprietary product containing horse chestnut.[49]

A proprietary product containing horse chestnut (together with phenopyrazone and cardiac glycoside-containing plant extracts) has been associated with the development of a drug-induced autoimmune disease called "pseudolupus syndrome" in Germany and Switzerland.[50,51] The individual components in the product responsible for the syndrome were not established.

Contraindications, Warnings
Aescin in horse chestnut binds to plasma protein and may affect the binding of other drugs. Horse chestnut should be avoided by patients with existing renal or hepatic impairment.

Pregnancy and Lactation
The safety of horse chestnut during pregnancy and lactation has not been established. In view of the pharmacologically active constituents present in horse chestnut, use during pregnancy and lactation is best avoided.

Lemon Verbena
Herbal Use
Lemon verbena has been used for the treatment of diarrhea, intestinal colic, indigestion, fever, and asthma.

Side Effects, Toxicity
None documented for lemon verbena. Terpene-rich volatile oils are generally regarded as an irritant and may affect the kidney during excretion.

Contraindications, Warnings
Individuals with existing renal disease should avoid excessive doses of lemon verbena in view of the possible irritant nature of the volatile oil.

Pregnancy and Lactation
Because of the lack of pharmacologic and toxicity data and the potential irritant nature of the volatile oil, excessive doses of lemon verbena are best avoided during pregnancy and lactation.

Licorice
Herbal Use
Licorice has been used for bronchitis, chronic gastritis, peptic ulcer, colic, and primary adrenocortical insufficiency.

Side Effects, Toxicity
Excessive or prolonged licorice ingestion has resulted in symptoms typical of primary hyperaldosteronism; namely, hypertension, sodium, chloride and water retention, hypokalemia, and weight gain. It also has resulted in low levels of plasma rennin activity, aldosterone, and antidiuretic hormone.[52,53]

Raised concentrations of atrial natriuretic peptide (ANP), which is secreted in response to atrial stretch and has vasodilating, natriuretic, and diuretic properties, have also been observed in healthy subjects following the ingestion of licorice. Individuals consuming between 10-45 g of licorice a day have exhibited raised blood pressure, together with a block of the aldosterone/rennin axis and electrocardiogram changes, which resolved one month after withdrawal of licorice.[52] Hypokalemic myopathy has also been associated with licorice ingestion.[54,55,56]

In addition, severe congestive heart failure and pulmonary edema have been reported in a previously healthy man who had ingested 700 g licorice over 8 days.[57] It has been noted that symptoms of hyperaldosteronism often resolve quickly, within a few days to two weeks, following the withdrawal of licorice, even in individuals who have ingested the substance for many years.[58]

Contraindications, Warnings

Numerous instances have been documented in which licorice ingestion has resulted in symptoms of primary hyperaldosteronism, such as water and sodium retention and hypokalemia. Licorice should therefore be avoided completely by individuals with an existing cardiovascular-related disorder, and ingested in moderation by other individuals. Hypokalemia is known to aggravate glucose intolerance, and licorice ingestion may therefore interfere with existing hypoglycemic therapy.

Pregnancy and Lactation

In view of the estrogenic and steroid effects associated with licorice, which may exacerbate pregnancy-related hypertension, excessive ingestion during pregnancy and lactation should be avoided.

St. John's Wort

Herbal Use

St. John's wort (SJW) traditionally has been used for wound healing, insomnia, rheumatism, and depression. It is most popular today for the treatment of mild to moderate depression and is widely used for this purpose, usually without medical guidance.

Contraindications, Warnings

SJW is usually well tolerated, but insomnia, dizziness, fatigue, restlessness, gastrointestinal upset, constipation, dry mouth, and allergy are reported as possible side effects.

A major emerging concern with SJW use is the numerous clinically significant herb–drug interactions that have been reported. SJW appears to be a major inducer of the cytochrome P450 3A4 (CYP3A4) enzyme system in the liver.[59,60] This first came to light following acute heart transplant rejection in a person taking cyclosporine and SJW.[60] The cyclosporine levels remained subtherapeutic until SJW was discontinued. Subsequently, more cases were reported in the literature, suggesting an interaction between SJW and tacrolimus in patients following renal transplantation.[61] SJW can adversely affect many other common medications, including nonsedating antihistamines, antifungals, chemotherapeutic agents, and calcium channel blockers.

Pregnancy and Lactation

SJW should be avoided in pregnant and breast-feeding women (it may increase uterine tone) and in children until its safety is further established.

CONCLUSION

Herbal medicines are being used by a large number of people because they are considered to be safe and effective substitute for conventional medicines. Often they may be taken in addition to conventional medicines. Therefore, treating physicians should be aware of any concomitant herbal products and understand the potential hazards associated with the product's use. The current lack of regulation and standardization is an important factor that complicates the use of these products. Herbal products can provide a useful alternative to conventional medicine in chronic non–life-threatening conditions, provided they are safe and of adequate quality.

PART II REFERENCES

1. Evans WC: *Trease and Evans Pharmacognosy*, 14th ed. London: WB Saunders, 1998.
2. Kessler RC et al: Long term trends in the use of complementary and alternative medical therapies in the United States, *Ann Intern Med* 135:262-68, 2001.
3. Eisenberg DM, Davis RB, Ettner SL et al: Trends in alternative medicine use in the United States, 1990-1997: Results of a follow up national survey, *JAMA* 280:1569-75, 1998.
4. Institute of Medical Statistics (IMS) Self Medication International. *Herbs in Europe*. London: IMS Self Medication International, 1998.
5. WHO: *A non regulatory situation of herbal medicines—a world wide review*. Geneva: WHO, 1998:1-45.
6. Vanherweghem, JL et al: Rapidly progressive interstitial renal fibrosis in young women: Association with slimming regimen including Chinese herbs, *Lancet* 341:135-39, 1993.
7. Cosyns JP et al: Chinese herbs nephropathy: A clue to Balkan endemic nephropathy, *Kidney Int* 45:1680-88, 1994.
8. Cosyns JP et al: Urothelial lesions in Chinese-herb nephropathy, *Am J Kidney Dis* 33:1011-17, 1999.
9. Charvill A: Investigation of formulated traditional Chinese medicines (TCM) and raw herbs for the presence of *Aristolochia* species, British Pharmaceutical Conference Science Proceedings 2001. London: Pharmaceutical Press, 2001:295.
10. Bisser NG, editor. *Herbal Drugs and Phytopharmaceuticals* (Wichtl M, ed., German edition). Stuttgart: Medpharm, 1994.
11. Miller L: Selected clinical consideration focusing on known and potential drug-herb interactions, *Arch Intern Med* 158:2200-11, 1998.
12. Brown R: Potential interactions of herbal medicines with antipsychotics, antidepressants, and hypnotics, *Eur J Herb Med* 3:25-28, 1997.
13. Boyle F: Herbal medicines can interfere with breast cancer treatment, *Med J Aust* 167:286, 1997.
14. Seigler DS: Plants of the northeastern United States that produce cyanogenic compounds, *Economic Bot* 30:395-407, 1976.
15. Bever BO, Zahnd GR: Plants with oral hypoglycemic action, *QJ Crude Drug Res* 17:139-96, 1979.
16. Kingwatanakul P, Alon US: Cranberries and urinary tract infection, *Child Hosp Q* 8:69-72, 1996.
17. Siciliano AA: Cranberry, *Herbalgram* 38:51-54, 1996.
18. Avorn J et al: Reduction of bacteriuria and pyuria after ingestion of cranberry juice, *JAMA* 271:751-54, 1994.
19. Jepson RG et al: Cranberries for preventing urinary tract infections (Cochrane Review). In: *The Cochrane Library*, Issue 1, 2000. Oxford: Update Software.
20. Foda MM et al: Efficacy of cranberry in prevention of urinary tract infection in a susceptible pediatric population, *Can J Urol* 2:98-102, 1995.

21. Walker EB et al: Cranberry concentrate: UTI prophylaxis, *J Family Pract* 45:167-68, 1997.
22. Kahn HD et al: Effects of cranberry juice on urine, *J Am Diet Assoc* 51:251-54, 1967.
23. Soloway MS, Smith RA: Cranberry juice as a urine acidifier, *JAMA* 260:1465, 1988.
24. Matsubara T et al: Antihypertensive actions of methylripariochromene A from Orthosiphon aristatus, an Indonesian traditional medicinal plant, *Biol Pharm Bull* 22:1083-88, 1999.
25. Rosenberg S et al: Serum IgE antibodies to psyllium in individuals allergic to psyllium and English Plantain, *Ann Allergy* 48:294-98, 1982.
26. Wilt TJ et al: *Serernoa repens* for treatment of benign prostatic hyperplasia. In: *The Cochrane Library*, Issue 3, 2001. Oxford: Update Software.
27. Ondrizek RR et al: Inhibition of human sperm motility by specific herbs used in alternative medicine, *J Assist Reprod Genet* 16:87-91, 1999.
28. Leape LL, Brennan TA, Laird N, et al: The nature of adverse events in hospitalized patients. Results of the Harvard Medical Practice Study II, *N Eng J Med* 324:277-84, 1991.
29. Malinow MR et al: Systemic lupus erythematosus-like syndrome in monkeys fed alfalfa sprouts: Role of a nonprotein amino acid, *Science* 216:415-17, 1982.
30. Alcocer-Varela J et al: Effects of L-canavanine on T cells may explain the induction of systemic lupus erythematosus by alfalfa, *Arthritis Rheum* 28:52-57, 1985.
31. Roberts JL, Hayashi JA: Exacerbation of SLE associated with alfalfa ingestion, *N Eng J Med* 208:1361, 1983.
32. Chang CH, Wang YM, Yang AH, Chiang SS: Rapidly progressive interstitial renal fibrosis associated with Chinese herbal medications, *Am J Nephrol* 21:441-48, 2001.
33. Lord GM, Tagore R, Cook T, Gower P, Pusey C: Nephropathy caused by Chinese herbs in the UK, *Lancet* 354:481-82, 1999.
34. Lord GM, Cook T, Arlt VM, Schmeiser HH, Williams G, Pusey CD: Urothelial malignant disease and Chinese herbal nephropathy, *Lancet* 358:1515-16, 2001.
35. Tsai CS, Chen YC, Chen HH, Cheng CJ, Lin SH: An unusual cause of hypokalemic paralysis: Aristolochic and nephropathy with fanconi syndrome, *Am J.Med Sci* 330:153-55, 2005.
36. Kelly KJ et al: Methemoglobinemia in an infant treated with the folk remedy glycerited asafetida, *Pediatrics* 73:717-19, 1984.
37. Anon: Boldo leaf oil, *Food Chem Toxicol* 20(Suppl B):643, 1982.
38. Hilepo JN et al: Acute renal failure caused by 'cat's claw' herbal remedy in a patient with systemic lupus erythematosus, *Nephron* 77:361, 1997.
39. Kraemer WJ, Volek JS: Creatine supplementation. Its role in human performance, *Clin Sports Med* 18:651-66, 1999.
40. Kuklo TR, Tis JE, Moores LK, Schaefer RA: Fatal rhabdomyolysis with bilateral gluteal, thigh, and leg compartment syndrome after the Army Physical Fitness Test. A case report, *Am J Sports Med* 28:112-16, 2000.
41. Robinson SJ: Acute quadriceps compartment syndrome and rhabdomyolysis in a weight lifter using high-dose creatine supplementation, *J Am Board Fam Pract* 13:134-37, 2000.
42. Sandhu RS, Como JJ. Scalea TS, Bets JM: Renal failure and exercise induced rhabdomyolysis in patients taking performance-enhancing compounds, *J Trauma* 53:761-63, 2002.
43. Koshy KM, Griswold E, Schneeberger EE: Interstitial nephritis in a patient taking creatine, *N Engl J Med* 340:814-15, 1999.
44. Pritchard NR, Kalra PA: Renal dysfunction accompanying oral creatine supplements, *Lancet* 351:1252-53, 1998.
45. Poortmans JR, Auquier H, Renaut V, Durussel A, Saugy M, Brisson GR: Effect of short-term creatine supplementation on renal responses in men, *Eur J Appl Physioal Occup Physiol* 76:566-67, 1997.
46. Poortmans JR, Francaux M: Long-term oral creatine supplementation does not impair renal function in healthy athletes, *Med Sci Sports Exerc* 31:1108-10, 1999.
47. Robinson TM, Sewell DA, Casey A, Steenge G, Greenhaff PL: Dietary creatine supplementation does not affect some hematological indices, or indices of muscle damage and hepatic and renal function, *Br J Sports Med* 34:284-88, 2000.
48. Grasso A, Corvaglia E: Two cases of suspected toxic tubulonephrosis due to aescine, *Gazz Med Ital* 135:581-84, 1976.
49. Takegoshi K et al: A case of Venoplant R induced hepatic injury, *Gastroenterol Japonica* 21:62-65, 1986.
50. Grob P et al: Drug-induced pseudolupus, *Lancet* 2:144-48, 1975.
51. Russell AS: Drug-induced autoimmune disease, *Clin Immunol Allergy* 1:57-76, 1981.
52. Forslund T et al: Effects to licorice on plasma atrial natriuretic peptide in healthy volunteers, *J Intern Med* 225:95-99, 1989.
53. Conn J et al: Licorice-induced pseudoaldosteronism. Hypertension, hypokalemia, aldosteronopenia, and suppressed plasma rennin activity, *JAMA* 205:492-96, 1968.
54. Cibelli G et al: Hypokalemic myopathy associated with licorice ingestion, *Ital J Neurol Sci* 5:463-66, 1984.
55. Bannister B et al: Cardiac arrest due to licorice-induced hypokalemia, *BMJ* 2:738-39, 1977.
56. Maresca MC et al: Low blood potassium and rhabdomyolysis. Description of three cases with different etiologies, *Minerva Med* 79:79-81, 1988.
57. Chamberlain TJ: Licorice poisoning, pseudoaldosteronism, heart failure, *JAMA* 213:1343, 1970.
58. Mantero F: Exogenous mineralocorticoid-like disorders, *Clin Endocrinol Metab* 10:465-78, 1981.
59. Bolley R, Zulke C, Kammerl M, Fischereder M, Kramer BK: Tacrolimus induced nephrotoxicity unmasked by induction of the CYP3A4 system with St. John's wort, *Transplantation* 73:1009, 2002.
60. Ahmed SM, Banner NR, Dubrey SW: Low cyclosporine A level due to St. John's wort in heart transplant patients, *J Heart Lung Transplant* 20:795, 2001.
61. Rocha G, Poli de Figueiredo CE, d Avila D, Saitovitch D: Depressive symptoms and kidney transplant outcome, *Transplant Proc* 33:3424, 2001.

CHAPTER 68

Extracorporeal Therapies for Poisoning

Guido Filler

INTRODUCTION

Each year a large number of children ingest toxins. Fortunately, the majority of these do not cause permanent damage to the child.[1] The task of the emergency physician is to discern which children are at risk and treat those children with appropriately aggressive therapy while minimizing intervention for the rest. In pediatric exposure cases, the toxin is usually identified. A careful toxic differential diagnosis will lead to a list of likely poisons in symptomatic patients without an identified exposure. Less than 0.05% of all toxic exposures require extracorporeal therapy. Nonetheless, the pediatric nephrologist clearly needs to be able to deal with situations that may benefit from extracorporeal removal of toxins.

Toxins most commonly removed by extracorporeal therapy include lithium, barbiturates, salicylates, and toxic alcohols. The potential benefit of the therapy must not be offset by the common complications of extracorporeal therapy, which include access-related problems, bleeding because of the need for anticoagulation, and hypotension because of extracorporeal blood volume. On the other hand, extracorporeal therapy may well be indicated to control metabolic complications such as metabolic acidosis.

Some drug intoxications require special extracorporeal treatment modalities, depending on the apparent volume of distribution of the toxin and the plasma protein binding. As such, these methods can be life saving. Phenobarbital and theophylline are removed most effectively by charcoal hemoperfusion, although convective clearance can be delivered with modern high-flux dialyzers. This chapter reviews the most common pediatric intoxications, the pharmacologic considerations of the choice of extracorporeal therapies, and common complications.

COMMON INTOXICATIONS

The projected incidence of intoxications in children is approximately 450 per 100,000 population.[2] The likelihood of poisoning differs with age. Intoxications are much more common in children under 6 years of age. Children may ingest a wide variety of toxins. Cosmetics and personal care products are the most common toxins, followed by cleaning products, analgesics, plants, cough and cold preparations, foreign bodies, topical agents, pesticides, vitamins, and hydrocarbons.[3]

Any child with an unexplained altered level of consciousness, respiratory distress, circulatory derangement, seizures, or metabolic abnormalities should be considered for toxic ingestion. Initial therapy of the poisoned child should follow the basic principles of advanced life support, including support of a patent airway and adequate oxygenation, ventilation, and circulation. Ingestion of certain substances requires agent-specific therapy, which may modify the standard resuscitative approach. Knowing the typical signs and symptoms of the common toxic syndromes can help with the identification of the unknown ingested agent.

INDICATIONS FOR ADMISSION AND EXTRACORPOREAL TREATMENTS

According to the American Association of Poison Control Centers (AAPCC), a total of 1.2 million poisonings of children younger than 6 years were reported over a 5-year period, of which 132,055 required treatments in a medical facility.[4] Of these, extracorporeal treatments were utilized in less than 0.05% of cases, with hemodialysis accounting for approximately 90% of interventions. Table 68-1 lists some more common toxins for which extracorporeal removal may be efficacious. Most of these interventions have to commence soon after diagnosis and require 24-hour availability of pediatric nephrologists and other critical care specialists, as well as suitable dialysis equipment, nursing and technician support, and reference laboratory personnel to monitor the efficacy of the treatment.

Only a small proportion of these ingestions face a potentially fatal outcome. For instance, from 1995 to 1998 out of 1.08 million ingestions of toxic substances 56 of these poisonings were fatal. Principal agents involved with fatal poisonings among children less than 6 years of age have been analgesic products (19%), cleaning products (10%), electrolytes and minerals (10%), and hydrocarbons (10%)—as well as antidepressant drugs, insecticides and pesticides, cosmetics and personal care products, stimulants, and a variety of other poisons.[2]

Clearly, a potentially fatal outcome warrants the employment of extracorporeal methods to improve the clearance of the toxin. According to Pond,[5] employing extracorporeal techniques to remove toxins should be considered in cases with a potentially unfavorable outcome—especially if the total body elimination of the toxin can be increased by 30%

TABLE 68-1 Typical Toxins for Which Extracorporeal Therapy Should Be Considered

Toxin	Serum Concentration	Molecular Weight (Daltons)	Volume of Distribution (L/kg)	Plasma Protein Binding
Ethylene glycol*	>50 mg/dl	62	0.6-0.7	Negligible
Lithium†	N/A	74	0.8	Negligible
Methanol‡	>50 mg/dl	32	0.6-0.7	Negligible
Phenobarbital§	N/A	232	0.50-0.88	50%
Salicylates¶	Acute: >100 mg/dl	138	0.15–>0.30 (increases with increasing levels)	50%-90% (decreases with increasing levels)

* Source: Pond SM: Extracorporeal techniques in the treatment of poisoned patients, *Med J Aust* 154:617-22, 1991.
† Source: Garella S: Extracorporeal techniques in the treatment of exogenous intoxications, *Kidney Int* 33:735-54, 1988.
‡ Source: Judge BS. Differentiating the causes of metabolic acidosis in the poisoned patient, *Clin Lab Med* 26:31-48, vii, 2006.
§ Source: Chebrolu SB, Hariman A, Eggert CH, Patel S, Kjellstrand CM, Ing TS: Phosphorus-enriched hemodialysis for the treatment of patients with severe methanol intoxication, *Int J Artif Organs* 28:270-74, 2005.
¶ Source: Agarwal SK, Tiwari SC, Dash SC: Spectrum of poisoning requiring haemodialysis in a tertiary care hospital in India, *Int J Artif Organs* 16:20-22, 1993.

or more. In addition, at least one of the following criteria should be met in order to consider extracorporeal blood purification systems for the removal of a toxin.[6]

- Blood levels or ingested quantities exist that are generally associated with severe or lethal toxicity.
- Clinical evidence of severe and potentially life-threatening toxicity exists, including hypotension, coma, refractory metabolic acidosis, respiratory depression, dysrhythmias, or cardiac decomposition.
- The clinical condition is deteriorating with supportive care.
- The ingested toxin has serious delayed effects that can be diminished with enhanced clearance.
- The natural removal mechanism is impaired.

For some types of intoxications, hemodialysis may result in removal of the toxin and in correction of important complications of the intoxication (such as metabolic acidosis).[7] It is important to consider the potential complications of blood purification methods for the treatment of these patients. For instance, severe methanol intoxication (which clearly serves as an indication for extracorporeal therapy) can be aggravated by treatment-induced hypophosphatemia.[8] Intoxicated patients may be profoundly hypotensive, and the outcome may depend more on adequate management of this complication than on the institution of extracorporeal treatment methods.[9]

MAXIMIZE LESS INVASIVE METHODS FIRST

All less invasive active methods for detoxification should be exhausted before considering extracorporeal treatments. These include oral sorbents, urine alkalization, and forced diuresis.

Oral Sorbents

Oral sorbents (particularly activated charcoal) contribute significantly to the management of poisoning by shortening drug half-life through interruption of enterohepatic circulation of specific agents. This applies particularly in the case of enterohepatic recirculation of drugs that undergo hepatic conjugation, excretion in the bile, and subsequent reabsorption because some drug can be deconjugated by the bowel flora. A good example is phenobarbital.[10]

Based on experimental and clinical studies, multiple-dose–activated charcoal should be considered if a patient has ingested a life-threatening amount of carbamazepine, dapsone, phenobarbital, quinine, or theophylline.[11] Unless a patient has an intact or protected airway, the administration of multiple-dose–activated charcoal is contraindicated. It should not be used in the presence of an intestinal obstruction. The need for concurrent administration of cathartics remains unproven and is not recommended. In particular, cathartics should not be administered to young children because of the potential for laxatives to cause fluid and electrolyte imbalance.

Urine Alkalinization

Urine alkalinization emphasizes that urine pH manipulation rather than a diuresis is the prime objective of treatment. The terms *forced alkaline diuresis* and *alkaline diuresis* should therefore not be used. The principle is based on the fact that most drugs are weak acids or bases in solution. They exist in both nonionized and ionized form. The nonionized molecules are usually lipid soluble and diffuse across the cell membrane by nonionic diffusion, whereas the ionized form usually does not penetrate lipid membranes. In the tubule, many drugs undergo passive tubular reabsorption.

This process involves a bidirectional movement of drugs across the renal tubular epithelium. Especially in the loop of Henle, a favorable concentration gradient is created for net absorption of dissolved materials back into the blood stream. This reabsorption requires little energy and is restricted to lipid-soluble drugs that undergo partial ionization of weak acids. Increasing the pH of urine increases the degree of ionization of weak acids and reduces passive reabsorption. Urine alkalinization is a treatment regimen that increases poison elimination by the administration of intravenous sodium bicarbonate to produce urine with a pH ≥7.5. Urine alkalinization increases elimination of chlorpropamide in urine (dissociation constant [pK_a] 4.8), 2,4-dichlorophenoxyacetic acid (pK_a 2.6), diflunisal, fluoride, mecoprop, methotrexate (pK_a 5.5), phenobarbital (pK_a 7.2), and salicylate (pK_a 3.0).[12-14]

Urine Alkalinization with Diuretics

This is what used to be called forced alkaline diuresis, and it is indicated for the following drugs: phenobarbital (levels >10 mg/dl), barbital (levels >10 mg/dl), and salicylates (levels >50 mg/dl).[15] Forced alkaline diuresis has also been shown to benefit the treatment of 2,4-dichlorophenoxyacetic acid poisoning.[16]

Although the opposite of this approach would theoretically apply to weak base in solution (and one could coin the phrase "forced acid diuresis," which can increase the excretion of drugs such as amphetamines, phenylcyclidine [1-(1-phenylcyclohexyl)piperidine], and quinine), this approach has been abandoned because of the risk of myoglobinuria and the risk of acute renal failure.[17] Altering urinary pH for better clearance of the toxin has to take into account whether the drug exposure itself poses a risk for renal failure; for example, angiotensin-converting enzyme (ACE) inhibitors, which normally are excreted by the kidneys. In utero exposure to ACE inhibitors may result in acute renal failure at birth, thus impairing the biological drug-removal mechanism.

PHARMACOLOGIC CONSIDERATIONS

Before the description of the various blood purification methods for the treatment of poisoning, pharmacologic considerations must be reviewed in order to guide the choice of modality. In particular, the factors favoring drug removal have to be considered. In vivo, the kidney clears substances by both convective clearance and active tubular transport. With regular hemodialysis, solute (and drug) clearance is achieved by diffusive clearance.

Only medications or toxins with low plasma protein binding and a volume of distribution similar to the blood volume (small volume of distribution) can be easily dialyzed with regular hemodialysis. In addition, the ability to dialyze a certain solute (or drug) depends on its size and its lipid solubility.[19] Normally, drugs with a high plasma protein binding (such as vancomycin) cannot be removed with hemodialysis utilizing only diffusive clearance.

Modern high-flux dialyzers have a larger pore size and allow for some convective clearance. For instance, vancomycin clearance was negligible with conventional hemodialysis—whereas there is substantial clearance with high-flux dialysis.[20] Although reviewed elsewhere,[21-22] the main characteristics of the dialyzability of a drug or toxin are briefly reviewed here. It is important to consider the age-dependent changes during childhood.[23]

Size and Charge

With diffusive clearance, small molecules move more rapidly across a concentration gradient. Charge will also affect the clearance. The best clearance will be achieved for small molecules similar to urea (molecular weight = 60 Daltons).

Plasma Protein Binding

The semipermeable dialysis membrane is designed to prevent the loss of large quantities of plasma proteins into the dialysate. Therefore, drugs that are heavily protein bound are not removed by dialysis. Although plasma protein binding is an important factor for the dialysis of a toxin, it is important to point out that some drugs do not saturate the binding sites at the usual pharmacologic concentrations.

Others demonstrate an increase in the ultrafiltrable fraction at high concentrations. This is noted with salicylate poisoning, which is therefore an ideal dialyzable drug despite its high plasma protein binding in lower concentrations.[24] Clearance of drugs that have a high plasma protein binding can be improved using continuous methods[25]—such as continuous venovenous hemofiltration (CVVH)[26] or hemodiafiltration (CVVHDF)[27]—where convective clearance prevails.

Volume of Distribution

The volume of distribution (VD), also known as apparent volume of distribution, is a pharmacologic term used to quantify the distribution of a drug throughout the body after oral or intravenous dosing. It is defined as the volume in which the amount of drug would need to be uniformly distributed to produce the observed blood concentration. VD may be increased by renal failure (due to fluid retention) and liver failure (due to altered body fluid and protein binding).

Conversely, it may be decreased in dehydration. Acetylsalicylic acid has a low volume of distribution and is basically distributed in blood, whereas digoxin has a high volume of distribution and is distributed into intravascular space as well as fat and muscle. Hemodialysis removes only the toxins in the intravascular space. As a rule of thumb, drugs with a volume of distribution of less than 1 L/kg can be removed effectively.

Certain drugs (such as acetaminophen and lithium) have a low plasma protein binding and a relatively low volume of distribution and are therefore easily dialyzable. Lithium is ideal for hemodialysis because it is not soluble in lipids. It is freely distributed in whole-body water, and does not have any plasma protein binding. Its apparent volume of distribution is low (0.8 L/kg), resembling total body water.

It is not present in the dialysate, providing for a continuous concentration gradient both for peritoneal dialysis and hemodialysis. Its clearance is proportional to the blood flow rate, and the modality of dialysis does not really matter.[28] Drugs of larger molecular weight (such as amitriptyline) have a large volume of distribution and are somewhat lipid soluble. Of them, 96.4% are albumin bound. Such drugs are very poorly dialyzable. Table 68-2 lists some data for common drugs, including the volume of distribution and the percentage plasma protein binding.

Based on these considerations, the following drugs can be removed by dialysis: alcohols (ethanol, ethylene glycol, isopropanol, and methanol); analgesics (acetaminophen, colchicine, and salicylates); most antibiotics (amoxicillin, clavulanic acid, penicillin, and ticarcillin), most cephalosporins (aminoglycosides, metronidazole, nitrofurantoin, tetracycline, ciprofloxacin, and imipenem); antiviral medications (acyclovir, foscarnet, and ganciclovir); sedatives and anticonvulsants (barbiturates, carbamazepine, chloral hydrate, and primidone); beta blockers; ACE inhibitors; solvents (acetone, camphor, thiols, and trichloroethylene); and drugs such as lithium, theophylline, paraquat, aniline, boric acid, chromic acid, chlorates, diquat, and thiocyanate.[29]

TABLE 68-2 **Pharmacological Parameters for Common Drug Poisonings**

Drug	Volume of Distribution (L/kg)	Volume of Distribution (Liters in a 70-kg person)	Plasma Protein Binding (%)
Acetaminophen	1.1	77	2-3
Acetylsalicylic acid	0.1-0.2	7-14	50-90
Amitriptyline	15	1050	95
Cyclophosphamide	0.79	55	12
Diazepam	0.95	67	97
Digoxin	6.8	476	2
Digitoxin	0.61	43	93
Ethanol	0.43	30	N/A
Phenobarbital	0.7	49	51
Phenytoin	0.54	38	90
Prednisone	1	70	70-95
Theophylline	0.33-0.74	23-52	59

(From Vande Walle JG, Raes AM, Dehoorne J, Mauel R: Use of bicarbonate/lactate-buffered dialysate with a nighttime cycler, associated with a daytime dwell with icodextrin, may result in alkalosis in children, *Adv Perit Dial* 20:222-25, 2004.)

EXTRACORPOREAL THERAPY

Apart from general considerations regarding the pharmacology of the drug or toxin to be removed, special consideration must be given to smaller children with regard to the choice of extracorporeal therapy. Many centers cannot offer all therapies to very young infants. Limitations may apply because of difficulties with regard to access, minimum blood flow, need to blood prime systems, and so on. The pediatric nephrologist must weigh the potential benefits of a proposed extracorporeal blood purification method against possible downsides. In many centers, peritoneal dialysis (PD) is the method of choice for infants—but there are many limitations.

This chapter cannot deal with all of these in depths and the author refers the reader to the respective sections elsewhere in the book. The pediatric nephrologist must base the therapeutic recommendation on the specific pharmacologic/toxicologic needs of the patient, and on patient suitability and availability of the respective treatment methods in each given center.

In infants, acute PD is probably the most rapid approach[30] (albeit of limited use for a variety of toxins). However, recent advances (especially with widespread availability of continuous methods such as CVVH) may soon broaden its use across all age ranges—providing excellent clearance even for toxins with a higher degree of plasma protein binding.[31]

PERITONEAL DIALYSIS

As pointed out, PD is much less efficient than hemodialysis as far as removal of toxins is concerned. However, it is used for situations in which the feasibility of hemodialysis is limited. A good example is in utero exposure to ACE inhibitors, resulting in postnatal acute renal failure.[32] Lisinopril is only cleared by the kidneys. PD is able to provide for some clearance in anuric patients, allowing for some removal of the drug and thereby improving the outcome.

One major limitation of PD is the fact that until recently the solutions were all lactate based, which precludes its use in patients with lactic acidosis. Several countries do not have the more modern bicarbonate-based PD solutions available.[33] The use of these new bicarbonate-based solutions may also be associated with significant metabolic alkalosis.[34,35] On the other hand, this makes PD an excellent treatment modality for toxin-induced metabolic acidosis.

The current consensus is that PD is an acceptable alternative treatment modality for toxin-induced acute renal failure, but its use for detoxification is limited and the required 30% increase of clearance is often not achievable at the usually prescribed rates of 10 ml/kg every hour.[23] Only drugs such as lithium would be good candidates for PD, but ingestion in infants is less likely. Therefore, peritoneal dialysis can be life saving (but only in specific circumstances).[36]

HEMODIALYSIS

Hemodialysis is the most widely used method for blood purification for the treatment of intoxications. Every pediatric dialysis center should offer hemodialysis with appropriate neonatal or infant tubing, as well as suitable dialyzers to avoid disequilibrium. The consequences of therapy-induced hypophosphatemia have already been discussed.[13] The reader may refer to the various chapters in this book for the technical details.

To maximize the effect, acute hemodialysis should be initiated as soon as possible after the indication is decided. Pediatric nephrology units therefore have to provide around-the-clock coverage with both a dialysis nurse and physician. In some centers, pediatric intensivists provide continuous methods (such as CVVH). The choice of renal replacement therapy (RRT) modality depends on the clinical setting,

TABLE 68-3 **Toxic Agents Removed by High-Flux HD or CVVH and to a Lesser Degree by Regular HD**
Aminoglycosides
Atenolol
Boric acid
Bromide
Carbamazepine
Chloral hydrate (trichloroethanol)
Diethylene glycol
Ethanol
Ethylene glycol
Isopropranolol
Magnesium
Metformin
Methotrexate*
Sotalol
Thallium
Valproic acid

* Should be definitively removed by high-flux hemodialysis.

vascular access, availability of equipment, and experience of the staff.

For drugs such as barbiturates, ethylene glycol, lithium, methanol, salicylates, theophylline, and monobutyl ether, either regular hemodialysis or CVVH can be considered—and the choice should be based on local availability. Drugs with a higher plasma protein binding can be dialyzed efficiently with modern high-flux dialyzers.[37-39] Table 68-3 lists some drugs for which either high-flux hemodialysis or CVVH should be considered.

Most of these patients are ordinarily treated in intensive care units. The choice of access should follow the general guidelines for acute renal failure in children and youth. Jugular dual lumen catheters with free-floating tips are preferred in our unit, but the choice of catheters depends on local availability and expertise. For neonates, two single lumen #5 French catheters may have to be considered. It is important to ensure that the dialysis does not inflict additional harm to the patient.

The choice of blood flow and dialyzer will depend on patient size and local availability. Monitoring of blood levels is important to check the efficacy of the extracorporeal treatment. The nephrologist should calculate the desired drug clearance and should be knowledgeable about the normal toxin half-life in order to prescribe a dialysis prescription that enhances the drug clearance by at least 30%. Patients without uremia should be treated differently than patients with uremia because of the osmotic load in uremia that may lead to disequilibrium with potentially severe complications such as brain edema.[40]

If urea is normal or only mildly elevated, a blood flow of up to 8 ml/kg/minute can be prescribed. For significant uremia owing to intoxication-associated acute renal failure, local protocols will apply. In general, a blood flow of 2 to 3 ml/kg/minute would be chosen in these patients. If available, the blood levels of the toxin should be plotted against time after initiation of dialysis on semilogarithmic paper to monitor the progress of the dialysis—and the dialysis prescription should be adjusted to achieve the desired clearance. The levels are not always indicative of the toxicity. A good example is the fact that lithium levels may not necessarily reflect the outcome in an acute setting.[41]

Clinical features of toxicity are more important than a spot lithium level.[42] In general, patients will be oversampled. Poison control centers are a most valuable ally in the management of these patients. Their value has also been recognized recently in developing nations.[43] It is recommended that case-specific guidelines be requested from the poison control center before implementing any extracorporeal therapy. The duration of treatment should be based on achieving the set targets (e.g., reduction of the levels by 50%). Based on the drug clearance, this may take a long time—and the choice of acute hemodialysis or CVVH should be based on patient stability (tolerance of variability of extracorporeal volume due to discontinuous nature of acute intermittent hemodialysis) and expected duration of treatment.

Acute methanol poisoning would rarely be treated with CVVH, whereas severe methotrexate intoxication may require more long-term treatment and therefore CVVH owing to rebound from other tissues and compartments after discontinuation.[44,45] This depends on the volume of distribution and transfer rates from tissues that may affect the efficacy of the removal, because only the intravascular space can be cleared with hemodialysis.

HEMOPERFUSION

Hemoperfusion is similar to hemodialysis, although the blood passes through a cartridge containing either charcoal or a resin that absorbs the toxin directly. This is different from the diffusive clearance with regular hemodialysis or even convective clearance with high-flux hemodialysis or CVVH. Hemoperfusion effectively eliminates substances that are adsorbed by activated charcoal (or resin). This is a method that should be considered for life-threatening intoxications with substances that are lipid-soluble or have a high molecular weight, making it unlikely that they are filtered through a hollow dialysis fiber.

Phenobarbital[46] and theophylline[47] are effectively removed by activated charcoal hemoperfusion. It was recently shown that conventional hemodialysis could also significantly lower toxic phenobarbital levels.[48] Hemoperfusion provides a higher theophylline clearance rate than hemodialysis. However, hemodialysis appears to have comparable efficacy in reducing the morbidity of severe theophylline intoxication and is associated with a lower rate of procedural complications.

Although regular hemodialysis machines can be used for hemoperfusion, this technique is not as readily available as hemodialysis. Cartridges are not stocked in many pediatric nephrology centers, and familiarity with the technique is limited. The author used the technique previously in a large mid-European center. Complications occur frequently, including hypotension, thrombocytopenia, leukopenia, and electrolyte disturbances.[49]

The priming volume of the cartridges may significantly contribute to the common complication of hypotension. Thrombocytopenia is less common with more modern cartridges.[50] Although some positive reports appear occasionally, especially for amitriptyline,[51] few studies have compared high-flux hemodialysis with hemoperfusion. Before embarking on this therapy in children, the indication should be thoroughly discussed with the poison control center. The pharmacokinetics of most compounds and the overriding importance of supportive care relegate the technique to one of minor importance.[52]

CONTINUOUS EXTRACORPOREAL METHODS

By contrast to hemoperfusion, we will see an increasing use of continuous extracorporeal methods such as CVVH/D. Continuous methods have several advantages, including filters with a larger pore size (up 50,000 Daltons) and better tolerability for unstable patients. This is especially beneficial for drugs/toxins with high transfer rates from nonblood compartments or ongoing rebound due to continued gastrointestinal absorption.

There is growing evidence that for critically ill children with acute renal failure CVVH/D is beneficial and early initiation is indicated, especially in cases with significant fluid overload. This applies to patients with early multiorgan system failure and risk of death, which is not offset by the minimal relative cost of CVVH/D provision because of the potential for improved outcome with initiation of CVVH/D at lesser degrees of fluid overload.[53] Unstable patients tolerate CVVH/D much better than intermittent hemodialysis.[54]

Despite the theoretical advantage, there have been very few studies documenting its usefulness for intoxications.[55] We have certainly used CVVH successfully in children in our center with acute methotrexate poisoning. With continuous methods, the problem of rebound toxicity as the drug reenters the intravascular space becomes insignificant. However, we have encountered problems in delivering adequate clearance and occasionally exceeded turnover rates of 1000 ml/m^2/hour.

Plasmapheresis

Plasmapheresis or plasma exchange removes toxins with high plasma protein binding, but only from the intravascular compartment. Plasma concentrations of toxins are lowered by the plasma volume exchanged. Plasma exchange can enhance elimination of toxins of the following drugs: phenytoin, mercury, paraquat, vanadate, propranolol, maprotiline, tobramycin, amanita phalloides, verapamil, and diltiazem. The method is ineffective for vancomycin, organophosphate agents, thyroxin, digoxin, gentamicin, carbamazepine, and tacrolimus.[56,57]

This method should be considered for removal of drugs such as phenytoin, which cannot be removed by hemodialysis or hemoperfusion. Many centers rely on plasma exchange being performed by centrifugal separators provided by blood services. In our center, pediatric nephrologists perform the plasma exchange using a CVVH machine.[58] For technical details, we suggest the technical paper recently published by Ciechanska et al.[59]

In short, we used the CVVH setup but utilized a plasma filter such as the Asahi plasmaflo, the Baxter Bellco MPS 0.5 m^2, or the plasmaflux PSu2S filter by Fresenius. Either fresh frozen plasma or 5% albumin was used as replacement fluid. The use of the pediatric setup of a CVVH machine in combination with plasma filters allows for child-specific extracorporeal volumes and blood flow rates.

Exchange Transfusion

Exchange transfusion is normally used in newborns for severe immunologic hyperbilirubinemias. In essence, blood is removed from the patient repeatedly—followed by transfusion of a similar quantity from a donor. The procedure can theoretically be used for situations involving hemoglobin toxicity. This may be helpful for parathion, acetaminophen, very high iron levels, caffeine, methyl salicylate, propafenone, ganciclovir, acyclovir, methemoglobin producers, lead, pine oil, and theophylline,[60] but the literature remains scarce.[61]

Liver or Albumin Dialysis

Extracorporeal liver assistance methods that use an albumin dialysate (MARS system)[62] can be used to treat liver failure in patients with hepatic encephalopathy by removing protein-bound and water-soluble toxins. This method can be used in children of all ages, even in infants.[63] Especially for intoxications with amanita phalloides[64,65] and paracetamol,[66] this therapy can be life saving. The method is not widely available yet, and is usually only offered in centers with a liver transplant program.

Recently, a few centers reported on new methods for albumin-enhanced CVVH (e.g., Goldstein's group from Houston, Texas).[67] This group added 25% albumin to a commercially available CVVH replacement solution to make a final albumin concentration of 45 g/L, which resulted in a 48% improvement in carbamazepine clearance.

COMPLICATIONS

It is important to be mindful of the potential for complications. The risk of employing extracorporeal blood purification methods must not exceed the risks of the toxin itself. The complications of extracorporeal elimination encountered most frequently are related to vascular access, hypotension, blood loss, hematomas, metabolic disequilibria, and mechanical problems such as air embolism. In the case of hemoperfusion, they are hypocalcaemia, thrombocytopenia, and leukopenia.

There are very little clinical data available that cite the frequencies of these complications in the pediatric setting. To minimize these complications, the use of these methods should be limited to specialized centers with well-trained intensive care units and 24-hour availability of pediatric nephrology services. Timely implementation of the therapy, when indicated, is critical.

REFERENCES

1. Bond GR: The poisoned child: Evolving concepts in care, *Emerg Med Clin North Am* 13:343-55, 1995.
2. Shannon M: Ingestion of toxic substances by children, *N Engl J Med* 342:186-91, 2000.
3. Litovitz TL, Klein-Schwartz W, Caravati EM, Youniss J, Crouch B, Lee S: 1998 annual report of the American Association of Poison Control Centers Toxic Exposure Surveillance System, *Am J Emerg Med* 17:435-87, 1999.
4. Watson WA, Litovitz TL, Rodgers GC Jr., Klein-Schwartz W, Youniss J, Rose SR, et al: 2002 annual report of the American Association of Poison Control Centers Toxic Exposure Surveillance System, *Am J Emerg Med* 21:353-421, 2003.
5. Pond SM: Extracorporeal techniques in the treatment of poisoned patients, *Med J Aust* 154:617-22, 1991.
6. Garella S: Extracorporeal techniques in the treatment of exogenous intoxications, *Kidney Int* 33:735-54, 1988.
7. Judge BS: Differentiating the causes of metabolic acidosis in the poisoned patient, *Clin Lab Med* 26:31-48, vii, 2006.
8. Chebrolu SB, Hariman A, Eggert CH, Patel S, Kjellstrand CM, Ing TS: Phosphorus-enriched hemodialysis for the treatment of patients with severe methanol intoxication, *Int J Artif Organs* 28:270-74, 2005.
9. Agarwal SK, Tiwari SC, Dash SC: Spectrum of poisoning requiring haemodialysis in a tertiary care hospital in India, *Int J Artif Organs* 16:20-22, 1993.
10. Alkhamis KA, Wurster DE: Study of multiple-component adsorption on the surface of activated carbon using a model system of benzyl alcohol and phenobarbital, *Pharm Dev Technol* 8:127-33, 2003.
11. American Academy of Clinical Toxicology; European Association of Poisons Centres and Clinical Toxicologists. Position statement and practice guidelines on the use of multi-dose activated charcoal in the treatment of acute poisoning, *J Toxicol Clin Toxicol* 37:731-51, 1999.
12. Proudfoot AT, Krenzelok EP, Vale JA: Position paper on urine alkalinization, *J Toxicol Clin Toxicol* 42:1-26, 2004.
13. Winchester JF: Active methods for detoxification. In LM Haddad, MW Shannon, JF Winchester (eds.), *Clinical management of poisoning and drug overdose, third edition*. Philadelphia: W. B. Saunders 1998:175-88.
13. Winchester JF. Active Methods for Detoxification. In: Haddad LM, Shannon MW, Winchester JF. Clinical management of poisoning and drug overdose. 3rd edition. W.B. Saunders Co, Philadelphia, PA, U.S.A, 1998. PP 175-188.
14. Proudfoot AT, Krenzelok EP, Brent J, Vale JA: Does urine alkalinization increase salicylate elimination? If so, why? *Toxicol Rev* 22:129-36, 2003.
15. Pierce RP, Gazewood J, Blake RL Jr.: Salicylate poisoning from enteric-coated aspirin: Delayed absorption may complicate management, *Postgrad Med* 89:61-64, 1991.
16. Prescott LF, Park J, Darrien I: Treatment of severe 2,4-D and mecoprop intoxication with alkaline diuresis, *Br J Clin Pharmacol* 7:111-16, 1979.
17. Penn AS, Rowland LP, Fraser DW: Drugs, coma, and myoglobinuria, *Arch Neurol* 26:336-43, 1972.
18. Filler G, Wong H, Condello AS, Charbonneau C, Sinclair B, Kovesi T, et al: Early dialysis in a neonate with intrauterine lisinopril exposure, *Arch Dis Child Fetal Neonatal Ed* 88:F154-F156, 2003.
19. Maher JF: Principles of dialysis and dialysis of drugs, *Am J Med* 62:475-81, 1977.
20. Touchette MA, Patel RV, Anandan JV, Dumler F, Zarowitz BJ: Vancomycin removal by high-flux polysulfone hemodialysis membranes in critically ill patients with end-stage renal disease, *Am J Kidney Dis* 26:469-74, 1995.
21. Pacifici GM, Viani A: Methods of determining plasma and tissue binding of drugs: Pharmacokinetic consequences, *Clin Pharmacokinet* 23:449-68, 1992.
22. Pinder M, Bellomo R, Lipman J: Pharmacological principles of antibiotic prescription in the critically ill, *Anaesth Intensive Care* 30:134-44, 2002.
23. Routledge PA: Pharmacokinetics in children, *J Antimicrob Chemother* 34(A):19-24, 1994.
24. Furst DE, Tozer TN, Melmon KL: Salicylate clearance, the resultant of protein binding and metabolism, *Clin Pharmacol Ther* 26:380-89, 1979.
25. Agostini M, Bianchin A: Acute renal failure from organophosphate poisoning: A case of success with haemofiltration, *Hum Exp Toxicol* 22:165-67, 2003.
26. Yu C, Liu Z, Gong D, Ji D, Li L: The monocyte dysfunction induced by acute tetramine poisoning and corrected by continuous blood purification, *Arch Toxicol* 79:47-53, 2005.
27. Dargan PI, Giles LJ, Wallace CI, House IM, Thomson AH, Beale RJ, et al: Case report: Severe mercuric sulphate poisoning treated with 2,3-dimercaptopropane-1-sulphonate and haemodiafiltration, *Crit Care* 7:R1-R6, 2003.
28. Peces R, Pobes A: Effectiveness of haemodialysis with high-flux membranes in the extracorporeal therapy of life-threatening acute lithium intoxication, *Nephrol Dial Transplant* 16:1301-03, 2001.
29. Winchester JF: Active methods for detoxification. In LM Haddad, MW Shannon, JF Winchester (eds.), *Clinical management of poisoning and drug overdose, third edition*. Philadelphia: W. B. Saunders 1998:183.
30. Bunchman TE: Acute peritoneal dialysis access in infant renal failure, *Perit Dial Int* 16(1):S509-S511, 1996.
31. Parekh RS, Bunchman TE: Dialysis support in the pediatric intensive care unit, *Adv Ren Replace Ther* 3:326-36, 1996.
32. Bhatt-Mehta V, Deluga KS: Fetal exposure to lisinopril: neonatal manifestations and management, *Pharmacotherapy* 13:515-18, 1993.
33. Fischbach M, Terzic J, Chauve S, Laugel V, Muller A, Haraldsson B: Effect of peritoneal dialysis fluid composition on peritoneal area available for exchange in children, *Nephrol Dial Transplant* 19:925-32, 2004.
34. Vande Walle JG, Raes AM, Dehoorne J, Mauel R: Use of bicarbonate/lactate-buffered dialysate with a nighttime cycler, associated with a daytime dwell with icodextrin, may result in alkalosis in children, *Adv Perit Dial* 20:222-25, 2004.
35. Nau B, Schmitt CP, Almeida M, Arbeiter K, Ardissino G, Bonzel KE, et al: for the European Pediatric Peritoneal Dialysis Study Group. BIOKID: Randomized controlled trial comparing bicarbonate and lactate buffer in biocompatible peritoneal dialysis solutions in children [ISRCTN81137991], *BMC Nephrol* 5:14, 2004.
36. Walsh I, Wasserman GS, Mestad P, Lanman RC: Near-fatal caffeine intoxication treated with peritoneal dialysis, *Pediatr Emerg Care* 3:244-49, 1987.
37. Tapolyai M, Campbell M, Dailey K, Udvari-Nagy S: Hemodialysis is as effective as hemoperfusion for drug removal in carbamazepine poisoning, *Nephron* 90:213-15, 2002.
38. Kielstein JT, Schwarz A, Arnavaz A, Sehlberg O, Emrich HM, Fliser D: High-flux hemodialysis: An effective alternative to hemoperfusion in the treatment of carbamazepine intoxication, *Clin Nephrol* 57:484-86, 2002.
38. Kielstein JT, Schwarz A, Arnavaz A, Sehlberg O, Emrich HM, Fliser D. High-flux hemodialysis–an effective alternative to hemoperfusion in the treatment of carbamazepine intoxication. Clin Nephrol. 2002;57:484-486.
39. Koh KH, Tan HH: High-flux haemodialysis treatment as treatment for carbamazepine intoxication, *Med J Malaysia* 61:109-11, 2006.
40. Keswani SC: Central pontine and extrapontine myelinolysis owing to disequilibrium syndrome, *J Child Neurol* 19:79-80, 2004.
41. Chen KP, Shen WW, Lu ML: Implication of serum concentration monitoring in patients with lithium intoxication, *Psychiatry Clin Neurosci* 58:25-29, 2004.
42. Nagappan R, Parkin WG, Holdsworth SR: Acute lithium intoxication, *Anaesth Intensive Care* 30:90-92, 2002.
43. Laborde A: New roles for poison control centres in the developing countries, *Toxicology* 198:273-77, 2004.

44. Kepka L, De Lassence A, Ribrag V, Gachot B, Blot F, Theodore C, et al: Successful rescue in a patient with high dose methotrexate-induced nephrotoxicity and acute renal failure, *Leuk Lymphoma* 29:205-09, 1998.
45. Ekstrom PO, Andersen A, Warren DJ, Giercksky KE, Slordal L: Determination of extracellular methotrexate tissue levels by microdialysis in a rat model, *Cancer Chemother Pharmacol* 37:394-400, 1996.
46. Lindberg MC, Cunningham A, Lindberg NH: Acute phenobarbital intoxication, *South Med J* 85:803-07, 1992.
47. Shannon MW: Comparative efficacy of hemodialysis and hemoperfusion in severe theophylline intoxication, *Acad Emerg Med* 4:674-78, 1997.
48. Jacobs F, Brivet FG: Conventional haemodialysis significantly lowers toxic levels of phenobarbital, *Nephrol Dial Transplant* 19:1663-64, 2004.
49. Jacobsen D, Frederichsen PS, Knutsen KM, Sorum Y, Talseth T, Odegaard OR: Clinical course in acute self-poisonings: A prospective study of 1125 consecutively hospitalised adults, *Hum Toxicol* 3:107-16, 1984.
50. Singh SM, McCormick BB, Mustata S, Thompson M, Prasad GV: Extracorporeal management of valproic acid overdose: A large regional experience, *J Nephrol* 17:43-49, 2004.
51. Donmez O, Cetinkaya M, Canbek R: Hemoperfusion in a child with amitriptyline intoxication, *Pediatr Nephrol* 20:105-07, 2005.
52. Webb D: Charcoal haemoperfusion in drug intoxication, *Br J Hosp Med* 49:493-96, 1993.
53. Goldstein SL, Currier H, Graf CD, Cosio CC, Brewer ED, Sachdeva R: Outcome in children receiving continuous venovenous hemofiltration, *Pediatrics* 107:1309-12, 2001.
54. Filler G: Acute renal failure in children: aetiology and management, *Paediatr Drugs* 3:783-92, 2001.
55. van Bommel EF, Kalmeijer MD, Ponssen HH: Treatment of life-threatening lithium toxicity with high-volume continuous venovenous hemofiltration, *Am J Nephrol* 20:408-11, 2000.
56. Nenov VD, Marinov P, Sabeva J, Nenov DS: Current applications of plasmapheresis in clinical toxicology, *Nephrol Dial Transplant* 18(5):v56-v58, 2003.
57. Mokrzycki MH, Kaplan AA: Therapeutic plasma exchange: Complications and management, *Am J Kidney Dis* 23:817-27, 1994.
58. Franke D, Zimmering M, Wolfish N, Ehrich JH, Filler G: Treatment of FSGS with plasma exchange and immunoadsorption, *Pediatr Nephrol* 14:965-69, 2000.
59. Ciechanska E, Segal L, Wong H, Chretien C, Feber J, Filler G: Plasma exchange using a continuous venovenous hemofiltration machine in children, *Blood Purif* 23:440-45, 2005.
60. Orlowski JM, Hou S, Leikin JB: Extracorporeal removal of toxins. In TB Erickson, WR Ahrens, SE Aks, CR Baum, LJ Ling (eds.), *Pediatric toxicology: Diagnosis and management of the poisoned child*. New York: McGraw-Hill 2005:137.
61. Osborn HH, Henry G, Wax P, Hoffman R, Howland MA: Theophylline toxicity in a premature neonate: Elimination kinetics of exchange transfusion, *J Toxicol Clin Toxicol* 31:639-44, 1993.
62. Tissieres P, Sasbon JS, Devictor D: Liver support for fulminant hepatic failure: Is it time to use the molecular adsorbents recycling system in children? *Pediatr Crit Care Med* 6:585-91, 2005.
63. Trittenwein G, Boigner H, Mostafa G, Burda G, Muhl A, Amann G, et al: Bridging to transplantation in acute liver failure in a 7-month-old infant, *Wien Klin Wochenschr* 118:298-301, 2006.
64. Shi Y, He J, Chen S, Zhang L, Yang X, Wang Z, et al: MARS: Optimistic therapy method in fulminant hepatic failure secondary to cytotoxic mushroom poisoning; A case report, *Liver* 22(2):78-80, 2002.
65. Rubik J, Pietraszek-Jezierska E, Kaminski A, Skarzynska A, Jozwiak S, Pawlowska J, et al: Successful treatment of a child with fulminant liver failure and coma caused by *Amanita phalloides* intoxication with albumin dialysis without liver transplantation, *Pediatr Transplant* 8:295-300, 2004.
66. Koivusalo AM, Yildirim Y, Vakkuri A, Lindgren L, Hockerstedt K, Isoniemi H: Experience with albumin dialysis in five patients with severe overdoses of paracetamol, *Acta Anaesthesiol Scand* 47:1145-50, 2003.
67. Askenazi DJ, Goldstein SL, Chang IF, Elenberg E, Feig DI: Management of a severe carbamazepine overdose using albumin-enhanced continuous venovenous hemodialysis, *Pediatrics* 113:406-09, 2004.

CHAPTER 69

Pediatric Interventional Radiology

Joao Guilherme Amaral and Bairbre Connolly

INTRODUCTION

Minimally invasive techniques have revolutionized medicine in recent years. Procedures that required a large incision are now performed with external image guidance methods [fluoroscopy, sonography, computed tomography (CT)] or video cameras (laparoscopy, endoscopy, cystoscopy) through a small skin incision. The outcomes of these percutaneous techniques are comparable to or better than open surgical techniques. In addition, these new techniques are less invasive and more cost effective—with shorter recovery times.

This evolution holds true in the diagnosis and management of renal and genitourinary diseases in children. This chapter addresses some of the most common procedures the pediatric interventional radiologist can offer in the renal and genitourinary system, including the following.

- Renal biopsies
- Percutaneous nephrostomies
- Ureteral stenting and dilatation
- Renal angioplasty

The chapter also addresses other interventional procedures (such as gastrostomies and central venous access) that play a role in supportive management of children with renal disease. The indications, contraindications, technique, results, and complications of each procedure are examined. The descriptions in this chapter reflect the current practice in our interventional suites. This practice may vary in other centers.

RENAL BIOPSY

Percutaneous renal needle biopsies are common procedures performed by the interventional radiologist. Iversen and Brun were the first to describe a percutaneous renal biopsy technique using an aspiration needle and placing the patient in a sitting position. In 1954, Kark and Muehrcke described the use of the cutting Vim-Silverman needle on patients in the prone position—with a substantial improvement in their success rate.[1,2] Since then, the technique has evolved and the use of real-time image guidance and automated devices has become standard practice in most interventional departments.

Percutaneous renal biopsy is a safe, inexpensive, and effective tool that provides histologic diagnosis with minimal invasiveness. The main advantages of a pediatric interventional radiologist performing this procedure are expertise in image interpretation and noninvasive image guidance skills.

Sonography is usually the imaging method of choice for guidance in renal biopsies in children. It is readily available, radiation free, and user friendly. It has excellent image resolution due to reduced subcutaneous tissues in children. In addition, it provides multiplanar and real-time visualization of the needle during the biopsy and is not affected by or dependent on renal function.[3] CT or CT fluoroscopy are reserved for rare but special circumstances in which kidney visualization is limited or inadequate with sonography (e.g., patients with severe scoliosis).

Although optimum or adequate visualization is important, it alone does not guarantee or ensure adequate renal biopsy samples. The use of automated devices or biopsy guns helps obtain consistent cores of tissue. These devices are special needles that have a notched central stylet and an outer cutting cannula. After the central stylet is advanced, tissue enters the notch. A semicylindrical tissue core is then cut off by advancement of the outer cannula. Automated devices are fast and easy to use.[4] In addition, although of smaller diameter (18 gauge) than other biopsy systems (14 or 16 gauge), these automated devices usually provide sufficient tissue for diagnosis. The smaller gauge is associated with less renal trauma and a potential reduction of bleeding complications.[5,6]

Adequate specimens for histologic diagnosis can be obtained in 91% to 99% of renal biopsies in children.[6-12] In fact, Fenenberg and colleagues reported in a large series of 1081 renal biopsies in children over a 27-year period that the advent of ultrasound and automated biopsy devices increased biopsy adequacy from 69% to 92%.[13] The size of the biopsy needle was one of the concerns regarding sample adequacy, but several studies have shown that 18-gauge devices provide adequate renal cores for pathologic diagnosis.[10,14]

Diffuse parenchymal renal disease (presenting as nephritic syndrome, nephrotic syndrome, or acute or chronic renal failure) is the most common indication for biopsies in native kidneys, whereas exclusion of rejection is the most common indication in transplant kidneys. Depending on protocols or trials, currently renal tumors such as Wilm's are frequently not biopsied because primary complete resection is preferred to avoid tract seeding. However, in cases of massive tumors that may benefit from neoadjuvant chemotherapy before surgery[15] and in cases of bilateral renal tumors (Figure 69-1) or suspicion of benign masses (e.g., angiomyolipomas) a biopsy is sometimes warranted. The most important contraindication to any renal or renal tumor biopsy is an uncorrect-

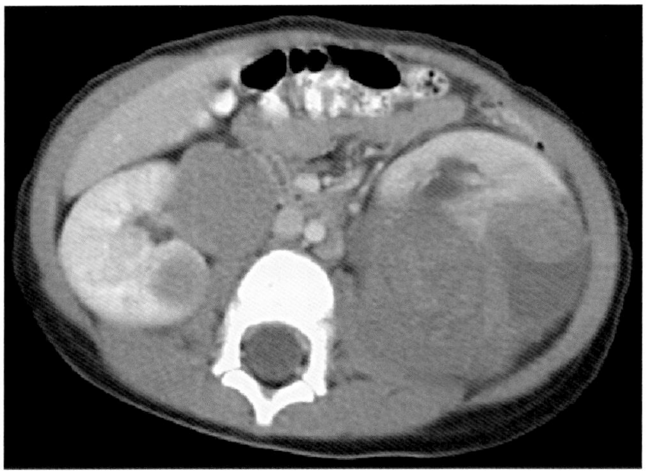

Figure 69-1 Three-year-old girl with bilateral renal tumors. This child had sonographic-guided biopsies performed on the left kidney, confirming the diagnosis of Wilms' tumor prior to chemotherapy.

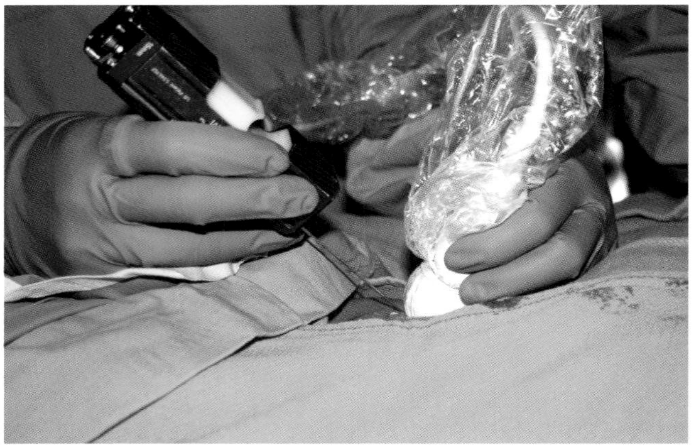

Figure 69-2 Sonographic-guided biopsy with "freehand" technique. Note that the needle of the biopsy gun is in the same imaging plane as the sonography probe.

able coagulation abnormality. Severe hypertension is a relative contraindication because it increases the risk of complications postbiopsy. Such complications are bleeding, renal damage, and arteriovenous fistula formation.

The day before the procedure, the interventional radiologist (or person performing the biopsy) ideally should see the patient and family in a clinic visit. This is an excellent opportunity to explain the procedure and its risks and benefits and to obtain informed consent. This also affords the patient and family an opportunity to meet the physician performing the procedure and to ask questions. All patients are then assessed to determine if they are suitable for sedation or require general anesthesia. A bleeding history is obtained, and a coagulation profile and complete blood count are ordered in all patients.

The patient's blood is typed and screened in case a transfusion is necessary. Acceptable values for renal biopsy are a normal partial thromboplastin time (PTT) for patient's age; international normalized ratio (INR), the standardized reporting of prothrombin time (<1.3); and platelets above $100,000 \times 10^6$/L. Abnormal values require correction. It is our practice to perform a mapping sonography to verify the presence of both kidneys and the absence of renal pelvis dilatation, and to mark the probable biopsy site on the skin.

On the day of the procedure, a urine sample is obtained to assess the presence of gross or microscopic hematuria prebiopsy. Local anesthetic cream is applied to the skin for approximately 20 to 60 minutes, intravenous access is obtained, laboratory values are checked, and baseline vital signs are recorded. The child is placed in a prone position with a roll under the abdomen. Most patients are sedated by an interventional radiology nurse who constantly monitors the vital signs (blood pressure, heart rate, oximetry, electrocardiogram, respiratory rate). Antibiotic prophylaxis is not routinely used unless the patient requires endocarditis prophylaxis. The skin is then prepared and draped in a sterile fashion.

The entire procedure is performed under real-time sonographic guidance using a "freehand" technique or needle guidance system. We use the former technique, in which one hand controls the needle and the other controls the ultrasound transducer (Figure 69-2). This technique gives greater flexibility to the operator but requires more expertise. The alternative method is to use needle guides attached to the transducer. The subcutaneous tissues and muscle planes are infiltrated with local anesthetic (lidocaine 1% buffered with sodium bicarbonate – concentration = 9 : 1) and a small incision is made on the skin.

The biopsy needle is then advanced under sonographic guidance to the edge of the lower pole of the kidney to obtain a maximum amount of cortex and to avoid the central sinus and the main renal vessels. The renal biopsy is then performed with an 18-gauge spring-loaded automated side-cutting needle. In our practice, we use a Bard Magnum reusable core biopsy system. Two passes are performed, obtaining cortex and medulla of the kidney (Figure 69-3). Care is taken not to transgress the renal pelvis, to avoid gross hematuria or urinoma formation.

After the biopsy, manual compression is applied for approximately 5 minutes at the biopsy site—and a repeated ultrasound is done to see if there is a perinephric hematoma. If active bleeding is noticed (Figure 69-4), manual compression is reapplied at the bleeding site, directed by sonography. If no bleeding or a small contained hematoma is seen, the patient is positioned supine and a sandbag is placed under the site of the biopsy to maintain pressure.

Bed rest is recommended for at least 6 hours. Vital signs are monitored for 6 to 8 hours. The urine is monitored for the presence of macroscopic hematuria. Intravenous fluids and diet are managed by the referring nephrologist. Pain is generally controlled with mild analgesics such as acetaminophen or low doses of opioids. Antiemetic medications are prescribed if the patient develops nausea or vomiting.

Patients are monitored for at least 8 hours in the hospital, and a complete blood count is done 4 to 6 hours postprocedure to check hemoglobin levels. If the patient is stable, has voided at least two times, and has no complications after 8

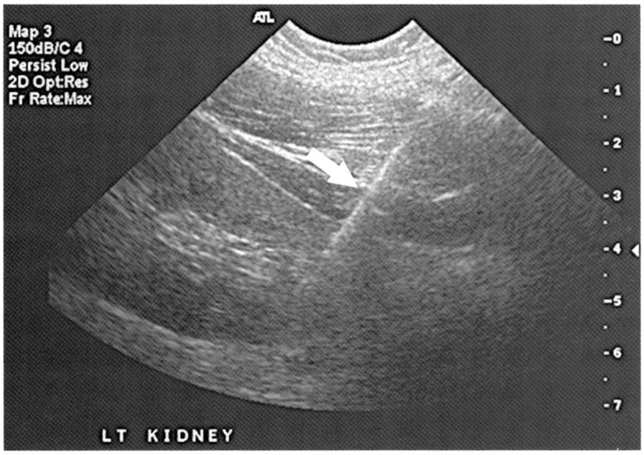

Figure 69-3 Fourteen-year-old girl with systemic lupus erythematosus undergoing a renal biopsy. Note needle *(arrow)* at the lower pole of the left kidney. Biopsy obtained predominantly from the cortex of the kidney showing lupus nephritis.

hours, he/she may be discharged.[3] If a significant hemoglobin drop is detected or if gross hematuria occurs, clinical evaluation is complemented by an ultrasound to assess for perinephric or retroperitoneal bleed. These patients remain on bed rest in the hospital overnight. The patient's vital signs (blood pressure, heart rate) continue to be closely monitored. If hemodynamic instability develops, the patient is properly resuscitated with intravenous fluids, kept nil by mouth, and again imaged with ultrasound or CT. In cases of uncontrollable active bleeding or growing pseudoaneurysm, an angiogram and embolization are performed to control the bleeding. The last recourse is a surgical intervention and possible nephrectomy.

Patients are advised to avoid sports contact or too much activity for 2 weeks, and to return to the hospital if there is any change in clinical status or development of gross hematuria. Patients are also provided with contact phone numbers (nephrologist and interventional radiologist on call) in case of an emergency, and a follow-up phone call is made the day after the biopsy to assess any changes or concerns.

Overall, complication rates of 1% to 21%[3,13,16-19] are reported in the literature after renal biopsies. Pain is not infrequent. Bohlin and colleagues reported an incidence of painful body movements in 37% of children submitted to a renal biopsy.[7] Therefore, pain and discomfort should be addressed in all children—especially in younger children for whom pain is difficult to assess. Bleeding is the most commonly reported complication. It can present as hematuria or retroperitoneal hemorrhage (Figure 69-4). In the majority of cases, bleeding is minor and requires no treatment. Transient macroscopic hematuria is seen in 0.8% to 12% of patients.[3,7,12,13,20,21] It usually lasts for 2 days and has no lasting effects on patients.

Retroperitoneal small perinephric hematomas, detected by sonography, are not uncommon[7] and are probably present in almost all patients. However, only a few are symptomatic.[13] Significant bleeding requiring transfusion, endovascular intervention, or surgery occurs in 0.3% to 0.6%.[3,13,20] Arteriovenous fistulae (Figure 69-5) are detected in 4% to 18% of cases, but most are asymptomatic[22] and resolve spontaneously (Figure 69-6). Infections are rare and occur generally in patients with urinary infection prior to the biopsy.[10] For elective renal biopsies, the presence of infection is usually a contraindication. The mortality rate from a renal biopsy is estimated at 0.08% to 0.1%.[13,23]

Renal biopsies in infants are more challenging due to the increased mobility of the kidney and its superficial nature and lack of supporting surrounding tissues. In our experience, general anesthesia is typically required in children less than 2 years of age.

PERCUTANEOUS NEPHROSTOMY

Percutaneous nephrostomy (PCN) is a procedure that creates a communication between the skin and the renal collecting system. Godwin and colleagues were the first to describe this procedure, in 1955.[24] Since then, PCN has supplanted surgery as the primary procedure for temporary drainage of an obstructed collecting system. It provides low-pressure drainage of the upper urinary system, enabling treatment of urosepsis and improvement in renal function prior to definitive therapy of the underlying obstructive condition.

PCN is a fundamental urinary tract access technique.[25,26] It may be the definitive procedure or a first step prior to more complex procedures. The most common indication is rapid relief of a hydronephrotic collecting system due to ureteropelvic junction (UPJ) obstruction (Figure 69-7), UPJ obstruction with a single functioning kidney, ureterovesical junction (UVJ) obstruction, obstruction after pyeloplasty, obstruction after lithotripsy, posterior urethral valves (PUV), primary obstructing megaureter, or external compression of ureters (e.g., solid tumors, lymphoma).[27] Other important indications include the following:

- Drainage of an infected collecting system (pyonephrosis), reducing the risk of sepsis.
- PCN is also performed to divert urine from the renal collecting system in order to heal distal fistulas, urinomas, or leakages (Figure 69-8).
- To divert urine in cases of hemorrhagic cystitis.
- To create a percutaneous tract for further intervention in the kidney and collecting system (nephrolithotomy, antegrade ureteral stent insertion, ureteral dilatation, retrieval of foreign bodies, endopyelotomy for UPJ obstruction, urothelial brush biopsy).
- To infuse medications (e.g., antifungal, antibacterial, antitumor drugs) directly in the collecting system, reducing systemic drug effects.
- To assess the potential for recovery in a chronically obstructed kidney (a substantial increase in renal plasma flow within 10 days after decompression of an obstructed kidney is a reliable predictor of recovering renal function).[28]

The only contraindications are uncorrectable bleeding diathesis, clotting deficiency, and unfavorable anatomy. However, if the coagulopathy is caused by urosepsis urinary drainage may be necessary before the bleeding abnormality is corrected. Severe electrolyte changes (hyperkalemia, metabolic acidosis) are also a relative contraindication and should be treated before PCN and may even require emergent hemodialysis.

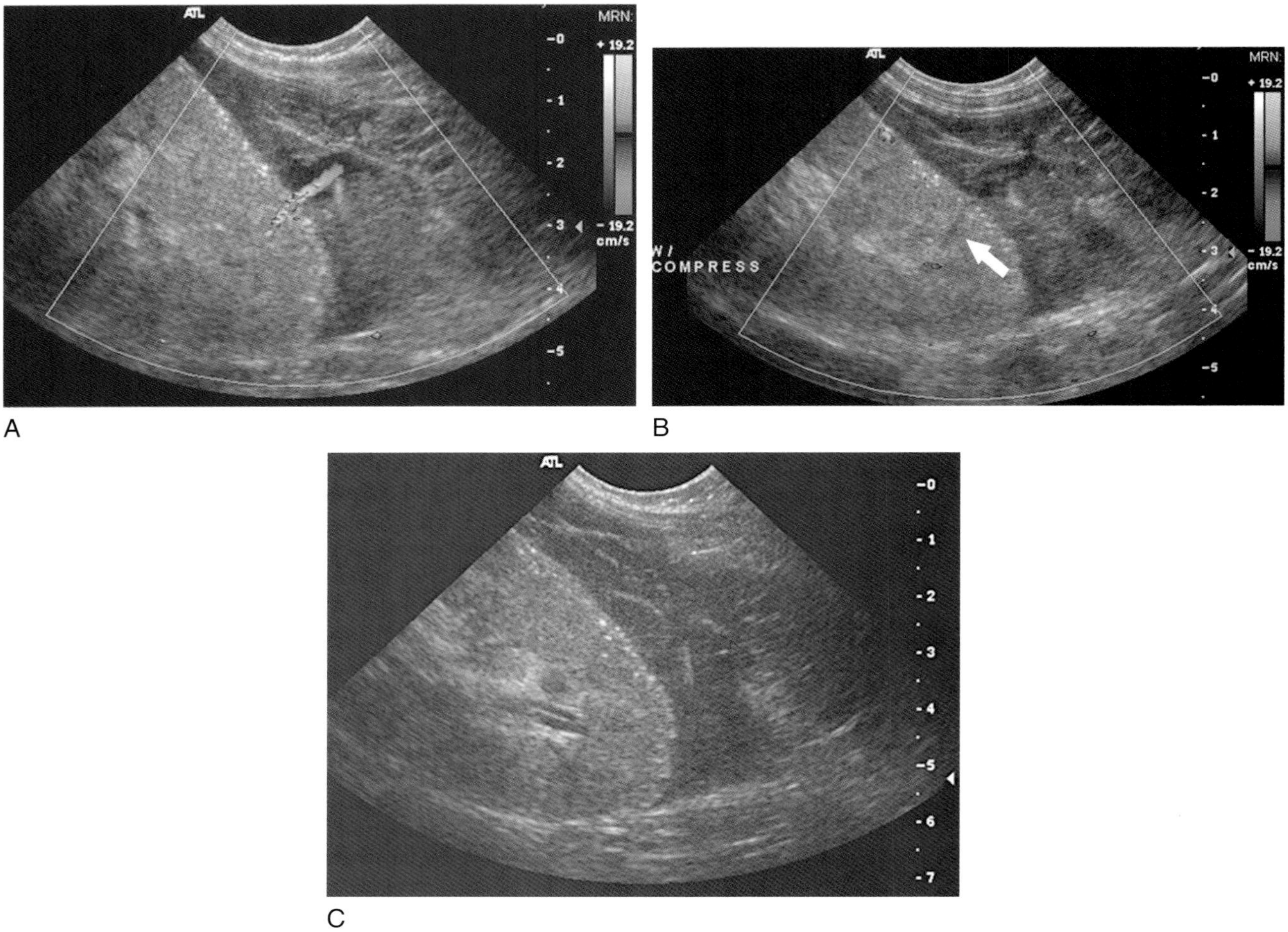

Figure 69-4 Sixteen-year-old boy with untreated transposition of the great vessels. **A,** Sonography immediately postrenal biopsy shows active bleeding on color Doppler images from an intrarenal vessel into an expanding perinephric hematoma. **B,** Spontaneous arrest of active bleeding after direct compression on the biopsy site under sonographic guidance. Note biopsy tract *(arrow)* with no active bleeding. **C,** Residual large perinephric/retroperitoneal hematoma 1 day later. Patient did not require any intervention. Pathology: chronic glomerular and interstitial vessel damage related to chronic venous hypertension and endothelial damage.

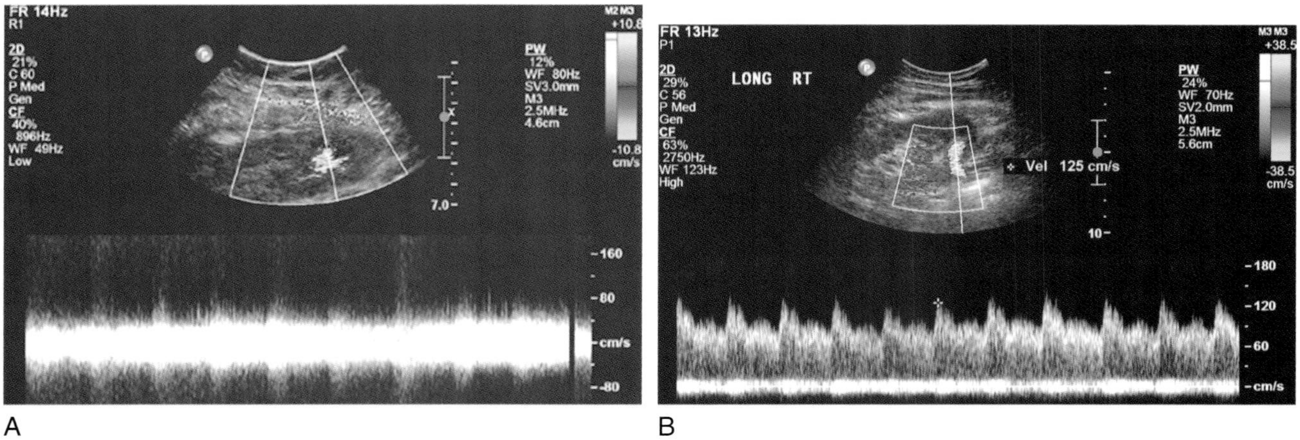

Figure 69-5 Fifteen-year-old boy postrenal transplant for chronic renal failure secondary to bilateral renal vein thrombosis at birth. **A,** Pulsed and color Doppler image showing turbulent flow in the lower pole of the transplant kidney after a renal biopsy, in keeping with an arteriovenous fistula. **B,** Pulsed and color Doppler image demonstrating arterialization of the efferent vein.

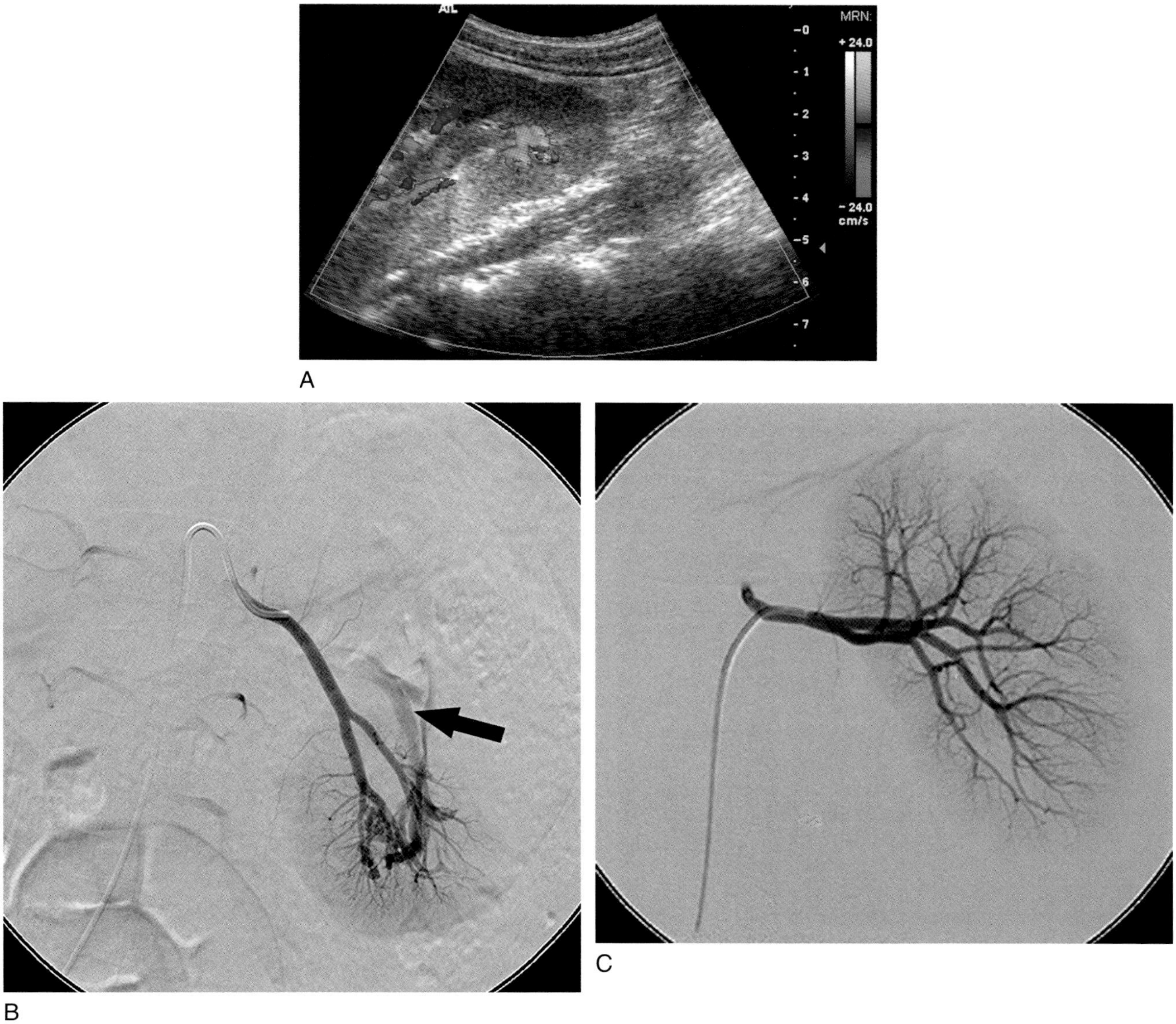

Figure 69-6 Nine-year-old boy with acute renal failure and hypertension due to vasculitis. **A,** Color Doppler sonographic image of an incidental pick up of an arteriovenous fistula of the lower pole of the left kidney, following a renal biopsy. **B,** Angiogram showing an arteriovenous fistula with early draining vein *(arrow)*. **C,** Follow-up angiogram 6 months later, showing spontaneous resolution of the arteriovenous fistula.

Placement of nephrostomies in dilated collecting systems has a high success rate, ranging between 98% and 100%.[29-38] Success rates in nondilated collecting systems are slightly lower, in the range of 85% to 90%.[39] Patients with dilated collecting systems complicated with urosepsis or azotemia have an almost immediate response after PCN drainage. Pain and fever generally improve in 24 to 48 hours.[40] In addition, the mortality rate from gram-negative septicemia in patients with urinary obstruction reduces fivefold after drainage.[41] Patients with impending renal failure may return to normal or almost normal renal function on average within a week after drainage.[42]

Preprocedural evaluation includes a clinical history to identify a potential bleeding tendency, complete blood count, platelets, PTT, and INR to assess bleeding risk.[43-45] The use of routine blood tests is controversial, and some authors believe a careful clinical history of bleeding disorders, renal failure, liver disease, and use of antiplatelet drugs and anticoagulants is sufficient to perform the procedure.[32] In our practice, we routinely use laboratory blood tests to assess bleeding risk. Accepted values include an INR <1.3, a normal PTT for age, and a minimum platelet count >50,000 × 10^9/L in the emergency situation.[46]

Abnormal coagulation parameters may require correction with fresh frozen plasma, vitamin K, or platelets. If the patient is on heparin infusion, discontinuation for at least 2 hours is recommended. If the patient is on low-molecular-weight heparin, discontinuation for 12 hours is required. If the patient is taking aspirin or other drugs that interfere with platelet function (nonsteroidal antiinflammatories, beta-

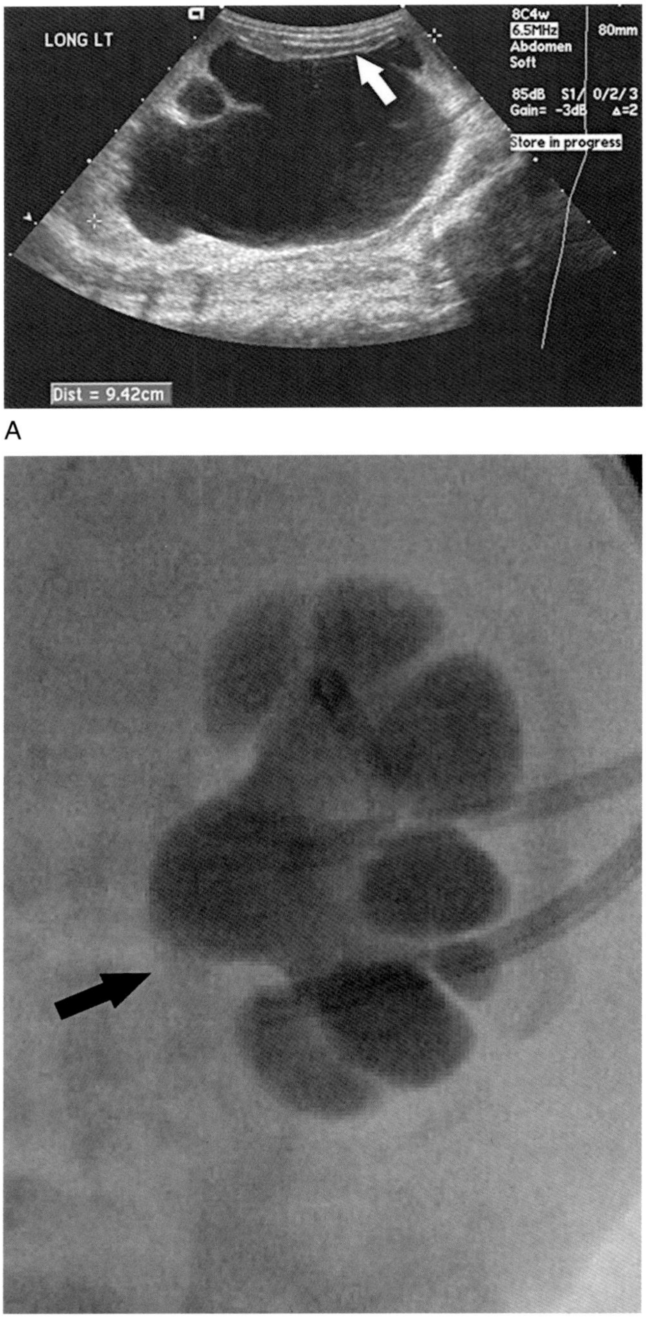

A

B

Figure 69-7 Neonate with ureteropelvic junction obstruction presented in renal failure and required emergent nephrostomy. **A,** Sonographic image showing thinned renal parenchyma *(white arrow)* with significant pelvicaliceal dilatation. **B,** Nephrostogram showing a dilated renal pelvis with an area of narrowing in the region of the ureteropelvic junction *(black arrow)* Note nephrostomy tube in situ and external catheter of central venous line overlying the image.

lactam antibiotics) and the PCN is elective, the procedure is postponed for 5 to 7 days.

Urea, creatinine, urinalysis results, and urine culture and sensitivity are reviewed—as well as any previous imaging studies [sonography, CT, magnetic resonance imaging (MRI), nuclear medicine]. In children with complex abnormal anatomy (scoliosis, congenital malformation) and in situations of poor visualization of the kidney, cross-sectional images are recommended before PCN to determine the relationship of the kidney to the colon, small bowel, spleen, liver, gallbladder, and pleura.

Antibiotic prophylaxis is used in all patients. Common urinary pathogens include *E. coli*, *Proteus*, *Klebsiella*, and enterococcus. Therefore, a broad-spectrum antibiotic is administered less than 2 hours before the procedure. The timing of administration is very important because the risk of infection-related complications increases fivefold if the antibiotics are given more than 3 hours prior to the procedure.[47] Some authors suggest that antibiotics be continued for 24 to 48 hours in patients with a low risk for developing sepsis and for 48 to 72 hours in high-risk groups (diabetics, struvite stones, urinary tract obstruction, urinary tract instrumentation, indwelling catheters).[45] High-risk cardiac patients require specific endocarditis prophylaxis.

In our practice, most nephrostomy procedures are performed under general anesthesia. However, other centers have used conscious sedation and local anesthesia to perform nephrostomies successfully.[26,27,48] The patient is placed in a prone or prone-oblique position with the ipsilateral side elevated 20 to 30 degrees, and the access site is mapped using sonography. A posterolateral approach (needle 30 to 45 degrees with respect to the table surface) is preferred to avoid vital structures such as colon, liver, or spleen.[25] The skin is prepped and draped in a sterile fashion.

The subcutaneous tissues are infiltrated with local anesthetic to minimize discomfort after the procedure, and a small skin incision (5 mm) is made to facilitate access. The Brodel's plane of least vascularity (renal artery division into major anterior and posterior branches at the junction of the anterior 2/3 and posterior 1/3 of an axial view of the kidney) is identified using color Doppler sonography, and under real-time sonographic guidance a calyx is punctured through the renal parenchyma. Direct puncture of the renal pelvis or infundibulum is avoided to minimize the chance of interlobar and main renal vessel damage.[49] It also reduces the chance of urine leak or loss of access due to lack of supporting parenchyma.[4,26]

Alternatively, fluoroscopic guidance alone or CT and CT fluoroscopy can be used as imaging guidance methods when a radio-opaque calyceal calculus is present or when the pelvicaliceal system is opacified by contrast (intravenous or retrograde injections). Caution should be exercised regarding radiation exposure and contrast nephropathy, especially in children, when using CT and fluoroscopy.

Access is obtained with a small-gauge needle (usually 22-gauge Chiba Hi-lighter). In nondilated systems, the use of an intravenous fluid bolus or diuretic agents may be helpful[50] to distend the collecting system and facilitate renal access. The needle's stylet is removed, and a small urine sample is obtained and sent for culture and sensitivity. Care should be taken not to completely decompress the collecting system, because renal access may be accidentally lost. A minimal amount of contrast is then injected to confirm the needle's position in the renal pelvis. A 0.018-inch stainless steel Mandril wire or nitinol guidewire is then advanced under

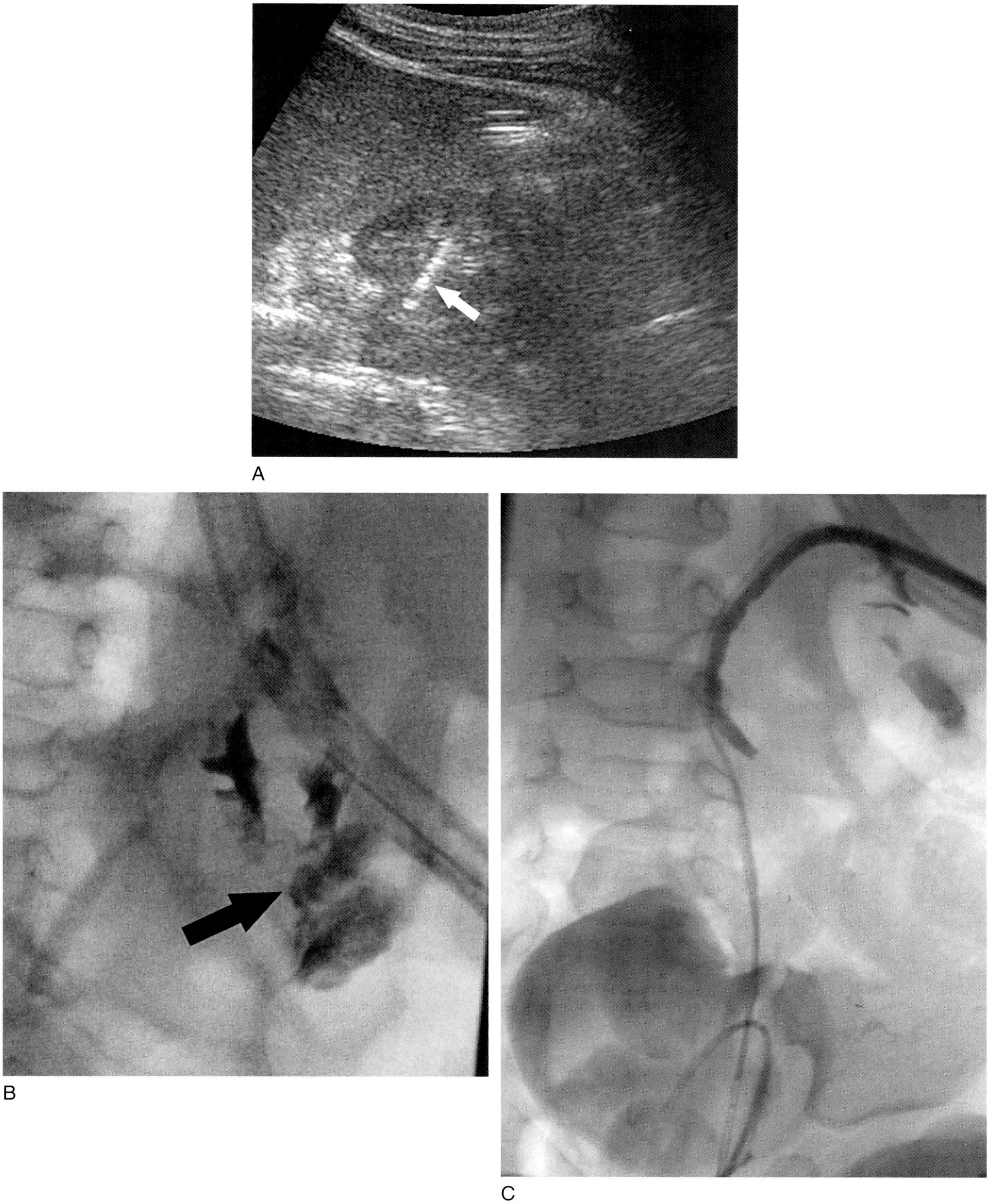

Figure 69-8 Two-year-old patient with multiple Wilms' tumors involving both kidneys. Urine leak post partial resection of the right kidney. Image-guided urinary diversion to treat urine leak. **A,** Sonographic transverse view of the kidney with needle *(arrow)* in the medullary region of an empty collecting system. **B,** Contrast injected in the renal pelvis with perinephric extravasation from the lower pole of the kidney *(arrow)* into the area of the Jackson Pratt drain. **C,** Number 8 French external nephrostomy and internal double J stent placed to divert urine from the pelvicaliceal fistula.

fluoroscopic guidance into the ureter or left coiled in the renal pelvis.[26] A Neff set or an Accustick introduction system is then used to upsize the tract, and a 0.035-inch or 0.038-inch guidewire (Benston, Amplatz, superstiff Amplatz, Glidewire) is positioned in the ureter or renal pelvis.

Alternatively, initial access is obtained directly with a 19-gauge BSDN needle or a 16-gauge angiocatheter—and a 0.035-inch guidewire (Benston, Amplatz, Glidewire) is advanced into the renal pelvis. This approach has the advantage of minimizing the number of tract manipulations, which reduces the risk of losing renal access or forming perinephric urinomas. The main disadvantage is that a larger access needle is required, increasing the risk of bleeding complications. Koral and colleagues[27] advocate this technique in neonates and young children with dilated collecting systems due to the risk of rapid decompression or dissection of the renal pelvis during serial tract dilatations. It is important to remember that PCN in neonates and young infants is more challenging than in the older child.

The tract is then dilated progressively with fascial dilators (e.g., Coons dilators) up to the appropriate French size, and finally a nephrostomy tube is advanced and placed in the renal pelvis. Once the tube is safely in the collecting system, the inner trocar and the guidewire may be removed and the retention mechanism reformed. A small amount of contrast is then injected to confirm the tube's position (Figure 69-9).

Multiple nephrostomy tube designs are available, differing mainly in the type of retention mechanism. The two basic shapes are a Malecot (tulip tip) and a locking pigtail tip (Figure 69-10). Malecot catheters retract slightly after insertion, allowing the sides to flare out beyond the external diameter of the catheter. Pigtail-locking catheters have a distal loop that is reformed by pulling a string after tube insertion in the renal pelvis. Tube size is chosen at the discretion of the interventional radiologist. Neonates are generally drained with a number 5 or 6 French drain. Older children are drained with numbers 8 to 12 French drains, depending on the characteristics of the fluid drained.

In addition to the tube check, a diagnostic nephrostogram may be indicated. When performing the nephrostogram, the system should not be overdistended—to lessen the risk of renal rupture (i.e., Figure 69-11). If there are any signs of infection, a nephrostogram is not performed to reduce the chance of bacteremia and sepsis. The nephrostomy tube is left open for drainage, the patient is treated with antibiotics, and the nephrostogram is deferred for 48 to 72 hours.

Vital signs are routinely checked for 6 to 8 hours, and then according to the patient's clinical status. Patients are kept on bed rest for 6 hours. Diet is allowed as tolerated, always starting with clear fluids because some patients have nausea and vomit after the anesthetic or sedation. Pain and fever are treated symptomatically, and antibiotics are continued for 24 to 72 hours postprocedure. Input and output from the nephrostomy is monitored. Following relief of obstruction, a post-obstructive diuresis may develop (and should be anticipated). It is our practice to flush the tube with 5 cc of normal saline every 8 hours to maintain tube patency.

If the patient develops gross hematuria or drainage of blood through the PCN, a nephrostogram is done to assess any communication between the tube and a major vessel (artery or vein). Most PCN are inpatient procedures. However, in a selected group of children and adolescents they can be performed as outpatient procedures. Candidates should have no signs of infection, no coexistent medical problem, and adequate renal function prior to the procedure. In addition, parents should be capable of caring for the PCN tube and have easy access to medical care near their homes.[48]

Overall, 10% of patients will develop a minor or major complication after PCN.[38] The reported mortality rate of PCN is approximately 0.2%.[39] Hemorrhage requiring transfusion is reported in 1% to 2.4% of cases,[29,30] generally due to renal artery pseudoaneurysms[51] or arteriovenous fistulas.[52] Most hemorrhages are self-limited and need no intervention. Some patients will require transfusion of blood or blood products (fresh frozen plasma [FFP], platelets) to help stop the bleeding. In uremic patients, desmopressin may be used to improve platelet function. If gross blood drains through the nephrostomy or large clots are seen in the nephrostogram, the PCN should be flushed with cold saline. The nephrostomy catheter may need to be upsized (at least 2 French sizes) in an attempt to tamponade the source of bleeding. Angiography and embolization should be considered in patients with persistent or recurrent bleeding after 3 to 5 days of PCN insertion. Finally, if the hematocrit drops without gross hematuria cross-sectional imaging (US, CT) is recommended to assess retroperitoneal bleeding.[53] Sepsis after PCN is reported in 0.5% to 3.5% of all cases.[29,30,33,41] However, if pyonephrosis is considered separately as the indication, 7% of the patients will develop sepsis despite appropriate antibiotic prophylaxis.[40,54,55] Other major complications include pneumothorax (1%),[29] pleural effusion, pneumonia, air embolism,[56] inadvertent injury to adjacent organs (colon,[57] duodenum, spleen), and peritonitis.

Minor complications are not uncommon, including microscopic hematuria (which usually clears within 48 hours), pain, fever, perirenal hematoma, self-limited urine extravasation, and catheter-related problems. Catheter dislodgement rates range from 1% to 30%,[29,30] depending on the length of time the PCN is necessary. Blockage may occur in 1% of patients. Flushing the tube regularly and high fluid intake may help prevent this complication.

NEPHROSTOMY TRACT DILATATION FOR ENDOUROLOGIC PROCEDURES

Image-guided percutaneous nephrostomy is a bridging technique for a variety of urinary tract interventions. Small nephrostomy tracts created for simple drainage (numbers 6 to 12 French) must be enlarged to at least numbers 20 to 24 French diameters to accommodate endourologic equipments. Nephrostomy tract dilatation is generally performed before percutaneous nephrolithotomy (using methods such as mechanical, laser fiber, or ultrasonic lithotriptor), and in some centers percutaneous pyeloplasty for UPJ obstructions. The main contraindication to tract dilatation is bleeding diathesis.

It is important to keep the child's size in mind when choosing the diameter of the sheath because disproportionate dilatation of the tract may lead to renal rupture or fracture. Close communication between the interventional radiologist and the urologist performing the endourologic procedure is

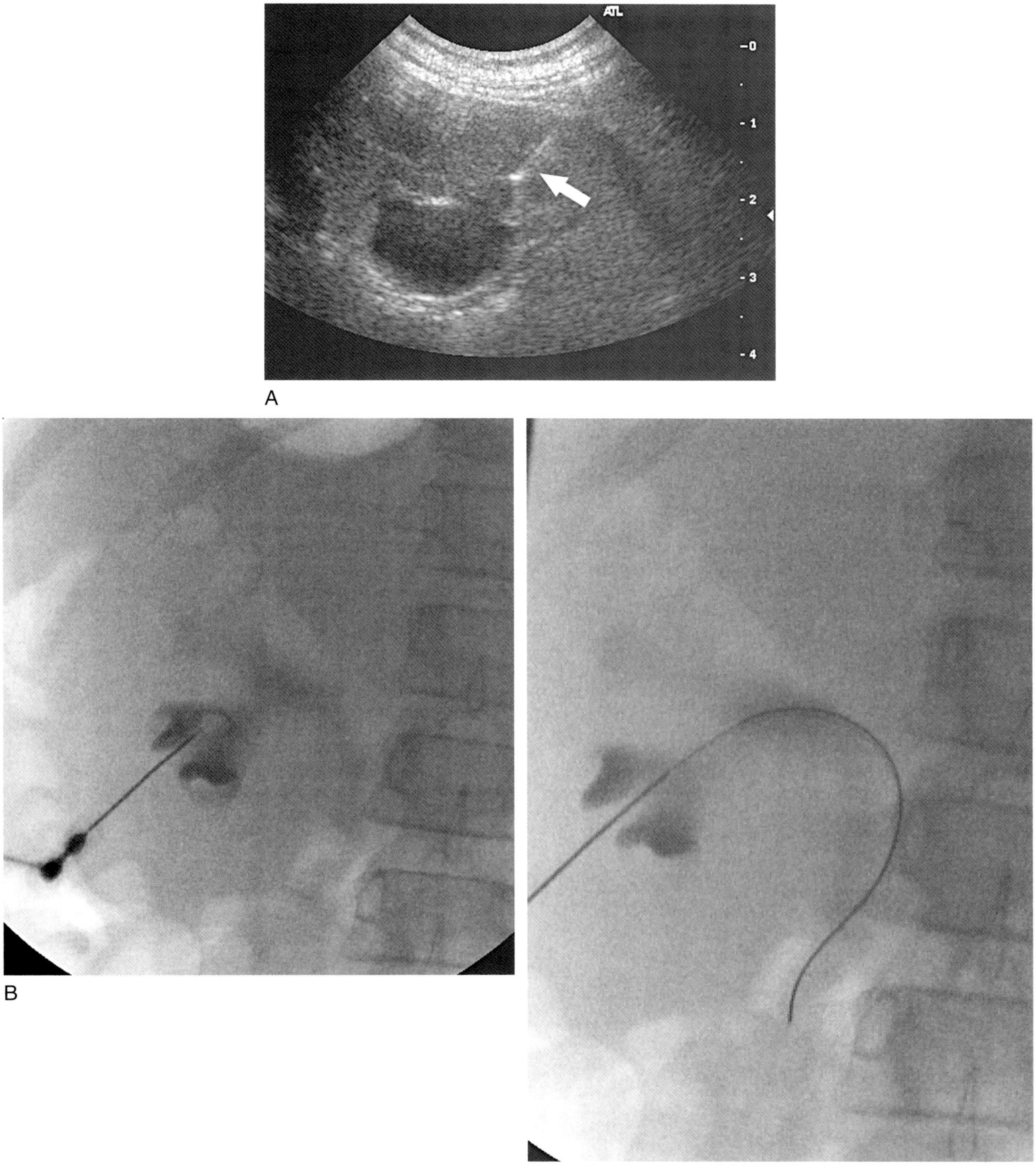

Figure 69-9 Nephrostomy procedure. **A,** The dilated renal pelvis is accessed through a calyx with a needle *(arrow)* under sonographic guidance. **B,** Contrast is injected confirming pelvic position. **C,** A guidewire is advanced into the pelvis and directed into the ureter, if possible.

Continued

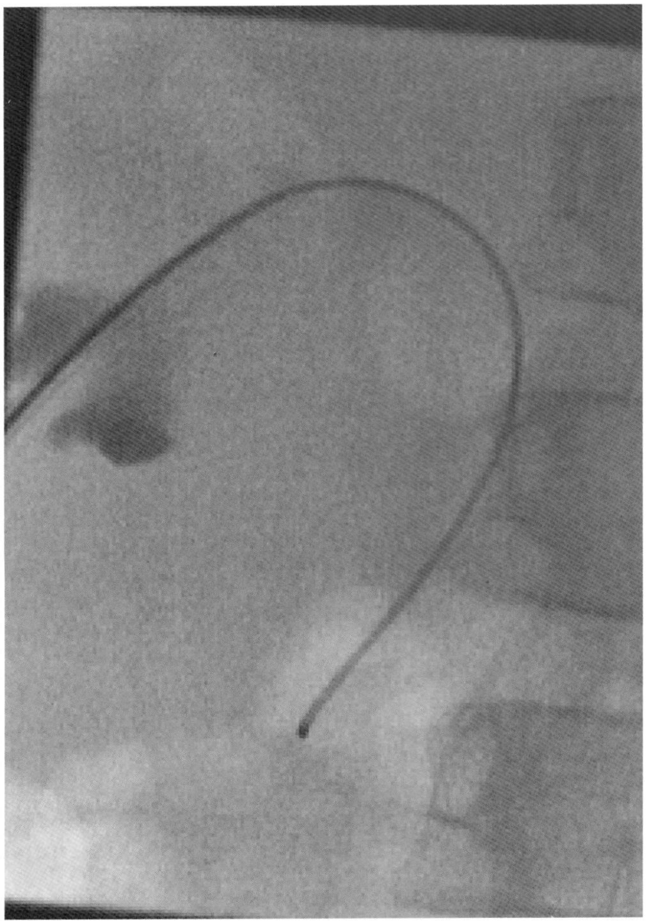

D

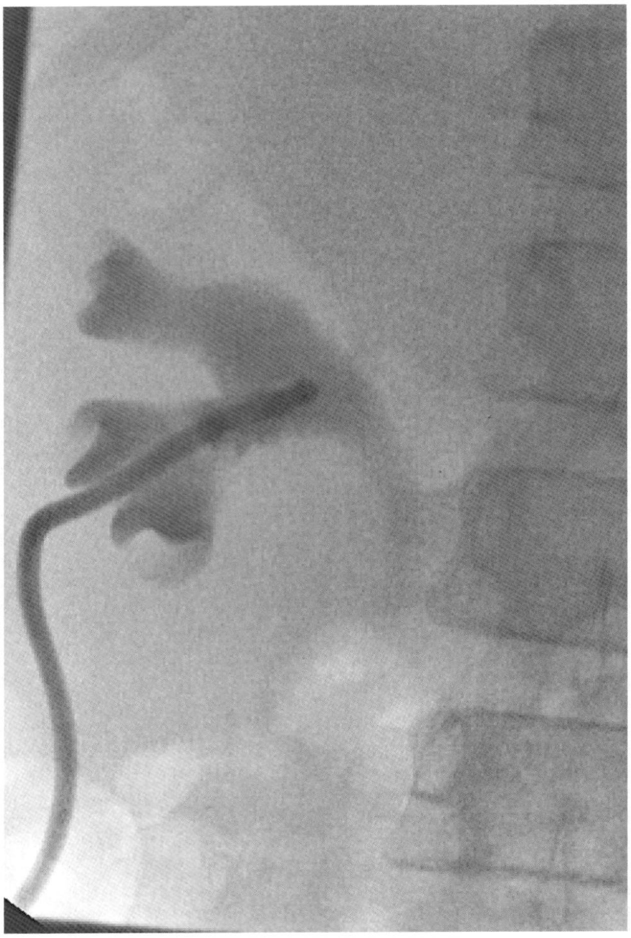

E

Figure 69-9, cont'd **D,** The skin and paraspinal muscle are dilated with fascial dilators. **E,** Nephrostomy tube is inserted into the renal pelvis.

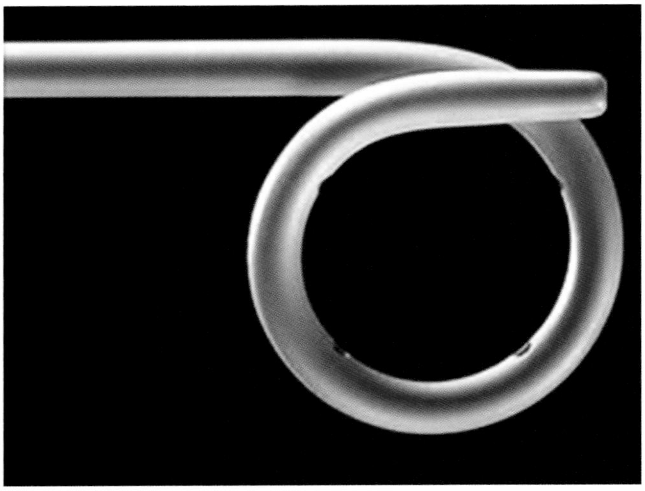

A

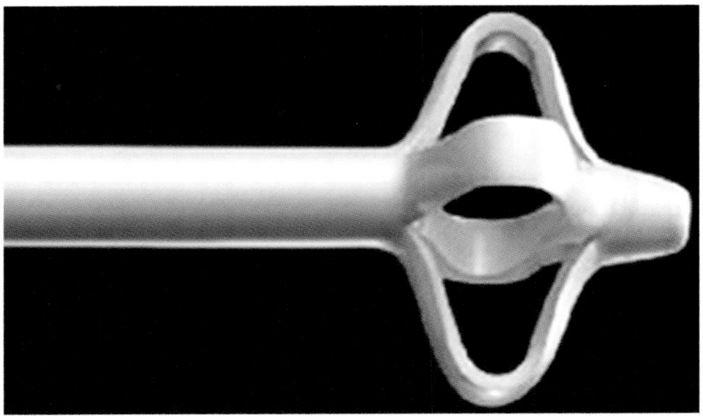

B

Figure 69-10 Nephrostomy tubes with different retention mechanisms: **A,** Pig-tail, **B,** Malecot.

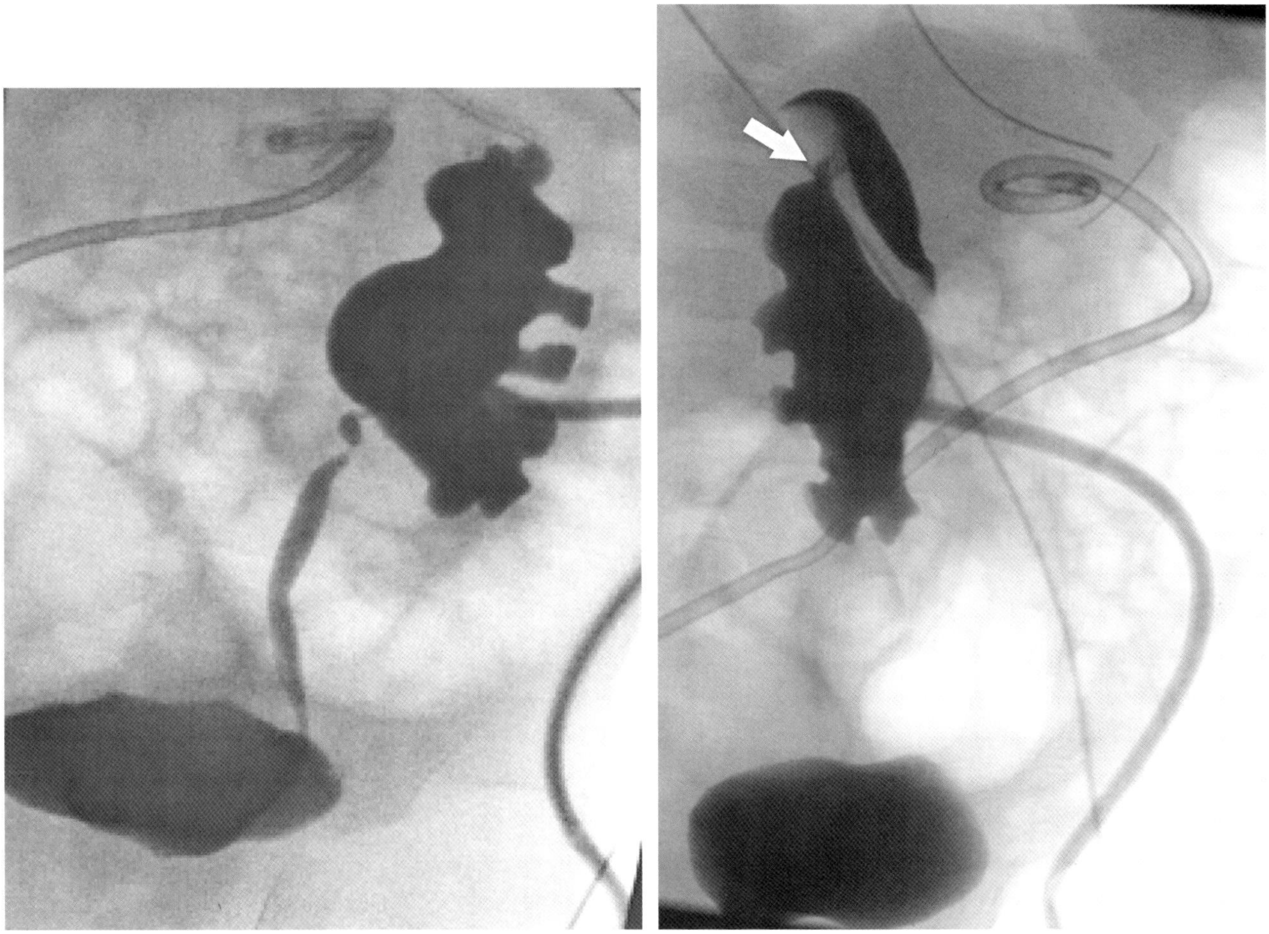

Figure 69-11 **A,** Nephrostogram showing ureteropelvic junction narrowing. **B,** Renal pelvis (calyceal) rupture *(arrow)* during forceful nephrostogram in a patient with ureteropelvic junction stenosis.

imperative to determine the best access route. It is usually adequate to enter the system in the middle pole calyx. However, some procedures require access into the superior pole of the kidney, which may pose significant technical challenges and complications such as transgression of the pleural space, potential lung trauma, and pneumothorax formation.

After access is obtained into the renal pelvis (percutaneous nephrostomy technique), if possible a stiff guidewire (Rosen, Nitinol, Amplatz) is advanced into the renal pelvis and negotiated into the ureter. Two techniques can be applied to create the nephrocutaneous tract. One approach is the use of incremental fascial dilators (e.g., Coons dilators) that gradually dilate the tract to the predetermined diameter over a stiff guidewire. Another approach is the one-step technique, in which a high-pressure noncompliant angioplasty balloon (e.g., Nephromax) (i.e., Figure 69-12) is advanced over the guidewire, a single tract dilatation is performed, and an introducer sheath is advanced over the inflated balloon.

We prefer this technique because radial stationary forces instead of longitudinal shear forces are applied in the tract, which reduces the risk of guidewire kinking or loss of access during serial dilatations. Davidoff and colleagues reviewed both methods and showed that the use of balloon tract dilators led to less renal hemorrhage and lower transfusion rates than serial dilators.[58]

However, this procedure is not free of risks, and renal trauma, hemorrhage, and loss of access are potential complications during tract dilatation. Another potential complication is balloon fracture (Figure 69-12), with a residual part of the balloon left in the collecting system—which requires interventional snaring or surgical removal.

URETERAL STENTING AND DILATATION

Ureteral dilatation and stenting are well-established procedures for managing ureteral obstruction of different etiologies and for managing urinary fistulas. Ureteral dilatation was first described by Doormashkin in 1926, but it only became popular in the early 1980s—after the development of angioplasty and drainage catheters. Ureteral narrowing may be caused by intrinsic or extrinsic ureteral lesions. Iatrogenic

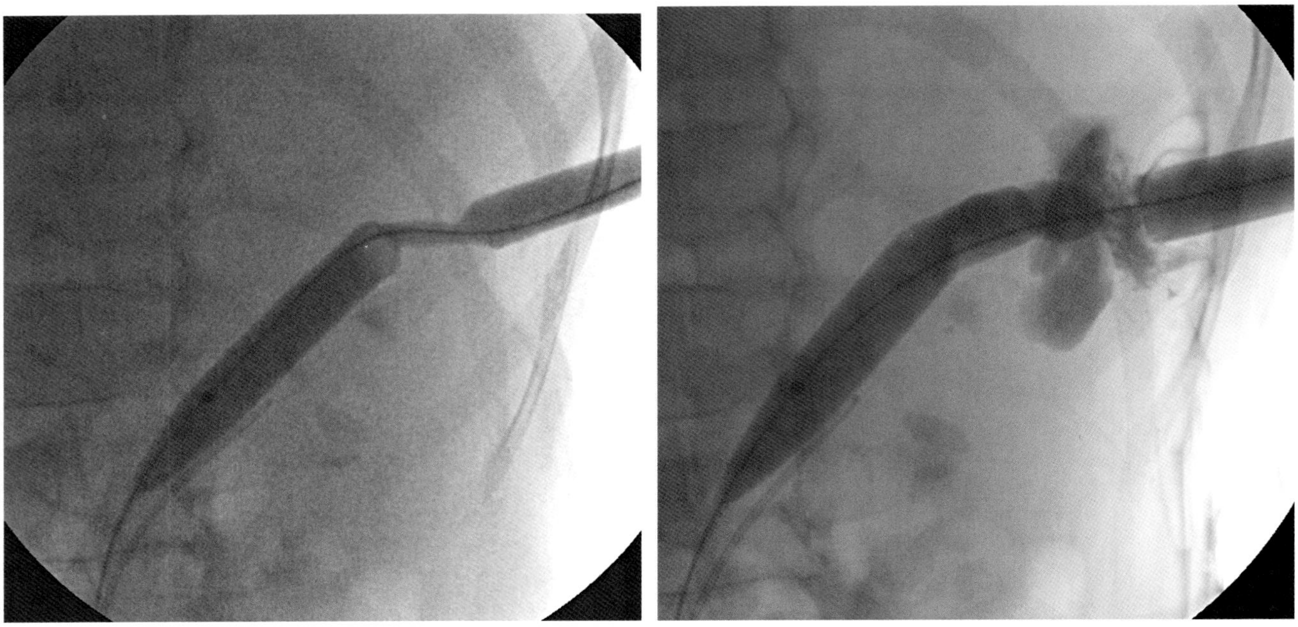

A B

Figure 69-12 Patient with hyperoxaluria requiring endoscopic lithotripsy. **A,** Fascial dilatation with high-pressure nephrostomy balloon catheter (NephroMax) to allow insertion of nephroscope. Note a waist in the balloon as it is inflated and dilates the fascial plane. **B,** NephroMax balloon burst and contrast extravasation into the fascial planes.

trauma (ureteral meatotomy, ureteroscopy, ureterolithotomy, urinary diversion, renal transplant) is considered the most common cause of intrinsic strictures (Figure 69-13). Congenital abnormalities (UPJ obstruction, UVJ obstruction, primary megaureter), chronic ureteral calculus, trauma, chronic inflammation (e.g., tuberculosis, schistosomiasis), and urothelial tumors are other causes of intraluminal ureteral stricture. External compression by malignancies (e.g., lymphoma, pelvic rhabdomyosarcoma) is the main cause of extrinsic compression.

Stents provide relief to the urinary collecting system and maintain ureteral caliber after trauma, edema, or interventions such as lithotripsy and surgery. Temporary internal (double J) or internal/external (nephroureterostomy) stents are preferred in the pediatric population. Metallic stents are generally not used in children due to their fixed permanent size in a growing child and difficulties with removal.

The preferred route of stent insertion in the ureter is retrograde (per urethra) through a cystoscope. This is the least invasive method, and no external tubes are left in the child. However, in some circumstances (such as ureteral dissection, a procedure following ureteral reimplantation, ureteral tortuosity, or urinary tract anomaly) the narrowing cannot be crossed and an antegrade (percutaneous) route through a nephrostomy is necessary. The antegrade approach is also preferred after a percutaneous procedure is performed (e.g., nephrostomy, nephrolithotripsy, endopyelotomy) because the access is already available and there is no risk of contamination as a result of the urethral access.

Percutaneous ureteral dilatation or stenting should not be performed in the presence of an active infection or in patients with a bleeding diathesis that cannot be corrected. Stent insertion should be questioned in patients with small, irritable bladders (e.g., neurogenic bladder, tuberculosus cystitis, hemorrhagic cystitis, radiation cystitis) because the stent may cause intolerable bladder irritation.

Preprocedural measures and renal access are similar to those for percutaneous nephrostomy (see percutaneous nephrostomy section). The middle renal calyx is the preferred access site because it provides a direct route to the UPJ, which allows the pushing forces to be directed to the UPJ (facilitating the subsequent manipulation of guidewires and catheters). The tract between the skin and the collecting system is then sequentially dilated with fascial dilators. A peel-away sheath, at least 1 French size larger than the stent, is advanced over the guidewire and positioned in the renal pelvis. A second guidewire is then inserted through the peel-away sheath for security purposes and is clamped to the drapes ("safety wire").

A directional catheter (JB-1, Berenstein) is then used to catheterize the proximal ureter and perform a ureterogram delineating the location and extension of ureteral obstruction or stenosis. The catheter is then advanced over a guidewire and used to negotiate the area of narrowing. Initially, attempts are made to cross the stricture with an atraumatic 0.035-inch guidewire (e.g., Bentson) or a hydrophilic-coated guidewire ("glidewire"). Tight strictures may require digital subtracted roadmaps and a 0.016-inch or 0.018-inch guidewire to be crossed. The catheter is then advanced into the bladder and the guidewire is exchanged for a stiff or superstiff guidewire (e.g., Amplatz, superstiff Amplatz, Rosen).

Noncompliant angioplasty balloons are used to dilate strictures. The balloon should be 1 to 2 mm wider than the expected normal ureteral diameter and longer than the length

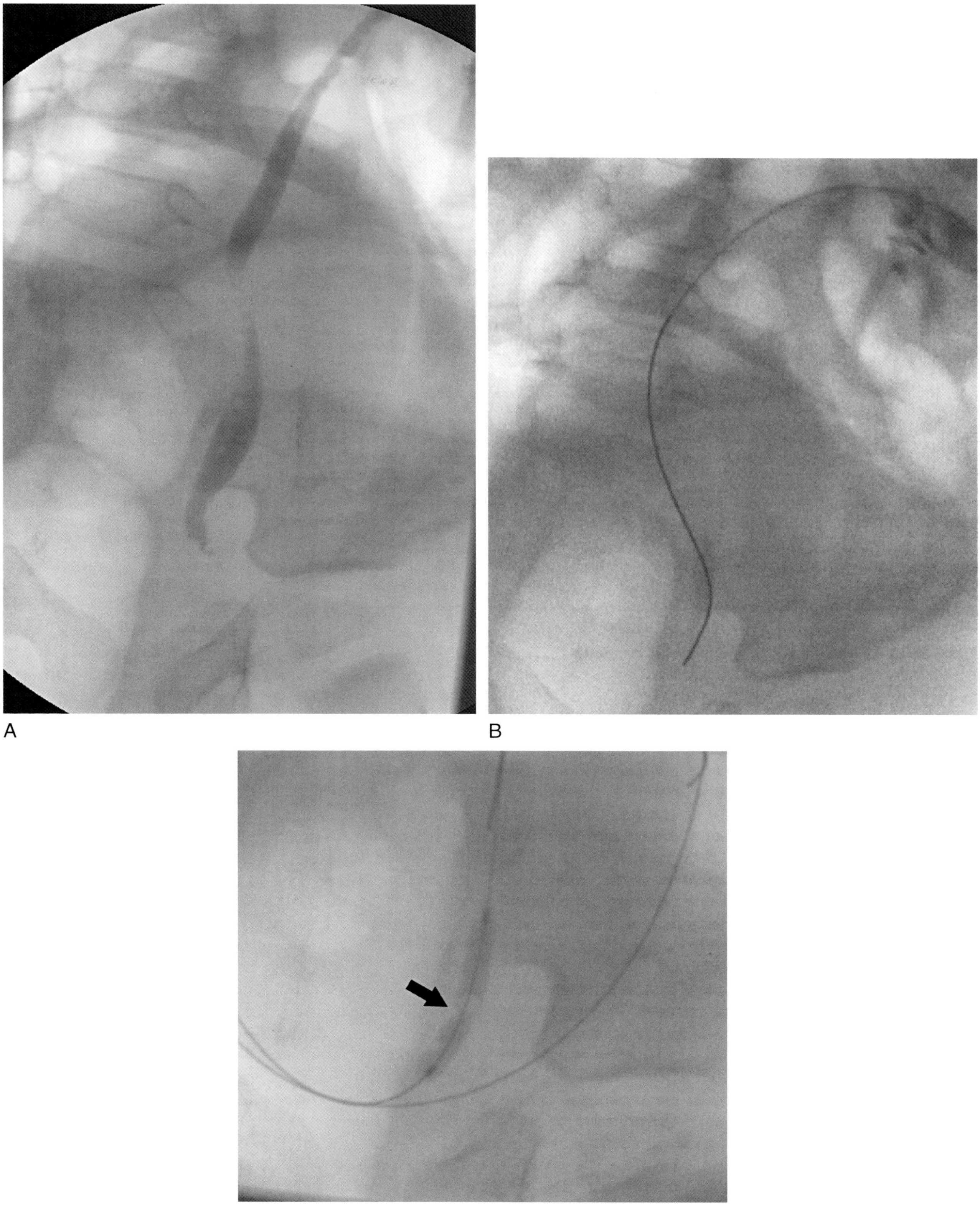

A B C

Figure 69-13 Ureteral trauma and dissection post-cystoscopy. **A,** Contrast stops in the distal ureter and does not flow into the bladder. **B,** Wire advanced into the bladder with difficulty. **C,** Balloon positioned in the area of dissection showing a waist *(arrow)*.

Continued

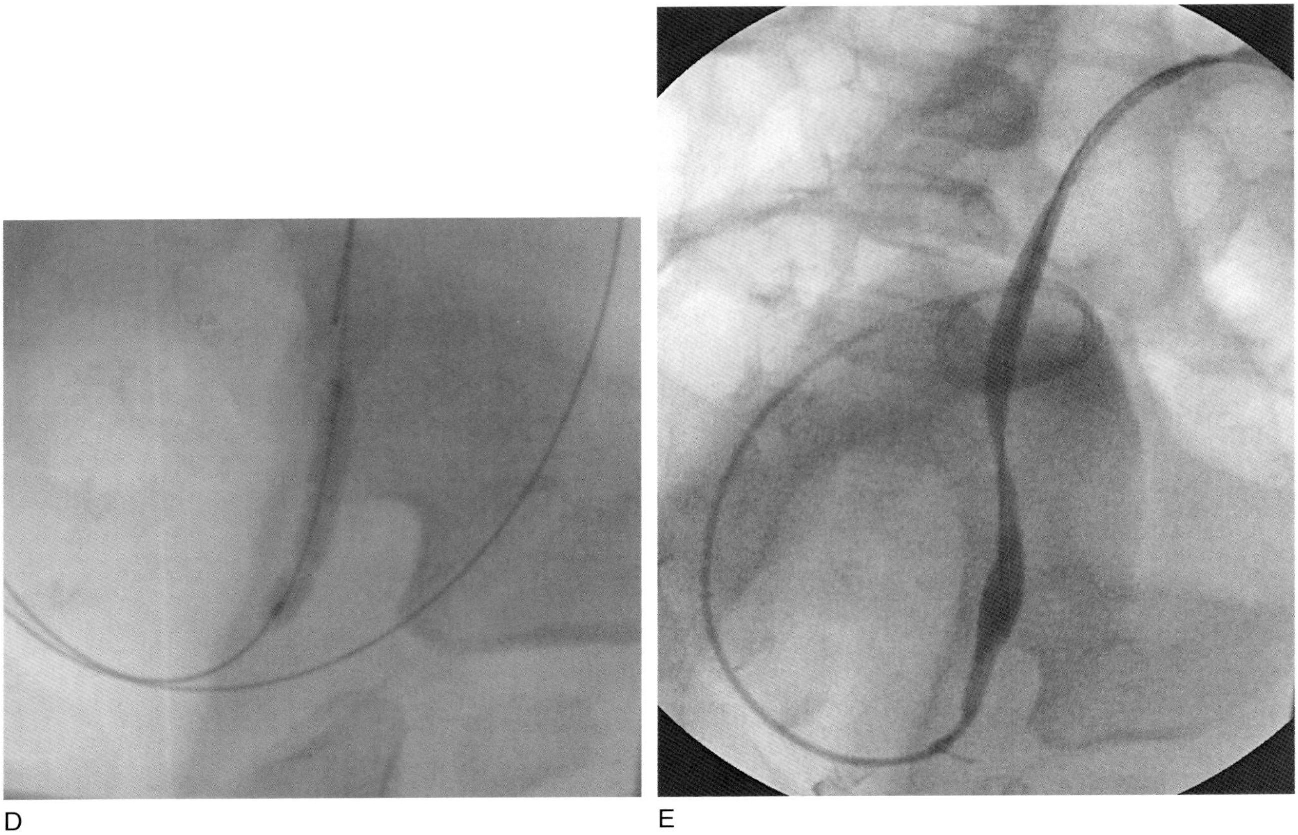

Figure 69-13, cont'd **D,** Balloon dilated almost completely effacing the waist. **E,** Double J internal stent inserted to maintain patency of the ureter.

of the stricture. Long strictures may require multiple dilatations. The angioplasty balloon is positioned at the level of the stricture and dilated using diluted contrast (50% saline + 50% nonionic contrast) under fluoroscopic guidance (Figure 69-14). The goal is to efface any "waist" noted in the balloon. No set protocol is available in the literature,[59] but in our practice we gently inflate the balloon three times for 30 to 60 seconds each time. Pressure syringes can be used for better control of the inflation pressures during dilatation, potentially decreasing the risk of balloon rupture. In noncompliant strictures, a cutting angioplasty balloon may be used. The use of cutting balloons is relatively new, and their efficacy and indications are still to be determined.

After dilating the stricture, a postdilatation ureterogram is performed to exclude ureteral rupture. The guidewire should be left crossing the stricture to secure access. In some cases, due to edema, the degree of narrowing appears even worse than on the predilatation ureterogram. However, this should not be discouraging. There is no consensus in the literature regarding the necessity for temporary stenting postdilatation. In our practice, we prefer leaving a stent across the area of dilatation.

The directional catheter is then readvanced into the bladder and the ureteral length is measured. The appropriate-length stent is then chosen and advanced over the guidewire into the renal pelvis and bladder. Internal or double J stents and internal/external or nephroureteral stents can be used to provide urinary drainage and diversion. Double J (internal) stents (Figure 69-15) are preferred because they are not externally visible, are less likely to be dislodged, and are easier to care for postprocedure. However, most of these stents cannot be cut and shorter lengths for small children may not be available. In addition, they are more difficult to remove (requiring a cystoscopy).

In contrast, nephroureteral (internal/external) stents (Figure 69-16) have some advantages because they can be tailored to length, can be flushed to maintain patency, and can be removed easily through the skin on an outpatient basis. This should be considered, especially in patients that require the stent for only a short time (e.g., post stone removal, edema) and in patients in whom cystoscopy is a challenging procedure (e.g., neurogenic bladder, augmented bladder). The main disadvantage is that a tube (and sometimes a drainage bag) is left outside the patient.

A nephrostomy tube is inserted in patients with internal stents and left for 24 to 48 hours. If the urine clears and no problems occur, the nephrostomy is removed under fluoroscopic guidance to avoid inadvertent ureteral stent removal. A sterile dressing is applied on the skin and the patient is followed clinically. Recently, Patel and colleagues reported their experience after ureteral stenting without a postprocedural nephrostomy tube in a selected population (absence of infection, atraumatic procedure with minimal amount of clot in the renal pelvis, good ureteral flow of contrast on a nephrostogram postureteral stenting) with a clinical success of 83%.[60] Despite their excellent results, in our practice we still

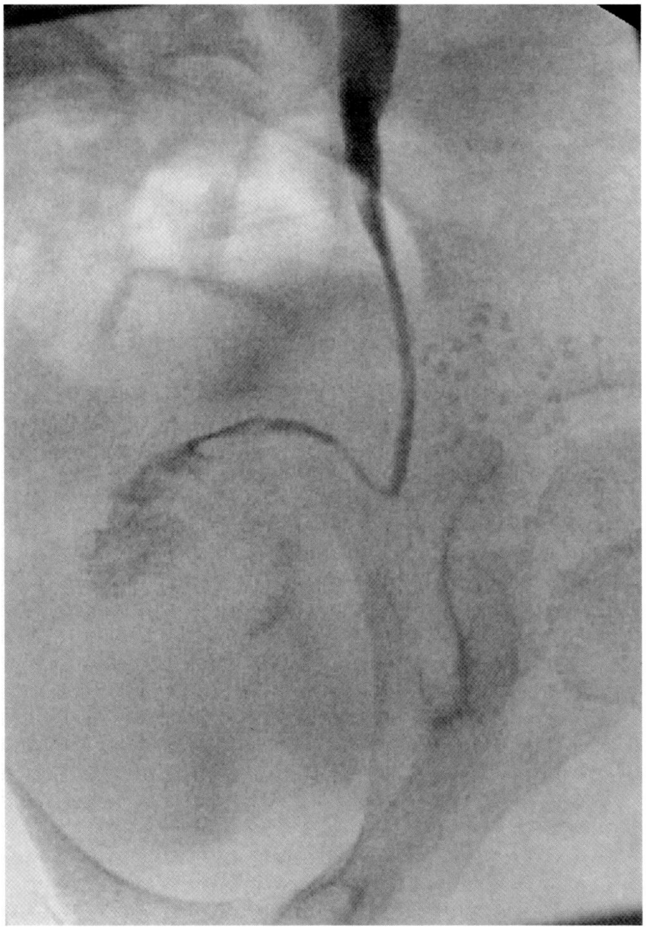

A

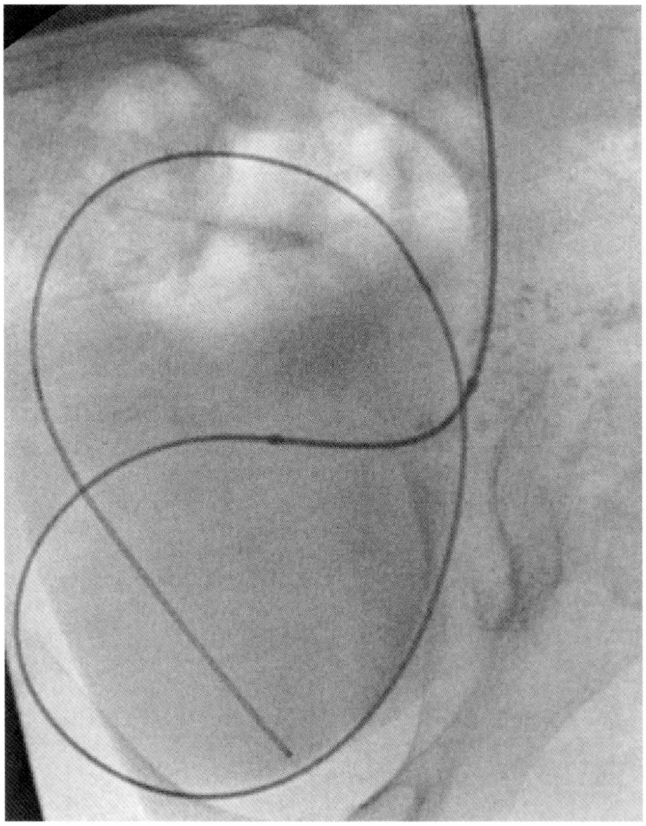

B

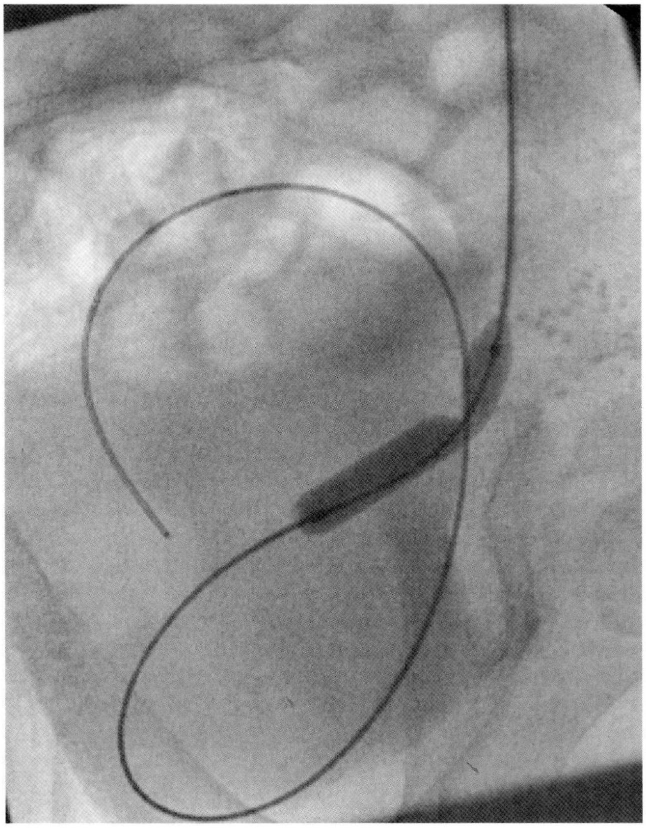

C

Figure 69-14 Eight-year-old patient postureteral implantation due to vesicoureteral reflux. Ureterovesical junction (UVJ) dilatation. **A,** Nephrostogram showing narrowing at the level of the UVJ. **B,** Wire crossing the UVJ. **C,** Partial inflation of angioplasty balloon showing a waist.

Continued

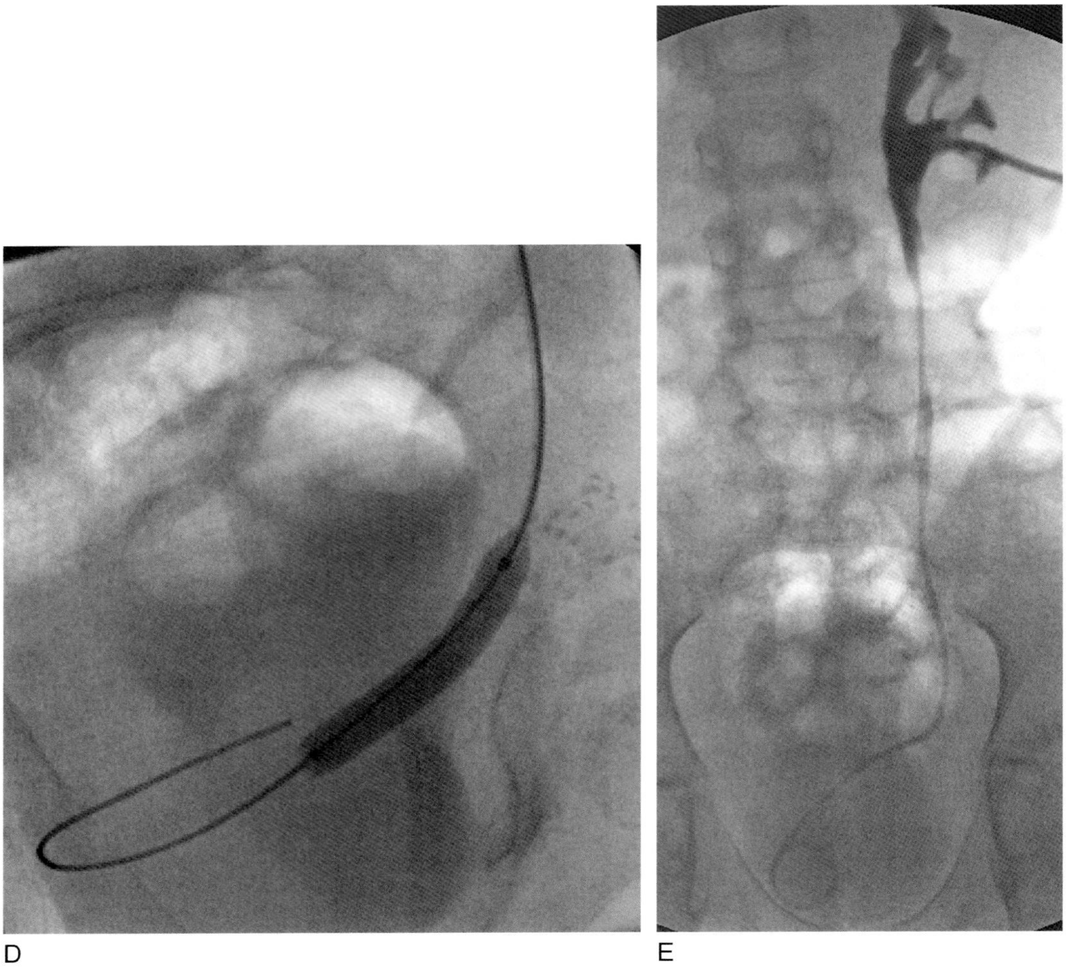

Figure 69-14, cont'd **D,** Effacement of the waist as the UVJ stricture is dilated. **E,** Double J internal stent placed across the UVJ.

prefer leaving a nephrostomy in place to maintain access to the renal pelvis for 24 to 48 hours.

If the urine is bloody or infected, stent placement should be deferred until the urine clears. In difficult cases and in cases of tight strictures where the stent cannot be easily advanced, an exchange guidewire can be inserted into the bladder and snared through the urethra. By controlling both ends of the wire ("body floss technique"), greater forces can be applied and the stent generally can be successfully placed.[61,62]

It is controversial how long the stent should remain in place, but experimental studies show that at least 6 weeks of stenting are required to allow proper ureteral muscle healing.[63] However, the length of time the stent is required also varies according to the underlying etiology of the ureteral narrowing. In general, stents placed due to edema can be removed in 5 to 7 days—whereas other strictures may require 2 to 8 weeks for adequate healing and maintenance of the ureteral diameter.

Percutaneous management of an isolated ureteral stricture is often effective. Overall, 50% to 65% of all benign strictures respond favorably to one attempt at balloon dilatation.[4] The success of the procedure, however, depends on the cause, length, location, and duration of the stricture. Ureteral ischemia and fibrosis are factors that lead to reduced success rates of balloon dilatation. Endoscopic incision by the urologist is suggested in these situations.[64]

Antegrade ureteral stent insertion is successful in 88% to 96% of cases.[60,65,66] Failures are generally related to marked ureteral tortuosity, fibrosis, tumor encasement, or angled nephrostomy access. However, in unsuccessful cases subsequent attempts made some days after nephrostomy drainage are generally successful because the ureter is less dilated and acute inflammation and edema from ureteral manipulations have resolved.[4] Regarding long-term stent patency, stents used in intrinsic obstructions function better than those used in extrinsic obstructions. Patency rates in intrinsic obstructions are close to 100%, whereas in extrinsic obstructions they range between 55% and 65%.[67-69]

Ureteral dilatation may result in ureteral rupture, dissection, or submucosal hematoma. Ureteral tears generally seal spontaneously after 72 hours if adequate proximal drainage is provided.[26] Stents can become a nidus for infection, and may be encrusted or obstructed by blood or purulent material. Patients should be encouraged to maintain a high fluid intake to dilute the urine, and infections should be treated aggressively. There is no consensus in the literature regarding the

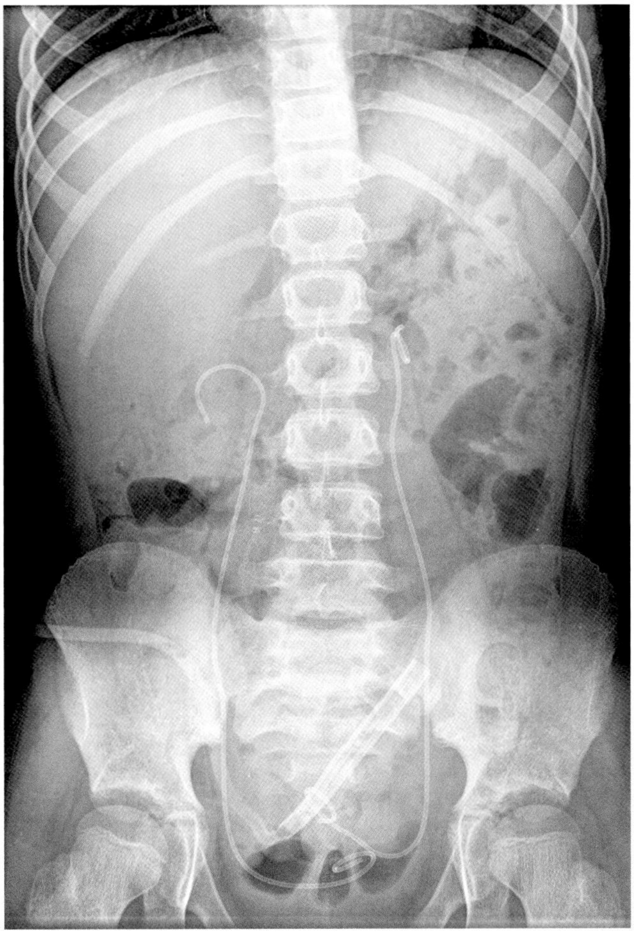

Figure 69-15 Bilateral double J stents post bladder augmentation and bilateral ureteral reimplantation in an 8-year-old patient with bladder exstrophy.

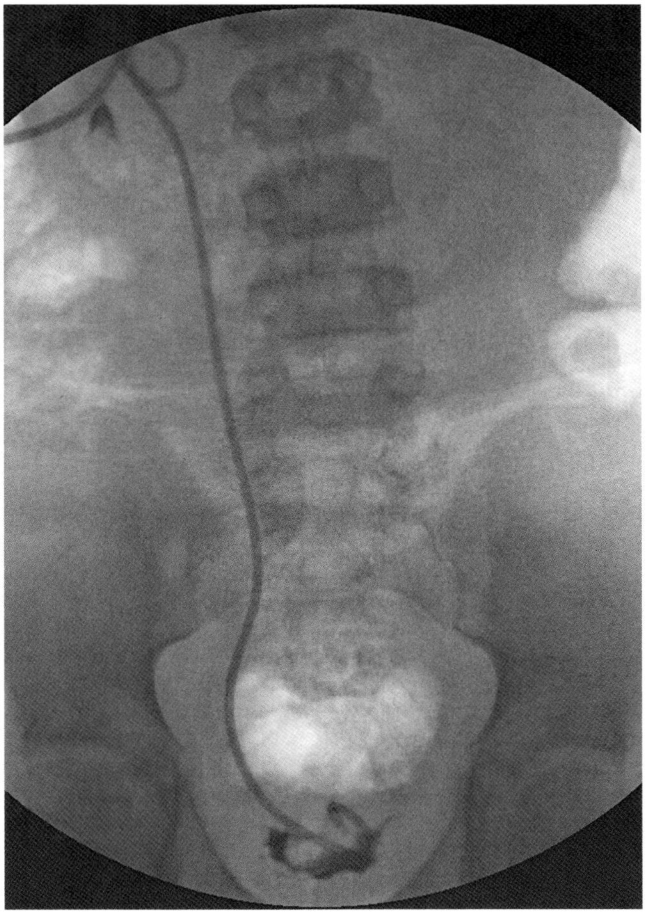

Figure 69-16 Patient with right kidney stone requiring multiple percutaneous lithotripsies. Internal/external stent left in the right kidney and ureter for future access and proper drainage of the renal pelvis.

ideal timing for stent replacement in those patients requiring a long-term stent, but most authors suggest 9 to 12 weeks as the time limit for stent permanence in a patient.[4,26]

Stents may also fracture or migrate distally into the bladder. Both situations require stent removal and replacement. If inappropriately measured, the stent may migrate (short stents) or may irritate the bladder (long stents)—causing voiding symptoms. Proximal migration may cause ureteral, renal pelvis, or calyceal perforation—resulting in urinomas or even erosion into renal vessels with catastrophic hemorrhage. Uretero arterial fistulas where the ureter crosses the iliac artery have also been reported in patients with indwelling stents. These are dangerous if not suspected and proactively treated.[70,71]

RENAL ANGIOGRAPHY AND ANGIOPLASTY

Renovascular disease accounts for approximately 10% of all cases of hypertension in children. Renal artery stenosis (RAS) with parenchymal hypoperfusion leads to increased production of renin/angiotensin/aldosterone and subsequently to hypertension. However, despite this etiology, systemic plasma renin levels are not elevated in all patients.[72] The most common etiology of RAS in childhood is fibromuscular dysplasia (FMD) (Figure 69-17), with bilateral or segmental disease and involvement of the small intrarenal arteries.[73] Other causes include neurofibromatosis,[72] arteritis (e.g., Takayasu's,[74] polyarteritis nodosa[75]), middle aortic syndrome, and Williams syndrome (mental retardation, hypercalcemia, ocular defect, elfin facies, aortic supravalvular stenosis, abdominal aortic hypoplasia, and RAS).

When a child is clinically diagnosed as hypertensive, appropriate renal imaging is mandatory. The suggested initial modality is sonography to exclude diffuse renal parenchymal disease, renal tumors, and adrenal tumors (e.g., pheochromocytoma). Color-flow duplex and Doppler sonography are very useful in the assessment of renal vasculature because 95% of main renal arteries are identified with these methods. When RAS is present, color-flow duplex images show turbulence and Doppler scans detect peak systolic velocities higher than 180 cm/second at the area of narrowing.

Doppler scans may also demonstrate a "tardus parvus" waveform in the intraparenchymal renal arteries with a delayed systolic upstroke. In a review of 71 children with hypertension, Connolly and colleagues (data presented at the 47th Annual Meeting of the Society for Pediatric Radiology, Savannah, 2004) showed that grayscale changes did not

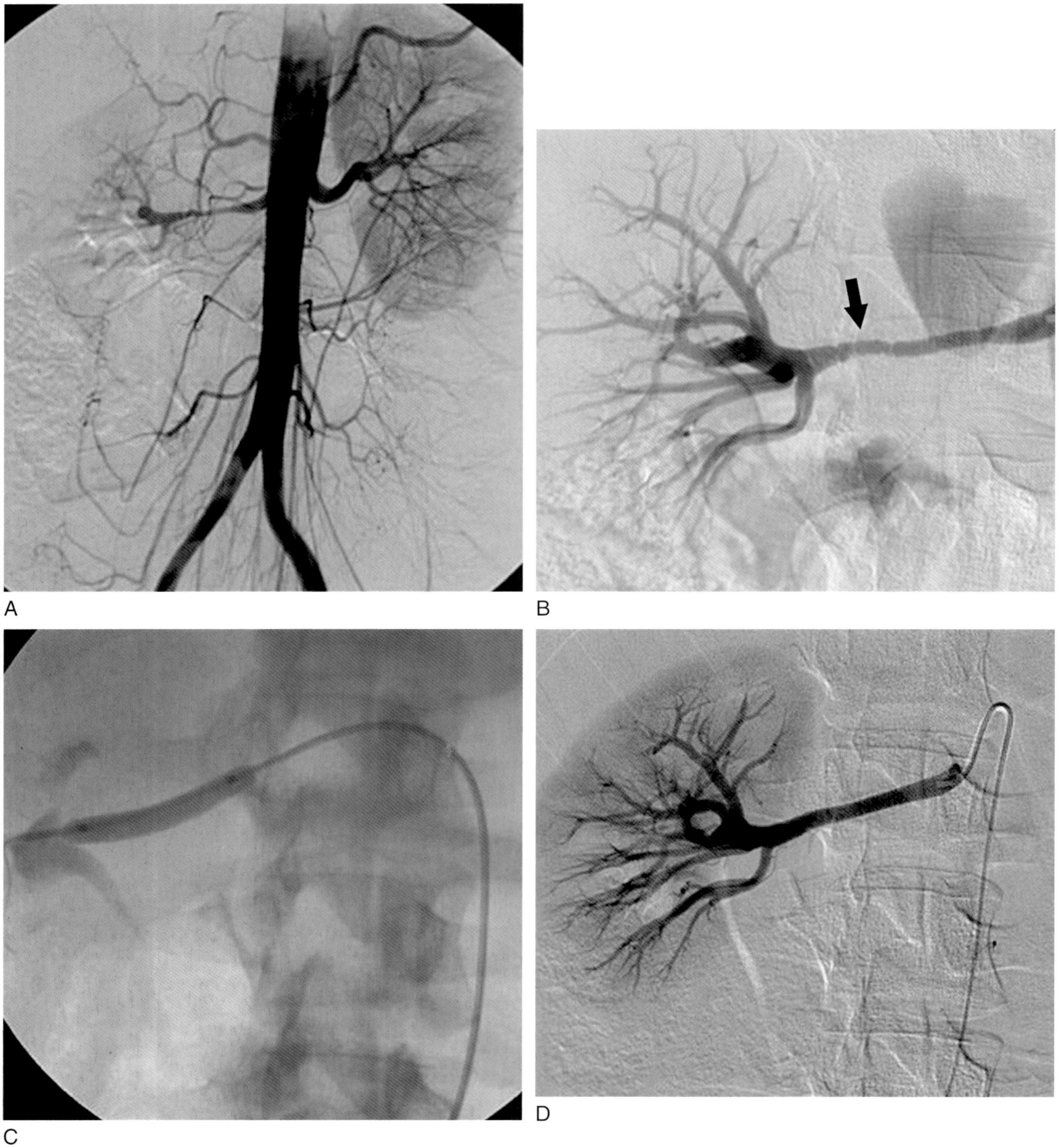

Figure 69-17 Fourteen-year-old patient with hypertension due to right renal artery stenosis. **A,** Aortogram showing right renal artery stenosis with delayed nephrogram. **B,** Note the "beaded" appearance *(arrow)* on the mid portion of the right main renal artery suggestive of FMD. **C,** Balloon angioplasty of the area of stenosis. **D,** Right renal angiogram postangioplasty showing significant improvement and normal diameter of the right renal artery.

predict RAS on angiography. However, Doppler changes were highly predictive of RAS on angiography (OR = 4.42; p = 0.01). Nuclear medicine studies can be very useful in providing functional information of the kidneys.

A decrease in glomerular filtration of certain agents such as technecium^{99m} mercaptoacetyltriglycine (MAG3), particularly following the administration of angiotensin-converting enzyme inhibitors, is suggestive of proximal RAS.

Multidetector CT angiography, MRI, and magnetic resonance angiography (MRA) are noninvasive modalities that provide high-resolution anatomic images and sensitive and specific diagnosis of main RAS. A good contrast bolus is

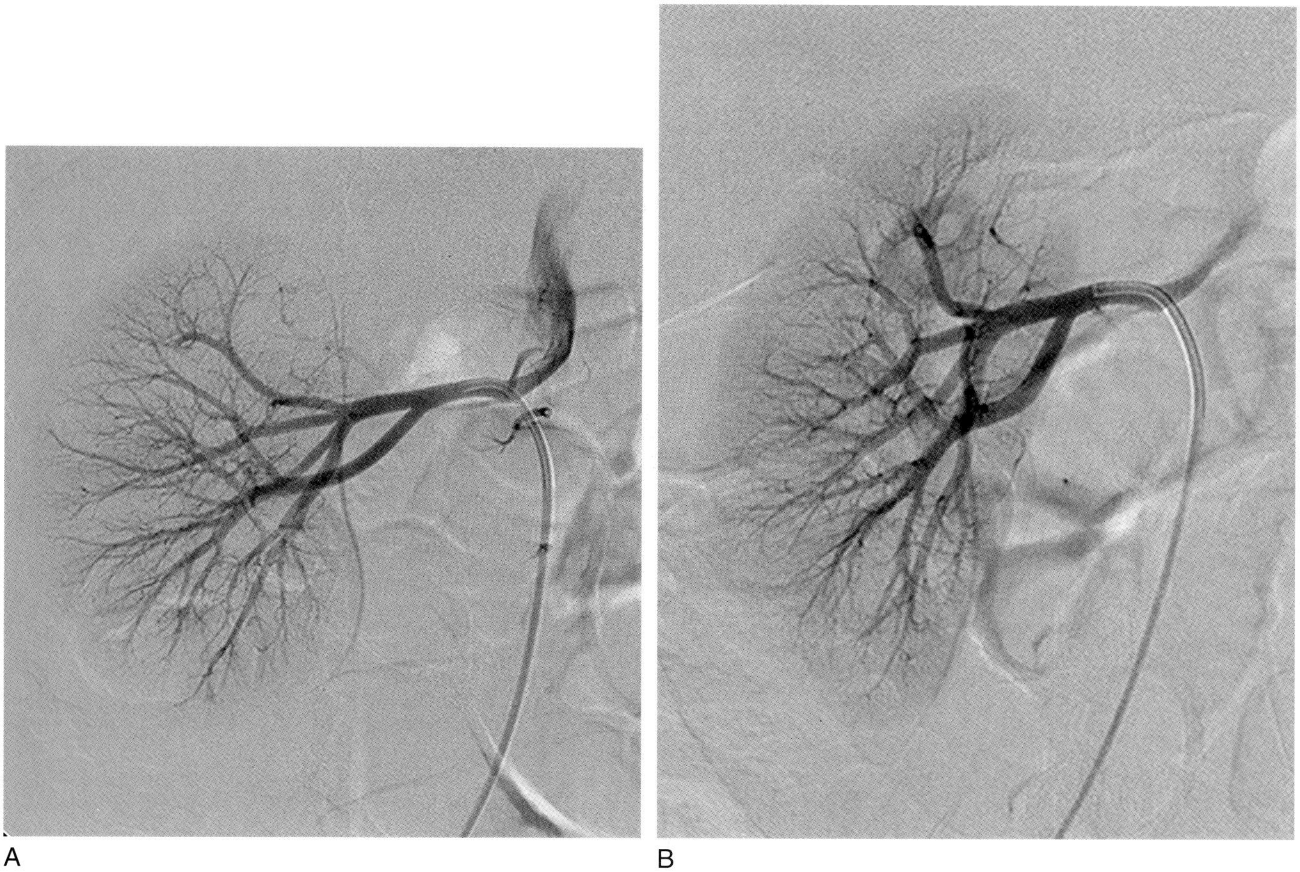

Figure 69-18 Normal right renal angiogram in patient with hypertension. **A,** Right anteroposterior view of the right kidney. **B,** Left posteroanterior view of the right kidney.

essential for CTA and MRA. One of the advantages of these methods includes the additional anatomic information related to surrounding tissues.

Unfortunately, a large percentage of children with renovascular hypertension have intrarenal disease (up to 76%)—which currently can only be adequately assessed with conventional angiography due to the resolution capabilities of noninvasive methods. Conventional angiography still is the gold standard technique for assessment of small renal vessels, despite its invasiveness. However, despite careful screening prior to referral 70% of renal angiograms in our center were normal.

In children, most angiograms are performed under general anesthesia. Peripheral pulses and perfusion are checked on both extremities before the procedure. Under sterile conditions, the femoral artery is accessed using sonographic guidance and a vascular sheath is introduced. In some cases, according to the anatomic origin of the renal arteries the brachial or axillary arteries are accessed. The child is then systemically heparinized with 100 units of heparin/kg to a maximum of 5000 units. The least amount of nonionic contrast is used to minimize the risk of contrast nephropathy (maximum dose = 5-6 ml/kg; depends on the duration of the procedure).

Vascular spasm is treated with intraarterial injections of nitroglycerine (1-3 μg/kg per injection) if needed. Intravenous injections of glucagon are given to optimize image quality and to avoid image degradation from bowel peristalsis. Attention must be paid to serum glucose, particularly if the child is medicated with beta blockers. A flush aortogram and selective renal artery angiogram (anteroposterior and oblique views) are performed. At least two oblique views of the kidneys are obtained to better evaluate the intraparenchymal vessels (Figure 69-18). Reduction of more than 75% of the intraluminal diameter of the renal artery, presence of collateral vessels, and decrease in renal mass indicate a hemodynamically significant disease.

Occasionally, direct sampling of plasma renin levels from the renal veins is helpful in establishing the diagnosis of renovascular hypertension. The femoral vein is accessed (side opposite the arterial access for angiogram to reduce the chance of arteriovenous fistula formation), and venous samples are withdrawn from each renal vein and from the suprarenal and infrarenal inferior vena cava. Renin levels from one kidney 1.5 times higher than the contralateral kidney and differences between the infrarenal and suprarenal inferior vena cava renin concentration are highly suggestive of renovascular hypertension. Occasionally, lateralization of renin results can direct a more detailed angiography of the involved kidney.

If an RAS is confirmed on angiography, a curved long sheath (number 6 French) or a large directional catheter (number 5

French) is then positioned in the aorta at the renal artery ostium. A nontraumatic guidewire (e.g., 0.035-inch Benston, 0.014-inch soft platinum tip) is gently advanced and managed across the stenosis. A catheter may be advanced over the wire to measure pressures in the prestenotic and poststenotic segments of the renal artery. However, due to the smaller size of vessels in children it may not always be possible to measure pressures. An angioplasty balloon is then advanced over the wire and positioned in the region of the narrowing.

In general, 2-mm to 6-mm angioplasty balloons are used to dilate the stenotic area. After dilatation, an angiogram is performed through the outer sheath to assess vessel patency and any potential complications (such as renal artery dissection or rupture). During the entire procedure, the guidewire is left crossing the area of narrowing. If an arterial rupture or arterial dissection with flow compromise to the kidney occurs, a covered stent may be placed in the artery. In emergency situations, an angioplasty balloon is inflated across the area of arterial rupture and the patient is explored surgically.

Success rates varying from 62% to 94% have been reported for renal angioplasty in children.[73,76-79] The reported angioplasty success rate is variable because it depends on the etiology of the RAS and how angioplasty success is defined in each study (angiographic success or clinical success). Patients with FMD have a high clinical success rate after angioplasty (see Figure 69-17). Tegtmeyer and colleagues reviewed 66 adults with FMD and showed a 92% success in a mean follow-up of 39 months.[80] RAS seen in patients with neurofibromatosis appear to be very fibrous, and often have a poor response to angioplasty (Figure 69-19).

In our center, 15 children with RAS of different etiologies were treated with angioplasty during a period of 10 years. Angioplasty was considered successful if the number of antihypertensive medications decreased without an increase in dosage of any of the medications, if the dosage of the same medications decreased, or if blood pressure decreased by at least one major percentile for age. Initial success was achieved in 89% of cases. The success rate, however, fell to 57% at 6 months and 50% at 1 year postangioplasty (data presented at the 47th Annual Meeting of the Society for Pediatric Radiology, Savannah, 2004). Shroff and colleagues reviewed the outcome of 33 children after percutaneous transarterial angioplasty (PTA) and showed improvement in blood pressure in 55% of patients. These authors also showed a high rate of restenosis (37%) in all children who had arterial stents inserted.

Complications are not common but can be very serious, including renal artery thrombosis, renal artery dissection, renal artery rupture (may require artery reimplantation or nephrectomy), renal infarction, renal failure, and death. Complications can also occur at the site of arterial access (hematomas, pseudoaneurysm, arteriovenous fistulas) and with the devices used during angioplasty (balloon rupture). Overall, complications are present in 13% of patients. However, major complications account for only 3%.[4,25] Shroff and colleagues, in a pediatric series, reported an 18% incidence of complications.[73]

GASTROINTESTINAL ACCESS

Gastrostomy tubing is a percutaneous enteral access that provides a conduit for long-term nutrition. Since its introduction in 1981, percutaneous radiologic gastrostomy has become a widely accepted procedure.[81] Using sonography and fluoroscopy as guiding tools, interventional radiologists ensure correct placement of gastrostomy or gastrojejunostomy tubes with lower morbidity and fewer major complications than percutaneous endoscopic or surgical techniques.[82-86]

Children with chronic renal disease may require a gastrostomy tube to help their growth. In our practice, these children are referred for an image-guided percutaneous retrograde gastrostomy tube insertion. Gastrostomies are indicated in children who require nutritional support because of failure to thrive, in children who are unable to feed orally, and in children who have excessively high caloric demands. There are only a few contraindications to gastrostomy tube insertion, including an uncorrectable coagulopathy or an unfavorable anatomy that precludes safe access to the stomach. In our experience, the presence of a peritoneal dialysis catheter is not a contraindication to a gastrostomy tube insertion—although the distance separating the insertion sites on the abdominal wall should be maximized.

Patients are first assessed by the enterostomy service (pediatrician, radiologist, and gastrostomy nurse) to determine the appropriateness of the procedure. If deemed appropriate, procedures are performed under sedation, general anesthesia, or local anesthetic alone. The position of the lower edge of the liver and spleen are marked on the skin with a surgical marker using sonographic guidance. The colon is then identified using diluted barium injected per rectum under fluoroscopic control. All children receive antibiotic prophylaxis. Glucagon is given to provide gastroparesis and pyloric constriction.

The stomach is inflated with air through a nasogastric tube to choose a site for placement of a gastrostomy tube. The chosen site for puncture is infiltrated with local anesthesia, and the stomach is punctured with an 18-gauge needle loaded with a pediatric retention suture. Contrast is injected to confirm the needle's intragastric position, and the retention suture is deployed into the stomach with a 0.035-inch straight guidewire. A fascial dilator is then used to dilate the tract to the same size as the gastrostomy tube. The dilator is removed and the gastrostomy tube of chosen size (numbers 8 to 12 French) is introduced over the guidewire. The position is checked with contrast to confirm placement and to identify any leaks (Figure 69-20).

Patients are kept "nil per os" for approximately 12 hours. Maintenance intravenous fluids are prescribed by the nephrology team. The nasogastric and the new gastrostomy tubes are left open for drainage to decompress the stomach and to reduce the risk of peritoneal spillage. When bowel sounds are present, gastric feedings are started slowly through the gastrostomy and increased as tolerated.

Wollman and colleagues[83] conducted an institutional evaluation and metaanalysis of the literature of radiologic, endoscopic, and surgical gastrostomy in adults without abdominal wall defects. Major complications occurred less frequently after radiologic gastrostomy (5.9%) compared to percutaneous endoscopic gastrostomy (PEG) (9.4%). Surgical gastrostomy had a significantly higher complication rate than both of these procedures (19.9%; $p < 0.001$). Radiologic gastrostomy also had significantly fewer tube-related complications than PEG (12.1% versus 16.0%). The authors concluded that

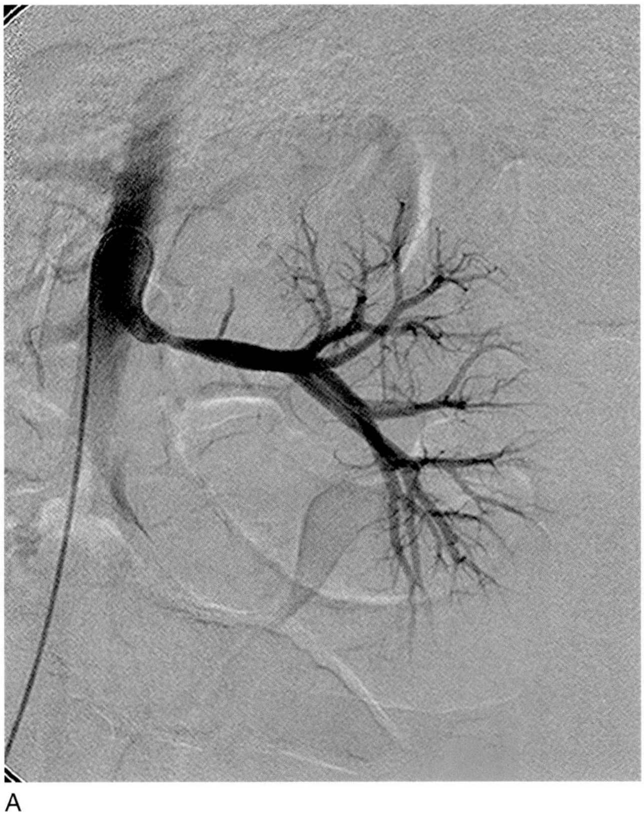

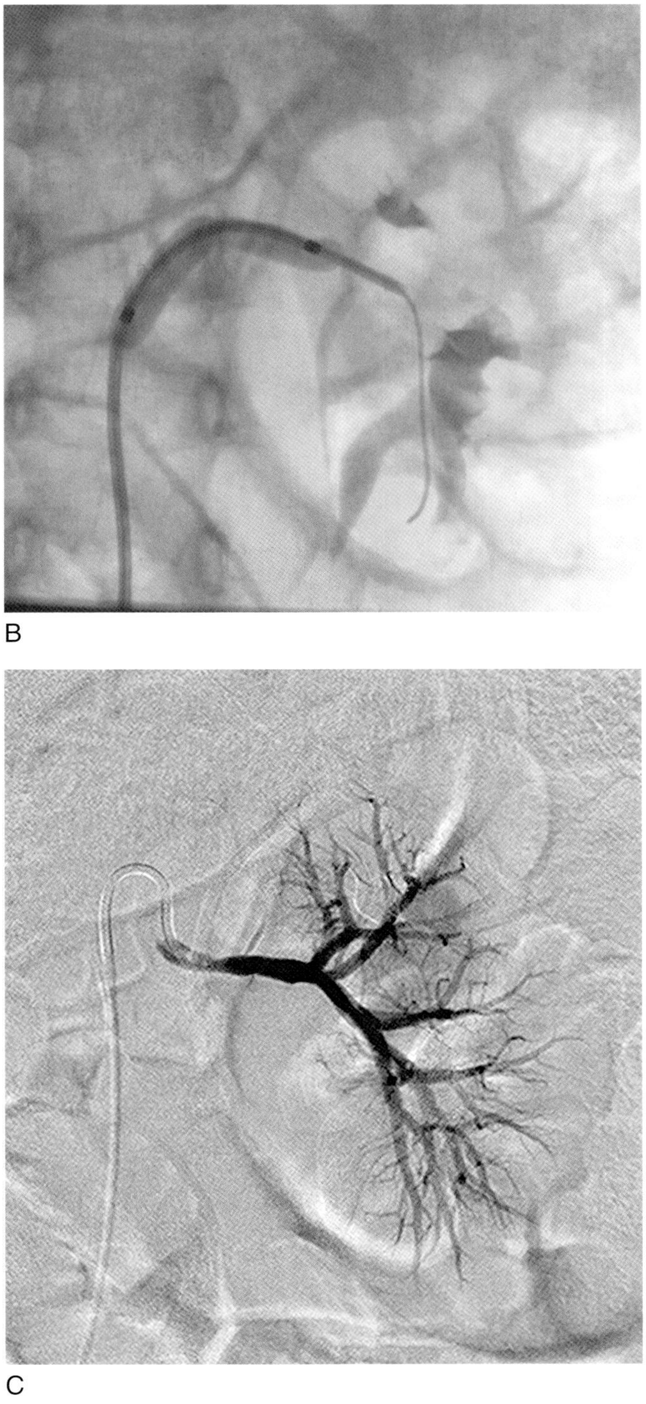

Figure 69-19 Four-year-old patient with neurofibromatosis type I, presenting with hypertension. **A,** Renal angiogram shows narrowing of the proximal portion of the left renal artery. **B,** Angioplasty attempted three times with no significant improvement. **C,** Residual narrowing of the left renal artery.

radiologic gastrostomy was associated with a higher success rate than PEG and less morbidity than either PEG or surgery.

The most serious complication associated with percutaneous gastrostomy is peritonitis. Friedman and colleagues, in a review of gastrostomies in our institution, reported a 3% incidence of peritonitis—with one case resulting in death (0.4%).[86] Minor complications include skin infection/irritation and granulation tissue formation around the insertion site. Family and patients should be warned that tube maintenance issues such as tube blockage, breakage, leakage, or dislodgement are common and may require a tube exchange.

CENTRAL VENOUS ACCESS

Vascular access for hemodialysis has been discussed in another chapter. However, in our center our team of interventional radiologists provides central venous access for many renal patients. Therefore, we include some comments about techniques offered by the interventionalist that can facilitate central venous access.

Central venous access can be very useful for fluid management, parenteral nutrition, and hemodialysis. The choice of vascular device depends on the type and length of treatment. Large-bore catheters that accommodate large volumes/minute are necessary for hemodialysis, and small-bore catheters are sufficient for medications, fluids, and parenteral nutrition. The use of sonography guidance to access the vascular system is a great advantage. Successful entry is obtained on the first pass, and the vessel is seldom transected (Figure 69-21). This reduces the risk of complications such as the following:

- Bleeding and hematoma with resulting venous compression.
- The chance of an arteriovenous fistula creation and venous dissection.
- Patient discomfort is diminished because less access attempts are necessary.

In addition, sonography allows assessment of venous patency and potential collaterals available for venous access in patients with thrombosis. Fluoroscopy is also useful because it allows visualization and control of the guidewire during manipulations in the heart. It also permits proper measurement of the vascular access device, avoiding malpositioning (Figure 69-22). Finally, the use of devices such as micropuncture needles and vascular dilators also helps to reduce complications and increase the success of vascular access.

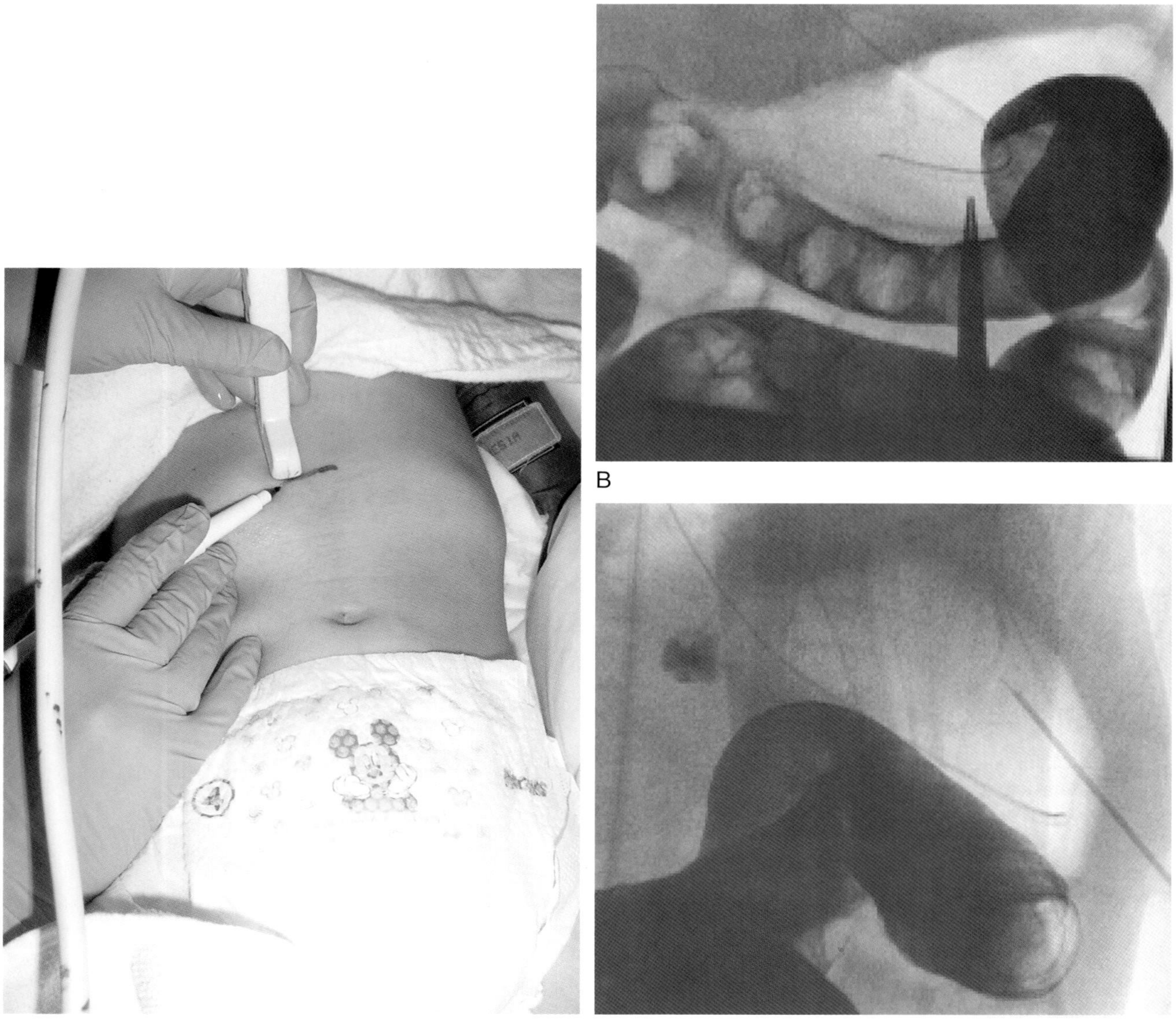

A B C

Figure 69-20 Gastrostomy tube insertion. **A,** Liver and spleen edges marked on the skin with sonographic guidance. **B,** Transverse colon delineated with barium and stomach inflated through a nasogastric tube. **C,** Stomach punctured under fluoroscopic guidance.

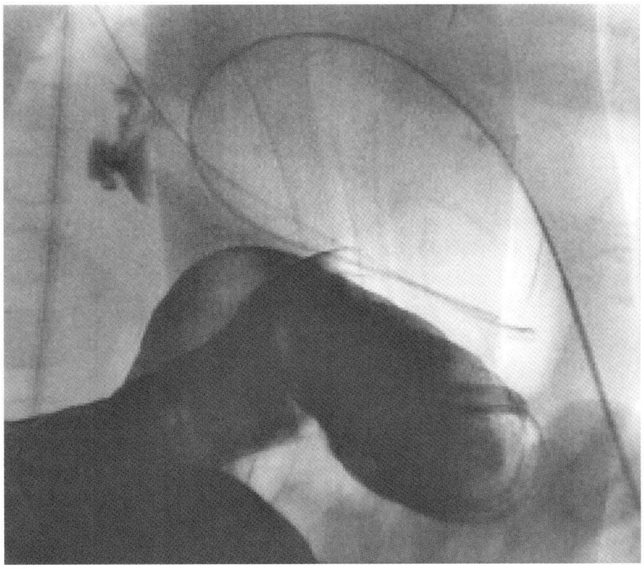

D

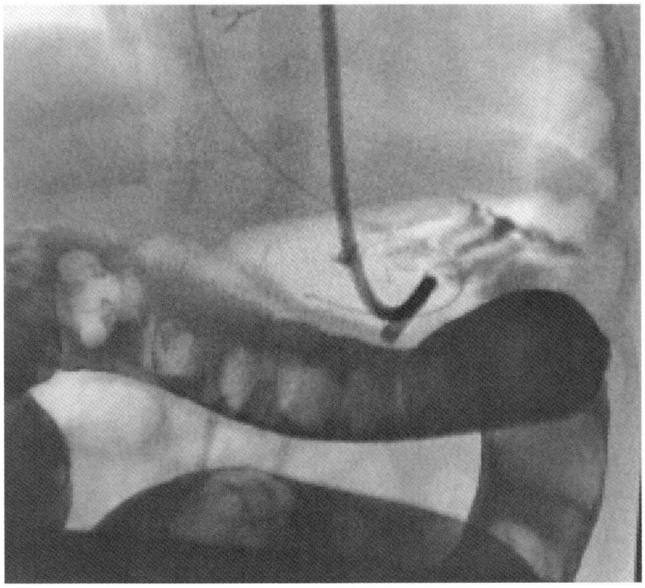

E

Figure 69-20, cont'd **D,** Gastrostomy tube advanced over a wire into the stomach. **E,** Gastrostomy in place, clear from colon.

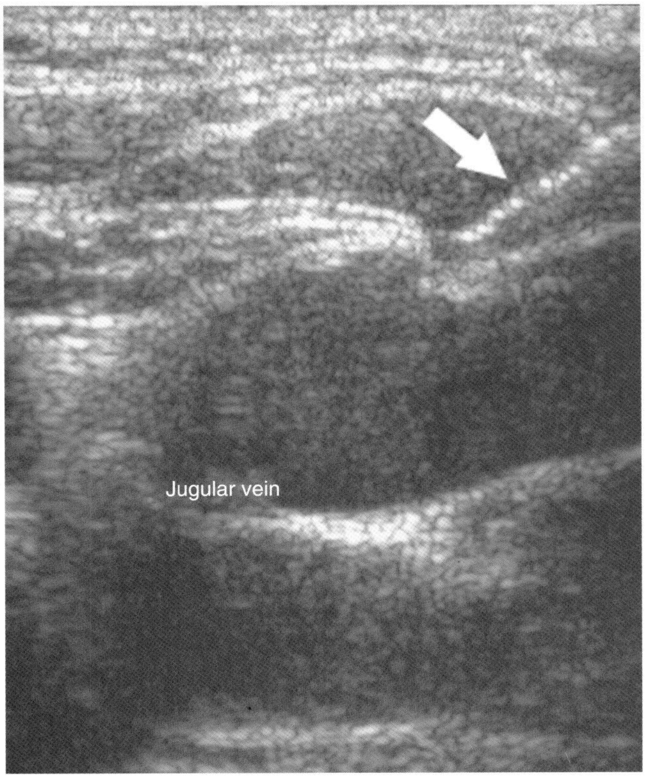

A

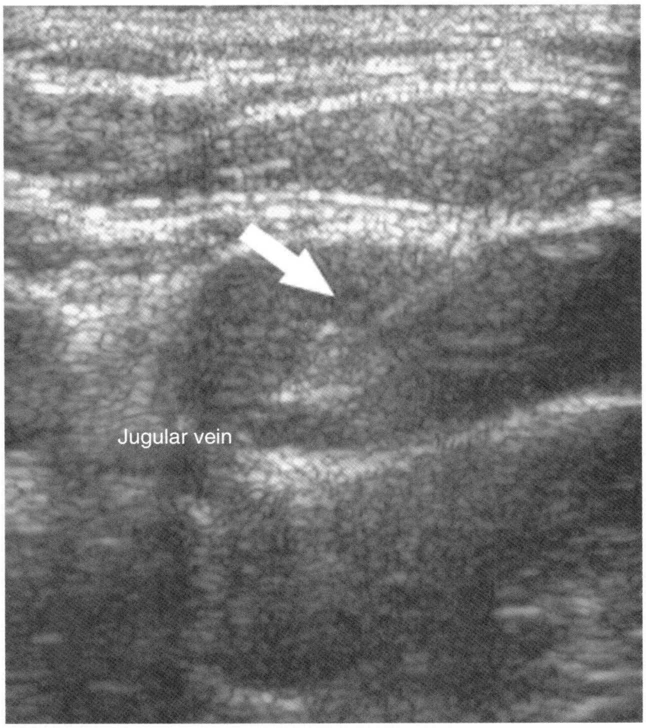

B

Figure 69-21 Sonographic-guided vascular access. **A,** Needle *(arrow)* indenting the lateral wall of the jugular vein. **B,** Needle *(arrow)* in the lumen of the jugular vein.

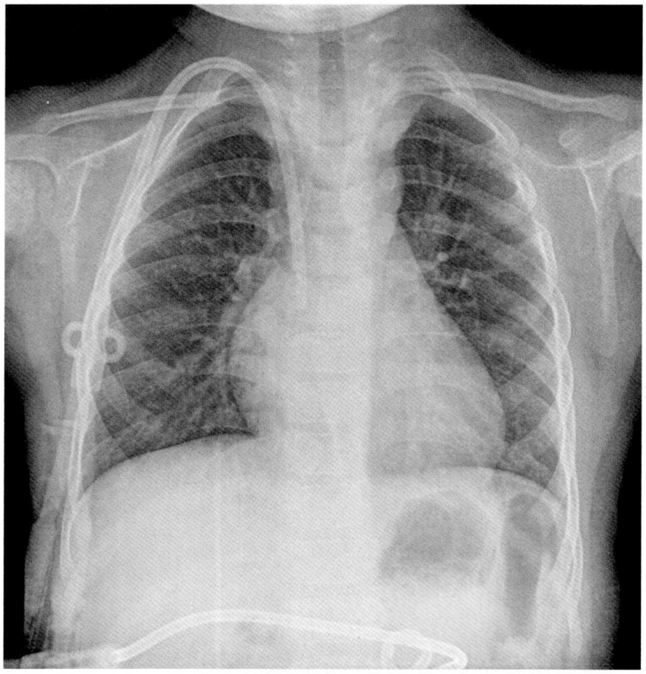

Figure 69-22 Patient with renal insufficiency requiring hemodialysis. Central venous catheter in proper position, with tip at the level of the right atrium/superior vena cava junction.

REFERENCES

1. Dodge WF, Daeschner CW Jr., Brennan JC, Rosenberg HS, Travis LB, Hopps HC: Percutaneous renal biopsy in children: I. General considerations, *Pediatrics* 30:287-96, 1962.
2. Fogazzi GB, Cameron JS: The early introduction of percutaneous renal biopsy in Italy, *Kidney Int* 56:1951-61, 1999.
3. Sinha MD, Lewis MA, Bradbury MG, Webb NJ: Percutaneous real-time ultrasound-guided renal biopsy by automated biopsy gun in children: Safety and complications, *J Nephrol* 19:41-44, 2006.
4. Baum SPM: *Abrams' angiography interventional radiology, second edition*. Philadelphia: Lippincott Williams & Wilkins 2006:669-97.
5. Kim D, Kim H, Shin G, et al: A randomized, prospective, comparative study of manual and automated renal biopsies, *Am J Kidney Dis* 32:426-31, 1998.
6. Webb NJ, Pereira JK, Chait PG, Geary DF: Renal biopsy in children: Comparison of two techniques, *Pediatr Nephrol* 8:486-88, 1994.
7. Bohlin AB, Edstrom S, Almgren B, Jaremko G, Jorulf H: Renal biopsy in children: indications, technique and efficacy in 119 consecutive cases, *Pediatr Nephrol* 9:201-03, 1995.
8. Kamitsuji H, Yoshioka K, Ito H: Percutaneous renal biopsy in children: Survey of pediatric nephrologists in Japan, *Pediatr Nephrol* 13:693-96, 1999.
9. Nammalwar BR, Vijayakumar M, Prahlad N: Experience of renal biopsy in children with nephrotic syndrome, *Pediatr Nephrol* 21:286-88, 2006.
10. Kersnik Levart T, Kenig A, Buturovic Ponikvar J, Ferluga D, Avgustin Cavic M, Kenda RB: Real-time ultrasound-guided renal biopsy with a biopsy gun in children: Safety and efficacy, *Acta Paediatr* 90:1394-97, 2001.
11. Bachmann H, Heckemann R, Olbing H: Percutaneous renal biopsy in children under guidance of ultrasonic real time technique, *Int J Pediatr Nephrol* 5:175-78, 1984.
12. Sweet M, Brouhard BH, Ramirez-Seijas F, Kalia A, Travis LB: Percutaneous renal biopsy in infants and young children, *Clin Nephrol* 26:192-94, 1986.
13. Feneberg R, Schaefer F, Zieger B, Waldherr R, Mehls O, Scharer K: Percutaneous renal biopsy in children: A 27-year experience, *Nephron* 79:438-46, 1998.
14. Sahney S, Mohan GC: Renal biopsy in infants and children, *Am J Kidney Dis* 23:31-32, 1994.
15. Saarinen UM, Wikstrom S, Koskimies O, Sariola H: Percutaneous needle biopsy preceding preoperative chemotherapy in the management of massive renal tumors in children, *J Clin Oncol* 9:406-15, 1991.
16. Cozens NJ, Murchison JT, Allan PL, Winney RJ: Conventional 15 G needle technique for renal biopsy compared with ultrasound-guided spring-loaded 18 G needle biopsy, *Br J Radiol* 65:594-97, 1992.
17. Bogan ML, Kopecky KK, Kraft JL, et al: Needle biopsy of renal allografts: Comparison of two techniques, *Radiology* 174:273-75, 1990.
18. Mostbeck GH, Wittich GR, Derfler K, et al: Optimal needle size for renal biopsy: In vitro and in vivo evaluation, *Radiology* 173:819-22, 1989.
19. Christensen J, Lindequist S, Knudsen DU, Pedersen RS: Ultrasound-guided renal biopsy with biopsy gun technique—efficacy and complications, *Acta Radiol* 36:276-79, 1995.
20. Hergesell O, Felten H, Andrassy K, Kuhn K, Ritz E: Safety of ultrasound-guided percutaneous renal biopsy-retrospective analysis of 1090 consecutive cases, *Nephrol Dial Transplant* 13:975-77, 1998.
21. Sateriale M, Cronan JJ, Savadler LD: A 5-year experience with 307 CT-guided renal biopsies: Results and complications, *J Vasc Interv Radiol* 2:401-07, 1991.
22. Riccabona M, Schwinger W, Ring E: Arteriovenous fistula after renal biopsy in children, *J Ultrasound Med* 17:505-08, 1998.
23. Schow DA, Vinson RK, Morrisseau PM: Percutaneous renal biopsy of the solitary kidney: A contraindication? *J Urol* 147:1235-37, 1992.
24. Goodwin WE, Casey WC, Woolf W: Percutaneous trocar (needle) nephrostomy in hydronephrosis, *J Am Med Assoc* 157:891-94, 1955.
25. Kandarpa K AJ: *Handbook of interventional radiologic procedures*, third edition, Philadelphia: Lippincott Williams & Wilkins 2002:278-301.
26. Fotter R: *Pediatric uroradiology*, Berlin: Springer-Verlag 2001:377-93.

27. Koral K, Saker MC, Morello FP, Rigsby CK, Donaldson JS: Conventional versus modified technique for percutaneous nephrostomy in newborns and young infants, *J Vasc Interv Radiol* 14:113-16, 2003.
28. Gupta DK, Chandrasekharam VV, Srinivas M, Bajpai M: Percutaneous nephrostomy in children with ureteropelvic junction obstruction and poor renal function, *Urology* 57:547-50, 2001.
29. Farrell TA, Hicks ME: A review of radiologically guided percutaneous nephrostomies in 303 patients, *J Vasc Interv Radiol* 8:769-74, 1997.
30. Lee WJ, Patel U, Patel S, Pillari GP: Emergency percutaneous nephrostomy: Results and complications, *J Vasc Interv Radiol* 5:135-39, 1994.
31. Lee WJ, Mond DJ, Patel M, Pillari GP: Emergency percutaneous nephrostomy: Technical success based on level of operator experience, *J Vasc Interv Radiol* 5:327-30, 1994.
32. Gray RR, So CB, McLoughlin RF, Pugash RA, Saliken JC, Macklin NI: Outpatient percutaneous nephrostomy, *Radiology* 198:85-88, 1996.
33. Stanley P, Diament MJ: Pediatric percutaneous nephrostomy: experience with 50 patients, *J Urol* 135:1223-26, 1986.
34. Ball WS Jr., Towbin R, Strife JL, Spencer R: Interventional genitourinary radiology in children: A review of 61 procedures, *AJR Am J Roentgenol* 147:791-96, 1986.
35. Winfield AC, Kirchner SG, Brun ME, Mazer MJ, Braren HV, Kirchner FK Jr.: Percutaneous nephrostomy in neonates, infants, and children, *Radiology* 151:617-19, 1984.
36. O'Brien WM, Matsumoto AH, Grant EG, Gibbons MD: Percutaneous nephrostomy in infants, *Urology* 36:269-72, 1990.
37. Irving HC, Arthur RJ, Thomas DF: Percutaneous nephrostomy in paediatrics, *Clin Radiol* 38:245-48, 1987.
38. Ramchandani P, Cardella JF, Grassi CJ, et al: Quality improvement guidelines for percutaneous nephrostomy, *J Vasc Interv Radiol* 12:1247-51, 2001.
39. Reznek RH, Talner LB: Percutaneous nephrostomy, *Radiol Clin North Am* 22:393-406, 1984.
40. Camunez F, Echenagusia A, Prieto ML, Salom P, Herranz F, Hernandez C: Percutaneous nephrostomy in pyonephrosis, *Urol Radiol* 11:77-81, 1989.
41. Lang EK, Price ET: Redefinitions of indications for percutaneous nephrostomy, *Radiology* 147:419-26, 1983.
42. Pappas P, Stravodimos KG, Mitropoulos D, et al: Role of percutaneous urinary diversion in malignant and benign obstructive uropathy, *J Endourol* 14:401-05, 2000.
43. Silverman SG, Mueller PR, Pfister RC: Hemostatic evaluation before abdominal interventions: An overview and proposal, *AJR Am J Roentgenol* 154:233-38, 1990.
44. Rapaport SI: Assessing hemostatic function before abdominal interventions, *AJR Am J Roentgenol* 154:239-240, 1990.
45. Cochran ST, Barbaric ZL, Lee JJ, Kashfian P: Percutaneous nephrostomy tube placement: An outpatient procedure? *Radiology* 179:843-47, 1991.
46. Payne CS: A primer on patient management problems in interventional radiology, *AJR Am J Roentgenol* 170:1169-76, 1998.
47. Classen DC, Evans RS, Pestotnik SL, Horn SD, Menlove RL, Burke JP: The timing of prophylactic administration of antibiotics and the risk of surgical-wound infection, *N Engl J Med* 326:281-86, 1992.
48. Hogan MJ, Coley BD, Jayanthi VR, Shiels WE, Koff SA: Percutaneous nephrostomy in children and adolescents: Outpatient management, *Radiology* 218:207-10, 2001.
49. Sampaio FJ, Zanier JF, Aragao AH, Favorito LA: Intrarenal access: 3-dimensional anatomical study, *J Urol* 148:1769-73, 1992.
50. Gupta S, Gulati M, Suri S: Ultrasound-guided percutaneous nephrostomy in non-dilated pelvicaliceal system, *J Clin Ultrasound* 26:177-79, 1998.
51. Cope C, Zeit RM: Pseudoaneurysms after nephrostomy, *Am J Roentgenol* 139:255-61, 1982.
52. Harris RD, Walther PC: Renal arterial injury associated with percutaneous nephrostomy, *Urology* 23:215-17, 1984.
53. Cronan JJ, Dorfman GS, Amis ES, Denny DF Jr.: Retroperitoneal hemorrhage after percutaneous nephrostomy, *AJR Am J Roentgenol* 144:801-03, 1985.
54. Yoder IC, Pfister RC, Lindfors KK, Newhouse JH: Pyonephrosis: Imaging and intervention, *AJR Am J Roentgenol* 141:735-40, 1983.
55. Yoder IC, Lindfors KK, Pfister RC: Diagnosis and treatment of pyonephrosis, *Radiol Clin North Am* 22:407-14, 1984.
56. Cadeddu JA, Arrindell D, Moore RG: Near fatal air embolism during percutaneous nephrostomy placement, *J Urol* 158:1519, 1997.
57. LeRoy AJ, Williams HJ Jr., Bender CE, Segura JW, Patterson DE, Benson RC: Colon perforation following percutaneous nephrostomy and renal calculus removal, *Radiology* 155:83-85, 1985.
58. Davidoff R, Bellman GC: Influence of technique of percutaneous tract creation on incidence of renal hemorrhage, *J Urol* 157:1229-31, 1997.
59. Chang R, Marshall FF, Mitchell S: Percutaneous management of benign ureteral strictures and fistulas, *J Urol* 137:1126-31, 1987.
60. Patel U, Abubacker MZ: Ureteral stent placement without postprocedural nephrostomy tube: Experience in 41 patients, *Radiology* 230:435-42, 2004.
61. Mitty HA: Ureteral stenting facilitated by antegrade transurethral passage of guide wire, *AJR Am J Roentgenol* 142:831-32, 1984.
62. D'Souza R, Tait P, Thomson RW, Trewhella M: Case report: An alternative approach to stenting the obstructed ureter, *Br J Radiol* 66:460-61, 1993.
63. Lee CK, Smith AD: Role of stents in open ureteral surgery, *J Endourol* 7:141-44, 1993.
64. Hafez KS, Wolf JS Jr.: Update on minimally invasive management of ureteral strictures, *J Endourol* 17:453-64, 2003.
65. Watson GM, Patel U: Primary antegrade ureteric stenting: Prospective experience and cost-effectiveness analysis in 50 ureters, *Clin Radiol* 56:568-74, 2001.
66. Dyer RB, Regan JD, Kavanagh PV, Khatod EG, Chen MY, Zagoria RJ: Percutaneous nephrostomy with extensions of the technique: Step by step, *Radiographics* 22:503-25, 2002.
67. Docimo SG, Dewolf WC: High failure rate of indwelling ureteral stents in patients with extrinsic obstruction: Experience at 2 institutions, *J Urol* 142:277-79, 1989.
68. Yossepowitch O, Lifshitz DA, Dekel Y, et al: Predicting the success of retrograde stenting for managing ureteral obstruction, *J Urol* 166:1746-49, 2001.
69. Chung SY, Stein RJ, Landsittel D, et al: 15-year experience with the management of extrinsic ureteral obstruction with indwelling ureteral stents, *J Urol* 172:592-95, 2004.
70. Batter SJ, McGovern FJ, Cambria RP: Ureteroarterial fistula: Case report and review of the literature, *Urology* 48:481-89, 1996.
71. Vandersteen DR, Saxon RR, Fuchs E, Keller FS, Taylor LM Jr., Barry JM: Diagnosis and management of ureteroiliac artery fistula: Value of provocative arteriography followed by common iliac artery embolization and extraanatomic arterial bypass grafting, *J Urol* 158:754-58, 1997.
72. McTaggart SJ, Gulati S, Walker RG, Powell HR, Jones CL: Evaluation and long-term outcome of pediatric renovascular hypertension, *Pediatr Nephrol* 14:1022-29, 2000.
73. Shroff R, Roebuck DJ, Gordon I, et al.: Angioplasty for renovascular hypertension in children: 20-year experience, *Pediatrics* 118:268-75, 2006.
74. McCulloch M, Andronikou S, Goddard E, et al: Angiographic features of 26 children with Takayasu's arteritis, *Pediatr Radiol* 33:230-35, 2003.
75. Brogan PA, Davies R, Gordon I, Dillon MJ: Renal angiography in children with polyarteritis nodosa, *Pediatr Nephrol* 17:277-83, 2002.
76. Mali WP, Puijlaert CB, Kouwenberg HJ, et al: Percutaneous transluminal renal angioplasty in children and adolescents, *Radiology* 165:391-94, 1987.
77. Casalini E, Sfondrini MS, Fossali E: Two-year clinical follow-up of children and adolescents after percutaneous transluminal angioplasty for renovascular hypertension, *Invest Radiol* 30:40-43, 1995.
78. Tyagi S, Kaul UA, Satsangi DK, Arora R: Percutaneous transluminal angioplasty for renovascular hypertension in children: Initial and long-term results, *Pediatrics* 99:44-49, 1997.
79. Courtel JV, Soto B, Niaudet P, et al: Percutaneous transluminal angioplasty of renal artery stenosis in children, *Pediatr Radiol* 28:59-63, 1998.

80. Tegtmeyer CJ, Selby JB, Hartwell GD, Ayers C, Tegtmeyer V: Results and complications of angioplasty in fibromuscular disease, *Circulation* 83:I155-61, 1991.
81. Preshaw RM: A percutaneous method for inserting a feeding gastrostomy tube, *Surg Gynecol Obstet* 152:658-60, 1981.
82. Chait PG, Weinberg J, Connolly BL, et al: Retrograde percutaneous gastrostomy and gastrojejunostomy in 505 children: A 4 1/2-year experience, *Radiology* 201:691-95, 1996.
83. Wollman B, D'Agostino HB, Walus-Wigle JR, Easter DW, Beale A: Radiologic, endoscopic, and surgical gastrostomy: an institutional evaluation and meta-analysis of the literature, *Radiology* 197:699-704, 1995.
84. Ozmen MN, Akhan O: Percutaneous radiologic gastrostomy, *Eur J Radiol* 43:186-95, 2002.
85. Towbin RB, Ball WS Jr., Bissett GS III: Percutaneous gastrostomy and percutaneous gastrojejunostomy in children: Antegrade approach, *Radiology* 168:473-76, 1988.
86. Friedman JN, Ahmed S, Connolly B, Chait P, Mahant S: Complications associated with image-guided gastrostomy and gastrojejunostomy tubes in children, *Pediatrics* 114:458-61, 2004.

Index

References are to pages. Pages followed by an "f" indicate figures; "t," tables.